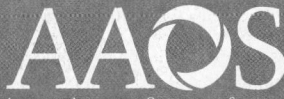

AAOS

AMERICAN ACADEMY OF ORTHOPAEDIC SURGEONS

TWELFTH E



ANNIVERSARY

# Emergency

## Care and Transportation of the Sick and Injured

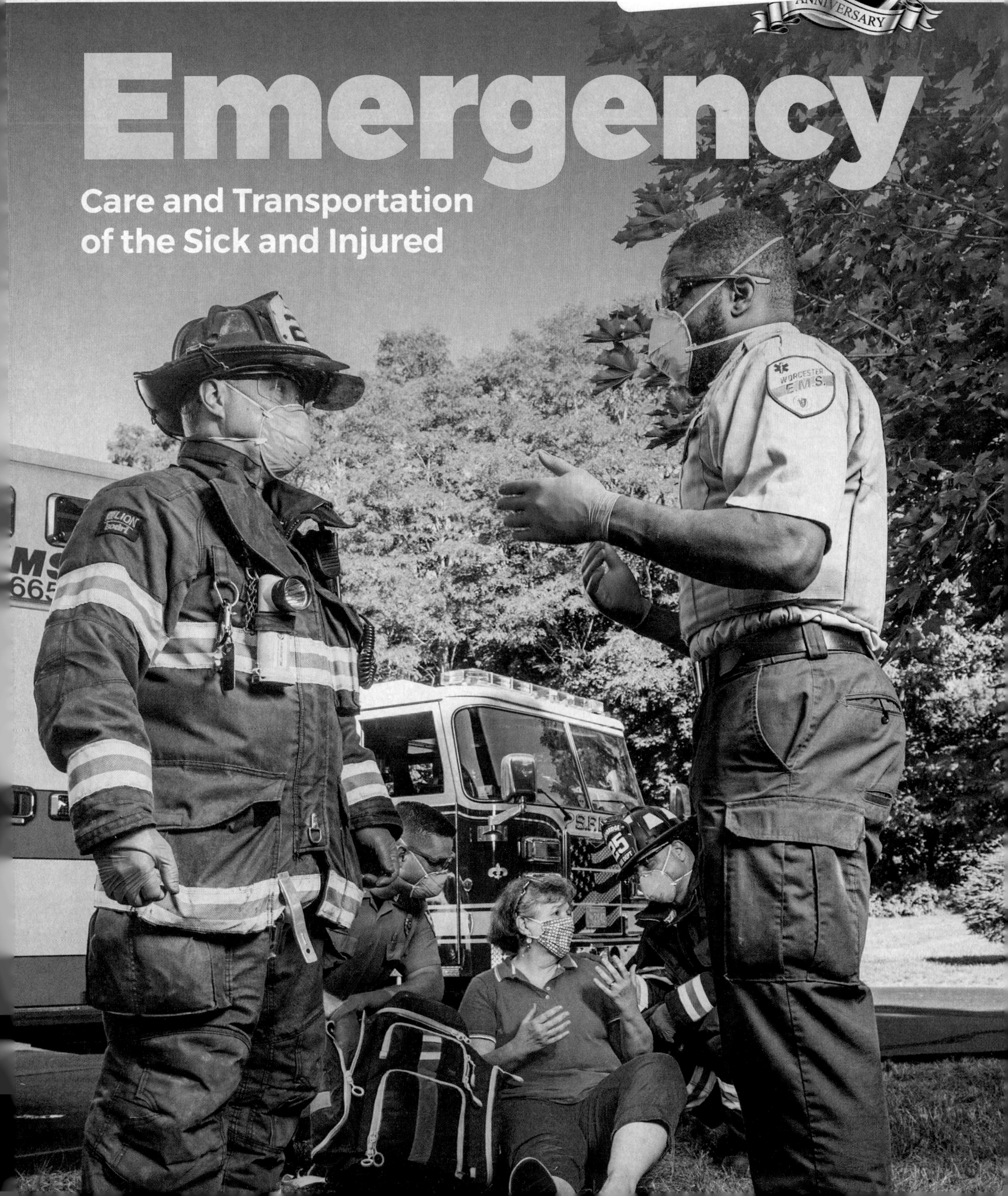

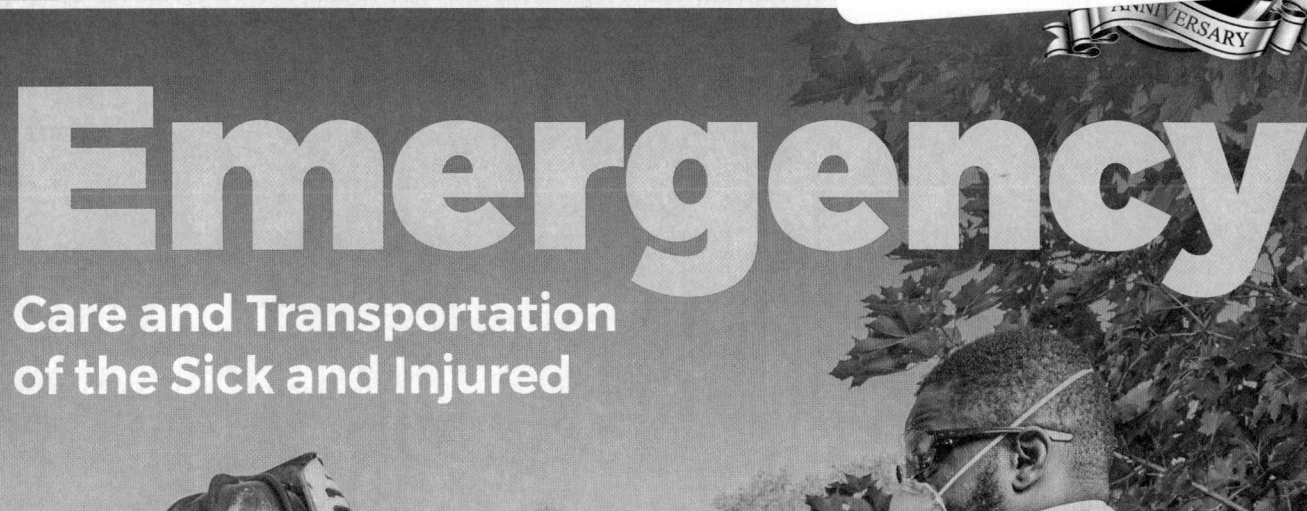

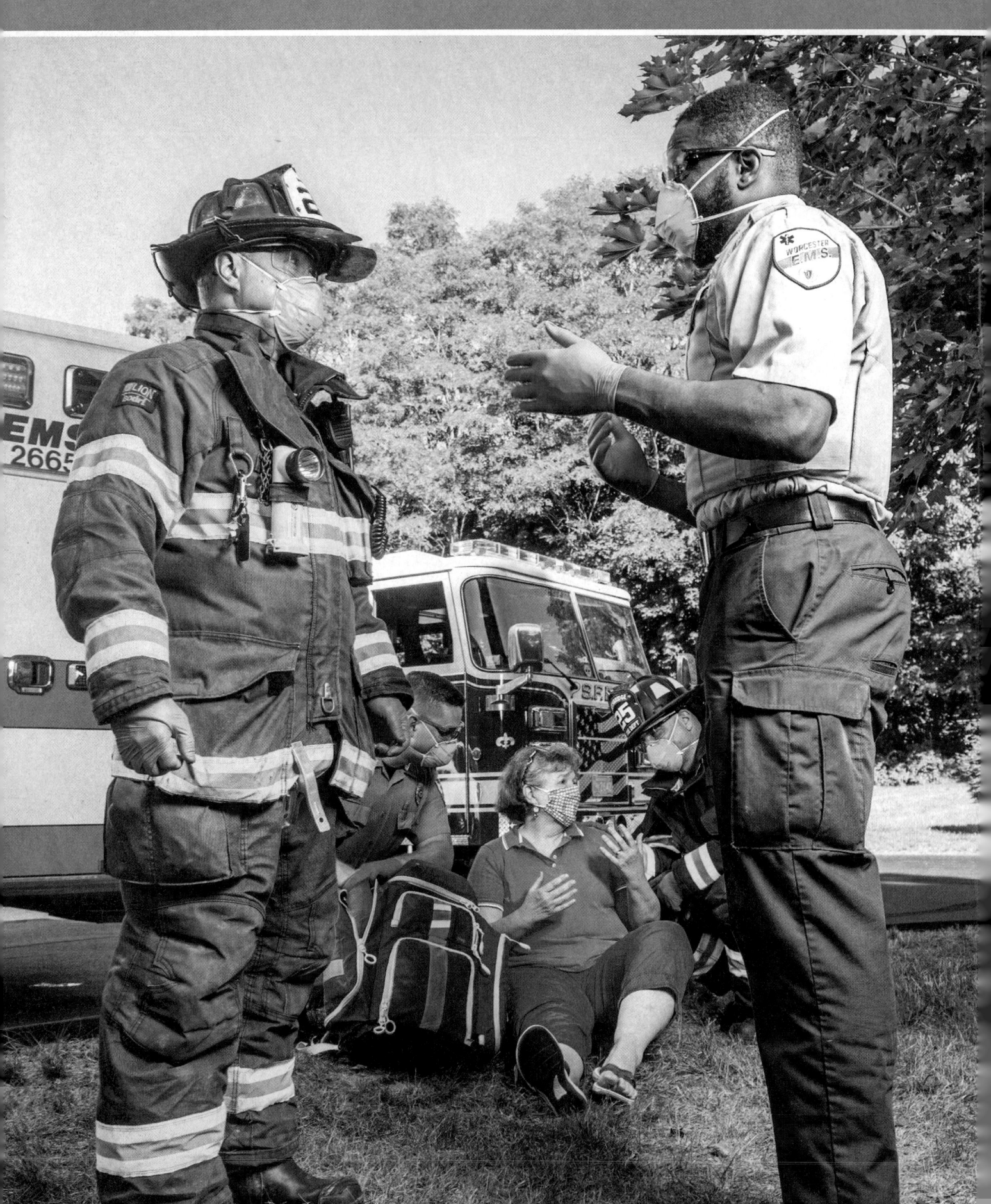

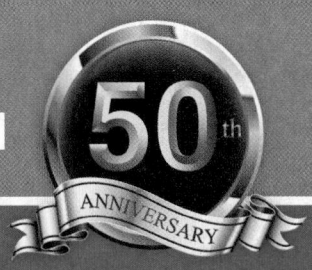

**TWELFTH EDITION**

# Emergency

## Care and Transportation of the Sick and Injured

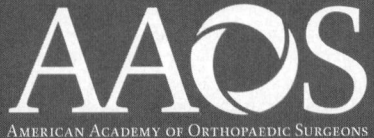

American Academy of Orthopaedic Surgeons

Series Editor:

**Andrew N. Pollak, MD, FAAOS**

Coeditor:

**Alfonso Mejia, MD, MPH, FAAOS**

Lead Editors:

**Dennis Edgerly, MEd, EMT-P**

**Kim D. McKenna PhD, MEd, RN, EMT-P**

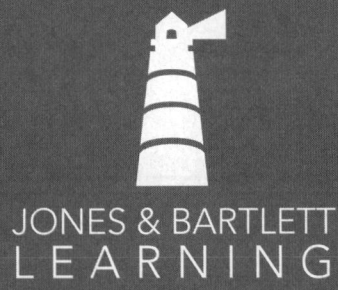

JONES & BARTLETT
LEARNING

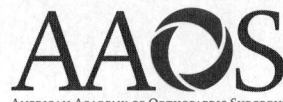
American Academy of Orthopaedic Surgeons

*World Headquarters*
Jones & Bartlett Learning
25 Mall Road
Burlington, MA 01803
978-443-5000
info@jblearning.com
www.jblearning.com
www.psglearning.com

Jones & Bartlett Learning books and products are available through most bookstores and online booksellers. To contact the Jones & Bartlett Learning Public Safety Group directly, call 800-832-0034, fax 978-443-8000, or visit our website, www.psglearning.com.

978-1-284-24383-3 (Hardcover)

**Production Credits**
President, Professional Eduction: Timothy McClinton
VP, Product Management: Christine Emerton
Director, Product Managment: Jonathan Epstein
Director, Content Management: Donna Gridley
Product Manager: Carly Mahoney
Content Strategist: Barbara Scotese
Content Strategist: Tiffany Sliter
Content Coordinator: Paula-Yuan Gregory
Content Coordinator: Andrew LaBelle
VP, International Sales: Matthew Maniscalco
Sales: Phil Charland
Sales Director: Brian Hendrickson
Marketing Director: Brian Rooney

Director, Project Management: Jenny Corriveau
Project Manager: Lori Mortimer
Senior Project Specialist: Dan Stone
Senior Digital Project Specialist: Angela Dooley
VP, Manufacturing: Therese Connell
Composition: S4Carlisle Publishing Services
Senior Media Development Editor: Troy Liston
Rights Specialist: Rebecca Damon
Cover Design: Scott Moden
Text Design: Scott Moden
Cover Image (Title Page): © Jones & Bartlett Learning
Printing and Binding: LSC Communications

**Library of Congress Cataloging-in-Publication Data**
Names: Pollak, Andrew N., editor. | Mejia, Alfonso,
 editor. | McKenna, Kim, editor. | Edgerly, Dennis, editor. | American
 Academy of Orthopaedic Surgeons, issuing body.
Title: Emergency care and transportation of the sick and injured/edited
 by Andrew N. Pollak, Alfonso Mejia, Kim D. McKenna, Dennis Edgerly.
Description: Twelfth edition. | Burlington, Massachusetts: Jones &
 Bartlett Learning, [2021] | Includes bibliographical references and
 index.
Identifiers: LCCN 2020013605 | ISBN 9781284204308 (paperback)
Subjects: MESH: Emergency Medical Services | Emergency Treatment |
 Transportation of Patients
Classification: LCC RA975.5.E5 | NLM WX 215 | DDC 362.18--dc23
LC record available at https://lccn.loc.gov/2020013605

6048

Printed in the United States of America
28 27 26 25 24   10 9 8 7 6

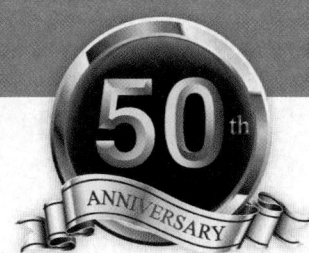
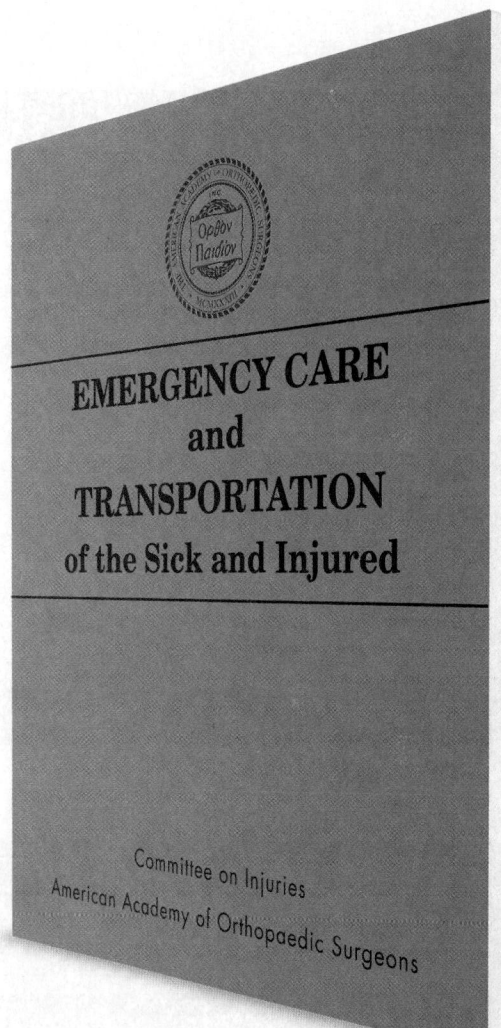
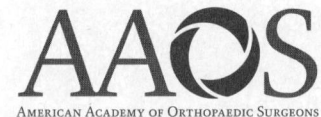
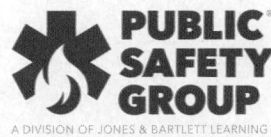

# Brief Contents

**SECTION 1** Preparatory    1

1   EMS Systems    2
2   Workforce Safety and Wellness    30
3   Medical, Legal, and Ethical Issues    85
4   Communications and Documentation    117
5   Medical Terminology    164
6   The Human Body    189
7   Life Span Development    253
8   Lifting and Moving Patients    273
9   The Team Approach to Health Care    319

**SECTION 2** Patient Assessment    337

10   Patient Assessment    338

**SECTION 3** Airway    415

11   Airway Management    416

**SECTION 4** Pharmacology    493

12   Principles of Pharmacology    494

**SECTION 5** Shock and Resuscitation    529

13   Shock    530
14   BLS Resuscitation    555

**SECTION 6** Medical    603

15   Medical Overview    604
16   Respiratory Emergencies    627
17   Cardiovascular Emergencies    675
18   Neurologic Emergencies    723
19   Gastrointestinal and Urologic Emergencies    755
20   Endocrine and Hematologic Emergencies    777
21   Allergy and Anaphylaxis    803
22   Toxicology    821
23   Behavioral Health Emergencies    853
24   Gynecologic Emergencies    881

**SECTION 7** Trauma    899

25   Trauma Overview    900
26   Bleeding    933
27   Soft-Tissue Injuries    961
28   Face and Neck Injuries    1005
29   Head and Spine Injuries    1039
30   Chest Injuries    1091
31   Abdominal and Genitourinary Injuries    1117
32   Orthopaedic Injuries    1145
33   Environmental Emergencies    1199

**SECTION 8** Special Patient Populations    1241

34  Obstetrics and Neonatal Care    1242

35  Pediatric Emergencies    1281

36  Geriatric Emergencies    1349

37  Patients With Special Challenges    1391

**SECTION 9** EMS Operations    1421

38  Transport Operations    1422

39  Vehicle Extrication and Special Rescue    1463

40  Incident Management    1485

41  Terrorism Response and Disaster Management    1527

Glossary    1561

Index    1605

# Contents

**SECTION 1** Preparatory     1

## 1 EMS Systems     2

Introduction     3
EMT Training: Focus and Requirements     6
Licensure Requirements     6
Overview of the EMS System     7
   History of EMS     7
Levels of Training     9
   Public Basic Life Support and Immediate Aid     10
   Emergency Medical Responder     10
   Emergency Medical Technician     11
   Advanced Emergency Medical Technician     11
   Paramedic     11
Components of the EMS System     12
   Public Access     12
   Human Resources     13
   Medical Direction     14
   Legislation and Regulation     14
   Integration of Health Services     15
   Mobile Integrated Health Care and Community Paramedicine     15
   Information Systems     15
   Evaluation     16
   System Finance     18
   Education Systems     18
   Prevention and Public Education     19
   EMS Research     20
Roles and Responsibilities of the EMT     21
   Professional Attributes     22

## 2 Workforce Safety and Wellness     30

Introduction     31
General Health, Wellness, and Resilience     31
   Wellness and Stress Management     32
   Sleep     35
   Disease Prevention and Health Promotion     36
   Balancing Work, Family, and Health     38
Infectious and Communicable Diseases     38
   Routes of Transmission     38
   Risk Reduction and Prevention for Infectious and Communicable Diseases     41
   Immunity     51
   General Postexposure Management     53
Scene Safety     54
   Scene Hazards     55
   Scenes of Violence     60
   Protective Clothing: Preventing Injury     61
Caring for Critically Ill and Injured Patients     65

   Techniques for Communicating With the Critical Patient     65
   Locating and Notifying Family Members     66
   Injured and Critically Ill Children     66
   Coping With the Death of a Child     66
   Helping the Family     67
Death and Dying     67
   The Grieving Process     68
   What Can the EMT Do?     68
   Assisting Patient and Family Members     69
Stress Management on the Job     69
   Posttraumatic Stress Disorder     71
   Burnout     72
   Compassion Fatigue     72
   Responder Risk for Suicide     72
   Emotional Aspects of Emergency Care     73
   Stressful Situations     74
Workplace Issues     75
   Cultural Diversity on the Job     75
   Sexual Harassment     76
   Substance Abuse     77
   Injury and Illness Prevention     77

## 3 Medical, Legal, and Ethical Issues     85

Introduction     86
Consent     86
   Expressed Consent     87
   Implied Consent     88
   Involuntary Consent     88
   Minors and Consent     88
   Forcible Restraint     89
The Right to Refuse Treatment     90
Confidentiality     91
   Health Insurance Portability and Accountability Act     91
   Social Media     93
Advance Directives     93
Physical Signs of Death     95
   Presumptive Signs of Death     95
   Definitive Signs of Death     95
   Medical Examiner Cases     96
Special Situations     97
   Organ Donors     97
   Medical Identification Insignia     97
Scope of Practice     98
Standards of Care     98
   Standards Imposed by Local Custom     98
   Standards Imposed by Law     98
   Professional or Institutional Standards     99
   Standards Imposed by Textbooks     100
   Standards Imposed by States     100
Duty to Act     100

Negligence                                                      101
Abandonment                                                     101
Assault and Battery and Kidnapping                              102
Defamation                                                      102
Good Samaritan Laws and Immunity                                103
Records and Reports                                             104
Special Mandatory Reporting Requirements                        104
   Abuse of Children, Older People, and Others   104
   Injury During the Commission of a Felony      104
   Drug-Related Injuries                         104
   Childbirth                                    105
   Other Reporting Requirements                  105
   Scene of a Crime                              105
   The Deceased                                  105
Ethical Responsibilities                                        106
The EMT in Court                                                107

**4 Communications and Documentation          117**

Introduction                                                    118
Therapeutic Communication                                       119
   Age, Culture, and Personal Experience         120
   Nonverbal Communication                       120
   Verbal Communication                          122
Written Communications and Documentation                        133
   Patient Care Report                           134
   Types of Forms                                137
   Standardized Narrative Formats                138
   Reporting Errors                              142
   Documenting Refusal of Care                   143
   Special Reporting Situations                  146
Communications Systems and Equipment                            146
   Base Station Radios                           146
   Mobile and Portable Radios                    147
   Repeater-Based Systems                        147
   Digital Equipment                             148
   Cellular/Satellite Telephones                 148
   Other Communications Equipment                149
Radio Communications                                            150
   Responding to the Scene                       151
   Communicating With Medical Control
     and Hospitals                     153
   Maintenance of Radio Equipment                156

**5 Medical Terminology          164**

Introduction                                                    165
Anatomy of a Medical Term                                       165
   Word Roots                                    165
   Prefixes                                      165
   Suffixes                                      166
   Combining Vowels                              166
Word Building Rules                                             168
Plural Endings                                                  168
Special Word Parts                                              168
   Numbers                                       168
   Colors                                        169
   Positions and Directions                      169
Common Direction, Movement, and
   Position Terms                                170
   Directional Terms                             170
   Movement Terms                                172
   Other Directional Terms                       172
   Anatomic Positions                            173
Breaking Terms Apart                                            174

Abbreviations and Symbols                                       174
   Abbreviations                                 174
   Symbols                                       175
Master Tables                                                   176

**6 The Human Body          189**

Introduction                                                    190
Topographic Anatomy                                             190
   The Planes of the Body                        190
From Cells to Systems                                           191
The Skeletal System: Anatomy                                    191
   Bones                                         191
   Joints                                        192
   The Axial Skeleton                            193
   The Appendicular Skeleton                     195
   The Pelvis                                    196
   The Lower Extremities                         196
The Skeletal System: Physiology                                 197
The Musculoskeletal System: Anatomy                             197
   Skeletal Muscle                               198
The Musculoskeletal System: Physiology                          198
The Respiratory System: Anatomy                                 198
   The Upper Airway                              198
   The Lower Airway                              200
   Mechanics of Breathing                        201
The Respiratory System: Physiology                              203
   Respiration                                   203
   Ventilation                                   206
   Characteristics of Normal Breathing           207
   Inadequate Breathing in Adults                207
The Circulatory System: Anatomy                                 207
   The Heart                                     208
   Arteries                                      211
   Capillaries                                   213
   Veins                                         213
   Blood Composition                             214
   The Spleen                                    215
The Circulatory System: Physiology                              215
   Normal Circulation in Adults                  215
   Inadequate Circulation in Adults              216
   The Function of Blood                         217
   Nervous System Control of the Cardiovascular
     System                            218
The Nervous System: Anatomy and Physiology                      220
   The Central Nervous System                    220
   The Peripheral Nervous System                 223
The Integumentary System (Skin): Anatomy                        224
The Integumentary System (Skin): Physiology                     225
The Digestive System: Anatomy                                   226
   The Abdomen                                   226
   Mouth                                         228
   Oropharynx                                    228
   Esophagus                                     228
   Stomach                                       228
   Pancreas                                      228
   Liver                                         228
   Small Intestine                               229
   Large Intestine                               229
   Appendix                                      229
   Rectum                                        229
The Digestive System: Physiology                                229
The Lymphatic System: Anatomy and Physiology                    230
The Endocrine System: Anatomy and Physiology                    230
The Urinary System: Anatomy and Physiology                      232

The Genital System: Anatomy and Physiology 233
  The Male Reproductive System and Organs 233
  The Female Reproductive System and Organs 234
Life Support Chain 235
Pathophysiology 236
  Respiratory Compromise 236
  Shock 238
  Alteration of Cellular Metabolism 240

**7  Life Span Development    253**

Introduction 254
  Vital Signs 254
Neonates (Birth to 1 Month) and Infants
  (1 Month to 1 Year) 254
  Physical Changes 254
  Psychosocial Changes 257
Toddlers (1 to 3 Years) and Preschoolers
  (3 to 6 Years) 258
  Physical Changes 258
  Psychosocial Changes 260
School-Age Children (6 to 12 Years) 260
  Physical Changes 260
  Psychosocial Changes 260
Adolescents (12 to 18 Years) 261
  Physical Changes 261
  Psychosocial Changes 262
Early Adults (19 to 40 Years) 263
  Physical Changes 263
  Psychosocial Changes 263
Middle Adults (41 to 60 Years) 263
  Physical Changes 263
  Psychosocial Changes 264
Older Adults (61 Years and Older) 264
  Physical Changes 264
  Psychosocial Changes 267

**8  Lifting and Moving Patients    273**

Introduction 274
The Wheeled Ambulance Stretcher 275
Backboards 276
Moving and Positioning the Patient 276
Body Mechanics 277
  Anatomy Review 277
Principles of Safe Reaching and Pulling 280
Principles of Safe Lifting and Carrying 282
  Patient Weight 282
  Lifting and Carrying a Patient on a Backboard
    or Stretcher 284
  Moving a Patient With a Stair Chair 287
  Moving a Patient on Stairs With a Stretcher 289
  Loading a Wheeled Stretcher Into an Ambulance 290
Directions and Commands 291
Emergency Moves 294
Urgent Moves 295
  Rapid Extrication Technique 295
Nonurgent Moves 300
  Direct Ground Lift 300
  Extremity Lift 302
  Transfer Moves 302
Geriatrics 307
Bariatrics 307
Additional Patient-Moving Equipment 309
  Bariatric Stretchers 309
  Pneumatic and Electronic Powered Wheeled
    Stretchers 309
  Binder Lift 309

Portable/Folding Stretchers 310
Flexible Stretchers 310
Short Backboards 311
Vacuum Mattresses 311
Basket Stretchers 311
Neonatal Isolettes 312
Decontamination 312
Patient Positioning 312
Personnel Considerations 313

**9  The Team Approach to Health Care    319**

Introduction 320
An Era of Team Health Care 321
  Community Paramedicine and Mobile Integrated
    Healthcare Teams 321
  Differences Among Teams 321
Types of Teams 321
  Regular Teams 321
  Temporary Teams 322
  Special Teams 322
Groups Versus Teams 322
  Groups 322
Dependent, Independent, and Interdependent
  Groups 323
  Dependent 323
  Independent 323
  Interdependent 323
Effective Team Performance 323
  A Shared Goal 323
  Clear Roles and Responsibilities 323
  Diverse and Competent Skill Sets 323
  Effective Collaboration and Communication 325
  Supportive and Coordinated Leadership 325
Transfer of Patient Care 326
  General Guidelines 327
BLS and ALS Providers Working Together 328
  Where BLS Care Ends and ALS Care Begins 328
Assisting With ALS Skills 328
Critical Thinking and Clinical Decision Making
  in EMS 329
  Stages of the Decision-Making Process 329
  Decision Traps 330
Troubleshooting Team Conflicts 331

**SECTION 2 Patient Assessment    337**

**10  Patient Assessment    338**

Introduction 342
Scene Size-up 343
  Ensure Scene Safety 344
  Determine Mechanism of Injury/Nature
    of Illness 345
  Take Standard Precautions 347
  Determine Number of Patients 348
  Consider Additional/Specialized Resources 349
Primary Assessment 350
  Form a General Impression 351
  Scan for Signs of Uncontrolled External Bleeding 352
  Assess Level of Consciousness 352
  Assess the Airway 354
  Assess Breathing 355
  Assess Circulation 357
  Performing a Rapid Exam to Identify Life Threats 361
  Determine Priority of Patient Care and Transport 363

| | |
|---|---|
| History Taking | 366 |
| Investigate the Chief Complaint (History of Present Illness) | 367 |
| Obtain SAMPLE History | 369 |
| Secondary Assessment | 377 |
| Systematically Assess the Patient—Secondary Assessment | 378 |
| Systematically Assess the Patient—Focused Assessment | 379 |
| Assess Vital Signs Using the Appropriate Monitoring Device | 401 |
| Reassessment | 405 |
| Repeat the Primary Assessment | 405 |
| Reassess Vital Signs | 405 |
| Reassess the Chief Complaint | 406 |
| Recheck Interventions | 406 |
| Identify and Treat Changes in the Patient's Condition | 406 |
| Reassess Patient | 406 |

## SECTION 3 Airway    415

### 11 Airway Management    416

| | |
|---|---|
| Introduction | 417 |
| Anatomy of the Respiratory System | 418 |
| Anatomy of the Upper Airway | 418 |
| Anatomy of the Lower Airway | 420 |
| Physiology of Breathing | 423 |
| Ventilation | 424 |
| Oxygenation | 427 |
| Respiration | 427 |
| Pathophysiology of Respiration | 428 |
| Factors in the Nervous System | 429 |
| Ventilation/Perfusion Ratio and Mismatch | 429 |
| Factors Affecting Pulmonary Ventilation | 429 |
| Factors Affecting Respiration | 430 |
| Circulatory Compromise | 431 |
| Patient Assessment | 431 |
| Recognizing Adequate Breathing | 432 |
| Recognizing Abnormal Breathing | 432 |
| Assessment of Respiration | 434 |
| Opening the Airway | 439 |
| Head Tilt–Chin Lift Maneuver | 440 |
| Jaw-Thrust Maneuver | 441 |
| Opening the Mouth | 442 |
| Suctioning | 442 |
| Suctioning Equipment | 443 |
| Techniques of Suctioning | 444 |
| Basic Airway Adjuncts | 446 |
| Oropharyngeal Airways | 446 |
| Nasopharyngeal Airways | 449 |
| Maintaining the Airway | 449 |
| Supplemental Oxygen | 451 |
| Supplemental Oxygen Equipment | 451 |
| Procedures for Operating and Administering Oxygen | 455 |
| Hazards of Supplemental Oxygen | 457 |
| Oxygen-Delivery Equipment | 457 |
| Nonrebreathing Masks | 458 |
| Nasal Cannulas | 458 |
| Partial Rebreathing Masks | 459 |
| Venturi Masks | 459 |
| Tracheostomy Masks | 459 |
| Humidification | 460 |

| | |
|---|---|
| Assisted and Artificial Ventilation | 460 |
| Assisting Ventilation in Respiratory Distress/Failure | 461 |
| Artificial Ventilation | 461 |
| Continuous Positive Airway Pressure | 469 |
| Mechanism | 469 |
| Indications | 470 |
| Contraindications | 470 |
| Application | 470 |
| Complications | 473 |
| Stomas and Tracheostomy Tubes | 474 |
| Foreign Body Airway Obstruction | 474 |
| Recognition | 475 |
| Emergency Medical Care for Foreign Body Airway Obstruction | 476 |
| Dental Appliances | 477 |
| Facial Bleeding | 477 |
| Assisting With ALS Airway Procedures | 477 |
| Assisting With Placement of Advanced Airways | 477 |

## SECTION 4 Pharmacology    493

### 12 Principles of Pharmacology    494

| | |
|---|---|
| Introduction | 495 |
| How Medications Work | 495 |
| Medication Names | 497 |
| Routes of Administration | 498 |
| Medication Forms | 501 |
| Tablets and Capsules | 501 |
| Solutions and Suspensions | 501 |
| Metered-Dose Inhalers | 502 |
| Topical Medications | 502 |
| Transcutaneous Medications | 502 |
| Gels | 503 |
| Gases for Inhalation | 503 |
| General Steps in Administering Medication | 503 |
| Medication Administration Cross-Check Procedure | 505 |
| Medication Administration and the EMT | 506 |
| Medications Used by EMTs | 507 |
| Oral Medications | 507 |
| Sublingual Medications | 511 |
| Intramuscular Medications | 513 |
| Intranasal Medications | 515 |
| Inhalation Medications | 515 |
| Patient Medications | 518 |
| Implications for EMS Providers | 519 |
| Medication Errors | 522 |

## SECTION 5 Shock and Resuscitation    529

### 13 Shock    530

| | |
|---|---|
| Introduction | 531 |
| Pathophysiology | 531 |
| Perfusion | 531 |
| Causes of Shock | 534 |
| Types of Shock | 534 |
| Cardiogenic Shock | 534 |
| Obstructive Shock | 536 |
| Distributive Shock | 537 |

Hypovolemic Shock                                      539
The Progression of Shock                               540
Patient Assessment for Shock                           540
    Scene Size-up                                      540
    Primary Assessment                                 541
    History Taking                                     542
    Secondary Assessment                               542
    Reassessment                                       542
Emergency Medical Care for Shock                       543
    Treating Cardiogenic Shock                         543
    Treating Obstructive Shock                         546
    Treating Septic Shock                              546
    Treating Neurogenic Shock                          546
    Treating Anaphylactic Shock                        546
    Treating Psychogenic Shock                         546
    Treating Hypovolemic Shock                         547
    Treating Shock in Older Patients                   548

**14  BLS Resuscitation                                555**

Introduction                                           556
Elements of BLS                                        557
The Components of CPR                                  559
Assessing the Need for BLS                             560
    Basic Principles of BLS                            561
Automated External Defibrillation                      561
    AED Usage in Children                              562
    Special AED Situations                             562
Positioning the Patient                                562
Check for Breathing and a Pulse                        563
    Provide External Chest Compressions               563
    Proper Hand Position and Compression
       Technique                                       563
Opening the Airway and Providing Artificial
    Ventilation                                        566
    Opening the Airway in Adults                       566
    Recovery Position                                  567
    Breathing                                          568
    Provide Artificial Ventilations                    568
One-Rescuer Adult CPR                                  569
Two-Rescuer Adult CPR                                  571
    Switching Positions                                571
Devices and Techniques to Assist Circulation           573
    Active Compression-Decompression CPR               573
    Impedance Threshold Device                         575
    Mechanical Piston Device                           575
    Load-Distributing Band CPR or Vest CPR             576
Infant and Child CPR                                   577
    Determining Responsiveness                         578
    Check for Breathing and a Pulse                    579
    Airway                                             582
    Provide Rescue Breathing                           583
Interrupting CPR                                        583
When Not to Start CPR                                   584
When to Stop CPR                                        586
Foreign Body Airway Obstruction in Adults              587
    Recognizing Foreign Body Airway Obstruction       587
    Removing a Foreign Body Airway Obstruction
       in an Adult                                     588
Foreign Body Airway Obstruction in Infants
    and Children                                       590
    Removing a Foreign Body Airway Obstruction
       in a Child                                      590
    Removing a Foreign Body Airway Obstruction
       in Infants                                      591

Special Resuscitation Circumstances                    593
    Opioid Overdose                                    593
    Cardiac Arrest in Pregnancy                        593
Grief Support for Family Members and Loved Ones        594
Education and Training for the EMT                      595
Education and Training for the Public                   595

**SECTION 6** Medical                                  603

**15  Medical Overview                                 604**

Introduction                                           605
Types of Medical Emergencies                           605
Patient Assessment                                     605
    Scene Size-up                                      606
    Primary Assessment                                 607
    History Taking                                     608
    Secondary Assessment                               609
    Reassessment                                       611
Management, Transport, and Destination                 611
    Scene Time                                         611
    Type of Transport                                  611
    Destination Selection                              613
Infectious Diseases                                    613
    General Assessment Principles                      613
    General Management Principles                      613
    Epidemic and Pandemic Considerations               613
Common or Serious Communicable Diseases                614
    Influenza                                          614
    Herpes Simplex                                     614
    HIV Infection                                      614
    Hepatitis                                          615
    Meningitis                                         618
    Tuberculosis                                       618
    Whooping Cough                                     619
    Methicillin-Resistant *Staphylococcus aureus*      619
    Global Health Issues                               620
    Travel Medicine                                    620
Conclusion                                             621

**16  Respiratory Emergencies                          627**

Introduction                                           628
Anatomy of the Respiratory System                      628
Physiology of Respiration                              629
Pathophysiology                                        631
    Carbon Dioxide Retention and Hypoxic Drive         631
Causes of Dyspnea                                      633
    Upper or Lower Airway Infection                    634
    Acute Pulmonary Edema                              638
    Chronic Obstructive Pulmonary Disease              639
    Asthma, Hay Fever, and Anaphylaxis                 642
    Spontaneous Pneumothorax                           644
    Pleural Effusion                                   644
    Obstruction of the Airway                          645
    Pulmonary Embolism                                 645
    Hyperventilation                                   646
    Environmental/Industrial Exposure                  647
Patient Assessment                                     648
    Scene Size-up                                      648
    Primary Assessment                                 648
    History Taking                                     651
    Secondary Assessment                               653
    Reassessment                                       655
Emergency Medical Care                                 656

Metered-Dose Inhaler and Small-Volume Nebulizer 656
Administration of an MDI 659
Administration of a Small-Volume Nebulizer 659
Treatment of Specific Conditions 662
Upper or Lower Airway Infection 662
Acute Pulmonary Edema 662
Chronic Obstructive Pulmonary Disease 663
Asthma, Hay Fever, and Anaphylaxis 663
Spontaneous Pneumothorax 664
Pleural Effusion 664
Obstruction of the Airway 664
Pulmonary Embolism 664
Hyperventilation 664
Environmental/Industrial Exposure 665
Foreign Body Aspiration 665
Tracheostomy Dysfunction 665
Asthma 665
Cystic Fibrosis 666

**17  Cardiovascular Emergencies      675**

Introduction 676
Anatomy and Physiology 677
Circulation 679
Pathophysiology 684
Atherosclerosis 684
Acute Coronary Syndrome 685
Cardiogenic Shock 688
Congestive Heart Failure 688
Hypertensive Emergencies 690
Patient Assessment 692
Scene Size-up 692
Primary Assessment 692
History Taking 693
Secondary Assessment 695
Reassessment 696
Emergency Medical Care for Chest Pain
or Discomfort 696
Administering Nitroglycerin 697
Cardiac Monitoring 699
Placing the Electrodes 699
Performing Cardiac Monitoring 700
Reviewing the ECG Tracing 702
Heart Surgeries and Cardiac Assistive Devices 703
Automatic Implantable Cardiac Defibrillators 704
External Defibrillator Vest 704
Left Ventricular Assist Devices 704
Cardiac Arrest 705
Automated External Defibrillation 705
Emergency Medical Care for Cardiac Arrest 710
Preparation 710
Performing Defibrillation 711

**18  Neurologic Emergencies      723**

Introduction 724
Anatomy and Physiology 724
Pathophysiology 725
Headache 726
Stroke 727
Types of Stroke 728
Signs and Symptoms of Stroke 730
Conditions That May Mimic Stroke 731
Seizures 732
Causes of Seizures 733
The Importance of Recognizing Seizures 734
The Postictal State 735

Syncope 735
Altered Mental Status 735
Causes of Altered Mental Status 736
Patient Assessment 737
Scene Size-up 737
Primary Assessment 738
History Taking 739
Secondary Assessment 741
Reassessment 744
Emergency Medical Care 745
Headache 747
Stroke 747
Seizure 748
Altered Mental Status 749

**19  Gastrointestinal and Urologic
Emergencies      755**

Introduction 756
Anatomy and Physiology 756
The GI System 756
Additional Abdominal Organs 757
The Genital System 757
The Urinary System 757
Pathophysiology 758
Abdominal Pain 759
Causes of Acute Abdomen 760
Urinary System 764
Kidneys 764
Female Reproductive Organs 765
Other Organ Systems 765
Patient Assessment 766
Scene Size-up 766
Primary Assessment 767
History Taking 768
Secondary Assessment 768
Reassessment 770
Emergency Medical Care 770
Dialysis Emergencies 771

**20  Endocrine and Hematologic
Emergencies      777**

Introduction 778
Endocrine Emergencies 778
Anatomy and Physiology 778
Pathophysiology 780
Patient Assessment of Diabetes 786
Scene Size-up 786
Primary Assessment 786
History Taking 787
Secondary Assessment 787
Reassessment 788
Emergency Medical Care for Diabetic
Emergencies 791
Giving Oral Glucose 791
The Presentation of Hypoglycemia 792
Seizures 792
Altered Mental Status 792
Misdiagnosis of Neurologic
Dysfunction 792
Relationship to Airway Management 793
Hematologic Emergencies 793
Anatomy and Physiology 793
Pathophysiology 793

Patient Assessment of Hematologic Disorders    796
  Scene Size-up    796
  Primary Assessment    796
  History Taking    796
  Secondary Assessment    797
  Reassessment    797
Emergency Medical Care for Hematologic
  Disorders    797

**21 Allergy and Anaphylaxis    803**

Introduction    804
Anatomy and Physiology    804
Pathophysiology    804
Common Allergens    806
  Insect Stings    806
Patient Assessment of an Immunologic Emergency    808
  Scene Size-up    808
  Primary Assessment    808
  History Taking    809
  Secondary Assessment    810
  Reassessment    811
Emergency Medical Care of Immunologic
  Emergencies    812
  Epinephrine    813

**22 Toxicology    821**

Introduction    822
Identifying the Patient and the Poison    822
How Poisons Enter the Body    824
  Inhaled Poisons    826
  Absorbed and Surface Contact Poisons    827
  Ingested Poisons    828
  Injected Poisons    829
Patient Assessment    830
  Scene Size-up    830
  Primary Assessment    831
  History Taking    831
  Secondary Assessment    832
  Reassessment    832
Emergency Medical Care    833
Specific Poisons    834
  Alcohol    834
  Opiates and Opioids    836
  Sedative-Hypnotic Drugs    837
  Abused Inhalants    838
  Hydrogen Sulfide    839
  Sympathomimetics    839
  Synthetic Cathinones (Bath Salts)    840
  Marijuana    841
  Hallucinogens    841
  Anticholinergic Agents    842
  Cholinergic Agents    842
  Miscellaneous Drugs    843
Food Poisoning    843
Plant Poisoning    846

**23 Behavioral Health Emergencies    853**

Introduction    854
Myth and Reality    854
Defining a Behavioral Crisis    855
The Magnitude of Mental Health Disorders    856
Pathophysiology    856
  Organic    857
  Functional    857
Safe Approach to a Behavioral Crisis    857

Patient Assessment    857
  Scene Size-up    857
  Primary Assessment    858
  History Taking    859
  Secondary Assessment    860
  Reassessment    861
Acute Psychosis    862
  Schizophrenia    863
Delirium    863
Excited Delirium    864
Restraint    864
  Risks Associated With Patient Restraint    864
  The Process of Restraining a Patient    865
  Performing Patient Restraint    866
The Potentially Violent Patient    868
Suicide    869
Posttraumatic Stress Disorder and Returning
  Combat Veterans    871
  Signs and Symptoms of PTSD    871
  Caring for the Combat Veteran    873
Medicolegal Considerations    873
  Consent    873
  Limited Legal Authority    874

**24 Gynecologic Emergencies    881**

Introduction    882
Anatomy and Physiology    882
Pathophysiology    884
  Pelvic Inflammatory Disease    884
  Sexually Transmitted Diseases    885
  Vaginal Bleeding    885
Patient Assessment    886
  Scene Size-up    886
  Primary Assessment    886
  History Taking    887
  Secondary Assessment    887
  Reassessment    889
Emergency Medical Care    889
Assessment and Management of Specific Conditions    889
  Pelvic Inflammatory Disease    889
  Sexual Assault and Rape    890

**SECTION 7 Trauma    899**

**25 Trauma Overview    900**

Introduction    901
Energy and Trauma    901
MOI Profiles    904
Blunt and Penetrating Trauma    904
Blunt Trauma    904
  Vehicular Crashes    904
  Car Versus Pedestrian    911
  Car Versus Bicycle    911
  Car Versus Motorcycle    911
  Falls    912
Penetrating Trauma    913
Blast Injuries    915
  Tissues at Risk    917
Multisystem Trauma    918
  Golden Principles of Prehospital Trauma Care    919
Patient Assessment    920
  Injuries to the Head    920
  Injuries to the Neck and Throat    920

Injuries to the Chest                                    921
Injuries to the Abdomen                                  921
Management: Transport and Destination                   922
Scene Time                                              922
Destination Selection                                   922
Type of Transport                                       924
Special Considerations                                  926

**26  Bleeding                                           933**

Introduction                                            934
Anatomy and Physiology of the Cardiovascular
System                                                  934
The Heart                                               935
Blood Vessels and Blood                                 935
Pathophysiology and Perfusion                           937
External Bleeding                                       938
The Significance of External Bleeding                   938
Characteristics of External Bleeding                    938
Internal Bleeding                                       940
Mechanism of Injury for Internal Bleeding               940
Nature of Illness for Internal Bleeding                 940
Signs and Symptoms of Internal Bleeding                 940
Patient Assessment for External and Internal
Bleeding                                                941
Scene Size-up                                           941
Primary Assessment                                      942
History Taking                                          942
Secondary Assessment                                    943
Reassessment                                            944
Emergency Medical Care for External Bleeding            944
Wound Packing and Hemostatic Dressings                  946
Tourniquets                                             949
Junctional Tourniquets                                  951
Splints                                                 951
Pelvic Binder                                           951
Bleeding From the Nose, Ears, and Mouth                 951
Emergency Medical Care for Internal Bleeding            955

**27  Soft-Tissue Injuries                              961**

Introduction                                            962
Anatomy and Physiology of the Skin                      962
Anatomy                                                 963
Physiology                                              964
Pathophysiology of Closed and Open Injuries             964
Closed Injuries                                         965
Open Injuries                                           966
Patient Assessment of Closed and Open Injuries          970
Scene Size-up                                           970
Primary Assessment                                      971
History Taking                                          973
Secondary Assessment                                    974
Reassessment                                            974
Emergency Medical Care for Closed Injuries              976
Emergency Medical Care for Open Injuries                976
Abdominal Wounds                                        977
Impaled Objects                                         978
Neck Injuries                                           978
Bites                                                   980
Burns                                                   981
Pathophysiology of Burns                                982
Complications of Burns                                  982
Burn Severity                                           983
Patient Assessment of Burns                             986
Scene Size-up                                           986
Primary Assessment                                      986

History Taking                                          987
Secondary Assessment                                    988
Reassessment                                            989
Emergency Medical Care for Burns                        989
Management of Specific Burns                             991
Dressing and Bandaging                                  997
Sterile Dressings                                       998
Bandages                                                998

**28  Face and Neck Injuries                           1005**

Introduction                                           1006
Anatomy and Physiology                                 1006
The Eye                                                1008
Injuries of the Face and Neck                          1009
Soft-Tissue Injuries                                   1010
Dental Injuries                                        1010
Patient Assessment                                     1011
Scene Size-up                                          1011
Primary Assessment                                     1011
History Taking                                         1012
Secondary Assessment                                   1013
Reassessment                                           1014
Emergency Medical Care                                 1015
Emergency Medical Care for Specific Injuries           1016
Injuries of the Eyes                                   1016
Injuries of the Nose                                   1027
Injuries of the Ear                                    1028
Facial Fractures                                       1030
Dental Injuries                                        1031
Injuries of the Cheek                                  1031
Injuries of the Neck                                   1031
Laryngeal Injuries                                     1033

**29  Head and Spine Injuries                          1039**

Introduction                                           1040
Anatomy and Physiology                                 1040
Nervous System                                         1040
How the Nervous System Works                           1043
Skeletal System                                        1044
Head Injuries                                          1045
Scalp Lacerations                                      1046
Skull Fracture                                         1046
Traumatic Brain Injuries                               1048
Intracranial Pressure                                  1049
Concussion                                             1051
Contusion                                              1051
Other Brain Injuries                                   1051
Spine Injuries                                         1052
Patient Assessment                                     1053
Scene Size-up                                          1053
Primary Assessment                                     1054
History Taking                                         1056
Secondary Assessment                                   1057
Reassessment                                           1060
Emergency Medical Care of Head Injuries                1061
Managing the Airway                                    1062
Circulation                                            1062
Emergency Medical Care of Spinal Injuries              1064
Managing the Airway                                    1064
Spinal Motion Restriction of the Cervical Spine        1064
Preparation for Transport                              1067
Supine Patients                                        1067
Sitting Patients                                       1075
Standing Patients                                      1077
Spinal Motion Restriction Devices                      1078

Helmet Removal                                      1079
  Preferred Method                         1081
  Alternative Method                       1083

**30  Chest Injuries                               1091**

Introduction                                        1092
Anatomy and Physiology                              1092
Mechanics of Ventilation                            1094
Injuries of the Chest                               1095
  Signs and Symptoms of Chest Injury      1096
Patient Assessment                                  1097
  Scene Size-up                           1097
  Primary Assessment                      1098
  History Taking                          1099
  Secondary Assessment                    1100
  Reassessment                            1101
Complications and Management of Chest Injuries      1102
  PPE in Chest Injuries                   1102
  Pneumothorax                            1102
  Hemothorax                              1105
  Cardiac Tamponade                       1105
  Rib Fractures                           1107
  Flail Chest                             1107
Other Chest Injuries                                1108
  Pulmonary Contusion                     1108
  Other Fractures                         1108
  Traumatic Asphyxia                      1109
  Blunt Myocardial Injury                 1109
  Commotio Cordis                         1109
  Laceration of the Great Vessels         1110

**31  Abdominal and Genitourinary Injuries      1117**

Introduction                                        1118
Anatomy and Physiology of the Abdomen               1119
  Abdominal Quadrants                     1119
  Hollow and Solid Organs                 1119
Abdominal Injuries                                  1121
  Closed Abdominal Injuries              1121
  Open Abdominal Injuries                 1122
  Hollow Organ Injuries                   1123
  Solid Organ Injuries                    1124
Patient Assessment of Abdominal Injuries            1125
  Scene Size-up                           1125
  Primary Assessment                      1125
  History Taking                          1126
  Secondary Assessment                    1127
  Reassessment                            1129
Emergency Medical Care of Abdominal Injuries        1129
  Closed Abdominal Injuries               1129
  Open Abdominal Injuries                 1129
Anatomy of the Genitourinary System                 1131
Injuries of the Genitourinary System                1133
  Injuries of the Kidneys                 1133
  Injuries to the Urinary Bladder         1133
  Injuries of the External Male Genitalia 1134
  Injuries of the Female Genitalia        1134
Patient Assessment of the Genitourinary System      1135
  Scene Size-up                           1135
  Primary Assessment                      1135
  History Taking                          1136
  Secondary Assessment                    1136
  Reassessment                            1137
Emergency Medical Care of Genitourinary Injuries    1137
  Kidneys                                 1137
  Urinary Bladder                         1137

External Male Genitalia                             1137
Female Genitalia                                    1138
Rectal Bleeding                                     1138
Sexual Assault and Rape                             1138

**32  Orthopaedic Injuries                       1145**

Introduction                                        1146
Anatomy and Physiology of the Musculoskeletal
  System                                  1146
  Muscles                                 1146
  The Skeleton                            1148
Musculoskeletal Injuries                            1151
  Mechanism of Injury                     1151
  Fractures                               1152
  Dislocations                            1155
  Sprains                                 1156
  Strain                                  1157
  Amputations                             1158
  Complications                           1158
  Assessing the Severity of Injury        1158
Patient Assessment                                  1159
  Scene Size-up                           1159
  Primary Assessment                      1159
  History Taking                          1161
  Secondary Assessment                    1161
  Reassessment                            1162
Emergency Medical Care                              1163
  Splinting                               1164
  Transportation                          1169
Specific Musculoskeletal Injuries                   1169
  Injuries of the Clavicle and Scapula    1169
  Dislocation of the Shoulder             1171
  Fracture of the Humerus                 1172
  Elbow Injuries                          1173
  Fractures of the Forearm                1175
  Injuries of the Wrist and Hand          1176
  Fractures of the Pelvis                 1178
  Dislocation of the Hip                  1179
  Fractures of the Proximal Femur         1180
  Femoral Shaft Fractures                 1181
  Injuries of Knee Ligaments              1187
  Dislocation of the Knee                 1187
  Fractures About the Knee                1188
  Dislocation of the Patella              1188
  Injuries of the Tibia and Fibula        1189
  Ankle Injuries                          1189
  Foot Injuries                           1190
  Sprains and Strains                     1191
  Amputations                             1191
Compartment Syndrome                                1191

**33  Environmental Emergencies                  1199**

Introduction                                        1200
Factors Affecting Exposure                          1201
Cold Exposure                                       1202
  Hypothermia                             1203
  Local Cold Injuries                     1205
Assessment of Cold Injuries                         1206
  Scene Size-up                           1206
  Primary Assessment                      1207
  History Taking                          1207
  Secondary Assessment                    1208
  Reassessment                            1208
General Management of Cold Emergencies              1209
  Emergency Care of Local Cold Injuries   1210

Cold Exposure and You                          1210
Heat Exposure                                  1210
   Heat Cramps                                 1211
   Heat Exhaustion                             1211
   Heatstroke                                  1212
Assessment of Heat Emergencies                 1213
   Scene Size-up                               1213
   Primary Assessment                          1213
   History Taking                              1214
   Secondary Assessment                        1214
   Reassessment                                1214
Management of Heat Emergencies                 1215
   Heat Cramps                                 1215
   Heat Exhaustion                             1215
   Heatstroke                                  1217
Drowning                                       1218
   Spinal Injuries in Submersion Incidents     1218
   Recovery Techniques                         1220
   Resuscitation Efforts                       1220
Diving Emergencies                             1220
   Descent Emergencies                         1220
   Emergencies at the Bottom                   1222
   Ascent Emergencies                          1222
Assessment of Drowning and Diving Emergencies  1223
   Scene Size-up                               1223
   Primary Assessment                          1223
   History Taking                              1224
   Secondary Assessment                        1224
   Reassessment                                1224
Emergency Care for Drowning or Diving
   Emergencies                                 1225
   Other Water Hazards                         1226
   Prevention                                  1226
High Altitude                                  1226
Lightning                                      1227
   Emergency Medical Care                      1227
Bites and Envenomation                         1228
   Spider Bites                                1228
   Hymenoptera Stings                          1229
   Snake Bites                                 1230
   Scorpion Stings                             1233
   Tick Bites                                  1234
Injuries From Marine Animals                   1235


**SECTION 8** Special Patient
Populations                                    1241

**34  Obstetrics and Neonatal Care            1242**

Introduction                                   1243
Anatomy and Physiology of the Female
   Reproductive System                         1243
Normal Changes in Pregnancy                    1246
Complications of Pregnancy                     1247
   Diabetes                                    1247
   Hypertension in Pregnancy                   1247
   Bleeding                                    1248
   Abortion                                    1250
   Abuse                                       1250
   Substance Abuse                             1250
Special Considerations for Trauma and Pregnancy 1251
   Maternal Cardiac Arrest                     1252
   Assessment and Management                   1252
Cultural Value Considerations                  1252

Teenage Pregnancy                              1253
Patient Assessment                             1253
   Scene Size-up                               1253
   Primary Assessment                          1253
   History Taking                              1254
   Secondary Assessment                        1254
   Reassessment                                1255
Stages of Labor                                1255
Normal Delivery Management                     1256
   Preparing for Delivery                      1256
   The Delivery                                1258
   Postdelivery Care                           1264
Neonatal Assessment and Resuscitation          1265
   Additional Resuscitation Efforts            1266
   The Apgar Score                             1269
Complicated Delivery Emergencies               1270
   Breech Delivery                             1270
   Presentation Complications                  1271
   Spina Bifida                                1272
   Multiple Gestation                          1272
   Premature Birth                             1273
   Postterm Pregnancy                          1273
   Fetal Death                                 1273
Postpartum Complications                       1274

**35  Pediatric Emergencies                   1281**

Introduction                                   1284
Communication With the Patient and the Family  1284
Growth and Development                         1284
   The Infant                                  1285
   The Toddler                                 1286
   The Preschool-Age Child                     1287
   School-Age Years                            1288
   Adolescents                                 1289
Anatomy and Physiology                         1290
   The Respiratory System                      1290
   The Circulatory System                      1292
   The Nervous System                          1292
   The Gastrointestinal System                 1292
   The Musculoskeletal System                  1292
   The Integumentary System                    1293
Patient Assessment                             1293
   Scene Size-up                               1293
   Primary Assessment                          1294
   History Taking                              1303
   Secondary Assessment                        1304
   Reassessment                                1306
Respiratory Emergencies and Management         1308
   Airway Obstruction                          1308
   Asthma                                      1310
   Pneumonia                                   1311
   Croup                                       1311
   Epiglottitis                                1311
   Bronchiolitis                               1312
   Pertussis                                   1312
   Airway Adjuncts                             1313
   Oxygen Delivery Devices                     1316
   Cardiopulmonary Arrest                      1319
Circulation Emergencies and Management         1320
   Shock                                       1320
   Bleeding Disorders                          1322
Neurologic Emergencies and Management          1322
   Altered Mental Status                       1322
   Seizures                                    1322
   Meningitis                                  1323

Gastrointestinal Emergencies and Management      1324
Poisoning Emergencies and Management             1325
   Dehydration Emergencies and Management     1326
Fever Emergencies and Management                 1327
   Febrile Seizures                          1328
Drowning Emergencies and Management              1328
Pediatric Trauma Emergencies and Management      1329
   Physical Differences                      1329
   Psychological Differences                 1329
   Injury Patterns                           1329
   Injuries to Specific Body Systems         1330
   Burns                                     1333
   Injuries of the Extremities               1335
   Pain Management                           1335
Disaster Management                              1335
Child Abuse and Neglect                          1336
   Signs of Abuse                            1336
   Symptoms and Other Indicators of Abuse    1338
   Sexual Abuse                              1338
Sudden Unexpected Infant Death and Sudden
   Infant Death Syndrome                     1339
   Patient Assessment and Management         1339
   Scene Assessment                          1340
   Communication and Support of the Family
     After the Death of a Child             1340
   Apparent Life-Threatening Event           1342
   Brief Resolved Unexplained Event          1342

**36  Geriatric Emergencies**                    **1349**

Introduction                                     1350
Generational Considerations                      1350
Communication and Older Adults                   1351
   Communication Techniques                  1351
Common Complaints and the Leading Causes
   of Death in Older People                  1352
Changes in the Body                              1352
Changes in the Respiratory System                1353
   Anatomy and Physiology                    1353
   Pathophysiology                           1353
Changes in the Cardiovascular System             1354
   Anatomy and Physiology                    1354
   Pathophysiology                           1354
Changes in the Nervous System                    1357
   Anatomy and Physiology                    1357
   Pathophysiology                           1358
Changes in the Gastrointestinal System           1360
   Anatomy and Physiology                    1360
   Pathophysiology                           1360
Changes in the Renal System                      1362
   Anatomy and Physiology                    1362
   Pathophysiology                           1362
Changes in the Endocrine System                  1363
   Anatomy and Physiology                    1363
   Pathophysiology                           1363
Changes in the Immune System                     1363
Changes in the Musculoskeletal System            1364
   Anatomy and Physiology                    1364
   Pathophysiology                           1364
   Changes in Skin                           1365
Toxicology                                       1365
Behavioral Emergencies                           1367
   Depression                                1367
   Suicide                                   1367
The GEMS Diamond                                 1368
Special Considerations in Assessing a Geriatric
   Medical Patient                           1368
   Scene Size-up                             1369

Primary Assessment                               1370
History Taking                                   1371
Secondary Assessment                             1372
Reassessment                                     1372
Trauma and Geriatric Patients                    1374
   Anatomic Changes and Fractures            1374
   Environmental Injury                      1375
Special Considerations in Assessing Geriatric
   Trauma Patients                           1375
   Scene Size-up                             1375
   Primary Assessment                        1376
   History Taking                            1376
   Secondary Assessment                      1377
   Reassessment                              1377
Assessment of Falls                              1378
Response to Nursing and Skilled Care Facilities  1379
Dying Patients                                    1380
   Advance Directives                        1380
Elder Abuse and Neglect                          1381
   Assessment of Elder Abuse                 1382
   Signs of Physical Abuse                   1383

**37  Patients With Special Challenges**          **1391**

Introduction                                     1392
Developmental Disability                          1393
   Autism Spectrum Disorder                  1394
   Down Syndrome                             1394
   Patient Interaction                       1395
Sensory Disabilities                             1396
   Visual Impairment                         1396
   Hearing Impairment                        1397
Physical Disabilities                            1400
   Cerebral Palsy                            1400
   Spina Bifida                              1401
   Paralysis                                 1402
Bariatric Patients                               1402
   Interaction With Patients With Obesity    1402
   Interaction With Patients With Morbid Obesity  1402
Patients With Medical Technology Assistance      1403
   Tracheostomy Tubes                        1403
   Home Oxygen                               1405
   Mechanical Ventilators                    1405
   Apnea Monitors                            1407
   Internal Cardiac Pacemakers               1408
   Ventricular Assist Devices                1408
   External Defibrillator Vest               1408
   Central Venous Catheter                   1409
   Gastrostomy Tubes                         1409
   Shunts                                    1410
   Vagus Nerve Stimulators                   1410
   Colostomies, Ileostomies, and Urostomies  1410
Patient Assessment Guidelines                    1411
Home Care                                        1411
Hospice Care and Terminally Ill Patients         1411
Poverty and Homelessness                         1412

**SECTION 9** EMS Operations                     1421

**38  Transport Operations**                     **1422**

Introduction                                     1423
Emergency Vehicle Design                         1424
Phases of an Ambulance Call                      1426
   The Preparation Phase                     1426
   The Dispatch Phase                        1436

En Route to the Scene                        1437
Arrival at the Scene                         1437
The Transfer Phase                           1440
The Transport Phase                          1440
The Delivery Phase                           1441
En Route to the Station                      1442
The Postrun Phase                            1442
Defensive Ambulance Driving Techniques       1443
Driver Characteristics                       1443
Safe Driving Practices                       1444
Air Medical Operations                       1453
Helicopter Medical Evacuation Operations     1454
Establishing a Landing Zone                  1455
Landing Zone Safety and Patient Transfer     1456
Special Considerations                       1458
Medevac Issues                               1458

**39 Vehicle Extrication and Special
Rescue                                       1463**

Introduction                                 1464
Safety                                       1464
Vehicle Safety Systems                       1464
Fundamentals of Extrication                  1465
Preparation                                  1466
En Route to the Scene                        1466
Arrival and Scene Size-up                    1467
Hazard Control                               1469
Support Operations                           1470
Gaining Access                               1470
Emergency Care                               1472
Removal of the Patient                       1473
Transfer of the Patient                      1474
Termination                                  1475
Specialized Rescue Situations                1475
Technical Rescue Situations                  1475
Search and Rescue                            1476
Trench Rescue                                1477
Tactical Emergency Medical Support           1477
Structure Fires                              1479

**40 Incident Management                     1485**

Introduction                                 1486
National Incident Management System          1486
Incident Command System                      1487
ICS Roles and Responsibilities               1488
Communications and Information Management    1490
Mobilization and Deployment                  1491
EMS Response Within the ICS                  1491
Preparedness                                 1491
Scene Size-up                                1492
Establishing Command                         1493
Communications                               1493
The Medical Branch of Incident Command       1493
Triage Supervisor                            1493
Treatment Supervisor                         1493
Transportation Supervisor                    1494
Staging Supervisor                           1494
Physicians on Scene                          1495
Rehabilitation Supervisor                    1495
Extrication and Special Rescue               1495
Morgue Supervisor                            1495
Mass-Casualty Incidents                      1496

Triage                                       1497
Triage Categories                            1498
Triage Tags                                  1499
START Triage                                 1499
JumpSTART Triage for Pediatric Patients      1500
Triage Special Considerations                1501
Destination Decisions                        1501
Disaster Management                          1502
Introduction to Hazardous Materials          1503
Recognizing a Hazardous Material             1503
Occupancy and Location                       1504
Senses                                       1504
Containers                                   1505
The Department of
    Transportation Marking System            1508
Other Considerations                         1510
Identification                               1513
Hazmat Scene Operations                      1514
Classification of Hazardous Materials        1516
Personal Protective Equipment Level          1516
Caring for Patients at a Hazmat Incident     1517

**41 Terrorism Response and Disaster
Management                                   1527**

Introduction                                 1528
What Is Terrorism?                           1528
Active Shooter Events                        1529
Weapons of Mass Destruction                  1531
Chemical Terrorism/Warfare                   1531
Biologic Terrorism/Warfare                   1532
Nuclear/Radiologic Terrorism                 1532
EMT Response to Terrorism                    1532
Recognizing a Terrorist Event (Indicators)   1532
Response Actions                             1533
Chemical Agents                              1535
Vesicants (Blister Agents)                   1535
Pulmonary Agents (Choking Agents)            1536
Nerve Agents                                 1537
Metabolic Agents (Cyanides)                  1540
Biologic Agents                              1542
Viruses                                      1543
Bacteria                                     1544
Neurotoxins                                  1545
Other EMT Roles During a Biologic Event      1548
Radiologic/Nuclear Devices                   1549
What Is Radiation?                           1549
Sources of Radiologic Material               1549
Radiologic Dispersal Devices                 1550
Nuclear Energy                               1551
Nuclear Weapons                              1551
Symptomatology                               1551
Medical Management                           1551
Protective Measure                           1552
Incendiary and Explosive Devices             1552
Mechanisms of Injury                         1552

**Glossary                                   1561**

**Index                                      1605**

# Skill Drills

| | | |
|---|---|---|
| **Skill Drill 2-1** | Proper Glove Removal Technique | 44 |
| **Skill Drill 2-2** | Managing a Potential Exposure | 49 |
| **Skill Drill 8-1** | Performing the Power Lift | 279 |
| **Skill Drill 8-2** | Performing the Diamond Carry | 285 |
| **Skill Drill 8-3** | Performing the One-Handed Carry | 286 |
| **Skill Drill 8-4** | Using a Stair Chair | 288 |
| **Skill Drill 8-5** | Carrying a Patient on Stairs | 289 |
| **Skill Drill 8-6** | Loading a Stretcher Into an Ambulance | 292 |
| **Skill Drill 8-7** | Performing the Rapid Extrication Technique | 297 |
| **Skill Drill 8-8** | Performing the Direct Ground Lift | 301 |
| **Skill Drill 8-9** | Performing the Extremity Lift | 303 |
| **Skill Drill 8-10** | Performing the Direct Carry | 304 |
| **Skill Drill 8-11** | Using a Scoop Stretcher | 306 |
| **Skill Drill 8-12** | Logrolling a Patient on the Ground | 308 |
| **Skill Drill 10-1** | Performing a Rapid Exam to Identify Life Threats | 362 |
| **Skill Drill 10-2** | Performing the Secondary Assessment | 379 |
| **Skill Drill 10-3** | Obtaining Blood Pressure by Auscultation | 391 |
| **Skill Drill 10-4** | Obtaining Blood Pressure by Palpation | 393 |
| **Skill Drill 10-5** | Assessing Neurovascular Status | 396 |
| **Skill Drill 10-6** | Assessing Blood Glucose Level | 403 |
| **Skill Drill 11-1** | Performing Pulse Oximetry | 436 |
| **Skill Drill 11-2** | Positioning the Unconscious Patient | 440 |
| **Skill Drill 11-3** | Suctioning a Patient's Airway | 445 |
| **Skill Drill 11-4** | Inserting an Oral Airway | 447 |
| **Skill Drill 11-5** | Inserting an Oral Airway With a 90° Rotation | 448 |
| **Skill Drill 11-6** | Inserting a Nasal Airway | 450 |
| **Skill Drill 11-7** | Placing an Oxygen Cylinder Into Service | 455 |
| **Skill Drill 11-8** | Performing One-Rescuer Bag-Mask Ventilations | 465 |
| **Skill Drill 11-9** | Using CPAP | 471 |
| **Skill Drill 14-1** | Performing Chest Compressions | 564 |
| **Skill Drill 14-2** | Performing One-Rescuer Adult CPR | 570 |
| **Skill Drill 14-3** | Performing Two-Rescuer Adult CPR | 572 |
| **Skill Drill 14-4** | Performing Infant Chest Compressions | 580 |
| **Skill Drill 14-5** | Performing CPR on a Child | 581 |
| **Skill Drill 14-6** | Removing a Foreign Body Airway Obstruction in an Unresponsive Child | 592 |
| **Skill Drill 16-1** | Assisting a Patient With a Metered-Dose Inhaler | 660 |
| **Skill Drill 16-2** | Assisting a Patient With a Small-Volume Nebulizer | 661 |
| **Skill Drill 17-1** | Administering Nitroglycerin | 698 |
| **Skill Drill 17-2** | Performing Cardiac Monitoring | 700 |
| **Skill Drill 17-3** | Using an AED | 711 |
| **Skill Drill 21-1** | Using an EpiPen Auto-injector | 815 |
| **Skill Drill 23-1** | Restraining a Patient | 867 |
| **Skill Drill 26-1** | Controlling External Bleeding | 947 |
| **Skill Drill 26-2** | Packing a Wound | 948 |
| **Skill Drill 26-3** | Applying a Commercial Tourniquet | 950 |
| **Skill Drill 26-4** | Controlling Epistaxis | 953 |
| **Skill Drill 26-5** | Controlling Internal Bleeding | 955 |
| **Skill Drill 27-1** | Stabilizing an Impaled Object | 979 |
| **Skill Drill 27-2** | Caring for Burns | 990 |

**Skill Drill 28-1**  Removing a Foreign Object From Under the Upper Eyelid        1018

**Skill Drill 28-2**  Stabilizing a Foreign Object Impaled in the Eye        1020

**Skill Drill 28-3**  Controlling Bleeding From a Neck Injury        1033

**Skill Drill 29-1**  Performing Manual In-Line Stabilization        1065

**Skill Drill 29-2**  Application of a Cervical Collar        1066

**Skill Drill 29-3**  Securing a Patient to a Long Backboard        1068

**Skill Drill 29-4**  Placing a Patient on a Full-Body Vacuum Mattress        1071

**Skill Drill 29-5**  Securing a Patient Found in a Sitting Position        1075

**Skill Drill 29-6**  Removing a Helmet        1082

**Skill Drill 32-1**  Caring for Musculoskeletal Injuries        1163

**Skill Drill 32-2**  Applying a Rigid Splint        1166

**Skill Drill 32-3**  Applying a Vacuum Splint        1168

**Skill Drill 32-4**  Splinting the Hand and Wrist        1177

**Skill Drill 32-5**  Applying a Hare Traction Splint        1183

**Skill Drill 32-6**  Applying a Sager Traction Splint        1186

**Skill Drill 33-1**  Treating for Heat Exhaustion        1216

**Skill Drill 33-2**  Stabilizing a Suspected Spinal Injury in the Water        1221

**Skill Drill 34-1**  Delivering the Newborn        1260

**Skill Drill 35-1**  Positioning the Airway in a Pediatric Patient        1298

**Skill Drill 35-2**  Inserting an Oropharyngeal Airway in a Pediatric Patient        1314

**Skill Drill 35-3**  Inserting a Nasopharyngeal Airway in a Pediatric Patient        1315

**Skill Drill 35-4**  One-Person Bag-Mask Ventilation on a Pediatric Patient        1319

**Skill Drill 35-5**  Immobilizing a Pediatric Patient        1331

**Skill Drill 35-6**  Immobilizing a Patient in a Car Seat        1332

# Preface

Although we were often painfully reminded during the course of the COVID-19 pandemic of the importance of personal protective equipment (PPE) in our profession, readers may notice some variability throughout this textbook with regard to the types of PPE worn by providers and others as they care for patients. There are several explanations for this.

Prior to 2020, the level of PPE commonly worn by all providers during patient encounters typically included gloves. Eye protection was added during situations when the risk of a splash was high or when there was significant risk of aerosolization of material that could potentially come in contact with the eyes. For example, eye protection was typically worn while caring for patients who were bleeding significantly, when performing airway-related procedures, and during maternity calls. It was added on calls when there was a perceived high risk of being splashed with a potentially contaminated body fluid. In the post–COVID-19 era, however, use of eye protection has become more common.

In addition, masks are now standard equipment for all interpersonal encounters, let alone patient encounters. At various times throughout the pandemic, masks have been required in public places such as grocery stores. Social distancing guidelines mandate the use of masks in public. Simple face masks or cloth masks are considered mandatory both to decrease the risk of infection for the person wearing the mask and to decrease the risk associated with viral shedding that is a known consequence of infection, even in asymptomatic hosts. In other words, people with no symptoms can still be infected with the virus and shed the virus, and thus they are capable of transmitting it to others. To make it safer for people to be around those individuals, asking everyone to wear a mask in public can make the environment safer.

Furthermore, when caring for COVID-19 patients or those who have overt symptoms such as fever or cough, a higher level of protection is recommended, such as an N95 mask or even a powered air-purifying respirator (PAPR) system. There is some variability in that recommendation, with many agencies using N95 masks for all patient encounters given the increased level of protection they afford and the degree to which asymptomatic individuals who could transmit the disease to others are pervasive in the population.

As of the time of the development of this text, however, the pandemic situation was actively evolving. We have tried throughout the text to make the language follow best available knowledge and practice as of the time that the text was developed. However, the science in this area is evolving rapidly, as is clinical practice. It is likely that some or even much of what is included in this textbook with regard to PPE recommendations may be partially or completely outdated by the time it is published. We will attempt to make supplemental material available that reflects the most up-to-date knowledge.

Revising the illustrations and images throughout the book is much more difficult. Organizing photo shoots has been dramatically hindered by necessary social distancing restrictions. For this reason, in order to get the best information to students as soon as possible, we made efforts to edit certain images associated with perceived high-risk procedures, such as aerosol-generating procedures. Furthermore, we added N95 masks and appropriate eye protection to all new images that were created for this textbook. However, we were not able to update all of the photos to reflect new practice guidelines. It is certainly our hope that by the time the next edition is published, our knowledge of best practices with regard to PPE will be more settled, and there will be greater consistency in the appearance of PPE in images throughout the text.

Until then, however, please accept our apologies for any inconsistencies in the use of PPE in the images and skill drills throughout this book. It is absolutely our intention to teach students the best practices with regard to PPE so that their risk of becoming infected and transmitting infection to their patients and others is minimized to the greatest degree possible.

**Andrew N. Pollak, MD, FAAOS**
Series Editor

# Acknowledgments

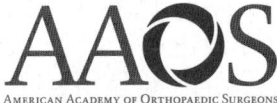

The American Academy of Orthopaedic Surgeons would like to acknowledge the editors and authors of previous editions of *Emergency Care and Transportation of the Sick and Injured,* as well as the reviewers of the new 12th edition.

## Series Editor

**Andrew N. Pollak, MD, FAAOS**
The James Lawrence Kernan Professor and Chairman, Department of Orthopaedics, University of Maryland School of Medicine
Chief of Orthopaedics, University of Maryland Medical System
Director, Shock Trauma Go Team, R. Adams Cowley Shock Trauma Center
Medical Director, Baltimore County Fire Department
Special Deputy US Marshal
Baltimore, Maryland

## Coeditor

**Alfonso Mejia, MD, MPH, FAAOS**
Program Director, Orthopedic Surgery Residency Program
Vice Head, Department of Orthopedic Surgery
University of Illinois College of Medicine
Medical Director
Tactical Emergency Medical Support Physician
South Suburban Emergency Response Team
Chicago, Illinois

## Lead Editors

**Dennis Edgerly, MEd, EMT-P**
Arapahoe Community College
Littleton, Colorado

**Kim D. McKenna, PhD, RN, EMT-P**
St. Charles County Ambulance District
St. Peters, Missouri

## Authors

**Matthew Adams, AHS, LP, NRP, FP-C**
*Chapters 38–41*
Flight Paramedic
Memorial Hermann Life Flight
Houston, Texas

**Andrew Bartkus, JD, MSN, RN, NRP, CEN, CCRN, CFRN, Esq.**
*Chapter 12*
Emergency Department Director
Sandoval Regional Medical Center
Rio Rancho, New Mexico

**Bruce Butterfras, MSEd, LP**
*Chapters 16–18*
Assistant Professor, Director of Bachelor Degree and SAFD Initial Education Programs
Department of Emergency Health Sciences
The University of Texas Health Science Center at San Antonio
San Antonio, Texas

**Chris Coughlin, PhD, NRP**
*Chapters 25–29*
Department Chair, Public Safety
Sciences
Glendale Community College
Glendale, Arizona

**David L. Dalton, BS, EMTP**
*Chapters 6, 7, 31, 32*
Captain
St. Charles County Ambulance
District
St. Peters, Missouri

**Rommie L. Duckworth, MS, LP**
*Chapters 1–5*
Captain/EMS Coordinator
Ridgefield Fire Department
Ridgefield, Connecticut

**Dennis Edgerly, MEd, EMTP**
*Chapters 15, 33*
Director EMS Academy
Arapahoe Community College
Littleton, Colorado

**Wm. Travis Engel, DO, MSc,
NRP, FP-C, CCP-C**
*Chapters 34, 37*
Pediatric Critical Care Medicine
Fellow
Children's Mercy Hospital
Kansas City, Missouri

**Michael Kaduce, MPS, NRP**
*Chapters 8, 10, 13, 14, 30, 36*
EMT Program Director
UCLA Center for Prehospital Care
David Geffen School of Medicine
Los Angeles, California

**Kim D. McKenna, PhD,
RN, NRP**
*Chapter 9*
St. Charles County Ambulance
District
St. Peters, Missouri

**Stephen J. Rahm, NRP**
*Chapter 11*
Chief, Office of Clinical
Direction
Co-Chair, Centre for Emergency
Health Sciences
Spring Branch, Texas

**Brittany Williams, DHSc,
RRT-ACCS, NPS, AE-C,
REMT-P**
*Chapters 19–24, 35*
Professor Respiratory Care,
Director Clinical Education
Santa Fe College
Gainesville, Florida

# Ancillary Authors

**Sharon Fralonardo
Chiumento, BSN, EMT-P**
Gates Volunteer Ambulance
Service
Rochester, New York

**Stephen J. Rahm, NRP**
Centre for Emergency Health
Sciences
Spring Branch, Texas

**Christopher Touzeau, MS,
FNP-C, NRP**
Gaithersburg, Maryland

**Bryan Ware, BS, EMT-P**
Beulah Fire Protection and
Ambulance District
Beulah, Colorado

**Brittany Williams, DHSc,
RRT-ACCS, NPS, AE-C,
REMT-P**
Santa Fe College
Gainesville, Florida

# Reviewers

**Riley S. Abrahamson,
NREMT**
Phillips County Ambulance
Service
Malta, Montana

**Lisa Aiken, AAS, NRP**
Central Virginia Community
College
Lynchburg, Virginia

**Eric W. Allmon, EdD, NRP**
Ivy Tech Community College
Fort Wayne, Indiana

**Jamie J.Barton, CCEMT-P,
EMT-P, NYS CIC**
Wilton Emergency Inc.
Saratoga Springs, New York

**Patricia Binion, SEI**
Skagit Valley College
Mt. Vernon, Washington

**Stephen Blackburn, AAS,
Paramedic**
Fayetteville Technical
Community College/Wayne
County EMS
Goldsboro, North Carolina

**Graeme A. Bockrath,
NREMT-P**
TECC Instructor, EMS Instructor
Apollo Career Center; Four
County Career Center
Lima, Ohio; Archbold, Ohio

**Gary Bonewald, MEd, LP**
Wharton County Junior College
Wharton, Texas

**Rick Busch, AEMT, EMSI**
Four County Career Center
Archbold, Ohio

**Bill Camarda, MS, NRP, FP-C**
Bennington Rescue
Bennington, Vermont

**Karen Case, AEMT, SEI**
Chewelah Rural Training
Program
Chewelah, Washington

**Fred D. Chambers,
Paramedic**
Retired Captain
Houston Fire Department
Houston, Texas

**Joy Cherry, NREMT-P, BS
EMS, MEd**
Central New Mexico
Community College
Albuquerque, New Mexico

**Robert Conklin, MPA, NRP, MICP**
Joint Base McGuire-Dix-Lakehurst Fire and Emergency Services
Sayreville, New Jersey

**Jon S. Cooper, MS, NRP**
Howard Community College
Columbia, Maryland

**Chris Credle, PhD, EMT-P, NCOEMS**
Level II Paramedic Instructor
Wake County Public Schools: Public Safety Tech Programs
Garner, North Carolina

**Julia Cusimano, EMT-P, EMSI**
Clark State Community College
Springfield, Ohio

**Sylvia Davis, NREMT-P, Kansas-P, IC, FF, AHA, BLSCRP, ACLS, PALS, BS**
Butler Community College;
McConnell AFB EMS Education Department
Andover, Kansas

**Brandy Debarge, EMT-P, I/C**
Patriot Ambulance, Inc.
Chelmsford, Massachusetts

**Melissa Doak, NRP, LTEMS**
York County Fire & Life Safety
Yorktown, Pennsylvania

**Alicia Elder, NREMT-P, PI, RN**
Lutheran EMS
Warsaw, Indiana

**Ronald B. Estanislao, BA, NRP, FP-C, NCEE**
Boston University
Boston, Massachusetts

**Joseph Gilles, MS, NRP**
Associate Professor of EMS/Fire Science
College of DuPage
Glen Ellyn, Illinois

**Lee Gillum, MPH, Lic-P, EMS-CC**
Montgomery County Hospital District EMS
Conroe, Texas

**Tony W. Gilmer**
Training Captain and Ambulance Board Member
Klickitat County Fire District #3
Husum, Washington

**Rusty Gilpin, MEd, NRP**
Gordon Cooper Technology Center
Shawnee, Oklahoma

**Jennifer L. Hervey, EMT-B, EMT-I, LGI, NAEMT-I,**
CEO, Owner
Twin Valley EMT Training Center
HoneyBrook, Pennsylvania

**Rick Hilinski, BA, EMT-P**
CCAC Public Safety Institute
Pittsburgh, Pennsylvania

**Mikka House-Moore, BS, NRP, AEMD**
Tulsa Technology Center
Tulsa, Oklahoma

**Donald Hutchinson, NREMT-P**
Northeastern Technical College
Wallace, South Carolina

**Joseph Itzkowitz, CCEMT-P, NRP**
Emergency Care Programs
Brooklyn, New York

**Scott Jaeggi, Paramedic**
Rio Hondo College Fire Academy
Santa Fe Springs, California

**Dorothy Jensen, AEMT**
Hinsdale Ambulance Service
Hinsdale, Montana

**Eugene W. Johnson Jr., FF/EMT-B**
Special Operations Educator, EMS Educator, NAEMT Instructor
HAZMAT Response Solutions LLC
Atlantic City, New Jersey

**Heidi Johnson, EMSI**
Washington Ambulance Association, Inc.
Washington Depot, Connecticut

**Ryan M. Johnson, NRP, C-NPT**
Emergency Care Professionals
Breese, Illinois

**Michael A. Kaduce, MPS, NRP**
EMT Program Director
UCLA Center for Prehospital Care
Los Angeles, California

**William Kane, BA, NRAEMT, WEMT, I/C**
The Kane Schools, Wild & Rescue Medicine
Fryeburg, Maine

**Jared Kimball, NRP BA**
Tulane University
New Orleans, Louisiana

**Jeffrey Lawley, BA, NRP, PI**
Ivy Tech Community College
Valparaiso, Indiana

**Lawrence Linder, MA, MS, NRP**
Hillsborough Community College, EMS Programs
Ruskin, Florida

**Gary Lingel, EMT-P, SEI**
EMTC
Arlington, Washington

**Douglas J. Lowe**
Director of Medical Programs
Federal Strategies
Fredericksburg, Virginia

**Katie J. Lyman, PhD, ATC, NREMT**
Jamestown Area Ambulance
Jamestown, North Dakota

**Scott McCormack, EMT-P**
Richlands Fire Rescue
Cedar Bluff, Virginia

**John R. McFarland, MS, EMT-P, PI**
Jay County High School
Portland, Indiana

**Kerry McKee, Paramedic I/C, APEMS, KVCC, EMCC**
Director
Vinalhaven Ambulance
Vinalhaven, Maine

**Kristen McKenna, MA, NRP**
University of South Alabama
Mobile, Alabama

**Terry Mendez, EdM, CCEMT-P**
Western Nevada College
Carson City, Nevada

**David Lynn Moseley, Paramedic**
Roanoke Rapids High School
Roanoke Rapids, North Carolina

**Melissa Osborne, BA, CCEMT-P, NRP**
EMS-Instructor
Ambulance Service of Manchester
Manchester, Connecticut

**Robert L. Painter, MS, EFO, NRP**
Tulsa Community College
Tulsa, Oklahoma

**Matthew Patrick, EMT-B**
Pittsburgh Public Schools
Pittsburgh, Pennsylvania

**Leo Pernesky Jr, Paramedic**
Jefferson County EMS
Punxsutawney, Pennsylvania

**Jared Priddy, NRP**
Lord Fairfax Community College
Winchester, Virginia

**Michael Pruitt, MPA, NRP**
Carilion Clinic Patient Transportation
Rocky Mount, Virginia

**Christopher T. Ryther, MS, NRP**
American River College
Sacramento, California

**Lindsey Schaaf, NRP**
Bowman Ambulance
Bowman, North Dakota

**Stephanie Scheib, MS, Paramedic**
Instructor/Coordinator
Mobile Medical Response, Inc.
Saginaw, Michigan

**Jeb Sheidler, DMSc, PA-C, ATC, NRP, TP-C**
Executive Director of Trauma/Emergency Management
Lutheran Hospital of Indiana
Lima, Ohio

**Sandra Sokol, NREMT-P**
Assistant Chief
Dale City Volunteer Fire Department
Charles Town, West Virginia

**Craig Spector**
EMT Instructor, Owner of CPR Heart Starters Safety Training
CPR Heart Starters Safety Training
Warrington, Pennsylvania

**Celia Sporer, PhD**
Emergency Care Programs
Cedarhurst, New York

**Nate Strobel, SEI**
Captain
South King County Fire Training Consortium
King County, Washington

**David M. Tauber, BS, NRP, FP-C, NCEE, NH I/C**
Advanced Life Support Institute
Conway, New Hampshire

**Rachel S. Trigg, Paramedic, RN, AAS, BSEd**
Assistant Professor
Emergency Medical Services, Southwest Tennessee Community College
Cordova, Tennessee

**William Vaughan, MAS, RN/MICP, CFRN**
Flight Nurse
Atlantic Air Ambulance
Netcong, New Jersey

**Mark Von Stein, EMT-P**
EMS Professor
Broward College
Davie, Florida

**Benjamin Vu, EMT-P, BS**
Mt. San Antonio College EMT Program
Walnut, California

**Amy Wasko, EMT-P**
Lead Instructor
College of DuPage
Glen Ellyn, Illinois

**Joseph Welsh**
Life-Savers, Inc.
Louisville, Kentucky

**R. Greg West, MEd, EMS I/C**
North Shore Community College
Danvers, Massachusetts

**Justin Whitehead, NRP-EMS-I, FFII, FI, FSI**
Assistant Chief
Pleasant Township Fire
South Vienna, Ohio

**Alexandra Williams**
Dutchess Community College
Poughkeepsie, New York

**Crystal Youmans, NREMT-P**
SC Midlands Regional EMS; Calhoun County EMS
West Columbia, South Carolina; Saint Matthews, South Carolina

# Photoshoot Acknowledgments

We would like to thank the following people and institutions for their collaboration on the photo shoots for this project. Their assistance was greatly appreciated.

## Technical Consultants

**Jonathan Epstein**
Director, EMS Product Management
Public Safety Group
Jones & Bartlett Learning
Burlington, Massachusetts

**Kim D. McKenna, PhD, RN, EMT-P**
St. Charles County Ambulance District
St. Peters, Missouri

**Richard A. Nydam, AS, NREMT-P**
Training and Education Specialist
EMS UMass Memorial Paramedics/Worcester EMS
Worcester, Massachusetts

**Andrew N. Pollak, MD, FAAOS**
The James Lawrence Kernan Professor and Chairman, Department of Orthopaedics, University of Maryland School of Medicine
Chief of Orthopaedics, University of Maryland Medical System
Director, Shock Trauma Go Team, R. Adams Cowley Shock Trauma Center
Medical Director, Baltimore County Fire Department
Special Deputy US Marshal
Baltimore, Maryland

## Institutions

UMass Memorial Paramedics—Worcester EMS
Worcester, Massachusetts

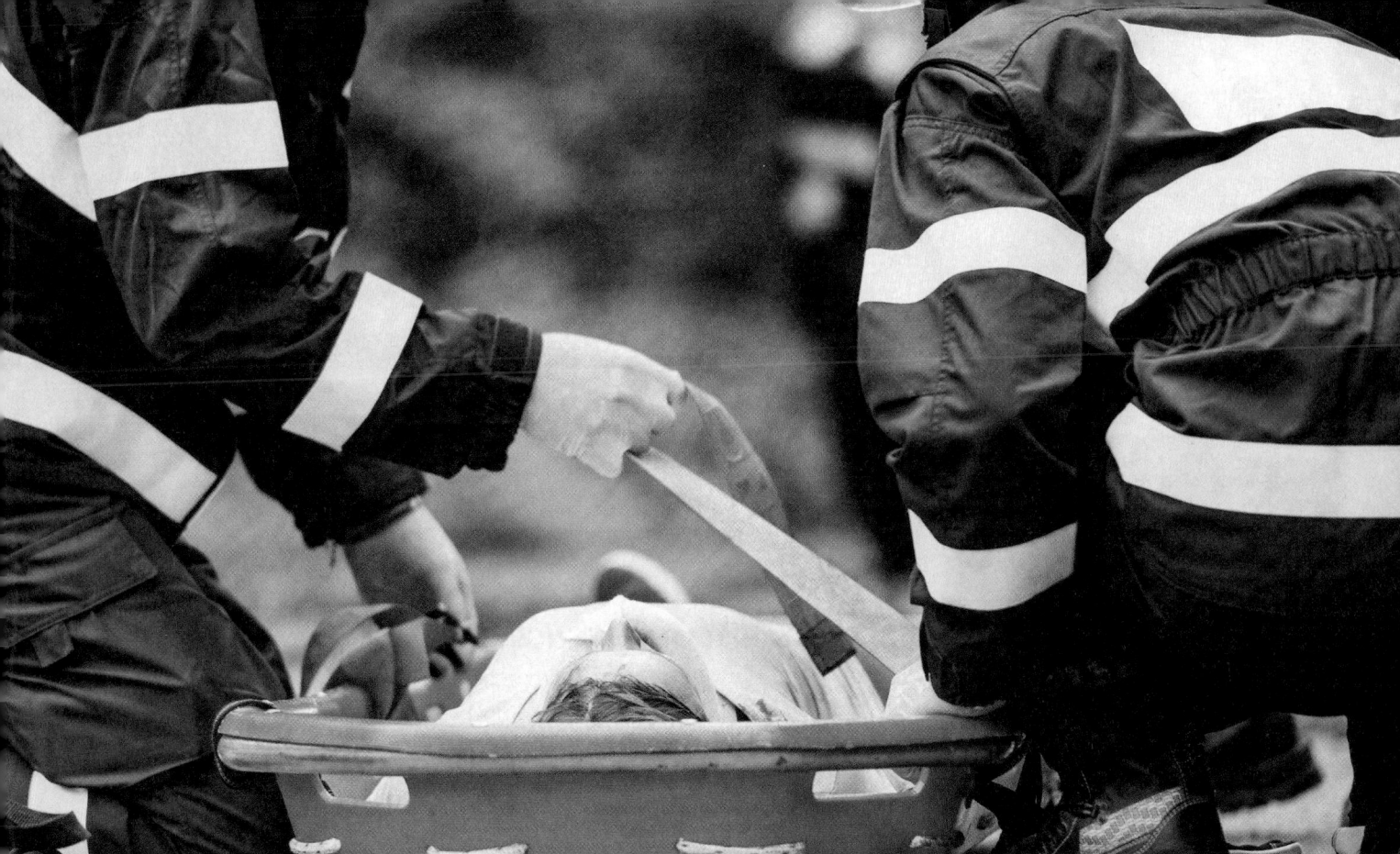

# SECTION

# 1

# Preparatory

1   EMS Systems

2   Workforce Safety and Wellness

3   Medical, Legal, and Ethical Issues

4   Communications and Documentation

5   Medical Terminology

6   The Human Body

7   Life Span Development

8   Lifting and Moving Patients

9   The Team Approach to Health Care

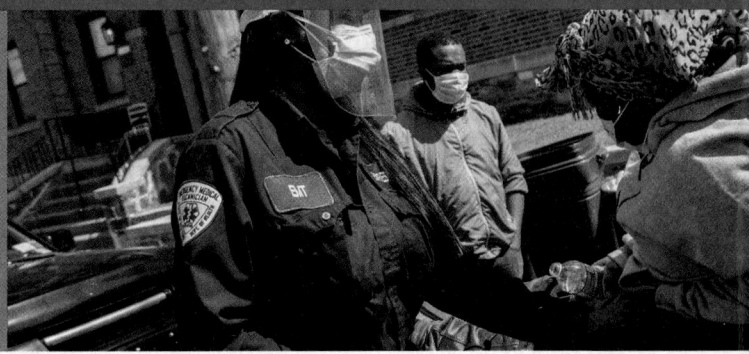

# Chapter 1

# EMS Systems

## NATIONAL EMS EDUCATION STANDARD COMPETENCIES

### Preparatory
Applies fundamental knowledge of the emergency medical services (EMS) system, safety/well-being of the emergency medical technician (EMT), medical/legal, and ethical issues to the provision of emergency care.

### Emergency Medical Services (EMS) Systems
- EMS systems (pp 12–21)
- History of EMS (pp 7–9)
- Roles/responsibilities/professionalism of EMS personnel (pp 21–23)

- Quality improvement (p 16)
- Patient safety (pp 17–18)

### Research
- Impact of research on EMS care (pp 20–21)
- Data collection (pp 20–21)
- Evidence-based decision making (pp 20–21)

### Public Health
Uses simple knowledge of the principles of illness and injury prevention in emergency care.

## KNOWLEDGE OBJECTIVES

1. Define emergency medical services (EMS) systems. (p 3)
2. Name the four levels of EMT training and licensure. (pp 4–7)
3. Describe EMT licensure criteria; include how the Americans With Disabilities Act (ADA) applies to employment as an EMT. (pp 4–7)
4. Discuss the historical background of the development of the EMS system. (pp 7–9)
5. Describe the levels of EMT training in terms of sets of knowledge, skills, and attitudes needed for each of the following: EMR, EMT, AEMT, and paramedic. (pp 9–11)
6. Recognize the presence of other first responders at a scene with EMS training, some knowledge of first aid, or merely good

intentions, and their need for direction. (pp 10–11)
7. Explain the guiding principles of EMS Agenda 2050. (p 12)
8. Describe how medical direction in an EMS system works and the EMT's role in the process. (p 14)
9. Define mobile integrated health care and community paramedicine. (p 15)
10. Explain the purpose of the EMS continuous quality improvement (CQI) process. (p 16)
11. Characterize the EMT's role in disease and injury prevention and public education in the community. (pp 19–20)
12. Describe the roles and responsibilities of the EMT. (pp 21–23)

13. Describe the attributes an EMT is expected to possess. (pp 22–23)

14. Explain the impact of the Health Insurance Portability and Accountability Act (HIPAA) on patient privacy. (p 23)

## SKILLS OBJECTIVES

There are no skills objectives for this chapter.

# Introduction

You are about to enter an exciting field. As an emergency medical technician (EMT), you will be a critical part of the emergency medical services (EMS) system. EMS is a team of health care professionals who are responsible for and provide emergency care and transportation to the sick and injured (FIGURE 1-1). While not every call for care will involve a life-threatening emergency, the compassion, professionalism, and skill you bring will have a tremendous positive impact on each patient you encounter.

This course is the initial step in acquiring the critical knowledge, skills, and abilities (KSAs) you will use to help with emergency and nonemergency prehospital medical problems (FIGURE 1-2). The National EMS Scope of Practice Model describes the four levels of EMS practice. The National EMS Education Standards outline the knowledge and competencies that should be taught to students in each of these four levels of EMS practice. This education incorporates all the KSAs needed to become a competent, entry-level EMT. Education must continue long past the end of this course as you refine your KSAs, learn the details of working in a particular part of the health care system, and grow and adapt to keep up with the health care industry overall. For any role in emergency services and health care, education must continue throughout your career.

The next step is certification. This process verifies that a provider meets the minimum required KSA competencies for safe and effective emergency operations and patient care. Such exams often use a variety of testing instruments such as multiple-choice questions, skills stations, and simulated emergency calls. They are typically conducted or regulated by a state or military agency or by the National Registry of EMTs (NREMT). The NREMT is a nongovernmental, not-for-profit organization whose mission is to provide a valid, uniform process to assess the KSAs for competent EMS practice. Almost all states require NREMT certification for candidates to be eligible for a license to practice.

Although not all states use the NREMT testing process, EMS certification exams may be informed

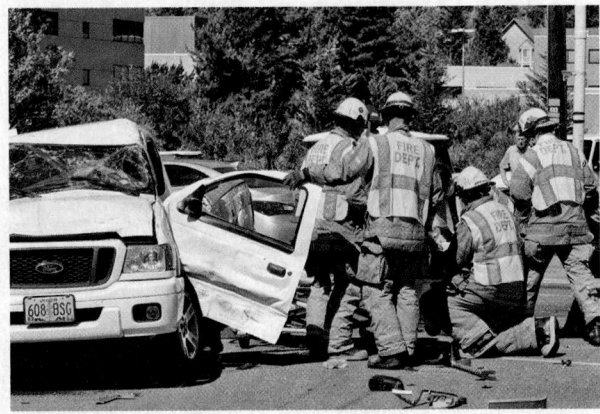

FIGURE 1-1 As an EMT, you are part of a larger team that responds to a variety of calls and provides a wide range of prehospital emergency care.

© tfoxfoto/iStock/Getty.

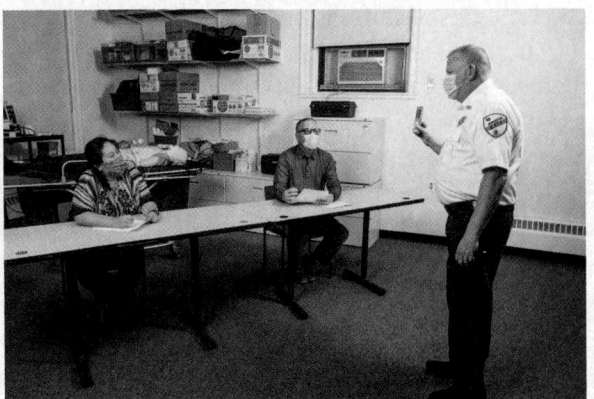

FIGURE 1-2 In the classroom, you will learn both didactic and practical skills to prepare you for various types of calls.

© Jones & Bartlett Learning.

by the NREMT's EMS Practice Analysis. Approximately every 5 years, the NREMT surveys EMS providers of all levels from across the United States to understand the current real-world practice of out-of-hospital emergency care and to help create a blueprint for valid certification exams. In 2019 the Practice Analysis also pulled data from the National EMS Information System (NEMSIS) to get a real picture of the types of calls and interventions EMS personnel in the United States encounter in actual practice. In effect, the Practice Analysis attempts to answer the question, "What is most important for EMS providers to know and be able to do to deliver safe and effective care?" From this information, the current Practice Analysis determines the certification test plan for each level of EMS provider. The test plan lays out an approximate percentage of questions on each topic that students will encounter on NREMT certification exams.

After successfully completing the certification process, the provider is typically eligible for licensure, the legal authority to practice in his or her state. Although some states still refer to this phase as certification, for the purposes of this textbook, the term *licensure* will be used.

Obtaining licensure in a state does not grant an EMT an unrestricted right to practice. The next phase of becoming a health care provider is credentialing. Credentialing is the verification process of a health care provider's qualifications. Credentialing may be a local or regional process, and it is typically directed and overseen by a physician medical director. In some cases, EMTs may be specifically credentialed to perform either fewer or additional techniques in their area or to work in certain types of care systems.

In most states, people who work in emergency medical care are categorized into four licensure levels, each with a different scope of practice and each requiring different types of education and training. The licensure levels are emergency medical responder (EMR), emergency medical technician (EMT), advanced EMT (AEMT), and paramedic. An EMR has basic emergency care and operations training, and is focused on managing the emergency scene and initiating immediate life-saving care before the ambulance arrives. EMRs may also perform roles under the direction of providers with more advanced training.

An EMT has additional depth and breadth of training in basic emergency care and transportation of sick and injured patients. Although not always the first to arrive, EMTs most commonly focus on initial stabilization of the scene and fundamental emergency care. EMTs are the primary link between the emergency scene and the health care system.

An AEMT has additional preparation beyond the EMT level that includes training and education in specific aspects of advanced life support (ALS), such as intravenous (IV) therapy, advanced airway management, and the administration of certain emergency medications. The AEMT's primary focus is on more advanced assessment techniques and selected emergency interventions known to improve patient outcomes.

Paramedics have the greatest breadth and depth of education and training among emergency care providers. Their preparation focuses on ALS assessment; diagnostic and treatment tools and techniques, such as interpretation of heart rhythms; advanced airway management; and emergency pharmacology. Paramedics function as part of a collaborative response, working under medical direction with EMS providers of other levels to help extend the reach of the health care system.

The standards for prehospital emergency care and the people who provide it are governed by the

## YOU are the Provider

You are working as a new EMT and are on duty with an EMT driver and a paramedic partner. You are in the process of checking the ambulance when you are dispatched to a report of a 48-year-old woman with back pain. You and your crew proceed to the scene, approximately 6 miles away.

1. How do your roles and responsibilities as an EMT compare to those of other EMS provider certification/licensure levels?

2. How do the National Scope of Practice Model and the National EMS Education Standards affect your ability to assess and treat a patient?

laws of each state and are typically regulated by an office of EMS operating under the state's department of health. Although the specific training and licensure requirements vary from state to state, almost every state's requirements follow or exceed the guidelines recommended in the current National Highway Traffic Safety Administration (NHTSA) EMS Education Standards.

In 2020, the National Registry of Emergency Medical Technicians launched the National EMS-ID number system. An EMS-ID is a 12-digit identification number issued at no charge to all EMS professionals, from EMR to paramedic, and to students entering the profession. The number is automatically generated by the National Registry when a person creates an account. For EMS providers with an existing account, an EMS-ID is retroactively created. Unlike the number issued by the National Registry (NR Number) when an individual becomes certified, EMS-IDs do not change as the person's certification level changes. Thus, the various certification numbers a person may obtain in his or her career are all tied back to the single EMS-ID.

This textbook covers the practices and skills identified in the NHTSA National EMS Education Standards. It also covers the information needed for EMTs to perform the skills outlined in the NHTSA 2019 National EMS Scope of Practice Model.

To supplement the required core content, this text includes additional information to help you understand and apply the knowledge and skills included in the EMT course. The goal is to apply the KSAs identified in this text to work in the field as an effective emergency responder and caregiver. To achieve this goal, it is essential that you complete the assigned reading before each class. Simply attending class will not adequately prepare you to demonstrate the KSAs needed to complete each part of the course. Each class builds your ability to apply previous information. It is vital that you complete the readings and assignments to help you understand subsequent lessons and, ultimately, to be able to apply those lessons in real-world emergency situations. This approach is pivotal to your success in this course.

In class, your instructor will review the key parts of the reading assignment and clarify and expand on them. He or she will answer any questions you have and clarify any points you or others do not yet understand how to apply. Unless you

### TABLE 1-1 Study Tips

- Determine the time of day when you can most effectively study.
- Make, and stick to, a study schedule that will allow you to master the information in small, digestible chunks.
- Find a place that is free from distractions and interruptions.
- Do not remain on call for work, family, or other obligations during study time.
- Turn off your devices so you are not taken out of the study zone by unnecessary alerts.
- Find a study group or partner. Work to help each other, and keep each other accountable.
- Before you begin, specify your study objectives. If necessary, write down specific questions you have about the material.
- Before reading an entire section, give it a quick overview to understand what you will be studying and how it will be presented.
- Study the most challenging information first, while you still have the most mental energy and drive.
- Group topics into manageable chunks to study.
- Think about each key learning point in terms of how you would explain it clearly to someone who was not in the class.
- Focus on learning and applying the information, not on exam grades.
- Consider making simple flowcharts or diagrams to better understand disease processes, assessment and care priorities, and decision making.
- Take advantage of additional learning tools, such as quizzes, simulations, or case studies, that allow you to test your knowledge and identify gaps in your learning.

© Jones & Bartlett Learning.

carefully read the assignment and take notes before coming to class, you will not fully understand or benefit from the classroom presentations and discussions. Creating your own tools, such as flashcards, study questions, scenarios, and outlines, will help you retain important information. It will also help you take better notes during class (**TABLE 1-1**).

In addition to textbook readings, EMT programs typically include a variety of learning activities, including the following:

1. Case presentations
2. Question-and-answer sessions
3. Small-group debates and discussions
4. Purposeful practice of practical (hands-on) skills with feedback

5. Putting-it-all-together patient care scenarios and simulations
6. Clinical experience to observe and participate in real EMS and in-hospital patient care

Using a variety of learning activities in class and in study sessions does not just make sessions more interesting; these strategies advance your knowledge from the most fundamental levels of learning, such as memorizing and understanding information, to applying this information. Further, this course breaks the information into chunks so you can evaluate and apply the right KSAs on actual EMS calls.

## EMT Training: Focus and Requirements

Some of the subjects discussed in this textbook include:

- **Scene size-up.** Scene size-up involves getting an overview of the situation at hand and an awareness of the presence and level of safety threats. During scene size-up, you must gain a big-picture perspective of the call, determine whether it is safe to proceed, determine whether additional resources are needed, and identify the initial approach to mitigate the emergency.
- **Patient assessment.** Patient assessment is the foundation of any EMS call. Using your understanding of anatomy, physiology, and the pathophysiology of diseases, you will perform effective assessment techniques to determine what is wrong with your patient and identify life threats.
- **Treatment.** As an EMT, you will identify the need for and prioritize patient care. In some cases, you may work to improve patient oxygenation and ventilation. In others, you will control bleeding or assist patients during childbirth. In addition to hands-on skills, you will learn how to treat patients who are in emotional crisis, and how to calm patients to relieve some of their anxiety.
- **Transport.** Most patients need to be transported to a facility. This could mean a hospital, clinic, or other medical care facility. You will learn how to transport patients with a wide variety of illnesses and injuries.
- **EMS as a career.** Most of you are taking this course because you want to help people. To ensure all EMS providers have a long, healthy

### Words of Wisdom

#### The Star of Life

The National Highway Traffic Safety Administration (NHTSA) recognized the need for a symbol that would represent EMS as a critical public service and created the *Star of Life*. NHTSA holds priority rights to the use of this registered certification mark.

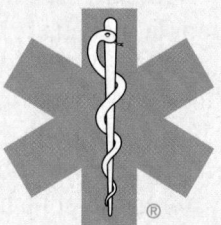

Adapted from the personal Medical Identification Symbol of the American Medical Association, each bar on the Star of Life represents an EMS function:

1. Detection
2. Reporting
3. Response
4. On-scene care
5. Care in transit
6. Transfer to definitive care

The serpent and staff in the symbol portray the staff of Asclepius, an ancient Greek physician deified as the god of medicine. Overall, the staff represents medicine and healing, with the skin-shedding serpent being indicative of renewal.

The Star of Life has become synonymous with emergency medical care around the globe. This symbol can be seen as a means of identification on ambulances, emergency medical equipment, patches or apparel worn by EMS providers, and materials such as books, pamphlets, manuals, reports, and publications that either have a direct application to EMS or were generated by an EMS organization. It also appears on road maps and highway signs indicating the location of or access to qualified emergency medical care.

Adapted from US National Highway Traffic Safety Administration. http://www.ems.gov.

career, it is important for you to learn how to take care of yourself. Job stressors and successful ways to cope with them will be discussed.

## Licensure Requirements

To be recognized and function as an EMT, you must meet certain requirements. The specific requirements differ from state to state. Ask your instructor or your state EMS official about the requirements in your state. Generally, the criteria to be licensed and employed as an EMT include the following:

- High school diploma or equivalent
- Proof of immunization against certain communicable diseases
- Successful completion of a background check and drug screening
- Valid driver's license
- Successful completion of a recognized health care provider basic life support (BLS)/cardiopulmonary resuscitation (CPR) course
- Successful completion of a state-approved EMT course
- Successful completion of a state-recognized written certification examination (usually NREMT)
- Successful completion of a state-recognized practical certification examination
- Compliance with other state, local, and employer provisions

The **Americans With Disabilities Act (ADA)** of 1990 protects people who have a disability from being denied access to programs and services that are provided by state or local governments and prohibits employers from failing to provide full and equal employment to the disabled. In addition, Title I of the ADA protects EMTs with disabilities seeking gainful employment under many circumstances. Employers with a certain number of employees are required to adjust processes so that a candidate with a disability can be considered for the position, and when possible, modify the work environment or how the job is normally performed. This allows EMTs who can perform the functional job skills with reasonable accommodations the opportunity to pursue a career in EMS.

One of the primary responsibilities of each state is to ensure the safety of its residents. As such, states have requirements prohibiting people with certain legal infractions from becoming EMS providers. The specific legal exclusions, either misdemeanors and/or felonies, are created on a state-by-state basis. Contact your state EMS office for more information.

## Overview of the EMS System
### History of EMS

As an EMT, you will join a long tradition of people who provide emergency medical care to their fellow human beings. With the early use of motor vehicles in warfare, volunteer ambulances were organized and personnel went overseas to provide care for the wounded in World War I. During World War II, the military trained special corpsmen to provide care in the field and bring the casualties to aid stations staffed by nurses and physicians. In the Korean War, this evolved into the field medic and rapid helicopter evacuation to nearby Mobile Army Surgical Hospital units, where immediate surgical interventions could be performed. Many advances in the immediate care of trauma patients resulted from the casualty experiences in the Korean and Vietnam Wars.

Unfortunately, emergency care of the injured and ill at home had not progressed to a similar level. As recently as the 1960s and early 1970s, emergency ambulance service and care varied widely across the United States. In some places, it was provided by well-trained advanced first aid personnel who had well-equipped, modern ambulances. In a few urban areas, it was provided by hospital-based ambulance services that were staffed with interns and early forms of prehospital care providers. In many areas, the only emergency care and ambulance service was provided by the local funeral home using a hearse that could be converted to carry a cot and serve as an ambulance. In other places, the police or fire department used a station wagon that carried a cot and a first aid kit. In most cases, these vehicles were staffed with a driver and an attendant who had some basic first aid training. In the few areas where a commercial ambulance was available to transport the ill, it was usually similarly staffed and served primarily as a means to transport the patient to the hospital.

Many communities did not have formal provisions for prehospital emergency care or transportation. Injured people were given basic first aid by police or fire personnel at the scene and were transported to the hospital in a police or fire officer's car. Customarily, patients with an acute illness were transported to the hospital by a relative or neighbor and were met by their family physician or

### Special Populations

EMS systems must be capable of handling many different types of patients and situations. These can include obstetric, pediatric, and geriatric emergencies. Assessment techniques, treatment procedures, and other aspects of EMS care vary between children, adults, and older people.

an on-call hospital physician, who assessed them and then summoned any specialists and operating room staff who were needed. Except in large urban centers, most hospitals did not have the emergency department (ED) staff available today.

EMS as we know it today had its origins in 1966 with the publication of *Accidental Death and Disability: The Neglected Disease of Modern Society.* This report, prepared jointly by the Committees on Trauma and Shock of the National Academy of Sciences/National Research Council, revealed to the public and Congress the serious inadequacy of prehospital emergency care and transportation in many areas. As a result, Congress mandated that two federal agencies address these issues. Seeing early EMS as essentially an emergency transportation service, the National Highway Traffic Safety Administration (NHTSA), under the US Department of Transportation (DOT), was directed to enact the Highway Safety Act of 1966, and the Department of Health, Education, and Welfare (now known as the Department of Health and Human Services [DHHS]) was directed to enact the Emergency Medical Services Development Act of 1973, creating funding sources and programs to develop improved systems of prehospital emergency care. This history is why EMS is administrated at the federal level through the DOT and not the DHHS.

In the early 1970s, the DOT developed and published the first curriculum to serve as the guideline for EMT training. To support the EMT course, the American Academy of Orthopaedic Surgeons prepared and published the first EMT textbook—*Emergency Care and Transportation of the Sick and Injured*—in 1971, often called the Orange Book for its original trademark orange cover. Through the 1970s, following the recommended guidelines, each state developed the necessary legislation, and the EMS system expanded throughout the United States. During the same period, emergency medicine became a recognized medical specialty, and the fully staffed EDs that we know today became the accepted standard of care.

In the late 1970s, the DOT developed a recommended National Standard Curriculum for the education and training of paramedics and identified a part of the course to serve for EMTs.

During the 1980s, many areas enhanced the EMT National Standard Curriculum by adding EMTs with advanced levels of training who could provide key components of ALS care and advanced life-saving procedures. The availability of paramedics and ALS-level care on calls that require or benefit from advanced care has grown steadily in recent years. In addition, with the evolution in training and technology, the EMT and AEMT can now perform a number of important advanced skills in the field that were formerly reserved for only the paramedic.

This growth and sophistication of the EMS system did not come without its drawbacks. As each state sought to create a system that would meet the needs of its citizens, the definitions of EMS providers began to vary from state to state. For example,

## YOU are the Provider

You arrive at the scene, ensure it is safe to enter, and make contact with the patient, a 48-year-old woman. She is sitting on her couch, is in obvious distress, and states her pain has been intermittent for about a month. She tells you and your crew that it is uncomfortable for her to walk. You assess the patient as your partner prepares to take her vital signs.

| Recording Time:   0 Minutes | |
|---|---|
| Appearance | Grimacing; obvious pain |
| Level of consciousness | Conscious and alert |
| Airway | Open; clear of secretions or foreign bodies |
| Breathing | Adequate rate and depth |
| Circulation | Radial pulse, normal rate and rhythm; skin is pink, warm, and dry |

**3.** Does this patient need any treatment at the scene that can be provided by an EMT?

EMTs were allowed to administer medications in some states, while in other states they were not.

In the 1990s, NHTSA began an examination of EMS from a national perspective. With the counsel of EMS providers, physicians, fire chiefs, nurses, state administrators, educators, and other interested professionals, NHTSA created the EMS Agenda for the Future. This important document established a plan to standardize the levels of EMS education and EMS providers in an effort to ensure a more seamless delivery of EMS care across the country. In 2019, NHTSA revised this document and published EMS Agenda 2050.

The skills you learn and the scope of practice EMTs now enjoy are part of this national movement toward an EMS system that meets the needs of an ever-changing health care industry through a safe and efficient method.

## Levels of Training

At the federal level, NHTSA brings in experts from around the country to create the National EMS Scope of Practice Model. This document provides overarching guidelines for the minimum skills each level of EMS provider should be able to accomplish. **TABLE 1-2** shows some of the guidelines from that model.

Because licensure is a state function, laws are enacted at the state level to regulate how EMS providers will operate, and they are then executed by the state-level EMS administrative offices that control licensure. Finally, the local medical director

**TABLE 1-2** Examples From the Interpretive Guidelines: National EMS Scope of Practice Model

**Note:**
- An EMT can provide all of the skills listed in the EMR level.
- An AEMT can provide all of the skills listed in the EMR and EMT levels.
- A paramedic can provide all of the skills listed in the EMR, EMT, and AEMT levels.

| Examples of Airway/Ventilation/Oxygenation Skills | | | |
|---|---|---|---|
| **EMR** | **EMT** | **AEMT** | **Paramedic** |
| Oral airway | Nasal airway | Supraglottic airway | Endotracheal intubation |
| Bag-mask device | CPAP | Tracheobronchial suctioning | Cricothyrotomy |
| Upper airway suctioning | Pulse oximetry | $ETCO_2$ monitoring | Airway obstruction removal by direct laryngoscopy |
| Nasal cannula | Oxygen humidifiers | | High-flow nasal cannula |
| **Examples of Cardiovascular/Circulation Skills** | | | |
| Manual CPR | Mechanical CPR | | Cardioversion, electrical |
| Auto-/semiautomatic defibrillation | Telemetry monitoring devices | | Manual defibrillation |
| **Examples of Medication Administration Routes** | | | |
| Intramuscular auto-injector | Oral | Subcutaneous | Transdermal |
| Intranasal, premeasured | Sublingual | Intravenous | Rectal |

*Abbreviations:* CPAP, continuous positive airway pressure; CPR, cardiopulmonary resuscitation; $ETCO_2$, end-tidal carbon dioxide.

*Note:* The 2019 National EMS Scope of Practice Model serves as a foundation for states to build their own model. It is intended to illustrate the operation of each level of EMS provider and the progression from one level to another. It is not inclusive of every skill a state may allow.

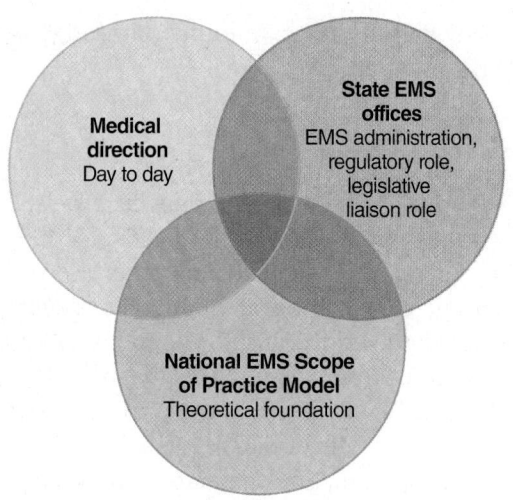

**FIGURE 1-3** Hierarchies of the 2019 National EMS Scope of Practice Model.

© Jones & Bartlett Learning.

should provide regular oversight and support to EMS personnel (**FIGURE 1-3**). For example, the medications that will be carried on an ambulance or where patients are transported are the day-to-day operational concerns on which the medical director, and often state, regional, or local EMS advisory boards, will have direct input.

The national guidelines are intended to ensure consistent delivery of EMS across the country. The only way a medical director can allow an EMT to perform a skill is if the state has already approved that skill. The medical director can limit the scope of practice but cannot expand it beyond state law. Expanding the scope of practice requires state approval.

You can download the complete list of approved skills in the National EMS Scope of Practice Model at www.ems.gov.

## Public Basic Life Support and Immediate Aid

With the development of EMS and increased awareness of the need for immediate emergency care, millions of laypeople have been trained in BLS/CPR. In addition to CPR, many people take first aid courses as well as other task-specific courses such as Stop the Bleed that focus on bleeding control and other simple skills that may be required to provide immediate essential care. These courses are designed to train people so those in the

workplace—teachers, coaches, child care providers, and others—can provide the necessary critical care in the minutes before EMTs or other responders arrive at the scene.

One of the most dramatic developments in prehospital emergency care is the increased availability of automated external defibrillators (AEDs) deployed in public places for use by untrained members of the general public. These devices, some no larger than a cell phone, detect treatable life-threatening cardiac dysrhythmias (ventricular fibrillation and ventricular tachycardia) and deliver the appropriate electrical shock to the patient without the need for a trained health care operator.

In addition to professional EMRs, EMTs often encounter a variety of people on the scene who are eager to help. You will encounter members of the public trained in first aid and CPR, physicians and nurses, and other well-meaning people with or without prior training and experience. Identified and used properly, these people can provide valuable assistance. At other times, they can interfere with operations and even create problems or danger for themselves or others. It will be your task in your initial scene size-up to identify the various people on the scene and orchestrate well-meaning attempts to assist.

## Emergency Medical Responder

Because the presence of a person who is trained to initiate BLS and other urgent care cannot be ensured, the EMS system includes immediate care by EMRs, such as law enforcement officers, firefighters,

### Street Smarts

Whether you accept or reject offers of assistance from nonaffiliated people on-scene, communication is key. Trained health care providers and emergency responders expect professional courtesy, even if you decide to decline assistance. Use clear verbal and nonverbal communication to accept or reject offers of help, and, if you are accepting help, be sure to give clear directions to those providing it. If you are rejecting help, be professional and polite, but firm. Being professional is always the right thing to do, and it is what you would prefer to see when viewing any recordings of your interactions with the public.

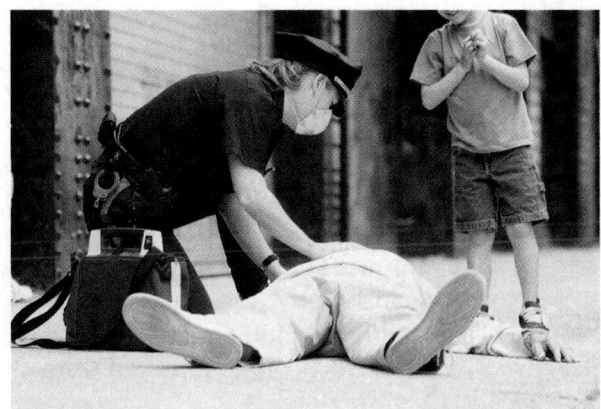

**FIGURE 1-4** Emergency medical responders, such as law enforcement officers, are trained to provide immediate basic life support until EMTs arrive on the scene.

© Hunterstock/Thinkstock.

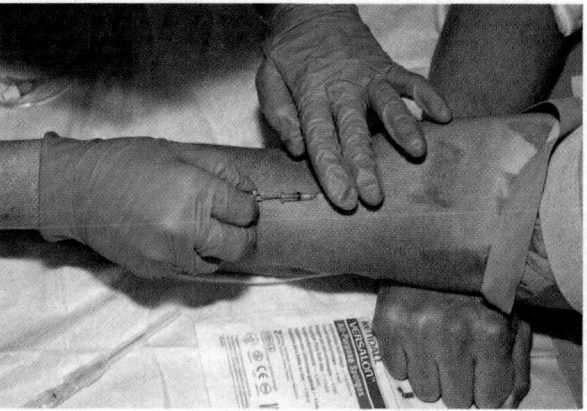

**FIGURE 1-5** Paramedic education and training cover a wide range of advanced life support skills.

© Jones & Bartlett Learning. Courtesy of MIEMSS.

park rangers, ski patrollers, or other organized rescuers who often arrive at the scene before the ambulance and EMTs (**FIGURE 1-4**). EMR training provides these people with the skills necessary to initiate immediate care and work with the EMTs on their arrival. The EMR course focuses on providing immediate care with limited equipment prior to the arrival of an ambulance. It also familiarizes students with the additional procedures, equipment, and packaging techniques that EMTs may use and that EMRs may be called on to assist.

## Emergency Medical Technician

EMS courses are competency-based. That is, the courses are designed to help students reach a level at which they can apply their KSAs to meet the minimum performance required to practice at their level of certification. The time to achieve this competence varies depending on factors that include prior student experience, program resources, or EMS educators' teaching methods. Thus, the total hours it may take to complete each level of the program will vary and is sometimes determined by state law. Although EMR courses are estimated to take approximately 50 to 80 hours, EMT courses may require approximately 150 to 200 hours to provide the essential knowledge and skills required to provide basic emergency care in the field. On arrival at the scene, you and any other EMTs who have responded should assume responsibility for the

assessment and care of the patient and follow the proper packaging and transport of the patient to the ED, if appropriate.

## Advanced Emergency Medical Technician

The AEMT course is designed to add knowledge and skills in specific aspects of ALS to providers who have been trained and have experience in providing emergency care as EMTs. These additional skills include IV and intraosseous (IO) therapy, use of advanced airway adjuncts, and the knowledge and skills necessary to administer a limited number of medications. The AEMT course ranges between 200 and 400 hours. The purpose of this level of EMS provider is to deliver an expanded range of skills beyond the EMT. In some parts of the United States, the availability of paramedics is limited. AEMTs help to fill the gap by providing limited ALS care in regions where paramedics are not available.

## Paramedic

The paramedic completes an extensive course of education and training that significantly increases knowledge and mastery of basic skills and covers a wide range of ALS skills (**FIGURE 1-5**). This course ranges from 1,000 to well over 2,000 hours, divided between classroom and internship training. Increasingly, this training is offered within the context of an associate's degree or bachelor's degree college program.

| TABLE 1-3 EMS Agenda 2050 Components of an EMS System |
|---|
| **A People-Centered EMS System** |
| 1. Comprehensive, quality, convenient care |
| 2. Evidence-based clinical care |
| 3. Efficient, well-rounded care |
| 4. Preventive care |
| 5. Comprehensive and easily accessible patient records |

© Jones & Bartlett Learning.

# Components of the EMS System

EMS Agenda 2050 is a multidisciplinary, national review of all aspects of EMS delivery. The goal is to develop a more cohesive and consistent system across the country. The document features five key aspects of a people-centered EMS system, as outlined in (**TABLE 1-3**).

The vision of EMS Agenda 2050 is that a people-centered EMS system is one in which people receive comprehensive, quality care in the most comfortable and convenient place. This care is based on sound research focused on producing the right outcomes. In this people-centered system, patients who need it will receive transport that is safe and efficient (not necessarily at a high rate of speed or with lights and sirens). Care in a people-centered system will focus not only on life-saving interventions, but also on reducing physical, emotional, and psychological suffering. Such EMS systems will be an integrated part of a larger health care system focused on proactively preventing injuries and illnesses rather than reactively responding to treat them. EMS clinicians will have access to and be able to contribute to a patient's comprehensive medical record, allowing not only improvements of treatment for individual patients, but also updates in prevention, diagnosis, and treatments as our understanding and technology advance.

The EMS Agenda 2050 guiding principles include an EMS system design that is as follows:

- Inherently safe and effective, so the entire system from start to finish is designed to minimize exposure to injury, infections, illness, or stress
- Integrated and seamless, where EMS is fully integrated with all other aspects of health care and is engaged with other emergency services and within the communities in which they operate
- Reliable and prepared, ensuring EMS care is delivered consistently and compassionately and is guided by sound research at all times, by all EMS providers, at all levels, or from all agencies
- Socially equitable, so that access to care and the quality of care are not determined by a patient's age, socioeconomic status, gender, ethnicity, or where they live
- Sustainable and efficient, meaning systems must be fiscally responsible, providing value to the community with a minimum of waste and a maximum of accountability
- Adaptable and innovative, evolving to meet the changing needs of the people whom they serve by continuously evaluating new tools and techniques, education programs, and system designs

## Public Access

Easy access to help in an emergency is essential. In most of the country, an emergency communication center that dispatches fire, police, rescue, and EMS units can be reached by dialing 9-1-1. At the communication center, trained dispatchers obtain the necessary information from the caller and, following dispatch protocols, dispatch the ambulance crew and other equipment and responders that may be needed (**FIGURE 1-6**). This communication center is called a public safety access point.

In an enhanced 9-1-1 system, the address of the caller is displayed on a screen. Most emergency communication centers are equipped with special equipment allowing people with speech or hearing disabilities to communicate with the dispatcher via a keyboard and text messages. In some areas, rather than 9-1-1, a different special published emergency number may be used to call for EMS. Mobile apps are playing an evolving role in allowing laypeople trained in CPR to be alerted of a cardiac arrest in their area and connecting them with the location of the nearest public AED.

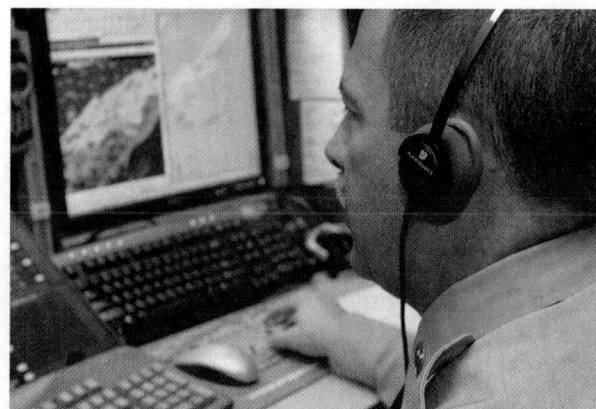

**FIGURE 1-6** Trained dispatchers obtain information about the call and then send responders to the scene as needed.

© Jones & Bartlett Learning. Courtesy of MIEMSS.

A system called **emergency medical dispatch (EMD)** assists dispatchers in providing callers with vital instructions to help them deal with a medical emergency until EMS crews arrive. Dispatchers are trained and provided scripts to help them relay relevant instructions to the callers. The system helps dispatchers select appropriately resourced units to respond to a request for assistance. It is the dispatcher's duty to relay all relevant and available information to the responding crews in a timely manner. Keep in mind that current technology does not typically allow the dispatcher to directly see what is going on at the scene; therefore, it is not uncommon for you to find the reality of the call quite different from the dispatch information.

Using the information provided by the caller, the dispatcher will select the appropriate parts of the emergency system that need to be activated. Over one-half of EMS support is provided by a governmental entity such as a fire agency (about 45%) or other nonfire governmental agency (20%). Private services deliver about one-fourth of EMS support. Other models seen less frequently include hospital-based programs and Native American tribal services.

## Human Resources

The human resources component deals with people. Who delivers the care? How are these people compensated for their time and energy? What is the role that volunteer providers play? How do other members of the medical community interact with and participate within the EMS world? These are some of the questions discussed within the component of human resources.

One of the goals of EMS Agenda 2050 is to encourage the creation of EMS systems that provide an environment where talented people want to work and can turn their passion into a rewarding career. Several objectives need to be accomplished to help make a career in EMS a lasting one. Efforts are

## YOU are the Provider

Your partner records the patient's vital signs on the patient care report as you ask the patient additional questions regarding her back pain. She tells you her lower back began hurting about a month ago; however, she has never been evaluated by a physician. She denies injuring her back. She further denies any other symptoms or past medical history.

| Recording Time: 4 Minutes | |
| --- | --- |
| **Respirations** | 16 breaths/min; regular and unlabored |
| **Pulse** | 88 beats/min; strong and regular |
| **Skin** | Pink, warm, and dry |
| **Blood pressure** | 126/66 mm Hg |
| **Oxygen saturation (Spo$_2$)** | 99% (on room air) |

Your assessment of the patient's back does not reveal any obvious deformities, swelling, or bruising, and her vital signs are stable. The patient requests you take her to the hospital.

**4.** How is patient care integrated across health systems when a patient is transported to the hospital?

being made to ensure that EMS providers can move from one state to another more seamlessly. One of the functions of the National EMS Scope of Practice Model is to create stable foundations on which each level of EMS provider is grounded. The net effect is to encourage a more consistent definition of "what is an EMT" so providers can move more freely about the country. National Registry certification often facilitates licensure in other states. The Interstate Commission for EMS Personnel Practice aims to increase the ability of EMS providers to practice in other states through the Recognition of EMS Personnel Licensure Interstate CompAct (REPLICA). REPLICA is not a form of EMS licensure reciprocity. It simply extends a privilege for EMS personnel from member states to practice on a short-term or intermittent basis under approved circumstances in other member states.

## Medical Direction

Each EMS system has a physician **medical director** who authorizes the EMTs in the service to provide medical care in the field. Although in some systems the individual EMTs may not regularly encounter their medical director, in virtually all systems the appropriate care for each injury, condition, or illness encountered in the field is determined by the medical director and is described in a set of written standing orders and protocols. Standing orders are part of protocols, and they designate what the EMT is required to do for a specific complaint or condition. Providers are not required to consult medical direction before implementing standing orders.

The medical director is the ongoing working liaison between the medical community, hospitals, and the EMTs in the service. If treatment problems arise or different procedures should be considered, they are referred to the medical director for his or her decision and action. To ensure the proper training standards are met, the medical director determines and approves the continuing education and training that are required of each EMT in the service.

**Medical control** is provided either off-line (indirect) or online (direct), as authorized by the medical director. Online medical control consists of direction given over the phone or radio directly from the medical director or a designated physician such as a base station physician at a receiving hospital. The

medical direction can be transferred by the physician's designee; it does not have to be transferred by the physician himself or herself. Off-line medical control consists of standing orders, training, and supervision authorized by the medical director. Each EMT must know and follow the protocols developed by his or her medical director.

The service's protocols will identify an EMS physician or other designee, usually at a local hospital, who can be reached by radio or telephone for medical control during a call. This is a type of direct online medical control. On some calls, once the ambulance crew has initiated any immediate urgent care and gives their radio report, the online medical control physician may either confirm or modify the proposed treatment plan or may prescribe any additional special orders that the EMTs are to follow for that patient. The point at which the EMTs should give their radio report or obtain online medical direction will vary.

## Legislation and Regulation

Although each EMS system, medical director, and training program has latitude, their training, protocols, and practices must conform to the EMS legislation, rules, regulations, and guidelines adopted by each state. The state EMS office is responsible for authorizing, auditing, and regulating all EMS, training institutions, courses, instructors, and providers within the state. In most states, the state EMS office obtains input from an advisory committee made up of representatives of the services, service medical directors, medical associations, hospitals, training programs, instructors' associations, EMT associations, and the public in that state.

At the local level, each EMS system operates in a designated **primary service area** in which it is responsible for the provision of prehospital emergency care and the transportation of the sick and injured to the hospital. Typically, each EMS function is administered by a senior EMS official. Daily operations and overall direction of the service are provided by an appointed chief executive officer and several other officers who serve under him or her. To provide clear guidelines, most services have written operating procedures and policies. When you join a service, you are expected to learn and follow them.

## Integration of Health Services

EMS does not work in a vacuum. EMS personnel travel to people's homes and to vehicle crashes and other scenes where illness and injury occur. Once on scene, they deliver care and transport the patient to a care facility. Integration of health services means that the prehospital care you administer is coordinated with the care administered at the hospital. When you deliver a patient to the ED you are simply transferring that patient to another care provider. The excellent care that you began should be continued in the ED. This component helps to decrease errors, to increase efficiencies, and, most of all, to ensure the patient receives comprehensive continuity of care.

Some EMS systems have collaborated with local hospitals to improve patient outcomes associated with time-sensitive treatment like heart attacks, trauma, and stroke. This is accomplished through special training in the EMS system and certain hospital departments. For example, when paramedics determine a patient is experiencing a heart attack, they alert the ED. In turn, the personnel in the ED notify the cardiac catheterization team. In other cases, you may be directed to transport the patient directly to a cardiac specialty center capable of providing the necessary intervention. As a result, the key personnel are ready to begin critical treatments as soon as the patient arrives at the hospital. Similar activities take place for stroke and trauma patients.

## Mobile Integrated Health Care and Community Paramedicine

Mobile integrated health care (MIH) is a method of delivering health care that utilizes the prehospital spectrum of care resources. It has evolved with the goal of facilitating improved access to health care at an affordable price. In the MIH model, health care is provided within the community, rather than at a physician's office or hospital. An integrated team of health care professionals, including EMS providers, delivers health care services in the community, and connects patients with other valuable resources such as social services. An advantage of this model is that it offers access to care for patients within communities who may have limited medical resources, and leads to better service for those who are homebound or disabled.

This new branch of health care is causing the evolution of additional training levels for EMS providers. The developing field of community paramedicine involves experienced paramedics who receive advanced education and training to equip them to provide services within a community. In addition to the patient care services a paramedic would typically provide, services provided by community paramedics may include performing health evaluations, monitoring chronic illnesses or conditions, obtaining laboratory samples, administering immunizations, and serving as a patient advocate.

## Information Systems

EMS is not unlike any other profession in today's world. Without computers, the job would be much more difficult. An information system allows EMS providers to efficiently document the care that has been delivered. Once that information is stored electronically, it can be used to improve care. For example, how many times has a department seen patients with chest pain? What is the average on-scene time for major trauma patients? How many AED runs has the department had? These questions and many more can be answered using the information gathered from computerized medical records.

This information is used for a variety of purposes. It can be used to construct educational sessions for the department. Data from ambulance activity logs may be used to justify hiring more personnel. Examining the types of patients and their frequency can provide the foundation for the purchase of new equipment and guide continuing education sessions. This information can also be combined with other database resources, such as from a hospital, to determine patient outcomes. Departments from around the country are sending

### Street Smarts

A patient may experience only once what you may witness hundreds of times. Understand and be empathetic to the patient's anxiety. Although it may not appear to be an emergency to you, it is considered an emergency by your patient and his or her family members. Treat them with respect. Your patients and their family members will always remember how you acted when you were with them.

information to Washington, DC, so a national snapshot of EMS activities can be obtained. Information gathered by NEMSIS can be found at www.nemsis.org. This information will be used to better plan for the needs of EMS systems today and in the future.

## Evaluation

In any EMS system, there are several individuals and organizations that are responsible for ensuring that high-quality care is being provided. The office of EMS in each state, along with the licensing bureau, works to ensure that only EMS providers who meet the minimum standards are licensed to provide care to the public. The medical director is responsible for maintaining quality control, ensuring that all staff members under his or her supervision meet appropriate medical care standards on each call. Chief officers and supervisors for each EMS function are responsible for ensuring delivery of quality care under their watch. Finally, each individual EMS provider is responsible for maintaining high-quality care for his or her own practice.

A commitment to quality does not mean that an EMS agency should have a punitive culture where errors are treated by shame and blame. A more productive approach to managing quality is to adopt a Just Culture. Just Culture is a strategy that promotes a learning culture that holds employees accountable for behavioral choices by balancing fairness and accountability. At the same time, these agencies focus on identifying risks within their system and attempt to design it for safety. This encourages trust within the agency and promotes reporting of errors and mishaps so their causes can be found and measures developed to prevent them from occurring in the future.

## Continuous Quality Improvement

Continuous quality improvement (CQI) is a quality management process that encourages team members at every level of the health care system to ask, "How are we doing now?" and "What can we do to be better?" CQI is a proactive process of development capitalizing on strengths and addressing challenges.

The CQI process is an essential element of any organization where the consequences of failure are potentially very harmful to either the patient, the team, or the community. In order to prevent failures, high consequence business such as EMS or

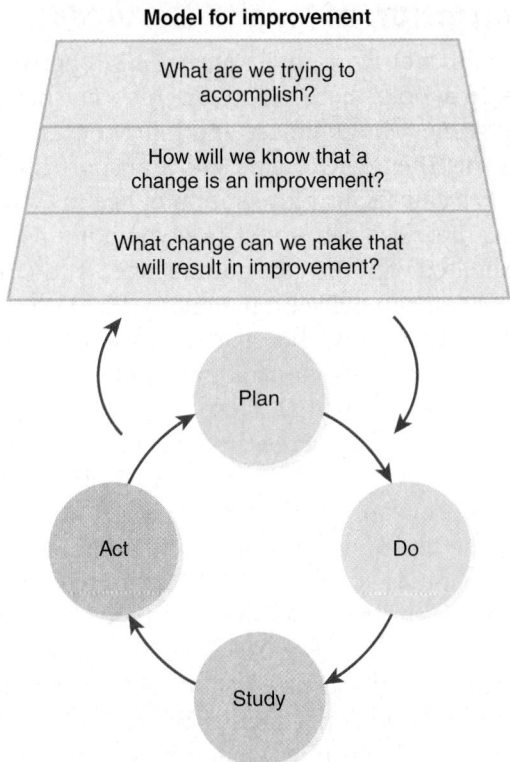

**FIGURE 1-7** Plan-do-study-act cycle.

Reproduced with permission from "Model for improvement." Boston, Massachusetts: Institute for Healthcare Improvement; 2020. Available at http://www.ihi.org/resources/Pages/HowtoImprove/default.aspx.

the airline industry strive to be high reliability organizations (HROs). To be an HRO means that the organization has a commitment to teamwork, a culture of safety, and a commitment to CQI in an effort to prevent errors.

In CQI, information is gathered about processes, performance, and outcomes. Evaluation of this information generates ideas to improve performance and efficiency, these ideas are tried and also evaluated, and the cycle continues. This cycle is known as plan-do-study-act (**FIGURE 1-7**). The *plan* phase involves gathering and analyzing information, such as run forms, call data, outcomes data, or information from crews and others. Analysis of this data may lead to ideas to improve the level of care, efficiency, or outcomes. The *do* phase then enacts these ideas. The *study* phase evaluates any significant positive or negative changes that resulted from the implementation of the new idea. If the change is positive, then a larger part of the EMS system adopts the change in the *act* phase. At every level, CQI is a learning and improvement process rather than simply a way to punish identified problems.

## Patient Safety

Another function of the evaluation process is to determine ways to limit or eliminate human error and improve patient safety. During the delivery of EMS, as with any occupation, there are times when errors can happen. Driving to the scene can be hazardous. As you are lifting and moving a patient, the patient can be dropped. Communicating with other EMTs or transferring the patient to the ED presents circumstances where errors can happen. Remember, errors can occur at any point during the call, and they can result in harm to the patient, the public, and you.

Errors are not inevitable, though. If the circumstances of the errors are understood, it may be possible to eliminate or at least minimize them.

There are many ways to examine medical errors. This textbook focuses on errors from three possible sources—as a result of a rules-based failure, a knowledge-based failure, or a skills-based failure (or any combination of these). For example, does the EMT have the legal right to administer the particular medication that the patient needs? Has the medical director given permission to administer the drug? If not, a rules-based failure has occurred if the EMT administers the medication. Does the EMT know all of the pertinent information about the medication being delivered? If not, a breakdown at this point, such as the administration of the wrong medication, would be referred to as a knowledge-based failure. Is the equipment operating and being used properly? If not, a skills-based error has occurred. Attitudes, including bias, can contribute to all of these types of errors, and an error can come from multiple sources.

Limiting errors requires the efforts of both the EMS agency and EMS personnel. Agencies need to have clear protocols, which are detailed plans that describe how certain patient issues, such as chest pain or shortness of breath, are to be managed. These protocols need to be understood by all EMTs within the service.

The environment can also contribute to errors. Are there ways to limit distractions? How do we

## YOU are the Provider

The patient is placed onto the stretcher in a position of comfort using pillows to support the uncomfortable areas of her back, and loaded into the ambulance. You and the paramedic are in the back with the patient coaching her to relax as your EMT partner drives to the hospital. You reassess the patient shortly after you begin transport to the hospital.

| Recording Time: 12 Minutes | |
| --- | --- |
| **Level of consciousness** | Conscious and alert |
| **Respirations** | 16 breaths/min; regular and unlabored |
| **Pulse** | 90 beats/min; strong and regular |
| **Skin** | Pink, warm, and dry |
| **Blood pressure** | 120/62 mm Hg |
| **Spo$_2$** | 97% (on room air) |

Within a few minutes, the patient tells you her back pain has begun to subside.

**5.** What safety concerns apply to this call and what are some ways to address those concerns?

improve lighting so EMTs can see well? How organized is the equipment? Can the EMT find what he or she needs in a timely manner? Environmental considerations can be managed using many approaches. Sometimes the solution is as easy as ensuring flashlights are available on all ambulances. Consider having police assistance on certain types of EMS calls or getting the assistance of an EMS supervisor. Perhaps a new type of equipment bag will provide better organization. Typically, when trying to reduce environmental factors regarding errors, this means having the right people with the right equipment in place.

EMTs can also help to reduce errors. Your job is to protect the patient from harm and to deliver high-quality medical care. This is one of your most important responsibilities. You are a patient care advocate—you speak for patients on their behalf. Keeping this responsibility in mind will help you to limit errors.

There are other ways errors can be reduced. When you are about to perform a skill, ask yourself, "Why am I doing this?" Knowing the reason for your actions gives you time to reflect and make a more informed decision. Even within EMS, rarely do you have to act so quickly that you do not have a moment to consider what it is you are doing and why. If you have considered what to do and cannot come up with a solution, ask for help. Talk with your partner, contact medical control, or call your EMS supervisor.

Another way to help limit medical errors is to use checklists and reference sheets. These can help keep you from missing key steps or key information, especially in times where your task load is high or the environment is particularly difficult to work in. Emergency physicians have many reference materials available to them. Physicians recognize they cannot memorize everything, so referencing a book or an Internet resource helps ensure the accuracy of their memory. Apps are also available for some checklists.

Finally, after a troublesome call, sit down and talk. Talk with your partner and/or your supervisor. Discussing the events that just happened provides an excellent avenue for learning. Your discussions can help lead to changes in protocol, how equipment is stocked, or even the purchase of new equipment.

## System Finance

All EMS departments need a funding system that allows them to continue to provide care; however, the type of system needed depends on many variables.

Departments may have paid personnel, volunteer personnel, or a mix of both. Financial resources are available for EMS departments through taxation, fee for service, paid subscription, donations, federal/state/local grants, fundraisers, or combinations of these resources. Which financial system is used depends on the needs and makeup of each EMS department.

How are EMTs involved with the financial side of EMS? You may think the financial activities belong to those who work in the office. Proper documentation by the EMS provider can significantly impact an agency's ability to process medical insurance claims, provide eligibility for financial grants for training or equipment, and provide evidence of competent practices. You may be asked to gather insurance information from patients, secure signatures on certain documents such as **Health Insurance Portability and Accountability Act (HIPAA)** notifications, or obtain written permission from patients to bill their health insurance company. All of these steps are important to the health care process as well as the viability of the EMS organization for which you work or volunteer.

Also, as the health care system in the United States evolves, billing is changing at every level. In 2020, the Centers for Medicare and Medicaid Services (CMS) implemented a pilot program in a small group of EMS agencies, known as Emergency Triage, Treat, and Transport (ET3). Rather than an EMS system getting paid only for transportation to an ED, ET3 strives to reimburse EMS systems for providing the right patient with the right care at the right time. This program allows transport to EDs for patients who need that level of care but also sets up a payment model for patient transport to alternative destinations, such as urgent care centers or doctors' offices, or on-scene treatment with no transport.

## Education Systems

Your education and training will be conducted by many knowledgeable EMS educators. In most states, the instructors who are responsible for coordinating and teaching the EMT course and continuing education courses are approved and licensed by the state EMS office or agency. In some states, to be credentialed to teach, an instructor must have extensive medical and educational training and teach for a designated period while being observed and supervised by an experienced instructor.

Paramedic programs, and in the future AEMT training programs, must adhere to national standards established by the CAAHEP (Commission on Accreditation of Allied Health Education Programs) and its EMS review branch, the CoAEMSP (Committee on Accreditation for the Emergency Medical Services Professions).

When you no longer have the structured learning environment that is provided in your initial training course, you must assume responsibility for directing your own study and learning. As an EMT, you are required to attend a specified number of hours of continuing education approved for EMTs each year to maintain, update, and expand your knowledge and skills. In many services, the required hours are provided by the training officer and medical director. In addition, most EMS education programs and hospitals offer a number of regular continuing education opportunities in each region. You may also attend state and national EMS conferences to help keep you current about local, state, and national issues affecting EMS. Because there are many levels of licensing, you should ensure that the continuing education you receive is approved for the EMT. You may decide to remain an EMT or to achieve a higher level of training and certification, but whatever you choose, the key to being a good EMT and providing high-quality care is your commitment to continual learning and increasing your knowledge and skills.

Knowledge and skills that are learned in any profession weaken when they are not used on a continual basis. Consider the steps involved in CPR, for example. If you have not used these skills since your original training, it is unlikely you will perform CPR proficiently. Frequent continuing education, refresher courses, simulations, and computer-based or manikin-based self-education exercises are measures you can take to maintain your skills and knowledge.

## Prevention and Public Education

The next two components of the EMS system are closely associated with each other. Prevention and public education are aspects of EMS where the focus is on public health. Public health examines the health needs of entire populations with the goal of preventing health problems. Although there are many definitions possible for public health, the prevention of health problems seems to provide a good overarching framework.

Health care in the United States is currently in a state of flux. The high-tech, on-demand style of care that is prevalent has two major drawbacks. One, it is very expensive. In the United States, according to the CMS, as of 2018 more than 17.7% of the US gross domestic product was accounted for by health care. Two, it may not deliver a better product. The US government reports people born in the United States have an average life expectancy of 79 years. There are 29 other countries where people live longer. If we are spending such large sums on health care, shouldn't we be living longer?

What needs to be addressed is the concept of prevention. The concept of prevention applies to both the patient and the EMS provider. Eating right, exercising, and using other stress management techniques can help prevent medical emergencies. It may seem strange, but the goal of education should be to create an environment where the need for EMS is decreased.

The focus of the public health arm of health care is prevention. Public health is proactive and works to prevent illness and injury. A good example of public health at work is in the common product, salt. In the United States, most table salt is sold with the additive iodine. It was discovered years ago that a condition known as goiter (abnormally large thyroid gland) is caused by a decrease in iodine levels within people's diets. The solution was to add this important element into a commonly used food source. Today, goiters are rare within the United States. **TABLE 1-4** demonstrates other significant accomplishments of the public health system.

EMS is able to work with public health agencies on both primary and secondary prevention strategies. Primary prevention focuses on strategies that will prevent the event from ever happening. Poliomyelitis (polio) was a devastating disease that caused death and disability for thousands of Americans in the early 1900s. A vaccine was developed to prevent the disease. In the span of one generation, the disease was virtually eliminated. Vaccinations

**TABLE 1-4** Examples of Public Health Accomplishments

| | |
|---|---|
| Vaccination programs | Clean drinking water |
| Fluoridation of water supplies | Seat belt laws |
| Helmet laws | Tobacco use laws |
| Sewage systems | Restaurant inspections |
| Formation of the Food and Drug Administration | Prenatal screenings |

© Jones & Bartlett Learning.

are a good example of primary prevention within public health.

There are several ways EMTs can contribute to primary prevention efforts. You can become involved in programs that educate the community about pool safety and car seat installation or in-home safety and fall prevention programs for older adults. Other opportunities include teaching first aid and CPR to various groups within your area. Remember, small actions can lead to big differences!

In a **secondary prevention** strategy, the event has already happened. The question is, how can we decrease the effects of the event? Helmets and seat belts do not prevent the accident from happening, yet they do prevent serious injuries from occurring due to the accident. The next time you drive down a major roadway, take note of the construction of the guardrails. There have been significant changes in guardrail construction over the years as more information has become available on what happens during a vehicle collision.

As an EMT, you may also be involved in the surveillance of illnesses and injuries. Information from the patient care reports that are generated by EMS personnel can be used to determine if a serious, widespread condition exists. For example, EMS reports can provide statistical information to the local government about collisions. Injury surveillance data can be used to determine ways to improve a dangerous intersection, to prevent crashes from ever happening, or to limit the severity of injuries to drivers.

As discussed earlier, you can help educate the public. People may not understand why an accident has happened. A parent allows her 5-year-old child to ride a bicycle without wearing a helmet. The child

falls and cuts the top of her head. You can work with the parents professionally, respectfully, and kindly to help educate them on how to prevent this injury from occurring in the future.

Teaching people how to perform compression-only CPR, how to help a choking victim, or how to stop serious bleeding are all aspects of public education. Public education increases public respect for EMS. When people understand what it means to work on an ambulance and provide care to the sick and injured, they are more likely to consider EMS a vital part of the public health care system. This change in attitude can be powerful and lead to increased EMS funding and greater respect for EMS as a profession.

## EMS Research

Why do EMTs perform the skills they do? How many ambulances does a city need? Should we remain on the scene and stabilize the patient or should we rapidly transport the patient? These questions and thousands more like them help determine the shape and impact of EMS on the community. The answers to these questions are derived from research and application of the scientific method. In the early days of EMS, expert opinion guided which tools and techniques EMS providers employed. While EMS care at the time was provided with the best information available, virtually all aspects of health care today utilize **evidence-based medicine (EBM)**. EBM is focused on procedures that have proven useful in improving patient outcomes. While not every aspect of EMS has enough research to be truly evidence-based, many EMS systems and states now consult the *National Model EMS Clinical Guidelines* from the National Association of State EMS Officials. These treatment guidelines are based on a review of current research and expert consensus. All aspects of the EMT role are currently being researched, not only within the academic community, but increasingly within the practitioner community, as every EMT has something to contribute to improving the role.

As an EMT, you will be involved in research through gathering data from every call you go on. Additionally, you may be involved in a specific research project. For example, you may be part of a study to determine how much oxygen should be given to patients with shortness of breath. Your job is to carefully follow the research protocol and record all of the pertinent information about these patients. The information gathered is analyzed by others to answer these questions and the results are shared with the rest of the EMS community to change patient care practices. Modern medical practice is based on such research.

It is important to stay current on the latest advances in health care. On a regular basis, the International Liaison Committee on Resuscitation (ILCOR), along with its member, the American Heart Association, update guidelines based on current medical evidence. The ILCOR guidelines are an excellent example of evidence-based medical decision making in progress. These changes occur as results of research become available.

## Roles and Responsibilities of the EMT

As an EMT, you will often be the first health care professional to assess and treat the patient; as such, you have certain roles and responsibilities (**TABLE 1-5**) and are expected to possess certain attributes (**TABLE 1-6**). The guiding principle for EMS personnel is "everything you do needs to be done with the patient in mind." What is in the best

**TABLE 1-5** Roles and Responsibilities of the EMT

- Keep vehicles and equipment ready for an emergency.
- Ensure the safety of yourself, your partner, the patient, and bystanders.
- Operate the emergency vehicle.
- Be an on-scene leader.
- Evaluate the scene.
- Call for additional resources as needed.
- Gain patient access.
- Perform a patient assessment.
- Give emergency medical care to the patient while awaiting the arrival of additional medical resources.
- Give emotional support to the patient, the patient's family, and other responders.
- Maintain continuity of care by working with other medical professionals.
- Resolve emergency incidents.
- Uphold medical and legal standards.
- Ensure and protect patient privacy.
- Give administrative support.
- Constantly continue your professional development.
- Cultivate and sustain community relations.
- Give back to the profession.

© Jones & Bartlett Learning.

## YOU are the Provider

The patient's condition has remained stable throughout transport. After reassessing her, the paramedic asks you to call in your patient report to the receiving facility. Your estimated time of arrival is 8 minutes.

**Recording Time: 19 Minutes**

| | |
|---|---|
| **Level of consciousness** | Conscious and alert |
| **Respirations** | 14 breaths/min; regular and unlabored |
| **Pulse** | 70 beats/min; strong and regular |
| **Skin** | Pink, warm, and dry |
| **Blood pressure** | 118/60 mm Hg |
| **Spo$_2$** | 98% (on room air) |

You deliver the patient to the ED in stable condition and give your verbal report to a staff nurse. The patient thanks you and your crew for taking such good care of her. You depart the hospital and return to service. On the way back to the station, the paramedic reviews your call and your performance.

**6.** What is the purpose of reviewing an EMS call?

**TABLE 1-6** Professional Attributes of EMTs

| Attribute | Description |
| --- | --- |
| Integrity | Consistent adherence to a code of honest behavior |
| Empathy | Aware of and thoughtful toward the needs of others |
| Self-motivation | Able to discover problems and solve them without direction |
| Appearance and hygiene | Uses persona to project a sense of trust, professionalism, knowledge, and compassion |
| Self-confidence | A state of being in which you know what you know *and* know what you do not know; able to ask for help |
| Time management | Able to perform or delegate multiple tasks, ensuring efficiency and safety |
| Communications | Able to understand others and have them understand you |
| Teamwork and diplomacy | Able to work with others and to know your place within a team; able to communicate while giving respect to the listener |
| Respect | Places others in high regard or importance; understands others are more important than self |
| Patient advocacy | Constantly keeps the needs of the patient at the center of care |
| Careful delivery of care | Pays attention to detail; makes sure what is being done for the patient is done as safely as possible |

© Jones & Bartlett Learning.

interest of the patient? This approach is referred to as being a patient advocate.

Often, patient outcomes depend on the care you provide in the field and your identification of patients who need prompt transport. You are responsible for all aspects of EMS, from the preparation of the equipment, to the delivery of care, to providing a good example for others within the community.

## Professional Attributes

As an EMT, whether you are paid or a volunteer, you are a health care professional. Part of your responsibility is to make sure patient care is given a high priority without endangering your own safety or the safety of others. Another part of your responsibility to yourself, other EMTs, the patient, and other health care professionals is to maintain a professional appearance and manner at all times. Appearance, including uniforms, hair length, and tattoos, are usually regulated by the policies of your department (**FIGURE 1-8**). Your attitude and behavior

must reflect that you are knowledgeable and sincerely dedicated to serving anyone who is injured or in an acute medical emergency. A professional appearance and manner help to build confidence and ease the patient's anxiety. You are expected to perform under pressure with composure and self-confidence. Patients and families who are under stress need to be treated with understanding, respect, and compassion.

Most patients will treat you with respect and appreciation, but some will not. Some patients are uncooperative, demanding, unpleasant, ungrateful, and verbally abusive. You must be nonjudgmental and overcome your instincts to react poorly to such behavior. Remember, when people are hurt, ill, under stress, frightened, despondent, under the influence of alcohol or drugs, or feel threatened, they will often react with inappropriate behavior, even toward those who are trying to help and care for them. Every patient, regardless of his or her attitude, is entitled to compassion, respect, and the best care that you can provide.

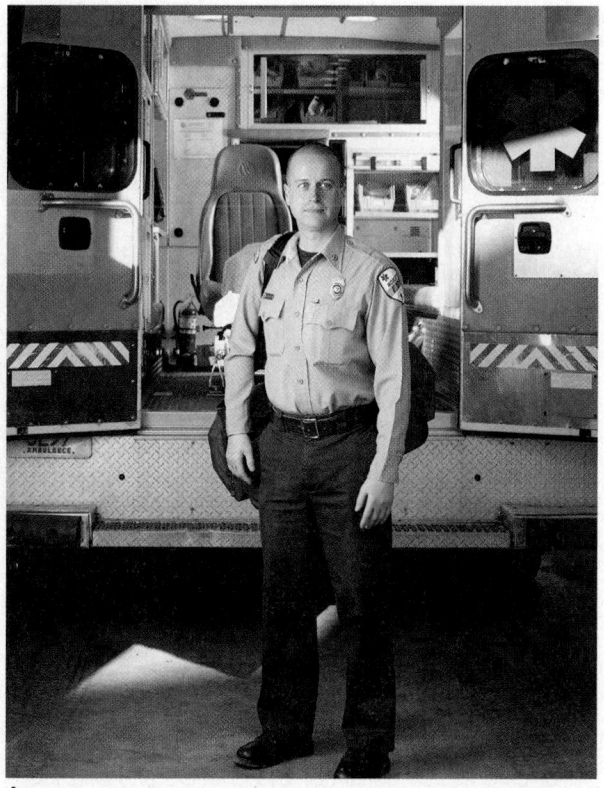 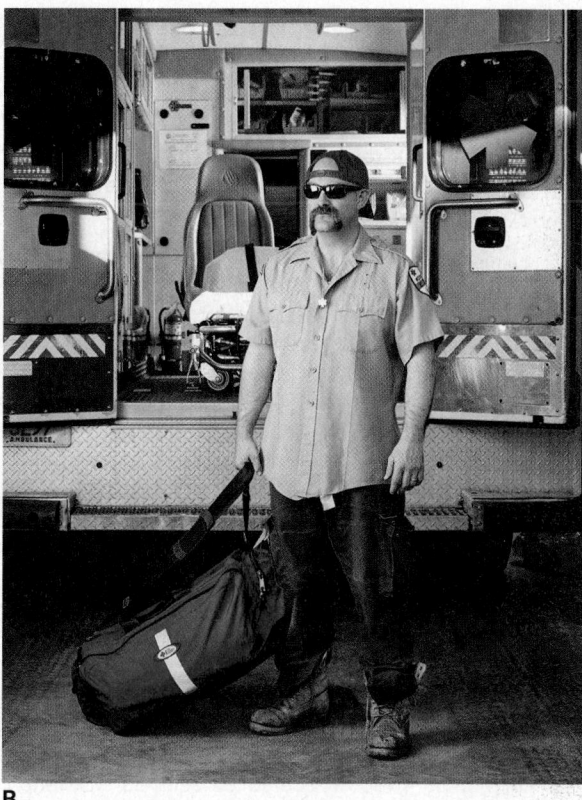

A  B

**FIGURE 1-8 A.** A professional appearance and demeanor help build confidence and ease patient anxiety. **B.** An unprofessional appearance may promote distrust and create the perception of incompetence.

© Jones & Bartlett Learning.

### Street Smarts

Professionalism extends beyond appearance and the activities you perform on a daily basis. As a professional, you have a responsibility to your partner, colleagues, patients, and profession to maintain a current level of knowledge.

Most people in this country can obtain proper routine medical care when they are ill and are supported by relatives and friends who will help to take care of them. However, when you are called to a home for a medical problem that is clearly not an emergency, remember that for some patients, calling an ambulance and being transported to the ED is the only way for them to obtain medical care.

As a new EMT, you will be given a lot of advice and training from the more experienced EMTs with whom you serve. Some may voice a callous disregard for some types of patients. Do not be influenced by the unprofessional attitude of these providers, regardless of how experienced or skilled they appear.

As a health care professional and an extension of physician care, you are bound by patient confidentiality. You should not discuss your findings or any disclosures made by the patient with anyone but those who are treating the patient or in limited situations, as required by law, the police, or other social agencies. When discussing a call with others, you should be careful to avoid revealing any information that might disclose the name or identity of patients you have treated. Be careful not to gossip about calls and patients with others, even in your own home. The protection of patient privacy has drawn national attention since the passage of HIPAA. You should be familiar with the requirements of this legislation, especially as it applies to your particular practice.

## YOU are the Provider SUMMARY

**1. How do your roles and responsibilities as an EMT compare to those of other EMS provider certification/licensure levels?**

EMRs, EMTs, AEMTs, and paramedics responding to the same call may have different levels of education, training, and scopes of practice, or may even work for different agencies, which may alter their specific roles somewhat. However, all levels of EMS personnel share the same fundamental roles and responsibilities—providing *safe and effective* emergency medical care to the sick and injured, and in many cases, transporting patients to an appropriate medical facility. The EMT curriculum provides more depth than that of the EMR, including increased knowledge of anatomy, physiology and pathophysiology, more comprehensive assessment skills, and additional treatment options to stabilize patients initially and provide fundamental care. For more severely ill or injured patients, more advanced assessment and treatment options may be needed by an AEMT who has additional knowledge and skills, including invasive techniques such as intravenous access, advanced airways, as well as additional medications that can be administered. A paramedic has an even greater scope of practice with more in-depth knowledge, diagnostic skills, and advanced treatment, electrical therapy, and medication options.

**2. How do the National Scope of Practice Model and the National EMS Education Standards affect an EMT's ability to assess and treat a patient?**

The National EMS Scope of Practice Model describes four levels of EMS practice, each with a different scope of practice and each requiring different types of education and training. The National EMS Education Standards outline the knowledge and competencies that should be taught to students in each of these four levels of EMS practice. These documents serve as a national framework from which the foundation of each state's scope of practice is developed, and help to determine the roles and responsibilities of EMS providers in the locality or agency where they serve. This initial education will be enhanced by a provider's experience and contact with patients, by reflecting on those experiences, and by feedback received from others.

**3. Does this patient need any treatment at the scene that can be provided by an EMT?**

Your role is to take care of patients whether the situation is what you would personally consider an

emergency or not. You should assume an emergency exists until a thorough and accurate assessment by someone qualified to distinguish an emergent medical condition from a nonemergent condition proves otherwise. In addition to repeating the patient's vital signs and reassessment as needed, and providing comfort measures, there is no immediate treatment that can be provided by an EMT. If the patient is transported to the hospital, an EMT will also need to consider methods to most safely and comfortably move, carry, and transport the patient.

**4. How is patient care integrated across health systems when a patient is transported to the hospital?**

Delivering excellent and compassionate care and providing transportation to a higher level of care should be the norm. When a patient is transported to a hospital, the responsibility for the assessment and treatment of the patient started at the scene is transferred to a higher level of care. This integration of care can be enhanced by complete and detailed communication of information from the scene and of history gathered by EMS personnel to the receiving staff. This may start before arrival with prenotification when appropriate or by consultation with online medical direction about treatment options. Verbal reports to hospital staff on arrival at the hospital pass along essential details that may help staff to make preliminary decisions about laboratory tests, radiologic studies, or the need for immediate treatment. In addition, your report provides information about the treatment given before arrival and the results of that treatment. Your verbal report can then be followed by a more complete and detailed written report with additional details or explanations.

**5. What safety concerns apply to this call and what are some ways to address those concerns or to avoid errors?**

Safety concerns and the possibility of errors affecting the safety of the patient occur in many ways on EMS calls. Safe transport is a major issue that needs to be considered during every phase of the call. Following traffic laws related to driving an emergency vehicle, proper restraint of driver and all passengers with appropriate seat belts or ambulance cot straps, avoiding distractions, and caution when moving through traffic can all contribute to safe transport. Similarly, proper lifting and carrying techniques, including the appropriate use of equipment and having sufficient manpower to safely lift and move a patient,

## YOU are the Provider SUMMARY *continued*

are essential to prevent injury to the patient and the crew. It is essential that EMS providers maintain current knowledge about the treatments they provide through continuing education and skill practice. Familiarity with current protocols and policies can also decrease errors, as well as carefully considering whether a treatment is appropriate or needed in the current circumstances. It can be beneficial to refer to tools such as copies of protocols or to discuss treatment choices with medical direction or a crew member in order to avoid errors. Communication errors can occur as well, especially in chaotic environments, as information can be misunderstood or inadvertently not communicated to other crew members or hospital staff. To help avoid miscommunication, talk in a clear, concise manner in common language and verify directions or medical orders by repeating them back to the sender so that both parties know that the information was correctly received.

**6. What is the purpose of reviewing an EMS call?**

A review of an EMS call can provide feedback regarding how you cared for the patient and met his or her physical and emotional needs. It should not be punitive or fault-finding; it is an educational tool to enhance your patient care skills. EMTs must be open to constructive criticism; this is how you learn and become more skilled emergency care providers. Informal reviews are ideal learning opportunities because information about the call is still fresh. Later formal critiques, such as those that are conducted as part of the CQI process, are designed to ensure that safe and effective patient care is consistently provided by all EMS providers in the system. This review may lead to changes and analysis of their effects on patient care at a system level. Formal CQI may also be used to provide feedback to an individual provider or crew, which may include positive reinforcement or recommendations for improvement.

### EMS Patient Care Report (PCR)

| Date: 9-30-19 | Incident No.: 010109 | Nature of Call: Back pain | | Location: 325 Blossom Ave. | |
|---|---|---|---|---|---|
| Dispatched: 0720 | En Route: 0720 | At Scene: 0723 | Transport: 0735 | At Hospital: 0750 | In Service: 0801 |

#### Patient Information

| Age: 48 Sex: F Weight (in kg [lb]): 64 kg (141 lb) | Allergies: None Medications: Ibuprofen Past Medical History: None Chief Complaint: Back pain |
|---|---|

#### Vital Signs

| Time: 0727 | BP: 126/66 | Pulse: 88 | Respirations: 16 | Spo$_2$: 99% |
|---|---|---|---|---|
| Time: 0735 | BP: 120/62 | Pulse: 90 | Respirations: 16 | Spo$_2$: 97% |
| Time: 0742 | BP: 118/60 | Pulse: 70 | Respirations: 14 | Spo$_2$: 98% |

#### EMS Treatment (circle all that apply)

| Oxygen @ ___ L/min via: NC  NRM  Bag mask | Assisted Ventilation | Airway Adjunct | CPR |
|---|---|---|---|
| Defibrillation | Bleeding Control | Bandaging | Splinting | Other: (Comfort care) |

## YOU are the Provider SUMMARY *continued*

| Narrative |
|---|

Unit 1 dispatched emergency to a private residence for back pain.

Chief Concern: Lower back pain

History: 48-year-old woman reports lower back pain, which has been present for the past month. She denied injuring her back; she further denied any other symptoms or past medical history. Medications include ibuprofen for pain. The patient stated she has not been evaluated by a physician for her back pain; however, because it has progressively worsened, she called 9-1-1.

Assessment: On arrival at the scene, found the patient sitting on the couch in her living room. She was conscious and alert; her airway was patent; and her breathing was adequate. Assessment of patient's back revealed no gross evidence of deformity, swelling, or bruising. Pulse, sensory, and motor functions were grossly intact in all extremities.

Treatment (Rx): Obtained vital signs. En route, patient expressed her pain had begun to subside. Reassessment revealed that she remained conscious and alert with stable vital signs. Provided reassurance and reassessment throughout remainder of transport.

Transport: Placed patient onto stretcher and placed her in position of comfort, loaded her into the ambulance, and began nonemergency transport to the hospital. Delivered patient to ED without incident and gave verbal report to staff nurse.

**End of report**

# Prep Kit

## Ready for Review

- The standards for prehospital emergency care and the providers who deliver it are governed by the laws in each state and are typically regulated by a state office of EMS.
- Ambulances in EMS systems are staffed by EMTs who have been trained to the EMT, AEMT, or paramedic level according to recommended national standards and have been licensed by the state they serve.
- An EMT has training in basic emergency care knowledge, skills, and attitudes, focusing on initial care and transport of patients that includes identification, assessment, and treatment of many emergency and nonemergency conditions.
- An AEMT has training in specific aspects of ALS care, such as IV therapy and the administration of certain emergency medications.
- A paramedic has extensive training in ALS, including endotracheal intubation, emergency pharmacology, cardiac monitoring, and other advanced assessment and treatment skills.

- EMRs, such as law enforcement officers, firefighters, park rangers, ski patrollers, or other organized rescuers often arrive at the scene before the ambulance and EMTs.
- After the EMTs size up the scene and assess the patient, they provide the emergency care and transport that is indicated based on their findings and ordered by their medical director in the service's standing orders and protocols or by the physician who is providing online medical direction.
- The National EMS Scope of Practice Model, developed by NHTSA, provides overarching guidelines as to what skills each level of EMS provider should be able to accomplish.
- EMS Agenda 2050 is a multidisciplinary, national review of all aspects of EMS delivery that provides a framework for the creation of improved, people-centered systems of care.
- You will often be the first health care professional to assess and treat the patient; as such, you have certain roles and are expected to possess certain attributes.

- EMT attributes include compassion and motivation to reduce suffering, pain, and mortality in those who are injured or acutely ill; a desire to provide each patient with the best possible care; commitment to obtain the knowledge and skills that this position requires; and the drive to continually increase your knowledge, skills, and ability.
- The EMT course that you are now taking will present the information and skills that you will need to pass the required certification examination needed to become a licensed EMT.
- Once you have completed the course, you must assume responsibility for directing your own study through continuing education provided by your service's training officer and medical director or through other opportunities available to you. Your commitment to continued learning is the key to being a good EMT.
- Throughout your career, seek new certifications and roles that will broaden your abilities and experience. Mobile integrated health care, including the role of community paramedic, is an example of how EMS roles are evolving.
- As a health care professional and as someone who functions as a physician extender, you are bound by patient confidentiality.

## Vital Vocabulary

**advanced EMT (AEMT)** An individual who has training in specific aspects of advanced life support, such as intravenous therapy, and the administration of certain emergency medications.

**advanced life support (ALS)** Advanced life-saving procedures, some of which are now being provided by the EMT.

**Americans With Disabilities Act (ADA)** Comprehensive legislation that is designed to protect people with disabilities against discrimination.

**automated external defibrillator (AED)** A device that detects treatable life-threatening cardiac dysrhythmias (ventricular fibrillation and ventricular tachycardia) and delivers the appropriate electrical shock to the patient.

**certification** A process in which a person, an institution, or a program is evaluated and recognized as meeting certain predetermined standards to provide safe and ethical care.

**community paramedicine** A health care model in which experienced paramedics receive advanced training to equip them to provide additional services in the prehospital environment, such as health evaluations, monitoring of chronic illnesses or conditions, and patient advocacy.

**continuous quality improvement (CQI)** A system of internal and external reviews and audits of all aspects of an EMS system aiming at improving outcomes.

**credentialing** An established process to determine the qualifications necessary to be allowed to practice a particular profession, or to function as an organization.

**emergency medical dispatch (EMD)** A system that assists dispatchers in selecting appropriate units to respond to a particular call for assistance and provides callers with vital instructions until the arrival of EMS crews.

**emergency medical responder (EMR)** A first trained professional, such as police officer, firefighter, lifeguard, or other rescuer, who may arrive first at the scene of an emergency to provide initial medical assistance.

**emergency medical services (EMS)** A multidisciplinary system that represents the combined efforts of several professionals and agencies to provide prehospital emergency care to the sick and injured.

**emergency medical technician (EMT)** An individual who has training in basic life support, including automated external defibrillation, use of a definitive airway adjunct, and assisting patients with certain medications.

**evidence-based medicine (EBM)** An approach to medicine where decisions are based on well-conducted research, classifying recommendations based on the strength of the scientific evidence; also called science-based medicine.

**Health Insurance Portability and Accountability Act (HIPAA)** Federal legislation passed in 1996. Its main effect in EMS is in limiting availability of patients' health care information and penalizing violations of patient privacy.

**intravenous (IV) therapy** The delivery of medication directly into a vein.

**licensure** The process whereby a competent authority, usually the state, allows people to perform a regulated act.

**medical control** Physician instructions given directly by radio or cell phone (online/direct) or indirectly by protocol/guidelines (off-line/indirect), as authorized by the medical director of the service program.

**medical director** The physician who authorizes or delegates to the EMT the authority to provide medical care in the field.

**mobile integrated health care (MIH)** A method of delivering health care that involves providing health care within the community rather than at a physician's office or hospital.

**National EMS Scope of Practice Model** A document created by the National Highway Traffic Safety Administration (NHTSA) that outlines the skills performed by various EMS providers.

**paramedic** An individual who has extensive training in advanced life support, including endotracheal intubation, emergency pharmacology, cardiac monitoring, and other advanced assessment and treatment skills.

**primary prevention** Efforts to prevent an injury or illness from ever occurring.

**primary service area** The designated area in which the EMS agency is responsible for the provision of prehospital emergency care and transportation to the hospital.

**public health** The branch of medicine that is focused on examining the health needs of entire populations with the goal of preventing health problems.

**public safety access point** A call center, staffed by trained personnel who are responsible for managing requests for police, fire, and ambulance services.

**quality control** Oversight by the medical director to ensure the appropriate medical care standards are met by EMTs on each call.

**secondary prevention** Efforts to limit the effects of an injury or illness that you cannot completely prevent.

# References

1. American Academy of Orthopaedic Surgeons. *Emergency Care and Transportation of the Sick and Injured.* Chicago, IL: American Academy of Orthopaedic Surgeons; 1971.

2. Caffrey SM, Barnes LC, Olvera DJ. Joint position statement on degree requirements for paramedics. *Prehosp Emerg Care.* 2019;23(3):434-437. https://doi.org/10.1080/10903127.2018.1519006

3. Centers for Medicare and Medicaid Services. Emergency Triage, Treat, and Transport (ET3) Model—Frequently Asked Questions. https://innovation.cms.gov/initiatives/et3/faq.html. Published November 18, 2019. Accessed February 6, 2020.

4. Centers for Medicare and Medicaid Services. National Health Expenditure Data. cms.gov/Research-Statistics-Data-and-Systems/Statistics-Trends-and-Reports/NationalHealthExpendData/NationalHealthAccounts Historical. Updated December 17, 2019. Accessed March 5, 2020.

5. Choi BY, Blumberg C, Williams K. Mobile integrated health care and community paramedicine: an emerging emergency medical services concept. *Ann Emerg Med.* 2016;67(3):361-366. https://doi.org/10.1016/j.annemergmed.2015.06.005

6. Cone D, Brice JH, Delbridge TR, Myers JB. *Emergency Medical Services: Clinical Practice and Systems Oversight.* Hoboken, NJ: John Wiley & Sons; 2014.

7. Cumbie TA. The mandatory accreditation of emergency medical services paramedic programs in the United States: a workforce perspective. *All Theses and Dissertations.* https://dune.une.edu/theses/180. Published 2018. Accessed February 6, 2020.

8. Dainty KN, Vaid H, Brooks SC. North American public opinion survey on the acceptability of crowdsourcing basic life support for out-of-hospital cardiac arrest with the PulsePoint mobile phone app. *JMIR MHealth UHealth.* 2017;5(5):e63. https://doi.org/10.2196/mhealth.6926

9. Davis D, Davis ME, Jadad A, et al. The case for knowledge translation: shortening the journey from evidence to effect. *BMJ.* 2003;327(7405):33-35. https://doi.org/10.1136/bmj.327.7405.33

10. Edemekong P, Haydel M, Slowik J, Sharma S, Dalal B. Health Insurance Portability and Accountability Act (HIPAA). StatPearls.com. https://knowledge.statpearls.com/chapter/sleep/22897/. Published 2019. Accessed February 6, 2020.

11. Faul M, Aikman SN, Sasser SM. Bystander intervention prior to the arrival of emergency medical services: comparing assistance across types of medical emergencies. *Prehosp Emerg Care.* 2016;20(3):317-323. https://doi.org/10.3109/10903127.2015.1088605

12. Goolsby C, Jacobs L, Hunt R, et al. Stop the Bleed Education Consortium: education program content and delivery recommendations. *J Trauma Acute Care Surg.* 2018;84(1):205-210. https://doi.org/10.1097/TA.0000000000001732

13. Gordon M, Gibbs T. STORIES statement: publication standards for health care education evidence synthesis. *BMC Medicine.* 2014;12(1):143. https://doi.org/10.1186/s12916-014-0143-0

14. Harvey JC. The Emergency Medical Service Systems Act of 1973. *JAMA.* 1974;230(8):1139-1140. https://doi.org/10.1001/jama.1974.03240080021019

15. International Association of Fire Chiefs. Joint position statement opposition to proposed degree requirements for accredited paramedic programs. https://www.iafc.org/docs/default-source/1ems/iafc-iaff-nfpa-nvfc-joint-position-statement-on-paramedic-education-requirements-12-30-18.pdf?sfvrsn=b588800d_2. Published December 30, 2018. Accessed February 6, 2020.

16. Interstate Commission for EMS Personnel Practice. EMS Compact. https://www.emscompact.gov/. Accessed February 6, 2020.

17. Lerner EB, Weik T, Edgerton EA. Research in prehospital care: overcoming the barriers to success. *Prehosp Emerg Care.* 2016;20(4):448-453. https://doi.org/10.3109/10903127.2014.980480

18. Magruder KM, McLaughlin KA, Borbon DLE. Trauma is a public health issue. *European J Psychotraumatol.* 2017;8(1):1375338. https://doi.org/10.1080/20008198.2017.1375338

19. National Academy of Sciences and National Research Council. *Accidental Death and Disability: The Neglected Disease of Modern Society.* Washington, DC: National Academies Press; 1966. https://doi.org/10.17226/9978

20. National Association of State EMS Officials. *National EMS Scope of Practice Model.* https://nasemso.org/projects/ems-scope-of-practice/. Published February 2019. Accessed February 6, 2020.

21. National Association of State EMS Officials. *National Model EMS Clinical Guidelines.* https://nasemso.org/projects/model-ems-clinical-guidelines/. Published January 5, 2019. Accessed February 6, 2020.

22. National Fire Protection Association, Technical Committee on Fire Service Occupational Safety and Health. *NFPA 1561, Standard on Emergency Services Incident Management System.* Quincy, MA: NFPA; 2008.

23. *National Geographic* staff. If you're an average American, you'll live to be 78.6 years old. *National Geographic.* https://www.nationalgeographic.com/culture/2018/12/life-expectancy-united-states/. Published 2018. Accessed February 6, 2020.

24. National Highway Traffic Safety Administration. *Emergency Medical Technician–Ambulance: National Standard Curriculum.* ems.gov. https://www.ems.gov/pdf/education/Emergency-Medical-Technician/EMT_Ambulance_1984.pdf. Published 1984. Accessed February 6, 2020.

25. National Highway Traffic Safety Administration. *Emergency Medical Technician–Basic: National Standard Curriculum.* ems.gov. https://www.ems.gov/pdf/education/Emergency-Medical-Technician/EMT_Basic_1996.pdf. Published 1996. Accessed February 6, 2020.

26. National Highway Traffic Safety Administration. *Emergency Medical Technician—Paramedic: National Standard Curriculum.* ems.gov. https://www.ems.gov/pdf/education/Emergency-Medical-Technician-Paramedic/Paramedic_Inst_Lessons_1985.pdf. Published 1985. Accessed February 6, 2020.

27. National Highway Traffic Safety Administration. *EMT-Paramedic: National Standard Curriculum.* ems.gov. https://www.ems.gov/pdf/education/Emergency-Medical-Technician-Paramedic/Paramedic_1998.pdf. Published 1998. Accessed February 6, 2020.

28. National Highway Traffic Safety Administration. *National EMS Education Standards.* ems.gov. https://www.ems.gov/pdf/National-EMS-Education-Standards-FINAL-Jan-2009.pdf. Published 2009. Accessed February 6, 2020.

29. National Highway Traffic Safety Administration. *EMS Agenda 2050: A People-Centered Vision for the Future of Emergency Medical Services* (p. 58). Washington, DC: National Highway Traffic Safety Administration. ems.gov. https://www.ems.gov/projects/ems-agenda-2050.html. Published 2019. Accessed February 6, 2020.

30. National Learning Consortium. *Continuous quality improvement (CQI) strategies to optimize your practice* (p. 20). healthit.gov https://www.healthit.gov/sites/default/files/tools/nlc_continuousqualityimprovement primer.pdf. Published 2013. Accessed February 6, 2020.

31. National Registry of Emergency Medical Technicians. *2014 Practice Analysis.* National Registry of Emergency Medical Technicians website. https://content.nremt.org/static/documents/2014%20NATIONAL%20EMS%20PRACTICE%20ANALYSIS.pdf. Published 2015. Accessed March 2, 2020.

32. Pollack RA, Brown SP, Rea T, et al. Impact of bystander automated external defibrillator use on survival and functional outcomes in shockable observed public cardiac arrests. *Circulation.* 2018;137(20):2104-2113. https://doi.org/10.1161/CIRCULATIONAHA.117.030700

33. Shapiro GL, Smith R, Callaway DW, Bobko JP. Leveraging bystanders as medical force multipliers during MCIs. JEMS.com. https://www.jems.com/2016/08/01/leveraging-bystanders-as-medical-force-multipliers-during-mcis/. Published August 2, 2016. Accessed February 6, 2020.

34. Taymour RK, Abir M, Chamberlin M, et al. Policy, practice, and research agenda for emergency medical services oversight: a systematic review and environmental scan. *Prehosp Disaster Med.* 2018;33(1):89-97. https://doi.org/10.1017/S1049023X17007129

# Chapter 2

# Workforce Safety and Wellness

## NATIONAL EMS EDUCATION STANDARD COMPETENCIES

### Medicine
Applies fundamental knowledge to provide basic emergency care transportation based on assessment findings for an acutely ill patient.

### Infectious Diseases
Awareness of
- How to decontaminate equipment after treating a patient (pp 50–51)

Assessment and management of
- How to decontaminate the ambulance and equipment after treating a patient (pp 50–51)

### Preparatory
Applies fundamental knowledge of the emergency medical services (EMS) system, safety/well-being of the emergency medical technician (EMT), medical/legal, and ethical issues to the provision of emergency care.

### Workforce Safety and Wellness
- Standard safety precautions (pp 41–49)
- Personal protective equipment (pp 38, 41–49, 61–65)
- Stress management (pp 32–35, 69–75)
  - Dealing with death and dying (pp 67–69)
- Prevention of response-related injuries (pp 54–61)
- Prevention of work-related injuries (pp 54–61, 77)
- Lifting and moving patients (p 35)
- Disease transmission (pp 38–40)
- Principles of wellness and resilience (pp 31–38)

## KNOWLEDGE OBJECTIVES

1. Explain the steps that contribute to wellness and resilience and their importance in managing stress. (pp 31–38)
2. Differentiate infectious disease and communicable disease. (p 38)
3. Identify the risks and hazards of sleep deprivation in EMS. (pp 35–36)
4. State the routes of disease transmission. (pp 38–40)
5. Describe the specific routes of transmission and the steps to prevent and/or deal with an exposure to hepatitis, tuberculosis, or human immunodeficiency virus (HIV)/acquired immunodeficiency syndrome (AIDS). (pp 38–49)
6. Apply the standard precautions used in treating patients to prevent infection. (pp 41–49)
7. Explain the steps to take for personal protection from airborne and bloodborne pathogens. (pp 41–49)
8. Demonstrate proper handwashing techniques. (pp 41–43)
9. Explain the ways in which immunity to infectious diseases is acquired. (pp 51–53)
10. Summarize postexposure management of exposure to patient blood or body fluids,

PHOTO: © AAron Ontiveroz/MediaNews Group/The Denver Post/Getty Images.

including completing a postexposure report. (pp 53–54)

11. Discuss the steps necessary to determine scene safety and to prevent work-related injuries at the scene. (pp 54–61)

12. Describe the different types of protective clothing worn to prevent injury. (pp 61–65)

13. Differentiate issues concerning care of the dying patient, death, and the grieving process of family members. (pp 67–69)

14. Recognize the physiologic, physical, and psychological responses to stress. (pp 69–70)

15. Explain posttraumatic stress disorder (PTSD) and steps that can be taken, including critical incident stress management, to decrease the likelihood that PTSD will develop. (pp 71–72)

16. Identify the emotional aspects of emergency care. (pp 73–74)

17. Recognize the stress inherent in many situations, such as mass-casualty scenes. (pp 74–75)

18. Recognize the possibility of violent situations and the steps to take to deal with them. (pp 60–61)

19. Identify behavioral emergencies. (pp 60–61)

20. Discuss workplace issues such as cultural diversity, sexual harassment, and substance abuse. (pp 75–77)

21. Identify resources for positive mental health and suicide prevention. (pp 72–73)

## SKILLS OBJECTIVES

1. Demonstrate how to properly remove gloves. (p 44, Skill Drill 2-1)

2. Demonstrate the steps necessary to take to manage a potential exposure situation. (p 49, Skill Drill 2-2)

# Introduction

Work as an emergency responder carries with it a level of increased risk compared to other professions. EMTs often work under demanding, strenuous, and rapidly changing circumstances. As part of their work, EMTs may be exposed to infectious disease, occupational injury, physical violence, and more. They may be called on to respond to scenes of sudden tragedy and violence, and during the course of caring for others, they themselves may suffer physical, mental, or emotional harm.

Recent years have brought an improved understanding of the threats and stressors that affect EMTs, including sleep deprivation, physical violence, compassion fatigue, posttraumatic stress disorder, and responder suicide. Recent studies have found that 84% of first responders have experienced traumatic events on the job and that 34% have received a formal diagnosis of a mental health disorder such as depression or posttraumatic stress disorder. Moreover, the rate among EMTs and paramedics of either contemplating or committing suicide is far higher than the rate among other adult Americans. Although such concerns for EMS providers have always existed, they are now being discussed more openly. As an EMT, you must care for yourself—not just physically, but also mentally and emotionally—before you can expect to care for your patients.

As part of your training, you will learn how to recognize threats to your health, safety, and well-being and that of your partners and your patients. You will also learn how, when possible, you can avoid such hazards, protect yourself and others from them, or minimize their effect. Finally, you will learn how best to manage the mental, physical, and emotional health conditions that result from operating in emergency environments and caring for the sick and injured.

# General Health, Wellness, and Resilience

Although most people might think of health simply as the absence of disease or physical injury, we now understand that health is a complex interaction between physical, mental, and emotional conditions. Because they are intertwined, chronic physical, mental, or emotional stresses can worsen or increase the chances of developing combinations of physical, mental, or emotional health conditions. Fortunately, the opposite is also true. Supporting good physical, mental, and emotional health can significantly lower the risk of chronic and acute health problems.

## Wellness and Stress Management

In daily life we often use the word *stress* to describe difficult, harmful, or negative conditions. In fact, not all reactions to stress are negative. A stressor that produces a positive response is called **eustress**. One example might be a dispatch to a high-speed motor vehicle collision. Characteristics of eustress following such a dispatch may include increased focus, energy in the short term, and, in the long term, increased job satisfaction and self-image from performing well under a challenging situation. In contrast, **distress** is stress that produces negative responses. For example, the same motor vehicle collision may result in short-term feelings of being overwhelmed, increased anxiety, and loss of focus, along with numerous long-term psychological and physiologic difficulties (**TABLE 2-1**).

| TABLE 2-1 Examples of Events Likely to Cause Distress or Eustress | |
|---|---|
| **Distress** | **Eustress** |
| Death of a family member or friend | Receiving a promotion |
| Divorce | Taking a vacation |
| Financial problems | Moving |
| Interpersonal conflict | Participating in a culture of challenge and debate |
| Health issues | Undertaking a physical fitness regimen |
| Responding to a scene of violence | Receiving an award or recognition |
| Responding to a mass-casualty incident | Giving birth |
| Responding to the death of a child | Taking a new certification class |
| Illness or injury of a friend or coworker | Taking a new job or joining a new organization |

© Jones & Bartlett Learning.

## Strategies for Wellness and Resilience

Understanding how stress affects you physically, mentally, and emotionally can help you manage the effects of distress. Stress may be experienced in the short term as a single, isolated event, or it may be a chronic or long-term issue. Likewise, how a person responds to a stressor can depend greatly on factors such as the person's overall mood, health, and other sources of stress that may be present at the same time. Because so many factors come into play, different people will react differently to the same stressors. Moreover, a person may react differently to the same stressor under different circumstances. While one EMT may not be adversely affected by the stress of a difficult emergency call, his or her partner on the same call may experience serious aftereffects. Also, although an EMT may be able to handle a certain amount of stress one day, he or she may not have the capacity to handle that much stress on another day or in other circumstances.

A significant challenge is that one source of distress can often lead to another. An EMT experiencing personal issues at home may become more sensitive to stressors at work. The troubles at work can, in turn, lead to more distress at home, leading to a vicious cycle that can be difficult to break. A key goal of workforce safety and wellness is to set yourself up for success by creating conditions that can help you better deal with stress in both the short term and the long term.

**Wellness** is the active pursuit of a state of good health. It is crucial for EMS providers to understand that they must work to maintain their wellness in the same way that they must work to maintain their knowledge, skills, and attitudes to be effective emergency responders. Wellness is multifaceted. Maintaining good physical fitness is important, but by itself it is not enough to ensure wellness for an EMS provider.

**Resilience** is the capacity of an individual to cope with and recover from distress. Although some people tend to be more resilient than others, a person's resilience may change. The following practices can help increase resilience:

- Eat a healthy and well-balanced diet.
- Ensure a minimum of 7 to 9 hours of sleep per day.
- Strengthen positive relationships with close family and friends.

- Build relationships with peers and colleagues.
- Incorporate daily stretching, movement, and exercise.
- Build habits of mindfulness and positivity.

The term *stress management* refers to the tactics that have been shown to alleviate or eliminate stress reactions (**TABLE 2-2**).

A clue to the management of stress comes from the fact that it is not the event itself but the individual's reaction to it that determines how much it will strain the body's resources.

### Words of Wisdom

Attitudes toward wellness are as important as knowledge and behaviors. An EMT can know the right way to deal with stress, but this knowledge will not help if the person's attitude is, "That doesn't apply to me. I'm fine."

The following sections provide some suggestions for how to prevent the effects of stress from adversely affecting you.

## Nutrition

As an EMT, you have little control over what stressors you will face on the job on any given day. Consequently, stress in one form or another is an unavoidable part of your life. Just as you would study for a test, dress properly for a day of snow skiing, or train for a sporting event, you should physically prepare your body for stress. Physical conditioning and proper nutrition are the two variables over which you have control. Muscles and bones will weaken without sufficient activity. Regular, well-balanced meals are essential to provide the nutrients that are necessary to keep your body

**TABLE 2-2** Strategies to Manage Stress

- Minimize or eliminate stressors as much as possible.
- Change partners to avoid a negative or hostile personality.
- Change work hours.
- Change the work environment.
- Cut back on overtime.
- Change your attitude about the stressor.
- Talk about your feelings with people you trust.
- Seek professional counseling if needed.
- Do not obsess over frustrating situations that you are unable to change, such as relapsing alcoholics and nursing home transfers; focus on delivering high-quality care.
- Try to adopt a more relaxed, philosophical outlook.
- Expand your social support system beyond your coworkers.
- Develop friends and interests outside emergency services.
- Minimize the physical response to stress by using various techniques, including:
  - Periodic stretching or yoga
  - Slow, deep breathing
  - Regular physical exercise (150 min per week, including cardiovascular effort)
  - Progressive muscle relaxation
  - Meditation
  - Limit intake of caffeine, alcohol, and tobacco use

fueled (**FIGURE 2-1**). Vitamin-mineral preparations that provide a balanced mix of all the nutrients may be necessary to supplement a less than perfectly balanced diet.

The physical exertion and stress that are a part of your job require a high energy output. If you do not have a ready source of fuel, your performance may be less than satisfactory. This can be dangerous

## YOU are the Provider

You became a certified EMT less than 6 months ago and have been working a shift of 24 hours on and 48 hours off. You receive a call at 0840 hours to 6 Catoonah Street for an unconscious child who is not breathing. You and your paramedic partner respond to the scene; a law enforcement EMR unit is dispatched at the same time. This is your first call involving a critically ill child.

**1.** How can you psychologically prepare yourself for this call?

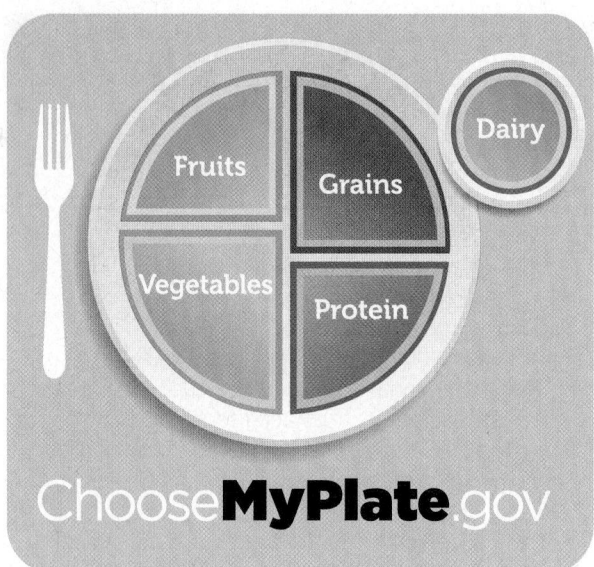

**FIGURE 2-1** The USDA's MyPlate icon emphasizes healthy portions of vegetables, fruits, grains, proteins, and dairy.

Courtesy of the USDA Center for Nutrition Policy and Promotion.

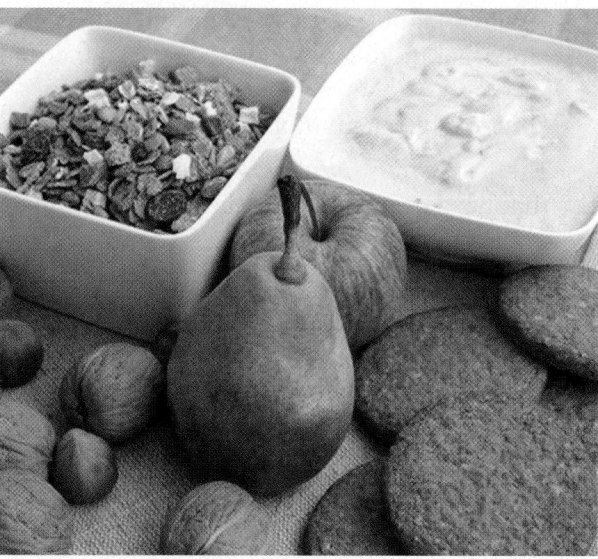

**FIGURE 2-2** Carry a supply of high-energy food with you so you can maintain your energy levels.

© Monika Adamczyk/ShutterStock.

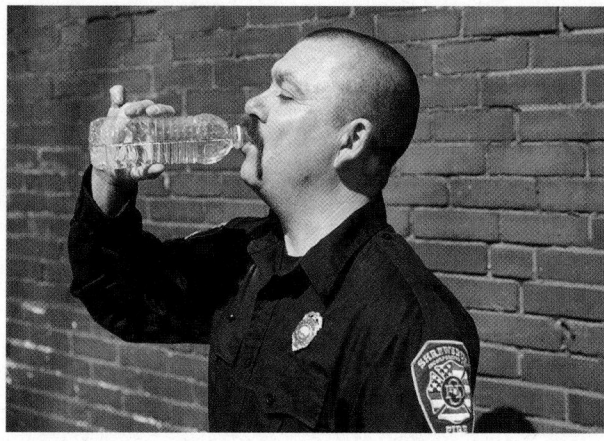

**FIGURE 2-3** Maintain an adequate fluid intake by drinking plenty of water or other nonalcoholic, caffeine-free fluids.

© Jones & Bartlett Learning.

for you, your partner, and your patients. Therefore, it is important for you to understand and follow the guidelines of good nutrition.

In general, you should limit your total consumption of sugar, fats, sodium, and alcohol. These foods are quickly absorbed and converted to fuel by the body. However, simple sugars also stimulate the body's production of insulin, which reduces blood glucose levels. For some people, eating a lot of sugar can actually result in lower energy levels.

Complex carbohydrates are comparable to simple sugars in their ability to produce energy. Complex carbohydrates such as pasta, rice, and vegetables are among the safest, most reliable sources for long-term energy production. However, some carbohydrates take hours to be converted into usable body fuel. The proteins in meat, fish, chicken, beans, and cheese can also take several hours to convert to energy.

Fats are also easily converted to energy, but eating too much fats, or eating the wrong fats, can lead to obesity, cardiac disease, and other long-term health problems. Consumption of fats should be limited to 10% of calories and should focus on monounsaturated and polyunsaturated fats while avoiding saturated fats or trans fats. It is also important to limit cholesterol intake and salt (sodium) intake.

Carry an individual supply of your own high-energy food to help you maintain your energy levels

(**FIGURE 2-2**). Eating several small, healthy meals throughout the day can keep your energy resources at constant high levels and help you cope with the stresses inherent in EMS work. However, overeating may reduce your physical and mental performance. After a large meal, the blood that is needed for the digestive process is not available for other activities.

You must also maintain an adequate fluid intake (**FIGURE 2-3**). Hydration is important for proper functioning. Fluids can be easily replenished by drinking any nonalcoholic, caffeine-free fluid. Water is generally the best fluid available because the body absorbs it faster than any other fluid. Avoid fluids that contain high levels of sugar. These can actually slow the rate of fluid absorption by the body and cause abdominal discomfort. One indication of adequate hydration is frequent urination. Infrequent urination or urine that has a deep yellow color indicates dehydration.

## Exercise and Relaxation

Regular exercise will enhance the benefits of maintaining good nutrition and adequate hydration. When you are in good physical condition, you can handle job stress more easily. Regular exercise will increase your strength and endurance. To maintain good health, you should engage in at least 30 minutes of physical activity at least 5 days per week. Exercise should be moderate or vigorous to have good health benefits. In other words, you should break a sweat (**FIGURE 2-4**).

Your exercise routine should involve aspects of cardiovascular endurance, muscular strength building, and muscle flexibility. Endurance will ensure your cardiovascular system is able to provide your muscles and brain with needed oxygen. Strength and flexibility building ensures the body is able to handle the requirements that you will place on it by lifting patients, performing CPR, and moving heavy equipment.

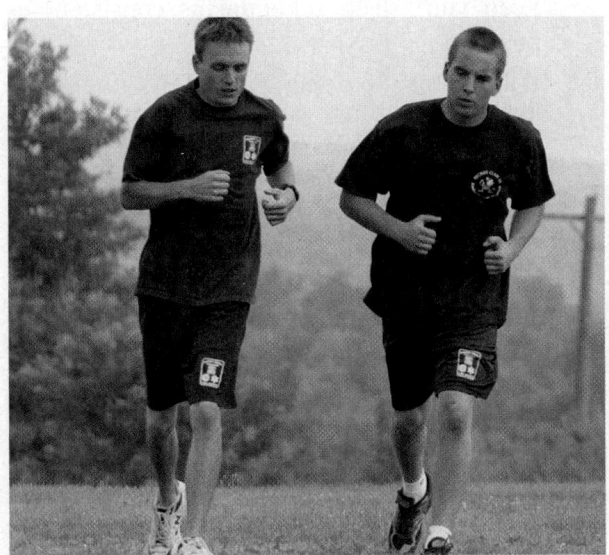

**FIGURE 2-4** A regular program of exercise will increase strength and endurance.

© Jones & Bartlett Learning. Courtesy of MIEMSS.

Remember, if you do not use it, you will lose it. Plan activities ahead of time and use strategies that make your exercise sessions convenient. Is there a gym or exercise facility near your home or on your route to work? Is there a walking path or a running track? Where possible, join or gather a group of other people to exercise with you. This can increase your chances of exercising consistently, increase your enjoyment of exercising, and build enjoyable social relationships, which can also increase your resilience.

## Safe Lifting Practices

We have already discussed the physical requirements of being an EMT. Lifting 125 lb (57 kg) can be difficult if you do not exercise regularly. Lifting is one of the things you will do often, so safe lifting techniques are critical to your health and well-being. Back injuries are common in EMS work. Chapter 8, *Lifting and Moving Patients*, discusses good techniques for lifting and moving that can decrease your risk of injury. For your health and well-being, remember these tips:

- Preplan the move.
- Bend your legs, not your waist.
- Keep the weight close to your body.
- Lift straight up, using your legs, not your back.

## Sleep

Because of the nature of shift work and the intensity and "around-the-clock" nature of emergency medical care, many EMS practitioners find themselves chronically fatigued and experiencing sleep deprivation issues. The National Sleep Foundation and the American Academy of Sleep Medicine recommend that adults sleep a minimum of 7 to 9 hours per night. Research has found that half of EMS personnel get less than 6 hours of sleep per 24 hours and report severe mental and physical fatigue. In the short term, such fatigue can lead to medical errors, vehicle crashes, and other harm to patients, bystanders, and EMS providers. In the long term, such sleep deprivation can lead to hypertension, sleep apnea, respiratory issues, diabetes, depression, and other medical conditions. Sleep deprivation and fatigue issues can increase stress, and, in turn, increased stress can contribute to sleep deprivation and fatigue issues. These problems may be compounded in EMS systems where workload is particularly high.

Evidence-based guidelines for fatigue management have been developed under the US Department of Transportation through the National Association of State EMS Officials. They include the following recommendations:

- Fatigue/sleepiness survey instruments should be used to measure and monitor fatigue among EMS personnel.
- EMS personnel should work shifts shorter than 24 hours in duration.
- EMS personnel should have access to caffeine to help stave off fatigue.
- EMS personnel should have the opportunity to nap while on duty to mitigate fatigue.
- EMS personnel should receive education and training to mitigate fatigue and fatigue-related risks.

Recommendations for individual providers to combat fatigue include the following:

- Get an adequate duration (more than 7 hours) and quality of sleep.
- Where allowed, take 20- to 30-minute naps or rest breaks during shift work.
- Increase physical exercise such as stretching, walking, and jogging in place.
- Be careful about caffeine consumption. Caffeine can increase alertness but is not a replacement for sleep and in large quantities can contribute to cardiac dysrhythmias, seizures, and increased stress and anxiety.
- Engage in mental exercise, such as having a conversation or playing a game.

Of course, the most effective way to combat fatigue is to ensure good sleep in the first place.

Productive sleep is as important as eating well and exercise in the maintenance of good health. Sleep should be regular and uninterrupted. Recommendations to improve sleep quality include the following:

- Avoid caffeine, alcohol, nicotine, and other chemicals that interfere with sleep for at least 4 hours before bedtime.
- Ensure your sleep environment is dark, quiet, and cool. If necessary, use blackout shades or an eye mask to block light, or earplugs or devices that produce "white noise" to reduce noise.
- Exercise early, but with enough time to relax before you try to fall asleep.
- If you nap, nap early. Avoid naps before your regular sleep.
- Avoid heavy presleep meals.
- Balance fluid intake. Stay hydrated, but avoid overhydration; you don't want your sleep to be interrupted by trips to the bathroom.
- Establish a calming presleep routine. This could include taking a bath, reading a book, or practicing meditation or relaxation exercises.
- Sleep when truly tired. If not asleep after approximately 20 minutes, try additional calming presleep activities rather than "fighting" to get to sleep.
- Don't watch the clock before bed or if you wake up in the middle of your sleep cycle.
- Keep your sleep schedule as consistent as possible.
- Where possible, expose yourself to natural light during your waking hours to maintain healthy sleep–wake cycles.

## Disease Prevention and Health Promotion

Another aspect of wellness involves disease prevention and health promotion. Strictly speaking, although both of these efforts involve personal practices and medical services, disease prevention focuses more on medical care and prevention to avoid or reduce the effect of disease on an individual. Health promotion is more focused on personal practices and social habits to improve one's health.

Examples of disease prevention include preventive and postexposure vaccinations, dental hygiene services, disease screening, and education and counseling relating to physical, mental, and emotional health risks. Examples of health promotion include education about and support for proper diet and nutrition, physical exercise, tobacco and vaping cessation, and use of mental health and substance abuse services.

## Smoking, Vaping, or Chewing Nicotine

If you don't already use tobacco or vape, don't start. Use of tobacco products produces many of the most horrible cardiovascular and lung disasters that you will confront during your career. Use of smokeless tobacco (dry or moist snuff) is associated with cancers of the throat, mouth, and pancreas. Vaping has been shown to produce significant negative effects on the cardiovascular and respiratory systems. It has been cited as the cause of death for dozens of users, from a condition termed e-cigarette, or vaping product, use-associated lung injury.

When trying to quit using products containing nicotine, several strategies may help, including the following:

- Create a plan that addresses the challenges that may trigger you to smoke, chew, or vape.
- Set a quit date, preferably within 2 weeks of setting your plan.
- Tell friends, family, and coworkers your plan to quit.
- Remove tobacco and vaping products from your home, car, and work, and, where possible, avoid places where they may be present.
- Talk to your doctor about other resources that may be available to help you quit.

## Alcohol Abuse

Acceptable alcohol consumption is described to be one drink per day for women and two drinks per day for men. Definitions of excessive drinking are shown in **TABLE 2-3**. In most cases, people who drink excessively are not necessarily alcoholics or have a diagnosis of alcohol substance use disorder; however, they may still experience adverse effects.

According to the **Centers for Disease Control and Prevention (CDC)**, excessive alcohol use causes approximately 88,000 deaths per year in

**TABLE 2-3** Definitions of Excessive Drinking

| | Binge Drinking | Heavy Drinking |
|---|---|---|
| Men | 5 or more drinks during a single occasion | 15 or more drinks per week |
| Women | 4 or more drinks during a single occasion | 8 or more drinks per week |

Data From: National Center for Chronic Disease Prevention and Health Promotion, Division of Population Health. Alcohol use and your health. Centers for Disease Control and Prevention website. http://www.cdc.gov/alcohol/pdfs/alcoholyourhealth.pdf. Accessed March 5, 2020.

the United States with an economic cost of more than $200 billion per year. Approximately 75% of the total cost of alcohol abuse is attributed to binge drinking.

Some studies have touted the health benefits related to moderate consumption of alcohol, such as improved heart health from drinking red wine. The CDC notes that no one should start drinking or drink more frequently based on potential reported health benefits. Although these benefits may exist, increased alcohol use may adversely affect other body systems, including the cardiovascular, hepatic, immune, and central nervous systems. Excessive alcohol use may also increase the risk of the development of various cancers, including those of the mouth, throat, breast, esophagus, and liver.

## Drug Use

Both prescription medications and illegal, or illicit, drugs may be abused or misused. Both are potentially dangerous and may lead to numerous additional health problems. According to the CDC, drug abuse costs the United States more than $190 billion annually in lost work productivity, health care, and crime.

Illicit drug use is both illegal and unhealthy, typically resulting in a snowball effect of bad outcomes. Many EMS agencies drug test their employees. Those who test positive for illegal drugs, or even for prescription drugs when a bona fide medical use cannot be verified by a physician, face suspension and/or dismissal. Therefore, avoid all illegal drugs; take only those drugs prescribed for you personally by a physician, and take them only as directed. In certain cases, even a drug prescribed by a physician should not be taken if the EMT plans to work. The benefits of the drug versus the chance that its effects could impair the performance and safety of the EMT, the crew, the patient, and the public must always be considered. If any type of restricted scheduled or narcotic drug is prescribed (usually while you are off duty), be sure to notify your employer of the situation.

## Balancing Work, Family, and Health

As an EMT, you will often be called to assist the sick and injured at any time of the day or night. Unfortunately, there is no way to predict the timing of illness, injury, or interfacility transfer. Volunteer EMTs may often be called away from family or friends during social activities. Shift workers may be required to be apart from loved ones for long periods of time. You should never let the job interfere excessively with your own needs. Find a balance between work and family; you owe it to yourself and to your family. It is important to make sure you have the time that you need to relax with family and friends.

It is also important to realize that coworkers, family, and friends often may not understand the stress caused by responding to EMS calls. As a result of a "bad call," you might not feel like going out to a movie or attending a planned family event. In these situations, help from a formal peer support group or critical incident stress management team, or information sessions conducted by your EMS unit's employee assistance program may assist you in resolving these issues.

When possible, rotate your schedule to give yourself time off. If your EMS system allows you to move from station to station, rotate to reduce or vary your call volume. Take vacations to lower stress and improve your physical health so you will be able to better respond the next time you are needed. If at any point you feel the stress of work is more than you can handle, seek help. You may want to discuss your stress informally with your family or coworkers. Help from more experienced team members can be invaluable. You may also want to get help from peer counselors or other professionals. Seeking help does not make you weak in the eyes of others. Rather, it shows that you are in control of your life.

## Infectious and Communicable Diseases

As an EMT, you will be called on to treat and transport patients with a variety of infectious or communicable diseases. An **infectious disease** is a medical condition caused by the growth and spread of harmful organisms within the body. A **communicable disease** is a disease that can be spread from one person or species to another. Immunizations, simple handwashing, and other protective techniques can dramatically reduce the health care provider's risk of **infection**.

Familiarize yourself with the following terminology related to infectious diseases. A **pathogen** is a microorganism that is capable of causing disease in a susceptible host. **Contamination** is the presence of pathogens or foreign bodies on or in objects such as dressings, water, food, needles, wounds, or a patient's body. **Exposure** is a situation in which a person has had contact with blood, body fluids, tissues, or airborne particles in a manner that may allow disease transmission to occur. **Personal protective equipment (PPE)** is protective equipment that an individual wears to prevent exposure to a pathogen or other hazardous condition.

### Words of Wisdom

All communicable diseases are infectious, but not all infectious diseases are easily communicable. For example, *Salmonella* is an infectious bacterium that causes food poisoning, but the infection is not communicable to others. Hepatitis B is an infectious disease that is communicable to others. Airborne- or droplet-spread infectious diseases such as COVID-19 are particularly dangerous because they are easily spread to others.

## Routes of Transmission

Whereas all infections result from an abnormal invasion of body spaces and tissues by germs, different germs use different means of attack, or mechanisms of transmission. **Transmission** is the way an infectious disease is spread. There are several ways infectious diseases can be transmitted: contact (direct or indirect), aerosolized (in droplets), foodborne, and vector-borne (transmitted through insects or parasitic worms).

Contact transmission is the movement of an organism from one person to another through physical touch. There are two types of contact transmission: direct and indirect.

**Direct contact** occurs when an organism is moved from one person to another through touching without any intermediary.

The scenario of a vehicle crash can help you understand how transmission occurs through direct contact. The driver of the vehicle has **hepatitis** B and is bleeding uncontrollably from an arm injury. The EMT caring for the patient will need to make contact with the blood to control the patient's bleeding. The EMT has a small unnoticed cut on her own arm and accidentally makes direct contact between the patient's bleeding arm and her own cut arm. As she touches the patient, the hepatitis B virus moves from the victim's blood into the EMT's body through the cut on her arm, thus infecting her (**FIGURE 2-5**). This is an example of direct contact, where blood is the vehicle. **Bloodborne pathogens** are microorganisms that are present in human blood and can cause disease in humans. Another example of direct contact is sexual transmission. Patients who are infected with the **human immunodeficiency virus (HIV)** can transfer the virus to their partners during sexual intercourse.

**Indirect contact** involves the spread of infection from the patient with an infection to another person through an inanimate object. The object

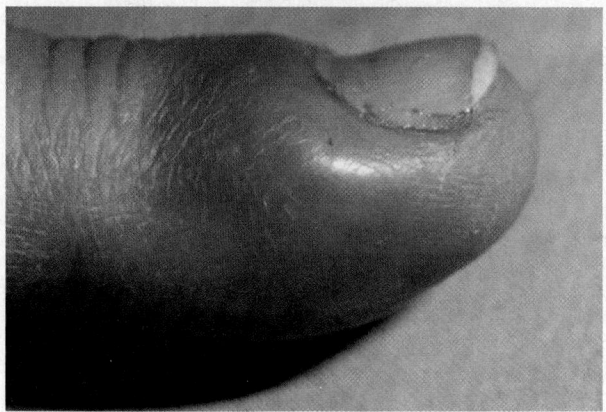

**FIGURE 2-5** Finger infection resulting from not wearing gloves during contact with a patient.
© DermQuest.com. Used with permission of Galderma S.A.

> ### Words of Wisdom
>
> Fungi are small, plantlike organisms such as yeast. Fungi cause many common conditions such as athlete's foot and jock itch. Protozoa are single-cell, animal-like microorganisms. Protozoa cause malaria. Helminths are worms such as roundworms, pinworms, and hookworms. These worms are parasites that can infect people and cause serious health problems.

that transmits the infection is called a *fomite*. Using the same patient from the previous example, as the EMT was caring for the patient, some blood got onto the ambulance stretcher. If the stretcher is not properly cleaned afterward, the virus remains on the stretcher and can be transmitted to someone else days later.

Needlesticks are another example of how infection spreads through indirect contact. In this case, the virus moves from the patient to the needle to the health care provider. This route of transmission was more common many years ago before the advent of safety equipment such as needleless intravenous systems.

**Airborne transmission** involves spreading an infectious agent through mechanisms such as droplets or dust. The common cold is caused by a type of virus called coronavirus that moves from person to person by coughing and sneezing. Interestingly, when a person sneezes, the moisture from the airway moves forcefully and quickly through a narrow opening. If the moisture droplets are large, they travel short distances and can be involved in direct contact transmission. If the moisture droplets are tiny, they are turned into an airborne particle and can float in the air for long distances. Sneezing can actually transmit disease through direct contact *and* airborne routes (**FIGURE 2-6**). When the virus lands on a surface, it can survive for some period of time. If someone touches the surface and then touches his or her face or mouth, infection can also occur via indirect contact. A type of coronavirus known as SARS-CoV-2 is responsible for the disease known as COVID-19. Its transmission is via the same routes as the coronavirus that causes the common cold.

Because of airborne transmission, it is unsanitary to use your hands to cover a cough or sneeze

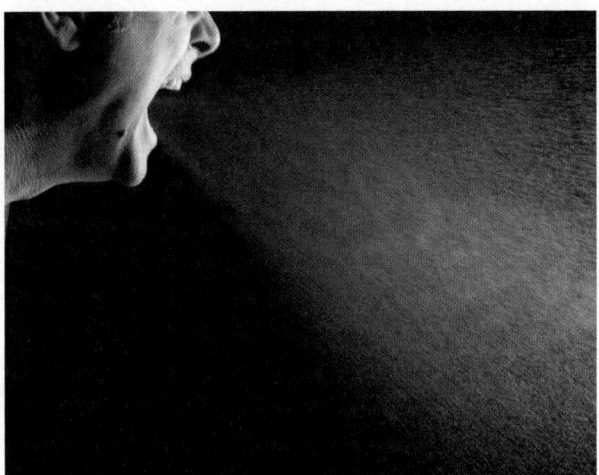

**FIGURE 2-6** Coughing and sneezing create droplets and aerosols.

© James Klotz/ShutterStock.

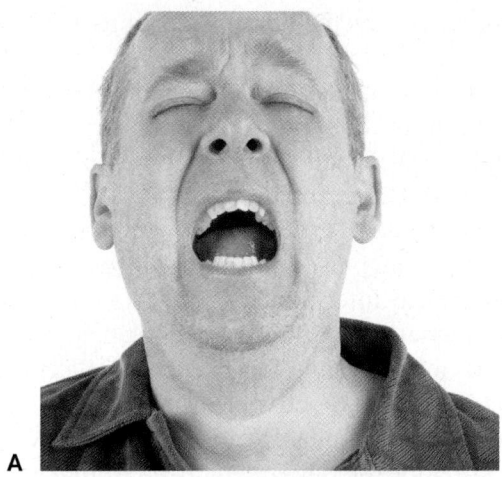

A

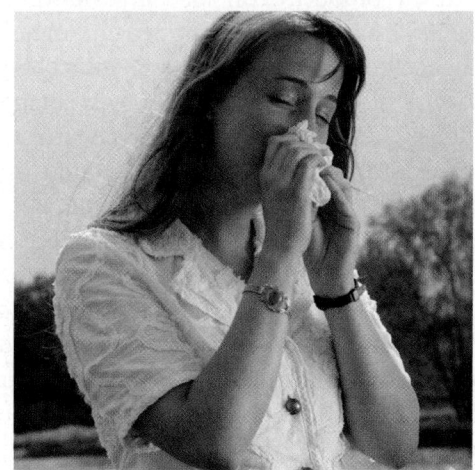

B

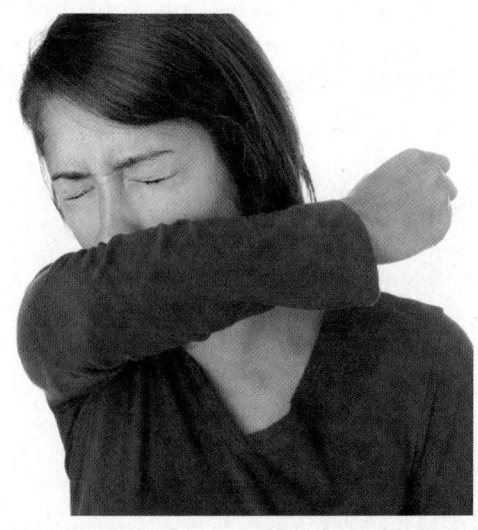

C

**FIGURE 2-7** Coughing and sneezing techniques. **A.** Poor coughing and sneezing technique allows for spread of germs. **B.** Acceptable coughing and sneezing technique limits the spread of germs somewhat. **C.** Best coughing and sneezing technique minimizes the extent to which germs can spread.

**A:** © Denis Pepin/ShutterStock; **B:** © Zsolt Biczó/Dreamstime.com; **C:** © Sebarnes/Dreamstime.com.

because the organisms travel onto your hands. If you then touch a cellphone, doorknob, or a patient, the organisms will travel. Using a tissue when coughing or sneezing is better for controlling the spread of organisms, but you then have a piece of paper full of organisms. One of the best techniques to avoid contaminating your hands is to cough or sneeze into your arm. Because you do not touch objects with your inner arms, the risk of moving organisms to an object or person is reduced (**FIGURE 2-7**). The organisms are trapped in the fabric and will eventually die.

**Foodborne transmission** involves the contamination of food or water with an organism that can cause disease. When food is prepared, it is important to ensure raw meats do not come into contact with other foods to prevent the spread of bacteria. It is also important that food is prepared and stored properly at all times to minimize the possibility of illness. Proper cleaning of food preparation surfaces before and after use also helps to decrease the likelihood of transmitting foodborne bacteria.

**Vector-borne transmission** involves the spread of infection by animals or insects that carry an organism from one person or place to another. The Black Death in Europe and Asia in the Middle Ages killed more than 25 million people. This bacterial disease was caused by infected fleas that live on rats. As the rats moved, so did their fleas, carrying the bubonic plague. Other vector-borne diseases include rabies and Lyme disease.

## Risk Reduction and Prevention for Infectious and Communicable Diseases

### Standard Precautions

The **Occupational Safety and Health Administration (OSHA)** develops and publishes guidelines concerning reducing hazards in the workplace. It is also responsible for enforcing these guidelines. OSHA requires all EMTs to be trained in handling bloodborne pathogens and in approaching a patient who may have an infectious or communicable disease. Training must be provided for issues including blood and body fluid precautions, airborne precautions, and contamination precautions.

Because health care workers are exposed to so many different types of infections, the CDC developed a set of **standard precautions** for health care workers to use in treating patients. Standard precautions are protective measures designed to prevent health care workers from coming into contact with objects, blood, body fluids, and other potential risks that could lead to exposure to germs. The CDC recommendation from 2016 is to assume that every person is potentially infected or can spread an organism that could be transmitted in the health care setting; therefore, you must apply **infection control** procedures—procedures to reduce infection in patients and health care personnel. OSHA refers to the same concept using the term *universal precautions*. **TABLE 2-4** summarizes the CDC recommendations. You must also notify your **designated officer** if you are exposed.

---

### Words of Wisdom

In some cases when standard N95 masks are not available or long periods of care for a highly infectious patient are needed, a powered air-purifying respirator (PAPR) may be used. A PAPR provides positive airflow into a loose-fitting hood or tight-fitting facepiece through a filter or cartridge powered by a battery. Although these devices are often more comfortable to work in than the standard goggles and masks, they are expensive, take considerable room to store, and require special training. PAPRs may also limit the EMT's ability to have a full field of vision and to hear using a stethoscope. Because of these facts, the PAPR is typically only deployed to special response teams in EMS systems rather than being readily available on every ambulance.

---

### Donning and Doffing Full PPE

Putting on (donning) and taking off (doffing) the full complement of PPE in a consistent sequence is essential to reduce the risk of contamination. Although there are some variations, and additional PPE used in certain situations, the most common components of PPE are a mask, eyewear or full face shield, gloves, and gown. To ensure proper donning and doffing, the EMT should have a partner observe and assist with the process. Always don the PPE in the same order based on your departmental policies. Regardless of the process used to doff PPE, the mask is the last PPE to be removed.

#### Donning PPE

Apply the gown and secure the ties at the neck and waist. Then put on the N95 mask and assure there is a tight seal. Don appropriate wraparound eyewear, googles or full face shield next, to protect your eyes. Gloves are donned last. Be sure to pull the cuffs up and over the sleeves of your gown.

#### Doffing PPE

Remove PPE carefully to assure you do not contaminate yourself. Take off the gloves as described previously and discard. Remove eye protection from the back, tilting it forward to remove and then decontaminate it later. Next, remove the gown by reaching around and untying it or breaking the ties. Then pull your arms out while pulling the gown inside out, being careful not to touch the contaminated side of the gown. Discard the gown and then clean your hands with an alcohol-based hand sanitizer. To remove the mask, reach around the back and pull the bottom strap over your head and then remove the top strap to pull the mask away from your face and then discard it. Clean your hands again thoroughly.

### Proper Hand Hygiene

Proper handwashing is the simplest yet most effective way to control disease transmission (**FIGURE 2-8**). You should always wash your hands before and after contact with a patient, even if you wear gloves. The longer the germs remain with you, the greater the chance they will get through your barriers. Any breaks in the skin such as tiny cuts and abrasions are potential access points for pathogens. Although soap and water are not protective

**TABLE 2-4** Standard Precautions for the Care of All Patients, Including Those With Confirmed or Suspected COVID-19, in All Health Care Settings—Centers for Disease Control and Prevention

| Component | Recommendations |
|---|---|
| Hand hygiene | • After touching blood, body fluids, secretions, excretions, or contaminated items<br>• Immediately after removing gloves<br>• Between patient contacts<br>For patients with confirmed or suspected COVID-19 or other highly communicable diseases, perform hand hygiene using an alcohol-based hand rub before putting on gloves. |
| **Personal Protective Equipment (PPE)** | |
| Gloves | • For touching blood, body fluids, secretions, excretions, or contaminated items<br>• For touching mucous membranes and nonintact skin<br>For patients with confirmed or suspected COVID-19 or other highly communicable diseases, a pair of clean, nonsterile gloves is required for all patient contact. |
| Gown | • During procedures and patient care activities when contact of the EMT's clothing/exposed skin to blood, body fluids, secretions, excretions, or contaminated items is anticipated.<br>For patients with confirmed or suspected COVID-19 or other highly communicable diseases, a gown is required for all patient contact. |
| Mask, eye protection, face shield | • During procedures and patient care activities likely to generate splashes or sprays of blood, body fluids, secretions, or excretions. Examples include suctioning or endotracheal intubation<br>For patients with confirmed or suspected COVID-19 or other highly communicable respiratory diseases, N95 or higher respirators, or powered air-purifying respirators (PAPRs), are preferred but N95 facemasks, are an acceptable alternative if respirators are not available. A face shield or goggles are required. |
| **Patient Care Environment** | |
| Soiled patient care equipment | • Wear gloves<br>• Handle in a manner that prevents transfer of microorganisms to others and to the environment<br>• Practice hand hygiene |
| Environmental controls | • Have procedures for the routine care, cleaning, and disinfection of environmental surfaces<br>• Pay special attention to frequently touched surfaces within the ambulance (handrails, seats, cabinets, doors) |
| Textiles and laundry | • Handle in a manner that prevents transfer of microorganisms to others and to the environment |
| Needles and other sharp objects | • Do not recap, bend, break, or hand-manipulate used needles<br>• Use safety features when available (needleless intravenous systems)<br>• Place sharps in puncture-resistant containers |
| **Special Circumstances** | |
| Patient resuscitation | • Use a resuscitation bag or other ventilation devices to prevent contact with mouth and oral secretions |
| Respiratory hygiene/ cough etiquette | • Instruct symptomatic patients to cover mouth/nose when sneezing or coughing<br>• Place surgical mask on patient<br>• If mask cannot be used, maintain special separation (> 6 feet, 2 meters [> 1 m]) if possible |

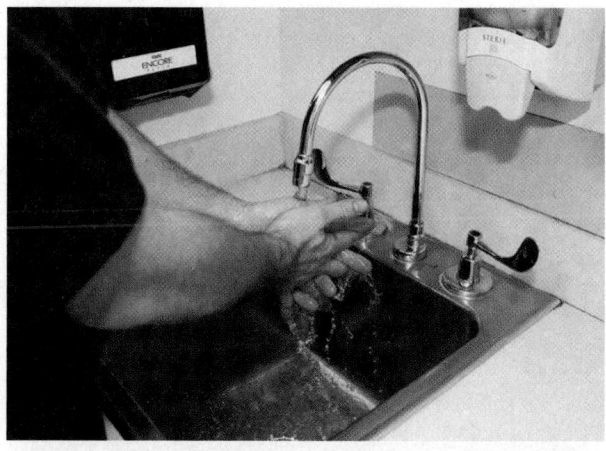

**FIGURE 2-8** When washing your hands, rub your hands together for at least 20 seconds to work up a lather. Pay particular attention to your fingernails, the areas between fingers, and the back of the hands.

© Jones & Bartlett Learning. Courtesy of MIEMSS.

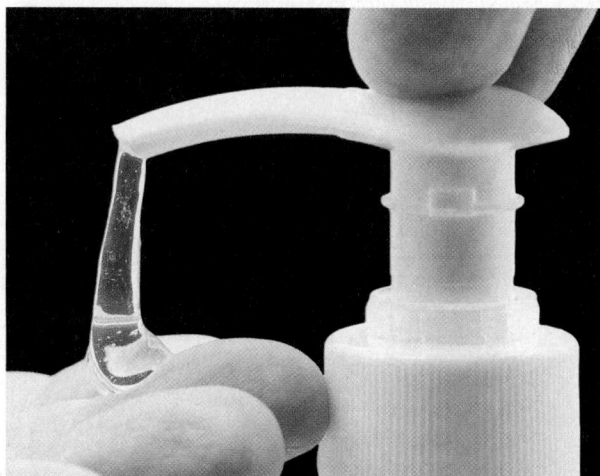

**FIGURE 2-9** Use a waterless handwashing solution if running water is not available. Be sure to wash your hands with soap and water once you arrive at the hospital.

© Svanblar/ShutterStock.

in all cases, in certain cases they provide excellent protection against further transmission from your skin to others.

Rinse your hands using warm water. If running water is not available, you may use waterless handwashing substitutes (**FIGURE 2-9**). These solutions can prevent many potential bacterial infections. If you use a waterless substitute in the field, make sure you wash your hands using soap and water at the hospital. Finally, dry your hands with a paper towel, and use the paper towel to turn off the faucet.

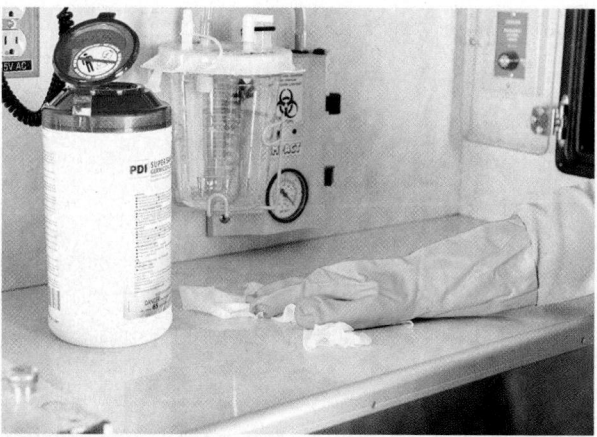

**FIGURE 2-10** Use heavy-duty utility gloves to clean the unit. You should not use lightweight latex or vinyl gloves for cleaning.

© Jones & Bartlett Learning.

## Gloves

Gloves and eye protection are the minimum standard for all patient care if there is any possibility of exposure to blood or body fluids. Vinyl, nitrile, and latex gloves provide adequate protection. Your department may prefer one type of glove over the other, or you may have the freedom to choose for yourself. You should evaluate each situation and choose the glove that works best. (Some patients and EMTs are allergic to latex. If you suspect you are allergic, consult your supervisor for options.) Vinyl gloves may be best for situations with minimal patient contact or nonsterile procedures, and nitrile or latex gloves may be best for invasive procedures where sterility is required. Change gloves if they have been exposed to motor oil, gasoline, or any petroleum-based product. Do not use petroleum jelly with latex gloves. Wear double gloves if there is substantial bleeding. You may also wear double gloves if you will be exposed to large volumes of other body fluids. Be sure to change gloves as you move from patient to patient. For cleaning and disinfecting the ambulance, you should use heavy-duty utility gloves (**FIGURE 2-10**). You should never use lightweight latex or vinyl gloves for cleaning.

Removing used latex or nitryl gloves requires following a methodical technique to avoid contaminating yourself with the materials on the outside of the gloves (**SKILL DRILL 2-1**).

1.  Begin by partially removing one glove. With your other gloved hand, pinch the first glove at

## Skill Drill 2-1 Proper Glove Removal Technique

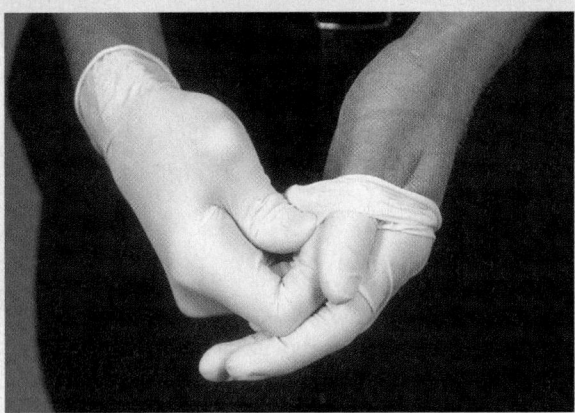

### Step 1

Partially remove the first glove by pinching at the wrist. Be careful to touch only the outside of the glove.

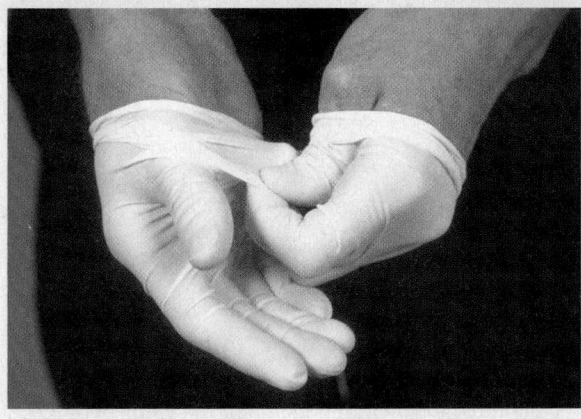

### Step 2

Remove the second glove by pinching the exterior with your partially gloved hand.

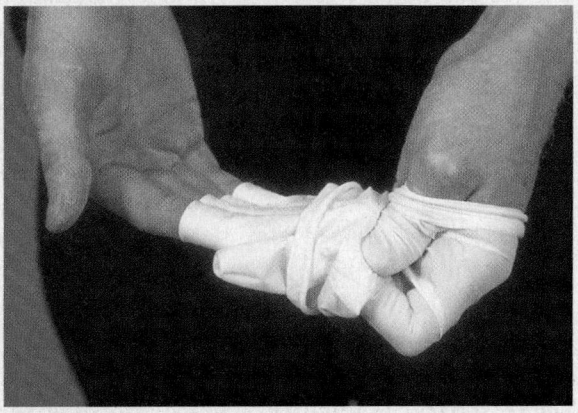

### Step 3

Pull the second glove inside out toward the fingertips.

© Jones & Bartlett Learning.

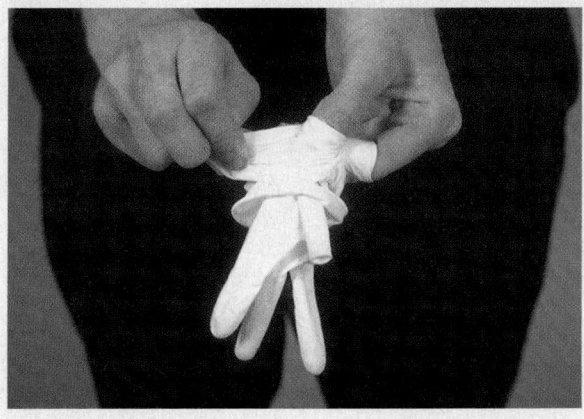

### Step 4

Grasp both gloves with your free hand, touching only the clean, interior surfaces.

the wrist—being certain to touch only the outside of the first glove—and start to roll it back off your hand, inside out. Leave the exterior of the fingers on that first glove exposed (**Step 1**).

2. Use the gloved fingers to pinch the wrist of the second glove and begin to pull it off, rolling it inside out toward the fingertips as you did with the first glove (**Step 2**).

3. Continue pulling off the second glove until you can pull the second hand free (**Step 3**).

4. With your now-ungloved second hand, grasp the exposed inside of the first glove and pull it free of your first hand and over the now-loose second glove. Be sure that you touch only clean, interior surfaces with your ungloved hand (**Step 4**).

Gloves are the most common type of PPE. In many EMS rescue operations, you must also protect your hands and wrists from injury. You may wear puncture-proof leather gloves, with latex gloves underneath. This combination will allow you free use of your hands with added protection from blood and body fluids. Remember that soiled latex or nitryl gloves are considered medical waste and must be properly disposed. Leather gloves must be treated as contaminated material until they can be properly decontaminated.

## Eye Protection and Face Shields

Eye protection is important in case blood or airborne droplets toward your eyes (**FIGURE 2-11**). Blood splatters are a significant possibility in most trauma situations, and airborne droplets can cause disease transmission in many viral infections such as COVID-19. Wearing goggles or a full face shield is your best protection. Providers who wear prescription eyeglasses will also need additional protection for their eyes. Prescription eyeglasses offer little side protection and are not considered appropriate for PPE. Contact lenses do not offer any added protection from splashing. Face shields will also provide good eye protection (**FIGURE 2-12**).

## Gowns

Occasionally, you may need to wear a gown. A gown provides protection from extensive blood or other body fluids splatter. Gowns may be worn in situations such as aerosol-generating procedures such as endotracheal intubation, field delivery of a baby, or major trauma. Your department will likely have a policy regarding gowns. Be sure you know your local policy. There are times when a change of uniform is preferred because trying to clean off contaminants is difficult and sometimes impossible without professional cleaning and disinfection or disposing of the uniform entirely.

## Masks, Respirators, and Barrier Devices

Wearing masks is a complex issue. You should wear a standard surgical mask if blood or body fluid spatter is a possibility. If you suspect a patient has an airborne- or droplet-spread disease such as tuberculosis or influenza, or in situations such as the COVID-19 pandemic, place a surgical mask on the patient and a particulate air respirator, such as an N95 mask, on yourself (**FIGURE 2-13**). Protective eyewear using safety glasses with side shields, goggles, or a full face shield is also needed. If the patient needs oxygen, place a nonrebreathing mask instead of a surgical mask on the patient and set the oxygen flow rate at 10 to 15 L/min. Do not place a particulate respirator on the patient; it is unnecessary and uncomfortable. A simple surgical mask will reduce the risk of transmission of germs from the patient into the air. Use of a particulate respirator should

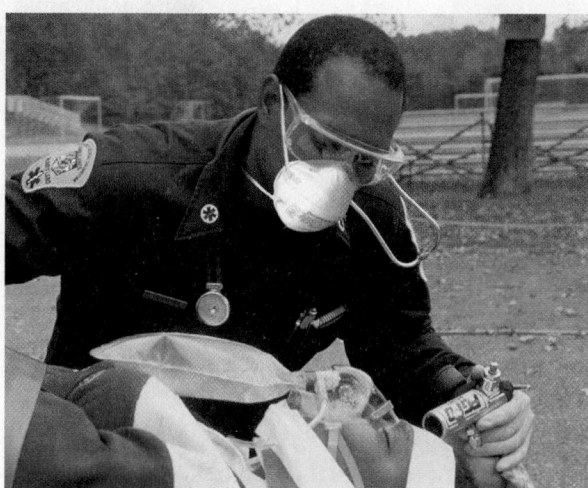

**FIGURE 2-11** Wear eye protection with side shields to prevent blood splatter or airborne droplets from getting into your eyes.
© Jones & Bartlett Learning. Courtesy of MIEMSS.

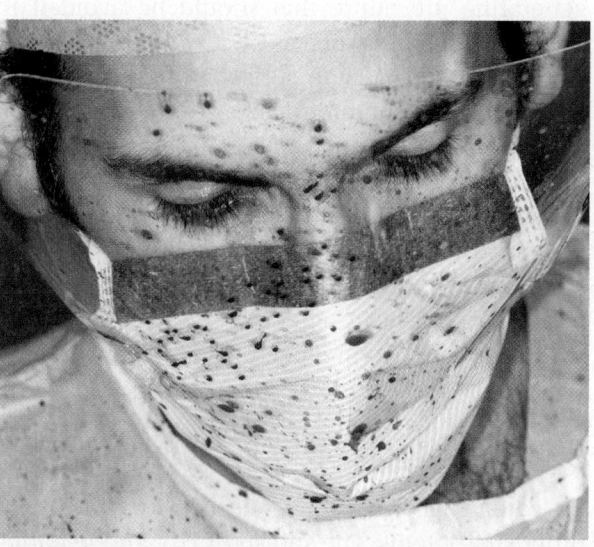

**FIGURE 2-12** The surgical mask/face shield combination.
© Dr. P. Marazzi/Science Source.

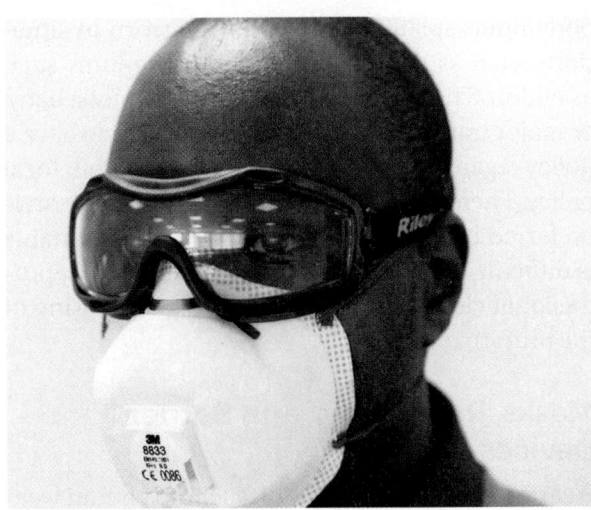

**FIGURE 2-13** Wear a particulate respirator to protect yourself from airborne disease transmission.

© European Centre for Disease Prevention and Control (ECDC) 2020.

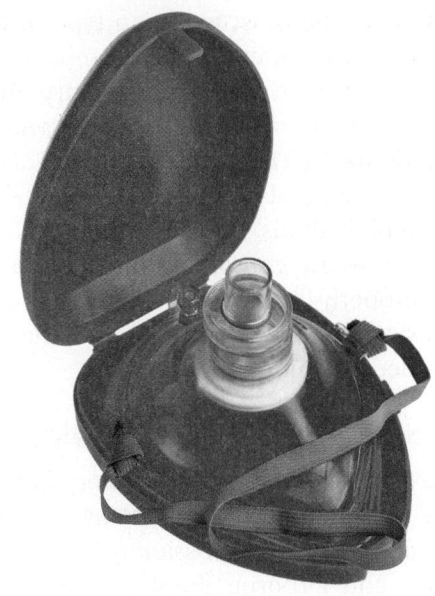

**FIGURE 2-14** Barrier devices such as a pocket mask provide protection when providing mouth-to-mask ventilation. These devices should not be used, however, if there is active community spread of virus by airborne route.

© Bart J/ShutterStock.

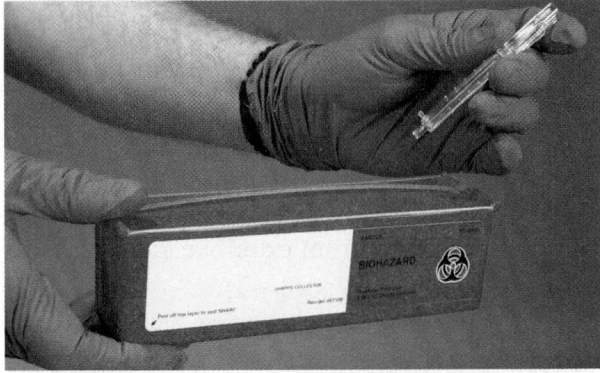

**FIGURE 2-15** Properly dispose of sharps in a closed, rigid, marked container.

© Jones and Bartlett Publishers. Courtesy of MIEMSS.

comply with OSHA standards, which state facial hair, such as long sideburns or a mustache, will prevent a proper fit. Particulate respirators must be fit-tested to ensure their efficacy.

Although there are no documented cases of disease transmission to rescuers as a result of performing unprotected mouth-to-mouth resuscitation on a patient with an infection, you should use a pocket mask (**FIGURE 2-14**). Neither mouth-to-mouth nor mouth-to-mask resuscitation are recommended in a situation where there is an active community spread of a virus that can be transmitted by airborne route. Bag-mask ventilation is an aerosol-generating procedure that should be avoided in epidemic scenarios such as COVID-19.

Remember, outside surfaces of these devices are considered contaminated after they have been exposed to the patient. You must make sure gloves, masks, gowns, and all other PPE items that have been exposed to infectious processes or blood are properly disposed of according to local guidelines. If you are stuck by a needle, get blood or body fluids in your eye, or have significant body fluid contact with the patient, immediately report the incident to your supervisor.

## Proper Disposal of Sharps

Be careful when handling needles, scalpels, and other sharp items. The spread of HIV and hepatitis in the health care setting can usually be traced back to careless handling of sharps.

- Do not recap, break, or bend needles. Even the most careful providers may expose themselves through an accidental needlestick.
- Dispose of all sharp items that have been in contact with human secretions in approved, closed, rigid containers (**FIGURE 2-15**).

## Employer Responsibilities

Your employer cannot guarantee a 100% risk-free environment. The risk of being exposed to a communicable disease is a hazard of your job. You have a right to know about diseases that may pose a risk to you. Remember, though, your risk for infection is not high; however, OSHA regulations, especially for private and federal agencies, require that all employees be offered a workplace environment that reduces the risk for exposure. Note that in some states that have their own OSHA plans, state and municipal employees must also be covered.

In addition to OSHA guidelines, other national guidelines and standards, including those from the CDC and National Fire Protection Agency Infection Control Standard 1581, address reducing the risk of exposure to bloodborne pathogens (disease-causing organisms) and airborne diseases. These agencies set a standard of care for all fire and EMS personnel and apply whether you are a full-time paid employee or a volunteer. It is your responsibility to know your department's infection control plan and to use it (**TABLE 2-5**).

**TABLE 2-5** Components of an Infection Control Plan

**Determination of Exposure Risk**

- Determines who is at risk for ongoing contact with blood and other body fluids
- Creates a list of tasks that pose a risk for contact with blood or other body fluids
- Includes PPE required by OSHA

**Education and Training**

- Explains why a qualified individual is required to answer questions about communicable diseases and infection control, rather than relying on packaged training materials
- Allows for an instructor able to train EMTs regarding bloodborne and airborne pathogens, such as hepatitis B and C, HIV, syphilis, and tuberculosis
- Ensures the instructor provides appropriate education, which is the best means for dispelling many myths surrounding these issues

**Personal Protective Equipment**

- Lists the PPE offered and why it was selected
- Lists how much equipment is available and where to obtain additional PPE
- States when each type of PPE is to be used for each risk procedure

**Cleaning and Disinfection Practices**

- Describes how to care for and maintain vehicles and equipment
- Identifies where and when cleaning should be performed, how it is to be done, what PPE to use, and what cleaning solution to use
- Addresses medical waste collection, storage, and disposal

**Tuberculin Skin Testing/Fit Testing**

- Addresses how often employees should undergo skin testing
- Addresses how often fit testing should be done to determine the proper-size mask to protect the EMT from airborne disease transmission
- Addresses all issues dealing with particulate respirator masks

**Hepatitis B Vaccine Program**

- Describes the vaccine offered, its safety and efficacy, record keeping, and tracking
- Addresses the need for postvaccine antibody titers to identify patients who do not respond to the initial three-dose vaccination series

**Postexposure Management**

Identifies who to notify when an exposure occurs, forms to be filled out, where to go for treatment

*(continues)*

**TABLE 2-5** Components of an Infection Control Plan (*continued*)

**Compliance Monitoring**

- Addresses how the service or department evaluates employee compliance with each aspect of the plan
- Ensures employees understand what they are to do and why it is important
- States that noncompliance should be documented
- Indicates what disciplinary action to take in the face of continued noncompliance

**Communication of Hazards to Employees and Training**

Ensures all employees (including volunteers) who have risk of occupational exposure to bloodborne pathogens receive initial and annual training by a designated person that includes the following elements:

- A copy and explanation of the OSHA bloodborne pathogen standard
- An explanation of the individual service's exposure control plan and how to obtain a copy
- An explanation of methods to recognize tasks and other activities that may involve exposure to blood and OPIM, including what constitutes an exposure incident
- An explanation of the use and limitations of engineering controls, work practices, and PPE
- An explanation of the types, uses, location, removal, handling, decontamination, and disposal of PPE
- An explanation of the basis for PPE selection
- Information on the hepatitis B vaccine, including information on its efficacy, safety, and method of administration; description of the benefits of being vaccinated; and assurance that the vaccine will be offered free of charge
- Information on the appropriate actions to take and persons to contact in an emergency involving blood or OPIM
- An explanation of the procedure to follow if an exposure incident occurs, including the method of reporting the incident and the medical follow-up that will be made available
- Information on the postexposure evaluation and follow-up that the employer is required to provide for the employee following an exposure incident
- An explanation of the signs and labels and/or color coding required by the standard and used at this facility
- An opportunity for interactive questions and answers with the person conducting the training session

**Record Keeping**

Lists all records to keep, how confidentiality will be maintained, and how, when, and by whom records can be accessed, including the following:

- Dates of training sessions
- Summary of the contents of the training sessions
- Names and qualifications of those conducting training
- Names and job titles of those attending training
- Occupational exposure records
- OSHA records of all exposures
- Sharps injury logs

Abbreviations: HIV, human immunodeficiency virus; OPIM, other potentially infectious material; OSHA, Occupational Safety and Health Administration; PPE, personal protective equipment.

© Jones & Bartlett Learning.

## Establishing an Infection Control Routine

Infection control should be an important part of your daily routine. Follow the steps in **SKILL DRILL 2-2** to manage potential exposure situations:

1. En route to the scene, make sure that PPE is out and available (**Step 1**).

2. On arrival, identify and address safety hazards, then perform a rapid scan of the patient, noting whether any blood or body fluids are present.

3. Select the proper PPE according to the tasks you are likely to perform. Typically, gloves and protective eyewear will be used for all patient contacts (**Step 2**). A disposable gown, and

## Skill Drill 2-2 Managing a Potential Exposure

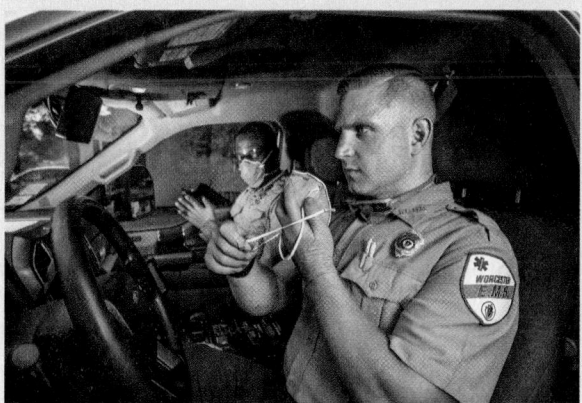

### Step 1

En route to the scene, make sure that PPE is out and available.

© Jones & Bartlett Learning.

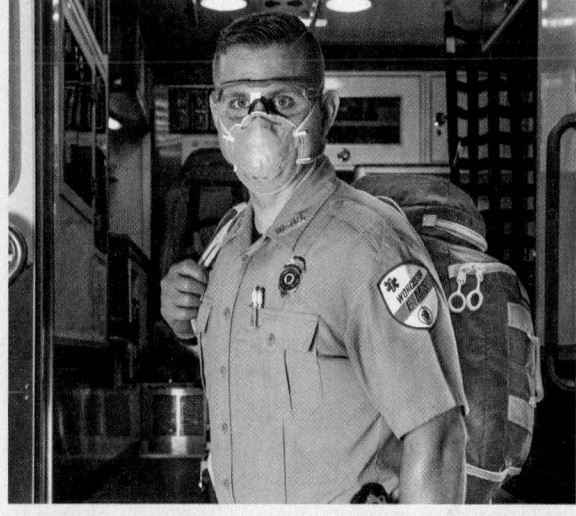

### Step 2

On arrival, identify and address safety hazards, then perform a rapid scan of the patient, noting whether any blood or body fluids are present. Select the proper PPE according to the tasks you are likely to perform. Typically, gloves and protective eyewear will be used for all patient contacts.

masks are often required during epidemic or pandemic situations, and the type of mask will depend on the transmission mode of the relevant pathogen.

4. Change gloves or remove the topmost layer of gloves if wearing multiple layers of gloves.
5. Wash hands or at the very least use hand sanitizer between patients; don PPE as quickly as possible to minimize time spent before initiating care. Remove gloves and other gear after contact with the patient, unless you are in the patient compartment. Remember that good hand hygiene is always necessary.
6. Limit the number of people who are involved in patient care if there are multiple injuries and a substantial amount of blood at the scene.
7. If you or your partner is exposed while providing care, try to relieve one another as soon as possible so that you can seek care, including basic first aid care such as cleaning and

dressing a wound. Notify the designated officer and report the incident. This will also help to maintain confidentiality for both the patient and for you.

### Words of Wisdom

Aerosol-generating procedures (AGPs) are treatments that increase the risk for transmission of infections that are spread through the air or by droplets. During AGP treatments, small particles and droplets from the patient's respiratory tract become airborne. Nearby EMTs or paramedics who are not wearing appropriate PPE can inhale those particles or droplets or get them into their eyes or mouth, exposing themselves to virus or bacteria. When a patient has an infectious respiratory disease or in situations of community spread of communicable diseases, AGPs pose a high risk for caregivers. Examples of AGPs include CPR and some basic and advanced airway procedures.

## Cleaning and Decontaminating the Ambulance and Equipment

Be sure to routinely clean the ambulance after each run and on a daily basis. Cleaning is an essential part of the prevention and control of communicable diseases, ensuring removal of surface organisms that may remain in the unit. You should clean your unit as quickly as possible so it can be returned to service. Address the high-contact areas, including surfaces that were in direct contact with the patient's blood or body fluids or surfaces that you touched while caring for the patient after having contact with the patient's blood or body fluids. More information about decontaminating the ambulance can be found in Chapter 38, *Transport Operations.*

Whenever possible, cleaning should be done at the hospital. If you clean the unit back at the station, make sure you have a designated area with good ventilation. Any medical waste should be placed in a red biohazard bag and disposed of at the hospital whenever possible. Any contaminated equipment that is left with the patient at the hospital should be cleaned by hospital staff or placed in a red bag for transport and cleaning at the station.

You can use a bleach and water solution at a 1:10 dilution to clean the unit. The solution you mix should not have a strong odor of bleach if mixed correctly. A hospital-approved disinfectant that is effective against *Mycobacterium tuberculosis* also can be used. Use the cleaning solution in a bucket or use a pistol-handled spray container. Do not use alcohol or aerosol spray products to clean the unit. Pay attention to disinfectant directions.

Bleach solutions and most disinfectant agents will require air drying to be effective. Do not routinely go back over sprayed surfaces and dry them. Allow the sprayed surfaces to air dry unless otherwise indicated in the product directions.

Remove contaminated linen and place it into an appropriate bag for handling. Each hospital may have a different system for handling contaminated linen; you should learn hospital or department protocols (**FIGURE 2-16**).

Any reusable medical equipment should be properly cleaned and sterilized per your department's standard operating procedures. Keep in mind that in hospitals entire departments are devoted to sterilizing medical instruments. Proper sterilization requires the right tools and the right skills, so always carefully follow your department's procedures.

Learn the regulations defining medical waste in your area. The disposal of infectious waste, such as needles, sharps, and heavily soiled dressings, may vary from hospital to hospital and from state to state.

## YOU are the Provider

You arrive at the scene, enter the residence, and find two EMRs performing CPR on the child, a 4-year-old girl. The child's mother tells you that when she went to wake up her daughter, she was unconscious and not breathing. She called 9-1-1 and started CPR. Your partner quickly assesses the child and asks you to open the jump kit.

| Recording Time:   0 Minutes | |
|---|---|
| **Appearance** | Cyanotic; motionless |
| **Level of consciousness** | Unconscious and unresponsive |
| **Airway** | Small amount of vomitus in her mouth |
| **Breathing** | Absent |
| **Circulation** | Carotid pulse absent; skin cool and cyanotic |

With CPR continuing, your partner prepares the cardiac monitor and asks you to suction the child's mouth and manage her airway. You quickly and effectively accomplish your assigned task, but notice that your hands are shaking somewhat, you are breathing rapidly, and can feel your heart racing.

**2.** What is stress? How does it manifest?

**3.** What phase of the stress response are you experiencing right now?

becomes infected with the hepatitis A virus may be ill for several weeks, but because immunity will develop, the person will not get the illness again; however, sometimes the immunity is only partial. Partial immunity protects against new infections. But pathogens that remain in the body from the first illness still may be able to cause the same disease again when the body is stressed or has some impairment in its immune system. For example, tuberculosis can cause a mild, unnoticeable infection before the body builds up a partial immunity. If the infection is never treated, the infection may be reactivated when immunity is weakened; however, these people are protected against a new infection from another person.

Humans seem unable to mount an effective immune response to some infections, such as HIV, which is an infection with the human immunodeficiency virus that can progress to AIDS.

Although hepatitis A immunization is not required by OSHA, you may want to be vaccinated as a preventive measure. Hepatitis A vaccination is not necessary if you have had hepatitis A in the past. All these vaccines are effective and rarely cause side effects.

Remember, germs that cause no symptoms in one person may cause serious illness in another.

## Immunizations

As an EMT, you are at risk for acquiring an infectious or communicable disease. Using basic protective measures can minimize the risk. You are responsible for protecting yourself, so take an active role in achieving that goal.

Prevention begins by maintaining your personal health. Annual health examinations should be required for all EMS personnel. A history of all your childhood infectious diseases should be recorded and kept on file. Childhood infectious diseases include chickenpox, mumps, measles, rubella, and whooping cough. You must be immunized against these diseases unless you already had the disease or have previously been vaccinated against it.

OSHA has developed requirements for protection from occupational exposure to bloodborne pathogens and needlesticks. Each employer whose employees may reasonably be expected to come in contact with blood or other potentially infectious materials must create an infection control plan

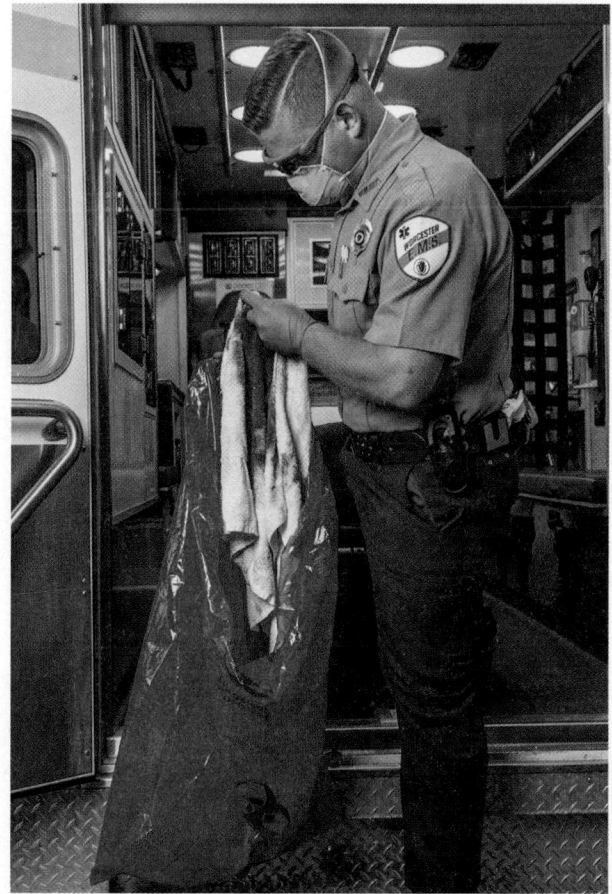

**FIGURE 2-16** Contaminated linen and other wastes should be bagged appropriately and disposed of according to your local protocols.

© Jones & Bartlett Learning.

## Immunity

Even if pathogens do reach you, you are not necessarily at risk for infection. For example, you may be **immune**, or resistant, to those particular germs. Immunity is a major factor in determining whether a **host** (the organism or the individual who is attacked by the infecting agent) will become ill from a particular germ (**TABLE 2-6**). One way to gain immunity from many diseases is to be immunized, or vaccinated, against them. Vaccinations have nearly eliminated some childhood diseases, such as measles and polio.

Another way in which the body becomes immune to a disease is when it recovers from an infection from that germ. Afterward, the body's immune system recognizes and repels that pathogen when it shows up again. After healthy people are exposed, lifelong immunity to many common pathogens will develop. For example, a person who contracts and

**TABLE 2-6** Immunity to Infectious Diseases

| Type of Immunity | Characteristics | Examples | Comments |
|---|---|---|---|
| Lifelong | The illness will not recur. | Measles<br>Mumps<br>Polio<br>Rubella<br>Hepatitis A<br>Hepatitis B | Infection or vaccination provides long-term immunity from getting a new infection. A live vaccine is required only for measles. |
| Partial | The person who has recovered from a first infection is unlikely to get a new infection from another person but illness may develop from germs that lie dormant from the initial infection. | Chickenpox<br>Tuberculosis | Infection provides lifelong immunity to the patient from acquiring a new infection, but the original illness may reoccur, or it may reoccur in a different way. In the case of chickenpox, which is caused by the herpes zoster virus, an infection may reoccur years later in the form of shingles. |
| None | Exposure confers no protection from reinfection. The infection may wear down the patient's resistance. | Gonorrhea<br>Syphilis<br>Human immunodeficiency virus infection | No vaccine is available. Repeated infections are common. For example, there is effective immediate treatment for gonorrhea, and the germs may be eradicated; however, reinfection is likely if the high-risk practices continue (eg, unprotected sex). For syphilis, the lack of immunity allows the germs to continue to cause damage within the host. |
| Other/unknown | Some viruses change from year to year, making it difficult to develop vaccines or innate immunity. | Influenza | Although a vaccine is available for influenza, researchers must predict which strains will be prevalent a year or more in advance. This means that if a new strain occurs, the vaccine will not provide full protection in the community |
| | In other cases virus strains are new, and little is known about them. | COVID-19 | COVID-19 is a new virus, which presents many unknowns. Initially there will be no vaccine. Additionally, it takes time to know if having the disease or getting the vaccine confers temporary or lifelong immunity. |

© Jones & Bartlett Learning.

designed to minimize occupational exposure. As part of these requirements, employers are required to offer the hepatitis B vaccine at no cost to employees with risk of occupational exposure. Employees who decline the vaccine must sign a waiver indicating their refusal to take the vaccine and may later decide to take the vaccine at the employer's expense. Furthermore, the CDC recommends the following immunizations for health care workers:

- Hepatitis B (required by OSHA)
- Influenza (yearly)
- Measles, mumps, and rubella (MMR) (typically one-time vaccination)
- Varicella (chickenpox) vaccine or having had chickenpox
- Tetanus, diphtheria, pertussis (Tdap) (every 10 years)

Most of these vaccinations are given to infants and children as part of their routine series of immunizations. It is imperative that you keep all these vaccinations up to date to help protect you as well as your family and patients. Health care workers who are routinely exposed to meningitis (often those who work in an institutional setting) should receive one dose of meningococcal vaccine.

In December 2020, vaccines for SARS-CoV-2 (COVID-19) were approved for emergency use authorization by the FDA.

You should also have a skin test for tuberculosis before you begin working as an EMT. The purpose of this test is to identify anyone who has been exposed to tuberculosis in the past. Testing should be repeated yearly.

If you know you will be transporting a patient who has a communicable disease, you have a definite advantage. This is when information in your health record will be valuable. If you have already had the disease or been vaccinated, you are not at risk. However, you will not always know whether a patient has a communicable disease. Therefore, you should always follow standard precautions if there is the possibility of exposure to blood or other body fluids.

## General Postexposure Management

The likelihood of you becoming infected during routine patient care is low. In the event that you are exposed to blood or other body substances despite all of your precautions, there are still measures that you can take to protect your health. If you are exposed to a patient's blood or body fluids, you should first turn over patient care to another EMS provider. When it is safe to do so, clean the exposed area with soap and water. If your eyes were exposed, rinse them with water for at least 20 minutes as soon as possible.

Next, activate your department's infection control plan. This usually involves contacting a supervisor or your department's infection control officer to assist you. This person will help you to navigate the postexposure protocols.

You will need to be screened to determine whether there was a significant exposure to possible bloodborne pathogens. Just because you were exposed to a patient's blood or body fluids does not mean that there is a risk of infection. Typically, you will need a follow-up evaluation by a physician to determine whether a significant exposure occurred. If the exposure was significant, blood may be drawn from both you and the patient to determine whether any infectious agents were present.

You will have to complete an exposure report. Questions in the report may include: When did the event happen? What were you doing when you were exposed? What PPE were you wearing? What did you do after you were exposed? Completing this paperwork will help relay critical information to the right people, resulting in help for you and possibly new protocols to help prevent another incident in the future.

Time is important! If you are exposed, let your supervisor or infection control officer know immediately. Some diseases will act quickly, whereas others may lay dormant for a long time. The best way to reduce your risk of contracting a work-related disease is through early activation of your department's infection control plan.

In the case of diseases spread in the air or by droplets, you may not realize you have been exposed to the disease until the hospital notifies you. If you were wearing full PPE including gloves, gown, eye protection, and N95 mask, no further follow-up may be needed. In other cases, specific postexposure care or prophylaxis may be indicated. In the event that you have been exposed to a highly communicable airborne disease such as COVID-19 without proper PPE, you may be required to quarantine for a predetermined period of time (usually 14 days). During that time public health officials may require you to report your temperature and other symptoms daily.

## Postexposure Prophylaxis and Treatment for Significant Exposure

The last defense for an EMT who has a significant exposure to an infectious disease is postexposure preventive measures or treatment. Unfortunately, these are not available for all diseases and are only offered if an investigation determines that you have had a significant exposure. Postexposure treatment for HIV includes treatment with a specific combination of antiviral medications. In the case of hepatitis B exposure, you will be tested to see if you already have antibodies if you have been vaccinated for the disease. If you have antibodies, no treatment is needed. If you do not have antibodies, you will receive an injection with hepatitis B immune globulin, which contains antibodies that will attack the virus in your body. However, this injection only confers temporary protection, so it is followed up with the series of three hepatitis B immunization shots. There is no treatment to prevent you from getting hepatitis C infection after an exposure.

Postexposure treatment for tuberculosis will not begin unless your tuberculin skin test is positive during the monitoring period. In those cases a long period of treatment with oral antituberculin medicines will begin.

There are very few infectious exposures for which you will receive antibiotics. Significant exposure to pertussis and some types of bacterial meningitis would be included.

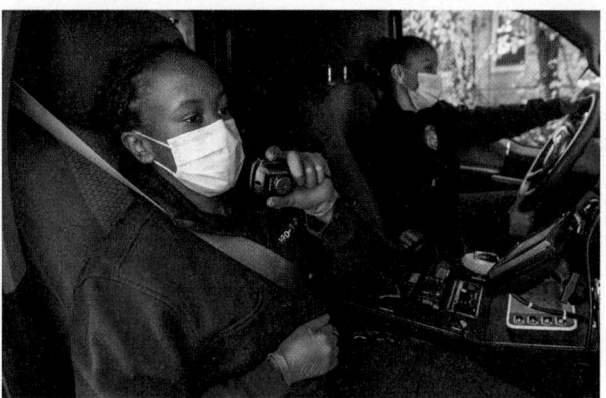

**FIGURE 2-17** Wear seat belts whenever you are riding in the ambulance, including when you are responding on a call.

© Jones & Bartlett Learning.

### Street Smarts

You should be aware of the procedures you are required to follow if you are involved in an exposure during your clinical or field experience. If you don't know, ask your instructor.

## Scene Safety

The personal safety of all those involved in an emergency situation is very important. In fact, it is so important that it is best that you internalize the steps necessary to preserve personal safety so your actions become automatic. A scene that appears safe initially can develop into a hazardous situation at any moment. Take care to notice any suspicious person or activity at the scene, because your first priority must be your own safety. A second accident at the scene or an injury to you or your partner creates more problems. Delays in emergency medical care for patients increase the burden on other EMTs and may result in unnecessary injury or death.

You should begin protecting yourself as soon as you are dispatched. Before you leave the scene, begin preparing yourself mentally and physically. Make sure you wear seat belts (including both the lap belt and shoulder harness) en route to the scene. Also make sure to wear seat belts and shoulder harnesses at all times during transport unless patient care makes it impossible (**FIGURE 2-17**). Many EMS units have mandatory seat belt policies for the driver at all times, for all EMTs during transit to the scene, and for anyone who is riding with a patient. Don the appropriate PPE prior to departing the ambulance.

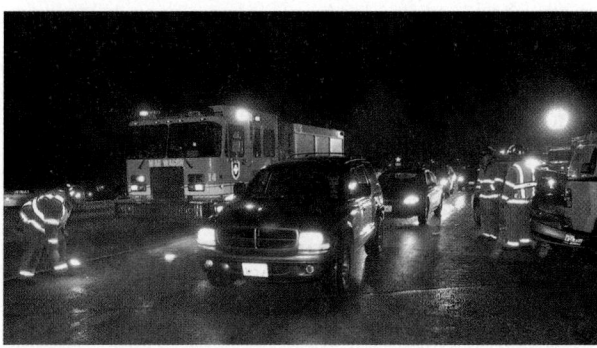

**FIGURE 2-18** Make sure the crash scene is well marked to prevent a second crash that may damage the ambulance or result in injury to you, your partner, or the patient.

© Glen E. Ellman.

### Safety Tips

An important safety measure is to always wear seat belts in the ambulance, including when you are en route to the scene and during transport.

Protecting yourself at the scene is also very important. A second accident may damage the ambulance and may result in injury to you or your partner, or additional injury to the patient. The scene must be well marked (**FIGURE 2-18**). If law enforcement has not already done so, you should make sure the proper warning devices are placed at a sufficient distance from the scene to properly warn, slow, and divert oncoming traffic. This will alert motorists coming from both directions that a

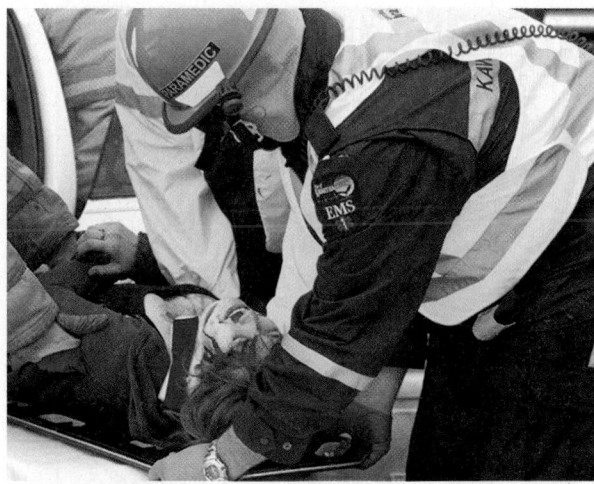

**FIGURE 2-19** The American National Standards Institute (and International Safety Equipment Association) require EMS personnel to wear reflective vests or clothing that meets class 2 or 3 standards on roadways. You can also wear emblems or clothing to help make you more visible at night and improve your safety in the dark.

© Murray Wilson/Fotolia.com.

crash has occurred. When you must work in a traffic lane, park a heavy vehicle such as a fire engine (if available) in a position that blocks traffic in the lane where you are working. Park the ambulance at a safe but convenient distance from the scene. Before attempting to access patients who are trapped in a vehicle, check the vehicle's stability. Then take any necessary measures to secure it. Do not rock or push on a vehicle to find out whether it will move. This can overturn the vehicle or send it crashing into a ditch. If you are uncertain about the safety of a crash scene, wait for appropriately trained personnel to arrive before approaching. It may not be your primary responsibility to ensure safe management of traffic flow, vehicle stabilization, and similar tasks, but it is always your responsibility to see that it has been properly accomplished.

When working at night, you must have plenty of light. Poor lighting increases the risk of injury to both you and the patient. It also results in poor emergency medical care. Wearing a reflective vest or clothing will help to make you more visible at night and decrease your risk of injury (**FIGURE 2-19**).

## Scene Hazards

In the course of your career as an EMT, you will be exposed to many hazards. Some situations will be life threatening. In these cases, you must be properly protected, or you must take steps to avoid the hazard completely.

## Hazardous Materials

Your safety is the most important consideration at a hazardous materials incident. Upon your arrival, you should look at the scene and try to read any labels, placards, and identification numbers from a distance, perhaps using binoculars. Placards are used on transportation vehicles and buildings, and labels are used on individual packages containing hazardous materials. The placards or labels are colored and diamond-shaped (**FIGURE 2-20**). You should never approach any object marked with a placard or label. Remember, some hazardous materials may not be properly marked.

Specially trained and equipped hazardous materials responders will handle disposal of materials and removal of patients. You should not begin caring for patients until they have been moved away from the scene and are decontaminated or the scene is safe for you to enter.

### Safety Tips

All types of things can injure you when you are caring for patients. Your best protection against being injured is to carefully size up the scene and constantly check for potential hazards. Don't be foolish and blindly rush in before conducting a proper assessment.

The US Department of Transportation's *Emergency Response Guidebook* (ERG) is an important resource when dealing with a hazardous materials incident (**FIGURE 2-21**). The ERG lists common hazardous materials and the proper procedures for scene control and the emergency care of patients. Some state and local government agencies may also have information about hazardous materials commonly present in their areas. A paper or electronic copy of the ERG and other information relevant to your area should be available in your unit. Smartphone and tablet apps with hazmat resource materials are also available. Using these references, you should be able to begin proper emergency management as soon as the hazardous material is identified. Do not go into an area and risk exposure to yourself or your partner.

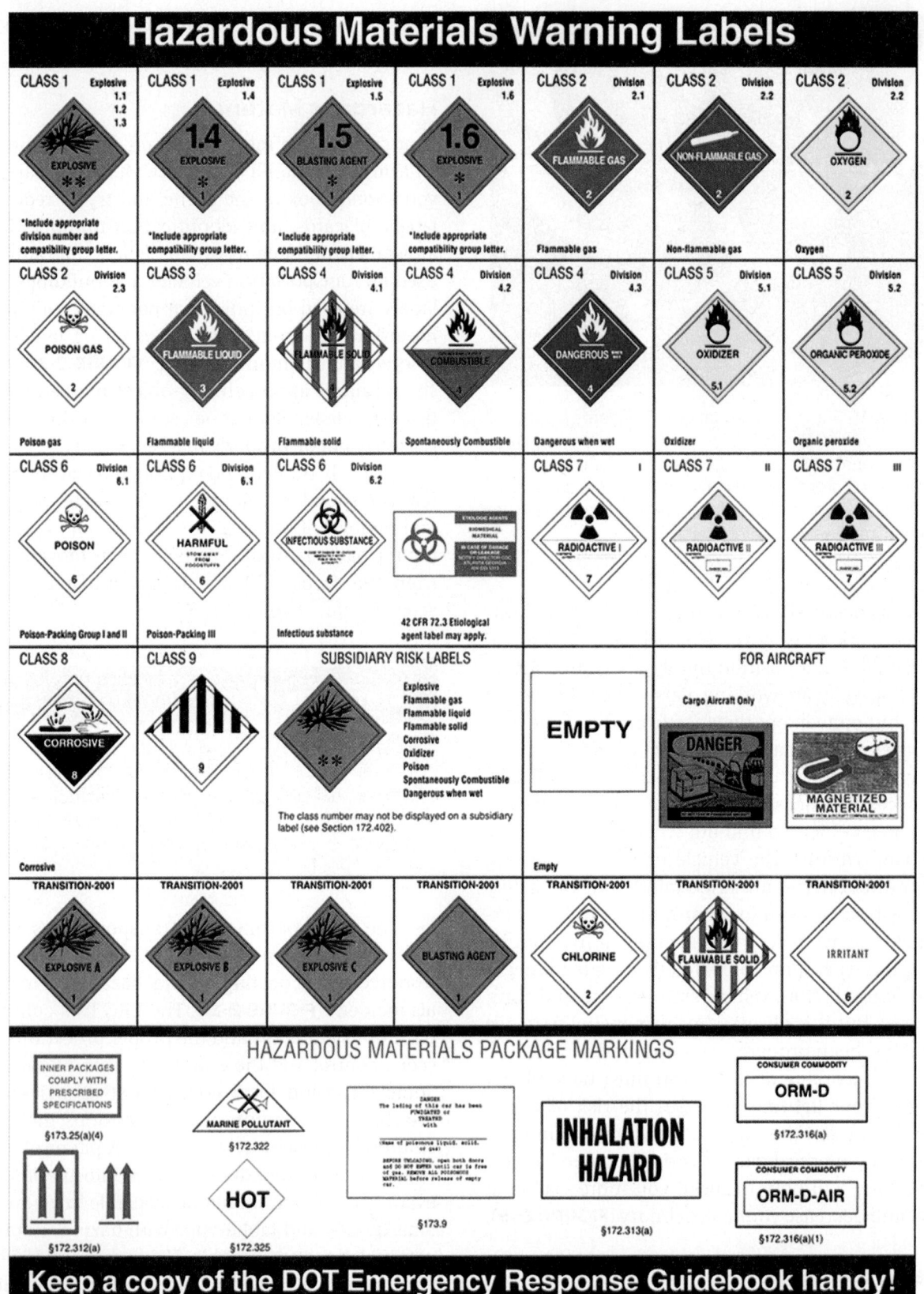

**FIGURE 2-20** Hazardous materials safety placards and labels are colored and diamond-shaped.

Courtesy of the U.S. Department of Transportation.

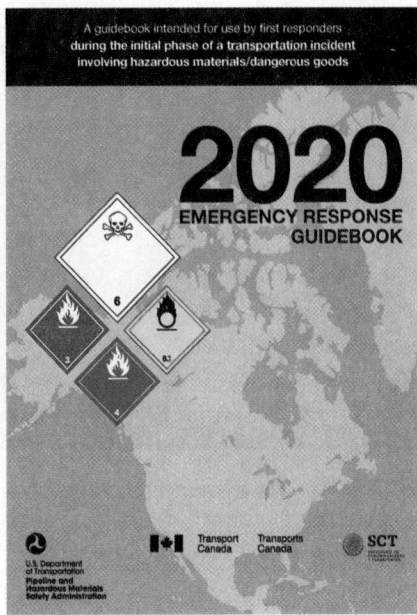

**FIGURE 2-21** The US Department of Transportation's *Emergency Response Guidebook* lists many hazardous materials and the proper procedures for scene control and emergency care of patients.

Courtesy of the US Department of Transportation.

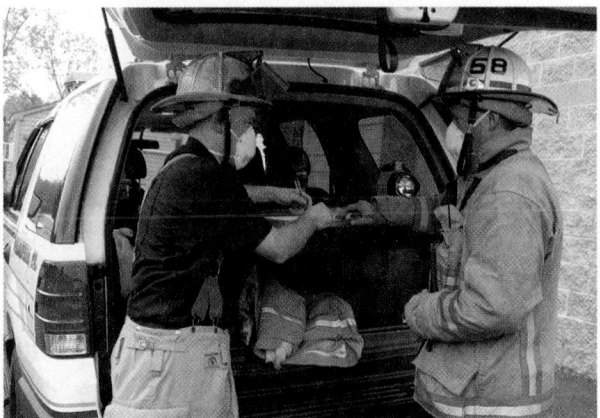

**FIGURE 2-22** Wear a helmet made of a certified electrical nonconductor material, making sure that the chin strap is fastened securely.

© Jones & Bartlett Learning. Photographed by Glen E. Ellman.

The following are general guidelines you should follow when dealing with scenes involving hazardous materials:

- Do not enter the scene if there is evidence of hazardous materials.
- Remain upwind and uphill of the scene.
- Keep your distance. This may mean retreating if you become aware of the true nature of the situation.
- Quickly contact dispatch.
- Request additional resources.
- Do not enter the scene until instructed by trained hazardous materials responders.

## Electricity

Electrical shock can be produced by human-made sources (power lines) or natural sources (lightning). No matter the source, you must evaluate the risk to you and your patient before you begin patient care.

### Power Lines

Do not touch downed power lines. Dealing with power lines is beyond the scope of EMT training. You should mark off a danger zone around the downed lines. Energized, or live, power lines, especially high-voltage lines, behave in unpredictable ways. You need in-depth training to operate the equipment that is used in an electrical emergency. The equipment has specific storage needs and requires careful cleaning. Dirt or other contaminants can make this equipment useless or dangerous.

At the scene of a motor vehicle crash, above-ground and below-grade power lines may become hazards. Disrupted overhead wires are usually a visible hazard. You must be very careful even if you do not see sparks coming from the lines. Visible sparks are not always present in charged wires. The area around downed power lines is always a danger zone. This danger zone extends well beyond the immediate accident scene.

Use the utility poles as landmarks for establishing the perimeter of the danger zone. The danger zone must be a restricted area. The safety zone is one span of the utility pole's distance. Only emergency personnel, equipment, and vehicles are allowed inside this area. Do not approach downed wires or touch anything with which downed wires are in contact until qualified personnel have concluded that no risk of electrical injury exists. This may mean you are unable to access a severely injured victim of a motor vehicle crash even though you can see and talk to the victim.

If you must enter this type of situation, be sure to wear the proper protective equipment according to the type of incident. A helmet and turnout gear (**FIGURE 2-22**) are typically required, but you cannot count on turnout gear for protection from electrical hazards. Other protective equipment may be needed.

### Lightning

Lightning is a complex natural phenomenon. It is untrue that lightning never strikes in the same place twice.

Lightning is a threat in two ways: through a direct hit and through ground current. After the lightning bolt strikes, the current drains along the earth, following the most conductive pathway. Although you should avoid high ground to avoid a direct strike, to avoid being injured by a ground current stay away from drainage ditches, moist areas, small depressions, and wet ropes. If you are involved in a rescue operation, you may need to delay rescue until the storm passes. Recognize the warning signs just before a lightning strike. As your surroundings become charged, you may feel a slight tingling sensation on your skin, or your hair may even stand on end. In this situation, a strike may be imminent. Move immediately to the lowest possible area.

If you are caught in an open area, make yourself the smallest possible target for a direct hit or for ground current. To avoid being hit by the initial strike, stay away from projections from the ground, such as a single tree. Drop all equipment, particularly metal objects, that project above your body. Avoid fences and other metal objects. These structures can transmit current from the initial strike over a long distance. Position yourself in a low crouch. This position exposes only your feet to the ground current. If you sit, both your feet and your buttocks are exposed. Place an object made of nonconductive material, such as a blanket, under your feet. Get inside a car or your unit, if possible, as vehicles will protect you from lightning.

### Fire

You will often be called to the scene of a fire. Therefore, you should understand some basic information about fire, if you do not know it already. There are seven common hazards in a fire:

- Smoke
- Oxygen deficiency
- High temperatures
- Toxic gases
- Building collapse
- Equipment
- Explosions

Smoke is made up of particles of tar and carbon. These particles irritate the respiratory system

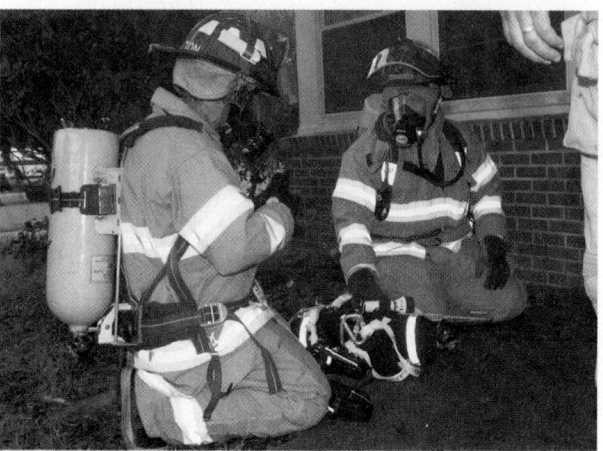

**FIGURE 2-23** EMTs who are also firefighters should be trained in the use of self-contained breathing apparatus and have it available if working near fire scenes.

© Courtesy of Lance Cpl. Brian Kester/U.S. Marines.

on contact. Most smoke particles are trapped in the upper respiratory system, but many smaller particles enter the lungs. Some smoke particles not only irritate the airway, but may also be deadly. If you are a firefighter, you will have a self-contained breathing apparatus to use at fire scenes (**FIGURE 2-23**).

Fire consumes oxygen. Particularly in confined spaces, fire may consume most of the available oxygen. This will make breathing difficult for anyone in that space. The high ambient temperatures in a fire can result in thermal burns and damage to the respiratory system. Breathing air that is heated above 120°F (49°C) can damage the respiratory system.

A typical building fire emits a number of toxic gases, including carbon monoxide, cyanide, and carbon dioxide. Carbon monoxide is a colorless, odorless gas that is responsible for more fire deaths each year than any other by-product of combustion. Carbon monoxide combines with the hemoglobin in your red blood cells about 200 times more readily than does oxygen. It blocks the ability of the hemoglobin to transport oxygen to your body tissues. Cyanide is a product of the combustion of many materials that burn. Inhaling cyanide prevents cells from using oxygen. In sufficiently high concentrations, it causes signs and symptoms of shock and severe hypoxia leading to death. Carbon dioxide is also a colorless, odorless gas. Exposure causes increased respirations, dizziness, and sweating. Breathing concentrations of carbon dioxide greater than 10% to 12% will result in death within a few minutes.

During and after a fire, there is always a possibility that all or part of the burned structure will collapse. Often, there are no warning signs. As an EMS provider, you should never enter a burning building without proper protective gear, breathing apparatus, and approval. Always follow the instructions of the incident commander and safety officer at the scene, and never undertake any task (ie, enter a burning structure or initiate search and rescue) unless you have been properly trained to do so. Hasty entry into a burning structure may result in serious injury and possibly death. Once inside a burning building, you are subject to an uncontrolled, hostile environment. Fires are not selective about their victims. You must be extremely cautious whenever you are near a burning structure or one in which a fire has just been placed under control.

Fuel and fuel systems of vehicles that have been involved in crashes are also a hazard. Although this rarely happens, any leaking car fuel may ignite under the right conditions. If you see or smell a fuel leak, or if people are trapped in the vehicle, you must coordinate appropriate fire protection equipment. Gasoline and other auto fluids are considered hazardous materials.

Make sure you are properly protected if there is or has been a fire in the vehicle. Wear appropriate respiratory protection and thermal protection because the smoke from a vehicle fire contains many toxic by-products. The use of appropriate protective gear at a crash scene can reduce your risk of injury. Avoid using oxygen in or near a vehicle that is smoking, smoldering, or leaking fuel.

## Vehicle Crashes

Vehicle crashes are common events for EMS providers. These environments provide some of the most unstable and potentially lethal situations you will face. Traffic hazards are the first risk to consider. As you drive your ambulance to the scene of the crash, it is important to keep several things in mind. What is the flow of traffic near and around the crash? How will you safely leave and move about the scene? Ideally, you should park your ambulance in a manner where you can easily leave the scene. Keep in mind that additional fire, rescue, and police vehicles may also be parked in the same area or they may be blocking your exit. Hydraulic and hose lines are just two examples of common blockages you may encounter.

If you are the first to arrive at the scene, use the ambulance itself as a shield to protect the scene. The ambulance can be relocated for easier exit once additional help arrives. Park at least 100 ft (30.5 m) away from all crash sites.

As you approach the scene, be very conscious about the flow of traffic. If needed, request assistance to control traffic. Traffic control will help ensure a safe scene as you work with patients.

How is the vehicle positioned? Is it stable? Cars and trucks can come to rest in a wide array of positions. As the center of gravity of the vehicle is raised, its ability to fall onto you increases. The standard approach for all vehicle crashes should be for firefighters to first stabilize the vehicle to ensure safety for the passengers and any EMS providers.

Identify any other hazards such as fluids leaking from the vehicles, which can be flammable. Fluids, dirt, sand, gravel, glass, and other materials on or around the roadway may cause slip and driving hazards. Additional hazards include power lines. Downed lines can generate lethal electrical charges many feet away from vehicle crashes. If there are lines down, you should assume they are power lines and do not approach. Call for additional resources to manage this hazard. Be aware that most electric companies will not shut down power to the grid. Although this seems like a logical solution, many injuries can be caused by an unscheduled power outage. If people in their homes are on ventilators or other life-saving medical devices, this could create another emergency situation if the power were shut off.

With proper equipment and training, you may enter the vehicle. If the vehicle is still running, put it in park and turn off the ignition. If the airbag has not deployed, there is a risk that it may accidently activate while you are in the vehicle. Likewise, alternative-fuel vehicles, including hybrid or electric vehicles and vehicles powered by propane, natural gas, or fuel cells, present their own unique hazards when damaged in collisions. Although it may not be your primary job to resolve all of the hazards associated with every type of vehicle, it is important for you to be aware of issues and seek to identify clues such as marked warnings, smoke or smells in or around the vehicle, or other signs of danger. When you identify a concern, speak up to your partner and other emergency response colleagues.

Your personal clothing will help you to remain safe while working in and around a vehicle crash.

The risk of injuries from glass and sharp metal objects cannot be underestimated. If you are working inside the vehicle, make sure you have sufficient protective gear.

## Scenes of Violence

Sometimes EMTs will be at a scene where a clearly dangerous situation is under way, such as an assault, a shooting, a hostage situation, a riot, or other disturbance. Assessment of the scene should begin while you are en route. Once on scene or at your staging location, continue your assessment using your personal observations—what you see and hear—as well as information that you can gather from other responders. Your safety and that of your team is of primary concern. You must thoroughly understand the risks of each environment you enter. Whenever you are in doubt about your safety, do not put yourself at risk.

## Mass Violence

Scenes of mass violence such as shootings or bombings, civil disturbances, and large gatherings of hostile or potentially hostile people can create many hazards for EMS personnel. Several agencies will respond to large civil disturbances. In these instances, it is important for you to know who is in command and will be issuing orders (**FIGURE 2-24**). In some cases, especially if the violence has only just occurred, other responders may not be aware of the

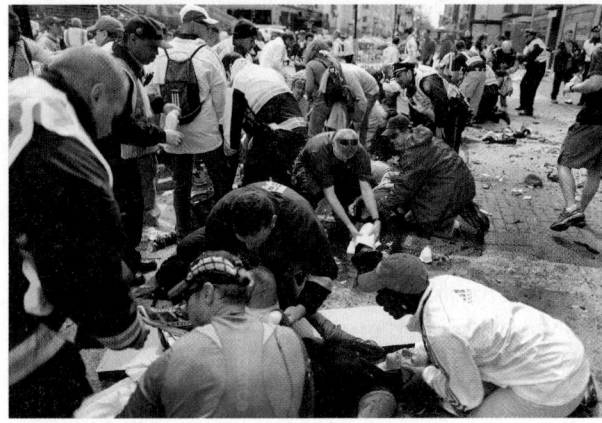

**FIGURE 2-24** Several agencies may respond to a scene that involves a large number of people, such as the Boston Marathon bombings on April 15, 2013. It is important for you to know who is in command and will be issuing orders.
© John Tlumacki/The Boston Globe/Getty Images.

situation. In other cases, the dispatch information may not reflect the potential for violence at all. In these situations you should call for law enforcement immediately if they are not already present.

It is not unusual to find yourself on a call where the potential for violence is present but is not immediately clear. You must remain vigilant for the potential for violence at all times. As part of your scene size-up, evaluate the scene for the potential for violence. When appropriate, allow law enforcement personnel to secure the scene before you approach; they have the necessary experience and expertise

## YOU are the Provider

Your partner coordinates effective, high-quality CPR with a responding police officer. You place a semiautomatic defibrillator, but it reads, "No shock advised. Continue CPR." The child's mother, who is standing back watching your efforts, is crying and keeps yelling at you, "Why isn't my daughter waking up! Why aren't you saving her!"

| Recording Time: 5 Minutes | |
|---|---|
| **Respirations** | Absent |
| **Pulse** | Absent |
| **Skin** | Cool and cyanotic |
| **Blood pressure** | Not obtainable |
| **Oxygen saturation (Spo$_2$)** | Not obtainable |

**4.** How should you respond to the mother?

**5.** What stage of the grieving process is the mother experiencing?

in handling these situations. They may ask you to stage, to remain in a safe location, until the scene is more secure and you can proceed. Remember, addressing your personal safety is your first task. You must attempt to understand the risks of each environment you enter. Whenever you are in doubt about your safety, do not put yourself at risk.

At scenes involving projectiles such as bullets, bottles, and rocks, you may need to find protection. When approaching the scene, look for areas of concealment or cover. **Cover** involves the tactical use of an impenetrable barrier for protection, whereas **concealment** involves hiding behind objects to limit a person's ability to see you. Do not depend on someone else for your safety. Remember, you and your partner must be protected from the dangers at the scene before you can provide patient care.

A crime scene often poses potential problems for EMS personnel. Perpetrators may be on the scene or reappear and threaten you, your partner, or the patient. Bystanders or family members may interfere with your emergency medical care. Be sure you have adequate assistance from the appropriate public safety agency in these situations. If you believe an event is a crime scene, you must attempt to maintain the chain of evidence. Do not disturb the scene unless it is absolutely necessary in caring for the patient.

### Violence Against Responders

In some cases, emergency responders might be the direct target of violence. The rate of violence-related injuries with work loss for emergency responders is 22 times higher than the overall rate for other employees in the United States. Ensuring health and wellness in the face of violence against EMS providers demands strategies of prevention and strategies of protection.

Recommendations for the prevention of violence include the following:

- Training and practice in identifying scenes of potential violence
- Training and practice in deescalation strategies and techniques
- Training and practice to improve interpersonal communications
- Practice in ongoing scene assessment
- Dispatch identification and alerting of past or potential threats of violence

Recommendations for protection against violence include the following:

- Training and practice in self-defense and escape techniques
- Training and practice in physical and chemical restraint techniques
- Fitting and use of body armor
- Training and practice in operations with law enforcement personnel

EMTs who experience physical or verbal violence should report this on the appropriate incident form. Follow your state laws and department policies to report instances of physical assault.

### Protective Clothing: Preventing Injury

Wearing protective clothing and other appropriate gear is critical to your personal safety. Become familiar with the protective equipment that is available to you. Then you will know what clothing and gear are needed for the job. You will also be able to adapt or change items as the situation and environment change. Remember, protective clothing and gear provide protection only when they are in good condition. It is your responsibility to inspect your clothing and gear. Learn to recognize how wear and tear can make your equipment unsafe. Be sure to inspect equipment before you use it; ideally, this is done before reaching the scene so care is not delayed.

Clothing that is worn for rescue must be appropriate for the activity and the environment where the activity will take place. For example, turnout gear worn for firefighting may be too restrictive for working in a confined space. In every situation involving blood and/or other body fluids, follow standard precautions. You must protect yourself and your patient by wearing gloves and eye protection, as well as any additional protective clothing that may be needed. EMS coats should provide a barrier to body fluids if they were purchased after 1998.

### Safety Tips

The American National Standards Institute requires all EMS providers to wear a high-visibility public safety vest while on or near the roadway.

## Cold Weather Clothing

When dressing for cold weather, you should wear several layers of clothing. Multiple layers provide much better protection than a single thick cover. You have more flexibility to control your body temperature by adding or removing a layer. Cold weather protection should consist of at least the following three layers:

1. A thin inner layer (sometimes called the transport layer) next to your skin. This layer pulls moisture away from your skin, keeping you dry and warm. Underwear made of polypropylene or polyester material works well. Wool is the best natural fiber. The goal is to wick moisture away from the skin.
2. A thermal middle layer of bulkier material for insulation. Wool has been the material of choice for warmth, but newer materials, such as polyester fleece, are also commonly used.
3. An outer layer that resists chilling winds and wet conditions, such as rain, sleet, or snow. The two top layers should have zippers to allow you to vent some body heat if you become too warm.

When choosing protective clothing, you should pay attention to the type of material from which it is made. Cotton should be avoided in cold, wet environments. Cotton tends to absorb moisture, causing chilling from wetness. However, cotton is appropriate in warm, dry weather because it absorbs moisture and pulls heat away from the body.

As an outer layer in cold weather, you might consider plastic-coated nylon, as it provides good waterproof protection. However, it can also hold in body heat and perspiration, which makes you wet both inside and out. Newer, less airtight materials allow perspiration and some heat to escape while the material retains its water resistance. Avoid flammable or meltable synthetic materials anytime there is any possibility of fire.

## Turnout Gear

Turnout gear, or bunker gear, is a fire service term for protective clothing designed for use in structural firefighting environments (**FIGURE 2-25**). Turnout gear provides some protection by using different layers of fabric or other material to provide

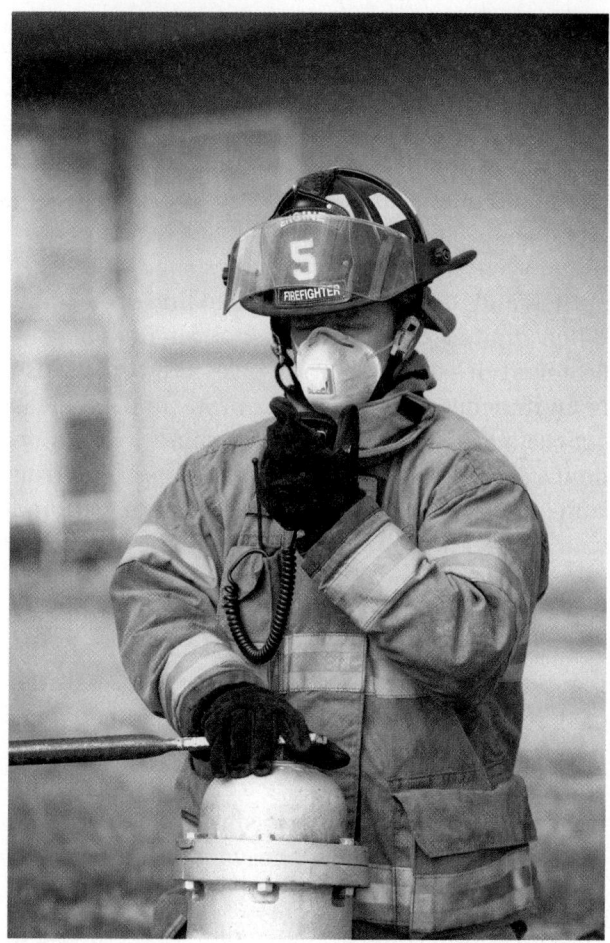

**FIGURE 2-25** Turnout gear, or bunker gear, is protective clothing designed for use in firefighting.
© Jones & Bartlett Learning. Photographed by Glen E. Ellman.

protection from the heat of fire. It also helps to reduce trauma from impact or cuts and keeps water away from the body. Like most protective clothing, turnout gear adds weight and reduces range of motion to some degree.

The exterior fabrics provide increased protection from cuts and abrasions. They also act as a barrier to high external temperatures. In cold weather, an insulated thermal inner layer of material that helps to retain body heat is recommended.

Turnout gear or a bunker jacket provides minimal protection from electrical shock. However, it does protect you from heat, fire, possible flashover, and flying sparks. The front opening of the jacket should be fastened, and the jacket should be worn with the collar up and closed in front to protect your neck and upper chest. Proper fit is important so that you can move freely.

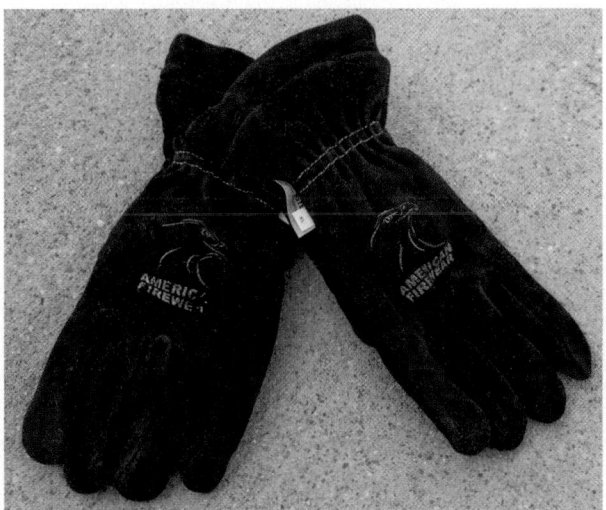

**FIGURE 2-26** Firefighting gloves protect your hands and wrists from heat, cold, and injury.

© Jones & Bartlett Learning. Photographed by Glen E. Ellman.

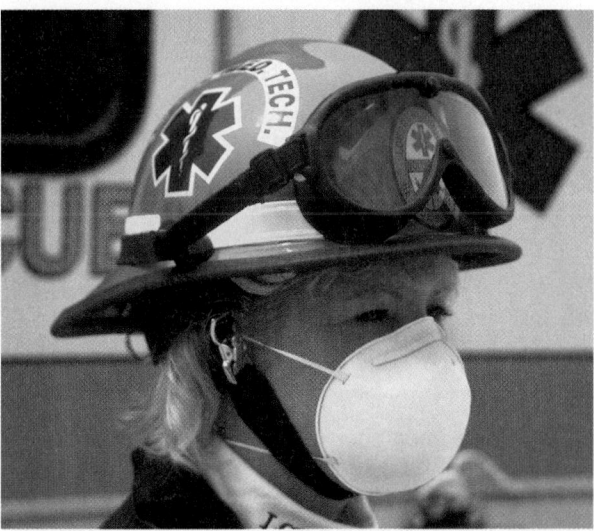

**FIGURE 2-27** A helmet with top and side impact protection.

© Jones & Bartlett Learning. Courtesy of MIEMSS.

## Gloves

Firefighting gloves provide the best protection from heat, cold, and cuts (**FIGURE 2-26**). However, these gloves reduce manual dexterity. In addition, firefighting gloves will not protect you from electrical hazards. In rescue situations, you must be able to freely use your hands to operate rescue tools, provide patient care, and perform other duties. Wearing puncture-proof leather gloves and latex gloves underneath will permit free use of your hands and offer added protection from both injury and body fluids.

### Words of Wisdom

Keep in mind that gloves or gear contaminated with blood or other potentially infectious materials can cross-contaminate equipment, patients, other responders, and you.

## Helmets

You should wear a helmet anytime you are working in a fall zone. A fall zone is an area where you are likely to encounter falling objects. The helmet should provide top and side impact protection. It should also have a secure chin strap (**FIGURE 2-27**). Objects will often fall one after another. If the strap

is not secure, the first falling object may knock off your helmet. This leaves your head unprotected as the remaining objects fall.

Construction-type helmets are not well suited for rescue situations. They offer minimal impact protection and have inadequate chin straps. Modern fire helmets offer impact protection. However, the projecting brim at the back of the neck may get in your way in a rescue situation. In cold weather, a great loss of body heat occurs if you are not wearing a hat or helmet. An insulated hat made from wool or a synthetic material can be pulled down over the face and the base of the skull to reduce heat loss in extremely cold weather.

You should always wear a helmet with a chin strap and face shield in situations involving electrical hazards. The shell of the helmet should be made of a certified electrical nonconductor. The chin strap should not stretch. In fact, it should fasten securely so the helmet stays in place if you are knocked down or a power line hits your head. You should also be able to lock the face shield on the helmet. This will protect your face and eyes from power lines and flying sparks. A standard fire turnout helmet should meet all of these needs.

## Boots

Boots should protect your feet. They should be water resistant, fit well, and be flexible so that you

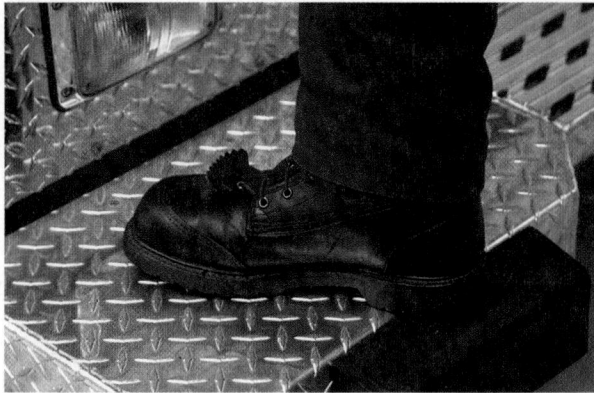

**FIGURE 2-28** Boots should cover and protect your ankles, keeping out stones, debris, and snow. Steel-toed boots are preferred.

© Jones & Bartlett Learning. Courtesy of MIEMSS.

can comfortably walk long distances. If you will be working outdoors, you should choose boots that cover and protect your ankles, keeping out stones, debris, and snow. Steel-toed boots are preferred (**FIGURE 2-28**). In cold weather, your boots must also protect you from the cold. Leather is one of the best materials for boots. However, other materials, such as any waterproof, windproof, and breathable fabrics, are also very good. The soles of your boots must provide traction. Lug-type soles may grip well in snow, but they become very slippery when caked with mud.

Properly fitted boots and shoes are extremely important, because a minor annoyance can develop into a disabling injury. Painful blisters may develop if your feet slip around inside your boots, so make sure you have enough room to wiggle your toes.

Boots should be puncture-resistant, protect the toes, and provide foot support. It may be difficult to obtain a good fit with firefighting boots; shoe inserts or sock layering may be needed to ensure a comfortable fit. Make sure the tops of your boots are sealed off to keep rain, snow, glass, or other materials from getting into your boots. Moisture increases blistering—wool or wicking socks help prevent feet from becoming wet.

Socks will keep your feet warm and provide some cushioning for you as you walk. In cold weather, two pairs of socks are generally preferable to one thick pair. A thin sock next to the foot helps to wick perspiration away to a thicker outer sock. This tends to keep your feet warmer, drier, and generally more comfortable. When you purchase

new shoes or boots, you may want to try them on while wearing the two pairs of socks to ensure a proper fit.

## Eye Protection

The human eye is very fragile, and permanent loss of sight can occur from minor injuries. You need to protect your eyes from blood and other body fluids, foreign objects, plants, insects, and debris from extrication. You may wear eyeglasses with side shields during routine patient care.

However, when tools are being used during extrication, you should wear a face shield or goggles. In these instances, prescription eyeglasses do not provide adequate protection. In snow or white sand, particularly at higher altitudes, you must protect your eyes from ultraviolet exposure. Specially designed eyeglasses or goggles can provide this. In addition, your eye protection must be adaptable to the weather and the physical demands of the task. It is critical that you have clear vision at all times.

### Words of Wisdom

Remember to wear your face shield or goggles at helicopter landing and takeoff zones on emergency scenes. The aircraft rotors often cause large amounts of dirt and debris to become airborne, posing a risk for eye injury.

## Ear Protection

Exposure to loud noises for long periods of time can cause permanent hearing loss. Certain equipment, such as helicopters, some extrication tools, and sirens, produces high levels of noise. Wearing soft foam industrial-type earplugs usually provides adequate protection.

## Skin Protection

Your skin needs protection against sunburn while you are working outdoors. Long-term exposure to the sun increases the possibility of skin cancer. It may be considered simply an annoyance, but sunburn is a type of burn injury. In reflective areas such as sand, water, and snow, your risk of sunburn increases. Protect your skin by applying sunscreen with a minimum sun protection factor of 15.

## Hair, Rings, and Jewelry

You need to be careful when wearing long, unsecured hair, loose rings, and jewelry. For example, these items can become caught in machinery during extrication. Due to the multitude of unusual situations in which EMTs may find themselves, many EMS agencies have restrictive policies regarding hair, rings, and jewelry. You should neatly secure long hair, limit the number of rings worn, and wear only a watch on the wrist.

## Body Armor

Some EMS responders wear body armor on-shift for personal protection from firearms. Several types of body armor are available, offering different features and levels and types of protection. They range from soft, lightweight, and flexible to hard-plated armor that is heavier and bulkier. Lighter vests are commonly worn concealed under a uniform shirt or jacket. The larger, heavier vests are typically worn on the outside of a uniform. Often, lighter body armor for daily wear differs from the heavier, higher levels of protection that are worn for response to scenes of violence. It is important to know what level of protection your body armor provides and to store it properly to ensure it retains its ability to protect you.

# Caring for Critically Ill and Injured Patients

When you are caring for a critically ill or injured patient, the patient needs to know who you are and what you are doing. Let the patient know you are attending to his or her immediate needs and these are your primary concerns at this moment (**FIGURE 2-29**). As soon as possible, explain to the patient what is going on. Confusion, anxiety, and other feelings of helplessness will be decreased if you keep the patient informed from the start. Never assume a patient cannot hear you. Avoid making unprofessional comments during resuscitation, and treat all patients with dignity and respect.

## Techniques for Communicating With the Critical Patient

Patients who are dying as a result of trauma, an acute medical emergency, or a terminal disease

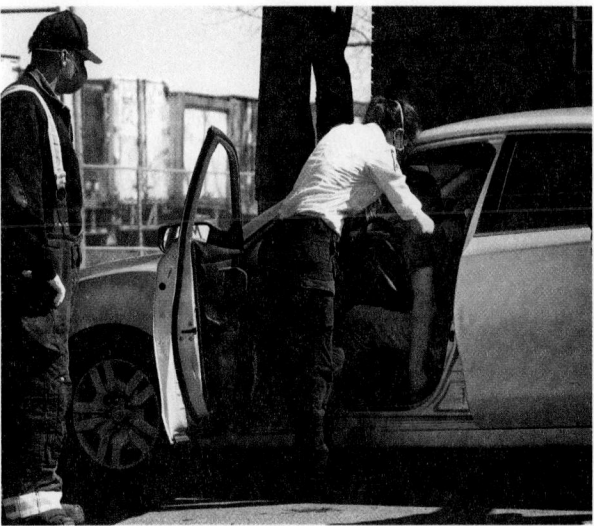

**FIGURE 2-29** Let the patient know immediately that you are there to help.
© Jessica Rinaldi/Boston Globe/Getty Images.

will feel threatened. That threat may be related to their concern about survival. These concerns may involve feelings of helplessness, disability, pain, and separation. Saying the wrong thing may further distress the patient or the patient's family. Knowing how to effectively communicate in these situations can bring the patient needed comfort, which may in turn allow you to provide better care.

## Avoid Sad and Grim Comments

EMTs, other safety personnel, family members, and bystanders must avoid making grim comments about a patient's condition. Remarks such as "This is a bad one" or "The leg is badly damaged. I think he'll lose it" are inappropriate. These remarks may upset or increase the patient's anxiety and compromise possible recovery outcomes. This is especially true for a patient who may be able to hear but cannot respond.

## Orient the Patient

You should expect a patient to be disoriented in an emergency situation. The aura of the emergency situation—lights, sirens, smells, and strangers—is intense. The impact and effect of injuries or acute illness may cause the patient to be confused or unsettled. It is important for you to orient the patient to his or her surroundings (**FIGURE 2-30**). Use brief, concise statements such as, "Mr. Rosa, you've had

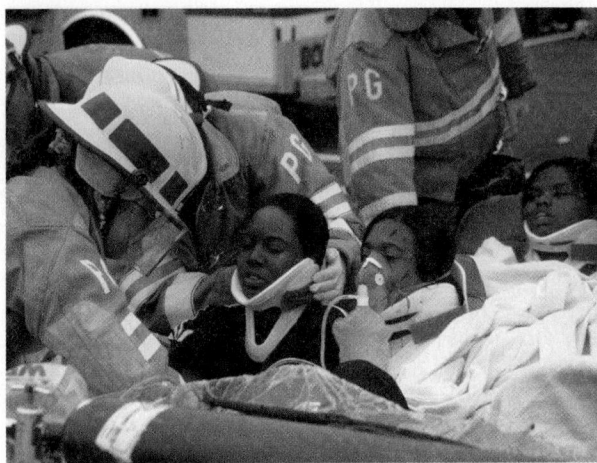

**FIGURE 2-30** Emergency situations can be confusing and frightening to patients.

© Tom Carter/age fotostock.

an accident, and I am now splinting your arm. I'm Mike Short of Ridgefield EMS. I'll be caring for you."

### Be Honest

When approaching any patient, you must decide how much information each patient is able to understand and accept. You should be honest without further alarming the patient or giving unnecessary information or information that may not be understood. Simply explain what you are doing and allow the patient to be part of the care being given; this can relieve feelings of helplessness as well as some of the fear.

### Allow for Hope

In trauma and acute medical conditions, patients may ask you whether they are going to die. At these times, you may feel at a loss for words. You may also know, on the basis of past experience or in view of the seriousness of the current situation, that the prognosis is poor. However, it is not your decision to tell the patient that he or she is dying. If there is the slightest chance of hope remaining, you want that message transmitted in your attitude and in the statements you make to the patient.

### Locating and Notifying Family Members

Many patients will be concerned and ask you to notify their family or others close to them. The patient

may not be able to assist you in doing this. In these cases, you should make sure an appropriate and responsible person makes an effort to locate the desired persons. Assuring the patient that someone is going to make these notifications may be an important aspect of the patient's care because it will help to calm the patient.

### Injured and Critically Ill Children

Injured and critically ill children who have life-threatening conditions should be cared for the same as any adult patient would, insofar as assessing airway, breathing, and circulation and addressing immediate life threats (XABCs). Due regard should be given to variations in height, weight, and size when providing emergency medical care to pediatric patients. Because of the increased commotion and the extraordinary nature of the emergency scene for a child, it is important that a relative or responsible adult accompany the child at all times to relieve anxiety and assist in care as appropriate.

### Coping With the Death of a Child

The death of a child is a tragic and dreaded event. It will not be unusual for you to think about the fact that the dead or dying child still has a lot more to do in life and should have many more years to live. In our society, we often assume only older people are supposed to die. Many people are unprepared for what they will feel when a child dies. You may think about your own children, related children, and children of close friends.

Answering the difficult questions of your own mortality will help you deal with the death of a child. Still, the death of a child will never be an easy subject to talk about. This will be especially so for the child's family, and as an EMT involved in a call that involves the death of a child, you will also likely experience stress.

One of your responsibilities may be to help the family through the initial period after the death. As an EMT, until more definitive and professional help can be arranged, you may be in the best position to help the family begin to cope with their loss. How a family initially deals with the death of a child will affect its stability and endurance. You can help a family through their initial period of grief and provide information about follow-up counseling and support services that are available.

## Helping the Family

Whether the child has just died in your presence or was dead when you arrived, acknowledging the death is important. This should be done in a private place, even if that is inside an ambulance. Often, the parents cannot believe the death is real, even if they have been preparing for it, as in the case of a terminal illness such as leukemia.

Reactions vary, but shock, disbelief, and denial are common emotions and reactions. Some parents show little emotion at the initial news. If it is possible and appropriate, find a place where the mother and father can hold or touch the child. This is important in the parents' grieving process; it helps to lessen the sense of disbelief and makes the death real. Even if the parents do not ask to see the child, you should tell them that they may do so; however, this may not be possible if it is a crime scene. Your decision in permitting the parents to see the child may require some discretion on your part. For example, in the case of a traumatic death in which there is significant disfigurement of the body, the decision whether to see the child might have to be delayed. The delay may involve waiting for support services or contacting the family physician or others who can help the parents through this difficult situation. This situation may also involve preparing the parents for what they will see and the changes brought on by rigor mortis or asphyxiation, for example.

Sometimes, you do not need to say much. In fact, silence can sometimes be more comforting than words. You can express your own sorrow. Do not overload grieving parents with a lot of information; at this point, they cannot handle it. Nonverbal communication, such as holding a hand or touching a shoulder, may be more valuable. Let the family's actions be your guide to what is appropriate. If you sense the parents want to talk, it is important for you to encourage them to talk about their feelings.

> **Street Smarts**
>
> Patients don't care what you know until they know that you care. Patients will judge your treatment based on how you care for them.

## Death and Dying

Death can occur in the hospital, a hospice facility, or convalescent home, at the workplace, or on the highway, and death is likely to occur either quite suddenly or after a prolonged illness. Illness can be much more drawn-out and much more removed

---

### YOU are the Provider

The child is placed onto the stretcher and loaded into the ambulance. Her mother is secured in the front seat of the ambulance. One of the first responders drives the ambulance so that both you and your partner can continue attending to the child. With resuscitative efforts continuing, you depart the scene and proceed to the hospital. The child's condition is reassessed en route.

| Recording Time: 11 Minutes | |
| --- | --- |
| Level of consciousness | Unconscious and unresponsive |
| Respirations | Absent |
| Pulse | Absent |
| Skin | Cool and cyanotic |
| Blood pressure | Not obtainable |
| Spo$_2$ | Not obtainable |

**6.** How can poorly managed stress affect your physical well-being?

**7.** How can you mitigate the stress associated with the job?

from daily life. Life support systems and impersonal care remove the whole experience of death from most people's awareness. The mobility of families also makes it less likely there will be extended family support when death does occur.

You may have painful personal experience with death. No matter what the frequency of response to emergency calls, death is something that every EMT will face at some point. For some of you, it may be infrequent. Others, in urban settings, may see death many times in responding to motor vehicle crashes, drug overdoses, suicides, or homicides. You may have to deal with the mass-casualty incident of an airplane crash or a hazardous materials incident. In all of these situations, coming to grips with your thoughts, understanding, and adjustment to death is not only important personally, but also a function of delivering emergency medical care.

## The Grieving Process

Everyone working as an EMT will experience grief at one time or another. This section discusses how to handle patient grief, as well as how to cope with your own grief that may result from a difficult call.

The death of a human being is one of the most difficult events for another human being to accept. For a relative or close friend of the deceased, it is even more difficult. Emotional responses to the loss of a loved one or friend are appropriate and should be expected. In fact, it is expected you will feel emotional about the death of a patient. Feelings and emotions are part of the grieving process. All of us experience these feelings after a stressful situation that causes us personal pain.

In 1969, Dr. Elisabeth Kübler-Ross published *On Death and Dying*, which revealed her theory on the stages of grief people go through. They are as follows:

1. **Denial.** Refusing to accept diagnosis or care, unrealistic demands for miracles, or persistent failure to understand why there is no improvement.
2. **Anger, hostility.** Projecting bad news onto the environment and commonly in all directions, at times almost at random. The person lashes out. Someone must be blamed, and those who are responsible must be punished. This is usually an ugly phase, and it may even be inappropriately directed toward the EMT.
3. **Bargaining.** Attempting to negotiate a favorable outcome for good behavior or promising to change. "I promise to be a 'perfect patient' if only I can live until 'x' event."
4. **Depression.** Internalizing anger, hopelessness, and the desire to die. It rarely involves suicidal threats, complete withdrawal, or giving up long before the illness seems terminal. The patient is usually silent.
5. **Acceptance.** Accepting the impending death of the patient, or accepting the death of a loved one.

The stages may follow one another, they may occur simultaneously, or a person may jump back and forth between stages. The stages may last different amounts of time.

Even though the event (death) has not yet happened, the patient knows that it will happen. The patient has no control over this process. The patient will die whether or not he or she is ready to die. As an EMT, you may encounter situations in which the patient is close to death, and you may need to provide reassurance and emotional care.

## What Can the EMT Do?

As patients and bystanders are grieving, you can do helpful things and make simple suggestions. Ask whether there is anything that you can do that will be of help, such as calling a relative or religious advisor. Provide gentle and caring support. Reinforcing the reality of the situation is important. This can be accomplished by merely saying to a grieving person, "I am so sorry for your loss." It is not important that you have a well-rehearsed script, for it is not likely that your exact words or consolations will be remembered. Being honest and sincere are important.

Some statements of consolation tend to be trite. Although these statements may be said with the intention of making the person feel better about a situation, they can also be viewed as an attempt to diminish the person's grief. The grieving person needs to be validated. Statements like these can indicate our inability to comprehend the profound sadness of grief because you have not experienced that kind of loss. If you have not experienced a death, it is okay to say so; do not pretend you have.

Attempts to take grief away too quickly are not good. If you do not know how the person really feels,

| TABLE 2-7 Words of Comfort When Responding to Grief |
|---|
| • I'm sorry for your loss. |
| • It is okay to be angry. |
| • It must be hard to accept. |
| • That must be painful for you. |
| • Tell me how you are feeling. |
| • If you want to cry, it's okay. |
| • People really cared for . . . |

you should not say so. People may be offended by responses that give advice or explanations about the death. Statements such as "Oh, you shouldn't feel that way" are judgmental. If you judge what the grieving person is feeling, it is likely that he or she will stop talking with you. People feel what people feel. Remember, anger is a stage of grieving. The anger may be directed at you. The anger seems irrational to everyone except the person grieving; therefore, it is necessary that you maintain a professional attitude and let the person grieve in his or her own way (**TABLE 2-7**).

Statements and comments that suggest action on your part are generally helpful. These statements imply a sense of understanding; they focus on the grieving person's feelings. It is not necessary to go into an extensive discussion. All you need to do is be sincere and say, "I am so sorry for your loss. I just want you to know that I am thinking about you." What people really appreciate is somebody who will listen to them. Simply ask, "Would you like to talk about how or what you are now feeling?" Then accept the response.

## Assisting Patient and Family Members

There is no right or wrong way to grieve. Each person will experience grief and respond to it in his or her own way. Family members may express rage, anger, and despair. Many people will be rational and cooperative. Their concerns will usually be relieved by your calm, efficient manner. Your actions and words, even a simple touch, can communicate caring. Although you must treat all patients with respect and dignity, use special care with dying patients and their families. Be concerned about their privacy and their wishes, and let them know you

take their concerns seriously. However, it is best to be honest with patients and their families; do not give them false hope.

## Stress Management on the Job

EMS is a high-stress job. Understanding the causes of stress and knowing how to deal with stress are critical to your job performance, health, and interpersonal relationships. To prevent stress from negatively affecting your life, you need to understand what stress is, its physiologic effects, what you can do to minimize these effects, and how to deal with stress on an emotional level.

Stress is the effect of stressors on your physical and mental well-being. Stressors include emotional, physical, and environmental situations or conditions that may cause a variety of physiologic, physical, and psychological responses. The body's response to stress begins with an alarm response, followed by a stage of reaction and resistance. These stages are followed by recovery, or, if the stress is prolonged, exhaustion. This three-stage response is referred to as the **general adaptation syndrome**.

The physiologic responses involve the interaction of the endocrine and nervous systems, resulting in chemical and physical responses. This is commonly known as the fight-or-flight response. Positive stress, such as exercise, as well as negative forms of stress, such as shift work, long hours, or the frustration of losing a patient, all have the same physiologic manifestations. These responses include the following:

- Increased respirations and heart rate
- Increased blood pressure
- Constricted venous vessels near the skin surface (causes cool, clammy skin)
- Dilated pupils
- Tensed muscles
- Increased blood glucose levels
- Perspiration
- Decreased blood flow to the gastrointestinal tract

Situations that are stressful for EMS providers include the following:

- Dangerous situations
- Physical and psychological demands

- Critically ill or injured patients
- Dead and dying patients
- Overpowering sights, smells, and sounds
- Multiple-patient situations
- Angry or upset patients, family, or bystanders
- Unpredictability and demands of EMS
- Noncritical/nonemergency patients

As you examine this list, you will see some situations are clearly stressful: a car crash where a child is killed or a terrorist attack. Other situations may seem confusing—you may ask yourself why caring for noncritically ill patients would be considered stressful. You will need to manage several patients, and one person's definition of an emergency may be quite different from that of another. As you begin your career in EMS, you may envision that all of your calls will be exciting life-and-death calls where you are able to save lives. In reality, most patients are not critically ill and the care they need can become rather routine. This can create stress in people who are unable to make the transition from the TV image of emergency medicine to its reality.

## Words of Wisdom

Not all of the patients you care for will be critically ill or injured. This does not mean that they do not need care, only that they need a different type of care. A thoughtful word or a hand on a shoulder can be powerful medicine. Care for each person, regardless of his or her complaint, as a person. This is what it means to be a caregiver.

Reactions to stress can be categorized as acute, delayed, or cumulative. **Acute stress reactions** occur during a stressful situation. You feel nervous and excited, and your ability to focus increases. This focus can be very helpful in managing a crisis situation. But if the stress of the situation becomes too great, you are at risk of being caught up in the emotional and physical reactions to stress. Picture stress as a wave in the ocean. If the crest of the wave is too high, you can potentially become overwhelmed and drown. If stress goes unrecognized and is not relieved, you can be overcome by it.

**Delayed stress reactions** manifest after the stressful event. During the crisis, you are able to focus and function, but after things have calmed down, you may be left with nervous, excited energy that continues to build and becomes a distraction. With both acute and delayed reactions, the important question to ask yourself is: How did you manage these feelings during the stressful event? Were you able to continue, managing the stress well and taking it in stride? Or, were you unable to manage the stress well, resulting in a delayed stress reaction?

**Cumulative stress reactions** are the most important to understand. After the stressful event is over, are you able to shake off the effects? Are you still tired? Cumulative stress occurs when you are exposed to prolonged or excessive stress. You fight to remain in control and you are successful, but you are starting to grow tired. Now the next stressful situation occurs. Each time, you find it harder to recover because the effects of the previous stress are tiring.

Cumulative stress can cause physical symptoms such as fatigue, changes in appetite, gastrointestinal problems, or headaches. It may cause insomnia or hypersomnia, irritability, inability to concentrate, and hyperactivity or underactivity. Additionally, it may present with psychological reactions such as fear, dull or nonresponsive behavior, depression, guilt, oversensitivity, anger, irritability, and frustration. A fast-paced lifestyle compounds these effects by not allowing a person to rest and recover after periods of stress. Prolonged or excessive stress has been proven to be a strong contributor to heart disease, hypertension, cancer, alcoholism, and depression.

Many people are subject to cumulative stress, whereby insignificant stressors accumulate to create a larger stress-related problem. In the emergency services environment (EMS personnel, law enforcement officers, firefighters), stressors may also be sudden and severe. Some events are unusually stressful or emotional, even by EMS standards. These acute severe stressors result in what is referred to as critical incident stress. Events that can trigger critical incident stress include the following:

- Mass-casualty incidents
- Serious injury or traumatic death of a child
- Crashes with injuries caused by an emergency services provider while traveling to or from a call
- Death or serious injury of a coworker in the line of duty

# Posttraumatic Stress Disorder

**Posttraumatic stress disorder (PTSD)** may develop after a person has experienced a psychologically distressing event. It is characterized by reexperiencing the event and overresponding to stimuli that recall the event. Stressful events in EMS are sometimes psychologically overwhelming. Some of the symptoms include depression, startle reactions, flashback phenomena, and dissociative episodes (eg, amnesia of the event).

A process called **critical incident stress management (CISM)** was developed to address acute stress situations and potentially decrease the likelihood that PTSD will develop after such an incident (**FIGURE 2-31**). The process theoretically is used to confront the responses to critical incidents and defuse them, directing the emergency services personnel toward physical and emotional equilibrium. CISM can occur formally, as a debriefing for those who were on scene. In such situations, trained CISM teams of peers and mental health professionals may facilitate this. Additionally, CISM can occur at an ongoing scene in the following circumstances:

- When personnel are assessed for signs and symptoms of distress while resting
- Before reentering the scene
- During a scene demobilization in which personnel are educated about the signs of critical incident stress and given a buffer period to collect themselves before leaving

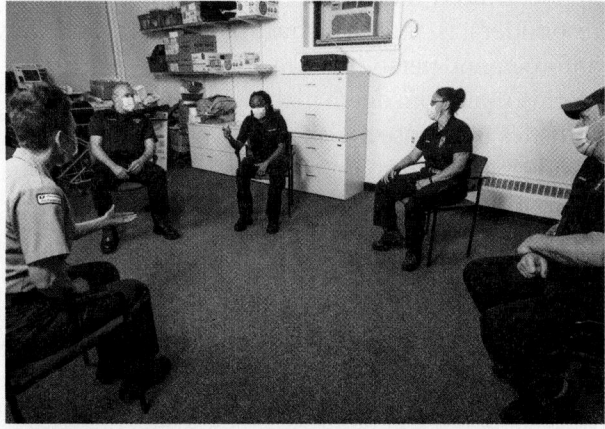

**FIGURE 2-31** Critical incident stress management is sometimes used to help providers manage stress.
© Jones & Bartlett Learning. Courtesy of MIEMSS.

Defusing sessions are the first to occur. These sessions are held during the event or immediately afterward. A group informally discusses events that they experienced together. Defusing sessions are designed to educate the participants as to the expectations over the next few days and give guidance on proper techniques to manage the feelings they may be experiencing. One example is to discourage drinking alcohol during this stressful time.

Debriefing sessions are held within 24 to 72 hours of a major incident. These meetings are held by a CISM team consisting of peers and mental health professionals. At the debriefing session, pent-up emotions can be properly expressed. It is more likely you will be ready to express your emotions more freely a few days following the event.

One of the important rules associated with the debriefing session is to not turn it into an operational critique. No one is right. No one is wrong. No one is to blame. Only emotions about the specific event are to be relayed. These debriefing sessions may have to be repeated at a later time.

CISM programs are located throughout the United States. You can locate a CISM in your area via the Internet, or it can be requested through your employer. The International Critical Incident Stress Foundation is dedicated to limiting the effects of stress on EMS providers through education and support services. For more information, go to the Foundation's website at www.icisf.org.

CISM is a helpful service for many providers, but it is not effective for everyone. Some providers are not receptive to helped by openly discussing psychologically traumatic memories with peers. If an EMT does not wish to participate in the CISM program, other services such as an employee assistance program or departmental peer support should be offered. When the individual's behavior is noticeably different after the event and CISM is not an option, private counseling by a mental health professional may be valuable.

## Burnout

**Burnout** is a term first coined in the 1970s to describe a combination of exhaustion, cynicism, and reduced performance resulting from long-term job stresses in health care and other high-stress professions. Like other negative aspects of distress, burnout affects not only the personal well-being of the EMT, but also the well-being of his or her colleagues and patients, through increased errors and decreased performance. In addition to the sources of stress mentioned, too much time at work or volunteering, and excessive nonpatient care administrative tasks have been specifically identified as contributors to burnout.

Burnout can result in increased major medical errors, increased likelihood of being involved in a lawsuit, increased rates of health care–associated infection, and increased patient mortality. In addition, burnout contributes to decreases in work morale, overall work effort, effective teamwork, and patient satisfaction, and an increase in job turnover.

## Compassion Fatigue

Sometimes described as "the cost of caring," **compassion fatigue** is common among those who work in health care and disaster and emergency services. Compassion fatigue, also known as secondary stress disorder, is a disorder characterized by gradual lessening of compassion over time. It differs from PTSD in that PTSD is caused by direct exposure to a traumatic incident or series of traumatic incidents, whereas compassion fatigue is a reaction to caring for others who have experienced trauma. Symptoms of compassion fatigue include the following:

- High absenteeism
- Difficult relationships with colleagues and coworkers
- Inability to work in teams
- Aggressive behavior toward patients
- Strong negative attitudes toward work
- Lack of empathy for patients
- Judgmental attitude toward patients
- Preoccupation with nonwork issues while on duty
- Other symptoms of increased stress

| TABLE 2-8 Warning Signs of Cumulative Stress |
|---|
| • Irritability toward coworkers, family, and friends |
| • Inability to concentrate |
| • Difficulty sleeping, increased sleeping, or nightmares |
| • Feelings of sadness, anxiety, or guilt |
| • Indecisiveness |
| • Loss of appetite (gastrointestinal disturbances) |
| • Loss of interest in sexual activities |
| • Isolation |
| • Loss of interest in work |
| • Increased use of alcohol |
| • Recreational drug use |
| • Physical symptoms such as chronic pain (headache, backache) |
| • Feelings of hopelessness |

© Jones & Bartlett Learning.

Supporting patients in emergency situations is difficult. It is stressful for them and for you. You are vulnerable to all the stresses that go with your profession. It is critical that you recognize the signs of cumulative stress so it does not interfere with your work or life away from work, including your family life. The signs and symptoms of cumulative stress may not be obvious at first. Rather, they may be subtle, and they may not be present all of the time (**TABLE 2-8**).

## Responder Risk for Suicide

Whereas suicide is the 10th leading cause of death in the United States, the rate among emergency responders is much higher. Firefighters and law enforcement personnel are more likely to die by suicide than from death in the line of duty. Although statistics like these are shocking, it must be kept in mind that suicides are estimated to be highly underreported, meaning that actual rates of suicide among responders are likely even higher.

Job stress is widely considered to be the largest contributing factor to suicide. In addition, the stigma of mental illness can keep responders from taking action to help others or to seek help themselves. In professions where being tough, brave, and reliable under any circumstances are key virtues, it can be extremely challenging for responders to seek help to cope with stress and trauma. It is crucial for

EMTs to recognize the signs of stress and trauma not only in friends and colleagues, but also in themselves. Moreover, it is crucial to seek consultation and assistance. Many emergency response organizations offer their own access to stress management and mental health services along with peer support teams and employee assistance programs. In addition, numerous national services are available to first responders. The Code Green Campaign is a mental health and advocacy organization for first responders. Its website directs those in need of emotional support to many resources, including the following:

- Fire/EMS Helpline (Share the Load): www.crewcarelife.com/crisis-support/, 1-888-731-FIRE (3473)
- National Suicide Prevention Lifeline: https://suicidepreventionlifeline.org, 1-800-273-TALK (8255)
- Center for Firefighter Behavioral Health: www.cffbh.org
- Safe Call Now: www.safecallnow.org

## Emotional Aspects of Emergency Care

At times, even the most experienced health care provider has difficulty overcoming personal reactions and proceeding without hesitation. You may have patients who need to be removed from life-threatening situations, or you need to provide life support measures to patients who are severely injured. You may also be called on to recover human remains from highway accidents, aircraft disasters, or explosions (**FIGURE 2-32**). In all of these situations, you must be calm and act responsibly as a member of the EMS team. You must also realize that

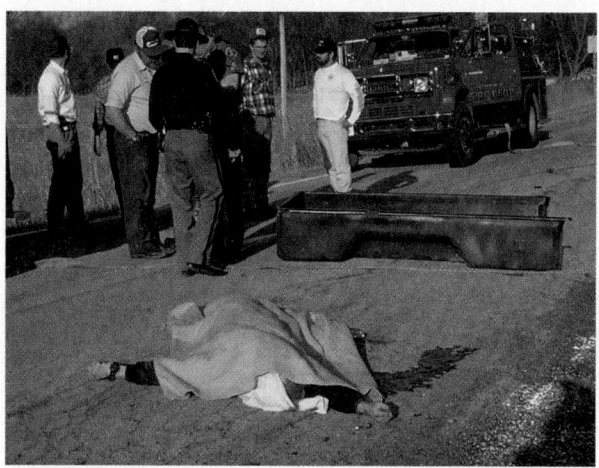

**FIGURE 2-32** As an EMT, you may be asked to recover and remove bodies from incident sites.

© James Schaffer/PhotoEdit, Inc.

# YOU are the Provider

Full resuscitative efforts are continued en route; however, the child has failed to respond to appropriate treatment. The child is reassessed, and a radio report is called in to the receiving facility.

| Recording Time: 18 Minutes | |
|---|---|
| **Level of consciousness** | Unconscious and unresponsive |
| **Respirations** | Absent |
| **Pulse** | Absent |
| **Skin** | Cool and cyanotic |
| **Blood pressure** | Not obtainable |
| **Spo$_2$** | Not obtainable |

The child is delivered to the emergency department (ED) and care is transferred to the attending physician. After an additional 15-minute period of resuscitative efforts in the ED, the child is pronounced dead. Later that evening, you find your partner in his dorm; he is crying and tells you he does not want to talk right now.

**8.** Does the death of a child affect the EMT differently than the death of an adult? If so, how?

**9.** How can you help your partner?

even though your personal emotions must be kept under control, these are normal feelings. You must deal with these feelings. The struggle to remain calm in the face of horrible circumstances contributes to the emotional stress of the job.

## Stressful Situations

Many situations, such as mass-casualty scenes; serious vehicle crashes; excavation cave-ins; house fires; infant and child trauma; amputations; abuse of an infant, child, spouse, or older person; or the death of a coworker or other public safety personnel will be stressful for everyone involved. During these situations, you must exercise extreme professional care in both your words and your actions at the scene. Words that do not seem important, or that are said jokingly, may hurt someone. Conversations at the scene must be professional. You should not say, "Everything will be all right," or "There is nothing to worry about." A person who is trapped in a wrecked car, hurting from head to foot and worried about a loved one, knows that all is not well. What will reassure the patient is your calm and caring approach to the emergency situation. Whether you are a brand-new EMT or a seasoned veteran, patients expect you to bring some sense of order and stability to the terrifying chaos that has suddenly engulfed them. Briefly explain your plan of action to assist the patient in the crisis. Inform the patient that you need his or her help and the assistance of family members or bystanders to carry out your plan of action.

How a patient reacts to injury or illness may be influenced by certain personality traits. Some patients may become highly emotional over what may seem to be a minor problem. Others may show little or no emotion, even after serious injury or illness. Many other factors influence how a patient reacts to the stress of an EMS incident. Among these factors are the following:

- Socioeconomic background
- Fear of medical personnel
- Alcohol or substance use disorders
- History of chronic disease
- Mental disorders
- Reaction to medication
- Age
- Nutritional status

- Feelings of guilt
- Past experience with illness or injury

You are not expected to always know why a patient is having an unusual emotional response. However, you can quickly and calmly assess the actions of the patient, family members, and bystanders. This assessment will help you to gain the confidence and cooperation of everyone at the scene. In addition, you should use a professional tone and show courtesy, along with sincere concern and efficient action. These simple considerations will go far to relieve worry, fear, and insecurity on the part of everyone involved. Your calm reassurance will inspire confidence and cooperation. Compassion is also important, but you must be careful. Your professional judgment takes priority over compassion. For example, suppose a screaming child with no obvious life-threatening injuries is covered with another patient's blood. This frightened child appeals to your sense of compassion and thus gets your attention. In the meantime, an unconscious, nonbreathing adult nearby could die from lack of care.

### Special Populations

When children are seriously ill or injured, family members and other people at the scene may be frantic. You should remain calm and confident in your skills because this may be all that is needed to provide reassurance to those at the scene.

Patients must be given the opportunity to express their fears and concerns. You can easily relieve many of these concerns at the scene. Usually, patients are concerned about the safety or well-being of others who are involved in the accident and about the damage or loss of personal property. Your responses must be discreet and diplomatic, giving reassurance when appropriate. If a loved one has been killed or critically injured, you should wait, if possible, until clergy or the ED staff can give the patient the news. They can provide the necessary psychological support the patient needs after receiving this type of news.

Some patients, especially children and older adults, may be terrified or feel rejected when separated from family members by uniformed EMS providers. Other patients may not want family members to share their stress, see their injury, or witness their pain. It is usually best if parents are transported with their children and relatives accompany older patients. Medical attention for a child often requires adult consent. Treatment may be delayed if a caregiver is not transported with the child.

Religious customs or needs of the patient must also be respected. Some people will cling to religious medals or charms, especially if you make any attempt to remove them. Other people will express a strong desire for religious counsel, baptism, or last rites if death is imminent. You must try to accommodate these requests. Some people have religious convictions that strongly oppose the use of medications, blood, and blood products. If you obtain such information about your patient, it is imperative that you report it to the next level of care.

In the event of a death, you must handle the body with respect and dignity. It must be exposed as little as possible. Learn your local regulations and protocols about moving the body or changing its position, especially if you are at a possible crime scene. Even in these situations, CPR and appropriate treatment must be given unless there are obvious signs of death.

## Workplace Issues

As our society grows more culturally diverse, so do EMS workplaces. You are required to provide an equal standard of care to all patients and also need to be able to work efficiently and effectively with other health care professionals from a variety of different backgrounds.

## Cultural Diversity on the Job

For many years, EMS and public safety have been dominated by Caucasian men. Currently 75% of EMS personnel are male and 85% identify as non-minority. The proactive EMT understands the benefits of a culturally diverse workforce to eliminate disparities in patient care. Socially equitable care is one of the EMS Agenda 2050 principles. EMTs should expect to work alongside coworkers with varying backgrounds, attitudes, beliefs, and values and to accept their differences.

Cultural diversity in EMS allows you to enjoy the benefits of accentuating the skills of a broad range of people. When you accept each coworker as an individual, the need to fit them into rigid roles is eliminated. To be more sensitive to cultural diversity issues, you must first be aware of your own cultural background. Ask yourself, "What are my own issues relative to race, color, religion, and ethnicity?" Because culture is not restricted to different nationalities, you should also consider age, disability, sex, sexual orientation, marital status, work experience, and education.

In sports, you play to your team's strengths. For example, in football, offensive lines have a fast side and a strong side, and they run plays toward either side depending on the situation. As part of an effective EMS team, you can make it part of your team's culture to play to your strengths.

Each individual is different, and you should communicate with coworkers and patients in a way that is sensitive to everyone's needs (**FIGURE 2-33**). Look at cultural diversity as an asset, and make the most of the differences among people in EMS, thus improving our ability to provide optimum patient care. As the public safety workplace becomes more culturally diverse, changes may occur that could be considered disruptive.

Alternatively, failure to diversify the workforce in the face of a culturally diverse patient population can lead to cultural incompetence. Diversity is an effective way to strengthen a public safety workforce. It is important to strive for cultural competency with coworkers as well as patients. Your ultimate goal should be cultural humility. This requires that you remain curious about others and continuously reflect on your viewpoints with an open mind. This process will allow you to constantly

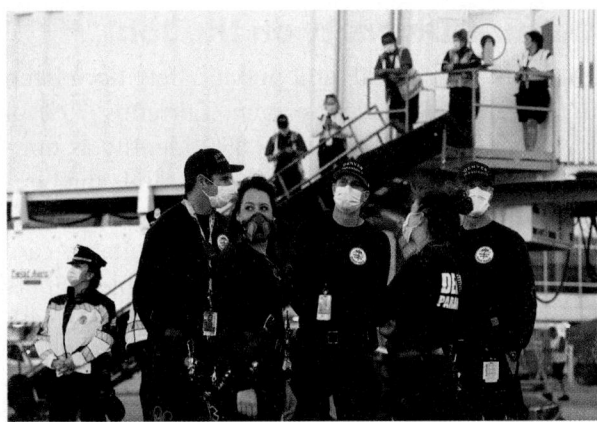

**FIGURE 2-33** Communicate with coworkers in a way that is sensitive and respectful to individual differences.

© Helen H. Richardson/MediaNews Group/The Denver Post via Getty Images/Contributor/Denver Post/Getty Images.

monitor your attitudes toward others, remain aware of your biases, and adapt your viewpoints if needed. It is sometimes difficult to be open and accepting of others who are different from yourself. To achieve cultural humility, you must first recognize the differences between yourself and those of other cultures, accept the differences, and in some cases adapt your behaviors based on them. This process is difficult for some, requiring much self-awareness and self-reflection, but it can yield rich rewards.

### Your Effectiveness as an EMT

To be an effective EMT, you need to discover the diverse cultural needs of your coworkers, as well as your patients and their families. Although it is unrealistic to expect you to become a cross-cultural expert with knowledge about all ethnicities, you should learn how to relate effectively.

Teamwork is essential in public safety and EMS. To work effectively as a team, you need to communicate to resolve cultural diversity issues.

When you are working with patients or calling the hospital on the radio, other EMTs may be sensitive to how you treat patients from their cultural group. Therefore, when referring to patients, you should use the appropriate language. Do not use terms such as, "cripple," "deformed," "drunk," "crazy," and "retard" to describe patients. The word "handicapped" even has a negative connotation. Instead, use the term "disabled," and describe the specific disability.

You might want to consider taking multilingual training classes. This will not only be useful in communicating with your coworkers; it will also help improve communication with your patients and sensitize you to the cultural richness of the people who are using the language.

Even the perception of discrimination can weaken morale and motivation and negatively affect the goal of EMS. Therefore, to achieve the benefits of cultural diversity in the EMS workplace, you must understand how to communicate effectively with coworkers from various backgrounds.

### Sexual Harassment

The number of reports of sexual harassment has increased in recent years because of increased scrutiny, along with guilty verdicts that have encouraged others to bring lawsuits concerning conduct that previously would have gone unchallenged.

*Sexual harassment* is any unwelcome sexual advance, request for sexual favors, or other verbal or physical conduct of a sexual nature when submitting is a condition of employment, submitting or rejecting is a basis for an employment decision, or such conduct substantially interferes with performance and/or creates a hostile or offensive work environment. Remember, even an overheard conversation can be construed as sexual harassment.

There are two types of sexual harassment: quid pro quo (the harasser requests sexual favors in exchange for something else, such as a promotion) and hostile work environment (jokes, touching, leering, requests for a date, talking about body parts).

Sexual harassment incidents include complaints of a hostile work environment. Remember, the intent of the harasser does not matter. What matters is the perception of the act and the effect the behavior has on someone else. For many years, it was not uncommon to walk into a fire station and see sexually suggestive posters, calendars, or cartoons and to hear sexual jokes or comments. This situation has changed because it is not acceptable professional practice.

Because EMTs and other public safety professionals depend on each other for their safety, it is especially important for you to develop nonadversarial relationships with coworkers. If you are concerned about a particular behavior, it may be helpful to ask yourself these questions: "Would I do or say this in front of my spouse, significant other, or parents?" "Would I want my family members to be exposed to this behavior?" "Would I want my behavior videotaped and shown on the evening news?"

If you have been harassed, you should report it according to local policy and procedure and keep notes of what happened and what was said.

## Substance Abuse

Drug and alcohol use in the workplace causes an increase in accidents and tension among workers, but most important, it can lead to poor treatment decisions. EMS personnel who use or abuse substances such as alcohol or marijuana are more likely to have problems with their work habits, and their driver's licenses may be revoked as a result. They may be absent from work more often than other workers. If the use of drugs or alcohol has occurred within hours before the start of their shift, the ability of EMS personnel to render emergency medical care may be diminished because of mental or physical impairment. Because of the seriousness of substance abuse, or misuse, many EMS systems now require personnel to undergo periodic random tests for illegal drug use and have "for cause" testing when it is believed that individuals are under the influence of alcohol or drugs. If you observe a coworker who appears impaired, it is your responsibility to immediately report to a supervisor. Covering for this type of behavior is not appropriate and has the potential to cause irreversible harm.

As a member of the EMS team, you are responsible for responding to the community's emergency medical needs. Hazards in the EMS workplace are many. If you or one of the members of your team has an alcohol or other drug problem, these risks are increased. Furthermore, drug use that occurs off the job does not necessarily decrease the risk if a team member is showing up at work still under the influence of a substance. Although it varies from state to state, a drug-related or alcohol-related arrest can result in the revocation of some or all driving privileges and even loss of EMT licensure.

---

### Safety Tips

Trust is your business. You will be given the privilege—and it is a privilege—to care for patients in their time of highest need. You must demonstrate that trust through consistent professionalism. Remember, you have support to help you make the right choice: your partner, your supervisor, your family.

---

Employee assistance programs are often available for EMS personnel. These agencies are contracted with the EMS department to provide a wide array of mental health, substance abuse, crisis management, and counseling services. Talk with your supervisor about resources that are available at your EMS department. Early intervention is the best bet to ensure a safe, alcohol- and drug-free workplace.

## Injury and Illness Prevention

According to the Bureau of Labor Statistics, approximately 4.1 million serious injuries and 4,500 deaths occur in US workplaces, with a direct cost of more than $50 billion each year. EMS providers visit EDs for work-related injuries and exposures over 20,000 times each year. As an EMT, you are most at risk for sprains and strains, exposures to blood and body fluids, and falls. Simple measures such as practicing safe lifting, using appropriate PPE, and wearing slip-resistant footwear can reduce the incidence of these visits.

Many companies, as well as EMS departments, have established injury and illness prevention programs to determine workplace hazards and implement a plan to mitigate those hazards. Each injury and illness prevention program should involve management and workers and include hazard identification, prevention, and control; education and training; and program evaluation.

Data show that injury and illness prevention programs pay dividends for the companies that implement them. Find out if your company has an injury and illness prevention program and learn how you can participate.

## YOU are the Provider SUMMARY

**1. How can you psychologically prepare yourself for this call?**

Regardless of your years of experience in EMS, you must prepare yourself psychologically and logistically when responding to *every* call.

You will experience anxiety during your response to the scene; this is a normal human reaction to a stressful event. The key is to recognize this and to remain focused on the critical tasks that lie ahead. Instead of reacting negatively, channel your anxiety into a positive psychological drive that will make you even more determined to provide the best emergency medical care possible.

You and your partner should have a plan; clearly delineate each of your roles when you arrive at the scene. Discuss the skills and interventions that may need to be performed, the equipment that will be required, and whether additional resources will be needed. Doing so will help minimize confusion at the scene and the psychological stress it causes.

**2. What is stress? How does it manifest?**

Stress is the body's physiologic response to any type of demand—good or bad—and is triggered by one or more stressors. A stressor is any emotional, physical, or environmental situation that causes a variety of physiologic, physical, and psychological responses. Although eustress prompts helpful reactions such as excitement and positivity, distress prompts negative reactions such as anxiety and self-destructive behaviors.

The body's response to stress begins with an alarm response. When stress is placed on the body—in this case, attempting to resuscitate a child in cardiac arrest—the nervous system releases adrenaline into the bloodstream, causing the fight-or-flight response. The alarm response is followed by a phase of reaction and resistance, and then recovery, or, if the stress is prolonged and ineffectively managed, exhaustion. This three-stage response to stress is called the general adaptation syndrome.

**3. What phase of the stress response are you experiencing right now?**

You are in an acutely stressful situation—attempting to resuscitate a child in cardiac arrest—and are experiencing the alarm response. Your nervous system is releasing adrenaline into the bloodstream, which is triggering the fight-or-flight response and causing your symptoms (eg, sweating, heart racing). As a result, your body has responded with a burst of energy that allows you to carry out your assigned task of suctioning the child's mouth and managing her airway (the "fight" response). If you were experiencing the "flight" response, you would either freeze or try to escape the situation altogether. The ability to effectively do your job—despite experiencing the symptoms of stress—indicates you are able to work under pressure.

**4. How should you respond to the mother?**

Anger is often expressed by very demanding behavior and/or yelling. In this case, anger is a predictable response given the seriousness of the situation.

Clearly, the situation looks grim, so in a calm, professional, and caring manner, reassure her that, although the situation is serious, you and your team are doing everything possible to save her child's life. Be honest, do not give her false hope, and do not make promises you cannot deliver. Your actions and words, even a simple touch, can communicate caring.

**5. What stage of the grieving process is the mother experiencing?**

The child's mother is actually simultaneously experiencing two stages of the grieving process—denial and anger. There are five stages of the grieving process: denial, anger, bargaining, depression, and acceptance. Not all people grieve in this order, and not all people experience all stages of the grieving process in the same way.

A person in denial refuses to accept the seriousness of the situation, makes unrealistic demands for miracles, or persistently fails to understand why there is no improvement in his or her loved one's condition.

Anger is usually the ugliest stage of the grieving process. During this phase, the person lashes out—usually at the EMS provider. Someone must be blamed, and those who are responsible must be punished. Anger often manifests as hostility toward the provider. Some people may become physically abusive, in which case law enforcement should be summoned to the scene.

**6. How can poorly managed stress affect your physical well-being?**

Most people can respond to sudden stress for a short time. However, prolonged or poorly managed stress can quickly drain the body of its reserves. This leaves it depleted of key nutrients, weakened, and more susceptible to disease.

In addition to the emotional damage that poorly managed stress can cause (eg, depression, guilt, persistent anxiety), it has been proven to be a strong contributor to heart disease, hypertension, cancer, alcoholism, and drug abuse, among other conditions.

**7. How can you mitigate the stress associated with the job?**

Before you can manage stress, you must first recognize its signs and symptoms and identify the stressors involved. Some stressors can be changed or eliminated altogether; others cannot. Caring for critically sick or injured patients is difficult. It is stressful for them, but also for you. It is critical to recognize the manifestations of stress so it does not interfere with your job or personal life.

The signs of chronic stress are not always obvious at first—they may be subtle, and they may not be present all the time. Warning signs include irritability toward coworkers, family, and friends; difficulty concentrating; insomnia, hypersomnia, or nightmares; anxiety; indecisiveness; loss of appetite; decreased sex drive; and loss of interest in work.

There are many useful and healthy strategies for managing stress; they may involve changing a few habits or your attitude. Behavioral tactics that have been shown to alleviate or eliminate the body's stress response include changing or eliminating the stressors (this is not always possible, especially in EMS), changing work hours, cutting back on overtime, changing your attitude about the stressor, developing a social network that does not involve your coworkers, and spending more time with your family.

There are also a number of exercises you can use to minimize the physical response to stress, such as periodic stretching; slow, deep breathing; regular physical exercise; and progressive muscle relaxation. If you are experiencing difficulty managing the stress associated with your job, you should consider seeing a professional counselor.

The key to successful stress management is to find a strategy that works for *you* and to use that strategy frequently and consistently. Remember, the signs of stress are not always present; you may not feel stressed, despite the fact that you are.

**8. Does the death of a child affect the EMT differently than the death of an adult? If so, how?**

The death of any patient is a tragic event. However, in our society, we often assume only older people are supposed to die, so most people are unprepared for what they will feel when a child's death does occur—including EMS personnel. It is common for EMS providers to feel they did not do everything possible for the child, despite the fact that they indeed provided their best resuscitative efforts.

It is normal to feel sadness and depression following the death of a child; however, unlike the death of an older person, these feelings are often more profound. Children only account for approximately 10% of all EMS calls; therefore, the death of a child—expected or not—often catches the EMT off guard, resulting in a greater degree of stress and anxiety compared to what is experienced following the death of an adult.

**9. How can you help your partner?**

Your partner's behavior is consistent with a critical incident stress reaction. Many people are prone to cumulative stress. In the emergency services field, stressors are often sudden and more severe; therefore, many events are unusually stressful or emotional, even by emergency services standards.

So, how do you help your partner? If he or she does not wish to talk, do not force the issue. He or she needs time to collect his or her thoughts and to grieve—just like the parents. However, you should reassure your partner that you are willing to listen; some people experience relief just by talking to a coworker, family member, or friend. In other cases, your partner may need to speak to a counselor.

You should alert your supervisor to your partner's crisis. If your partner is not emotionally fit to provide safe and effective emergency care, he or she should be replaced for the rest of the shift. In some cases, a grieving EMT or paramedic will become angry if his or her crisis is reported to the supervisor. However, you should reassure your partner that you reported the incident out of concern for his or her physical and emotional well-being. EMS personnel do not just look out for each other during an EMS call; they should also look out for each other after the call—even if it is just as a "sounding board."

## YOU are the Provider SUMMARY *continued*

### EMS Patient Care Report (PCR)

| **Date:** 5-19-20 | **Incident No.:** 020109 | **Nature of Call:** Child not breathing | | **Location: 6** Catoonah Street | |
|---|---|---|---|---|---|
| **Dispatched:** 0840 | **En Route:** 0841 | **At Scene:** 0847 | **Transport:** 0859 | **At Hospital:** 0912 | **In Service:** 0935 |

#### Patient Information

| **Age:** 4 | **Allergies:** None |
|---|---|
| **Sex:** F | **Medications:** None |
| **Weight (in kg [lb]):** 19 kg (42 lb) | **Past Medical History:** None |
| | **Chief Complaint:** Cardiopulmonary arrest |

#### Vital Signs

| **Time:** 0847 | **BP:** Unobtainable | **Pulse:** Absent | **Respirations:** Absent | **Spo$_2$:** Unobtainable |
|---|---|---|---|---|
| **Time:** 0852 | **BP:** Unobtainable | **Pulse:** Absent | **Respirations:** Absent | **Spo$_2$:** Unobtainable |
| **Time:** 0858 | **BP:** Unobtainable | **Pulse:** Absent | **Respirations:** Absent | **Spo$_2$:** Unobtainable |
| **Time:** 0901 | **BP:** Unobtainable | **Pulse:** Absent | **Respirations:** Absent | **Spo$_2$:** Unobtainable |
| **Time:** 0905 | **BP:** Unobtainable | **Pulse:** Absent | **Respirations:** Absent | **Spo$_2$:** Unobtainable |
| **Time:** 0909 | **BP:** Unobtainable | **Pulse:** Absent | **Respirations:** Absent | **Spo$_2$:** Unobtainable |
| **Time:** 0912 | **BP:** Unobtainable | **Pulse:** Absent | **Respirations:** Absent | **Spo$_2$:** Unobtainable |

#### EMS Treatment (circle all that apply)

| **Oxygen @ ___ L/min via:**<br><br>NC    NRM    Bag mask | | **Assisted Ventilation** | **Airway Adjunct** | (CPR) |
|---|---|---|---|---|
| **Defibrillation** | **Bleeding Control** | **Bandaging** | **Splinting** | **Other:** (AED) |

#### Narrative

9-1-1 dispatch for an un conscious child not breathing.

Chief Complaint: Cardiopulmonary arrest

History: The child's mother stated when she went to wake up her child, she was unconscious, unresponsive, and not breathing; she called 9-1-1 and began CPR. The mother denies her child has any significant past medical history or drug allergies. She further denies any recent trauma or potentially toxic ingestion.

Assessment: On arrival, EMS found a 4-year-old girl pulseless and apneic.

Treatment (Rx): Two EMRs performing CPR on arrival. EMS providers took over CPR. EMS applied an automated external defibrillator. AED advised no-shock and CPR was immediately resumed. After 2 minutes of CPR, confirmed effective by observation and carotid pulse, reassessment revealed the child remained apneic and pulseless. Cardiac monitor was applied, revealing asystole. Paramedic performed resuscitative efforts at the scene for approximately 12 minutes, and then loaded the child into the ambulance and began transport.

Transport: The child's mother accompanied her to the hospital and was secured in the passenger's seat of the ambulance. Continued CPR and appropriate medication therapy en route. The child's condition remained unchanged; she remained apneic and pulseless and the electrocardiogram continued to show asystole. Delivered the child, whose condition remained unchanged, to the ED staff and gave verbal report to the attending physician. Provided emotional support to the child's mother and then returned to service.

**End of report**

# Prep Kit

## Ready for Review

- Your health and wellness are the foundation for your career; without these, you cannot provide care. Wellness includes your mental, physical, and social well-being.
- Components of wellness include protecting yourself from communicable diseases and scene hazards; maintaining proper nutrition; getting sufficient exercise, relaxation, and sleep; refraining from use of tobacco and inappropriate use of drugs and alcohol; and taking time to relax, engage with others, and enjoy life.
- Every patient encounter should be considered potentially dangerous. It is essential that you take all available precautions to minimize exposure and risk to scene hazards and infectious and communicable diseases.
- A communicable disease is any disease that can be spread from person to person or animal to person.
- Infectious diseases can be transmitted by contact (direct or indirect), or they can be airborne, foodborne, or vector-borne.
- Even if you are exposed to an infectious disease, your risk of becoming ill is small.
- Whether or not an acute infection occurs depends on several factors, including the amount and type of infectious organism and your resistance to that infection.
- You can take several steps to protect yourself against exposure to infectious diseases, including:
  - Keeping up to date with recommended vaccinations
  - Following standard precautions at all times
  - Handling all needles and other sharp objects with great care
- Because it is often impossible to tell which patients have infectious diseases, you should avoid direct contact with the blood and body fluids of all patients.
- You should know what to do if you are exposed to an airborne or bloodborne disease. Your department's designated officer will be able to help you follow the protocol set up in your area.
- Infection control should be an important part of your daily routine. Be sure to follow the proper steps when dealing with potential exposure situations.
- If you think you may have been exposed to an infectious disease, see your physician (or your employer's designated physician) immediately.
- Scene hazards include potential exposure to the following:
  - Hazardous materials
  - Electricity
  - Fire
- At a hazardous materials incident, your safety is the most important consideration. Never approach an object labeled with a hazardous materials placard or label. Use binoculars to read the placards or labels from a safe distance.
- Do not begin caring for patients until they have been moved away from the scene and decontaminated by the hazardous materials team or the scene has been made safe for you to enter.
- Wearing protective clothing and specialized gear is another important component in preventing injury.
- Part of your role is to know how to care for critically ill and injured patients. Becoming familiar with interpersonal communication techniques to use in these situations will allow you to communicate with patients and their families in an optimal way.
- You will encounter death, dying patients, and the families and friends of those who have died. Your appropriate response to grief can have a significant effect on those with whom you work.
- Recognizing the signs of stress is important for all EMTs. When signs of stress such as fatigue, anxiety, or anger; feelings of hopelessness, worthlessness, or guilt; and other such indicators are present, behavioral problems can develop.

- Violent situations can create many hazards for EMS personnel. If you see the potential for violence during a scene size-up, call for additional resources.

- Common workplace issues include cultural diversity, sexual harassment, and substance abuse. You should know what to do to avoid or address these situations.

## Vital Vocabulary

**acute stress reactions** Reactions to stress that occur during a traumatic situation.

**aerosol-generating procedure** Treatments that increase the risk for transmission of infections that are spread through the air or by droplets; CPR is an example.

**airborne transmission** The spread of an organism via droplets or dust.

**bloodborne pathogens** Pathogenic microorganisms that are present in human blood and can cause disease in humans. These pathogens include, but are not limited to, hepatitis B virus and human immunodeficiency virus (HIV).

**burnout** A combination of exhaustion, cynicism, and reduced performance resulting from long-term job stresses in health care and other high-stress professions.

**Centers for Disease Control and Prevention (CDC)** The primary federal agency that conducts and supports public health activities in the United States. The CDC is part of the US Department of Health and Human Services.

**communicable disease** A disease that can be spread from one person or species to another.

**compassion fatigue** A stress disorder characterized by gradual lessening of compassion over time.

**concealment** The use of objects to limit a person's ability to see you.

**contamination** The presence of infectious organisms on or in objects such as dressings, water, food, needles, wounds, or a patient's body.

**cover** The tactical use of an impenetrable barrier for protection.

**critical incident stress management (CISM)** A process that confronts the responses to critical incidents and defuses them, directing the emergency services personnel toward physical and emotional equilibrium.

**cumulative stress reactions** Prolonged or excessive stress.

**delayed stress reactions** Reactions to stress that occur after a stressful situation.

**designated officer** The individual in the department who is charged with the responsibility of managing exposures and infection control issues.

**direct contact** Exposure or transmission of a communicable disease from one person to another by physical contact.

**distress** A negative response to a stressor.

**eustress** A beneficial response to a stressor.

**exposure** A situation in which a person has had contact with blood, body fluids, tissues, or airborne particles in a manner that suggests disease transmission may occur.

**foodborne transmission** The contamination of food or water with an organism than can cause disease.

**general adaptation syndrome** The body's response to stress that begins with an alarm response, followed by a stage of reaction and resistance, and then recovery or, if the stress is prolonged, exhaustion.

**hepatitis** Inflammation of the liver, usually caused by a viral infection, that causes fever, loss of appetite, jaundice, fatigue, and altered liver function.

**host** The organism or individual that is attacked by the infecting agent.

**human immunodeficiency virus (HIV)** Acquired immunodeficiency syndrome (AIDS) is caused by HIV, which damages the cells in the body's immune system so that the body is unable to fight infection or certain cancers.

**immune** The body's ability to protect itself from acquiring a disease.

**indirect contact**  Exposure or transmission of disease from one person to another by contact with a contaminated object.

**infection**  The abnormal invasion of a host or host tissues by organisms such as bacteria, viruses, or parasites, with or without signs or symptoms of disease.

**infection control**  Procedures to reduce transmission of infection among patients and health care personnel.

**infectious disease**  A medical condition caused by the growth and spread of small, harmful organisms within the body.

**Occupational Safety and Health Administration (OSHA)**  The federal regulatory compliance agency that develops, publishes, and enforces guidelines concerning safety in the workplace.

**pathogen**  A microorganism that is capable of causing disease in a susceptible host.

**personal protective equipment (PPE)**  Protective equipment that blocks exposure to a pathogen or a hazardous material.

**posttraumatic stress disorder (PTSD)**  A delayed stress reaction to a prior incident. Often the result of one or more unresolved issues concerning the incident, and may relate to an incident that involved physical harm or the threat of physical harm.

**resilience**  The capacity of an individual to cope with and recover from distress.

**standard precautions**  Protective measures that have traditionally been developed by the CDC for use in dealing with objects, blood, body fluids, and other potential exposure risks of communicable disease.

**transmission**  The way in which an infectious disease is spread: contact, airborne, by vehicles, or by vectors.

**vector-borne transmission**  The use of an animal to spread an organism from one person or place to another.

**wellness**  The active pursuit of a state of good health.

## References

1. Barber E, Newland C, Young A, Rose M. Survey reveals alarming rates of EMS provider stress and thoughts of suicide. *JEMS* website. https://www.jems.com/2015/09/28/survey-reveals-alarming-rates-of-ems-provider-stress-and-thoughts-of-suicide/. Published September 28, 2015. Accessed March 6, 2020.

2. Centers for Disease Control and Prevention, National Center for Emerging and Zoonotic Infectious Diseases, Division of Healthcare Quality Promotion. Infection control basics. CDC website. https://www.cdc.gov/infectioncontrol/basics/index.html. Reviewed January 5, 2016. Accessed March 6, 2020.

3. Centers for Disease Control and Prevention, National Institute for Occupational Safety and Health. EMS providers: how to stay safe on the job. https://www.ems.gov/pdf/workforce/Provider-Resources/NIOSH_EMS_Provider_Safety_Infographic.pdf. Accessed March 6, 2020.

4. Collingwood J. The relationship between mental and physical health. PsychCentral website. https://psychcentral.com/lib/the-relationship-between-mental-and-physical-health/. Updated October 8, 2018. Accessed March 6, 2020.

5. Compassion Fatigue Awareness Project. https://compassionfatigue.org/. Published 2017. Accessed March 6, 2020.

6. Division of Sleep Medicine, Harvard Medical School. Twelve simple tips to improve your sleep. Healthy Sleep website. http://healthysleep.med.harvard.edu/healthy/getting/overcoming/tips. Reviewed December 18, 2007. Accessed March 6, 2020.

7. Dyrbye LN, Shanafelt TD, Sinsky CA, et al. Burnout among health care professionals: a call to explore and address this underrecognized threat to safe, high-quality care. *NAM Perspectives*. https://doi.org/10.31478/201707b. Published July 5, 2017. Accessed March 6, 2020.

8. Gormley MA, Crowe RP, Bentley MA, Levine R. A national description of violence toward emergency medical services personnel. *Prehosp Emerg Care*. 2016;20(4):439-447.

9. Grant L, Kinman G. Emotional resilience in the helping professions and how it can be enhanced: health and social care education. *J Health Soc Care Ed*. 2015;3(1):3(1):23-34.

10. Hayeman M, Dill J, Douglas R. Police officers and firefighters are more likely to die by suicide than in line of duty. Ruderman Family Foundation website. https://rudermanfoundation.org/white_papers/police-officers-and-firefighters-are-more-likely-to-die-by-suicide-than-in-line-of-duty/. Accessed March 6, 2020.

11. Khalsa S, Barnes L, Audet R, et al. The impact of cultural humility in prehospital healthcare delivery and education a position paper from the National Association of EMS Educators (NAEMSE). *Prehosp Emerg Care*. 2020;27:1-5. doi:10.1080/10903127.2019.1709001.

12. Maguire BJ, Browne M, O'Neill BJ, Dealy MT, Clare D, O'Meara P. International survey of violence against EMS personnel: physical violence report. *Prehosp Disaster Med.* 2018;33(5):526-531.

13. National Association of Emergency Medical Technicians. 2016 Mental Health Survey Report. http://www.naemt.org/docs/default-source/ems-health-and-safety-documents/mental-health-grid/2016-naemt-mental-health-report-8-14-16.pdf. Published 2016. Accessed March 6, 2020.

14. National Association of Emergency Medical Technicians. New guide to building an effective EMS wellness and resilience program. http://www.naemt.org/WhatsNewALLNEWS/2019/01/18/new-guide-to-building-an-effective-ems-wellness-and-resilience-program. Published January 18, 2019. Accessed March 6, 2020.

15. National Highway Traffic Safety Administration. EMS Agenda 2050: envision the future. EMS.gov website. http://emsagenda2050.org. Accessed March 6, 2020.

16. Patterson PD, Higgins JS, Dongen HPAV, et al. Evidence-based guidelines for fatigue risk management in emergency medical services. *Prehosp Emerg Care.* 2018;22(Suppl 1):89-101.

17. Patterson PD, Weaver MD, Guyette FX. Studying sleep health and fatigue in EMS. EMS1.com website. https://www.ems1.com/ems-products/consulting-management-and-legal-services/articles/studying-sleep-health-and-fatigue-in-ems-3narld42peye9MHM/. Updated August 2, 2017. Accessed March 6, 2020.

18. Reith TP. Burnout in United States healthcare professionals: a narrative review. *Cureus.* 2018;10(12):e3681. https://doi.org/10.7759/cureus.3681

19. Rutherford B, Krueger GP. General effects of EMS fatigue. Markel Specialty website. https://www.markelinsurance.com/resources/medical-transportation/general-effects-of-ems-fatigue. Published 2019. Accessed March 6, 2020.

20. Simon S. How to quit smoking. American Cancer Society website. https://www.cancer.org/latest-news/how-to-quit-smoking.html. Published January 2, 2020. Accessed March 6, 2020.

21. University of Phoenix. Majority of first responders face mental health challenges. https://www.phoenix.edu/about_us/media-center/news/uopx-releases-first-responder-mental-health-survey-results.html. Published April 18, 2017. Accessed March 6, 2020.

22. US Fire Administration. Preventing suicide among first responders. https://www.usfa.fema.gov/operations/infograms/080819.html. Published August 8, 2019. Accessed March 6, 2020.

23. US Fire Administration. Violence against EMS responders. https://www.usfa.fema.gov/current_events/083117.html. Published August 31, 2017. Accessed March 6, 2020.

24. Vigil NH, Grant AR, Perez O, et al. Death by suicide—the EMS profession compared to the general public. *Prehosp Emerg Care.* 2019;23(3):340-345.

25. World Health Organization. Health promotion and disease prevention through population-based interventions, including action to address social determinants and health inequity. http://www.emro.who.int/about-who/public-health-functions/health-promotion-disease-prevention.html. Accessed March 6, 2020.

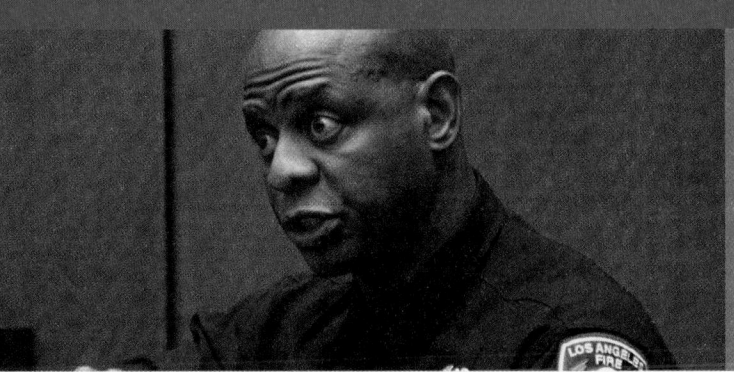

# Medical, Legal, and Ethical Issues

## NATIONAL EMS EDUCATION STANDARD COMPETENCIES

### Preparatory

Applies fundamental knowledge of the emergency medical services (EMS) system, safety/well-being of the emergency medical technician (EMT), medical/legal, and ethical issues to the provision of emergency care.

### Medical/Legal and Ethics

- Consent/refusal of care (pp 86–90)

- Confidentiality (p 91)
- Advance directives (pp 93–95)
- Tort and criminal actions (pp 101–103)
- Evidence preservation (p 105)
- Statutory responsibilities (pp 103–104)
- Mandatory reporting (pp 104–105)
- Ethical principles/moral obligations (pp 106–107)
- End-of-life issues (pp 95–97)

## KNOWLEDGE OBJECTIVES

1. Define consent and how it relates to decision making. (p 86)
2. Compare expressed consent, implied consent, and involuntary consent. (pp 87–88)
3. Discuss consent by minors for treatment or transport. (p 88)
4. Describe local EMS system protocols for using forcible restraint. (pp 89–90)
5. Discuss the EMT's role and obligations if a patient refuses treatment or transport. (pp 90–91)
6. Describe the relationship between patient communications, confidentiality, and the Health Insurance Portability and Accountability Act (HIPAA). (pp 91–92)
7. Discuss the importance of do not resuscitate (DNR) orders and local protocols as they relate to the EMS environment. (pp 93–95)
8. Describe the physical, presumptive, and definitive signs of death. (pp 95–96)
9. Explain how to manage patients who are identified as organ donors. (p 97)
10. Recognize the importance of medical identification devices in treating the patient. (p 97)
11. Discuss the scope of practice and standards of care. (pp 98–100)
12. Describe the EMT's legal duty to act. (p 100)
13. Discuss the issues of negligence, abandonment, assault and battery, and kidnapping and their implications for the EMT. (pp 101–103)
14. Explain the reporting requirements for special situations, including abuse, drug- or felony-related injuries, childbirth, and crime scenes. (pp 104–105)

15. Define ethics and morality and their implications for the EMT. (pp 106–107)

16. Describe the roles and responsibilities of the EMT in court. (pp 107–109)

## SKILLS OBJECTIVES

There are no skills objectives for this chapter.

# Introduction

A basic medical, legal, and ethical principle of emergency care is to first do no further harm. As an EMT, you will have the opportunity to do considerably more for your patients than simply preventing further injury. A thorough understanding of medical, legal, and ethical issues related to EMS is essential. EMTs are better positioned to avoid professional legal problems when they act in good faith, follow an appropriate standard of care, and provide compassionate care.

EMTs provide **emergency medical care**—that is, immediate care or treatment—and are often the first link in the chain of prehospital care. As the scope and nature of emergency medical care becomes more complex, litigation involving participants in EMS systems will likely increase. Providing competent emergency medical care that conforms to the scope and standard of care will help you to avoid both civil and criminal actions.

You must also consider ethical issues. As an EMT, should you stop and treat patients who were involved in an automobile crash while you are en route to another emergency call? Should you begin CPR on a patient who, according to the family, has terminal cancer? Should you begin treatment on a child with obvious signs of death because the parents are begging you to do something? Consider the following situations:

- While transporting a patient to the hospital, he states, "I don't want to go to the hospital anymore. You have to let me out."
- As you begin treating a child you suspect might be the victim of abuse, a parent commands you to stop.
- Your partner takes out his phone to post a comment on his social media account about the last emergency call.

What should you do? Even when emergency medical care is properly rendered, there are still times when you may be sued by a patient who seeks compensation. Administrative action, such as suspension of your state EMT license, may be brought against you for failure to abide by the regulations of your state EMS agency. For these reasons, you must understand the various legal aspects of emergency medical care.

# Consent

Typically, consent is required from every conscious adult before care can be started. A person receiving care must give permission, or **consent**, for treatment. An adult who is conscious, rational, and capable of making informed decisions has a legal right to refuse care, even though this person may be ill or injured. A patient may also consent to some aspects of care and deny consent for others. If the patient refuses care, you may not care for the patient. In fact, doing so may be grounds for both criminal and civil action. Consent can be expressed (actual) or implied.

The foundation of consent is decision-making capacity. **Decision-making capacity** is the ability of a patient to understand the information you are providing, coupled with the ability to process that information and make an informed choice regarding medical care. It is important to keep in mind that the law allows the patient to make choices that may seem medically unsound and that might endanger the patient's life. The right of a patient to make decisions concerning his or her health is known as **patient autonomy**. The terms *decision-making capacity* and *competence* are often used interchangeably but there is a distinction: Competence is generally regarded as a legal term and determinations regarding competence are typically made by a court of law, whereas decision-making capacity is the term more commonly used in health care to determine whether or not a patient is capable of making health care decisions.

The following factors should be considered when determining a patient's decision-making capacity:

- Is the patient's intellectual capacity impaired by mental limitation or any type of dementia?
- Is the patient of legal age (18 years old in most states)?
- Is the patient impaired by alcohol or drug intoxication or serious injury or illness?
- Does the patient appear to be experiencing significant pain?
- Does the patient have a significant injury that could distract him from a more serious injury? (For example, a significant non–life-threatening injury can cause extreme pain and distract the patient from neck pain, which could indicate a potentially more serious problem.)
- Are there any apparent hearing or visual problems?
- Is a language barrier present? Do you and your patient speak the same language?
- Does the patient appear to understand what you are saying? Does he or she ask rational questions that demonstrate an understanding of the information you are trying to share?

You should be familiar with various types of consent. These include expressed consent, implied consent, and involuntary consent.

## Expressed Consent

**Expressed consent** (or actual consent) is the type of consent given when the patient specifically acknowledges that he or she wants you to provide care or transport. Expressed consent may be verbal or nonverbal. For example, if you ask a patient if you can check his or her blood pressure and the patient says yes, that is verbal consent; if the patient nods yes or extends an arm to you, the patient is expressing consent nonverbally.

To be valid, the consent the patient provides must be **informed consent**, which means that you explained the nature of the treatment being offered, along with the potential risks, benefits, and alternatives to treatment, as well as potential consequences of refusing treatment. Often, the prehospital environment requires that consent be obtained more quickly than in the hospital setting. Paramedics will often provide additional information if advanced life support (ALS) interventions are necessary. In such cases, there is a greater potential for side effects and other adverse responses associated with drug administration and other forms of advanced care.

Informed consent is valid if given verbally, but it may be difficult to prove at a later point in time. Rarely do EMS providers have patients sign a consent form, so it is always advisable to document consent in your run report. Having someone witness the patient's consent may be helpful if the issue of consent is later challenged in court.

Remember, a patient may agree to certain types of emergency medical care but not to others. The patient's right to refuse treatment is discussed later in this chapter.

## Street Smarts

Rather than specifically saying, "We would like your consent," the EMT can work the consent into the conversation more casually. For example, the EMT may say, "We're from the ambulance. We're here to take care of you. We would like to check your blood pressure and check you over. Are you okay with that?"

## YOU are the Provider

At 1720 hours, you are dispatched to a grocery store at 1175 N. Main Street for a man with a severe headache. You respond to the scene, which is located only a few miles away. The weather is clear, the temperature is 90°F (32°C), and the traffic is heavy.

1. Why is it essential that you obtain consent to treat the patient once you arrive?
2. Should you assess the patient's competency or decision-making capacity once you arrive?

## Implied Consent

When a person is unconscious or otherwise incapable of making a rational, informed decision about care and unable to give consent, the law assumes that the patient would consent to care and transport to a medical facility if he or she were able to do so (**FIGURE 3-1**). Patients who are intoxicated by drugs or alcohol, mentally impaired, or suffering from certain conditions such as head injury might be included in this category. The legal principle that allows treatment under such circumstances is called implied consent. Implied consent applies only when a serious medical condition exists and should never be used unless there is a threat to life or limb. For this reason, the principle of implied consent is known as the emergency doctrine. Sometimes what represents a serious threat may be unclear. This may result in legal proceedings and a medicolegal judgment, which should be supported by your best efforts to obtain consent and a thoroughly documented run report. In most instances, the law allows a spouse, a close relative, or next of kin to give consent for an injured person who is unable to do so, and you should make every effort to obtain consent from an available relative before treating based on implied consent; however, treatment should never be delayed when the patient has imminently life-threatening injuries. It is also important to understand that if a patient being treated based on implied consent were to regain

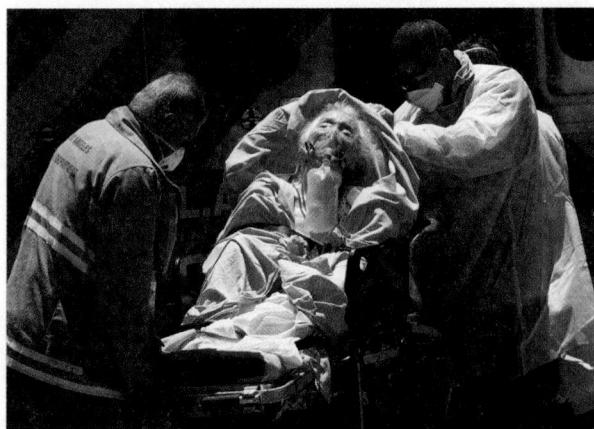

**FIGURE 3-1** When a serious threat to life exists and the patient is unconscious or otherwise unable to give consent, the law assumes that the patient would give consent to care and transport to the hospital.

© Genaro Molina/Los Angeles Times/Getty Images.

consciousness and appear capable of making an informed decision, the doctrine of implied consent would no longer apply. This often occurs with calls involving diabetic emergencies, overdoses, syncope, and seizures.

## Involuntary Consent

Assisting patients who are mentally ill, developmentally delayed, or who are in behavioral (psychological) crisis is complicated. An adult patient who is mentally incompetent is not able to give informed consent. From a legal perspective, this situation is similar to those involving minors. Consent for emergency care should be obtained from someone who is legally responsible for the patient, such as a guardian or conservator. In many cases, however, such permission will not be readily obtainable. Many states have protective custody statutes allowing such a person to be taken, under law enforcement authority, to a medical facility. Under certain conditions, law enforcement and prison officials are legally permitted to give consent for any individual who is incarcerated or has been placed under arrest. However, a prisoner who is conscious and capable of making decisions does not necessarily surrender the right to make medical decisions and may refuse care. Know the provisions in your area and involve online medical control in the process.

## Minors and Consent

Because a minor might not have the wisdom, maturity, or judgment to give consent, the law requires that a parent or legal guardian, when available, give consent for treatment or transport (**FIGURE 3-2**). In every state, when a parent cannot be reached to provide consent, health care providers are allowed to give emergency care to a child. In some states, a minor can consent to receive medical care, depending on the minor's age and maturity. A great deal of confusion surrounds the issue of emancipated minors. Emancipated minors are people who, despite being under the legal age in a given state (in most cases the age is 18 years), can be legally treated as adults based on certain circumstances. For example, many states consider minors to be emancipated if they are married, if they are members of the armed services, or if they are parents. A minor who

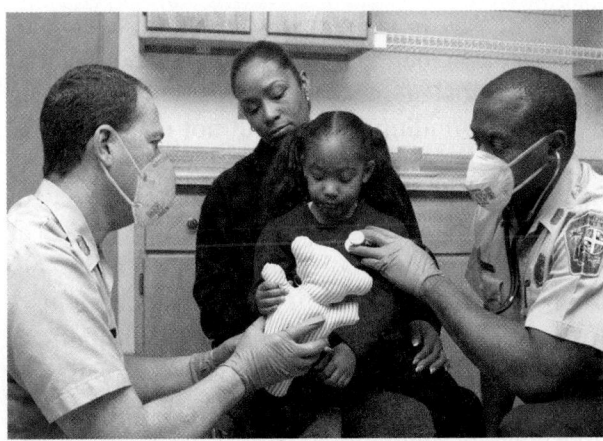

**FIGURE 3-2** The law requires that a parent or a legal guardian give consent for treatment or transport of a minor. However, you must never withhold life-saving care.

© Jones & Bartlett Learning. Courtesy of MIEMSS.

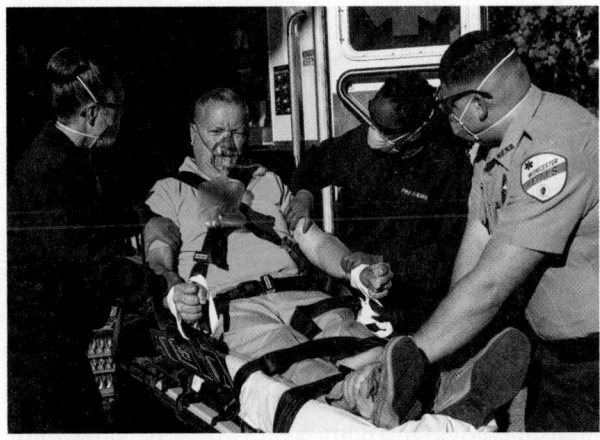

**FIGURE 3-3** Be sure that you know the local laws about forcible restraint of a patient. In some states, only a police officer has the authority to restrain a patient.

© Jones & Bartlett Learning.

is a parent may also give consent for his or her own child. In addition, a minor is usually considered emancipated if living away from and no longer relying on his or her parents for support. A court may issue an order declaring a minor to be emancipated but this is not commonly seen. You should know your state's laws concerning the issues surrounding emancipation.

If a minor is injured and requires medical treatment in a school or camp setting, teachers and school officials may act **in loco parentis**, which means in the position or place of a parent, and can legally give consent for treatment of the minor if a parent or guardian is not available. You should still attempt to obtain consent from a parent or legal guardian whenever possible; however, if a true emergency exists and the parent or legal guardian is not available, the consent to treat the minor is implied, just as with an adult. You must never withhold life-saving care for a minor because a person authorized to provide consent is not available.

It is important to reach the parent or guardian as quickly as possible. Even though life-saving interventions will not be delayed, it is possible that other interventions at the hospital could be delayed until consent is obtained. Follow local protocol or consult medical control to determine if someone acting in loco parentis will need to accompany the child during transport and be present at the receiving hospital until a parent or guardian arrives.

## Forcible Restraint

**Forcible restraint** is sometimes necessary when you are confronted with a patient who is in need of medical treatment and transportation but is combative and presents a significant physical risk of danger to himself or herself, rescuers, or others (**FIGURE 3-3**). Such behavior may result from an underlying psychiatric or behavioral condition, the effects of drugs, or a medical condition such as a head injury or hypoxia. Typically, you should consult medical control for authorization to restrain or contact law enforcement personnel who have the authority to restrain people. In some states, only a police officer may forcibly restrain an individual. You should be knowledgeable about local laws. Restraint without legal authority exposes you to potential civil and criminal penalties. Restraint may be used only in circumstances of risk to the patient or others. When a patient is combative and poses a risk to the rescuer, it is advisable to wait for law enforcement to arrive on scene before attempting to treat the patient. See Chapter 23, *Behavioral Health Emergencies*, for a complete discussion of the use of restraint.

Your service should have clearly defined protocols to deal with situations involving restraint. Restraints should be considered only if the patient has a medical condition that appears serious or if he or she suffers from an apparent behavioral disorder that poses a risk to the patient or others. Verbal deescalation should always be attempted prior to considering physical restraints. The patient's decision-making capacity should be assessed and thoroughly documented. After restraints are applied, they should not be removed en route unless they pose a risk to the patient, even if the patient promises to behave. Appropriate safe strategies for restraint should be used to minimize the risk of harm to the patient. It is essential that you protect the patient's airway and monitor the patient's respiratory and circulatory status while restrained to avoid asphyxia, aspiration, and other complications. Consider calling for ALS backup to provide chemical pharmacologic restraint, as this may be safer than physical restraint depending on the situation

## The Right to Refuse Treatment

Adults who are conscious, alert, and appear to have decision-making capacity have the right to refuse treatment or withdraw from treatment at any time, which is supported by the principle of autonomy. This is true even if doing so may result in death or serious injury. Such patients present you with a dilemma. Should you provide care against their will? Should you leave them alone? Calls involving refusal of treatment pose a risk of litigation in EMS and require you to proceed cautiously. You must be familiar with local policies regarding refusal of care. In all such cases, you should involve online medical control and document this consultation. A patient's decision to either accept or refuse treatment should be based on information that you provide. This information should include your assessment of what might be wrong with the patient, a description of the treatment that you think is necessary, any possible risks of treatment, the availability of alternative treatments, and the possible consequences of refusing treatment. Be sure that the patient understands everything that you say and encourage the patient to ask questions. All of this information should be included in your patient care report (PCR). Many jurisdictions have preprinted refusal forms to ensure that all of these items are documented or acknowledged.

When treatment is refused, you must assess the patient's ability to make an informed decision. Ask and repeat questions, assess the patient's answers, and observe the patient's behavior. If the patient appears confused or delusional, you cannot assume that the decision to refuse is an informed

refusal. Patients who have attempted suicide or conveyed suicidal intent should not be regarded as having normal mental capacity. Remember, a single assessment finding usually will not enable you to determine whether the patient is capable of making an informed decision about health care. As with most medical conditions, it is the constellation of findings that will support your conclusion. *When in doubt, providing treatment is usually a much more defensible position than failing to treat a patient.* Contact medical direction when you are unsure. Do not endanger yourself to provide care, and use the assistance of law enforcement if necessary to ensure your own safety.

Before leaving the scene where a patient has refused care, you should again encourage the patient, up to three times if the situation allows, to permit treatment. Remind the patient to call 9-1-1 if he or she changes his or her mind or the condition worsens. Advise the patient to contact a personal physician as soon as possible. It is essential for you to ask the patient to sign a refusal of treatment form and to thoroughly document all refusals. Your documentation should include any assessment findings that you were able to make and all efforts that you made to obtain consent. Your documentation should also include a description of possible consequences of refusing treatment and transport. The patient's signature should be witnessed by a family member or police officer to help protect you from a later claim for negligence or abandonment. Both of these terms are discussed later in this chapter. A signed patient refusal form does not guarantee your protection against legal action; however, it can help defend you when legal actions arise. Also, it is wise, and often required by local protocol, that you notify medical control of your actions; medical control can help guide your decisions.

You may also be faced with a situation in which a parent refuses to permit treatment of an ill or injured child. In this situation, you must consider the emotional effect of the emergency on the parent's judgment. As with most cases of refusal, you can usually resolve the situation with patience and calm persuasion. You may also need the help of others, such as your supervisor, ALS personnel, medical control, or law enforcement officials.

When you are not able to persuade the patient, guardian, or parent to proceed with treatment, you must obtain the signature of the individual who is refusing treatment on an official release form that acknowledges refusal. Document any assessment findings, the emergency care that you provided, your efforts to obtain consent, your consultation with medical control, and the responses to your efforts. You should also obtain a signature from a witness to the refusal. Make every effort to have a responsible person, such as a police officer, serve as a witness to these events. Retain the documents with your records—they will be important in the event a legal claim is filed later. If the patient refuses to sign a release form, inform medical control and thoroughly document the situation and the refusal. In some cases, parents who have refused medical care for a child have been charged with child neglect. You might be called as a witness in such cases and you must be sure that all documentation is thorough and accurate. Remember, your safety is your first priority. Act in the best interest of your patient, but do not place yourself in danger attempting to care for a patient who is refusing care.

## Confidentiality

Communication between you and the patient is considered confidential and generally cannot be disclosed without permission from the patient or a court order. Confidential information includes the patient history, assessment findings, and treatment provided. Disclosure of such information other than to those providers directly involved in the care of the patient without proper authorization may result in liability for **breach of confidentiality**. In most states, records may be released when a legal subpoena is presented or the patient signs a written release. Patient information may also be shared with third-party billing personnel; this is not considered a breach of confidentiality.

## Health Insurance Portability and Accountability Act

HIPAA is the acronym for the Health Insurance Portability and Accountability Act of 1996. Although this act had many aims, the section of the act that most affects EMS relates to patient privacy. The aim

### Words of Wisdom

When a patient, parent, or guardian refuses treatment or transport, protect yourself with both a thorough PCR and official refusal documentation. Have the patient or other refusing party sign the form, document what you have done to ensure an informed refusal, and note the involvement of medical control in the situation. Be sure to submit the refusal form with your PCR if it is not already part of the PCR.

## YOU are the Provider

On arriving at the scene, you find the patient, a 32-year-old man, sitting on the sidewalk outside the grocery store. He is grabbing both sides of his head, but looks up and acknowledges your presence. You begin to assess the patient as your partner opens the jump kit and prepares to take his vital signs.

| Recording Time: 0 Minutes | |
| --- | --- |
| Appearance | Grabbing both sides of his head; in obvious pain |
| Level of consciousness | Conscious and alert |
| Airway | Open; clear of secretions or foreign bodies |
| Breathing | Increased respiratory rate; adequate depth |
| Circulation | Radial pulses bilaterally strong and regular; skin pink, warm, and dry |

Without talking to the patient, your partner begins to take his blood pressure and applies the pulse oximeter to his finger.

**3.** Are you legally authorized to treat this patient? Why or why not?

**4.** How does informed consent differ from implied consent?

of this section of the act is to strengthen laws for the protection of the privacy of health care information and to safeguard patient confidentiality. It provides guidance on what types of information is protected, the responsibility of health care providers regarding that protection, and the penalties for breaching that protection.

HIPAA considers all patient information that you obtain in the course of providing medical treatment to a patient to be **protected health information (PHI)**. This includes not only medical information, but also any information that can be used to identify the patient. As an EMT, you have an obligation to guard all PHI from unlawful disclosure, either written or verbal. Safeguards to protect this information include departmental security measures to prevent HIPAA violations, such as rules to prohibit sharing of passwords or log-in credentials to systems that contain PHI; proper measures to dispose of documents or other records that contain PHI; and rules to never leave electronic devices or patient reports that contain PHI unattended. PHI must also be maintained when two or more patients, who may or may not be family, are in close proximity of each other, such as in the back of an ambulance,

When an EMT's role provides access to PHI of patients other than those for whom the EMT provided care, those records may be accessed only if there is a legitimate business reason to do so. Records of celebrities, the EMTs own medical records, or the records of family members may never be viewed without appropriate permission granted by the department privacy and security officer, as specified in policy.

## Words of Wisdom

Do *not* use a personal electronic device, such as a cell phone, to capture information from a call. Digital images such as photos of a patient's injuries or vehicle, or recordings made by crew members during a patient call, are considered PHI and a confidential part of the patient report. *Never* post PHI on social media.

PHI may be disclosed for purposes of treatment, payment, or operations. This means you are permitted to report your assessment findings and treatment to other health care providers directly involved in the care of the patient. Information may be used for internal quality improvement and training programs, but all identifying information must first be removed. There are also certain situations when you may be legally mandated to report your findings, such as in the case of child abuse or when you receive a subpoena. In most situations, except for treatment purposes, only the minimum amount of information necessary should be released. Failure to abide by the provisions of the HIPAA laws can result in civil and/or criminal action against your response agency and against you personally. Each EMS system is required to have a policy and procedure manual and a privacy officer who can answer questions. You can expect to receive further training on how this act affects your specific response agency.

It cannot be overstated that any sharing of private or protected information, whether it is directly sharing images or recordings or verbally relaying information, is a serious violation of HIPAA and ethical principles, even when done privately. In situations where responders or care providers casually share information, such as in face-to-face conversations at the station or in social media postings, the communications may feel private. The fact remains, however, that private and protected information must remain between the patient and the caregiver only. Information about emergency calls may be used under special circumstances for purposes such as education and quality improvement, but all identifying and private information must first be removed.

The general public is often permitted by law to record identifying and protected patient information and images. For example, while it would be unethical and illegal for a responding EMT to take a picture of a severely injured patient while caring for the person at a motor vehicle collision, if the collision takes place on a public road and in public view, members of the general public can, and often will, record the incident. In most of these situations, EMTs, and even law enforcement officers, cannot order members of the public to stop recording, confiscate their phones or cameras, or otherwise interfere with the public.

## Street Smarts

Often a polite request made to members of the public to respect patient privacy is sufficient to stop them from filming or photographing at public scenes.

## Social Media

Although unauthorized sharing of private and protected patient information is never permitted, sharing personal opinions about work and non–work-related topics via social media is a complex and controversial topic. Whether such sharing is appropriate depends greatly on the nature of the information and the circumstances (eg, who is sharing it, how, when, and where?).

In general, if an EMT uses agency-supplied equipment to record or distribute information, or records or distributes information while in the course of his or her duties (including volunteering), the agency likely owns the images and information. In many states, the agency must follow requirements to control and store this content and, in some cases, release it to the public on request. Moreover, if EMTs associate themselves with their agency, such as showing a logo, wearing their uniform, or specifically identifying their agency, they may not be able to express their private views in the same way that other members of the general public could. There are no absolute recommendations when it comes to social media, but the following advice may help EMTs avoid serious ethical or legal issues:

- Unless you are operating as an official spokesperson for your agency, avoid logos, uniforms, vehicles, or other markings that associate you with your agency while off duty.
- Conduct yourself online with the same professionalism that you do while on duty.
- Respect your patients, their friends and family, bystanders, colleagues, and the organization for which you work both in person and online.
- Recognize that free speech does not mean every person has a right to say anything under any circumstances and without repercussions.

## Advance Directives

As an EMT, you will respond to calls in which a patient is dying from an illness. When you arrive at the scene, you may find that family members do not want you to try to resuscitate the patient. Without valid written documentation from a physician, such as an advance directive or a **do not resuscitate (DNR) order** (also known as a "do not attempt resuscitation" order), you may be placed in a very difficult position. A **competent** patient is able to make rational decisions about his or her well-being. An **advance directive** is a written document that specifies medical treatment for a competent patient, should he or she become unable to make decisions. Advance directives are most commonly used when a patient becomes comatose. An advance directive is often referred to as a living will but may also be referred to as a **health care directive**. Not all advance directives are directions to withhold care. Such care may include nutrition and medication for pain.

DNR orders give you permission not to attempt resuscitation (**FIGURE 3-4**). Laws differ from state to state, so be familiar with your state's requirements to determine whether the DNR order will be honored; however, to be valid, DNR orders must meet the following requirements:

- Clear statement of the patient's medical problem(s)
- Signature of the patient or legal guardian
- Signature of one or more physicians or other licensed health care providers
- In some states, DNR orders contain an expiration date. DNR orders with expiration dates must be dated in the preceding 12 months to be valid.

You may also encounter Physician Orders for Life-Sustaining Treatment (POLST) and Medical Orders for Life-Sustaining Treatment (MOLST) forms when caring for patients with terminal illnesses. These explicitly describe acceptable interventions for the patient in the form of medical orders. These forms must be signed by an authorized medical provider in order to be valid; this may be a physician, physician assistant, or nurse practitioner, and varies by state. If you encounter these documents, contact medical control for guidance.

Some patients may have named surrogates to make decisions for them regarding their health care in the event that they are incapacitated and unable to make such decisions for themselves. Such designations may be referred to as a **durable power of attorney for health care** or **health care proxy**. There are many different types of powers of attorney and not all are authorized to exercise medical decision making. When presented with a power of attorney at the scene of a medical emergency, you must read it carefully to ascertain its meaning and validity. If there is any question, you

PREHOSPITAL MEDICAL CARE DIRECTIVE
(side one)
IN THE EVENT OF CARDIAC OR RESPIRATORY ARREST, I REFUSE ANY RESUSCITATION MEASURES INCLUDING CARDIAC COMPRESSION, ENDOTRACHEAL INTUBATION AND OTHER ADVANCED AIRWAY MANAGEMENT, ARTIFICIAL VENTILATION, DEFIBRILLATION, ADMINISTRATION OF ADVANCED CARDIAC LIFE SUPPORT DRUGS AND RELATED EMERGENCY MEDICAL PROCEDURES.

Patient: _____ Date: _____
(Signature or mark)

Attach recent photograph here or provide all of the following information below:
Date of Birth _____
Sex _____ Race _____     PHOTO
Eye Color _____
Hair Color _____
Hospice Program (if any)_____
Name and telephone number of patient's physician _____

(side two)
I have explained this form and its consequences to the signer and obtained assurance that the signer understands that death may result from any refused care listed above (on reverse side).

_____ Date_____
(Licensed health care provider)

I was present when this was signed (or marked). The patient then appeared to be of sound mind and free from duress.

_____ Date_____
(Witness)

**Outside the Hospital Do-Not-Resuscitate Identification Card**

Patient's Full Name_____
I affirm that I have authorized an Outside the Hospital Do-Not-Resuscitate Order for this patient and have documented the grounds for the order in this patient's medical file.

**Attending Physician Signature**_____
**Attending Physician (print)**_____
**Address**_____ **Phone**_____
**Date**_____

I, _____,
(name)
authorize emergency medical services personnel to withhold or withdraw cardiopulmonary resuscitation from me in the event I suffer cardiac or respiratory arrest.

I understand this means that if my heart stops beating or I stop breathing, no medical procedure to restart heart function or breathing will be instituted.

I understand that I may revoke this order at any time.
**Patient or Patient's Representative**
**Signature**_____
**Date**_____

**A**     **B**

**FIGURE 3-4 A.** An example of a wallet-sized DNR order. **B.** An example of a pocket-sized DNR order.

should contact online medical control for assistance. Do not delay emergency care while efforts to interpret the power of attorney are made. Keep in mind that a patient who remains conscious and competent does not surrender the right to make medical decisions. The person named in the power of attorney or health care proxy is only authorized to make decisions when the patient is no longer capable of doing so.

Remember, DNR does not mean "do not treat." Even in the presence of a DNR order, you are still obligated to provide supportive measures (oxygen, pain relief, and comfort) to a patient who is not in cardiac arrest. Each agency, in consultation with its medical director and legal counsel, must develop a protocol to follow in these circumstances.

The number of hospice (end of life) home health programs is growing, so you may be faced with these situations often. Specific guidelines vary from state to state, but the following four statements may be considered general guidelines:

1. Patients have the right to refuse treatment, including resuscitative efforts, provided that they are able to communicate their wishes.
2. A written order from a physician is required for DNR orders to be valid in a health care facility.
3. You should periodically review state and local protocols and legislation regarding advance directives.
4. When you are in doubt or the written orders are not present, you have an obligation to resuscitate.

When presented with an advance directive, you should never become annoyed with family members and allow yourself to wonder, "Why did they bother to call 9-1-1 if they don't want us to do anything?" The patients, and their families, should be treated with the utmost respect and empathy. If information and support is what they called you for, be sure to provide it—it is part of your job.

## Physical Signs of Death

Determination of the cause of death is the medical responsibility of a physician. There are both definitive and presumptive signs of death. In many states, death is defined as the absence of circulatory and respiratory function. Many states have also adopted brain death provisions; these provisions refer to irreversible cessation of all functions of the brain and brainstem. Questions often arise as to whether to begin basic life support. In the absence of physician orders, such as DNR orders, the general rule is: If the body is still intact and there are no definitive signs of death, initiate emergency medical care.

Hypothermia is a general cooling of the body in which the internal body temperature becomes abnormally low. People have survived hypothermic incidents with temperatures as low as 64°F (18°C). In cases of hypothermia, the patient should not be considered dead until he or she is warm and dead. When the patient's condition is unclear, or if you are unsure if you should initiate care, it is best to begin CPR immediately and contact medical control for guidance. Remember, not all incidents of hypothermia occur outdoors; for example, an older patient in a home without heat or who has been lying on a cold floor could be hypothermic.

## Presumptive Signs of Death

Most medicolegal authorities will consider the presumptive signs of death that are listed in **TABLE 3-1** adequate, particularly when they follow a severe trauma or occur at the end stages of long-term illness such as cancer or other prolonged diseases. More evidence is typically needed in cases of sudden death due to hypothermia, acute poisoning, or cardiac arrest.

## Definitive Signs of Death

Definitive or conclusive signs of death that are obvious and clear to even nonmedical people include the following:

- Obvious mortal damage, such as decapitation
- **Dependent lividity**: blood settling to the lowest point of the body, causing discoloration of the skin (**FIGURE 3-5**)

**TABLE 3-1** Presumptive Signs of Death

- Unresponsiveness to painful stimuli
- Lack of a carotid pulse or heartbeat
- Absence of chest rise and fall
- No deep tendon or corneal reflexes
- Absence of pupillary reactivity
- No systolic blood pressure
- Profound cyanosis
- Lowered or decreased body temperature

© Jones & Bartlett Learning.

## YOU are the Provider

Your partner reports that the patient's blood pressure is very high. The patient tells you that he has "blood pressure problems" and experiences a bad headache whenever he does not take his Prinivil—the medication he takes. He does not want to go to the hospital and tells you that the clerk called 9-1-1, not him.

| Recording Time: 4 Minutes | |
|---|---|
| **Respirations** | 24 breaths/min; regular and unlabored |
| **Pulse** | 110 beats/min; strong and regular |
| **Skin** | Pink, warm, and dry |
| **Blood pressure** | 200/110 mm Hg |
| **Oxygen saturation (Spo₂)** | 98% (on room air) |

**5.** What should you do when a patient refuses treatment and/or transport?

**6.** What questions should you ask yourself to help determine whether you can transport this patient against his will?

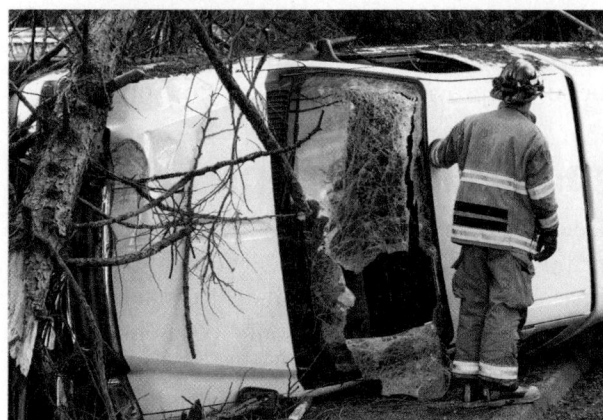

**FIGURE 3-6** When trauma is a factor or the death involves an unusual or a suspected criminal situation, the medical examiner must be notified.

© TFoxFoto/Shutterstock.

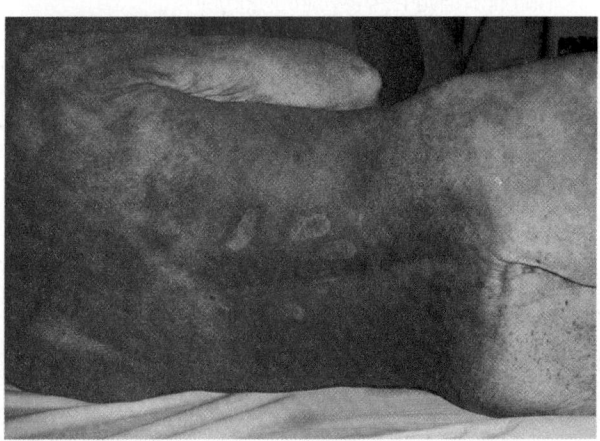

**FIGURE 3-5** Dependent lividity is an obvious sign of death caused by discoloration of the body from pooling of the blood to the lower parts of the body.

© American Academy of Orthopaedic Surgeons.

- **Rigor mortis**, the stiffening of body muscles caused by chemical changes within muscle tissue. It develops first in the face and jaw, gradually extending downward until the body is in full rigor. The rate of onset is affected by the body's ability to lose heat to its surroundings. The rate of heat loss in a thin body is faster than in a fat body. A body on a tile floor has faster heat loss than a body wrapped up in a blanket in a bed. Rigor mortis occurs sometime between 2 and 12 hours after death

- **Algor mortis**, refers to the cooling of the body until it matches the ambient temperature.
- **Putrefaction** (decomposition of body tissues). Depending on temperature conditions, this occurs sometime between 40 and 96 hours after death

## Medical Examiner Cases

Involvement of the medical examiner, or the coroner in some states, depends on the nature and scene of the death. In most states, when trauma is a factor or the death involves suspected criminal or unusual situations such as hanging or poisoning, the medical examiner must be notified (**FIGURE 3-6**). When the medical examiner or coroner assumes responsibility of the scene, that responsibility supersedes all others at the scene, including the family's. The following are a few examples of deaths that may be considered medical examiner cases:

- When the person is dead on arrival (DOA; sometimes referred to as dead on scene [DOS])
- Death without previous medical care or when the physician is unable to state the cause of death
- Suicide
- Violent death
- Poisoning, known or suspected
- Death resulting from unintentional injuries
- Suspicion of a criminal act
- Infant and child deaths

You should make every attempt to limit your disturbance of a scene involving a death. Once you have adequately determined death based on local protocols, remove yourself from the scene. This is especially important if there is anything potentially suspicious about the death.

If emergency medical care has been initiated, be sure to keep thorough notes of what was done or found. These records may be important during a subsequent investigation.

In such instances, there is no urgent reason to move the body. The only immediate action that is required of you is to cover the body and prevent its disturbance. Local protocol will determine your ultimate action in these instances.

## Special Situations
### Organ Donors

You may be called to a scene involving a potential organ donor. Consent to organ donation is voluntary and knowing. Consent is evidenced by either a donor card or a driver's license indicating that the individual wishes to be a donor (**FIGURE 3-7**). You may need to consult with medical control when faced with this situation.

In specific circumstances, a patient who is not successfully resuscitated may be a potential organ donor. Certain centers can procure organs, including the kidneys and liver, in certain situations. These situations typically occur after in-hospital cardiac arrest but may be associated with certain specific out-of-hospital cardiac arrest situations that occur near specialized centers. Be aware of your local centers and their protocols and capabilities.

You should treat a potential organ donor in the same way that you would any other patient needing treatment. Use all means necessary to keep that patient alive. Organs that are often donated, such as a kidney, heart, or liver, need oxygen at all times; you must give oxygen to the possible donor or the organs will be damaged and become useless.

Remember, your priority is to save the patient's life. Be sure to learn what the specific protocols are in your area regarding special situations such as organ donation.

## Medical Identification Insignia

Many patients will carry important medical identification and information, often in the form of a bracelet, necklace, key chain, or card that identifies patient history information. This may include a DNR order or information related to medications taken, allergies, diabetes, epilepsy, or some other serious condition (**FIGURE 3-8**). Some patients wear medical bracelets with a USB flash drive, which contains pertinent patient information, such as drug interactions, allergies, or emergency contact information. This information is often stored as a PDF file that can be read on most computers.

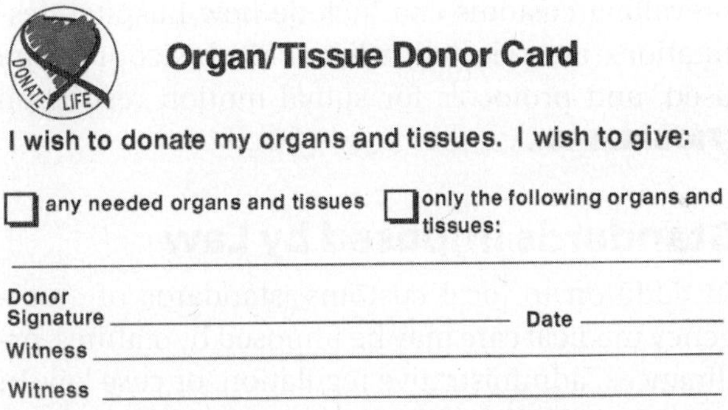

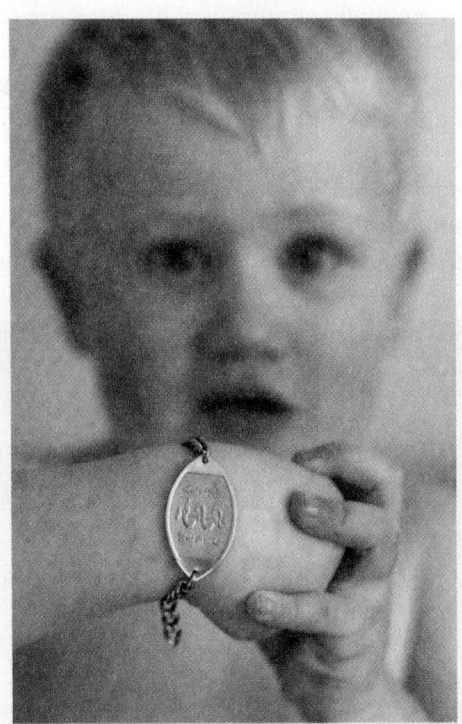

**FIGURE 3-8** The patient may be carrying a medical identification card or wearing a bracelet or necklace that indicates important medical information and possible DNR orders. In the case of MedicAlert, the EMS provider can obtain stored patient history information from the MedicAlert Foundation.

© Lucas Oleniuk/Contributor/Toronto Star/Getty Images.

---

**Organ/Tissue Donor Card**

I wish to donate my organs and tissues. I wish to give:

☐ any needed organs and tissues ☐ only the following organs and tissues:

_____

Donor
Signature _____ Date _____

Witness _____

Witness _____

**FIGURE 3-7** The patient may be carrying a donor card or driver's license indicating that he or she wishes to be an organ donor.

Courtesy of the U.S. Department of Health and Human Services.

## Scope of Practice

The scope of practice, which is most commonly defined by state law, outlines the care you are legally able to provide for the patient. Your medical director further defines the scope of practice by developing protocols and standing orders. The medical director gives you the legal authorization to provide patient care through telephone or radio communication (online) or standing orders and protocols offline. It is your responsibility as an EMT to know your scope of practice and follow it. You and other EMS personnel have a responsibility to provide proper, consistent patient care and to report problems, such as possible liability or exposure to infectious disease, to your medical director immediately.

If you carry out procedures for which you are not authorized, you are practicing outside your scope of practice, which may be considered negligence or, in some states, even a criminal offense. The scope of practice should not be confused with the standard of care.

## Standards of Care

The law generally requires you be concerned about the safety and welfare of others when your behavior or activities have the potential for causing others injury or harm (**FIGURE 3-9**). The manner in which you must act or behave as an EMT is called a standard of care.

Standard of care is established in many ways, among them local customs, statutes, ordinances,

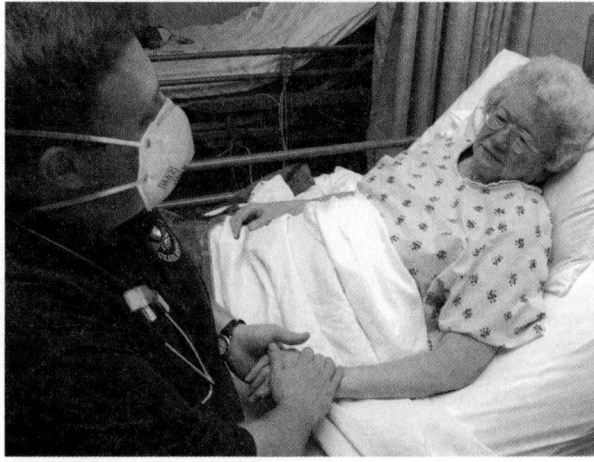

**FIGURE 3-9** Act or behave toward others in a way that shows your concern about their safety and welfare.

© Jones & Bartlett Learning. Courtesy of MIEMSS.

protocols, medical literature, textbooks, administrative regulations, and case law. In addition, professional or institutional standards have a bearing on determining the adequacy of your conduct.

## Standards Imposed by Local Custom

The standard of care is how a reasonably prudent person with similar training and experience would act under similar circumstances, with similar equipment, and in a similar place. For example, the conduct of an EMT who is employed by an ambulance service is judged in comparison with the expected conduct of other EMTs from comparable ambulance services in the same geographic area. These standards are often based on local protocols.

As an EMT, you will not be held to the same standard of care as physicians or other more highly trained professionals. In addition, your conduct must be judged in light of the given emergency situation, taking into certain factors including the following:

- Scene safety
- General confusion at the scene of the emergency
- The needs of other patients
- The type of equipment available

In this context, an emergency is a serious situation, such as an injury or an illness that arises suddenly, threatens the life or welfare of a person or group of people, and requires immediate intervention.

Prevailing customs within a community are important elements in determining the standard of emergency care within that community. This means the accepted standard of care can change from one community to another. Examples of prevailing customs can include how hospital destinations are selected, when EMS helicopters are used, and protocols for spinal motion restriction (**FIGURE 3-10**).

## Standards Imposed by Law

In addition to local customs, standards of emergency medical care may be imposed by statutes, ordinances, administrative regulation, or case law. In many jurisdictions, violating one of these standards is said to create presumptive negligence. Therefore, you must become familiar with the particular

Chapter 3 Medical, Legal, and Ethical Issues**   **99**

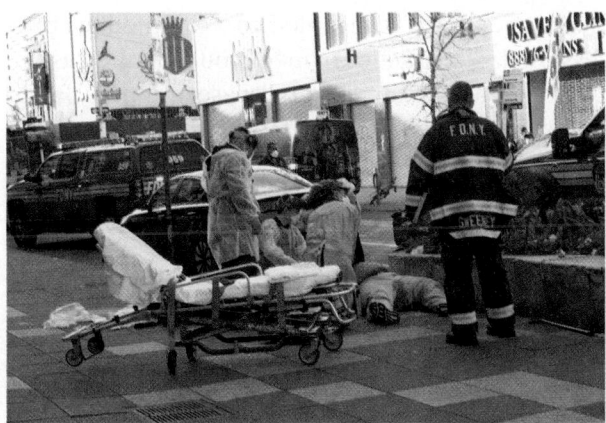

**FIGURE 3-10** In emergency situations, you will care for those with potentially life-threatening injuries or illnesses by practicing a standard of care—the accepted level of care expected in your profession for your level of training.

© SOPA Images/LightRocket/Getty Images.

legal standards that may exist in your state. In many states, this may take the form of treatment protocols published by a state agency.

## Professional or Institutional Standards

In addition to standards imposed by law, professional or institutional standards may be admitted as evidence in determining the adequacy of an EMT's conduct. Professional standards include recommendations published by organizations and societies that are involved in emergency medical care. Institutional standards include specific rules and procedures of the EMS system, ambulance service, or organization with which you are affiliated.

Two notes of caution: First, you must be familiar with the standards of your organization. Second, if you are involved in formulating standards for a particular agency, they should be reasonable and realistic so that they do not impose an unreasonable burden on EMTs. Regardless, providing the best emergency medical care should be every EMT's goal.

Many standards of care may be imposed on you. State health department regulations usually govern the scope and level of training. Court decisions have resulted in case law defining standards of care. Professional standards are also imposed. For example, the International Liaison Committee on Resuscitation (ILCOR), along with its member the American Heart Association (AHA), updates the standard for basic life support and CPR on a regular basis (**FIGURE 3-11**).

Ordinary care is a minimum standard of care. In general, it is expected that any EMT who offers

## YOU are the Provider

The patient consents to EMS treatment and transport after you tell him he could be experiencing a serious medical emergency. You place the patient onto the stretcher. While loading the patient in the ambulance, the clerk asks, "What's wrong with him? Did I do the right thing?"

| Recording Time: 10 Minutes | |
| --- | --- |
| **Level of consciousness** | Conscious and alert |
| **Respirations** | 22 breaths/min; regular and unlabored |
| **Pulse** | 104 beats/min; strong and regular |
| **Skin** | Pink, warm, and dry |
| **Blood pressure** | 194/108 mm Hg |
| **Spo$_2$** | 99% |

En route to the hospital, you dim the lights in the ambulance, apply a cool compress to his forehead, and ensure that he is in a comfortable position. You then obtain his patient information and medical history.

**7.** Does HIPAA affect the medical care you provide to your patients? What information are you allowed to discuss with family members, bystanders, the media, and others?

**8.** How do you respond to the clerk's question in a professional manner without violating HIPAA regulations?

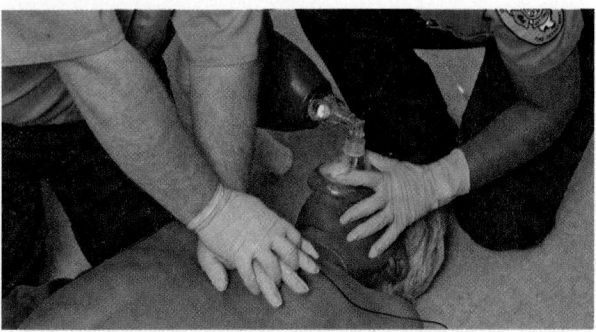

**FIGURE 3-11** Many standards of care are imposed on you as an EMT. If you deviate from these standards, legal action may be taken against you. Learn the standards of care for your level and organization.

© Jones & Bartlett Learning. Courtesy of MIEMSS.

assistance will exercise reasonable care and act prudently. If you act reasonably, according to the accepted standard, the risk of a civil lawsuit is small. If you apply the standard practices you have been trained to use, you can likely avoid liability. For example, various organizations have defined standards for performing CPR. If you deviate from these standards, you may be liable for civil and possibly criminal prosecution. In addition, state regulatory agencies that oversee EMS operations can sanction EMS personnel for deviating from the standard of care.

## Standards Imposed by Textbooks

In the course of a lawsuit, an attorney will often ask an EMT if he or she recognizes various textbooks as being authoritative works in the field of EMS. Because almost all EMS textbooks follow standards published by the National Highway Transportation Safety Administration (NHTSA), these textbooks are often recognized as contributing to, but not completely defining, the standard of care that is followed by EMTs. Local protocols or state standards may differ from material presented in textbooks. When such differences occur, you are bound to follow local protocols.

## Standards Imposed by States
### Medical Practices Act

In some states, EMS personnel are exempt from the licensure requirements of the Medical Practices Act because an EMT is regarded as a nonmedical professional. The practice of medicine is defined as the diagnosis and treatment of disease or illness. EMTs and others in the prehospital care chain assess the need for life support and begin care. Some states, however, have adopted legislation that establishes the scope of practice for EMS providers. Therefore, as an EMT you must be aware of the standards established by legislation in your state so you can be sure to provide care that is consistent with those standards.

## Certification and Licensure

Some states provide certification, licensure, or credentialing of people who perform emergency medical care. Once certified, you are obliged to conform to the standards that are generally recognized nationally by various registry groups and provide an important link in nationwide EMS. You must ensure that your certification or licensure remains current and that your skill levels are kept up to date. For more information on certification and licensure, see Chapter 1, *EMS Systems*.

## Duty to Act

**Duty to act** is an individual's responsibility to provide patient care. Responsibility comes from either statute or function. A bystander is under no obligation to assist a stranger in distress and therefore has no duty to act. For an EMT, there may be a duty to act in certain instances, including the following:

- You are charged with emergency medical response.
- Your service or department's policy states that you must assist in any emergency.

Once your ambulance responds to a call or treatment is begun, you have a legal duty to act. In most cases, if you are off duty and happen to see a motor vehicle crash, you are not legally obligated to stop and assist patients. There may be some circumstances where this is not true, and you should be familiar with the laws and policies that apply in your service area. If you choose to intervene while off duty, you must continue to provide competent care until an equal or higher medical authority assumes care of the patient.

# Negligence

Negligence is the failure to provide the same care that a person with similar training would provide in the same or a similar situation. It is deviation from the accepted standard of care that may result in further injury to the patient. Determination of negligence is based on the following four factors:

1. **Duty.** The EMT has an obligation to provide care and to do so in a manner that is consistent with the standard of care established by training and local protocols.
2. **Breach of duty.** There is a breach of duty when the EMT does not act within an expected and reasonable standard of care.
3. **Damages.** There are damages when a patient is physically or psychologically harmed in some noticeable way.
4. **Causation.** There must be a reasonable cause-and-effect relationship between the breach of duty and the damages suffered by the patient. This is often referred to as proximate causation. An example is dropping the patient during lifting, causing a fracture of the patient's leg. If an EMT has a duty and breaches it, thereby causing harm to a patient, the EMT, the agency, and/or the medical director may be sued for negligence if that breach of duty was the direct cause of the patient's injury.

All four elements must be present for the legal doctrine of liability to apply and for a plaintiff to prevail in a lawsuit against an EMS system or provider. It is also possible for an EMT or an EMS system to be held liable even when the plaintiff is unable to clearly demonstrate how an injury occurred, under the theory of res ipsa loquitur. An EMT could be held liable under this theory if it can be shown that an injury occurred, that the cause of the injury was in the control of the EMT, and that such injuries generally do not occur unless there is negligence. For example, you and your partner are called to the home of a man with diabetes who has lapsed into unconsciousness. You find the patient lying on a couch with no visible signs of trauma. While loading the patient into the ambulance, your partner slips and the stretcher drops, causing the patient to sustain a facial laceration. The patient later files a lawsuit against you for negligence. Because the patient was unconscious, he is unable to describe exactly how he sustained a facial laceration. Under the theory of res ipsa loquitur, the patient may prevail in his lawsuit by showing that he was under your care, that he suffered an injury, and that his injury would not have occurred unless there was negligence.

In rare cases, the plaintiff may be able to establish liability by using the theory of negligence per se. This is a theory that may be used when the conduct of the person being sued is alleged to have occurred in clear violation of a statute. For example, if you were to perform an ALS skill, such as the intravenous administration of a cardiac medication that resulted in injury to a patient, the plaintiff might allege that this was negligence per se. In that case, the plaintiff would not have to establish the circumstances surrounding your conduct. There would be no need to show that the administration of the medication was inappropriate for the patient because you clearly exceeded your scope of practice.

All forms of negligence come under the general category known as torts. Torts are simply defined as civil wrongs. They are not within the jurisdiction of US criminal courts. Examples of other tort actions are lawsuits for defamation of character and invasion of privacy.

# Abandonment

Abandonment is the unilateral termination of care by the EMT without the patient's consent and without making any provisions for continuing care by a medical professional who is competent to provide care for the patient. Once care is started, you have assumed a duty that must not stop until an equally competent medical provider assumes responsibility. Failure to perform that duty is a serious legal and ethical matter that exposes the patient to harm and can result in civil action against you.

For example, suppose you arrive at the scene of a single-car crash and begin care of two injured patients. A passerby tells you of a two-car crash farther down the road in which five people are injured. You turn over care of the two injured patients from the first crash to the passerby, who is not a trained emergency care provider, and leave to go to the second crash. Abandonment may have occurred because you did not turn care of the patients over to a person who is trained and competent to provide emergency care that meets the needs of the two patients. Consider the following general questions when you are faced with making a decision such as this one:

- What problems may develop from your actions?
- How might the patient's condition worsen if you leave?
- Does the patient need care?
- Are you neglecting your duty to your patient?
- Is the person assuming care capable of providing the level of care needed by the patient?
- Are you abandoning the patient if you leave the scene?
- Are you violating a standard of care?
- Are you acting prudently?

Surprisingly, abandonment may also take place in the emergency department (ED) where you drop off your patient. A part of your obligation as an EMT is to provide appropriate hospital personnel with a report of your assessment findings, the care you provided, and any changes in patient status that occurred during transport to the hospital. The failure to do so could result in a delay in treatment or a misdiagnosis. In such a case, a claim for abandonment could be filed against the EMT who failed to provide the report.

## Assault and Battery and Kidnapping

**Assault** is defined as unlawfully placing a person in fear of immediate bodily harm. Threatening to restrain a patient who does not want to be transported could be considered assault. **Battery** is defined as unlawfully touching a person; this includes providing emergency care without consent. Assault and battery can be either civil or criminal in nature. Civil lawsuits for battery are common in health care. To sustain a criminal case of assault or battery, it is generally necessary to prove the intent to cause harm. The element of intent is rarely present in the case of an EMS provider; therefore, criminal cases of assault and/or battery are rare. **Kidnapping** is the seizing, confining, abducting, or carrying away of a person by force. In theory, this might include a situation where a patient is transported against his or her will. In reality, criminal charges of kidnapping

are almost unheard of in EMS because the EMT is almost always acting in a good-faith effort to provide care to the patient. It is far more likely that an EMT could be the target of a civil lawsuit for **false imprisonment**. This is defined as the unauthorized confinement of a person that lasts for an appreciable period of time. Consider a patient who rescinds consent during transport and demands to be let out of the ambulance. If you refuse, you may be accused of false imprisonment.

Serious legal problems may arise in situations in which a patient has not given consent for treatment. Battery could be considered if you apply a splint to a suspected fracture of the lower leg, or use an EpiPen on a patient without the patient's consent. Under such circumstances, a patient might file a lawsuit for assault, battery, false imprisonment, or all three. Criminal charges are possible but far less likely. To protect yourself from these charges, make sure that you obtain expressed consent or that the situation allows for implied consent. Consult your medical director or service attorney if you have questions or doubt about a specific situation.

> ### Words of Wisdom
>
> The best way to ensure you make good ethical decisions is to make the welfare of your patient your top priority.

## Defamation

As an EMT, you should also be aware of the laws involving defamation. **Defamation** is the communication of false information that damages the reputation of a person. Defamation that is in writing is referred to as **libel**, and defamation that is spoken is known as **slander**. A legal claim for defamation could arise out of a false statement on a run report, inappropriate comments made on social media or during "station house" conversations, or sharing "war stories" with friends, relatives, or neighbors. To avoid liability for such a claim and to protect the confidentiality of patients, you must only communicate information about your patients to authorized people, and you should be sure that the information contained in your run reports and other documentation is accurate and relevant. There is no reason to post information about your patient on social media. You should never comment on your patient's personal information when it is not relevant to your assessment or treatment of the patient.

## Good Samaritan Laws and Immunity

All states have adopted **Good Samaritan laws**, which are based on the common law principle that when you reasonably help another person, you should not be liable for errors and omissions that are made in giving good-faith emergency care. These laws, however, apply to Good Samaritans, and are not intended for people who are at work being compensated for doing a job, and do not necessarily protect you from a lawsuit. The laws apply when you are off duty. Good Samaritan provisions vary significantly from state to state. Good Samaritan statutes in some jurisdictions provide immunity from a lawsuit while others provide an affirmative defense if you are sued for rendering care. In most cases, they do not prohibit the filing of a lawsuit, nor do they pertain to acts that could be considered wanton,

gross, or willful negligence. To be protected by the provisions of a Good Samaritan law, several conditions must generally be met:

1. You acted in good faith in rendering care.
2. You rendered care without expectation of compensation.
3. You acted within the scope of your training.
4. You did not act in a grossly negligent manner.

**Gross negligence** is defined as conduct that constitutes a willful or reckless disregard for a duty or standard of care.

Another group of laws grants immunity from liability to official EMS providers, such as EMTs, in some circumstances. These laws, which vary from state to state, do not provide immunity when injury or damage is caused by gross negligence or willful misconduct. In most cases, immunity statutes apply to EMS systems that are considered governmental agencies. This concept is known as sovereign immunity, and it usually provides limitations on liability; immunity is not complete.

Most states have also adopted specific laws granting special privileges to EMS personnel, authorizing them to perform certain medical procedures. Many states also grant partial immunity to EMTs and physicians and nurses who give emergency instructions to EMS personnel via radio or

## YOU are the Provider

While reassessing the patient, he admits to using cocaine. You complete your reassessment and then call in your radio report to the receiving facility. The patient's blood pressure has improved, and he tells you that his headache is not as bad as it was before.

| Recording Time: 15 Minutes | |
|---|---|
| Level of consciousness | Conscious and alert |
| Respirations | 18 breaths/min; regular and unlabored |
| Pulse | 90 beats/min; strong and regular |
| Skin | Pink, warm, and dry |
| Blood pressure | 166/94 mm Hg |
| Spo$_2$ | 99% |

You deliver the patient to the ED and give your oral report to the receiving nurse. After completing your PCR, you and your partner return to service.

**9.** Should you report the patient's use of illegal substances to law enforcement personnel? Why or why not?

**10.** Why is it a good idea to have the receiving nurse sign your PCR acknowledging the transfer of care?

other forms of communication. Consult your medical director or state EMS agency for more information about the laws in your area.

## Records and Reports

Because EMS providers are in a position to observe and gather information about diseases, injuries, and emergency events, an obligation to compile such information and report it to certain agencies may be imposed. Even if there is no such requirement, you should compile a complete and accurate record of all incidents in which you have contact with sick or injured patients. A complete and accurate record of an emergency medical incident is an important safeguard against legal complications. The absence of a record, or a substantially incomplete record, increases the likelihood that you may have to testify on memory alone. This can prove to be wholly inadequate and embarrassing in the face of aggressive cross-examination.

You should consider the following two general rules regarding reports and records:

- If an action or procedure is not recorded on the written report, it was not performed.
- An incomplete or untidy report is evidence of incomplete or inexpert emergency medical care.

You can avoid both of these potentially dangerous presumptions by compiling and maintaining accurate reports and records of all events and patients. PCRs also help the EMS system evaluate individual and service provider performance. These reports are an integral part of most quality assurance programs. Data extraction from PCRs is also used to conduct prehospital emergency care research, which may improve patient outcomes.

The National EMS Information System (NEMSIS) is a tool for the EMS profession. NEMSIS provides the ability to collect, store, and share standardized EMS data throughout the United States. This incredibly useful database can be used to improve the speed and accuracy of data collection. NEMSIS could, for example, provide early warning of a disease outbreak.

## Special Mandatory Reporting Requirements
### Abuse of Children, Older People, and Others

All states have enacted laws to protect abused children, and some have added other protected groups such as the older population and at-risk adults. Most states have a reporting obligation for certain people, ranging from physicians to any person. You must be aware of the requirements of the law in your state. Such statutes frequently grant immunity from liability for libel, slander, or defamation of character to the individual who is obligated to report, even if the reports are subsequently shown to be unfounded, as long as the reports are made in good faith.

### Injury During the Commission of a Felony

Many states have laws requiring the reporting of any injury that is likely to have occurred during the commission of a crime, such as gunshot wounds, knife wounds, or poisonings. Again, you must be familiar with the legal requirements of your state.

### Drug-Related Injuries

In some instances, drug-related injuries must be reported. These requirements may affect how you approach documenting the care of a patient. However, it should be stressed that the US Supreme Court has held that drug addiction, in contrast to drug possession or sale, is an illness and not a crime. Therefore, an injury that results from a drug overdose may not be within the definition of an injury resulting from a crime.

Some states, by statute, specifically establish confidentiality and excuse certain specified people from reporting drug cases, either to a government agency or to a minor's parents, if, in the opinion of those people, withholding reporting is necessary

**Street Smarts**

Most lawsuits take years to unfold. If you are called to testify in 2 or 3 years for a case that may have seemed routine, your documentation, particularly how you told the story in the narrative, may provide your only memory of the call when you are on the stand.

for the proper treatment of the patient. Once again, you must be familiar with the legal requirements of your state.

## Childbirth

Many states require that anyone who attends at a live birth in any place other than a licensed medical facility report the birth. As before, you must be familiar with state requirements.

## Other Reporting Requirements

Other reporting requirements may include burns (in children under a certain age), attempted suicides, dog bites, certain communicable diseases, assaults, domestic violence, and sexual assault or rape.

---

### Special Populations

Elder abuse is as prominent as child abuse in our society. Do not forget to be observant and report any suspicious signs or symptoms to the proper authorities.

---

Most EMS agencies require that exposures to specific communicable diseases be reported. You may be asked to transport certain patients in restraints, which may also need to be reported. Each of these situations can present significant legal problems. You should learn your local protocols regarding these situations.

Not only do the events that need to be reported vary significantly from state to state but so do the methods and procedures by which such reporting must take place. For example, although all states require that suspected child abuse be reported, some states require that the report be filed with law enforcement, others with a designated child protection agency, and yet others with the ED. There are often time-sensitive provisions associated with reporting statutes. As has been noted earlier, it is important that you become familiar with reporting requirements of your state. Failure to report may result in disciplinary action, suspension of your privileges to practice as an EMT, a fine, or even criminal prosecution.

## Scene of a Crime

If there is evidence at an emergency scene that a crime may have been committed, in most cases you must notify the dispatcher immediately so that law enforcement authorities can respond. Such circumstances should not stop you from providing life-saving emergency medical care to the patient; however, your safety is a priority, so you must ensure that the scene is safe to enter. At times, you may have to transport the patient to the hospital before law enforcement arrives. While emergency medical care is being provided, you must be careful not to disturb the scene of the crime any more than absolutely necessary. Notes and drawings should be made of the position of the patient and of the presence and position of any weapon or other objects that may be valuable to the investigating officers. If possible, do not cut through holes in clothing that were caused by weapons or gunshot wounds. Avoid walking through blood and try to avoid leaving footprints in the dirt or grass at or near a crime scene. When a sexual assault is suspected, try to persuade the victim not to shower or clean himself or herself. You should confer periodically with local authorities and be aware of their wishes regarding actions you should take at the scene of the crime. It is best if these guidelines can be established by protocol.

---

### Words of Wisdom

State laws vary regarding whether EMS personnel must report rape or sexual assault. In some states, the decision to report these crimes lies with the patient. Note that suspected sexual abuse of children or older adults and domestic abuse must be reported in most states.

---

## The Deceased

In most states, EMTs do not have the authority to pronounce a patient dead. If there is any chance that life exists or that the patient can be resuscitated, you must make every effort to save the patient at the scene and during transport. However, at times death is obvious. If a victim is clearly dead and the scene of the emergency may be where a crime was committed, do not move the body or disturb the scene.

# Ethical Responsibilities

In addition to legal duties, you have certain ethical responsibilities as a health care provider. These responsibilities are to yourself, your patients, your coworkers, and the public. **Ethics** is the philosophy of right and wrong, of moral principles, and of ideal professional behavior. It is often referred to as the study of morality. **Morality** is a code of conduct that can be defined by society, religion, or a person, affecting character and conscience and the definition of right versus wrong. An entire field of ethics known as **bioethics** has evolved over the past several decades that addresses issues that arise in the practice of health care. Many such issues have drawn national attention, such as those dealing with the termination of life support, rationing of medical resources, and physician-assisted suicide. Ethical issues are present in nearly every EMS incident. As an EMT, you will be expected to conduct yourself in a manner that is consistent with the standards of your profession and to keep the best interests of your patients at the forefront of your conduct and decision making. The manner in which principles of ethics are incorporated into professional conduct is known as **applied ethics**.

You will encounter ethical dilemmas in the course of your employment that can be challenging to resolve. Examples might include the following:

- Your partner arrives at work smelling of alcohol.
- You are called to the scene of a belligerent driver who has seriously injured several children after causing a crash while drag racing.
- You are dispatched to a 9-1-1 call for chest pain. Your partner recognizes the address and tells you not to use the lights and siren because this is a "frequent flyer" who constantly calls 9-1-1 to get attention.
- You respond to the home of an older woman in cardiac arrest. One relative hands you DNR paperwork and states the patient did not want to be resuscitated. Another relative demands that you do everything possible to save the patient.
- One of your coworkers is unable to attend a training session and asks you to sign him in, stating, "You know I would do it for you."

The manner in which you respond to each of these circumstances requires you to evaluate and apply your own moral standards as well as those of your profession. Obviously, these choices can be difficult at times, particularly in those cases where your own personal standards of right and wrong do not necessarily agree with the standards of your profession. You know you should report that your partner may be intoxicated while on duty, even if he is a good friend. You might also want to honor the patient's DNR wishes, but medical control may order you to initiate care based on the family's request.

Your behavior both on and off the job is a reflection of your personal ethical standards. News stories that depict EMS personnel engaging in any immature or illegal activities serve to lessen the public's confidence in the services EMTs provide. Illegal drug use or selling drugs, inappropriate use of emergency vehicles, inappropriate visitors entertained at the station, and use of alcohol on duty can have a negative effect on the EMT and on EMS in general and should be strictly forbidden.

If you care about your patients, your coworkers, and the EMS system as a whole, you also may not stand by silently and watch as other EMS providers engage in misbehavior. Misconduct should be promptly reported to the appropriate chain of command. Similarly, you are obligated to report medical errors you make or witness to the medical director or another appropriate person as soon as possible.

EMS providers should establish their own ethical standards and monitor the ethical behavior of their members. How can you make sure that you are acting ethically, especially with all the decisions you have to make in the field? First, you should consider all options available to you and the consequence of each option. Have decisions been made in the past regarding a similar situation? Can an existing policy or rule be applied? How will the consequences of your decision provide the greatest benefit in view of all the alternatives? Involve online medical control in your decision making (**TABLE 3-2**).

You must meet your legal and ethical responsibilities while caring for your patients' physical and emotional needs. Patient needs will vary depending on the situation, and you must be prepared to offer whatever physical and emotional support is necessary. In most cases that you will encounter as an EMT, there will be a rule, a law, or a policy that will guide your decision making and your actions. As a professional, you are bound to follow all such policies, rules, and laws even in those rare

| TABLE 3-2 Ethical Decision-Making Checklist | | |
|---|---|---|
| | **Yes** | **No** |
| Is the decision in the best interests of the patient? | ❏ | ❏ |
| Is the decision based on logic and reason rather than emotion? | ❏ | ❏ |
| Does the decision protect the patient's rights? | ❏ | ❏ |
| Would you agree to the same decision if you were the patient? | ❏ | ❏ |
| Would you make the same decision again in similar circumstances? | ❏ | ❏ |
| Can you defend this decision to others? | ❏ | ❏ |

© Jones & Bartlett Learning.

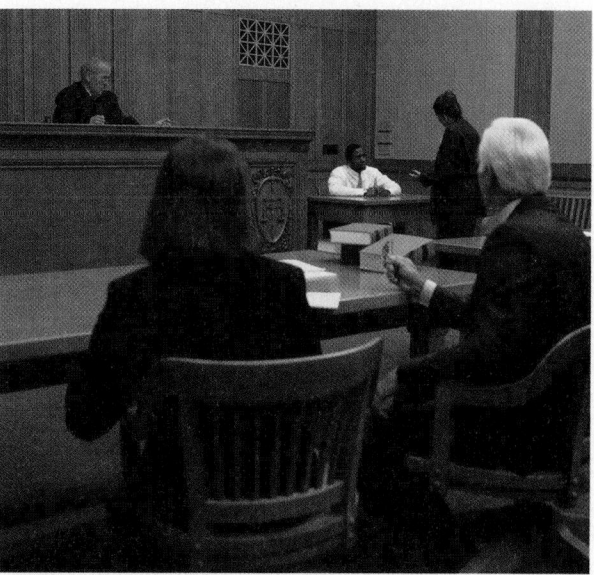

**FIGURE 3-12** Court discussions will be based on your documentation. Make sure your documentation is thorough and accurate.

© Brand X Pictures/Creatas.

circumstances where your own personal sense of morals might lead you to a different result. In short, your professional ethics trump personal morals while on duty.

One unquestionable responsibility you have is honest reporting. Remember, absolute honesty in reporting is essential. You must provide a complete and accurate account of the events and the details of all patient care and professional duties.

## The EMT in Court

As an EMT, there are several different circumstances that might cause you to end up in court, either as a witness or a defendant in a civil lawsuit or as a witness or defendant in a criminal case. Regardless of the circumstances, being in court is often stressful. As a witness in a civil case, you may be called to testify about the condition of the plaintiff when you arrived at the scene of a crash and about the treatment that you provided. In a criminal case, you may be asked to describe a crime scene or the injuries that you found when you examined a crime victim, or to testify concerning any admissions or statements made to you by a criminal defendant.

Whenever you are subpoenaed to testify in any court proceeding, you should immediately notify the director of your service and legal counsel. As

a witness you should remain neutral during your testimony. You are simply there to provide the facts as you observed them and not to take sides. Many of the questions that you will be asked likely will be based on the documentation you wrote at the time of the incident. Be sure to review your run report prior to your court appearance (**FIGURE 3-12**).

As a defendant in either a civil or criminal proceeding, your involvement will obviously be far more significant and the outcome will have far greater personal consequences. In either case, you will definitely require the assistance of an attorney. In a civil lawsuit, where you are being sued in your capacity as an employee or volunteer of an EMS system, your service or its insurance company generally will provide you with legal counsel.

A civil lawsuit begins with the service of a summons and complaint. The complaint sets forth the details of the plaintiff's case and provides the theory on which the plaintiff is relying to recover a judgment against you and your service. If served with a summons, you must bring this to the attention of the head of your service immediately, because the complaint must be responded to within a set period of time that is usually within 20 to 30 days. The response to the complaint is called an answer and it will generally deny the claims established in the complaint and set forth one or more defenses on behalf of you and your service. A defense is essentially a reason why the plaintiff should not recover a judgment against you. Depending on the nature of the case filed against you, the type of EMS system that you work for, and the state where you work, there may be different possible defenses available to you. These may include the defenses of statute of limitations, immunity, or contributory negligence.

The **statute of limitations** is the time within which a claim must be initiated. For example, in many states, a claim for negligence must be initiated within 3 years of the event that led to injury. A case initiated beyond the 3-year period would be barred by the statute of limitations. In such a case, your attorney would include the defense of statute of limitations in the answer that is filed in response to the complaint. In most states the statute of limitations is different for children. States often specify an extended period to file these cases as well as a maximum age by which a claim must be filed. For example, an injury that occurred when a child was 12 years old may not have to be filed until that child's 21st birthday in some states.

Another possible defense is that of governmental immunity. **Governmental immunity** generally applies only to EMS systems that are operated by municipalities or other governmental entities. If your service is covered by immunity, it may mean that in some cases, particularly when an emergency situation exists, you cannot be sued at all or it may limit the amount of the monetary judgment that the plaintiff may recover. State laws vary significantly on both the statute of limitations and immunity, and you should understand the laws that apply in your state.

**Contributory negligence** is a legal defense that may be raised when the defendant thinks that the conduct of the plaintiff somehow contributed to any injuries or damages that were sustained by the plaintiff. For example, you are treating a patient with chest pain and you think that the administration of aspirin is indicated. You ask the patient if he is allergic to aspirin and he says no. Shortly after you administer the aspirin, the signs and symptoms of a severe allergic reaction develop in the patient. Later in the hospital, the doctor advises you that the patient's medical chart history indicates that the patient has an allergy to aspirin. The patient states that he forgot he was allergic to aspirin. In this case, the defense of contributory negligence might be raised because it was the patient's forgetfulness and his denial of an aspirin allergy that contributed to his allergic reaction.

The next phase of the case is known as **discovery**, and it is an opportunity for both sides to obtain information that will enable the attorneys to have a better understanding of the case and assist in negotiating a possible settlement or in preparing for trial. Discovery may include interrogatories, depositions, requests for production of documents, and physical examinations. **Interrogatories** are written questions that each side sends to the other, and **depositions** are oral questions asked of parties and witnesses under oath. On completion of the discovery phase, the parties may try to negotiate a possible settlement. Most cases are settled and do not go to trial. If a settlement is not able to be negotiated, the case will be set for trial. It is not uncommon for a case to take several years to get to trial.

At trial, each side will have an opportunity to present evidence that includes testimony of witnesses and documents such as medical reports and your run report. Witnesses may include experts such as physicians. Once both sides have concluded presenting evidence, a judge or jury will render a decision or verdict. If a judgment is rendered against you or your service, the plaintiff may be awarded compensatory or punitive damages:

1. **Compensatory damages.** These damages are intended to compensate the plaintiff for the injuries he or she sustained, including economic damages such as medical bills, damages to personal property, or lost earnings, and noneconomic damages such as physical or emotional pain and suffering.
2. **Punitive damages.** Punitive damages are not commonly awarded in negligence cases and

## Street Smarts

When you provide testimony in any phase of a lawsuit, it is best to be brief. Answer only the specific question that is asked based on your review of the patient report or your vivid memories of the incident. It is perfectly acceptable to answer "I don't know" or "I can't recall" if you are unsure. Opinions and elaborations subject you to challenges by the attorneys and can make you and your testimony seem less believable to the judge or jury.

are reserved for those cases where the defendant has acted intentionally or with a reckless disregard for the safety of the public.

In most cases, if a judgment is rendered against you, your service or its insurance carrier will pay the judgment.

It is also possible that you could be arrested and charged with a criminal offense arising out of your employment as an EMS provider. Although these are rare occurrences, EMTs have been charged with crimes, including theft of patient property, assault or sexual assault on a patient, operating a vehicle while under the influence of drugs or alcohol, manslaughter, and various drug-related offenses. Obviously, any arrest is considered very serious because a conviction could lead to imprisonment, the imposition of fines, and possible loss of the ability to practice as an EMT. Any EMT charged with a criminal offense should immediately secure the services of a highly experienced criminal attorney.

# YOU are the Provider SUMMARY

**1. Why is it essential that you obtain consent to treat the patient once you arrive?**

Consent is required from every conscious adult before care can be started. The adult patient who is conscious, rational, and capable of making informed decisions has a legal right to refuse care. The patient does not forfeit this right simply because you disagree or because it may not be the best medical decision. The law allows the patient to make choices that may seem medically unsound and might even endanger his or her own life. Failing to honor a competent adult patient's right to refuse care or transport may be grounds for both criminal and civil action against you.

**2. Should you assess the patient's competency or decision-making capacity once you arrive?**

Your role is to assess the patient's decision-making capacity. Although the terms *competence* and *decision-making capacity* are often thought of interchangeably, there is a distinction. Competence is typically determined by a court of law, whereas decision-making capacity refers to whether a patient is capable of making a rational decision. Assessing a patient's decision-making capacity can often be complicated in the prehospital setting, and you may require the assistance of medical control to make the best decision.

**3. Are you legally authorized to treat this patient? Why or why not?**

At this point, you have not obtained consent from the patient to begin treating him; in fact, you have not even introduced yourself. Under most circumstances, you may not begin treatment of a mentally competent adult until he or she has given you permission, or consent, to do so. If the patient has decision-making capacity—that is, the patient is conscious, alert, not under the influence of drugs or alcohol, and of legal age (18 years in most states)—you cannot legally provide care without the patient's consent, even if the patient is obviously sick or injured. Providing care without the patient's consent may be grounds for both criminal and civil action, such as assault and battery.

**4. How does informed consent differ from implied consent?**

A patient's consent must be informed, which means you have explained the nature of the treatment being offered, including the potential risks, benefits, and alternatives to treatment, as well as any potential consequences of refusing treatment.

Implied consent is based on the legal assumption that a critically ill or injured patient, who is physically unable to give consent (ie, unconscious, under the influence of drugs or alcohol), would consent to EMS treatment and transport if he or she were physically able to do so. Consent to treat is also implied when caring for a minor whose parents or caregivers are unable to be located; a minor cannot legally consent to or refuse medical care.

**5. What should you do when a patient refuses treatment and/or transport?**

When a patient refuses treatment and/or transport, it is not unreasonable to ask why he or she does not wish to be treated. Many people refuse treatment because of financial concerns or the fact that they are scared. In this case, you should explain that his high blood pressure and severe headache could indicate bleeding in the brain or some other potentially life-threatening condition and that only a physician can diagnose his problem. Do not be afraid to advise the patient that his refusal could ultimately result in death if you believe it is true. This is not a scare tactic; it is the truth and the patient has a right to hear it.

If, despite your best efforts to obtain consent to treat, a mentally competent adult still refuses, there is little else you can legally do. You should, however, inform medical control of the situation. In some cases, the physician may wish to speak directly to the patient.

**6.** **What questions should you ask yourself to help determine whether you can transport this patient against his will?**

When a patient refuses treatment, you must assess the patient's decision-making capacity. Is the patient's mental condition impaired? Is the patient under the influence of drugs or alcohol? Is the patient of legal age? Is the patient a danger to himself/herself or others? These are but a few of the questions that must be answered.

In this case, there is no evidence that has been uncovered thus far that the patient's decision-making capacity is impaired, and although he needs medical attention for his headache and blood pressure, you cannot legally force him to accept it, nor can you transport him against his will.

The best course of action is to ensure that the patient is aware of the potential consequences of his refusal—namely, death—and contact medical control to apprise him or her of the situation.

**7.** **Does HIPAA affect the medical care you provide to your patients? What information are you allowed to discuss with family members, bystanders, the media, and others?**

HIPAA has many aims; however, the section of the act that most directly affects EMS relates to patient privacy. *Confidential patient information* includes patient history, assessment findings, treatment, etc. HIPAA provides guidance on what types of information are protected, the responsibility of health care providers regarding that protection, and penalties for breaching that protection. Confidential information can be shared under certain conditions, such as for continuity of care and for billing purposes. *You should not allow HIPAA to affect the medical care that you provide to a patient.*

You must be very careful about what you discuss with family members, bystanders, the media, etc. You must protect the patient's confidential information. There may be times when this is difficult, especially with concerned family members. When in doubt about what to share, simply provide reassurance that everyone is doing his or her best for the patient.

**8.** **How do you respond to the clerk's question in a professional manner without violating HIPAA regulations?**

This is a great opportunity to praise a conscientious bystander who did the right thing. Thank the clerk, but do not provide him with any confidential patient information. For example, "You did the right thing during a stressful situation and we appreciate it. We are required to protect the patient's privacy, but I want to reassure you we will take excellent care of the patient from here."

**9.** **Should you report the patient's use of illegal substances to law enforcement personnel? Why or why not?**

The patient's use of cocaine is pertinent medical information that may have an effect on the care he receives at the hospital; therefore, it should be included in your PCR and your oral report to the receiving facility. However, the US Supreme Court has held that drug use or addiction (in contrast to possession or sale) is an illness and not a crime. Therefore, you are not legally required to report the patient's admitted use of these substances to law enforcement personnel. If you are in doubt, consult with your EMS medical director. More important, you must be familiar with the reporting requirements of the state in which you function as an EMT.

**10.** **Why is it a good idea to have the receiving nurse sign your PCR acknowledging the transfer of care?**

Sign-off is important for several reasons. It ensures that an equal or higher medical authority has accepted care of the patient from you. It also provides a record of who accepted care of the patient in the event there are any questions later. Failure to appropriately transfer care at the receiving hospital may be considered abandonment. Your documentation should show that you have met this obligation.

## YOU are the Provider SUMMARY *continued*

### EMS Patient Care Report (PCR)

| Date: 4-19-20 | Incident No.: 040109 | Nature of Call: Headache | | Location: 1175 N. Main St. | |
|---|---|---|---|---|---|
| Dispatched: 1720 | En Route: 1721 | At Scene: 1736 | Transport: 1743 | At Hospital: 1748 | In Service: 1801 |

#### Patient Information

| | |
|---|---|
| Age: 32<br>Sex: M<br>Weight (in kg [lb]): 91 kg (200 lb) | Allergies: None<br>Medications: Prinivil<br>Past Medical History: Hypertension<br>Chief Complaint: Severe headache |

#### Vital Signs

| Time: 1735 | BP: 200/110 | Pulse: 110 | Respirations: 24 | Spo$_2$: 98% |
|---|---|---|---|---|
| Time: 1741 | BP: 194/108 | Pulse: 104 | Respirations: 22 | Spo$_2$: 99% |
| Time: 1747 | BP: 166/94 | Pulse: 90 | Respirations: 18 | Spo$_2$: 99% |

#### EMS Treatment (circle all that apply)

| Oxygen @ ___ L/min via:<br><br>NC   NRM   Bag mask | Assisted Ventilation | Airway Adjunct | CPR |
|---|---|---|---|
| Defibrillation | Bleeding Control | Bandaging | Splinting | Other: Dimmed lights, position of comfort |

#### Narrative

9-1-1 dispatch for a man with a severe headache.

Chief Complaint: Severe headache

History: Patient states that his headache began a few hours earlier and that he has not taken his prescribed antihypertensive medication. No trauma was involved in this incident. Past medical history significant for hypertension. He denies loss of consciousness, nausea, or any other symptoms.

Assessment: On arrival at the scene, found the patient, a 32-year-old man, sitting on the sidewalk outside convenience store, grabbing his head in pain. He was conscious and alert; his airway was patent, and his breathing was adequate. Obtained vital signs and performed further assessment, which was unremarkable.

Treatment (Rx): Patient was initially hesitant to consent to EMS treatment and transport. However, after the potential complications of his refusal were explained to him, he agreed to EMS treatment and transport.

Transport: Placed patient onto stretcher, loaded him into the ambulance, dimmed the lights, and placed him in a position of comfort. Began transport to the hospital and monitored his condition en route. Patient admitted to using cocaine, but he did not think this was contributing to his condition. Patient remained conscious and alert during transport and stated that his headache was improving. Reassessment of his vital signs revealed that his blood pressure had improved. Delivered patient to emergency department staff and gave oral report to charge nurse.

**End of report**

# Prep Kit

## Ready for Review

- Under most circumstances, consent is required from every conscious adult before care can be started. The foundation of consent is decision-making capacity.
- You should never withhold life-saving care unless a valid DNR order is present.
- Because a minor might not have the wisdom, maturity, or judgment to give consent, the law requires that a parent or legal guardian give consent for treatment or transport.
- Adults who are conscious and alert and who appear to have decision-making capacity have the right to refuse treatment or withdraw from treatment at any time, even if doing so may result in serious injury or death.
- You should include all information pertaining to patient refusals in your PCR.
- Communication between you and the patient is considered confidential and generally cannot be disclosed without permission from the patient or a court order.
- Advance directives, living wills, or health care directives are most commonly used when a patient becomes comatose. Physician Orders for Life-Sustaining Treatment and Medical Orders for Life-Sustaining Treatment forms explicitly describe acceptable interventions for the patient in the form of medical orders.
- There are both definitive and presumptive signs of death. In many states, death is defined as the absence of circulatory and respiratory function.
- Consent to organ donation is evidenced by either a donor card or a driver's license indicating that the individual wishes to be a donor.
- Standard of care is established in many ways, among them local customs, statutes, ordinances, protocols, textbooks,

administrative regulations, and case law. The scope of practice outlines the care you are able to provide for the patient.
- Once your ambulance responds to a call or treatment is begun, you have a legal duty to act. In most cases, if you are off duty and happen to see a motor vehicle crash, you are not legally obligated to stop and assist patients.
- Determination of negligence is based on the following four factors: duty, breach of duty, damages, and causation. All four elements must be present for the legal doctrine of negligence to apply and for a plaintiff to prevail in a lawsuit against an EMS system or provider.
- Abandonment is the termination of care without the patient's consent and without making provisions for the transfer of care to a medical professional with skills at the same level or at a higher level than your own skills. Abandonment is legally and ethically a serious act. Always try to obtain a signature on your PCR from the person accepting transfer of care.
- Assault is defined as unlawfully placing a person in fear of immediate bodily harm. Battery is unlawfully touching a person; this includes providing emergency care without consent. To protect yourself from these charges, be sure to obtain expressed consent whenever possible.
- To avoid liability for defamation, you must only communicate information about your patients to authorized people and you should be sure that the information contained in your run reports and other documentation is accurate and relevant.
- Good Samaritan laws are based on the common law principle that when you reasonably help another person, you should

not be liable for errors and omissions that are made in giving good faith emergency care. Whereas some laws provide Good Samaritan protection for anyone who stops to render aid, others only provide protection for people with medical training.

- Records and reports are important; make sure that you compile a complete and accurate record of each incident. The courts consider an action or procedure that was not recorded on the written report as not having been performed, and an incomplete or untidy report is considered evidence of incomplete or inexpert medical care.

- You should know what the special reporting requirements are involving abuse of children, older adults, and others; injuries related to crimes; drug-related injuries; and childbirth.
- You must meet your legal and ethical responsibilities while caring for your patients' physical and emotional needs.
- As an EMT, there are several different circumstances that might cause you to end up in court, either as a witness or a defendant in a civil lawsuit or as a witness or defendant in a criminal case.

## Vital Vocabulary

**abandonment** Unilateral termination of care by the EMT without the patient's consent and without making provisions for transferring care to another medical professional with the skills and training necessary to meet the needs of the patient.

**advance directive** Written documentation that specifies medical treatment for a competent patient should the patient become unable to make decisions; also called a living will or health care directive.

**algor mortis** Cooling of the body after death until it matches the ambient temperature.

**applied ethics** The manner in which principles of ethics are incorporated into professional conduct.

**assault** Unlawfully placing a patient in fear of bodily harm.

**battery** Unlawfully touching a patient or providing emergency care without consent.

**bioethics** The study of ethics related to issues that arise in health care.

**breach of confidentiality** Disclosure of information without proper authorization.

**compensatory damages** Damages awarded in a civil lawsuit that are intended to restore the

plaintiff to the same condition that he or she was in prior to the incident.

**competent** Able to make rational decisions about personal well-being.

**consent** Permission to render care.

**contributory negligence** A legal defense that may be raised when the defendant thinks that the conduct of the plaintiff somehow contributed to any injuries or damages that were sustained by the plaintiff.

**decision-making capacity** Ability to understand and process information and make a choice regarding appropriate medical care.

**defamation** The communication of false information about a person that is damaging to that person's reputation or standing in the community.

**dependent lividity** Blood settling to the lowest point of the body, causing discoloration of the skin; a definitive sign of death.

**depositions** Oral questions asked of parties and witnesses under oath.

**discovery** The phase of a civil lawsuit where the plaintiff and defense obtain information from each other that will enable the attorneys to have a better understanding of the case and which will assist in negotiating a possible settlement or in preparing for trial. Discovery includes depositions, interrogatories, and demands for production of records.

**do not resuscitate (DNR) order** Written documentation by a physician giving permission to medical personnel not to attempt resuscitation in the event of cardiac arrest.

**durable power of attorney for health care** A type of advance directive executed by a competent adult that appoints another individual to make medical treatment decisions on his or her behalf, in the event that the person making the appointment loses decision-making capacity.

**duty to act** A medicolegal term relating to certain personnel who either by statute or by function have a responsibility to provide care.

**emancipated minor** A person who is under the legal age in a given state but, because of other circumstances, is legally considered an adult.

**emergency** A serious situation, such as injury or illness that threatens the life or welfare of a person or group of people and requires immediate intervention.

**emergency doctrine** The principle of law that permits a health care provider to treat a patient in an emergency situation when the patient is incapable of granting consent because of an altered level of consciousness, disability, the effects of drugs or alcohol, or the patient's age.

**emergency medical care** Immediate care or treatment.

**ethics** The philosophy of right and wrong, of moral duties, and of ideal professional behavior.

**expressed consent** A type of consent in which a patient gives verbal or nonverbal authorization for provision of care or transport.

**false imprisonment** The confinement of a person without legal authority or the person's consent.

**forcible restraint** The act of physically preventing an individual from initiating any physical action.

**Good Samaritan laws** Statutory provisions enacted by many states to protect citizens from liability for errors and omissions in giving good-faith emergency medical care, unless there is wanton, gross, or willful negligence.

**governmental immunity** Legal doctrine that can protect an EMS provider from being sued or that may limit the amount of the monetary judgment that the plaintiff may recover; generally applies only to EMS systems that are operated by municipalities or other governmental entities.

**gross negligence** Conduct that constitutes a willful or reckless disregard for a duty or standard of care.

**health care directive** A written document that specifies medical treatment for a competent patient, should he or she become unable to make decisions. Also known as an advance directive or a living will.

**health care proxy** A type of advance directive executed by a competent adult that appoints another individual to make medical treatment decisions on his or her behalf in the event that the person making the appointment loses decision-making capacity. Also known as a durable power of attorney for health care.

**implied consent** Type of consent in which a patient who is unable to give consent is given treatment under the legal assumption that he or she would want treatment.

**informed consent** Permission for treatment given by a competent patient after the potential risks, benefits, and alternatives to treatment have been explained.

**in loco parentis** Refers to the legal responsibility of a person or organization to take on some of the functions and responsibilities of a parent.

**interrogatories** Written questions that the defense and plaintiff send to one another.

**kidnapping** The seizing, confining, abducting, or carrying away of a person by force, including transporting a competent adult for medical treatment without his or her consent.

**libel** False and damaging information about a person that is communicated in writing.

**medicolegal** A term relating to medical jurisprudence (law) or forensic medicine.

**morality** A code of conduct that can be defined by society, religion, or a person, affecting character, conduct, and conscience.

**negligence** Failure to provide the same care that a person with similar training would provide.

**negligence per se** A theory that may be used when the conduct of the person being sued is alleged to have occurred in clear violation of a statute.

**patient autonomy** The right of a patient to make informed choices regarding his or her health care.

**protected health information (PHI)** Any information about health status, provision of health care, or payment for health care that can be linked to an individual. This is interpreted rather broadly and includes any part of a patient's medical record or payment history.

**proximate causation** When a person who has a duty abuses it, and causes harm to another individual, the EMT, the agency, and/or the medical director may be sued for negligence.

**punitive damages** Damages that are sometimes awarded in a civil lawsuit when the conduct of the defendant was intentional or constituted a reckless disregard for the safety of the public.

**putrefaction** Decomposition of body tissues; a definitive sign of death.

**res ipsa loquitur** When the EMT or an EMS system is held liable even when the plaintiff is unable to clearly demonstrate how an injury occurred.

**rigor mortis** Stiffening of the body muscles; a definitive sign of death.

**scope of practice** Most commonly defined by state law; outlines the care that the EMT is able to provide for the patient.

**slander** False and damaging information about a person that is communicated by spoken word.

**standard of care** Written, accepted levels of emergency care expected by reason of training and profession; written by legal or professional organizations so that patients are not exposed to unreasonable risk or harm.

**statute of limitations** The time within which a case must be commenced.

**torts** Wrongful acts that give rise to a civil lawsuit.

# References

1. AARP. Advance directive forms. http://www.aarp.org/caregiving/financial-legal/free-printable-advance-directives/. Accessed February 27, 2020.
2. American College of Emergency Physicians EMS Committee. *Ethical Questions in Emergency Medical Services: Controversies and Recommendations*. https://www.acep.org/globalassets/uploads/uploaded-files/acep/clinical-and-practice-management/ems-and-disaster-preparedness/ethical---ems---info-paper.pdf. Published October 2012. Accessed February 27, 2020.
3. American Medical Association. Confidentiality. https://www.ama-assn.org/delivering-care/ethics/confidentiality. Accessed February 27, 2020.
4. American Medical Association. Informed consent. https://www.ama-assn.org/delivering-care/ethics/informed-consent. Accessed February 27, 2020.
5. American Medical Association. Privacy in health care. https://www.ama-assn.org/delivering-care/ethics/privacy-health-care. Accessed February 27, 2020.
6. American Medical Association. Professionalism in relationships with media. https://www.ama-assn.org/delivering-care/ethics/professionalism-relationships-media. Accessed February 27, 2020.
7. Center for Medicare and Medicaid Services. Advance directives and long-term care. Medicare.gov website. https://www.medicare.gov/manage-your-health/advance-directives-long-term-care. Accessed February 27, 2020.
8. Erbay H. Some ethical issues in prehospital emergency medicine. *Turkish J Emerg Med.* 2016;14(4):193-198.
9. National Association of Emergency Medical Technicians. Code of ethics and EMT oath. https://www

.naemt.org/about-ems/emt-oath. Accessed February 27, 2020.

10.  Ogilvie WA, Furin M, Lopez RA, Goldstein S. EMS, legal and ethical issues. National Center for Biotechnology Information website (StatPearls). http://www.ncbi.nlm .nih.gov/books/NBK519553/. Updated August 30, 2018. Accessed February 27, 2020.

11.  Torabi M, Borhani F, Abbaszadeh A, Atashzadeh-Shoorideh F. Experiences of pre-hospital emergency medical personnel in ethical decision-making: a qualitative study. *BMC Med Ethics.* https://doi.org/10.1186 /s12910-018-0334-x. Published December 18, 2018. Accessed February 27, 2020.

12.  US Department of Health and Human Services. Your rights under HIPAA. HHS.gov website. https://www.hhs .gov/hipaa/for-individuals/guidance-materials-for -consumers/index.html. Reviewed January 21, 2020. Accessed February 27, 2020.

13.  Wolfberg D. Pro bono: is reporting rape an EMS obligation? *JEMS* website. https://www.jems.com/2015/06/05 /pro-bono-is-reporting-rape-an-ems-obligation/. Published June 15, 2015. Accessed February 27, 2020.

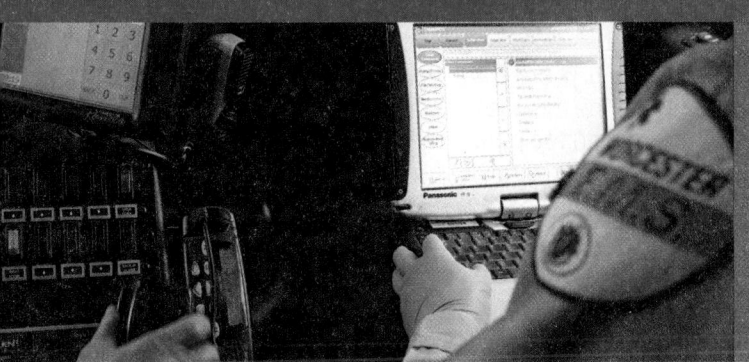

# Chapter 4

# Communications and Documentation

## NATIONAL EMS EDUCATION STANDARD COMPETENCIES

### Preparatory

Applies fundamental knowledge of the emergency medical services (EMS) system, safety/well-being of the emergency medical technician (EMT), and medical/legal and ethical issues to the provision of emergency care.

### Therapeutic Communication

Principles of communicating with patients in a manner that achieves a positive relationship
- Interviewing techniques (pp 122–126)
- Adjusting communication strategies for age, stage of development, patients with special needs, and differing cultures (pp 120, 127–131)
- Verbal defusing strategies (pp 120–123)
- Family presence issues (pp 123–126)

### EMS System Communication

Communication needed to
- Call for resources (pp 151–153)
- Transfer care of the patient (pp 153–156)

- Interact within the team structure (pp 151–153)
- EMS communication system (pp 146–151)
- Communication with other health care professionals (pp 153–156)
- Team communication and dynamics (pp 131–133, 153–156)

### Documentation

- Recording patient findings (pp 134–146)
- Principles of medical documentation and report writing (pp 134–146)

### Medical Terminology

Uses foundational anatomical and medical terms and abbreviations in written and oral communication with colleagues and other health care professionals.

## KNOWLEDGE OBJECTIVES

1. Describe the factors and strategies to consider for therapeutic communication with patients. (pp 119–133)
2. Discuss the techniques of effective verbal communication. (pp 122–133)
3. Explain the skills that should be used to communicate with family members, bystanders, people from other agencies, and hospital personnel. (pp 122–133)

4. Discuss special considerations in communicating with older people, children, patients who are hard of hearing, visually impaired patients, and non–English-speaking patients. (pp 127–131)
5. Describe the use of written communications and documentation. (pp 133–146)
6. State the purpose of a patient care report (PCR) and the information required to complete it. (pp 134–143)

7. Explain the legal implications of the PCR. (pp 142–143)
8. Describe how to document refusal of care, including the legal implications. (pp 143–146)
9. Discuss state and/or local special reporting requirements, such as for gunshot wounds, dog bites, and abuse. (p 146)
10. Describe the basic principles of the various types of communications equipment used in EMS. (pp 146–150)
11. Describe the use of radio communications, including the proper methods of initiating and terminating a radio call. (pp 150–151)
12. List the correct radio procedures in the following phases of a typical call: initial receipt of call, en route to call, on scene, arrival at hospital (or point of transfer), and return to service. (pp 151–153)
13. List the proper sequence of information to communicate in radio delivery of a patient report. (pp 153–156)

## SKILLS OBJECTIVES

1. Demonstrate the techniques of successful cross-cultural communication. (p 120)
2. Demonstrate completion of a PCR. (pp 134–143)
3. Demonstrate how to make a simulated, concise radio transmission with dispatch. (pp 150–153)

# Introduction

**Communication** is the transmission of information from one person to another—whether it is written, verbal, or nonverbal (through body language). Effective communication is an essential component of prehospital care and is necessary to achieve a positive relationship with patients, coworkers, and others in the health care industry.

Verbal communication skills are vitally important for EMTs. Your verbal skills will enable you to gather information from the patient and bystanders. These skills will also make it possible for you to effectively coordinate with the variety of responders who are often present at the scene. Excellent verbal communication is also an integral part of transferring the patient's care to the nurses and physicians at the hospital.

**Documentation** is the written or electronically recorded portion of your patient care interaction that becomes part of the patient's permanent medical record. It serves many purposes, including demonstrating that the care delivered was appropriate and within the scope and practice of the providers involved. Documentation also provides an opportunity to communicate the patient's story to others who may participate in the patient's care in the future. Adequate reporting and accurate records ensure the continuity of patient care. Complete patient records also facilitate transfer of care, transfer of responsibility, and help comply with requirements of health departments and law enforcement agencies, as well as fulfill your organization's administrative needs. Reporting and record-keeping duties are an essential aspect of patient care, although they are performed only after the patient's condition has been stabilized. Documentation in the field drives both funding and research for EMS. Seat belts are a prime example. Studies gathered from record keeping in the 1970s showed that patients have a significantly higher survival rate if seat belts are used during motor vehicle crashes. Armed with this information, laws were passed to enforce seat belt usage, and huge amounts of money were spent on educating the public. Fast forward to the present—research on the data collected in the National Emergency Medical Services Information System (NEMSIS) and on data in other commercial documentation systems that can link prehospital records to hospital discharge outcomes is rapidly expanding the knowledge base about what EMS providers actually do on a day-to-day basis and on what treatment measures really make a difference.

Computer, radio, and telephone communications link you and your team with other members of the EMS, fire, and law enforcement communities. This link helps the entire team to work together more effectively and provides an important layer of safety and protection for each member of the team. You must know what your system can and cannot do, and you must be able to use your system efficiently and effectively.

This chapter describes the factors and strategies that you need to be an effective communicator, discusses a variety of effective methods of verbal communication, and provides guidelines for appropriate written documentation of patient care. The chapter concludes by identifying the kinds of communication equipment that are used, along with standard radio operating procedures and protocols. The roles of the Federal Communications Commission in EMS are also described.

## Therapeutic Communication

How do we communicate? This simple question can be surprisingly complex because there are many things to consider during communication (**TABLE 4-1**). **Therapeutic communication** uses various communication techniques and strategies, both verbal and nonverbal, to encourage patients to express how they are feeling and to achieve a positive relationship with the patient. This section will discuss the factors and strategies that are necessary for therapeutic communication.

People communicate in a variety of ways, such as through eye contact, body position, and facial expressions. Factors such as culture and age need to be taken into consideration during communication. Patients with special needs may require you to consider alternative forms of communication. For example, if your patient is deaf and you cannot communicate using sign language, you may need to communicate by having the patient write down his or her feelings.

| TABLE 4-1 Factors and Strategies to Consider During Communication | |
| --- | --- |
| Age | Eye contact |
| Body language | Facial expression |
| Clothing | Sex |
| Culture | Posture |
| Education | Voice tempo |
| Environment | Volume |

© Jones & Bartlett Learning.

### Words of Wisdom

The Shannon–Weaver communication model was developed to assist in the mathematical theory of communication for Bell Telephone Labs in the late 1940s (**FIGURE 4-1**). Shannon and Weaver were trying to figure out the math involved in sending information through telephone lines. After its creation, it quickly became apparent that this model had application in areas other than math. Social scientists adopted this model, and it remains a valuable tool in understanding the variables involved in human communication. In the communication model, the sender must take a thought, encode it into a message, and send the message to the receiver. The receiver then decodes the message and sends feedback to the sender.

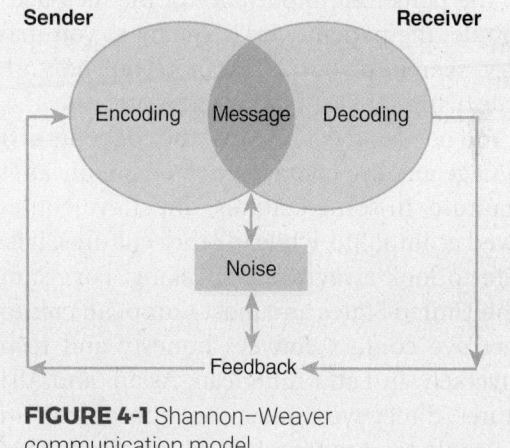

**FIGURE 4-1** Shannon–Weaver communication model.

© Jones & Bartlett Learning.

# Age, Culture, and Personal Experience

The thoughts of people are greatly influenced by their personal experiences. For example, an older person who often experiences significant pain may view pain as more of an inconvenience than a problem. A child who has limited experience with pain would likely react much differently. People from various cultures are taught to handle illness, injury, and pain differently. Some cultures encourage people to express their emotions; others see it as a sign of weakness. These social and personal influences will shape how people communicate.

Patients may talk, make gestures, or write a note to express how they are feeling. "I am so sorry to bother you, but my chest hurts a little." "Hey! What took you so long? My chest is killing me! Are you going to help me or what?" Both of these messages talk about pain, but they also have much more information within them.

The tone, pace, and volume of the language will tell you about the mood of the person who is communicating. These clues also provide some insight into the perceived importance of the message. For example, the patient who is yelling at you may be angry, scared, or both. Take note not only of the words being spoken, but how they are said.

You need to recognize that the concepts of body language and eye contact are often greatly affected by culture. In some cultures, direct eye contact is viewed as impolite, while in other cultures, it is impolite to look away while speaking. For example, in the United States and most European countries, direct eye contact conveys honesty and respect. Conversely, in Latin American, Asian, and African cultures, direct eye contact conveys confrontation.

People tend to translate the messages they receive using their own worldview. **Ethnocentrism** occurs when you consider your own cultural values as more important when you are interacting with people of a different culture. If you are North American, for example, you might think that a patient is hiding something, afraid, or untrustworthy if the patient looks away from you while you are talking. These conclusions may be true if the two people communicating are from a North American culture. All aspects of communication—eye contact, social distances, body language, and even touching—have a cultural foundation. In Thailand, for example, the touching of the head is reserved for those who are very intimate. This cultural belief can present a problem for you if the patient's head is bleeding. By being aware that in Thai culture touching the head is very personal, you will know to ask permission, if at all possible, before doing so. Even during life-threatening emergencies, it is important to recognize and respect others' cultures.

**Cultural imposition** takes this idea to an extreme. Some health care providers may consciously or subconsciously force their cultural values onto their patient because they believe their values are better. For example, consider a child who is brought to the emergency department (ED) with red marks on his back from a traditional Asian healing practice called coining—rubbing hot coins on the child's back as a treatment for medical illness. The parents explain to the physician that the coining helped for a short time, but now the child seems to be getting sicker. The physician responds angrily to the parents, accusing them of potential abuse and insisting that their practices are harmful (although they are not). This accusation reflects cultural imposition.

## Nonverbal Communication

### Facial Expressions, Body Language, and Eye Contact

Eye contact and body language are powerful communication tools. Consider how dogs interact. When two dogs meet for the first time, they look at each other. The position of the head, shoulders, tail, and back all help dogs communicate. Before they get any closer, the dogs need to understand their new relationship. Who is dominant? Will you hurt me? These questions must be answered quickly.

People communicate using a similar technique. The body language we consciously or subconsciously choose provides more information than words alone. Consider the images in **FIGURE 4-2**. Without any words, the mood of each of these people should be clear.

Patients can become hostile toward EMS providers. When you are treating a potentially hostile patient, it is important that you understand and be aware of your own body language. People tend to react to anger with anger. If you are dealing with an angry patient, you must stay calm and try to defuse the situation before it escalates. Consider the following steps:

1. **Assess the safety of the scene.** Decide whether you need to call law enforcement. Make sure

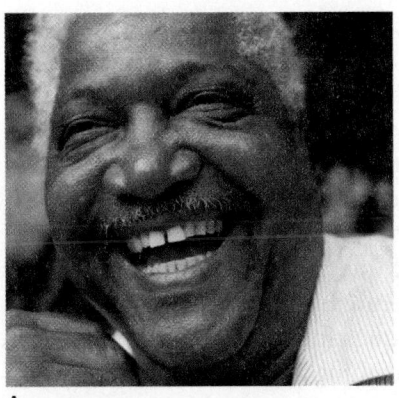
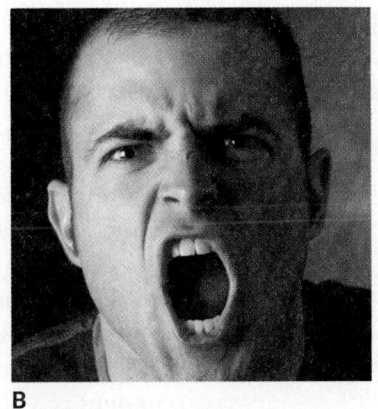
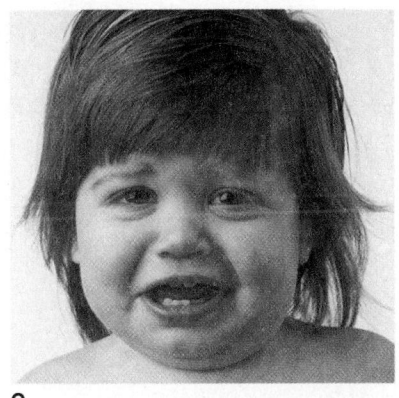

**A**                **B**                **C**

**FIGURE 4-2** The effectiveness of body language. **A.** Happy. **B.** Angry. **C.** Sad.

A, C: © Photodisc; B: © Photodisc/Thinkstock.

that you have sufficient backup to ensure the safety of the patient and your crew.

2. **Do not assume an aggressive posture.** Be aware that if you cross your arms, clench your fists, or place your hands on your hips, it sends a message (whether intentional or not) that you are impatient, uninterested, or asserting a position of authority. Instead, stand with your palms facing out; this communicates openness and acceptance and allows for quick movement, if necessary.

3. **Make good eye contact, but do not stare.**

4. **Speak calmly, confidently, and slowly.** With your backup clearly visible, advise the patient what needs to be done, or provide the patient with limited, acceptable choices. "Sir, I need you to sit on the ambulance cot now. Would you like to sit on the cot or can we help you to the cot?"

5. *Never* threaten the patient, either verbally or physically. Personal safety should be your primary concern when caring for any patient, but this is especially true with patients who display hostile behavior.

Remember, it is important for you to be attentive to facial expressions, body language, and eye

contact—your own and your patient's. These physical cues will help you and your patient to truly understand the message being sent. Additional techniques you can use to calm a patient and establish a therapeutic rapport will be discussed later in this chapter.

## Words of Wisdom

EMTs must always be dressed professionally. The first impression you make may be influenced by your appearance. Caring for your uniform may improve that impression and enhance your ability to establish trust and rapport with your patients. You are sending the message that you care without speaking a word.

## Physical Factors

Various physical factors affect communication, which are referred to as noise. **Noise** is anything that dampens or obscures the true meaning of the message. Literal noise, or sounds in the environment, can make it difficult to understand the patient or for the patient to understand you. Lighting, distance, or physical obstacles are other factors that may affect your communication.

Cultural norms often dictate the amount of space, or proximity, between people when communicating (**TABLE 4-2**). The degree to which people feel comfortable depends on with whom they are communicating. As a person gets closer, a greater sense of trust must be established. When you finally enter someone's intimate space, there must be a high sense of trust.

## Street Smarts

When both you and the patient must wear masks, important nonverbal communication cues are lost. If you make a joke, you may need to say, "I'm smiling under my mask" so the patient doesn't misinterpret your comment. Masks also make it difficult to communicate with patients who are hard of hearing and have come to rely on reading lips to compensate for their hearing loss.

| TABLE 4-2 Guidelines for Personal Space in the United States | | |
|---|---|---|
| **Space** | **Distance** | **Description** |
| Intimate | Less than 18 in. (46 cm) | Whispering, touching; must be invited |
| Personal | 18 in. to 4 ft (46 cm–1.2 m) | Conversations with close friends or family |
| Social | 4 to 10 ft (1.2 m–3.0 m) | Conversations with acquaintances |
| Public | 10 to 25 ft (3.0–7.6 m) | Interacting with strangers |

© Jones & Bartlett Learning.

Understanding how communication works and the importance of effective communication is important when gathering information from the patient. Your communication skills will be put to the test when you communicate with patients and/or families in emergency situations. Remember that someone who is sick or injured is scared and might not understand what you are doing or saying. Therefore, your gestures, body movements, and attitude toward the patient are critically important in gaining the trust of both patient and family.

## Verbal Communication

As an EMT, you must master many communication skills, including those associated with radio operations and written communications. Skilled verbal communication with the patient and family, bystanders, and the rest of the health care team is an essential part of high-quality patient care and transport. You must be able to listen effectively to fully understand the nature of the scene and the patient's problem. You must also be able to organize your thoughts to quickly and accurately verbalize instructions to the patient, bystanders, and other health care professionals.

One of the most fundamental aspects of what EMTs do is to ask patients questions. There are two types of questions: **Open-ended questions** are ones in which a patient needs to provide some level of detail to give an answer, whereas **closed-ended questions** can be answered in short or single-word responses. When first approaching your patient, you should use open-ended questions. "What seems to be bothering you today?" Open-ended questions allow a free flow of conversation. They let the patient direct you to what is bothering him or her.

Closed-ended questions are important to use when patients are unable to provide long or complete answers to questions. Perhaps the patient is having severe breathing problems, or maybe the patient is a child who is scared and does not know what to say. In situations for which thoughtful answers are not possible, closed-ended questions that invite a "yes" or "no" answer are appropriate and are particularly useful when assessing a patient's condition. "Are you having trouble breathing? Do you take medications for your heart?"

With closed-ended questions, however, it is possible for you to miss important issues if pertinent questions are not asked. Imagine how many ways a person can be sick or injured. Now imagine trying to come up with a single yes/no question for each sickness or injury. Closed-ended questions typically provide limited information, and you should consider the answers to these questions as only a starting point toward understanding the patient's condition.

Before beginning your interview with the patient, determine which provider will lead the interview. This will ensure that you and your partner do not ask questions at the same time or ask repetitive questions. When you are asking questions of the patient, be conscious of how many questions you are asking. "How are you doing today? Have you been feeling ill?" This common approach actually asks the patient two kinds of questions, one open-ended and one closed-ended. Often the patient will respond with a simple "yes." To avoid this situation, it is best to ask a single question, wait for an answer, and then proceed to another question.

There are many powerful communication tools you can use when trying to obtain information from patients. Sometimes patients will hide information, either consciously or unconsciously, due to fear or confusion. The techniques in **TABLE 4-3** provide you with strategies that will assist you in gathering patient information. They can be helpful to use not only with patients who are willing to share, but with those who are resistant to sharing information.

| Communication Technique | Definition | Example |
|---|---|---|
| Facilitation | Encourage the patient to talk more or provide more information. | EMT: "I am listening to you. Can you tell me more about that?" |
| Pause | Do not speak. | Give the patient space and time to think and respond. |
| Reflection | Restating a patient's statement made to you to confirm your understanding. | Patient: "I am so depressed that I could die." EMT: "I understand that you are feeling depressed." |
| Empathy | Be sensitive to the patient's feelings and thoughts. | Use eye contact and, if appropriate, touching to reinforce communication; adjust tone of voice and pace to allow for open communication. |
| Clarification | Ask the patient to explain what he or she meant by an answer. | Patient: "I just feel sick." EMT: "Can you tell me how you are feeling sick? What feels wrong?" |
| Confrontation | Make the patient who is in denial or in a mental state of shock focus on urgent and life-critical issues. | Patient: "I am having pain in my chest, my back has been hurting me, and I ran out of my blood pressure medication." EMT: "We will talk about your medicines in a moment. Please tell me about your chest pain." |
| Interpretation | Restate the patient's complaint to confirm your understanding. | EMT: "If I understand correctly, you have been feeling pain for the past 3 days, and it has gotten worse today." Patient: "That's right." |
| Explanation | Provide factual information to support a conversation. | Patient: "I do not understand what is happening." EMT: "We have checked your blood sugar and blood pressure and don't see anything we need to immediately treat." |
| Summary | Provide the patient with an overview of the conversation and the steps you will take. | EMT: "We will be taking you to the emergency department to care for your chest pain. I will be giving you some medication that should make you feel better." |

**TABLE 4-3** Therapeutic Communication Techniques

© Jones & Bartlett Learning.

When you interview the patient, consider using touch to communicate caring and compassion. Touch is a powerful tool; therefore, keep in mind that it should be used consciously and sparingly (**FIGURE 4-3**). Many people will be uncomfortable with a stranger touching them suddenly. If you are going to touch the patient, approach slowly and touch the patient's shoulder or arm respectfully. You can consider holding the patient's hand. This allows you to touch the patient, showing you care about what he or she is telling you, and also allows you to remain at a slight distance.

Avoid touching the patient's torso, chest, or face simply as a means of communication, because these areas are often viewed as intimate. Also, to touch these areas, you will need to get closer to the patient, potentially invading the patient's intimate space. **TABLE 4-4** provides other tips on what to avoid when communicating with patients.

The presence of family, friends, and bystanders during your interview of the patient can be valuable. Sometimes, however, well-meaning family members will speak for the patient, and, at times, you may need to ask the family member to allow the

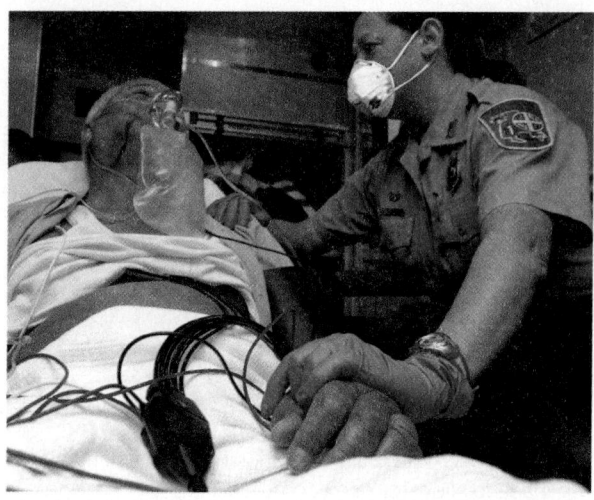

**FIGURE 4-3** Using touch conveys a sense of caring and compassion.

© Jones & Bartlett Learning.

patient to answer. Ultimately, you will need to assess the situation and determine whether the additional people are helping you care for the patient or hindering your efforts. Do not be afraid to ask others to step outside or step aside for a moment while you talk with the patient. It is generally best

**TABLE 4-4** Interview Techniques to Avoid

| Improper Technique | Example | Rationale |
|---|---|---|
| Provide false hope or reassurance. | EMT: "It will be okay." "This is nothing to worry about." | You do not know that everything will be okay. |
| Give unsolicited advice. | EMT: "Well, if I were you, I wouldn't have called the ambulance at all." | This demeans the patient and makes you seem arrogant, rather than helpful. |
| Ask leading or biased questions. | EMT: "Are you telling me that this cut is the only reason you called the ambulance?" | Your patient deserves respectful communication. It is inappropriate for you to suggest to the patient that an ambulance was not needed, even if that is what you believe. |
| Talk too much. | The EMT talks to the patient without really listening to the patient, simply going through the motions. | When the patient provides you information, you need to consider the information and guide the conversation toward a goal. |
| Interrupt the patient. | Patient: "Well, I was having trouble breathing last month and …" EMT: "Can we move on to how you are feeling now?" | You may seem bored or annoyed that the patient is taking up your time. |
| Use "why" questions. | EMT: "Why did you call the ambulance today?" | "Why" questions often appear to accuse the listener. You may seem annoyed that the patient called 9-1-1. |
| Use authoritative language. | EMT: "Tell me what is wrong with you." "Just give me the details." | This language does not encourage open communication. |
| Speak in professional jargon. | EMT: "I think we need to take you to the ED stat. We will give you ASA and NTG en route. Any questions?" | This type of communication confuses the patient. Most patients do not understand medical jargon. |

© Jones & Bartlett Learning.

to keep families together, but in cases where a family member is not helpful, consider giving him or her a task to do, such as gathering medications or clothing. This task can transform the person from a hindrance into a valuable aide. Take into account how the patient will feel without his or her loved ones nearby. Separating them may make the patient more anxious.

These 10 Golden Rules will help you to calm and reassure your patient and provide a therapeutic rapport:

1. **Make and keep eye contact with your patient.** Give the patient your undivided attention. This will let the patient know that he or she is your top priority. Look the patient straight in the eye to establish a **rapport**. Establishing a rapport is building a trusting relationship with your patient. This will make caring for the patient much easier.

2. **Provide your name and use the patient's proper name.** Introduce yourself and your partner. If your department provides you with a name tag, wear it. Ask the patient what he or she wishes to be called. Avoid using terms such as "honey" or "dear." Use a patient's first name only if the patient is a child or the patient asks you to use his or her first name. Rather, use a courtesy title, such as "Mr. Peters," "Mrs. Smith," or "Ms. Butler." If you do not know the patient's name, refer to the patient as "sir" or "ma'am."

3. **Tell the patient the truth.** Even if you have to say something very unpleasant, telling the truth is better than lying. Lying will destroy the patient's trust in you and decrease your own confidence. You might not always tell the patient everything, but if the patient or a family member asks a specific question, you should answer truthfully. A direct question deserves a direct answer. If you do not know the answer to a patient's question, say so. For example, a patient may ask, "Am I having a heart attack?" To which you would answer, "I don't know, but we will certainly get more information at the hospital. Right now, I am caring for you just like I would care for someone who is having a heart attack."

4. **Use language that the patient can understand.** Do not talk up or down to the patient in any way. Avoid technical medical terms that the patient might not understand. For example, ask the patient whether he or she has a history of "heart problems." This will usually result in more accurate information than if you ask about "previous episodes of myocardial infarction" or a "history of cardiomyopathy."

5. **Be careful what you say about the patient to others.** You need to understand the relationship between the person you are talking with (such as a bystander) and the patient. Ask the patient if it is okay for you to talk with this person. While speaking to others, ensure that you leave the general area of the patient if you must have a confidential conversation. Be mindful that sharing patient information may be a Health Insurance Portability and Accountability Act (HIPAA) violation. Do not talk about the patient in front of him or her; to do so gives the impression that the patient has no choice in his or her medical care. This is easy to forget when the patient has impaired cognitive (thought) processes or has difficulty communicating.

6. **Be aware of your body language.** Nonverbal communication is extremely important in dealing with patients (**FIGURE 4-4**). In stressful situations, patients may misinterpret your gestures and movements. Be particularly careful not to appear frustrated or threatening. Instead, position yourself at the same level or at a lower level than the patient when practical.

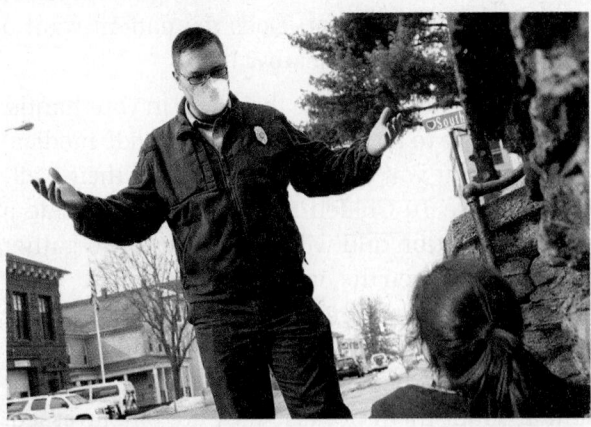

**FIGURE 4-4** Watch your body language, because patients may misinterpret your gestures, movements, and stance.
© Jones & Bartlett Learning.

Remember that you should always conduct yourself in a calm, professional manner.

7. **Always speak slowly, clearly, and distinctly.** Pay close attention to your tone of voice.

8. **If the patient is hard of hearing, face the person so that he or she can read your lips.** Try lowering or raising the tone of your voice; some people who are hard of hearing can hear certain pitches better than others. Do not shout at a person who is hard of hearing. Shouting will make it harder for the patient to hear you and may frighten the patient. Never assume that an older patient is hard of hearing or otherwise unable to understand you. Also, never use "baby talk" with older patients or with anyone other than infants. If you are unable to communicate with the patient, have your partner try. Another technique is to have the patient put the stethoscope in his or her ears while you speak softly into the diaphragm to help amplify the sound.

9. **Allow time for the patient to answer or respond to your questions.** Do not rush a patient unless there is immediate danger. Sick and injured people may not be thinking clearly and may need time to answer even simple questions. This is especially true when treating older patients.

10. **Act and speak in a calm, confident manner while caring for the patient.** Make sure you attend to the patient's comfort and needs. Try to make the patient physically comfortable and relaxed. Find out whether the patient is more comfortable sitting or lying down. Is the patient cold or hot? Does the patient want a friend or relative nearby?

Patients literally place their lives in your hands. They deserve to know that you can provide medical care and that you are concerned about their well-being. These 10 Golden Rules will help provide a good foundation and will make it easier to gather information when the patient wants to talk.

Sometimes, you need to gather information from a reluctant audience. Patients may be defensive about their problems and may not want to talk about them because they are embarrassed. They may direct the conversation away from the true problem. With these patients, start the conversation as usual. Introduce yourself. Be open and compassionate. If you find yourself not getting any real answers, then consider one of the techniques described in Table 4-3.

## Emotional Intelligence

**Emotional intelligence** is the ability to understand and manage your own emotions and properly respond to others' emotions. Sometimes referred to as people skills, emotional intelligence can help EMTs defuse conflict, build a rapport, communicate more effectively, and manage difficult situations. Emotional intelligence is commonly understood to have five attributes.

1. **Self-awareness.** The ability to recognize your own emotions and how they affect your thoughts and behavior.

2. **Self-regulation.** The ability to control impulsive emotions and behaviors and to manage emotions in positive ways.

3. **Motivation.** The ability to motivate yourself and others in a positive direction, often deferring short-term rewards for long-term success.

4. **Empathy.** The ability to understand the concerns, emotions, and needs of others by picking up on communication and social cues and clues.

5. **Social skills.** The ability to develop and maintain positive rapport and relationships through effective communications.

Think of people in your life whom you consider kind, caring, and exceptional listeners. These are people with high emotional intelligence. They can identify, understand, and manage their own emotions and the emotions of others.

As an EMT, you should seek to understand and improve your own emotional intelligence. Consider the following tips:

- Assess how you react to stressful situations. Do you become upset by every little frustration, such as delays, people not performing tasks correctly, or things not going your way? Try to manage your frustration, and work on staying calm and in control when faced with minor irritations.

- Practice mindfulness. Purposely focus your attention on the current moment, without blame and judgment of yourself or others. Doing so can help calm and focus you and make you more aware of the situation around you.

- Take responsibility for your actions. Don't be quick to immediately blame or attack others if things don't go your way. Acknowledge your own role in the situation.
- Consider how your actions will affect others before you take those actions. Think about how your words and actions will make others feel.

When communicating in difficult situations, especially when high levels of emotion are involved, a communication method known as the behavioral change stairway model may be helpful. This five-step model was developed by the Federal Bureau of Investigation to manage hostage negotiations quickly and effectively. It can be adapted to most crisis communications. Each step should be followed in order, as each step builds on the previous step or steps to help improve communications, build rapport, and deescalate crisis situations.

1. **Employ active listening.** Carefully listen to what the other person has to say, and let the person know you are doing so. Acknowledge what the person is saying, and do not interrupt, disagree, or give commands.
2. **Display empathy.** Use your emotional intelligence to understand the patient's perspective. You do not have to agree with the person or condone his or her actions, but you have to understand where the person is coming from and what the person wants.
3. **Build a rapport.** Once you have listened to the person and understand where he or she is coming from, it is much easier, especially in a crisis, to empathize with the person and "speak the person's language."
4. **Exert influence.** Look at realistic solutions to move the situation forward in a positive way. Understanding the person's perspective along with your own needs, consider how you can move forward in a way the person will understand. Initiate behavior change: Propose a solution that makes sense to the other person and is acceptable to you.

## Communicating With Older Patients

In 2018 about 49 million people, representing 16% of the US population, were older than 65 years; this population is expected to reach 22% by 2050.

Thus, EMS providers can expect an ever-increasing number of encounters with people in this age category. However, a person's actual age might not be the most important factor in classifying a person as geriatric. It is more important to determine a person's functional age. The functional age relates to the person's ability to function in daily activities, mental state, health status, and activity pattern.

As an EMS provider, when you enter a scene to care for an older patient, you have been called because a person needs help. What you say and how you say it has an effect on the patient's perception of the call. You should present yourself as competent, confident, and caring. You must take charge of the situation, but do so with compassion. You are there to listen and act on what you learn. Do not limit your assessment to the obvious problem. Often, older patients who express that they are not well, or who are overly concerned about their health or general condition, are at risk for a serious decline in their physical, emotional, or psychological state.

In general, older people think clearly, can give you a clear medical history, and are able to answer your questions appropriately (**FIGURE 4-5**). Do not assume that an older patient is senile or confused. Conversely, communicating with some older patients is extremely difficult, and you may encounter hostility, irritability, and, in some cases confusion.

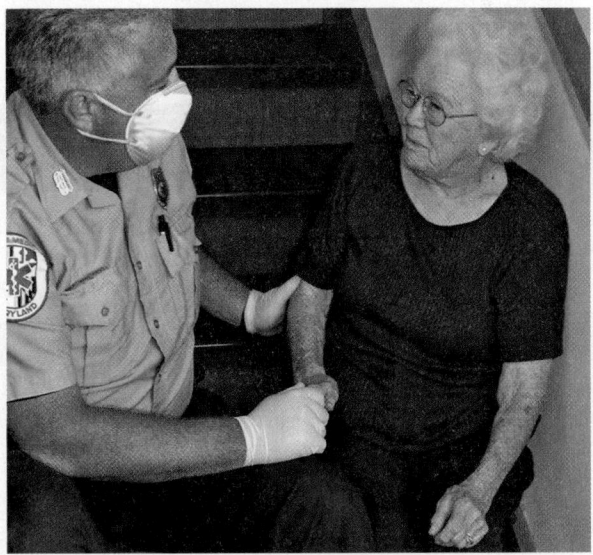

**FIGURE 4-5** You need a great deal of compassion and patience when caring for older patients. Never assume that a patient is senile or confused.

Do not assume this to be normal behavior for an older patient. These signs may be caused by lack of oxygen (hypoxia); brain injury, including a stroke; unintentional drug overdose; infection; abnormal blood glucose level; or even insufficient perfusion (circulation of blood and, therefore, nutrients to the cells). Never attribute altered mental status to old age. In addition, your older patients may have difficulty hearing or seeing you. Therefore, you need great patience and compassion when you are called on to care for such a patient. Think of the patient as someone's grandmother or grandfather—or even as yourself when you reach that age.

## Words of Wisdom

Remember that not all older patients are cognitively impaired. Be careful to assess each patient's individual abilities.

Approach an older patient slowly and calmly. Allow plenty of time for the patient to respond to your questions. Watch for signs of confusion, anxiety, or impaired hearing or vision. The patient should feel confident that everything possible is being done for him or her.

Some older patients who have chronic diseases such as diabetes may not feel much pain. When these patients fall or are injured, they may report no pain. In addition, older patients might not be fully aware of important changes in their body systems. Therefore, be especially vigilant for objective changes—no matter how subtle—in their condition.

If appropriate, help the patient pack a few personal items before leaving for the hospital. Be sure to locate hearing aids, eyeglasses, or dentures before departure if such items will significantly improve the patient's stay. If you do so, you should document on the patient care report (PCR) that these items accompanied the patient to the hospital and the person to whom they were given in the ED. Older patients are often worried about the safety of their home, valuable items, and pets. Take the time to share these concerns with the person assuming care of the patient at the hospital.

### Communicating With Children

Everyone who is thrust into an emergency situation becomes frightened to some degree. However, fear is probably most obvious and severe in children. Children may be frightened by your uniform, the ambulance, and the number of people who have suddenly gathered around. Even a child who says little may be very much aware of all that is going on.

Familiar faces and objects will help to reduce this fright. Let a child keep a favorite toy, doll, or security blanket to give the child some sense of control and comfort. Having a family member or

## YOU are the Provider

You arrive at the scene and find the patient, an 83-year-old woman, sitting on the couch in her living room. She is conscious and alert and tells you that she started having lightheadedness and nausea about an hour ago. As you begin your assessment, you note that she has hearing aids in both ears.

| Recording Time: 0 Minutes | |
| --- | --- |
| Appearance | Calm; no obvious distress |
| Level of consciousness | Conscious and alert |
| Airway | Open; clear of secretions or foreign bodies |
| Breathing | Normal rate and depth; regular |
| Circulation | Radial pulses strong and regular; skin circulation assessed as adequate by examination of mucous membranes inside the inner lower eyelid and capillary refill with skin warm and dry |

3. How can you maximize successful communication with a patient who is hard of hearing?

4. Should your general approach to the assessment process be any different for this patient versus a younger patient? Why or why not?

friend nearby is also helpful. When not impractical due to the child's condition, it is often helpful to let the parent or a guardian hold the child during your evaluation and treatment. However, you will have to make sure this person will not upset the child or prevent the child from telling you important information. Sometimes, adult family members are not helpful because they become too upset by what has happened, or the child will not share important information in front of them. An overly anxious parent or relative can make things worse. Be careful about selecting the proper adult for this role. A child may not be able to communicate verbally, but the child's appropriate or inappropriate reaction to the environment or situation can communicate a great deal of information about his or her level of consciousness and condition.

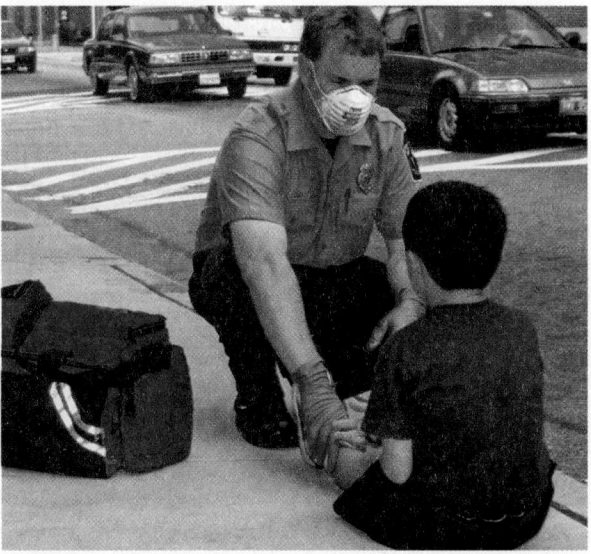

**FIGURE 4-6** Maintain eye contact with a child to let the child know that you are there to help and that you can be trusted.

© Jones & Bartlett Learning. Courtesy of MIEMSS.

Children can easily see through lies or deceptions, so you must always be honest with them. Explain to the child as often as necessary why certain things are happening. If treatment will hurt, such as applying a splint, tell the child ahead of time.

Respect a child's modesty. Children are often embarrassed if they have to undress or be undressed in front of strangers. This anxiety often intensifies during adolescence. When a wound or site of injury has to be exposed, try to do so out of the sight of strangers, and when appropriate be sure to have a parent or guardian present. Again, it is extremely important to tell the child what you are doing and why you are doing it.

You should speak to a child in a professional, yet friendly way. When speaking to a child, make sure to use an appropriate tone and vocabulary. A child should feel reassured that you are there to help in every way possible. Maintain eye contact with a child, as you would with an adult, to let the child know that you are there to help and that you can be trusted (**FIGURE 4-6**). It is helpful to position yourself at the child's eye level so you do not appear to tower above the child.

## Communicating With Patients Who Are Deaf or Hard of Hearing

Patients who are hard of hearing are usually not ashamed or embarrassed by their disability. You must be able to communicate with patients who are hard of hearing so you can provide necessary or even life-saving care.

Most patients who are hard of hearing have normal intelligence and can easily understand what is going on around them, provided you can successfully communicate with them. Most patients who are hard of hearing can read lips to some extent. Therefore, you should place yourself in a position so the patient can see your lips. Many patients who are hard of hearing have hearing aids to help them communicate. Be careful that hearing aids are not lost during an accident or fall. Hearing aids may also be forgotten if the patient is confused or ill. Look around for one in the immediate area, or ask the patient or the family about use of a hearing aid.

Remember the following five steps to efficiently communicate with patients who are hard of hearing:

1. **Have paper and a pen available.** This way, you can write down questions and the patient can write down answers, if necessary. Be sure to print so that your handwriting is not a communication barrier.
2. **If the patient can read lips and you need to remove your mask, have a clear barrier mask ready to use. You should face the patient and speak distinctly at a normal pace.** Do not cover your mouth or mumble. If it is dark, consider shining a light on your face.
3. **Never shout.** This will not help the patient hear you and may frighten the patient.
4. **Be sure to listen carefully, ask short questions, and give short answers.** Remember that although many patients who are hard of hearing can speak distinctly, some cannot.
5. **Learn some simple phrases in sign language.** For example, knowing the signs for "sick," "hurt," and "help" may be useful if you cannot communicate in any other way (**FIGURE 4-7**).

## Communicating With Visually Impaired Patients

Like patients who are hard of hearing, visually impaired and blind patients have usually accepted and learned to deal with their disability. Of course, visually impaired patients are not necessarily completely blind. Many can perceive light and dark or can see shadows or movement. Ask the patient whether he or she can see at all. Also remember, as with other patients who have disabilities, you should expect visually impaired patients to have normal intelligence.

As you begin caring for a visually impaired patient, explain everything you are doing in detail as you are doing it. Be sure to stay in physical contact with the patient as you begin your care. Place your hand lightly on the patient's shoulder or arm, and try to avoid sudden movements. If the patient can walk to the ambulance, guide him or her by placing his or her hand on your arm, taking care not to rush. Transport eyeglasses and any mobility aids, such as a cane, with the patient to the hospital. A visually impaired person may have a guide dog. Guide dogs are easily identified by their special harnesses (**FIGURE 4-8**). Guide dogs are trained to not leave their masters and to not respond to strangers. A visually impaired patient who is conscious can tell you about the dog and give instructions for its care.

If the patient is stable, bring the guide dog to the hospital in the back of the ambulance with the patient because it will help to alleviate some of the stress for both the patient and the dog. If the patient is unstable, the dog is injured or unruly, or for other

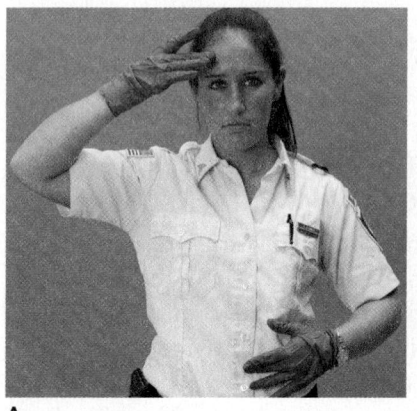 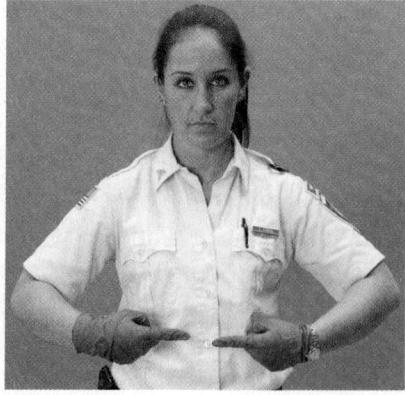 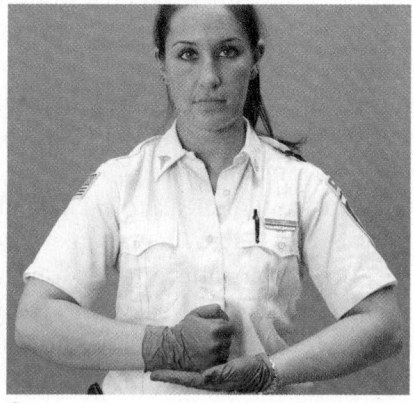

A B C

**FIGURE 4-7** Learn simple phrases in sign language. Signing requires movement and is best learned by attending a sign language class. **A.** Sick. **B.** Hurt. **C.** Help.

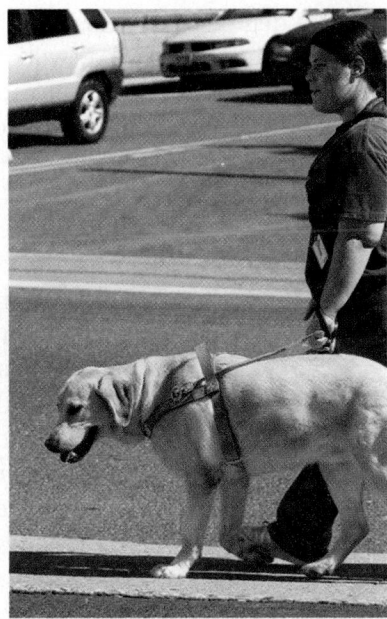

**FIGURE 4-8** A guide dog is easily identified by its special harness.

Courtesy of the Guide Dog Foundation for the Blind. Photographed by Christopher Appoldt.

show the pronunciation of these terms are available. If the patient does not speak any English, use a smartphone app or website to help you translate, or find an interpreter. In an emergency, it may be necessary to have a family member or friend translate until a professional interpreter is located. Also, remember to request a translator at the hospital while providing the radio report if the patient's language is known. Hospitals must have professional foreign language interpreters in-house or on-call for this purpose.

> **Street Smarts**
>
> When communicating with the help of an interpreter, look at the patient as you ask questions and listen to the interpreter's answers. Keeping your eyes on the patient allows you and the patient to interpret body language that accompanies verbal communication and maintains the relationship with the patient.

safety or patient care reasons it is inappropriate to transport the dog, then you should make arrangements for the care of the dog. Contact your supervisor for assistance. The exact method for managing a patient with a guide dog (or other medical care animal) will be outlined in your department's policies and procedures. Follow your local protocols.

## Communicating With Non–English-Speaking Patients

Part of patient care includes obtaining a medical history from the patient. You cannot skip this step simply because the patient does not speak English. Most patients who do not speak English fluently will still know certain important words or phrases.

Your first step is to find out how much English the patient can speak. Use short, simple questions and simple words whenever possible, and avoid difficult medical terms. You can help patients better understand if you point to specific parts of the body as you ask questions. Speaking louder will not increase a patient's ability to understand you.

In many areas, particularly large urban centers, major segments of the population do not speak English. Your job will be much easier if you learn some common words and phrases in their language, especially common medical terms. Pocket cards that

## Mission-Critical Communications

**Mission-critical communications** are any communications where disruption will result in the failure of the task at hand. Although mission-critical communications will change from industry to industry, many of the problems encountered as well as recommendations to help avoid errors and improve effectiveness can be employed by EMS providers.

A concept central to mission-critical communications is the shared **mental model**. A mental model is the picture individuals have in their head of "what's going on." Even though individuals on a team may be in different roles, seeing different things from different perspectives, for any team to work effectively together, all members must share a mental model. The goal of mission-critical communications is an efficient, effective, and error-free transfer of the mental model. When providers have different ideas of "what's going on," situational awareness fails and problems begin.

For an individual health care provider or a team to build a mental model, the following sequence of four questions must be answered:

1. What is the focused priority for the patient? (What is the crux of the problem?)
2. What is the history of prior care? (What got us to this point?)

3. What is the patient's current state? (Where are we right now?)
4. What are the patient's immediate needs? (What is the very next thing that needs to happen?)

Answering these four questions quickly and efficiently will not just help avoid errors and misunderstandings, but will provide a handoff that allows receiving clinicians to continue forward progress in patient care rather than spend time with unnecessary questions and clarifications or, even worse, begin the patient interview and assessment essentially from scratch.

## Patient Care Handover

Patient care is a coordinated effort among numerous providers, from bystanders and first responders to paramedics, from primary care physicians to ED nurses, and beyond. Effective communication between the EMT and other health care professionals is a cornerstone of efficient, effective, and appropriate patient care. Nowhere is communication more important than during patient care **handover**, often called handoff. Patient care handover is the transfer of pertinent patient information and the responsibility for the patient's care. It often involves the physical movement of the patient and associated equipment.

Even on a single emergency call, an EMT may be involved in numerous patient care handovers. For example, a first responder or primary-care medical provider may hand over patient care on arrival of an EMT, the EMT may hand over care on arrival of a paramedic, and the EMT–paramedic team may hand over care to the ED staff. As common as this occurrence may be, it is a hazardous one. The American College of Emergency Physicians has called patient handover "the most dangerous point in a patient's ED journey," and the World Health Organization has identified communication during patient handover as a critical failure point that can cause "serious breakdowns in the continuity of care, inappropriate treatment, and potential harm to the patient." Furthermore, communication failures between reporting providers and receiving providers are a major source of medical liability for providers and organizations, accounting for 30% of malpractice claims in all health care sectors, including EMS.

Although the degree of control that EMTs may have over the system in which they work will vary, a five-point method can be used by providers both when giving and when receiving the handover report in virtually all situations.

### Giving the Handover Report

- **Initiate eye contact.** When handing over patient care, responsibility, and information, it is critical to begin by making eye contact with the person to whom the patient is being transferred. Eye contact helps identify that the handover is beginning, and which individuals are reporting and receiving. It sends the message, "We are communicating now, you and I."
- **Manage the environment.** Whenever possible, try to minimize noise, interruptions, and distractions by, for example, momentarily turning down a radio, stopping nonpriority activities, or moving to a quieter area to give the report. Avoid moving the patient during the handover report so that the attention of both you and the person receiving the report is focused on the patient information.
- **Ensure the ABCs.** If there is priority critical care that must be initiated or continued, it must be immediately conveyed and addressed by the receiving clinician or team (the doctor, nurse, or whomever will be taking responsibility for the patient). Such care includes life-saving interventions that are either needed immediately (eg, the placement of an endotracheal tube) or that must be continued (eg, CPR) for the patient to survive. The full handover report may be delayed until after the immediate life threat is addressed.
- **Provide a structured report.** Research on mission-critical communications has shown that the use of a structured format greatly improves efficiency and reduces errors. Numerous standardized report formats exist. Although not inherently superior to other structured formats, SBAR (which stands for situation, background, assessment, and recap/Rx) is widely used in hospitals and is likely to be well understood by a variety of health care providers. The mnemonic is sometimes modified slightly to SBAT when used in EMS:
  - Situation (a concise statement of the problem)

- Background (relevant, brief information about the patient situation)
- Assessment (your assessment findings and what you think)
- Treatment (care that has been provided to the patient)

- **Provide documentation.** The verbal report should consist of the patient's priority conditions, prior care, current state, and immediate needs. The numerous other patient details should be transferred via a paper or electronic report. Avoid clouding the handover with information that is not immediately critical.

Consider the following example of a structured report that uses the SBAT format to focus on priority issues, prior care, current state, and immediate needs (**FIGURE 4-9**):

S   This is a trauma alert. We have a hypotensive 28-year-old female involved in a motor vehicle collision with an unstable pelvis and right-side open tibia/fibula fracture.

B   Patient was struck by a motor vehicle at approximately 35 mph approximately 20 minutes ago.

A   She is conscious and alert but slow to respond. Vital signs are BP, 88/48; pulse, 124 and irregular; respirations, 24; and $Sao_2$, 96%. Head to toe finds injuries to the pelvis and the left leg as well as minor abrasions, but no other significant findings. Her only significant medical history is asthma.

T   We applied oxygen and stabilized her pelvis and left leg, and both have good distal PMS. Do you have any questions?

### Receiving the Handover Report

- **Maintain eye contact.**
- **Manage the environment.** Many hospitals now establish a moment of silence during trauma, cardiac, stroke, sepsis, and other alerts and critical patient situations. Although this is not always possible for the EMT receiving the handover in the field, attempt to pause during the report so you can focus on key information.
- **Ensure understanding.** Once you have received the handover report, ask questions as necessary to clarify and correct any issues.
- **Summarize.** This is *not* a repeat of the entire handover report, but a summary of the receiving clinician's mental model. This mental model summary is stated aloud so that the reporting provider and members of the receiving team can ask questions or correct any errors to ensure the shared mental model is correct.
- **Gather supplementary patient documentation.**

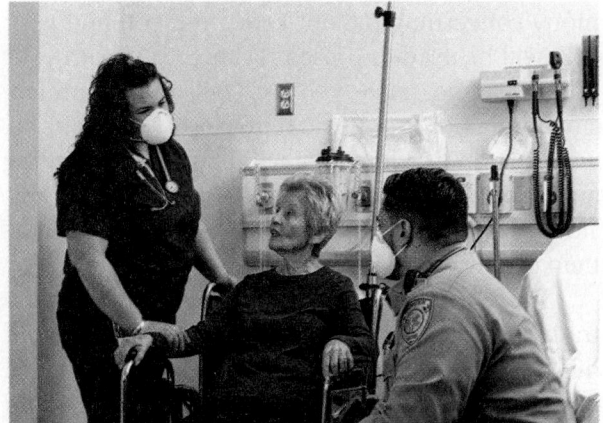

**FIGURE 4-9** Once you arrive at the hospital, a staff member will take a patient handover report and responsibility for the patient from you.
© Jones & Bartlett Learning.

# Written Communications and Documentation

The **patient care report (PCR)**, also known as a prehospital care report, is the legal document used to record all aspects of the care your patient received, from initial dispatch to arrival at the hospital. Either term can be used, and both are acceptable. You may be able to complete the report en route to the hospital if the trip is long enough and the patient needs minimal care. Usually, you will finish the report after you have transferred care of the patient to an ED staff member. There are two types of PCRs: written and electronic (ePCRs), which will be discussed later in this chapter.

The information you collect during a call becomes part of the PCR, and that information is ultimately entered into a data pool. NEMSIS has been collecting prehospital care information for research purposes since the early 1970s. NEMSIS

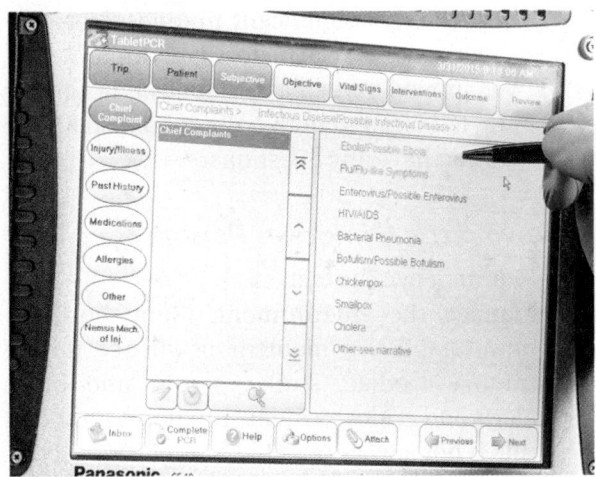

**FIGURE 4-10** The minimum data set includes patient and administrative information, including narrative components and checkboxes.

© Jones & Bartlett Learning.

has identified specific data points (uniform components) needed to enable communication and comparison of EMS runs between agencies, regions, and states. The minimum data set includes both narrative components and checkboxes (**FIGURE 4-10** and **FIGURE 4-11**). The NEMSIS website (www.nemsis.org) provides the national data set and interesting facts about delivery of EMS within the United States.

Because EMS systems track their own time, make sure that your watch is synchronized with dispatch time at the beginning of the shift, if that is procedure. Another way you can manage this information is to contact the dispatcher and have him or her provide you with the time. Either way, it is important to be able to keep close track of time. Accurate documentation will depend on it.

You will begin gathering patient information as soon as you reach the patient. Continue collecting information as you provide care until you arrive at the hospital.

## Patient Care Report

As discussed, a PCR helps ensure efficient continuity of patient care. This report describes the nature of the patient's injuries or illness at the scene and the initial treatment you provide. Although this report might not be read immediately at the hospital, it may be referred to later for important information. The report serves the following six functions:

1. Transfer of information and continuity of care
2. Compliance and legal documentation
3. Administrative information
4. Reimbursement
5. Education
6. Data collection for quality improvement and research

A good PCR documents any changes in the patient's condition on arrival at the hospital. It is critical that you document everything in the clearest manner possible because the report serves multiple purposes. The information in the report will help to prove that you have provided a standard of care and, in some instances, shows you have properly handled unusual or uncommon situations. Both objective and subjective information is included in this report.

The following are examples of information collected on a PCR:

- Chief complaint or chief concern
- Mechanism of injury or nature of illness
- Level of consciousness (according to the AVPU scale) or mental status
- Vital signs
- Initial and ongoing assessment
- Patient demographics (age, sex, ethnic background)
- Transport information (how the patient was moved, reason for destination choice)

Should you ever be called on to provide testimony concerning patient care, both you and your PCR will be used to present evidence. As with your personal appearance, your PCR will reflect a professional or a nonprofessional image. A neat, concise, well-written document—including correct spelling and grammar—will reflect good patient care. Consider the adage, "If the report looks sloppy, the patient care was also sloppy."

These reports also provide valuable administrative information, such as that used for patient billing. Information included in PCRs can be used to evaluate response times, equipment usage, and other areas of administrative responsibility. The following are examples of administrative information gathered from a PCR:

- Time the incident was reported
- Time the EMS unit was notified

- Time the EMS unit arrived at the scene
- Time the EMS crew makes contact with the patient.
- Time the EMS unit left the scene
- Time the EMS unit arrived at the receiving facility
- Time the patient care was transferred
- Time unit was back in service

It is standard procedure to use military time in EMS documentation. With military time, each time is unique; for example, 12 noon cannot be confused with 12 midnight. Military times are shown in **TABLE 4-5**.

Data may be obtained from the PCR to analyze causes, severity, and types of illness or injury requiring emergency medical care. These reports may also be used in an ongoing program for evaluation of the quality of patient care. All reports are periodically reviewed by your system to make sure trauma triage and/or other prehospital care criteria have been met.

There are many requirements of a PCR (**TABLE 4-6**). Often, these requirements vary from jurisdiction to jurisdiction, mainly because different agencies obtain information from them. Although no universally accepted form exists, certain uniform data points are common in all areas.

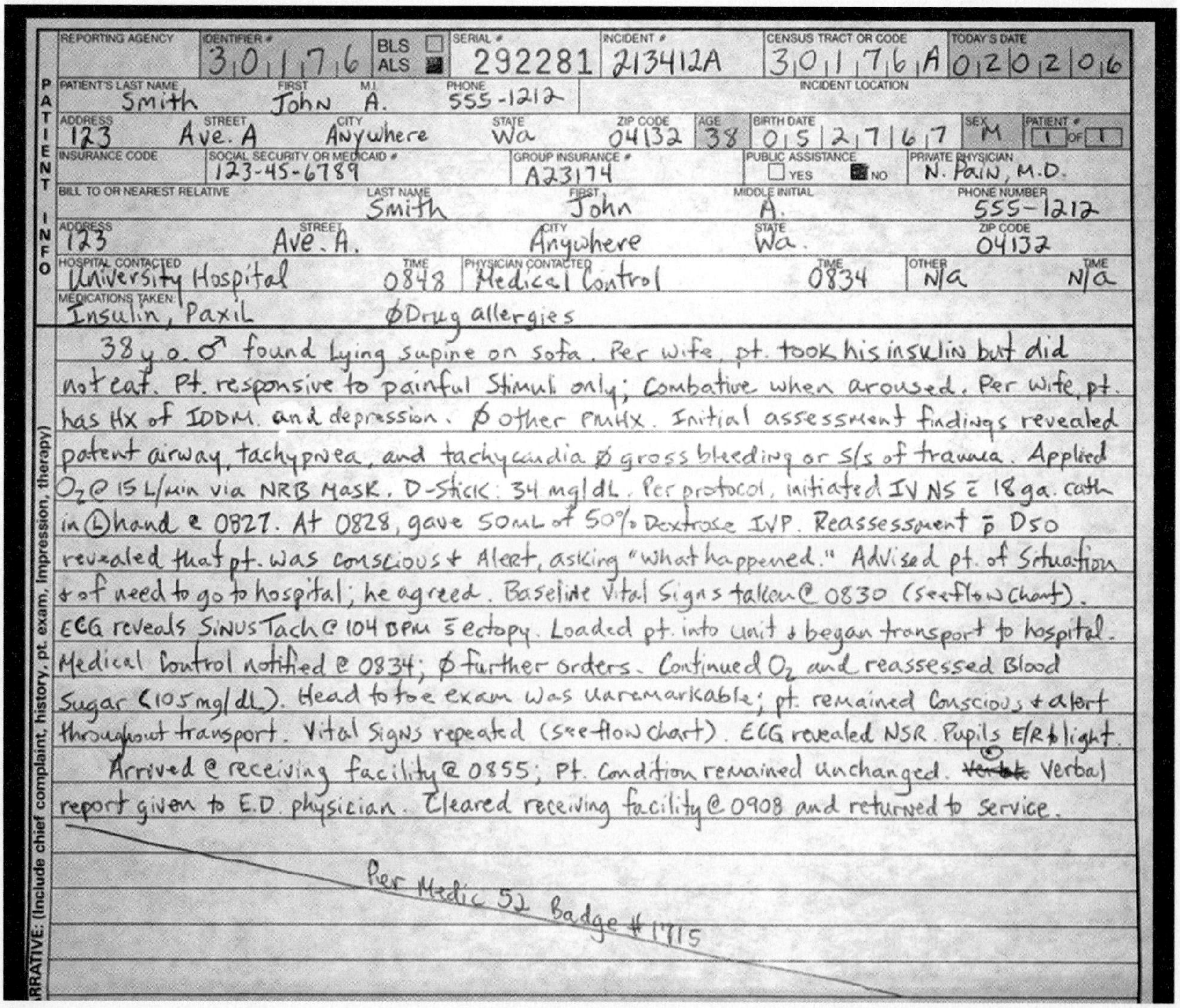

PATIENT INFO

REPORTING AGENCY | IDENTIFIER # 3 0 1 7 6 | BLS ☐ ALS ■ | SERIAL # 292281 | INCIDENT # 213412A | CENSUS TRACT OR CODE 3 0 1 7 6 A | TODAY'S DATE 02 02 06

PATIENT'S LAST NAME Smith | FIRST John | M.I. A. | PHONE 555-1212 | INCIDENT LOCATION

ADDRESS 123 | STREET Ave. A | CITY Anywhere | STATE Wa | ZIP CODE 04132 | AGE 38 | BIRTH DATE 05 27 67 | SEX M | PATIENT # 1 OF 1

INSURANCE CODE | SOCIAL SECURITY OR MEDICAID # 123-45-6789 | GROUP INSURANCE # A23174 | PUBLIC ASSISTANCE ☐ YES ■ NO | PRIVATE PHYSICIAN N. Pain, M.D.

BILL TO OR NEAREST RELATIVE | LAST NAME Smith | FIRST John | MIDDLE INITIAL A. | PHONE NUMBER 555-1212

ADDRESS 123 | STREET Ave. A. | CITY Anywhere | STATE Wa. | ZIP CODE 04132

HOSPITAL CONTACTED University Hospital | TIME 0848 | PHYSICIAN CONTACTED Medical Control | TIME 0834 | OTHER N/a | TIME N/a

MEDICATIONS TAKEN: Insulin, Paxil ØDrug allergies

NARRATIVE: (Include chief complaint, history, pt. exam, Impression, therapy)

38 y.o. ♂ found lying supine on sofa. Per wife, pt. took his insulin but did not eat. Pt. responsive to painful stimuli only; combative when aroused. Per wife, pt. has Hx of IDDM. and depression. Ø other PMHX. Initial assessment findings revealed patent airway, tachypnea, and tachycardia Ø gross bleeding or S/s of trauma. Applied $O_2$ @ 15 L/min via NRB Mask. D-Stick: 34 mg/dL. Per protocol, initiated IV NS c̄ 18 ga. cath in Ⓛ hand @ 0827. At 0828, gave 50mL of 50% Dextrose IVP. Reassessment p̄ D50 revealed that pt. was conscious + Alert, asking "what happened." Advised pt. of situation + of need to go to hospital; he agreed. Baseline Vital Signs taken @ 0830 (see flow chart). ECG reveals Sinus Tach @ 104 BPM s̄ ectopy. Loaded pt. into unit + began transport to hospital. Medical Control notified @ 0834; Ø further orders. Continued $O_2$ and reassessed Blood Sugar (105 mg/dL). Head to toe exam was unremarkable; pt. remained conscious + alert throughout transport. Vital Signs repeated (see flow chart). ECG revealed NSR. Pupils E/R to light.

Arrived @ receiving facility @ 0855; Pt. condition remained unchanged. ~~Verbal~~ Verbal report given to E.D. physician. Cleared receiving facility @ 0908 and returned to service.

Per Medic 52 Badge #1715

A

**FIGURE 4-11** Filing a PCR is a critical part of your responsibilities as an EMT. **A.** Proper documentation.

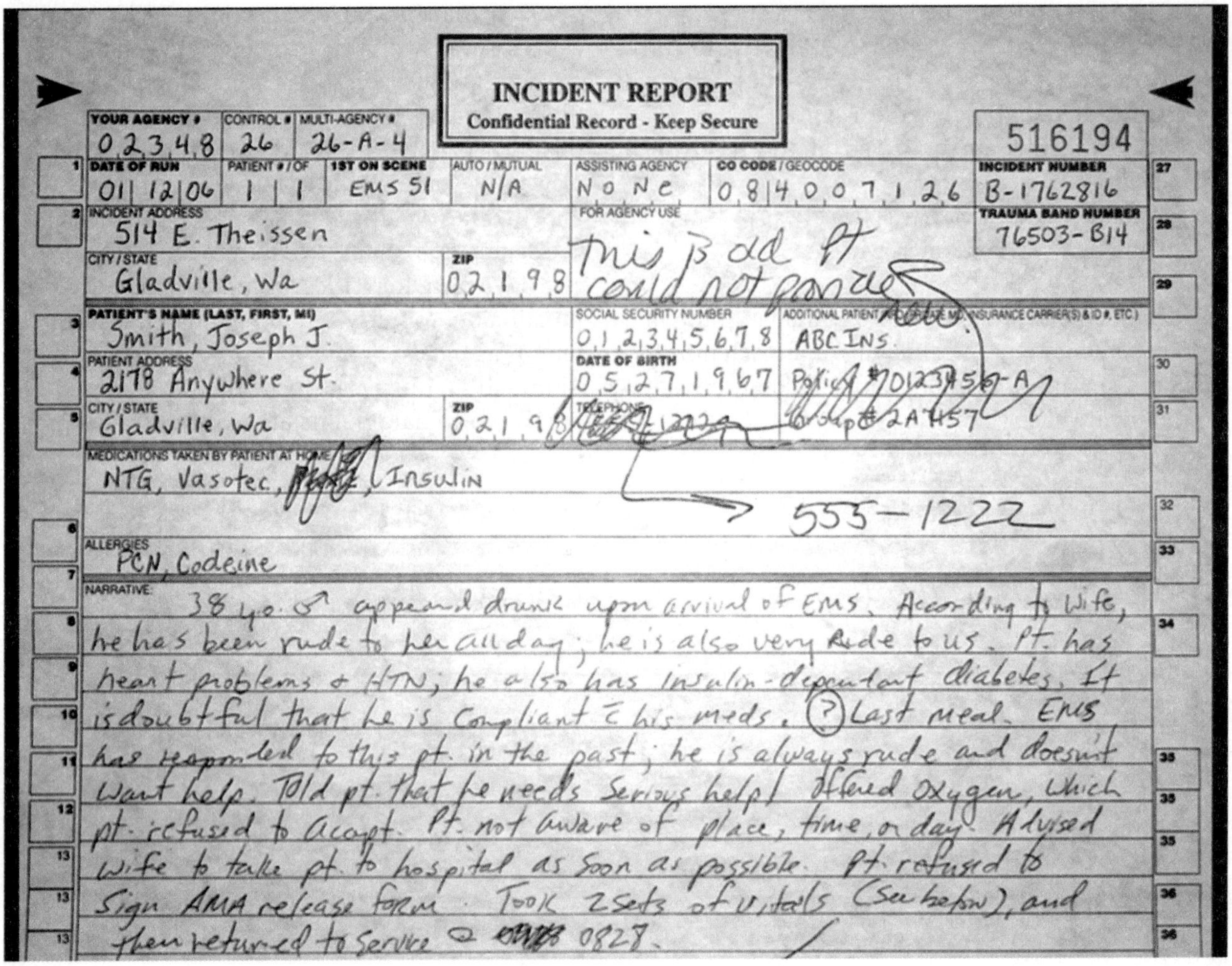

**B**

**FIGURE 4-11 B.** Improper documentation. *(Continued)*

© Jones & Bartlett Learning.

**TABLE 4-5** Military Times

| Regular Time | Military Time | Regular Time | Military Time |
|---|---|---|---|
| Midnight | 0000 | Noon | 1200 |
| 1:00 AM | 0100 | 1:00 PM | 1300 |
| 2:00 AM | 0200 | 2:00 PM | 1400 |
| 3:00 AM | 0300 | 3:00 PM | 1500 |
| 4:00 AM | 0400 | 4:00 PM | 1600 |
| 5:00 AM | 0500 | 5:00 PM | 1700 |
| 6:00 AM | 0600 | 6:00 PM | 1800 |
| 7:00 AM | 0700 | 7:00 PM | 1900 |
| 8:00 AM | 0800 | 8:00 PM | 2000 |
| 9:00 AM | 0900 | 9:00 PM | 2100 |
| 10:00 AM | 1000 | 10:00 PM | 2200 |
| 11:00 AM | 1100 | 11:00 PM | 2300 |

© Jones & Bartlett Learning.

**TABLE 4-6** Sample Uniform Components of a Patient Care Report

- Patient's name, gender, date of birth, and address
- Dispatched as (When was the ambulance called? What was the nature of the call as reported by the dispatcher?)
- Chief complaint or chief concern
- Location of the patient when first seen (including specific details, especially if the incident is a car crash or when criminal activity is suspected)
- Rescue and treatment given before your arrival
- Signs and symptoms found during your patient assessment
- Care and treatment given by you at the site and during transport
- Response to treatment
- Vital signs
- SAMPLE history (Signs and symptoms, Allergies, Medications, Pertinent past medical history, Last oral intake, Events leading up to the illness or injury)
- Changes in vital signs and condition
- Additional orders received from the hospital
- Name of person receiving the patient report
- Date of the call
- Time of the call
- Location of the call
- Time of dispatch
- Time of arrival at the scene
- Time of leaving the scene
- Time of arrival at the hospital
- Patient's insurance information
- Names and/or certification numbers of the EMTs who responded to the call
- Name of the transport destination
- Type of run to the scene: emergency or routine

© Jones & Bartlett Learning.

The benefits of collecting such information are significant, one being that national trends can be detected. For example, approximately 15% of the nation's EMS calls involve children ages birth to 9 years. Of those patients, 3% have a respiratory complaint. Such information is invaluable.

Finally, PCRs are used by individual agencies to determine patterns of EMS responses. Busy times and high call-volume areas can be predictive, and a thorough review of PCRs can set the stage for scheduling shifts and for system status management, including where units are placed or where new stations should be built.

## Types of Forms

Most PCRs are completed in an electronic format often referred to as an ePCR (**FIGURE 4-12**). Although the features of ePCR software and services vary greatly, virtually all are designed to comply with NEMSIS data collection requirements. Some ePCRs will be initially completed on a computer, tablet, or other device and then uploaded to a local or state database, while other ePCRs will collect and record each page or even each data field as it is entered. Electronic PCRs have several advantages over the written forms. For example, ePCRs allow you to transmit patient information directly to hospital computers for review by the physician, pharmacy, and other professionals providing patient care and may be directly integrated with the patient's electronic medical record.

In cases where there is a temporary failure of Internet connectivity or where ePCRs have not yet been fully implemented, the PCR may be completed on a paper form, which can be uploaded later. When using paper forms, fill in the boxes completely and avoid making stray marks on the sheet.

The narrative section of the PCR is arguably the most important portion. Here you will describe all of the facts related to the EMS call. The narrative should tell the story and present a clear, detailed picture of what you found, what you did, and how it affected the patient's condition. Be sure to include significant negative findings and important

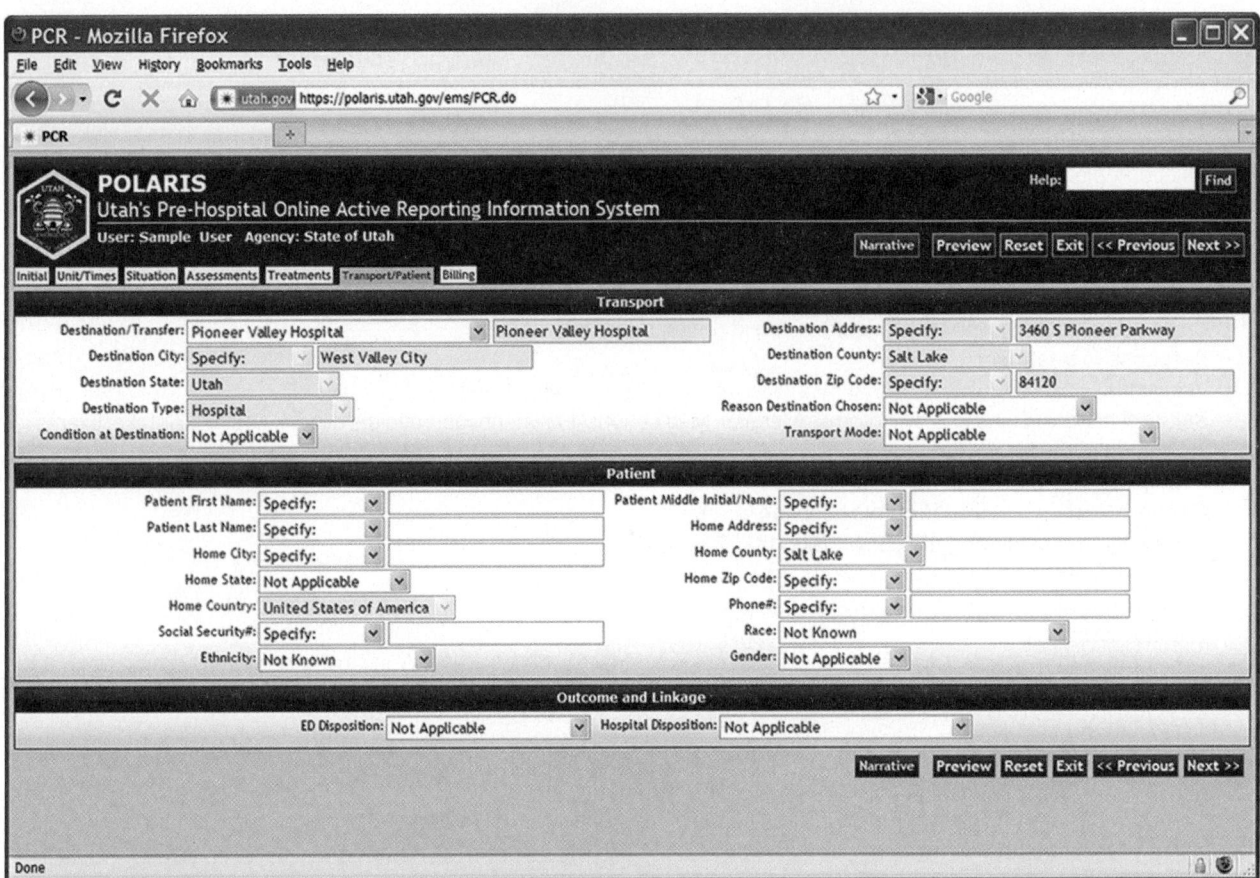

**FIGURE 4-12** An electronic PCR (ePCR).

Courtesy of the Utah Department of Health.

observations about the scene. Make sure what you write is not an opinion, but is factually based on findings. For example, you may write, "The patient admits to drinking today" or "The patient smelled of alcohol." These are clear descriptions that do not make any judgments about the patient's condition. However, stating "the patient was drunk" is a personal judgment that may not be supportable. Choose your words carefully and thoughtfully. Your job is to reproduce the important facts of the EMS call in writing. Although some ePCRs can automatically generate narratives from previously entered data, such automatically generated documentation is virtually always a starting point only and should not be considered complete or substitute for a fully written narrative.

## Standardized Narrative Formats

Many EMS systems require the use of a standardized format to document care. Using one of these methods can ensure that important information is not omitted. Further, the standardized format allows others who consult your patient report, such as physicians, billing clerks, or administrators, to find information within it quickly. The two most common narrative formats used in health care are CHART and SOAP.

### CHART Method

CHART stands for Chief complaint, History and physical examination, Assessment, Treatment (Rx), and Transport. This method's strength is that it groups the care and treatment into smaller, logical sections, which makes it easier to locate specific assessments or care without reading the entire report. Its weakness is that it is somewhat difficult to learn.

To document a narrative using CHART, begin with the dispatch information. For example, your report may open with, "Unit 4 dispatched from headquarters for [dispatch code] to a [location]."

Use a specific location type, such as residence, roadway, or health care institution, rather than simply saying "scene."

Next, review each letter of the CHART abbreviation, as follows:

C  **Chief complaint** or **chief concern.** This section states the condition most urgently requiring EMS intervention. For example, a patient may complain of a headache (chief complaint), but you are most concerned because it is evident the person has signs of possible stroke, such as paralysis on one side (chief concern).

H  **History.** The history includes details relating to the current event and the patient's medical history prior to this event. These details come from the patient or others on scene, from dispatch, or from the patient record.

A  **Assessments.** Describe all assessments you perform on the patient, including vital signs and the physical examination.

R  **Treatments (Rx).** The *R* in CHART comes from the medical abbreviation for treatment. This section details all interventions that were performed.

T  **Transport.** This final section explains how the patient was moved to the ambulance and possibly why the person was moved in that way; how the patient was transported (eg, how the person was positioned and secured); whether emergency lights and sirens were used; where the patient was taken, including the room number; and the person to whom the report was given and care was transferred (eg, nurse Jones).

## SOAP Method

The SOAP framework is another common method to structure documentation of the narrative.

S  **Subjective.** This section includes information provided by the patient or others on the scene, such as the chief complaint, events leading up to the incident, mechanism of injury, and past medical history.

O  **Objective.** The objective section includes details you gather primarily through patient assessment, such as vital signs, physical exam findings, and other measurements, such as blood glucose or oxygen saturation.

A  **Assessment.** Summarize key findings in the assessment section. If appropriate, provide your impression of what the patient's problem might be (eg, possible fractured lower leg or possible stroke).

P  **Plan.** Within the plan area, document treatment provided for the patient.

The SOAP method is fairly simple to learn, and when it is completed, it provides a means for the reader to review the assessment and management.

Regardless of the method used, the PCR's narrative section should include the following information:

- Time of events
- Assessment findings
- Emergency medical care provided
- Changes in the patient after treatment
- Observations at the scene
- Final patient disposition
- Refusal of care
- Staff person who continued care

In written documentation, avoid radio codes and abbreviations. Remember, EMS personnel are not the only people who will be reading this document. Other hospital and billing personnel will need to read the document and note the source of the information. Be sure to spell words correctly, especially medical terms. If you do not know the correct spelling of a particular word, find out how to spell it or use another word. Be sure to record the time with all assessment findings. **TABLE 4-7** provides guidelines on how to write the narrative portion of your report. Whether you completed a medical or trauma assessment, the assessment-based approach follows each step of the assessment or assessments as a guideline to narrative writing.

Remember that the report form itself—and all the information in it—is considered a confidential document, as are all formal and informal notes that contain protected patient information. Be sure you are familiar with federal, state, and local laws concerning confidentiality. All prehospital forms must be handled with care and stored in an appropriate manner once you have completed them. After you have completed a report, distribute copies to the appropriate locations, according to state and local protocol. In most instances, a copy of the report will remain at the hospital and will become part of the patient's medical record.

| TABLE 4-7 How to Write a Narrative Report | |
|---|---|
| Standard precautions | Were standard precautions initiated? If so, state which precautions were used and why. |
| Scene safety | Did you have to make your scene safe? If so, what did you do and why did you do it? Did this create a delay in patient care? |
| NOI/MOI | Simply state. |
| Number of patients | Record only when more than one patient is present; "This is patient 2 of 3." |
| Additional help | Did you call for help? If so, state why, at what time, and what time the help arrived. Was transport delayed? |
| Initial general impression | Simply record, if not already documented on the PCR. |
| Level of consciousness | Be sure to report LOC, any changes in LOC, and at what time changes occurred. |
| Chief complaint | Note and quote pertinent statements made by the patient and/or bystanders. This includes any pertinent denials; "Patient denies chest pain..." |
| Life threats | List all interventions and how the patient responded; "Assisted ventilations with $O_2$ (15 L/min) at 20 BPM with no change in LOC." |
| ABCs | Document what you found, and again, any interventions performed. |
| Oxygen | Record if $O_2$ was used, how it was applied, and how much was administered. |
| Primary, secondary, patient history, or reassessment | State the type of assessment used and any pertinent findings; "Secondary assessment revealed unequal pupils, crepitus to right ribs, and an apparent closed fracture of left tibia." |
| SAMPLE/OPQRST | Note and quote any pertinent answers. |
| Vital signs | Your service may want you to record vital signs in the narrative portion, as well as other places in the PCR. |
| Medical direction | Quote any orders given to you by medical control and who gave them. |
| Management of secondary injuries/treat for shock | Report all patient interventions, at what time they were completed, and how the patient responded. |
| Receiving facility | Document the name of the facility, the area of the facility where the patient was delivered, and the room number (if known). |
| Transfer of care | Record the name of the staff person who received your report and took over patient care, as well as the time. |

Abbreviations: ABCs, airway, breathing, and circulation; LOC, level of consciousness; MOI, mechanism of injury; NOI, nature of illness; OPQRST, mnemonic used to facilitate the evaluation of a patient's pain: onset, provocation or palliation, quality, region/radiation, severity, and timing of pain; PCR, patient care report; SAMPLE, mnemonic used to determine signs and symptoms, allergies, medications, pertinent past history, last oral intake, and events leading up to the injury or illness.

Reprinted with permission. Courtesy of Jay C. Keefauver.

Depending on the requirements of the EMS system in which you work, you may not have the time to complete the full PCR while at the hospital; some EMS systems allow for shorter handover notes to be left at the hospital. The full report can then be completed at the station or transmitted electronically.

## Documenting Medical Necessity

Medicare and Medicaid payers will reimburse for ambulance transport only if the services are documented as being medically necessary. *Medically necessary* means it would have been unsafe or impossible to transport the patient by any other means.

The following scenarios constitute medical necessity:

- The patient was transported in an emergency situation (eg, as a result of an accident, injury, or acute illness) and could not be transported by other means.
- The patient needed to be restrained to prevent injury to self or others.
- The patient required oxygen or other emergency treatment during transport to the nearest appropriate facility.
- The patient was unconscious or in shock.
- The patient exhibited signs and symptoms of acute respiratory distress or cardiac distress such as shortness of breath or chest pain.
- The patient exhibited signs and symptoms that indicated the possibility of acute stroke.
- The patient needed to remain immobile because of a fracture that had not been stabilized or the possibility of a fracture.
- The patient experienced severe hemorrhage.
- The patient was confined to a bed before and after the ambulance trip. For a patient to be considered bed-confined, the person must be unable to get up from bed without assistance, unable to ambulate, and unable to sit in a chair or a wheelchair.

Medical necessity also applies to the level of care provided for the patient. For example, it would be inappropriate to document that advanced life support interventions were provided to a patient who did not need them. It is therefore crucial to clearly document the patient's dispatch-reported condition, the actual patient condition the EMT found on scene, EMS

treatments and services rendered and the patient's response to those treatments, and an objective report of the patient's appearance and mental status.

Another essential element to ensure your EMS agency is appropriately reimbursed for services provided is signatures. Every attempt should be made to obtain appropriate signatures from the patient or guardian.

### Health Information Exchanges

Some EMS systems use a **health information exchange (HIE)** to improve sharing of data between EMS and other health care providers. HIEs allow EMS providers to access relevant health data (eg, past medical problems, medications, allergies, end-of-life decisions), avoid unnecessary duplication of effort in data entry, and view patient outcomes related to hospital care. HIEs allow EMTs to contribute to and access electronic health information on both a regular basis and during times of disaster, when accurate patient medical records may be destroyed or difficult to obtain.

Most HIEs follow the SAFR framework to improve patient care by giving health care providers rapid and universal access to accurate patient medical information:

- **Search.** EMS providers in the field can search for hospital and other records that will help them make treatment and transport decisions.
- **Alert.** Hospitals are notified of incoming EMS patients with automated systems that populate ED dashboards with information entered by EMS in the field.
- **File.** The data in EMS electronic patient care reports are incorporated directly into patients' longitudinal health records.
- **Reconcile.** Feedback on outcomes and other hospital data are provided to EMS agencies for billing and quality improvement.

## Reporting Errors

Everyone makes mistakes. If you leave something out of a report or record information incorrectly, do not try to cover it up. Rather, write down what did or did not happen and the steps that were taken to correct the situation. Falsifying information on the PCR may result in suspension and/or revocation of your certification or license, and also may have legal implications. More important, falsifying information results in poor patient care, because other health care providers have a false impression of assessment findings or the treatment given. For example, if you did not give the patient oxygen, do not document that the patient was given oxygen.

Document only the vital signs that were obtained. A classic case of improper documentation occurs with patients experiencing cardiac arrest. Consider this scenario. Under "Vital Signs," an EMT documents: pulse 0 beats/min, respirations 0 breaths/min, and blood pressure 0/0 mm Hg. What the EMT implied by documenting in that manner was the actual application of a blood pressure cuff—inflating it and deflating it while listening for a pulse. Someone reviewing the PCR after the call may ask why the EMT took the time to check the blood pressure on a patient who did not have a pulse, instead of performing CPR.

What if the wrong drug or the wrong dose is given to a patient? What if the patient is accidentally dropped? Unfortunately, these things can and do happen. It is important that you document the event. Do not lie or cover it up by withholding the information. In your narrative, provide a factual account of what happened. For example: "Ordered: one sublingual nitroglycerin. Given: two sublingual nitroglycerin. Patient blood pressure checked following administration. No changes noted" or "While loading the patient into the ambulance, the patient was dropped. Patient was on the ambulance cot when it fell a total of 4 feet. Patient was not thrown off cot. Patient was assessed after being dropped and reported feeling scared and having neck pain. Hospital advised."

If you discover an error as you are completing a handwritten report, draw a single horizontal line through the error, initial it, and write the correct information next to it (**FIGURE 4-13**). Do not try to erase or cover the error with correction fluid. This may be interpreted as an attempt to cover up a mistake.

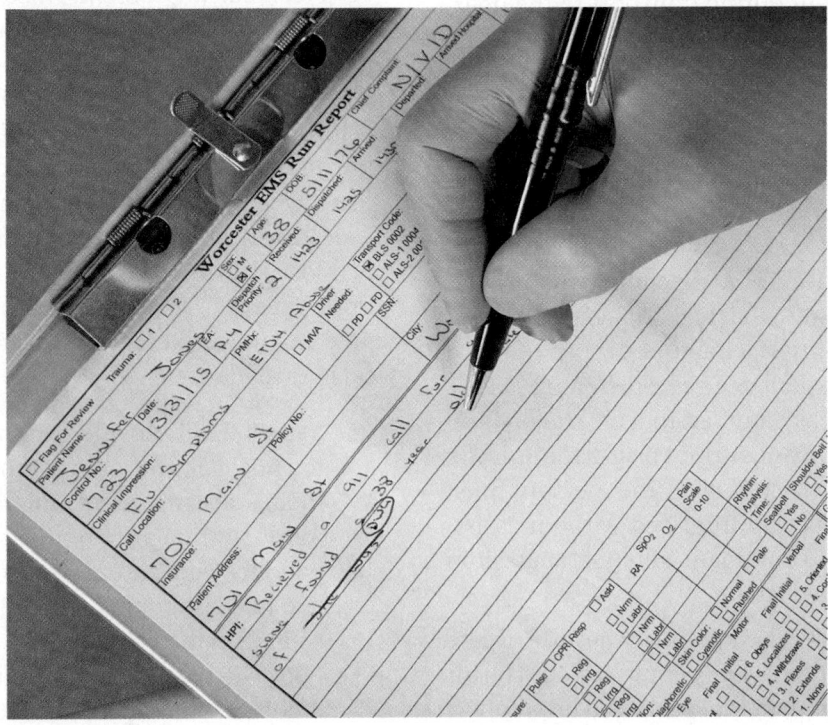

**FIGURE 4-13** If you make a mistake on a handwritten report, the proper way to correct it is to draw a single horizontal line through the error, initial it, and write the correct information next to it.

If an error is discovered after you submit your report, follow the same process. Make sure to add a note with the correct information. If you accidentally left out information, begin the new section with the word "addendum," add the new information, and then add the date and your initials. When using a paper system, you may be able to add addendums using specific addendum forms. If you are using an electronic documentation system, refer to the system's direction as to how to make an amendment to the original document. Most electronic systems will allow for amendments that are date stamped but will prevent erasure in a completed document.

## Documenting Refusal of Care

Refusal of care is an important potential source of litigation in EMS; therefore, thorough documentation is crucial. As discussed in Chapter 3, *Medical, Legal, and Ethical Issues*, competent adult patients with decision-making capacity have the right to refuse treatment and, in fact, must specifically provide permission for treatment to be initiated. If you are not able to persuade the patient to proceed with treatment, document any patient assessment findings, emergency medical care given, your efforts to obtain consent, and the patient's response to your efforts. Have the patient sign a refusal form (**FIGURE 4-14**). You should also have a family member, police officer, or bystander sign the form as a witness. If the patient refuses to sign the refusal form, have a family member, police officer, or bystander sign the form verifying that the patient refused to sign. Inform online medical control when patients refuse care.

Even if a patient refuses care, you must complete the PCR. You will need to document the advice you gave regarding the risks associated with refusal of care. Report clinical information, such as the level of consciousness (LOC), showing the competency of the person refusing care. Note pertinent patient comments and any medical advice given to the patient by the physician or medical control through phone or radio. Also include a description of the care that you wished to provide for the patient. There are many local variations of requirements for patient refusals. **TABLE 4-8** provides a reasonable list of items that should be included within the PCR of a patient refusal.

Refusal of care pertains not only to patients who do not wish to be transported to the hospital, but also to those who refuse a certain aspect of care. For example, a patient involved in a car crash who has neck pain may wish to be treated and transported but refuses to allow you to apply a cervical collar. In these instances, you should carry out all other medical care and document that the patient refused application of a cervical collar. Just because the patient refuses a cervical collar is no reason to deny oxygen. The same is true for the patient who wishes to use a local hospital when the injuries dictate transport to a trauma facility. Anytime a patient refuses any part of the standard treatment, it needs to be documented in the PCR.

## YOU are the Provider

As your partner takes the patient's vital signs, you ask the patient further questions regarding her chief complaint. She denies any other complaints or past medical history and tells you that she only takes vitamins. Her blood glucose level is obtained at 112 mg/dL.

| Recording Time: 5 Minutes | |
| --- | --- |
| **Respirations** | 20 breaths/min; regular and unlabored |
| **Pulse** | 68 beats/min; strong and regular |
| **Skin** | Adequate circulation; skin warm and dry |
| **Blood pressure** | 122/62 mm Hg |
| **Oxygen saturation (Spo$_2$)** | 98% (on room air) |

**5.** What techniques can facilitate the process of interviewing an older patient?

# Patient Initiated Refusal of EMS

Patient Name: Doe, John          Primary Care Giver: John Smith, NREMT-P

Agency: BALTIMORE COUNTY FIRE DEPARTMENT  Incident#: 1122141          eMEDS#: 00314105399

Unit #: Medic 14          Inc Date Entered: 11/22/2016          Inc Time Entered: 1824 hrs

I (or my guardian) have been informed regarding the state of my present physical condition to the extent I allowed an examination, and I (or my guardian) hereby refuse to accept such medical care and/or transportation as recommended by representatives of the EMS System above.

I (or my guardian) do hereby for myself, my heirs, executors, and administrators and assigns forever release and fully discharge said EMS system, its officers, employees, medical consultants, hospitals, borrowed servants or agents from any and all conceivable liability that might arise from this refusal of care and/or transportation, and I (and my guardian) therefore agree to hold them completely harmless. I (or my guardian) have been informed that a refusal of care and/or transportation for an evaluation may cause me to suffer PAIN, DISABILITY, LOSS of FUNCTION, WORSENING of my CONDITION, or even DEATH as a result of my illness/injury. As a competent adult, I (or my guardian) fully understand all of the above, and am/is capable of determining a rational decision on my own behalf.

*Providers: When encountering a patient who is attempting to refuse EMS treatment or transport, access his or her condition, and record whether the patient screening reveals any lack of medical decision-making capability (1-3,4a or b) or high risk criteria (5-8).*

| | |
|---|---|
| 1) Medical Capacity: Was the patient disoriented to person? If yes, transport | ☐ Yes ☑ No |
| 2) Medical Capacity: Was the patient disoriented to place? If yes, transport | ☐ Yes ☑ No |
| 3) Medical Capacity: Was the patient disoriented to time? If yes, transport | ☐ Yes ☑ No |
| 4) Medical Capacity: Was the patient disoriented to situation? If yes, transport | ☐ Yes ☑ No |
| 5) Medical Capacity: Did the patient show altered level of consciousness? If yes, transport | ☐ Yes ☑ No |
| 6) Medical Capacity: Alcohol or drug ingestion by history or exam with slurred speech? If yes, transport | ☐ Yes ☑ No |
| 7) Medical Capacity: Alcohol or drug ingestion by history or exam with unsteady gait? If yes, transport | ☐ Yes ☑ No |
| 8) Medical Capacity: Patient does not understand the nature of illness and potential for bad outcome? If yes, transport | ☐ Yes ☑ No |
| 9) At Risk Criteria (Abnormal vital signs): For adults. Pulse greater than 120 or less than 60? If yes, consult | ☐ Yes ☑ No |
| 10) At Risk Criteria (Abnormal vital signs): For adults. Systolic BP less than 90? If yes, consult | ☐ Yes ☑ No |
| 11) At Risk Criteria (Abnormal vital signs): For adults. Respirations greater than 30 or less than 10? If yes, consult | ☐ Yes ☑ No |
| 12) At Risk Criteria (Abnormal vital signs): For minor/pediatric patients. Age inappropriate HR? If yes, consult | ☐ Yes ☑ No |
| 13) At Risk Criteria (Abnormal vital signs): For minor/pediatric patients. Age inappropriate RR? If yes, consult | ☐ Yes ☑ No |
| 14) At Risk Criteria (Abnormal vital signs): For minor/pediatric patients. Age inappropriate BP? If yes, consult | ☐ Yes ☑ No |
| 15) At Risk Criteria: Serious chief complaint (chest pain, SOB, syncope)? If yes, consult | ☐ Yes ☑ No |
| 16) At Risk Criteria: Head injury with history of loss of consciousness? If yes, consult | ☐ Yes ☑ No |
| 17) At Risk Criteria: Significant MOI or high suspicion of injury? If yes, consult | ☐ Yes ☑ No |

**FIGURE 4-14** Even though competent adult patients with decision-making capacity have the right to refuse medical treatment, ask them if they would be willing to sign a refusal form to document their informed refusal.

| | |
|---|---|
| 18) At Risk Criteria: For minor/pediatric patients. ALTE, significant past medical history, or suspected intentional injury? If yes, consult | ☐ Yes ☑ No |
| 19) At Risk Criteria: Provider impression is that the patient requires hospital evaluation? If yes, consult | ☐ Yes ☑ No |
| 20) Providers: Did you perform an assessment (including exam) on this patient? If yes to # 20, skip to # 22 | ☐ Yes ☑ No |
| 21) Providers: If unable to examine, did you attempt vital signs? | ☐ Yes ☑ No |
| 22) Providers: Did you attempt to convince the patient or guardian to accept transport? | ☐ Yes ☑ No |
| 23) Providers: Did you contact medical direction for patient still refusing service? | ☐ Yes ☑ No |
| 24) Patient: The patient or his or her representative refuses EMS examination. | ☐ Yes ☑ No |
| 25) Patient: The patient or his or her representative refuses EMS treatment. | ☐ Yes ☑ No |
| 26) Patient: The patient or his or her representative refuses EMS transport. | ☐ Yes ☑ No |

**Patient Signature:** **Printed Name:**

**Patient Phone:** **Date:** 18:24 11/24/2016

**Patient Address:**

## Initial Disposition

| | | |
|---|---|---|
| Patient Refused Exam ☑ | Patient Refused Treatment ☑ | Patient Refused Transport ☑ |
| Patient Accepted Exam ☐ | Patient Accepted Treatment ☐ | Patient Accepted Transport ☐ |
| Auth. Decision Maker (ADM) Refused Exam ☐ | Auth. Decision Maker (ADM) Refused Treatment ☐ | Auth. Decision Maker (ADM) Refused Transport ☐ |

## Intervention

Attempt to Convince Patient ☑ Attempt to Convince Family Member/Auth. Decision Maker (ADM) ☐ Contact Medical Direction ☑ Contact Law Enforcement ☐ None of the Above Available ☐

**AMA Contact Medical Direction Facility** St Elsewhere Hospital

## Final Disposition

| | | |
|---|---|---|
| Patient Refused Exam ☐ | Patient Refused Treatment ☐ | Patient Refused Transport ☑ |
| Patient Accepted Exam ☑ | Patient Accepted Treatment ☑ | Patient Accepted Transport ☐ |
| Auth. Decision Maker (ADM) Refused Exam ☐ | Auth. Decision Maker (ADM) Refused Treatment ☐ | Auth. Decision Maker (ADM) Refused Transport ☐ |

## Provide in the patient's own words why he/she refused the above care/service:

"Patient reports that despite the damage to his vehicle, he has only a small laceration on his finger and no other symptoms. He eventually agreed to allow EMS to evaluate him and provide a bandage for a small finger laceration (index finger, right hand). He agreed to follow up with his primary care MD later today. When offered transport to the hospital he indicated, "No. thanks. I will be fine." Discussed plan with Dr Smith at St Elsewhere ED who agreed with plan and recommended reiterating to Mr Smith the importance of close follow-up with his primary care MD for tetanus prophylaxis and consideration of laceration care to include sutures.

Inc. Date: 11/22/2016 Patient Name: Doe, John BALTIMORE COUNTY FIRE DEPARTMENT Page: 2

Incident #: 1122141 Date Printed: 11/24/2016 18:24

**FIGURE 4-14** *(Continued)*

| TABLE 4-8 Components of a Thorough Patient Refusal Document |
|---|

Complete assessment

Evidence the patient has the decision-making capacity to make a rational, informed decision

Discussion with the patient as to what care/transportation EMS recommends

Discussion with the patient as to what may happen if the patient does not allow care or transportation. Typically these consequences should be listed and clear to include the possibility of severe illness/injury or death if care or transportation is refused.

Discussion with family/friend/bystanders to try to encourage the patient to allow care

Discussion with medical direction according to local protocol

Providing the patient with other alternatives: going to see his or her family doctor, having a family member drive him or her to the hospital

Willingness of EMS to return if the patient changes his or her mind

Signatures: Have a family member, police officer, or bystander sign the form as a witness. If the patient refuses to sign the refusal form, have a family member, police officer, or bystander sign the form verifying that the patient refused to sign.

If the patient refused care or did not allow a complete assessment, document that the patient did not allow for proper assessment, and document whatever assessments were completed.

© Jones & Bartlett Learning.

## Special Reporting Situations

In some situations, you may be required to file special reports with appropriate authorities. These situations may involve gunshot wounds, dog bites, certain infectious diseases, or suspected physical or sexual abuse. Learn your local requirements for reporting these incidents. Failure to report them may have legal consequences. It is important that the report be accurate, objective, and submitted in a timely manner.

Another special reporting situation is a mass-casualty incident (MCI). The local MCI plan should have some means of temporarily recording important medical information (such as a triage tag that can be used later to complete the form). The standard for completing the form in an MCI is not the same as for a typical call. Your local plan should have specific guidelines. MCIs are discussed in Chapter 40, *Incident Management*.

## Communications Systems and Equipment

Radio and telephone communications link you and your team with other members of the EMS, fire, and law enforcement communities. This link helps the entire team to work together more effectively and provides an important layer of safety and protection for each member of the team. You must know what your system can and cannot do, and you must be able to use your system efficiently and effectively. You must be able to send precise, accurate reports about the scene, the patient's condition, and the treatment that you provide.

As an EMT, you must be familiar with two-way radio communications and have a working knowledge of the mobile and handheld portable radios that are used in your unit. You must also know when to use them and what to say when you are transmitting.

## Base Station Radios

The dispatcher usually communicates with field units by transmitting through a fixed radio base station that is controlled from the dispatch center. A **base station** is any radio hardware containing a transmitter and receiver that is located in a fixed place. The base station may be used by an operator speaking into a microphone that is connected directly to the equipment. It also works remotely through telephone lines or by radio from a communications center. Base stations may include dispatch centers, fire stations, ambulance bases, or hospitals.

A two-way radio consists of two units: a transmitter and a receiver. Some base stations may have more than one transmitter and/or more than one receiver. They may also be equipped with one multichannel transmitter and several single-channel receivers. A **channel** is an assigned frequency or frequencies used to carry voice and/or data communications. Regardless of the number of transmitters and receivers, they are commonly called *base radios* or *stations*. Base stations usually have more power (often 100 watts or more) and higher, more efficient antenna systems than mobile or portable radios. This increased broadcasting range allows the base station operator to communicate with field units and other stations at much greater distances.

The base radio must be physically close to its antenna. Therefore, the actual base station cabinet and hardware are commonly found on the roof of a tall building or at the bottom of an antenna tower. The base station operator may be miles away in a dispatch center or hospital, communicating with the base station radio by dedicated lines or special radio links. A **dedicated line**, also known as a *hotline*, is used for specific point-to-point contact. This type of phone, typically located within an ED, is not on the main switchboard. EMS personnel are able to call the number directly without being placed on hold or transferred. This type of line makes recording medical command conversations much easier.

## Mobile and Portable Radios

In the ambulance, you will use both mobile and portable radios to communicate with the dispatcher and/or medical control. An ambulance will often have more than one mobile radio, each on a different frequency (**FIGURE 4-15**). One radio may be used to communicate with the dispatcher or other public safety agencies. A second radio is often used for communicating patient information to medical control.

A mobile radio is installed in a vehicle and usually operates at lower power than a base station. Most **VHF (very high frequency)** mobile radios operate between 30 and 300 MHz. **UHF (ultra-high frequency)** mobile radios operate between 300 MHz and 3,000 MHz. Radios that operate at 800 MHz are increasingly common in EMS systems. These systems provide a great amount of system flexibility without the need for vast numbers of frequencies. What was once accomplished with 30 separate frequencies can be done with fewer than 10. Mobile antennas are much closer to the ground than base station antennas, so communications from the unit are typically limited to 10 to 15 miles over average terrain.

Portable radios are handheld devices that operate at 1 to 5 watts of power. Because the entire radio can be held in your hand, when in use, the antenna is often no taller than you. The transmission range of a portable radio is more limited than that of mobile or base station radios. Portable radios are essential in helping to coordinate EMS activities at the scene of an MCI. They are also helpful when you are away from the ambulance and need to communicate with dispatch, another unit, or medical control (**FIGURE 4-16**).

## Repeater-Based Systems

A **repeater** is a special base station radio that receives messages and signals on one frequency and then automatically retransmits them on a second frequency. Because a repeater is a base station (with a large antenna), it is able to receive lower power

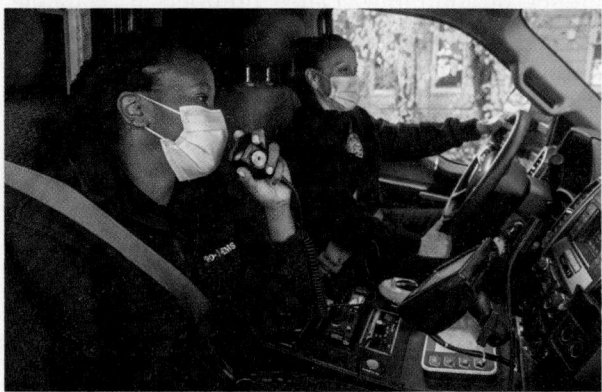

**FIGURE 4-15** Some ambulances have more than one mobile radio to allow communications with hospitals, mutual aid jurisdictions, and other agencies.

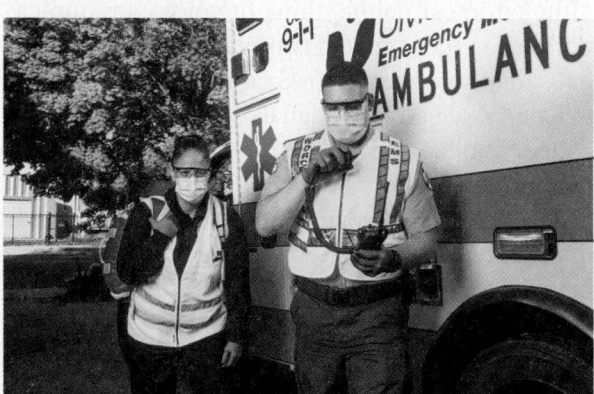

**FIGURE 4-16** A portable radio is essential if you need to communicate with the dispatcher or medical control when you are away from the ambulance.

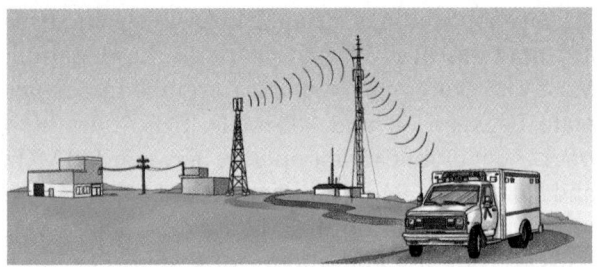

**FIGURE 4-17** A message is sent from the control center to the transmitter by a landline. The radio carrier wave is picked up by the repeater for rebroadcast to outlying units. Return radio traffic is picked up by the repeater and rebroadcast to the control center.

© Jones & Bartlett Learning.

signals, such as those from a portable radio, from a long distance away. The signal is then rebroadcast with all the power of the base station (**FIGURE 4-17**). EMS systems that use repeaters usually have outstanding systemwide communications and are able to get the best signal from portable radios. There are also mobile repeaters that may be found in ambulances or placed in various areas around an EMS system area.

At times, you may be able to communicate with a base station radio, but you will not be able to hear or transmit to another mobile unit that is also communicating with that base. Repeater base stations eliminate such problems. They allow two mobile or portable units that cannot reach each other directly to communicate through the repeater, using its greater power and antenna.

## Digital Equipment

Although most people think of voice communications when they think of two-way radios, digital signals are also a part of EMS communications. With telemetry, electronic signals are converted into coded, audible signals. These signals can then be transmitted by radio or telephone to a receiver with a decoder at the hospital. The decoder converts the signals back into electronic impulses that can be displayed on a screen or printed. New technology also allows for digital telemetry. For example, data from cardiac monitors can be transmitted via Bluetooth-enabled mobile devices to a monitoring center, where physicians can review the data and quickly contact patients, if needed. Rhythm strips and 12-lead ECGs are transmitted to the hospital to identify abnormal heart rhythms and critical cardiac information such as ST-segment elevation myocardial infarction (STEMI) alerts, allowing informed treatment decisions to be made during the prehospital phase. Digital signals are also used in some types of paging and tone alerting systems because they transmit faster than spoken words and allow more choices and flexibility.

## Cellular/Satellite Telephones

Whereas dispatchers communicate with field units by transmitting through a fixed radio base station, it is common for EMTs to communicate with receiving facilities by cellular telephone. These telephones are effectively low-power portable radios that communicate through a series of interconnected repeater stations called *cells* (hence the name *cellular*). Cells are linked by a sophisticated computer system and connected to the telephone network. Another option is a satellite phone, or satphone. These phones use a satellite, instead of a cell, to receive and relay the signals.

Many cellular systems make equipment and air time available to EMS systems at little or no cost as a public service. The public is often able to call 9-1-1 or other emergency numbers on a cellular telephone free of charge. However, this easy access may result in overloading and jamming of cellular systems in mass-casualty and disaster situations. To overcome this problem, the federal government funded the FirstNet program. States that participate in this program have priority access to high-speed broadband cellular data transmission during high-use events.

When using these systems, ensure that a reference of commonly called numbers is available. Local hospitals, poison control, police services, and the number to the dispatcher should be readily available. Cellular and satellite systems also have areas of bad reception. As an EMT, it is important to be aware of any areas in which your equipment will not work.

As with all repeater-based systems, a cellular or satellite telephone is useless if the equipment fails, if there is a loss of power, or if it is damaged by severe weather or other circumstances.

A scanner is a radio receiver that searches or scans across several frequencies, stops whenever it receives a radio broadcast on that frequency, and continues once the message is complete. Although cellular and satellite telephones are more private than most other forms of radio communications, keep in mind that these telephones use digital signals, which makes eavesdropping difficult but not impossible. Therefore, you must always be careful to appropriately respect patient privacy and to speak in a professional manner every time you use any form of an EMS communications system.

## Other Communications Equipment

Ambulances and other field units are usually equipped with an external public address system. This system may be a part of the siren or the mobile radio. The intercom between the cab and the patient compartment may also be a part of the mobile radio. These components do not involve radio wave transmission, but you must understand how they work and practice using them before you really need them.

EMS systems may use a variety of two-way radio hardware. Some systems operate VHF equipment in the **simplex** (push to talk, release to listen) mode. In this mode, radio transmissions can occur in either direction but not simultaneously. When one party transmits, the other can only receive. Once one party finishes transmitting, the other party can then reply. Other systems conduct **duplex** (simultaneous talk–listen) communications on UHF frequencies and cellular telephones. In the full duplex mode, radios can simultaneously transmit and receive communications on one channel. This is sometimes called pair of frequencies. A third possible configuration for a communications system is **multiplex**. This design utilizes two or more frequencies, which enables more than one transmission to occur simultaneously and provides for the transmission of both audio and data signals via separate channels. This type of system is what allows paramedics to transmit a patient's electrocardiogram to the hospital from the scene or back of the ambulance. Many VHF and UHF channels, commonly called **MED channels**, are reserved exclusively for EMS use. However, hundreds of other commercial, local government, and fire services frequencies are also used for EMS communications.

**Trunking**, or 800-MHz, systems take advantage of the latest technologies in communications. Instead of being assigned to one or two frequencies, in a trunking system many frequencies are assigned to a group.

As the radio conversation begins, a computer selects the next open frequency and you begin talking. When you speak a second time, you will likely be speaking on a different frequency because the computer is constantly monitoring for frequency load and reassigning transmissions to unused frequencies. These systems allow for greater traffic without greater numbers of frequencies. Therefore, you do not need to worry about being able to transmit or receive. In a trunking system, the computer will switch you to another channel without you being aware and you will operate the radio as you normally do.

Any large-scale emergency requires cooperative efforts from several agencies, such as law enforcement, fire departments, and EMS. At times more than one jurisdiction is involved and effective communication between all of those involved becomes challenging. An **interoperable communications system** allows all agencies involved to share valuable information with each other in real time. This system utilizes a voice-over-Internet protocol format to connect landlines, cell phones, and computers to create a seamless, reliable exchange of information between all parties.

Another type of communication system is a **mobile data terminal (MDT)** (**FIGURE 4-18**). An MDT is a small computer terminal inside the ambulance or other vehicle that directly receives data from the dispatch center. MDTs allow for greatly expanded communication capabilities. Instead of asking the dispatcher to confirm whether he said 11345 Main Street or 11354 Main Street, you look at the terminal where the address is displayed. Satellite communications can track your progress to the scene and can provide important scene information, such

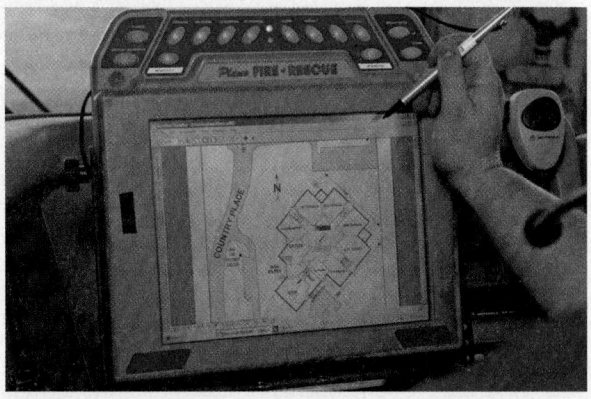

**FIGURE 4-18** A mobile data terminal.
© Jones & Bartlett Learning. Courtesy of MIEMSS.

as known violent calls to this address, the nature of those calls, and the number of times the ambulance has been called.

Your ability to effectively communicate with other units or medical control depends on how well the weaker radio can talk back. Base and repeater station radios often have higher antennas and much greater power than mobile or portable units do. This increased power ensures that signals are generally heard and understood from a far greater distance than the signal produced from a mobile unit. Remember, when you are at the scene, you may be able to clearly hear the dispatcher or hospital on your radio, but you may not be heard or understood when you transmit.

Even small changes in your location can significantly affect the quality of your transmission. Also, remember that the location of the antenna is critically important for clear transmission. Commercial aircraft flying at 37,000 feet can transmit and receive signals over hundreds of miles, yet their radios have only a few watts of power. The power comes from their antenna positioned at 37,000 feet.

The success of communications depends on the efficiency of your equipment. A damaged antenna or microphone often prevents high-quality communications. Check the condition and status of your equipment at the start of each shift, and then correct or report any problems.

# Radio Communications

All radio operations in the United States, including those used in EMS systems, are regulated by the **Federal Communications Commission (FCC)**. The FCC has jurisdiction over interstate and international telephone and telegraph services and satellite communications—all of which may involve EMS activity.

The FCC has five principal EMS-related responsibilities:

1. **Allocate specific radio frequencies for use by EMS providers.** Modern EMS communications began in 1974. At that time, the FCC assigned 10 MED channels in the 460- to 470-MHz (UHF) band to be used by EMS providers. These UHF channels were added to the several VHF frequencies that were already available for EMS systems. However, these VHF frequencies had to be shared with other special emergencies uses, including school buses and veterinarians.

2. **License base stations and assign appropriate radio call signs for those stations.** An FCC license is usually issued for 5 years, after which time it must be renewed. Each FCC license is granted only for a specific operating group. Often, the longitude and latitude (locations) of

---

## YOU are the Provider

The patient wishes to be evaluated at the hospital and agrees to EMS transport, is placed on the stretcher, and is loaded into the ambulance. You cover her with a blanket to keep her warm and proceed to a hospital located 15 miles away. En route, you reassess her condition.

| Recording Time: 11 Minutes | |
| --- | --- |
| **Level of consciousness** | Conscious and alert |
| **Respirations** | 20 breaths/min; regular and unlabored |
| **Pulse** | 74 beats/min; strong and regular |
| **Skin** | Adequate circulation; skin warm and dry |
| **Blood pressure** | 118/60 mm Hg |
| **Spo$_2$** | 98% (on room air) |

The patient's condition remains unchanged since your initial encounter. You contact the receiving facility and provide them with a radio report.

**6.** What are the components of a radio report to the hospital?

**7.** How does the handover report differ from the radio report?

the antenna and the address of the base station determine the call signs.

3. **Establish licensing standards and operating specifications for radio equipment used by EMS providers.** Before it can be licensed, each piece of radio equipment must be submitted to the FCC by its manufacturer for type acceptance, based on established operating specifications and regulations.

4. **Establish limitations for transmitter power output.** The FCC regulates broadcasting power to reduce radio interference between neighboring communications systems.

5. **Monitor radio operations.** This includes making spot field checks to help ensure compliance with FCC rules and regulations.

The FCC's rules and regulations are written in technical and legal language and fill many volumes. Only a small section (part 90, subpart B) deals with EMS communication issues. You are not responsible for reading these detailed and often confusing documents. For appropriate guidance on technical issues, contact your EMS system supervisor. In fact, many EMS systems look to radio and telephone communications experts for advice on technical issues.

## Responding to the Scene

EMS communication systems may operate on several frequencies and use different frequency bands. Some EMS systems may even use different radios for various purposes. However, all EMS systems depend on the skill of the dispatcher. The dispatcher receives the first call to 9-1-1. You are part of the team that responds to calls once the dispatcher notifies your unit of an emergency.

The dispatcher has several important responsibilities during the alert and dispatch phase of EMS communications. The dispatcher must do all of the following:

- Properly screen and assign priority to each call (according to predetermined protocols).
- Select and alert the appropriate EMS response unit or units.
- Dispatch and direct EMS response unit or units to the correct location.
- Coordinate the EMS response unit or units with other public safety services until the incident is over.

- Provide emergency medical instructions to the telephone caller (according to predetermined protocols) so that essential care (eg, CPR) may begin before the EMTs arrive.

When the first call to 9-1-1 comes in, the dispatcher must judge its relative importance to begin the appropriate EMS response using emergency medical dispatch protocols. First, the dispatcher must find out the exact location of the patient and the nature and severity of the problem. The dispatcher asks for the caller's telephone number, the patient's name and age, and other information, as directed by local protocol. Next, the dispatcher asks for some description of the scene, such as the number of patients or special environmental hazards.

Using this information, the dispatcher will assign the appropriate EMS response unit or units based on local protocols and the following factors:

- Dispatcher's determination of the nature and severity of the problem (Many emergency medical dispatch systems will determine this automatically based on a caller's answers to a defined series of questions.)
- Anticipated response time to the scene
- Level of training (EMR, EMT, AEMT, paramedic) of available EMS response unit or units
- Need for additional EMS units, fire suppression, rescue, a hazardous materials team, air medical support, or law enforcement

The dispatcher's next step is to alert the appropriate EMS response unit or units (**FIGURE 4-19**).

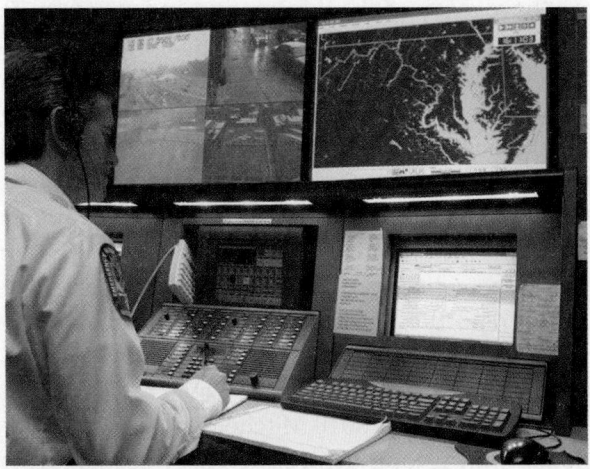

**FIGURE 4-19** You will be assigned to a call by the dispatcher.

© Jones & Bartlett Learning. Courtesy of MIEMSS.

Alerting these units may be done in a variety of ways. The dispatcher may use the dispatch radio system to contact units. Dedicated lines (hotlines) between the control center and the EMS station may also be used.

The dispatcher may also page EMS personnel. Pagers are commonly used in EMS operations to alert on-duty and off-duty personnel. **Paging** involves the use of a coded tone or digital radio signal and a voice or display message that is transmitted to pagers (beepers) or desktop monitor radios. Paging signals may be sent to alert specific personnel or may be blanket signals that activate all pagers in the EMS service. Pagers and monitor radios are convenient because they are usually silent until their specific paging code is received. Alerted personnel contact the dispatcher to confirm the message and receive details of their assignments.

Once EMS personnel have been alerted, they must be properly dispatched and sent to the incident. Every EMS system should use a standard dispatching procedure. The dispatcher should give the responding unit or units the following information:

- Nature and severity of the injury, illness, or incident
- Exact location of the incident
- Number of patients
- Responses by other public safety agencies
- Special directions or advisories, such as adverse road or traffic conditions, severe weather reports, or potential scene hazards
- Time at which the unit or units are dispatched

Your unit must confirm with the dispatcher that you have received the information and are en route to the scene. Local protocol will dictate whether it is the job of the dispatcher or your unit to notify other public safety agencies that you are responding to an emergency. In some areas, the ED is also notified when an ambulance responds to an emergency.

You should report any problems during your response to the dispatcher. You should also inform the dispatcher when you have arrived at the scene. The arrival report to the dispatcher should include any obvious details that you see during scene size-up. For example, you might say, "Dispatcher, BLS Unit Two is on scene at 3010 Mitchell Street. It is a blue house with a long driveway." This information is particularly useful if additional units are responding to the same scene.

All radio communications during dispatch, as well as during other phases of operations, must be brief and easily understood. Speak in plain English and do not use code words in your transmissions. The use of 10-codes is specifically discouraged because their meanings vary by jurisdiction, which increases the possibility for misunderstanding a transmission. Your tone and pace should be slow, relaxed, and clear. You do not need to use excessively polite language. Also, avoid wordiness. An example of an excessively wordy communication is: "Good morning dispatch, this is Ambulance 6-3-1. We are responding to 381 South Main Street. Have a good day." Although it sounds pleasant (and you should try to foster a good working environment with the dispatcher), it wastes radio time. Remember, the dispatcher's job is to field hundreds of calls per hour; therefore, you only need to report important information so that the dispatcher can focus on what to do next. **TABLE 4-9** lists common instances for which EMS providers will need to use the radio to communicate with dispatch.

| TABLE 4-9 Typical EMS Communications With Dispatch | |
|---|---|
| **Phase of EMS Call** | **EMS Unit Communication** |
| Initial receipt of call | Acknowledge call |
| | Respond to the call |
| En route to call | Request assistance with directions, when needed |
| | Request additional resources, when needed |
| On scene | Report arrival at scene |
| | Check in; often a system will require EMS units to transmit every 10–20 minutes as a safety measure |
| | Request additional resources, when needed |
| | Report leaving scene |
| Arrival at hospital (or point of transfer) | Notify dispatch of arrival at point of transfer |
| Return to service | Notify dispatch when the unit is available for another call |
| Miscellaneous | Some systems require EMS units to notify dispatch anytime they are not in station |

© Jones & Bartlett Learning.

| TABLE 4-10 Tips When Using EMS Radio Communications |
| --- |
| Turn radio on and adjust volume. |
| Ensure a clear frequency before speaking. |
| To speak, use the press-to-talk button, and wait 1 second before speaking. |
| Hold the microphone 2 to 3 in. (5–8 cm) from your mouth. |
| Address the unit you are calling, and provide the name of your unit. |
| The unit you call will signal that you can begin your transmission. |
| Use a clear and calm voice and speak at a reasonable pace. |
| Keep the transmission brief. |
| Use clear text. |
| Avoid the use of codes or agency-specific terms. |
| Avoid using slang or unapproved abbreviations. |
| Do not use useless or meaningless phrases, such as "be advised." |
| Limit saying "please," "thank you," and "you're welcome." |
| When transmitting numbers, such as an address, provide both the number and the individual digits (ie, "Respond to 1381, 1-3-8-1, Main Street"). |
| Remember that the airwaves are public and the use of scanners is popular. |
| Do not use names; protect the privacy of patients. |
| Remain objective and impartial in describing patients. |
| Never use profanity; always be professional. |
| Use the words "affirmative" and "negative" instead of "yes" or "no." |
| Use the standard format for transmission of information. |
| When you are finished transmitting, indicate this by saying "over." |
| Do not provide a diagnosis of the patient's problem. |
| Use EMS frequencies only for EMS communications. |
| Monitor background noise. |

© Jones & Bartlett Learning.

**TABLE 4-10** lists tips for using the radio. Although these may change slightly from department to department, they provide a good foundation from which to begin.

## Communicating With Medical Control and Hospitals

The principal reason for radio communication is to facilitate communication between you and medical control (and the hospital). Medical control may be located at the receiving hospital, at another facility, or sometimes even in another city or state. You must, however, consult with medical control to notify the hospital of an incoming patient, request advice or receive orders, or advise the hospital of special situations.

It is important to plan and organize your radio communication before you push the transmit button. Remember, a concise, well-organized report is the best method of accurately and thoroughly describing the patient and his or her medical condition to the providers who will be receiving the patient. It also demonstrates your competence and professionalism to all who hear your report. Well-organized radio communications with the hospital will engender confidence in the receiving facility's physicians and nurses, as well as others who are listening. In addition, the patient and family will be comforted by your organization and ability to communicate clearly. A well-delivered radio report puts you in control of the information, which is correct procedure.

Hospital notification is the most common type of communication between you and the hospital. The purpose of these calls is to notify the receiving facility of the patient's chief complaint and condition (**FIGURE 4-20**). On the basis of this information, the ED is able to appropriately prepare staff and equipment to receive the patient. This is primarily a one-way form of communication. You are telling the ED what to expect. You are not asking for advice or orders; you are simply notifying them.

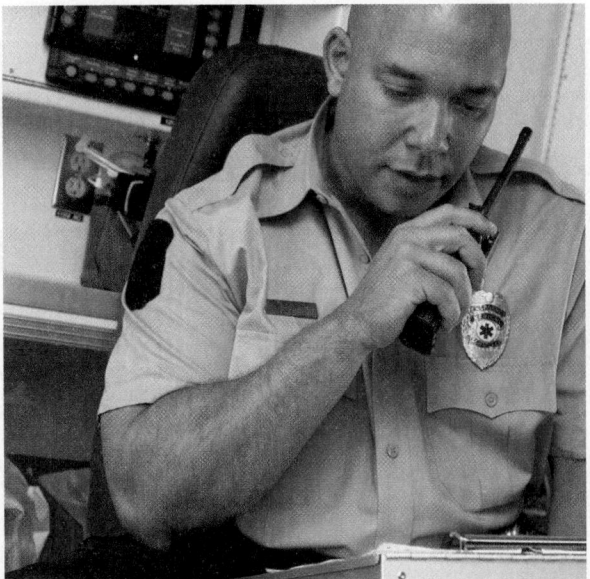

**FIGURE 4-20** The patient report should be given in an objective, accurate, and professional manner.

© Jones & Bartlett Learning. Courtesy of MIEMSS.

## Giving the Patient Report

The patient report should follow a standard format established by your EMS system. The report commonly includes the following 10 elements:

1. Your unit identification and level of services. Example: "Columbus Fire 2-BLS."
2. Any special "alert" indicated by the patient's status or care. For example, a patient suffering from a severe traumatic injury will be a "trauma alert," or a heart attack may call for a "cardiac alert."
3. The receiving hospital and your estimated time of arrival. Example: "Columbus Community Hospital, ETA 10 minutes," or "patient transport code" according to local protocols.
4. The patient's age and sex. Example: "An 86-year-old woman." The patient's name should not be given over the radio because it may be overheard. This would be a violation of the patient's privacy.
5. The patient's chief complaint or your chief concern regarding the patient's problem and its severity. Example: "Patient reports severe pelvic and less severe back pain."
6. A brief history of the patient's current problem. Example: "Patient fell into bathtub at 0300 this morning and wasn't able to get out." Other important history information that may pertain to the current problem should also be included, such as "The patient has diabetes and takes insulin."
7. A brief report of physical findings. This report should include level of consciousness, the patient's general appearance, pertinent abnormalities noted, and vital signs. Example: "The patient is alert and oriented, has adequate circulation based on examination of mucous membranes inside the inner lower eyelid and capillary refill, and is cold to the touch. We noted crepitus in the pelvic girdle. Her blood pressure is 112/84, pulse is 72, and respirations 14."
8. A brief summary of the care given and any patient response. Example: "We have applied a cervical collar. She still has pulse, motor, and sensory function distally in all four extremities."
9. A brief description of the patient's response to the treatment provided.
10. Determine whether the receiving facility has any additional questions or orders.

Be sure you report all patient information in an objective, accurate, and professional manner. Remember that people with scanners are listening. You could be successfully sued for slander if you describe a patient in a way that injures the patient's reputation.

## The Role of Medical Control

The delivery of EMS involves an impressive array of assessments, stabilization, and treatments. In

## YOU are the Provider

With an estimated time of arrival at the hospital of 20 minutes, you reassess the patient and note that her condition has remained unchanged.

**Recording Time: 16 Minutes**

| | |
|---|---|
| Level of consciousness | Conscious and alert |
| Respirations | 18 breaths/min; regular and unlabored |
| Pulse | 72 beats/min; strong and regular |
| Skin | Adequate circulation; skin warm and dry |
| Blood pressure | 120/60 mm Hg |
| SpO$_2$ | 99% (on room air) |

You arrive at the hospital and give your handover report to the charge nurse. After answering the nurse's questions, you complete your PCR and return to service.

**8.** What functions does the PCR serve?

some cases, you may assist patients in taking medications. AEMTs and paramedics go beyond this level by initiating medication therapy based on the patient's presenting signs. For logical, ethical, and legal reasons, the delivery of such sophisticated care must be done in association with physicians. For this reason, every EMS system needs input and involvement from physicians, including your system or department medical director, providing medical direction (medical control) for your EMS system. Medical control is either offline (indirect) or online (direct), as authorized by the medical director. Medical control guides the treatment of patients in the system through protocols, direct orders, advice, and post-call review.

Depending on how the protocols are written, you may need to call medical control for direct orders (permission) to administer certain treatments, to determine the transport destination of patients, or to be allowed to stop treatment and/or not transport a patient. In these cases, the radio or cellular phone provides a vital link between you and the expertise available through the base physician.

To maintain this link 24 hours per day, 7 days per week, medical control must be readily available on the radio at the hospital or on a mobile or portable unit when you call (**FIGURE 4-21**). In most areas, medical control is provided by the physicians who work at the receiving hospital. However, many variations have developed across the country. For example, some EMS units receive medical direction from one hospital even though they are taking the patient to another hospital. In other areas, medical direction may come from a freestanding center or even from an individual physician. Regardless of your system's design, your link to medical control is vital to maintain the high quality of care your patients require and deserve.

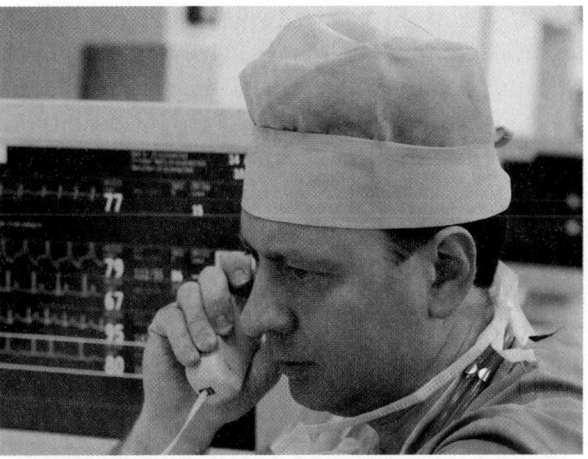

**FIGURE 4-21** Medical control must be readily available on the radio or telephone at the hospital.
© Andrei Malov/Dreamstime.com.

## Calling Medical Control

You can use the radio in your unit or a portable radio to call medical control. A cellular telephone can also be used. Regardless of the type of communication, you should use a channel that is relatively free of other radio traffic and interference and one that is recorded. Medical command communications create medicolegal requirements that such conversations should be recorded. There are several ways to control access on ambulance-to-hospital channels. In some EMS systems, the dispatcher monitors and assigns appropriate, clear medical control channels. Other EMS systems rely on special communications operations, such as centralized medical emergency dispatch or resource coordination centers, to monitor and allocate the medical control channels.

Because of the large number of EMS calls to medical control, your radio report must be precise and well organized and must only contain important information. In addition, because you need specific directions on patient care, the information that you provide to medical control must be accurate. Remember, the physician on the other end bases his or her instructions on the information you provide.

### Words of Wisdom

Some EMS systems assign roles in their units: a primary person to speak on the radio and a primary person to administer patient care. In these systems, all members of the crew must communicate closely to make this process work. EMTs are involved in every role, but the partial division of responsibilities can be efficient and effective. This approach is most common in systems that use extensive online medical control.

### Words of Wisdom

Orders that are unclear or seem inappropriate or incorrect should be respectfully questioned. Do not blindly follow an order that does not make sense to you.

As discussed earlier, you should use proper medical terminology when giving your report. Never use codes when communicating with medical control unless you are directed by local protocol to do so. Most medical control systems handle many EMS agencies and will most likely not know your unit's special codes or signals.

To ensure complete understanding, once you receive an order from medical control, such as an order for a medication or the denial of a request for a particular treatment, you must repeat the order back, word for word, and then receive confirmation. This helps to eliminate confusion and the possibility of poor patient care. Orders that are unclear or seem inappropriate or incorrect should be questioned. Do not blindly follow an order that does not make sense to you. The physician may have misunderstood or may have missed part of your report. In that case, the physician may not be able to respond appropriately to the patient's needs. The role of medical control will be discussed further in Chapter 12, *Principles of Pharmacology*.

## Information About Special Situations

Depending on your system's procedures, you may initiate communication with one or more hospitals to advise them of an extraordinary call or situation. For instance, a small rural hospital may be better able to respond to multiple victims of a highway crash if it is notified when the ambulance is first responding. At the other extreme, an entire hospital system must be notified of any disaster, such as a plane or train crash, as early as possible to enable activation of its staff call-in system. These special situations may also include hazardous materials situations, rescues in progress, MCIs, or any other situation that could require special preparation on the part of the hospital. In some areas, mutual aid frequencies may be designated in MCIs so that responding agencies can communicate with one another on a common frequency.

When notifying the hospital of any special situations, keep the following in mind: The earlier the notification, the better. You should ask to speak to the charge nurse or physician in charge, as this person is best able to mobilize the resources necessary to respond. Also, whenever possible, provide an estimate of the number of people who may be transported to the facility. Be sure to identify any conditions the patient or patients may have that require special needs, such as burns or hazardous

materials exposure, to assist the hospital in preparation. In many cases, hospital notification is part of a larger disaster or hazardous materials plan. Follow the plan for your system.

## Maintenance of Radio Equipment

Similar to all other EMS equipment, radio equipment must be serviced by properly trained and equipped personnel. Remember that the radio is your lifeline to other public safety agencies (which function to protect you), as well as to medical control, and it must perform under emergency conditions. Radio equipment that is operating properly should be serviced at least once per year. Any equipment that is not working properly should be immediately removed from service and sent for repair. Outdated equipment should be removed from service as new equipment becomes available.

When you are beginning your shift, it is typical to check the ambulance to ensure that it is ready to go. You cannot assume that the crew before you left the ambulance well stocked and in operational readiness. The radio is an important component that needs to be checked to ensure that it is operating correctly and using the correct frequency.

Sometimes, radio equipment will stop working during a run. Your EMS system must have several backup plans and options for this scenario. The goal of a backup plan is to make sure you can maintain contact when the usual procedures do not work. Fortunately, there are quite a few options.

The simplest backup plan relies on written standing orders. **Standing orders** are written documents that have been signed by the EMS system's medical director. These orders outline specific directions, permissions, and sometimes prohibitions regarding patient care. By their very nature, standing orders do not require direct communication with medical control. When properly followed, standing orders or formal protocols have the same authority and legal status as orders given over the radio. They exist to one extent or another in every EMS system and can be applied to all levels of EMS providers. Other backup plans can involve using a cell phone and calling the ED directly. The problem with this approach is that the conversation may not be recorded. Medical command conversations are often recorded for the purpose of quality improvement.

## YOU are the Provider SUMMARY

**1. What information should you ask the dispatcher to obtain from the caller?**

A "sick person" could be anyone from a patient with the flu to a patient in cardiac arrest. What you do when you arrive at the scene, such as donning appropriate PPE, may be modified by information from the caller if there is a potential of significant infectious disease. You may also need to delay entry to the scene if there are environmental concerns such as an unusual odor or the possibility of carbon monoxide that would need a fire department dispatch. For all you know, the patient could be experiencing a psychiatric crisis with a potential for violence, in which case law enforcement should be dispatched to secure the scene before your arrival.

After determining the nature of the patient's illness and gathering information that will maximize your own safety, your next priority is to determine if the patient is conscious and breathing adequately or if respirations may be compromised. Try to ascertain the patient's age and sex, if possible. Although you will truly not know what you are dealing with until you arrive at the scene and assess the patient, you should capitalize on the fact that the dispatcher still has the caller on the phone. The more information you obtain prior to arrival at the scene, the better prepared you will be to care for the patient.

**2. Why is effective communication between the responding EMS unit and the dispatcher so important?**

Effective communication between the dispatcher and the EMS unit is important because accurate, thorough communication results in quicker and more effective care for the patient at the scene. Once you respond to a scene, you will confirm with the dispatcher that you are en route. Should there be any delay in your unit's response, your communication with the dispatcher allows adjustments to the response as needed.

During an emergency call, you will communicate with the dispatcher regarding any problems. Depending on your local protocol, the dispatcher will inform other public agencies that you are responding, and coordinate efforts with them to ensure that needed resources are mobilized.

If the dispatcher remains on the line with the caller, additional information about changes in the patient's condition may be available while you are responding. The dispatcher can also relay any information from other responders that arrive before your unit related to the patient's condition or scene concerns.

**3. How can you maximize successful communication with a patient who is hard of hearing?**

First, determine the degree of the patient's hearing loss; her hearing aids may allow her to hear normally. Do not assume she is totally deaf. Remember, most patients who are hard of hearing have a normal intelligence level. Provided you successfully communicate with them, they usually understand what is going on around them. In some cases, placing a stethoscope in the patient's ears and talking slowly and precisely into the diaphragm of the stethoscope may amplify the sound enough if a hearing aid is not working or is not available.

Many patients who are hard of hearing can read lips to some extent; therefore, you should position yourself where the patient can see your lips. Even if they do not read lips, they can receive communication clues from your facial expressions or head motions. Never shout in the ear of a patient who is hard of hearing. Listen carefully, ask short questions, and give short answers whenever possible.

If your efforts to verbally communicate with the patient are unsuccessful, write down your questions on paper and ask the patient to write down her response. Print legibly, so your handwriting is not a communication barrier.

You can ask a family member or friend at the scene to interpret if he or she knows sign language. Learn some simple phrases in sign language, such as "hurt," "sick," and "help" in case you cannot communicate in any other way.

**4. Should your general approach to the assessment process be any different for this patient versus a younger patient? Why or why not?**

As a result of the natural process of aging, some older patients may not react to pain the same as younger patients. An older person who has fallen, for example, may not report any pain, despite the presence of an obvious injury.

Assess the patient just as you would a younger patient; however, you may need to allow extra time for her to answer your questions. As with any patient, she should feel confident that everything possible is being done for her. If the patient seems confused or has difficulty communicating, you should not assume that the cause is age-related. A change from the patient's normal status may be due to a medical cause such as a low oxygen or low blood glucose level.

**5. What techniques can facilitate the process of interviewing an older patient?**

Many of the same techniques used to interview younger patients can be used effectively to interview older patients. When interviewing an older patient, however, patience is even more important. Identify yourself; do not assume that an older person—or any person for that matter—knows who you are. Remain aware of how you present yourself; frustration and impatience can be conveyed through body language.

Look directly at an older patient and speak slowly and distinctly. Do not increase the volume of your voice based on the assumption that the patient is hard of hearing. After asking the patient a question, allow her ample time to answer it and then actively listen to her response. As with any patient, show respect. Refer to her as Mrs. or Miss unless she asks to be addressed otherwise.

Do not talk about the patient in front of her; doing so gives the impression that she has no choice in her medical care. This may escalate her fear of losing independence.

**6. What are the components of a radio report to the hospital?**

The purpose of the radio report is to inform the receiving facility that you are transporting to its location and to provide an overview of the patient's condition so it can adequately prepare to receive the patient. Your radio report to the receiving hospital should be concise: brief in length, yet comprehensive in scope. Identify your EMS system and unit number and then advise the nurse or physician that you are prepared to give a radio report with any appropriate alerts. After he or she confirms being able to hear you, begin your radio report with the patient's age, sex, chief complaint, or chief concern, and level of consciousness. Next, provide a brief elaboration of the patient's chief complaint (eg, the history of present illness), your assessment findings, pertinent history, initial vital signs, and the most recent set of vital signs. Summarize any treatment that you provided and the patient's response, if any, to your treatment, or any other changes in the patient's condition since you made contact. Finally, give the hospital your estimated time of arrival and transport mode.

**7. How does the handover report differ from the radio report?**

Patient care transfer occurs during your handover report, not your radio report. Once a hospital staff member is ready to take responsibility for the patient, you should provide that person with a formal oral report of the patient's condition.

The following components may be included in your handover report, depending on the process at the receiving hospital:

- **Situation.** The patient's name and the chief complaint or chief concern
- **Background.** A brief description of the nature of the problem and pertinent history
- **Assessment.** Key assessment findings and any changes in the patient's condition
- **Treatment.** Treatment provided to the patient prior to arrival

**8. What functions does the PCR serve?**

In addition to your radio and handover reports, you should complete a formal PCR before you leave the hospital or shortly thereafter depending on your local jurisdictional protocol. There are two types of PCRs: written and electronic. A copy of the report, whether written or transmitted electronically, must be left at the hospital at some point.

The PCR describes the nature of the patient's injuries or illness at the scene, the treatment you provided initially and en route, vital signs, and the patient's condition on arrival at the hospital. The PCR serves the following functions:

1. Transfer of information and continuity of care
2. Compliance and legal documentation
3. Administrative information
4. Reimbursement
5. Education
6. Data collection for quality improvement and research

The information in the PCR confirms that you provided proper patient care. In some cases, it also shows that you properly handled unusual or uncommon situations. You should include both objective (what you find) and subjective (what the patient tells you) information in the PCR. A well-written, neat, and concise PCR—including correct spelling and grammar—reflects good patient care. If the report looks sloppy, the care you provided may be assumed to have been the same.

**YOU** are the Provider **SUMMARY** *continued*

## EMS Patient Care Report (PCR)

| **Date:** 4-16-20 | **Incident No.:** 030109 | **Nature of Call:** Sick person | | **Location:** 514 E. Bandera St. | |
|---|---|---|---|---|---|
| **Dispatched:** 0610 | **En Route:** 0610 | **At Scene:** 0616 | **Transport:** 0627 | **At Hospital:** 0650 | **In Service:** 0705 |

### Patient Information

| | |
|---|---|
| **Age:** 83 <br> **Sex:** F <br> **Weight (in kg [lb]):** 50 kg (110 lb) | **Allergies:** None <br> **Medications:** Vitamins <br> **Past Medical History:** None <br> **Chief Complaint:** Lightheadedness and nausea |

### Vital Signs

| **Time:** 0621 | **BP:** 122/62 | **Pulse:** 68 | **Respirations:** 20 | **Spo$_2$:** 98% |
|---|---|---|---|---|
| **Time:** 0627 | **BP:** 118/60 | **Pulse:** 74 | **Respirations:** 20 | **Spo$_2$:** 98% |
| **Time:** 0632 | **BP:** 120/60 | **Pulse:** 72 | **Respirations:** 18 | **Spo$_2$:** 99% |

### EMS Treatment (circle all that apply)

| Oxygen @ ___ L/min via: <br><br> NC   NRM   Bag mask | | Assisted Ventilation | Airway Adjunct | CPR |
|---|---|---|---|---|
| **Defibrillation** | **Bleeding Control** | **Bandaging** | **Splinting** | **Other:** Blood glucose assessment, blanket for warmth |

### Narrative

Dispatched for a "sick person."

Chief complaint: Lightheadedness and nausea

History: Only medications are vitamins; no prescribed medications or known drug allergies. The patient reported lightheadedness and nausea that had started approximately 1 hour earlier. Patient denied chest pain, shortness of breath, abdominal pain, headache, or significant medical problems.

Assessment: Arrived on scene to find the patient, an 83-year-old woman, sitting on the couch in her living room. She was conscious and alert; her airway was patent and her breathing was adequate Assessment did not reveal any gross abnormalities. Her blood glucose level was 112 mg/dL. Obtained vital signs.

Treatment (Rx): Prepared patient for transport. Patient was assisted to sit on the ambulance cot for movement to the ambulance. Applied blanket because the patient stated she was cold.

Transport: Began transport and monitored patient's mental status and vital signs en route. Her condition remained unchanged. The patient wears hearing aids in both ears but was easy to communicate with. Arrived at the hospital and transferred patient care without incident. Oral report was given to staff nurse Asad. Returned to service at 0705.

**End of report**

# Prep Kit

## Ready for Review

- For effective communication to occur, the sender must take a thought, encode it into a message, and send the message to the receiver. The receiver then decodes the message and sends feedback to the sender. A breakdown at any of these steps can interfere with the intended message.
- Many verbal and nonverbal factors and strategies are necessary for therapeutic communication.
- Excellent communication skills are crucial in relaying pertinent information to the hospital before arrival.
- Remember that people who are sick or injured may not understand what you are doing or saying. Therefore, your body language and attitude are important in gaining the trust of both the patient and family. You must also take special care of people such as children, older adults, patients who are hard of hearing, patients who are visually impaired, and non–English-speaking patients.
- As an EMT, you must have excellent verbal communication skills. You should be able to interact with the patient and any family members, friends, or bystanders.
- You must aim to complete a patient care report before you leave the hospital. This is a vital part of providing emergency medical

care and ensuring the continuity of patient care. This information guarantees the proper transfer of responsibility, complies with the requirements of health departments and law enforcement agencies, and fulfills your agency's administrative needs.
- Radio and telephone communications link you and other members of the EMS, fire, and law enforcement communities. This enables your entire team to work together more effectively.
- Understand and be able to use different forms of communication. Be familiar with two-way radio communications and have a working knowledge of mobile and handheld portable radios. You must know when to use them and what type of information you can transmit.
- Know what your communication system can and cannot handle. You must be able to communicate effectively by sending precise, accurate reports about the scene, the patient's condition, and the treatment that you provide.
- Remember, the lines of communication are not always exclusive; therefore, speak in a professional manner at all times and protect patient privacy.
- Your reporting and record-keeping duties are essential, but they should never come before the care of a patient.

## Vital Vocabulary

**base station** Any radio hardware containing a transmitter and receiver that is located in a fixed place.

**cellular telephone** A low-power portable radio that communicates through an interconnected series of repeater stations called cells.

**channel** An assigned frequency or frequencies that are used to carry voice and/or data communications.

**chief complaint** The reason a patient called for help; also, the patient's response to questions such as "What's wrong?" or "What happened?"

**chief concern** The condition requiring the most urgent intervention as determined by the provider's assessment of the patient; it is not always the same as the chief complaint.

**closed-ended questions** Questions that can be answered in short or single-word responses.

**communication** The transmission of information to another person—verbally or through body language.

**cultural imposition** When one person imposes his or her beliefs, values, and practices on another because he or she believe his or her ideals are superior.

**dedicated line** A special telephone line that is used for specific point-to-point communications; also known as a *hotline*.

**documentation** The recorded portion of the EMT's patient interaction, either written or electronic. This becomes part of the patient's permanent medical record.

**duplex** The ability to transmit and receive simultaneously.

**emotional intelligence** The ability to understand and manage one's own emotions and properly respond to the emotions of others.

**ethnocentrism** When a person considers his or her own cultural values as more important when interacting with people of a different culture.

**Federal Communications Commission (FCC)** The federal agency that has jurisdiction over interstate and international telephone and telegraph services and satellite communications, all of which may involve EMS activity.

**handover** The transfer of pertinent patient information and the responsibility for the patient's care; often involves the physical movement of the patient and associated equipment; also known as handoff.

**health information exchange (HIE)** A system that allows EMS providers to access relevant health data (eg, past medical problems, medications, allergies, end-of-life decisions), avoid unnecessary duplication of effort in data entry, and view patient outcomes related to hospital care.

**interoperable communications system** A communication system that uses voice-over-Internet protocol (VoIP) technology to allow multiple agencies to communicate and transmit data.

**MED channels** VHF and UHF channels that the Federal Communications Commission has designated exclusively for EMS use.

**mental model** The picture an individual has in his or her head of "what's going on" in a given situation.

**mission-critical communications** Any communications where disruption will result in the failure of the mission at hand.

**mobile data terminal (MDT)** A small computer terminal inside the ambulance that directly receives data from the dispatch center.

**multiplex** The ability to transmit audio and data signals through the use of more than one communications channel.

**noise** Anything that dampens or obscures the true meaning of a message.

**open-ended questions** Questions for which the patient must provide detail to give an answer.

**paging** The use of a radio signal and a voice or digital message that is transmitted to pagers ("beepers") or desktop monitor radios.

**patient care report (PCR)** The legal document used to record all patient care activities. This report has direct patient care functions but also administrative and quality control functions. PCRs are also known as *prehospital care reports*.

**rapport** A trusting relationship that you build with your patient.

**repeater** A special base station radio that receives messages and signals on one frequency and then automatically retransmits them on a second frequency.

**scanner** A radio receiver that searches or scans across several frequencies until the message is completed; the process is then repeated.

**simplex** Single-frequency radio; transmissions can occur in either direction but not simultaneously; when one party transmits, the other can only receive, and the party that is transmitting is unable to receive.

**standing orders** Written documents, signed by the EMS system's medical director, that outline specific directions, permissions, and sometimes prohibitions regarding patient care; also called *protocols*.

**telemetry** A process in which electronic signals are converted into coded, audible signals;

these signals can then be transmitted by radio or telephone to a receiver with a decoder at the hospital.

**therapeutic communication** Verbal and nonverbal communication techniques that encourage patients to express their feelings and to achieve a positive relationship.

**trunking** Telecommunication systems that allow a computer to maximize utilization of a group of frequencies.

**UHF (ultra-high frequency)** Radio frequencies between 300 and 3,000 MHz.

**VHF (very high frequency)** Radio frequencies between 30 and 300 MHz; the VHF spectrum is further divided into high and low bands.

# References

1. Al-Fedaghi S. A conceptual foundation for the Shannon–Weaver model of communication. *Int J Soft Comput* 2012;7(1):12-19.
2. Bonvillain N. *Language, Culture, and Communication: The Meaning of Messages*. 8th ed. Lanham, MD: Rowman & Littlefield; 2019.
3. California Emergency Medical Services Authority. Health information exchange. https://emsa.ca.gov/hie/. Published 2019. Accessed March 17, 2020.
4. Centers for Medicare and Medicaid Services. Provider compliance tips for ambulance services. https://www.cms.gov/Outreach-and-Education/Medicare-Learning-Network-MLN/MLNProducts/Downloads/ProviderComplianceTipsforAmbulanceServicesEmergentandNonEmergent-ICN909409-TextOnly.pdf. Published December 2017. Accessed March 17, 2020.
5. Codier E, Codier D. A model for the role of emotional intelligence in patient safety. *Asia-Pacific J Oncol Nurs* 2015;2(2):112-117.
6. CRICO Strategies. *Malpractice Risks in Communication Failures 2015 Annual Benchmarking Report*. Cambridge, MA: Risk Management Foundation of the Harvard Medical Institutions; 2016:22.
7. Daley K, Campbell SC. *Simulation Scenarios for Nursing Educators: Making It Real*. 3rd ed. New York, NY: Springer Publishing Company; 2017.
8. Duckworth R. Five ways to perfect the patient handoff. *EMS World*. https://www.emsworld.com/article/12257122/five-ways-to-perfect-the-patient-handoff. Published September 14, 2016. Accessed March 17, 2020.
9. Duckworth R. Hard times for soft skills. *Rescue Digest*. http://www.rescuedigest.com/2015/06/15/hard-times-for-soft-skills/. Published June 15, 2015. Accessed March 17, 2020.
10. Duckworth R. How to use the FBI's Behavioral Change Stairway Model to influence like a pro. EMS1.com. https://www.ems1.com/ems-training/articles/how-to-use-the-fbis-behavioral-change-stairway-model-to-influence-like-a-pro-c5W8CNGj5tuZZ0Av/. Published May 14, 2018. Accessed March 17, 2020.
11. Fitzpatrick D, Maxwell D, Craigie A. The feasibility, acceptability and preliminary testing of a novel, low-tech intervention to improve pre-hospital data recording for pre-alert and handover to the emergency department. *BMC Emerg Med* 2018;18(1):16.
12. Fitzpatrick D, McKenna M, Duncan EAS, Laird C, Lyon R, Corfield A. Critcomms: a national cross-sectional questionnaire based study to investigate prehospital handover practices between ambulance clinicians and specialist prehospital teams in Scotland. *Scand J Trauma Resusc Emerg Med* 2018;26. https://doi.org/10.1186/s13049-018-0512-3
13. General Devices. Patient handoffs continue to present challenges and risk to hospitals. https://general-devices.com/patient-handoffs/. Published April 16, 2018. Accessed March 17, 2020.
14. Gillet A, Ghuysen A, Bonhomme S, D'Orio V, Nyssen SA. Cognitive support for a better handoff: does it improve the quality of medical communication at shift change in an emergency department? *Eur J Emerg Med* 2015;22:192-198.
15. Goldberg SA, Porat A, Strother CG, et al. Quantitative analysis of the content of EMS handoff of critically ill and injured patients to the emergency department. *Prehosp Emerg Care* 2017;21(1):14-17.
16. James MK, Clarke LA, Simpson RM. Accuracy of prehospital trauma notification calls. *Am J Emerg Med* 2018. https://doi.org/10.1016/j.ajem.2018.06.058
17. Kalyani NM, Fereidouni Z, Sarvestani RS, Shirazi HZ, Taghinezhad A. Perspectives of patient handover among paramedics and emergency department members: a qualitative study. *Emergency* 2017;5(1):e76. https://www.ncbi.nlm.nih.gov/pmc/articles/PMC5703753/
18. Meisel ZF, Shea JA, Peacock NJ. Optimizing the patient handoff between emergency medical services and the emergency department. *Ann Emerg Med* 2015;65(3):310–317.e1. https://doi.org/10.1016/j.annemergmed.2014.07.003
19. National Association of EMS Physicians. The EMS-ED handoff: a critical moment in patient care. http://www.naemsp-blog.com/emsmed/2017/7/27/the-ems-ed-handoff-a-critical-moment-in-patient-care. Published July 27, 2017. Accessed March 17, 2020.
20. Nether K. The art of handoff communication [blog]. The Joint Commission. https://www.centerfortransforminghealthcare.org/en/why-work-with-us/blogs/patient-safety/2017/12/the-art-of-handoff-communication/. Published December 7, 2017. Accessed March 17, 2020.

21. Nickson C. Communication in a crisis [blog]. *Life in the Fast Lane*. https://lifeinthefastlane.com/ccc /communication-in-a-crisis/. Updated March 20, 2019. Accessed March 17, 2020.

22. Office of the National Coordinator for Health Information Technology. Emergency medical services (EMS) data integration to optimize patient care. https://www.healthit .gov/sites/default/files/emr_safer_knowledge_product _final.pdf. Published January 2017. Accessed March 17, 2020.

23. Panchal AR, Gaither JB, Svirsky I, Prosser B, Stolz U, Spaite DW. The impact of professionalism on transfer of care to the emergency department. *J Emerg Med* 2015;49(1):18-25.

24. Rural Health Information Hub. Demographic changes and aging population. https://www.ruralhealthinfo.org /toolkits/aging/1/demographics. Accessed March 17, 2020.

25. Statistica. Share of old age population (65 years and older) in the total US population from 1950 to 2050. https://www.statista.com/statistics/457822/share-of -old-age-population-in-the-total-us-population/. Accessed June 3, 2020.

26. US Census Bureau. Facts for features: older Americans month: May 2017. https://www.census.gov/newsroom /facts-for-features/2017/cb17-ff08.html. Published April 10, 2017. Accessed March 17, 2020.

27. US Department of Health and Human Services, Office of the Chief Technology Officer. EMS to HIE innovation. https://www.hhs.gov/cto/projects/ems-to-hie-innovation /index.html. Published October 18, 2018. Accessed March 17, 2020.

28. Wurster F. Mnemonic device helps patient hand-offs. *JEMS*. https://www.jems.com/2011/05/31/mnemonic -device-helps-patient-hand-offs/. Published May 31, 2011. Accessed March 17, 2020.

# Chapter 5

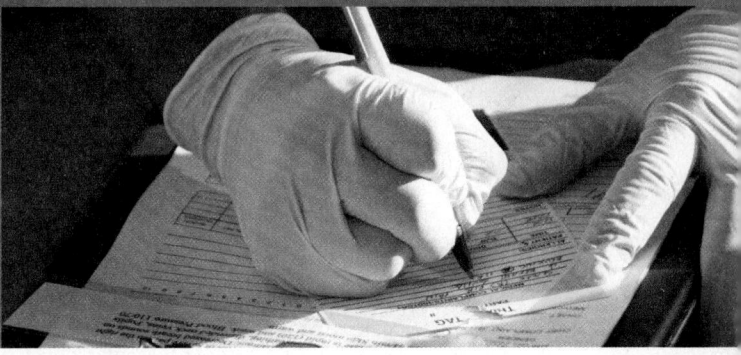

# Medical Terminology

## NATIONAL EMS EDUCATION STANDARD COMPETENCIES

### Medical Terminology

Uses foundational anatomical and medical terms and abbreviations in written and oral communication with colleagues and other health care professionals.

## KNOWLEDGE OBJECTIVES

1. Explain the purpose of medical terminology. (p 165)
2. Identify the four components of a medical term. (p 165)
3. Describe the following directional terms: anterior (ventral), posterior (dorsal), right, left, superior, inferior, proximal, distal, medial, lateral, superficial, and deep. (pp 170–173)
4. Describe the prone, supine, Fowler, and semi-Fowler positions of the body. (pp 173–174)
5. Break down the meaning of a medical term based on the components of the term. (p 174)
6. Identify error-prone medical abbreviations and symbols. (pp 174–175)
7. Interpret selected medical abbreviations and symbols. (pp 174–175)

## SKILLS OBJECTIVES

There are no skills objectives for this chapter.

# Introduction

As an EMT, it is essential that you have a strong working knowledge of medical terminology. Understanding key terms, abbreviations, and symbols is important for effective communication and documentation. Understanding how terms are formed and the definitions for the various parts of a medical term will help you determine the meaning of an unknown term by breaking the word apart. Once you understand medical terminology, you will be able to communicate more effectively with other members of the EMS, health care, and public safety system.

# Anatomy of a Medical Term

Medical terms are composed of distinct parts that perform specific functions. Changing or deleting any of those parts can significantly change the function (or meaning) of a word. Components of medical terms include the following:

- **Word root**—the foundation of the word
- **Prefix**—what occurs before the word root
- **Suffix**—what occurs after the word root
- **Combining vowel**—a vowel that joins one or more word roots to other components of a term

How the parts of a term are combined determines its meaning. Accurate spelling, especially when some words are pronounced almost the same way, is essential in medical terminology. For example, the suffix *-phasia* means speaking, whereas *-phagia* means eating or swallowing. The prefix *dys-* means difficult or painful. Combining those two parts, *dysphasia* means difficulty speaking, while *dysphagia* means difficulty eating or swallowing. These are very different terms and the two words, although spelled differently, sound almost identical. Likewise, the terms *ilium* and *ileum* are pronounced exactly the same, but refer to different

anatomic parts. The ilium is the largest bone of the pelvis, and the ileum is the last part of the small intestine. Knowing anatomy and the context of how these words are used will help you correctly determine (and spell) the term in a given situation.

## Word Roots

The main part or stem of a word is called a word root. Some books use the term *word root*; others use *root word*. Both terms mean the same thing. A word root conveys the essential meaning of the word and frequently indicates a body part, organ, or organ system. Most terms have at least one word root, and some have more than one word root. Adding a prefix or suffix to the word root creates a term. Changing the prefix or suffix will change the meaning of the term.

A frequently used medical abbreviation is CPR, which stands for cardiopulmonary resuscitation. *Cardiopulmonary* breaks down as follows: *cardio* is a word root meaning "heart," and *pulmon* is a word root meaning "lungs." By performing CPR, you introduce air into the lungs and circulate blood by compressing the heart to resuscitate the patient. Some word roots may also be used as prefixes or suffixes for other terms.

Examples of some word roots are shown in **TABLE 5-1**. See the tables at the end of this chapter for additional common word roots. Combining forms are discussed later in the chapter.

## Prefixes

A prefix is the part of a term that appears at the beginning of a word. It generally describes location and intensity. Prefixes are frequently found in general language (ie, *auto*pilot, *sub*marine, *tri*cycle), as well as in medical and scientific terminology. Not all medical terms have prefixes.

A prefix gives the word root a specific meaning. When a medical word contains a prefix, the meaning of the word is altered. For example, *pnea* is the word root for breathing. Adding the prefix *a-* (without), *brady-* (slow), or *tachy-* (rapid) to a word creates three very different terms:

- a/pnea—without breathing
- brady/pnea—slow breathing
- tachy/pnea—rapid breathing

By learning to recognize a few of the more commonly used medical prefixes, you can figure out the meaning of terms that may not be immediately familiar to you. Some common prefixes are shown in **TABLE 5-2**. See the tables at the end of the chapter for additional common prefixes.

## Suffixes

Suffixes are placed at the end of words and usually indicate a procedure, condition, disease, or part of speech.

A commonly used suffix is *-itis*, which means "inflammation." When this suffix is paired with the word root *arthro-*, meaning joint, the resulting word is arthritis, an inflammation of the joints.

Some common suffixes are listed in **TABLE 5-3**. See the tables at the end of this chapter for more common suffixes.

## Combining Vowels

A combining vowel is the part of a term that connects a word root to a suffix or another word root. In most cases, the combining vowel is an *o*; however, it may also be an *i* or an *e*. A combining vowel

**TABLE 5-1** Common Word Roots in Medical Terminology

| Root | Meaning | Example | Definition of Example |
|------|---------|---------|-----------------------|
| cardi | heart | tachycardia | fast heart rate |
| hepat | liver | hepatomegaly | enlargement of the liver |
| nephr | kidney | nephropathy | disease of the kidney |
| neur | nerves | neurologist | physician who specializes in diseases of the nervous system |
| psych | mind | psychology | study of the mind |
| thorac | chest | thoracic | pertaining to the chest or thorax |

© Jones & Bartlett Learning.

**TABLE 5-2** Common Prefixes in EMS

| Prefix | Meaning | Example | Definition of Example |
|--------|---------|---------|-----------------------|
| hyper- | over, excessive, high | hyperventilation | fast ventilations |
| hypo- | under, below normal | hypoperfusion | below-normal blood flow to vital organs |
| tachy- | rapid, fast | tachycardia | fast heart rate |
| brady- | slow | bradypnea | slow breathing |
| pre- | before | prenatal | occurring before birth |
| post- | after, behind | postsurgical | occurring after surgery |

© Jones & Bartlett Learning.

## YOU are the Provider

It is almost the end of your shift when you get a call for a routine transfer from the nursing home to the hospital for a 79-year-old woman with constipation and abdominal pain. She has not had any gastroenteritis symptoms including vomiting or diarrhea. On your arrival, you are met by a nurse who informs you the patient is new to the facility. She hands you the medical record, which includes the following information:

Patient Hx: AAA; HTN; CHF; AMI in 2010; GERD; and type 1 DM.

Your patient is pale and her skin is wet. When you gently palpate her abdomen, you feel a pulsating mass in the area of her umbilicus. Your partner has placed a nonrebreathing oxygen mask on the patient at 12 L/min and obtained vital signs.

**1.** What can you determine about the patient's medical history based on the abbreviations in the record?

is usually used when joining a suffix that begins with a consonant or when joining another word root. For example, take the term *gastroenterology*, the study of diseases of the stomach and small intestines:

- gastr/o + enter/o + logy
- stomach + small intestines + the study of

In this term, *gastr* and *enter* are both word roots, *-logy* is the suffix, and *o* is the combining vowel (used twice). The combining vowel helps ease the pronunciation of the term. Without the vowel, the term would be rather difficult to pronounce—*gastrenterlogy*.

Refer to the tables at the end of this chapter for combining vowels associated with common word roots. A combining vowel shown with the word root is called a combining form. Here are a few of the most common combining forms you will see:

- cardi/o (heart)
- gastr/o (stomach)
- hepat/o (liver)
- arthr/o (joint)
- oste/o (bone)
- pulmon/o (lungs)

**TABLE 5-3** Common Suffixes in Medical Terminology

| Suffix | Meaning | Example | Definition of Example |
|---|---|---|---|
| -al | pertaining to | syncopal | pertaining to syncope |
| -algia | pertaining to pain | arthralgia | joint pain |
| -ectomy | surgical removal of | appendectomy | surgical removal of the appendix |
| -ic | pertaining to | diaphoretic | pertaining to diaphoresis |
| -itis | inflammation | epiglottitis | inflammation of the epiglottis |
| -logy | study of | cardiology | the study of the heart |
| -logist | specialist | pulmonologist | specialist in diseases of the lung |
| -megaly | enlargement | cardiomegaly | enlargement of the heart |
| -meter | measuring instrument | sphygmomanometer | instrument to measure blood pressure |
| -oma | tumor (usually referring to cancer) | lymphoma | cancer of the lymphatic system |
| -pathy | disease | nephropathy | diseases of the kidneys |

© Jones & Bartlett Learning.

## YOU are the Provider

Advanced life support (ALS) assistance is 15 minutes away, so after administering oxygen you prepare the patient for transport. En route to the hospital, you call with a report:

"EMT 123 to Regional Medical Center. We are en route to your facility with a 79-year-old woman reporting abdominal pain that started 2 hours ago. History of abdominal aortic aneurysm, hypertension, congestive heart failure; acute myocardial infarction in 2010, gastroesophageal reflux disease, and type 1 diabetes. Patient's skin is pale and wet and there is a pulsing mass in the periumbilical area. Blood pressure is 80/50 mm Hg; pulse 108 beats/min; respirations 24 breaths/min. Patient is on nonrebreathing mask at 12 L/min. Our ETA is 10 minutes."

**2.** How could a misunderstanding of the medical terminology or abbreviations affect patient care?

**3.** What other abbreviations could have been used in this report?

## Word Building Rules

When building or taking apart a medical term, it is helpful to understand some basic rules. The following summarizes the rules covered thus far:

1. The prefix is always at the beginning of a term; however, not all terms will have a prefix.
2. The suffix is always at the end of the term.
3. When a suffix begins with a consonant, a combining vowel is used between the word root and suffix to make pronunciation easier.
4. When a term has more than one word root, a combining vowel must be placed between the two word roots, even if the second root begins with a vowel.

## Plural Endings

To change a term from a singular to plural form, certain rules apply. In some cases, you simply add an *s* to the word (lung becomes lungs). However, for some medical terms, making the plural form is more complicated. Rules you may encounter when converting terms from singular to plural are:

1. Singular words that end in *a* change to *ae* when plural.
   - Example: vertebra becomes vertebrae.
2. Singular words that end in *is* change to *es* when plural.
   - Example: diagnosis becomes diagnoses.
3. Singular words that end in *ex* or *ix* change to *ices*.
   - Example: apex becomes apices.
4. Singular words that end in *on* or *um* change to *a*.
   - Examples: ganglion becomes ganglia, ovum becomes ova.
5. Singular words that end in *us* change to *i*.
   - Example: bronchus becomes bronchi.

## Special Word Parts

As already described, prefixes appear at the beginning of a word, before the word root. Prefixes used to indicate numbers, colors, and directions are described in the following sections. Look at the prefixes, meanings, and examples. Can you think of other terms using the same prefix with another root? Do you see how it changes the meaning?

### Numbers

Several prefixes are used to indicate if a term involves a number such as one-half, or one or two or more parts or sides. Common prefixes for numbers are listed in **TABLE 5-4**.

**TABLE 5-4** Common Number Prefixes

| Prefix | Meaning | Example | Definition of Example |
|---|---|---|---|
| uni- | one | unilateral | one side |
| dipl- | two; double | diplopia | double vision |
| null- | none | nullipara | never given birth |
| primi- | first | primigravida | pregnant for the first time |
| multi- | many | multiparous | giving birth to more than one offspring at a time |
| bi- | two | bilateral | pertaining to both sides |
| tri- | three | trigeminy | irregular heartbeat of two normal beats followed by one premature beat |
| quad- | four | quadriplegic | paralysis of all four extremities |
| tetra- | four | tetralogy of Fallot | congenital defect involving four anatomic abnormalities of the heart |

| Prefix | Meaning | Example | Definition of Example |
|---|---|---|---|
| quint- | five | quintipara | five pregnancies resulting in five live births |
| sext- | six | sextuplets | six offspring of the same pregnancy |
| sept- | seven | septuplets | seven offspring of the same pregnancy |
| oct- | eight | octigravida | pregnant for the eighth time |
| nona- | nine | nonan | occurring on the ninth day |
| deca- | ten | decagram | measurement of 10 grams |
| semi- | half; partial | semiconscious | partially conscious |
| hemi- | half; one sided | hemiplegia | paralysis on one side of the body |
| ambi- | both | ambidextrous | able to use either hand equally well |
| pan- | all, entire | pandemic | a worldwide epidemic |

© Jones & Bartlett Learning.

**TABLE 5-5** Word Roots That Describe Color

| Root | Meaning | Example | Definition of Example |
|---|---|---|---|
| cyan/o | blue | cyanosis | blue discoloration of the skin |
| leuk/o | white | leukocyte | white blood cells that fight infection |
| erythr/o | red | erythrocyte | red blood cells that contain hemoglobin to carry oxygen |
| cirrh/o | yellow-orange | cirrhosis | inflammation of the liver causing yellow-orange pigmentation of the liver |
| melan/o | black | melena | black, tarry stool typically caused by upper gastrointestinal bleeding |
| poli/o | gray | poliomyelitis | acute viral disease that attacks the motor neurons of the central nervous system (brain and spinal cord) |
| alb | white | albino | person lacking skin pigmentation (very white hair, very pale skin, and nonpigmented iris) |
| chlor/o | green | chlorophyll | green pigment in leaves used in photosynthesis |

© Jones & Bartlett Learning.

## Colors

Several word roots are used to describe color. The most common include those listed in **TABLE 5-5**.

## Positions and Directions

Prefixes can also be used to describe a position, direction, or location. The most common include those listed in **TABLE 5-6**.

**TABLE 5-6** Prefixes That Describe Position

| Prefix | Meaning | Example | Definition of Example |
|---|---|---|---|
| To/From | | | |
| ab- | away from | abduction | away from the point of reference |
| ad- | to, toward | adduction | toward the center |
| Above/Below/Around | | | |
| de- | down from, away | decay | to waste away |
| circum- | around, about | circumferential burn | a burn around an entire area (arm, chest, abdomen, etc) |
| peri- | around | pericardium | sac around the heart |
| trans- | across, through, beyond | transvaginal | across or through the vagina |
| epi- | above, upon, on | epigastric | above or over the stomach |
| supra- | above, over | suprasternal notch | top of the sternum |
| retro- | behind | retroperitoneal | area behind the peritoneum |
| sub- | under, beneath | subcutaneous | beneath the skin |
| infra- | below, under | infraclavicular | below the clavicle |
| para- | near, beside, beyond, apart from | parasternal | beside the sternum |
| contra- | against, opposite | contraindicated | something that is not indicated |
| Outside/Inside | | | |
| ecto- | out, outside | ectopic pregnancy | pregnancy where the embryo attaches outside of the uterus |
| endo- | within | endoscopy | examining inside someone's body (with an endoscope) |
| extra- | outside, in addition | extraneous | outside the organism and not belonging to it |
| intra- | inside, within | intrauterine | within the uterus |
| ipsi- | same | ipsilateral | on or affecting the same side |

© Jones & Bartlett Learning.

# Common Direction, Movement, and Position Terms

## Directional Terms

When discussing where an injury is located or how pain radiates in the body, you need to know the correct directional terms (**FIGURE 5-1**). **TABLE 5-7** provides the basic terms used in medicine. Notice how directional terms are paired as opposites.

## Right and Left

The terms *right* and *left* refer to the patient's right and left sides, not to your right and left sides.

## Superior and Inferior

The **superior** part of the body, or any body part, is the portion nearer to the head from a specific reference point. The part nearer to the feet is the **inferior** portion. These terms are also used to describe the relationship of one structure to another when both structures are part of the trunk or head. For example, the xyphoid is superior to the umbilicus and inferior to the mandible.

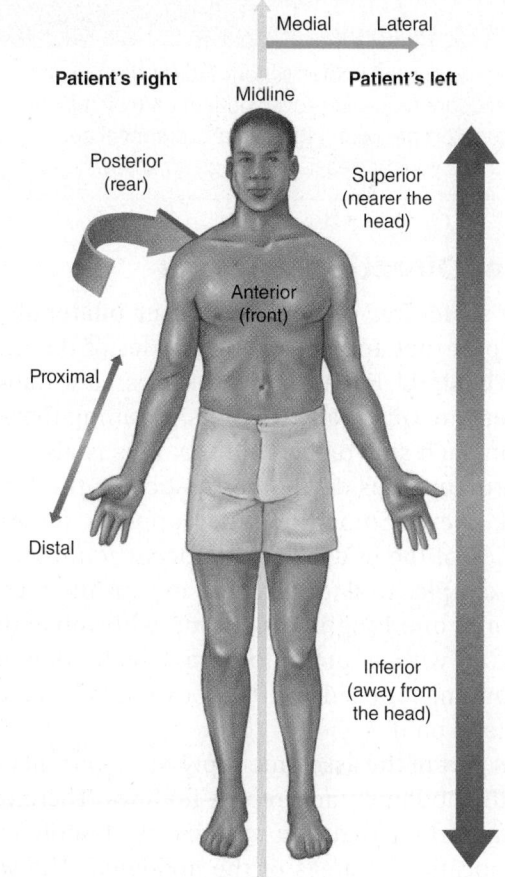

**FIGURE 5-1** Directional terms indicate distance and direction from the midline.

© Jones & Bartlett Learning.

## Lateral and Medial

Parts of the body that lie farther from the midline are called **lateral** (outer) structures. The parts that lie closer to the midline are called **medial** (inner) structures. For example, the thigh has medial (inner) and lateral (outer) surfaces. In general terms, *lateral* means side. For example, lying on the left side is called left lateral recumbent. Something that occurs on both sides is referred to as *bilateral*. When describing the location of an injury, the terms *medial* and *lateral* help pinpoint an exact location. For example, the patient has a 2-inch (5-cm) laceration on the medial aspect of the thigh (toward the inside).

## Proximal and Distal

The terms *proximal* and *distal* are used to describe the relationship of any two structures on an extremity. **Proximal** describes structures that are closer to the trunk. **Distal** describes structures that are farther from the trunk or nearer to the free end of the extremity. For example, the elbow is distal to the shoulder and proximal to the wrist and hand.

## Superficial and Deep

**Superficial** means closer to or on the skin. **Deep** means farther inside the body or tissue and away from the skin. For example, a superficial burn involves only the top layer of skin, similar to a sunburn. An abrasion is a superficial wound, similar to scraping your knee, whereas a deep laceration involves a cut deeper into the tissue such as with a knife.

**TABLE 5-7** Directional Terms

| Common Term | Directional Term | Definition |
|---|---|---|
| Front and back | Anterior (ventral) Posterior (dorsal) | The front surface of the body The back surface of the body |
| Right and left | Right Left | The patient's right The patient's left |
| Top and bottom | Superior Inferior | Closest to the head Closest to the feet |
| Closest and farthest | Proximal Distal | Closest to the point of attachment Farthest from the point of attachment |
| Middle and side | Medial Lateral | Closest to the midline Farthest from the midline |
| In and out | Deep Superficial | Farthest from the surface of the skin Closest to the surface of the skin |

© Jones & Bartlett Learning.

## Ventral and Dorsal

**Ventral** refers to the belly side of the body, or the anterior surface of the body. **Dorsal** refers to the spinal side of the body, or the posterior surface of the body, including the back of the hand. These terms are used less frequently than the terms **anterior** (the front surface of the body) and **posterior** (the back surface of the body). An easy way to remember *dorsal* is to think of the dorsal fin on a dolphin, which is on its back (posterior) side.

> ### Street Smarts
>
> It's easy to recall *dorsal* if you think of a fish's dorsal fin, which is on its back.

## Palmar and Plantar

The front region of the hand is referred to as the palm or **palmar** surface. The bottom of the foot is referred to as the **plantar** surface.

## Apex

The **apex (plural apices)** is the tip of a structure. For example, the apex of the heart is the bottom (inferior portion) of the ventricles in the left side of the chest.

## Movement Terms

The following terms relate to movement (**FIGURE 5-2**):

- **Flexion** is decreasing the angle of the joint.
- **Extension** is increasing the angle of the joint.
- **Adduction** is motion toward the midline.
- **Abduction** is motion away from the midline.

> ### Words of Wisdom
>
> Using the correct anatomic terminology in your patient care report improves patient care by making the report more useful to hospital personnel and enhances your professional image as an EMT.

## Other Directional Terms

Many structures of the body occur bilaterally. A body part that appears on both sides of the midline is **bilateral**. For example, the eyes, ears, hands, and feet are bilateral structures, meaning there is one on each side of the midline. This is also true for structures inside the body, such as the lungs and kidneys. Something that appears on only one side of the body is said to occur *unilaterally*. For example, unilateral chest expansion means that only one lung is expanding with inhalation (such as with a pneumothorax). Pain that occurs on only one side of the body could be called unilateral pain.

As part of the assessment process, you will palpate the abdomen and report findings. Therefore, it is important that you are able to describe the exact location of areas of the abdomen. The way to describe the sections of the abdominal cavity is by **quadrants**. Imagine two lines intersecting at the umbilicus, dividing the abdomen into four equal areas (**FIGURE 5-3**). These are referred to as the right upper quadrant, left upper quadrant, right lower

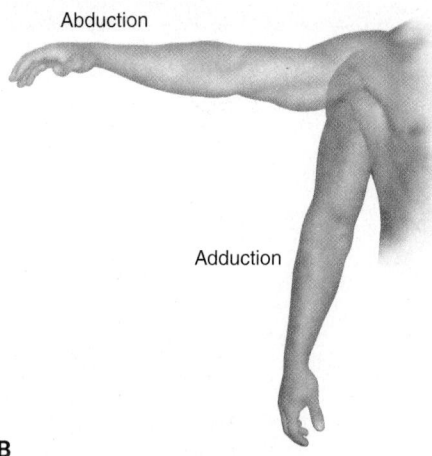

**A**

**B**

**FIGURE 5-2 A.** Flexion and extension at the elbow. **B.** Adduction and abduction at the shoulder.

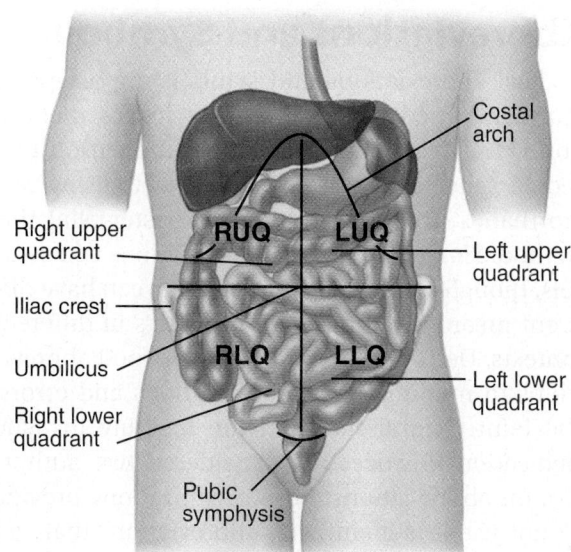

**FIGURE 5-3** The abdomen is divided into four quadrants. RUQ indicates right upper quadrant; LUQ, left upper quadrant; RLQ, right lower quadrant; and LLQ, left lower quadrant.

© Jones & Bartlett Learning.

quadrant, and left lower quadrant. Remember that here, too, right and left refer to the patient's right and left, not yours.

It is important to learn all of these terms and concepts so you can describe the location of any injury or assessment findings. When you use these terms properly, any other medical personnel who care for the patient will know immediately where to look and what to expect.

## Anatomic Positions

There are many terms used to describe the position of the patient on your arrival or during transport to the emergency department (**FIGURE 5-4**).

### Prone and Supine

These terms describe the position of a body. The body is in the **prone** position when lying face down; the body is in the **supine** position when lying faceup.

### Fowler Position

The **Fowler position** was named after a US surgeon, George R. Fowler, MD, at the end of the 19th century. Dr. Fowler placed his patients in a semi-reclining position with the head elevated to help them breathe easier and to control the airway. A patient who is sitting upright is therefore said to be in the

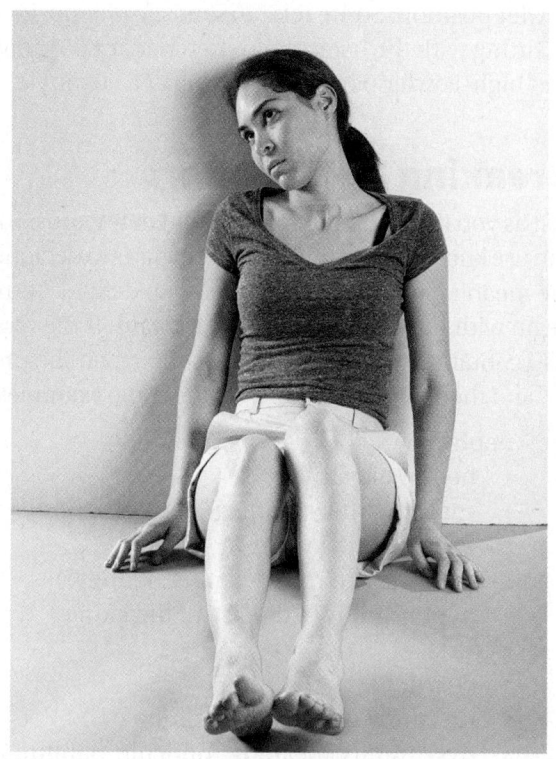

A

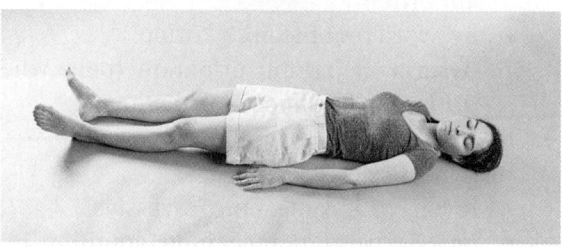

B

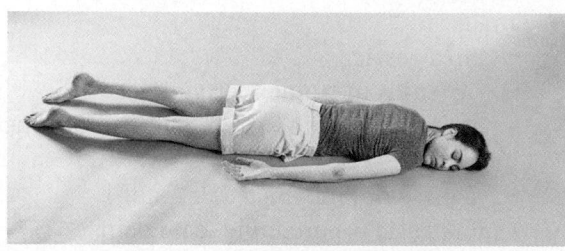

C

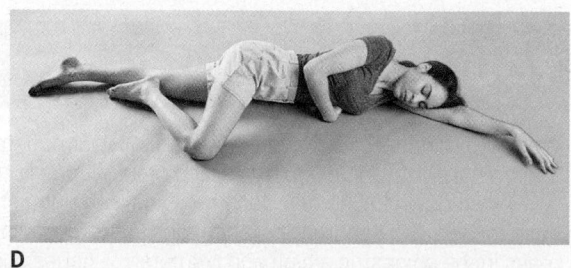

D

**FIGURE 5-4 A.** Fowler position. **B.** Supine. **C.** Prone. **D.** Recovery position.

**A-D:** © Jones & Bartlett Learning.

Fowler position. Some refer to semi-Fowler position as sitting with the back of the stretcher at a 45° angle and high-Fowler position as sitting at a 90° angle.

## Breaking Terms Apart

Just as you use parts of terms to build new words, you can use knowledge of the meaning of parts to decipher the meaning of a term. When trying to define a term, begin with the suffix and work backward. If the term also contains a prefix, define the suffix, then the prefix, and then the word root. Here are some examples:

- nephropathy
  - nephr/o/pathy
  - -pathy (suffix meaning "disease")
  - o (combining vowel)
  - nephr (word root meaning "kidney")
  - nephropathy = disease of the kidney
- dysuria
  - dys/ur/ia
  - -ia (suffix meaning "condition of")
  - dys- (prefix meaning "difficult, painful, or abnormal")
  - ur (word root meaning "urine")
  - dysuria = painful urination (pain when urinating) or difficulty urinating
- hyperemesis
  - hyper/emesis
  - hyper- (prefix meaning "excessive")
  - emesis (word root meaning "vomiting")
  - hyperemesis = excessive vomiting
- analgesic
  - an/alges/ic
  - -ic (suffix meaning "pertaining to")
  - an- (prefix meaning "without" or "absence of")
  - alges (word root meaning "pain")
  - analgesic = pertaining to no pain

## Abbreviations and Symbols

Medical abbreviations and symbols are a type of shorthand used to communicate in the medical world. They came about for the same reason that people send text messages and tweets using text shorthand—you can communicate faster using this method. Similarly, medical abbreviations and symbols, though somewhat standardized, can have different meanings to different providers in different contexts. Use only commonly understood abbreviations to minimize misinterpretations and errors. The Joint Commission and the Institute for Safe Medication Practices are considered two authorities on abbreviations; both organizations provide do-not-use lists identifying abbreviations that can lead to errors.

### Abbreviations

*Abbreviation* is an umbrella term for any word or phrase that has been shortened so that it may be spoken or written more concisely. You will encounter various types of abbreviations in the health care field. The simplest type is the omission of a portion of the word or phrase, such as when someone says "prep" instead of "prepare" or "cath lab" instead of "catheter laboratory." Other common types of abbreviations are initialisms and acronyms. When you shorten a word or phrase using an initialism, you pick representative letters from the full term and pronounce each letter separately. For example, *emergency medical technician* becomes *EMT*, pronounced "E-M-T." When you use an acronym, you are shortening several words, usually using the first letter of each word, to make a shorter term that is pronounced as its own word. For example, the SAMPLE acronym represents several words that are pronounced as a single word, "sample." Note that

## YOU are the Provider

Within 30 minutes of arriving at the hospital, your patient receives a CT scan that confirms a diagnosis of ruptured abdominal aortic aneurysm (AAA), and preparations for immediate surgery are underway.

You sit down to carefully document your care, and start with: "EMT123 arrived to find a 79 yo female, AO, supine in hospital bed. CC: Periumbilical abdominal pain. Skin is pale and wet. On palpation, noted a pulsing midline abdominal mass in the epigastric region approximately 2 inches superior to the umbilicus."

**4.** What do the abbreviations in this portion of the report mean?

you will also encounter a combination of different types of abbreviations. For example, DCAP-BTLS is pronounced "D-cap-B-T-L-S," and USAR (which stands for "urban search and rescue") is pronounced "U-sar."

When using abbreviations on patient care reports, remember to use only standard, accepted abbreviations to avoid confusion and errors. Misunderstandings will occur if everyone involved in the emergency care of a patient does not understand the meaning of abbreviations. For this reason, some agencies limit the use of abbreviations. See the tables at the end of this chapter for a list of commonly used abbreviations. This list is intended to help you decipher documents written by other health care professionals. Before using any abbreviations in your own reports, be familiar with accepted use of abbreviations in your local jurisdiction or service area.

### Words of Wisdom

Medical professionals use many medical terms, abbreviations, and symbols. The material in this chapter provides only a small sample. You may find it helpful to invest in a phone app or pocket reference guide to assist you when you encounter unfamiliar terms.

## Symbols

Like abbreviations, symbols are sometimes used as a shortcut in communication and documentation. As with abbreviations, it is important to use only the symbols that are widely understood and accepted (**TABLE 5-8**).

**TABLE 5-8** Common Symbols

| | |
|---|---|
| 1° | first, first degree, primary |
| 2° | secondary, second degree |
| ↑ | increase(d) |
| ↓ | decrease(d) |
| ® | right |
| © | left |
| μ | micro |
| α | alpha |
| β | beta |
| ~ | approximately |
| N | normal |
| ×2 | times two |
| / | per |
| ≠ | not equal |
| > | greater than |
| < | less than |
| ? | questionable, possible |
| Δ | change |
| — | negative |
| ♀ | female |
| ♂ | male |

*Note:* The forward slash mark ("/") is included for explanatory purposes, but its use is not recommended by the Institute for Safe Medication Practices.

© Jones & Bartlett Learning.

## YOU are the Provider

Knowing that the abbreviations related to the patient's history point to severe cardiovascular disease helps direct the assessment and subsequent field impression to abdominal aortic aneurysm. The ability to call in the report using common abbreviations helps save precious time so you can return to the care of your patient. However, excessive or inappropriate use of abbreviations can lead to confusion and errors. Using medical terminology correctly to document the call increases your professionalism as an EMT. In addition to abbreviations, other types of medical terminology convey information to the medical staff taking over the care of your patient.

**5.** What other medical terms or word parts, such as prefixes, were used in this case?

## Master Tables

**TABLES 5-9** through **5-12** provide a thorough reference list of common word roots, combining forms, prefixes, suffixes, and abbreviations.

### Street Smarts

When transferring a patient from another health care facility, there may be terms or abbreviations you do not understand on the transfer paperwork. Take a moment to ask the meaning of these terms so you can fully understand the patient's condition. Never repeat abbreviations that you are unfamiliar with in your own documentation or written communications as the chance of miscommunication is high.

### TABLE 5-9 Common Word Roots and Combining Forms

| Root | Meaning | Root | Meaning |
|------|---------|------|---------|
| abdomin/o | abdomen | bil/i | bile |
| acou/o | hear | blast/o | germ, bud, developing cell |
| aden/o | gland | blephar/o | eyelid |
| adip/o | fat | brachi/o | arm |
| alb/o | white | bronch/i | airway, bronchus |
| alges/o | pain | bucc/o | cheek |
| andr/o | man, male | burs/o | pouch or sac |
| angi/o | vessel | calc/i | calcium |
| angin/o | blood vessel | capn/o | carbon dioxide |
| ankyl/o | fused, stiff | carcin/o | cancer |
| anter/o | front | cardi/o | heart |
| aort/o | aorta | carp/o | wrist |
| append/o | appendix | cartil/o | cartilage, gristle |
| arteri/o | artery | caud/o | tail |
| arthr/o | joint | cec/o | blind intestine, cecum |
| asthen/o | weak | cel/o | hernia, protrusion |
| atel/o | incomplete | cent/e | to puncture (a body cavity) |
| ather/o | fat | cent/i | one-hundredth or 100 |
| atri/o | atrium | cephal/o | head |
| audi/o | to hear | cerebr/o | brain, cerebrum |
| aur/o | ear | cervic/o | neck |
| aut/o | self | chol/e | bile |
| bacteri/o | bacteria | chondr/o | cartilage |
| bi | life; also two | chrom/o | color |

| Root | Meaning | Root | Meaning |
|------|---------|------|---------|
| chron/o | time | electr/o | electricity |
| cirrh/o | yellow-orange | embol/o | a plug |
| cleid/o | clavicle | embry/o | embryo |
| col/o | colon | emesis | vomit |
| colp/o | vagina | emmetr/o | according to measure |
| condyl/o | knuckle of a joint | encephal/o | brain |
| cor/o | pupil | enter/o | small intestine |
| corne/o | cornea | episi/o | vulva |
| cost/o | rib | erythr/o | red |
| crani/o | cranium, skull | esthesi | sensation or perception |
| crin/o | to secrete | febr | fever |
| cubitus | elbow | flex | bend |
| cutane/o | skin | foramen | opening |
| cyan/o | blue | fract | break |
| cycl/o | circle or cycle | gastr/o | stomach |
| cyst/o | bladder | gest | carry, produce, congestion |
| cyt/o | cell | glyc/o | sugar, sweet |
| derm(at)/o | skin | gno | know |
| digit | finger or toe | gyn/o | woman, female |
| dipl/o | two, double | hem(at)/o | blood |
| dips/o | thirst | hepat/o | liver |
| disk/o | flat shape, intervertebral disk | heter/o | other, different |
| dist/o | distant, away | hom/o | the same |
| diverticul/o | diverticulum, a small blind pouch | hydr/o | water |
| dors/o | back | idi/o | person, self |
| duct/o | lead, move | lact/o | milk |
| duoden/o | duodenum | leuk/o | white |
| ech/o | to bounce, sound | lingu/o | tongue |
| ede | swelling | mal/o | abnormal, bad |
| elast/o | change shape | medi/o | middle |

*(continues)*

**TABLE 5-9** Common Word Roots and Combining Forms (*continued*)

| Root | Meaning | Root | Meaning |
|------|---------|------|---------|
| melan/o | black, dark | pur, py | pus |
| men/o | month, menstruation | pyr/o | fire, heat |
| mening/o | usually refers to the meninges | quadr/o; quar | four |
| myel/o | marrow or spinal cord | ren/o | kidney |
| my/o | muscle | rhin/o | nose |
| nephr/o | kidney | sangui(n)o | blood |
| neur/o | nerve | scler/o | hard |
| ocul/o | eye | sebum | fatty secretion of the sebaceous glands |
| ophthalm/o | eye | | |
| oste/o | bone | sect/o | cut |
| ot/o | ear | sept/o | wall, divider; also seven |
| ov/o | egg | serum | clear portion of blood |
| palpate | to examine by touch | sinus | cavity, channel, or hollow space |
| path/o | disease | som(at) | body |
| ped/o | child or foot | spir/o | coil, to breathe |
| percuss | to examine by striking | stern/o | sternum (breastbone) |
| phag/o | eat | stomat/o | mouth |
| pharyng/o | throat | thorac/o | chest |
| phot/o | light | tom/o | cut |
| pleur/o | rib, side | toxic/o | poisonous |
| pneum(at)/o | lungs, air | trich/o | hair |
| pneumo(n)/o | lung | ur/o | urine |
| pod(i) | foot | uter/o | uterus, womb |
| pseud/o | false | varic/o | dilated vein |
| psych/o | mind | vas/o | blood vessel |
| pto | fall | viscer/o | internal organs |
| ptyal/o | saliva | xen/o | foreign (material) |
| pulmon/o | lungs | xer/o | dry |

## TABLE 5-10 Common Prefixes

| Prefix | Meaning | Prefix | Meaning |
|---|---|---|---|
| a- | without, lack of | mega- | large |
| ab- | away from | meta- | after, change |
| ad- | to, toward | micro- | small |
| an- | without, lack of | mono- | one, single |
| ana- | up, back, again | multi- | many |
| ante- | before, forward | neo- | new |
| anti- | against, opposed to | noct- | night |
| auto- | self | nulli- | none |
| bi- | two | olig(o)- | little, deficient |
| brady- | slow | ortho- | straight or normal |
| circum- | around, about | pan- | all, entire |
| contra- | against, opposite | para- | near, beside, beyond, apart from |
| de- | down from, away | per- | through |
| di- | twice, double | peri- | around |
| dia- | through, completely | poly- | many |
| dys- | difficult, painful, abnormal | post- | after, behind |
| ect(o)- | out, outside | pre- | before |
| end(o)- | within | primi- | first |
| epi- | upon, over, above | pro- | before, in front of |
| eu- | easy, good, normal | quadr(i)- | four |
| ex(o)- | outside, away from | re- | back |
| extra- | outside, in addition | retro- | backward, behind |
| hemi- | half | semi- | half, partial |
| hyper- | over, excessive, high | sub- | under, below |
| hypo- | under, below normal | super- | above, excessive, or more than normal |
| in- | in, into, not, without | supra- | above, upper |
| infra- | below, under | sym- | together, joined |
| inter- | between | syn- | together, joined |
| intra- | inside, within | tachy- | rapid, fast |
| ipsi- | same | tetra- | four |
| iso- | equal | trans- | across, through, beyond |
| macro- | large | tri- | three |
| mal- | bad or abnormal | uni- | one |

## TABLE 5-11 Common Suffixes

| Suffix | Meaning | Suffix | Meaning |
|---|---|---|---|
| -al | pertaining to | -oma | tumor |
| -algia | pertaining to pain | -osis | pertaining to a disease process (*see also* -sis) |
| -asthenia | weakness | | |
| -blast | immature cell | -ostomy | surgical creation of an opening |
| -cele | pertaining to a tumor or swelling | -pathy | disease or a system for treating disease |
| -centesis | pertaining to puncturing an organ or body cavity, often to drain excess fluid or obtain a sample for analysis | -phagia | pertaining to eating or swallowing |
| | | -phasia | pertaining to speech |
| | | -phobia | pertaining to an irrational fear |
| -cyte | cell | -plasty | plastic surgery |
| -ectomy | surgical removal of | -plegia | paralysis |
| -emesis | vomiting | -pnea | pertaining to breathing |
| -emia | pertaining to the presence of a substance in the blood | -ptosis | drooping |
| -esthesia | pertaining to sensation or perception | -rrhage | abnormal or excessive flow or discharge |
| -genic | causing | -rrhagia | abnormal or excessive flow or discharge |
| -gram | record | -rrhaphy | suture of; repair of |
| -graph | a record or the instrument used to create the record | -rrhea | flow or discharge |
| | | -scope | instrument for examination |
| -ia | condition of | -scopy | examination with an instrument |
| -ic | pertaining to | -sis | a process, action, or condition (*see also* -osis) |
| -itis | inflammation | | |
| -lysis | decline, disintegration, or destruction | -stasis | slowing or stopping of the normal flow of a fluid, such as blood |
| -megaly | enlargement of | | |
| -meter | measuring instrument | -taxis | order, arrangement of |
| -ology | science or study of | -trophic | pertaining to nutrition |

© Jones & Bartlett Learning.

## TABLE 5-12 Common Abbreviations*

| Abbreviation | Meaning | Abbreviation | Meaning |
|---|---|---|---|
| A&P | anatomy and physiology | ABC, ABCs | airway, breathing, circulation |
| ā | before | ac | before meals |
| AAA | abdominal aortic aneurysm | ACLS | advanced cardiac life support |
| abd | abdomen | ADL, ADLs | activity/activities of daily living |

| Abbreviation | Meaning |
| --- | --- |
| ad lib | as desired |
| AED | automated external defibrillator |
| AF, A-fib | atrial fibrillation |
| AICD | automated implantable cardioverter defibrillator |
| AIDS | acquired immunodeficiency syndrome |
| AK | above the knee |
| AKA | above-the-knee amputation |
| ALTE | apparent life-threatening event |
| AMA | against medical advice |
| amb | ambulatory |
| AMI | acute myocardial infarction |
| ant | anterior |
| AO × 4, A/O × 4 | alert and oriented to person, place, time, and self |
| AP | anteroposterior, front-to-back, action potential, angina pectoris, anterior pituitary, arterial pressure |
| ARDS | adult respiratory distress syndrome |
| ASA | aspirin (acetylsalicylic acid) |
| ASHD | arteriosclerotic or atherosclerotic heart disease |
| BGL | blood glucose level |
| bid/b.i.d./BID | twice daily |
| BKA | below-the-knee amputation |
| BLS | basic life support |
| BM | bowel movement |
| BP, B/P | blood pressure |
| BPM | beats per minute |
| BRUE | brief resolved unexplained event |
| BS | blood sugar, breath sounds, bowel sounds, bachelor of science (degree) |
| BSA | body surface area |
| BVM | bag-valve mask |
| bx | biopsy |

| Abbreviation | Meaning |
| --- | --- |
| c̄ | with |
| °C | degrees Celsius (centigrade) |
| CA | cancer, cardiac arrest, chronologic age, coronary artery, cold agglutinin |
| CABG | coronary artery bypass graft |
| CAD | coronary artery disease |
| CBC | complete blood cell count |
| CC or C/C | chief complaint |
| CCU | coronary care unit |
| C diff | *Clostridium difficile* |
| CHF | congestive heart failure |
| cm | centimeter |
| CN | cyanide |
| CNS | central nervous system |
| c/o | complaining of |
| CO | cardiac output, carbon monoxide |
| $CO_2$ | carbon dioxide |
| COLD | chronic obstructive lung disease |
| COPD | chronic obstructive pulmonary disease |
| CP | chest pain, chemically pure, cerebral palsy |
| CPAP | continuous positive airway pressure |
| CPR | cardiopulmonary resuscitation |
| CRNA | certified registered nurse anesthetist |
| CRT | capillary refill time, cathode ray tube |
| CSF | cerebrospinal fluid |
| CT | computed tomography |
| CVA | cerebrovascular accident |
| DM | diabetes mellitus |
| DNR | do not resuscitate |
| DOA | dead on arrival |
| DOE | dyspnea on exertion |
| DON | director of nursing |

*(continues)*

**TABLE 5-12** Common Abbreviations* (*continued*)

| Abbreviation | Meaning | Abbreviation | Meaning |
|---|---|---|---|
| DPT | diphtheria and tetanus toxoids and pertussis vaccine, doctor of physical therapy | GSW | gunshot wound |
| | | gtt | drop(s) |
| DSD | dry sterile dressing | GTT | glucose tolerance test |
| DtaP | diphtheria and tetanus toxoids and acellular pertussis vaccine | GU | genitourinary |
| | | gyn | gynecology |
| DTP | diphtheria and tetanus toxoids and pertussis vaccine | h | hour |
| | | H&P | history and physical |
| DTs | delirium tremens | HA, H/A | headache |
| DVT | deep vein thrombosis | Hb, Hgb | hemoglobin |
| Dx | diagnosis | HBV | hepatitis B virus |
| ECG | electrocardiogram | Hct | hematocrit |
| ED | emergency department, erectile dysfunction | HCV | hepatitis C virus |
| EDC | estimated date of confinement | HH | hiatal hernia |
| EEG | electroencephalogram | HIV | human immunodeficiency virus |
| EKG | electrocardiogram | $H_2O$ | water |
| ENT | ears, nose, and throat | HPI | history of present illness |
| EOC | Emergency Operations Center | HR | heart rate |
| ER | emergency room | hr | hour |
| ET, ETT | endotracheal, endotracheal tube | HTN | hypertension |
| ETA | estimated time of arrival | Hx | history |
| $ETCO_2$ | end-tidal carbon dioxide | I&O | intake and output |
| ETOH | ethyl alcohol | ICP | intracranial pressure |
| °F | degrees Fahrenheit | ICS | incident command system, intercostal space |
| $FIO_2$ | fraction of inspired oxygen | | |
| FBS | fasting blood sugar | ICU | intensive care unit |
| Fe | iron | IDDM | insulin-dependent diabetes mellitus |
| FHR | fetal heart rate | IM | intramuscular |
| FHx | family history | IMS | incident management system |
| fl. fld | fluid | IN | intranasal |
| fx | fracture | IO | intraosseous |
| GB | gallbladder | IUD | intrauterine device (contraceptive) |
| GCS | Glasgow Coma Scale | IV | intravenous |
| GERD | gastroesophageal reflux disease | JVD | jugular venous distention |
| GI | gastrointestinal | kg | kilogram |

| Abbreviation | Meaning |
|---|---|
| LE | lower extremity, left eye, lupus erythematosus |
| LLL | left lower lobe of the lung |
| LLQ | left lower quadrant of the abdomen |
| L/m, LPM | liters per minute |
| LMP | last menstrual period |
| LOC | level of consciousness, loss of consciousness |
| LUL | left upper lobe of the lung |
| LUQ | left upper quadrant of the abdomen |
| LVAD | left ventricular assist device |
| MAE | moves all extremities |
| MAEW | moves all extremities well |
| mg | milligram |
| MI | myocardial infarction |
| MICU | mobile intensive care unit; medical intensive care unit |
| min | minute |
| mL | milliliter |
| mm | millimeter |
| mm Hg | millimeters of mercury |
| MOI | mechanism of injury |
| MRI | magnetic resonance imaging |
| MRSA | methicillin-resistant *Staphylococcus aureus* |
| MVA | motor vehicle accident |
| MVC | motor vehicle crash |
| MVP | mitral valve prolapse |
| NA, N/A | not applicable |
| NAD | no apparent distress, no appreciable disease |
| NC | nasal cannula |
| NG | nasogastric |
| NICU | neonatal intensive care unit |

| Abbreviation | Meaning |
|---|---|
| NIDDM | non–insulin-dependent diabetes mellitus |
| NKA | no known allergies |
| NKDA | no known drug allergies |
| NP | nurse practitioner |
| NPA | nasopharyngeal airway |
| NPO | nil per os (nothing by mouth) |
| NRB, NRBM | nonrebreathing mask |
| NS | normal saline |
| NSR | normal sinus rhythm |
| NTG | nitroglycerin |
| N/V | nausea and vomiting |
| N/V/D | nausea, vomiting, and diarrhea |
| $O_2$ | oxygen |
| OB | obstetrics |
| OBS | organic brain syndrome |
| OD | overdose, right eye, optical density, outside diameter, doctor of optometry |
| OP | outpatient |
| OPA | oropharyngeal airway |
| OR | operating room |
| OS | left eye |
| OU | both eyes |
| oz | ounce |
| $\bar{p}$ | after |
| PA | physician assistant |
| pc | after meals |
| $Pco_2$ | partial pressure of carbon dioxide |
| PE | pulmonary embolism, physical examination |
| PEARL or PERL | pupils equal and reactive to light |
| PEARLA | pupils equal and reactive to light and accommodation |

*(continues)*

**TABLE 5-12** Common Abbreviations* (*continued*)

| Abbreviation | Meaning | Abbreviation | Meaning |
|---|---|---|---|
| PEARRL | pupils equal and round, regular in size, react to light | RUL | right upper lobe of the lung |
| ped or peds | pediatric | RUQ | right upper quadrant of the abdomen |
| PEEP | positive end-expiratory pressure | Rx | prescription |
| PERRL | pupils equal, round, and reactive to light | $\bar{s}$ | without |
| PID | pelvic inflammatory disease | $Sao_2$ | oxygen saturation |
| PMH | past medical history | SC | subcutaneous |
| PND | paroxysmal nocturnal dyspnea | SG | supraglottic |
| po | per os (by mouth) | SICU | surgical intensive care unit |
| PO | postoperative, post-op | SIDS | sudden infant death syndrome |
| PRN | pro re nata (as needed) | SL | sublingual |
| psi | pounds per square inch | SOB | shortness of breath |
| PSVT | paroxysmal supraventricular tachycardia | $Spo_2$ | saturation of peripheral oxygen |
| pt | patient | S/S, S&S | signs and symptoms |
| PT | physical therapy, prothrombin time | stat | immediately |
| PTA | prior to admission, plasma thrombo-plastin antecedent | STEMI | ST-segment elevation myocardial infarction |
| PTT | partial thromboplastin time | STI | sexually transmitted infection |
| PVC | premature ventricular contraction, polyvinyl chloride | subcut | subcutaneous |
| | | SVT | supraventricular tachycardia |
| PVD | peripheral vascular disease | sym or Sx | symptoms |
| q | every | T | temperature |
| RA | rheumatoid arthritis, right atrium | tab | tablet |
| RAD | reactive airway disease, right axis deviation | TB | tuberculosis |
| | | TBA | to be admitted, to be announced |
| RBC | red blood cell | tech | technician, technologist |
| Rh | Rhesus blood factor, rhodium | TIA | transient ischemic attack |
| RLL | right lower lobe of the lung | tid/t.i.d./TID | three times a day |
| RLQ | right lower quadrant of the abdomen | Tx | treatment |
| RN | registered nurse | UA | urinalysis |
| R/O | rule out | UE | upper extremity |
| ROM | range of motion, rupture of membranes | URI | upper respiratory infection |
| | | UTI | urinary tract infection |
| | | VD | venereal disease |

| Abbreviation | Meaning | Abbreviation | Meaning |
|---|---|---|---|
| VF/V-fib | ventricular fibrillation | WMD | weapon of mass destruction |
| VRE | vancomycin-resistant enterococcus | WNL | within normal limits |
| VS | vital signs | W/O | without |
| VT/V tach | ventricular tachycardia | wt | weight |
| W/ | with | x | except |
| WBC | white blood cell | yo; y/o | year old |

*Abbreviations are sometimes written with periods (for example, abd. and a.c.), and different capitalization might be used that may convey a different meaning. This table does not include all possible meanings. If you are uncertain, always ask the person using the abbreviation.

© Jones & Bartlett Learning.

# YOU are the Provider SUMMARY

**1. What can you determine about the patient's medical history based on the abbreviations in the record?**

You can determine that the patient has a significant past medical history. The record indicates the patient has had an abdominal aortic aneurysm, hypertension, congestive heart failure, acute myocardial infarction (heart attack), gastroesophageal reflux disease, and type 1 diabetes.

**2. How could a misunderstanding of the medical terminology or abbreviations affect patient care?**

When providing a verbal report to the hospital, it is important to be as succinct as possible. Using abbreviations may help you deliver the most information in the minimum amount of time. Time in an emergency can be critical, so providing a concise report of essential information may be valuable; however, conciseness should never come at the expense of clarity. There is no savings in a report that uses abbreviations but requires clarification or, worse, is misunderstood by a receiving provider.

**3. What other abbreviations could have been used in this report?**

You could use abbreviations when reporting most of the past medical history, but ensure that the abbreviations you use do not adversely affect the ability of other providers to understand them. Appropriate abbreviations that could have been used for this report include *AAA*, *CHF*, *AMI*, and *GERD*. Abbreviations are useful in written and verbal reports. Also, *LPM* could be used in place of *L/min* when documenting oxygen flow.

**4. What do the abbreviations in this portion of the report mean?**

The abbreviations in this report include *EMT* for Emergency Medical Technician, *AO* meaning "alert and oriented," and *CC* meaning chief complaint. The abbreviation *yo* is used for years old.

**5. What other medical terms or parts, such as prefixes, were used in this case?**

Word roots in this case include "gastro" (stomach) and "entero" (intestine), which are combined with the suffix "itis" (inflammation) in the word *gastroenteritis*. Additionally, "cardio" (heart) and "vas" (blood vessel) are word roots in the word *cardiovascular*. Some of the prefixes used in this case included "hyper" (high) in the word *hypertension* relating to the blood pressure, "peri" (around) in the word *periumbilical* related to the pain around the patient's umbilicus, and "epi" (above or over) in the word *epigastric* related to pain above the stomach. The directional term "superior" (above) and the directional term "supine" (lying flat on back) were also used in this case.

## EMS Patient Care Report (PCR)

| Date: 6-10-20 | Incident No.: 060109 | Nature of Call: Constipation and abdominal pain | | Location: Friends Acre Nursing Home, 322 Azalea Trail | |
|---|---|---|---|---|---|
| Dispatched: 1740 | En Route: 1741 | At Scene: 1747 | Transport: 1759 | At Hospital: 1809 | In Service: 1817 |

### Patient Information

**Age:** 79
**Sex:** F
**Weight (in kg [lb]):** 84 kg (185 lb)

**Allergies:** Sulfa, codeine, contrast dye
**Medications:** Lopressor, ASA, metoprolol, lisinopril, Pepcid AC, NovoLog insulin
**Past Medical History:** AAA, HTN, CHF, AMI in 2010, GERD, type 1 diabetes
**Chief Complaint:** Abdominal pain

### Vital Signs

| Time: 1749 | BP: 80/50 | Pulse: 128 | Respirations: 24 | SpO$_2$: 98% |
|---|---|---|---|---|
| Time: 1758 | BP: 86/54 | Pulse: 112 | Respirations: 24 | SpO$_2$: 97% |
| Time: 1808 | BP: 100/60 | Pulse: 108 | Respirations: 20 | SpO$_2$: 99% |

### EMS Treatment (circle all that apply)

| Oxygen @ _12_ L/min via:<br><br>NC (NRM) Bag mask | Assisted Ventilation | Airway Adjunct | CPR |
|---|---|---|---|
| Defibrillation | Bleeding Control | Bandaging | Splinting | Other: Position of comfort |

### Narrative

Dispatched for a female patient c/o constipation and abdominal pain.

Chief Complaint: Abdominal pain

History: Patient states the pain began suddenly approximately 20 minutes ago. Her medical history is significant for AAA, HTN, CHF, AMI in 2010, GERD, and type 1 diabetes. Patient denies chest pain, shortness of breath, nausea or vomiting, and any other symptoms. She further denies radiating and referred pain.

Assessment: On arrival at the scene, found the patient, a 79-year-old female, lying on her side in bed with her knees drawn up into her abdomen. She was conscious and alert; her airway was patent, and breathing adequate. Skin was pale and wet. She reports pain is 8 on scale of 1 to 10. She denies symptoms of gastroenteritis.

Treatment (Rx): Applied oxygen at 12 L/min via nonrebreathing mask and obtained vital signs. Further assessment of patient's abdomen revealed an anterior, periumbilical pulsating mass; it was point tender to palpation of the RUQ.

Transport: Patient was placed onto the stretcher in a position of comfort, loaded into the ambulance, and transported to the hospital. En route, continued to monitor patient's condition, which remained unchanged. Vital signs reassessed and noted above.

Reassessment: Shortly before arrival at the hospital, reassessment of the patient revealed that her vital signs were not stable and that her pain persisted. Transferred care of patient to receiving hospital without incident and gave verbal report to charge nurse. Departed the hospital and returned to service.

**End of report**

# Prep Kit

## Ready for Review

- Knowledge of medical terminology is essential for health care team members to effectively communicate and document calls.
- Understanding how terms are formed, and the definitions for the various parts of a medical term, will help you determine the meaning of an unknown term.
- Parts that can make up a word include the word root, prefix, suffix, and combining vowels. Not every part is included in every word. Each part can significantly change the meaning of a word.
- The word root is the stem of the word and conveys the core meaning. It frequently indicates a body part. Most terms have at least one word root.
- A prefix and/or suffix can be added to the word root to create a term. Changing the prefix or suffix will change the meaning of the term.
- A prefix is the part of a term that appears at the beginning of a word. It generally describes location and intensity.
- A suffix is placed at the end of a word to change the original meaning. In medical terminology, a suffix usually indicates a procedure, condition, disease, or part of speech.
- A combining vowel is the part of a term that connects a word root to a suffix or other word root to make it easier to pronounce.
- To make some terms plural, an *s* is added to the term. Other terms use other plural forms.
- Prefixes can also indicate numbers, colors, or direction.
- Directional terms indicate distance and direction from the midline. These include right, left, superior, inferior, lateral, medial, proximal, distal, superficial, deep, ventral, dorsal, palmar, plantar, and apex.
- Terms related to movement include flexion, extension, adduction, and abduction.
- Anatomic position refers to the position of the body—for example, the position the patient is in when you arrive on scene. Anatomic positions include prone, supine, and Fowler.
- Abbreviations and symbols are used as shorthand to communicate and document in a concise manner. To avoid potentially dangerous misinterpretation of your documentation, be sure to use only abbreviations that are commonly understood; avoid using abbreviations that are not recommended.

## Vital Vocabulary

**abduction** Motion of a limb away from the midline.

**adduction** Motion of a limb toward the midline.

**anterior** The front surface of the body; the side facing you in the standard anatomic position.

**apex (plural apices)** The pointed extremity of a conical structure.

**bilateral** A body part or condition that appears on both sides of the midline.

**combining vowel** The vowel used to combine two word roots or a word root and suffix.

**deep** Farther inside the body and away from the skin.

**distal** Farther from the trunk or nearer to the free end of the extremity.

**dorsal** The posterior surface of the body, including the back of the hand.

**extension** The straightening of a joint.

**flexion** The bending of a joint.

**Fowler position** An inclined position in which the head of the bed is raised.

**inferior** Below a body part or nearer to the feet.

**lateral** Parts of the body that lie farther from the midline; also called outer structures.

**medial** Parts of the body that lie closer to the midline; also called inner structures.

**palmar** The forward-facing part of the hand in the anatomic position.

**plantar** The bottom surface of the foot.

**posterior** The back surface of the body; the side away from you in the standard anatomic position.

**prefix** Part of a term that appears before a word root, changing the meaning of the term.

**prone** Lying face down.

**proximal** Closer to the trunk.

**quadrants** Describes the sections of the abdominal cavity, in which two imaginary lines intersect at the umbilicus, dividing the abdomen into four equal areas.

**suffix** The part of a term that comes after the word root, at the end of the term.

**superficial** Closer to or on the skin.

**superior** Above a body part or nearer to the head.

**supine** Lying face up.

**ventral** The anterior surface of the body.

**word root** The main part of a term that contains the primary meaning.

## References

1. Cimino JJ, Clayton PD, Hripcsak G, Johnson SB. Knowledge-based approaches to the maintenance of a large controlled medical terminology. *J Am Med Inform Assoc.* 1994;1(1):35-50.

2. Hamiel U, Hecht I, Nemet A, et al. Frequency, comprehension and attitudes of physicians towards abbreviations in the medical record. *Postgrad Med J.* 2018;94(1111):254-258.

3. Joint Commission International. Use of codes, symbols, and abbreviations. https://www.jointcommission international.org/standards/hospital-standards -communication-center/use-of-codes-symbols-and -abbreviations. Accessed February 27, 2020.

4. Schultz CH, Koenig KL, Whiteside M, Murray R; National Standardized All-Hazard Disaster Core Competencies Task Force. Development of national standardized all-hazard disaster core competencies for acute care physicians, nurses, and EMS professionals. *Ann Emerg Med.* 2012;59(3):196-208.e1.

5. Taber's Online. Medical abbreviations. https://www .tabers.com/tabersonline/.//view/Tabers-Dictionary /767492/all/Medical_Abbreviations?refer=true. Accessed February 27, 2020.

6. Tariq RA, Sharma S. Inappropriate medical abbreviations. NCBI website (StatPearls). http://www.ncbi.nlm.nih.gov /books/NBK519006/. Updated June 24, 2019. Accessed February 27, 2020.

7. Thompson CL, Pledger LM. Doctor–patient communication: is patient knowledge of medical terminology improving? *Health Commun.* 1993;5(2):89-97.

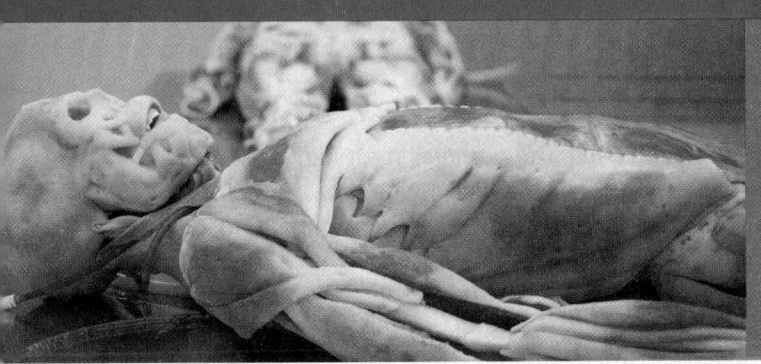

# Chapter 6

# The Human Body

## NATIONAL EMS EDUCATION STANDARD COMPETENCIES

### Preparatory

Applies fundamental knowledge of the emergency medical services (EMS) system, safety/well-being of the emergency medical technician (EMT), medical/legal and ethical issues to the provision of emergency care.

### Anatomy and Physiology

Applies fundamental knowledge of the anatomy and function of all human systems to the practice of EMS.

### Pathophysiology

Applies fundamental knowledge of the pathophysiology of respiration and perfusion to patient assessment and management.

## KNOWLEDGE OBJECTIVES

1. Identify the body's topographic anatomy, including the anatomic position and the planes of the body. (pp 190–191)
2. Identify the anatomy and physiology of the skeletal system. (pp 191–197)
3. Describe the anatomy and physiology of the musculoskeletal system. (pp 197–198)
4. Discuss the anatomy and physiology of the respiratory system. (pp 198–207)
5. Discuss the anatomy and physiology of the circulatory system. (pp 207–220)
6. Discuss the anatomy and physiology of the nervous system. (pp 220–224)
7. Describe the anatomy and the physiology of the integumentary system. (pp 224–226)
8. Explain the anatomy and physiology of the digestive system. (pp 226–230)
9. Describe the anatomy and physiology of the lymphatic system. (p 230)
10. Discuss the anatomy and physiology of the endocrine system. (pp 230–232)
11. Describe the anatomy and physiology of the urinary system. (pp 232–233)
12. Discuss the anatomy and physiology of the genital system. (pp 233–234)
13. Describe the life support chain, aerobic metabolism, and anaerobic metabolism. (pp 235–236)
14. Define pathophysiology. (p 236)

## SKILLS OBJECTIVES

There are no skills objectives for this chapter.

**PHOTO:** Courtesy of SynDaver Labs.

# Introduction

As an EMT, having a clear understanding of human anatomy, physiology, and pathophysiology is essential. **Anatomy** is a field of study that focuses on the physical *structure* of the body and its systems. **Physiology** goes a step further, examining the normal *functions and activities* of these biologic components. **Pathophysiology** is the study of functional *changes* that accompany a particular disease or syndrome. This chapter provides basic information about the many structures and functions of the body and its parts.

# Topographic Anatomy

Many anatomic landmarks on the surface of the body are easy to identify. It is not too difficult to find the **umbilicus** (navel) or the lower tip of the breastbone. In much the same way that "X marks the spot" on a map where something hidden can be found, these surface structures—the body's **topographic anatomy**—help guide the EMT to the locations of internal features that lie beneath. Understanding these external-to-internal relationships is fundamental to an effective patient assessment.

Directional terminology ensures consistency and clarity of communication between providers. Imagine being on scene with a trauma patient and calling the emergency department to report your findings. When the nurse answers the phone, you need to relay the specific location of your patient's injury as clearly and concisely as possible. And the nurse, in turn, must be able to quickly and accurately interpret your description, virtually "seeing" what *you* see. How will you accomplish this task?

Begin by imagining the patient standing in the **anatomic position**, with palms and feet facing toward you. This position is a frame of reference used by all health care providers. In addition, directional terms are always presented from the patient's

perspective (eg, the *patient's* right leg), as opposed to the EMT's point of view. To illustrate, imagine you are face to face with a patient complaining of pain in his left arm. From your point of view, the affected arm is on the right; but from the patient's point of view, the arm is on the left. Both perspectives are accurate, but when reporting the information to another health care provider, you would refer to the affected limb as "the *patient's* left arm."

## The Planes of the Body

Another approach used when describing a particular location on the patient's body is to divide the body into anatomic planes. These imaginary straight-line divisions begin with three main axes (**FIGURE 6-1**). The **coronal (frontal) plane** runs vertically through the body and divides it into front

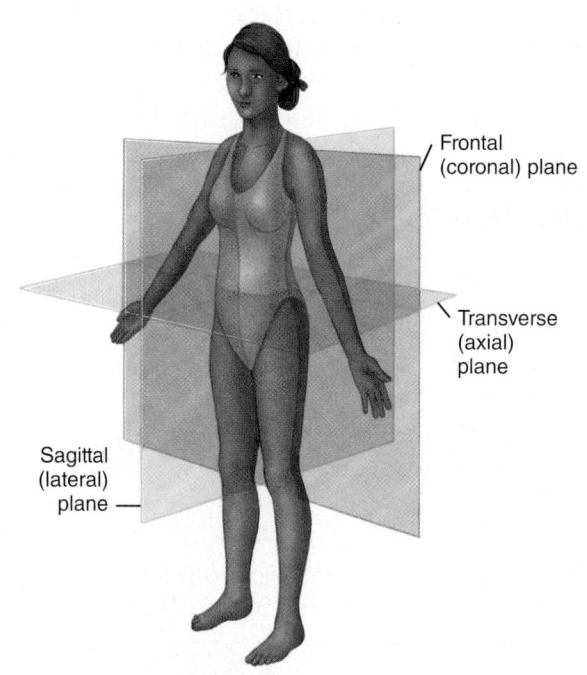

**FIGURE 6-1** Anatomic planes of the body.
© Jones & Bartlett Learning.

---

## YOU are the Provider

At 1740 hours, you are dispatched to 322 Azalea Trail for a 60-year-old man with severe abdominal pain. The weather is overcast, the traffic is heavy, and your response time to the scene is approximately 6 minutes.

**1.** How will knowledge of anatomy and physiology help you provide appropriate patient care?

**TABLE 6-1** Planes of the Body

| Plane of the Body | Description |
|---|---|
| Coronal (frontal) | Front and back |
| Transverse (axial) | Top and bottom |
| Sagittal (lateral) | Left and right |
| Midsagittal (midline) | Left and right (equal halves) |

© Jones & Bartlett Learning.

and back sections. The **sagittal (lateral) plane** also runs vertically, but divides the body into left and right sections. It is worth noting that these left and right sections do not necessarily need to be divided equally; however, a subtype of the sagittal plane—the **midsagittal (midline) plane**—divides the body into equal left and right halves. Your nose and umbilicus are found along this midline. Last, the **transverse (axial) plane** divides the body horizontally into top and bottom sections. These planes help you to identify the location of internal structures and understand the relationships between and among the organs (**TABLE 6-1**).

## From Cells to Systems

*Cells* are the foundation of the human body. Billions of cells compose the human body. Every organ, every body part, and every structure can be reduced to individual cells. Cells that share a common function grow close to each other, forming tissues. Groups of tissues that perform similar or interrelated jobs form organs. Organs with similar functions work together to comprise the different body systems discussed in this chapter.

## The Skeletal System: Anatomy

The **skeletal system** serves many functions, but some of the most obvious are to (1) provide structural support to bear the body's weight, (2) establish a framework to attach soft tissues and internal organs, and (3) protect vital organs such as the heart and lungs. In addition, the red marrow found within the internal cavities of many bones produces red blood cells.

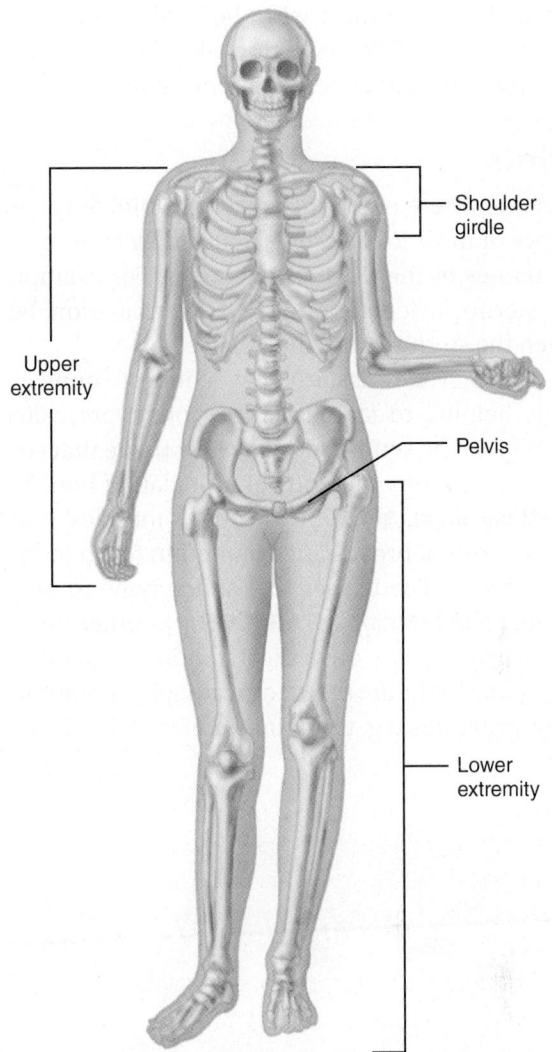

**FIGURE 6-2** The 206 bones of the skeleton give the body its form, protect the vital organs, and allow the body to move. The axial skeleton runs in a straight line from the skull to the base of the spine (ie, the coccyx, or tailbone). The appendicular skeleton is made up of the arms and legs and their points of attachment to the axial skeleton (ie, the shoulder and pelvis).

© Jones & Bartlett Learning.

## Bones

The 206 bones that compose the skeletal system are divided between the axial and appendicular skeletons (**FIGURE 6-2**). The **axial skeleton** forms the longitudinal axis of the body, from the skull to the tailbone, or **coccyx**. It includes the skull, facial bones, **thoracic cage**, and vertebral column. The **appendicular skeleton** comprises the upper and lower extremities (ie, arms and legs) and the points by which they connect with the axial skeleton (eg, the shoulder). The pelvis includes portions from both the axial and appendicular skeletons.

## Joints

A **joint** is where two bones meet (**FIGURE 6-3**). The names of most joints are formulated by combining the names of these adjoining bones. For example, the sternoclavicular joint is the articulation between the sternum and the clavicle.

The fibrous tissues that connect bone to bone, helping to stabilize these joints, are called **ligaments**. The semirigid yet flexible tissue that covers and cushions the ends of articulating bones is called **cartilage**. Aided by the body's muscles, most joints permit a broad range of motion (eg, bending at the knee). The tissues that attach bone to muscle are called **tendons** (**TABLE 6-2**). In other joints, called **symphyses**, only slight motion is possible. Last, some joints are fused to create solid, immobile, bony structures (eg, the cranial bones of the skull).

The bone ends of a joint are held together by a fibrous sac called the **joint capsule**. This sac is composed of connective tissue (connecting bone to bone). At certain points around the joint, the capsule is lax and thin, permitting movement. In other areas, it is thick and resists stretching and bending. For example, while a joint such as the **sacroiliac joint** is virtually surrounded by tough, thick ligaments and will therefore have little motion, the shoulder, having fewer ligaments, is free to move in

**TABLE 6-2** Support Structures Within the Skeletal System

| Name | Function |
| --- | --- |
| Ligament | Connects bone to bone |
| Tendon | Connects muscle to bone |
| Cartilage | Cushion between bones |

© Jones & Bartlett Learning.

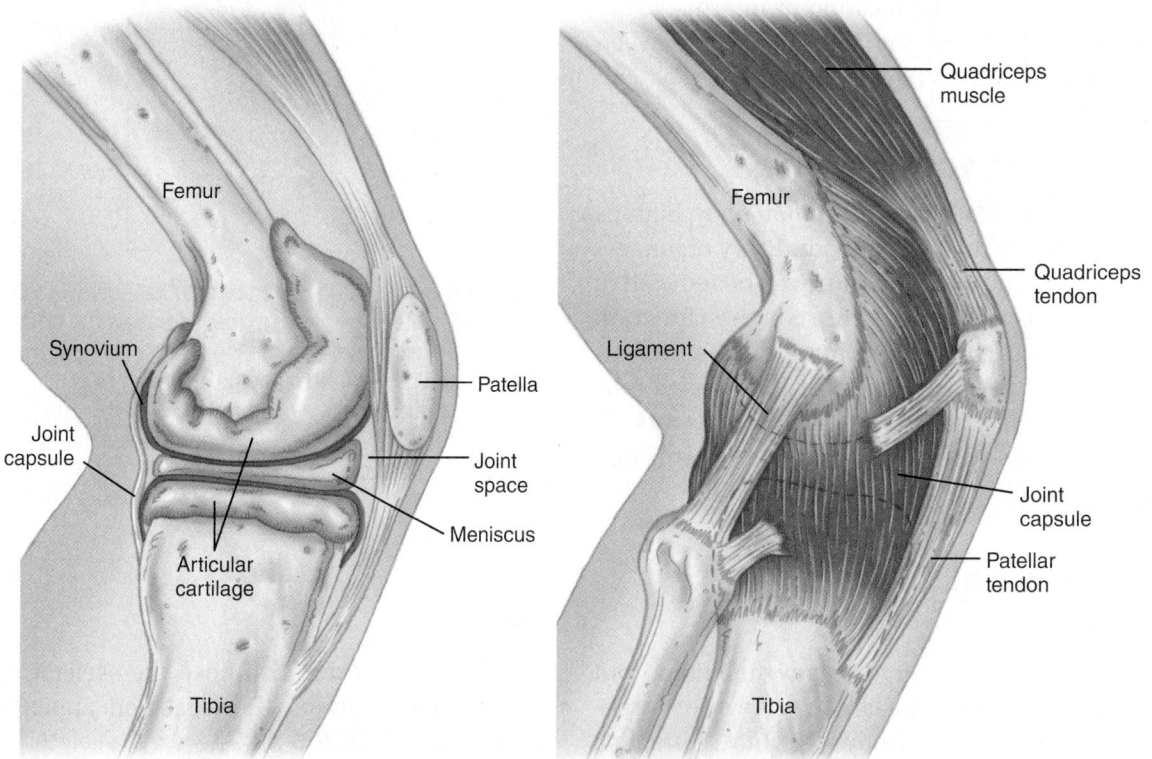

**FIGURE 6-3** A joint consists of bone ends, a fibrous joint capsule, synovial membranes, and ligaments. The degree to which a joint can move is determined by how the ligaments hold the bone ends and by the configuration of the bones themselves.

© Jones & Bartlett Learning.

almost any direction (and will, as a result, be more susceptible to dislocation). In moving joints, the ends of the bones are covered with a thin layer of cartilage known as **articular cartilage**. This cartilage is a pearly white substance that allows the ends of the bones to glide easily. On the inner lining of the joint capsule is the **synovial membrane**. This special tissue is responsible for making a thick lubricant called **synovial fluid**. This oil-like substance allows the ends of the bones to glide over each other as opposed to rubbing and grating over each other.

The degree to which a joint can move is determined by the extent to which the ligaments hold the bone ends together and also by the configuration of the bone ends themselves. The shoulder joint is a **ball-and-socket joint**, which allows rotation and bending (**FIGURE 6-4**). The finger joints, elbow, and knee are **hinge joints**, with motion restricted to **flexion** (bending) and **extension** (straightening) (**FIGURE 6-5**). Rotation is not possible because of the shape of the joint surfaces and the strong restraining ligaments on both sides of the joint. Although the amount of motion varies from joint to

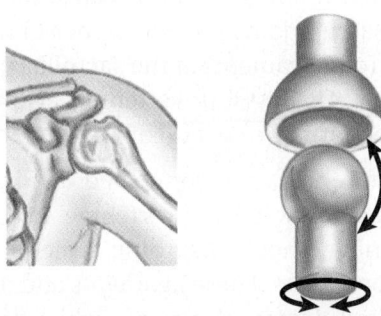

**FIGURE 6-4** The shoulder is an example of a ball-and-socket joint.

© Jones & Bartlett Learning.

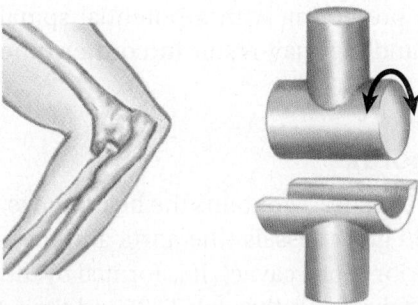

**FIGURE 6-5** The elbow joints are hinge joints, which allow motion in only one plane (flexion and extension).

© Jones & Bartlett Learning.

joint, all joints have a definite limit beyond which motion cannot occur. When a joint is forced beyond this limit, damage to some structure must occur. Either the bones that form the joint will break, or the supporting capsule and ligaments will be disrupted.

## The Axial Skeleton

### The Skull

The skull consists of 28 bones divided into three groups: the cranium, the facial bones, and three small bones in the ear. The **cranium** comprises the **frontal bones**, **temporal bones**, **parietal bones**, **occipital bone**, ethmoid bone, and sphenoid bone. Fused together, these bones encase and protect the brain (**FIGURE 6-6**).

At the base of the cranium, a large opening called the **foramen magnum** (Latin for "great opening") serves as the passageway for the spinal cord to connect with the brain and descend into the spinal, or vertebral column.

The 14 facial bones include the upper jawbones (**maxillae**), the lower jawbone (**mandible**), and the cheek bones (**zygomas**). The **orbit**, or eye socket, is not a bone itself; it is a cavity formed by the joining of multiple facial bones. The upper third of the nose is made up of the very short *nasal bones* that form the bridge of the nose; the remaining two-thirds consist of flexible cartilage.

### The Spinal Column

The **vertebral column** (or spinal column) consists of 33 **vertebrae**. The vertebrae can be divided into five sections, with each vertebra labeled according to its respective section and numbered from the top down (**FIGURE 6-7**).

- **Cervical spine.** The first seven vertebrae (C1 through C7) in the neck form the cervical spine. The skull rests on and attaches to both the first cervical vertebra (the atlas) and the second cervical vertebra (the axis). The vertebrae fit together but move separately, allowing the head to turn in multiple directions.
- **Thoracic spine.** The next 12 vertebrae make up the thoracic spine. One pair of ribs is attached to each of the thoracic vertebrae.
- **Lumbar spine.** The next five vertebrae form the lumbar spine.

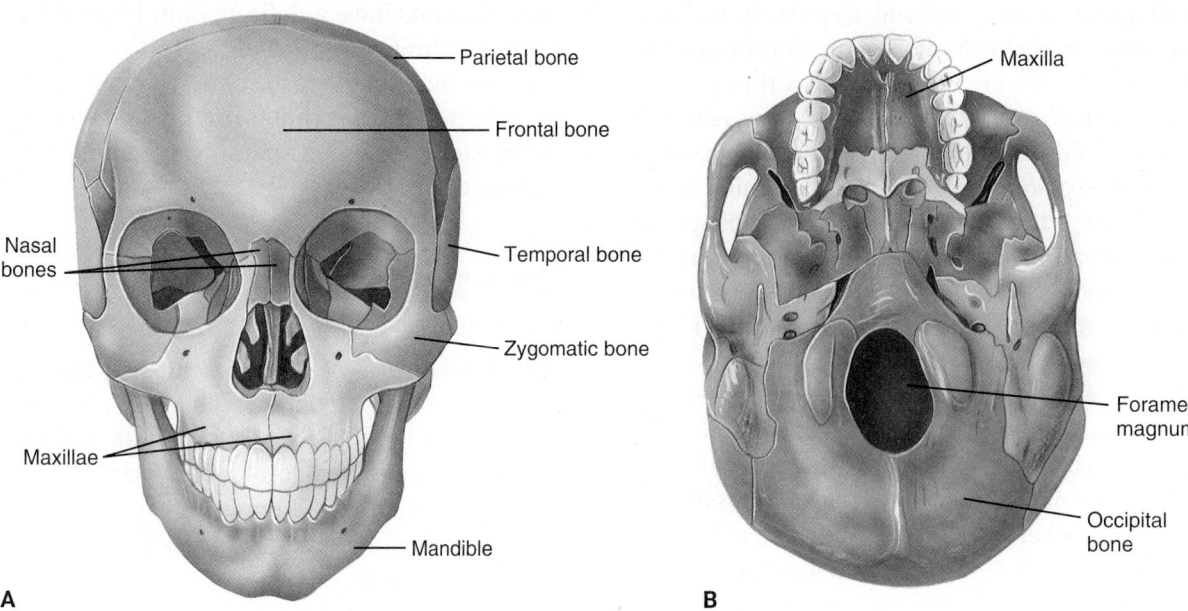

**FIGURE 6-6** The skull. **A.** Anterior view. **B.** Inferior view.

© Jones & Bartlett Learning.

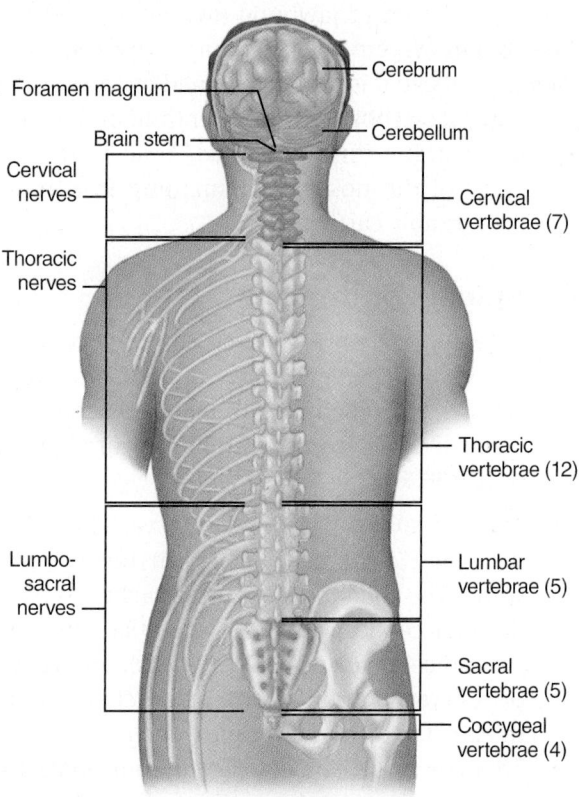

**FIGURE 6-7** The vertebral column is composed of 33 bones divided into five sections.

© Jones & Bartlett Learning.

- **Sacrum.** The five sacral vertebrae are fused together to form one bone called the sacrum. The sacrum joins the iliac bones of the pelvis via strong ligaments at the sacroiliac joints.
- **Coccyx.** The last four vertebrae, also fused together, form the coccyx, or tailbone.

The vertebrae are connected by ligaments, and the gaps between the vertebrae are occupied by cushioning, shock-absorbing structures called **intervertebral disks**. These ligaments and disks permit a limited degree of motion, while preventing any extreme movement that might harm the spinal cord. An injury to the vertebrae or the tissues between them has the potential to cause spinal cord damage. Use caution when assessing and treating patients presenting with a potential spinal injury, as mishandling may result in cord or other nerve damage.

## The Thorax

The **thorax** (chest) contains the heart, lungs, esophagus, and great vessels (the aorta and the superior and inferior venae cavae). It is formed by the 12 thoracic vertebrae (T1 through T12) and their 12 pairs of ribs.

Midline on the anterior surface of the chest is the **sternum** (breastbone). The sternum has three main

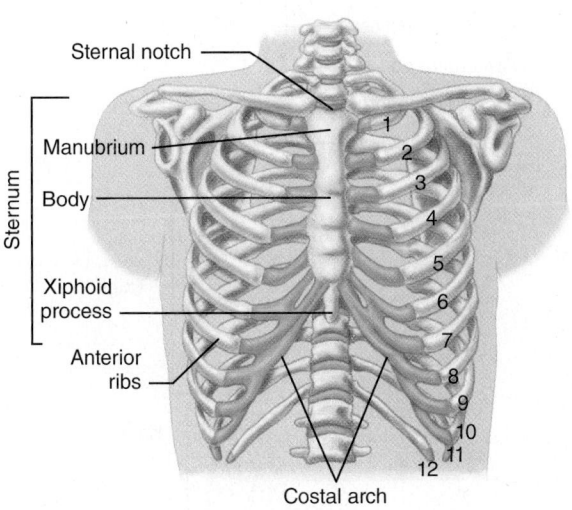

**FIGURE 6-8** The thorax.

© Jones & Bartlett Learning.

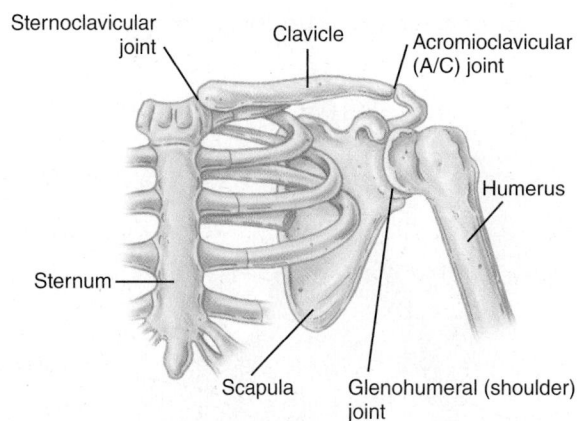

**FIGURE 6-9** The bones of the shoulder girdle include the clavicle and scapula.

© Jones & Bartlett Learning.

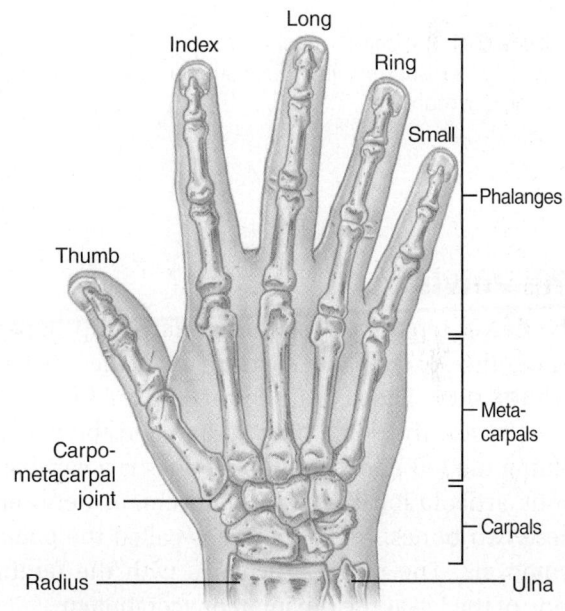

**FIGURE 6-10** The major bones in the wrist and hand include the carpals, the metacarpals, and the phalanges.

© Jones & Bartlett Learning.

parts: the manubrium, the body, and the xiphoid process. The **manubrium** is the uppermost section. The superior edge of the manubrium forms a landmark called the *sternal notch.* Immediately inferior to the manubrium is the sternal *body,* the largest bony section of the sternum. Last, the inferior tip of the sternum is formed by a narrow, cartilaginous structure called the **xiphoid process** (**FIGURE 6-8**).

## The Appendicular Skeleton
### Upper Extremities

The upper extremities (ie, arms) extend distally from the **pectoral girdle** (shoulder), which comprises the **clavicle** (ie, collarbone) and the **scapula** (shoulder blade) (**FIGURE 6-9**). The medial end of the clavicle articulates with the manubrium of the sternum; this is the only joint that directly connects the shoulder girdle and the axial skeleton. The clavicle's lateral end articulates with the scapula. The scapula is supported and positioned by skeletal muscles and has no bony or ligamentous connections to the thoracic cage.

The scapula articulates with the proximal head of the **humerus**, the single bone of the upper arm. Distally, the humerus articulates with the two bones that make up the forearm: the **radius** on the lateral, or thumb, side and the **ulna** on the medial, or little finger, side.

At their distal ends, the radius and ulna articulate with the proximal row of wrist bones, via a modified ball-and-socket joint (**FIGURE 6-10**). The eight bones that form the wrist are called **carpals**. Extending from the carpals are five **metacarpals**, which form the palm of the hand. The metacarpals in turn articulate with the bones of the fingers, or **phalanges**. The thumb is composed of two phalanges (proximal and distal); the remaining four digits each contain three phalanges (proximal, middle, and distal).

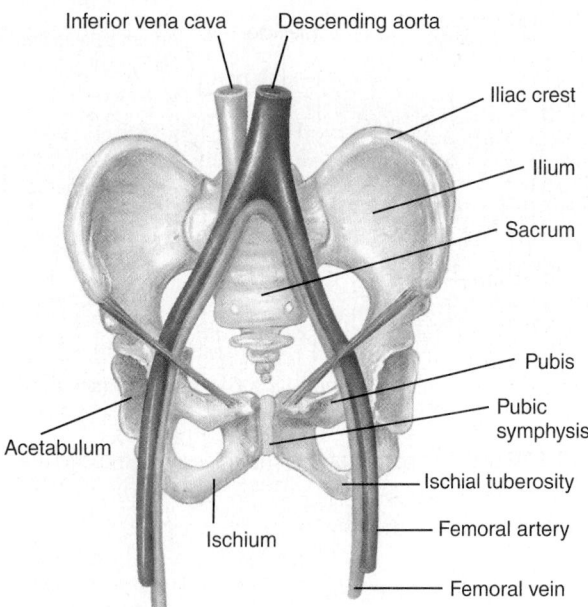

**FIGURE 6-11** The pelvis is a closed, bony ring that consists of the sacrum, ilium, ischium, pubis, acetabulum, and pubic symphysis.

© Jones & Bartlett Learning.

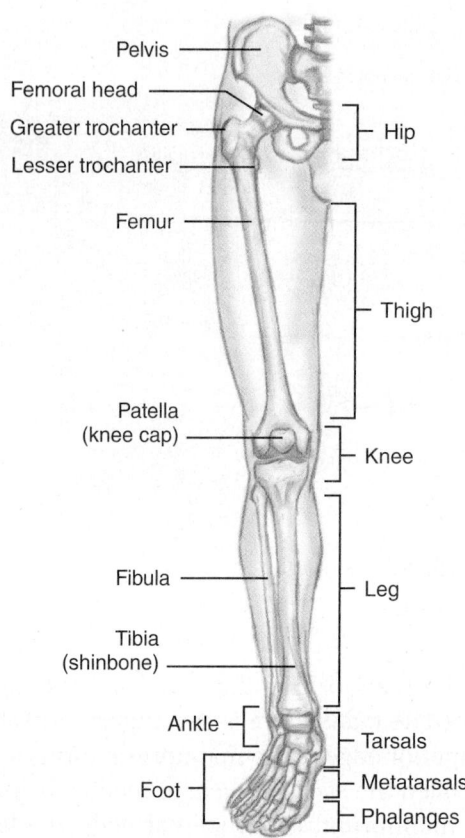

**FIGURE 6-12** The major parts of the lower extremities include the femur, femoral head, greater and lesser trochanters, patella, tibia, and fibula.

© Jones & Bartlett Learning.

## The Pelvis

The **pelvic girdle** consists of two large hip bones called the **coxae**, the sacrum, and the coccyx (**FIGURE 6-11**). Each coxa is formed by the fusion of three bones: the **ilium**, the **ischium**, and the **pubis**. Joining the left and right pubic bones is a cartilaginous articulation that limits movement between these two bones; this structure is called the **pubic symphysis**. The pelvis articulates with the femur bone of the leg at the hip joint, or **acetabulum**.

## The Lower Extremities

The **femur** (thighbone) is the longest and one of the strongest bones in the body. The femur's rounded superior end is referred to as the **femoral head**. The femoral head articulates with the acetabulum of the pelvic girdle by a ball-and-socket joint. Immediately inferior and lateral to the head is the narrowed femoral neck. A projection called the **greater trochanter** is located proximal to the femoral head and neck on the lateral side of the femur. A second projection, called the **lesser trochanter**, is found on the medial side of the femur, just inferior to the femoral neck (**FIGURE 6-12**). Both trochanters

serve as anchor points for the major muscles of the thigh.

At the inferior end of the femur, a hinge joint commonly referred to as the knee connects the femur to the bones of the lower leg. The anterior side of the knee is covered by a specialized bone called the **patella** (kneecap). The lower leg comprises two bones: the tibia and the fibula. The larger of the two, the **tibia** (shinbone), articulates with the inferior end of the femur at the knee joint. It is positioned on the medial side of the lower leg and can be palpated along its entire length on the anterior surface of the leg, just beneath the skin. The smaller **fibula** lies on the lateral side of the lower leg. The ankle joint includes protrusions from the broadened distal ends of the tibia and fibula. On the lateral side, the fibula's lateral **malleolus** can be palpated. On the medial side, the prominence from the distal tibia is called the medial malleolus.

## Ankle and Foot

The foot comprises the tarsals, metatarsals, and phalanges. The seven tarsals include the large calcaneus, or heel bone, and the talus. The distal ends of the tibia and fibula articulate with the talus to form the ankle. The hinge joint of the ankle allows flexion and extension of the foot (**FIGURE 6-13**).

The five metatarsal bones form the middle of the foot. The bottom surface of the foot is referred to as the plantar surface, while the top of the foot is described as the dorsum or dorsal surface. The five toes are formed by 14 phalanges, with two in the great toe and three in each of the remaining toes.

### Safety Tips

As you gain a better understanding of the anatomy and physiology of the body, remember that these systems work together, not in isolation. A person who falls and breaks a leg may appear to have an isolated bone injury. But is there bleeding inside the leg? Is there damage to the nerves, tendons, or ligaments? Has the injury disrupted the skin, creating a risk for infection? A seemingly simple illness or injury can involve several body systems, not all of which are obvious at first glance. Always perform a thorough patient assessment.

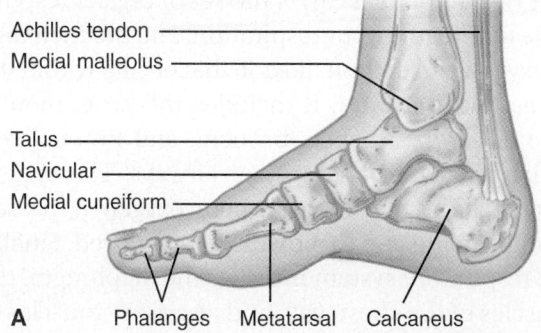

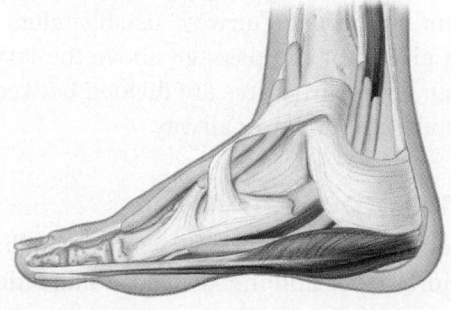

Achilles tendon
Medial malleolus
Talus
Navicular
Medial cuneiform
**A**    Phalanges    Metatarsal    Calcaneus
**B**

**FIGURE 6-13 A.** The surface landmarks of the foot, including the talus, the calcaneus, and the phalanges. **B.** Soft tissue of the ankle.

© Jones & Bartlett Learning.

## The Skeletal System: Physiology

The skeletal system is responsible for several functions: It gives the body shape, provides protection of fragile organs, and allows for movement. Another function of the skeletal system is the storage of calcium. Associated with and in reaction to the normal stress from daily activity, the bones are continually broken down and rebuilt. Calcium is essential to the formation of hard, resilient bones. It is also vital to the function and well-being of other body systems. The heart, muscles, and nervous system are a few examples.

The skeletal system also plays a crucial role in the creation of various types of blood cells and components. As the need arises (eg, existing blood cells die), specialized cells present in the marrow can be transformed into red blood cells, white blood cells, and platelets.

## The Musculoskeletal System: Anatomy

Muscle is a form of tissue that facilitates movement. The human body contains three types of muscle: skeletal, smooth, and cardiac (**FIGURE 6-14**). Skeletal muscle, so named because it attaches to the bones of the skeleton, accounts for the bulk of human muscle mass. Because of its characteristic striped appearance, skeletal muscle is often referred to as *striated* muscle. It is also known as voluntary muscle because its movements are under our conscious control.

By contrast, the activities of smooth muscle and cardiac muscle do not require conscious thought. You do not, for example, need to "make" your heart beat. For this reason, smooth and cardiac muscle are recognized as involuntary muscle. Smooth muscle is found within blood vessels and the intestines. When you hear your stomach growling, you are in fact hearing the rhythmic smooth muscle contractions of the intestines. Cardiac muscle is unique from other muscle types in that it can generate its own electrical impulses.

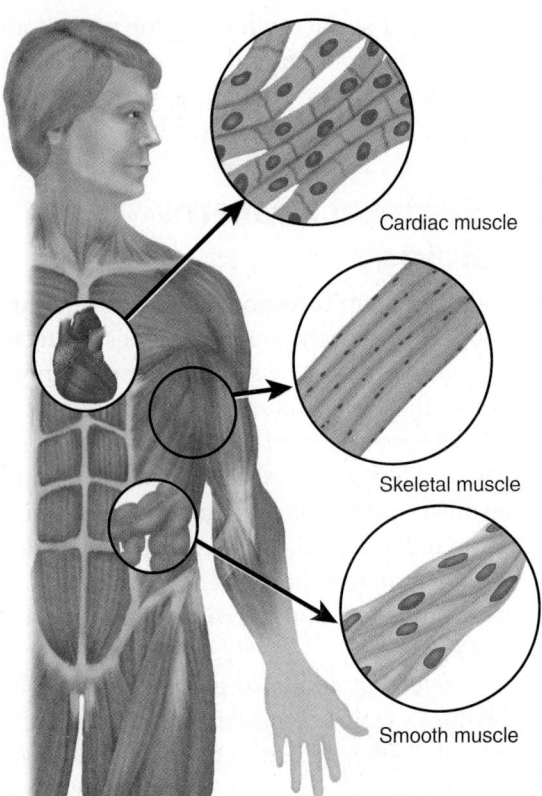

Cardiac muscle

Skeletal muscle

Smooth muscle

**FIGURE 6-14** The three types of muscle are skeletal, smooth, and cardiac.

© Jones & Bartlett Learning.

## Skeletal Muscle

As the name implies, *musculoskeletal* is a term that refers to a partnership between bone and muscle. Thus, whenever we discuss the musculoskeletal system, we acknowledge this synergistic relationship. Voluntary movements, such as walking, raising your hand, and nodding your head, would not be possible otherwise.

In most instances, a given motion—no matter how small—requires the simultaneous participation of multiple muscles. Skeletal muscles often function in *antagonistic pairs*. The muscles of the upper arm include the biceps muscle, which is located on the anterior aspect of the humerus. This muscle bends the elbow by moving the lower part of the arm toward the head. If the muscle were working alone, you would have little control over the speed of that movement. The way the body achieves control and fine movement is to have the biceps compete against another muscle group. The biceps competes with the triceps muscle, which is the three-headed muscle of the back of the arm that functions to

straighten the elbow. Without the triceps, you would slap yourself in the face every time you bend your arm. Conversely, the biceps works to slow the movement of the triceps as the arm is extended.

There are more than 600 muscles in the musculoskeletal system. **FIGURE 6-15** and **TABLE 6-3** show the major muscles, their locations, and their functions.

## The Musculoskeletal System: Physiology

The musculoskeletal system has several functions. One of these is the production of heat. When a person is cold, shivering begins. This involuntarily shaking of the muscles generates heat, thereby maintaining *homeostasis* (the body's self-regulating process for preserving internal balance, or equilibrium, in order to survive). Muscles also protect underlying structures, such as the internal organs. For example, the intestines are protected by the rectus abdominis muscles.

## The Respiratory System: Anatomy

The respiratory system is the set of organs responsible for breathing, or respiration, and the exchange of oxygen and carbon dioxide that occurs within the lungs (**FIGURE 6-16**). It includes the nose, mouth, throat, larynx, trachea, bronchi, and bronchioles, which are all air passages or airways. The system also includes the lungs, where oxygen is passed into the blood and carbon dioxide removed. Finally, the respiratory system includes the diaphragm, the muscles of the chest wall, and accessory muscles of breathing, which permit normal respiratory movement. In this text, "airway" usually refers to the upper airway or the passage above the larynx (voice box). These structures are divided between the upper airway and lower airway.

### The Upper Airway

The structures of the upper airway are located anteriorly at the midline. In descending order, they include the following:

- **Nasopharynx.** Upper section of the pharynx that connects with the nasal cavity above the soft palate

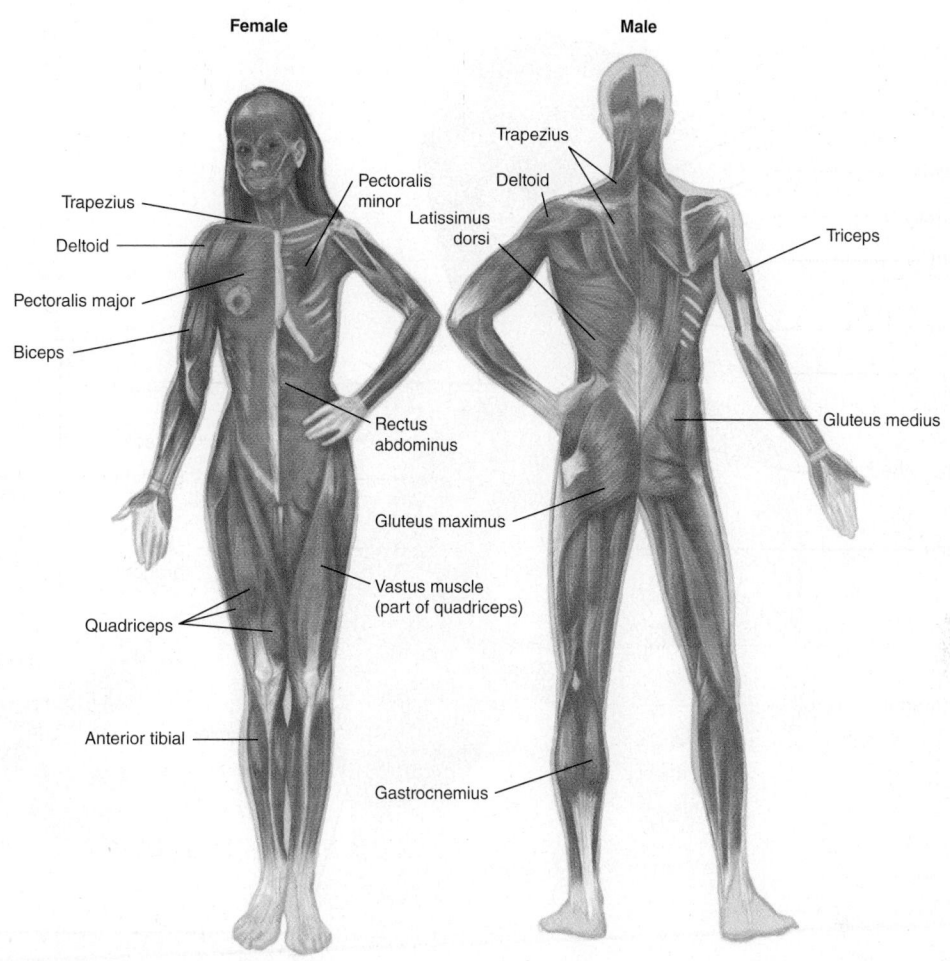

**FIGURE 6-15** The major muscle groups.
© Jones & Bartlett Learning.

**TABLE 6-3** Muscles: Locations and Functions

| Muscle Name | Location | Function |
|---|---|---|
| Biceps | Anterior, humerus | Flexes lower arm |
| Triceps | Posterior, humerus | Extends lower arm |
| Pectoralis | Anterior, thorax | Flexes and rotates arm |
| Latissimus dorsi | Posterior, thorax | Extends and rotates arm |
| Rectus abdominis | Anterior, abdomen | Flexes and rotates spine |
| Tibialis anterior | Anterior, tibia | Points foot toward head |
| Gastrocnemius | Posterior, tibia | Points foot away from head |
| Quadriceps (four separate muscles) | Anterior, femur | Extends lower leg |
| Biceps femoris | Posterior, femur | Flexes lower leg |
| Gluteus (three separate muscles) | Posterior, pelvis/buttocks | Extends and rotates thigh |

© Jones & Bartlett Learning.

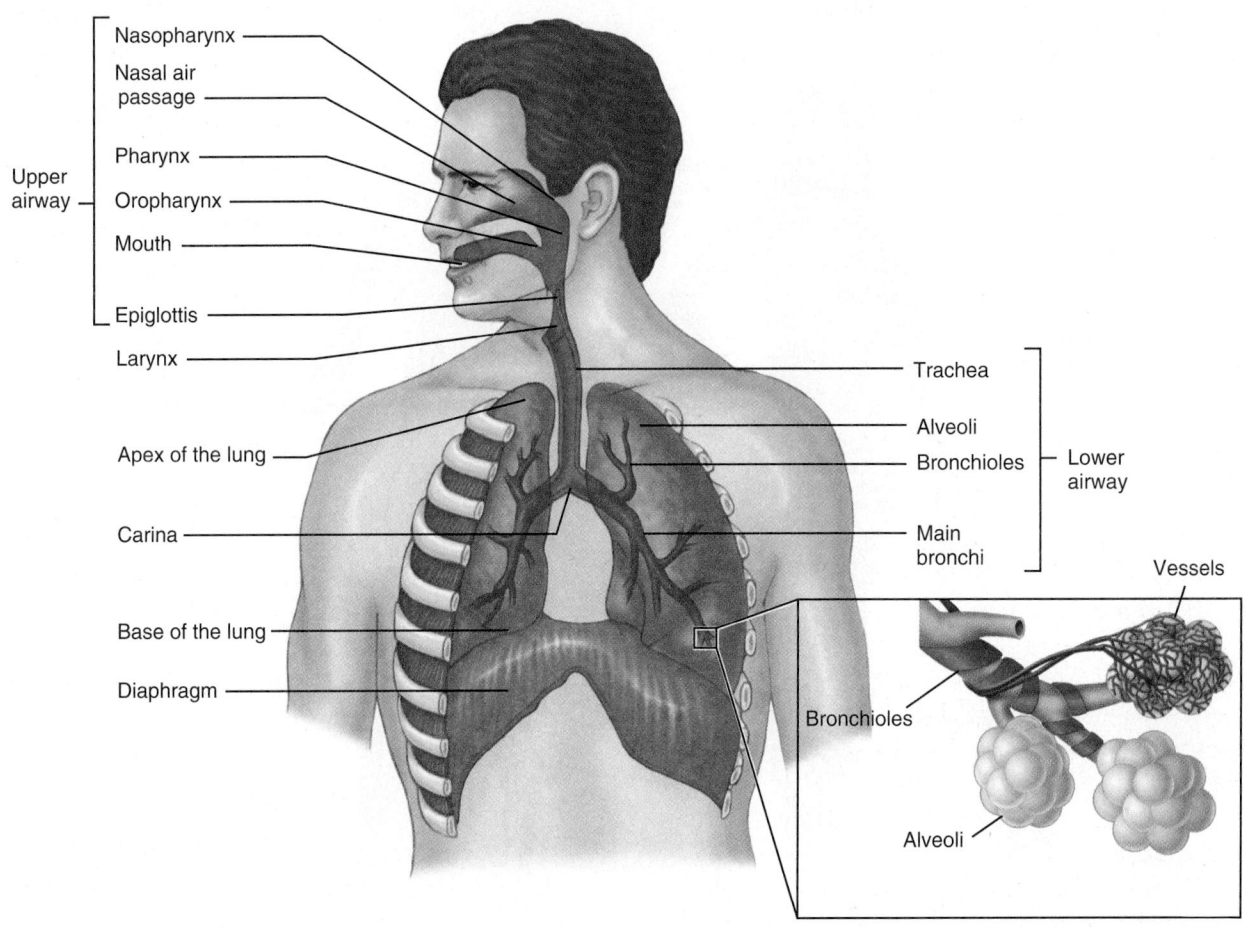

**FIGURE 6-16** The respiratory system consists of all structures of the body that contribute to the process of breathing.

© Jones & Bartlett Learning.

- Oropharynx. Section of the pharynx at the back of the throat, from the soft palate to the U-shaped hyoid bone near the base of the tongue
- Laryngopharynx
- Larynx (voice box)

At the base of the larynx, the vocal cords (ie, glottis) mark the transition point from the upper airway to the lower airway.

The nose and mouth lead to the oropharynx. The pharynx is composed of the nasopharynx, oropharynx, and the laryngopharynx. The nostrils lead to the nasopharynx (above the roof of the mouth and soft palate), and the mouth leads to the oropharynx. The nasal passages and nasopharynx warm, filter, and humidify air as you breathe. Air enters through the mouth more rapidly and directly. As a result, it is less moist than air that enters through the nose.

Food, liquids, and air all can travel through the oropharynx, but on reaching the laryngopharynx they must diverge, with food/liquids continuing posteriorly into the esophagus, while air proceeds to the anteriorly positioned larynx (voice box) and **trachea** (windpipe). The larynx does not tolerate any solid or liquid material, and any contact will result in a violent episode of coughing and spasm of the vocal cords. To help keep food and liquid out of the trachea while permitting air to pass, a thin, leaf-shaped flap (the **epiglottis**) covers the larynx during swallowing and then lifts open to allow for air passage during breathing.

## The Lower Airway

Structures of the lower airway include the trachea, the bronchial tree (main stem bronchi and bronchioles), the alveoli, and the lungs themselves.

The **thyroid cartilage** (Adam's apple), which tends to be more visible in men, is in the anterior midline portion of the neck. This cartilage is the anterior part of the larynx. Tiny muscles open and close the vocal cords and control tension on them. Sounds are created as air is forced past the vocal cords, making them vibrate. The pitch of the sound changes as the cords open and close. You can feel the vibrations if you place your fingers lightly on the larynx as you speak or sing. The vibrations of air are shaped by the tongue and muscles of the mouth to form understandable sounds. Immediately below the thyroid cartilage is the palpable **cricoid cartilage**.

Between the thyroid and cricoid cartilage lies the **cricothyroid membrane**, which can be felt as a depression in the midline of the neck just inferior to the thyroid cartilage. Below the cricoid cartilage is the trachea. The trachea is approximately 5 inches (13 cm) long and is a semirigid, enclosed air tube made up of rings of cartilage that are open in the back. The rings of cartilage keep the trachea from collapsing when air moves into and out of the lungs. Air and other gases enter the trachea and proceed to the lungs.

The two lungs are held in place by the trachea, the arteries and veins, and the pulmonary ligaments. Each lung is divided into lobes. The right lung has three lobes: upper, middle, and lower. The left lung has two: an upper lobe and a lower lobe. Each lobe is divided further into segments

The lungs are supplied air by the right and left main stem bronchi, which are two tubes that branch from the trachea at a structure called the carina (see Figure 6-16). Each bronchus enters its respective lung and branches into smaller and smaller airways called bronchioles. The bronchioles end in about 700 million tiny, grapelike clusters of air sacs called **alveoli**. It is within these alveolar sacs that oxygen and carbon dioxide are exchanged between the lungs and the bloodstream (**FIGURE 6-17**).

The respiratory structures covered thus far serve as a pathway by which air can reach the alveoli. The alveoli are referred to as the functional units of the respiratory system. The walls of the alveoli contain a network of tiny blood vessels (pulmonary capillaries) that carry carbon dioxide from the body to the lungs (for removal through exhalation) and oxygen from the lungs to the body.

## Mechanics of Breathing

For air to flow in and out of the lungs, the lungs must be able to expand and relax. The lungs cannot accomplish this on their own, because they are without muscle tissue. However, an effective mechanism

## YOU are the Provider

When you arrive at the scene, you find the patient lying on his side on the floor of his bedroom. His knees are drawn up to his abdomen, and he is in severe pain. He also says he feels like he might vomit. As you assess the patient, your partner opens the jump kit and prepares to begin treatment.

| Recording Time:   0 Minutes | |
| --- | --- |
| Appearance | Restless; diaphoretic; in severe pain |
| Level of consciousness | Conscious and alert |
| Airway | Open; clear of secretions and foreign bodies |
| Breathing | Increased rate; adequate depth |
| Circulation | Radial pulses present and strong; skin cool and clammy |

The patient tells you that the pain is in the right upper side of his abdomen and that it began suddenly about 20 minutes ago.

**2.** On the sole basis of the patient's chief complaint, which organ or organs should you suspect is/are the cause of his condition?

**3.** What additional questions should you ask to gather more information about his chief complaint?

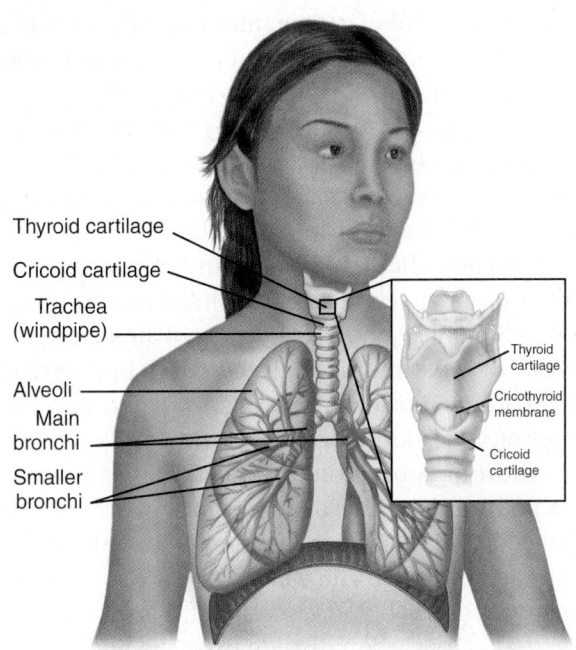

**FIGURE 6-17** The lungs contain millions of air sacs (alveoli), which lie at the ends of air passages. Small blood vessels surround the alveoli, allowing for gas exchange.

© Jones & Bartlett Learning.

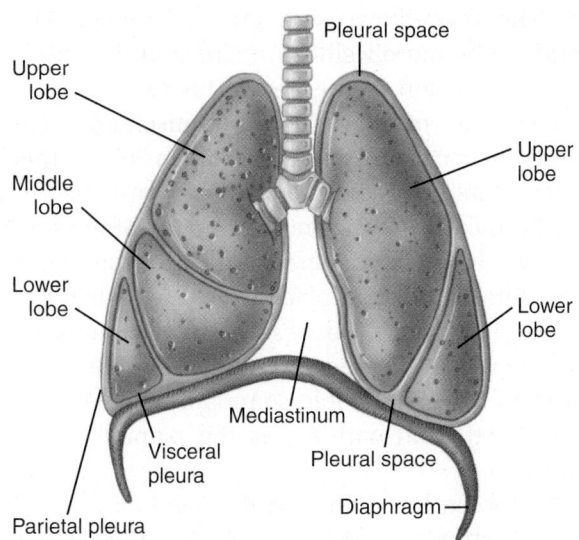

**FIGURE 6-18** The pleura lining the chest wall and covering the lungs is an essential part of the breathing mechanism. The pleural space is not an actual space until blood or air leaks into it, causing the pleural surfaces to separate.

© Jones & Bartlett Learning.

is in place to ensure that the lungs follow the motion of the chest wall, expanding and contracting with it. Covering each lung is a layer of smooth, glistening tissue called **pleura** (**FIGURE 6-18**). Another layer of pleura lines the inside of the chest cavity. The two layers are called visceral pleura (covering the lungs) and parietal pleura (lining the chest wall). Between these two layers is a small amount of fluid that permits smooth gliding of the tissues. This is similar in concept to how joints work.

Between the parietal pleura and the visceral pleura is the **pleural space**, called a potential space because under normal conditions, the space does not exist. These two layers are usually sealed tightly to one another by a thin film of fluid. When the chest wall expands, the lung is pulled with it and made to expand by the force exerted through these closely applied pleural surfaces. When blood or air leaks into the pleural space, however, the surfaces separate.

## Muscles of Breathing

There are several muscles involved in making the lungs expand and contract. The primary muscle of breathing is the **diaphragm**. The diaphragm is

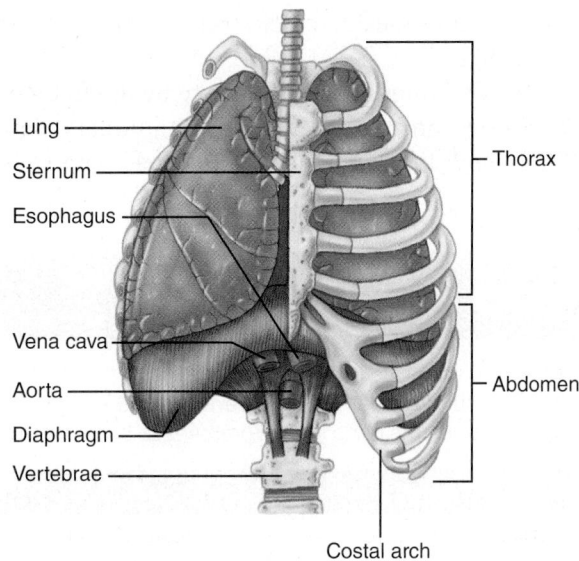

**FIGURE 6-19** The dome-shaped diaphragm divides the thorax from the abdomen. It is pierced by the great vessels and the esophagus.

© Jones & Bartlett Learning.

unique because it has characteristics of voluntary (skeletal) and involuntary (smooth) muscles. It is a dome-shaped muscle that divides the thorax from the abdomen and is pierced by the great vessels and the esophagus (**FIGURE 6-19**). It acts like a voluntary muscle when you take a deep breath, cough, or hold your breath. You control these variations in the way you breathe.

However, unlike other skeletal or voluntary muscles, the diaphragm performs an automatic function. Breathing continues during sleep and at all other times. Even though you can hold your breath or temporarily breathe faster or slower, you cannot continue these variations in breathing pattern indefinitely. When the concentration of carbon dioxide becomes too high, automatic regulation of breathing resumes. Therefore, although the diaphragm looks like voluntary skeletal muscle and is attached to the skeleton, it behaves, for the most part, like an involuntary muscle.

The other muscles involved in breathing are the neck (cervical) muscles, the intercostal muscles, the abdominal muscles, and the pectoral muscles. During inhalation, the diaphragm and intercostal muscles contract. When the diaphragm contracts, it moves down slightly, enlarging the thoracic cage from top to bottom. When the intercostal muscles contract, they move the ribs up and out. These actions combine to enlarge the chest cavity in all dimensions. As the volume of the chest cavity increases, pressure in the cavity falls and air rushes into the lungs. This is referred to as negative-pressure breathing because air is essentially sucked into the lungs. This part of the cycle is active, requiring the muscles to contract.

During exhalation, the diaphragm and the intercostal muscles relax. Unlike inhalation, exhalation does not normally require muscular effort. As these muscles relax, all dimensions of the thorax decrease, and the ribs and muscles assume a normal resting position. When the volume of the chest cavity decreases, air in the lungs is compressed into a smaller space. Pressure is increased, and air is pushed out through the trachea. This phase of the cycle is passive.

The process of breathing is typically easy and requires little muscular effort. But, now imagine breathing through a straw and suddenly the diameter of the straw decreases. The smaller the diameter of the straw, the more effort you will have to exert to move air. As the resistance in the airway increases, you will begin to use accessory muscle groups, namely your abdominal and pectoral muscles, to assist the diaphragm in moving that air.

### Words of Wisdom

When you assess a patient, make sure you assess both sides of the patient. It may seem like a waste of time to assess the left arm when the right arm is the one that is injured. However, you need to compare the sides to see whether there are differences. An abnormality on one arm may be normal if the same abnormality is found on the other arm. This idea of comparing sides applies to the respiratory system as well. You need to listen to both sides of the chest to evaluate the patient's lung sounds. Lung sounds can change on only one side of the chest, or they can change on both sides of the chest. Use all information you obtain from both sides of the body to help you make your patient care decisions.

## The Respiratory System: Physiology

The function of the respiratory system is to provide the body with oxygen and eliminate carbon dioxide. The exchange of oxygen and carbon dioxide takes place in the lungs and in the tissues. It is a complicated process that occurs automatically unless the airways or the lungs become diseased or damaged. There are two separate yet interdependent overall functions of the respiratory system: ventilation and respiration.

**Ventilation** is simply the movement of air between the lungs and the environment. It requires chest rise and fall. You are providing artificial ventilation when you assist a patient who is not breathing with a bag-mask device—a large bag filled with air that, when squeezed, pushes air out one end. The typical device holds approximately 1,000 to 1,200 mL of air. Bag-mask devices are designed to rapidly reinflate and allow you to control the amount of air that is moved to achieve chest rise and fall in any given patient. Artificial ventilation is provided in the hope that your patient will resume respiration. **Respiration** is the process of gas exchange. Respiration provides the much-needed oxygen to cells and removes the waste product carbon dioxide. This exchange of gases also helps to control the pH of the blood.

### Respiration

As blood travels through the body, it delivers oxygen and nutrients to cells. At the capillaries, the oxygen

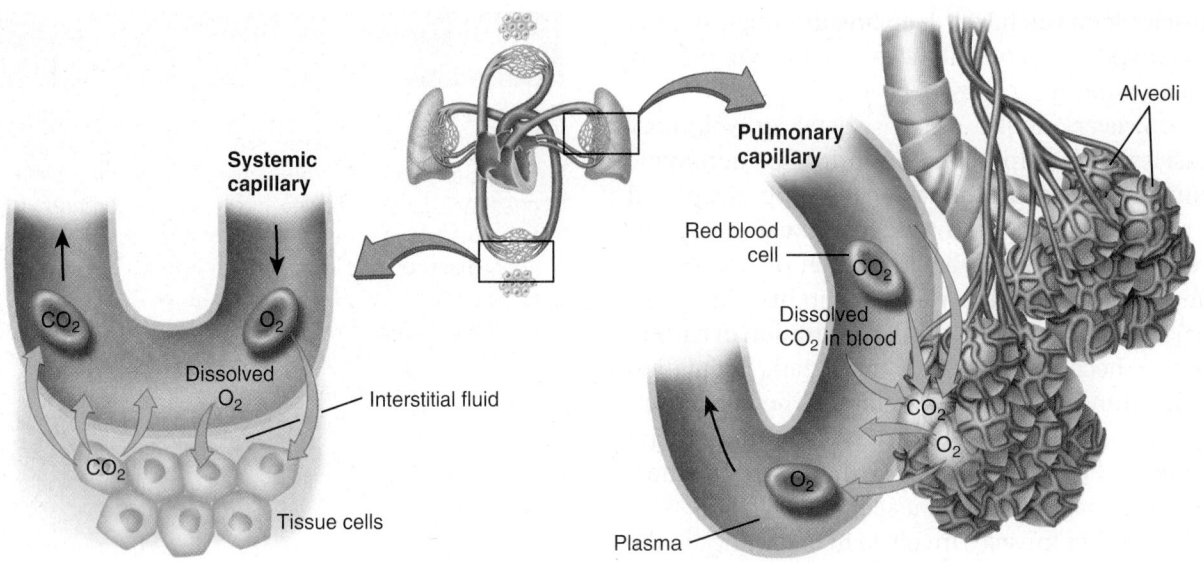

**FIGURE 6-20** In the capillaries, oxygen ($O_2$) passes from the blood to the tissue cells, and carbon dioxide ($CO_2$) and waste pass from the tissue cells to the blood.

© Jones & Bartlett Learning.

is off-loaded from red blood cells. It passes through the thin capillary wall and enters the tissue cells, where it is used to produce energy. Carbon dioxide and cell wastes are transported in the reverse, leaving the cells, crossing the capillary walls, and entering the bloodstream (**FIGURE 6-20**).

Each time you take a breath, the alveoli receive a supply of oxygen-rich air. Recall that the oxygen then passes into a network of pulmonary capillaries, which are located in the walls of the alveoli. The walls of the capillaries and the alveoli are extremely thin. Thus, air in the alveoli and blood in the capillaries are only separated by two thin layers of tissue.

Oxygen and carbon dioxide pass rapidly across these thin tissue layers by diffusion. **Diffusion** is a passive process in which molecules move from an area with a higher concentration of molecules (oxygen in the air) to an area of lower concentration (oxygen in the bloodstream). There are more oxygen molecules in the alveoli than in the blood. Therefore, the oxygen molecules move from the alveoli into the blood. Because there are more carbon dioxide molecules in the blood than in the inhaled air, carbon dioxide moves from the blood into the alveoli. This process is completely passive—nature does all the work.

The blood does not use all the inhaled oxygen as it passes through the body. Exhaled air contains

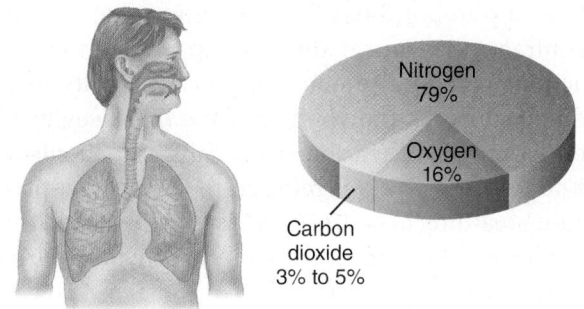

**FIGURE 6-21** The components of exhaled air include oxygen, carbon dioxide, and nitrogen.

© Jones & Bartlett Learning.

16% oxygen and 3% to 5% carbon dioxide; the rest is nitrogen (**FIGURE 6-21**).

## The Chemical Control of Breathing

The brain—specifically, the brainstem—controls breathing. The nerves in this area act as sensors for the level of carbon dioxide in the blood and subsequently the spinal fluid. The brain automatically controls breathing if the level of carbon dioxide or oxygen in the arterial blood is too high or too low. In fact, adjustments can be made in just one breath. For these reasons, you cannot hold your breath indefinitely or breathe rapidly and deeply indefinitely.

Breathing occurs as the result of a buildup of carbon dioxide, which causes the pH to decrease in the **cerebrospinal fluid (CSF)**. CSF is a colorless fluid in and around the brain and spinal cord that cushions these structures and filters out impurities and toxins. The cells are constantly working to eliminate carbon dioxide to regulate the acid–alkaline balance of the body. When the level of carbon dioxide becomes too high, a slight change occurs in the pH (the measure of acidity) of the CSF. The medulla oblongata (a portion of the brainstem), which is sensitive to pH changes, stimulates the phrenic nerve, sending a signal to the diaphragm to increase its rate of contraction. As the diaphragm becomes more active, the respiratory rate and tidal volume increase (discussed later in this chapter). As minute volume increases, more carbon dioxide is exhaled. The primary reason you breathe is to lower your level of carbon dioxide, not to increase your level of oxygen.

The body also has a backup system to control respiration called the **hypoxic drive**. When the oxygen level falls, this system will also stimulate breathing. There are areas in the brain, the walls of the aorta, and the carotid arteries that act as oxygen sensors. These sensors are easily satisfied by minimal levels of oxygen in the arterial blood. Therefore, the backup system, the hypoxic drive, is much less sensitive and less powerful than the carbon dioxide sensors in the brainstem.

## The Nervous System Control of Breathing

The exact way breathing occurs is complicated and also poorly understood by science. It is known that the medulla oblongata is primarily responsible for initiating the ventilation cycle and is primarily stimulated by high carbon dioxide levels. The function of the medulla is to keep you breathing without having to think about it. The medulla helps control the rhythm of breathing, initiates inspiration, sets the base pattern for respirations, and sends signals down the phrenic nerve to the diaphragm, triggering it to contract.

The pons, another area within the brainstem, has two areas, both of which help augment respirations during emotional or physical stress. The pons is involved in changing the depth of inspiration, expiration, or both. The medulla and the pons work together to help you get the right amount of air when you need it. The anatomy and physiology of the nervous system are discussed in more detail later in this chapter.

## Special Populations

The anatomy of the respiratory system in children is proportionally smaller and less rigid than in adults (**FIGURE 6-22**). A child's nose and mouth are much smaller than those of an adult. The larynx, cricoid cartilage, and trachea are smaller, softer, and more flexible as well. This makes the mechanics of breathing much more delicate. A child's pharynx is also smaller and less deeply curved. The tongue takes up proportionally more space in a child's mouth than in an adult's mouth.

These anatomic differences are important for you to understand. For example, the smaller larynx of a child becomes obstructed more easily. The chest wall in children is softer. Therefore, children depend more heavily on the diaphragm for breathing. You will notice that a child's abdomen moves in and out considerably with each breath, especially in an infant. Infants younger than 1 month do not know how to breathe through their mouth. Smaller children also have proportionally larger heads compared with the rest of their body. This will affect the way you treat a suspected spinal injury. Carefully consider these differences as you assess and treat an infant or a child.

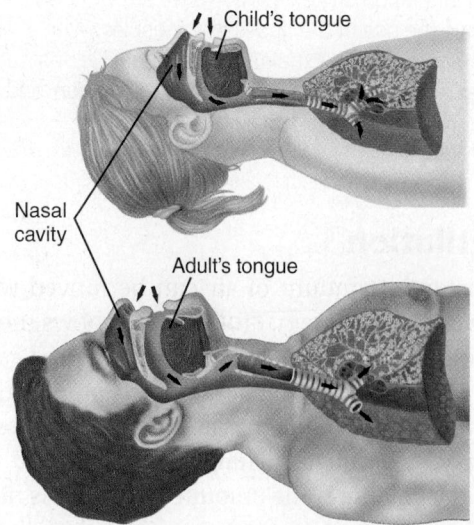

**FIGURE 6-22** The respiratory system of a child is proportionally smaller and less rigid than that of an adult.

## Special Populations

Normal breathing patterns in infants and children are essentially the same as those in adults. However, infants and children breathe faster than adults. An infant who is breathing normally will have respirations of 30 to 60 breaths/min. A child will have respirations of 12 to 40 breaths/min. Like adults, infants and children who are breathing normally will have smooth, regular inhalation and exhalation, equal breath sounds, and regular rise and fall movements on both sides of the chest.

Breathing problems in infants and children often appear the same as breathing problems in adults. Signs such as increased respirations, an irregular breathing pattern, unequal breath sounds, and unequal chest expansion indicate breathing problems in adults and children. Other signs that an infant or child is not breathing normally include the following:

- Muscle retractions, in which the muscles of the chest and neck are working extra hard in breathing
- Nasal flaring, in which the nostrils flare out as the child breathes
- Seesaw respirations in infants, in which the chest and abdominal muscles alternately contract to look like a seesaw
- Grunting with each exhalation to keep the small airways open

Exhalation becomes active when infants and children have trouble breathing. Normally, inhalation alone is the active, muscular part of breathing, as described earlier. However, with labored breathing, both inhalation and exhalation are hard work and involve the use of the accessory muscles. With labored breathing, exhalation is not passive. Instead, air is forced out of the lungs during exhalation, and the child will often begin to wheeze.

## Ventilation

A substantial amount of air can be moved within the respiratory system. **FIGURE 6-23** shows the typical volumes. An adult man has a total lung capacity of 6,000 mL (equivalent to three 2-liter bottles of soda). An adult woman has about one-third less total capacity because the lung size is smaller.

**Tidal volume** is the amount of air that is moved into or out of the lungs during a single breath, generally 500 mL in an adult. **Inspiratory reserve volume** is the deepest breath you can take after a normal breath. Conversely, **expiratory reserve volume** is

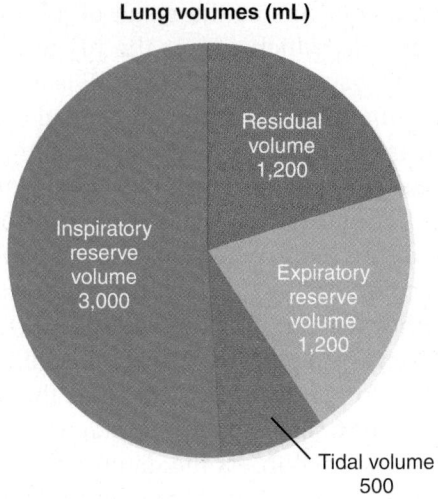

Lung volumes (mL)

**FIGURE 6-23** Lung volumes.

© Jones & Bartlett Learning.

the maximum amount of air that you can forcibly breathe out after a normal breath. Gas remains in the lungs after exhalation simply to keep the lungs open. This is the **residual volume**. A loss of residual volume occurs when a person is hit in the chest and has the "wind knocked out" of him or her.

**Dead space** is the portion of the respiratory system that has no alveoli, and, therefore, little or no exchange of gas between air and blood occurs. The mouth, trachea, bronchi, and bronchioles are all considered dead space. When you ventilate a patient with any device, you create more dead space. Gas must first fill the device before it can be moved into the patient.

When you assess your patient, you need to accurately determine whether he or she is having trouble breathing. Often, EMTs will look at the patient's respiratory rate; this rate, however, provides only part of the information that is needed. The depth of each breath is critical information to know when assessing ventilation. **Minute volume** is another measure used to assess ventilation; it is the amount of air that moves in and out of the lungs in 1 minute.

$$\text{Minute Volume} = \text{Respiratory Rate} \times \text{Tidal Volume}$$

This calculation helps you to determine if a patient is breathing adequately. While riding in the ambulance it will be difficult to determine the patient's exact tidal volume, but you will be able to estimate it. Consider the scenario of a patient who is breathing at a normal rate of 20 breaths/min. Yet, when you look at the patient's chest, it is barely moving. When you feel for air movement out of the mouth, you find very little movement. The patient is in trouble and needs your assistance now! Even though the patient's respiratory rate is normal, the amount of air being moved is inadequate. The minute volume is too low, and the patient needs ventilatory assistance. Always evaluate the amount of air being moved with each breath when assessing a patient's respirations.

## Characteristics of Normal Breathing

You can think of a normal breathing pattern as a bellows system. Normal breathing should appear easy, not labored. As with a bellows that is used to move air to start a fire, breathing should be a smooth flow of air moving into and out of the lungs.

Normal breathing has the following characteristics:

- A normal rate and depth (tidal volume)
- A regular rhythm or pattern of inhalation and exhalation
- Clear, audible breath sounds on both sides of the chest
- Regular rise and fall movement on both sides of the chest
- Movement of the abdomen

## Inadequate Breathing in Adults

An awake and alert adult speaking to you in full sentences, usually has no immediate airway or breathing problem. An adult who is not breathing well may appear to be working hard to breathe. Labored breathing is characterized by significant effort and may require the use of accessory muscles in the chest, neck, and abdomen. The person may also be breathing much slower (fewer than 12 breaths/min) or much faster (more than 20 breaths/min) than normal. An adult at rest who is breathing normally will have respirations of 12 to 20 breaths/min (**TABLE 6-4**).

Other signs that a person is not breathing normally include the following:

- Muscle retractions above the clavicles, between the ribs, and below the rib cage, especially in children

**TABLE 6-4** Normal Respiratory Rate Ranges

| | |
|---|---|
| Adults | 12 to 20 breaths/min |
| Children | 12 to 40 breaths/min |
| Infants | 30 to 60 breaths/min |

Data adapted from *Pediatric Advanced Life Support*, 2012, the American Heart Association.

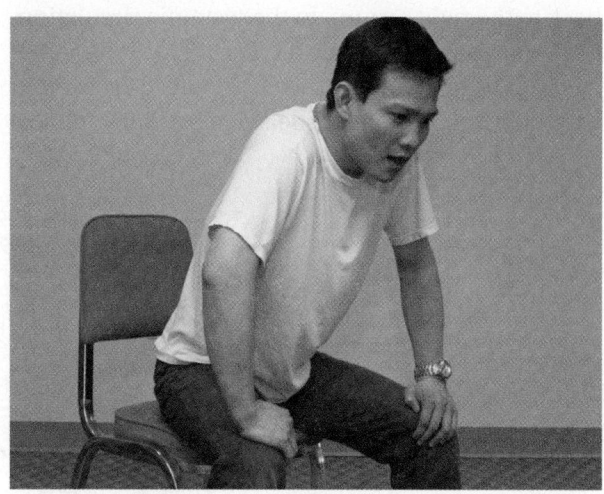

**FIGURE 6-24** A patient in the tripod position will sit leaning forward on outstretched arms with the head and chin thrust slightly forward.

© Jones & Bartlett Learning. Courtesy of MIEMSS.

- Pale or cyanotic (blue) skin
- Cool, damp (clammy) skin
- Tripod position (**FIGURE 6-24**), a position in which the patient leans forward onto two arms

A patient in cardiac arrest may appear to be breathing. These occasional, gasping breaths are called agonal gasps and occur when the respiratory center in the brain continues to send signals to the breathing muscles. However, these gasps are inadequate because they come at a slow rate and are generally shallow. Patients with agonal gasps need artificial ventilations and, most likely, chest compressions. Both topics will be discussed in later chapters.

## The Circulatory System: Anatomy

The circulatory system is a complex arrangement of connected tubes, including the arteries, arterioles, capillaries, venules, and veins (**FIGURE 6-25**). Another name for this system is the cardiovascular (heart/blood vessels) system. The circulatory system is entirely closed, with capillaries connecting arterioles and venules. There are two circuits in the body: the systemic circulation in the body and the pulmonary circulation in the lungs. The systemic circulation, the circuit in the body, carries oxygen-rich blood from the left ventricle through the body and back to the right atrium. In the systemic circulation, as blood passes through the tissues and organs, it gives up oxygen and nutrients and absorbs cellular wastes and carbon dioxide. Many cellular wastes

are eliminated in passages through the liver and kidneys. The pulmonary circulation, the circuit in the lungs, carries oxygen-poor blood from the right ventricle through the lungs and back to the left atrium. In the pulmonary circulation, as blood passes through the lungs, it is refreshed with oxygen and gives up carbon dioxide.

## The Heart

The **heart** is a hollow muscular organ approximately the size of a clenched fist. It is made of a specialized muscle tissue called cardiac muscle or **myocardium**

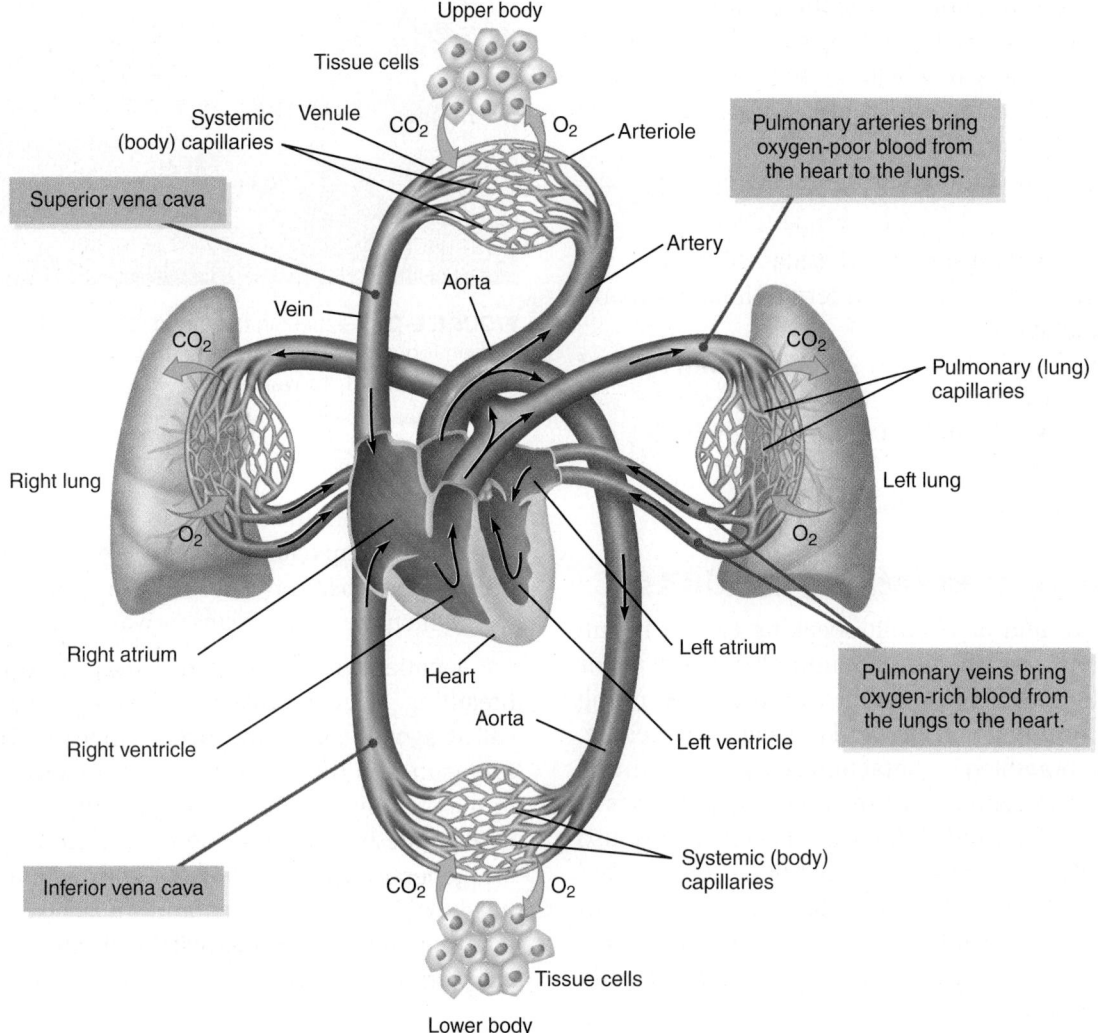

**FIGURE 6-25** The circulatory system includes the heart, arteries, veins, and interconnecting capillaries. The capillaries are the smallest vessels and connect venules and arterioles. At the center of the system, and providing its driving force, is the heart. Blood circulates through the body under pressure generated by the two sides of the heart.

and works as two paired pumps; the left side is more muscular. A wall called the septum divides the heart down the middle into right and left sides. Each side of the heart is divided again into an upper chamber (atrium) and a lower chamber (ventricle). The left side of the heart, which pumps blood to the body, is a high-pressure pump; the right side supplies blood to the lungs and is a low-pressure pump.

The heart is an involuntary muscle. As such, it is under the control of the autonomic nervous system. However, it has its own electrical system and continues to function even without its central nervous system control. It is also unlike skeletal and smooth muscle in its requirement for a continuous supply of oxygen and nutrients, as it cannot function on anaerobic metabolism.

The heart must function continuously from birth to death and has developed special adaptations to meet the needs of this continuous function. It can tolerate a serious interruption of its own blood supply for only a few seconds before the signs of a heart attack develop. Thus, its blood supply is rich and well distributed.

## Circulation

The heart muscle's blood supply comes from the aorta. The aorta has two branches at its base that form the left and right coronary arteries. These arteries supply the heart muscle with oxygenated blood (**FIGURE 6-26**).

The right side of the heart receives blood from the veins of the body (**FIGURE 6-27A**). The blood enters from the superior and inferior venae cavae into the right atrium and then passes through the tricuspid valve to fill the right ventricle. After the right ventricle is filled, the tricuspid valve closes to prevent backflow as the right ventricular muscle contracts. Contraction of the right ventricle causes blood to flow through the pulmonic valve into the pulmonary artery and the pulmonary circulation.

The left side receives oxygenated blood from the lungs through the pulmonary veins into the left atrium, where the blood passes through the mitral valve into the left ventricle (**FIGURE 6-27B**). Contraction of this most muscular of the pumping chambers pumps the blood through the aortic valve into the aorta and then to the arteries of the body.

The flow of blood through the four heart chambers is governed by one-way valves. The valves prevent the backflow of blood and keep it moving through the circulatory system in the proper direction. The chordae tendineae are thin bands of fibrous tissue that attach to the valves in the heart and prevent them from inverting. When a valve controlling the filling of a heart chamber is open, the other valve allowing it to empty is shut, and vice versa. Normally, blood moves in only one direction through the entire system.

## Normal Heartbeat

In the normal adult, the resting heartbeat may range from 60 to 100 beats/min. A well-conditioned athlete may have a normal resting heart rate (HR) of 45 to 60 beats/min. During vigorous physical activity, the heart rate may rise to as fast as 180 beats/min until the activity stops. At each beat, 70 to 80 mL of blood is ejected from the adult heart. The amount of blood moved in one beat is called the stroke volume (SV). In 1 minute, the entire blood volume of 5 to 6 L is circulated through all the vessels. The amount of blood moved in 1 minute is called the cardiac output (CO). Cardiac output is equal to heart rate times stroke volume. Mathematically, cardiac output can be expressed as follows:

$$CO = HR \times SV$$

For example: 70 beats/min $\times$ 75 mL/beat = 5,250 mL/min or 5.25 L/min.

## Electrical Conduction System

A network of specialized tissue with the capacity to conduct electrical current runs throughout the heart. The flow of electrical current through this network causes smooth, coordinated contractions of the heart. These contractions produce the pumping action of the heart. Each mechanical contraction of the heart is associated with two electrical processes. The first is depolarization, during which the electrical charges on the surface of the muscle cell change from positive to negative. The second is repolarization, during which the heart returns to its resting state and the positive charge is restored to the surface.

When the heart is working normally, the electrical impulse begins high in the atria at the sinoatrial node, then travels to the atrioventricular node and bundle of His, and moves through the Purkinje fibers to the ventricles. This movement produces a

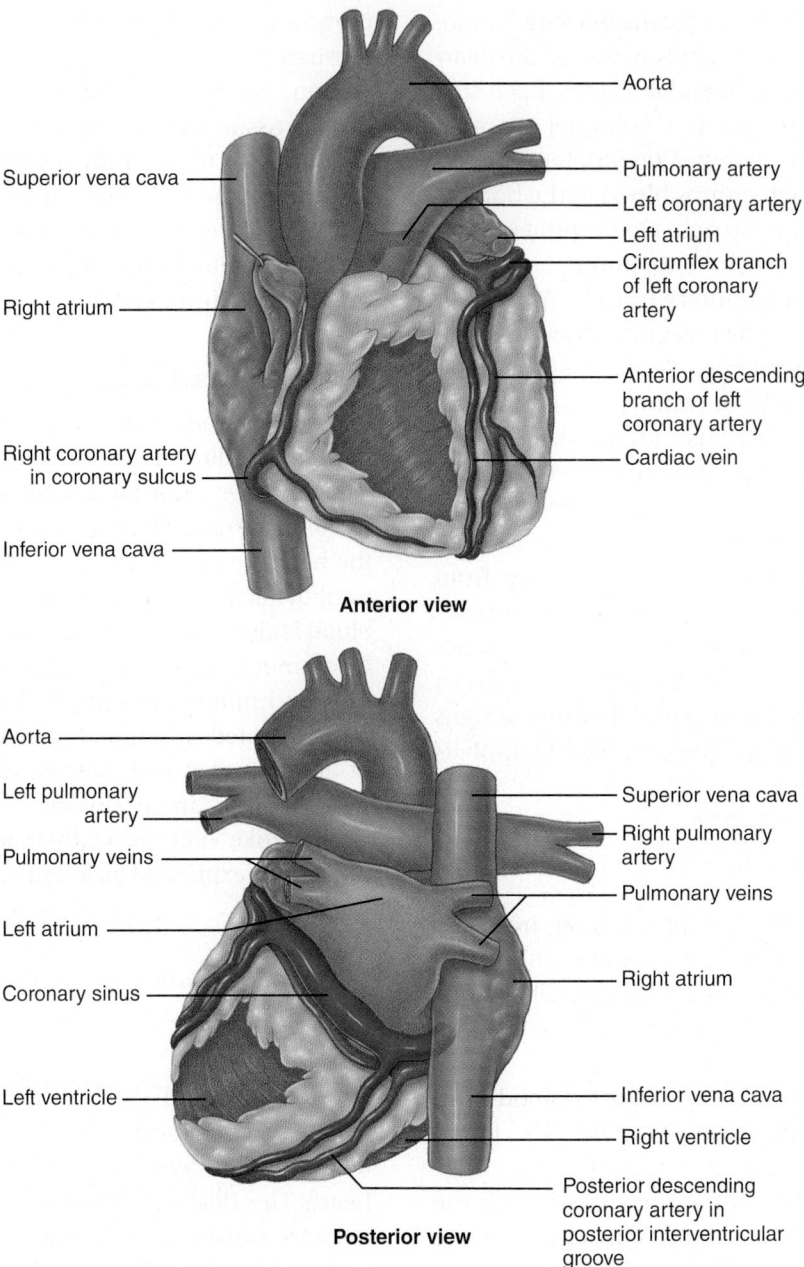

**FIGURE 6-26** Two main coronary arteries supply the heart with blood.

smooth flow of electricity through the heart, which depolarizes the muscle and produces a coordinated pumping contraction. Just as the walls of the heart can be injured when deprived of blood flow and oxygen, if areas of the heart's conduction system are deprived of blood flow and oxygen, serious abnormalities of the heart's rate, rhythm, and coordinated contraction can occur. Simply put, when the conduction system is injured, the heart will not beat properly. This may lead to dangerously low blood pressure, which, if untreated, can result in the patient experiencing a loss of consciousness or cardiac arrest. Blood pressure is discussed later in the chapter.

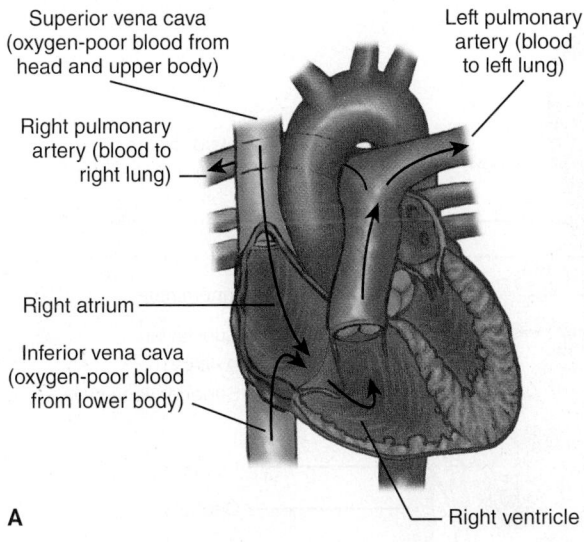

- Superior vena cava (oxygen-poor blood from head and upper body)
- Left pulmonary artery (blood to left lung)
- Right pulmonary artery (blood to right lung)
- Right atrium
- Inferior vena cava (oxygen-poor blood from lower body)
- Right ventricle

**A**

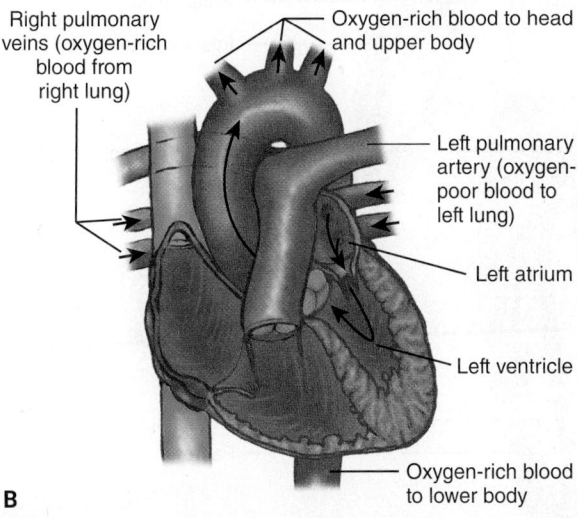

- Right pulmonary veins (oxygen-rich blood from right lung)
- Oxygen-rich blood to head and upper body
- Left pulmonary artery (oxygen-poor blood to left lung)
- Left atrium
- Left ventricle
- Oxygen-rich blood to lower body

**B**

**FIGURE 6-27 A.** The right (lower pressure) side of the heart pumps blood from the body through the lungs. **B.** The left (higher-pressure) side of the heart pumps oxygen-rich blood to the rest of the body.

© Jones & Bartlett Learning.

## Words of Wisdom

Many of the abnormal cardiac rhythms associated with cardiac arrest can be effectively treated with defibrillation. Therefore, any patient in cardiac arrest should have an AED applied as soon as possible.

## Arteries

The arteries carry blood from the heart to all body tissues (**FIGURE 6-28**). They branch into smaller arteries and then into arterioles. The arterioles, in turn, branch into the vast network of capillaries. The walls of an artery are made of fine, circular muscle tissue. Some arteries are made of fine circular muscle and elastic tissue.

Arteries contract to accommodate loss of blood volume and increase blood pressure. Blood is supplied to tissues as they need it. For example, the digestive system is supplied with more blood after you eat a meal. The leg muscles are more heavily supplied when jogging. Some tissues need a constant blood supply, especially the heart, kidneys, and brain. Other tissues, such as the muscles in the extremities, the skin, and intestines, can function with less blood when at rest. The ability to respond to the needs of the body is possible because of the way arteries are constructed. The middle layer of the artery is the **tunica media**, formed from smooth muscles that can contract and dilate to change the diameter of the blood vessel.

The **aorta** is the main artery leaving the back left side of the heart; it carries freshly oxygenated blood to the body. This blood vessel is found just in front of the spine in the chest and abdominal cavities. The aorta has many branches that supply the body's vital organs. The coronary arteries supply the heart; the carotid arteries supply the head; the hepatic arteries supply the liver; the renal arteries supply the kidneys; and the mesenteric arteries supply the digestive system. The aorta divides at the level of the umbilicus into the two common iliac arteries that lead to the lower extremities. All branches of the aorta ultimately become arterioles leading into the body's capillary network.

The **pulmonary artery** begins at the right side of the heart and carries oxygen-depleted blood to the lungs. It divides into finer and finer branches until it meets with the pulmonary capillary system located in the thin walls of the alveoli. These arteries are the only ones in the body that carry oxygen-depleted blood.

Arteries branch into smaller arteries and then into arterioles. **Arterioles** are the smallest branches of an artery leading to the vast network of capillaries.

**Major arteries**

**Major veins**

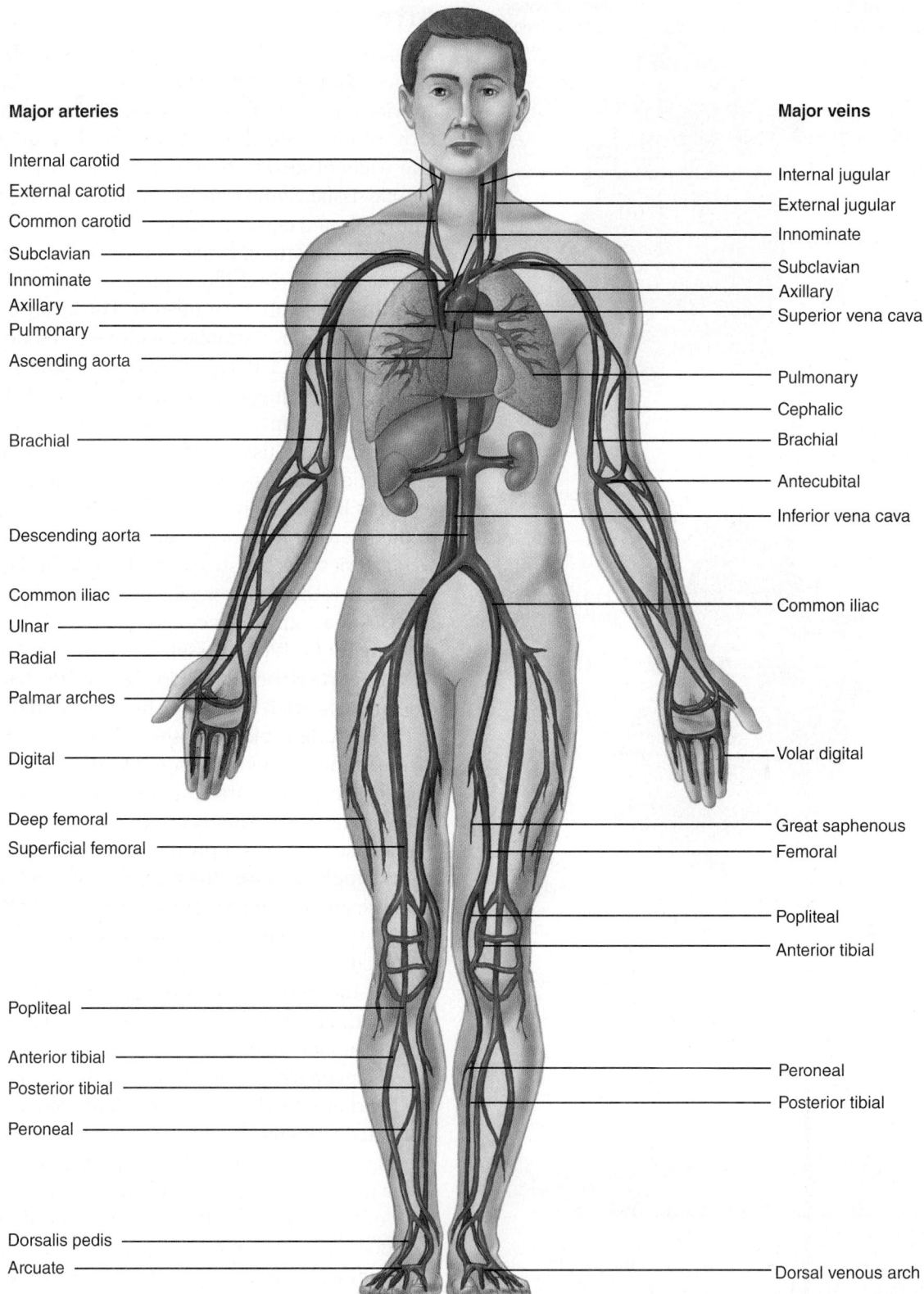

Internal carotid
External carotid
Common carotid
Subclavian
Innominate
Axillary
Pulmonary
Ascending aorta

Brachial

Descending aorta

Common iliac
Ulnar
Radial
Palmar arches

Digital

Deep femoral
Superficial femoral

Popliteal

Anterior tibial
Posterior tibial

Peroneal

Dorsalis pedis
Arcuate

Internal jugular
External jugular
Innominate
Subclavian
Axillary
Superior vena cava

Pulmonary
Cephalic
Brachial
Antecubital
Inferior vena cava

Common iliac

Volar digital

Great saphenous
Femoral

Popliteal
Anterior tibial

Peroneal
Posterior tibial

Dorsal venous arch

**FIGURE 6-28** The main arteries supply blood to a vast network of smaller arteries and arterioles. Venules deliver oxygen-poor blood to the veins that return blood to the heart.

The **pulse**, which is palpated most easily at the neck, wrist, or groin, is created by the forceful pumping of blood out of the left ventricle and into the major arteries. It is present throughout the entire arterial system. It can be felt most easily where the larger arteries near the skin can be pushed against a solid structure, such as a bone or large muscle (**FIGURE 6-29**). Pulses and their locations are listed in **TABLE 6-5**.

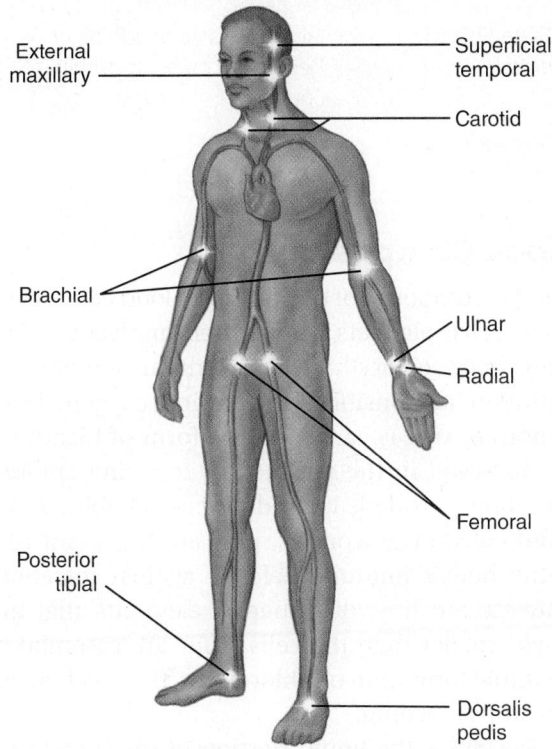

External maxillary

Superficial temporal

Carotid

Brachial

Ulnar

Radial

Femoral

Posterior tibial

Dorsalis pedis

**FIGURE 6-29** The central and peripheral pulses can be felt where the large arteries are near the skin.

© Jones & Bartlett Learning.

## Capillaries

In the body, there are billions of cells and billions of capillaries. **Capillary vessels** are fragile divisions of the arterial system that allow contact between the blood and the cells of the tissues. Oxygen and other nutrients pass from blood cells and plasma in the capillaries to the individual tissue cells through the thin wall of the capillary. Carbon dioxide and other metabolic waste products pass in a reverse direction from the tissue cells to the blood to be carried away. Blood in arteries is characteristically bright red, because its hemoglobin is rich in oxygen. Blood in the veins is dark blue-red, because it has passed through a capillary bed and given up its oxygen to the cells. Capillaries connect directly at one end with the flow-regulating arterioles and at the other with the venules.

Capillaries allow blood to move through them a single cell at a time.

## Veins

Once oxygen-depleted blood passes through the network of capillaries, it moves to the venules, which are the smallest branches of the veins. The blood returns to the heart via a network of larger and larger veins. Veins have much thinner walls than arteries and are generally larger in diameter. The veins become larger and larger and ultimately form two major vessels, called the superior and inferior venae cavae. These two veins lie just to the right of the spine and collect blood just before it enters the heart. Because pressure generated by the

| **TABLE 6-5** Pulses | | |
|---|---|---|
| **Central Versus Peripheral** | **Pulse Name** | **Location Where Felt** |
| Central pulses | **Carotid artery** pulse | At the upper portion of the neck |
| | **Femoral artery** pulse | In the groin |
| Peripheral pulses | **Radial artery** pulse | At the wrist at the base of the thumb |
| | **Brachial artery** pulse | On the medial aspect of the arm, midway between the elbow and shoulder |
| | **Posterior tibial artery** pulse | Posterior to the medial malleolus |
| | **Dorsalis pedis artery** pulse | On the top of the foot |

© Jones & Bartlett Learning.

heart dissipates as blood passes through the capillaries, venous blood flow is assisted by gravity, skeletal muscle contraction, and intrathoracic pressure changes from breathing. One-way flow in the veins is governed by valves within the veins.

The **superior vena cava** carries blood returning from the head, neck, shoulders, and upper extremities. Blood from the abdomen, pelvis, and lower extremities passes through the **inferior vena cava**. The superior and inferior venae cavae join at the right atrium of the heart. The right ventricle receives blood from the right atrium and pumps it through the pulmonary arteries into the lungs. The venae cavae, aorta, and pulmonary arteries and veins are collectively known as the great vessels.

Recall that the body's ability to change blood flow is critical to survival. The body constricts blood vessels to change the size of the total blood volume container. A smaller container that has the same amount of liquid as the original container means a higher liquid pressure.

The state of the blood vessels—how dilated or constricted they are—is referred to as the **systemic vascular resistance (SVR)**. SVR is the resistance to blood flow within all blood vessels except the pulmonary vessels. The pathophysiology section of this chapter will discuss how various types of shock affect container size. In some types of shock, blood vessels dilate, the container becomes too large, and the patient's blood pressure falls dramatically (**TABLE 6-6**).

**TABLE 6-6** Effects of Blood Vessel Diameter on Blood

| State | Effects |
|---|---|
| Constricted blood vessel | Decreased size of container<br>Increased pressure within container |
| Normal diameter | Balance of size and pressure |
| Dilated blood vessel | Increased size of container<br>Decreased pressure within container |

© Jones & Bartlett Learning.

## Blood Composition

Blood is composed of plasma, red blood cells, white blood cells, platelets, and protein molecules. **Red blood cells**, or erythrocytes, contain **hemoglobin**, a protein responsible for carrying oxygen. Most carbon dioxide is carried in the form of bicarbonate dissolved in the plasma, while a tiny amount of carbon dioxide is carried by hemoglobin. **White blood cells**, or leukocytes, play an important role in the body's immune defense against infection. **Platelets** are tiny, disc-shaped elements that are much smaller than the cells. They are essential in the initial formation of a blood clot, the mechanism that stops bleeding.

**Plasma** is the liquid portion of the blood that carries the blood cells, hormones, and nutrients.

## YOU are the Provider

Your partner obtains and records the patient's vital signs and then gives him supplemental oxygen while you complete your assessment. The patient tells you he has a history of gallbladder problems. Based on your assessment and the patient's medical history, you suspect that the gallbladder is the origin of his pain.

| Recording Time: 2 Minutes | |
|---|---|
| **Respirations** | 24 breaths/min; adequate depth |
| **Pulse** | 110 beats/min; strong and regular |
| **Skin** | Pink, warm, and moist |
| **Blood pressure** | 142/82 mm Hg |
| **Oxygen saturation (Spo$_2$)** | 98% |

**4.** What additional symptoms would you expect the patient to experience based on the function of the gallbladder?

About 99% of its composition is water and proteins. Its composition can be broken down as follows:

- **Water:** Constitutes 92% of plasma.
- **Proteins:** Constitute 7% of the plasma. The majority of this protein is albumin, which has a role in controlling the movement of water into and out of the circulation. Also include clotting factors, enzymes, and some hormones.
- **Oxygen:** Very little oxygen is dissolved in the plasma; most is bound to the hemoglobin found in red blood cells.
- **Carbon dioxide:** Transported as bicarbonate in the plasma.
- **Nitrogen:** Accounting for roughly 78% of the air we breathe, this gas is dissolved within the plasma.
- **Nutrients:** Fuel for the cells.
- **Cellular wastes:** Lactic acid, carbon dioxide, etc.
- **Others:** Hormones, other cellular products.

## The Spleen

The spleen is a solid organ located under the rib cage in the left upper quadrant of the abdomen. Although it is a lymphatic organ, it plays an important supportive role for the circulatory system. Red blood cells have a life span of about 120 days. As they age and degrade, they are filtered from the bloodstream and digested in the spleen and liver. Hemoglobin is then recycled.

Because its tissue is delicate and due to its position directly under flexible ribs (with very little soft tissue to cushion it), the spleen is one of the most frequently injured abdominal organs after blunt trauma. And because it is so highly vascular, an injured spleen can produce significant internal bleeding.

## The Circulatory System: Physiology

**Blood pressure (BP)** is the force of circulating blood against the walls of the arteries. This pressure wave keeps the blood moving through the body. When the left ventricle of the heart contracts, it pumps blood into the aorta. This phase in the cardiac cycle is called **systole**. The pressure inside the arteries during this time is referred to as the systolic blood pressure. The time between contractions when the ventricle is relaxed and refilling with blood is called **diastole**. The resting pressure in the arteries during this phase is the diastolic blood pressure. The values of the systolic and diastolic pressures are measured with a **sphygmomanometer** (blood pressure cuff) and are expressed numerically in millimeters of mercury (mm Hg). Blood pressure is displayed as the systolic number over the diastolic number. Additional cardiovascular values of importance are shown in **TABLE 6-7**.

The average adult has approximately 6 L of blood. Children have 2 to 3 L, depending on age and size. Infants have about 300 mL. Thus, while the loss of a relatively small amount of blood might be insignificant for an adult, an equal amount of blood loss in an infant could be fatal.

## Normal Circulation in Adults

In all healthy people, the circulatory system is automatically adjusted and readjusted constantly so that 100% of the capacity of the arteries, veins, and capillaries holds 100% of the blood at that moment. All of the vessels are never fully dilated or constricted. The size of arteries and veins is controlled by the nervous system, according to the amount of blood that is available and many other factors, to keep blood pressure normal at all times. Under the condition of normal pressure, with a system that can hold just 100% of the blood available, all parts of the system will have adequate blood supply all the time.

**Perfusion** is the circulation of blood in an organ or tissue. When perfusion is adequate, the cells' metabolic needs are met. Blood enters an organ or tissue through the arteries and leaves it through the veins (**FIGURE 6-30**). Loss of normal blood pressure is an indication that blood is no longer circulating efficiently to every organ in the body. (However, a "good blood pressure" does not indicate that it is reaching all parts of the body.) There are many

---

### Words of Wisdom

When multiple systems are affected (ie, systemic), the terms *shock* and *hypoperfusion* may be used interchangeably. However, hypoperfusion can also be limited to a specific region of the body, such as an arm, perhaps from an arterial occlusion (blockage). By contrast, shock is always systemic. In short, shock is a state of *systemic* hypoperfusion.

**TABLE 6-7** Cardiovascular Values

| Name | Description | Comments/Notes |
|---|---|---|
| Systolic blood pressure | Pressure within the arteries when the heart is contracting; left ventricular force | Indicates heart pumping effectiveness<br>Indicates blood available to the heart |
| Diastolic blood pressure | Pressure within the arteries when the heart is at rest | Indicates adequate cardiac relaxation and pressure in the arteries between heartbeats<br>Indicates amount of blood within blood vessels |
| Pulse pressure | Difference between systolic blood pressure and diastolic blood pressure | Relationship between systolic and diastolic pressures; provides information about the body's response to stress |
| Preload | Amount of blood returning to the heart | Too little preload and blood pressure falls<br>Too high preload and the heart cannot move blood effectively |
| Afterload | Pressure to be overcome when left ventricle contracts (pressure within the aorta) | Diastolic pressure is the same as afterload |
| Stroke volume (SV) | Amount of blood moved with one contraction of the heart (left ventricle) | Weak left ventricle moves less blood per beat than a strong left ventricle |
| Cardiac output (CO) | Amount of blood moved in 1 minute | $CO = SV \times HR$ |
| Systemic vascular resistance (SVR) | Resistance to blood flow within all of the blood vessels (excluding the pulmonary vessels) | The higher the SVR, the smaller the container; therefore, the higher the pressure of blood within the vessel |

© Jones & Bartlett Learning.

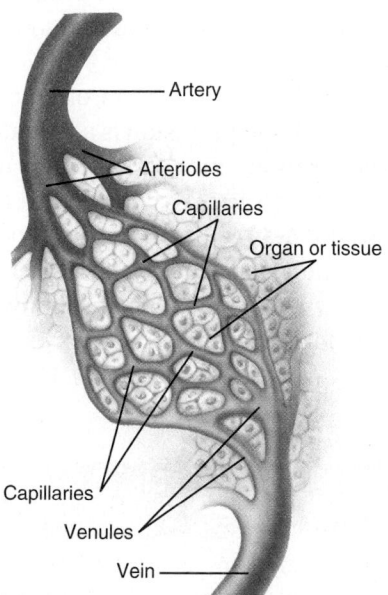

**FIGURE 6-30** Blood enters an organ or tissue through the arteries and leaves through the veins. This process, called perfusion, provides adequate blood flow to the tissue to meet the cells' needs.

© Jones & Bartlett Learning.

reasons for loss of blood pressure. The result in each case is the same: Organs, tissues, and cells are no longer adequately perfused or supplied with oxygen and fuel, and wastes accumulate. Under these conditions, cells, tissues, and whole organs may die. **Hypoperfusion** (inadequate perfusion) affecting the entire body is called **shock**.

## Inadequate Circulation in Adults

When a patient has a small amount of blood loss, the arteries, veins, and heart automatically adjust to the smaller volume. The adjustment occurs to maintain adequate pressure throughout the circulatory system and maintain circulation for every organ. The adjustment occurs rapidly after the loss, usually within minutes. Specifically, the vessels constrict to provide a smaller bed for the reduced volume of blood to fill, and the heart pumps more rapidly to circulate the remaining blood more efficiently. As the blood pressure falls, the pulse increases to keep the cardiac output constant at 5 to 6 L per minute. If the loss of blood is too great, the adjustment fails, and the patient goes into shock. One measure of perfusion that can detect shock and that is often displayed on automated blood pressure monitors is mean arterial pressure (MAP). The mean arterial pressure indicates the average arterial pressure during systole and diastole. This can be expressed by the following formula, in which MAP is mean arterial pressure, HR is heart rate, SV is stroke volume, and SVR is systemic vascular resistance:

$$MAP = (HR \times SV) \times SVR$$

Since heart rate (HR) times stroke volume (SV) equals cardiac output (CO), this can also be written as:

$$MAP = CO \times SVR$$

**FIGURE 6-31** illustrates this formula.

## The Function of Blood

Most blood is unevenly distributed throughout the body. Approximately 30% of blood is found within the heart, arteries, and capillaries. Seventy percent of blood is found within the veins and venules. This may seem confusing, but if you remember that the heart and arteries are high-pressure systems and veins are low-pressure systems, it becomes clearer. As blood pressure falls, blood flow slows down and there is more blood in the veins. The blood flows away from the left ventricle and moves back to the right atria.

Consider the movement of blood and its ultimate function of perfusion. You know that capillaries are the smallest portions of the circulatory system, where materials are able to exit and enter the bloodstream. Nutrients move from the capillaries into the **interstitial space** (space between the cells) and into the **intracellular space** (within the cell). Wastes move from the cells through the interstitial space and into the capillaries.

Inside the capillary, two main forces are at work: hydrostatic pressure and oncotic pressure. **Hydrostatic pressure** occurs as fluid pushes against the vessel walls to force fluid out of the capillary. **Oncotic pressure** is the opposing force and occurs because proteins in the blood plasma cause water to be pulled into the capillary by diffusion.

The movement of fluid into and out of the capillaries occurs as follows. Blood flows into the arterial

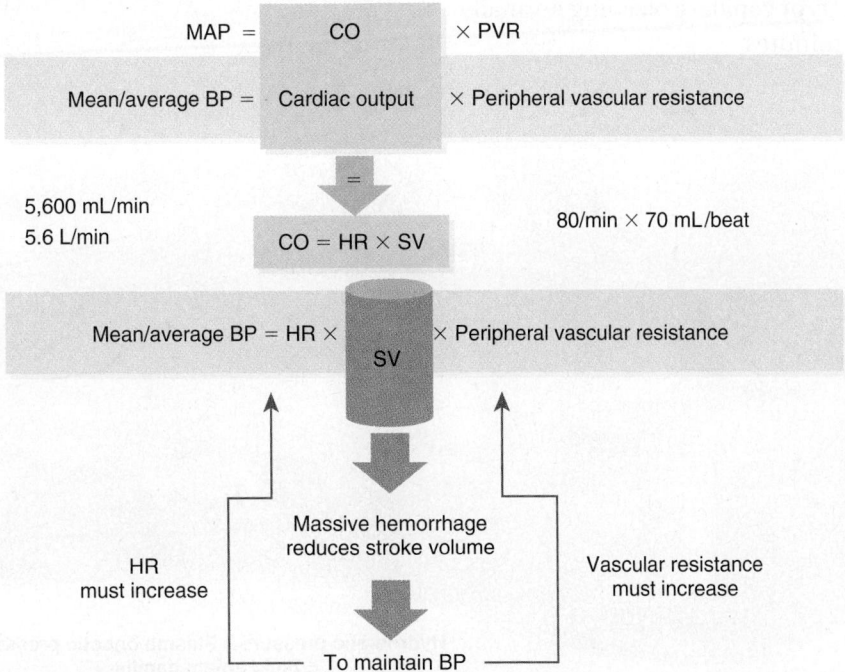

**FIGURE 6-31** Significant blood loss results in reduced stroke volume (SV). To compensate, the body increases heart rate (HR) and systemic vascular resistance to maintain mean arterial pressure (MAP).

side of the capillary. Water is forced out because the pressure is high. At the same time, water is trying to enter the capillary. Pressure on the arterial side is higher, so the hydrostatic pressure is also higher, and water, carrying nutrients, leaves the capillary and enters the interstitial space. The hydrostatic pressure is greatly diminished, however, by the time the fluid reaches the venous side because the effort of pushing the fluid out of the capillary decreased its force. This decrease in pressure is beneficial because oncotic pressure is still pulling fluid into the capillary and the pressure is higher. Water, with all of the wastes from the cells, enters the venous side of the capillary. These wastes are then carried away (**FIGURE 6-32**).

Another function of blood is the ability to clot. Coagulation, or clotting, occurs as the result of a complex chemical process that creates small fibers near the injured blood vessel, trapping red blood cells. This chemical process involves platelets and clotting factors that are in the bloodstream. **TABLE 6-8** outlines the major functions of the blood.

Blood under pressure will gush or spurt intermittently from an artery. When blood comes from a vein, it flows in a steady stream. From capillaries, blood will ooze at many tiny individual points. Clotting after venous or capillary bleeding normally takes from 6 to 10 minutes.

## Nervous System Control of the Cardiovascular System

The nervous system, discussed next, has direct effects on the cardiovascular system. The sympathetic nervous system sends commands to the adrenal glands (which sit atop the kidneys) where two

**TABLE 6-8** Functions of the Blood and the Components of Blood in Use

| Function | Component of the Blood in Use |
|---|---|
| Fights infection | White blood cells |
| Transports oxygen | Red blood cells (hemoglobin) |
| Transports carbon dioxide | Plasma |
| Controls (buffers) pH | Chemicals within the plasma |
| Transports wastes and nutrients | Plasma (water) |
| Clotting (coagulation) | Platelets and clotting factors in the plasma |

© Jones & Bartlett Learning.

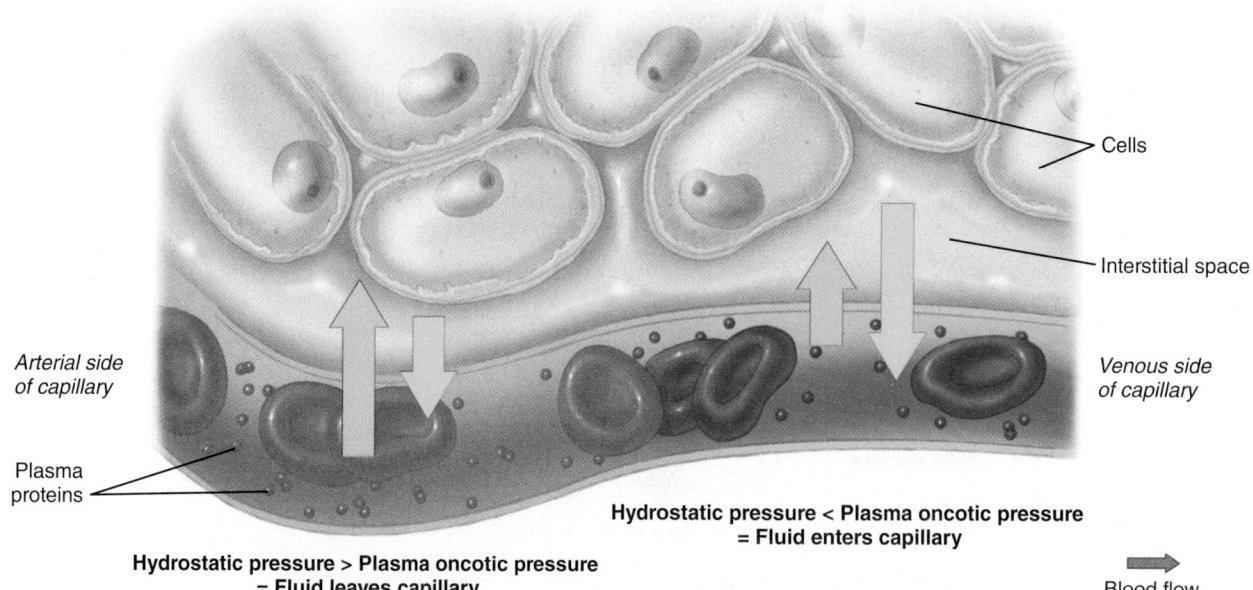

Arterial side of capillary

Plasma proteins

**Hydrostatic pressure > Plasma oncotic pressure = Fluid leaves capillary**

**Hydrostatic pressure < Plasma oncotic pressure = Fluid enters capillary**

Cells

Interstitial space

Venous side of capillary

Blood flow

**FIGURE 6-32** Fluid movement from capillaries to interstitial space and back.

hormones, **epinephrine** (also known as adrenaline) and **norepinephrine** (also known as noradrenaline), are secreted to stimulate the heart and blood vessels. The release of epinephrine and norepinephrine affects receptors within the heart and blood vessels and improves the ability to cope with stress, known as the fight-or-flight reaction. Two types of receptors within the heart and blood vessels will be discussed next so you can understand how the nervous system controls the circulatory system.

The heart and blood vessels have **alpha-adrenergic receptors** and **beta-adrenergic receptors** within them. **Adrenergic** simply means related to the adrenal gland, where epinephrine and norepinephrine are made. The alpha-adrenergic receptors are found in the blood vessels. When stimulated, the blood vessels constrict, thereby increasing blood pressure. The beta-adrenergic receptors are found in the heart and lungs. When beta-1 receptors are stimulated, they cause the heart to increase its rate and also squeeze harder with each contraction. This increases cardiac output. When beta-2 receptors are stimulated, the bronchi in the lungs dilate. This allows more air to be inhaled and exhaled; therefore, more oxygen is available to the cells of the body. Together, the alpha- and beta-adrenergic receptors prepare the body for fight or flight.

The parasympathetic nervous system also has effects on the cardiovascular system. When stimulated, this system causes the heart to slow and beat more weakly. Although the sympathetic and parasympathetic divisions function in opposition to each other, this opposition is considered complementary rather than antagonistic. The net effect is a dynamic body able to respond quickly for fight or flight (**TABLE 6-9**).

The brain needs to know how the body is performing so that adjustments in the pressure exerted by circulating blood can be made. How is the brain alerted to what is happening at the feet, the liver, or the heart? Signals are sent through the nervous system from special pressure sensors (baroreceptors) spread throughout the body, which allow the brain to receive information about blood pressure. Remember, the main function of the cardiovascular system is to perfuse blood throughout the body. The main locations for these pressure receptors are found in the arch of the aorta and the carotid arteries. By measuring the pressure in these two locations, the body can ensure that the most vulnerable and most important cells get oxygen.

With this information, the brain is able to act to maintain perfusion. To see the system in action, you may want to try this test. Kneel down to the floor. Now, as fast as you can, jump up. Did you pass out? Most likely you did not pass out because these systems with their pressure sensors are designed to maintain perfusion.

When you jumped up quickly, gravity was relocating the blood out of your brain. The baroreceptors detected the decrease in blood pressure at the carotid arteries. A signal was sent to the brain. The brain understood the implication of low blood pressure and immediately turned on the sympathetic nervous system. The blood vessels contracted, and the heart rate increased. The heart pumped harder. Your blood pressure returned to normal and may even have gone slightly high. Again, the

**TABLE 6-9** Nervous System Effects on the Cardiovascular System

| Portion of Nervous System | Receptor | Stimulation Area | Effect When Stimulated |
|---|---|---|---|
| Sympathetic nervous system | Alpha-1 | Blood vessels | Constricted blood vessels; skin becomes pale, cool, clammy |
| | Beta-1 | Heart | Increased heart rate |
| | | | Increased force of heart contraction |
| | Beta-2 | Lungs | Bronchodilation |
| Parasympathetic nervous system | Muscarinic | Heart | Decreased heart rate<br>Decreased force of contraction |

baroreceptors detected this change. Signals were sent to the brain. The sympathetic nervous system was turned off. The parasympathetic nervous system was turned on. The heart rate slowed, and the force of the heart's contractions weakened. All of this happened in a fraction of a second. That is how responsive the cardiovascular system can be.

## The Nervous System: Anatomy and Physiology

The **nervous system** is perhaps the most complex organ system within the human body. It comprises the brain, spinal cord, and thousands of nerves spread throughout the body. This system has many functions, such as the control of breathing, heart rate, and blood pressure. However, what makes the nervous system so special is that it allows the performance of higher-level activity. Reading a good book, enjoying music, having a discussion with a friend, and even watching television require the brain to engage memory, understanding, and thought. This is where the true complexity of the nervous system is revealed.

The nervous system is divided into two main portions: the **central nervous system (CNS)** (the brain and spinal cord) and the **peripheral nervous system (PNS)** (the nerves outside of the brain and spinal cord that link the CNS to various organs throughout the body).

The peripheral nervous system can be further divided into the somatic and autonomic nervous systems. The **somatic nervous system** regulates activities over which we have voluntary control, such as walking, talking, and writing. The **autonomic nervous system** controls those functions that occur autonomously (ie, automatically), including digestion, dilation and constriction of blood vessels, sweating, and other involuntary actions (**FIGURE 6-33**).

## The Central Nervous System
### Brain

The **brain** controls all functions of the body, and it assembles and interprets the information received through the body's various senses. It stores information in memory; it controls thought, speech, movement of skeletal muscle, and involuntary

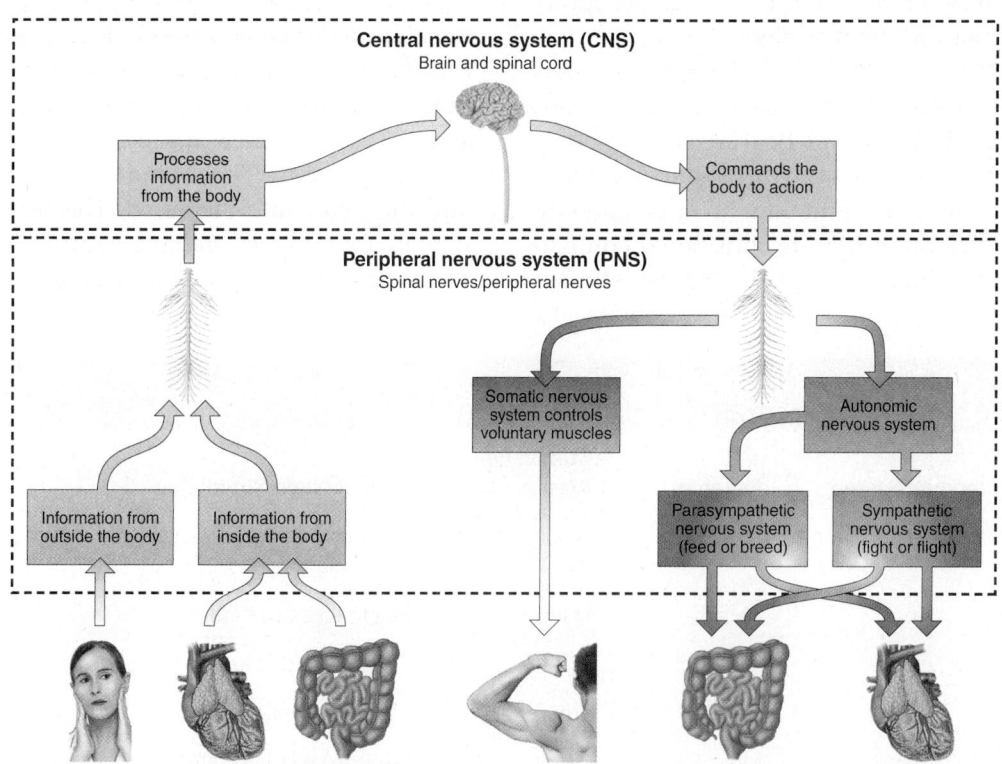

**FIGURE 6-33** The basic configuration of the nervous system.

© Jones & Bartlett Learning.

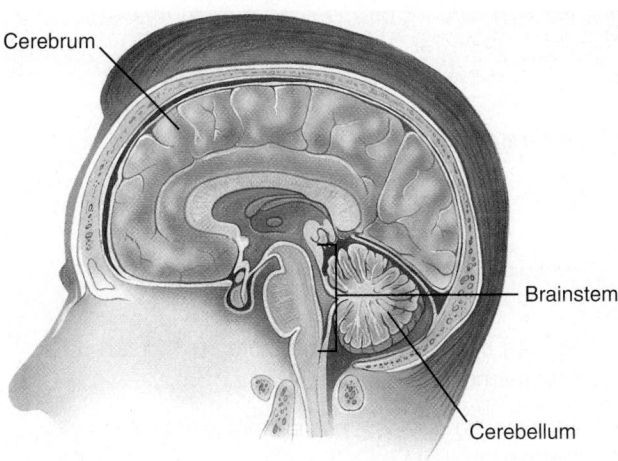

**FIGURE 6-34** The brain lies well protected within the skull. Its major subdivisions are the cerebrum, the cerebellum, and the brainstem.

© Jones & Bartlett Learning.

processes such as heart and breathing rates. The brain is subdivided into several components, all of which have specific roles. Three major subdivisions of the brain are the cerebrum, the cerebellum, and the brainstem (**FIGURE 6-34**).

The **cerebrum** accounts for the largest portion of the brain (about three-fourths). Its surface, the cortex, is made up of **neurons** (nerve cell) bodies, which give it a gray-brown color (thus the reason why the cerebrum is sometimes called the gray matter). The cerebrum is responsible for higher brain functions, such as interpreting what we see, hear, or feel; encoding and decoding speech; reasoning and learning; controlling precise muscle movements (ie, fine motor control); and managing emotions.

The cerebrum can be divided into right and left halves, or hemispheres. These hemispheres can be further divided into lobes. In general, control of one side of the body belongs to the hemisphere on the opposite side (eg, the left hemisphere controls the movements of the right leg). Each hemisphere has four lobes: frontal, parietal, temporal, and occipital. No single lobe operates entirely on its own; complex relationships exist between them and with other parts of the brain. However, each lobe has a certain set of duties for which it is recognized as having the greatest degree of control. For example, personality, judgment, planning, problem solving, concentration, and self-awareness all are attributed to the frontal lobe. The parietal lobe controls our

recognition of spatial relationships and it integrates sensory information received from the body to form our perception of the world around us. The occipital lobe is responsible for vision. Taste, hearing, and our ability to understand words all are functions of the temporal lobe.

Located beneath the cerebrum is the **cerebellum**, a structure that controls balance, muscle coordination, and posture. Without the cerebellum, highly specialized muscular activities such as writing would be impossible.

Deep within the cranium, the well-protected **brainstem** acts as a relay center connecting the cerebrum and cerebellum to the spinal cord. It is the most primitive part of the CNS, controlling virtually all involuntary, life-sustaining functions, such as heart rate, breathing, temperature regulation, digestion, vomiting, swallowing, coughing, and the wake/sleep cycle. The brainstem comprises the **midbrain**, the **pons**, and the **medulla oblongata**.

One noteworthy feature within the brainstem is a network of neurons called the **reticular activating system (RAS)**. One of its functions is to regulate consciousness. When stimulated, it wakes the cerebral cortex. Without the RAS, wakefulness and awareness would not be possible. When someone experiences a concussion from a head injury, the immediate loss of consciousness is due to a momentary interruption in the RAS. Much like a computer having to reboot, the RAS must "reboot" for the patient to regain conscious awareness.

The brain has many other anatomic elements, all of which have important functions. **TABLE 6-10** summarizes several key components of the nervous system and their functions.

### Cerebrospinal Fluid

In addition to filtering out impurities and toxins, CSF absorbs shocks. When significant forces are applied to the head, CSF allows the brain to shift inside the skull without being damaged. Some skull fractures may allow CSF to leak from the ears or nose. This is considered a significant finding. Refer to Chapter 29, *Head and Spine Injuries*, for more information.

### Circulation in the Head

The brain requires a constant flow of oxygenated blood. Blood is supplied to the head through the

**TABLE 6-10** Structures of the Nervous System and General Functions

| System | Major Structure | Subdivision | General Function |
|---|---|---|---|
| Central nervous system | Brain | Occipital lobe | Vision and storage of visual memories |
| | | Parietal lobe | Sense of touch and texture; storage of those memories |
| | | Temporal lobe | Hearing, smell, and language; storage of sound and odor memories |
| | | Frontal lobe | Voluntary muscle control and storage of those memories |
| | | Prefrontal area | Judgment and predicting consequences of actions, abstract intellectual functions |
| | | Limbic system | Basic emotions, basic reflexes (eg, chewing, swallowing) |
| | | Diencephalon (thalamus) | Relay center; filters important signals from routine signals |
| | | Diencephalon (hypothalamus) | Emotions, temperature control, interface with endocrine system (hormone control) |
| | Brainstem | Midbrain | Level of consciousness, reticular activating system, muscle tone, and posture |
| | | Pons | Respiratory patterning and depth |
| | | Medulla oblongata | Heart rate, blood pressure, respiratory rate |
| | Spinal cord | | Reflexes, relays information to and from body |
| Peripheral nervous system | Cranial nerves | | Brainstem to head and neck; special peripheral nerves that connect directly to body parts |
| | Peripheral nerves | | Brain to spinal cord to body part; receive stimulus from body, send commands to body |

© Jones & Bartlett Learning.

carotid arteries, which can be palpated on either side of the neck. Deoxygenated blood drains from the head via the internal and external jugular veins.

## Spinal Cord

The **spinal cord** is an extension of the brainstem (**FIGURE 6-35**). The opening at the base of the cranium, which allows the brain and cord to connect, is called the foramen magnum. The spinal cord then travels downward, encased within the vertebral column, through a passageway called the spinal canal.

The spinal canal is formed by the openings that run vertically through the middle of adjoining vertebrae. The cord terminates at the level of the second lumbar vertebra (L2).

The cord contains nerve cell bodies, but a larger portion is composed of extensions from those bodies that facilitate communication between neurons. Before connecting with the brain, nerve fibers from the spinal cord cross over from one side to the other. This accounts for the fact that many actions taking place on one side of the body are controlled by the cerebral hemisphere on the opposite side. The primary function of the spinal cord is to transmit messages between the brain and the body. These messages are passed along the nerve fibers as electrical impulses, moving quickly from one nerve to the next.

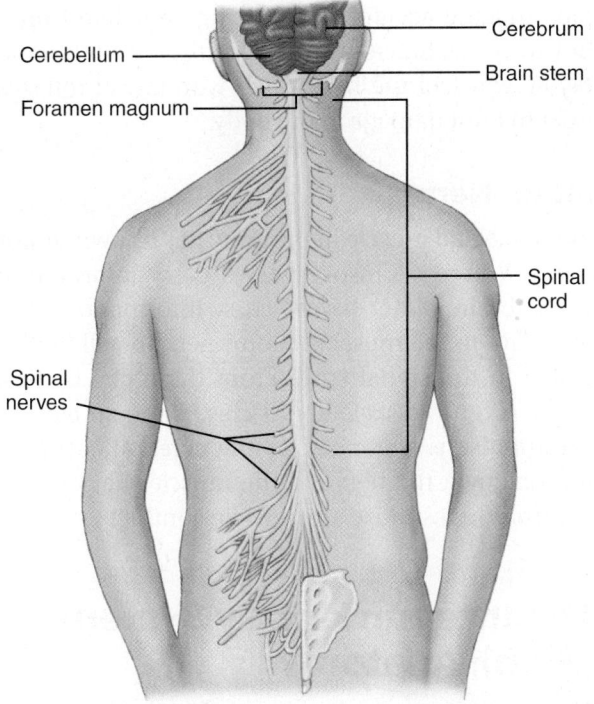

**FIGURE 6-35** The spinal cord is a continuation of the brainstem. It exits the skull at the foramen magnum and extends down to the level of the second lumbar vertebra.

© Jones & Bartlett Learning.

Labels in figure:
- Cerebellum
- Cerebrum
- Brain stem
- Foramen magnum
- Spinal cord
- Spinal nerves

## The Peripheral Nervous System

The PNS is divided into the somatic nervous system and the autonomic nervous system. The autonomic nervous system, in turn, is divided between the sympathetic and parasympathetic nervous systems. The **sympathetic nervous system** is responsible for the fight-or-flight reaction that enables us to respond under stress. This reaction generally increases activity within the body. When stimulated, the sympathetic nervous system increases blood flow to the skeletal muscles, increases heart and respiratory rates, dilates the pupils, increases production and use of energy, dilates respiratory passageways, and causes sweating.

By contrast, the **parasympathetic nervous system** tends to slow the body's activities or return the body to its resting state. Effects include pupil constriction, promotion of digestive system activities, constriction of airway passages, and reduction of heart rate and force of contraction.

There are two types of nerves used in the peripheral nervous system: sensory nerves and motor nerves.

### Sensory Nerves

**Sensory nerves** are complex. They can be found in the eyes, ears, skin, muscles, joints, lungs, and other organs. When a sensory cell is stimulated, it

---

## YOU are the Provider

You prepare the patient for transport. He remains conscious and alert, but is still experiencing severe pain. Shortly after loading him into the ambulance and departing the scene, you perform a reassessment.

| Recording Time: 12 Minutes | |
| --- | --- |
| Level of consciousness | Conscious and alert |
| Respirations | 24 breaths/min; adequate depth |
| Pulse | 112 beats/min; strong and regular |
| Skin | Pink, warm, and moist |
| Blood pressure | 138/88 mm Hg |
| Spo$_2$ | 97% |

You allow the patient to assume a position of comfort, which seems to help with his pain. With an estimated time of arrival at the hospital of 10 minutes, you call in your radio report.

**5.** How does knowledge of anatomy, physiology, and medical terminology facilitate communication with other health care professionals?

transmits a message to the brain. There are many different kinds of sensory nerves. Some detect heat or cold, while others relay information about position, motion, pressure, pain, balance, light, taste, smell, or some other sensation. Every sensory nerve uses specialized nerve endings unique to its type, so that it perceives and communicates information about a single type of sensation. Most sensory nerves must carry information to the brain via the spinal cord. Others take information to the brain directly, without having to go through the spinal cord first.

One example of a nerve with a direct line of communication with the brain that bypasses the spinal cord is the optic nerve. Its nerve endings are found in the retina of the eye. When stimulated by light, the optic nerve carries visual information from the eye straight to the occipital lobe of the brain, where it is interpreted. It does not pass through the spinal cord.

By contrast, when sensory nerve endings in the extremities are stimulated, they transmit the impulses along a peripheral nerve to the spinal cord. The information is then conducted up the spinal cord, passing from one neuron to the next, until it reaches the parietal lobe of the cerebrum.

In many cases, sensory information cannot be acted on until the brain has received and decoded the message sent by the sensory nerves. The brain must then reply with a command, telling the body how to respond. In other cases, certain stimuli can evoke a physical response even before the message reaches the brain. In such instances, the impulse is intercepted by a nearby motor nerve, which promptly initiates physical movement. For example, imagine accidentally placing your hand on a hot stove. Technically, you will withdraw your hand *before* you feel the heat. Such withdrawal reflexes exist to limit damage to the body.

## Motor Nerves

Every skeletal muscle in the body has its own motor nerve. Whereas sensory nerves carry information *to* the brain, **motor nerves** carry information *from* the brain to the muscles. Motor neuron cell bodies reside in the spinal cord. From these cell bodies, **axons** extend to skeletal muscles. When an electrical impulse is generated by the cerebral cortex, it travels down the nerve to the muscle that neuron controls. In response, the muscle contracts.

## The Integumentary System (Skin): Anatomy

The cutaneous membrane, or skin, is the largest single organ in the body. It has two major components: the epidermis and the dermis. Beneath these layers is **subcutaneous tissue** (**FIGURE 6-36**).

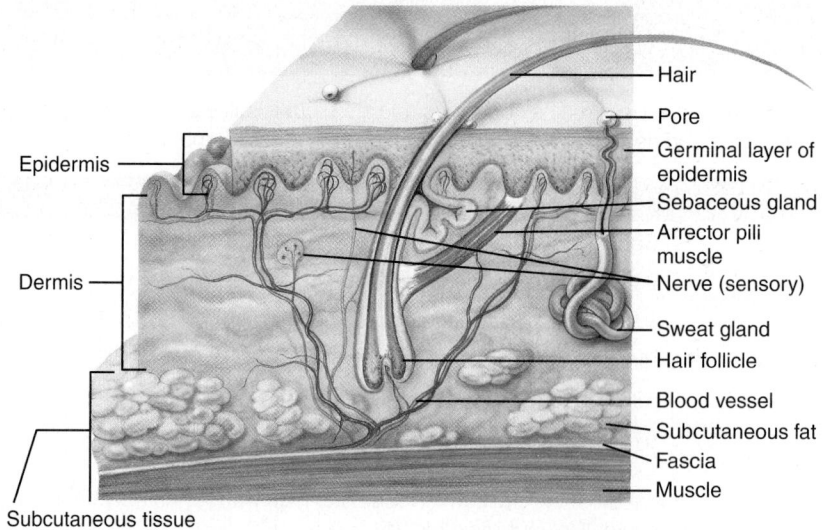

Epidermis

Dermis

Subcutaneous tissue

Hair
Pore
Germinal layer of epidermis
Sebaceous gland
Arrector pili muscle
Nerve (sensory)
Sweat gland
Hair follicle
Blood vessel
Subcutaneous fat
Fascia
Muscle

**FIGURE 6-36** The layers of the skin can be divided between the epidermis and the dermis. Below the skin is a layer of subcutaneous tissue.

The outermost layers that make up the skin's surface are known collectively as the **epidermis** (*epi-* is a prefix meaning "above"). The epidermis forms a watertight barrier that provides considerable protection, keeping microorganisms from getting inside the body while preventing fluid from escaping. Its thickness varies depending on its location on the body. On the soles of the feet and the palms of the hands, the back, and the **scalp**, the skin is quite thick, while in other areas it is only two or three cells thick.

Epidermal cells are arranged in multiple layers. The innermost layer, called the **germinal layer**, continuously produces new cells that gradually ascend through the other skin layers. The germinal layer also contains cells that produce pigment granules, which give the skin its color. In time, germinal layers reach the exposed surface layer, called the **stratum corneum**. Whereas the germinal layer is supplied with blood, the stratum corneum is not. Thus, the cells of the corneum are dead and are continually shed and replaced by new cells arriving from the layers below. The journey from the germinal layer to the surface takes about 4 weeks.

Located beneath the epidermis, the **dermis** is home to the **sweat glands**, sebaceous (oil) glands, hair follicles, blood vessels, and nerve endings. Sweat reaches the surface of the skin by way of small pores, or ducts, that pass from sweat glands in the dermis and up through the epidermis. Sweat helps to cool the body.

**Hair follicles** are small organs that produce hair. As hair grows, it passes along a shaft, ultimately reaching and emerging from the epidermal surface. Connected to the hair is a small muscle that pulls the hair into an erect position when triggered by certain stimuli (eg, cold air or fright). Hairs grow and are shed according to a hair growth cycle. Adjacent to hair follicles, **sebaceous glands** secrete an oily substance called sebum along the hair follicles to the skin surface. Sebum seals the surface, waterproofing the skin and preventing it from drying and cracking.

Blood vessels provide nutrients and oxygen to the skin. The blood vessels lie in the dermis. Small branches extend up to the germinal layer. A complex array of nerve endings also lies in the dermis. These specialized nerve endings are sensitive to environmental stimuli; they respond to these stimuli and send impulses along the nerves to the brain.

Beneath the skin, immediately under the dermis and attached to it, lies the subcutaneous tissue. The subcutaneous tissue is composed largely of fat, which serves as an insulator for the body and a reservoir that stores energy. The amount of subcutaneous tissue varies greatly from individual to individual. The subcutaneous layer helps to anchor the skin to the structures below (eg, the muscles and skeleton). As you age, the loss of subcutaneous tissue causes a reduction in support for the skin, resulting in wrinkles.

While skin covers the entire external surface of the body, it does not cover the various openings to the body such as the mouth, nose, anus, and vagina. Instead, these structures are lined with mucous membranes. **Mucous membranes** are quite similar to skin in that they provide a protective barrier against bacterial invasion. However, they differ from skin in that they secrete **mucus**, a watery substance that lubricates and keeps them moist. A continuous mucous membrane lines the entire length of the gastrointestinal tract, from mouth to anus.

## The Integumentary System (Skin): Physiology

The skin serves multiple functions. Chief among these are to (1) protect the body from the environment, (2) maintain normal body temperature, and (3) transmit sensory information (ie, touch, pain, pressure, and temperature) from the environment to the brain.

The protective functions of the skin are numerous. Water makes up a large portion of the body. This water contains a delicate balance of chemical substances in solution. The skin is watertight and serves to keep this balanced internal solution intact. The skin also protects the body from the invasion of infectious organisms: bacteria, viruses, and fungi. These organisms are everywhere and are routinely found lying on the skin surface. However, they typically do not penetrate the skin unless it is broken by injury; thus, the skin provides a constant protection against outside invaders.

The major organ for regulation of body temperature is the skin. Blood vessels in the skin constrict when the body is in a cold environment and dilate when the body is in a warm environment. In a cold environment, constriction of the blood vessels shunts the blood away from the skin to decrease the amount of heat radiated from the body surface. When the outside environment is hot, the vessels in the skin dilate, bringing blood closer to the surface. The skin becomes flushed (red), and heat radiates from the body surface.

Also, in a hot environment, sweat is secreted to the skin surface from the sweat glands. Evaporation of the sweat causes the body temperature to fall because water absorbs heat as it evaporates. Sweating alone is not as effective in reducing body temperature; evaporation of the sweat must also occur.

Information from the environment is carried to the brain through a rich supply of sensory nerves that originate in the skin. Nerve endings that lie in the skin are adapted to perceive and transmit information about heat, cold, external pressure, pain, and the position of the body in space. The skin thus recognizes any changes in the environment. The skin also reacts to pressure, pain, and pleasurable stimuli.

## The Digestive System: Anatomy

The digestive system, also called the gastrointestinal system, is composed of the gastrointestinal tract (stomach and intestines), mouth, salivary glands, pharynx, esophagus, liver, gallbladder, pancreas, rectum, and anus. The function of this system is digestion: the processing of food that nourishes the individual cells of the body. Most of the organs of this system are found within the abdomen.

### The Abdomen

The abdomen is the second major body cavity; it contains the major organs of digestion and excretion. The diaphragm separates the thorax from the abdominal cavity. Anteriorly and posteriorly, thick muscular abdominal walls create the boundaries of this space. Inferiorly, the abdomen is separated from the pelvis by an imaginary plane that extends from the pubic symphysis through the sacrum (**FIGURE 6-37**). Some organs lie in the abdomen and the pelvis, depending on the posture of the patient.

The simplest and most common method of describing the portions of the abdomen is by quadrants, the four equal areas formed by two imaginary lines that intersect at right angles at the umbilicus. On the anterior abdominal wall, the quadrants thus formed are the right upper, right lower, left upper,

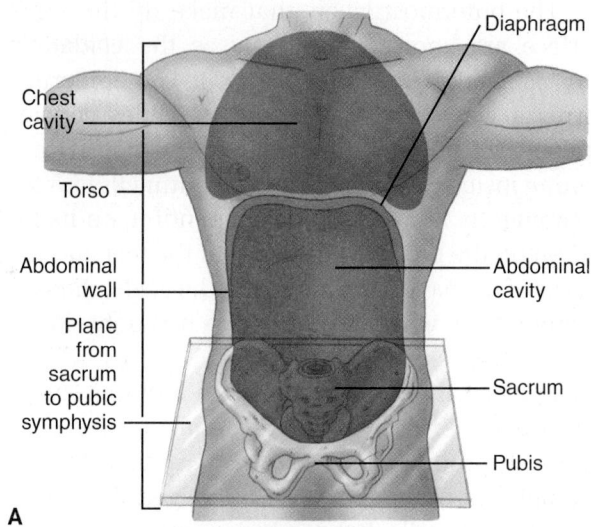

A

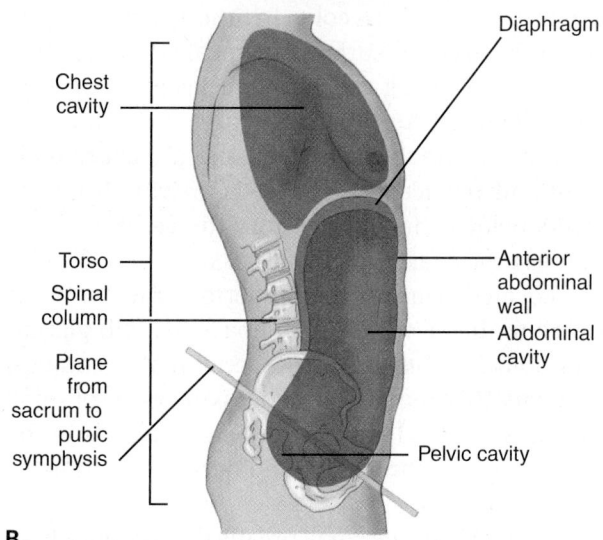

B

**FIGURE 6-37** The boundaries of the abdomen are the anterior and posterior abdominal cavity walls, the diaphragm, and an imaginary plane from the pubic symphysis to the sacrum. The region below the plane is called the pelvic cavity. **A.** Anterior view. **B.** Lateral view.

© Jones & Bartlett Learning.

and left lower (**FIGURE 6-38**). Pain or injury in a given quadrant usually arises from or involves the organs that lie in that quadrant. This simple means of designation will allow you to identify injured or diseased organs that require emergency attention.

### Organs and Vascular Structures

In the right upper quadrant (RUQ), the major organs are the liver, the gallbladder, and a portion of the colon. Most of the liver lies in this quadrant, and immediately in front of the 9th to 11th ribs. The spleen is frequently injured, especially when these ribs are fractured.

The right lower quadrant (RLQ) contains two portions of the large intestine: the **cecum**, the first portion into which the small intestine (ileum) opens, and the ascending colon. The **appendix** is a small, tubular structure that is attached to the lower border of the cecum. In the left lower quadrant (LLQ) lie the descending and the sigmoid portions of the colon.

Several organs lie in more than one quadrant. The small intestine, for instance, occupies the central part of the abdomen around the umbilicus, and parts of it lie in all four quadrants. The pancreas lies just behind the abdominal cavity on the posterior abdominal wall in both upper quadrants. The large intestine also traverses the abdomen, beginning in the RLQ and ending in the LLQ as it passes through all four quadrants. The urinary bladder lies just behind the pubic symphysis in the middle of the abdomen and, therefore, lies in both lower quadrants and also in the pelvis.

The kidneys and pancreas are called **retroperitoneal** organs because they lie behind the abdominal cavity (**FIGURE 6-39**). They are above the level of the umbilicus, extending from the 11th rib

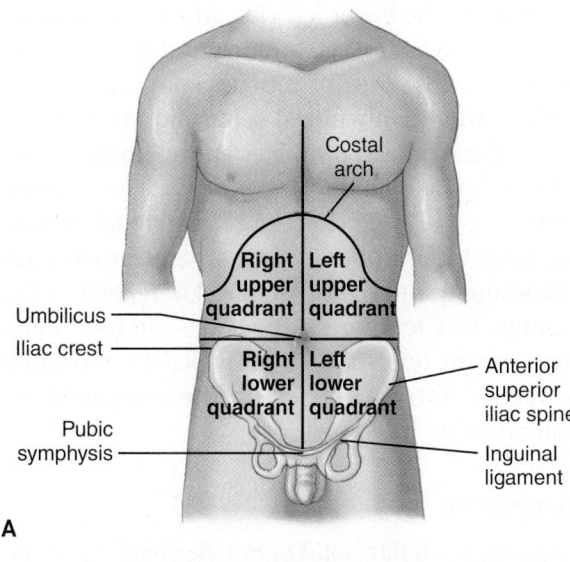

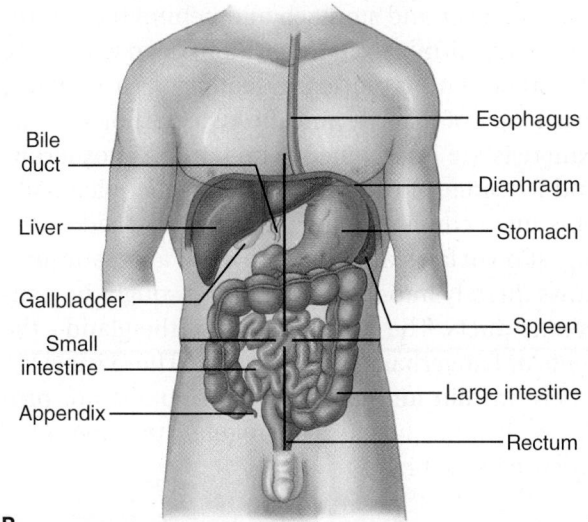

**FIGURE 6-38 A.** In the abdomen, quadrants are the easiest system for identifying areas. Major bony landmarks are also shown. **B.** Several of the organs in the abdomen lie in more than one quadrant.

© Jones & Bartlett Learning.

almost entirely under the protection of the 8th to 12th ribs. The liver fills the entire anteroposterior depth of the abdomen in this quadrant. Therefore, the liver is at risk for injuries in this area.

In the left upper quadrant (LUQ), the major organs are the stomach, the spleen, and a portion of the colon. The spleen is almost entirely under the protection of the left rib cage, whereas the stomach may sag well down into the left lower quadrant when full. The spleen lies in the lateral and posterior portion of this quadrant, under the diaphragm

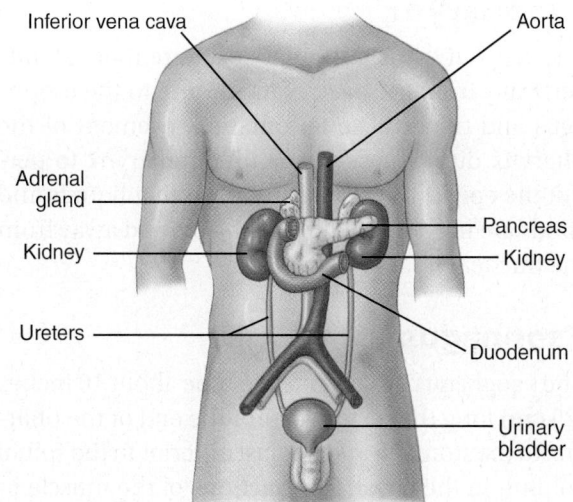

**FIGURE 6-39** The major organs of the retroperitoneal space lie behind the abdominal cavity, above the level of the umbilicus, and extend from the 11th rib to the 3rd lumbar vertebra. The bladder, inferior vena cava, and aorta also lie in this space.

© Jones & Bartlett Learning.

to the third lumbar vertebra on each side. The kidneys are approximately 5 inches (13 cm) long and lie just anterior to the costovertebral angle, which is the junction between the posterior aspect of the lower portion of the rib cage and the spine.

## Mouth

The mouth consists of the lips, cheeks, gums, teeth, and tongue. A mucous membrane lines the mouth. The roof of the mouth is formed by the hard and soft palates. The hard palate is a bony plate lying anteriorly; the soft palate is a fold of mucous membrane and muscle that extends posteriorly from the hard palate into the throat. The soft palate is designed to hold food that is being chewed within the mouth and to help initiate swallowing.

## Salivary Glands

There are two sets of salivary glands, one set on each side of the mouth under the tongue, and the other set in front of each ear. They produce nearly 1.5 L of saliva daily. Saliva is approximately 98% water. The remaining 2% is composed of mucus, salts, and organic compounds. Saliva serves as a binder for the chewed food that is being swallowed and as a lubricant within the mouth. Saliva also contains certain digestive enzymes.

## Oropharynx

The oropharynx is a tubular structure that extends vertically from the back of the mouth to the esophagus and trachea. An automatic movement of the pharynx during swallowing lifts the larynx to permit the epiglottis to close over it so that liquids and solids are moved into the esophagus and away from the trachea.

## Esophagus

The esophagus is a collapsible tube about 10 inches (25 cm) long that extends from the end of the pharynx to the stomach and lies just anterior to the spinal column in the chest. Contractions of the muscle in the wall of the esophagus propel food through it to the stomach. Liquids pass with very little assistance.

## Stomach

The stomach is a hollow organ located in the left upper quadrant of the abdominal cavity, largely protected by the lower left ribs. Muscular contractions in the wall of the stomach and gastric juice, which contains a lot of mucus, convert ingested food to a thoroughly mixed semisolid mass, called chyme. The stomach produces approximately 1.5 L of gastric juice daily for this process. The primary function of the stomach is to receive food in large quantities intermittently, store it, and provide for its movement into the small bowel in regular, small amounts. In 1 to 3 hours, the semisolid food mass derived from one meal is propelled by muscular contraction into the duodenum, the first part of the small intestine.

## Pancreas

The pancreas, a flat, solid organ, lies below and behind the liver and stomach and behind the peritoneum. It is firmly fixed in position, deep within the abdomen, and is not easily damaged. It contains two kinds of glands, and the two portions of the pancreas are intertwined. One portion is exocrine, and it secretes nearly 2 L of pancreatic juice daily. This juice contains many enzymes that aid in the digestion of fat, starch, and protein. Pancreatic juice flows directly into the duodenum through the pancreatic ducts. The other portion of the gland—the islets of Langerhans—is endocrine. These islets are where insulin and glucagon (hormones) are produced. Insulin and glucagon regulate the amount of glucose in the blood.

## Liver

The liver is a large, solid organ that takes up most of the area immediately beneath the diaphragm in the right upper quadrant and also extends into the left upper quadrant. It is the largest solid organ in the abdomen and has several functions. Poisonous substances produced by digestion are brought to the liver and rendered harmless. Factors that are necessary for blood clotting and for the production of normal plasma are formed here. Between 0.5 and 1 L of bile is made by the liver daily to assist in the normal digestion of fat. The liver is the primary organ for the storage of sugar or starch for immediate use by the body for energy. It also produces many of the factors that aid in the proper regulation of immune responses. The liver is fragile and, because of its size, relatively easily injured. Blood flow in the liver is high, because all of the blood that is pumped to the gastrointestinal tract passes into the liver, through the portal vein, before it returns to the heart. In addition, the liver has a generous arterial blood supply of its own. Ordinarily, approximately 25% of the cardiac output of blood (1.5 L) passes through the liver each minute.

### Bile Ducts

The liver connects with the intestine by way of the bile ducts. The gallbladder is a small pouch extending from the bile ducts that serves as a reservoir and concentrating organ for bile produced in the liver. Together, the bile ducts and the gallbladder form the biliary system. The gallbladder discharges stored and concentrated bile into the duodenum through the common bile duct. The presence of food in the duodenum triggers a contraction of the gallbladder to empty it. The gallbladder usually contains about 60 to 90 mL of bile.

### Small Intestine

The small intestine is the major hollow organ of the abdomen. The cells lining the small intestine produce enzymes and mucus to aid in digestion. Enzymes from the pancreas and the small intestine carry out the final processes of digestion. More than 90% of the products of digestion (amino acids, fatty acids, and simple sugars), together with water, ingested vitamins, and minerals, are absorbed across the wall of the lower end of the small intestine into veins to be transported to the liver. The small intestine is composed of the duodenum, the jejunum, and the ileum. The duodenum, which is about 12 inches (30 cm) long, is the part of the small intestine that receives food from the stomach. Here, food is mixed with secretions from the pancreas and liver for further digestion. Bile, produced by the liver and stored in the gallbladder, is emptied as needed into the duodenum. Bile is green-black, but through changes during digestion, it gives feces its typical brown color. Its major function is in the digestion of fat. The jejunum and ileum together measure more than 20 feet (6 m) on average to make up the rest of the small intestine.

### Large Intestine

The large intestine, another major hollow organ, consists of the cecum, the colon, and the rectum. About 5 feet (1.5 m) long, it encircles the outer border of the abdomen around the small bowel. The major function of the colon, the portion of the large intestine that extends from the cecum to the rectum, is to absorb the final 5% to 10% of digested food and water from the intestine to form solid stool, which is stored in the rectum and passed out of the body through the anus.

### Appendix

Recall that the appendix is a tube that opens into the cecum (the first part of the large intestine) in the right lower quadrant of the abdomen. It is 3 to 4 inches (8 to 10 cm) long and may easily become obstructed and, as a result, inflamed and infected. Appendicitis, which is the term for this inflammation, is one of the major causes of severe abdominal distress.

### Rectum

The lowermost end of the colon is the rectum. It is a large, hollow organ that is adapted to store quantities of feces until it is expelled. At its terminal end is the anus, a 2-inch (5-cm) canal lined with skin. The rectum and anus are supplied with a complex series of circular muscles, called sphincters, that control, voluntarily and automatically, the escape of liquids, gases, and solids from the digestive tract. **TABLE 6-11** provides a summary of the organs and functions of the digestive system.

## The Digestive System: Physiology

Digestion of food, from the moment it is taken into the mouth until essential compounds are extracted and delivered by the circulatory system to nourish all cells in the body, is a complicated chemical process. In succession, different secretions, primarily enzymes, are added to the food by the salivary glands, the stomach, the liver, the pancreas, and the small intestine to convert the food into basic sugars, fatty acids, and amino acids. These basic products of digestion are carried across the wall of the intestine and transported through the portal vein to the liver. In the liver, the products are processed further and stored or transported to the heart through veins draining the liver. The heart then pumps the blood with these nutrients throughout the arteries to the capillaries, where

**TABLE 6-11** Digestive Organs and Functions

| Organ/Structure | Function |
| --- | --- |
| Mouth | Mechanically breaks down food; begins chemical breakdown with saliva |
| Esophagus | Moves food from the mouth to the stomach; muscular and vascular structure |
| Stomach | Performs mechanical and chemical breakdown of food: food in, chyme out |
| Small intestine: duodenum, jejunum, and ileum | Major site for chemical breakdown of food; major absorption of water, fats, proteins, carbohydrates, and vitamins |
| Large intestine | Water absorption; formation of feces; bacterial digestion of food |
| Anus/rectum | Last portion of large intestine; sphincter to control release of feces |
| Liver | Production of bile; assists with carbohydrate, protein, and fat metabolism of nutrients within the bloodstream; manufactures proteins for immune regulation and clotting; detoxification of blood; elimination of waste |
| Pancreas | Exocrine: produces enzymes for protein, carbohydrate, and fat breakdown within the duodenum<br>Endocrine: produces insulin and glucagon |
| Gallbladder | Storage of bile |

© Jones & Bartlett Learning.

the nutrients pass through the capillary walls to nourish the body's individual cells.

In normal routine activity, without any food or fluid ingestion at all, between 8 and 10 L of fluid is secreted daily into the gastrointestinal tract. This fluid comes from the salivary glands, stomach, liver, pancreas, and small intestine. In a healthy adult, about 7% of the body weight is delivered as fluid daily to the gastrointestinal tract. If significant vomiting or diarrhea occurs for more than 2 or 3 days, the person will experience a substantial alteration of body composition and become severely ill.

## The Lymphatic System: Anatomy and Physiology

The lymphatic system includes the spleen, lymph nodes, lymph, lymph vessels, thymus gland, and other components. It supports both the circulatory system and the immune system. Unlike the circulatory system, the lymphatic system has no pump and relies on muscle contractions and movements of the body for lymph to flow.

**Lymph** is a thin, straw-colored fluid that transports materials from the lymph tissue into the central venous circulation via the thoracic ducts. Lymph vessels form a network throughout the body. **Lymph nodes** are located in various places along the lymph vessels in the body. These tiny, oval-shaped structures filter lymph.

Together with the circulatory system, the lymphatic system helps to rid the body of toxins and other harmful materials. The spleen also plays an important role in the body's immune function. It houses immune cells that help eliminate infectious agents.

## The Endocrine System: Anatomy and Physiology

The brain controls the body through the nervous system using electrical impulses, and the endocrine system using hormones. The **endocrine system** is a complex message and control system that integrates many body functions. Endocrine glands release their hormones directly into the bloodstream (**FIGURE 6-40**). Epinephrine, norepinephrine, and insulin are examples of hormones. Each endocrine gland produces one or more hormones.

Each hormone has a specific effect on some organ, tissue, or process (**TABLE 6-12**). The brain controls the release of hormones by the endocrine glands. **Hormones** can have a stimulating or an inhibiting effect on the body's organs and systems. For example, when you are frightened, your brain stimulates the adrenal gland through a hormone to release epinephrine and norepinephrine. This increases your blood pressure and heart rate. The resulting increase in blood pressure and heart rate decreases the amount of hormone released by the adrenal gland. The brain then reduces the amount of stimulation to the **adrenal glands**. Thus, a new steady state is achieved at heightened levels of alertness. This cycle is known as a feedback loop, and it helps keep the body's systems and functions in balance (**FIGURE 6-41**).

Excesses or deficiencies in hormone levels cause various diseases. With endocrine diseases, specific body functions are increased, decreased, or absent. Type 1 diabetes mellitus is a common endocrine condition. Because production of the hormone insulin is deficient, the body is unable to use glucose normally. Glucose is the primary fuel of the body. Insulin is responsible for rapidly moving glucose

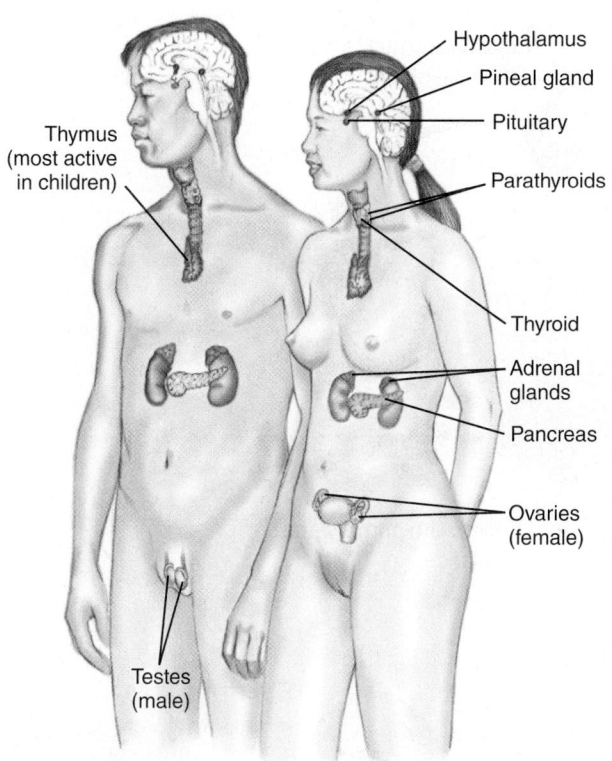

**FIGURE 6-40** The endocrine system controls the production and release of hormones in the body.

© Jones & Bartlett Learning.

## TABLE 6-12 Endocrine Glands

| Gland | Location | Function | Hormones Produced |
|---|---|---|---|
| Adrenal | Above the kidneys | Stress response, fight-or-flight reaction | Epinephrine, norepinephrine, cortisol, and others |
| Ovaries | Female pelvis (two glands) | Regulate sexual function, characteristics, and reproduction | Estrogen and others |
| Pancreas | Retroperitoneal space | Regulates glucose metabolism and other functions | Insulin, glucagon, and others |
| Parathyroid | Neck (behind and beside the thyroid) (three to five glands) | Regulates serum calcium | Parathyroid hormone |
| Pituitary | Base of skull | Regulates all other endocrine glands | Multiple, controls other endocrine glands |
| Testes | Male scrotum (two glands) | Regulate sexual function, characteristics, and reproduction | Testosterone and others |
| Thyroid | Neck (over the larynx) | Regulates metabolism | Thyroxine and others |

© Jones & Bartlett Learning.

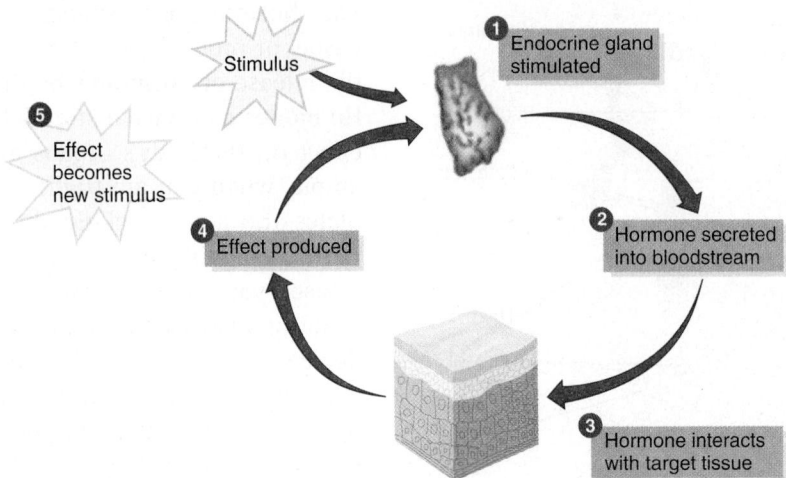

**FIGURE 6-41** The endocrine system is tightly controlled with primary and secondary feedback loops to keep body systems in balance.

© Jones & Bartlett Learning.

into cells; without insulin, glucose moves slowly. This creates a series of complications as the body struggles to find a more readily available fuel for its cells. People with diabetes begin to burn fats and proteins to create the glucose that cells require. Interestingly, the end result is higher and higher blood glucose levels as glucose accumulates, unable to be efficiently moved into the cells. Chapter 20, *Endocrine and Hematologic Emergencies*, discusses how high blood glucose levels affect the body.

## The Urinary System: Anatomy and Physiology

The **urinary system** controls the discharge of certain waste materials filtered from the blood by the kidneys. In the urinary system, the kidneys are solid organs; the ureters, bladder, and urethra are hollow organs (**FIGURE 6-42**). The main functions of the urinary system are (1) to control fluid balance in the body, (2) to filter and eliminate wastes, and (3) to control pH balance.

The body has two **kidneys** that lie on the posterior muscular wall of the abdomen behind the peritoneum in the retroperitoneal space. These organs rid the blood of toxic waste products and control its balance of water and salts. Blood flow in the kidneys is high. Nearly 20% of the output of blood from the heart passes through the kidneys each minute. Large vessels attach the kidneys directly to the aorta and the inferior vena cava. Waste products

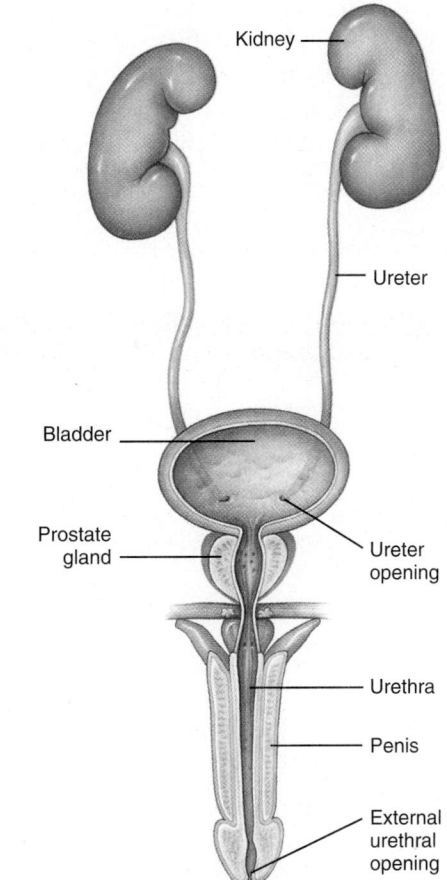

**FIGURE 6-42** The urinary system lies in the retroperitoneal (behind the peritoneum) space behind the organs of the digestive system. The urinary system in men and women includes the kidneys, ureters, bladder, and urethra. This diagram shows the male urinary system.

© Jones & Bartlett Learning.

and water are constantly filtered from the blood to form urine. The kidneys continuously concentrate this filtered urine by reabsorbing the water as it passes through a system of specialized tubes within them. The tubes finally unite to form the **renal pelvis**, a cone-shaped area within the kidney that collects urine and funnels it through the ureter into the bladder. Normally, each kidney drains its urine into one ureter through which the urine passes to the bladder.

A **ureter** passes from the renal pelvis of each kidney along the surface of the posterior abdominal wall behind the peritoneum to drain into the urinary bladder. The ureters are small (0.2 inch [0.5 cm] in diameter), hollow, muscular tubes. **Peristalsis**, a wavelike contraction of smooth muscle, occurs in these tubes to move the urine to the bladder.

The **urinary bladder** is located immediately behind the pubic symphysis in the pelvic cavity and is composed of smooth muscle with a specialized lining membrane. The two ureters enter posteriorly at its base on either side. The bladder empties to the outside of the body through the **urethra**. In a man, the urethra passes from the anterior base of the bladder through the penis. In a woman, the urethra opens in front of the vagina. A healthy adult forms 1.5 to 2 L of urine every day. This waste is extracted and concentrated from the 1,500 L of blood that circulates through the kidneys daily.

## The Genital System: Anatomy and Physiology

The **genital system** controls the reproductive processes. The male genitalia, except for the **prostate gland** and the **seminal vesicles**, lie outside the pelvic cavity. The female genitalia, with the exception of the clitoris and labia, are contained entirely within the pelvis. The male and female reproductive organs have certain similarities and, of course, basic differences. They produce sperm and egg cells and reproductive hormones and play a significant role in sexual intercourse and reproduction.

## The Male Reproductive System and Organs

The male reproductive system consists of the testicles, epididymis, vasa deferentia, prostate gland, seminal vesicles, and penis (**FIGURE 6-43**). Each **testicle** contains specialized cells and ducts; some of these produce male hormones, and others develop sperm. The hormones are absorbed directly into the bloodstream from the testicles. The sperm are immature and are moved from the testicles to the epididymis so they can develop. The sperm are carried through vasa deferentia (or vas deferens) to the seminal vesicles, where are stored. During ejaculation, they are passed through the urethra.

## YOU are the Provider

Shortly before arriving at the hospital, you reassess the patient. He remains conscious and alert and tells you that his pain is less severe than before. After transferring patient care to the attending physician, you later learn that the patient had an inflamed gallbladder, which was surgically removed.

| Recording Time: 20 Minutes | |
| --- | --- |
| **Level of consciousness** | Conscious and alert |
| **Respirations** | 20 breaths/min; adequate depth |
| **Pulse** | 90 beats/min; strong and regular |
| **Skin** | Pink, warm, and moist |
| **Blood pressure** | 132/80 mm Hg |
| **Spo$_2$** | 98% |

**6.** Should your documentation of an EMS call differ from your verbal communication with other health care professionals? Why or why not?

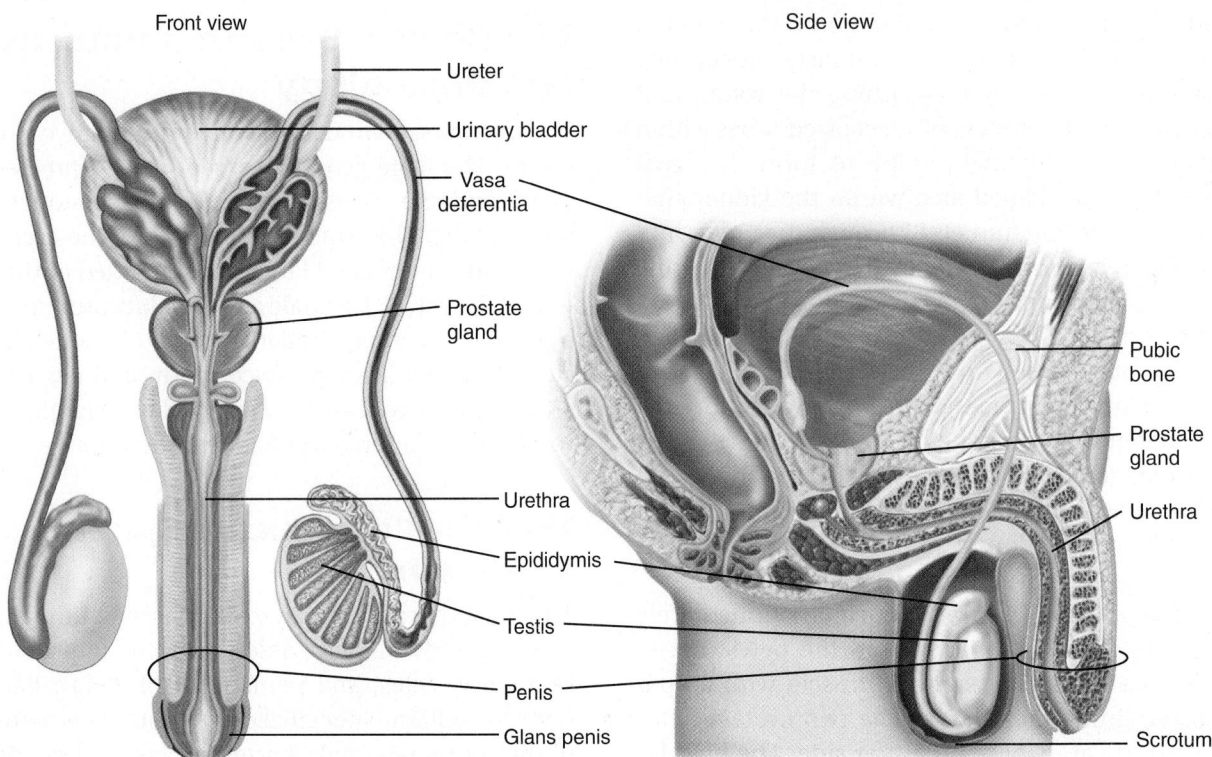

Front view

Side view

Ureter

Urinary bladder

Vasa
deferentia

Prostate
gland

Pubic
bone

Prostate
gland

Urethra

Urethra

Epididymis

Testis

Penis

Glans penis

Scrotum

**FIGURE 6-43** The male reproductive system consists of the testicles, epididymis, vasa deferentia, prostate gland, seminal vesicles, and penis.

© Jones & Bartlett Learning.

The function of the reproductive system is to reproduce. Sperm are able to join with an egg to form an embryo. In addition to reproduction, this system is responsible for the production of sex hormones. Many of the physical characteristics of men, such as increased muscle mass, body hair, and deep voice, are attributed to the powerful effects of the hormones released by the testes. Finally, the penis, though part of the reproductive system, is also part of the urinary system. Any damage or infection to the penis can cause problems within the urinary bladder and/or the kidneys.

## The Female Reproductive System and Organs

The female reproductive organs include the ovaries, fallopian tubes, uterus, cervix, and vagina (**FIGURE 6-44**). The ovaries, like the testicles, produce sex hormones and specialized cells for reproduction. The female sex hormones are absorbed directly into the bloodstream. A specialized ovum, or egg cell, matures and is released regularly during the adult woman's reproductive years. The ovaries release a mature egg approximately every 28 days. This egg travels through the fallopian tubes, where fertilization normally occurs. The fallopian tubes exit into the uterus.

The fallopian tubes (sometimes called uterine tubes) connect with the uterus and carry the ovum into the cavity of this organ. The uterus is pear-shaped and hollow, with muscular walls. The narrow opening from the uterus to the vagina is the cervix. The vagina (birth canal) is a muscular, distensible tube that connects the uterus with the vulva (the external female genitalia). The vagina receives the penis during sexual intercourse, when semen is deposited in it. The sperm in the semen may pass through the uterus and fertilize an egg, typically in the fallopian tube, resulting in pregnancy. Should the pregnancy come to completion at about 40 weeks, the neonate will pass through the vagina and be born. The vagina also channels the menstrual flow from the uterus out of the body.

The functions of the female reproductive system are similar to those of the male reproductive system: reproduction and hormone balance.

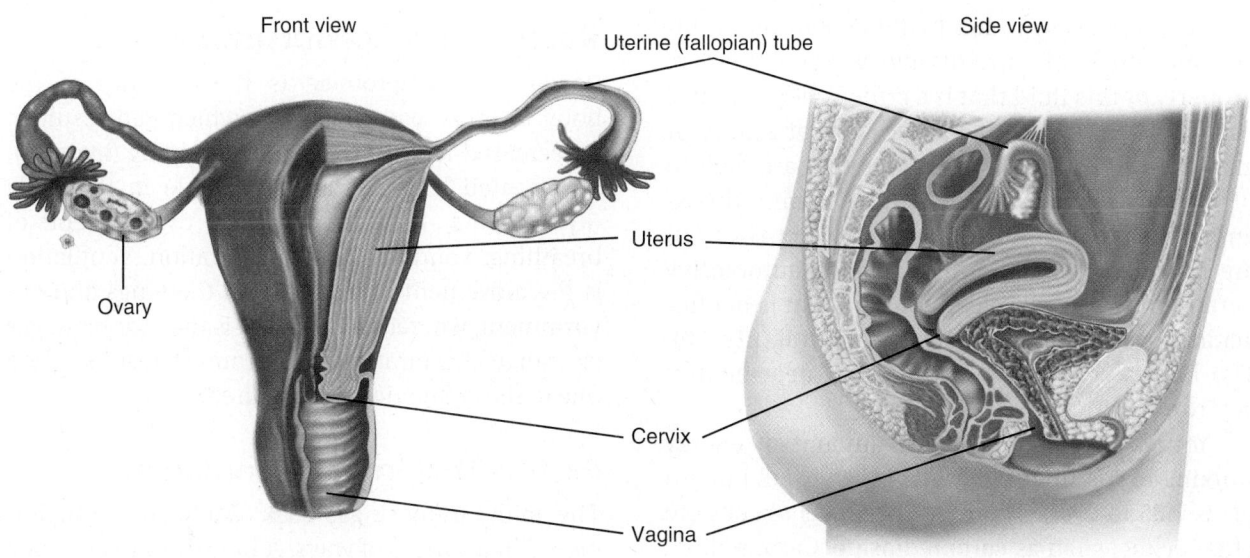

Front view                    Uterine (fallopian) tube                    Side view

Ovary

Uterus

Cervix

Vagina

**FIGURE 6-44** The female reproductive system consists of the ovaries, fallopian tubes, uterus, cervix, and vagina.

© Jones & Bartlett Learning.

## Life Support Chain

To perform their job, the body's cells, tissues, and organs, regardless of their function, all depend on the reliable supply of oxygen and nutrients and the removal of wastes. Oxygen is brought to the cells via the respiratory and circulatory systems. Nutrients are derived from the food we eat after the digestive system breaks it down into, among other things, glucose. The circulatory system then delivers these supplies while picking up and carrying away wastes through the process of perfusion. If interference occurs in this delivery system, cells will become damaged or die.

Cells use oxygen to turn available nutrients into chemical energy through the biochemical process of **metabolism**. **Adenosine triphosphate (ATP)** is used in energy metabolism and storage. Cells prefer to use oxygen for this process, referred to as **aerobic metabolism** (meaning "with air"), as doing so provides the cells with 15 times more ATP than is possible without oxygen. The waste products of aerobic metabolism are carbon dioxide and water.

In the absence of oxygen, most cells turn to a faster yet less efficient means of producing ATP called **anaerobic metabolism** (without air). The most well-known by-product of anaerobic metabolism is **lactic acid**, which is the material that causes muscle burning during anaerobic activities like weight lifting. Most cells can tolerate anaerobic metabolism for only about 1 to 3 minutes, and some specialized cells (such as the heart and brain) are unable to survive without a constant supply of oxygen. Brain cells, for example, begin to die after only 4 to 6 minutes without oxygen.

As lactic acid and other wastes accumulate around the cells, the area becomes toxic. Cells subjected to this toxic waste may die. Given enough time and a large enough number of affected cells, whole organs may fail, and the individual may go into cardiac arrest.

The main force enabling all of this movement of material—oxygen, waste, nutrients—is diffusion. Recall that when you breathe, oxygen moves from an area of higher concentration to one of lower concentration.

### Words of Wisdom

**Remember**
- When cells function with oxygen, they use aerobic metabolism.
  - They generate large amounts of ATP (cellular energy) and produce wastes of carbon dioxide and water.
- When cells function without oxygen, they use anaerobic metabolism.
  - They generate small amounts of ATP (cellular energy) and produce lactic acid as waste.

Cells are surrounded by fluid that allows for easy movement of nutrients and wastes. A physical property of this fluid that is a critical factor for cell survival is pH, which is the measure of acidity or alkalinity in a solution. Solutions that are high in pH (>7.0) are considered alkaline. A common example is soap. Solutions that are low in pH (<7.0) are considered acidic. Sulfuric acid in automotive batteries is one example. A solution that is neither acidic nor alkaline is considered neutral (pH 7.0). The body's cells want to exist in a near-neutral environment.

Your body spends a large amount of energy working to maintain a normal pH (normal human pH is 7.35 to 7.45). The waste products of cells are often acidic, such as carbon dioxide. Carbon dioxide is transported by combining with water to create *carbonic acid*, which is more soluble in the plasma. The plasma also contains sodium bicarbonate, which is alkaline and helps to buffer or neutralize the acidic waste products of cells.

The blood and lungs interact continuously to help to maintain the pH level in the body by controlling the level of carbon dioxide, and therefore the level of carbonic acid, in the blood. If the blood becomes acidic, the respiratory centers in the brainstem will increase breathing to "blow off" more carbon dioxide. If too much carbon dioxide is blown off, then the body can become too alkaline, which is what happens during hyperventilation.

# Pathophysiology

As mentioned previously, pathophysiology is the study of how normal physiologic processes are affected by disease. Many diseases can occur in patients and will result in calls to EMS. Some examples are diabetes (a disease of the pancreas), pneumonia (a disease of the lungs), and stroke (resulting from disease of the brain). Pathophysiologic changes that occur with specific diseases and trauma, respectively, are discussed in the chapters of Section 6, *Medical*, and Section 7, *Trauma*.

Respiratory compromise and shock are two common emergencies that you will likely encounter in your work as an EMT. This section provides an overview of respiratory compromise, shock, and alteration of cell metabolism as background for how the body responds to disease or injury.

## Respiratory Compromise

**Respiratory compromise** is the inability of the body to move gas effectively, which can result in a decreased level of oxygen in the body (**hypoxia**), an elevated level of carbon dioxide in the body (**hypercapnia**), or both. Recall the two concepts of breathing: ventilation and respiration. Ventilation is the movement of air between the lungs and environment, whereas respiration is the process of gas exchange. Respiratory compromise results when one of these functions is impaired.

## Factors That Impair Ventilation

The ability to move gas back and forth can be impaired in a variety of ways. A blocked airway is one example. If a person chokes on what he or she is eating, this will partially or completely block the movement of air through the trachea. The airway can also be blocked by foreign bodies (eg, toys, broken teeth), swelling in the airway, trauma to the mouth or neck, and swallowing blood or vomitus. The most common airway obstruction is blockage by the tongue. When a person is unconscious, the tongue relaxes and sags posteriorly in the mouth. The patient cannot "swallow his tongue," but the relaxed tongue may block the opening to the trachea. Fortunately, the airway can be easily opened with manual techniques. This will be discussed in later chapters.

Impairment of the muscles of breathing will impair the movement of gas into and out of the lungs. Neuromuscular diseases, such as cerebral palsy, can interfere with the ability of the brain to send signals to the diaphragm. Trauma can injure the phrenic nerve (the nerve that signals the diaphragm to contract and initiate inspiration) or damage the brainstem. If a patient's level of consciousness is too low, ventilatory problems can occur. This means that any condition that results in a loss of consciousness can have a direct effect on ventilation. For example, a soccer player who is unconscious after being struck in the head during a match may have impaired ventilation.

Ventilation can also be impaired when the lower airway is obstructed physiologically—for example, during an asthma attack. Early in an asthma attack, hyperventilation results in a decrease in the amount of carbon dioxide in the blood. As the patient fatigues, the level of carbon dioxide increases.

Contraction of muscles surrounding the lower airways prevents effective ventilation.

Ventilation can also be impaired by numerous other factors, including drug overdose (which depresses the CNS), trauma to the chest wall, and allergic reactions. These are discussed in their respective chapters in greater detail.

## Factors That Impair Respiration

Impairment of respiration (movement of gas at the cellular level) can also cause respiratory compromise.

A change in the atmosphere can interfere with a person's ability to breathe. The air you breathe is 21% oxygen, and the air you exhale is 16% oxygen. This means there is only a 5% margin of safety for oxygen concentration in the air you breathe. In certain situations—for example, in a fire—oxygen is displaced by another gas. When there is insufficient oxygen in the air, insufficient oxygen is inhaled. That means there is less oxygen in the alveoli to diffuse into the blood that passes by the lungs. If the cells of the body do not have enough oxygen delivered to them, they will not be able to function normally.

Respiration can also be impaired at high altitudes. At high altitudes, gas pressures change. The low atmospheric pressure of oxygen at high altitudes can impair oxygen movement into the blood.

### Words of Wisdom

There are two ways to express the amount of oxygen in the air: as a straight percentage or as a fraction of the inspired oxygen ($FIO_2$). $FIO_2$ is expressed as the decimal equivalent of the percentage of oxygen being delivered. Therefore, because oxygen makes up 21% of ambient room air, the $FIO_2$ of ambient room air is 0.21. The oxygen from a nonbreathing mask at 15 L/min is approximately 90%; therefore, the $FIO_2$ of the air from a nonrebreather mask at 15 L/min is approximately 0.9.

Respiration can also become compromised when movement of the gas across the cell membrane is impaired. If the patient has fluid in the alveoli, this fluid may prevent or hinder gas exchange. In pneumonia, mucus and pus form a barrier, preventing gas from accessing the alveoli. If the interstitial space (space between the cells in the lungs) is filled with fluid, this edema increases the distance from the capillary to the air in the alveoli. Because of the increased distance, it will take longer for the gas to move from inside the alveoli to inside the capillary. If one of the blood vessels bringing blood to the lungs is clogged, this will also affect the amount of gas that diffuses into and out of the blood.

## Ventilation/Perfusion Mismatch

One way to describe respiratory function and therefore to understand respiratory compromise is the ventilation/perfusion ratio. This measurement, also called the $\dot{V}/\dot{Q}$ ratio, describes how much gas is being moved effectively (ventilation) through the lungs and how much blood is flowing around the alveoli where gas exchange (perfusion) occurs. A mismatch occurs when one of those two variables is abnormal.

For example, in a patient with pulmonary embolism, a blood clot breaks off from a large vein and creates a sudden clog in one of the branches of the pulmonary arteries, preventing blood flow to the alveoli in the lung. A ventilated segment of the lung does not receive blood, and therefore gas is not exchanged. This results in a ventilation/perfusion mismatch, expressed as a change in the $\dot{V}/\dot{Q}$ ratio.

Another example is edema caused by pulmonary contusion, in which gas is unable to move effectively through the alveoli in a portion of the lung. Due to fluid bruising in a portion of the lung, blood passing through that portion does not undergo air exchange because there is no ventilation occurring in that portion of the lung. Therefore the "V" portion of the $\dot{V}/\dot{Q}$ ratio is impacted.

When either the "V" or the "Q" is impacted, respiratory compromise can occur.

## Effects of Respiratory Compromise on the Body

Regardless of the cause of impaired ventilation or respiration, the overall effect of respiratory compromise is the same.

- Oxygen levels throughout the body fall and carbon dioxide levels rise.
- The brain detects an increase in carbon dioxide levels.
- The body increases its respiratory rate to return the carbon dioxide levels to normal.

- If increased respiration does not occur or is not effective in returning the carbon dioxide levels to normal, the blood will become more acidic.
- Similarly, blood oxygen levels will begin to fall. This will cause the brain to issue further commands to breathe.

Decreased oxygen levels will force cells to move from aerobic metabolism to anaerobic metabolism. Remember, heart and brain cells cannot survive without a constant supply of oxygen and will die in minutes. Anaerobic metabolism generates a fraction of the needed energy, and cellular functions will be impaired. Recall that a by-product of anaerobic metabolism is lactic acid. If too much of this acid is created, the pH of the blood will drop further. If the pH becomes too low, cells will die.

If respiratory compromise is mild and gradual, the body can adapt. Complete anaerobic metabolism that is severe (ie, a complete lack of oxygen in the body) and that lasts more than 1 to 3 minutes can overwhelm the body's ability to adapt; if left untreated, it can exhaust the body's energy supplies and the patient may die (**TABLE 6-13**).

## Shock

Recall that shock (systemic hypoperfusion) is a condition in which organs and tissues receive an inadequate supply of blood and oxygen; in other words, they are poorly perfused. It can occur due to inadequacy of the central circulation (insufficient blood volume, or a heart that does not pump effectively) or of the peripheral circulation (inability of the body to control the size of the blood vessels).

Oxygen delivery is directly related to the concentration of red blood cells (and their hemoglobin concentration), the amount of oxygen being carried by the blood (oxygen saturation), and the pumping ability of the heart (cardiac output). Impairment in any one of these three areas will lead to impaired oxygen delivery and shock.

Impaired oxygen delivery causes cellular hypoxia (decreased amount of oxygen delivered to the cells), which leads to anaerobic metabolism, lactic acid production, and organ dysfunction.

Shock is categorized into several types depending on the cause. These types are defined in **TABLE 6-14**. They are discussed in more detail in Chapter 13, *Shock.*

### TABLE 6-13 Summary of Respiratory Compromise

| Category | Problem | Effect |
|---|---|---|
| Ventilation | Damage to the regulatory centers of the brain | Erratic breathing pattern and rate |
| | Inability to exhale effectively | Carbon dioxide builds up in blood |
| | Inability to inhale effectively | Oxygen levels in the blood decrease |
| | Injury to chest | Breathing depth decreases |
| | Obstruction of the airway | Decreased or absent movement of air |
| | Overdose/toxic exposure | Decreased level of consciousness leading to decreased breathing rate and depth |
| | Loss of consciousness | Breathing depth decreases |
| | Weakened respiratory muscles | Breathing depth decreases |
| Respiration | Fluid within the alveoli (pulmonary edema) | Prevents gas from entering the alveoli |
| | Mucus or infectious wastes | Prevent gas from entering the alveoli |
| | Impaired blood flow to the lungs (pulmonary embolism) | Affects blood flow to lung tissue where gas exchange occurs |
| Oxygenation | Decreased oxygen in the air breathed | Affects diffusion of gas |
| | Increased carbon dioxide in the air breathed | Affects diffusion of gas |
| | Toxins in the air breathed | Affect ability of oxygen to be carried effectively in blood |

**TABLE 6-14** Types of Shock

| Type | Description | Examples of Causes |
|---|---|---|
| Hypovolemic | Shock resulting from lack of blood volume<br>Circulating blood volume is inadequate to deliver sufficient oxygen and nutrients to the body | • Trauma (blood loss results in inability to transport oxygen and nutrients)<br>• Severe vomiting/diarrhea (substantial loss of water can lead to decreased circulating blood volume; there is less blood to transport oxygen and nutrients) |
| Cardiogenic | Shock associated with impaired heart function<br>Compromised heart function prevents wastes and nutrients from moving around the body effectively | • Weakened heart muscles as a result of myocardial infarction (heart attack) or other conditions<br>• Very fast or very slow heart rate (can prevent blood from moving effectively, blood pressure drops, and perfusion is diminished) |
| Obstructive | Shock resulting from blocked blood flow back to or through the heart | • Severe lung collapse (tension pneumothorax) (pushes on the vena cava, preventing it from returning blood to the heart)<br>• Accumulation of fluid in the sac surrounding the heart (prevents heart from filling)<br>• Large blood clot in pulmonary artery (pulmonary embolus) (can prevent right ventricle from pumping blood out of the heart into the lungs) |
| Anaphylactic | Shock resulting from severe allergic reaction | • Severe allergic reaction (blood vessels dilate, blood pressure drops, and perfusion decreases) |
| Septic | Shock resulting from severe infection. Blood vessels dilate and decreased blood pressure results; leads to dysfunction in multiple organ systems and death | • Severe infection (blood vessels dilate, blood pressure drops, and perfusion decreases) |
| Neurogenic | Shock resulting from injury to the nervous system.<br>For example, spinal cord injury may result in dilation of vessels (vasodilation) below the level of the injury | • High spinal cord injury (blood vessels dilate, blood pressure drops, and perfusion decreases) |

© Jones & Bartlett Learning.

## Effects of Shock on the Body

The effects of inadequate perfusion on the body are similar to those of respiratory compromise. The level of oxygen supplied to the tissues falls. This causes the cells to engage in anaerobic metabolism, which results in increased lactic acid production. A severe metabolic acidosis ensues, leading to increased levels of carbonic acid within the blood. Patients who can compensate increase their breathing rate and depth, thereby increasing their minute volume.

Baroreceptors detect the decreased blood pressure and initiate the release of epinephrine and norepinephrine. The heart rate will increase, the heart will beat more forcefully, and the blood vessels will constrict. The body's goal is to maintain blood pressure to the areas of the body that are unable to survive without oxygen: the brain and the heart.

Another compensatory mechanism, particularly with hypovolemic shock, is the movement of fluid outside of the cells and outside of the blood vessels (interstitial fluid) into the capillaries. This helps refill the blood vessels and restore some fluid volume so the heart has enough liquid to pump. However, in other forms of shock such as septic and anaphylactic shock, the capillaries leak and volume from the blood vessels (intravascular volume) moves into the interstitial space. This loss of vascular fluid means there is less blood returning to the heart to pump.

Ultimately the effect of all types of shock is decreased availability of fuel for the cells and impairment of cellular metabolism. Once a certain level of tissue hypoperfusion is reached, cell damage proceeds in a similar manner regardless of the underlying cause of the shock.

## Alteration of Cellular Metabolism

Impairment of cellular metabolism results in the inability to properly use oxygen and glucose at the cellular level.

As discussed, when there is inadequate oxygen, cells will create energy through anaerobic metabolism. Anaerobic metabolism serves as a temporary backup system to allow cells to function at low energy levels for a short time. Most cells are able to use alternative fuel supplies to help bridge the gap until perfusion is restored. For example, when a person is engaged in strenuous exercise, the demand for glucose by the muscles exceeds the available supply. The body begins to burn fats and turns them into glucose to meet this need.

However, anaerobic metabolism has some important drawbacks. Recall that the use of fats as an alternative fuel supply results in a buildup of lactic acid. This ultimately can result in metabolic acidosis. The process of anaerobic metabolism requires more energy than when using glucose for fuel. Therefore, there are more wastes to be removed, and the body must work harder. Other conditions resulting from anaerobic metabolism include decreased ability of the blood to effectively carry oxygen to the cells and overall decreased functioning of oxygen within the cell.

Although most cells are able to use alternative fuels, brain cells cannot. They rely on a constant supply of glucose to function. When perfusion is impaired, there is less glucose for cells to use. If the supply of available glucose is dramatically decreased, brain cells will quickly become damaged or die.

Cellular injury may, up to a point, be repairable if normal tissue perfusion is restored. When irreversible injury occurs, however, no treatment will help. Cell death is followed by necrosis, a process in which the cell breaks down. The cell membrane becomes abnormally permeable, leading to an influx of electrolytes and fluids. The cell and its components (organelles) swell and are ultimately destroyed, resulting in cell death.

Therefore, when perfusion is ineffective, it needs to be restored so that cells can return to a state of aerobic metabolism and life can continue. Many interventions you will perform as an EMT are aimed at improving conditions that can result in impaired perfusion.

## YOU are the Provider SUMMARY

**1. How will knowledge of anatomy and physiology help you provide appropriate patient care?**

Knowledge of anatomy and physiology is important for anyone who provides patient care—emergency or otherwise. When a patient reports pain to any part of the body, your knowledge of human anatomy will help you form a logical field impression—that is, what you believe to be the primary problem—regarding which organ or organs may be affected. Your knowledge of physiology will help you predict the negative effects the patient may experience based on the organ or organs affected. From this information, an appropriate treatment plan can be formulated and implemented.

Although you are not expected to diagnose a patient's condition, a strong fundamental knowledge of anatomy, physiology, and medical terminology will help you communicate the correct information to the emergency department physician or nurse.

**2. On the sole basis of the patient's chief complaint, which organ or organs should you suspect is/are the cause of his condition?**

The major organs in the right upper quadrant (RUQ) are the liver, gallbladder, and a portion of the large intestine (colon). Although your initial thoughts should focus on dysfunction of one or more of these organs, the patient's true problem may exist elsewhere in his abdomen and the pain just happens to be manifesting in his RUQ. Although your objectives are to recognize that the patient has an acute abdominal problem and to find and treat life-threatening conditions, you will need to ask additional questions to clarify his complaint. His answers to your questions will help you formulate a field impression.

**3. What additional questions should you ask to gather more information about his chief complaint?**

After determining why the patient called 9-1-1, ask the patient to elaborate on the complaint; this is called the history of present illness. The OPQRST mnemonic is a useful tool for this purpose.

The patient has already told you that his pain began suddenly 20 minutes ago, so the "O" and "T" in the OPQRST have been established. Ask him if anything makes his pain better or worse; patients with abdominal pain often draw their knees into their abdomen to take pressure off the abdominal muscles, which may provide them with slight relief from their pain. Ask the patient if the pain stays in the RUQ of his abdomen or moves/travels somewhere else; determine if he has referred pain by asking if he hurts anywhere else in addition to his RUQ. Assess the severity of his pain by using a 0 to 10 scale, with 0 being no pain and 10 being the worst pain ever experienced. Pain severity should be assessed frequently, especially after any interventions have been performed. Although chronic pain can indicate a serious underlying problem, you should be especially concerned that his pain began acutely.

Other questions to ask the patient should focus on common symptoms associated with abdominal pain, such as nausea and/or vomiting, diarrhea, and urinary difficulty, among others. When possible, try not to ask leading questions (ie, "Are you nauseated?"); instead, simply ask him if he has any other symptoms.

**4. What additional symptoms would you expect the patient to experience based on the function of the gallbladder?**

The gallbladder contracts only when food enters the duodenum; patients with inflammation of the gallbladder (cholecystitis) typically have pain in the RUQ within an hour or so after eating a meal. In many cases, the patient also reports referred pain to the right shoulder. Other symptoms of gallbladder disease include nausea, vomiting, and heartburn.

Most cases of cholecystitis occur when gallstones form and block the outlet of the gallbladder. In some cases, the gallstones spontaneously pass; however, if they do not, the patient experiences pain of varying intensity.

**5. How does knowledge of anatomy, physiology, and medical terminology facilitate communication with other health care professionals?**

As part of the health care team, everything you do should benefit the patient. An integral part of patient care is effective communication with other health care professionals. Your ability to speak the language of medicine will minimize communication barriers between you and other members of the health care team and therefore will directly benefit your patient.

Whether you are calling in your radio report from the ambulance or giving a verbal report at the hospital, the use of appropriate medical terminology ensures that the information you pass along is relevant and accurate.

Review human anatomy and physiology and medical terminology on a regular basis. Although the structure and function of the body and the terms used to describe it do not change, your ability to recall the information can deteriorate over time.

**6. Should your documentation of an EMS call differ from your verbal communication with other health care professionals? Why or why not?**

In general, your verbal communication and the patient care report (PCR) should reflect the same relevant and accurate information, although you may expand on some of the details in your written report. For example, a verbal report will likely only indicate one set of vital signs or any significant changes in the vital signs, whereas your PCR will usually have several sets of vital signs.

Similarly, your written report may expand on the list of medications or contain data on time that would not be included in a verbal report. However, both reports should contain any significant information about the patient, his condition, symptoms and history, treatments given, and any changes during the call. When possible, use proper medical terminology when documenting the patient's complaint, history of present illness, medical history, and any treatment provided in the prehospital setting. If you are unsure of the correct medical term to accurately describe a particular aspect of the patient's complaint or physical examination, use plain English.

## YOU are the Provider SUMMARY *continued*

The PCR is read by the personnel who assume patient care from you and may have a direct effect on future care that the patient receives. It also becomes part of the patient's permanent medical record. The use of proper medical terminology, coupled with an accurate depiction of the care you provided, will facilitate continuity of the patient's care.

### EMS Patient Care Report (PCR)

| Date: 6-10-20 | Incident No.: 050109 | Nature of Call: Abdominal pain | | Location: 322 Azalea Trail | |
|---|---|---|---|---|---|
| Dispatched: 1740 | En Route: 1741 | At Scene: 1747 | Transport: 1759 | At Hospital: 1809 | In Service: 1817 |

#### Patient Information

| | |
|---|---|
| **Age:** 60<br>**Sex:** M<br>**Weight (in kg [lb]):** 84 kg (185 lb) | **Allergies:** Sulfa, codeine, contrast dye<br>**Medications:** Zyrtec, Pepcid<br>**Past Medical History:** Gallbladder problems<br>**Chief Complaint:** Abdominal pain |

#### Vital Signs

| Time: 1749 | BP: 142/82 | Pulse: 110 | Respirations: 24 | Spo$_2$: 98% |
|---|---|---|---|---|
| Time: 1759 | BP: 138/88 | Pulse: 112 | Respirations: 24 | Spo$_2$: 97% |
| Time: 1808 | BP: 132/80 | Pulse: 90 | Respirations: 20 | Spo$_2$: 99% |

#### EMS Treatment (circle all that apply)

| Oxygen @ ___ L/min via:<br><br>NC   NRM   Bag mask | | Assisted Ventilation | Airway Adjunct | CPR |
|---|---|---|---|---|
| Defibrillation | Bleeding Control | Bandaging | Splinting | **Other:** Position of comfort |

#### Narrative

9-1-1 dispatch to a residence for a male patient with abdominal pain.

Chief Complaint: Abdominal pain

History: His past medical history is significant for gallbladder problems; no other medical history reported.

Assessment: On arrival at the scene, found the patient, a 60-year-old man, lying on his side on the floor of his bedroom with his knees drawn up into his abdomen. He was conscious and alert; his airway was patent, and his breathing was adequate with an initial Sao$_2$ 98%. Patient stated the pain (8 on a 0 to 10 scale) began suddenly approximately 20 minutes earlier.

Treatment (Rx): Obtained vital signs. Further assessment of patient's abdomen revealed that it was soft; however, it was point tender on palpation of the RUQ. Patient stated he had some nausea but denied chest pain, shortness of breath, vomiting, or any other symptoms. He further denied radiating and referred pain.

Transport: Lifted the patient onto the stretcher, allowed him to assume a position of comfort, loaded him into the ambulance, and began transport to the hospital. En route, continued to monitor patient's condition, which remained unchanged. Vital signs reassessed and noted above.

Shortly before arrival at the hospital, the patient stated that his pain had decreased in severity. Transferred care of patient to receiving hospital without incident and gave verbal report to charge nurse. Departed the hospital and returned to service.

**End of report**

# Prep Kit

## Ready for Review

- To properly care for your patients, you must have a thorough understanding of human anatomy and physiology so you can assess your patients' condition and communicate with hospital personnel and other health care providers.
- You must be able to identify superficial landmarks of the body and know what lies underneath the skin so that you can perform an accurate patient assessment.
- The skeleton gives the body its recognizable human form through a collection of bones, ligaments, tendons, and cartilage.
- The skeletal system provides protection for fragile organs, allows for movement, and gives the body its shape.
- The contraction and relaxation of the musculoskeletal system gives the body its ability to move.
- The respiratory system consists of all the structures of the body that contribute to the process of breathing. It includes the nose, mouth, throat, larynx, trachea, bronchi, and bronchioles.
- The function of the respiratory system is to provide the body with oxygen and eliminate carbon dioxide.
- The circulatory system is a complex arrangement of connected tubes, including the arteries, arterioles, capillaries, venules, and veins.
- The nervous system is perhaps the most complex organ system within the human body. It consists of the brain, spinal cord, and nerves.
- The skin is divided into two parts: the superficial epidermis, which is composed of several layers of cells, and the deeper dermis, which contains the specialized skin structures.
- The skin, the largest single organ in the body, has multiple functions, chiefly to protect

the body in the environment, to regulate the temperature of the body, and to transmit information from the environment to the brain.
- The digestive system is composed of the gastrointestinal tract (stomach and intestines), mouth, salivary glands, pharynx, esophagus, liver, gallbladder, pancreas, rectum, and anus.
- Digestion of food, from the moment it is taken into the mouth until essential compounds are extracted and delivered by the circulatory system to nourish all cells in the body, is a complicated chemical process.
- The lymphatic system is composed of the spleen, lymph nodes, lymph, lymph vessels, thymus gland, and other components. It supports the circulatory system and the immune system, and relies on muscle contractions and movements of the body for lymph to flow.
- The endocrine system is a complex message and control system that integrates many body functions.
- The urinary system controls the discharge of certain waste materials filtered from the blood by the kidneys.
- The genital system controls the reproductive processes by which life is created.
- Solutions that are high in pH (>7.0) are considered alkaline. Solutions that are low in pH (<7.0) are considered acidic. A solution that is neither acidic nor alkaline is considered neutral (pH 7.0).
- Pathophysiology is the study of how normal physiologic processes are affected by disease.
- Respiratory compromise is the inability of the body to move gas effectively. Respiratory compromise results when either ventilation or respiration is impaired.
- Shock is a condition in which organs and tissue receive an inadequate flow of blood and

oxygen, or perfusion. Impaired oxygen delivery causes cellular hypoxia, which in turn leads to anaerobic metabolism, lactic acid production, and organ dysfunction.

- Impairment of cellular metabolism results in the inability to properly use oxygen and

glucose at the cellular level. When irreversible cellular injury occurs, no treatment will help. Therefore, when perfusion is ineffective, it needs to be restored quickly.

## Vital Vocabulary

**abdomen**  The body cavity that contains many of the major organs of digestion and excretion. It is located below the diaphragm and above the pelvis.

**acetabulum**  The depression on the lateral pelvis where its three component bones join, in which the femoral head fits snugly.

**adenosine triphosphate (ATP)**  The nucleotide involved in energy metabolism; used to store energy.

**adrenal glands**  Endocrine glands located on top of the kidneys that release adrenaline when stimulated by the sympathetic nervous system.

**adrenergic**  Pertaining to nerves that release the neurotransmitter norepinephrine, or nor-adrenaline (eg, adrenergic nerves, adrenergic response); also pertains to the receptors acted on by norepinephrine.

**aerobic metabolism**  Metabolism that can proceed only in the presence of oxygen.

**agonal gasps**  Abnormal breathing pattern characterized by slow, gasping breaths, sometimes seen in patients in cardiac arrest.

**alpha-adrenergic receptors**  Portions of the nervous system that, when stimulated, can cause constriction of blood vessels.

**alveoli**  The air sacs of the lungs in which the exchange of oxygen and carbon dioxide takes place.

**anaerobic metabolism**  Metabolism that takes place in the absence of oxygen; the main by-product is lactic acid.

**anatomic position**  The position of reference in which the patient stands facing forward, arms at the side, with the palms of the hands forward.

**anatomy**  The study of the physical structure of the body and its components.

**aorta**  The main artery leaving the left side of the heart and carrying freshly oxygenated blood to the body.

**appendicular skeleton**  The portion of the skeletal system that comprises the arms, legs, pelvis, and shoulder girdle.

**appendix**  A small, tubular structure that is attached to the lower border of the cecum in the lower right quadrant of the abdomen.

**arterioles**  The smallest branches of arteries leading to the vast network of capillaries.

**articular cartilage**  A pearly layer of specialized cartilage covering the articular surfaces (contact surfaces on the ends) of bones in synovial joints.

**atrium**  One of the two upper chambers of the heart.

**autonomic nervous system**  The part of the nervous system that regulates functions, such as digestion and sweating, that are not controlled voluntarily.

**axial skeleton**  The part of the skeleton comprising the skull, vertebral column, and rib cage.

**axons**  Extensions of a neuron that carry impulses away from the nerve cell body to the dendrites (receivers) of another neuron.

**ball-and-socket joint**  A joint that allows internal and external rotation, as well as bending.

**beta-adrenergic receptors**  Portions of the nervous system that, when stimulated, can cause an increase in the force of contraction of the heart, an increased heart rate, and bronchial dilation.

**biceps** The large muscle that covers the front of the humerus.

**bile ducts** The ducts that convey bile between the liver and the intestine.

**blood pressure (BP)** The pressure that the blood exerts against the walls of the arteries as it passes through them.

**brachial artery** The major vessel in the upper extremities that supplies blood to the arm.

**brain** The controlling organ of the body and center of consciousness; functions include perception, control of reactions to the environment, emotional responses, and judgment.

**brainstem** The area of the brain between the spinal cord and cerebrum, surrounded by the cerebellum; controls functions that are necessary for life, such as respiration.

**calcaneus** The heel bone.

**capillary vessels** The tiny blood vessels between the arterioles and venules that permit transfer of oxygen, carbon dioxide, nutrients, and waste between body tissues and the blood.

**cardiac muscle** The heart muscle.

**cardiac output (CO)** A measure of the volume of blood circulated by the heart in 1 minute, calculated by multiplying the stroke volume by the heart rate.

**carotid artery** The major artery that supplies blood to the head and brain.

**carpals** Small bones that compose the wrist.

**cartilage** The smooth connective tissue that forms the support structure of the skeletal system and provides cushioning between bones; also forms the nasal septum and portions of the outer ear.

**cecum** The first part of the large intestine, into which the ileum opens.

**cellular metabolism** A set of chemical reactions that supplies cells with energy. Includes both anaerobic and aerobic metabolism.

**central nervous system (CNS)** The brain and spinal cord.

**cerebellum** One of the three major subdivisions of the brain, sometimes called the little brain; coordinates the various activities of the brain, particularly fine body movements.

**cerebrospinal fluid (CSF)** Fluid produced in the ventricles of the brain that flows in the subarachnoid space and bathes the meninges.

**cerebrum** The largest part of the three subdivisions of the brain, sometimes called the gray matter; made up of several lobes that control movement, hearing, balance, speech, visual perception, emotions, and personality.

**cervical spine** The portion of the vertebral column consisting of the first seven vertebrae that lie in the neck.

**chordae tendineae** Thin bands of fibrous tissue that attach to the valves in the heart and prevent them from inverting.

**chyme** The substance that leaves the stomach. It is a combination of all of the eaten foods with added stomach acids.

**circulatory system** The complex arrangement of connected tubes, including the arteries, arterioles, capillaries, venules, and veins, that moves blood, oxygen, nutrients, carbon dioxide, and cellular waste throughout the body.

**clavicle** The collarbone; it is lateral to the sternum and anterior to the scapula.

**coccyx** The last three or four vertebrae of the spine; the tail bone.

**coronal (frontal) plane** An imaginary plane where the body is divided into front and back parts.

**coxae** The hip bones (singular: coxa).

**cranium** The part of the skull that encloses the brain and is composed of eight bones.

**cricoid cartilage** A firm ridge of cartilage that forms the lower part of the larynx.

**cricothyroid membrane** A thin sheet of fascia that connects the thyroid and cricoid cartilages that make up the larynx.

**dead space** Any portion of the airway that does contain air and cannot participate in gas exchange, such as the trachea and bronchi.

**dermis** The inner layer of the skin, containing hair follicles, sweat glands, nerve endings, and blood vessels.

**diaphragm** A muscular dome that forms the undersurface of the thorax, separating the chest from the abdominal cavity. Contraction of this (and the chest wall muscles) brings air into the lungs. Relaxation allows air to be expelled from the lungs.

**diastole** The relaxation, or period of relaxation, of the heart, especially of the ventricles.

**diffusion** Movement of a gas from an area of higher concentration to an area of lower concentration.

**digestion** The processing of food that nourishes the individual cells of the body.

**dorsalis pedis artery** The artery on the anterior surface of the foot between the first and second metatarsals.

**endocrine system** The complex message and control system that integrates many body functions, including the release of hormones.

**enzymes** Substances designed to speed up the rate of specific biochemical reactions.

**epidermis** The outer layer of skin, which is made up of cells that are sealed together to form a watertight protective covering for the body.

**epiglottis** A thin, leaf-shaped valve that allows air to pass into the trachea but prevents food and liquid from entering.

**epinephrine** A substance produced by the body (commonly called adrenaline), and a drug produced by pharmaceutical companies that increases pulse rate and blood pressure; the drug of choice for an anaphylactic reaction.

**esophagus** A collapsible tube that extends from the pharynx to the stomach; muscle contractions propel food and liquids through it to the stomach.

**expiratory reserve volume** The amount of air that can be exhaled following a normal exhalation; average volume is about 1,200 mL in the average adult man.

**extension** The straightening of a joint.

**fallopian tubes** The tubes that connect each ovary with the uterus and are the primary location for fertilization of the ovum.

**femoral artery** The major artery of the thigh, a continuation of the external iliac artery. It supplies blood to the lower abdominal wall, external genitalia, and legs. It can be palpated in the groin area.

**femoral head** The proximal end of the femur, articulating with the acetabulum to form the hip joint.

**femur** The thighbone; the longest and one of the strongest bones in the body.

**fibula** The smaller of the two bones that form the lower leg, located on the lateral side.

**flexion** The bending of a joint.

**foramen magnum** A large opening at the base of the skull through which the brain connects to the spinal cord.

**frontal bones** The bones of the cranium that form the forehead.

**gallbladder** A sac on the undersurface of the liver that collects bile from the liver and discharges it into the duodenum through the common bile duct.

**genital system** The reproductive system in men and women.

**germinal layer** The deepest layer of the epidermis where new skin cells are formed.

**greater trochanter** A bony prominence on the proximal lateral side of the thigh, just below the hip joint.

**hair follicles** The small organs that produce hair.

**heart** A hollow muscular organ that pumps blood throughout the body.

**heart rate (HR)** The number of heartbeats during a specific time (usually 1 minute).

**hemoglobin** An oxygen-carrying protein found in red blood cells.

**hinge joints** Joints that can bend and straighten but cannot rotate; they restrict motion to one plane.

**hormones** Substances formed in specialized organs or glands and carried to another organ or group of cells in the same organism; they regulate many body functions, including metabolism, growth, and body temperature.

**humerus** The supporting bone of the upper arm.

**hydrostatic pressure** The pressure of water against the walls of its container.

**hypercapnia** An abnormally high level of carbon dioxide in the bloodstream; also called hypercarbia.

**hypoperfusion** A condition in which the circulatory system fails to provide sufficient circulation to maintain normal cellular function; also called shock.

**hypoxia** Deficient oxygen concentration in the tissues.

**hypoxic drive** A "backup system" to control respiration; senses drops in the oxygen level in the blood.

**ilium** One of three bones that fuse to form the pelvic ring.

**inferior vena cava** One of the two largest veins in the body; carries blood from the lower extremities and the pelvis and the abdominal organs to the heart.

**inspiratory reserve volume** The amount of air that can be inhaled after a normal inhalation; the amount of air that can be inhaled in addition to the normal tidal volume.

**interstitial space** The space in between the cells.

**intervertebral disks** Tough, elastic structures between adjoining vertebrae that act as shock absorbers.

**intracellular space** The space within a cell or cells.

**involuntary muscle** The muscle over which a person has no conscious control. It is found in many automatic regulating systems of the body.

**ischium** One of three bones that fuse to form the pelvic ring.

**joint** The place where two bones come into contact; also called an articulation.

**joint capsule** The fibrous sac that encloses a joint.

**kidneys** Two retroperitoneal organs that excrete the end products of metabolism as urine and regulate the body's salt and water content.

**labored breathing** The use of muscles of the chest, back, and abdomen to assist in expanding the chest; occurs when air movement is impaired.

**lactic acid** A metabolic by-product of the breakdown of glucose that accumulates when metabolism proceeds in the absence of oxygen (anaerobic metabolism).

**large intestine** The portion of the digestive tube that encircles the abdomen around the small bowel, consisting of the cecum, the colon, and the rectum. It helps regulate water balance and eliminate solid waste.

**lesser trochanter** The projection on the medial/superior portion of the femur.

**ligaments** Bands of fibrous tissue that connect bones to bones. Ligaments support and strengthen a joint.

**liver** A large, solid organ that lies in the right upper quadrant immediately below the diaphragm; it produces bile, stores glucose for immediate use by the body, and produces many substances that help regulate immune responses.

**lumbar spine** The lower part of the back, formed by the lowest five nonfused vertebrae; also called the dorsal spine.

**lymph** A thin, straw-colored fluid that carries oxygen, nutrients, and hormones to the cells and carries waste products of metabolism away from the cells and back into the capillaries so that they may be excreted.

**lymph nodes** Tiny, oval-shaped structures located in various places along the lymph vessels that filter lymph.

**malleolus** A rounded bony prominence on either side of the ankle; also called the ankle bone.

**mandible** The bone of the lower jaw.

**manubrium** The upper quarter of the sternum.

**maxillae** The upper jawbones that assist in the formation of the orbit, the nasal cavity, and the palate and hold the upper teeth.

**medulla oblongata** Nerve tissue that is continuous inferiorly with the spinal cord; serves as a conduction pathway for ascending and descending nerve tracts; coordinates heart rate, blood vessel diameter, breathing, swallowing, vomiting, coughing, and sneezing.

**metabolism** The biochemical processes that result in production of energy from nutrients within cells.

**metacarpals** Bones of the hand, situated between the carpals and phalanges.

**metatarsals** Bones of the foot, situated between the tarsals and phalanges.

**midbrain** The part of the brain that is responsible for helping to regulate the level of consciousness.

**midsagittal (midline) plane** An imaginary vertical line drawn from the middle of the forehead through the nose and the umbilicus (navel) to the floor, dividing the body into equal left and right halves.

**minute volume** The volume of air that moves in and out of the lungs per minute; calculated by multiplying the tidal volume and respiratory rate; also called minute ventilation.

**motor nerves** Nerves that carry information from the central nervous system to the muscles of the body.

**mucous membranes** The lining of body cavities and passages that communicate directly or indirectly with the environment outside the body.

**mucus** The watery secretion of the mucous membranes that lubricates the body openings.

**musculoskeletal system** The bones and voluntary muscles of the body.

**myocardium** The heart muscle.

**nasopharynx** The part of the pharynx that lies above the level of the roof of the mouth, or palate.

**nervous system** The system that controls virtually all activities of the body, both voluntary and involuntary.

**neurons** The functional units of the nervous system; also called nerve cells.

**norepinephrine** A neurotransmitter and drug sometimes used in the treatment of shock; produces vasoconstriction through its alpha-stimulator properties.

**occipital bone** The most posterior bone of the cranium.

**oncotic pressure** The pressure of water to move, typically into the capillary, as the result of the presence of plasma proteins.

**orbit** The eye socket, made up of the maxilla and zygoma.

**oropharynx** A tubular structure that extends vertically from the back of the mouth to the esophagus and trachea.

**ovaries** The primary female reproductive organs that produce an ovum, or egg, that, if fertilized, will develop into a fetus.

**pancreas** A flat, solid organ that lies below the liver and the stomach; it is a major source of digestive enzymes and produces the hormone insulin.

**parasympathetic nervous system** A subdivision of the autonomic nervous system, involved in control of involuntary functions, mediated largely by the vagus nerve through the chemical acetylcholine.

**parietal bones** The bones that lie between the temporal and occipital regions of the cranium.

**patella** The knee cap; a specialized bone that lies within the tendon of the quadriceps muscle.

**pathophysiology** The study of how normal physiologic processes are affected by disease.

**pectoral girdle** The supporting structure for the arms, which attaches the arms to the axial skeleton. It comprises the clavicles and scapulae; also called the shoulder girdle.

**pelvic girdle** The supporting structure for the legs, which serves to connect the legs to the axial skeleton.

**perfusion** The circulation of oxygenated blood within an organ or tissue in adequate amounts to meet the current needs of the cells.

**peripheral nervous system (PNS)** The part of the nervous system that consists of 31 pairs of spinal nerves and 12 pairs of cranial nerves; these may be sensory nerves, motor nerves, or connecting nerves.

**peristalsis** The wavelike contraction of smooth muscle by which the ureters or other tubular organs propel their contents.

**phalanges** The bones of the fingers and toes.

**physiology** The study of the normal functions of living organisms and their parts.

**plasma** A sticky, yellow fluid that carries the blood cells and nutrients and transports cellular waste material to the organs of excretion.

**platelets** Tiny, disc-shaped elements that are much smaller than the cells; they are essential in the initial formation of a blood clot, the mechanism that stops bleeding.

**pleura** The serous membranes covering the lungs and lining the thorax, completely enclosing a potential space known as the pleural space.

**pleural space** The potential space between the parietal pleura and the visceral pleura; described as "potential" because under normal conditions, the space does not exist.

**pons** An organ that lies below the midbrain and above the medulla and contains numerous important nerve fibers, including those for sleep, respiration, and the medullary respiratory center.

**posterior tibial artery** The artery just behind the medial malleolus; supplies blood to the foot.

**prostate gland** A small gland that surrounds the male urethra where it emerges from the urinary bladder; it secretes a fluid that is part of the ejaculatory fluid.

**pubic symphysis** A hard, bony, and cartilaginous prominence found at the midline in the lowermost portion of the abdomen where the two halves of the pelvic ring are joined by cartilage at a joint with minimal motion.

**pubis** One of three bones that fuse to form the pelvic ring.

**pulmonary artery** The major artery leading from the right ventricle of the heart to the lungs; carries oxygen-poor blood.

**pulmonary circulation** The flow of blood from the right ventricle through the pulmonary arteries and all of their branches and capillaries in the lungs and back to the left atrium through the venules and pulmonary veins; also called the lesser circulation.

**pulmonary veins** The four veins that return oxygenated blood from the lungs to the left atrium of the heart.

**pulse** The wave of pressure created as the heart contracts and forces blood out the left ventricle and into the major arteries.

**radial artery** The major artery in the forearm; it is palpable at the wrist on the thumb side.

**radius** The bone on the thumb side of the forearm.

**rectum** The lowermost end of the colon.

**red blood cells** Cells that carry oxygen to the body's tissues; also called erythrocytes.

**renal pelvis** A cone-shaped area that collects urine from the kidneys and funnels it through the ureter into the bladder.

**residual volume** The air that remains in the lungs after maximal expiration.

**respiration** The inhaling and exhaling of air; the physiologic process that exchanges carbon dioxide from fresh air.

**respiratory compromise** The inability of the body to move gas effectively.

**respiratory system** All the structures of the body that contribute to the process of breathing, consisting of the upper and lower airways and their component parts.

**reticular activating system (RAS)** Located in the upper brainstem; responsible for maintenance of consciousness, specifically one's level of arousal.

**retroperitoneal** Behind the abdominal cavity.

**sacroiliac joint** The connection point between the pelvis and the vertebral column.

**sacrum** One of three bones (sacrum and two pelvic bones) that make up the pelvic ring; consists of five fused sacral vertebrae.

**sagittal (lateral) plane** An imaginary line where the body is divided into left and right parts.

**salivary glands** The glands that produce saliva to keep the mouth and pharynx moist.

**scalp** The thick skin covering the cranium, which usually bears hair.

**scapula** The shoulder blade.

**sebaceous glands** Glands that produce an oily substance called sebum, which discharges along the shafts of the hairs.

**semen** Fluid ejaculated from the penis and containing sperm.

**seminal vesicles** Storage sacs for sperm and seminal fluid, which empty into the urethra at the prostate.

**sensory nerves** The nerves that carry sensations such as touch, taste, smell, heat, cold, and pain from the body to the central nervous system.

**shock** A condition in which the circulatory system fails to provide sufficient circulation to maintain normal cellular functions; also called hypoperfusion.

**skeletal muscle** Muscle that is attached to bones and usually crosses at least one joint; striated, or voluntary, muscle.

**skeletal system** The framework of the body, composed of bones and other connective tissues, that supports and protects internal organs and other body tissues.

**small intestine** The portion of the digestive tube between the stomach and the cecum, consisting of the duodenum, jejunum, and ileum.

**smooth muscle** Involuntary muscle; it constitutes the bulk of the gastrointestinal tract and is present in nearly every organ to regulate automatic activity.

**somatic nervous system** The part of the nervous system that regulates activities over which there is voluntary control.

**sphincters** Muscles arranged in circles that are able to decrease the diameter of tubes. Examples are found within the rectum, bladder, and blood vessels.

**sphygmomanometer** A device used to measure blood pressure.

**spinal cord** An extension of the brain, composed of virtually all the nerves carrying messages between the brain and the rest of the body. It lies inside of and is protected by the spinal canal.

**sternum** The breast bone.

**stratum corneum** The outermost or dead layer of the skin.

**stroke volume (SV)** The volume of blood pumped forward with each ventricular contraction.

**subcutaneous tissue** Tissue, largely fat, that lies directly under the dermis and serves as an insulator of the body.

**superior vena cava** One of the two largest veins in the body; carries blood from the upper extremities, head, neck, and chest into the heart.

**sweat glands** The glands that secrete sweat, located in the dermal layer of the skin.

**sympathetic nervous system** The adrenergic part of the autonomic peripheral nervous system responsible for the fight-or-flight response.

**symphyses** Joints that have grown together to form a very stable connection.

**synovial fluid** The small amount of liquid within a joint used as lubrication.

**synovial membrane** The lining of a joint that secretes synovial fluid into the joint space.

**systemic circulation** The portion of the circulatory system outside of the heart and lungs.

**systemic vascular resistance (SVR)** The resistance that blood must overcome to be able to move within the blood vessels; related to the amount of dilation or constriction in the blood vessel.

**systole** The contraction, or period of contraction, of the heart, especially that of the ventricles.

**tarsals** The group of bones situated between the lower leg bones (ie, tibia and fibula) and the metatarsal bones of the foot.

**temporal bones** The lateral bones on each side of the cranium; the temples.

**tendons** The fibrous connective tissue that attaches muscle to bone.

**testicle** A male genital gland that contains specialized cells that produce hormones and sperm.

**thoracic cage** The chest or rib cage.

**thoracic spine** The 12 vertebrae that lie between the cervical vertebrae and the lumbar vertebrae. One pair of ribs is attached to each of these vertebrae.

**thorax** The chest cavity that contains the heart, lungs, esophagus, and great vessels.

**thyroid cartilage** A firm prominence of cartilage that forms the upper part of the larynx; the Adam's apple.

**tibia** The shinbone; the larger of the two bones of the lower leg.

**tidal volume** The amount of air moved in and out of the lungs in one relaxed breath; about 500 mL for an adult.

**topographic anatomy** The superficial landmarks of the body that serve as guides to the structures that lie beneath them.

**trachea** The windpipe; the main trunk for air passing to and from the lungs.

**transverse (axial) plane** An imaginary line where the body is divided into top and bottom parts.

**triceps** The muscle in the back of the upper arm.

**tunica media** The middle and thickest layer of tissue of a blood vessel wall, composed of elastic tissue and smooth muscle cells that allow the vessel to expand or contract in response to changes in blood pressure and tissue demand.

**ulna** The inner bone of the forearm, on the side opposite the thumb.

**umbilicus** The navel; also called the belly button.

**ureter** A small, hollow tube that carries urine from the kidneys to the bladder.

**urethra** The canal that conveys urine from the bladder to outside the body.

**urinary bladder** A sac behind the pubic symphysis made of smooth muscle that collects and stores urine.

**urinary system** The organs that control the discharge of certain waste materials filtered from the blood and excreted as urine.

**vagina** The outermost cavity of a woman's reproductive tract; the lower part of the birth canal.

**ventilation** The movement of air between the lungs and the environment.

**ventricle** One of two lower chambers of the heart.

**vertebrae** The bones of the vertebral column.

**vertebral column** The structure formed by the 33 vertebrae, separated by intervertebral disks. It houses and protects the spinal cord; also called the spinal column.

**voluntary muscle** Muscle that is under direct voluntary control of the brain and can be contracted or relaxed at will; skeletal, or striated, muscle.

**$\dot{V}/\dot{Q}$ ratio** A measurement that examines how much gas is being moved effectively and how much blood is flowing around the alveoli where gas exchange (perfusion) occurs.

**white blood cells** Blood cells that have a role in the body's immune defense mechanisms against infection; also called leukocytes.

**xiphoid process** The narrow, cartilaginous lower tip of the sternum.

**zygomas** The quadrangular bones of the cheek, articulating with the frontal bone, the maxillae, the zygomatic processes of the temporal bone, and the great wings of the sphenoid bone.

## References

1. National Highway Traffic Safety Administration. *National Emergency Medical Services Education Standards*. DOT HS 811 077A. www.ems.gov/pdf/811077a.pdf. Published January 2009. Accessed February 6, 2020.

2. National Highway Traffic Safety Administration. *National Emergency Medical Services Education Standards. Emergency Medical Technician Instructional Guidelines*. DOT HS 811 077C. www.ems.gov/pdf/811077c.pdf. Published January 2009. Accessed February 6, 2020.

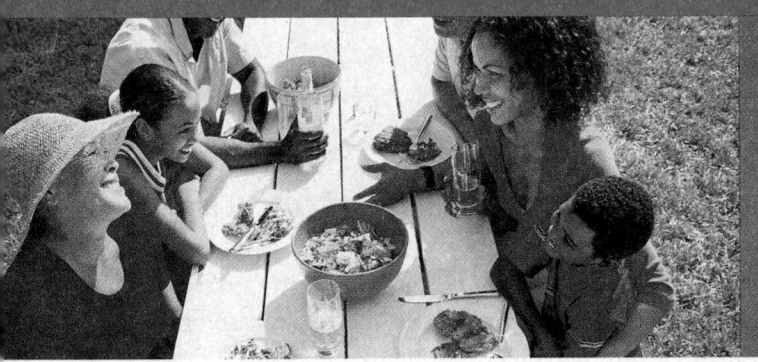

# Chapter 7

# Life Span Development

## NATIONAL EMS EDUCATION STANDARD COMPETENCIES

### Preparatory

Applies fundamental knowledge of the emergency medical services (EMS) system, safety/well-being of the emergency medical technician (EMT), medical/legal, and ethical issues to the provision of emergency care.

### Life Span Development

Applies fundamental knowledge of life span development to patient assessment and management.

## KNOWLEDGE OBJECTIVES

1. Know the terms used to designate the following stages of life: infants, toddlers and preschoolers, school-age children, adolescents (teenagers), early adults, middle adults, and older adults. (pp 254–264)
2. Describe the major physical and psychosocial characteristics of an infant's life. (pp 254–258)
3. Describe the major physical and psychosocial characteristics of a toddler's and preschooler's life. (pp 258–260)
4. Describe the major physical and psychosocial characteristics of a school-age child's life. (pp 260–261)

5. Describe the major physical and psychosocial characteristics of an adolescent's life. (pp 261–262)
6. Describe the major physical and psychosocial characteristics of an early adult's life. (p 263)
7. Describe the major physical and psychosocial characteristics of a middle adult's life. (pp 263–264)
8. Describe the major physical and psychosocial characteristics of an older adult's life. (pp 264–268)

## SKILLS OBJECTIVES

There are no skills objectives for this chapter.

# Introduction

As an EMT, you must be aware of the obvious and not-so-obvious changes a person undergoes physically and mentally at various stages of life and understand how some of these changes will substantially alter the way you perceive your patient's condition and, subsequently, how you manage his or her care. Vital signs are one example of such variations between age groups.

## Vital Signs

In general, the younger the person, the faster his or her pulse and respiratory rates should be. Finding a pulse rate of 140 beats/min and a respiratory rate of 60 breaths/min is usually normal for an infant. However, for a 30-year-old adult, the same values would likely signal the presence of a life-threatening condition. Normal blood pressure values also vary widely between different age groups, but unlike pulse and respiratory rates, blood pressure values tend to *increase* with age. **TABLE 7-1** lists approximate normal vital signs for various age groups.

# Neonates (Birth to 1 Month) and Infants (1 Month to 1 Year)

Unmatched by any other phase of life, the list of developmental changes occurring in the first year is long and substantial. These 12 months are often divided into two stages: neonate and infant. From birth to 1 month of age, a person is called a **neonate**. An in-depth discussion of the neonatal period is included in Chapter 34, *Obstetrics and Neonatal Care*. From 1 month to 1 year of age, a person is identified as an **infant** (**FIGURE 7-1**).

## Physical Changes
### Weight

At birth, a neonate usually weighs between 6 and 8 pounds (3 to 3.5 kg). The head accounts for about 25% of this weight. During the first week, a neonate's body weight decreases by 5% to 10%, due to fluid loss. By the second week, the neonate begins to gain weight. From there on, infants grow at a rate of about 1 ounce (30 g) per day, doubling their weight by 4 to 6 months and tripling it by the end of the first year.

| **TABLE 7-1** Vital Signs at Various Ages[a] | | | | |
|---|---|---|---|---|
| Age | Pulse Rate (beats/min) | Respirations (breaths/min) | Systolic Blood Pressure (mm Hg) | Temperature (°F) |
| Neonate (0 to 1 month) | 100 to 180 | 30 to 60 | 50 to 70 | 98 to 100 (37°C to 38°C) |
| Infant (1 month to 1 year) | 100 to 160 | 25 to 50 | 70 to 95 | 96.8 to 99.6 (36°C to 37.5°C) |
| Toddler (1 to 3 years) | 90 to 150 | 20 to 30 | 80 to 100 | 96.8 to 99.6 (36°C to 37.5°C) |
| Preschool age (3 to 6 years) | 80 to 140 | 20 to 25 | 80 to 100 | 98.6 (37°C) |
| School age (6 to 12 years) | 70 to 120 | 15 to 20 | 80 to 110 | 98.6 (37°C) |
| Adolescent (12 to 18 years) | 60 to 100 | 12 to 20 | 90 to 110 | 98.6 (37°C) |
| Early adult (19 to 40 years) | 60 to 100 | 12 to 20 | 90 to 130 | 98.6 (37°C) |
| Middle adult (41 to 60 years) | 60 to 100 | 12 to 20 | 90 to 130 | 98.6 (37°C) |
| Older adult (61 years and older) | 60 to 100 | 12 to 20 | 90 to 130 | 98.6 (37°C) |

[a]Vital sign ranges may vary in different sources.

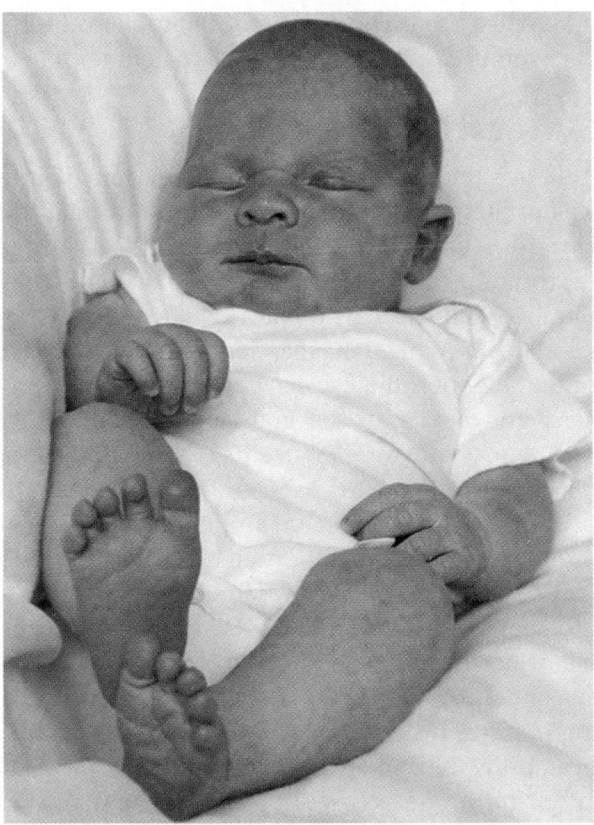

**FIGURE 7-1** An infant is 1 month to 1 year of age.

© Johanna Goodyear/ShutterStock.

## Cardiovascular System

Prior to birth, fetal blood supply comes from the mother via the placenta. During the birthing process, hormones and pressure changes help the neonate make the transition from fetal circulation to independent circulation. See Chapter 34, *Obstetrics and Neonatal Care*, for more information on fetal circulation.

## Pulmonary System

Prior to taking his or her first breath, a neonate's lungs have never been inflated. As such, a neonate's first breath is forceful and is facilitated in part by the chest's passage through the birth canal and the subsequent increase in intrathoracic pressure.

Neonates are primarily nose breathers. Infants younger than 6 months are particularly susceptible to nasal congestion, which can lead to viral upper respiratory infections. If you respond to a call for a baby choking, make sure the nasal passages are clear of mucus and other obstructions.

An infant's upper airway is quite different from that of an adult. The infant's tongue is larger in proportion to the size of the oral cavity, and the airway is proportionally shorter and narrower. As a result, airway obstruction is more common in infants than in older children and adults. Due to factors such as the proportionally oversized occiput, the increased

**YOU** are the Provider

You and your partner are outside washing the ambulance when a man in his 50s drives up to the front of the ambulance bay door. He requests that you check his vital signs, which your EMS system offers as part of its community outreach program. As your partner is retrieving the blood pressure cuff and stethoscope from the ambulance, the man tells you he is very lightheaded and needs to sit down because he thinks he might pass out. The time is 1310 hours according to the dispatch operator, who acknowledges that you have a walk-in patient.

1. How does a patient's age affect your assessment?
2. What are some physical differences between middle adults and older adults?

flexibility of the trachea, and the infant's limited or absent ability to reposition himself or herself, it is crucial that the EMT preserve the airway's patency through proper positioning. Hyperextending or hyperflexing the infant's head and neck can easily produce an airway obstruction.

The rib cage of an infant is less rigid and the ribs sit horizontally. This explains the distinctive diaphragmatic breathing (belly breathing) typically seen in infants.

When providing bag-mask ventilations to an infant, be aware that the infant's lungs are fragile. Forceful ventilations and overinflation increase pressure in the lungs and can result in pressure-induced trauma, referred to as **barotrauma**.

The muscles that infants use to breathe are immature, and the number of alveoli in their lungs is relatively low. Fortunately, the amount of oxygen they need is also relatively low. When stressed, however, their respiratory system's ability to compensate is limited. They can hold out for a short time, but without expedient support, infants struggling to breathe can quickly tire and become overheated

## Special Populations

When you are counting respirations in an infant, count the number of times the abdomen rises instead of concentrating solely on the chest rise.

and dehydrated. Thus, respiratory problems in the very young can quickly turn life threatening.

## Nervous System

Although the human nervous system is remarkably well established at birth, it has yet to fully mature. However, in a healthy, full-term infant, certain reflexes are present at birth. The **Moro reflex** (commonly called the startle reflex) is illustrated when neonates are caught off guard and startled, at which time they open their arms wide, spread their fingers, and appear to be grabbing for something. The **palmar grasp reflex** occurs when an object is placed into a neonate's palm and he or she instinctively closes his or her hand around the object. Two other reflexes play an important role in feeding. The **rooting reflex** is displayed when something touches the neonate's cheek and he or she intuitively turns his or her head in the direction of the touch. The **sucking reflex** is illustrated when a breastfeeding mother strokes her baby's lips with her nipple, prompting the child to latch on.

At birth, the bones of the cranium are not yet fully developed or fused together. Instead, the gaps between these bones are connected by relatively flexible fibrous tissue. These areas, called **fontanelles**, allow the newborn's head to change shape slightly as it passes through the narrow birth canal (**FIGURE 7-2**). In the months that follow, the fontanelles begin to shrink as the cranial bones

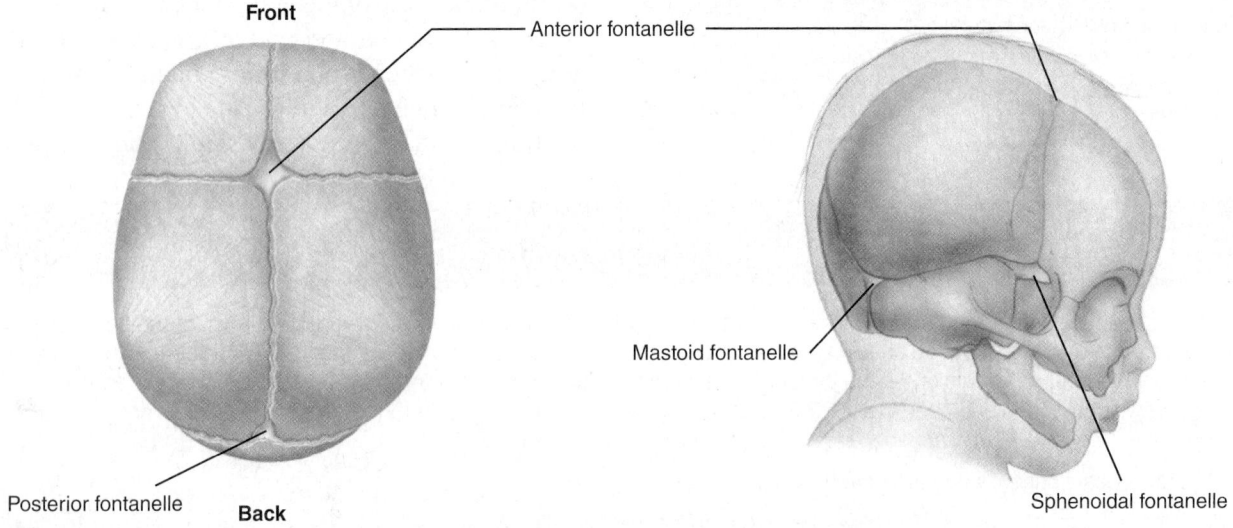

**FIGURE 7-2** Fontanelles.

© Jones & Bartlett Learning.

grow together and fuse, forming a unified, rigid structure. The posterior fontanelle normally closes by the third month. The anterior fontanelle closes between 9 and 18 months. When present, the fontanelles can provide the EMT with valuable information about the child's condition. For example, a depressed fontanelle may indicate dehydration, whereas a bulging fontanelle is often a sign that pressure inside the cranium has increased. Information on intracranial pressure is presented in Chapter 29, *Head and Spine Injuries.*

At birth, neonates are unable to do much without assistance. They cannot roll from their backs onto their abdomens, and their eyes are incapable of focusing on objects beyond a very short distance. However, by 2 months of age, infants can track objects with their eyes and recognize familiar faces. At 6 months, they can sit upright, and they begin to make cooing and babbling sounds. By the time an infant is 12 months of age, the infant can walk with minimal assistance and knows his or her name.

## Immune System

While still in the womb, the neonate's immune system is supported by the mother's antibodies, delivered through placental blood flow. Infants continue to carry some of this immunity. This passive immunity is further strengthened by antibodies contained in breast milk.

### Special Populations

Another development that occurs during infancy is the emergence of baby teeth. Teething (teeth breaking through the gums) can be painful and is sometimes accompanied by a low-grade fever.

## Psychosocial Changes

An infant's psychosocial development begins at birth and continues to advance as the infant interacts with, and reacts to, his or her environment. **TABLE 7-2** outlines typical ages at which major psychosocial changes are noticed.

For most infants, the primary method used to communicate distress is crying. Parents are often able to discern the reason for their child's crying by simply listening to the tone of those cries. They can distinguish between a cry of anger and one

**TABLE 7-2** Noticeable Characteristics at Various Ages

| Age | Characteristic |
|---|---|
| 2 months | Recognizes familiar faces; uses eyes to track objects and people |
| 3 months | Brings objects to the mouth; smiles and frowns |
| 4 months | Reaches arms out to people; drools |
| 5 months | Sleeps throughout the night; distinguishes family members from strangers |
| 6 months | Begins teething; sits upright; speaks one-syllable words |
| 7 months | Afraid of strangers; displays mood swings |
| 8 months | Responds to "no"; can sit alone; plays peek-a-boo |
| 9 months | Pulls self up to stand; explores objects by placing them in his or her mouth |
| 10 months | Responds to his or her name; crawls efficiently |
| 11 months | Begins to walk without assistance; becomes frustrated by restrictions |
| 12 months | Knows his or her name; walks |

© Jones & Bartlett Learning.

motivated by frustration, pain, fear, hunger, discomfort, or sleepiness. Another distinctive cry is one of distress, prompted by some unexpected event that has caused a situational crisis for the child.

The pace at which infants develop relationships with their parents or caregivers varies greatly from one child to the next. *Bonding*, the formation of a close, personal relationship, is generally fostered by a *secure attachment*, which results when the infant understands that his or her parents/caregivers will respond to his or her needs. Having this confidence that his or her parents will provide a "safety net" inspires the child to venture out and explore.

By contrast, *anxious-avoidant attachment* is the result of recurring rejection. Infants who acquire this form of attachment show little emotional response to their parents/caregivers and treat them as they would a stranger. These children may compensate by developing an isolated lifestyle wherein they avoid having to depend on the support and care of others.

In older infants, *separation anxiety* is common. Characterized by clingy behavior and fear of unfamiliar places and people, it typically reaches its peak between the ages of 10 and 18 months. Crying as a means of protest is normal at this age. As they grow accustomed to their homes and families, infants have an inherent need for a secure, stable environment. An environment that is too unpredictable may trigger feelings of despair, causing the child to become withdrawn. This experience may even lead to trust issues later in life.

**Trust versus mistrust** refers to the stage of psychosocial development beginning at birth and concluding at approximately 18 months of age. As the name implies, it is a time when children learn whether they can trust the people around them. Because infants depend entirely on their parents/caregivers, a crucial element in the formation of this trust is the quality of care the infant receives from them. When their needs are met consistently in a

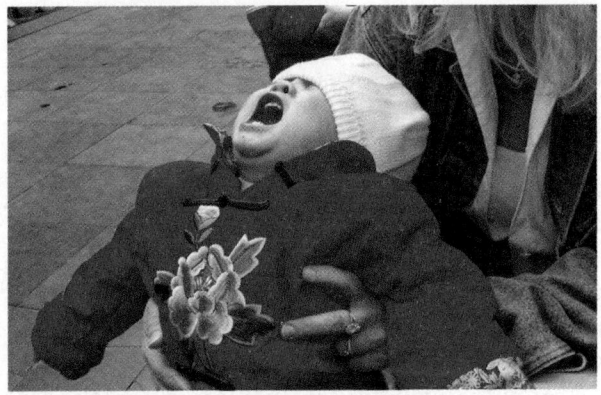

**FIGURE 7-3** Children develop a sense of mistrust if they perceive their parents or caregivers will not provide an organized, predictable environment.
© Scot Milless/ShutterStock.

stable environment, children learn to trust those responsible for their well-being. Conversely, if their parents/caregivers are inconsistent, emotionally unavailable, or rejecting, children may develop a sense of mistrust (**FIGURE 7-3**).

# Toddlers (1 to 3 Years) and Preschoolers (3 to 6 Years)
## Physical Changes

The cardiovascular system of a **toddler** (ages 1 to 3 years) or **preschooler** (ages 3 to 6 years) is not dramatically different from that of an adult (**FIGURE 7-4** and **FIGURE 7-5**).

## Special Populations

When caring for the very young, try to preserve as much of their routine as is reasonable. An easy way to achieve this is to keep family and familiar items nearby.

## YOU are the Provider

After sitting the man down in a chair inside your station, he tells you he has been stressed lately, although he does not know why, and he has had several episodes of lightheadedness over the past few days. He denies having chest pain, shortness of breath, or any other symptoms. As you are assessing the patient, your partner prepares to take his vital signs.

| Recording Time: 0 Minutes | |
| --- | --- |
| Appearance | Calm |
| Level of consciousness | Conscious and alert |
| Airway | Open; clear of secretions or foreign bodies |
| Breathing | Normal rate; adequate depth |
| Circulation | Radial pulses strong and regular; skin pink, warm, and dry |

**3.** What are some common psychosocial concerns experienced by middle-aged adults?

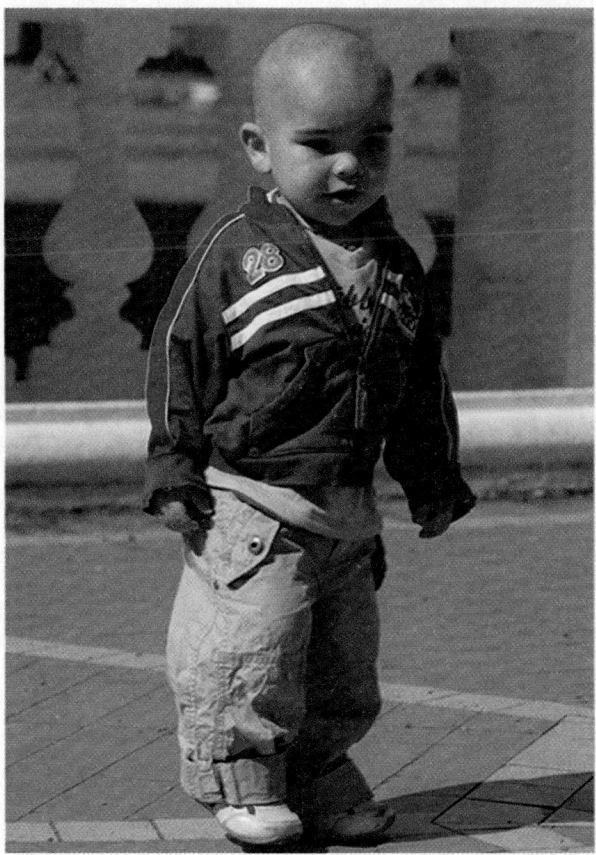

**FIGURE 7-4** A toddler is 1 to 3 years of age.

© EML/ShutterStock.

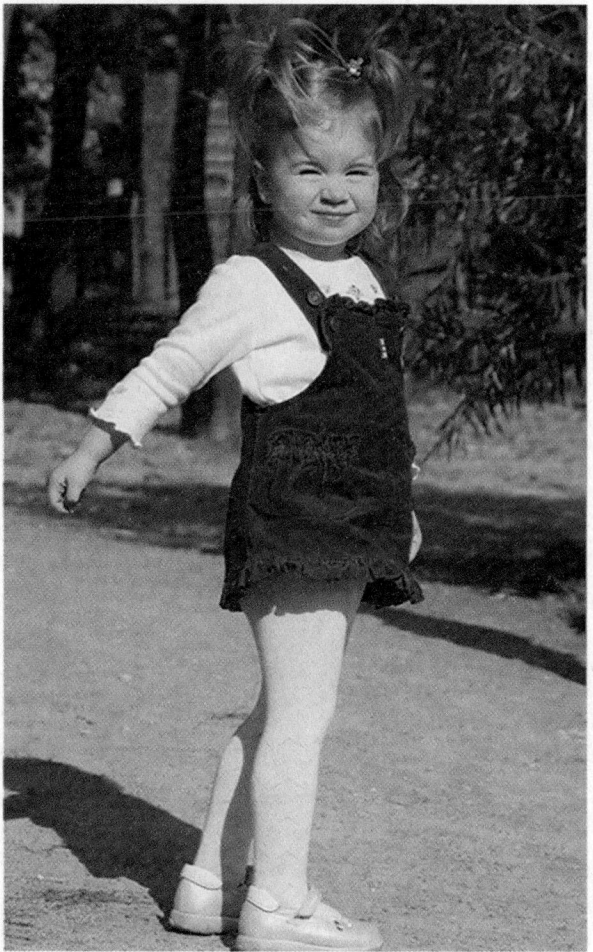

**FIGURE 7-5** A preschooler is 3 to 6 years of age.

© Maxim Bolotnikov/ShutterStock.

Their lungs continue to develop more terminal bronchioles and alveoli to meet the ever-increasing oxygen demands of their growing bodies. However, the musculature of their lungs is not well developed. This anomaly prevents them from sustaining deep or rapid respirations for an extended period of time.

One of the most important physiologic changes at this age is the loss of passive immunity. As toddlers spend more time around other children, they are exposed to a variety of viruses. Viral infections (colds) develop frequently, often manifesting with gastrointestinal distress or upper respiratory symptoms. In the process, however, these exposures initiate the development of antibodies, resulting in acquired immunity.

Neuromuscular growth also makes considerable progress at this age. By performing activities such as walking, running, jumping, and playing catch, toddlers and preschoolers learn to use their muscles and expansive nervous system (**FIGURE 7-6**). This

boost in physical activity supports an increase in muscle mass and bone density. The progression in how they play at this age demonstrates their transition from exclusively gross motor activity (eg, grabbing an object using the entire palm) to including fine motor skills (eg, picking up a crayon using only the thumb and forefinger). By the end of this stage, the weight of a preschooler's brain is roughly 90% of his or her adult weight.

Another milestone during this stage is the maturation of the renal system and the establishing of elimination patterns (ie, toilet training). Physiologically, by 12 to 15 months of age, toddlers possess the neuromuscular capability to control the bladder. However, many are not psychologically prepared until about 18 to 30 months of age. The average age when toddlers complete toilet training is 28 months.

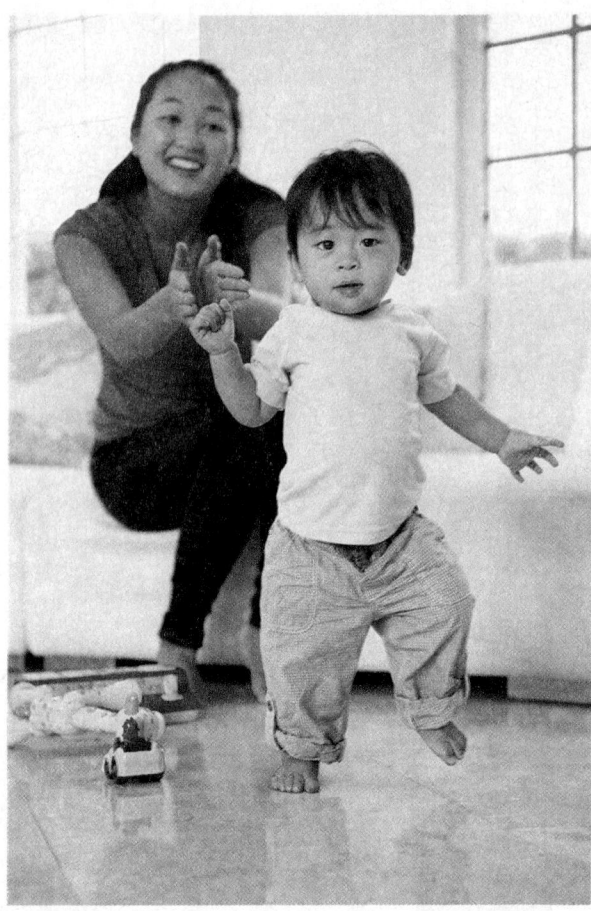

**FIGURE 7-6** A toddler learns to walk, one of the major milestones in life.
© monkeybusinessimages/iStock.

## Psychosocial Changes

The psychosocial challenge for this age group is sometimes referred to as autonomy versus shame and doubt. Through milestones such as speech development and toilet training, the child begins to attain a measure of self-sufficiency. However, toddlers and preschoolers are nevertheless very attached to their parents, deriving feelings of safety and security from their presence. Separation anxiety peaks between 10 and 18 months of age.

By 36 months of age, most children have mastered basic language skills, understanding full sentences by the time they are 3 or 4 years of age. As they progress further through this stage, they make a transition from using language solely for the purpose of communicating what they want, to using it creatively and playfully.

This is also the time when toddlers become more socially interactive with other children, playing games and, as a result, learning to control their own behavior, follow rules, and be competitive. Significant learning and development occur as the child observes other children. By age 18 to 24 months, toddlers begin to understand the concept of cause and effect. And by observing their role models, they also learn to recognize gender differences.

### Street Smarts

When responding to a severely sick or injured child, you may find a secondary patient on scene: a parent. For some, the sudden stress, fear, and uncertainty will be overwhelming, causing panic. The parent's distress can add to an already intense situation, making the task of treating the child much more difficult.

## School-Age Children (6 to 12 Years)

### Physical Changes

From ages 6 to 12 years, a **school-age** child's physical traits and functions continue to mature at a relatively rapid pace (**FIGURE 7-7**). Most gain about 4 pounds (2 kg) and grow 2.5 inches (6 cm) each year. Baby teeth are replaced by permanent teeth, and brain activity in both hemispheres increases significantly.

### Psychosocial Changes

School-age children experience substantial psychosocial growth. During this critical time in human development, children learn various types of reasoning. With **preconventional reasoning**, the child's moral compass is directed by external forces, such as parental discipline. Whether a given behavior is right or wrong is judged by its consequences: punishment or incentive. When children reach the level of **conventional reasoning**, their behavior is more motivated by the approval of peers and society. They still accept the rules set by authority figures, but now they do so primarily because they perceive those rules as necessary for positive relationships and acceptance. For children who reach the third level, **postconventional reasoning**, moral judgments are more abstract, with the individual beginning to follow an internalized moral compass

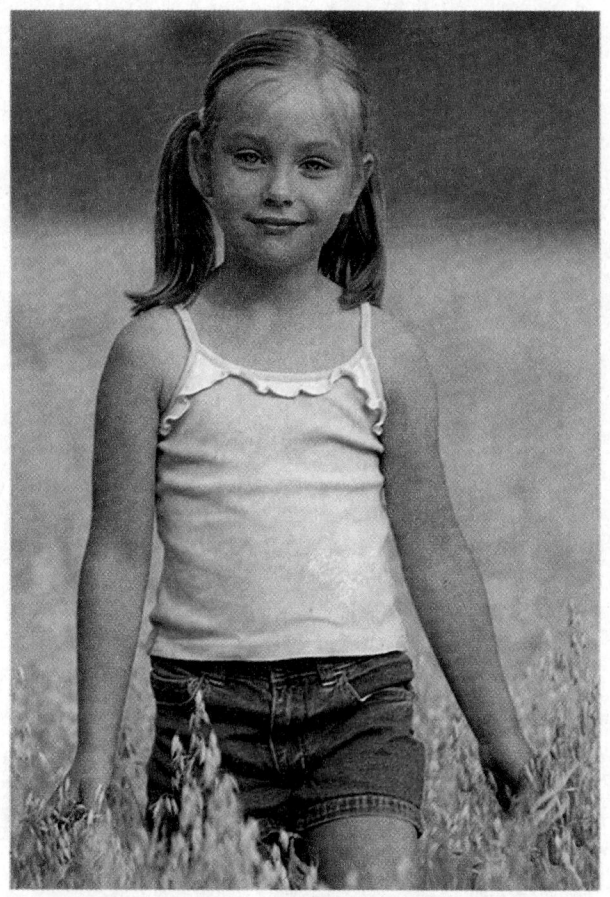

**FIGURE 7-7** A school-age child is 6 to 12 years of age.

© Trout55/ShutterStock.

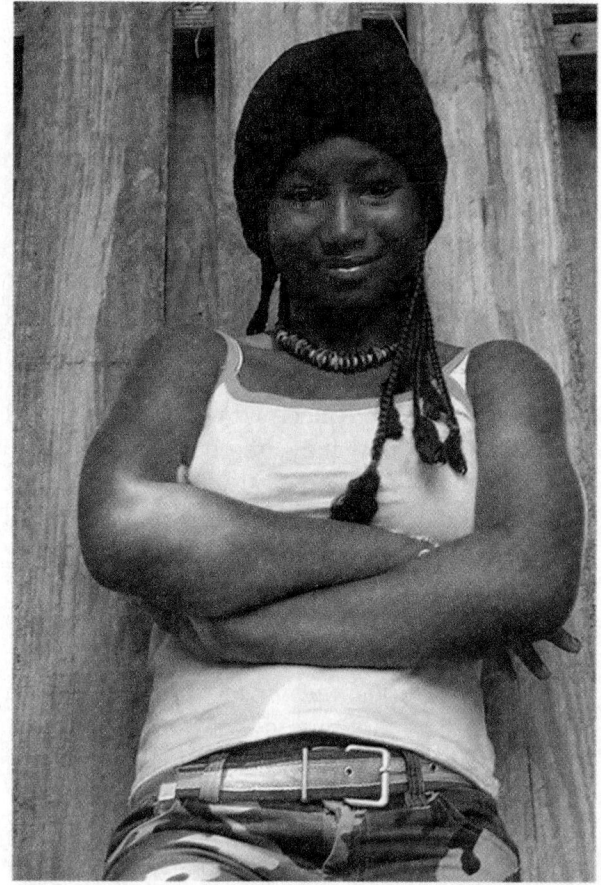

**FIGURE 7-8** An adolescent is 12 to 18 years of age.

© Jamie Wilson/ShutterStock.

(ie, conscience). This form of reasoning develops further during adolescence.

During this stage, school-age children begin to develop their self-concept and self-esteem. *Self-concept* is our perception of ourselves; *self-esteem* is how we feel about ourselves and how we fit in with our peers.

## Adolescents (12 to 18 Years)
### Physical Changes

In the **adolescent** (ages 12 to 18 years), vital signs begin to level off within the adult ranges, with a systolic blood pressure generally between 90 and 110 mm Hg, a pulse rate between 60 and 100 beats/min, and respirations that range from 12 to 20 breaths/min (**FIGURE 7-8**).

During the adolescent period, teens experience a 2- to 3-year growth spurt (ie, an increase in muscle and bone growth). Growth begins with the hands and feet, then moves to the long bones of the extremities, and finishes with growth of the torso. At the conclusion of the growth spurt, muscle mass and bone density have nearly reached adult levels. Girls tend to experience this growth at an earlier age than boys, finishing by about 16 years of age. Boys typically reach their growth peak by 18 years, generally becoming taller than girls.

Another important milestone of adolescence is the maturation of the endocrine and reproductive systems. Secondary sexual development begins, along with enlargement of the external reproductive organs. Pubic and axillary hair appear. Vocal sound changes in range and depth.

In girls, the deposit of adipose (fat) tissue causes the breasts and thighs to increase in size. Menstruation begins with *menarche*, the first menstrual bleeding; however, it is not uncommon for some girls to begin menstruation prior to adolescence. Along with these changes comes the capacity for reproduction. By the middle of adolescence, the male body can produce sperm, and the female body produces eggs (oocytes).

## Psychosocial Changes

Conflict between young people and their parents is common at this stage. In seeking to express their independence, adolescents may begin to distance themselves from parents and siblings, desiring privacy and personal space. Most begin spending more time with friends and struggling to create a sense of identity (**FIGURE 7-9**). While "trying on" different personas, they may begin dressing in a certain style of clothing that fits their desired personality. Self-consciousness increases, as both sexes become more concerned with their physical appearance and how they are perceived by peers. Multiple options for gender exist, allowing the adolescent to freely gender-identify. Many adolescents are fixated on their public image and terrified of being embarrassed.

At times, adolescence can be intensely emotional. Teenagers often find themselves caught between two worlds; they want to be treated like adults, yet they continue to want and need their parents' support. Rebellious behavior is common. Smoking, illicit drug use, unprotected sex, and other high-risk behaviors tend to peak at around age 14 to 16 years, along with antisocial behavior and peer pressure. Even without these particular manifestations, the adolescent's struggle toward independence can have devastating setbacks. Patience and support from family and friends are essential in assisting a young person's transition into adulthood.

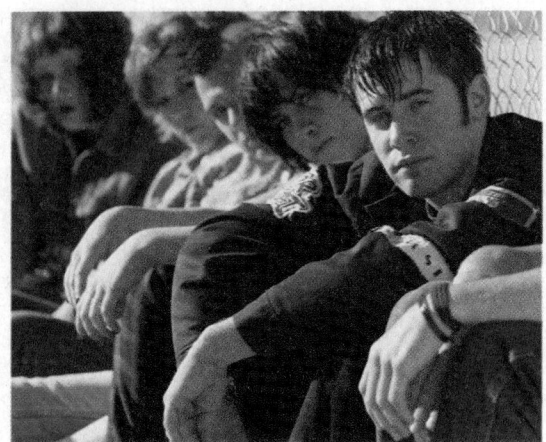

**FIGURE 7-9** Adolescents want to fit in and may struggle to create their identities.
© SW Productions/Jupiterimages.

At this age, young people develop a code of personal ethics, influenced in part by their parents' ethics and values and partly by their peers and personal experience.

### Special Populations

When you interview adolescents in the presence of their family, they may withhold certain information or even lie to protect their privacy or image. For this reason, you should attempt to ask more sensitive questions privately, where adolescents feel they can answer without constraint.

## YOU | are the Provider

As your partner takes the patient's vital signs, he tells you he and his wife are taking care of his father, who is 82 years old and has Alzheimer disease. He further tells you that, although this situation is very stressful for him, he does not want to put his father in a nursing home. He is still lightheaded and now reports a headache. You advise him he should be transported to the hospital via EMS, but he tells you he would rather drive himself.

| Recording Time: 5 Minutes | |
| --- | --- |
| **Respirations** | 14 breaths/min; regular and adequate |
| **Pulse** | 76 beats/min; strong and regular |
| **Skin** | Pink, warm, and dry |
| **Blood pressure** | 174/98 mm Hg |
| **Oxygen saturation (SpO$_2$)** | 98% (on room air) |

4. Are the patient's vital signs consistent with his age?

5. Why should you transport this patient to the hospital?

# Early Adults (19 to 40 Years)
## Physical Changes

Following adolescence, a person is classified as an **early adult** (age 19 to 40 years) (**FIGURE 7-10**). The vital signs of early adults do not vary greatly from those seen throughout adulthood. Ideally, the human pulse rate will average around 70 beats/min, the respiratory rate will stay in the range of 12 to 20 breaths/min, and the systolic blood pressure will be approximately between 90 and 120 mm Hg.

From about 19 to 25 years of age, men and women typically reach their physical peak. Lifelong habits and routines are established, whether healthy or unhealthy (eg, diet, exercise, tobacco use).

In the latter years of early adulthood, the effects of aging gradually become evident (ie, subtle wear and tear). Muscle strength decreases, and reflexes slow. The disks between vertebrae begin to settle, sometimes producing a decrease in height. Metabolism also decreases, while fatty tissue increases.

Thus, without adjusting his or her diet and level of activity accordingly, the early adult may experience unwanted weight gain, while simultaneously finding it more difficult to lose weight than in previous years.

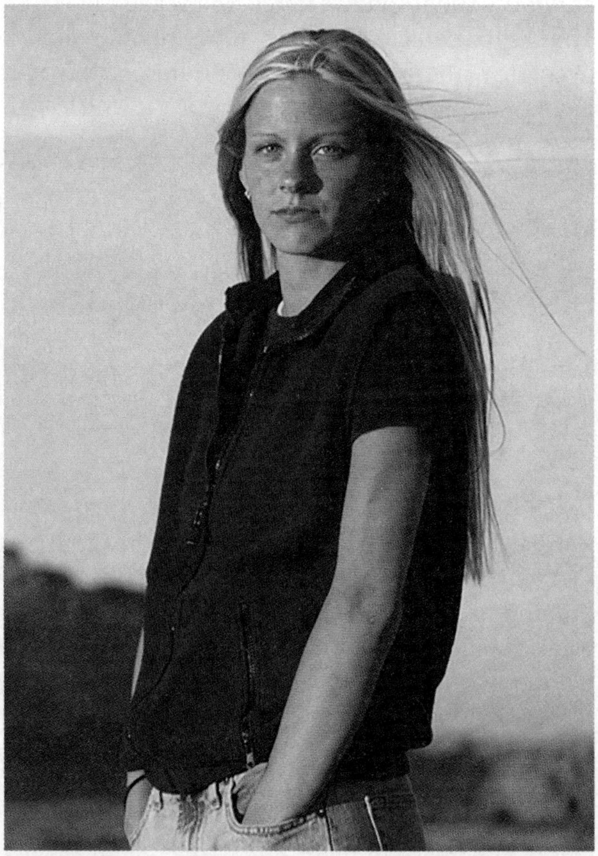

## Psychosocial Changes

Most early adults spend these years focusing on family and career—"settling down," getting married, starting a family, and striving for career achievement. Although immensely rewarding, these life events also bring about significant stress. Interestingly, despite the amount of stress and change, this age group enjoys one of the more stable periods of life psychologically.

# Middle Adults (41 to 60 Years)
## Physical Changes

For a **middle adult** (age 41 to 60 years) (**FIGURE 7-11**), the aging process continues to take its toll. Middle adults become more susceptible to vision and hearing loss, cardiovascular health becomes a growing

**FIGURE 7-10** An early adult is 19 to 40 years of age.
© Rubberball Productions.

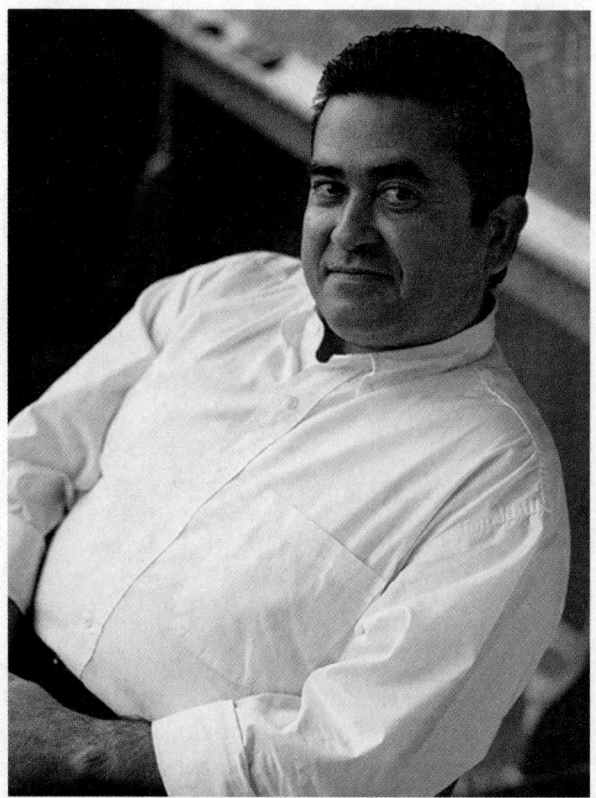

**FIGURE 7-11** A middle adult is 41 to 60 years of age.
© Ryan McVay/Photodisc/Getty Images.

concern, and the incidence of cancer increases. Women in their late 40s to early 50s enter menopause: the end of menstruation and the ability to reproduce.

Middle adults may experience increased cholesterol levels, decreased cardiac efficiency, and difficulties with weight control. However, many of the effects of aging can be diminished with proper exercise and a healthy diet.

Middle adults may also have conditions of which they are unaware, including diabetes and hypertension. Whereas the leading cause of death in all age groups younger than 44 years is unintentional injury, the leading cause of death in persons between ages 45 and 64 is cancer.

## Psychosocial Changes

The pressure to accomplish their professional and relational goals, the need to adjust after their adult children leave the home (ie, empty nest syndrome), and the worries that come with assessing whether they will have the financial means to retire are among the many psychosocial challenges facing the middle adult. However, they have the physical, emotional, and spiritual reserves needed to overcome these challenges, and their health is generally stable.

By this time, the parents of middle adults have become *older adults* (discussed in the next section), many of whom will require care and assistance in completing routine tasks of daily life. In the United States, many of these older adults receive such care at home, from family members. Therefore, in addition to supporting children departing for college, middle adults may experience an overlapping period during which they must also care for their aging parents.

## Older Adults (61 Years and Older)
### Physical Changes

Life expectancy is continually changing. In the early 1900s, the average human life expectancy was 47 years of age. In more modern times, that number has increased to approximately 78 years, with a maximum life expectancy of approximately 120 years. As a result, more and more people will live to become an older adult (age 61 years and older) (**FIGURE 7-12**). How long an individual lives

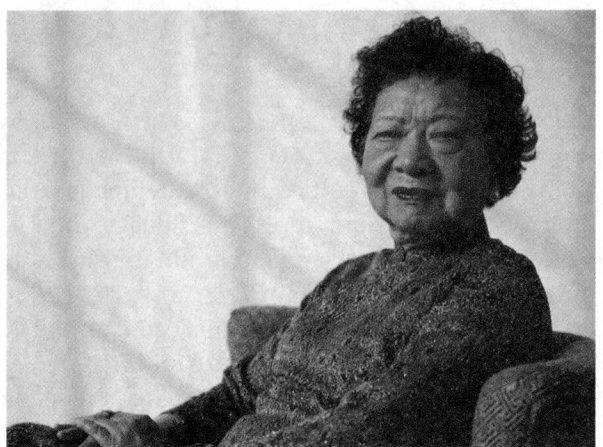

**FIGURE 7-12** An older adult is 61 years of age or older.
© Michael Matisse/Photodisc/Getty Images.

is determined by many factors, including his or her birth year and country of residence. These two factors correlate with advances in public health, enhanced awareness of healthy eating habits, improved attitudes toward exercise, and access to ever-advancing medical care. Currently, older adults are staying active longer than their ancestors. Thanks to medical advances, they are often able to overcome numerous medical conditions, but may need multiple medications to do so (**FIGURE 7-13**).

### Special Populations

Some older patients have physical, cognitive, and psychological barriers that impede their ability to communicate effectively. Proper assessment and management of this population will often depend on your ability to use patience when interviewing them.

## Cardiovascular System

Cardiac function declines with age, due in large part to atherosclerosis, a condition characterized by the buildup of cholesterol and calcium along the inner walls of blood vessels, resulting in the formation of plaque. As plaque accumulates, the flow of blood through the affected vessels becomes restricted or blocked entirely. More than 60% of people older than 65 years have atherosclerotic disease.

Additional cardiovascular effects of aging include a decrease in heart rate, a decline in cardiac output (the amount of blood pumped by the heart per minute), and diminished ability of the heart to

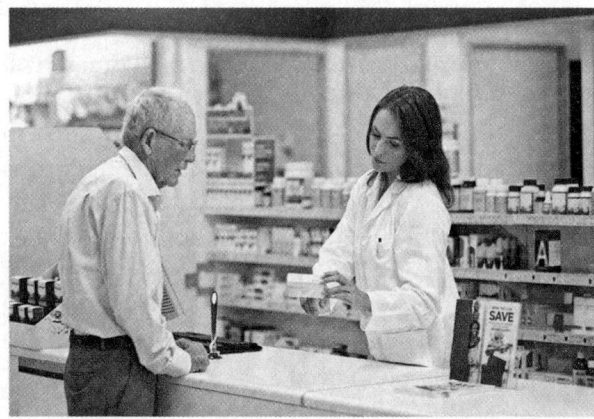

**FIGURE 7-13** Older people are often prescribed multiple medications to help them stay active.

© Yuri_Arcurs/iStock.

increase cardiac output to meet the body's demands. These changes translate into a heart that is less able to cope with exercise or disease. In the event of a life-threatening illness, the body typically preserves blood pressure by increasing the heart rate. However, because cardiac muscle tends to weaken with age, the increased rate may cause damage to the heart. Combined with atherosclerosis of sufficient severity, the damage could prove fatal.

Because the vascular system of the older adult becomes stiff, blood vessels are unable to dilate and contract as effectively. As a result, the diastolic blood pressure increases and the heart must work harder to overcome vascular resistance to move blood throughout the body. Over time, the increase in workload can be detrimental to the heart.

Human blood cells originate within bone marrow. But with advancing age, bone marrow is replaced by fatty tissue. Consequently, the loss of marrow equals a reduction in the body's ability to manufacture new blood cells. Alone, this change is not cause for alarm. However, in the presence of traumatic injury in which a relatively large volume of blood is lost quickly, the impeded ability to replace lost cells can have devastating effects.

## Respiratory System

In older adults, the airway increases in size. However, the surface area of the alveoli decreases, as do the elasticity of the lungs and the strength of the intercostal muscles and diaphragm. Together, these factors make breathing more laborious for older adults. By the time the older adult is 75 years old, his or her vital capacity (the volume of air moved during the deepest inspiration and expiration) has declined to about 50% of that of a young adult.

The chest becomes more rigid, yet more fragile. Instead of bending and flexing under stress, the calcified rib case is more susceptible to fracture. Normally, these changes in the respiratory system are gradual, often going unnoticed until the onset of a severe, life-threatening condition, in which case the lack of respiratory reserve becomes more pronounced.

## YOU are the Provider

After expressing your concern about the patient's health and advising him that driving himself to the hospital would not be safe, he agrees to be transported via EMS. You place the patient onto the stretcher, load him into the ambulance, and begin transport to a hospital located a short distance away. En route, you reassess his vital signs; assess his blood glucose level, which reads 100 mg/dL; and then call your radio report to the hospital.

| Recording Time: 11 Minutes | |
| --- | --- |
| Level of consciousness | Conscious and alert |
| Respirations | 14 breaths/min; regular and adequate |
| Pulse | 80 beats/min; strong and regular |
| Skin | Pink, warm, and dry |
| Blood pressure | 180/102 mm Hg |
| SpO₂ | 99% (on room air) |

**6.** What additional treatment, if any, does this patient require?

As the patient ages, the structures protecting the upper airway decrease in function. Cough and gag reflexes diminish along with the ability to clear secretions. The cilia that line the airway dwindle, and sensation within the airway declines, making it more difficult for the older adult to maintain upper airway patency. Thus, older adults are at greater risk of aspiration and airway obstruction.

When a younger patient inhales, the airway maintains its shape, allowing air to enter. As the smooth muscles of the lower airway weaken with age, strong inhalation can cause the walls of the airway to collapse inward, producing inspiratory wheezing, lower flow rates, and air trapping in the alveoli (incomplete expiration). Because of these reductions in function, and because the white blood cells of the airway are less aggressive toward invading organisms, the older patient is more susceptible to lung infections.

## Endocrine System

Endocrine function also declines with age. Glucose metabolism slows, while insulin production decreases. Sexually, men often continue to produce sperm long into their 80s (although the rigidity of the penis typically diminishes over time). The size of a woman's uterus and vagina decreases. Hormone production in both sexes gradually declines, and although sexual desire may lessen, it does not ordinarily cease entirely.

## Digestive System

Age-related changes in gastric and intestinal functions may inhibit nutritional intake and utilization. Tooth loss can make chewing more difficult; taste buds become less sensitive to salty and sweet foods; and food in general may be perceived as bland and flavorless, as the senses of smell and taste response begin to fade. A decrease in saliva secretion impairs the body's ability to break down complex carbohydrates. Similarly, gastric acid secretion diminishes. Peristalsis (the process by which intestinal contractions move food along the digestive tract) slows with age, sometimes resulting in constipation and/or suppressed feelings of hunger. And because blood flow to the intestines can drop by as much as 50%, the extraction of vitamins and minerals from digested food can also wane. Gallstones become increasingly common, and changes in the elasticity of the anal sphincter can lead to fecal incontinence.

## Renal System

Between the ages of 20 to 90 years, the kidneys will decrease in size by 20%, and their filtration capabilities will decline by as much as 50%. This is due in part to a decrease in blood supply to the nephrons of the kidneys. Nephrons filter blood within the kidney. In addition, the number of nephrons declines between the ages of 30 and 80 years. As a result of the changes, the renal system's ability to remove waste from the body declines, as does its ability to conserve fluids when needed.

## Nervous System

By the time a person is 80 years of age, the brain has decreased in weight by as much as 10% to 20%. Motor and sensory neural networks are slower and less responsive. However, the brain's metabolic rate and oxygen consumption remain unchanged. And although it is generally true that the infant brain has a larger number of neurons than its adult counterpart, the adult brain is much more flexible. This is because the number of interconnections between neurons increases with age. These connections produce redundancies within the brain that permit the loss of neurons without a loss of knowledge or skill. However, although cognitive function remains intact throughout most of older adulthood, mental function often declines in the 5 years immediately preceding death.

One consequence of the reduced number of neurons is the alteration of sleep patterns. Instead of sleeping through the night, the older adult may take a nap during the day and be awake late at night. It is not uncommon for older adults to develop a biphasic (two-phased) sleep cycle (eg, sleeping from 0100 to 0600 hours and then taking a nap from 1200 to 1500 hours).

Throughout life, the cranial vault is almost entirely occupied by the brain, the meningeal layers, and the cerebrospinal fluid between these layers. As such, there is virtually no empty space. However, in older adults, the age-related shrinkage of the brain creates a void between the brain and the outermost layer of the meninges. The resulting space gives the brain room to move inside the cranium (**FIGURE 7-14**). As such, any mechanism that causes a rapid or forceful shifting of the brain has the potential to result in the tearing of bridging veins. Subsequent bleeding into the open space may go unnoticed for some time.

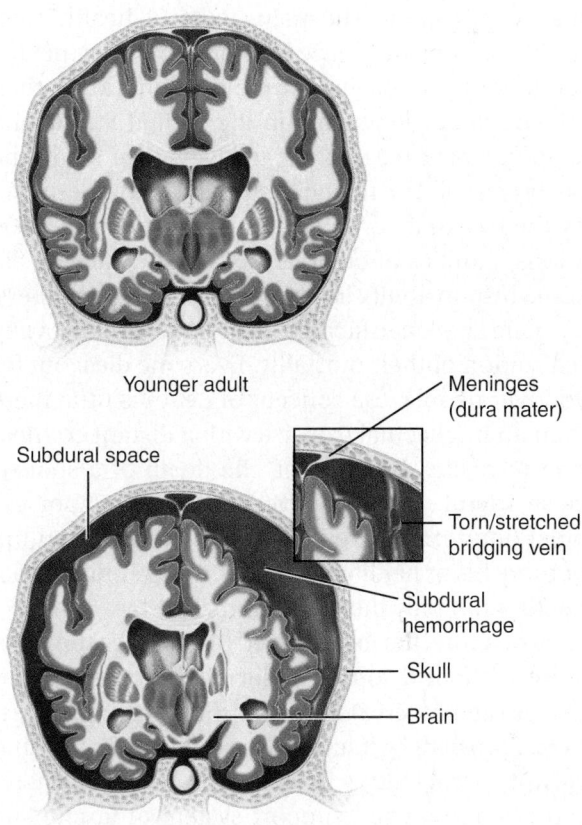

Younger adult

Subdural space

Meninges (dura mater)

Torn/stretched bridging vein

Subdural hemorrhage

Skull

Brain

Older adult

**FIGURE 7-14** Age-related atrophy or shrinkage of the brain creates space between the brain and dura mater (subdural space). When the bridging veins are stretched and torn, blood may accumulate in this area.

© Jones & Bartlett Learning.

The functioning of the peripheral nervous system slows with age. Sensations become diminished and may be misinterpreted. Nerve endings deteriorate, and the ability of the skin to sense the surroundings becomes hindered. Hot, cold, sharp, and wet objects all can create dangerous situations because the body cannot sense them quickly enough. Combined with prolonged reaction time and slower reflexes, these sensory alterations may

## Street Smarts

Some of your geriatric patients will present with confusion. The confusion may be the result of long-standing dementia, such as Alzheimer disease. At other times, it may be new and sudden. In either situation, you may find the patient unable to answer your questions. If the patient cannot answer your questions, you must determine how to obtain the information you need.

contribute to the higher incidence of falls and trauma in older adults.

## Sensory Changes

Pupillary reaction and ocular movements become more restricted with age. The pupils are generally smaller in older patients, and the opacity of the eye's lens diminishes visual acuity and causes the pupils to be sluggish in their reaction to light. Visual distortions are also common in older people. Thickening of the lens makes it more difficult for the eye to focus, especially at close range. Peripheral fields of vision narrow, and increased sensitivity to glare constricts the visual field.

In late adulthood, hearing loss is about four times more common than vision loss. Changes in several hearing-related structures may lead to a loss of high-frequency hearing or even deafness. Even so, although it is often assumed that all older adults have difficulty hearing and seeing, many older adults have remarkably good vision and hearing. Some may need eyeglasses or hearing aids, but this does not mean they are almost deaf or nearly blind.

## Psychosocial Changes

Statistics indicate that 95% of older adults live at home. They may have the assistance of family, friends, or home health care, but they are shown to be relatively healthy, active, and independent. The increasing number of older adults in the United States as a result of the baby boom of the 1940s through the 1960s has produced a need for additional assisted living facilities. These facilities allow older adults to live in campus-based communities with people in their own age group, while enjoying the independence and privacy of their own apartment and the security of nursing care, maintenance, and food preparation, if desired (**FIGURE 7-15**). Unfortunately, these facilities can be expensive.

An additional and important consequence of congregate living facilities is the proximity of the residents to one another. Although having people close to each other is advantageous from a social interaction standpoint, it limits the natural social distancing that occurs when people live completely independently. Residents of these communities interact with one another and with caregivers on a close, regular basis, which has the disadvantage of enhancing the spread of contagious diseases such as influenza virus and coronavirus. Furthermore,

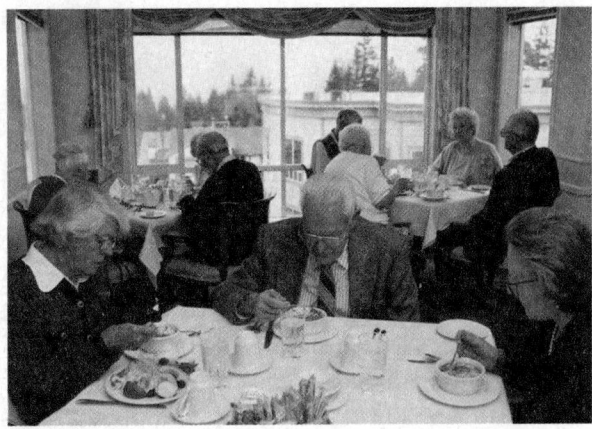

**FIGURE 7-15** A small percentage of older adults live in assisted living facilities.

© Keith Brofsky/Photodisc/Getty Images.

residents of these facilities are necessarily more susceptible to the consequences of these diseases. This helps explain the disproportionate effect that epidemics and pandemics associated with these diseases have on older adults living in continuing care, assisted living, and nursing home communities.

Few things in life cause more worry and stress than money problems. Older adults, in particular,

may worry about the rising cost of health care. At times, some may have to choose between paying for groceries or paying for medications. More than 50% of all single women in the United States who are 60 years of age or older are living at or below the poverty level. The financial struggle is compounded by the fact that currently, compared to past generations, families of older adults are less likely to assume responsibility for their aging family members.

One challenge facing older adults is the growing realization of their mortality. Everyone dies; but for younger people, the concept of death is little more than an intellectual exercise with a distant connection to reality. By contrast, the death of a spouse, close friend, or other loved one with whom the older adult may have shared one-half of a century or more his or her life, can be a strong reminder that death is not only inevitable, but close by.

For some, the loss of loved ones leaves the older adult without a source of social support, and this places them at greater risk of isolation and depression. Fortunately, many older adults are happy and actively participating in life. With good financial resources and a good support system of family and friends, adults in their 80s can enjoy life and continue to feel productive.

## YOU are the Provider SUMMARY

**1. How does a patient's age affect your assessment?**

The fundamental concepts of patient assessment are the same for all age groups. However, factors such as physical development, communication skills, behavior, and vital sign values vary with age.

Communication with the patient is an integral part of the patient assessment process, especially the history-taking phase. Depending on the patient's age, communication can be relatively easy or extremely difficult.

Certain medical conditions that are common in one age group are uncommon in others. Determining a patient's risk factors for disease is an important part of the history-taking process and affects your index of suspicion. For example, it is rare—although not impossible—for an otherwise healthy 8-year-old child with chest pain to be experiencing a cardiac problem because children generally have healthy hearts. However, you should be suspicious of a cardiac problem if a 55-year-old patient with a history of high blood pressure—a major risk factor for cardiovascular disease—has the same symptoms.

Older patients are more likely to have one or more chronic diseases that can be the origin of the

current problem (eg, chronic lung disease exacerbation), complicate the current problem (eg, respiratory infection in a patient with a history of asthma or chronic lung disease), or make the assessment process more difficult (eg, obtaining history in a patient with a medical problem with dementia). Older patients also frequently take medications that can affect assessment (eg, blood pressure medications that may keep pulses lower than would normally occur in response to disease or injury) or exacerbate symptoms (eg, too much insulin for the amount of food intake).

Understanding which illnesses are common in various age groups will help you formulate a plausible field impression—that is, what you believe is wrong with the patient based on your assessment findings and the patient's history.

**2. What are the physical differences between middle adults and older adults?**

Middle adults (41 to 60 years of age) have reached the halfway point in human life expectancy. However, provided they are otherwise healthy, their vital signs and physical abilities usually remain consistent with those of early adults. Their average pulse rate is 70 beats/min, their respiratory rate is between 12 and 20 breaths/min, and their systolic blood pressure is between 90 and 130 or 120 mm Hg.

The age-related physical changes that occur in older adults (61 years of age and older) are more pronounced than they are in middle adults and affect nearly every organ and organ system in the body.

The vital signs of older adults depend largely on their underlying health and are often affected by medications taken. In general, however, age-related vital sign changes include a decrease in heart rate and an increase in diastolic blood pressure. The elasticity of the lungs also decreases, forcing this group to rely more on their intercostal muscles to breathe. In addition, the ribs become more rigid due to calcification, which adds to their breathing difficulty.

Other physical changes that occur during late adulthood include a decrease in metabolism and insulin production, which can lead to diabetes, decreased gastrointestinal function, decreased taste bud sensation, decreased kidney size and filtration (kidney function declines by 50% from age 20 to age 90 years), nervous system changes (including a 10% to 20% decrease in brain weight by 80 years of age) and sensory and motor nerve deterioration, and vision and hearing loss, among others. Additionally, decreased muscle mass and strength in the elderly may alter body temperature regulation or cause problems with balance, leading to a higher risk of falls as compared with middle adults. Thinning bones due to osteoporosis also increase the risk of bone fractures in late adulthood.

The anatomic and physiologic changes that occur between middle and late adulthood must be taken into consideration during your assessment.

Keep in mind, however, that compared with middle adults, older adults often have fewer classic signs and symptoms of a wide variety of medical conditions. For example, pain sensation may be diminished due to nervous system decrease, fever may be less likely in infection due to diminished immune system function, or increased heart rate in response to a medical problem or trauma may not occur due to diminished heart function or medications being taken by older adults.

**3. What are some common psychosocial concerns experienced by middle adults?**

During middle adulthood, many people's concerns center on finances. This often causes stress and uncertainty.

A unique psychosocial concern in middle adults relates to their children and their parents. As their children move away from home—which forces them to readjust their lifestyle (empty nest syndrome)—their own parents are getting older and now need

care. Most middle adults prefer to care for their parents in their own home or in their parents' home; however, this often increases the stress and anxiety they are already experiencing from other factors such as finances or retirement.

**4. Are the patient's vital signs consistent with his age?**

The patient's heart rate and respiratory rate are consistent with his age. However, his blood pressure is not. A typical middle adult's systolic blood pressure ranges between 90 and 130 mm Hg; the diastolic blood pressure usually ranges between 70 and 80 mm Hg.

Ask the patient if he keeps a journal of his vital signs or if he has had his vital signs recently taken. If he knows, ask him what his blood pressure typically reads; clearly, hypertension cannot be diagnosed based on a single blood pressure reading. If he tells you his current blood pressure is consistent with what it normally reads, ask him if he is under a physician's care or being treated with any medication. If he is not, you should advise him to be evaluated by a physician; he may have hypertension and not be aware of it. Hypertension is often referred to as the silent killer, and a blood pressure of 174/98 mm Hg is abnormal at any age.

**5. Why should you transport this patient to the hospital?**

This patient should *not* drive himself to the hospital. He experienced a near-syncopal episode, which could indicate a variety of underlying medical conditions—some of them potentially life threatening. The patient is lightheaded, reports a headache, and is hypertensive. He should be informed that if he drives himself to the hospital, he could experience worsening of his lightheadedness or even a syncopal episode while driving; this would jeopardize not only his own safety but also the safety of other motorists.

Although the patient is of legal age and has the decision-making capacity to legally refuse EMS transport, you should make *every effort* to convince him to agree to EMS transport and advise him that his refusal could potentially result in death.

**6. What additional treatment, if any, does this patient require?**

Further treatment of this patient should be supportive. Continue to monitor his mental status and ABCs and make him comfortable. Dimming the lights in the back of the ambulance may provide him with some relief from his headache.

Remain alert for any changes in his neurologic status, such as slurred speech, unilateral weakness (weakness to one side of the body), or confusion, and contact the receiving facility if any changes are noted.

# YOU are the Provider SUMMARY *continued*

## EMS Patient Care Report (PCR)

| Date: 7-17-20 | Incident No.: 060109 | Nature of Call: Vital signs check | | Location: EMS Station 2 | |
|---|---|---|---|---|---|
| Dispatched: 1310 | En Route: 1310 | At Scene: 1310 | Transport: 1324 | At Hospital: 1330 | In Service: 1339 |

### Patient Information

**Age:** 50
**Sex:** M
**Weight (in kg [lb]):** 86 kg (190 lb)

**Allergies:** No known drug allergies
**Medications:** Vitamins
**Past Medical History:** None
**Chief Complaint:** Lightheadedness, fainting, headache

### Vital Signs

| Time: 1315 | BP: 174/98 | Pulse: 76 | Respirations: 14 | SpO$_2$: 98% |
|---|---|---|---|---|
| Time: 1321 | BP: 180/102 | Pulse: 80 | Respirations: 14 | SpO$_2$: 99% |

### EMS Treatment (circle all that apply)

| Oxygen @ ___ L/min via:<br><br>NC   NRM   Bag mask | | Assisted Ventilation | Airway Adjunct | CPR |
|---|---|---|---|---|
| Defibrillation | Bleeding Control | Bandaging | Splinting | **Other:** Blood glucose level |

### Narrative

50-year-old man presented to EMS Station 2 requesting vital signs check.

Chief Complaint: Lightheadedness, headache

History: He denies any past medical history and stated he only wanted his vital signs checked. He further denies any medication allergies and states he only takes vitamins. He stated he has been "stressed" about caring for his ill father and has experienced several episodes of lightheadedness over the past few days.

Assessment: On presentation, he was conscious and alert; his airway was patent and his breathing was adequate. Shortly after arrival, the patient stated he felt lightheaded and needed to sit down. Initial vital signs revealed an elevated blood pressure. After vital sign assessment, the patient reported a headache.

Treatment (Rx): No indication for supplemental oxygen. Reassessed his mental status; he remained conscious and alert.

Transport: Advised patient that because of his elevated blood pressure, syncopal episode, lightheadedness, and headache, EMS transport to the hospital for evaluation by a physician was wise. He stated he preferred to drive himself, because he did not think transport via ambulance was necessary. Advised patient that driving himself was unsafe because he could experience worsening of his lightheadedness or even a syncopal episode while driving. He was further advised that his signs and symptoms could signal a potentially life-threatening condition that only a physician could diagnose. After being informed of these potential consequences, the patient agreed to EMS transport. Placed patient onto the stretcher, loaded him into the ambulance, and began transport. The patient's condition remained unchanged en route. After dimming the lights in the back of the ambulance, he stated his headache improved slightly, but he was still lightheaded. Reassessed his vital signs and assessed his blood glucose level, which read 100 mg/dL. Duration of transport was uneventful, and the patient was delivered to the emergency department without incident. After giving verbal report to the charge nurse, Medic 2 returned to service.

**End of report**

# Prep Kit

## Ready for Review

- Each developmental stage is marked by different physical and psychosocial changes and characteristics; infants (1 month to 1 year) develop at a surprising rate.
- The vital signs of toddlers (ages 1 to 3 years) and preschoolers (ages 3 to 6 years) differ somewhat from those of an infant. During this stage, children learn to speak and express themselves.
- From ages 6 to 12 years, the school-age child's vital signs and body gradually approach those observed in adulthood. During this stage, children develop self-esteem.

- The vital signs of adolescents (ages 12 to 18 years) begin to level off within the adult ranges. Adolescents focus on creating their self-image.
- Early adults are 19 to 40 years old. Early adults focus on work and family.
- Middle adults are 41 to 60 years old. Middle adults focus on achieving life goals.
- Older adults are age 61 years and older. Older adults focus on their mortality and the mortality of friends and loved ones.
- Vital signs do not vary greatly throughout adulthood.

## Vital Vocabulary

**adolescent** A young person age 12 to 18 years.

**atherosclerosis** A disorder in which cholesterol and calcium build up inside the walls of blood vessels, eventually leading to partial or complete blockage of blood flow.

**barotrauma** Injury caused by pressure to enclosed body surfaces, for example, from too much pressure in the lungs.

**conventional reasoning** A type of reasoning in which a child looks for approval from peers and society.

**early adult** A young adult age 19 to 40 years.

**fontanelles** Areas where the neonate's or infant's skull has not fused together; usually disappear at approximately 18 months of age.

**infant** A young child age 1 month to 1 year.

**life expectancy** The average number of years a person can be expected to live.

**middle adult** An adult age 41 to 60 years.

**Moro reflex** An infant reflex in which, when an infant is caught off guard, the infant opens his or her arms wide, spreads the fingers, and seems to grab at things.

**neonate** A newborn age birth to 1 month.

**nephrons** The basic filtering units in the kidneys.

**older adult** An adult age 61 years or older.

**palmar grasp reflex** An infant reflex that occurs when something is placed in the infant's palm; the infant grasps the object.

**postconventional reasoning** A type of reasoning in which a child bases decisions on his or her conscience.

**preconventional reasoning** A type of reasoning in which a child acts almost purely to avoid punishment or to get what he or she wants.

**preschooler** A child age 3 to 6 years.

**rooting reflex** An infant reflex that occurs when something touches an infant's cheek, and the infant instinctively turns his or her head toward the touch.

**school age** A person who is 6 to 12 years of age.

**sucking reflex** An infant reflex in which the infant starts sucking when his or her lips are stroked.

**toddler** A child age 1 to 3 years.

**trust versus mistrust** The stage of development from birth to approximately 18 months of age, during which infants gain trust in their parents or caregivers if their world is planned, organized, and routine.

# References

1. Banerjee S. More Americans are entering poverty as they age. Next Avenue website. http://www.nextavenue.org /more-americans-are-entering-poverty-they-age/. Published June 18, 2012. Accessed April 23, 2020.

2. Chameides L, Samson RA, Schexnayder SM, et al. *Pediatric Advanced Life Support Provider Manual*. Dallas, TX: American Heart Association; 2015.

3. *National Emergency Medical Services Education Standards*. US Department of Transportation. National Highway Traffic Safety Administration. DOT HS 811 077A. January 2009. www.ems.gov/pdf/811077a.pdf. Accessed April 23, 2020.

4. *National Emergency Medical Services Education Standards. Emergency Medical Technician Instructional Guidelines*. US Department of Transportation. National Highway Traffic Safety Administration. DOT HS 811 077C. January 2009. www.ems.gov/pdf/811077c.pdf. Accessed April 23, 2020.

5. National Model EMS Clinical Guidelines: Version 2.2. National Association of State EMS Officials website. https://nasemso.org/wp-content/uploads/National-Model -EMS-Clinical-Guidelines-2017-PDF-Version-2.2.pdf. Updated January 5, 2019. Accessed April 23, 2020.

6. National Vital Statistics System, National Center for Health Statistics, Centers for Disease Control and Prevention. Ten leading causes of death by age group, United States—2012. Centers for Disease Control and Prevention website. http://www.cdc.gov/injury/wisqars /pdf/leading_causes_of_death_by_age_group_2012-a .pdf. Accessed April 23, 2020.

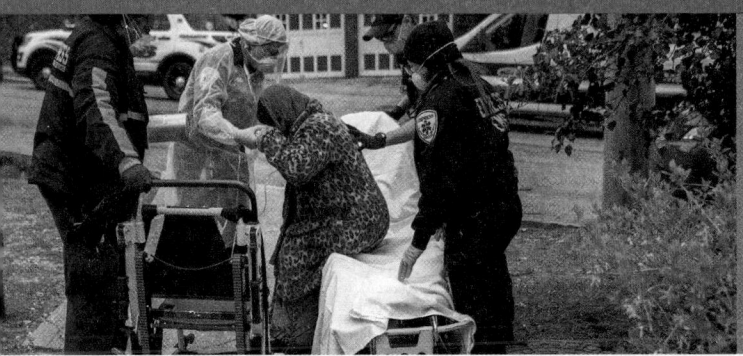

# Chapter 8

# Lifting and Moving Patients

## NATIONAL EMS EDUCATION STANDARD COMPETENCIES

### Preparatory

Applies fundamental knowledge of the EMS system, safety/well-being of the EMT, medical/legal and ethical issues to the provision of emergency care.

## KNOWLEDGE OBJECTIVES

1. Explain the need and use of the most common patient-moving equipment, the stretcher and backboard. (pp 274–276)
2. Explain the technical skills and general considerations required of EMTs during patient packaging and patient handling. (pp 276–277)
3. Define the term *body mechanics*. (p 277)
4. Discuss how following proper patient lifting and moving techniques can help prevent work-related injuries. (pp 276–277)
5. Identify how to avoid common mistakes when lifting and carrying a patient. (pp 278–280)
6. Explain the power grip and sheet or blanket methods for lifting a patient. (pp 280–282)
7. Explain the general considerations required of EMTs to safely move patients without causing the patient further harm and while protecting themselves from injury. (pp 282–287)
8. Explain how to carry patients safely on stairs, including the selection of appropriate equipment to aid in the process. (pp 287–289)
9. Describe specific situations in which an emergency move may be necessary to move a patient; include how each one is performed. (pp 294–295)

10. Describe specific situations in which an urgent move or rapid extrication may be necessary to move a patient; include how each one is performed. (pp 295–300)
11. Describe specific situations in which a nonurgent move may be necessary to move a patient; include how each one is performed. (pp 300–307)
12. Explain the special considerations and guidelines related to moving and transporting geriatric patients. (p 307)
13. Define the term *bariatrics*. (p 307)
14. Discuss the guidelines for lifting and moving bariatric patients. (pp 307–309)
15. Explain the need and use for additional patient-moving equipment (specialized); include examples. (pp 309–312)
16. Explain the importance of decontaminating equipment in the prevention of disease transmission. (p 312)
17. Describe proper positioning for the following conditions: (pp 312–313)
    - Unresponsive patients without suspected spine injury

- Patients with chest pain, discomfort, or difficulty breathing
- Patients with suspected spine injury
- Pregnant patients with hypotension
- Patients who are nauseated or vomiting

## SKILLS OBJECTIVES

1. Perform a power lift to lift a patient. (pp 279–280, Skill Drill 8-1)
2. Demonstrate a power grip. (p 280)
3. Demonstrate the body mechanics and principles required for safe reaching and pulling, including the technique used for performing log rolls. (pp 280–282)
4. Perform the diamond carry to move a patient. (pp 284–285, Skill Drill 8-2)
5. Perform the one-handed carry to move a patient. (pp 284–286, Skill Drill 8-3)
6. Perform a patient carry using a stair chair to move a patient down the stairs. (pp 287–288, Skill Drill 8-4)
7. Perform a patient carry to move a patient down the stairs on a backboard. (p 289, Skill Drill 8-5)
8. Demonstrate how to load a stretcher into an ambulance. (pp 291–292, Skill Drill 8-6)
9. Demonstrate how to perform an emergency or urgent move. (pp 294–300)
10. Perform the rapid extrication technique to move a patient from a vehicle. (pp 297–300, Skill Drill 8-7)
11. Perform the direct ground lift to lift a patient. (pp 300–301, Skill Drill 8-8)
12. Perform the extremity lift to move a patient. (pp 302–303, Skill Drill 8-9)
13. Perform the direct carry to move a patient. (pp 302–304, Skill Drill 8-10)
14. Demonstrate how to use the draw sheet method to transfer a patient onto a stretcher. (pp 304–305)
15. Use a scoop stretcher to move a patient. (pp 305–306, Skill Drill 8-11)
16. Demonstrate how to log roll a patient on the ground (pp 307–308, Skill Drill 8-12)

# Introduction

In the course of a typical call, you will have to move the patient several times to provide emergency medical care and transport. Once you have assessed the patient and provided emergency care, the patient is generally moved onto a stretcher. In most cases, you will have to lift and carry the patient to the stretcher, move the stretcher to the ambulance, and load the stretcher into the patient compartment. Upon arrival at the hospital, the patient must be removed from the ambulance, wheeled into the emergency department (ED), and transferred to the ED bed. To avoid injury to the patient, yourself, or your team, you need to learn how to lift and carry a patient properly, using proper body mechanics and a power grip.

To move a patient safely in the various situations that you may encounter in the field, it is necessary to learn how to perform emergency body drags and lifts, rapidly extricate a patient from a vehicle onto the stretcher, assist a patient from a chair or bed onto the stretcher, lift a patient from the floor onto the stretcher, and manually carry a patient up or down stairs. You and your team should know how to place a patient with a suspected spinal injury onto an immobilization device and how to package patients with and without suspected spinal injury. At times, you and your team may need to move a patient who is very heavy or carry a patient on a trail or across rugged terrain. Special techniques for loading and unloading the stretcher and transferring the patient from the stretcher to a bed in the ED are necessary.

Lifting and carrying are dynamic processes. Back injuries are the leading cause of injury that forces EMTs and paramedics to leave the profession. Learning the proper way to lift and move patients will help prevent you from suffering injury. You also need to know how to properly use patient-moving devices, such as a stretcher, stair chair, backboard, scoop stretcher, flexible stretcher, and any other equipment your service may carry. You must also know which device or combination of devices is appropriate for the current situation. This chapter will cover lifting, carrying, and reaching techniques as well as principles of moving patients, including emergency, urgent, and nonurgent moves, and the use of physical restraints to protect the patient and your team from further harm. In addition, different types of equipment and patient positioning will be discussed in detail.

## The Wheeled Ambulance Stretcher

The **wheeled ambulance stretcher** (also called an ambulance stretcher, gurney, litter, or cot) is the most commonly used device to transport patients. The wheeled ambulance stretcher is a specially designed stretcher that can be rolled along the ground and weighs between 40 and 145 lb (18 and 66 kg), depending on its design and features (**FIGURE 8-1**). Because of its weight, it is generally not taken up or down stairs or to other locations where the patient must be carried for any significant distance. Moving a patient by rolling, using a stretcher or other wheeled device, is preferred when the situation helps prevent injuries.

The modern stretcher is available in a number of different models, which may include different features. During your training, familiarize yourself with the specific features of the stretcher that your ambulance carries. You must know where to locate the controls to adjust and lock each feature and how each works.

The stretcher has a specific head end and foot end. The stretcher has a strong, rectangular, tubular metal main frame to which all of its other

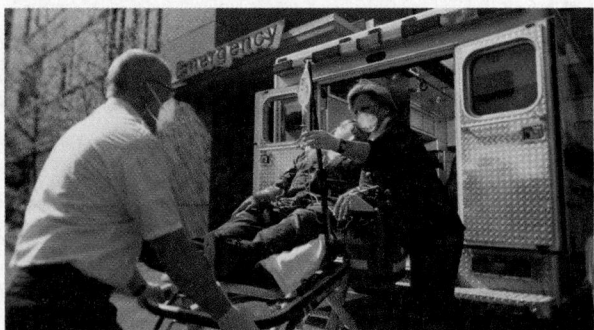

**FIGURE 8-1** The wheeled ambulance stretcher is specially designed to roll along the ground.

© Keith Brofsky/Photodisc/Getty Images.

parts are attached. The stretcher should be pulled, pushed, and lifted only by its main frame or handles, which are attached to the frame specifically for this purpose.

A retractable guardrail is attached along the central portion of the main frame of the stretcher at each side and is lowered out of the way when a patient is being loaded onto the stretcher. Once the patient has been properly placed on the stretcher, the handle is drawn up and locked in an elevated position perpendicular to the surface of the stretcher. The guardrail is not a restraint device and will not prevent the patient from falling off of the stretcher. The guardrail at each side can be lowered only if its locking handle is released.

The underside of the main frame of the stretcher is supported on a folding undercarriage that has a smaller, horizontal, rectangular frame and four large rubber casters at its bottom end. The folding undercarriage is designed so that the litter can be adjusted to any height from about 12 inches (30 cm) above the ground, which is the desired height when the stretcher is secured in the ambulance, to 32 to 36 inches (81 to 91 cm) above the ground, which is the desired height when the stretcher is being rolled. Because you are able to lock the stretcher at any height between its lowest height and its fully extended height, it can be locked at the same height as any bed or examining table to allow the patient to sit or be slid from one to the other. This permits you to transfer the patient without the need for any additional lifting. The controls for folding the undercarriage are designed so that the stretcher remains locked at its current height when the controls are not being activated. As an additional safety feature on most stretchers, the main frame must be slightly lifted to remove all weight from the undercarriage before it will fold, even if the control is pulled. Therefore, if the handle is accidentally pulled, the elevated stretcher will not suddenly drop. Controls for elevating and lowering most stretchers are located at the foot end. You and your partner must use the proper lifting mechanics to lift the wheeled ambulance stretcher.

The mattress on a stretcher is fluid resistant so that it does not absorb any type of potentially infectious material, including water, blood, or other body fluid. This also allows for easy cleaning and disinfecting.

Patients must always be secured with the straps on the stretcher. In the event of a crash while en route to the hospital, the straps help to protect the patient from further injury. Secure the patient to the wheeled ambulance stretcher as follows:

1. Secure the stretcher's safety belts over the patient's shoulders and around the patient's chest in a four-point harness fashion. They should be tight enough to keep the patient secured on the stretcher but not limit breathing.
2. Secure the stretcher's safety belt over the patient's abdomen.
3. Secure the stretcher's safety belt over the patient's thighs.
4. Secure the stretcher's safety belt over the patient's ankles.

## Backboards

A **backboard** is a long, flat board made of rigid, rectangular material (**FIGURE 8-2**). Backboards are also called long backboards, spine boards, trauma boards, or longboards. A backboard is used to temporarily restrict spinal motion in supine patients with potential neck and back injuries. Backboards can also be used to move patients out of awkward places.

Backboards are 6 to 7 feet long (approximately 2 m) and are commonly used for patients who are found lying down. Parallel to the sides and ends of the backboard are a number of long holes that are about 0.5 to 1 inch (1 to 2.5 cm) from the outer edge. These holes form handles and handholds so that the board can be easily grasped, lifted, and carried. The handles and adjacent holes also allow the patient to be secured to the board using straps located at each side and end of the backboard.

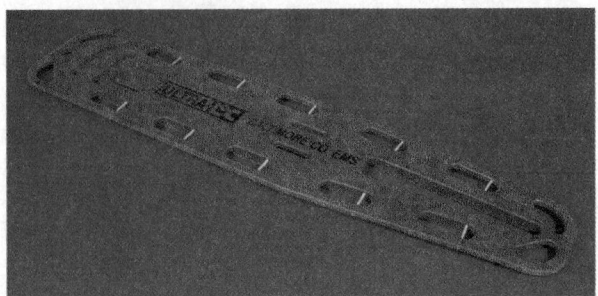

**FIGURE 8-2** A backboard is used to transfer patients who must be moved in a supine or immobilized position.

© Jones & Bartlett Learning. Courtesy of MIEMSS.

For many years, backboards were made of thick marine plywood whose surface was sealed with polyurethane or marine varnish. Newer backboards are made of lighter plastic materials that will not absorb blood or other infectious substances. Some services are moving away from backboard use due to injuries patients can receive after being secured to them for long periods and are instead using other devices, such as vacuum mattresses.

## Moving and Positioning the Patient

Every time you have to move a patient, special care must be taken so that neither you, your team, nor the patient is injured. Patient packaging and handling are technical skills that you will learn and perfect through repeated training and practice. Every year, a significant number of EMTs are injured when they attempt to lift and move patients. Even when you are lifting, moving, or transferring relatively lightweight patients, the need for proper body

**YOU** are the Provider

You are dispatched to a motor vehicle crash with an overturned vehicle. You arrive on scene to find a four-door sedan lying on the passenger side in a deep ditch. The vehicle is resting on a concrete pipe and a metal signpost. There are two patients, neither of whom appear to be restrained. The driver is an older man who is unresponsive. You note that his skin is ashen with cyanosis around his lips. He is crumpled in a semisupine position over the second patient. Only the top of the head of the passenger is visible, but she is alert and able to speak with you.

1. What immediate challenges do you face?
2. Why is knowledge of body mechanics important when lifting and moving a patient?
3. What other resources are needed?

mechanics should remain paramount. Occasionally injuries occur when proper lifting techniques are used; however, using proper body mechanics and maintaining physical fitness greatly reduces the chance of injury.

Moving a patient should be done in an orderly, planned, and unhurried manner. This approach will protect you and the patient from further injury and reduce the risk of worsening the patient's condition when he or she is moved. Therefore, practice each technique with your team often so that when you must move a patient, you can perform the move quickly, safely, and efficiently. You must also master the skills necessary for the use of all equipment and understand the advantages and limitations of each device before you use it in the field. After each patient transfer, you and your team should evaluate the appropriateness of the technique that you used, as well as your technical skill in completing the transfer. You must also be sure to maintain your equipment according to the manufacturer's instructions. Using clean, well-maintained equipment is a critical part of providing high-quality patient care.

After delivering the patient to the ED, you and your team must begin preparation for your next call by reviewing the positive points about the transport and discussing changes that would improve the next run. This process of evaluation should help you identify the following:

- Procedures that need more practice
- Equipment that needs to be cleaned or serviced
- Skills that you need to review or acquire

## Body Mechanics

### Anatomy Review

The shoulder girdle rests on the rib cage and is supported by the vertebrae that lie inferior to it. The arms are connected to and hang from the shoulder girdle. When a person stands upright, the individual weight-bearing vertebrae are stacked on top of each other and aligned over the sacrum. The sacrum is both the mechanical weight-bearing base of the spinal column and the fused central posterior section of the pelvic girdle. **Body mechanics** is the relationship between the body's anatomic structures and the physical forces associated with lifting, moving, and carrying—in other words, the ways in

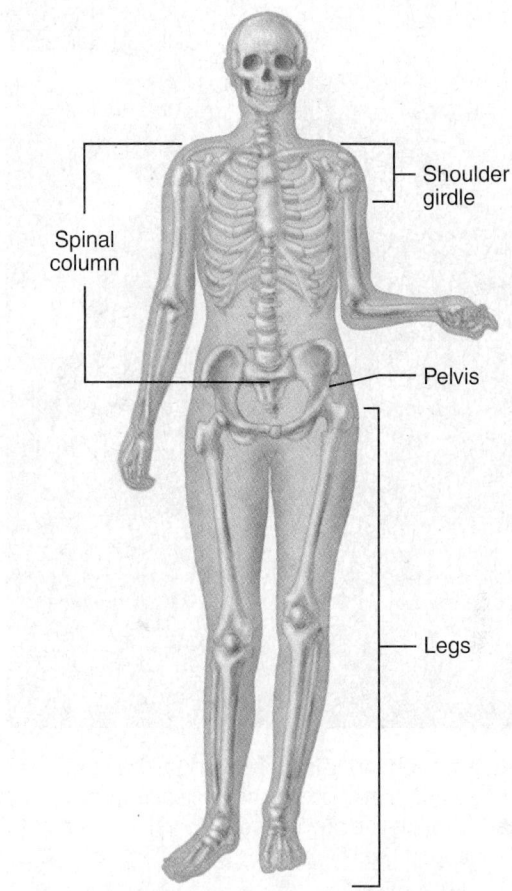

**FIGURE 8-3** When you stand upright, the weight of anything that you lift and carry in your hands is borne by the shoulder girdle, the spinal column, the pelvis, and the legs.

© Jones & Bartlett Learning.

which the body moves to achieve a specific action. Maintaining proper posture and body movement during daily activities is applying the use of body mechanics. Using good body mechanics while lifting and moving patients reduces your risk of injury.

When a person stands upright, the weight of anything being lifted and carried in the hands is reflected onto the shoulder girdle, the spinal column inferior to it, the pelvis, and then the legs (**FIGURE 8-3**). In lifting, if the shoulder girdle is aligned over the pelvis and the hands are held close to the legs, the force that is exerted against the spine occurs in an essentially straight line down the vertebrae in the spinal column. Therefore, with the back properly maintained in an upright position, little strain occurs against the muscles and ligaments that keep the spinal column in alignment, and

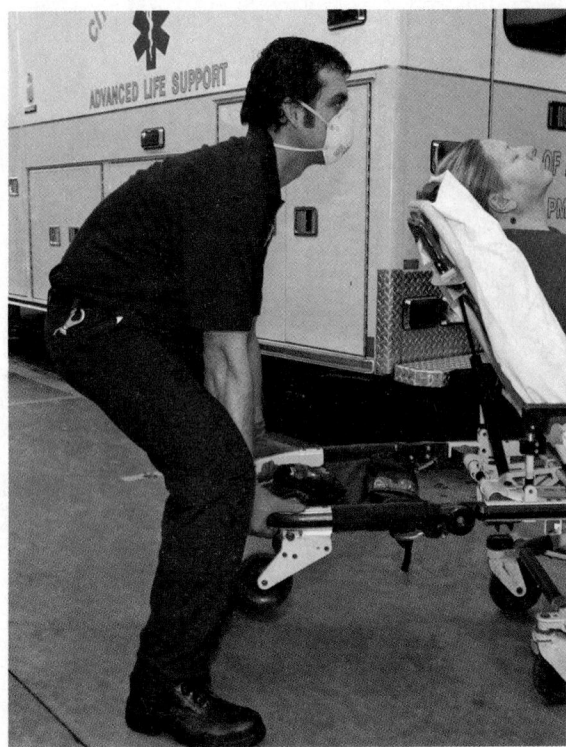

**FIGURE 8-4** If your body is properly aligned when you lift, the line of force exerted against the spine occurs in an essentially straight line down the vertebrae. In this way, the vertebrae support the lift.

© Jones & Bartlett Learning. Courtesy of MIEMSS.

significant weight can be lifted and carried without injury to the back (**FIGURE 8-4**). However, you may injure your back if you lift while leaning forward, or even if you lift while the back is straight, while you are bent significantly forward at the hips. With the back in either of these positions, the shoulder girdle lies significantly anterior to the pelvis, and the force of lifting is exerted primarily across, rather than down, the spinal column. When this occurs, the weight is supported by the muscles of the back and ligaments that run from the base of the skull to the pelvis, keeping the spinal column in alignment, rather than by each vertebral body and disk resting on those aligned below it. In addition, the upper spine and torso serve as a lever so that the force that is exerted against the muscles and ligaments in the lumbar and sacral regions, as a result of the mechanical advantage produced, is many times that of the combined weight of your upper body and the object you are lifting. Therefore, the first key rule of lifting is to always keep your back in a straight, upright (vertical) position, and lift without twisting.

Always face the patient and point your feet in the same direction. After lifting the patient, change the direction of your feet as opposed to twisting or turning from the waist.

When lifting, spread your legs approximately shoulder width apart, and place your feet so that your center of gravity is properly balanced between them. Your weight should be balanced on the balls of your feet, not your toes. Then, with the back held upright, bring your upper body down by bending the legs. Once you have properly grasped the patient or stretcher and made any necessary adjustments in the location of your feet, lift the patient by straightening your legs until you are in a standing position and then curling your arms up to waist height. If you still have not reached the desired height, reposition your legs so they are closer together and repeat the process. Because the leg muscles are regularly exercised by walking, climbing stairs, or running, they are well developed and strong. Therefore, as well as being the safest method, lifting by extending the properly placed flexed legs is also the most powerful way to lift. This method is appropriately called a **power lift**.

## Words of Wisdom

The stretcher is designed so that the patient's head is slightly higher than the feet. Always position the tallest EMTs at the head of the stretcher when lifting to offset this difference in the height of the stretcher.

One mistake to avoid while performing a lift is lifting a patient or other heavy object with your arms outstretched. Even if your back is held properly upright, adverse forces across the spinal column and leverage against the low back will occur if your hands are significantly anterior to the plane described by the front of the torso (the plane consists of the anterior torso and imaginary lines extended vertically above and below it). Whenever you lift or carry a patient, be sure to hold your arms so that your hands are almost adjacent to the plane described by your anterior torso, and always keep the weight that you are lifting as close to your body as possible.

Another rule to remember when lifting is to avoid placing lateral force across the spine and sideways leverage against the low back. If you lift with only one arm or with the arms extended more to one side than the other, more force will be exerted against one side of the shoulder girdle than the other, causing lateral force to be exerted across the spinal column. To prevent this, keep your arms approximately the same distance apart as when hanging at each side of the body, with the weight distributed equally and properly centered between them. If the weight is not balanced between both arms or properly centered between the shoulders when you are preparing to lift, turn and/or move

to the left or right until the weight is properly balanced and centered. To lift safely and produce the maximal power lift, take the following steps (**SKILL DRILL 8-1**):

1. Tighten your back in its normal upright position, and use your abdominal core muscles to lock it in a slight curve.
2. Spread your legs apart about 15 inches (38 cm), and bend your legs to lower your torso and arms.

## Skill Drill 8-1 Performing the Power Lift

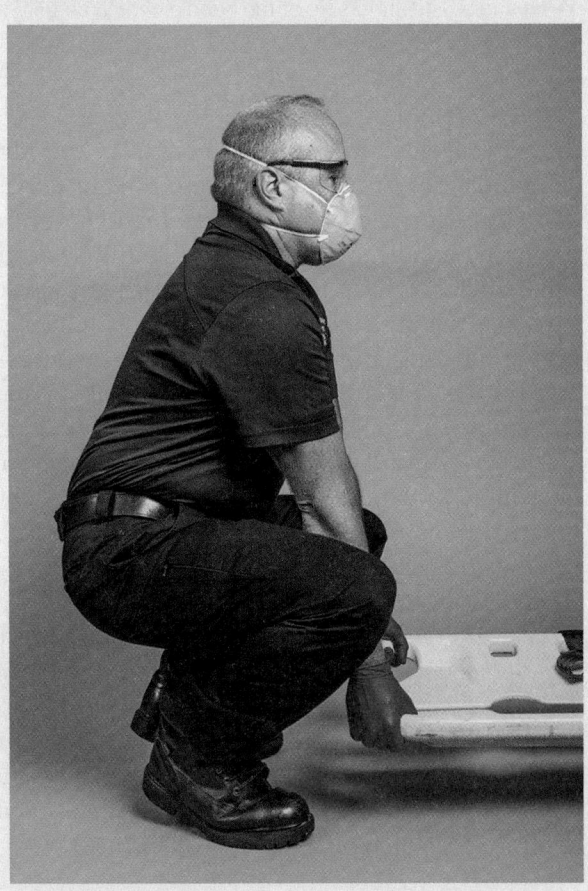

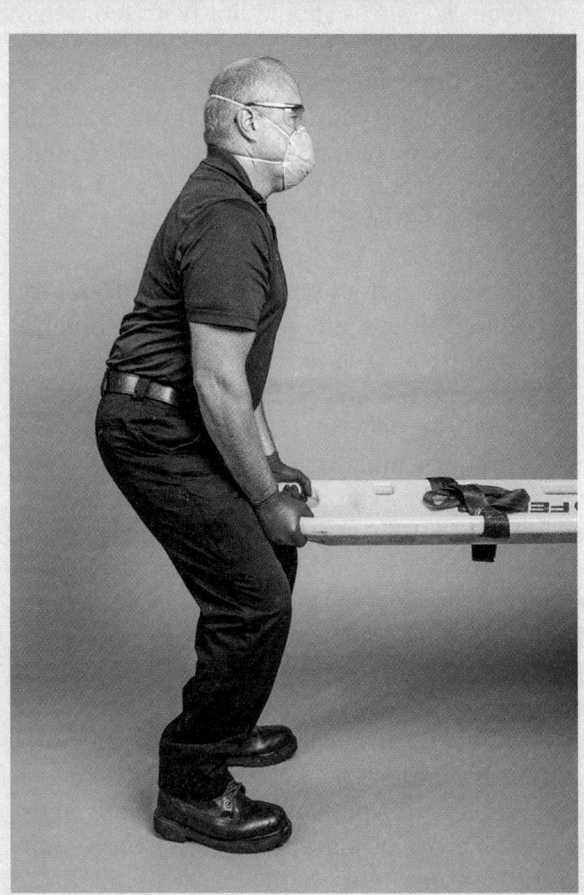

### Step 1
Lock your back in a slight curve. Spread and bend your legs. Grasp the backboard, palms up and just in front of you. Balance and center the weight between your arms.

### Step 2
Position your feet, straddle the object, and distribute your weight evenly. Lift by straightening your legs, keeping your back locked in.

3. With arms extended down each side of the body, grasp the stretcher or backboard with your hands held palm up and just in front of the plane described by the anterior torso and imaginary lines extending vertically from it to the ground.

4. Adjust your orientation and position until the weight is balanced and centered between both arms (**Step 1**).

5. Reposition your feet as necessary so that they are about 15 inches (38 cm) apart with one slightly farther forward and rotated so that you and your center of gravity will be properly balanced between them. Be sure to straddle the object, keep your feet flat, and distribute your weight to the balls of the feet or just behind them. The knees should not bend more than 90 degrees, nor extend past the toes.

6. With the arms extended downward, lift by straightening your legs until you are fully standing. Make sure your back is held upright and that your upper body comes up before your hips (**Step 2**).

Reverse these steps whenever you are lowering the stretcher. Always remember to avoid bending at the waist or twisting as you stand.

Your safety, as well as that of the other EMTs and the patient, depends on the use of proper lifting techniques and maintaining a proper hold when lifting or carrying a patient. If you do not have proper hold of the stretcher or of the patient in a body lift, you will not be able to bear a proper share of the weight, and there is an increased chance that you might suddenly lose your grasp with one or both hands. If you temporarily lose your grasp, the position and weight distribution of the stretcher will change suddenly, and the other team members must quickly overextend beyond a safe distance to avoid dropping the patient. As a result, sudden excessive force may be placed across each one's spine, causing low back injury.

You should use the **power grip** to get the maximum force from your hands and arms whenever you are lifting a patient (**FIGURE 8-5**). The arm and hand have their greatest lifting strength when facing palm up. Whenever you grasp a stretcher or backboard, your hands should be at least 10 inches (25 cm) apart. Each hand should be inserted under the handle with the palm facing up and the thumb extended upward. Next, advance the hand until the

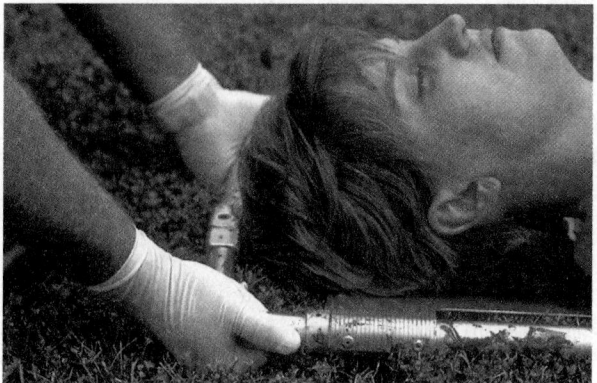

**FIGURE 8-5** To perform the power grip, grasp the handle of the stretcher or backboard with your palms up and your thumbs extending up. Make sure your hands are about 10 inches (25 cm) apart and that your fingers are all at the same angle. The underside of the handle should be fully supported by the palms of your hands.

© Jones & Bartlett Learning. Courtesy of MIEMSS.

thumb prevents further insertion and the cylindrical handle lies firmly in the crease of your curved palm. Curl your fingers and thumb tightly over the top of the handle. All your fingers should be at the same angle. To have the proper power grip, make sure that the underside of the handle is fully supported on your curved palm with only the fingers and thumb preventing it from being pulled sideways or upward out of the palm.

If you must lift the object higher once you have lifted by extending your legs, you will be able to "curl" the object higher by using your biceps to flex the arms while maintaining the power grip and weight supported in the palms.

Never grasp a stretcher or backboard with the hand placed palm down over the handle. When you are lifting with the palm down, the weight is supported by the fingers rather than the palm. This hand orientation places the tips of the fingers and thumb under the handle. If the weight forces them apart, your grasp on the handle will be lost.

## Principles of Safe Reaching and Pulling

The same basic body mechanics and principles apply to moving, lifting, and carrying a patient.

When you use a body drag to move a patient, your back should always be locked in a slight curve created by tightening your abdominal muscles, not curved laterally or bent laterally. It should be held in its normal upright position. Avoid any twisting so that the vertebrae remain in their normal alignment. When you reach overhead, avoid hyperextending your back. When you pull a patient who is on the ground, always kneel to minimize the distance that you will have to lean over (**FIGURE 8-6A**). To keep your reach within the recommended distance, reach forward and grasp the patient so that your elbows are just beyond the anterior torso (**FIGURE 8-6B**). When you pull a patient who is at a different height from you, bend your knees until your hips are just below the height of the plane across which you will be pulling the patient. During pulling, extend your arms no more than about 15 to 20 inches (38 to 50 cm) in front of your torso. Reposition your feet (or knees, if kneeling) so that the force of pull will be balanced equally between both arms and the line of pull will be centered between them (**FIGURE 8-6C**). Pull the patient by slowly flexing your arms. When you can pull no farther because your hands have reached the front of your torso, stop and move back another 15 to 20 inches (38 to 50 cm). Then, when properly positioned, repeat the steps. Alternate between pulling the patient by flexing your arms and then repositioning yourself so that your arms are again extended with your hands about 15 inches (38 cm) in front of your torso. By not moving yourself and the patient simultaneously, you will prevent undesirable jostling of the patient and the chance that sudden force will occur across your spine. You should also try to prevent injury to yourself by avoiding situations that involve strenuous effort lasting more than 1 minute.

If you must drag a patient across a bed, kneel on the bed to avoid reaching beyond the recommended distance. Then follow the steps described previously until the patient is within 15 to 20 inches (38 to 50 cm) of the bed's edge (see **FIGURE 8-6**). You can then complete the drag while standing at the side of the bed. Rather than dragging the patient by his or her clothing, use the sheet or blanket under the patient for this purpose. You can roll the bedding under the patient until it is about 6 inches (15 cm) wider than the patient. Pull on the rolled bedding smoothly and evenly to glide the patient to the bedside.

Transfer the patient from the stretcher to a bed in the ED or the patient's hospital room with a body drag. With the stretcher at the same height as the bed or slightly higher and held firmly against the bed's side, you and another EMT should kneel on

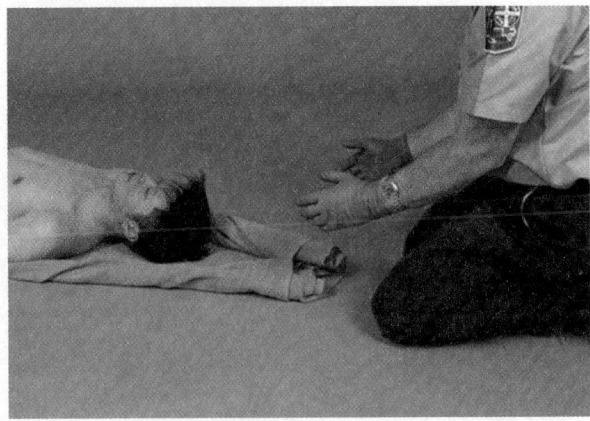

A

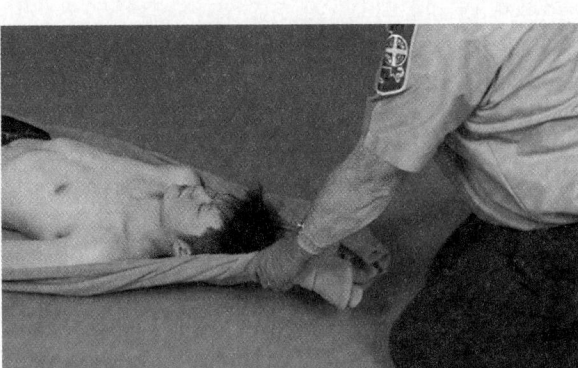

B

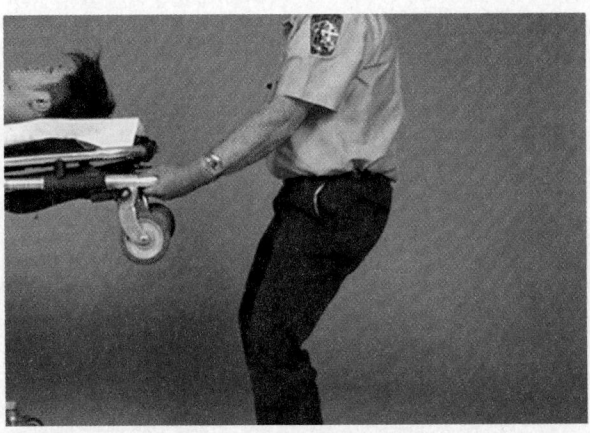

C

**FIGURE 8-6** Reaching and pulling safely. **A.** Kneel to pull a patient who is on the ground. **B.** When pulling, your elbows should only extend just beyond the anterior torso. **C.** Bend your knees to pull a patient who is at a different height than you are. Position your feet or knees to balance the force of pull.

A, B, C: © Jones & Bartlett Learning. Courtesy of MIEMSS.

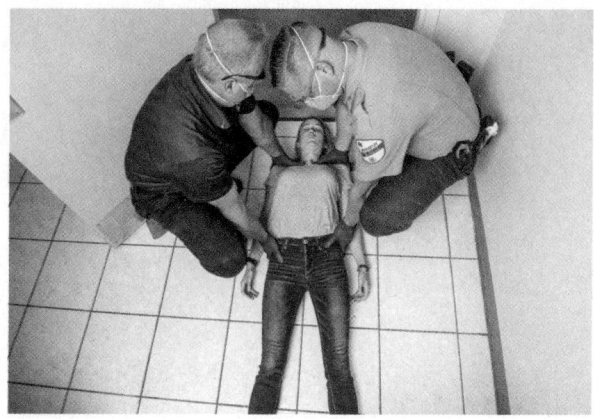

**FIGURE 8-7** A body drag with an EMT on each side of the patient.
© Jones & Bartlett Learning.

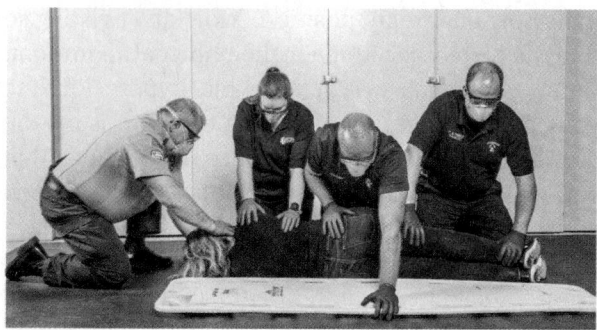

**FIGURE 8-8** Placing a patient onto a backboard.
© Jones & Bartlett Learning.

the hospital bed and, in the manner previously described, drag the patient in increments until he or she is properly centered on the bed. A third person may need to take both sides of the head to move the patient safely.

Sometimes during a body drag, you and another EMT may have to pull the patient with one of you on either side of the patient (**FIGURE 8-7**). You will have to alter the pulling technique to prevent pulling sideways and producing adverse lateral leverage against your lower back. Position yourself by kneeling just beyond the patient's shoulder and facing toward his or her groin. By extending one arm across and in front of your chest, you can grasp the armpit and, with your other arm extended in front and to the side of the patient's torso, the patient's belt. Then, by raising your elbows and flexing your arms, you can pull the patient with the line of force at the minimum angle possible.

### Words of Wisdom

When moving a patient, you may grab the patient's belt or belt loops to assist with the move.

Generally, when log rolling a patient onto his or her side, you will initially have to reach farther than 18 inches (46 cm) (**FIGURE 8-8**). To minimize this distance, kneel as close to the patient's side as possible, leaving only enough room so that your knees will not prevent the patient from being rolled. When you lean forward, keep your back straight and lean solely from the hips. Be sure to use your shoulder muscles to help with the roll. To minimize the amount of time you are extended like this and to support the patient's weight, roll the patient without stopping until the patient is resting on his or her side and braced against your thighs. Pulling toward you allows your legs to prevent the patient from rolling over completely and from rolling beyond the intended distance.

### Words of Wisdom

You will often be called upon to lift a patient in tandem with someone you have never worked with before. Pay attention to what each person is doing, and verbalize your actions to decrease the risk of dropping the patient or hurting one another. If you have the chance to practice lifts with a new partner prior to your first call together, do so.

## Principles of Safe Lifting and Carrying

Whenever possible, use a device that can be rolled to move a patient. However, in a situation where a wheeled device is not available, you must make sure that you understand and follow certain guidelines for carrying a patient on a stretcher. **TABLE 8-1** presents the guidelines.

### Patient Weight

You should estimate how much the patient weighs before you attempt to lift. Commonly, adult patients weigh between 120 and 220 lb (54 and 100 kg). Depending on your individual strength, you and another EMT may be able to safely lift an even heavier

**TABLE 8-1** Guidelines for Carrying a Patient on a Stretcher

- Estimate the weight of both the patient and the associated equipment to be lifted and gauge the limitations of your team's abilities.
- Coordinate your movements with those of the other team members while constantly communicating with them.
- Do not twist your body as you are carrying the patient.
- Keep the weight that you are carrying as close to your body as possible while keeping your back in a locked-in position.
- Do not bend at the waist; this could hyperextend your back. Instead, flex at the hips, and bend at the knees.

© Jones & Bartlett Learning.

## YOU | are the Provider

Due to the critical condition of the driver, you immediately request paramedic backup. Because of the position of the vehicle and the patients, you determine that the patients are entrapped and that the vehicle is potentially unstable. You ask dispatch to send a rescue unit to assist with stabilizing the vehicle and extricating the victims. You are able to look through the door and perform a primary assessment on the patients while waiting for further assistance.

**Patient 1 (the driver)**

| Recording Time: 0 Minutes | |
| --- | --- |
| Appearance | Motionless; ashen skin with cyanosis around the mouth |
| Level of consciousness | Unresponsive |
| Airway | Snoring respirations |
| Breathing | Increased rate; shallow depth |
| Circulation | Unable to reach patient to feel for pulse; no obvious bleeding |

**Patient 2 (the passenger)**

| Recording Time: 0 Minutes | |
| --- | --- |
| Appearance | Unable to visualize due to patient's position, but she is anxious and reports some pain to her back and right side |
| Level of consciousness | Alert and oriented |
| Airway | Open; clear of secretions and foreign bodies |
| Breathing | Unable to assess, but talking in complete sentences with no sounds of distress and she denies any dyspnea |
| Circulation | Unable to assess due to patient's position |

The passenger tells you that the driver, her husband, is normally on oxygen and the tube was pulled off during the crash. She thinks she may be sitting on the portable oxygen machine. She also thinks that she may have "cracked a rib or two" when she was thrown against the door. She begs you to please help her husband before it is too late.

4. Do you consider the driver to be in stable or unstable condition? Should you wait for further assistance or proceed to gain access to him?

5. Once you are able to gain access, what are your concerns for the use of proper body mechanics while removing these patients?

6. Once the driver is no longer entrapped, how will you attempt to remove him from the vehicle while maintaining spinal motion restriction?

patient. However, due to safety concerns, consider using four providers to lift when possible. There is more stability with a four-person carry, and the carry requires less strength. You should know how much you can comfortably and safely lift, and do not attempt to lift a proportional weight (the share of the weight that you will bear) that exceeds this amount. If you find that lifting the patient places a strain on you, stop the lift and lower the patient. You should then obtain additional help before again attempting to lift the patient. Be sure to communicate clearly and frequently with your partner and other providers whenever you are lifting a patient.

Protocols should include a method to rapidly summon additional help to lift and carry a heavy patient or, as in the case of a cardiac arrest, provide and maintain the necessary care in the field. In addition, you must know, or be able to find out, the weight limitations of the equipment you are using and how to handle patients who exceed those weight limitations. Special bariatric techniques, equipment, and resources are generally required to move any patient who weighs more than 350 lb (159 kg) to the ambulance (discussed later in the chapter). These resources should be called on when you arrive on scene and have assessed the situation.

## Lifting and Carrying a Patient on a Backboard or Stretcher

If a patient is supine on a backboard or is lying in a semi-Fowler position on the stretcher, his or her weight is not equally distributed between the two ends of the device. Between 68% and 78% of the body weight of a patient in a horizontal position is in the torso. Therefore, more of the patient's weight rests on the head half of the device than on the foot half.

A patient on a backboard or stretcher can be lifted and carried by four providers in a **diamond carry**, with one provider at the head end of the device, one at the foot end, and one at each side of the patient's torso (**FIGURE 8-9**). Follow these steps to perform the diamond carry (**SKILL DRILL 8-2**):

1.  To best balance the weight, the providers at each side should be located so that they are able to grasp the backboard or stretcher with one hand adjacent to the distal edge of the

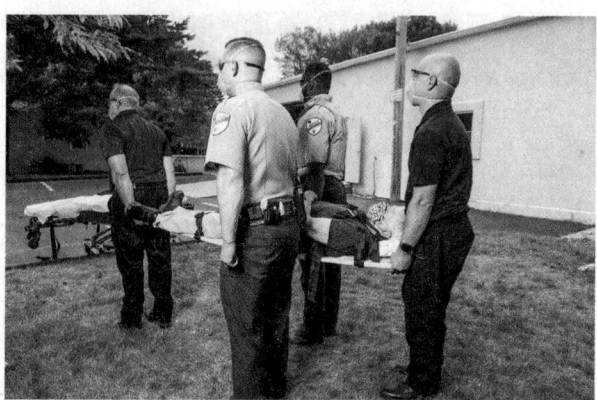

**FIGURE 8-9** The diamond carry requires four providers: one at the head of the backboard, one at the foot end, and one at each side of the patient's torso.

© Jones & Bartlett Learning.

patient's pelvis and the other hand located midthorax. All four providers lift the device while facing toward the patient (**Step 1**).
2.  The provider at each side should grasp the backboard or stretcher with the head-end hand (**Step 2**).
3.  The providers at each side turn toward the patient's feet. The provider at the foot end turns to face forward. All four providers should face the same direction and walk forward when carrying the patient (**Step 3**).

A patient on a backboard or stretcher should be carried feetfirst to place the lightest load on the provider at the patient's feet, who, to walk forward, must turn and grasp the handles with his or her back to the device. Carrying the patient feetfirst will also allow a conscious patient to see in the direction of movement, which may reduce anxiety.

It is important that you and your team use the correct lifting techniques to lift the stretcher. One method of lifting and carrying a patient on a backboard is the one-handed carry. With this method, four or more providers each use one hand to support the backboard so that they are able to face forward as they are walking. To perform the one-handed carry, follow the steps in **SKILL DRILL 8-3**:

1.  Before lifting the backboard, be sure that at least two providers are on each side of the backboard facing across from each other and using both hands (**Step 1**).

## Skill Drill 8-2 Performing the Diamond Carry

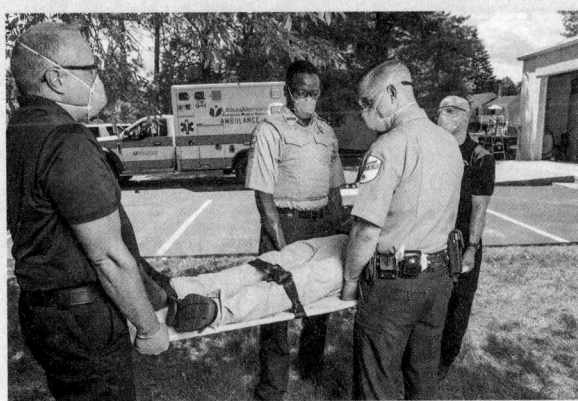

### Step 1
Position yourselves facing the patient.

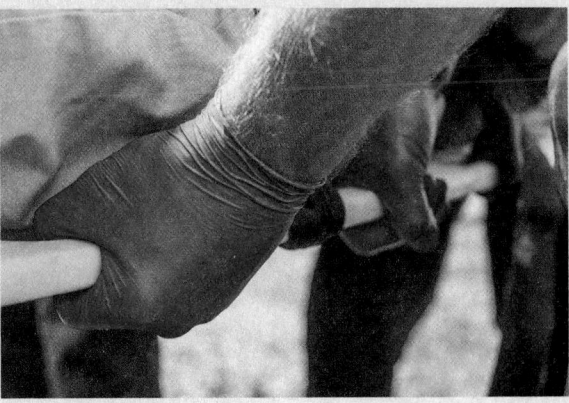

### Step 2
The providers at each side turn the head-end hand palm down and release the other hand.

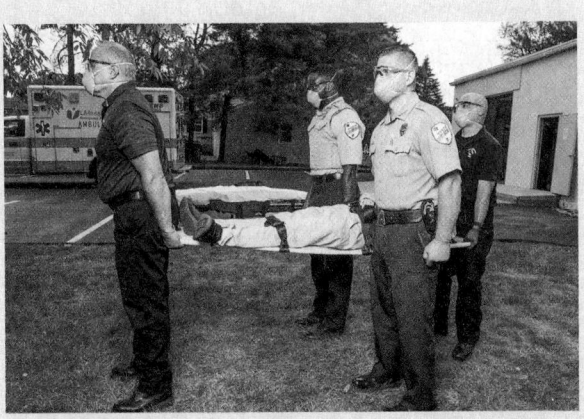

© Jones & Bartlett Learning.

### Step 3
The providers at each side turn toward the foot end. The provider at the foot end turns to face forward.

2. Lift the backboard to carrying height using correct lifting techniques, including a locked-in back (**Step 2**).
3. Once you have lifted the backboard to carrying height, you and your partners turn in the direction you will be walking and switch to using one hand (**Step 3**).

Be sure to pick up and carry the backboard with your back in the upright position. If you need to lean to either side to compensate for a weight imbalance,

you have probably exceeded your weight limitation. If this occurs, reevaluate the carry; you may need additional providers or else you might injure yourself or drop the patient.

In most instances, it is best if you push the head of the stretcher while your partner guides the foot of the stretcher. When the stretcher must be carried, it is best if four providers are available to carry it. One provider should be positioned at each corner of the stretcher to provide an even lift. If only two providers are available, or if limited space allows room for only

## Skill Drill 8-3 Performing the One-Handed Carry

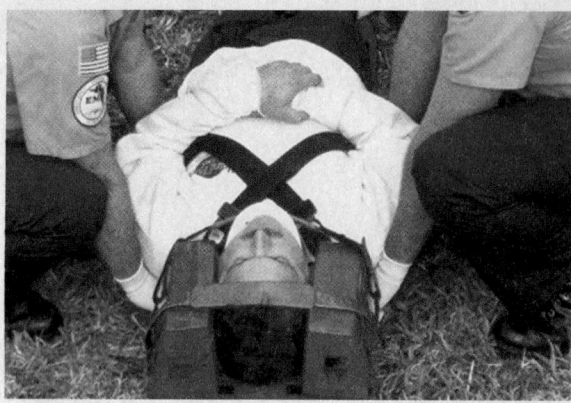

**Step 1**

Face each other and use both hands.

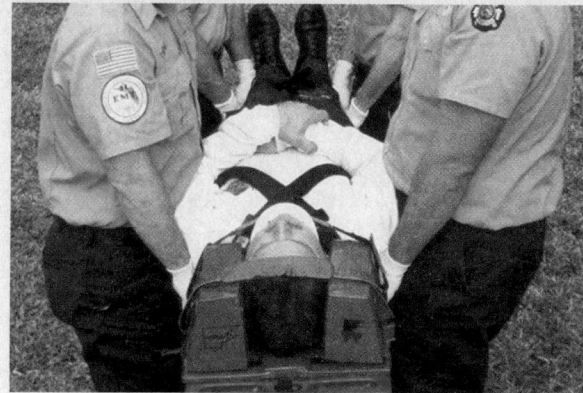

**Step 2**

Lift the backboard to carrying height.

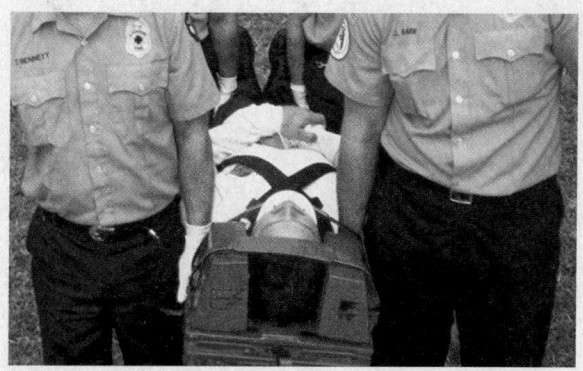

**Step 3**

Turn in the direction you will walk, and switch to using one hand.

© Jones & Bartlett Learning.

two providers to carry the stretcher, there is a risk that the stretcher will become unbalanced. In a two-person carry, the two providers should stand facing each other, with one person at the head end of the stretcher and the other at the foot end. With this type of carry, one provider will have to walk backward.

When you are rolling the wheeled ambulance stretcher, make sure that it is in the fully elevated position. If you are guiding the stretcher from the foot end, make sure your arms are held close to your body, and be careful to avoid reaching significantly behind you or hyperextending your

back (**FIGURE 8-10**). Recall that your back should be locked, straight, and untwisted. While you are walking and guiding the stretcher, bend slightly forward at the hips. As you walk, your legs are pulled back with your feet on the ground, your pelvis is moved forward, and the movement of the pelvis is transferred to the stretcher through your straight torso and firmly held arms. Try to keep the line of the pull through the center of your body by bending your knees.

Your partner should control the head end and assist you by pushing with his or her arms held with

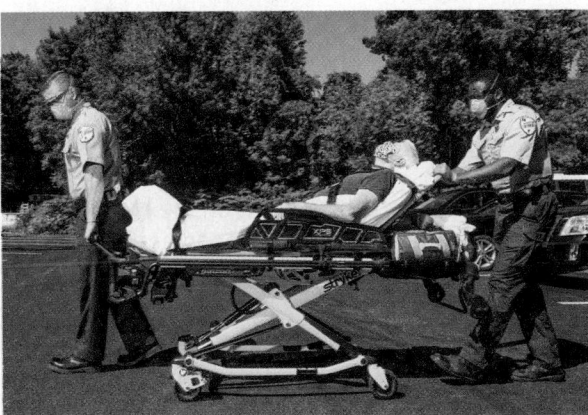

**FIGURE 8-10** Push the stretcher from the head end. If you are guiding the stretcher from the foot end, make sure your arms are held close to your body, and be careful to avoid reaching significantly behind you or hyperextending your back. Your back should be locked, straight, and untwisted.

© Jones & Bartlett Learning.

the elbows bent so that the hands are about 12 to 15 inches (30 to 38 cm) in front of the torso. To protect your elbows from injury, never push an object with your arms fully extended in a straight line and the elbows locked. When you push with the elbow bent but firmly held from bending further, the strong muscles of the arm serve as a shock absorber if the wheels or foot end of the stretcher strikes an obstacle that causes its progress to be suddenly slowed or stopped. Be sure that you push from the area of your body that is between the waist and shoulder. If the weight you are pushing is lower than your waist, push from a kneeling position. Remember not to push or pull from an overhead position.

## Moving a Patient With a Stair Chair

When you must carry a conscious patient up or down a flight of stairs or other significant incline, use a stair chair if the patient's condition allows him or her to be placed in a sitting position. A **stair chair** is a lightweight folding chair with a molded seat, adjustable safety straps, and fold-out handles at both the head and feet (**FIGURE 8-11**). Most models have rubber wheels in the back with casters in front so that they can roll along the floor and make turns. Some have a specially designed track to facilitate movement down steps with little lifting required. Stair chairs serve as an adjunct for moving a patient up or down stairs to the ground floor, where the prepared wheeled ambulance stretcher is waiting.

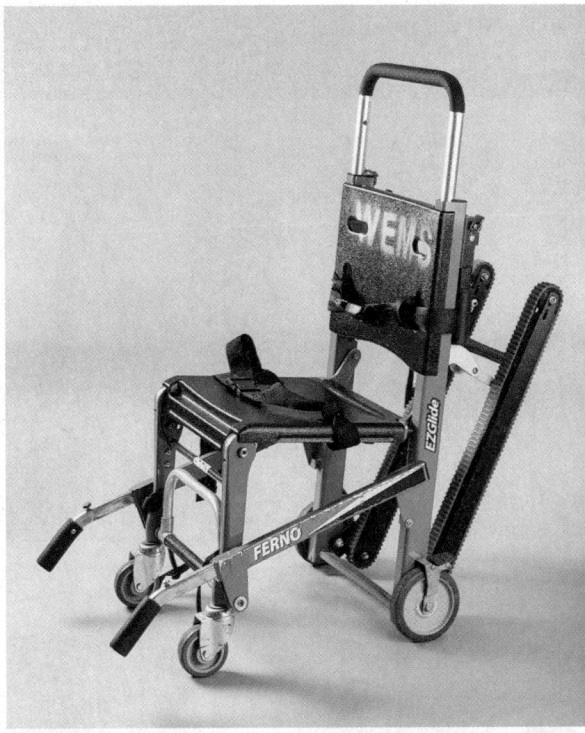

**FIGURE 8-11** A wheeled stair chair can be used to transfer a conscious patient up or down a flight of stairs.

© Jones & Bartlett Learning.

You can roll the stair chair on the floor until you reach the stairwell, and then both providers carry it (rather than roll and bump it) up or down the stairs. You will find this is one of the most useful tools in moving a patient.

When the patient is upstairs, you should take the wheeled ambulance stretcher to the ground floor landing and prepare it for the patient. Place it at the proper height, lower the side rails, turn down the cover sheet, and remove any equipment that you may have secured on the top. You should then take the stair chair upstairs and load the patient into it. Once reaching the bottom of the stairs, transfer the patient from the stair chair onto the stretcher.

Follow these steps to use a stair chair (**SKILL DRILL 8-4**):

1. Secure the patient to the stair chair with straps. At a minimum, use a lap belt at the hips and two straps around the chest. You will need to coach the patient to hold on to the chest straps tightly as to prevent the patient from grabbing on to the stair well or rails and throwing the team off balance.

## Skill Drill 8-4 Using a Stair Chair

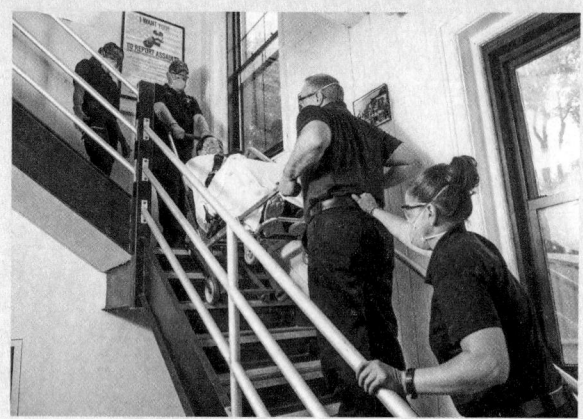

### Step 1

Position and secure the patient on the chair with straps. Take your places at the head and foot of the chair.

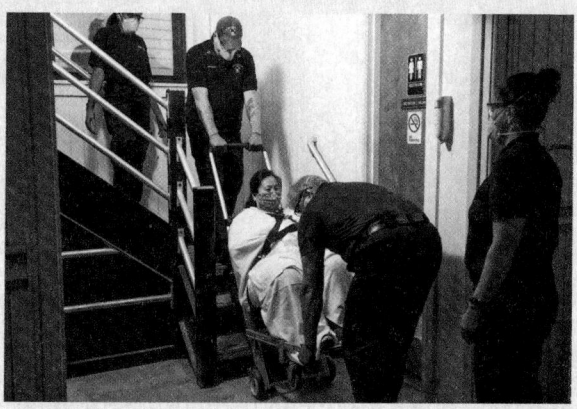

### Step 2

Lower the chair to roll on landings and for transfer to the stretcher.

© Jones & Bartlett Learning.

2. Take your places around the patient seated on the chair: one provider at the head end and one at the foot end (**Step 1**). The provider at the head will give directions to coordinate the lift and movement. If a third provider is on scene, he or she may precede you and your partner. Keeping his or her hand on the back of the second provider who is at the feet, the third provider can assist by opening doors and providing guidance and support. For lengthy carries, a third provider can also rotate into the carrying team to provide breaks for the other two.
3. When reaching landings and other flat intervals in the move, lower the chair to the ground and roll the chair to the next position. Upon reaching the ground level where the stretcher awaits, roll the chair into position next to the stretcher in preparation for transferring the patient (**Step 2**).

As with other carries, always remember to keep your back in a locked-in position and to flex at the hips, not the waist. Bend at the knees and keep the patient's weight and your arms as close to your body as possible. Twisting while carrying or moving a patient will increase your risk of injury. Try to avoid any unnecessary lifting and carrying of the patient. You may find that a log roll or a body drag will aid you in moving your patient onto the backboard or the stretcher. If these techniques will not harm or jeopardize your patient's condition, use one of these moves.

## Moving a Patient on Stairs With a Stretcher

When a patient is unresponsive, must be moved in a supine position, or must be immobilized, secure the patient onto a soft stretcher, backboard, or vacuum matress. Be sure that the patient is anatomically secured to the device so that he or she cannot slide significantly. Carry the patient on the backboard down the stairs to the prepared stretcher. When moving on stairs, more than half of a patient's weight is distributed to the head end of the device, so make sure the strongest provider is positioned at the head end. (Even with four or more providers carrying the patient, the strain on the provider at the head end will be increased when you must negotiate a narrow flight of stairs.) In carrying a patient up or down a flight of stairs, proportionally greater weight will also be distributed to the provider who carries the foot end when the device becomes angled because of the incline or decline. You should anticipate this and, in such cases, make sure the two strongest providers are positioned at the head and foot ends of the device. Because of the incline of the stairway, if one of the two strongest providers is considerably taller than the other, it will be easier if the shorter provider is at the head end and the taller provider is at the foot end. This minimizes bending while lifting and moving the patient. Once you reach the stretcher, place both the device and the patient on the stretcher; then secure both to the stretcher with additional straps.

To carry a patient on stairs on a backboard or vacuum mattress, follow the steps in **SKILL DRILL 8-5**:

1. Apply the straps to pass tightly across the upper torso over the shoulder and across the patient's chest, but not over the arms, to hold the patient in place while leaving the arms free. The strap is secured to the handles at both sides of the backboard or vacuum mattress so that it cannot slide toward the foot end of the device. Strap the patient securely to the device (**Step 1**).
2. When you carry the patient down stairs or an incline, make sure the backboard or vacuum mattress is carried with the foot end first so that the head end is elevated higher than the foot end. The straps will prevent the patient from sliding down or off the device (**Step 2**).

## Skill Drill 8-5 Carrying a Patient on Stairs

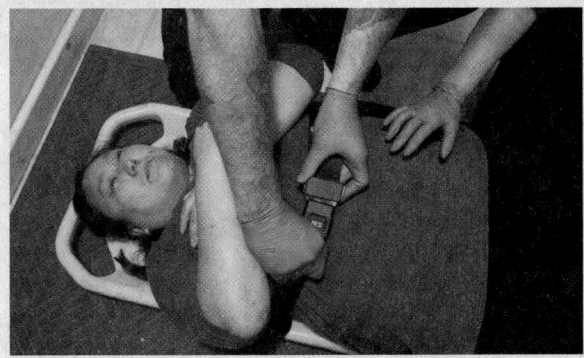

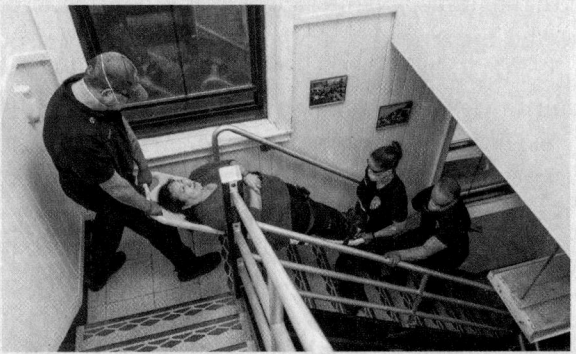

**Step 1**

Strap the patient securely. Make sure one strap is tight across the upper torso, under the arms, and secured to the handles to prevent the patient from sliding.

**Step 2**

Carry a patient down stairs with the foot end first, always keeping the head elevated. Unless the patient is completely conscious and cooperative, hands need to be secured for safety and to prevent the patient from grabbing onto the railing of the stairs or the patient's hands from falling off the side of the board.

## Words of Wisdom

When you encounter a patient in a confined space, such as a bathroom, it can pose a unique set of problems. Prior to moving a patient in a confined space, it is important to discuss the process with your fellow team members. Ensure that everyone agrees with the extrication plan and understands his or her role. Remember that communication with the crew, as well as the patient, will assist in minimizing potential problems.

## Street Smarts

Patients are commonly uneasy and scared as they are being carried, especially when they are being carried up or down stairs. Remember to talk with your patient continually while the move is taking place. Ask the patient to help by keeping arms in and holding still, and reassure him or her the EMS team is working safely.

## Loading a Wheeled Stretcher Into an Ambulance

Whenever a patient has been placed onto the stretcher, one EMT must hold the main frame to prevent movement. When the stretcher is elevated, the main frame and the patient extend considerably beyond the wheels at both the head end and foot end of the stretcher. Therefore, whenever a patient is on an elevated stretcher, you must ensure that it is held firmly between two hands at all times so that even if the patient moves, the stretcher cannot tip (**FIGURE 8-12**).

Inside the ambulance are strong clamps that fasten around the undercarriage when the stretcher is pushed into them. The clamps are located in a rack on the floor or side of the patient compartment, or through a center-mounted track system, and will hold the stretcher in place until they are released at the hospital. You can control and release the clamps with a single handle when standing on the ground at the open back doors of the ambulance when the stretcher is to be unloaded. The stretcher is designed to be rolled on flat surfaces. Ensure the intended travel path is free from debris and potential obstacles. If the patient must be moved over a lawn or other irregular surface, you must lift and

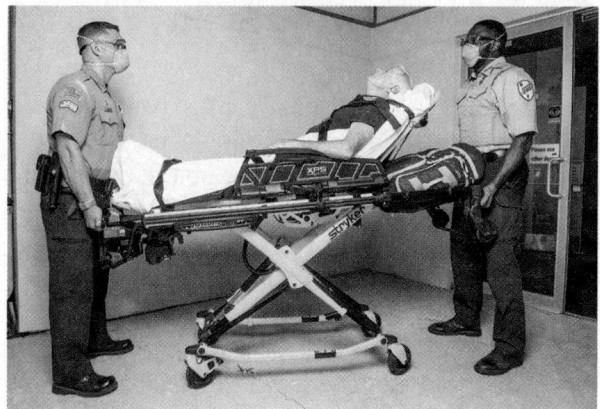

**FIGURE 8-12** Make sure that you hold the main frame of the stretcher when it is elevated so that even when the patient moves, the stretcher does not tip over.
© Jones & Bartlett Learning.

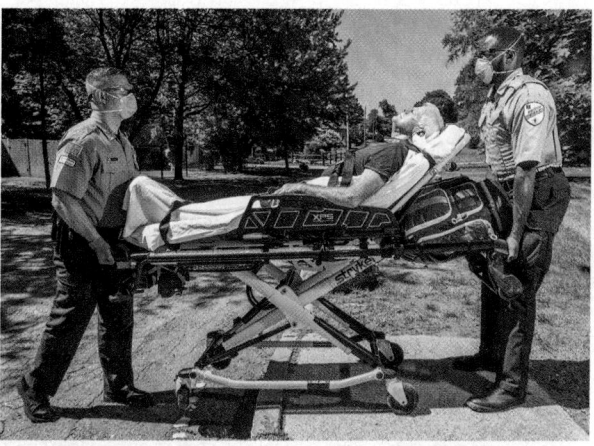

**FIGURE 8-13** You need not retract the undercarriage of the stretcher when lifting it over a curb, a single step, or an obstacle of similar height.
© Jones & Bartlett Learning.

carry the stretcher over the terrain. A four-person carry is much safer if the stretcher must be moved over rough ground.

If the loaded stretcher must be carried down a short flight of steps, be sure to first retract or raise the undercarriage; however, this is not necessary when the stretcher must be lifted over a curb, a single step, or an obstacle of a similar height (**FIGURE 8-13**).

When you reach the back of the ambulance, you and your partner will roll the front wheels onto the floor in the back of the ambulance, advancing the stretcher until the safety hook catches the stretcher. The EMT at the foot of the stretcher lifts and releases the undercarriage. The second EMT lifts the undercarriage with the wheels up to the level of the ambulance floor. Both EMTs then guide the stretcher into the locking mechanism in the back of the ambulance. Often the raising and lowering of the stretcher is done with a battery-powered motor; however, it is still important for you to maintain a firm grip on the stretcher. Newer automatically loading stretchers will manage the entire loading and unloading of the stretcher and only require the provider to operate the buttons on the stretcher.

An intravenous (IV) pole is attached to many stretchers. The IV pole can be unfolded or extended above the main frame to hold an IV bag above the patient while you move the stretcher to the ambulance. Some wheeled ambulance stretchers even include a carrier to hold a cardiac monitor or automated external defibrillator and portable oxygen unit. If the model you use does not include these features, you will have to secure the portable oxygen unit and cardiac monitor or automated external defibrillator to the top surface of the stretcher mattress at the patient's legs. If possible, remove these items before lifting the stretcher to avoid the excess weight. These items must be secured in the ambulance prior to departing the scene.

**TABLE 8-2** shows the guidelines that you must follow to load the stretcher into the ambulance.

Follow these steps to load the stretcher into an ambulance (**SKILL DRILL 8-6**).

1. Tilt the head end of the main frame upward, and place it into the patient compartment with the wheels on the floor. The two additional wheels that extend just below the head

end are attached to the main frame and will enable this movement. Ensure that the safety bar under the head of the stretcher catches on the hook prior to lifting the stretcher (**Step 1**).
2. With the patient's weight supported by these two head-end wheels and the EMT at the foot end of the stretcher, move to the side of the main frame and release the undercarriage lock to lift the undercarriage up to its fully retracted position. The wheels of the undercarriage and the two on the head end of the main frame will now be on the same level (**Step 2**).
3. Simply roll the stretcher the rest of the way into the back of the ambulance, where it will rest on all six wheels (**Step 3**).
4. Secure the stretcher in the ambulance with the strong clamps that fasten around the undercarriage when the stretcher is pushed into them. The clamps are located in a rack on the floor or side of the patient compartment (**Step 4**).

## Safety Tips

Choose one EMT to be the team leader and direct all movements to prevent confusion. He or she should explain the procedure in advance and verbalize instructions such as "We will lift on three" or "We will count to three and then lift."

## Directions and Commands

To safely lift and carry a patient, you and your team must anticipate and understand every move, and each move must be executed in a coordinated manner. Before any lifting is initiated, the team leader should indicate where each team member is to be located and rapidly describe the sequence of steps that will be performed to ensure the team knows what is expected. If you must lift and move the

**TABLE 8-2** Guidelines for Loading the Stretcher Into the Ambulance

- Make sure there are enough providers for sufficient lifting power.
- Follow the manufacturer's directions for safe and proper use of the stretcher.
- Make sure that all stretchers and patients are fully secured before the ambulance is moved.

© Jones & Bartlett Learning.

## Words of Wisdom

Remember that moving a patient is a dynamic process, and the team leader must be prepared to alter the sequence of moves as needed. Any alteration in the original established plan must be clearly vocalized to all EMS providers involved in the move.

## Skill Drill 8-6 Loading a Stretcher Into an Ambulance

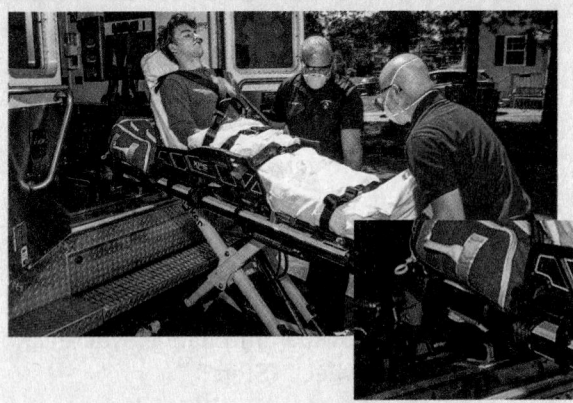

### Step 1

Lift the stretcher into the load position, and place it into the patient compartment with the wheels on the floor and the safety bar latched on the hook.

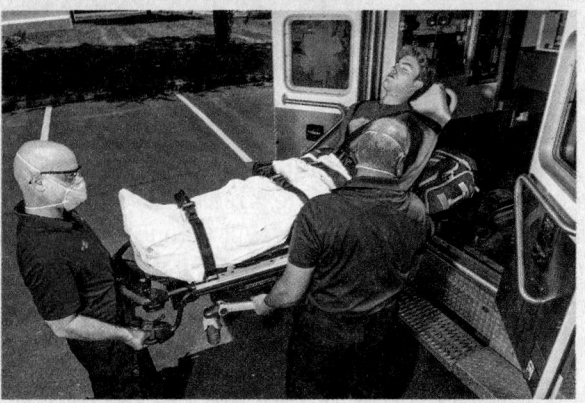

### Step 2

The second EMT on the side of the stretcher releases the undercarriage lock and lifts the undercarriage. Some newer powered stretchers lift the undercarriage with the push of a button.

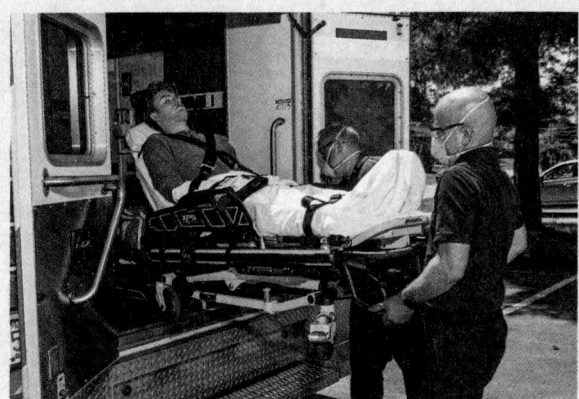

### Step 3

Roll the stretcher into the back of the ambulance.

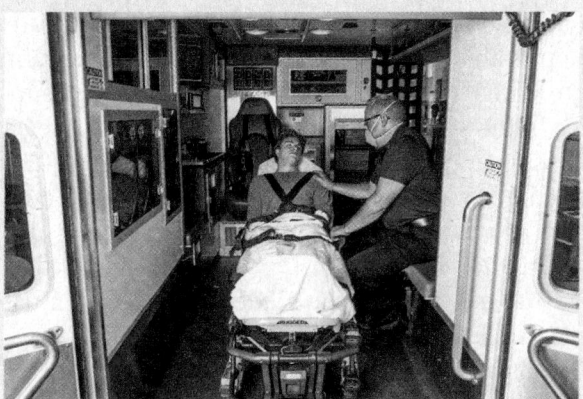

### Step 4

Secure the stretcher to the clamps mounted in the ambulance.

© Jones & Bartlett Learning.

patient through a number of separate stages, the team leader should first give an abbreviated overview of the stages, followed by a more detailed explanation of each stage just before it will occur.

Orders that will initiate the actual lifting or moving or any significant changes in movement should be given in two parts: a preparatory command and a command of execution. For example, if the team leader says, "All ready to stop. STOP!," the phrase "All ready to stop" will get your attention, identify who should act, and prepare you to act; the declarative "STOP!" will indicate the exact moment of execution. Commands of execution should be delivered in a louder voice. Often, a countdown is helpful when you need to lift a patient. To avoid confusion in using a countdown, the leader should always clarify whether "three" is to be a part of the preparatory command or whether it is to serve as the order to execute. He or she can say, "We're going to lift on three. One, two, THREE!" or "I'm going to count to three, and then we're going to lift. One, two, three, LIFT!"

You will often have to perform several additional steps to place the patient onto a backboard and/or carry him or her down a flight of stairs. You will also have to add a stop at the top of the stairway so that everyone can reposition before carrying the patient down the stairs. Repositioning usually requires lowering the backboard to the ground and lifting it again when all providers are in their proper places. If you are carrying the patient in a stair chair, the additional step occurs after you have descended the stairs and reached the stretcher. At that point,

you will have to assist or lift the patient from the stair chair onto the stretcher.

You should carefully plan ahead and select the methods that will involve the least amount of lifting and carrying. Remember to always consider whether there is an option that will cause less strain to you and the other providers.

## Safety Tips

Follow these rules to keep you and your patient safe:

- Minimize the number of total body lifts you have to perform.
- Coordinate every lift in advance.
- Minimize the total amount of weight you have to lift.
- *Never* lift with your back.
- Do not carry what you can put on wheels.
- Ask for help when you think it will be needed.

## YOU are the Provider

Once the vehicle has been stabilized by the fire department, you are able to gain access through the rear driver's-side door that is about halfway open. The vehicle is still lying on the passenger's side. A paramedic unit is standing by awaiting removal of the driver. You are able to wedge about half of a backboard through the doorway with a firefighter holding the other end, but there is no room inside for additional providers.

**Patient 1 (the driver)**

| Recording Time: 5 Minutes | |
| --- | --- |
| **Appearance** | Motionless; ashen skin with cyanosis around the mouth |
| **Level of consciousness** | Unresponsive |
| **Airway** | Snoring respirations |
| **Breathing** | Increased rate; shallow depth |
| **Circulation** | Weak and rapid radial pulse; no obvious bleeding |

**Patient 2 (the passenger)**

| Recording Time: 5 Minutes | |
| --- | --- |
| **Respirations** | Seem to be a little rapid, but still unable to visualize patient |
| **Pulse** | Unable to assess due to patient's position |
| **Skin** | Pink where visualized |
| **Blood pressure** | Unable to assess |
| **Oxygen saturation (Spo$_2$)** | Unable to assess |

**7.** What type of move is best for removing the driver?

**8.** What steps can you take to maximize safety while lifting a patient?

# Emergency Moves

When there is a potential for danger to you or the patient, use an emergency move to drag or pull a patient to a safe place before assessment and care are provided. The risk of serious harm or death due to fire, explosives, or hazardous materials, your inability to protect the patient from other hazards, or your inability to gain access to others in a vehicle who need life-saving care all are situations in which you should use an emergency move. In such conditions, protecting the cervical spine is secondary to rapidly getting your patient to safety.

The only other time you should use an emergency move is if you cannot properly assess the patient or provide critical emergency care because of the patient's location or position.

If you are alone and danger at the scene makes it necessary for you to use an emergency move, regardless of a patient's injuries, you should use a drag to pull the patient along the long axis of the body. Remember that it is impossible to remove a patient quickly from a vehicle while providing as much protection to the spine as would a spinal immobilization device such as a Kendrick extrication device (KED). However, if you follow certain guidelines during the move, you can usually remove a patient from a life-threatening situation without causing further injury to the patient.

You can move a patient on his or her back along the floor or ground by using one of the following methods:

- Pull on the patient's clothing in the neck and shoulder area (**FIGURE 8-14A**).
- If the shirt has buttons, the top two should be undone to prevent the patient from choking.
- Place the patient onto a blanket, coat, or other item that can be pulled (**FIGURE 8-14B**).
- Rotate the patient's arms so that they are extended straight on the ground beyond his or her head, grasp the wrists, and, with the arms

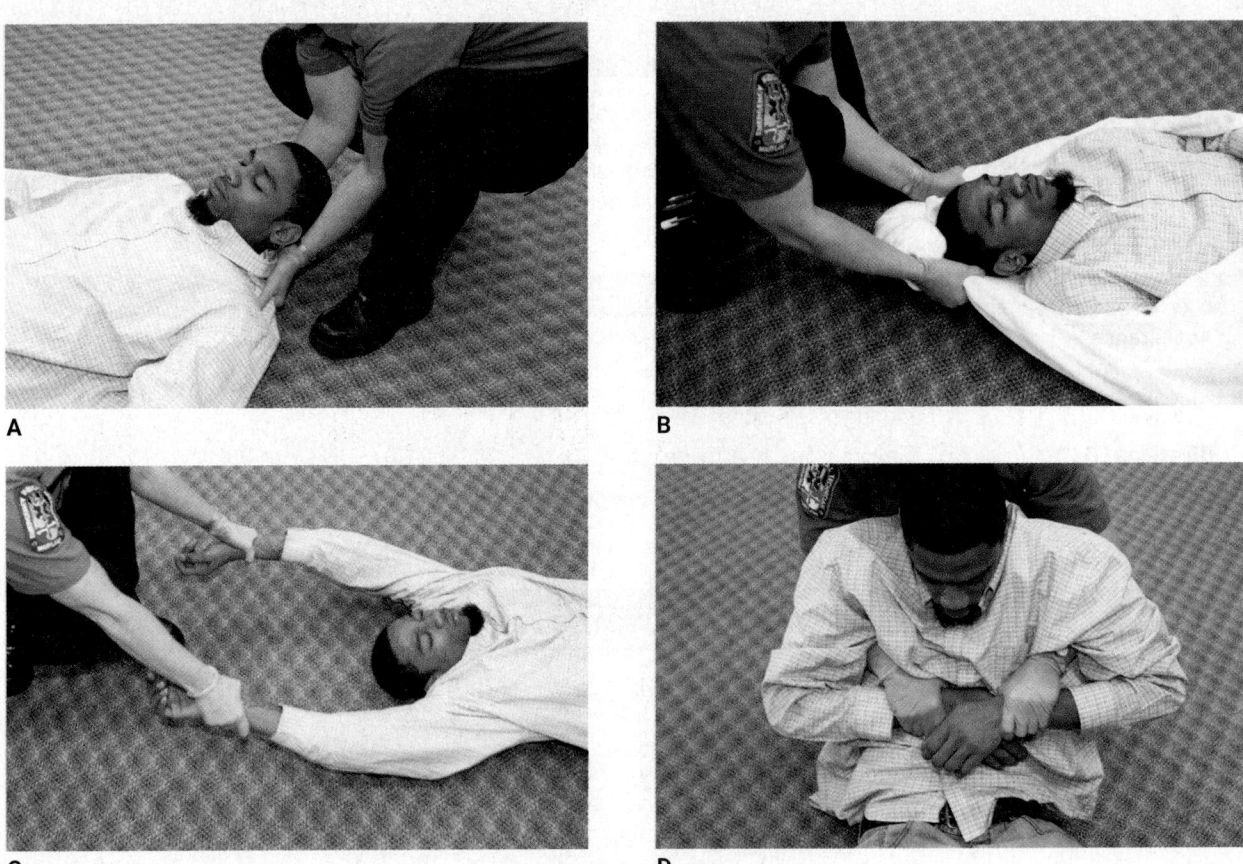

**A**

**B**

**C**

**D**

**FIGURE 8-14** Dragging methods. **A.** Emergency clothes drag. **B.** Blanket drag. **C.** Arm drag. **D.** Arm-to-arm drag.

elevated above the ground, drag the patient (**FIGURE 8-14C**).

- Place your arms under the patient's shoulders and through the armpits, and, while grasping your opposite wrist, drag the patient backward (**FIGURE 8-14D**).

If you are alone and must remove an unresponsive patient from a vehicle, first move the patient's legs so they are clear of the pedals and are against the seat. Then rotate the patient so that his or her back is positioned toward the open vehicle door. Next, place your arms through the armpits and support the patient's head against your body (**FIGURE 8-15A**). While supporting the patient's weight, drag the patient from the seat. If the legs and feet clear the vehicle easily, you can rapidly drag the patient to a safe location by continuing this method (**FIGURE 8-15B**). If the legs and feet do not clear the vehicle easily, you can slowly lower the patient until he or she is lying on his or her back next to the vehicle, clear the legs from the vehicle, and, as previously described, use a long-axis body drag to move the patient a safe distance from the vehicle.

You should use one-person techniques to move a patient only if an immediately life-threatening danger exists and you are alone or, because of the pressing nature of the danger, your partner is moving a second patient simultaneously. Additional one-provider drags, carries, and lifts are shown in **FIGURE 8-16**.

## Urgent Moves

An urgent move may be necessary to move a patient with an altered level of consciousness, inadequate ventilation, or shock (hypoperfusion). An extreme weather condition may also make an urgent move necessary. In some cases, patients must be urgently moved from the location or position in which they are found. When a patient who is sitting in a vehicle must be urgently moved, use the rapid extrication technique.

## Rapid Extrication Technique

The backboard, short backboard, and vest-type devices are known as spinal immobilization devices. Normally, you would use an extrication-type vest or short backboard device to immobilize a seated patient with a suspected spinal injury before removing the patient from the vehicle. (See Chapter 39, *Vehicle Extrication and Special Rescue*.) However, proper placement of either of these devices on the patient usually requires between 6 and 8 minutes, and in some cases even longer. By using the **rapid extrication technique** instead, the patient can be moved from sitting in the vehicle to supine, on a backboard if required, in 1 minute or less. However, the rapid nature of this type of extrication can potentially increase the risk of damage if the patient has a spinal injury. Because of this possible patient injury, all available options need to be considered

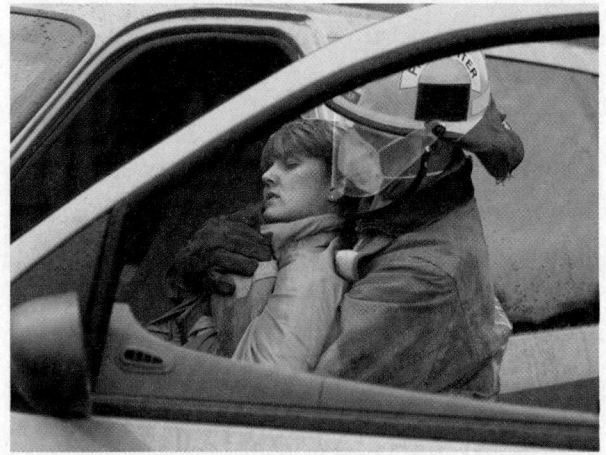
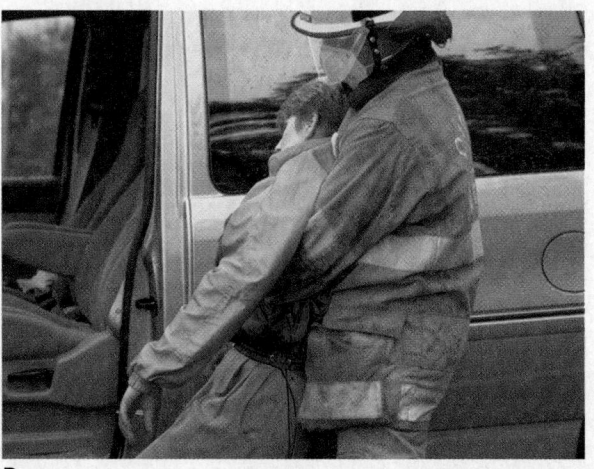

**A**  **B**

**FIGURE 8-15** One-person technique for moving an unresponsive patient from a vehicle. **A.** Grasp the patient under the arms. **B.** Lower the patient down into a supine position.

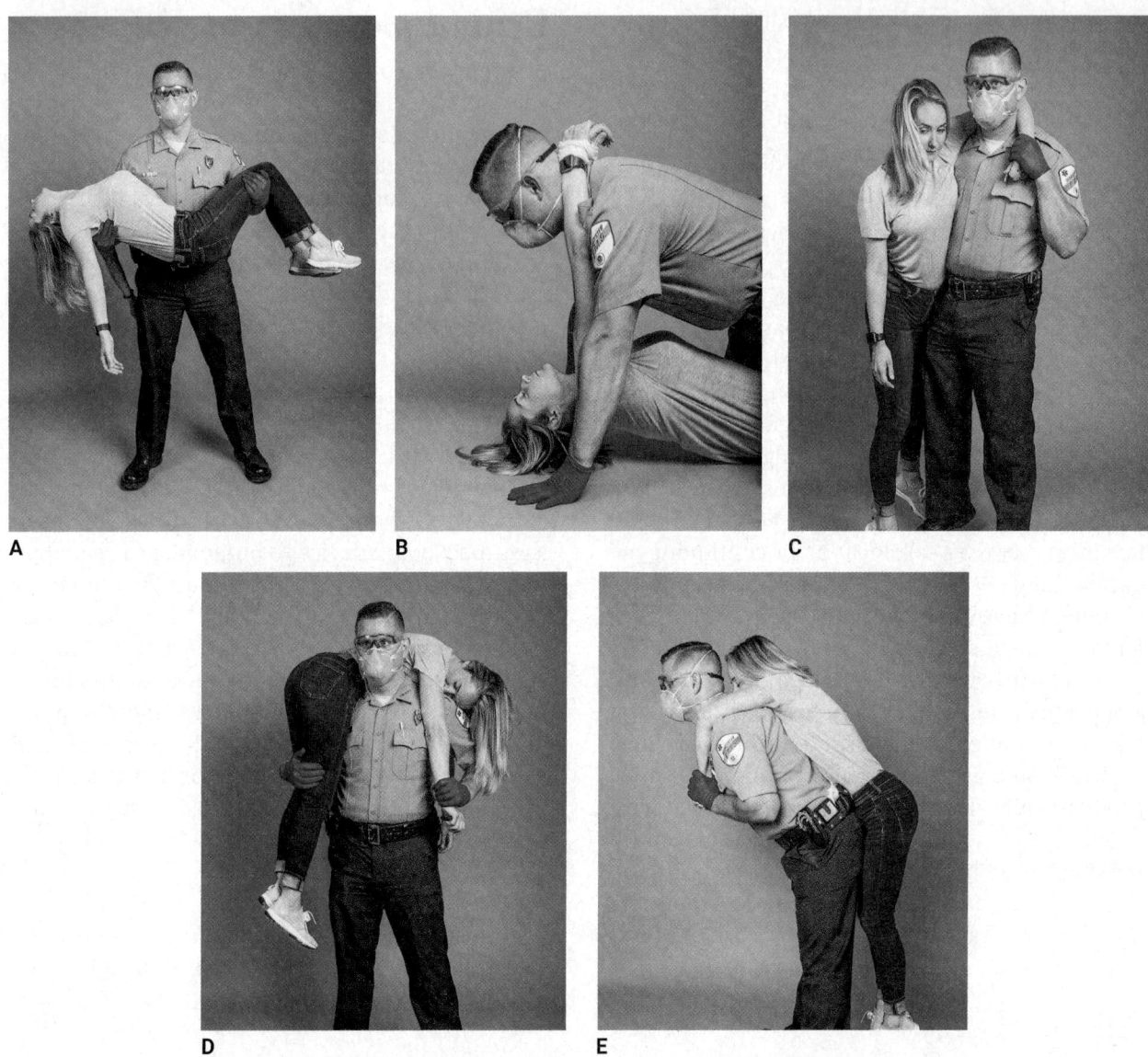

**FIGURE 8-16** One-person drags, carries, and lifts. **A.** Front cradle. **B.** Firefighter's drag. **C.** One-person walking assist. **D.** Firefighter's carry. **E.** Pack-strap carry.

**A-E:** © Jones & Bartlett Learning.

prior to performing a rapid extrication. **TABLE 8-3** describes the situations in which you should use the rapid extrication technique.

In such cases, the delay that occurs in applying immobilization devices is a contraindication. However, the manual support and stabilization that you provide when using the rapid extrication technique produce a greater risk of spine movement. Because of this increased risk, do not use the rapid extrication technique if no urgency exists. If the patient is able to stand and pivot to the stretcher, it is safer to have them do so.

**TABLE 8-3** Situations in Which to Use the Rapid Extrication Technique

- The vehicle or scene is unsafe.
- Explosives or other hazardous materials are on the scene.
- There is a fire or a danger of fire.
- The patient cannot be properly assessed before being removed from the vehicle.
- The patient has a life-threatening condition.
- The patient blocks your access to another seriously injured patient.

© Jones & Bartlett Learning.

The rapid extrication technique requires a team of three providers who are knowledgeable and practiced in the procedure. Take the following steps when using the rapid extrication technique (**SKILL DRILL 8-7**). Whether a backboard is used for this skill will depend on your local protocols. Here, use of a backboard is included.

1. The first provider applies manual in-line support of the patient's head and cervical spine

## Skill Drill 8-7 Performing the Rapid Extrication Technique

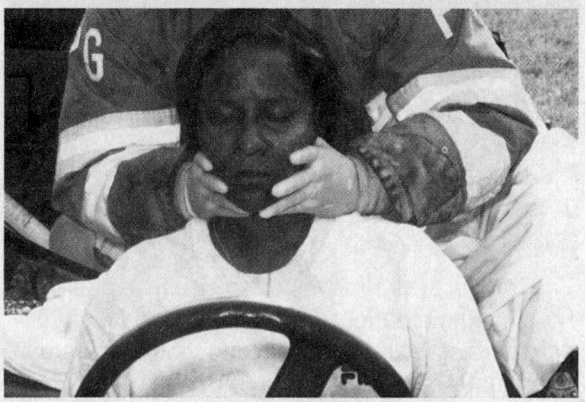

### Step 1
The first provider provides in-line manual support of the head and cervical spine.

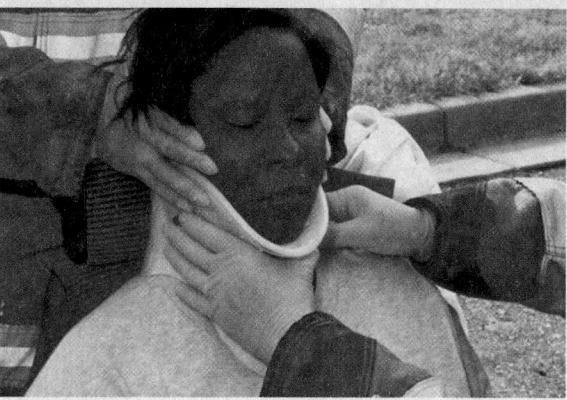

### Step 2
The second provider gives commands, applies a cervical collar, and performs the primary assessment.

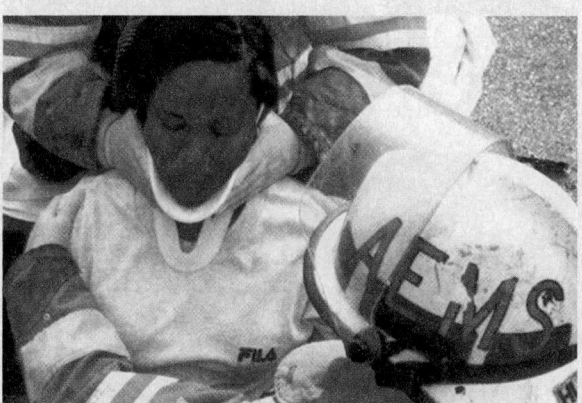

### Step 3
The second provider supports the torso. The third provider frees the patient's legs from the pedals and moves the legs together, without moving the pelvis or spine.

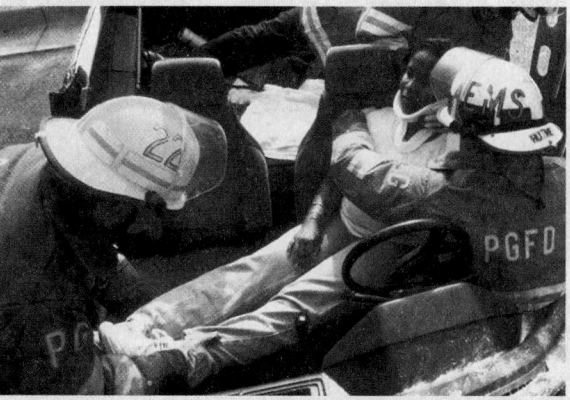

### Step 4
The second provider and the third provider rotate the patient as a unit in several short, coordinated moves. The first provider (relieved by the fourth provider as needed) supports the patient's head and neck during rotation (and later steps).

*(continues)*

## Skill Drill 8-7 Performing the Rapid Extrication Technique (*continued*)

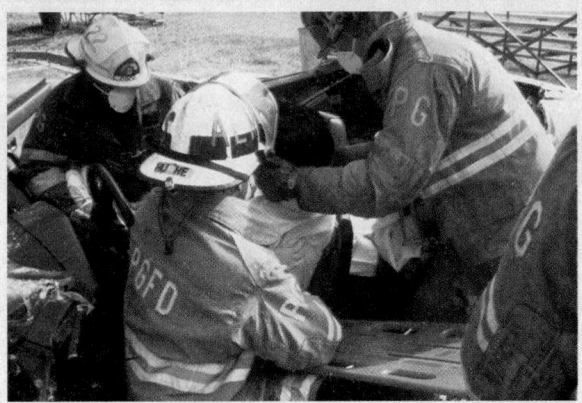

### Step 5

The first (or fourth) provider places the backboard on the seat against the patient's buttocks. (Use of a backboard may depend on local protocols.)

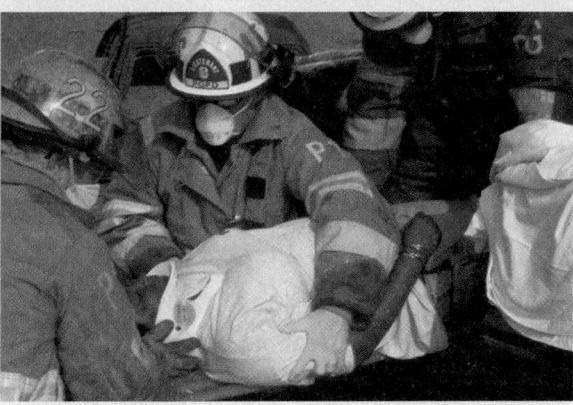

### Step 6

The third provider moves to an effective position for sliding the patient. The second and the third providers slide the patient along the backboard in coordinated 8- to 12-inch (20- to 30-cm) moves until the patient's hips rest on the backboard.

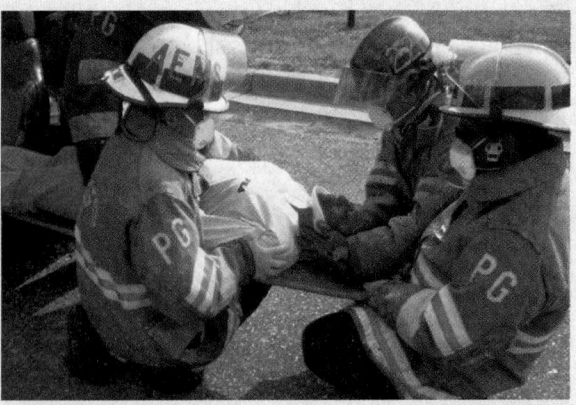

### Step 7

The third provider exits the vehicle and moves to the backboard opposite the second provider. They continue to slide the patient until the patient is fully on the backboard.

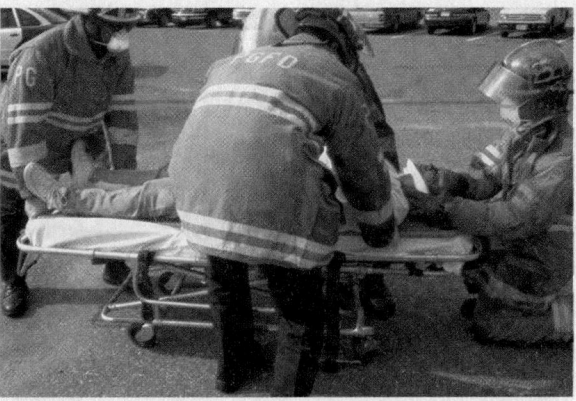

### Step 8

The first (or fourth) provider continues to stabilize the head and neck while the second provider and the third provider carry the patient away from the vehicle and onto the prepared stretcher.

from behind. Support may be applied from the side, if necessary, by reaching through the driver's-side doorway (**Step 1**).

2. The second provider serves as team leader and, as such, gives the commands until the patient is supine on the backboard. Because the second provider lifts and turns the patient's torso, he or she must be physically capable of moving the patient. The second provider works from the driver's-side doorway. If the first provider is also working from that doorway, the second provider should stand closer to the door hinges toward the front of the vehicle. The second provider applies a cervical collar and may perform the primary assessment (**Step 2**).

3. The second provider provides continuous support of the patient's torso until the patient is supine on the backboard. Once the second provider takes control of the patient's torso, usually in the form of a body hug, he or she should not let go of the patient for any reason. Some type of cross-chest shoulder hug usually works well, but you will have to decide what method works best for you on any given patient. You must remember that you cannot simply reach into the vehicle and grab the patient; this will only twist the patient's torso. You must rotate the patient as a complete unit.

4. The third provider works from the front passenger's seat and is responsible for rotating the patient's legs and feet as the torso is turned, ensuring that they are free of the pedals and any other obstruction. With care, the third provider should first move the patient's nearer leg laterally without rotating the patient's pelvis and lower spine. The pelvis and lower spine rotate only as the third provider moves the patient's second leg during the next step. Moving the nearer leg early makes it much easier to move the second leg in concert with the rest of the body. After the third provider moves the legs together, they should be moved as a unit (**Step 3**).

5. These initial steps of the rapid extrication technique direct the team to its starting positions and responsibilities. The first provider applies in-line support and stabilization of the head and neck. The second provider gives orders and supports the torso. The third provider moves and supports the patient's legs. The team is now ready to move the patient.

6. The patient is rotated 90 degrees so that the patient's back is facing out the driver's door and the feet are on the front passenger's seat. This coordinated movement is done in three or four short, quick "eighth turns." The second provider directs each quick turn by saying, "Ready, turn," or "Ready, move." Hand position changes should be made between moves.

7. In most cases, the first provider will be working from the back seat and will have removed the headrest (if possible). At some point, either because the doorpost is in the way or because he or she cannot reach farther from the back seat, the first provider will be unable to follow the torso rotation. At that time, the third provider should assume temporary in-line support of the head and neck until the first provider can regain control of the head from outside the vehicle. If a fourth provider is present, the fourth provider stands next to the second provider. The fourth provider takes control of the patient's head and neck from outside the vehicle without involving the third provider. As soon as the change has been made, the rotation can continue (**Step 4**).

8. Once the patient has been fully rotated, the backboard should be placed against the patient's buttocks on the seat. Do not try to wedge the backboard under the patient. If only three providers are present, be sure to place the backboard within arm's reach of the driver's door before the move so that the backboard can be pulled into place when needed. In such cases, the far end of the backboard can be left on the ground. When a fourth provider is available, the first provider exits the back seat of the vehicle, places the backboard against the patient's buttocks, and maintains pressure toward the interior of the vehicle from the far end of the backboard. (Note: When the door opening allows, some providers prefer to insert the backboard onto the seat before the patient is rotated.)

9. As soon as the patient has been rotated and the backboard is in place, the second provider and the third provider lower the patient onto the backboard while supporting the head and torso so that neutral alignment is maintained. The first provider holds the backboard until the patient is secured (**Step 5**).

10. Next, the third provider must move across the front seat to be in position at the patient's hips. If the third provider stays at the patient's knees or feet, he or she will be ineffective in helping to move the body's weight. The knees and feet follow the hips.

11. The fourth provider maintains manual in-line support of the head and now takes over giving the commands. The second provider maintains the direction of the extrication. The second provider stands with his or her back to the door, facing the rear of the vehicle. The backboard should be immediately in front of the third provider. The second provider grasps the patient's shoulders or armpits. Then, on command, the second provider and the third provider slide the patient 8 to 12 inches (20 to 30 cm) along the backboard, repeating this slide until the patient's hips are firmly on the backboard (**Step 6**).

12. At that time, the third provider gets out of the vehicle and moves to the opposite side of the backboard, across from the second provider. The third provider now takes control at the shoulders, and the second provider moves back to take control of the hips. On command, these two providers move the patient along the backboard in 8- to 12-inch (20- to 30-cm) slides until the patient is placed fully on the backboard (**Step 7**).

13. The first (or fourth) provider continues to maintain manual in-line support of the patient's head. The second provider and the third provider now grasp their side of the backboard and then carry it and the patient away from the vehicle onto the prepared stretcher nearby (**Step 8**).

In some cases, you will be able to rest the head end of the backboard on the stretcher while the patient is moved onto the backboard. In other situations, you will not be able to do this. Once the backboard and patient have been placed on the stretcher, begin life-saving treatment immediately. If you used the rapid extrication technique because the scene was dangerous, you and your team should immediately move the stretcher a safe distance away from the scene before you assess or treat the patient.

## Nonurgent Moves

When both the scene and the patient are stable, carefully plan how to move the patient. If your patient move is rushed or poorly planned, it may result in discomfort or injury to the patient, you, and/or your team. Before you attempt any move, the team leader must be sure that there are enough providers, any obstacles have been identified or removed, the proper equipment is available, and the procedure and path to be followed have been clearly identified and discussed. Remember, communication is the key to success.

In nonurgent situations, you and your team may choose one of several methods for lifting and carrying a patient and should coordinate your movements through direct verbal commands. Three general methods are presented here, which may serve as a basis for your plan. You may adapt these procedures to meet your needs on a case-by-case basis.

## Direct Ground Lift

The **direct ground lift** is used for patients with no suspected spinal injury who are found lying supine on the ground. Use this lift when you have to lift and carry the patient some distance to be placed on the stretcher. If you find the patient semiprone or lying on his or her side, first log roll the patient onto his or her back. Ideally, the direct ground lift should be performed by three providers; however, it can be done with only two. Perform the direct ground lift as follows (**SKILL DRILL 8-8**):

1. Take your places on one side of the patient with the first provider at the patient's head, the second provider at the patient's waist, and the third provider at the patient's knees. All providers kneel on one knee, preferably the same knee.

2. The patient's arms should be placed on his or her chest if possible (**Step 1**).
3. The first provider places one arm under the patient's neck and shoulders and cradles the patient's head. The first provider then places the other arm under the patient's low back.
4. The second provider places one hand under the patient's waist, and the other under the knees.

5. The third provider places one arm under the patient's knees and the other under the ankles.
6. On command, the team lifts the patient up to knee level as each provider rests an arm on his or her knee (**Step 2**).
7. As a team and on command, each provider rolls the patient in toward his or her chest. Again on command, the team stands and carries the patient to the stretcher (**Step 3**).

## Skill Drill 8-8 Performing the Direct Ground Lift

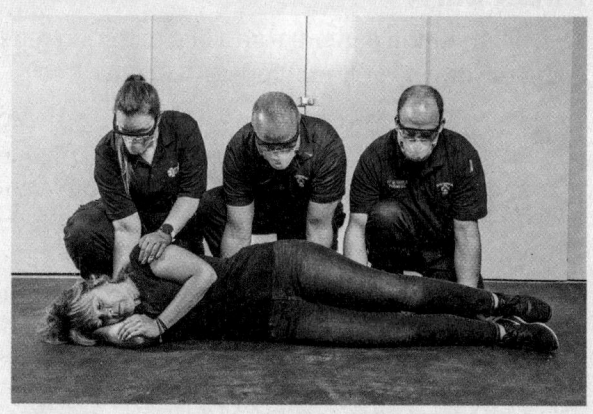

### Step 1

Line up on one side of the patient, with one provider at the head, one at the waist, and one at the patient's knees. Place a soft stretcher underneath the patient. All providers should be kneeling. Place the patient's arms on his or her chest, if possible.

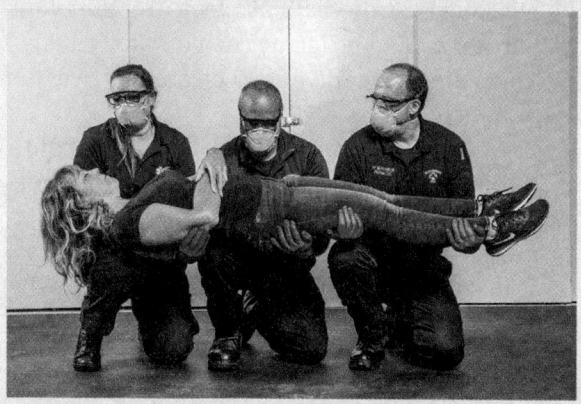

### Step 2

On command, lift the patient to knee level.

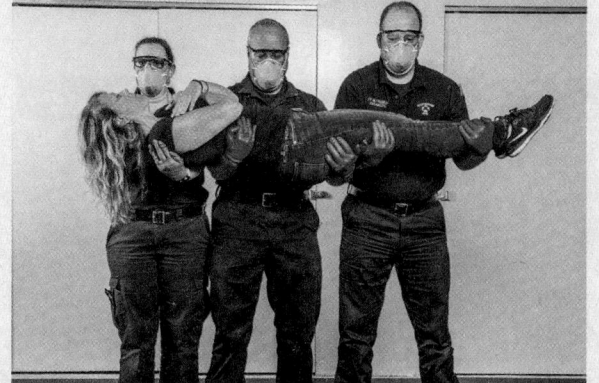

### Step 3

On command, roll the patient toward your chest, and then stand and carry the patient to the stretcher.

© Jones & Bartlett Learning.

*Note:* The steps are reversed to lower the patient onto the stretcher.

## Extremity Lift

The extremity lift may also be used for patients with no suspected extremity or spinal injuries who are supine or in a sitting position. The extremity lift may be especially helpful when the patient is in a very narrow space or there is not enough room for the patient and several EMTs to stand side by side. Perform the extremity lift as follows (**SKILL DRILL 8-9**):

1. Kneel behind the patient's head as your partner kneels at the patient's feet. You and your partner should be facing each other.
2. The patient's hands should be crossed over his or her chest.
3. Place one hand under each of the patient's armpits. Grasp the patient's wrists or forearms and pull the upper torso until the patient is in a sitting position (**Step 1**).
4. Your partner moves to a position between the patient's legs, facing in the same direction as the patient, and slips his or her hands under the patient's knees (**Step 2**).

5. As you give the command, stand fully upright and move the patient to the stretcher (**Step 3**).

You will be less likely to injure yourself if you bend at the hips and knees and use your legs for lifting. However, this lift and carry method increases pressure on the patient's chest, so the patient may be uncomfortable in this position.

## Transfer Moves

There are several ways to transfer the patient from a bed onto the stretcher.

## Direct Carry

Transfer a supine patient from a bed to the stretcher using the direct carry method (**SKILL DRILL 8-10**).

1. Position the stretcher parallel to the bed, facing the same direction as the bed. Prepare the stretcher by unbuckling the straps and removing any other items from it. Secure the stretcher to prevent movement.
2. Position yourself at the head of the bed facing toward the patient. Your partner should be positioned between the bed and the stretcher facing both you and the patient.

## YOU are the Provider

There is no easy way to remove the driver, but by bracing yourself through the seats you are able to grab his belt and pull him toward you. Once you get the patient's head and shoulders between the headrests, the firefighter helps pull him onto the backboard. As soon as he is secured on the backboard, several other providers help the firefighter pull the backboard out of the vehicle and transfer him to the waiting paramedic unit for evaluation, treatment, and transport. You now have access to the passenger, who is sitting waist-deep in water and still reporting pain in her back and right side. She tells you that she has a history of back pain and thinks she can move a little with help.

### Patient 2 (the passenger)

| Recording Time: 20 Minutes | |
| --- | --- |
| Level of consciousness | Alert and oriented |
| Respirations | 20 breaths/min; adequate depth |
| Pulse | 112 beats/min; strong and regular |
| Skin | Pink, cool, and moist |
| Blood pressure | 148/92 mm Hg |
| SpO$_2$ | 99% (on room air) |

**9.** How is a patient's weight distributed when he or she is on a carrying device? Why is it important to know this?

**10.** Considering her complaints and the fact that her condition is stable, what are your best options for removing the passenger?

## Skill Drill 8-9 Performing the Extremity Lift

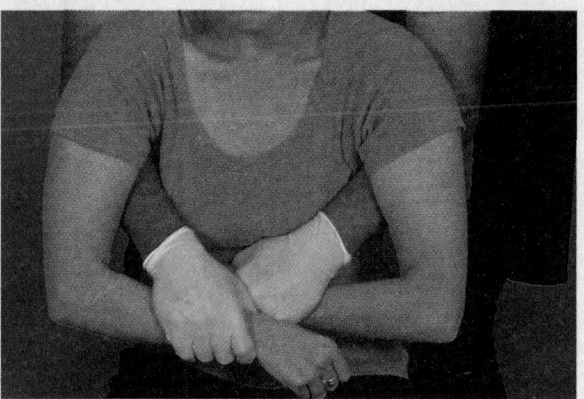

### Step 1

The patient's hands are crossed over the chest. Grasp the patient's wrists or forearms and pull the patient to a sitting position.

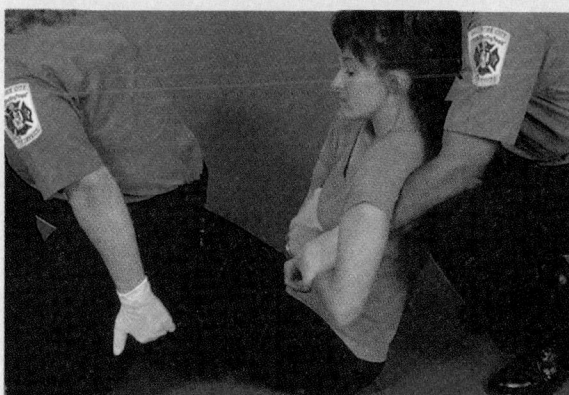

### Step 2

Your partner moves to a position between the patient's legs, facing in the same direction as the patient, and places his or her hands under the knees.

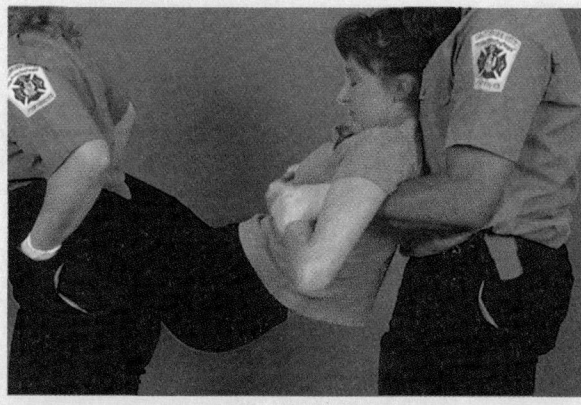

### Step 3

Rise to a crouching position. On command, lift and begin to move.

© Jones & Bartlett Learning. Courtesy of MIEMSS.

3. Slide your arms under the patient's neck and shoulders. Your partner should slide his or her hands under the patient's knees and lock them together or use them to grasp the posterior part of the patient's thighs (**Step 1**).

4. Lift the patient upward slowly and smoothly. Your partner should move the patient's knees from the left side of his body to the right to facilitate placing the patient onto the stretcher (**Step 2**).

5. Slowly carry the patient from the bed to the stretcher (**Step 3**).

6. Gently lower the patient onto the stretcher and secure with straps (**Step 4**).

This carry can also be performed with three providers. If a third provider is available, he or she can be positioned to support the patient's feet and legs from the bottom of the bed.

## Skill Drill 8-10 Performing the Direct Carry

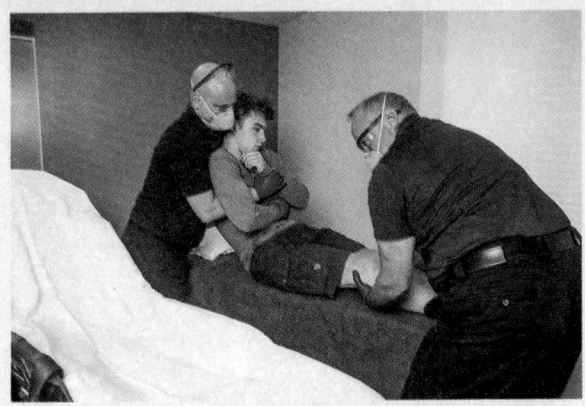

### Step 1

Position the stretcher parallel to the bed. Secure the stretcher to prevent movement. Face the patient while standing between the bed and the stretcher. Position your arms under the patient's neck and shoulders. Your partner should position his or her hands under the patient's knees.

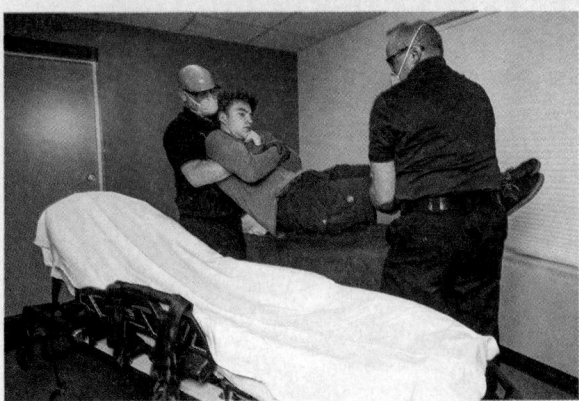

### Step 2

Lift the patient from the bed in a smooth, coordinated fashion.

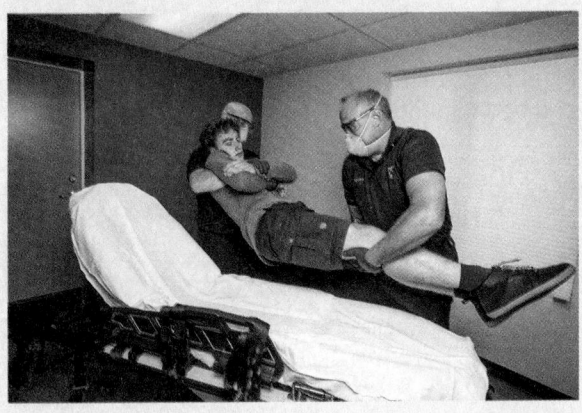

### Step 3

Slowly carry the patient to the stretcher.

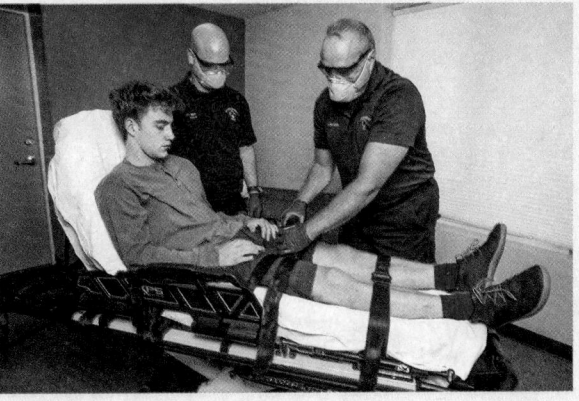

### Step 4

Gently lower the patient onto the stretcher and secure with straps.

© Jones & Bartlett Learning.

### Draw Sheet Method

To move the patient from a bed onto a stretcher, use the draw sheet method. Place the stretcher next to the bed, making sure it is at the same height or slightly lower than the bed and that the rails are lowered and straps are unbuckled. Be sure to hold or secure the stretcher to keep it from moving. Loosen the bottom sheet underneath the patient, or

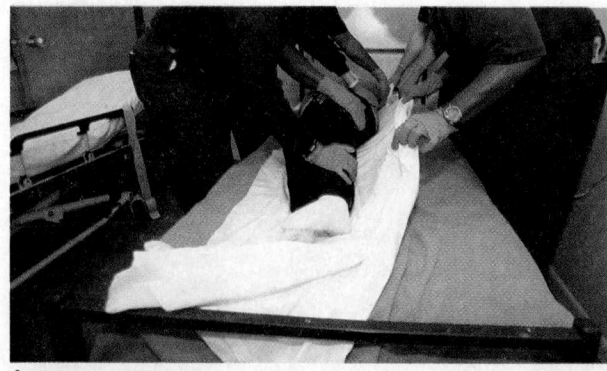

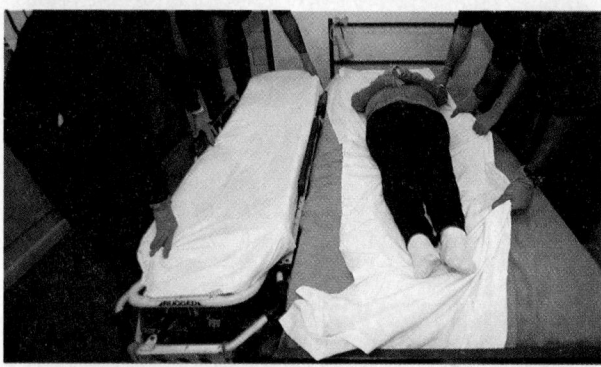

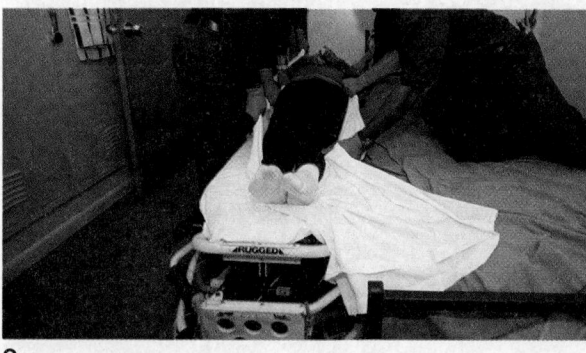

**FIGURE 8-17** The draw sheet method. **A.** Log roll the patient onto a sheet or blanket. **B.** Place the stretcher parallel to the bed. Secure the stretcher. Gently pull the patient to the edge of the bed. **C.** Transfer the patient to the stretcher.

A, B, C: © Jones & Bartlett Learning. Courtesy of MIEMSS.

log roll the patient onto a blanket (**FIGURE 8-17A**). Reach across the stretcher, and grasp the sheet or blanket firmly at the patient's head, chest, hips, and knees (**FIGURE 8-17B**). Gently slide the patient onto the stretcher (**FIGURE 8-17C**).

When lifting a patient by a sheet or blanket, center the patient on the sheet and tightly roll up

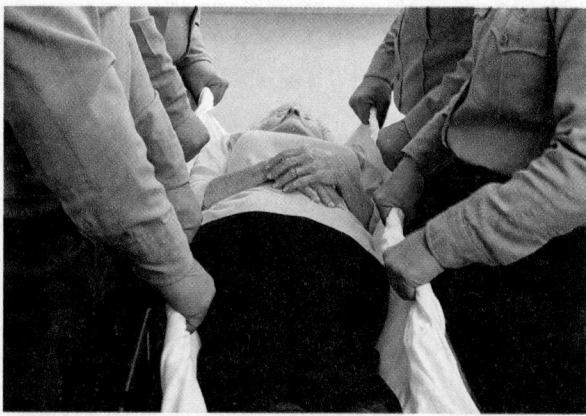

**FIGURE 8-18** When lifting a patient by a bed sheet, center the patient on the sheet and tightly roll up the excess fabric on each side. This produces a cylindrical handle that provides a strong way to grasp the fabric.

© Jones & Bartlett Learning.

the excess fabric on each side. This produces a cylindrical handle that provides a strong, secure way to grasp the fabric (**FIGURE 8-18**). Although sliding boards or other devices are not routinely carried on an ambulance, you may have access to these items in the hospital or at nursing homes that will assist you in sliding the patient from bed to stretcher or stretcher to bed with minimal effort.

## Safety Tips

A soft stretcher or slip mover and other such devices may be used to move patients from a bed onto a stretcher and are safer than the draw sheet method.

## Using a Scoop Stretcher

Another option when moving a patient is to use a scoop stretcher. With a scoop stretcher, the two halves of the device are inserted under each side of the patient, and the two sides are fastened together. Then the patient is lifted and carried to the nearby prepared stretcher. (Note that you can also log roll a patient onto a scoop stretcher that is already locked together.) To use a scoop stretcher, follow the steps in **SKILL DRILL 8-11**.

1. With the scoop stretcher separated, measure the length of the scoop and adjust to the proper length (**Step 1**).
2. Position the stretcher, one side at a time. Lift the patient's side slightly by pulling on the far

## Skill Drill 8-11 Using a Scoop Stretcher

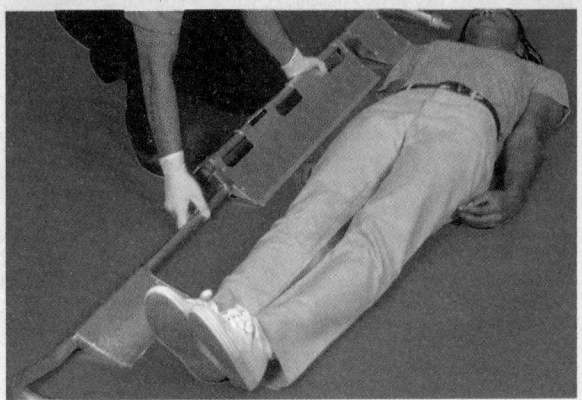

### Step 1
Adjust the length of the stretcher.

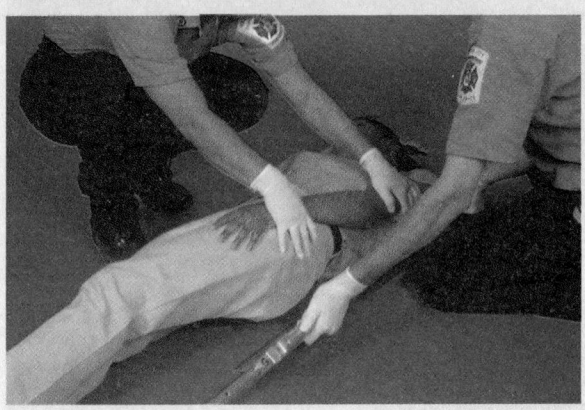

### Step 2
Lift the patient slightly and slide the stretcher into place, one side at a time.

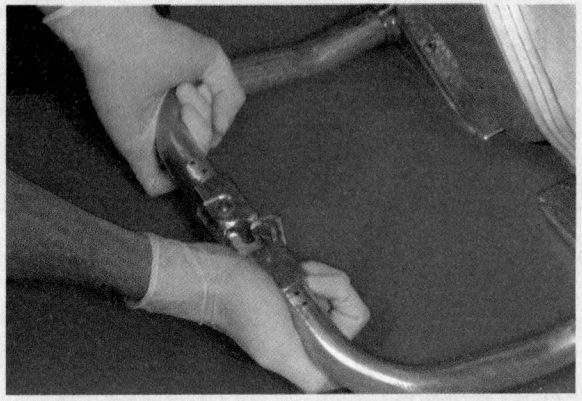

### Step 3
Lock the stretcher ends together, and avoid pinching both the patient and your fingers!

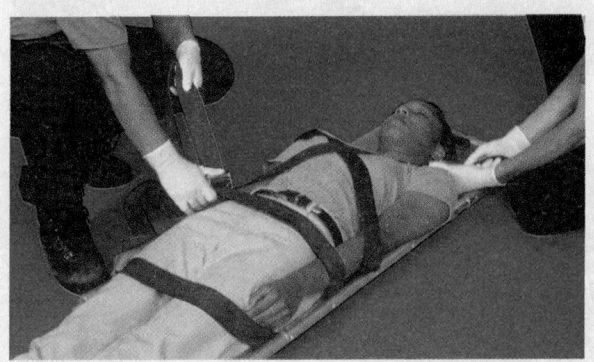

### Step 4
Secure the patient to the scoop stretcher, and transfer it to the stretcher.

© Jones & Bartlett Learning. Courtesy of MIEMSS.

hip and upper arm, while your partner slides the stretcher into place (**Step 2**).

3. Lock the stretcher ends together by engaging their locking mechanisms one at a time and continue to lift the patient slightly as needed to avoid pinching (**Step 3**).

4. Apply and tighten straps to secure the patient to the scoop stretcher before transferring to the stretcher (**Step 4**).

## Other Carries

Other carries are performed in the following manner:

- Place a backboard next to the patient, and, after using a log roll or slide to move the patient onto the backboard, secure the patient and lift and carry the backboard to the nearby prepared stretcher.

- Assist an able patient to the edge of the bed, and place the patient's legs over the side, helping the patient to sit up. Move the stretcher so that its foot end touches the bed near the patient. Help the patient to stand and rotate so that he or she can sit down on the center of the stretcher. Lift the patient's legs, and rotate them onto the stretcher while your partner lowers the patient's torso onto the stretcher.

To avoid the strain of unnecessary lifting and carrying, use the draw sheet method or assist an able patient to the stretcher whenever possible.

To move a patient from the ground or the floor onto the stretcher, use one of the following methods:

- Lift and carry the patient to the nearby prepared stretcher using a direct body carry.
- Use a log roll or long-axis drag to place the patient onto a backboard, and then lift and carry the backboard to the stretcher. Place both the backboard and the patient onto the stretcher.
- Use a scoop stretcher.
- Log roll the patient onto a blanket, centering the patient on the blanket and rolling up the excess material on each side (**SKILL DRILL 8-12**). Lift the patient by the blanket, and carry him or her to the nearby stretcher.

If a patient is sitting in a chair and cannot assist you, transfer the patient from the chair to a stair chair as described earlier in this chapter (**FIGURE 8-19**).

### Words of Wisdom

Ensure a thorough patient care report by including details of how you moved the patient. For example: "Moved patient to stretcher with draw sheet lift."

## Geriatrics

Most patients transported by EMS are older adults (geriatric patients). These patients will need to be moved, lifted, and carried frequently. The aging process is associated with multiple changes in the body, including the musculoskeletal system and the integumentary system (ie, the skin). As people age, they may become less flexible, and bones become more brittle. Using the extremities to move or carry a geriatric patient may cause the person a significant amount of pain or discomfort. In some older patients, pulling an arm or leg may cause a dislocation or fracture. The skin of a geriatric patient is thinner and more susceptible to tears and bruising. Be careful not to cause a skin tear when gripping an arm or leg. Chronic medical conditions such as rheumatoid arthritis may limit the patient's movement and are associated with pain. Some older patients cannot lie flat or straighten their arms. Extra padding and support may be necessary to transport some patients comfortably. EMTs must keep these considerations in mind as they prepare to move, lift, and carry geriatric patients. Do not cause additional injury or pain to your patient. See Chapter 36, *Geriatric Emergencies*, for a more detailed discussion of the concepts specific to moving and carrying geriatric patients.

## Bariatrics

Just fewer than half (42.4%) of the adults in the United States (more than 100 million people) are considered obese. The incidence of obesity is higher among adults aged 40 to 59 years (almost 45%) than among adults aged 20 to 39 years (40%) or adults aged 61 years or older (almost 43%). The incidence among children is also alarming; approximately 18% of all children and adolescents in the United States are classified as obese. The obesity rate has tripled compared to just one generation ago and continues to increase. In 2008, the estimated annual cost of medical care for patients with obesity in the United States was $147 billion, or approximately $1,429 higher for an obese person than for a person of normal weight. Obesity has reached epidemic proportions in the United States, and many programs are now aimed at teaching people from a young age the importance of exercise and a healthy diet.

Bariatrics is the branch of medicine concerned with the management (prevention or control) of obesity and allied diseases. It comes from the Greek words *baros*, weight, and *iatreia*, medical treatment. There is a direct correlation between the degree of obesity and the frequency and severity of health problems; therefore, the larger the patient, the more likely he or she will need emergency treatment and transportation. This issue is taking an increasing toll on the health of EMTs because back injuries account for the highest number of missed days of work and both temporary and permanent disability.

## Skill Drill 8-12 Logrolling a Patient on the Ground

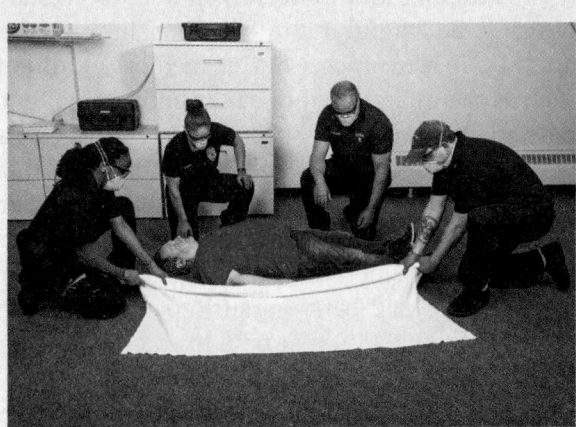

**Step 1**

Prepare the blanket by rolling it up by half.

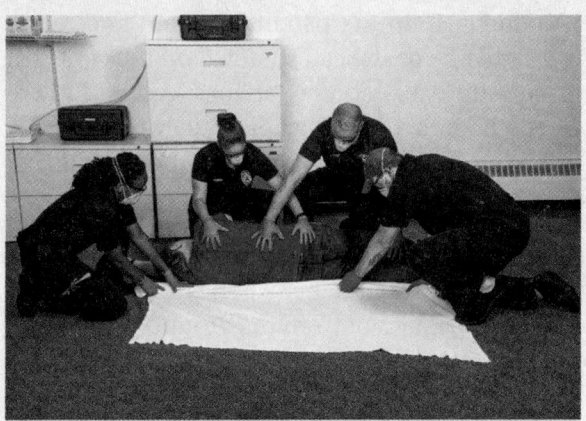

**Step 2**

Logroll the patient.

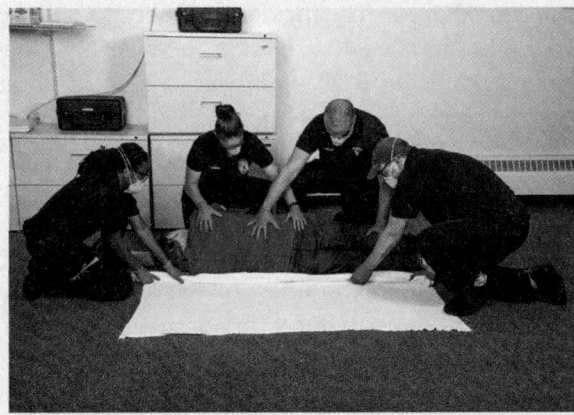

**Step 3**

Position the blanket that has been rolled up half way underneath the patient. Logroll the patient back onto the blanket and then in the opposite direction to unroll the blanket.

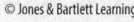
© Jones & Bartlett Learning.

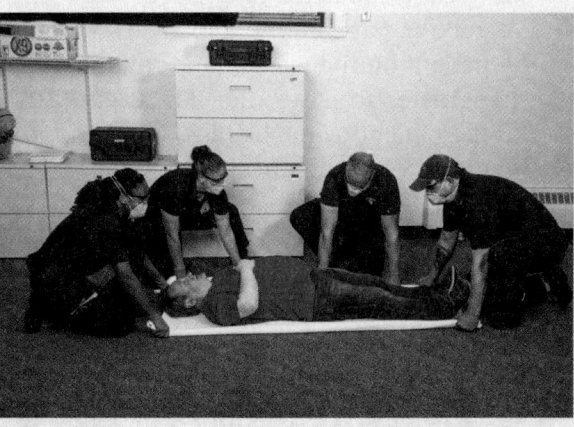

**Step 4**

Roll the patient back onto his or her back and roll up the ends of the blanket for lifting. Lift the blanket and transfer the patient to the stretcher.

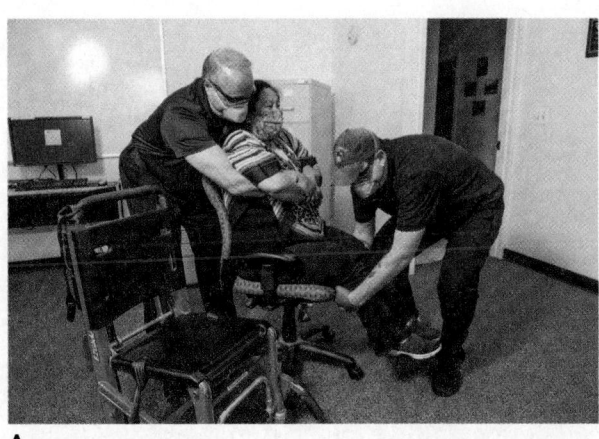

**A**

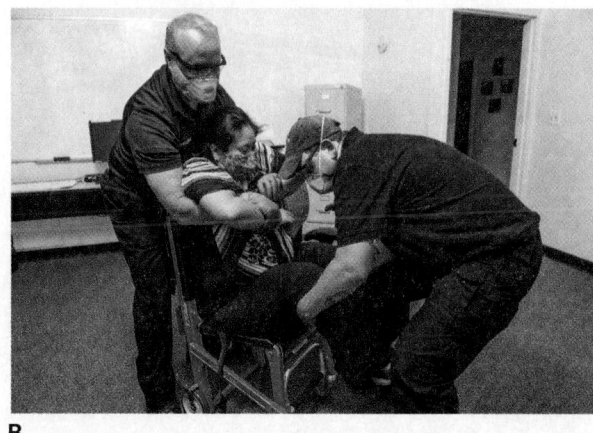

**B**

**FIGURE 8-19** Moving a patient from a chair to a stair chair. **A.** If present, any removable side pieces on the chair should be removed or placed in a position so they will not interfere. Slide your arms through the patient's armpits, and grasp the patient's crossed forearms. Your partner grasps the patient's legs at the knees. **B.** Gently lift the patient into the locked stair chair.

A, B: © Jones & Bartlett Learning.

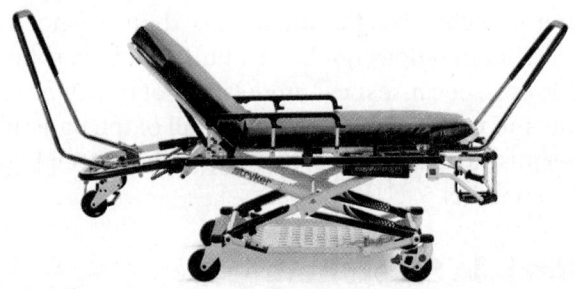

**FIGURE 8-20** A bariatric stretcher.

Courtesy of Stryker Medical, a division of Stryker Corporation.

# Additional Patient-Moving Equipment

## Bariatric Stretchers

Because of the weight and large girth of bariatric patients, they may not fit comfortably or safely on the standard wheeled stretcher. As a result, a specialized type of wheeled stretcher has been developed, called a bariatric stretcher (**FIGURE 8-20**). This type of stretcher is similar in design to the common wheeled stretcher; however, it has several differences. Bariatric stretchers typically have a wider patient surface area to allow for increased comfort, and in addition ensure the patient's dignity is maintained during transport. Bariatric stretchers also have a wider wheelbase, allowing for increased stability when rolling the patient over uneven terrain. Bariatric stretchers are sometimes equipped with optional features such as a tow package, which allows an ambulance-mounted winch to assist in loading the patient

into the ambulance, decreasing the potential for EMT back injuries. Another optional feature is telescoping side lift handles, which provide increased leverage when lifting with multiple providers. However, the most important feature of the bariatric stretcher is the increased weight-lifting capacity. Typical wheeled ambulance stretchers, depending on manufacturer ratings, allow for a maximum weight of 650 lb (295 kg). Bariatric stretchers are usually able to support maximum weight as high as 1600 (725 kg) pounds when rolled in the lowest position.

## Pneumatic and Electronic Powered Wheeled Stretchers

In an effort to decrease the potential for back injuries to EMS providers, manufacturers have developed pneumatic and electronic stretchers. Similar in appearance to conventional wheeled stretchers, electronic stretchers are battery operated and have electronic controls to facilitate raising and lowering of the undercarriage at the touch of a button (**FIGURE 8-21**). Some of these wheeled stretchers also have the ability to be loaded and unloaded from the ambulance by motor and thus only require the provider to control the equipment. These devices limit the risk of injury to providers and to the patient by removing the physical strain of the task.

## Binder Lift

A Binder Lift gives EMS providers another safe way to lift patients as a team to help prevent injuries.

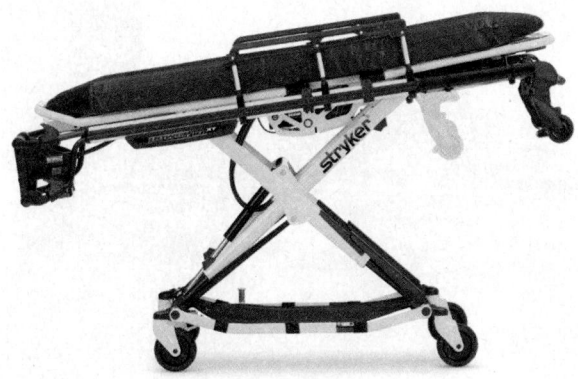

**FIGURE 8-21** An electronic stretcher.

Courtesy of Stryker Medical, a division of Stryker Corporation.

The binder is wrapped around patient's torso. The Binder Lift design has up to 25 handles for providers to use during the patient lift before moving the patient to a stair chair or stretcher.

## Portable/Folding Stretchers

A **portable stretcher** is a stretcher with a strong, rectangular, tubular metal frame and rigid fabric stretched across it (**FIGURE 8-22**). Portable stretchers do not have a second multipositioning frame or adjustable undercarriage. Some models have two wheels that fold down about 4 inches (10 cm)

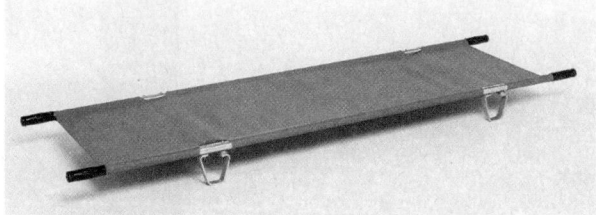

**FIGURE 8-22** A portable stretcher.

© Steve Gorton/Getty.

underneath the foot end of the frame and legs of a similar length that fold down from the head end at each side. The wheels make it easier to move the loaded stretcher. The legs should not be used as handles.

Some portable stretchers can be folded in half across the center of each side so that the stretcher is only half its usual length during storage. A portable stretcher weighs much less than a wheeled stretcher and does not have a bulky undercarriage. However, because most models do not have wheels, you and your team must support all of the patient's weight and any equipment along with the weight of the stretcher.

## Flexible Stretchers

Several types of flexible stretchers are available and can be rolled up across either the stretcher's width or

## YOU are the Provider

A cervical collar is applied and the passenger is secured to a KED. You are then able to remove her from the wreckage and onto a backboard. After loading her into the ambulance, you perform a complete assessment and transport her to the local trauma center for evaluation.

| Recording Time:   27 Minutes | |
| --- | --- |
| **Level of consciousness** | Alert and oriented |
| **Respirations** | 16 breaths/min; adequate depth |
| **Pulse** | 110 beats/min; strong and regular |
| **Skin** | Pink, warm, and moist |
| **Blood pressure** | 148/72 mm Hg |
| **Spo$_2$** | 100% (on room air) |

On arrival at the hospital, the patient tells you that she is still experiencing pain in her back, although it is not as severe and feels like "a pulled muscle." After moving her from the wheeled stretcher to the hospital bed, you give your verbal report to the staff nurse and return to service.

**11.** How can you minimize the risk of injury while moving a patient on a wheeled ambulance stretcher?

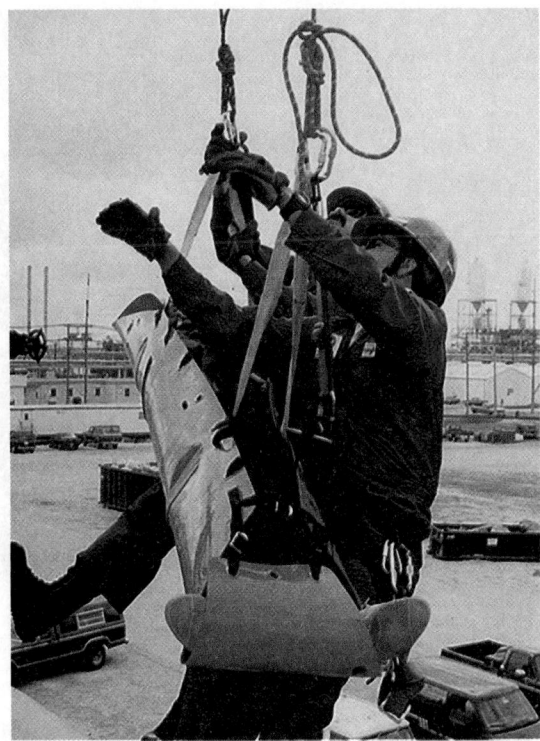

**FIGURE 8-23** A flexible stretcher.

© American Academy of Orthopaedic Surgeons.

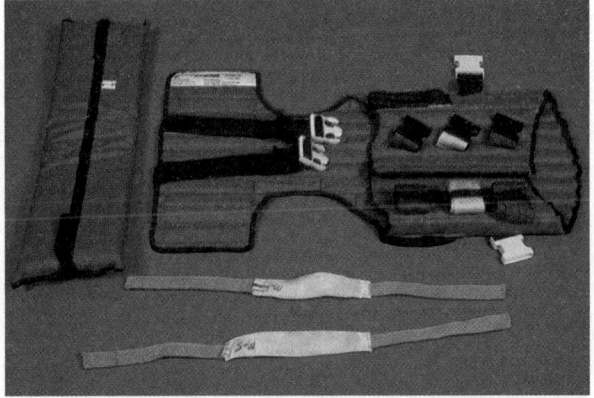

**FIGURE 8-24** The Kendrick extrication device (KED) is a vest-type immobilization device.

© Jones & Bartlett Learning. Courtesy of MIEMSS.

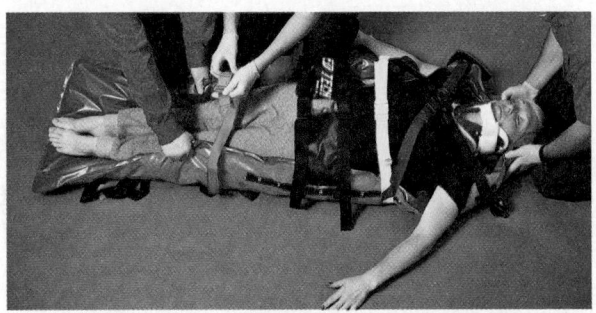

**FIGURE 8-25** The vacuum mattress fits snugly to the curvatures and contours of the body and limits pressure-point tenderness.

© Jones & Bartlett Learning. Courtesy of Glen Ellman.

length, so that the stretcher becomes a smaller, tubular package for storage and carrying (**FIGURE 8-23**). When you must carry the equipment a considerable distance from the nearest place that the ambulance can be located, this is an important consideration. A **flexible stretcher** forms a rigid stretcher that conforms around the patient's sides and does not extend beyond them. When these stretchers are extended, they are particularly useful when you must remove a patient from or through a confined space. Certain flexible stretchers can also be used if the patient must be belayed or rappelled by ropes.

## Short Backboards

You can use a short backboard to immobilize the torso, head, and neck of a seated patient with a suspected spinal injury until you can immobilize the patient on a backboard. Short backboards are 3 to 4 feet long (approximately 1 m). However, the wooden short backboard has generally been replaced with a vest-type device, such as the KED, that is specifically designed to immobilize the patient until he or she is moved from a sitting position to a supine position on a backboard (**FIGURE 8-24**).

## Vacuum Mattresses

Another alternative to the backboard is the vacuum mattress (**FIGURE 8-25**). With this device, the patient is placed on the mattress and the air is removed from the device, allowing it to mold around the patient. It fits snugly to the curvatures and contours of the body and limits pressure-point tenderness. Padding may be used for tender areas but is not required for most patients. The vacuum mattress is seen as equivalent to padding to secure the patient's neck and spine and is more comfortable for the patient than the long spine board. See Chapter 29, *Head and Spine Injuries*, for more information about the vacuum mattress.

## Basket Stretchers

Use a rigid **basket stretcher**, also called a Stokes litter, to carry a patient across uneven terrain from a

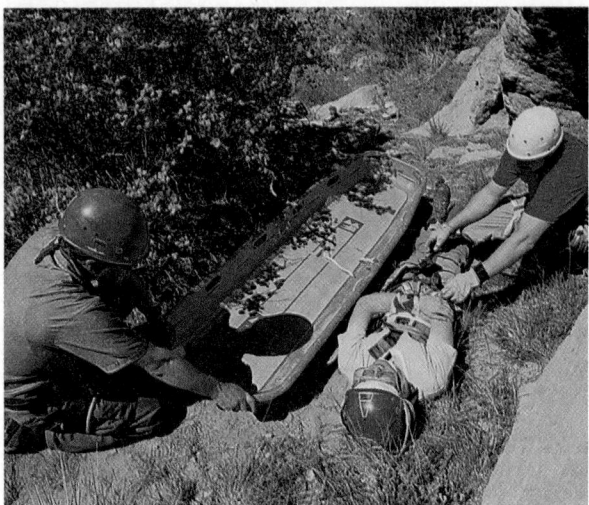

**FIGURE 8-26** A basket stretcher.

© Jones & Bartlett Learning. Courtesy of MIEMSS.

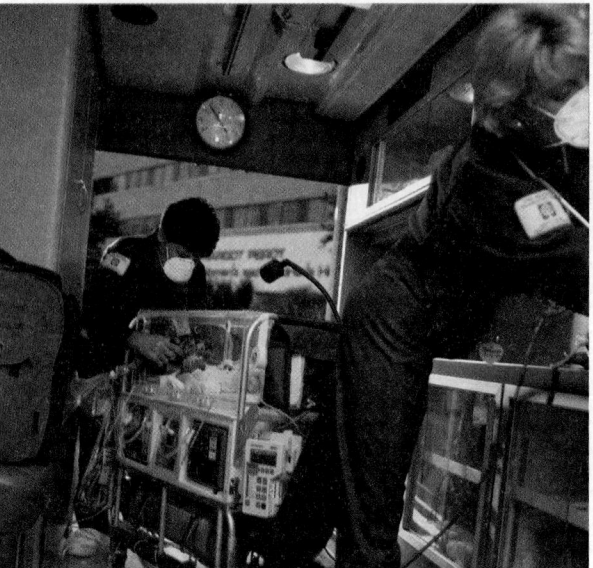

**FIGURE 8-27** Neonatal isolette.

© DreamPictures/Getty Images.

remote location that is inaccessible by ambulance or other vehicle (**FIGURE 8-26**). If you suspect that the patient has a spinal injury, first secure him or her on a backboard and then place the backboard into the basket stretcher. Once you have reached the ambulance and wheeled ambulance stretcher, you can remove the patient secured to the backboard from the basket stretcher and place the patient on the stretcher.

Basket stretchers are made of plastic with an aluminum frame or have a full steel frame that is connected by a woven wire mesh. The wire basket is uncomfortable for the patient unless the wire is padded. Either type can be used to carry a patient across fields, rough terrain, or trails or on a toboggan, boat, or all-terrain vehicle. Basket stretchers are also used for technical rope rescues and some water rescues. Not all basket stretchers are rated or appropriate for each of these specialized rescue uses.

## Neonatal Isolettes

When you need to transport a neonatal patient from one hospital to another, the common wheeled ambulance stretcher will not suffice. To safely transport a neonatal patient, the patient must be placed inside of an isolette, sometimes referred to as an incubator. The isolette keeps the neonatal patient warm with moistened air in a clean environment and helps to protect the infant from noise, drafts, infection, and excess handling. These specialized transport devices come in one of two forms: an isolette that is placed directly on top of the

wheeled stretcher and secured with seat belts or a free-standing isolette that is secured into the back of the ambulance, taking the place of the standard stretcher (**FIGURE 8-27**).

## Decontamination

It is essential that you decontaminate your equipment after each use to prevent the spread of disease—for your own safety, the safety of the EMTs using the equipment after you, and the safety of your patients. Just as you expect a hospital bed to be disinfected after the previous patient, so too with your stretcher and other transport equipment. Know and follow your local standard operating procedures for disinfecting equipment after each call.

## Patient Positioning

It is imperative while treating a patient that he or she be properly positioned based on the chief complaint. Certain patient conditions, such as head injury, shock, spinal injury, pregnancy, and obesity, call for special lifting and moving techniques. Although a patient with a potential spinal injury should be secured to restrict movement of the spine, a patient with no suspected injury reporting chest pain or respiratory distress should be placed in a position of comfort—typically a Fowler or semi-Fowler position—unless he or she is hypotensive. Patients who are in shock should be packaged and placed in a supine position. Patients in late stages of pregnancy should be positioned and transported on their left side if they are uncomfortable or hypotensive when supine. Place an unresponsive patient with no suspected spinal, hip, or pelvic injury into the recovery position by rolling the patient onto his or her side without twisting the body. Transport a patient who is nauseated or vomiting in a position of comfort, but ensure that you are positioned appropriately to manage and maintain a patent airway. Patients with obesity should be positioned the same as other patients with a similar condition; however, particular attention must be paid to ensure their dignity is maintained.

## Personnel Considerations

As an EMT, you will be required to assist in the movement of patients. In an effort to minimize injuries, prior to moving any patient, a complete plan needs to be developed and discussed among your team. Some questions to ask are the following:

- Am I physically strong enough to lift and move this patient?
- Is there adequate room to get the proper stance to lift the patient?
- Do I need additional providers for lifting assistance?

The answers to these questions need to be evaluated prior to moving your patient. Remember that injured EMTs cannot help anyone.

### Words of Wisdom

Restraints should never be punitive. Only apply restraints to patients who pose a threat to you, your team members, themselves, or bystanders, and follow local protocols for the use of restraints. If a restrained patient starts to spit, cover the patient's mouth with a simple face mask or surgical mask. Once restraints have been applied, never remove them until you arrive at the hospital and are requested to remove them by the hospital staff.

### Street Smarts

Lifting and moving patients is a large part of the job when working as an EMT or paramedic. It is important that you work to keep yourself in good physical shape. Weight training and stretching in addition to eating well and getting enough sleep will help you remain active and effective in the field.

## YOU are the Provider SUMMARY

**1. What immediate challenges do you face?**

Your first concern is for the stability and safety of the vehicle. Prior to attempting to physically access the patients, safety measures must be taken to stabilize the vehicle and prevent further rollover or collapse during the extrication process.

If the patients are not trapped, the vehicle is stabilized, and you decide to remove a patient yourself, the next consideration is the size of the patient. Does he or she weigh more than you and your partner can safely lift? There is also the consideration of working in an enclosed space that may not allow for additional providers to help with the initial movement of a patient.

Additionally, there are two patients and at least one is in critical condition. This further increases the stress on you and may lead to injury if the lift is not adequately planned. While your intention to help the patient is admirable, you must remember that you will be useless to the team and the patient if you are injured in the process.

**2. Why is knowledge of body mechanics important when lifting and moving a patient?**

Body mechanics describes the way you move your body. Posture is an important component in body mechanics. Good posture means the spine is in a neutral position. Knowing how your body moves will minimize the risk of a back injury when you are lifting or moving a patient. Always keep your back in a straight and upright position and lift without twisting.

**3. What other resources are needed?**

You already know the driver is unresponsive and showing signs of dyspnea with cyanosis. You also know that both patients are entrapped in the overturned vehicle, and extrication will be required. Therefore, immediately call for paramedic backup and a rescue unit, as well as lifting assistance. There will be a delay in care as the patients are extricated. Having advanced units standing by will decrease the time to definitive care. You will likely need a second ambulance, or if you are a long distance from a Level I trauma center, consider the use of air transport, if available. Ask the dispatcher for a fire or rescue response if it is not already on scene or en route to the scene. The rescuers can disconnect batteries and stabilize the vehicle and also may be needed to help extricate the patients.

Law enforcement should be dispatched for crowd control and to help with directing traffic around the scene to make it safe for everyone to work. Each agency has its own job to do, and the sooner each agency is dispatched, the quicker the patient will receive optimal care.

**4.  Do you consider the driver to be in stable or unstable condition? Should you wait for further assistance or go ahead and gain access to him?**

The condition of the driver is unstable due to his altered level of consciousness and cyanosis. Regardless, you must never enter a scene that is not safe. With the vehicle lying on its side in such a precarious position, any weight added could cause it to roll over and crush you or cause further injury to the patients. If you enter the vehicle in such a situation, you risk making the situation even more hazardous to vehicle occupants and to the rest of the rescue team. The vehicle must be stabilized prior to gaining access to the patients. Safety of the crew is paramount before any patient care is provided.

If the passenger is able to lift her arms and the tubing is long enough, it may be possible to toss a nonrebreathing mask into the vehicle and have her place and hold the mask over the face of her husband to provide him with oxygen before further treatment begins. Any further care will have to be postponed until the vehicle has been stabilized.

**5.  Once you are able to gain access, what are your concerns for the use of proper body mechanics while removing these patients?**

The overturned vehicle is a confined space that only allows for access by one EMT. This means that you must consider your lifting limits and think through what type of equipment may be utilized to place the least amount of physical stress on you. The patients may have to be moved in carefully planned stages. Try to use your legs to do most of the lifting, and try to keep your back as straight as possible within the limitations imposed.

**6.  Once the driver is no longer entrapped, how will you attempt to remove him from the vehicle while maintaining spinal motion restriction?**

Due to the mechanism of injury, spinal motion restriction for both patients is warranted. After gaining access, you will have to assess the situation and available space to see whether a backboard or scoop stretcher can be introduced through the back door of the vehicle or slid in from the driver's door if it is possible to open it. Careful movement of the car's seats may provide more space to work. If not, is there any other device that you may slide underneath the patient to assist with moving him? You can place an appropriately sized cervical collar on the patient, but remember that this does not provide stabilization of the neck unless someone is actually holding the head and neck in alignment and it provides no stabilization for the thoracic or lumbar spine. This is far from an ideal lifting situation, so you must proceed cautiously and try to manipulate his spine as little as possible, while recognizing that without gaining control of his airway and assisting with ventilations, he will die rapidly. This is a situation where an urgent move is required and time is of the essence. Be as careful as possible while expeditiously removing the patient.

**7.  What type of move is best for removing the driver?**

Due to the unstable condition of the patient, it is necessary to move him as quickly and safely as possible. Unfortunately, with such a confined space there is no way to utilize additional help to maintain spinal alignment. If the rescue team is able to wedge a backboard through the open door of the vehicle, it will give you a platform to stand or kneel on, as well as something on which to move the patient. The best options for moving the driver likely would be to use a clothes drag or to grab underneath his arms and pull him upward if you are able to reach that far. If the passenger is able to use her arms, she may be able to help push upward from his hips to assist you in moving him. He will have to be pulled between the headrests if there is no other access. In some vehicles it may be possible to remove the headrests. Make sure he is moved in small increments, using your arms to "curl" and repositioning often to protect your back. After his head and shoulders have been pulled though the seats, a second provider can possibly reach through far enough to help pull him onto the backboard and then assist in removing him and the backboard from the vehicle.

**8.  What steps can you take to maximize safety while lifting a patient?**

To safely lift and carry a patient, you and your team must anticipate and understand every move, and each move must be coordinated. To avoid confusion, which may result in one or more providers suddenly bearing an unexpected amount of weight, the team leader (typically the provider closest to the head of the patient) should call out all of the lifting commands.

The following general guidelines should be followed to maximize safety when lifting any patient:

- Keep your legs shoulder width apart.
- Keep your back in a straight, locked-in position.
- Keep the patient's weight as close to your body as possible.
- Bend at the knees, not the waist, when lifting.
- Avoid lifting and reaching at the same time.
- Avoid twisting your body as you are lifting.
- Lift with your palms facing up (power grip).
- Communicate with your partner (or team) at all times.

**9. How is a patient's weight distributed when he or she is on a carrying device? Why is it important to know this?**

To position your team accordingly, and thus minimize the potential for injury, it is important to know how a patient's weight is distributed when he or she is on a carrying device.

If a patient is supine on a backboard or a scoop stretcher or is in a semisitting position on an ambulance stretcher, his or her weight is not equally distributed between the two ends of the device. When a patient is in a horizontal position, between 68% and 78% of his or her weight is in the torso. Therefore, the strongest provider or providers should be positioned at the head end of the carrying device. However, you should still position the remaining providers so that each one—including the provider or providers at the patient's head—bears an equal amount of the patient's weight.

**10. Considering her complaints and the fact that her condition is stable, what are your best options for removing the passenger?**

An urgent move is not required because the patient's condition is stable. Think through the possibilities while you provide reassurance to the patient. She has the potential for spinal injuries because of the mechanism of injury and because she is reporting back pain. The best way to move a stable patient reporting neck or back pain is to use a short vest device such as a KED. Apply a cervical collar to the patient

and then position the KED behind the patient and have her thread the leg straps underneath her legs. Continuously remind the patient to hold her head still and try to move as little as possible because there is no room for another provider to hold cervical spine control. Once the device is positioned, you will have to lean through the seats to attach and secure the straps. Once secured, the patient can be moved as a unit. Pull her through the seats and onto the awaiting backboard where you will have additional assistance to remove her from the vehicle and transfer her onto the ambulance stretcher.

**11. How can you minimize the risk of injury while moving a patient on a wheeled ambulance stretcher?**

When you move a patient on a wheeled ambulance stretcher, make sure that it is elevated whenever possible, not lowered to the ground. If the stretcher is lowered to the ground, you will have to bend down and move the patient at the same time; this increases the potential for a back injury.

When the stretcher is elevated, the main frame and the patient are considerably higher than the wheels; this makes the stretcher top-heavy. Therefore, when you are moving a patient on an elevated stretcher, ensure that you hold the frame firmly between both of your hands at all times so that if the patient moves, the stretcher will not tip over.

If you are guiding the stretcher from the foot end, make sure your arms are held close to your body, and avoid reaching a great distance behind you or hyperextending your back. Your back should be locked, straight, and untwisted. To avoid hyperextending your elbows or injuring your shoulder, keep your elbows slightly flexed and use the muscles of your arms to pull.

If you are guiding the stretcher from the head end, push with your arms and bend your elbows so that your hands are about 12 to 15 inches (30 to 38 cm) in front of your torso. To protect your elbows from injury, avoid pushing the stretcher with your arms fully extended and your elbows locked. When you push with your elbows bent but firmly held from bending further, the strong muscles of your arms serve as a shock absorber if the wheels of the stretcher strike an obstacle, causing the stretcher to come to an abrupt stop.

## YOU are the Provider SUMMARY *continued*

### EMS Patient Care Report (PCR)

| Date: 09-20-20 | Incident No.: 013409 | Nature of Call: Motor vehicle crash | Location: 125 Parkview Place | |
|---|---|---|---|---|
| Dispatched: 0822 | En Route: 0822 | At Scene: 0828 | Transport: 0938 | At Hospital: 0947 | In Service: 0955 |

#### Patient Information

**Age:** 82
**Sex:** F
**Weight (in kg [lb]):** 69 kg (152 lb)

**Allergies:** Penicillin
**Medications:** Ibuprofen, lisinopril
**Past Medical History:** Chronic back pain, hypertension
**Chief Complaint:** Back pain, right side pain

#### Vital Signs

| Time: 0833 | BP: Unable to assess | Pulse: Unable to assess | Respirations: Unable to visualize | Spo$_2$: N/A |
|---|---|---|---|---|
| Time: 0912 | BP: 148/92 | Pulse: 112 | Respirations: 20 | Spo$_2$: 99% |
| Time: 0928 | BP: 148/72 | Pulse: 110 | Respirations: 16 | Spo$_2$: 100% |

#### EMS Treatment (circle all that apply)

| Oxygen © __ L/min via:  NC  NRM  Bag mask | Assisted Ventilation | Airway Adjunct | CPR |
|---|---|---|---|
| Defibrillation | Bleeding Control | Bandaging | Splinting | Other: KED and backboard |

#### Narrative

Dispatched to the scene of a motor vehicle crash where a sedan-type vehicle was found lying on the passenger's side in ditch.

Chief complaint: Back pain, right side pain

History: 82-year-old female unrestrained passenger with a history of chronic back pain was reporting pain to her back and right side.

Assessment: This patient was pinned underneath the male driver, who was unresponsive. Upon arrival, secondary units were requested to stabilize vehicle and a paramedic unit was requested for backup. Once the vehicle was stabilized the male patient was removed and turned over to the awaiting paramedic team. The woman was then able to be accessed. Patient was alert and oriented with no significant injuries noted on physical exam.

Treatment (Rx): A cervical collar was applied and a Kendrick extrication device (KED) was placed behind the patient, and, with her help, the device was secured around her body and legs. Using the KED, the patient was pulled up over the seats and onto an awaiting backboard. Once the patient was removed from the vehicle and secured to the backboard, she was loaded into the ambulance.

Transport: Vital signs were obtained and a secondary assessment was completed en route to the local trauma center. There were no significant injuries found and the patient remained stable during transport. Upon arrival at the trauma center, patient report was given to the receiving nurse Fields and the crew returned to service.

**End of report**

*Note:* The responding paramedic team provided documentation for the care of the male patient turned over upon removal from the wreckage.

# Prep Kit

## Ready for Review

- The wheeled ambulance stretcher and the backboard are the devices most commonly used to move and transport patients.
- It is best to move a patient on a device that can be rolled. However, if a wheeled device is not available, you must understand and follow certain guidelines for carrying a patient on a stretcher or backboard.
- Whenever you move a patient, you must take special care to avoid injury to you, your team, and the patient.
- The safety of you, your team, and the patient depends on the use of proper lifting techniques and maintaining a proper hold when lifting or carrying a patient. You must practice each technique with your team often so that you are able to perform the move quickly, safely, and efficiently.
- The same basic body mechanics apply for safe reaching, pulling, lifting, and carrying.
- Good body mechanics are important to prevent injuries, but are not always sufficient. Special devices and technology should be used when possible to further decrease your risk of injury.
- The first key rule of lifting is to always keep your back in an upright position and lift without twisting. You can lift and carry significant weight without injury as long as your back is in the proper upright position.
- Do not hyperextend your back when reaching overhead.
- The power lift is the safest and most powerful way to lift.
- Pushing is better than pulling.
- If you do not have a proper hold, you will not be able to bear your share of the weight, or you may lose your grasp with one or both hands and possibly cause a low back injury to one or more providers.
- When you must carry a patient up or down a flight of stairs or other significant incline, use a stair chair. The exception to this is when the patient is in cardiac arrest, must be moved in a supine position, or must have his or her spine immobilized during transport, in which case the patient will be moved on the stairs on a backboard.

- If you must carry a loaded backboard or stretcher up or down stairs or other inclines, be sure that the patient is tightly secured to the device to prevent sliding.
- Be sure to carry the backboard or stretcher foot end first so that the patient's head is elevated higher than the feet.
- Directions and commands are important parts of safe lifting and carrying.
- You must constantly coordinate your movements with those of the other team members and communicate with them.
- You and your team must anticipate and understand every move and execute it in a coordinated manner.
- The team leader is responsible for coordinating the moves.
- Try to use four providers for patient moves whenever resources allow.
- Know how much you can comfortably and safely lift and do not attempt to lift more than this amount.
- Rapidly summon additional help to lift and carry a weight that is greater than you are able to lift.
- Perform an urgent move if a patient has an altered level of consciousness or inadequate ventilation, if the patient is in shock, or during extreme weather conditions.
- Normally, you should move a patient with nonurgent moves, in an orderly, planned, and unhurried manner, selecting methods that involve the least amount of lifting and carrying.
- At times, you may have to use an emergency move to maneuver a patient before providing assessment and care.
- Other devices that are used to lift and carry patients include portable stretchers, flexible stretchers, backboards, basket stretchers (Stokes litters), and scoop stretchers.
- Training and practice are required to use all the equipment that is available to you.
- You will learn the technical skills of patient packaging and handling through practice and training.

## Vital Vocabulary

**backboard** A long, flat board made of rigid, rectangular material that is used to provide support to a patient who is suspected of having a hip, pelvic, spinal, or lower extremity injury; also called a spine board, trauma board, and longboard.

**bariatrics** A branch of medicine concerned with the management (prevention or control) of obesity and allied diseases.

**basket stretcher** A rigid stretcher commonly used in technical and water rescues that surrounds and supports the patient yet allows water to drain through holes in the bottom; also called a Stokes litter.

**body mechanics** The relationship between the body's anatomic structures and the physical forces associated with lifting, moving, and carrying; the ways in which the body moves to achieve a specific action.

**diamond carry** A carrying technique in which one provider is located at the head end of the stretcher or backboard, one at the foot end, and one at each side of the patient; each of the two providers at the sides uses one hand to support the stretcher or backboard so that all are able to face forward as they walk.

**direct ground lift** A lifting technique that is used for patients who are found lying supine on the ground with no suspected spinal injury.

**emergency move** A move in which the patient is dragged or pulled from a dangerous scene before assessment and care are provided.

**extremity lift** A lifting technique that is used for patients who are supine or in a sitting position with no suspected extremity or spinal injuries.

**flexible stretcher** A stretcher that is a rigid carrying device when secured around a patient but can be folded or rolled when not in use.

**portable stretcher** A stretcher with a strong, rectangular, tubular metal frame and rigid fabric stretched across it.

**power grip** A technique in which the stretcher or backboard is gripped by inserting each hand under the handle with the palm facing up and the thumb extended, fully supporting the underside of the handle on the curved palm with the fingers and thumb.

**power lift** A lifting technique in which the EMT's back is held upright, with legs bent, and the patient is lifted when the EMT straightens the legs to raise the upper body and arms.

**rapid extrication technique** A technique to move a patient from a sitting position inside a vehicle to supine on a backboard in less than 1 minute when conditions do not allow for standard immobilization.

**scoop stretcher** A stretcher that is designed to be split into two or four sections that can be fitted around a patient who is lying on the ground or other relatively flat surface; also called an orthopaedic stretcher.

**stair chair** A lightweight folding device that is used to carry a conscious, seated patient up or down stairs.

**wheeled ambulance stretcher** A specially designed stretcher that can be rolled along the ground. A collapsible undercarriage allows it to be loaded into the ambulance; also called an ambulance stretcher.

## References

1. Centers for Disease Control and Prevention. Adult obesity facts. https://www.cdc.gov/obesity/data /adult.html. Accessed April 22, 2020.

2. Centers for Disease Control and Prevention. Child overweight and obesity. https://www.cdc.gov/obesity /childhood/index.html. Accessed April 22, 2020.

3. Hales CM, Carroll MD, Fryar CD, Ogden CL. Prevalence of obesity and severe obesity among adults: United States, 2017–2018. National Center for Health Statistics, Centers for Disease Control and Prevention. https://www.cdc.gov/nchs/products/databriefs/db360.

htm. Published February 2020. Accessed March 18, 2020.

4. National Highway Traffic Safety Administration. *National Emergency Medical Services Education Standards.* DOT HS 811 077A. www.ems.gov/pdf/811077a.pdf. Published January 2009. Accessed June 14, 2020.

5. National Highway Traffic Safety Administration. *National Emergency Medical Services Education Standards. Emergency Medical Technician Instructional Guidelines.* DOT HS 811 077C. www.ems.gov/pdf/811077c.pdf. Published January 2009.Accessed June 14, 202.

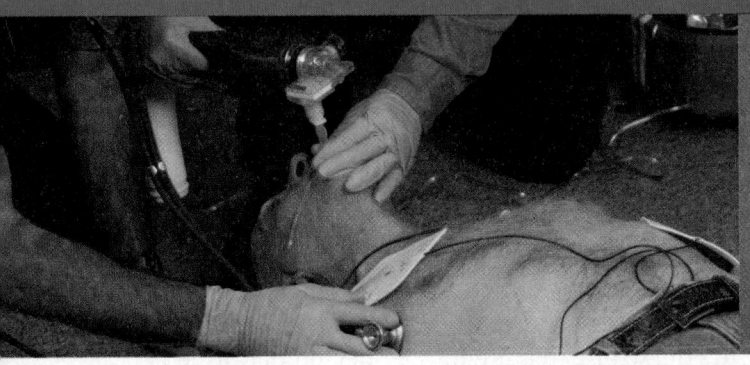

# Chapter 9

# The Team Approach to Health Care

## NATIONAL EMS EDUCATION STANDARD COMPETENCIES

Applies fundamental knowledge of patient safety to the provision of emergency care.

Applies fundamental knowledge of transferring patient care; how to interact within the team structure; and team communication and dynamics.

## KNOWLEDGE OBJECTIVES

1. Define continuum of care. (p 321)
2. List the five essential elements of a group. (p 322)
3. Explain the advantages of a team over a group; include the advantages of regularly training and practicing together. (pp 321–322)
4. List the five essential elements of a team. (pp 323–325)
5. Explain how crew resource management (CRM) can be useful in the prehospital environment. (pp 325–326)
6. List the five critical elements necessary to ensure effective transfer of patient care from one provider to another. (pp 326–328)
7. List the five steps a receiving health care provider should perform when taking a patient care report (PCR). (p 327)
8. Explain the stages of effective decision making. (pp 329–330)
9. Describe decision traps that can lead to decision-making errors. (p 330)
10. Describe the steps EMTs can take to troubleshoot interpersonal conflicts. (p 331)

## SKILLS OBJECTIVES

There are no skills objectives for this chapter.

# Introduction

As an EMT, you are a critical member of the emergency health care team that includes not only first responders, paramedics, and other EMTs, but also physicians, nurses, and other personnel who will help care for your patient throughout the duration of his or her injury or illness (**FIGURE 9-1**). You play a pivotal role by bringing emergency medicine into patients' homes, assisting with advanced patient care skills, and ensuring the effective transfer of patient care to emergency department (ED) staff when you arrive at the hospital.

One of the key goals of EMS Agenda 2050 is EMS systems that are designed to be inherently safe to minimize exposure to injury, infections, illness, or stress. As part of this effort, decisions should be made with the safety of all as a priority. In other words, EMS should have a culture of safety. Underpinning such a culture are elements such as data collection, just culture, coordinated support and resources, EMS education initiatives, EMS safety standards, and reporting and investigation of errors and near misses.

Just culture is an approach to leadership in organizations that balances fairness and accountability and encourages people to report errors and near misses. It focuses on risk management—that is, proactively identifying problems in the system that could lead to error or opportunities to improve safety. In a just culture, both the EMS system and individual providers are held accountable for overall safety.

In a just culture, behaviors associated with error or risk are categorized as human error, at-risk behavior, or reckless behavior. The EMS system considers human error to be a function of three factors: (1) a person intended to do the right thing but somehow committed an error, such as choosing the wrong treatment, (2) a person performed a skill incorrectly, or (3) a person meant to do something but did not follow through. In a just culture, the reasons for the error are investigated and the individual who committed the error is counseled or educated. At-risk behavior is conceptually different than this description of human error. At-risk behavior is when an EMT actively makes a choice to take a risk, believing that the potential adverse outcome is insignificant or that it was justified in the moment. This situation typically requires coaching and increased awareness. Reckless behavior involves a conscious disregard for a significant and unjustified risk, and it usually results in disciplinary action.

A positive culture of safety within an EMS system is linked to a decreased number of errors and near misses. Several common elements lead to both positive and negative safety cultures (**TABLE 9-1**).

## Words of Wisdom

When procedures that are established to promote safety are routinely ignored, noncompliance with the procedure becomes the norm in the EMS system. This process, known as normalization of deviance, increases risk to those working within the system. Examples include failure to wear appropriate eye protection and failure to follow checklists during procedures.

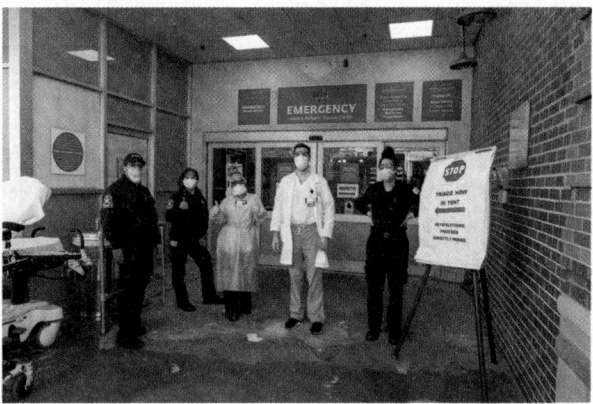

**FIGURE 9-1** As an EMT, you will work with various health care providers along the continuum of care.

© Pacific Press/Contributor/LightRocket/Getty Images.

**TABLE 9-1** Positive and Negative Attributes Contributing to a Culture of Safety

| Positive | Negative |
| --- | --- |
| Trust | Lack of communication |
| Teamwork | Taking shortcuts |
| Communication | Punishment |
| Sensitivity | Poor teamwork |
| Mutual support | Freelancing |

© Jones & Bartlett Learning.

As an EMT, you will need to do more than just acquire clinical knowledge and master necessary skills. You must also learn to be an effective team member. Essentially, this means communicating and collaborating with others who may have different backgrounds and levels of expertise than you have. By working as a team, emergency health care providers—from the first responders in the field to the physicians in the hospital—can improve patient and provider safety and deliver quality patient care. For basic life support (BLS) and advanced life support (ALS) providers to perform well together, each team member must share a common goal and demonstrate excellent communication skills. This chapter will provide an overview of the team health care approach and discuss how diversity among providers' backgrounds, skills, and abilities can strengthen a team. The chapter will also discuss how to assist with advanced skills and manage interpersonal conflict.

The positive effect of effective teamwork on the delivery of health care is highlighted by programs such as the World Health Organization's *Being a Team Player* and in the American Heart Association's *Chain of Survival*.

## An Era of Team Health Care

Currently, it is understood that for the delivery of EMS to be effective, health care providers must work together toward a unified goal of quality patient care. Historically, however, this was not always the case. Previous models of emergency care often consisted of providers who worked independently, passing the patient from one individual or group to the next. Gradually, emergency health care providers recognized that by working as a unified team from first patient contact to patient discharge, it was possible to improve individual and team performance, patient and provider safety, and, ultimately, patient outcomes. This concept is known as the **continuum of care**.

## Community Paramedicine and Mobile Integrated Healthcare Teams

**Community paramedicine** and **mobile integrated healthcare (MIH)** teams may be the best examples of the team concept of continuum of care. Recall that

in the MIH model, health care is provided within the community rather than at a physician's office or hospital. (See Chapter 1, *EMS Systems*, for more detail.) The success of MIH programs has shown that EMS providers, working as a unified team with in-hospital and other community health care providers, can improve patient outcomes, increase patient satisfaction, and reduce health care costs.

## Differences Among Teams

The structure and effectiveness of emergency health care teams differ from system to system. EMS providers may be trained as emergency medical responders (EMRs) or may be BLS- or ALS-certified. They may be volunteers, part-time employees, or full-time employees, and they may be based in police or fire departments, hospitals, or private agency settings. Multiple EMS agencies across different regions or response districts may respond to the same 9-1-1 call. Because of the variety of providers, agencies, and systems involved in each call, it may be difficult for all providers to function as one unified team. For instance, you may find it challenging to share patient assessment information and integrate newly arriving providers into ongoing care. Such challenges can be overcome by ensuring effective communication and mutual respect. In this case, as new responders arrive, it is helpful to think of them as "joining the team" as opposed to "taking over."

## Types of Teams

Depending on the EMS system in which you work, you may consistently interact with the same team members. Other systems may require emergency health care providers to assemble their teams "on the fly" for each individual call.

## Regular Teams

Some EMS systems rely on regular teams. In this model, EMTs consistently interact with the same partner or team and often develop a rapport with the other emergency health care providers and hospital staff with whom they frequently interact. Regular teams often train together. Team members who frequently train and work together are more likely to move smoothly from one step in the procedure to the next, performing as one seamless unit. By contrast, team members who train and work together less often may need more explicit verbal direction to accomplish their tasks, which can potentially lead to patient care delays.

## Temporary Teams

In this model, EMTs work with providers with whom they do not regularly interact or may not even know. This creates a special challenge. For a temporary team to function effectively, providers must work within an environment that supports and promotes collaboration rather than competition. It is crucial to have a clear understanding of the roles, responsibilities, and capabilities of each team member. One of the best ways to accomplish this is to train together when possible.

## Special Teams

Some EMS systems form special teams whose members have particular knowledge, skills, abilities, equipment, and/or training to serve a specialized role within the larger emergency health care team. Examples include the following:

- Fire Team
- Rescue Team
- Hazardous Materials (HazMat) Team
- Tactical EMS Team
- Special Event EMS Team
- EMS Bike Team
- In-Hospital Patient Care Technicians
- Mobile Integrated Health (MIH) Technicians

## Groups Versus Teams

Do not assume that any gathering of EMS providers responding together on a call is a team. True emergency response teams have better interaction, performance, and patient outcomes than groups of health care providers who do not share a team dynamic.

## Groups

The National Incident Management System (NIMS) defines a group as "The organizational level that divides the incident according to functional levels of operation. Groups perform special functions, often across geographic boundaries." When operating under NIMS, EMS providers often work as a group in this sense. In the context of this chapter, the term *group* is used in the more general sense.

You must be able to distinguish between a group of providers gathered together on an emergency call and a true team. In the context of EMS, a **group** consists of individual health care providers working independently to help the patient. Some examples of EMS groups are triage, treatment, and transport groups at a mass-casualty incident. In contrast, a **team** consists of a group of health care providers who are assigned specific roles and are working interdependently in a coordinated manner under a designated leader.

In 1945, the Research Center for Group Dynamics first defined the five essential elements of a group that people must share. These elements include:

- A common goal
- An image of themselves as "a group"
- A sense of continuity of the group (an understanding that the group may work together more than once, even in a slightly different configuration)
- A set of shared values (how the group wants to get things done)
- Different roles within the group (often self-assigned)

## YOU are the Provider

At 0905 hours, you are dispatched to a private home at 6 Catoonah Street for a 72-year-old man who is unresponsive. The dispatcher has no additional information to provide. An EMR crew from the fire department has been dispatched and will likely arrive before you. The weather is clear and sunny, the temperature is 82°F (27.8°C), and the traffic is light. Your response time to the scene is approximately 6 minutes.

**1.** How will you work together as a team with the EMRs?

**2.** How will members of this team decide who will perform each role?

Once a group has formed, the ability to function as a true emergency response team depends on the way in which its members work together.

# Dependent, Independent, and Interdependent Groups

## Dependent

In dependent groups, each individual is told what to do and often how to do it by his or her supervisor or group leader. Group members rely on the group leader for task assignments, troubleshooting, and virtually all decisions, thus limiting the group's ability to adapt and deliver critical medical care in an uncontrolled field environment.

## Independent

In independent groups, each individual is responsible for his or her own area (either a physical space or a set of tasks). Members of an independent group may receive support and guidance from a supervisor or group leader, but do not have to wait for an assignment before taking action as they would in a dependent group. Although independent group members may work on the same patient, each person is focused on individual goals (eg, starting an intravenous [IV] line, splinting an arm), rather than on working together to achieve a unified goal. The classic example of a poor outcome of independent group work is the perfectly splinted and packaged trauma patient who is dead on arrival at the ED due to an unrecognized and poorly managed airway.

## Interdependent

EMTs and other health care providers who work interdependently are functioning as a true team. Although each provider may still be assigned to a particular area or task, all of the providers in an interdependent group work together with shared responsibilities, accountability, and a common goal (the best possible patient outcome), as opposed to focusing on the goals of their respective individual areas.

# Effective Team Performance

Building on the five essential elements of a group, you will learn the five essential elements that health care providers must share to perform as an effective team.

## A Shared Goal

Every health care provider on the team, from EMT to paramedic to emergency physician, must be committed to a common goal—typically, the best possible patient outcome. Although this may seem like common sense, evidence of providers not working as a team can be heard in such alarming phrases as "Why take the time to splint the patient if they're only going to undo it in the ED?" and "There was no point in doing good CPR if the paramedic wasn't even trying to save the patient."

## Clear Roles and Responsibilities

To achieve a common goal, each provider must know what needs to be done and what is expected of him or her. An excellent example of this is the pit crew approach to CPR for cardiac arrest situations (**FIGURE 9-2**). The term originated in motor racing, in which teams of technicians rapidly assess and repair vehicles in a matter of seconds. Similarly, pit crew CPR consists of defining each intervention that needs to be addressed during cardiac arrest (compressions, defibrillation, airway management, vascular access, medications) and training providers *before* the call to rapidly identify, prioritize, and take over any areas that are not being addressed as soon as they arrive on scene. The effectiveness of pit crew CPR is dependent on defining clear roles and responsibilities among team members. Tasks are divided among team members based on their training and experience so that each person has a clearly defined job. It is an outstanding example of how training together can allow providers with different certifications from various agencies to rapidly come together as a team to improve outcomes for critically ill patients.

## Diverse and Competent Skill Sets

As discussed, EMS providers often have varying levels of certification or licensure. Think of these diverse backgrounds and skill sets not as obstacles, but as opportunities to fill roles and responsibilities within a high-performing team. Again, the best way for a team to be effective during an emergency call is to practice with one another and become familiar with each other's tools, techniques, capabilities, and preferences, so that each team member is competent *before* the call comes in.

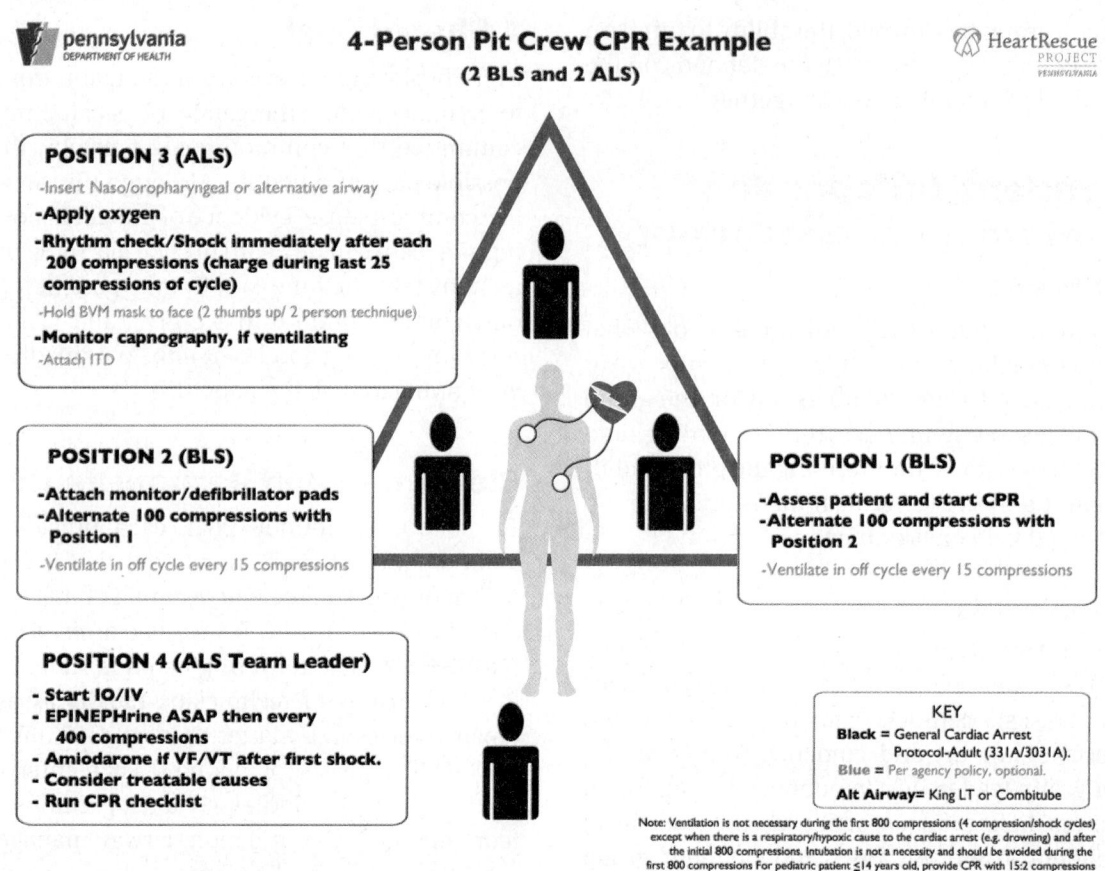

**FIGURE 9-2** Example of an overview of a four-person pit crew with two BLS providers that includes ALS providers. Although this example does not explicitly describe the pit crew model presented in the text, the same concepts can be applied to a BLS-only arrest. BLS providers may be in charge running the arrest or they may be participating in the arrest. Teamwork-oriented resuscitation can improve patient outcomes by minimizing the chance for error and improving team speed and efficiency.

Courtesy of University of Pennsylvania Perelman School of Medicine.

# YOU are the Provider

When you arrive on scene, a frantic bystander waves you inside. She tells you, "It's my husband! He isn't breathing!" As you walk to the front door, the fire officer meets you and tells you two EMRs are already inside caring for the patient. The scene is safe. As you enter the residence you find the patient, an older man, lying in a supine position on the floor of the living room. He is being ventilated with a bag-mask device by one EMR as another EMR performs a reassessment. As you approach the patient with your equipment bag, airway kit, and AED, the EMR looks up and tells you, "We've lost a pulse." He immediately starts chest compressions while you prepare the AED.

| Recording Time: 2 Minutes | |
|---|---|
| Appearance | Motionless |
| Level of consciousness | Unconscious and unresponsive |
| Airway | Open; maintained by fire department EMRs |
| Breathing | Absent; bag-mask ventilations at a rate of 1 breath every 5 seconds |
| Circulation | No pulse; skin cool and pale; CPR has been started |

**3.** Which roles will need to be assigned to perform cardiac arrest resuscitation?

**4.** The AED analyzes the patient's heart rhythm and advises you whether to deliver a shock. How can your team maximize patient perfusion and minimize "hands-off" time during this part of the cardiac arrest?

## Effective Collaboration and Communication

For team members to collaborate successfully, you must communicate effectively with one another. Four important elements of team communication include:

- **A clear message.** Speak calmly, confidently, and concisely so that the information delivered or the action requested is clear to your listeners. Be clear who you are speaking to by using names or ranks when giving direction, as opposed to just asking "someone" to do a task.
- **Closed-loop communication.** When a team member speaks, you should repeat the message back to him or her. This technique helps confirm that you heard and understand the message, and will act on it.
- **Courtesy.** All team members expect and deserve to be spoken to politely. "Please" and "thank you" do not take that much time.
- **Constructive intervention.** Sometimes it is necessary for you to respectfully question or correct team members (or the team leader) if you believe a mistake has been or is about to be made. This technique is not only allowed and encouraged—it is essential for effective team performance.

## Supportive and Coordinated Leadership

The **team leader** is the team member who provides role assignments, coordination, oversight, centralized decision making, and support for the team to accomplish their goals and achieve desired results. The team leader is often defined by policy, procedure, or statute. He or she may be the most senior provider in the group or the person with the highest level of certification. A team leader who simply commands others is not leading a team; he or she is simply directing a dependent group. A key differentiation between a team leader and a group leader is that a team leader helps the individual team members to do their jobs not only by providing support but also by working together with them and facilitating coordination. In this way, a team leader helps the team produce a better outcome than is possible with a simple group. Team leaders also foster communication and team dynamics using concepts such as crew resource management and team

situational awareness (the knowledge and understanding of one's surroundings and the ability to recognize potential threats to safety).

## Effective Team Membership

A team leader cannot manage an emergency call alone. Skilled team members are needed to ensure that critical calls are managed safely and effectively. Good team members communicate effectively; accept feedback; are good followers; have confidence, compassion, and maturity; maintain situational awareness; and use appreciative, or positive, inquiry to approach organization change. They use closed-loop communication, perform tasks accurately and in a timely manner, and then report progress on those tasks to the team leader. Good team members treat their fellow team members with respect, regardless of their rank or experience. It is a team member's responsibility to speak up immediately and suggest a corrective action if a harmful action is ordered or performed by others or if a procedure is not being performed but is indicated. Each person on the team is accountable for the safety and well-being of the patient and other crew members.

### Street Smarts

An essential component of teamwork is trust. Team members must be able to trust each other to do their best, do what is correct, and watch out for each other. Trust must be earned. As a team member, you must continually be diligent to maintain a good attitude, skill proficiency, and current knowledge.

## Crew Resource Management

Crew resource management (CRM) is a way for team members to work together with the team leader to develop and maintain a shared understanding of the emergency situation. CRM allows team members with different skill sets to collaborate and communicate, fulfill their roles and responsibilities, and achieve the shared goal of the best possible patient outcome (**FIGURE 9-3**). The concept of CRM says that each member is responsible for maintaining awareness of the current patient situation and sharing any critical information with the team leader. Likewise, the team leader is responsible for listening to any critical information provided by you or other team members, and incorporating it into his or her decision making.

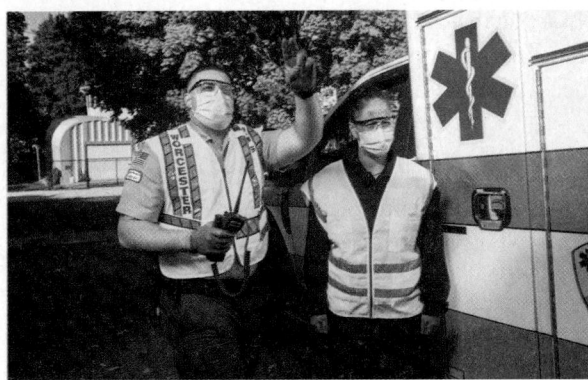

**FIGURE 9-3** Collaboration and communication are crucial aspects of crew resource management.
© Jones & Bartlett Learning.

In the noisy and often distracting environment in which EMS providers work, it is easy for errors to occur. Misunderstandings and misinterpretations may occur due to situational awareness failures. These failures are more likely when one or more emergency responders do not accurately perceive what is happening, such as when there is a lack of information. For example, on some calls, providers may not know crucial details of the patient's medical history, data may be hard to detect or interpret (eg, trying to hear lung sounds when it is noisy), or providers may fail to monitor data, such as forgetting to put on the pulse oximeter to measure the oxygen level.

Errors and miscommunication can occur when an EMT sends or receives a message. To reduce the incidence of errors on either end of the communication chain, providers should use closed-loop communication. In this system, each member confirms that a message has been received correctly so both parties know they share the same understanding. Here is an example of closed-loop communication: EMT Aziz says, "Let's go with 2 liters of oxygen." His partner Becky replies, "Got it. I'll put him on 10 liters of oxygen." Aziz recognizes immediately that his partner did not receive the message he intended and he responds, "No, not 10 liters. We need to go with 2 liters." His partner Becky then replies, "Got it. I'll put him on 2 liters of oxygen."

There are times when even the most seasoned EMS crew members lose situational awareness or make an error. When you believe there is an immediate or potential problem that must be brought to the attention of the team leader, first, get the attention of the crew member, then use the PACE mnemonic:

- **P** *Probe.* Look or ask to confirm the problem or make sense of the situation.
- **A** *Alert.* Communicate the problem to the team leader.
- **C** *Challenge.* If the issue is not corrected, then clearly challenge the team's current course of action that is leading to the problem and suggest an alternative plan. For example, "Lieutenant, I think this additional action should be taken. Do you agree?"
- **E** *Emergency.* If the problem is clear and critical (such as an immediate safety issue), then immediately communicate the emergency to the entire team. This is used when there is an imminent and serious danger.

If the other team member agrees that the original plan should be altered, it is essential for the leader to communicate the change to everyone else on the team.

The CRM concept does not mean you are free to ignore the chain of command within the incident command system or NIMS structure. It means you are empowered to provide the team leader and other team members with immediate feedback in the event of a potential threat to patient or crew safety. It means the team, as a whole, recognizes the importance of every individual's input and that the team is committed to creating open lines of communication. CRM empowers people to speak clearly and concisely when they detect a problem or potential problem.

## Words of Wisdom

It is essential to speak up when there is an error of omission (something not being done) or commission (something being done incorrectly or inappropriately). It is also important to avoid side conversations and commentary when managing a patient. Nonessential conversation can be distracting, creates unnecessary noise, and can lead to errors in patient care.

## Transfer of Patient Care

Although effective health care teams work together from first patient contact to patient discharge, clearly not all providers will be present throughout the entire continuum of care. At several points along the continuum, the patient's care will be transferred, or "handed off," from one unit of providers on the team to another. These transfers introduce the possibility of critical patient care errors, especially when they occur several times and in different settings along the continuum of care. Effective teams minimize the number of transfers during patient care, and adhere to strict and careful guidelines when such transfers are unavoidable.

Just like in a relay race, a proper transfer of patient care will allow the team to keep moving forward with patient care. When incorrect information is handed off, information is miscommunicated, or care is interrupted, the team is forced to move backward, resulting in a loss of valuable time and effort. For this reason, it is important for you to trust other team members—even those who work at different levels or for various agencies. For example, if an EMR reports a patient had a syncopal episode, but the patient is now alert, then do not assume the EMR's information is incorrect.

## General Guidelines

If possible, a single person—the team leader—should coordinate the patient's transfer of care and report the patient information. Whenever the verbal

transfer of care occurs, all team members should do their best to ensure the following:

1. **Uninterrupted critical care.** Whenever possible, the team member giving the report and the team member taking the report should hand off life-saving care (such as performing chest compressions) to another team member, allowing them to focus on the transfer of care.
2. **Minimal interference.** The transfer of patient care should occur in a location with the least interference possible. If the transfer takes place at the patient's side, it should not occur while the patient is being moved.
3. **Respectful interaction.** Each team member involved in the transfer must be respectful of members' different roles and recognize the importance of each role.
4. **Common priorities.** Both the team member giving the report and the team member taking the report must focus on their common priorities (critical assessment findings and patient care) vital for the best possible patient outcome.
5. **Common language or system.** Whenever possible, a mutually agreed-on and standardized patient handoff format should be used.

See Chapter 4, *Communications and Documentation*, for information on patient care reports (PCRs).

## YOU are the Provider

After the AED reanalyzes and advises a shock, you clear the patient and deliver the defibrillation, quickly directing the two EMRs to rotate compressors and continue CPR. As the EMRs continue compressions and bag-mask ventilations, the paramedics arrive.

| Recording Time: 12 Minutes | |
| --- | --- |
| Respirations | Absent; ventilations are being assisted |
| Pulse | Absent; fire department EMR performing CPR |
| Skin | Cool and cyanotic |
| Blood pressure | Not obtainable; the patient has no pulse |
| Oxygen saturation (Spo$_2$) | Not obtainable; the patient has no pulse |

While your partner gathers a medical history from the patient's wife and the fire officer collects the patient's medications, one of the paramedics asks you to assist her in setting up to intubate the patient.

**5.** When should you give the patient's medical history and medication list to the paramedic?

**6.** How should you respond if you notice that the EMR doing CPR is compressing at an inappropriate rate?

## BLS and ALS Providers Working Together

In the world of prehospital emergency care, BLS and ALS care cannot exist independently of each other. For example, if a patient experiences sudden cardiac arrest, then BLS care (high-quality CPR and defibrillation) are the core interventions around which ALS providers build their resuscitative efforts. It would be a mistake to think of BLS care as only the first steps of ALS care. As an EMT, you may begin BLS efforts early, but keep in mind that BLS efforts must continue throughout the continuum of care. To successfully stabilize and treat the patient's condition, you must carefully coordinate your efforts with the advanced tools and techniques used by ALS providers. Remember, excellent communication skills and teamwork are essential elements of emergency medicine. Each member of the EMS team must work in harmony with one goal in mind—high-quality patient care.

As mentioned previously, all team members, regardless of their level of licensure, are responsible for the safety of the patient, crew, and bystanders

on an EMS call. The skilled EMT may recognize a dangerous situation or possible error that others on scene have not noticed, even higher-level providers. It is essential for the EMT to speak up in such instances. In an effective EMS system, all members have the confidence to voice concerns, and all members have the professionalism to listen.

## Where BLS Care Ends and ALS Care Begins

Many patient care skills can be considered advanced; however, the tools and techniques that you can use as an EMT versus those that are reserved for ALS providers vary from system to system. What may be a paramedic-only skill in your EMS system may be common for an AEMT or EMT to perform in another.

It is your responsibility to understand what is allowed by the scope of practice, standard of care, and local protocols where you work. These topics are discussed in greater detail in Chapter 3, *Medical, Legal, and Ethical Issues*. If you work outside these bounds, such as performing a skill for which you are not authorized, then you risk legal liability. This liability is not reduced because you were unaware you were "not supposed to do that."

It is just as important to understand that, as a key part of the emergency team, there are many ways in which you can assist paramedics and other ALS providers with advanced procedures.

For an EMS team to effectively perform an advanced skill, its members should train and practice together. Although a good EMT knows what he or she is allowed to do in assisting with an advanced procedure, a great EMT has the foundational knowledge to understand the procedure. Most important, you must understand that when using any advanced tool or technique, the focus is always on achieving a goal (solving a clinical problem) rather than simply completing a procedure.

## Assisting With ALS Skills

As an EMT, there are many different ALS skills with which you may be able to assist. The exact list of ALS procedures and how they are to be performed will vary from system to system. In general, assisting follows a four-step process: (1) patient preparation, (2) equipment setup, (3) performing the procedure, and (4) continuing care. Specific steps to assist with advanced airway skills and vascular access are discussed in subsequent chapters.

# Critical Thinking and Clinical Decision Making in EMS

EMTs in some systems work with an EMT partner and are the primary decision makers on the ambulance. When a life threat occurs, the EMT must make critical decisions (often many) that can affect the patient's outcome. Effective decisions are based on sound up-to-date knowledge and the information provided from the patient, the patient's history, and physical examination. EMTs must use a series of steps to ensure the proper course of action is chosen. These steps occur throughout the call.

## Stages of the Decision-Making Process

### Prearrival

The decision-making process on many calls begins when the initial dispatch information is received. Knowing the nature of the emergency, especially when the call is low frequency and high risk, can help the EMT prepare, even before arriving on the scene. En route to the call, the EMT should mentally rehearse the steps in the care that may be needed. A leader should be clearly designated. Crew members can discuss their roles, what additional help may be needed, what equipment should be taken in, and what transport destination should be considered. For example, if the call is for a pediatric cardiac arrest, consider the ratio of compressions to ventilations needed and the size of equipment, such as the bag-mask device that will be used.

### Arrival

Provide the scene size-up and request additional resources as soon as possible. Position equipment in a standard location when possible so other responders can anticipate where to find supplies when needed. Assess and intervene for life threats immediately.

The EMT must first consider and treat life threats. When given information about the patient, EMTs should first rule out the worst-case scenario. The acronym ROWS (*r*ule *o*ut *w*orst-case *s*cenario) is sometimes used to remember this step.

## During the Call

Although the overall goals of the scene are to find and treat life threats and transport the patient to the appropriate facility, often many other small, short-term goals have to be achieved to accomplish these overall goals. The strategies the team leader uses to make decisions depend on the nature of the situation (**FIGURE 9-4**). The team leader must do the following:

1. **Gather data.** This begins with the dispatch information and continues when the EMT gathers the patient history and completes the physical examination.
2. **Interpret that data.** What do the data mean? Is there a clear pattern? Is more information needed?
3. **Develop a plan.** The EMT determines what treatment is needed based on the information at hand.
4. **Communicate the plan to the team and implement it.** During this time, the team leader reflects on whether it is the right choice and invites feedback from the team.
5. **Evaluate the effect of the decision.** During this phase, the patient and situation are reassessed. Based on this reevaluation, the team either continues with the plan or adjusts it.

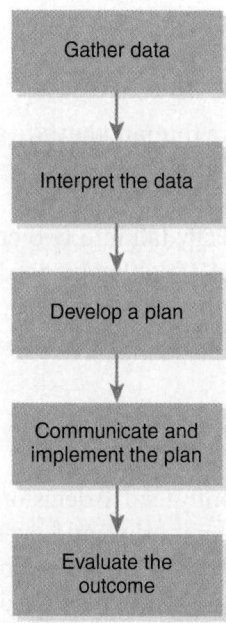

**FIGURE 9-4** Strategies the team leader can use to make decisions.

© Jones & Bartlett Learning.

For example, an EMT crew treating a patient with chest discomfort, possibly experiencing a heart attack, may make an initial determination to not administer oxygen because the patient is not short of breath. Reassessment reveals the patient is now experiencing mild shortness of breath. The EMT crew should change the initial treatment plan and administer oxygen.

## After the Call

After a stressful or complicated call, it is important to debrief and talk about what happened. If the team consists of an EMT and his or her partner, that discussion can be informal and happen during the cleanup after the call. Sometimes this is called a back-step debrief. For complex calls, a department may assemble the entire team to talk about the call. Formal debriefings may include the medical director, supervisory staff, and personnel from other departments. These should be structured to help everyone gain an understanding of what happened on the call (not everyone has the same perspective), what went well, and what opportunities exist for improvement. EMTs should listen to the feedback with an open mind. Moving from novice to expert practice means being willing to listen to suggestions for improvement and being willing to change.

## Decision Traps

Because EMTs are human, they are subject to mental blocks that can lead to errors in decision making. Although decision traps may come in many forms, they typically fall into two categories: those that cause the EMT to either overestimate or underestimate the probability of disease or injury and those that result in failure to consider all reasonable possibilities.

## Common Decision Traps in EMS

Traps that frequently lead to decision-making errors in EMS are bias, anchoring, and overconfidence.

Everyone has biases. Biases are fixed beliefs about something. Once established, they are hard to rethink. It can be harmful when an EMT remains locked into the bias and considers only one possible idea, ignoring or not seeking other data. For example, suppose a patient has fallen and has an altered level of consciousness. This patient is known to be an alcoholic and has an odor resembling alcohol on his breath. The EMT assumes he is drunk and while gathering the patient's history asks only questions that follow that path. As a result, the EMT fails to ask detailed questions about the nature of the fall or the patient's other signs and symptoms and misses the fact that the patient has sustained a head injury.

Another type of error, anchoring, occurs when the EMT settles on one possible cause of the patient's problems early (sometimes before the call) and fails to consider other options. For example, EMTs arrive to find a 24-year-old woman with a history of asthma who is short of breath. They quickly administer a breathing treatment and begin transport without completing their assessment. Due to their incomplete assessment, they fail to realize that, although the patient does have asthma, today she is having a life-threatening allergic reaction (anaphylaxis), and her condition worsens en route to the hospital.

Overconfidence is another decision trap that some EMTs fall into. It occurs when the EMT overestimates his or her ability. In this case, ability may apply to skills such as emergency driving, assessment, splinting, or decision making. Overconfidence may cause the EMT to ignore others when they disagree with a decision, resulting in actions that harm either the patient, the crew, or the public.

## Avoiding Decision Traps

The first step toward avoiding errors related to bias is developing a solid knowledge base and an organized approach to patient care that is consistent and thorough. EMTs must also recognize their blind spots—areas where they know biases exist, such as those related to intoxicated patients, obese patients, or older adults. Knowing those biases exist should set off an alarm on those calls, signaling the need to take extra care not to fall into a decision trap.

# Troubleshooting Team Conflicts

As outlined in this chapter, applying the principles of effective emergency health care teams will help to minimize interpersonal conflicts. However, because most emergency health care teams consist of highly trained, enthusiastic, and dedicated people, it is inevitable that conflict will arise from time to time. When conflict occurs, keep in mind the following five techniques:

- **The patient comes first.** Regardless of interpersonal conflicts that may arise, the patient's needs must always come first.
- **Do not engage.** If the problem causing the conflict does not directly and immediately affect patient care, then do not engage. Have the discussion after the call, when more positive communication may be possible.

- **Keep your cool.** Maintain your composure. If you feel that the conflict is over a critical component of patient care, then follow the PACE mnemonic discussed previously. If it is not, then begin by taking a deep breath and slowly counting to 10.
- **Separate the person from the issue.** If the conflict arises from the behavior of another team member and the conflict cannot be delayed or avoided, then focus on the behavior itself rather than the individual.
- **Choose your battles.** Remember, there is strength in the diversity of team members. Not everyone will work in exactly the same way, and that is a good thing. Avoid engaging in conflict over minor issues in patient care that center around one provider "style" over another.

## YOU are the Provider

The patient is intubated and has an IV line established. Before any medications are administered, the patient regains a pulse, even though he remains unconscious. You transport the patient to the local hospital, which is only a few minutes away. The paramedic gives a radio report while en route.

| Recording Time: 24 Minutes | |
|---|---|
| Level of consciousness | Unconscious and unresponsive |
| Respirations | 6 breaths/min (baseline); ventilations are being assisted |
| Pulse | 104 beats/min |
| Skin | Pale and cyanotic |
| Blood pressure | 104/80 mm Hg |
| Spo$_2$ | 92% (with assisted ventilation) |

On arrival, you bring the patient into the resuscitation room, where the ED team members await.

**7.** In the ED, if the paramedic is giving the handoff report, then who will ensure that patient care is continued during the transfer of care?

**8.** During the transfer of patient care, at what point is the EMS unit of the team relieved of responsibility for caring for the patient?

## YOU are the Provider SUMMARY

**1. How will you work together as a team with the EMRs?**

Because the EMRs will arrive at the scene before you, they will have begun patient care. When you arrive, begin by making contact with the EMR in charge while your partner assists the other EMRs. You should gather information about the patient's current condition as well as the care that has already been provided, so you understand the patient care priorities as well as which roles need to be filled and what tasks need to be completed. This information-gathering step will allow you to seamlessly integrate into the patient care team for the call already in progress.

**2. How will members of this team decide who will perform each role?**

Throughout the emergency call, provider roles and responsibilities will change as patient needs and available resources change. In some cases, certain roles will need to be filled by providers with specific levels of expertise or advanced certifications. In other cases, local protocol will require the highest-certified or most senior provider to be the team leader. Be aware that it will not always be necessary (and may even set the team back) for an arriving responder to take over simply because they have a higher certification. For example, if you arrive on this scene to find the patient in respiratory arrest with an EMR already providing ventilations, then it may not be helpful to stop the EMR and have him or her hand over the procedure. The most helpful way, assuming there are no higher patient priorities at that time, would be for you to step into another necessary but unfilled role or to verify that the ventilations by the EMR are adequately done and then focus on other procedures that need to be accomplished. In this case, you can check that compressions are being done correctly while you are applying the AED.

**3. Which roles will need to be assigned to perform cardiac arrest resuscitation?**

Depending on local protocol, the next role is to manage the patient's airway and breathing. If the person filling this role is a BLS provider, then he or she will utilize a bag-mask device, oxygen, and airway adjuncts as allowed by local protocol. If an ALS provider arrives, then he or she may assume this role from a BLS provider. In this scenario, this role has already been filled by the second EMR, but a paramedic may intubate or utilize another advanced airway. That paramedic may take over ventilations, but in most cases will have an EMT or EMR resume ventilation through the endotracheal tube or advanced airway. If advanced providers are available, the next function in a cardiac arrest would be to gain vascular access and administer medication. In this situation, one of the paramedics would fulfill this role.

If enough providers are available, then a fifth role is that of team leader, who directs the care given. His or her tasks include gathering patient history and assessment information from the family, bystanders, or the first responders, formulating a resuscitation plan, and coordinating all of the other roles. In some cases the team leader will change. In this case, you or your partner may have been the team leader making decisions about the resuscitation until ALS arrived. Often in medical situations, the paramedic will assume the team leader role after receiving the assessment, history, and treatment information already gathered by the previous providers on the scene. Other times, such as at trauma scenes, hazmat scenes, or mass-casualty incidents, a fire officer can fulfill this role until the patient is transported, when team leadership would likely be taken over by one of the transporting providers.

**4. The AED analyzes the patient's heart rhythm and advises you whether to deliver a shock. How can your team maximize patient perfusion and minimize "hands-off" time during this part of the cardiac arrest?**

The provider performing CPR (the EMR) should resume compressions immediately after the shock is delivered, without having to be directed to do so by the team leader.

In general, methods for minimizing hands-off time will depend greatly on the amount of training and practice the providers on the resuscitation team have had prior to the call. After any defibrillation, CPR should resume immediately after the shock is delivered, regardless of the patient's cardiac rhythm—unless the patient has obvious signs of circulation (such as movement, breathing, or speaking). In a well-coordinated team, all team members should understand this priority, even if the team members hold different levels of certification or are from different organizations. However, team members who have not practiced or worked together before are likely to wait until they are given specific direction from a team leader because they do not know what to expect next.

In cardiac resuscitation, this can lead to delays in the resumption of CPR, which negatively affects the patient's chances of successful resuscitation.

**5. When should you give the patient's medical history and medication list to the paramedic?**

As a single ALS provider arriving on scene of a cardiac resuscitation, the paramedic will have multiple roles that he or she may need to fill. The most obvious role is that of team leader. However, a dilemma the paramedic may face is that he or she may be the only one able to complete certain ALS-level tasks such as cardiac rhythm interpretation, obtaining vascular access, and medication administration.

As a result, the exact answer to this question will depend on the specifics of the situation. Generally, most ALS providers assuming the role of team leader on arrival will want an immediate report of priority patient concerns, priority assessment, medical history, and key interventions that have been performed. This brief, priority-only report is typically verbal, not written. Therefore, in this case, you should provide a verbal report to the paramedic as soon as possible on arrival.

Although not always possible, it is recommended that the full patient demographics, medical history, medication list, and other pertinent information be written down in a clear format and turned over to the paramedic team leader for additional reference, and then turned over to the team members on arrival at the ED.

**6. How should you respond if you notice that the EMR doing CPR is performing compressions at an inappropriate rate?**

If you notice that a member of the patient care team is not completing a task correctly, you have an obligation to speak up. It is inappropriate to allow known and witnessed errors to occur during a patient care event without offering input for correction. The CRM techniques discussed in this chapter provide a format for team members to appropriately and professionally interact to ensure the best patient care is being performed. Gain the attention of the person doing CPR or the team leader. State the concern as

you see it: "I believe the rate of compressions should be faster. Do you agree?" This allows team members to reflect on action and make corrections without placing blame or criticism.

**7. In the ED, if the paramedic is giving the handoff report, then who will ensure that patient care is continued during the transfer of care?**

It is important for other team members to avoid interrupting or causing interference with the handoff report. It is just as important for team members to ensure that priority treatments (think ABCs) are continued during the transfer of care until treatments are assumed by the receiving team members.

It is for this reason that many team-focused patient handoff protocols specify that all priority treatments must be completely taken over by the receiving team before the handoff report is given. This ensures that the team's complete attention can be given to the person (in this case, the paramedic) providing the report. Many protocols even include a specific, so-called moment of silence to ensure that the report is given only once and that all team members received the information. This is especially important during critical care handoffs such as this cardiac arrest, but this concept can also apply to severe trauma, and "alert" situations such as a heart attack, stroke, and sepsis.

**8. During the transfer of patient care, at what point is the EMS unit of the team relieved of responsibility for caring for the patient?**

It is crucial for team members to ensure that patient care continues through any transition of team members, from the time you arrive on scene to join the team to the moment you hand off care to your team members in the ED.

Once the handoff is complete, it is important for you to ask if your team members in the ED have any remaining questions or need anything else from you. Do not make assumptions. Ask explicit questions aloud, such as "Do you have any questions?" and "Is there anything else that you need from me?" You should receive a clear response from the team members to whom you are handing off patient care.

## EMS Patient Care Report (PCR)

| **Date:** 7-20-20 | **Incident No.:** 0101855 | **Nature of Call:** Unresponsive | | **Location:** 6 Catoonah St. | |
|---|---|---|---|---|---|
| **Dispatched:** 0905 | **En Route:** 0905 | **At Scene:** 0912 | **Transport:** 0937 | **At Hospital:** 0943 | **In Service:** 1034 |

### Patient Information

| | |
|---|---|
| **Age:** 72 | **Allergies:** Cipro |
| **Sex:** M | **Medications:** Atorvastatin |
| **Weight (in kg [lb]):** 90 kg estimated (198 lb) | **Past Medical History:** Chronic obstructive pulmonary disease |
| | **Chief Complaint:** Cardiac arrest |

### Vital Signs

| Time | BP | Pulse | Respirations | Spo$_2$ |
|---|---|---|---|---|
| **Time:** 0910 | **BP:** Unable to obtain | **Pulse:** 71 | **Respirations:** 8 | **Spo$_2$:** 82% |
| **Time:** 0912 | **BP:** N/A | **Pulse:** 0 | **Respirations:** 0 | **Spo$_2$:** N/A |
| **Time:** 0919 | **BP:** N/A | **Pulse:** 0 | **Respirations:** 0 | **Spo$_2$:** N/A |
| **Time:** 0937 | **BP:** N/A | **Pulse:** 0 | **Respirations:** 0 | **Spo$_2$:** N/A |
| **Time:** 0941 | **BP:** 104/80 | **Pulse:** 104 | **Respirations:** 6 baseline, ventilations assisted | **Spo$_2$:** 92%, ventilations assisted |

### EMS Treatment (circle all that apply)

| Oxygen @ 15 L/min via:<br><br>NC    NRM    (Bag mask) | | Assisted Ventilation | Airway Adjunct:<br>(OPA) | CPR |
|---|---|---|---|---|
| **Defibrillation** | **Bleeding Control** | **Bandaging** | **Splinting** | **Other:** (Assisted with ET intubation and vascular access) |

### Narrative

Unit 118-1 co-dispatched with fire department EMRs and paramedic unit to a private residence for a 72-year-old male "unresponsive patient."

Chief Complaint: Cardiac arrest

History: On arrival, patient was reported to be in respiratory arrest under care of EMRs. Patient history of COPD obtained from spouse. Paramedic arrival at 0915.

Assessment: On reassessment, patient found to be pulseless and apneic.

Treatment (Rx): CPR initiated by EMRs. AED applied by EMS. Shock advised and delivered. CPR continued rotating compressors every 2 minutes. EMS assisted with advanced airway placement and vascular access. Before medications were administered, patient regained pulse, but remained unconscious.

Transport: Patient moved onto a backboard for transport with assistance of EMRs in case CPR might be needed if patient arrested during transport. Paramedic gave radio report en route. Upon arrival at ED, care was assumed by ED staff. Verbal report was given to attending physician (team leader). Written patient history and medications were given to RN (resuscitation team recorder). ED staff confirmed no further questions. Transfer of care complete at 0935. Unit 118-1 cleared the hospital and returned to service at 1000 hrs.

**End of report**

# Prep Kit

## Ready for Review

- Just culture is an approach to leadership in organizations that balances fairness and accountability and encourages people to report errors and near misses. It focuses on risk management.
- Emergency health care providers must know how to work effectively as a unified team, from first patient contact to patient discharge. Ensuring consistent patient care across all team members is known as the continuum of care.
- Although some EMS systems allow EMTs to work together in regular teams, others require providers to assemble their teams "on the fly" for each call (temporary teams). It is especially important for team members to train and practice together if they are from different organizations.
- An effective team must work interdependently toward a shared goal (best possible patient outcome) instead of focusing on individual, task-based goals (such as splinting an arm or starting an IV line).
- An effective team must have clearly defined roles and responsibilities. The diverse and highly competent team members must communicate and collaborate efficiently under supported and coordinated leadership.

- An effective team must have a team leader to coordinate and guide decision making. For this system to work, every member must be responsible for maintaining individual situational awareness and conveying critical information to each other and to the team leader.
- For all emergency health care providers to work together successfully, they must be well versed in efficient patient handoff techniques.
- The ALS skills with which you may assist will vary from EMS system to EMS system, but you will generally follow a four-step process: (1) patient preparation, (2) equipment setup, (3) performing the procedure, and (4) continuing care.
- Effective decision making is an ongoing process that may be broken down into stages, according to factors that should be considered before arrival, on arrival, during the call, and after the call.
- EMTs must be aware of and avoid decision traps, such as bias, anchoring, and overconfidence, which can lead to decision-making errors.

## Vital Vocabulary

**community paramedicine** A health care model in which experienced paramedics receive advanced training to equip them to provide additional services in the prehospital environment, such as health evaluations, monitoring of chronic illnesses or conditions, and patient advocacy.

**continuum of care** The concept of consistent patient care across the entire health care team from first patient contact to patient discharge; working together with a unified goal results in improved individual and team performance,

better patient and provider safety, and improved patient outcome.

**crew resource management (CRM)** A set of procedures for use in environments where human error can have disastrous consequences. It empowers people within a team to communicate effectively with one another with a goal of improving team situational awareness, patient and crew safety, and overall communication.

**group** In the context of EMS, a collection of individual health care providers working independently to help the patient.

**mobile integrated healthcare (MIH)** A method of delivering health care that involves providing health care within the community rather than at a physician's office or hospital.

**situational awareness** Knowledge and understanding of one's surroundings and the ability to recognize potential risks to the safety of the patient or EMS team.

**team** In the context of EMS, a group of health care providers who are assigned specific roles and are working interdependently in a coordinated manner under a designated leader.

**team leader** The team member who provides role assignments, coordination, oversight, centralized decision making, and support for the team to accomplish their goals and achieve desired results.

## References

1. EMS Agenda 2050 Technical Expert Panel. *EMS Agenda 2050: A People-Centered Vision for the Future of Emergency Medical Services* (Report No. DOT HS 812 664). Washington, DC: National Highway Traffic Safety Administration; January 2019.

2. National Association of State EMS Officials. National Model EMS Clinical Guidelines: Version 2.2. https://nasemso.org/wp-content/uploads/National-Model-EMS-Clinical-Guidelines-2017-PDF-Version-2.2.pdf. Updated January 5, 2019. Accessed February 5, 2020.

3. National Highway Traffic Safety Administration. *National Emergency Medical Services Education Standards.* DOT HS 811 077A. www.ems.gov/pdf/811077a.pdf. Published January 2009. Accessed February 6, 2020.

4. National Highway Traffic Safety Administration. *National Emergency Medical Services Education Standards. Emergency Medical Technician Instructional Guidelines.* DOT HS 811 077C. www.ems.gov/pdf/811077c.pdf. Published January 2009. Accessed February 6, 2020.

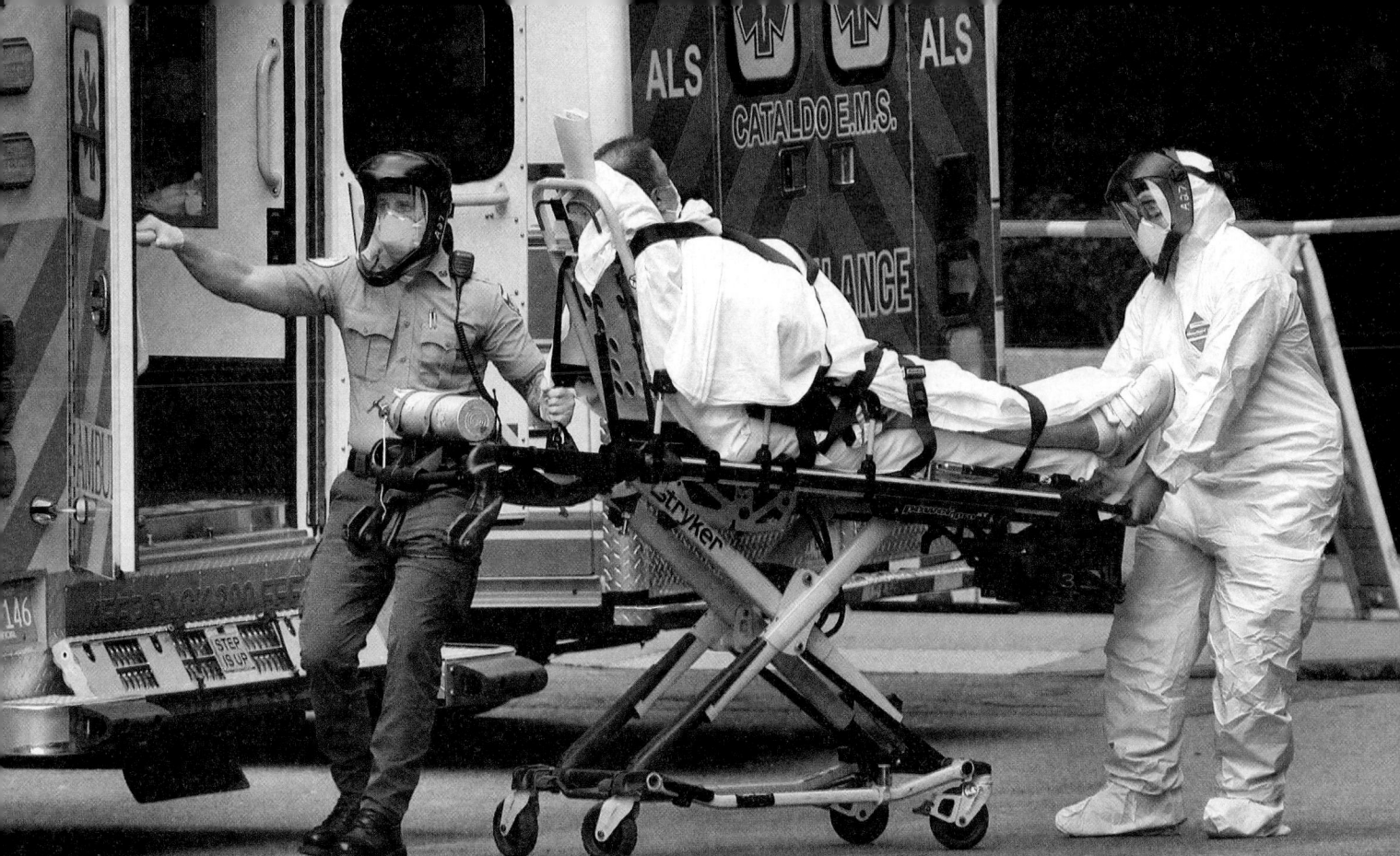

# SECTION

# 2

# Patient Assessment

**10** Patient Assessment

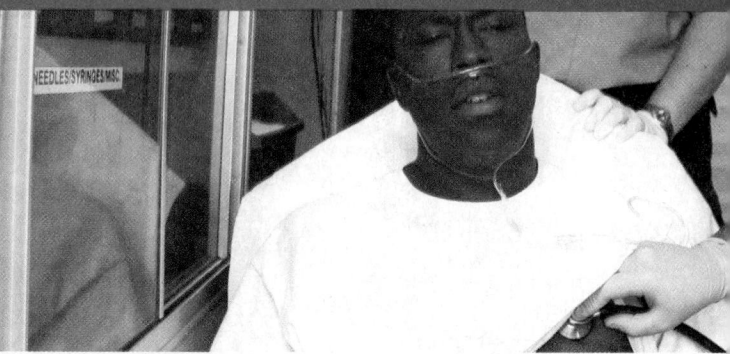

# Chapter 10

# Patient Assessment

## NATIONAL EMS EDUCATION STANDARD COMPETENCIES

### Assessment

Applies scene information and patient assessment findings (scene size-up, primary and secondary assessment, patient history, and reassessment) to guide emergency management.

### Scene Size-up

- Scene safety (pp 344–345)
- Scene management
  - Impact of the environment on patient care (pp 344–345)
  - Addressing hazards (p 345)
  - Violence (p 345)
  - Need for additional or specialized resources (p 349)
  - Standard precautions (pp 347–348)
  - Multiple patient situations (pp 348–349)

### Primary Assessment

- Primary assessment for all patient situations (pp 350–351)
  - Level of consciousness (pp 352–353)
  - ABCs (pp 354–361)
  - Identifying life threats (pp 352–353, 361–363)
  - Assessment of vital functions (pp 352–353, 357–358)
  - Initial general impression (p 351)
- Begin interventions needed to preserve life (pp 353–354, 360–363)
- Integration of treatment/procedures needed to preserve life (pp 363–365)

### History Taking

- Determining the chief complaint (pp 366–368)
- Mechanism of injury/nature of illness (pp 345–347)
- Associated signs and symptoms (pp 366–369)
- Investigation of the chief complaint (pp 367–369)
- Past medical history (pp 366–369)
- Pertinent negatives (p 369)

### Secondary Assessment

- Performing a rapid full-body scan (pp 377–379)
- Focused assessment of pain (pp 377–379, 383–401)
- Assessment of vital signs (pp 383–392, 401–404)
- Techniques of physical examination
  - Respiratory system (pp 383–387)
    - Presence of breath sounds (pp 385–387)
  - Cardiovascular system (pp 387–394)
  - Neurologic system (pp 394–398)
  - Musculoskeletal system (pp 399–401)
  - All anatomic regions (pp 398–401)

### Monitoring Devices

- Obtaining and using information from patient monitoring devices including (but not limited to)
  - Pulse oximetry (pp 401–402)
  - Noninvasive blood pressure (p 404)

### Reassessment

- How and when to reassess patients (p 405)
- How and when to perform a reassessment for all patient situations (pp 405–406)

# KNOWLEDGE OBJECTIVES

1. Identify the components of the patient assessment process. (p 342)

2. Explain how the different causes and presentations of emergencies will affect how EMTs perform each step of the patient assessment process. (p 342)

3. Discuss some of the possible environmental, chemical, and biologic hazards that may be present at an emergency scene, ways to recognize them, and precautions to protect personal safety. (pp 343–345)

4. Discuss the steps EMTs should take to survey a scene for signs of violence and protect themselves and bystanders from real or potential danger. (pp 343–345)

5. Describe how to determine the mechanism of injury (MOI) or nature of illness (NOI) at an emergency and the importance of differentiating trauma patients from medical patients. (pp 345–347)

6. List the minimum standard precautions that should be followed and personal protective equipment (PPE) that should be worn at an emergency scene, including examples of when additional precautions would be appropriate. (pp 347–348)

7. Explain why it is important for EMTs to identify the total number of patients at an emergency scene and how this evaluation relates to determining the need for additional or specialized resources, implementation of the incident command system (ICS), and triage. (pp 348–349)

8. Describe the principal goals of the primary assessment process, including how to identify and treat life threats and determine if immediate transport is required. (pp 350–351)

9. Explain the process of forming a general impression of a patient as part of primary assessment and the reasons why this step is critical to patient management. (p 351)

10. Explain the importance of assessing a patient's level of consciousness (LOC) to determine altered mental status and include examples of different methods used to assess alertness, responsiveness, and orientation. (pp 352–353)

11. Describe the assessment of airway status in patients who are both responsive and unresponsive, including examples of possible signs and causes of airway obstruction in each

case as well as the appropriate EMT response. (pp 354–355)

12. Describe the assessment of a patient's breathing status, including the key information EMTs must obtain during this process and the care required for patients who have adequate and inadequate breathing. (pp 355–357)

13. List the signs of respiratory distress and respiratory failure. (p 357)

14. Describe the assessment of a patient's circulatory status, including the different methods for obtaining a pulse and appropriate management depending on the patient's status. (pp 357–358)

15. Explain the variations required to obtain a pulse in infant and child patients compared with adult patients. (pp 357–358)

16. Describe the assessment of a patient's skin color, temperature, and condition, including examples of both normal and abnormal findings and the information this provides related to the patient's status. (pp 358–360)

17. Discuss the process of assessing and methods for controlling external bleeding. (pp 360–361)

18. Discuss the steps used to identify and subsequently treat life-threatening conditions that endanger a patient during an emergency. (pp 361–363)

19. List the steps EMTs should follow during the primary assessment of a trauma patient, including examples of abnormal signs and appropriate related actions. (pp 362–363)

20. Explain the process for determining the priority of patient care and transport at an emergency scene and include examples of conditions that necessitate immediate transport. (pp 363–365)

21. Discuss the importance of protecting a trauma patient's spine and identifying fractured extremities during patient packaging for transport. (pp 363–365)

22. Discuss the process of taking a focused history, its key components, and its relationship to the primary assessment process. (p 366)

23. Describe examples of different techniques EMTs may use to obtain information from patients during the history-taking process. (pp 368–376)

24. Discuss different challenges EMTs may face when taking a patient history on sensitive

topics and strategies that can be used to facilitate each situation. (pp 370–372)

25. Describe the purpose of a secondary assessment and a physical exam; include how to determine which aspects of the physical exam to use, and the steps. (pp 377–378)

26. Explain situations in which patients may receive a focused assessment, including examples by body system of what each focused assessment should include based on a patient's chief complaint. (pp 379–404)

27. List normal blood pressure ranges for adults, children, and infants. (p 394)

28. Explain the importance of performing a reassessment of the patient and the steps in this process. (pp 405–406)

## SKILLS OBJECTIVES

1. Demonstrate how to use the AVPU scale to test for patient responsiveness. (p 352)

2. Demonstrate how to evaluate a patient's orientation and document his or her status correctly. (pp 352–353)

3. Demonstrate the techniques for assessing a patient's airway, and correctly obtain information related to respiratory rate, rhythm, quality, and character of breathing, and depth of breathing. (pp 354–357)

4. Demonstrate how to assess a radial pulse in a responsive patient and an unresponsive patient. (pp 357–358)

5. Demonstrate how to assess a carotid pulse in an unresponsive patient. (pp 357–358)

6. Demonstrate how to palpate a brachial pulse in a child who is younger than 1 year. (pp 357–358)

7. Demonstrate how to obtain a pulse rate in a patient. (pp 357–358)

8. Demonstrate how to assess capillary refill in an adult or child older than 6 years. (p 360)

9. Demonstrate how to assess capillary refill in an infant or child younger than 6 years; include variations that would be required when assessing a newborn. (p 360)

10. Demonstrate how to perform a rapid exam during primary assessment of a patient. (pp 361–363, Skill Drill 10-1)

11. Demonstrate how to perform a secondary assessment. (pp 379–383, Skill Drill 10-2)

12. Demonstrate how to measure blood pressure by auscultation. (p 391, Skill Drill 10-3)

13. Demonstrate how to measure blood pressure by palpation. (p 393, Skill Drill 10-4)

14. Demonstrate how to test pupil reaction in response to light in a patient and document his or her status correctly. (pp 394–396)

15. Demonstrate the assessment of neurovascular status. (pp 396–397, Skill Drill 10-5)

16. Demonstrate the use of a pulse oximetry device to evaluate the effectiveness of oxygenation in the patient. (pp 401–402)

17. Demonstrate the use of electronic devices to assist in determining the patient's blood pressure in the field. (p 404)

18. Demonstrate how to assess a patient's blood glucose level. (p 403, Skill Drill 10-6)

# Patient Assessment

## Scene Size-Up

Ensure scene safety
Determine mechanism of injury/nature of illness
Take standard precautions
Determine number of patients
Consider additional/specialized resources

## Primary Assessment[a]

Form a general impression
Assess level of consciousness
Assess the airway: identify and treat life threats
Assess breathing: identify and treat life threats
Assess circulation: identify and treat life threats
Perform primary assessment
Determine priority of patient care and transport

## History Taking

Investigate the chief complaint (history of present illness)
Obtain SAMPLE history

## Secondary Assessment: Medical

Systematically assess the patient
- Secondary assessment and/or focused assessment
Assess vital signs using the appropriate monitoring device

## Secondary Assessment: Trauma

Systematically assess the patient
- Secondary assessment and/or focused assessment
Assess vital signs using the appropriate monitoring device

## Reassessment

Repeat the primary assessment
Reassess vital signs
Reassess the chief complaint
Recheck interventions
Identify and treat changes in the patient's condition
Reassess the patient
- Unstable patients: every 5 minutes
- Stable patients: every 15 minutes

---

[a]Identify and control life-threatening external hemorrhage before assessing the airway.

## Introduction

One of the most important skills that you can develop as an EMT is the ability to assess your patients. This skill is used in every patient encounter and is the basis for all treatment you will provide as an EMT. This chapter provides the framework and information necessary for you to be able to understand and conduct the patient assessment. The assessment process is divided into five main parts:

1. Scene size-up
2. Primary assessment
3. History taking
4. Secondary assessment
5. Reassessment

Although these steps represent a logical approach to patient assessment, the order in which they are performed may vary depending on the patient's condition and the environment in which you find the patient. For example, the same components of patient assessment used to evaluate a medical patient are used to assess a trauma patient; however, it may be necessary to change the order of some steps after scene size-up based on your findings and the need to prioritize the care of certain conditions. Regardless of the patient's complaint or the environment in which you find yourself, the key to effective patient assessment is to remain organized.

Rarely does one sign or symptom show you the patient's status or underlying problem. Rather, it is the combination of signs and symptoms that will direct the care you provide for your patient. A **symptom** is a subjective condition that the patient feels and tells you about. A **sign** is an objective condition that you can observe or measure. Therefore,

it is essential to have a basic understanding of the causes and presentations of commonly encountered emergencies, as this information can help you formulate a **field impression** (conclusion about the cause of the patient's condition after considering the situation, history, and examination findings) that will help you determine your priorities of care.

For example, a man with chest pain may be having a heart attack. Or, he may have a lung infection, a pulmonary embolism, or a simple strained muscle in the chest. He may also have sustained chest trauma. He describes the pain as crushing, radiating down the left arm and up into the jaw; he is pale and soaked in sweat; the episode began while he was shoveling snow; he has a history of coronary bypass surgery; and he has nitroglycerin in his pocket. On the basis of this information, it seems likely the patient is experiencing, and should be treated for, a myocardial infarction.

As an EMT, the treatment you will provide for most patients is based on symptoms, not an exact diagnosis. Many conditions may have similar signs and symptoms. As your career in EMS progresses, you may begin to formulate a list of potential conditions or injuries that patients may be experiencing as you treat them. Remember, it is essential to collect all pertinent information and be able to interpret how it fits together.

### Words of Wisdom

Although the steps of patient assessment represent a logical approach to the evaluation of a patient, the order in which they are performed is determined by the patient's condition.

## YOU are the Provider

At 1815 hours, you are dispatched to an apartment complex at 3820 121st Street for an unresponsive person. Law enforcement officers have been dispatched. The weather is overcast and rainy, the temperature is 62°F (16.7°C), and the traffic is light. Your response time to the scene is approximately 4 minutes.

**1.** What are the components of patient assessment?

**2.** Will your assessment of the patient differ if he or she is injured versus ill? If so, how?

# Patient Assessment

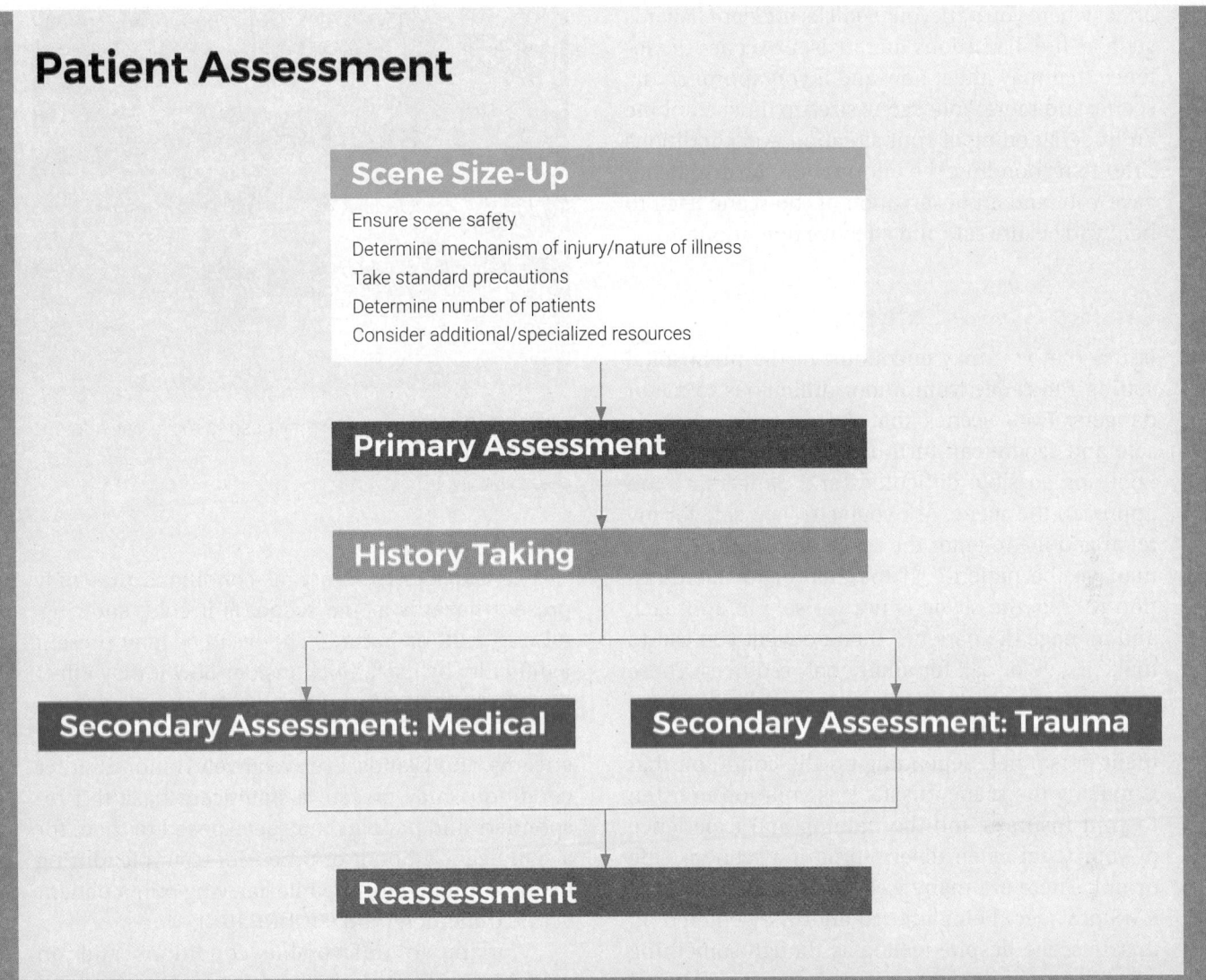

## Scene Size-up

**Scene size-up** refers to your evaluation of the conditions in which you will be operating. Although this will be the focus of your attention when you first arrive on scene, continuous **situational awareness** is necessary throughout the entire call to ensure safety. Situational awareness is paying attention to the conditions and people around you at all times and the potential risks those conditions or people pose.

For example, before you know the specific location of the incident, consider how the weather, time of day, currently available resources, and other incidents in the same response district may affect your ability to operate safely and effectively. Scene size-up is listed at the top of the assessment algorithm because it is the first thing you must consider, and it does not end when you move through the rest of the assessment process.

When you are alerted for an emergency call, the emergency medical dispatcher will provide you with some basic information about the request for your assistance. From the moment you are called into action until you reach your patient, you will consider a variety of things that will have an effect on how you operate on scene and provide patient care. These include road and traffic hazards that will affect where you park your vehicle; incident hazards such as fire, hazardous materials, or scenes of violence that may affect how and if you approach the scene; and more. Your scene size-up must combine an understanding of your situation and conditions prior to responding, the information the dispatcher gave you, and an observation of the scene itself to help you ensure safe and effective operations.

## Ensure Scene Safety

Issues that you may encounter in the prehospital setting can range from minor difficulties to major dangers. Even scenes that first appear relatively safe and secure can turn unsafe with little notice. Look for possible difficulties and dangers as you approach the scene. Ask yourself, "Is it safe for my team and me to enter the scene and approach and manage the patient?" If the answer to this question is, "No, the scene is not yet safe to approach and manage the patient," then do what you can to make it safe or call for additional resources. These resources may include firefighters, utility workers, hazardous materials technicians, or law enforcement personnel, depending on the condition that is making the scene unsafe. It is your job to listen to your instincts and the training and experience of your team when determining if a scene is safe or not. There are many well-documented cases of EMS providers being injured after they entered an unsafe scene despite feeling as though something was wrong.

Before you step out of your response vehicle, observe for issues such as uneven or unstable surfaces, water, mud, and ice on the ground. Remember, you have to gain access to a patient to provide care, typically while carrying gear and a stretcher with you. In addition, when you leave, you will be moving at least a 100-pound (45-kg) stretcher and possibly a patient weighing 200 pounds (90 kg) or more, as well as patient care equipment and the patient's personal belongings. If your footing was compromised going in, you are going to have an even more difficult time coming out.

Working on a roadway is particularly dangerous. Wear a high-visibility Class 2 or 3 safety vest and use appropriate safety precautions while responding to these incidents. See Chapter 2, *Workforce Safety and Wellness*, for further discussion of safe operations while working along a roadway.

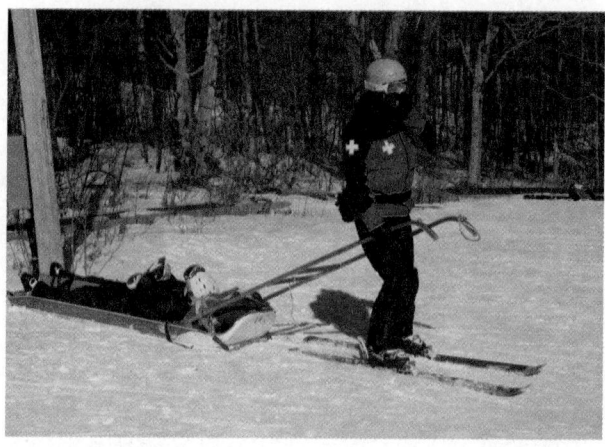

**FIGURE 10-1** At times, you may need to move patients out of areas with difficult terrain.
Courtesy of the National Ski Patrol.

Consider environmental conditions that may present hazards at the scene. Is it cold, snowing, raining, hot, or humid? The weather may present a difficulty by itself, but consider how it may affect the physical terrain you may encounter, such as wooded areas, hills, mountains, gorges, rivers, lakes, streams, and islands. Even relatively minor weather conditions may present a significant hazard if responders and patients may be exposed to them for a significant amount of time—for example, during a long approach to, or while carrying out, a patient across difficult terrain (**FIGURE 10-1**).

Working in unfavorable conditions and on unstable surfaces is a large part of prehospital care. Without knowing the infinite number of situations you may become involved in, a good rule to use when faced with a wide variety of possibilities is that any actions you may take to protect yourself (eg, heavy coats, rain gear, life jackets, air conditioned or heated vehicles) should also be considered for the patient. If you are putting on equipment to address environmental hazards and can safely do so, provide the patient with the same or similar equipment. If you move away from the scene to take cover from an environmental hazard, move the patient with you when possible. Taking your time to stay focused on what you are doing will go a long way in preventing injuries to yourself and your patients.

If appropriate, help protect bystanders from becoming patients as well. Many bystanders attempt to help during an emergency; always remember

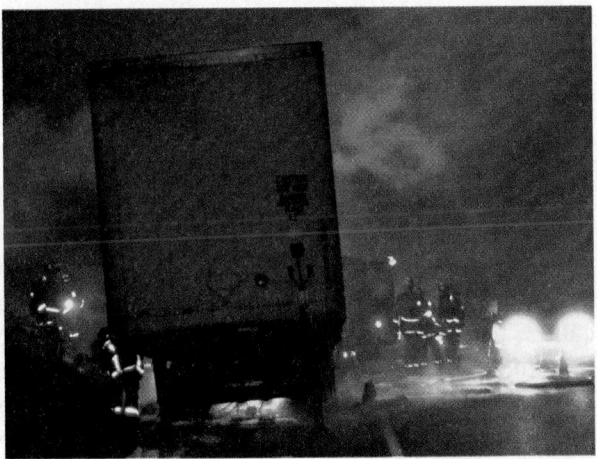

**FIGURE 10-2** Evaluate the scene for hazards as soon as you arrive.

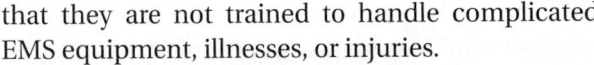
© Keith D. Cullom/www.fire-image.com.

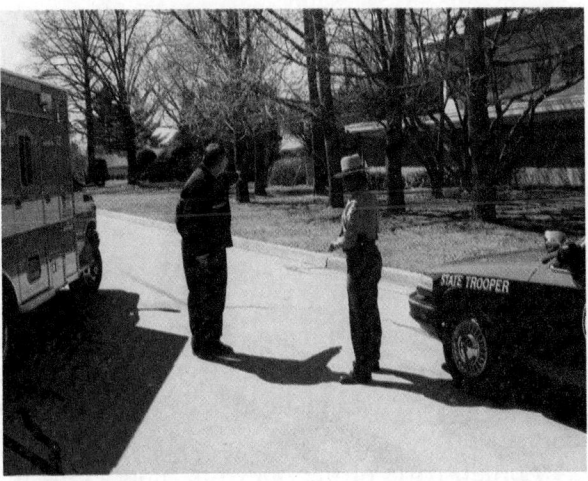

**FIGURE 10-3** If the scene is unsafe, request law enforcement support.

© Jones & Bartlett Learning. Courtesy of MIEMSS.

that they are not trained to handle complicated EMS equipment, illnesses, or injuries.

Hazards come in many different forms, shapes, and sizes. You may encounter environmental hazards; physical hazards (such as sharp metal and broken glass, or slip-and-fall hazards from leaking fluids at a motor vehicle crash); biohazards (such as blood and body fluids); chemical hazards (such as the release of a hazardous material); electrical hazards (such as downed power lines); water hazards; fires; explosions; and the threat of physical violence, to name a few (**FIGURE 10-2**).

You must be aware of scenes that have the potential for violence due to violent patients, distraught family members, angry bystanders, gangs, or unruly crowds. When you enter a patient's home, look around the immediate area. Do you see any weapons that the patient or others can access? Weapons may not be items typically associated with violence, such as a knife or gun; they can be household items such as a screwdriver or hammer, or other readily available objects sitting on the kitchen table or nightstand by the bed. Always be observant for such objects, and if they are not secured, make sure you place yourself between the patient and the potential danger, thus preventing possible access to the object. Request the assistance of law enforcement personnel if the scene presents the potential for violence (**FIGURE 10-3**). In some areas, law enforcement is dispatched with EMS on most calls. If this is not the approach used in your

area, you must request law enforcement assistance as soon as you think there may be danger. In some cases, you will need to quickly retreat from the scene until law enforcement arrives, or if you are not yet on the scene, stage at a safe location as defined by your local protocols until law enforcement advises that it is safe to proceed to the call. Responding to abandoned buildings and areas of known violence should raise your suspicions for the need for law enforcement.

An emergency scene is a dynamically changing environment and simply checking the safety of the scene once at the beginning of the call is not enough. As an EMT, you must remain aware of changes in your surroundings that may present safety hazards to you, your EMS team, the patient, or bystanders. Regardless of when the hazards present themselves, it is up to you to either make the scene safe, if you have the education and equipment to safely do so, or call for additional resources and move to a safe location.

## Determine Mechanism of Injury/Nature of Illness

Virtually all calls for assistance to which you may respond can be categorized as medical conditions, traumatic injuries, or both. Some emergency calls may involve a medical problem that leads to a traumatic injury, such as a patient who becomes weak and dizzy from a low blood glucose level, causing her to stumble, fall, and break her ankle. As an EMT, you will need to be able to identify the general classification and underlying issue or issues of the emergency to which you respond.

Traumatic injuries are the result of physical forces applied to the outside of the body, usually from an object striking the body or a body striking an object. These are generally classified according to the type or amount of force, how long it was applied, and where it was applied to the body. This is described as the **mechanism of injury (MOI)**. The MOI can be used as a guide to help you focus your assessment.

Certain parts of the body are more easily injured than others. The brain and the spinal cord are fragile and easy to injure. Fortunately, they are protected by the skull, the vertebrae, and several layers of soft tissues. The eyes are also easily injured. Even small forces on the eye may result in serious injury. The bones and certain organs are stronger and can absorb small forces without resulting significant injury. A good understanding of anatomy and physiology will help you identify times when the MOI may lead to injury to parts of the body not directly impacted. For example, consider a patient who has fallen off a roof, landing feetfirst. This patient's MOI would direct attention to possible injury to the feet. But significant energy likely transferred to other body areas and may have caused further injury in the patient's legs and pelvis, and even his or her spine.

Terms commonly associated with MOI include blunt trauma and penetrating trauma. With blunt trauma, the force of the injury occurs over a broad area, and the skin is sometimes not broken. However, the tissues and organs underneath the area of impact may be damaged. With penetrating trauma, the force of the injury occurs at the specific point of contact between the skin and the object. The object pierces the skin and creates an open wound that carries a higher potential for infection.

As an EMT, you will also care for patients who require EMS attention because of illnesses or conditions not caused by an outside force. For these patients with medical problems, you must examine the general type of illness the patient is experiencing, or the **nature of illness (NOI)**. An example of this would be a patient who tells you that he feels as if he cannot get enough air. This patient's NOI would be difficulty breathing and, like the MOI,

would help direct both your assessment and your care.

There are similarities between the MOI and the NOI. Both require you to search for clues about how the incident occurred or the problem developed. You must make an effort to determine the general type of illness, which is often best described by the patient's **chief complaint**, the most serious thing the patient is concerned about and the reason EMS was called. To quickly determine the NOI, talk with the patient, family, or bystanders about the problem. At the same time, use your senses to check the scene for clues as to the possible problem. You may see open or spilled medication containers, poisonous substances, or unsanitary living conditions. You may smell an unusual or strong odor, such as the odor of fresh paint in a closed room. You may hear a hissing sound, such as a leak from a home oxygen system. Keep these observations of the scene in mind as you begin to assess a medical patient.

Be aware of scenes with multiple patients who are exhibiting similar signs or symptoms. An example would be an older couple experiencing flu-like symptoms, headache, nausea, and vomiting. These symptoms may be indicative of carbon monoxide poisoning, which would also indicate an unsafe scene for you and your partner.

## The Importance of the MOI and NOI

Considering the MOI or NOI early can be of value in preparing to care for your patient. For example, when you begin to gather equipment from the unit, what would you take to treat a patient reporting chest pain? How would that equipment differ from the equipment used for a pedestrian struck by a vehicle? The appearance of the scene may also guide your preparation. Other MOIs may include falls, motor vehicle crashes, assaults, and industrial accidents. Examples of NOIs include seizures, heart attacks, diabetic problems, and poisonings. Family members, bystanders, or even law enforcement personnel may also provide important trauma or medical information to help you assist the patient.

You may be tempted to categorize your patient immediately as a trauma or medical patient. Remember, the fundamentals of a good patient assessment are the same despite the unique aspects of trauma and medical care. If an unconscious patient is found at the bottom of a ladder, did he or she fall off the ladder, strike his head, and become unconscious? Or did he or she experience a medical problem that caused him or her to have a loss of consciousness and then fall off the ladder? Early in the assessment, it can be difficult to identify with absolute certainty whether the problem is of a traumatic or medical origin. Although further assessment is needed to come to a conclusion, considering the MOI or NOI early will help you begin your assessment.

## Street Smarts

Although it is always a good idea to start formulating a plan as you respond to the call, it is important to note that there are times when the dispatch information does not match the NOI or MOI that you find on the scene. The EMT must be able to quickly adapt to that change and reframe his or her thinking about the call.

## Take Standard Precautions

Standard precautions and **personal protective equipment (PPE)** need to be considered and adapted to the prehospital task at hand. PPE includes clothing or specialized equipment that protects the wearer. The type of PPE used depends on the specific job duties required during a patient care interaction. For example, rescue personnel may wear PPE such as helmets, eye protection, boots, gloves, and turnout gear designed to protect them from injury when working to extricate a patient trapped in a damaged motor vehicle. Hazardous materials technicians may don a protective suit designed to prevent contamination by potentially lethal hazardous materials.

**Standard precautions** are protective measures that have traditionally been recommended by the Centers for Disease Control and Prevention (CDC) for use in dealing with objects, blood, body fluids, and other potential exposure risks of communicable disease. If you have a primary responsibility for patient care, you will need to follow standard precautions when assessing and treating the patient. They are required in every patient encounter. These measures may not provide absolute protection from exposure to infectious diseases or bloodborne pathogens, but they are the most effective way to reduce your risk of exposure. The concept of standard precautions assumes that all blood, body fluids, nonintact skin, and mucous membranes may pose a substantial risk of infection. This includes blood and other potentially infectious materials that are dried, because some diseases such as hepatitis can live for days outside the body. During a situation in which there is active community transmission of a virus that can be transmitted by airborne particles or aerosolized particles, this concept of standard precautions must be expanded to recognize the risk associated with non-bloodborne pathogens.

Take standard precautions before actual patient contact, often before you step out of your response vehicle (**FIGURE 10-4**). After you make contact with a patient, it may be too late to think about what precautions should have been considered. The use of standard precautions in EMS, including but not limited to consistent handwashing (with soap

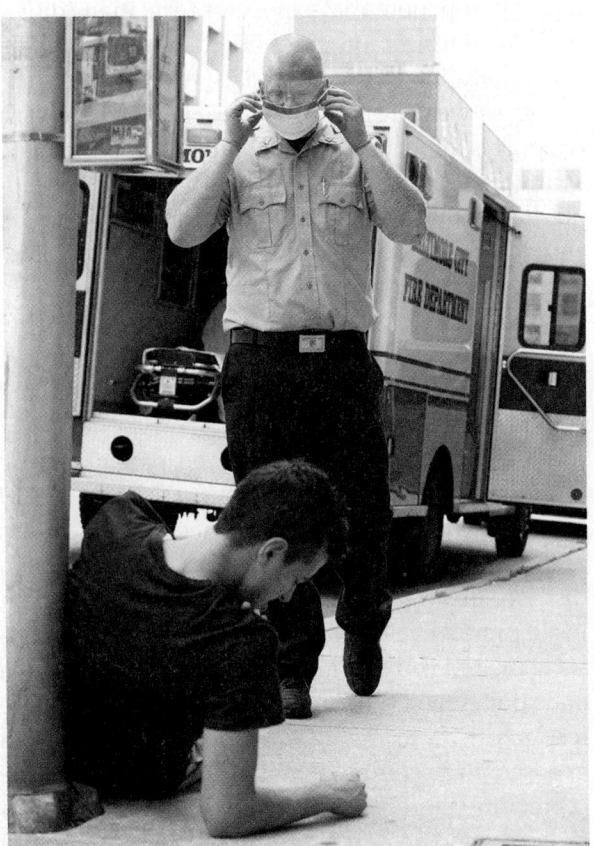

**FIGURE 10-4** Proper protective equipment is vital when you are called to a scene in which you may be exposed to infection or blood or other body fluids.

© Jones & Bartlett Learning. Courtesy of MIEMSS.

and water if possible or with alcohol-based hand cleansers if soap and water are not readily available) before and after care, gloves, eye protection, a mask, and a gown, may be dictated by local standards or protocols. At a minimum, gloves and eye protection must be in place before any patient contact. Remember that after contact with a patient, gloves may be contaminated by infectious materials, so avoid handling EMS equipment with the same gloves used during patient contact. Never touch your face or any areas of bare skin with gloves that have been in contact with a patient. The use of eye protection is recommended for patient encounters. Patients do not typically give you a warning before they vomit or have a seizure—events that pose a high risk of body fluids splashing into the eye. By wearing eye protection on calls, you will reduce the risk of eye injuries and blood or bodily fluid exposure. Standard eyeglasses may not offer enough protection because most are not designed with side splash guards. For that reason, eyewear should protect you from potential exposures from many different directions. Blood and body fluids that contain potentially infectious materials may become airborne, so wearing a mask if there is a risk of splash or spray is important. A patient displaying signs and symptoms such as coughing, stiff neck with headache, sore throat, or fever with shortness of breath should prompt you to don a mask if local standard precautions do not include a mask for all patient encounters. A mask will provide protection from some airborne diseases, but its level of protection will depend on the type of mask, a proper fit, and your ability to apply and wear it properly.

After making contact with the patient, if you discover a condition that warrants a higher level of PPE than you are using, do not hesitate to regroup and upgrade your protection. For example, if you discover in your primary assessment that a patient has a productive cough and a history of tuberculosis (TB), and you are not wearing an N95 mask, you and your crew should immediately don appropriate respiratory protection. If you suspect you have been exposed to a communicable disease without the protection of proper PPE, follow your local agency's protocols for postexposure reporting, testing, and prophylaxis.

## Words of Wisdom

Keep in mind that standard precautions are the infection prevention practices intended to reduce the risk of transmission of bloodborne and other pathogens from both identified and unrecognized sources of infection. These precautions include hand hygiene; use of PPE such as gloves, eye protection, gowns, and masks; safe injection practices; safe handling of potentially contaminated equipment and surfaces; and respiratory hygiene/cough etiquette. The term *standard precautions* has replaced terms for similar concepts, such as *body substance isolation*, and is promoted by both the CDC and World Health Organization (WHO).

## Determine Number of Patients

As part of the scene size-up, it is essential that you accurately identify the total number of patients. This evaluation is critical in determining your need for additional resources, such as firefighters, a specialized rescue group, a hazardous materials team, or additional ambulances. When there are multiple patients, use the **incident command system**, establish command, identify the number of patients, and then begin triage (**FIGURE 10-5**). The incident command system is a flexible system implemented to manage a variety of emergency scenes. Emergency

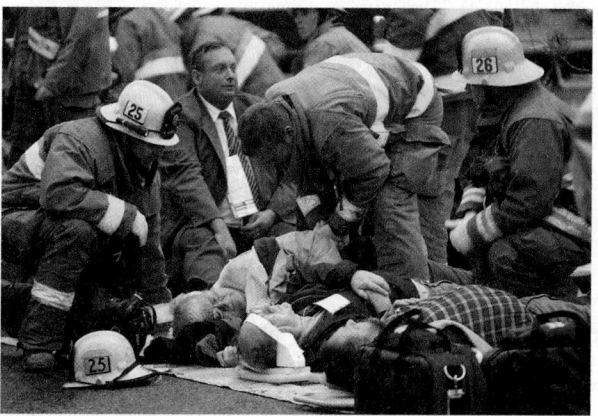

**FIGURE 10-5** With multiple patients, use the incident command system, call for additional resources, and then begin triage. A multiple casualty incident involving two trains that collided in 2005.

© David McNew/Getty Images News/Getty Images.

responders work in groups according to their function or assigned area, with the leader of each group reporting to the person in charge of the incident, the incident commander. **Triage** is the process of sorting patients based on the severity of their condition. Once all patients have been triaged, treatment and transport of these patients can begin. Usually the most experienced EMT is assigned to perform triage. This process helps allocate personnel, equipment, and resources to provide the most effective care to everyone. When many patients are present or there are more patients than the responding unit can effectively handle, put your mass-casualty plan into action, utilizing the incident command system and your local protocols. These topics are covered in Chapter 40, *Incident Management*.

## Consider Additional/Specialized Resources

Some trauma or medical situations may require more ambulances, whereas others may have a need for specialized resources. Basic life support units may be all that are needed for some patients; however, advanced life support (ALS) should be requested for patients with severe injuries or complex medical problems, depending on available resources and local protocols. ALS care may be provided by AEMTs or paramedics, depending on how your EMS system is set up. Air medical support or critical care response teams may be another resource for ALS in your area. Follow your local protocols in requesting ALS resources.

In addition to EMS and fire suppression, many resources such as hazardous materials management, technical rescue services including complex extrication from motor vehicle crashes, wilderness search and rescue, high-angle rope rescue, and water rescue are typically available through the fire department (**FIGURE 10-6**).

Law enforcement personnel may be needed to assist with traffic or scene control and should be the first to enter crime scenes and hostile environments.

If any situation presents itself as a danger to you, your partner, or your patient, you must retreat to a safe area. Be aware of the potential for danger

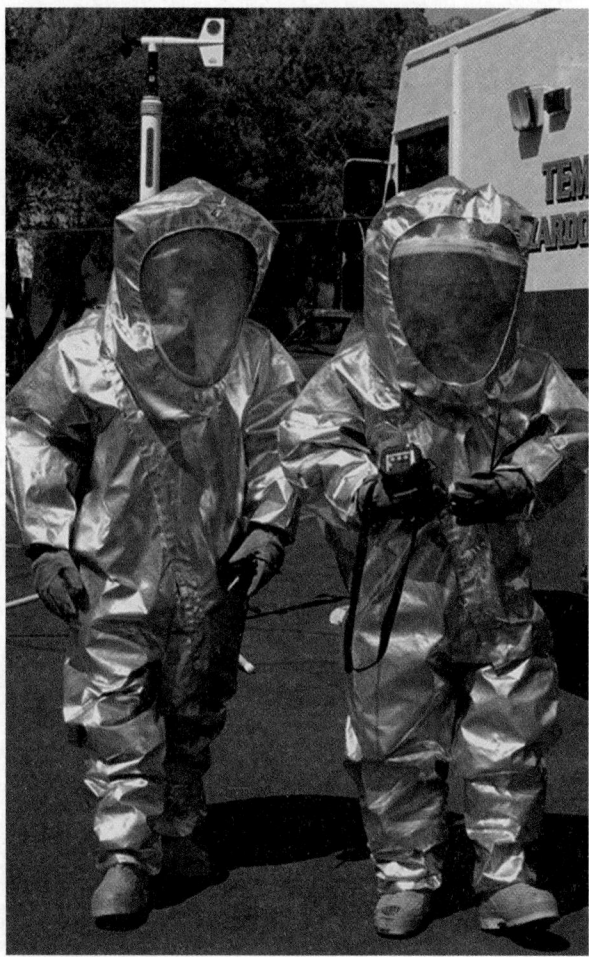

**FIGURE 10-6** Scenes involving toxic substances may require specially trained rescuers with extra protective equipment.

Courtesy of Tempe Fire Department.

at all times and understand when additional or specialized resources are required.

To determine if you require additional resources, ask yourself the following questions:

- Does the scene pose a threat to you, your patient, or others?
- How many patients are there?
- Do we have the resources to respond to their conditions?

Knowing how your EMS system is organized will help you determine the additional resources that may be required. The sooner these resources are identified, the sooner they can be requested.

# Patient Assessment

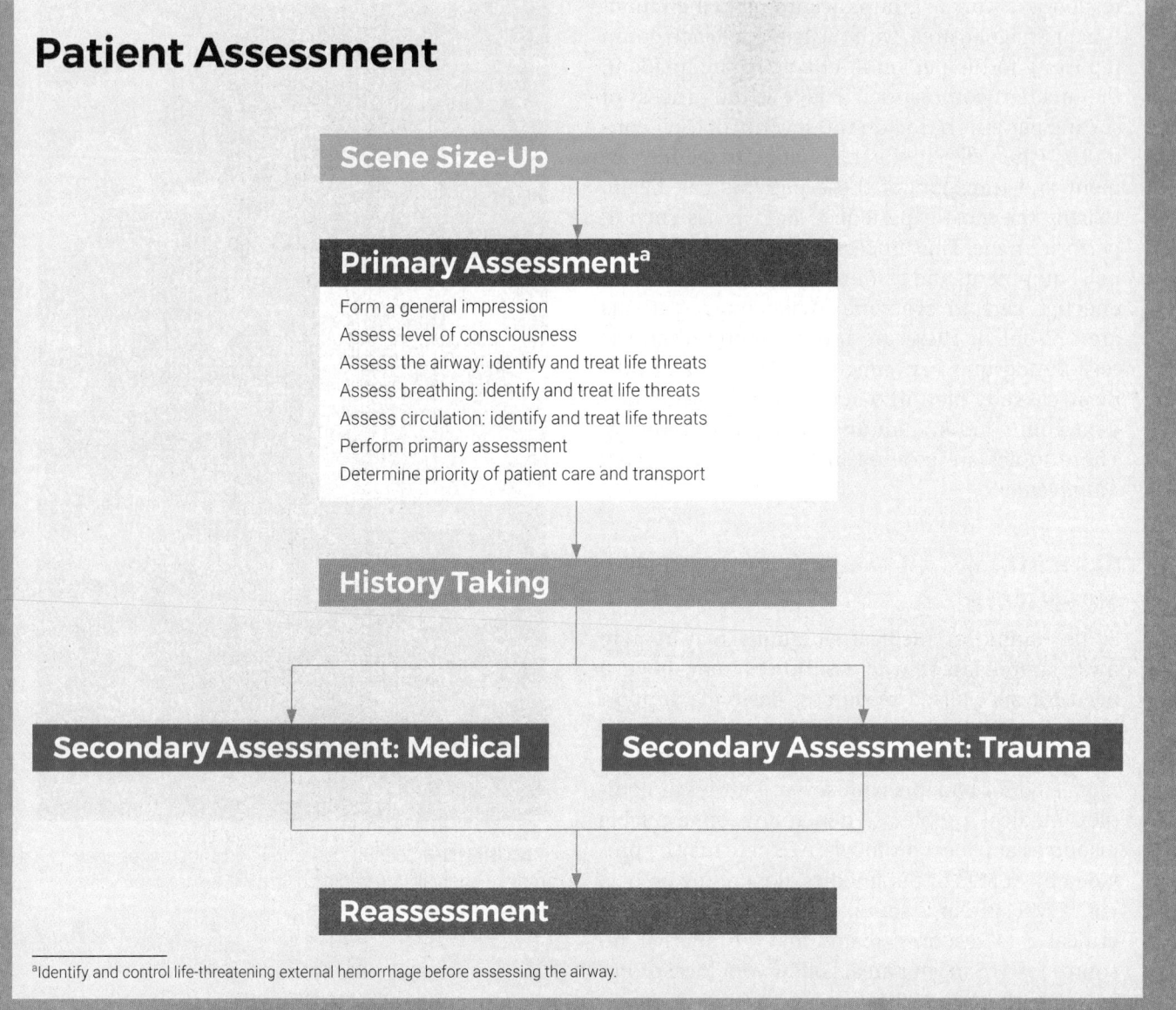

Scene Size-Up

Primary Assessment[a]

Form a general impression
Assess level of consciousness
Assess the airway: identify and treat life threats
Assess breathing: identify and treat life threats
Assess circulation: identify and treat life threats
Perform primary assessment
Determine priority of patient care and transport

History Taking

Secondary Assessment: Medical

Secondary Assessment: Trauma

Reassessment

[a]Identify and control life-threatening external hemorrhage before assessing the airway.

## Primary Assessment

During the scene size-up, you evaluated potential or actual scene hazards and threats, protected yourself and your team, and decided whether you needed additional resources. You also evaluated the dispatch information, the environment in which you are responding, and your initial view of the patient setting to begin to understand what happened and what action you should take. It is critical for these steps to be accomplished before you make direct contact and begin to focus on the patient. Nevertheless, the heart of patient assessment begins when you first greet the patient and begin the **primary assessment**.

The primary assessment has a single, all-important goal: to identify and begin treatment of immediate or imminent life threats. To do this, you must physically examine the patient and assess level of consciousness (LOC) and airway, breathing, and circulation (ABCs); however, this is not an in-depth physical exam or assessment of **vital signs**. These will be addressed later in the secondary assessment. During the primary assessment, you must identify signs of life threats and immediately work to correct them (**FIGURE 10-7**). From here you

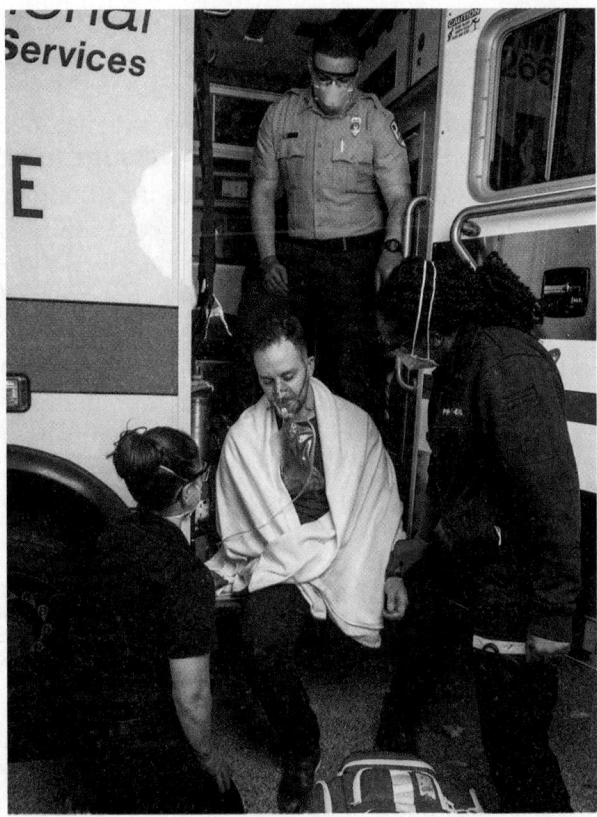

**FIGURE 10-7** A survey of the patient's airway, breathing, and circulatory status is used to establish whether the patient has a life-threatening condition(s) and what you should do about it.

© Jones & Bartlett Learning.

will be able to determine the priority of patient care and transport.

## Form a General Impression

Anytime you meet someone new, you form an initial general impression about that person. Forming the **general impression** of a patient is a similar process, but the focus is on rapid identification of potentially life-threatening problems. The general impression is formed to determine the priority of care and is the first part of your primary assessment. This includes noting things such as the person's age, sex, race, level of distress, and overall appearance, which may lead you to anticipate different problems. A woman of childbearing age who reports abdominal pain, for example, is susceptible to a significantly different spectrum of possible conditions than a middle-aged man with the same complaint because of both physiologic and anatomic differences.

Think of your general impression as an overall visual assessment, gathering information as you approach the patient. Make sure that the patient sees you coming to avoid surprising the patient or causing the patient to turn to see you, possibly making any injuries worse. Note the patient's position and whether the patient is moving or still.

Avoid standing over the patient. This helps to show respect for the patient and helps the patient feel comfortable and less threatened as you begin your assessment. Refer to the patient by name. The initial general impression continues during your introduction (**FIGURE 10-8**). Introduce yourself to the patient by stating something like, "Hi, I am Sam, an EMT with the fire department, and I am here to help you." After you introduce yourself, ask the patient about the chief complaint. Is the patient able to respond to your greeting easily and appropriately? The patient's response can give you insight into the LOC, airway patency, respiratory status, and overall circulatory status before you begin your examination. Sometimes life-threatening conditions are obvious even during the general impression. If a life-threatening condition is found, treat it immediately.

You will define your patient's condition as stable, potentially unstable, or unstable to direct further assessment and treatment. This determination must be made so that prehospital care providers can work together with an appropriate sense of urgency. However, you must constantly be aware of changes in the patient's condition.

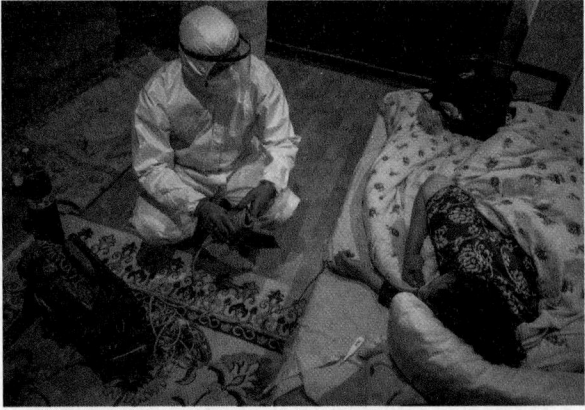

**FIGURE 10-8** As you approach the patient, form a general impression of his or her overall condition.

© Chris McGrath/Getty Images News/Getty Images.

## Scan for Signs of Uncontrolled External Bleeding

Uncontrolled external bleeding takes priority over other assessments. The determination of uncontrolled bleeding is somewhat subjective but is suggested by a large amount of bleeding that is squirting or gushing, has soaked through clothing, or is pooling under the patient. Life-threatening external bleeding should be controlled before the assessment proceeds.

## Assess Level of Consciousness

Early in your assessment, you will need to evaluate the patient's LOC. This will help you rapidly determine if the patient has a life-threatening injury and to what extent the patient will be able to provide reliable information about his or her own condition as well as follow your directions. The patient's LOC can tell you a great deal about his or her neurologic and physiologic status. The brain requires a constant supply of oxygen and glucose to function properly. In the primary assessment, you need to ascertain only the gross LOC.

The AVPU scale is used to assess a patient's LOC depending on how well he or she responds to external stimuli, including verbal stimuli (sound) and painful stimuli (such as pinching the trapezius muscle on top of the patient's shoulder). The **AVPU scale** tests a patient's **responsiveness** based on the following criteria:

**A** *Awake and alert.* The patient's eyes open spontaneously as you approach, and the patient appears to be aware of you and responsive to the environment. The patient is awake, appears to follow commands, and the eyes visually track people and objects.

**V** **Responsive to *verbal* stimuli.** The patient is not alert and awake. The patient's eyes do not open spontaneously. However, the patient's eyes do open when you speak to him or her, or the patient is able to respond in some meaningful way when spoken to—for example, by moaning, speaking, or moving. A patient who does not respond to your normal speaking voice but who responds when you speak loudly is responding to loud verbal stimuli.

**P** **Responsive to *pain*.** The patient does not respond to your questions but moves or cries out in response to painful stimulus. There are appropriate and inappropriate methods of applying a painful stimulus (**FIGURE 10-9**). Be aware that some methods may not give an accurate result if a spinal cord injury is present.

**U** ***Unresponsive.*** The patient does not respond spontaneously or to a verbal or painful stimulus. Unresponsive patients usually have no cough or gag reflex and lack the ability to protect their airway. If you are in doubt about whether a patient is truly unresponsive, assume the worst and treat appropriately.

---

### Words of Wisdom

When using the AVPU scale, be sure to note how the patient responded. Tap a patient who is hard of hearing with your fingers repeatedly. If the patient responds, note that the patient is hard of hearing but responds to being tapped.

---

To determine whether a patient who does not respond to verbal stimuli will respond to a painful stimulus, gently but firmly apply pressure or pinch the patient's tissue. Areas where this technique works best are on the sternum, posterior edge of the mandible (lower jaw), or the trapezius area (the muscle above the collar bone). Another effective technique is to apply upward pressure along the ridge of the orbital rim along the underside of the eyebrow (without applying any pressure to the eyeball). A patient who moans or withdraws is responding to the painful stimulus. Be sure to note the type and location of the stimulus and how the patient responded. Remember the point is not to cause as much pain as possible, but to see if the patient responds to or withdraws from the sensation of pain where you have caused it. Note that a patient who remains flaccid and does not move or make a sound is considered unresponsive.

For a patient who is alert or responsive to verbal stimuli, next evaluate orientation. **Orientation** tests a patient's mental status by checking his or her memory and thinking ability. The most common

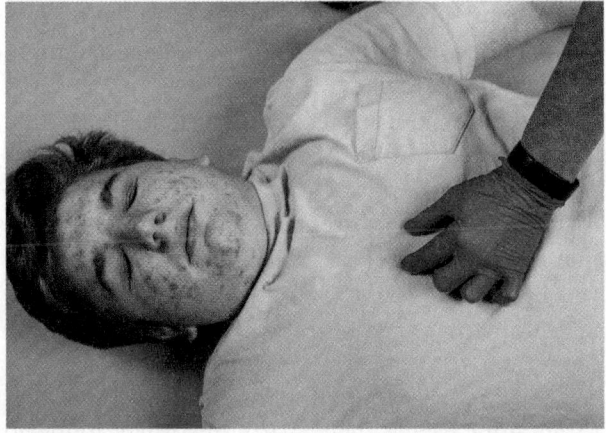

A

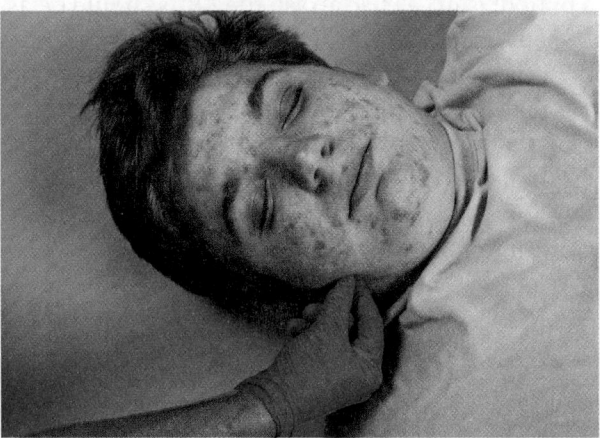

B

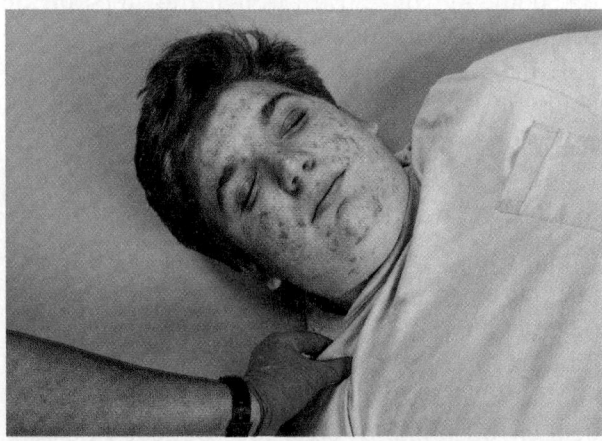

C

**FIGURE 10-9** Methods of gauging a patient's responsiveness to painful stimuli. **A.** Gently or firmly apply pressure on or pinch the patient's sternum. **B.** Gently but firmly apply pressure or pinch the posterior edge of the patient's mandible (lower jaw). **C.** Gently but firmly pinch the patient's trapezius muscle on top of the shoulder.

© Jones & Bartlett Leaning.

test evaluates a patient's ability to remember four things:

- **Person.** The patient is able to remember his or her name.
- **Place.** The patient is able to identify his or her current location.
- **Time.** The patient is able to tell you the current year, month, and day of the week.
- **Event.** The patient is able to describe what happened (the MOI or NOI).

These questions were not selected at random; it is paramount to assess for all four. They evaluate long-term memory (person and place), intermediate memory (place and time when asking year or month), and short-term memory (time when asking approximate day of the week and event). If the patient knows these facts, the patient is said to be "alert and fully oriented," "alert and oriented to person, place, time, and event," or "alert and oriented × 4." It is important to determine, if possible, the patient's normal mental status. A number of circumstances, including ongoing illness, history of stroke, traumatic brain injury, developmental delay, Alzheimer disease, and more, may cause a patient to have a baseline of not being fully alert and oriented. Any deviation from alert and oriented to person, place, time, and event, or from a patient's normal baseline is considered an **altered mental status**.

If you determine that the patient has any of the indicators for spinal motion restriction listed in **TABLE 10-1**, ensure that the unresponsive patient's cervical spine is manually stabilized by either you or another provider. If it is not possible to both manually stabilize the patient's cervical spine and continue your assessment to identify and correct life threats, do your best to ensure that the patient's spine remains in a stable position while you continue your primary assessment. You should complete your primary assessment prior to applying a cervical collar.

## Identify and Treat Life Threats

Your role as an EMT is to determine if a life threat is present and, if so, to quickly address it. A life-threatening condition can quickly lead to death; this rapid process may begin with the absence or loss of meaningful communication between you and the patient. In some cases, the patient is unconscious

**TABLE 10-1** Indications for Spinal Immobilization

| Either blunt or penetrating trauma with any of the following: | • Pain or tenderness on palpation of the neck or spine<br>• Patient report of pain in neck or back<br>• Paralysis or neurologic complaint (numbness, tingling, partial paralysis of the legs or arms) |
|---|---|
| Blunt trauma with any of the following: | • Altered mental status<br>• Intoxication (alcohol or drugs)<br>• Difficulty or inability to communicate |

**Distracting injury**
(Any injury that distracts the patient's attention from other injuries he or she may have, even severe injuries. An example is a painful femur or tibia fracture that prevents the patient from noticing back or neck pain.)

Adapted from National Association of Emergency Medical Technicians, American College of Surgeons. *PHTLS: Prehospital Trauma Life Support.* 9th ed. Burlington, MA: Jones & Bartlett Learning; 2019:298-301.

when you arrive. In other cases, a severely sick or injured person becomes less aware of his or her surroundings and stops being able to communicate. Unless an intervention occurs, loss of consciousness may follow. The patient will become totally unresponsive to external stimuli. In both situations, the muscles become slack, among them the muscles of the jaw, thus permitting the tongue to sag against the posterior part of the throat, obstructing the airway. When air can no longer enter the lungs, the patient stops breathing, cutting off the intake of oxygen and the release of carbon dioxide. The heart cannot continue to function without oxygen, and

## Words of Wisdom

Distracting injuries may prevent patients from reliably identifying neck or back pain associated with an unstable fracture. Therefore, all patients with a long bone fracture and a significant MOI warrant spinal immobilization.

it will soon stop beating. Starved of oxygen, brain cells begin to die within a few minutes, leading to irreversible brain damage.

There are only a few general conditions that cause sudden death: airway obstruction, respiratory failure, respiratory arrest, shock, severe bleeding, and cardiac arrest. Often these conditions are manageable or even reversible, but to address them you have to be able to recognize them quickly and take immediate steps to correct them. This is the purpose of the primary assessment.

In most cases, identifying and correcting life-threatening issues begins with the airway, followed by breathing and circulation (ABC). However, when a patient is in cardiac arrest, the ABCs should be assessed simultaneously in the interest of minimizing the time to first compression. Also, when a patient has life-threatening bleeding, it is more appropriate to first address the life threat posed by exsanguinating hemorrhage, following a sequence of circulation, airway, and breathing (CAB). In these cases, controlling life-threatening bleeding takes priority over airway and breathing concerns.

## Assess the Airway

An airway obstruction can result in partial or complete blockage of air movement into and out of the lungs and therefore inadequate **perfusion** of the entire body. As you move through the steps of the primary assessment, stay alert for signs of airway obstruction. To prevent death or permanent disability to your patient, ensure that the airway remains open (patent) and adequate.

## Responsive Patients

Patients of any age who are talking or crying have an open airway. However, watching and listening to how patients speak, particularly patients with respiratory problems, may provide important clues about the adequacy of their airway and the status of their breathing. A conscious patient who cannot speak or cry most likely has a severe airway obstruction.

If you identify an airway problem, stop the assessment process and work to clear the patient's airway. This may be as simple as positioning the patient so the air moves in and out, suctioning liquids from the airway, or removing an obvious foreign body from the patient's mouth; it may be as complex as abdominal thrusts or chest compressions to remove a foreign body from the airway. Although airway and breathing problems are not the same, their signs and symptoms often overlap. If your patient has signs of difficulty breathing or is not breathing, immediately take corrective actions using appropriate airway management techniques.

## Unresponsive Patients

With an unresponsive patient or a patient with a decreased LOC, immediately assess the patency of the airway. Unresponsive patients may have experienced a traumatic event. If there is a potential for trauma, use the jaw-thrust maneuver to open the airway. If you cannot obtain a patent airway using the jaw-thrust maneuver or if it can be confirmed that the patient did not experience a traumatic event, use the head tilt–chin lift maneuver to open and maintain a patent airway. This maneuver is described in Chapter 11, *Airway Management*. Another cause of airway obstruction in an unconscious patient could be relaxation of the tongue muscles, allowing the tongue to fall to the back of the throat. Address this first by positioning the airway, then by placing an oral or nasal airway. Dentures, blood clots, vomitus, mucus, food, and other foreign objects may also create an obstruction. These can be cleared with manual techniques and suctioning. These techniques are also described in Chapter 11, *Airway Management*. Once you have confirmed that the airway is clear, you can continue your assessment.

Signs of airway obstruction in an unconscious patient include the following:

- Obvious trauma, blood, or other obstruction
- Noisy breathing, such as snoring, bubbling, gurgling, crowing, stridor, or other abnormal sounds (Normal breathing is quiet.)
- Extremely shallow or absent breathing (Airway obstructions may impair breathing.)

If any of these conditions exist, the airway is considered inadequate and you should open it using the head tilt–chin lift maneuver, suction as necessary, and use an airway adjunct as necessary. If the patient's airway is not managed quickly and efficiently, the body will not be able to receive the oxygen needed to survive.

## Assess Breathing

A patient's breathing status is directly related to the adequacy of the patient's airway. Once you have made sure the patient's airway is open, confirm that the patient's breathing is present and adequate. A patient who is breathing without assistance is said to have **spontaneous respirations**, or spontaneous breathing.

## YOU are the Provider

When you arrive on scene, a police officer directs you to a poorly kept apartment on the second floor. The scene is safe. You find the patient, a young man, lying in a prone position on the floor in the kitchen. He was found by his neighbor, who became concerned when he did not answer the door. You carefully roll the patient to a supine position and begin your assessment. An engine company arrives to provide assistance.

| Recording Time: 0 Minutes | |
| --- | --- |
| Appearance | Pale; blood draining from the side of the mouth |
| Level of consciousness | Responsive to pain |
| Airway | Bloody secretions and vomitus in the mouth |
| Breathing | Slow, shallow, and gurgling |
| Circulation | Radial pulse slow and weak; skin cool and pale |

**3.** Is spinal motion restriction indicated? Why or why not?

**4.** Which of these assessment findings requires your *most* immediate attention?

As you assess the patient's breathing, ask yourself the following questions:

- Is the patient breathing?
- Is the patient breathing adequately?
- Is the patient hypoxic?

Positive-pressure ventilations should be performed for patients who are not breathing or whose breathing is too slow or too shallow. If the patient is breathing adequately but remains hypoxic, administer oxygen. The goal for oxygenation for most patients is an oxygen saturation of greater than 94%.

If a patient seems to develop difficulty breathing after your primary assessment, immediately reevaluate the airway. When respirations exceed 28 breaths/min with signs of distress or are fewer than 8 breaths/min, or are too shallow to provide adequate air exchange, consider providing positive-pressure ventilations with an airway adjunct. Remember that air exchange is the critical issue, not the number of breaths. Normal breathing is an effortless process that does not affect a patient's speech, posture, or positioning. Speech is a good indicator of whether a conscious patient is having difficulty breathing. A patient who can speak smoothly without unusual extra pauses is breathing normally. However, a patient who can speak only one word at a time, or must stop every two to three words to catch his or her breath, is having significant difficulty breathing. Normal respirations are not usually shallow or excessively deep. **Shallow respirations** can be identified by little movement of the chest wall (reduced tidal volume) or poor chest excursion. Deep respirations cause a significant rise and fall of the chest. Document when the patient's respirations are shallow or deep.

Observe how much effort is required for the patient to breathe. The presence of **retractions** (indentation above the clavicles and in the spaces between the ribs) or the use of **accessory muscles** of respiration is a sign of inadequate breathing. Accessory muscles include the neck muscles (sternocleidomastoid), the chest pectoralis major muscles, and the abdominal muscles. **Nasal flaring** and seesaw breathing in pediatric patients indicate inadequate breathing. A patient who can speak only two or three words without pausing to take a breath, a condition known as **two- to three-word dyspnea**, has a serious breathing problem.

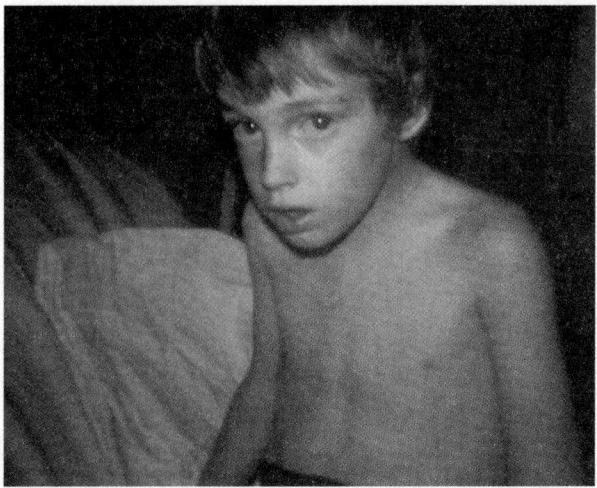

**FIGURE 10-10** A patient in the sniffing position sits upright with the head and chin thrust slightly forward.

Courtesy of Health Resources and Services Administration, Maternal and Child Health Bureau, Emergency Medical Service for Children Program.

Patients who are having marked difficulty breathing will instinctively assume a posture in which it is easier for them to breathe. There are two common postures that indicate the patient is trying to increase air flow. The first position is called the **tripod position**. In this position, a patient is sitting and leaning forward on outstretched arms with the head and chin thrust slightly forward; significant conscious effort is required for breathing. The second position is most commonly seen in children—the **sniffing position**. The patient sits upright with the head and chin thrust slightly forward, and the patient appears to be sniffing (**FIGURE 10-10**).

Breathing that becomes progressively more difficult requires progressively more effort. When you can see that effort, the patient's breathing is described as **labored breathing**. Initially, labored breathing is characterized by the patient's position, concentration on breathing, and the increased effort and depth of each breath. As breathing becomes more labored, accessory muscles in the chest and neck are used, and the patient may make grunting sounds with each breath. In infants and small children, nasal flaring and supraclavicular and intercostal retractions are commonly associated with labored breathing. Sometimes the patient may be gasping.

Infants and small children may have labored breathing for a sustained period, will then often

**TABLE 10-2** Signs of Respiratory Distress and Failure

| Respiratory Distress | Respiratory Failure |
|---|---|
| Agitation, anxiety, restlessness | Lethargy, difficult to rouse |
| Stridor, wheezing | Tachypnea with periods of bradypnea or agonal respirations |
| Accessory muscle use; intercostal retractions, neck muscle use (sternomastoid) | Inadequate chest rise/poor excursion |
| Tachypnea | Inadequate respiratory rate or effort |
| Mild tachycardia | Bradycardia |
| Nasal flaring, seesaw breathing, head bobbing | Diminished muscle tone |

© Jones & Bartlett Learning.

become exhausted, and finally will no longer have the strength to maintain the necessary energy to breathe. In infants and small children, cardiac arrest is generally caused by respiratory arrest.

Respiratory distress occurs when a person has difficulty breathing; therefore, the work of breathing is increased. Typically, a person in respiratory distress has an increase in respiratory effort and rate. Respiratory failure occurs when the blood is inadequately oxygenated or ventilation is inadequate to meet the oxygen demands of the body. Respiratory arrest is the ultimate result of respiratory failure if it is not corrected (**TABLE 10-2**).

## Assess Circulation

Assessing circulation helps you to evaluate how well blood is circulating to the major organs, including the brain, lungs, heart, kidneys, and the rest of the body. A variety of problems can impair circulation, including blood loss, shock, and conditions that affect the heart and major blood vessels. Circulation is evaluated by assessing the patient's mental status, pulse, and skin condition. The first step in evaluating any patient is to rapidly scan for, identify, and control severe external bleeding.

## Assess Pulse

With each heartbeat, the ventricles contract, forcefully ejecting blood from the heart and propelling it into the arteries. Often referred to as a heartbeat, the **pulse** is the pressure wave that occurs as each heartbeat causes a surge in the blood circulating through the arteries. The pulse is most easily felt at a pulse point where a major artery lies near the surface and can be pressed gently against a bone or solid organ.

Your first consideration when taking a pulse is to determine whether the patient has one. To determine if a pulse is present, you will need to **palpate** (feel) the pulse. Hold together your index and long fingers and place your fingertips over a pulse point. Press gently against the artery until you feel intermittent pulsations. In responsive patients who are older than 1 year, palpate the radial pulse at the wrist (**FIGURE 10-11A**). In unresponsive patients older than 1 year, palpate the carotid pulse in the neck (**FIGURE 10-11B**). When palpating the carotid pulse, place the fingertips of your index and long fingers in the center of the throat on the windpipe and then slide your fingers toward you into the groove between the trachea and the neck muscle. This positions your fingers directly over the carotid artery. Only gentle pressure on one side of the neck should be used. Never press on the carotid arteries on both sides of the neck at the same time. Palpating too hard can occlude the blood flow, especially in a patient who has poor perfusion or is hypotensive.

Sometimes, you may have to slide your fingertips a little to each side and press again until you feel a pulse. When palpating a pulse, do not use your thumb. If you do so, you may mistake the strong pulsing circulation in your thumb for the patient's pulse.

## Special Populations

In infants, the radial and carotid pulses are difficult to locate.

Palpate the brachial pulse, located at the medial area (inside) of the upper arm, in children younger than 1 year (**FIGURE 10-12**). With the infant lying

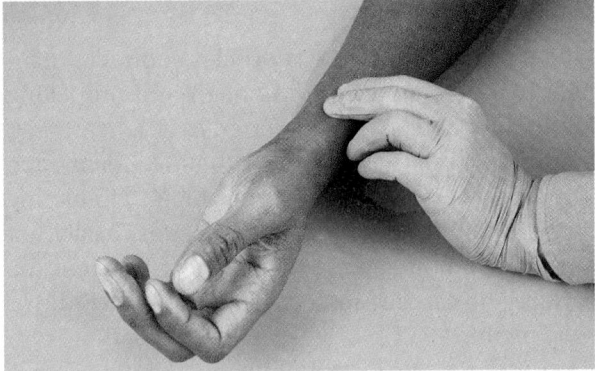

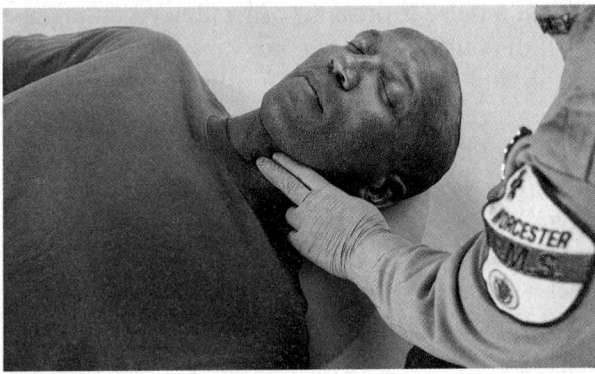

**FIGURE 10-11 A.** To palpate the radial pulse, place the tips of your index and long fingers over the radial artery, pressing gently until you feel intermittent pulsations. **B.** To palpate the carotid pulse, place the tips of your index and long fingers over the carotid artery, pressing gently until you feel intermittent pulsations.

**A, B:** © Jones & Bartlett Learning.

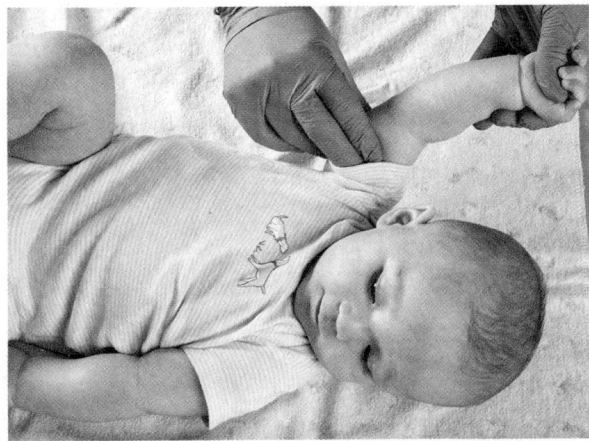

**FIGURE 10-12** To palpate the brachial pulse in an infant, press firmly along the brachial artery on the inside of the upper arm.

© Jones & Bartlett Learning.

supine, you can access the brachial pulse by elevating the arm over the infant's head. Because most infants have chubby arms, you need to press your adjacent fingertips firmly along the brachial artery, which lies parallel to the long axis of the upper arm, to be able to palpate the pulse.

If you cannot palpate a carotid pulse in an unresponsive patient, begin CPR. If an automated external defibrillator (AED) is available, turn it on and follow the voice prompts, following your local protocol. An AED is indicated for use on patients who have been assessed to be unresponsive and pulseless. More information about this is available in Chapter 14, *BLS Resuscitation*.

If the patient has a pulse but is not breathing, provide ventilations at a rate of 10 to 12 breaths/min for adults and 12 to 20 breaths/min for an infant or a child. Continue to monitor the pulse every 2 minutes to evaluate the effectiveness of your ventilations. If the patient becomes pulseless, start CPR and apply the AED. The apparent absence of a palpable pulse in a responsive patient is not caused by cardiac arrest. Therefore, never begin CPR or use an AED on a responsive patient.

With practice, you will be able to assess whether the pulse is too slow, too fast, or irregular without actually counting the pulsations. This will help to speed up your assessment of the ABCs and allow you to focus on finding other potentially life-threatening problems. A pulse rate that is too slow or too fast may change decisions related to transporting your patient. The pulse should be easily felt at the radial or carotid artery and have a regular rhythm. If it is difficult to feel or is irregular, the patient may have problems with his or her circulatory system that may need further evaluation later in your assessment.

## Skin Condition

The skin has many functions. It acts as insulation and protection from infection, helps maintain the water content of the body, and has a role in regulating body temperature by changing the amount of blood circulating through the surface of the skin.

Assessing the skin is one of the most important and most readily accessible ways of evaluating circulation and perfusion, blood oxygen level, and body temperature. Perfusion is assessed by evaluating a patient's skin color, temperature, moisture, and capillary refill. A normally functioning circulatory system perfuses the skin with oxygenated blood, allowing it to maintain a normal color, temperature, and moisture for the environment. Inadequate blood flow to the skin will result in abnormal findings such as pale, cool skin. This may be associated with hypoperfusion to the brain, lungs, heart, and kidneys. In most situations, hypoperfusion is caused by shock. The degree of hypoperfusion and how long it lasts will determine if a patient will sustain permanent injuries.

### Skin Color

Many blood vessels lie near the surface of the skin. The skin's color is determined by the blood circulating through these vessels and the amount and type of pigment that is present in the skin. In patients with deeply pigmented skin, changes in color may be apparent only in certain areas, such as the fingernail beds, the mucous membranes in the mouth, the lips, the underside of the arm and palm (which are usually less pigmented), and the conjunctiva of the eyes. The conjunctiva is the delicate membrane lining the eyelids, and it covers the exposed surface of the eye. In addition, the palms of the hands and soles of the feet should be assessed in infants and children.

Poor peripheral circulation will cause the skin to appear pale, white, ashen, or gray, possibly with a waxy translucent appearance similar to a white candle. Abnormally cold or frozen skin may also appear this way. When the blood is not properly saturated with oxygen, it appears blue. Therefore, in a patient with insufficient air exchange and low levels of oxygen in the blood, the blood and vessels appear blue, and the lips, mucous membranes, nail beds, and skin over the blood vessels appear blue or gray. This condition is called cyanosis (**FIGURE 10-13**).

High blood pressure may cause the skin to be abnormally flushed and red. A patient with a significant fever, heatstroke, sunburn, mild thermal burns, or other conditions in which the body is unable to properly dissipate heat will also appear to have red skin.

Changes in skin color may also result from chronic illness. Liver disease or dysfunction may cause jaundice, resulting in the patient's skin and sclera turning yellow. The sclera is the normally white portion of the eye and may show color changes even before skin color change is visible.

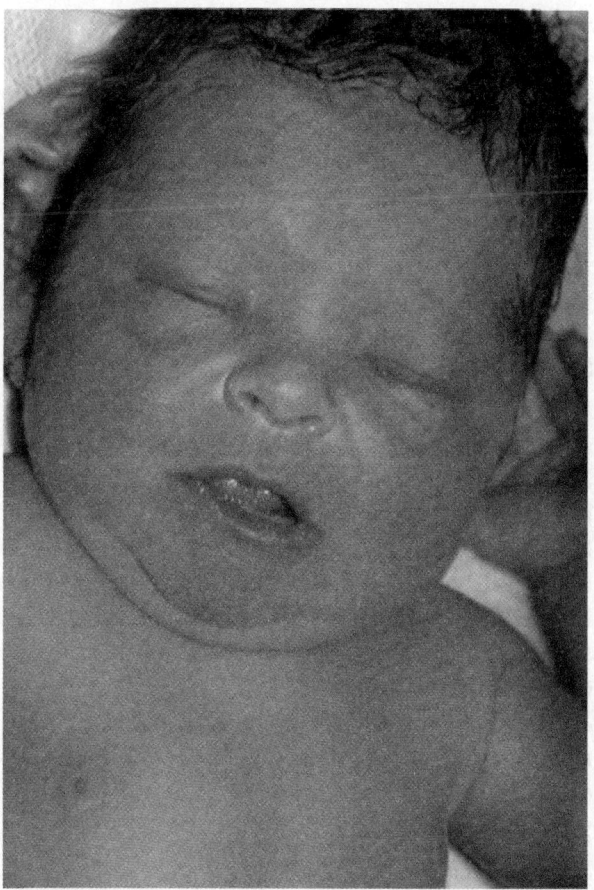

**FIGURE 10-13** Cyanosis occurs when the patient has low levels of oxygen in the blood.

© St. Bartholomew's Hospital, London/Photo Researchers, Inc.

### Skin Temperature

Normal skin temperature will be warm to the touch; normal body temperature is 98.6°F (37°C). Abnormal skin temperatures are hot, cool, cold, and clammy (moist). When the patient has a significant fever, sunburn, or hyperthermia, the skin feels hot to the touch. The skin will feel cool when the patient is in early shock, has mild hypothermia, or has inadequate perfusion. With poor perfusion, the body pulls blood away from the surface of the skin and diverts it to the core of the body. The result is cool, pale, clammy skin; in your primary assessment, this is a good indication of hypoperfusion and shock. The skin will feel cold when the patient is in profound shock, has hypothermia, or has frostbite.

In most cases it will initially be adequate to assess the patient's skin temperature by feeling the patient's forehead with the back of your gloved hand to see if it is excessively elevated or decreased. A more accurate temperature obtained with a thermometer during the vital signs assessment will often be helpful. In situations of viral pandemic or other active community transmission of viral illness, routine temperature screening will be extremely valuable. It is also important for some other cases such as environmental hypothermia or hyperthermia, infection, and septic shock.

### Skin Moisture

Dry skin is normal. Skin that is moist or wet from sweat, or excessively dry and hot suggests a problem. In the early stages of shock, the skin will become slightly moist. Skin that is only slightly moist but not covered excessively with sweat is described as clammy, damp, or moist. When the skin is bathed in sweat, such as after strenuous exercise or when the patient is in shock, the skin is described as wet or **diaphoretic.**

Because the skin's color, temperature, and moisture are often related signs, you should consider them together. When recording or reporting your assessment of the skin, first describe the color, then the temperature, and last, whether the skin is dry, moist (clammy), or wet. For example, you could say or write, "Skin: pale, cool, and clammy."

Again, these characteristics are important findings in your primary assessment because hypoperfusion can lead to serious consequences if treatment is delayed or ignored.

---

### Words of Wisdom

Remember to assess:

- Skin color
- Skin temperature
- Skin moisture

---

### Capillary Refill

**Capillary refill** is often evaluated in pediatric patients to assess the ability of the circulatory system to perfuse the capillary system in the fingers and toes. When evaluated in an uninjured limb, capillary refill time (CRT) may provide an indication of the pediatric patient's level of perfusion. It should be kept in mind, however, that especially in an adult patient, capillary refill can be affected by the

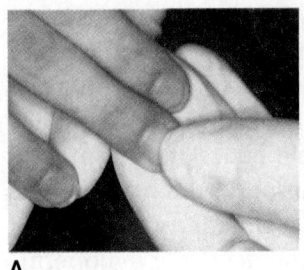 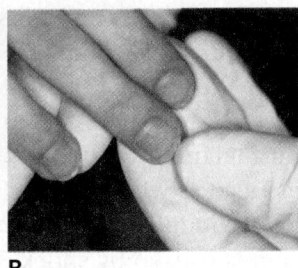

**A** **B**

**FIGURE 10-14 A.** To test capillary refill, gently compress the fingertip until it blanches. **B.** Release the fingertip, and count until it returns to its normal pink color.

**A., B:** © Jones & Bartlett Learning. Courtesy of MIEMSS.

patient's position, age, history as a smoker, history of medical problems such as diabetes, medications the patient is currently taking, and exposure to a cold environment (**hypothermia**) including frozen tissue (**frostbite**) and **vasoconstriction** (narrowing of a blood vessel). Injuries to bones and muscles of the extremities may cause local circulatory compromise, resulting in hypoperfusion of an extremity rather than hypoperfusion of the body in general.

To test capillary refill, place your thumb on the patient's fingernail with your fingers on the underside of the patient's finger and gently compress (**FIGURE 10-14A**). The blood will be forced from the capillaries in the nail bed. Remove the pressure applied against the tip of the patient's finger. The nail bed will remain blanched (white) for a brief period. As the underlying capillaries refill with blood, the nail bed will return to its normal pink color.

To assess capillary refill in newborns and young infants, press on the forehead, chin, or sternum.

With adequate perfusion, the color in the infant's or child's nail bed should be restored to its normal pink color within 2 seconds, or about the time it takes to say "capillary refill" at a normal rate of speech (**FIGURE 10-14B**). Report and document the CRT as normal (2 seconds or less). Suspect poor peripheral circulation when capillary refill takes more than 2 seconds or the nail bed remains blanched. In this case, report and document the CRT as delayed or "CRT > 2." Again, delayed capillary refill is not always considered an accurate indication of poor perfusion, particularly in adult patients.

### Assess and Control External Bleeding

Identify and immediately control major external bleeding. This step should occur before addressing airway or breathing concerns. In some cases, blood loss can be very rapid and can quickly result in shock or even death. Signs of blood loss include active bleeding from wounds and/or evidence of bleeding such as blood on the clothes or near the patient. Serious bleeding from a large vein may be characterized by steady blood flow. Bleeding from an artery is characterized by a spurting flow of blood. Often major blood loss is visible when approaching the patient. When you evaluate an unconscious patient, do a sweep for blood by quickly and lightly running your gloved hands from head to toe, pausing periodically to see if your gloves are bloody.

Controlling external bleeding is often very simple. Initially, direct pressure with your gloved hand and soon thereafter a sterile bandage over the wound will control bleeding in most cases. Direct pressure stops the bleeding and helps the blood to coagulate, or clot, naturally. Most minor bleeding can be adequately controlled by using direct pressure. When direct pressure is not quickly successful or whenever you encounter obvious arterial hemorrhage of an extremity, apply a tourniquet. More information about applying a tourniquet is found in Chapter 26, *Bleeding*.

## Performing a Rapid Exam to Identify Life Threats

A rapid head-to-toe exam is performed following the primary assessment. This exam is used to find any additional injuries. It is not a focused assessment and should take no more than 90 seconds. This assessment can identify other injuries that must be managed prior to transport.

To perform a rapid exam of the patient to identify life treats, follow the steps in **SKILL DRILL 10-1**. Remember, this should take no longer than 90 seconds!

1. Assess the head, looking and feeling for **DCAP-BTLS** (**TABLE 10-3**). You should also assess the patient's pupils (**Step 1**).
2. Assess the neck, looking and feeling for DCAP-BTLS, jugular venous distention, deviation of the trachea from midline in the neck, and spinal step-off or a vertebra that is not aligned with the rest (**Step 2**).
3. Assess the chest, looking and feeling for DCAP-BTLS, chest wall movement, crepitus, subcutaneous emphysema, and equal rise and fall. Listen to breath sounds on both sides of the patient's chest (**Step 3**).

## YOU are the Provider

Your partner begins assisting the patient's ventilations with high-flow oxygen while an EMT from the engine company obtains his vital signs. You ask the police officer to inspect the patient's apartment for anything suspicious. The officer on the engine tells you that the neighbor has no knowledge of the patient's medical history. The patient's blood glucose level is assessed and reads 108 mg/dL.

| Recording Time: 5 Minutes | |
|---|---|
| **Respirations** | 8 breaths/min and shallow (baseline); ventilations are being assisted |
| **Pulse** | 42 beats/min; weak and regular |
| **Skin** | Cool and pale |
| **Blood pressure** | 76/58 mm Hg |
| **Oxygen saturation (Spo$_2$)** | 95% (with assisted ventilation) |

Your primary assessment of the patient reveals no obvious signs of trauma, medical alert tags, or anything else that might explain his condition. The police officer did not find any pill bottles, drug paraphernalia, or anything else suspicious. His driver's license shows that he is 25 years old. You hear on the radio that a paramedic unit has just cleared a scene and is approximately 18 minutes away.

**5.** Does the patient require further treatment at the scene? If so, what?

**6.** Should you remain at the scene and wait for the paramedic unit? Why or why not?

## Skill Drill 10-1 Performing a Rapid Exam to Identify Life Threats

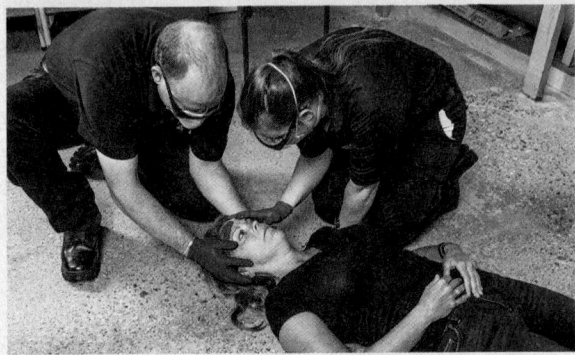

### Step 1

Assess the head. Have your partner maintain in-line spinal stabilization if indicated.

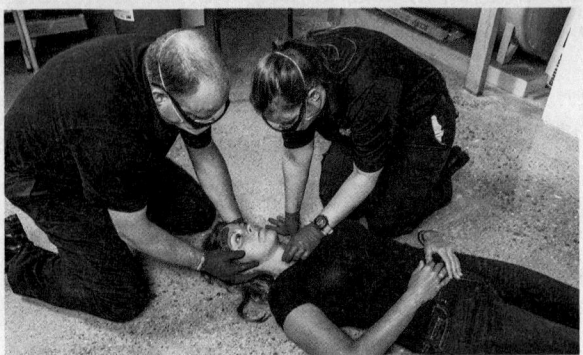

### Step 2

Assess the neck.

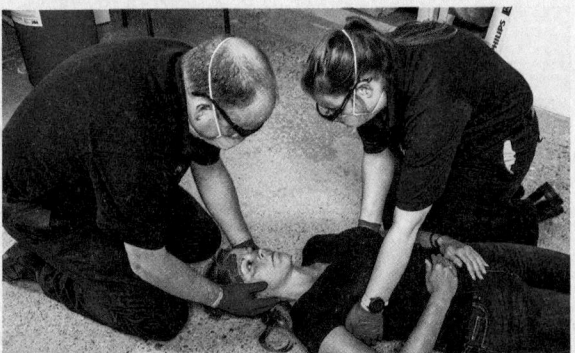

### Step 3

Assess the chest. Listen to breath sounds on both sides of the chest.

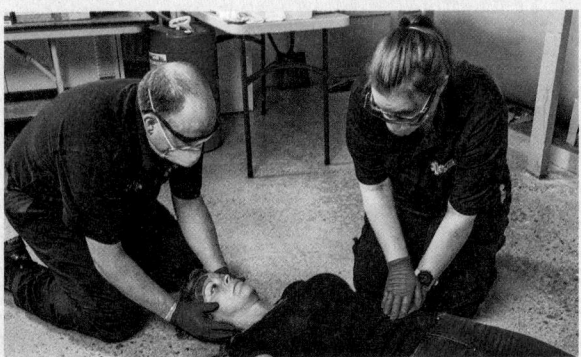

### Step 4

Assess the abdomen.

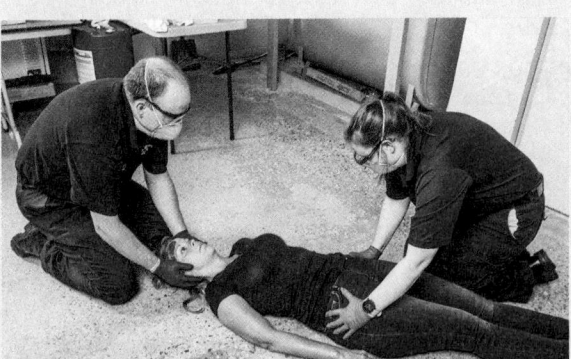

### Step 5

Assess the pelvis. If there is no pain, gently compress the pelvis downward and inward to look for tenderness and instability.

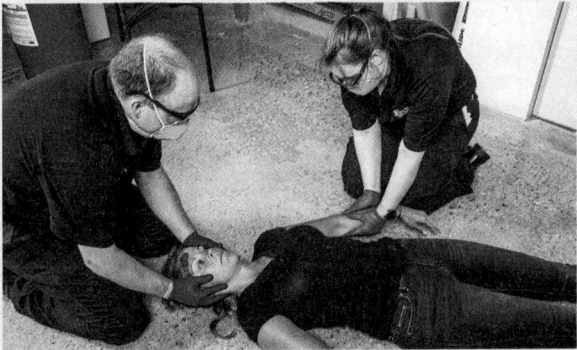

### Step 6

Assess all four extremities. Assess the pulse and motor and sensory function.

## Skill Drill 10-1 Performing a Rapid Exam to Identify Life Threats (*continued*)

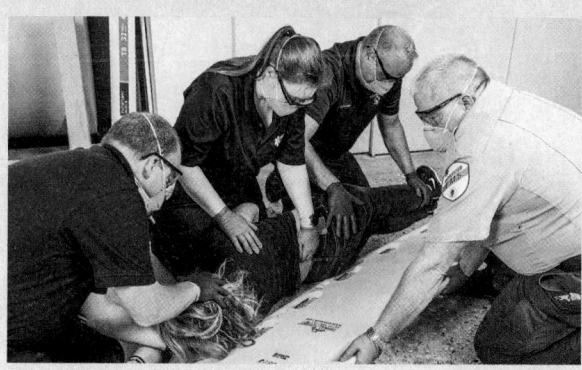

© Jones & Bartlett Learning.

### Step 7

Assess the patient's back and buttocks. If spinal immobilization is indicated, do so with minimal movement to the patient's spine by log rolling the patient in one motion.

---

### TABLE 10-3  The DCAP-BTLS Mnemonic

| | |
|---|---|
| D—Deformity | Misshapen body part (eg, the arm or leg is no longer straight) |
| C—Contusions | Bruising; a collection of blood under the skin |
| A—Abrasions | Loss or damage to the surface of the skin from rubbing or scraping |
| P—Punctures | A small penetration through the skin into the soft tissue |
| B—Burns | Redness, blisters, or white areas of skin |
| T—Tenderness | Pain when an area is palpated |
| L—Lacerations | A deep cut in the skin |
| S—Swelling | A raised or enlarged area of soft tissue on the surface of the body |

© Jones & Bartlett Learning.

4. Assess the abdomen, looking and palpating for DCAP-BTLS, rigidity (firm or soft), and distention (**Step 4**).
5. Assess the pelvis, looking for DCAP-BTLS. If there is no pain, gently compress the pelvis, placing your palms over the iliac crests and pressing downward and inward to look for tenderness and instability (**Step 5**).
6. Assess all four extremities, looking and palpating for DCAP-BTLS. Also assess bilaterally for distal pulses and motor and sensory function (**Step 6**).
7. Assess the back and buttocks, looking and feeling for DCAP-BTLS. In all trauma patients, maintain in-line stabilization of the spine while rolling the patient on his or her side in one motion (**Step 7**). It is particularly important that you check the patient's back before you load the patient for transport.

## Determine Priority of Patient Care and Transport

The primary assessment will assist you in determining transport priority (**FIGURE 10-15**). If you do not identify any injuries that require treatment or immediate transport when completing your assessment of the ABCs, you may find indications for immediate transport during your primary assessment of the patient's body. For example, you may identify an internal hemorrhage by the presence of a distended or firm abdomen or bilateral femoral fractures. These types of conditions are indications for immediate transport.

Would you consider your patient a high, medium, or low priority for transport? Priority designation is used to determine if a patient needs immediate transport or will tolerate a few more

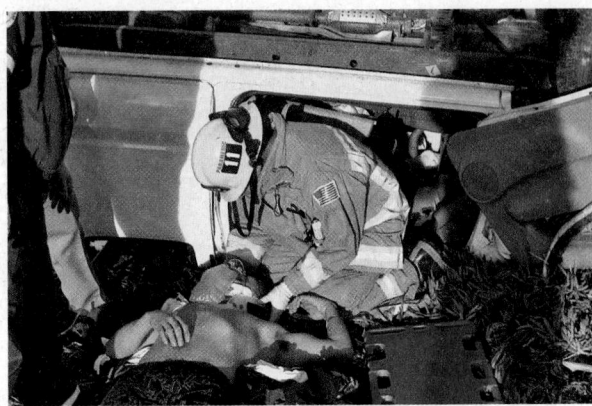

**FIGURE 10-15** Identifying priority patients.

© Keith D. Cullom/www.fire-image.com.

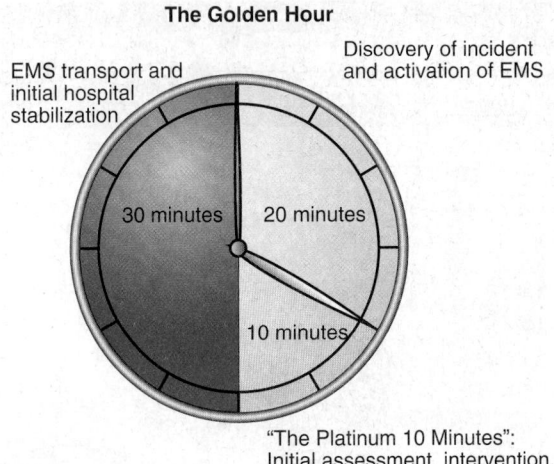

**The Golden Hour**

EMS transport and initial hospital stabilization

Discovery of incident and activation of EMS

30 minutes

20 minutes

10 minutes

"The Platinum 10 Minutes": Initial assessment, intervention, and packaging

**FIGURE 10-16** The Golden Hour, also called the Golden Period, is the time during which treatment of shock or traumatic injuries is most critical and the potential for survival is best.

© Jones & Bartlett Learning.

minutes on scene. Patients with any of the following conditions are examples of high-priority patients and should be transported immediately:

- Unresponsive
- Difficulty breathing
- Uncontrolled bleeding
- Altered LOC
- Severe chest pain
- Pale skin or other signs of poor perfusion
- Complicated childbirth
- Severe pain in any area of the body

Recognizing the need to transport serious trauma patients is of such importance that you may hear colleagues refer to the Golden Hour, also called the Golden Period. This refers to the time from injury to definitive care, during which treatment of shock and traumatic injuries must occur to maximize the patient's chance of survival (**FIGURE 10-16**). Over time, the body has increasing difficulty in compensating for shock and traumatic injuries. For this reason, you should spend as little time as possible on scene with patients who have sustained significant or severe trauma.

Some patients may benefit from remaining on scene and receiving continuing care. For example, an older patient with chest pain may be better served on scene by being administered nitroglycerin and waiting for an ALS vehicle than by immediate transport. When indicated, ALS support should be requested if a unit is not already en route to the scene. If ALS is delayed or farther away, coordinating a rendezvous may be a better decision

for a high-priority patient. It would also be important, for example, to apply splinting to a patient who has sustained an isolated injury to a bone, as relief from the pain is more important than immediate transport in an isolated injury. Your decision to stay on scene or transport immediately will be based on your patient's condition, the availability of more advanced help, the distance for which you must transport the patient, and your local protocols.

Correct identification of high-priority patients is an essential aspect of the primary assessment and helps to improve the outcome in some patients. Although initial treatment is important, it is essential to remember that immediate transport is one of the keys to the survival of patients who need immediate care that the EMT cannot provide. Transport should be initiated as soon as practical and possible.

Remember, the goal of your primary assessment is to identify and treat life threats, including management of ABCs, as quickly as possible. Measure vital signs precisely during the secondary assessment (discussed later), once time and life threats are less of an issue.

If the patient's condition is stable, reassess vital signs every 15 minutes until you reach the emergency department (ED). If the patient's condition is unstable, reassess vital signs every 5 minutes, or as often as the situation permits, looking for trends in the patient's condition.

Do not be falsely reassured by apparently normal vital signs. The body has amazing abilities to compensate for severe injury or illness, especially in children and young adults. Even patients who have experienced severe medical or traumatic conditions may initially exhibit fairly normal vital signs. However, the body's ability to compensate eventually decreases (decompensated shock), and the vital signs may deteriorate rapidly, especially in children. In fact, this tendency for the vital signs to fall rapidly as the patient decompensates is the reason that it is important to frequently recheck and record vital signs. Treating a patient for shock before the blood pressure drops increases your patient's chance to survive.

# Patient Assessment

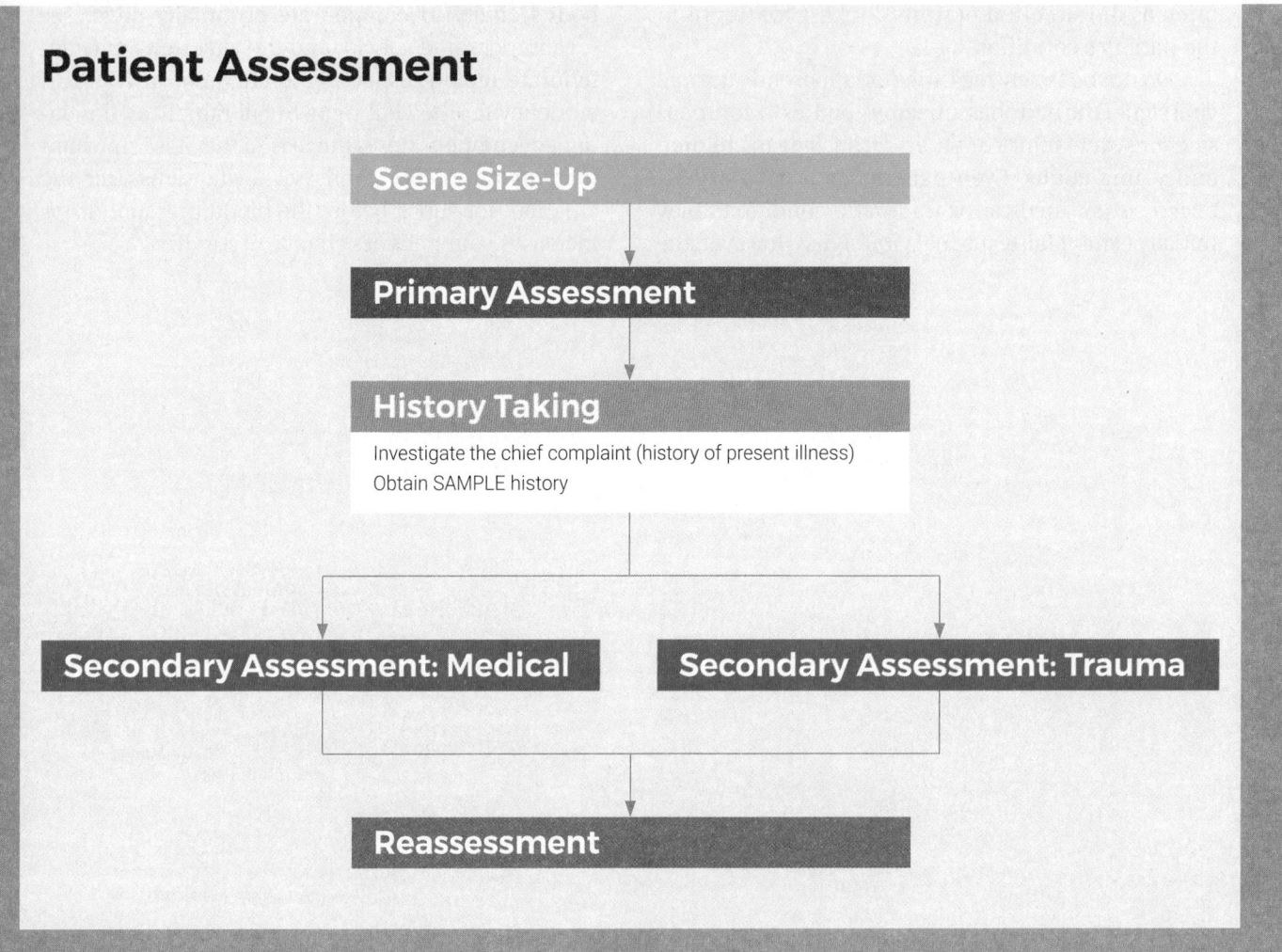

**Scene Size-Up**

**Primary Assessment**

**History Taking**

Investigate the chief complaint (history of present illness)
Obtain SAMPLE history

**Secondary Assessment: Medical**

**Secondary Assessment: Trauma**

**Reassessment**

## History Taking

Although history taking is listed after the primary assessment, it is an integral part of the assessment and should be initiated on scene simultaneously with other tasks, if possible. You may work with another responder, allowing one of you to ask questions of people in the vicinity, while the other initiates patient assessment. It is important to gather as much history as possible on scene from family, friends, and bystanders because this information may not be obtainable once transport is initiated. Also check for medical identification tags and paperwork to gain essential information concerning events leading up to the incident. If the patient is able to answer questions or a family member is transported in the ambulance with the patient, history taking can

be expanded while en route. Sometimes the history may be essential to determining patient treatment; however, transport should not be delayed in patients who are in unstable condition. **History taking** provides details about the patient's chief complaint and an account of the patient's signs and symptoms. It is important to document all information gathered during this phase of the assessment process. This includes demographic information, past medical history, and current health status of the patient. Be sure to document the following information:

- Date of the incident
- Patient's age
- Patient's sex
- Patient's race
- Past medical history, including any pertinent information about the patient's condition,

such as medical problems, traumatic injuries, and surgical procedures

- Patient's current health status, including diet, medications, drug use, living environment and hazards, physician visits, and family history

## Investigate the Chief Complaint (History of Present Illness)

The patient's chief complaint is the most serious thing the patient is concerned about (**FIGURE 10-17**) and is usually the reason EMS was dispatched. To investigate the chief complaint, begin by making introductions. Make the patient feel comfortable and obtain permission to treat. Then ask a few simple and direct questions. Refer to the patient as Mr., Ms., or Mrs., using the patient's last name. Open-ended questions such as "What seems to be the matter?" or "What is bothering you the most today?" will help determine the chief complaint. These questions and others can help to elicit a response that may determine the patient's highest concern. The response is usually expressed in the patient's own words with simple answers such as, "My chest hurts" or "I have been feeling weak." This is a good time to gather further information about the chief complaint and identify if there are any associated complaints. Use eye contact to encourage the patient to continue speaking, and repeat statements back to the patient to show that you understand the situation. Do not interrupt, and be empathetic toward the patient's situation. As discussed previously, the problems or feelings the patient reports

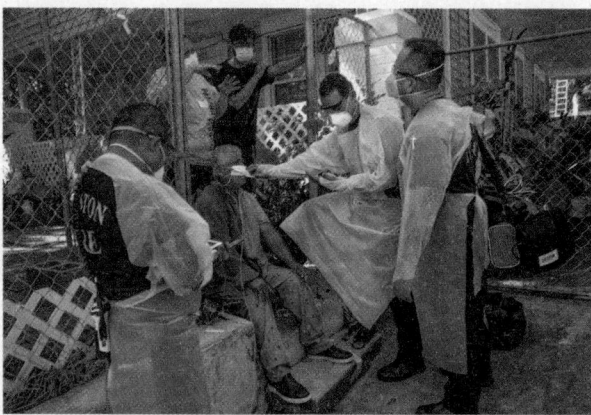

**FIGURE 10-17** The patient's initial response to the question "What's wrong?" isthe chief complaint.

© John Moore/Staff/Getty Images News/Getty Images.

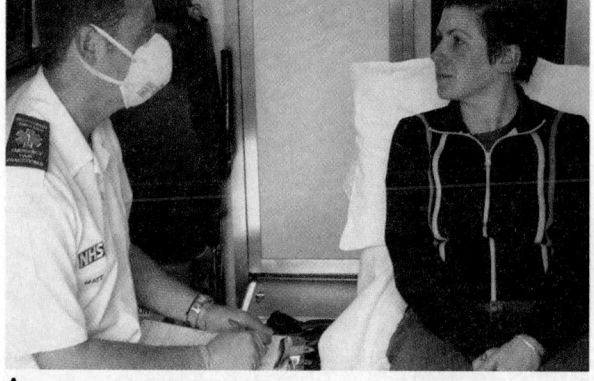

A

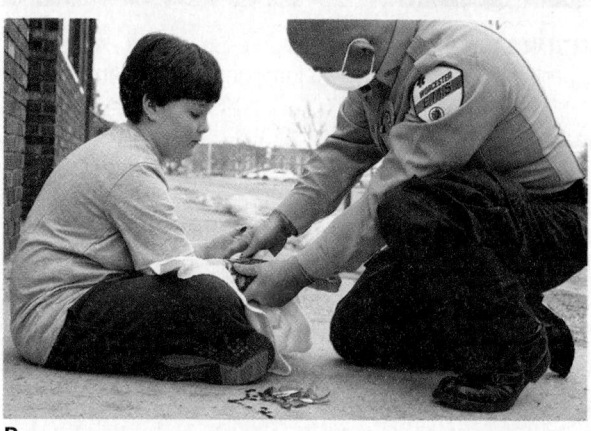

B

**FIGURE 10-18 A.** A symptom is a subjective condition that the patient feels and tells you about. **B.** A sign is an objective finding that you can detect by observing or examining the patient.

**A., B:** © Jones & Bartlett Learning. Courtesy of MIEMSS.

to you are the symptoms. Symptoms cannot be felt or observed by others. Signs are objective conditions that can be seen, heard, felt, smelled, or measured by you or others (**FIGURE 10-18**).

You must consider the wide range of age groups with which you will interact. Information from infants and children may come from a parent or caregiver. Some older patients may be slow to respond or have multiple complaints. Over time, every EMT develops his or her own particular method or style to obtain a patient's chief complaint and history.

## Street Smarts

Listen to how your coworkers ask questions during history taking of difficult patients and consider trying some of these approaches in the future.

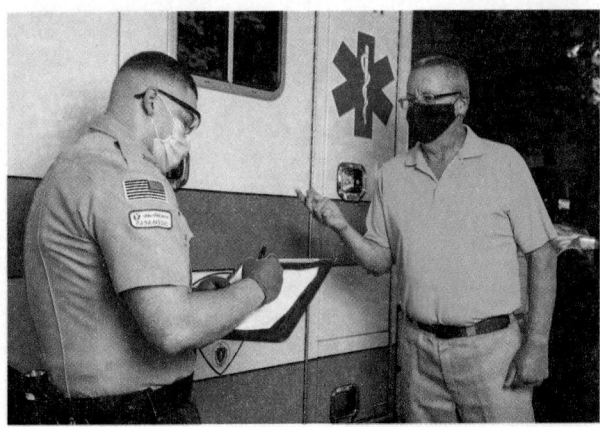

**FIGURE 10-19** If the patient is unresponsive, try to obtain a pertinent history or patient information from family or bystanders.

© Jones & Bartlett Learning. Courtesy of MIEMSS.

You will also gather information about the chief complaint from observable clues and information received from the original dispatch. If the patient is unresponsive, information about the patient, pertinent past medical history, and clues about the immediate incident may be obtained from family members present, a person who may have witnessed the situation, bystanders, medical alert jewelry, or other patient medical history documentation (**FIGURE 10-19**). Observable signs may include things such as the patient not being able to respond using full sentences and appearing to have some respiratory distress. These clues may indicate the patient's chief complaint is "difficulty breathing," or the clues may be part of a bigger problem that has to do with a lengthy history of cardiac problems.

For example, you are called to the home of an older man who fell. This information was provided by the dispatcher, and you can use it to help process all clues that may be presented in what appears to be a simple fall. You find the patient lying at the bottom of the stairs. How many stairs are there, are they carpeted, and is the floor concrete, wood, or tile? Additional observable clues are used to determine a chief complaint. You note that the patient has an obvious deformity to his right arm, and your initial general impression is a possible fracture. Is this the patient's chief complaint, or is this the result of another problem? The patient states he did fall, which is how the injury occurred, and he reports pain in the right arm. However, was the fall the

result of tripping on a step, or was it associated with a medical problem such as dizziness, vertigo, or a syncopal episode, all of which may have caused the fall? It is your responsibility to look at the possibilities and ask the appropriate questions to determine the patient's primary complaint.

## Street Smarts

In some cases, what the patient tells you is the chief complaint will not be your chief concern. For example, a patient with no prior medical history who has fallen says, "My wrist hurts," but you observe that her speech is slurred and she is not moving her right arm or leg. In this case, your chief concern will be possible stroke even though it is not her chief complaint.

Patient interaction sometimes occurs during the worst possible time in the patient's life. These are emergency situations in which patients are afraid and confused. Some patients assume this could be the end of their lives. Sorting through the clues from the emergency scene itself, from the patient's complaints, and from the patient's signs and symptoms and past medical history will assist you in understanding the cause of your patient's problem and enable you to make appropriate, timely decisions about your patient's care.

### OPQRST

You may find it helpful to use the **OPQRST** mnemonic for gathering additional information about a patient's history of present illness and current symptoms. Although OPQRST can be used most easily for questions about pain, it can be adapted to quantify other symptoms such as dizziness, nausea, or shortness of breath.

- **O** **Onset.** What were you doing when the symptoms began?
- **P** **Provocation/palliation.** Does anything make the symptoms better or worse? How are you most comfortable?
- **Q** **Quality.** What does the symptom feel like? Is it sharp, dull, crushing, tearing? Does it come in waves? Ask the patient to describe the symptom.
- **R** **Region/radiation.** Where do you feel the symptom? Does it move anywhere?

S **Severity.** On a scale of 0 to 10, with 0 being "nothing at all" and 10 being "the worst you can imagine," how would you rate your symptom?

T **Timing.** How long have you had the symptom? When did it start?

---

## Special Populations

Assessment of pain is important. According to studies by the American Academy of Pediatrics and the Society for Academic Emergency Medicine, a pain scale such as the Wong-Baker scale (discussed in Chapter 35, *Pediatric Emergencies*) may be helpful in assessing pain in children and patients with a developmental delay.

---

## Identify Pertinent Negatives

The process of gathering a patient's past medical history, history of present illness, and signs and symptoms is important, but sometimes just as important are the signs and symptoms that the patient does not have. These important negative findings are referred to as **pertinent negatives**. Often, a patient's complaint would be expected to be associated with other related findings. Examples include chest pain with shortness of breath, palpitations, and sweating or a severe allergic reaction with itching, hives, and trouble breathing. The absence of these findings is relevant, and should be reported and documented. Pertinent negatives are often helpful in identifying a patient's problem and choosing an appropriate treatment.

## Obtain SAMPLE History

As you obtain a patient history from medical and trauma patients, you will need to know some of the standard techniques for questioning patients. By obtaining a **SAMPLE history**, you will be able to gather important information from the patient. Use the mnemonic SAMPLE to obtain the following information:

S **Signs and symptoms.** What signs and symptoms occurred at the onset of the incident?

A **Allergies.** Is the patient allergic to any medication, food, or other substance? What reactions did the patient have to any of them?

If the patient has no known allergies, you should note this on the run report as "No known allergies."

M **Medications.** What medication is the patient prescribed? What dosage is prescribed? How often does the patient take the medication? What prescription, over-the-counter, and herbal medications has the patient taken in the last 12 hours? Are there medications the patient has been prescribed but is not taking? Does the patient take recreational drugs?

P **Pertinent past medical history.** Does the patient have any history of medical, surgical, or trauma occurrences? Is there important family history that should be known?

L **Last oral intake.** When and what did the patient last eat or drink? In women of childbearing age, the "L" in SAMPLE also represents *last menstrual period*.

E **Events leading up to the injury or illness.** What are the key events that led up to this incident? What occurred between the onset of the incident and your arrival? What was the patient doing when this illness started?

## Critical Thinking in Assessment

Assessment is the logical and ordered process of identifying problems and setting priorities to provide treatment, but it is important that this is not done robotically by the book. When providers do this, it is referred to as *cookbook medicine*—the process of going through steps in a process without considering other options.

Cookbook medicine does not work in emergency medical services because EMS work occurs in a dynamically changing and often chaotic environment. To provide quality patient care in this environment, you must become an expert in gathering, evaluating, and synthesizing information. This is called critical thinking; without it, you will find yourself confused and unable to manage any incident that does not appear exactly the same as described in the textbook.

### Gathering

The first step in gathering information involves seeking facts to help your clinical decision making and scene management. Gathering information is often a straightforward process of observing the scene and questioning the patient and bystanders. However, you may experience challenges in gathering information, such as patients who are uncooperative, are unconscious, or have communication barriers. Consider a scenario where you receive a call for a patient with a headache and flulike symptoms. The call occurs during cold weather flu season, so it is possible that this patient simply has a cold or flu. As you gather more information on scene, you learn that the patient believes that he got sick from his family and they are all experiencing the same signs and symptoms. The patient also tells you that the heater in their home is not working properly, leaving them with chills, and that he has been happy on the days that he has been able to make it into work because he feels much better there.

### Evaluating

The next step is to consider what the information gathered means. In the previous example, although it is possible this is simply a case of cold or flu moving from person to person within a household, you must use critical thinking skills and consider other conditions that would produce the same signs and symptoms. In this case, the same signs and symptoms might be caused by carbon monoxide. Several other elements of information that you have gathered point in that direction as well, including a malfunctioning heater, everyone in the house experiencing the same signs and symptoms, and that the patient feels better when out of the house.

### Synthesizing

The final step in critical thinking is putting together the information that you have gathered and validated, and synthesizing it into a plan to manage the scene and/or care for the patient. In the previous example, you may choose to continue your primary assessment of the patient while you direct your partner to reassure the bystanders and try to gather any additional information. You may also recommend the evacuation and evaluation of all occupants of the house, as well as calling for the fire department to test the house for carbon monoxide.

## Taking History on Sensitive Topics
### Alcohol and Drugs

The signs and symptoms a patient may have while under the influence of alcohol or drugs may be confusing, hidden, or disguised. Many patients who abuse alcohol and/or drugs may deny having any problems. Families, friends, and coworkers may be unaware that a patient has any drug or alcohol troubles because patients often hide their dependency from these same people. The reasons patients deny using alcohol or drugs can vary greatly. It may be out of fear of losing their employment or driver's license, worry about what friends may think about them, and embarrassment or insecurity about their disorder.

The history that you gather from a chemically dependent patient may be unreliable (**FIGURE 10-20**). If patients are not telling the people closest to them that they have a problem, you, as an outsider, may have even less success in obtaining information about a patient's current substance use disorder. The signs and symptoms of alcohol or drug use may be masked by the patient's presentation. Use all of your senses when providing patient care. You can assure patients whom you suspect are withholding information for fear of penalty that their privacy is protected and their honesty will improve the level of care you can provide.

Establish a strong rapport with your patients. Do not judge a patient who may have a chemical dependency, and be professional in your approach. Be honest and open. Above all, impress on

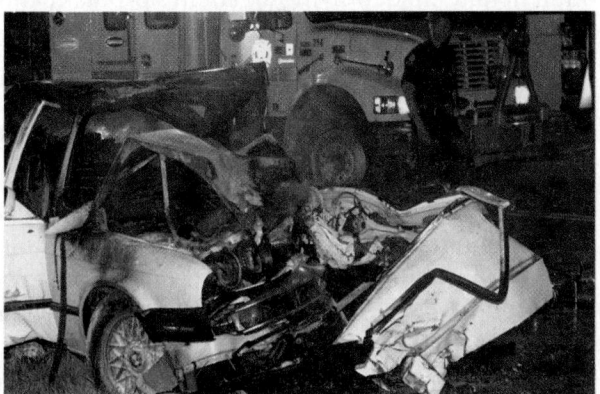

**FIGURE 10-20** Many vehicle crashes involve alcohol. In these cases, the patient history may not be reliable.

© Jack Dagley Photography/ShutterStock.

the patient that information received will be kept in confidence. Then and only then, a patient may open up to you and provide information that can be valuable in his or her assessment and treatment.

### Physical Abuse or Violence

All cases of suspected physical abuse or domestic violence must be reported to the appropriate authorities. Follow your state laws and local protocols when dealing with such cases. If you suspect a patient is a victim of physical abuse or domestic violence, do not accuse any person of being responsible for the situation. Instead, immediately involve law enforcement.

Because abuse and physical violence are very sensitive situations, look for hidden clues that such a situation exists. Information gathered at the scene, during the assessment process, and while transporting a patient may indicate violence or abuse.

What should you look for? When gathering a history, determine if the information provided by the patient and others present at the scene is inconsistent. Do you observe multiple injuries in various stages of healing? Are some bruises red, black, brown, or even green? In some cases, a victim of abuse or violence will not tell you what happened because of fear of further violence when EMS is not present. Victims may not answer your questions because the physical aggressor is still present and is answering questions for the patient. In these cases, separate the people present and interview both parties about the situation.

In cases of domestic violence, involvement can be extremely dangerous. If you determine that the emergency response is part of a domestic abuse situation, call law enforcement personnel immediately (**FIGURE 10-21**).

When involved with cases of physical abuse, be observant and open-minded, have a high index of suspicion, and be nonjudgmental. Documentation will be very important in cases of abuse and domestic violence. Your documentation should be an objective report of the facts. Avoid subjective, judgmental statements, and include any pertinent statements made by the patient or others present using quotation marks. Remember, these prehospital situations could possibly involve some type of legal process later on. You may be summoned

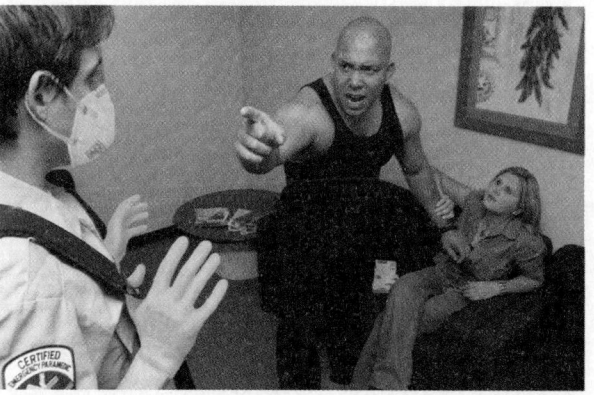

**FIGURE 10-21** Do not handle potentially violent calls alone. Summon law enforcement personnel.
© Jones & Bartlett Learning. Courtesy of MIEMSS.

several years later to provide testimony regarding what may have happened, which makes accurate and thorough documentation very important.

### Sexual History

Obtaining information about a patient's sexual history may be limited because a number of factors may influence the details a patient may reveal. Religious beliefs, cultural stereotypes, and society's expectations may have a major role in patients not revealing a very personal side of their life, including practices considered by some people to be bizarre or exotic. In addition, some patients find sharing information regarding their sexual history with others very uncomfortable.

When would information about a patient's sexual history become important? As an EMT, you will be involved in the care of female patients reporting lower abdominal pain. You should consider all women of childbearing years who are reporting lower abdominal pain to be pregnant unless ruled out by history or other information. There are several questions to ask when faced with this prehospital scenario:

- When was your last menstrual period?
- *If the patient is bleeding:* How many sanitary pads or tampons have you used?
- Do you have urinary frequency or burning?
- What is the severity of cramping, and are there any foul odors?
- Is there a possibility you may be pregnant?
- Are you using any form of birth control?

When dealing with a male patient, you must inquire about urinary symptoms:

- Is there pain associated with urination?
- Do you have any discharge, sores, or an increase in urination?
- Do you have burning or difficulty voiding?
- Has there been any trauma?

When appropriate, based on presenting symptoms, ask about the potential for sexually transmitted diseases. Gathering this information may be difficult and uncomfortable for the patient. Never be judgmental once this information is gathered. All patients should be, and expect to be, treated with compassion and respect. All information gathered from a patient for the purpose of determining a treatment plan is strictly confidential and should not be shared with others unless necessary in the process of treating a patient's medical or traumatic condition.

## Street Smarts

Remember that patients are and will continue to be diverse. Treat members of the LGBTQIAP communities with the standard of dignity and care you provide all patients.

## Special Challenges in Obtaining Patient History

Dealing with patient care, you will be faced with challenges, many of them new and difficult. Every patient interaction should be viewed as a new experience and handled as an educational opportunity as well.

### Silence

Dealing with patients who say very little or say nothing at all can be difficult and frustrating. Patience is extremely important when dealing with patients and their emergency crises. Patients may be thinking about how to answer you, getting the facts straight, or assessing your crew to determine if they feel comfortable answering you. Using a closed-ended question that requires a simple yes or no answer may work best in certain circumstances. Consider whether the silence is a clue to the patient's chief complaint.

Always look for visual signs in the patient's environment that may indicate why a patient is not communicating. In addition, look for nonverbal clues, including facial expressions that may show pain or fear. Is the patient distressed or intimidated by your presence? How is the patient sitting or standing? Is there a communication problem? Is there a language problem? There are many reasons a patient may be silent during the prehospital encounter. A good EMT will continue to assess the situation and determine a way to communicate with the patient.

### Overly Talkative

On the other end of the spectrum is the patient or bystander who is extremely talkative. Some people just talk a lot, and gathering details about their medical condition may be difficult if they talk around your question or you have a difficult time refocusing the patient's conversation. Some possible causes as to why a patient may be overly talkative could include excessive caffeine consumption; nervousness; ingestion of cocaine or methamphetamines; or some underlying psychological issue.

Once you have allowed a talkative patient a chance to express himself or herself, you must keep the patient focused on the questions presented. Have the patient stick to the facts, and clarify statements for the purpose of making sure the information you are gathering is correct. Remember that there is no such thing as too much information.

### Multiple Symptoms

Some patients present with multiple symptoms. Prioritize the patient's complaints as you would in triage; start with the most serious and end with the least serious. Always ask for additional information to determine why EMS was called. Do not limit the patient's complaints; doing so will hinder your ability to gather information.

Keep an open mind, and do not focus on just one complaint or detail to determine a treatment plan. Always remember there may be several possible medical or traumatic causes for a patient's chief complaint.

### Anxiety

When a person is involved in an emergency situation, it is natural for that person to appear excited or anxious. Many people have not been faced with a true emergency during their lifetime, and part of your job as an EMT will be to help provide calm to the situation. It is important to also consider the context of the situation and recognize that the anxiety you are observing may be a sign of a serious underlying medical condition. Your patient or bystander may be nervous, pacing, vocal, panicked, or, in some extreme cases, experiencing complete hysteria. It is your responsibility to deal not only with the emergency crisis at hand, but also with the people present who are having difficulties coping with the situation. Frequently, anxious patients can be observed in emergency scenes that involve many patients, such as during a disaster. Anxiety also can be observed or encountered during a routine EMS call when family members or patients are having difficulty coping.

Some anxious patients exhibit signs of psychological shock, such as pallor, diaphoresis, shortness of breath, numbness in the hands and feet, dizziness or lightheadedness, and even loss of consciousness. The patient may have no real medical complaint but may be hiding or concealing something such as physical abuse or a domestic situation that he or she wants to keep quiet. In any situation involving an anxious patient, be aware of verbal and nonverbal clues. Is the patient making sense during a verbal conversation? Anxiety can also be an early indicator of low blood glucose level, shock, or hypoxia. Perform the appropriate examination to rule out these potentially life-threatening causes early in your assessment.

During a crisis situation, reassure the patient that any nervous or anxious response is normal and can be overcome. It may be possible for you to control an anxious patient by simply smiling or using a delicate touch. Be confident in your approach and have a positive demeanor. In many patient care interactions, your presence may be all that is required to calm the patient. Remaining calm, and calming your patient, can help ensure you are getting accurate, complete information.

## Anger and Hostility

Every patient encounter has the potential for verbal hostility and physical violence, from a situation involving a 9-year-old boy who was hit by a vehicle to a 90-year-old grandmother experiencing chest pain. Emergency calls have a high potential for sudden violence because friends, family, or bystanders may direct their anger and rage toward you. Do not take this anger and frustration personally. More important, do not become angry yourself because anger feeds anger.

---

## YOU are the Provider

As you are packaging the patient and preparing to move him from his building, the paramedic unit is dispatched to another call. There are no other paramedic units in your district. You move the patient from his apartment and load him into the ambulance. With an EMT from the engine company assisting you in the back with the patient, you depart the scene and reassess the patient. The closest appropriate hospital is 25 minutes away.

| Recording Time: 12 Minutes | |
|---|---|
| Level of consciousness | Unconscious and unresponsive |
| Respirations | 6 breaths/min (baseline); ventilations are being assisted at a rate of 10 breaths/min |
| Pulse | 44 beats/min; weak and regular |
| Skin | Pale and cool; cyanosis noted around mouth |
| Blood pressure | 78/54 mm Hg |
| Spo$_2$ | 88% (with assisted ventilation) |

**7.** How has your patient's condition changed from the previous assessments?

**8.** What should you do in response to the patient's change in condition?

When handling potentially violent situations, remain calm, reassuring, and gentle. Always be observant. Be aware of nonverbal clues, such as posture, position, and facial expressions. Look at the patient and be aware of how the patient is positioned. Is the patient stiff, with hands clenched and feet wide apart? If this is the case and the patient steps forward quickly with one foot into a side (blade) position, it may indicate the patient has assumed a position to allow him or her to kick.

If the scene is not safe or secured, retreat until it is secured. Never remain alone in a room with a potentially violent or hostile patient. Understand that everything a patient can reach has the potential to be used as a weapon.

### Intoxication

When you gather a history from an intoxicated patient, be aware that the information may be difficult to get and also could be unreliable. An intoxicated patient may become impatient with you when he or she is trying to provide you with information. As the patient's impatience increases, so does his or her anger level. Do not put an intoxicated patient in a position where he or she feels threatened and has no way out. As in other emergency cases, the potential for violence and a physical confrontation is high when a patient is intoxicated.

During the assessment and treatment of a patient who has consumed alcohol, be accepting, diplomatic, objective, and nonjudgmental. Because of the intoxication, the patient may not be telling you everything about how he or she feels. Alcohol dulls a patient's senses, which will make it difficult for an intoxicated patient to inform you that something feels painful. Treat the patient with dignity and respect despite the intoxication.

### Street Smarts

When you think a patient is intoxicated, it is essential to complete a thorough assessment. The patient may instead be experiencing hypoglycemia, a head injury, or other life-threatening medical condition.

### Crying

A crying patient is a breathing patient. A patient who cries may be sad, in pain, or emotionally overwhelmed. No matter the reason for crying, you need to be calm, patient, reassuring, and confident, and to maintain a soft voice.

Your presence may make a crying patient feel more secure. In some extreme cases, additional verbal intervention will help the patient. As with all patients, treat a crying patient with respect and dignity.

### Depression

Depression is a common reason that patients call EMS. In fact, according to the WHO, depression is among the leading causes of disability worldwide. Some of the symptoms a patient with depression will have include sadness, a feeling of hopelessness, restlessness, and irritability. The patient may also have sleeping and eating disorders and a decreased energy level. Depression is a normal human response, but it can lead to harmful behavior. In the treatment of depression, be nonjudgmental and compassionate toward the patient's feelings. The most effective treatment in handling a patient's depression is being a good listener.

### Confusing Behavior or History

Patients sometimes provide more or additional history information to hospital personnel because they are embarrassed or frightened about telling the EMTs and they may feel more comfortable talking with hospital staff. Whatever the situation may be, there are medical causes that you must be aware of that can cause a patient to report a confusing history. Conditions such as hypoxia, stroke, diabetes, trauma, medications, and other drugs could alter a patient's explanation of events. One of the most common causes of confusion is hypoxia. It is not uncommon to encounter an older patient who has dementia, delirium, or Alzheimer disease. It is important to verify the normal mental status of each patient. Do not assume that because a patient is older he or she has one of these conditions.

Confused behavior is not a normal response. After you have properly assessed and treated any life threats, attempt to ask the patient again about the chief complaint or ask someone close to the patient, such as family members or friends, to provide additional details.

### Limited Cognitive Abilities

Cognitive disabilities can range from those that are barely recognizable to those that are severe. You should develop a method for dealing with a patient who has limited cognitive abilities. First, assume you can get an adequate history. Keep your questions simple, and limit the use of medical terms. Be alert for partial answers, and keep asking questions. In cases of patients with severely limited cognitive function, rely on family, caregivers, and friends to supply answers to your questions.

## Cultural Challenges

As an EMT, you are likely to provide care for patients from a variety of different backgrounds and cultures. Cross-cultural communication is an important skill for you to develop to provide proper medical care to all patients equally. Just as you may experience physical challenges in providing good field care, you might also need to overcome cultural and literacy barriers to provide proper prehospital services.

For example, you may obtain only a limited patient history if you ask questions using health care terminology. The patient may have limited understanding of medical language and have difficulty answering your questions. Or, you may encounter a female patient who can ride in the ambulance only in the presence of her husband or family member.

Strategies for overcoming cultural challenges include gaining an understanding of the cultures and patient backgrounds you might encounter on emergency calls; gaining the assistance of the patient's friends or family members; and enlisting the help of health care providers of the same culture or background.

## Language Barriers

We live in a country that is a melting pot of people with diverse nationalities. Not everyone speaks English. For example, you respond to a call for an older woman who fell at a nursing home. The emergency response seems pretty straightforward until you ask the patient what happened and she answers in French. If you don't speak the language, how will you ask the patient to describe what happened and what hurts? Keep in mind that some patients may have disabilities that make it difficult to understand them in any language.

To overcome language barriers, consider using interpreters, translation resources, and related mobile device apps. The best answer is to find an interpreter, but it is not always that simple. First, determine whether the patient speaks or understands any English by asking the patient or others who may be present. Start by introducing yourself by using your name. Determine whether the patient understands who you are. If the patient is able to respond by giving you his or her name, the patient has the ability to understand some English. Remember that increasing the volume of your questions will not increase the patient's understanding of what you are asking him or her. Keep questions straightforward and brief. Simple is best in these patient situations. Use of hand gestures may be helpful.

Be aware of the language diversity in your community. Some dispatch centers and most hospitals have set up programs within the institution that identify various employees who can speak different languages. Provide the hospital with advance notice that a non–English-speaking patient will be arriving. This will allow the hospital the opportunity to make arrangements for an interpreter.

Family and friends on the scene may temporarily interpret for you in an emergency.

## Hearing Problems

Hearing disabilities in patients range from very slight to total deafness. Hearing problems can make the process of obtaining an in-depth history difficult. When you are treating a patient who has a hearing loss, ask questions slowly and clearly. You may want to use a stethoscope to function like a hearing aid; have the patient place the stethoscope in his or her ears while you speak into the stethoscope bell, which will amplify the sound. Changing the pitch of your voice may also help the patient to hear you.

Often, a patient who has had a hearing disability for some time will have mastered the technique of reading lips. If the patient has a hearing aid, ask the patient to use it. Speak slowly and face-to-face with the patient. Some deaf patients will attempt to use sign language for communication. Learning simple sign language will help you in the communication process. Probably the simplest way to communicate with a patient who has a hearing deficit is to use a pencil and paper. Write uncomplicated questions that require simple yes or no answers. If the patient cannot see clearly and has glasses, ask the patient to put them on.

### Visual Impairments

Identify yourself verbally when you enter the home of a visually impaired patient who has called for help. Announcing yourself when entering a residence lets a patient know that help has arrived. Any response from the patient may help you safely locate the patient's whereabouts.

During the assessment and subsequent treatment of a patient who is visually impaired, it is important that you put any items that have been moved back into their previous position. Many visually impaired patients can move freely about their homes because they know exactly where everything is placed.

During the assessment and history-taking process, explain each step in your assessment of vital signs. Notify the patient when you prepare to lift and move him or her on the stretcher. Remember, you are a stranger to the patient, and an EMS vehicle is a foreign environment. A little communication can ease uncertainty in a visually impaired patient.

# Patient Assessment

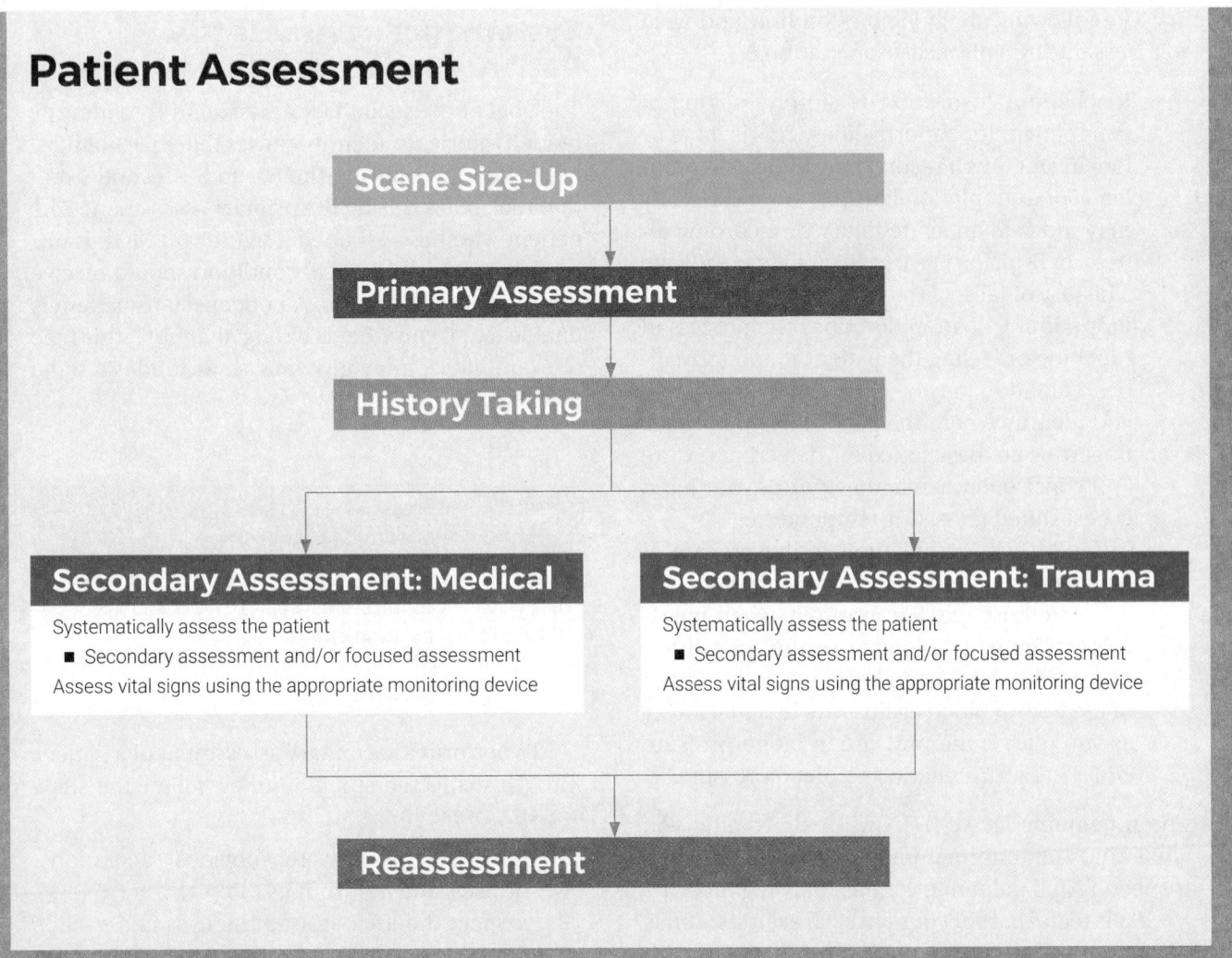

Scene Size-Up

↓

Primary Assessment

↓

History Taking

**Secondary Assessment: Medical**

Systematically assess the patient
- Secondary assessment and/or focused assessment

Assess vital signs using the appropriate monitoring device

**Secondary Assessment: Trauma**

Systematically assess the patient
- Secondary assessment and/or focused assessment

Assess vital signs using the appropriate monitoring device

↓

Reassessment

## Secondary Assessment

If the patient is in stable condition and has an isolated complaint, you may choose to perform the secondary assessment at the scene. If the secondary assessment is not performed at the scene, it is performed in the back of the ambulance en route to the hospital. However, you may not have time to perform a secondary assessment if you have to continually manage life threats that were identified during the primary assessment.

The purpose of the **secondary assessment** is to perform a systematic physical examination of the patient. The physical examination may be a systematic head-to-toe secondary assessment or an assessment that focuses on a certain area or system of the body, often determined by the chief complaint (a focused assessment). Circumstances will determine which aspects of the physical examination will be used.

## Words of Wisdom

Patients may feel vulnerable and exposed during a physical examination. Display compassion during this difficult time. It is also important to cover the patient as much as possible during your assessment to maintain the patient's modesty and body temperature.

The following are guidelines on how and what to assess during a physical examination:

- **Inspection.** Inspection is simply looking at your patient for abnormalities. This is done by looking for anything that may indicate a problem. For example, swelling in a lower extremity may indicate an acute injury or a chronic illness, or bruising in a certain area may indicate a history of falls.
- **Palpation.** Palpation describes the process of touching or feeling the patient for abnormalities. Palpation may be gentle or firmer to help you identify where the patient has pain. Your fingertips are best suited for detecting texture and consistency, while the back of your hand is best suited for noting temperature.
- **Auscultation.** Auscultation is the process of listening to sounds the body makes by using a stethoscope. For example, when measuring a patient's blood pressure, you listen (auscultate) with a stethoscope to the sound of the flow of blood against the brachial artery as you release the pressure in blood pressure cuff. This is auscultation of blood pressure.

The mnemonic DCAP-BTLS will help remind you what kinds of abnormal findings to look for when inspecting and palpating various body regions.

An integral part of your physical examination is to compare findings on one side of the body with the other side when possible. For example, if a patient reports a grating or grinding sensation in his or her arm or you note air bubbles under the skin that produce a crackling sound, check the other arm before determining that the sensation or noise is caused by fractured bone ends or joints rubbing together (crepitus). If one ankle appears swollen, look at the other. If one shoulder feels "out of joint," feel the other one to compare. When listening to breath sounds, listen to both sides of the chest. If possible, find out what conditions are new and which ones the patient has been experiencing for some time. Do not assume that just because a patient has a condition that is causing discomfort, it just happened. As you assess, ask what, if anything, has changed about the condition.

On some occasions, it may even be helpful to note odors during an examination. Odors can indicate anything from infections, to certain medical conditions, to scene safety threats.

## Systematically Assess the Patient—Secondary Assessment

The goal of the secondary assessment is to identify hidden injuries or identify causes that may not have been identified during the 60- to 90-second exam that took place during the primary assessment. Any patient who has sustained a significant MOI, is unconscious, or is in critical condition should receive this type of examination. An unconscious patient is unable to tell you what is wrong; therefore, this type of examination may give you clues to identify the problem.

### Street Smarts

The secondary survey may seem like repetition, but it is very easy to miss significant physical findings on the rapid first assessment.

To perform a secondary assessment of a patient with no suspected spinal injuries, follow the steps in **SKILL DRILL 10-2**:

1. Look at the face for obvious lacerations, bruises, and deformities (**Step 1**).
2. Inspect the area around the eyes and eyelids (**Step 2**).
3. Examine the eyes for redness and for contact lenses. Assess the pupils using a penlight (**Step 3**).
4. Look behind the patient's ears to assess for bruising (Battle sign) (**Step 4**).
5. Use the penlight to look for drainage of spinal fluid or blood in the ears (**Step 5**).
6. Look for bruising and lacerations about the head. Palpate for tenderness, depressions of the skull, and deformities (**Step 6**).
7. Palpate the zygomas for tenderness or instability (**Step 7**).
8. Palpate the maxillae (**Step 8**).
9. Check the nose for blood and drainage (**Step 9**).
10. Palpate the mandible (**Step 10**).
11. Assess the mouth and nose for cyanosis, foreign bodies (including loose teeth or dentures), bleeding, lacerations, and deformities (**Step 11**).
12. Check for unusual odors on the patient's breath (**Step 12**).

13. Look at the neck for obvious lacerations, bruises, and deformities. Observe for jugular vein distention (**Step 13**).

14. Palpate the back of the neck for tenderness and deformity (**Step 14**).

15. Look at the chest for obvious signs of injury before you begin palpation. Be sure to watch for movement of the chest with respirations (**Step 15**).

16. Gently palpate over the ribs to elicit tenderness. Avoid pressing over obvious bruises and fractures (**Step 16**).

17. Listen for breath sounds over the midaxillary and midclavicular lines (**Step 17**).

18. Listen also to breath sounds posteriorly at the bases and apices of the lungs (**Step 18**).

19. Look at the abdomen and pelvis for obvious lacerations, bruises, and deformities. Gently palpate the abdomen for tenderness. If the abdomen is unusually tense, describe the abdomen as rigid (**Step 19**).

20. Gently compress the pelvis from the sides to assess for tenderness (**Step 20**).

21. Gently press the iliac crests to elicit instability, tenderness, and/or crepitus (**Step 21**).

22. Inspect all four extremities for lacerations, bruises, swelling, deformities, and medical alert anklets or bracelets. Also assess distal pulses and motor and sensory function in all extremities (**Step 22**).

23. Assess the back for tenderness and deformities. Remember, if you suspect a spinal injury, maintain spinal motion restriction as you log roll the patient (**Step 23**).

## Systematically Assess the Patient—Focused Assessment

A **focused assessment** is generally performed on patients who have sustained nonsignificant MOIs or on responsive medical patients. This type of examination is typically based on the chief complaint. Your assessment can focus on a specific body part that has been affected, such as abrasions to the elbow, or to a particular body system that has been affected, such as the cardiovascular, respiratory, neurologic, musculoskeletal, integumentary, or genitourinary system. For example, a person with a laceration to the arm may need to have direct pressure applied. For a person reporting a headache, carefully and systematically assess the head and/or the neurologic system. The goal of a focused assessment is to focus your attention on the body part or systems affected by the priority problem or problems.

## Skill Drill 10-2 Performing the Secondary Assessment[a]

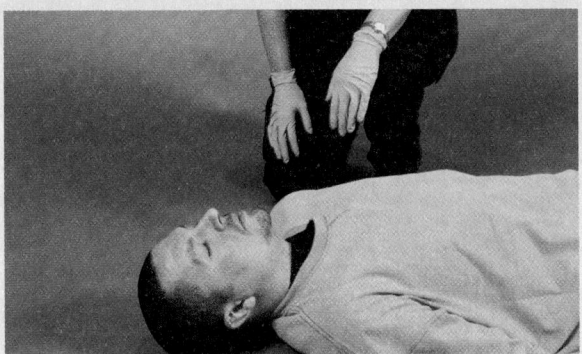

**Step 1**
Observe the face.

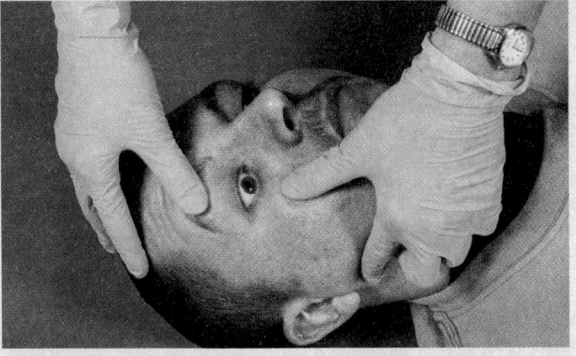

**Step 2**
Inspect the area around the eyes and eyelids.

*(continues)*

# Skill Drill 10-2 Performing the Secondary Assessment (*continued*)

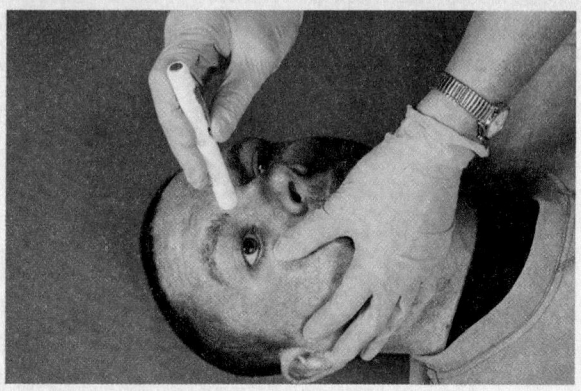

**Step 3**

Examine the eyes for redness and contact lenses. Check pupil function.

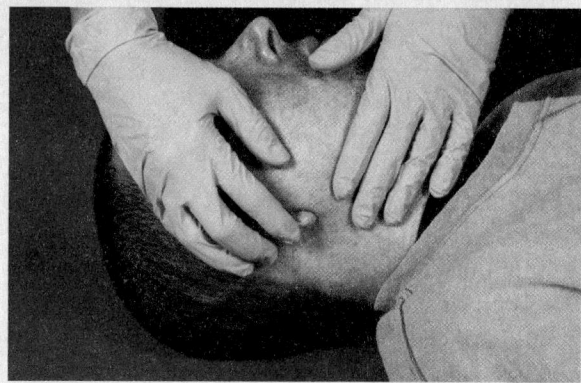

**Step 4**

Look behind the ears for Battle sign.

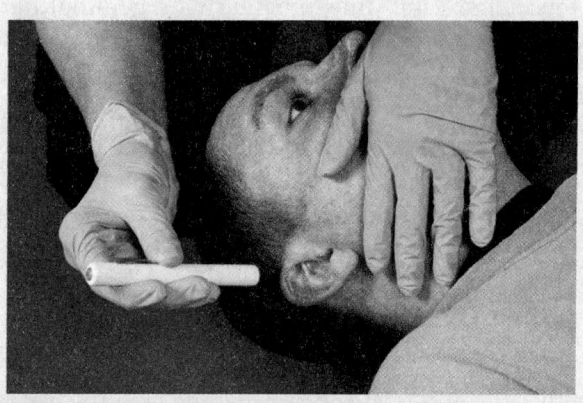

**Step 5**

Check the ears for drainage or blood.

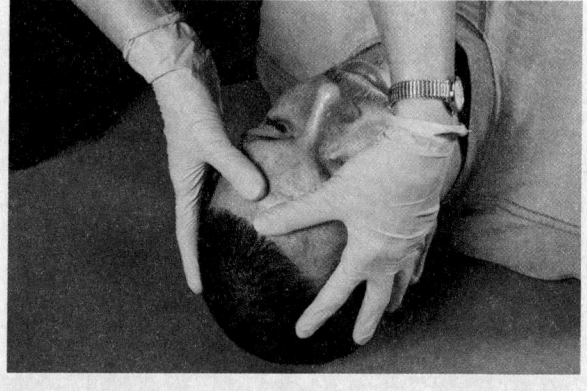

**Step 6**

Observe and palpate the head.

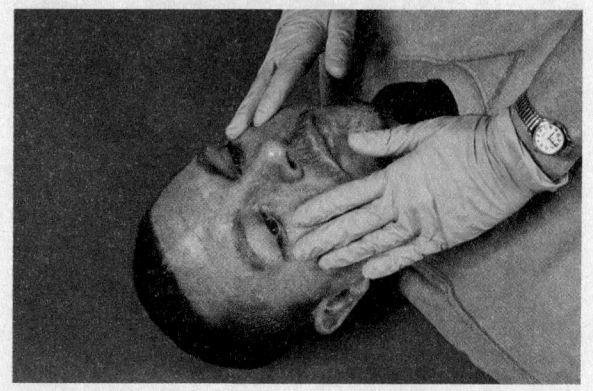

**Step 7**

Palpate the zygomas.

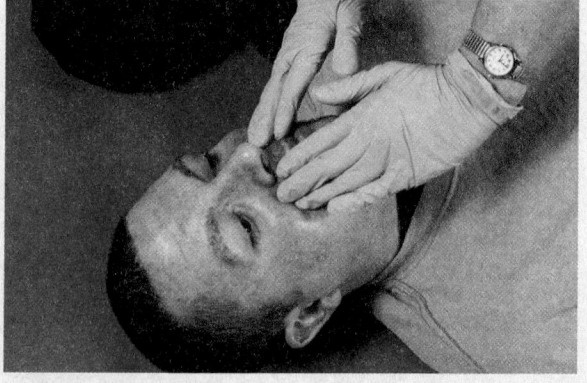

**Step 8**

Palpate the maxillae.

## Skill Drill 10-2 Performing the Secondary Assessment (*continued*)

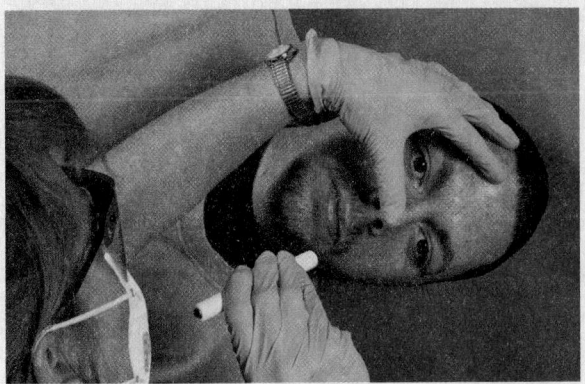

### Step 9

Check the nose for blood and drainage.

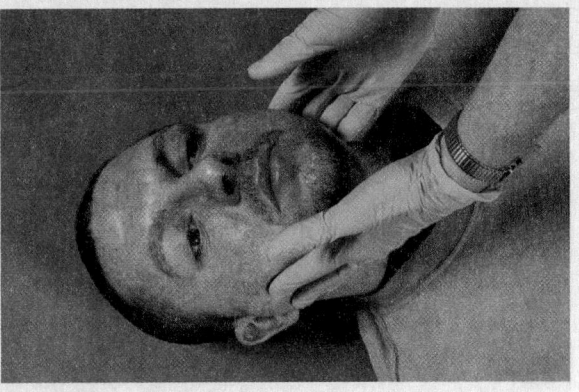

### Step 10

Palpate the mandible.

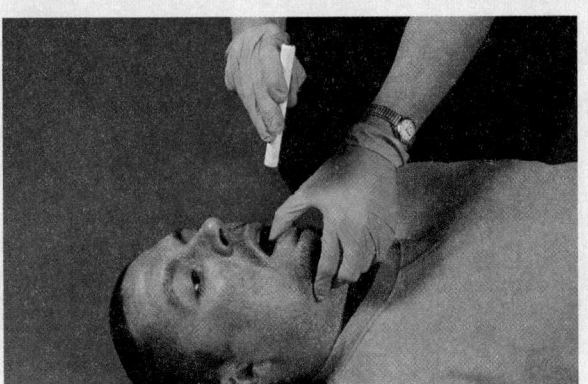

### Step 11

Assess the mouth and nose.

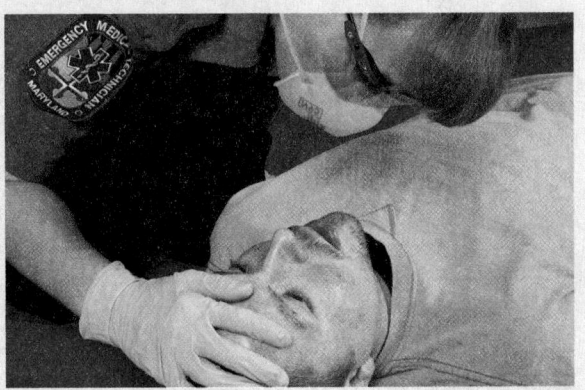

### Step 12

Check for unusual breath odors.

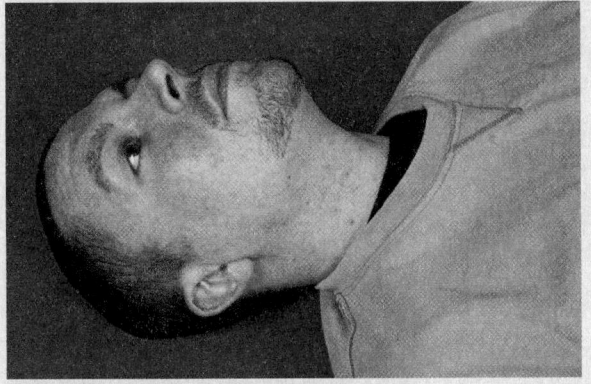

### Step 13

Inspect the neck. Observe for jugular vein distention.

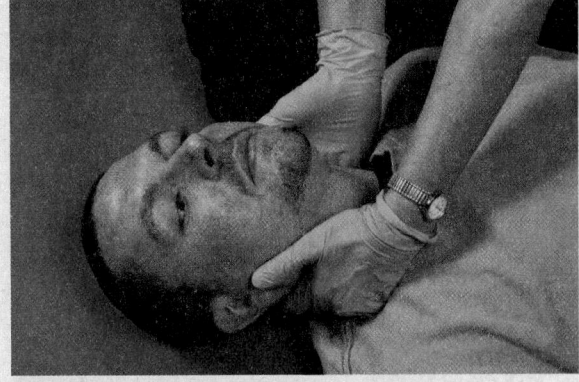

### Step 14

Palpate the front and back of the neck.

*(continues)*

## Skill Drill 10-2 Performing the Secondary Assessment (*continued*)

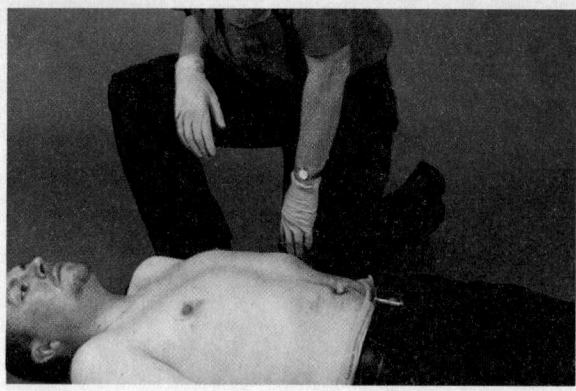

### Step 15

Inspect the chest, and observe breathing motion.

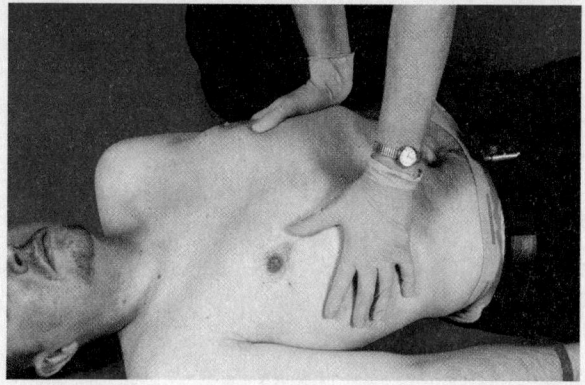

### Step 16

Gently palpate over the ribs.

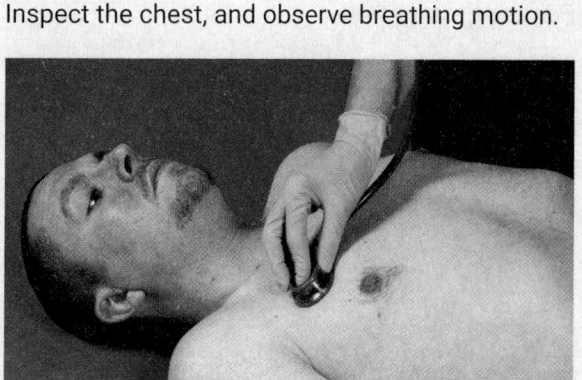

### Step 17

Listen to anterior breath sounds (midaxillary, midclavicular).

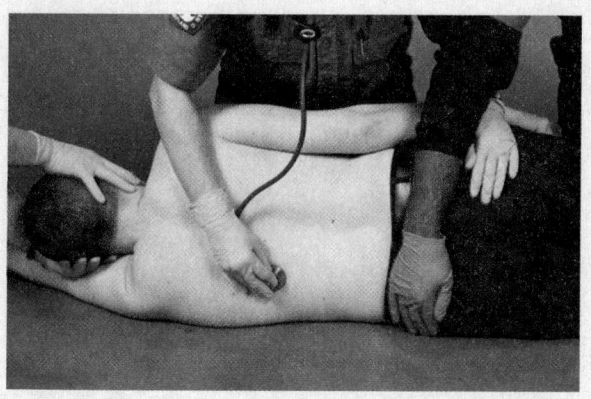

### Step 18

Inspect the back. Listen to posterior breath sounds (bases, apices).

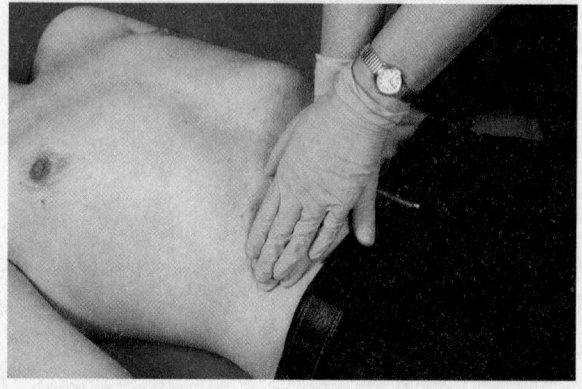

### Step 19

Observe and then palpate the abdomen and pelvis.

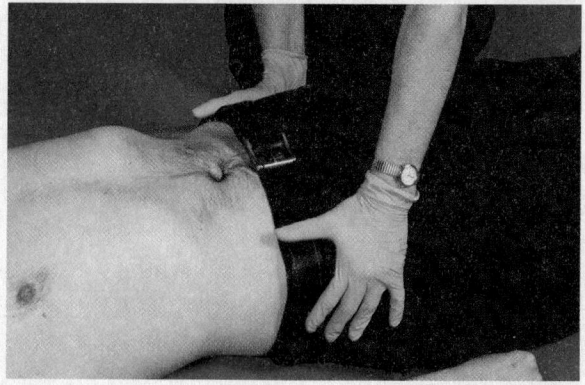

### Step 20

Gently compress the pelvis from the sides.

## Skill Drill 10-2 Performing the Secondary Assessment (*continued*)

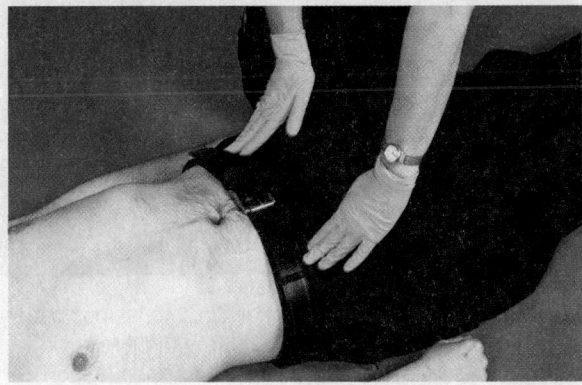

### Step 21

Gently press the iliac crests.

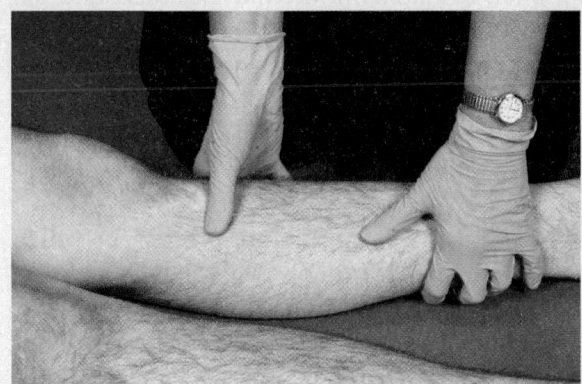

### Step 22

Inspect the extremities; assess distal circulation and motor and sensory function.

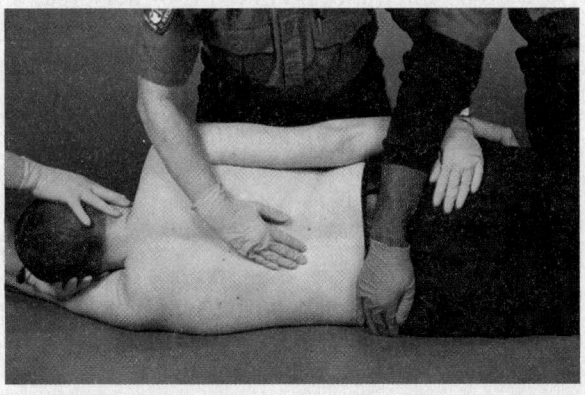

### Step 23

Log roll the patient, and inspect the back for tenderness or deformities.

aWhen performing a secondary assessment on a patient who has sustained significant trauma, maintain spinal motion restriction.

© Jones & Bartlett Learning. Courtesy of MIEMSS.

## Respiratory System

When the patient's chief complaint is focused on the respiratory system, you should have identified and managed life threats during the primary assessment. During the secondary assessment, you will perform an examination directed at obtaining clues that will help determine which treatment to perform and protocols to follow.

Expose the patient's chest. Look again for signs of airway obstruction, as well as trauma to the neck and/or chest. Inspect the chest for overall symmetry. Does the right side of the chest look like the left side? Listen carefully to breath sounds, noting abnormalities. Measure the respiratory rate, chest rise and fall (for tidal volume), and effort. Look for retractions. Is the patient using accessory muscles to help with breathing, and is there increased work of breathing?

For example, sounds of stridor, a brassy crowing sound prominent on inspiration, suggest a partially occluded upper airway caused by swelling. High-pitched crowing sounds may indicate an upper airway obstruction from a foreign body.

Each complete breath includes two distinct phases: inspiration and expiration. During inspiration (inhalation), the diaphragm and inter-costal muscles contract and the chest rises up and out, drawing oxygenated air into the lungs. During expiration (exhalation), the muscles relax and the chest returns to its original position, releasing air with an increased carbon dioxide level out of the lungs. Inhalation and exhalation occur in a 1:3 ratio over their duration; the active inhalation phase lasts one-third the amount of time of the passive exhala-tion phase.

Breathing is a continuous process in which each breath regularly follows the last with no nota-ble interruption. Breathing is normally a spontan-eous, automatic process that should occur without conscious thought, visible effort, marked sounds, or pain. You will assess breathing by *watching* the patient's chest rise and fall, *listening* to **breath sounds** with a stethoscope over each lung and, if the patient is unconscious, *feeling* for air through the mouth and nose during exhalation. Chest rise and breath sounds should be equal on both sides of the chest.

When assessing breathing, you must obtain the following information:

- Respiratory rate
- Rhythm: regular or irregular
- Quality of breathing
- Depth of breathing

## Respiratory Rate

The normal respiratory rate varies widely in adults, ranging from approximately 12 to 20 breaths/min. Children breathe at even faster rates. With prac-tice, you will be able to estimate the rate and note whether it is too fast or too slow. At times it may be important to count the number of respirations during your primary assessment either by listen-ing to breaths, observing the patient for chest rise, or gently placing a hand on the patient's chest and feeling for chest rise.

Respirations are determined by counting the number of breaths the patient takes in 30 seconds and multiplying by two. The result is the number of breaths per minute. For accuracy, count each breath at the same point in its cycle. This is most easily done by counting each peak chest rise. Although you can see peak chest rise, it is easier to place your hand on the patient's chest and feel it.

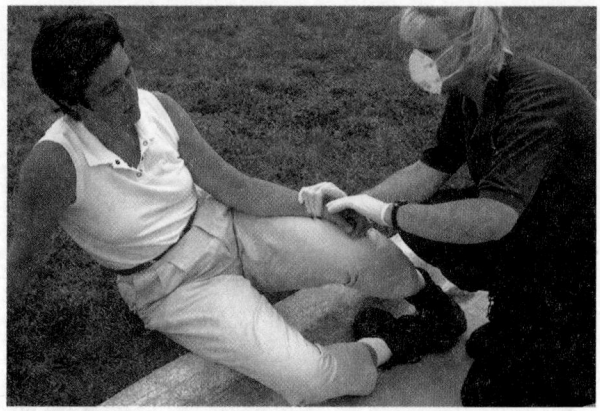

**FIGURE 10-22** Assess respirations in a conscious patient by first taking a radial pulse and then, without releasing the patient's wrist, counting the chest rise and fall for 30 seconds.

© Jones & Bartlett Learning.

However, be aware that a conscious patient who knows that you are evaluating his or her breathing will often override the automatic rate and depth by breathing more slowly and deeply. To prevent this from happening, check respirations in a conscious, alert patient without making the patient aware of what you are evaluating. This can be easily done by first taking a radial pulse and then, without re-leasing the wrist or otherwise suggesting a change, counting the chest rise that you see or feel as the patient's forearm rises and falls with the movement of the chest (**FIGURE 10-22**). If the patient coughs, yawns, sighs, or talks during the 30-second period, wait a few seconds and start again.

**TABLE 10-4** shows the normal range of respira-tory rates of patients who are at rest.

### Respiratory Rhythm

While counting the patient's respirations, also note the rhythm. If the time from one peak chest rise to the next is fairly consistent, respirations are con-sidered regular. If the respirations vary or the rate changes frequently, the respirations are considered irregular. When you document the vital signs, be sure to note whether the patient's respirations were regular or irregular.

### Quality of Breathing

It may be helpful to listen to breath sounds on each side of your patient's chest early in the primary assessment. This can help identify the quality of

**TABLE 10-4** Normal Ranges for Respirations

| Age | Range (breaths/min) |
|---|---|
| Adults | 12 to 20 |
| Adolescents (13 to 18 years) | 12 to 16 |
| School-aged children (6 to 12 years) | 18 to 30 |
| Preschoolers (4 to 5 years) | 22 to 34 |
| Toddlers (1 to 3 years) | 24 to 40 |
| Infants | 30 to 60 |

*Note:* Adult respiratory ranges are per the NHTSA 2009 EMT National EMS Education Standards. Pediatric ranges are modified from *Pediatric Advanced Life Support*, 2012, American Heart Association. Ranges presented in other sources may vary.

© Jones & Bartlett Learning.

air movement in both lungs. Decreased or absent breath sounds on one side of the chest and decreased movement in the rise and fall on one side indicate inadequate breathing.

Normal breathing is almost silent. In a quiet environment, you may hear only the sounds of air movement at the mouth and nose. Through a stethoscope, normal breath sounds include just the sound of air movement through the bronchi accompanied by a soft, low-pitched murmur. Breathing accompanied by other sounds may indicate a significant respiratory problem. A snoring sound may indicate an upper airway obstruction and is usually a result of the tongue blocking the airway. When the upper airway has a partial obstruction by a foreign body or swelling, you may hear stridor, a harsh, high-pitched, crowing sound. If you can hear bubbling or gurgling in the upper airway, the patient probably has fluid in those passages, potentially impeding the exchange of gases. Suction the patient's airway to clear the airway and reduce the risk of aspiration of fluid into the lungs. You may hear other sounds, such as wheezes, a whistling sound indicative of a mild lower airway obstruction. The presence of any of these abnormal sounds indicates that an airway or breathing problem exists. Remember that with a complete airway obstruction, the patient will not be able to move any air and will no longer be able to cough or talk. If you hear no sounds, the patient may not be moving any air at all and will require some action to clear the obstruction.

A patient who coughs up thick, yellow or green sputum (matter from the lungs) most likely has a respiratory infection. A patient with a chest injury may cough up blood or frothy white or pink foamlike sputum caused by blood and fluid mixing with air in the lungs. A patient with congestive heart failure may also cough up pink frothy sputum. The presence of either substance, regardless of its cause, indicates that an urgent, potentially critical cardiovascular and respiratory problem exists, possibly requiring oxygenation, ventilation, and other treatments. Without these treatments, the patient's condition may deteriorate rapidly to a point where the patient can no longer breathe.

## Depth of Breathing

The amount of air that the patient is exchanging depends on the rate and the tidal volume. **Tidal volume** is a measure of the amount of air that is moved into or out of the lungs during one breath. The depth of the breath determines whether the tidal volume is normal, less than normal, or greater than normal.

## Breath Sounds

The following describes how and where to listen to assess breathing:

- First, remember that you can almost always hear a patient's breath sounds better from the patient's back; therefore, if the patient's back is accessible, listen (auscultate) there. If you cannot, listen from the front and sides (**FIGURE 10-23**).
- Auscultate over the upper lungs (apices) at approximately 1 inch (2.5 cm) below the clavicle at the midclavicular line, the midlung fields at the third or fourth intercostal space from the patient's posterior, and the lower lungs (bases) at the sixth intercostal space, midaxillary line.
- Lift the clothing or slide the stethoscope under the clothing. If you listen over clothing, you will primarily hear the sound of the stethoscope sliding over the fabric because breath sounds are muted by clothing.
- Place the diaphragm of the stethoscope firmly against the skin to hear breath sounds.

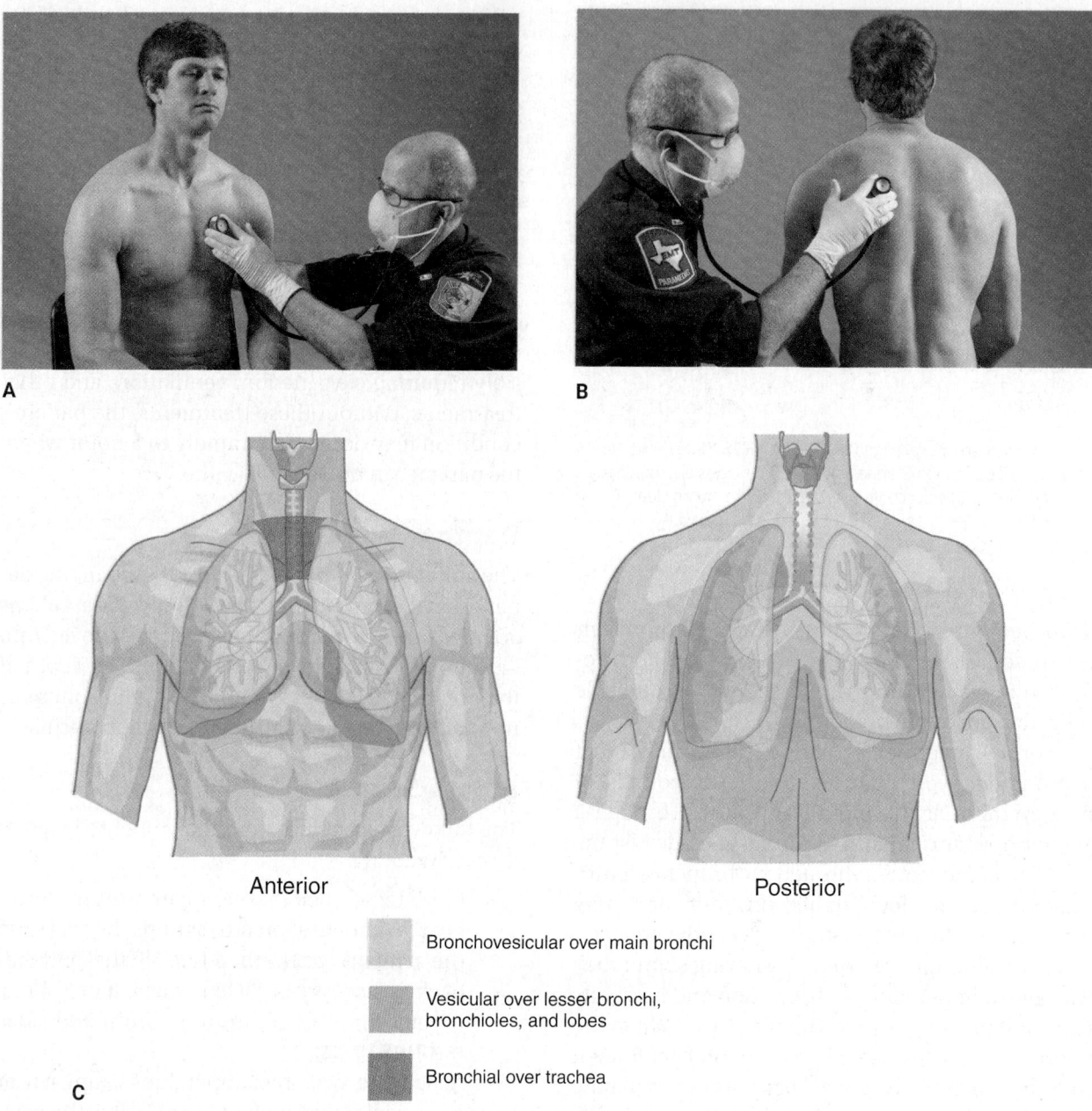

**FIGURE 10-23** Locations for auscultating breath sounds: both sides of the chest in multiple lung fields, as shown. **A.** Stethoscope position for auscultating the front of the chest. **B.** Stethoscope position for auscultating the back. **C.** Colors in illustration correspond to areas where sounds are heard.

A., B., C: © Jones & Bartlett Learning.

What are you listening for? You may be able to identify one of the following sounds:

- **Normal breath sounds.** These are clear and relatively quiet during inspiration and expiration. You will hear the air moving into and out of the lungs freely without obstruction.
- **Snoring breath sounds.** These usually indicate a simple, but potentially dangerous, upper airway

obstruction, usually caused by the tongue or a foreign body. Snoring is an upper airway sound and does not require a stethoscope to be heard.

- **Stridor.** This is often heard before even listening with a stethoscope and may indicate that the patient has an airway obstruction in the neck or upper part of the chest. Expect to hear a brassy, crowing sound that is most prominent on inspiration.

- **Wheezing breath sounds.** These suggest an obstruction or narrowing of the lower airways. Wheezing is a high-pitched whistling sound that is most prominent on expiration. Wheezing is a lower airway sound and is typically heard through auscultation.
- Crackles. Wet, crackling breath sounds (usually on both inspiration and expiration) may indicate fluid in the lungs. Crackles sound similar to the sound made by Rice Krispies when added to milk as the alveoli are popped open.
- Rhonchi. Congested breath sounds may suggest the presence of mucus or fluid in the lungs. Expect to hear low-pitched, noisy sounds that are most prominent on expiration. These lung sounds may be similar to those of blowing bubbles under water. The patient often reports a productive cough associated with these sounds.

You can determine the quality or character of respirations as you are counting the number of respirations. **TABLE 10-5** shows four ways in which the quality or character can be described. Use your sense of hearing to listen for breath sounds or use the preferred method of auscultation, listening with a stethoscope. Note any abnormal breath sounds and treat the patient accordingly.

Because the location of this complaint is the chest, carefully reevaluate the pulse rate, skin, and blood pressure (described in the next section). Inspect and palpate from the clavicles to the shoulder to the abdomen, and reassess breath sounds.

| TABLE 10-5 Characteristics of Respirations | |
|---|---|
| Normal | Breathing is neither shallow nor deep; it appears effortless<br>Equal chest rise and fall<br>No use of accessory muscles |
| Shallow | Decreased chest or abdominal wall motion |
| Labored | Increased breathing effort<br>Use of accessory muscles<br>Possible gasping<br>Nasal flaring, supraclavicular and intercostal retractions in infants and children |
| Noisy | Increase in sound of breathing, including snoring, wheezing, gurgling, crowing, grunting, and stridor |

© Jones & Bartlett Learning.

Note any abnormalities found and document those findings on the patient care report. With this information, you can develop a treatment plan and prioritize transport procedures.

## Cardiovascular System

When the patient's chief complaint is associated with chest pain or other discomfort, a physical examination should include looking, listening, and feeling for abnormalities in the patient's thoracic region. Look for trauma to the chest and listen for breath sounds. Consider the pulse and respiratory rate and the blood pressure. Pay particular attention to rate, quality, and rhythm. Consider your findings when assessing skin condition, which will allow you to determine how well the cardiovascular and respiratory systems are functioning. Check and compare distal pulses to determine any right- and left-side differences. Consider auscultation for abnormal heart sounds; however, keep in mind that obtaining these sounds may be difficult in a noisy prehospital setting. Always remember that a patient's chief complaint may have a medical cause or could be the result of trauma.

### Pulse Rate

After you have determined that a pulse is present, next determine its adequacy. This is done by assessing the pulse rate, pulse quality, and pulse rhythm. For an adult, the normal resting pulse rate should be between 60 and 100 beats/min and could be as much as 100 beats/min in older patients. In general, in pediatric patients, the younger the patient, the faster the pulse rate. In well-conditioned athletes or in people taking heart medications such as beta blockers, the pulse rate may be considerably lower. Remember, you can always ask patients if they know their normal or resting heart rate. **TABLE 10-6** shows the normal ranges of pulse rates for adults and children.

To obtain the pulse rate in most patients, count the number of pulses felt in a 30-second period and then multiply by two. A pulse that is weak and difficult to palpate, irregular, or extremely slow should be palpated and counted for a full minute. A pulse rate is counted as beats per minute.

In an adult patient, a pulse rate that is greater than 100 beats/min is described as tachycardia, and a rate of less than 60 beats/min is described as bradycardia.

| TABLE 10-6 Normal Ranges for Pulse Rate | |
|---|---|
| **Age** | **Range (beats/min)** |
| Adults and children (older than 10 years) | 60 to 100 |
| Preschoolers and school-aged children (2 years to 10 years) | 60 to 140 |
| Infants and toddlers (3 months to 2 years) | 100 to 190 |
| Infants (up to 3 months of age) | 85 to 205 |

Data From: *Pediatric Advanced Life Support*, 2015, American Heart Association, Dallas, TX.

## Pulse Quality

Always report the pulse quality whenever reporting or recording the pulse. The pulse is generally palpated at the radial or carotid arteries in adults and at the brachial artery in infants, because it is normally strong and easily palpable at these locations. Therefore, if the pulse feels to be at normal strength, describe it as being strong. Health care practitioners often describe a stronger-than-normal pulse as "bounding" and a pulse that is weak and difficult to feel as "weak" or "thready." With some experience, you will be able to easily make the necessary distinctions.

## Pulse Rhythm

When you are assessing the pulse, you must also determine whether the rhythm is regular or irregular. Regardless of the rate, the interval between each contraction should be the same, and the pulse should occur at a constant, regular rhythm. Document this rhythm as regular.

The rhythm is considered irregular if the heart periodically has an early or late beat or if a pulse beat is missed. If an irregular pulse is found in a patient with signs and symptoms that suggest a cardiovascular problem, the patient likely needs advanced cardiac assessment and life support. Therefore, depending on your protocols, you should call for ALS backup, arrange for an intercept by paramedics, or initiate prompt transport to definitive care. As with any deviation from expected findings, it is important to determine, if possible, if this irregular rhythm is new or if it represents either a normal or a chronic condition for the patient.

## Blood Pressure

Adequate blood pressure is necessary to maintain proper circulation and perfusion of the vital organs. **Blood pressure** is the pressure of circulating blood against the walls of the arteries. A decrease in the blood pressure may indicate one of the following:

- Loss of blood or its fluid components
- Loss of vascular tone and sufficient arterial constriction to maintain the necessary pressure even without any actual fluid or blood loss
- A cardiac pumping problem

When any of these conditions occurs and results in a drop in circulation, the body's compensatory mechanisms are activated, resulting in an increased heart rate and constriction of the arteries. Normal blood pressure is maintained, and by decreasing the blood flow to the skin and extremities, available blood volume is temporarily redirected to the vital organs so that they remain adequately perfused. However, as shock progresses, eventually the body's defense mechanisms can no longer keep up, and the blood pressure will fall. Decreased blood pressure is a late sign of shock and indicates that the patient is in the critical stage of decompensated shock. Any patient with a markedly low blood pressure has inadequate pressure to maintain proper perfusion of all vital organs and needs to have his or her blood pressure and perfusion restored to a normal level.

When the blood pressure becomes elevated, the body's defenses act to reduce it. Some people have chronically high blood pressure from progressive narrowing of the arteries that occurs with age, and during an acute episode, their blood pressure may increase to even higher levels. Head injury or any number of other conditions may also cause blood pressure to rise to very high levels. Abnormally high blood pressure may result in a rupture or other critical damage in the arterial system.

Blood pressure contains two key separate components: systolic pressure and diastolic pressure. **Systolic pressure** is the increased pressure that is caused along the artery with each contraction (systole) of the ventricles and the pulse wave that it produces. **Diastolic pressure** is the residual pressure that remains in the arteries during the relaxing phase of the heart's cycle (diastole), when the left ventricle is at rest. Systolic pressure represents the maximum pressure to which the arteries are subjected, and diastolic pressure represents the minimum amount of pressure that is always present in the arteries.

Blood pressure is measured in millimeters of mercury (mm Hg). Blood pressure is reported as a fraction in the form of systolic pressure over diastolic pressure. Therefore, if the patient's systolic pressure is 120 and the diastolic pressure is 80, you would record it as "BP 120/80 mm Hg." You would report the patient's blood pressure verbally as "120 over 80."

Avoid obtaining a blood pressure reading on an arm if the patient has an intravenous site or other medical device in place, such as an indwelling catheter or dialysis fistula; has had a mastectomy on that side; or has an injury to that arm. You can ask the patient if any of these exist if they are not visible, such as, a mastectomy. If a patient has chronic renal failure and is undergoing dialysis, ask if the patient has a fistula or any other reason that you should not take a blood pressure using that arm.

A blood pressure cuff with gauge (sphygmomanometer) contains the following components (**FIGURE 10-24**):

- A wide outer cuff designed to be fastened snugly around the entire arm or leg
- An inflatable wide bladder sewn into a portion of the cuff
- A ball-pump with a one-way valve that allows air to enter and a turn-valve that can be closed

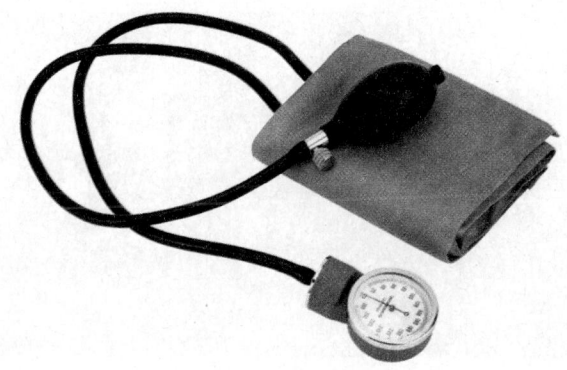

**FIGURE 10-24** A sphygmomanometer.
© WizData, Inc./ShutterStock.

or, when opened, will allow air to be released at a controlled speed from the cuff
- A pressure gauge calibrated in millimeters of mercury, which indicates the pressure that exists in the cuff that is being applied against the underlying artery

Most agencies carry at least three sizes of blood pressure cuffs: thigh, adult, and pediatric (**FIGURE 10-25**). A large adult cuff is also available. You must be sure to select the appropriate-size cuff. A cuff that is too small may result in falsely

## YOU are the Provider

Following the appropriate interventions, your patient's oxygenation and ventilation status have improved; however, he is still bradycardic, hypotensive, and unresponsive. Because there was no one at the scene to provide information regarding his medical history, you continue to treat him based on his signs and symptoms, perform a reassessment, and call in your radio report to the receiving facility.

**Recording Time: 20 Minutes**

| | |
|---|---|
| **Level of consciousness** | Unconscious and unresponsive |
| **Respirations** | 6 breaths/min (baseline); ventilations are being assisted at a rate of 12 breaths per minute. |
| **Pulse** | 38 beats/min; weak and regular |
| **Skin** | Pale and cool; cyanosis has resolved |
| **Blood pressure** | 84/56 mm Hg |
| **SpO$_2$** | 95% (with assisted ventilation) |

You reassess the patient again just before arriving at the ED and note that his condition is unchanged. He is immediately evaluated by the staff physician, who determines that he has overdosed on numerous drugs—including narcotics. After further treatment in the ED, he is admitted to the intensive care unit for close observation.

**9.** What components of the SAMPLE history, if any, can you obtain when your patient is unresponsive? How would you obtain the information?

**10.** Why is reassessing your interventions so important?

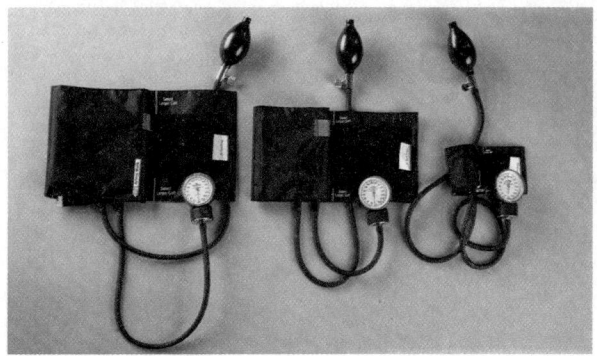

**FIGURE 10-25** Three sizes of blood pressure cuffs: thigh, adult, and pediatric.

© Jones & Bartlett Learning.

high readings; a cuff that is too large may result in falsely low readings. The normal size cuff is designed to wrap around the arm 1 to 1.5 times and take up two-thirds the length from the armpit to the crease in the elbow of most adults. Use a thigh cuff with patients who are obese or have exceptionally well-developed arm muscles or to take the blood pressure of the thigh in patients who have injuries in both arms. Use a small pediatric cuff with children and exceptionally small adults. Measure blood pressure in all patients older than 3 years.

Auscultation is the most common means of measuring a patient's blood pressure. A blood pressure cuff is applied to a patient's upper arm, allowing for the compression of the brachial artery when inflated. This compression creates turbulence and arterial vibrations that make sounds that can be heard using a stethoscope. These sounds are known as Korotkoff sounds. As the cuff is released, the blood flow returns to the artery, and Korotkoff sounds will be heard, denoting the systolic pressure. The disappearance of Korotkoff sounds indicates the diastolic pressure reading.

## Street Smarts

It is a good idea to ask patients if they know their normal pulse rate or blood pressure. Many people monitor heart rate with a smart watch and can readily provide this information. Very fit people and those taking medicines such as beta blockers may have a normal resting heart rate of less than 60 beats per minute. Likewise, a patient may know that his or her average blood pressure is very high or runs less than 90 mm Hg systolic. This baseline information helps you gauge whether the values you are finding are normal for your patient.

Follow the steps in **SKILL DRILL 10-3** to measure blood pressure by auscultation:

1. Follow standard precautions. Explain the procedure to the patient. Examine for a dialysis fistula, central lines, mastectomy, injury to the arm, or other reason to not use this arm to measure blood pressure. If any are present, use the other arm.
2. With the patient's arm exposed, free of clothing, and extended, and with the palm up, place the appropriate-size cuff so that it lies across the upper arm and is located with its distal edge about 1 inch (2.5 cm) above the antecubital space (the crease at the inside of the patient's elbow). Make sure the center of the inflatable bladder, which is usually marked by an arrow on the cuff, lies over the brachial artery. Next, wrap the ends so that the cuff surrounds the upper arm snugly but not tightly. Secure the cuff with the Velcro, making sure to rub your hand over the entire area where the two sides of the Velcro are in contact (**Step 1**).
3. Once the cuff has been properly secured around the upper arm, the arm should be held at about the same level as the heart. With your nondominant hand, palpate the brachial artery (in the antecubital fossa, the anterior aspect of the elbow) to determine where to place the stethoscope (**Step 2**).
4. Place the bell of the stethoscope over the artery and hold it firmly against the artery with the fingers of your nondominant hand. Hold the rubber ball-pump in the palm of your other hand and the turn-valve between your thumb and first finger (**Step 3**).
5. Close the valve tightly and pump the ball-pump until you no longer hear pulse sounds. Continue pumping to increase the cuff's pressure to 200 mm Hg. Next, slowly turn the valve, opening it until air is steadily escaping from the cuff and you see the needle of the gauge slowly drop. Watch the gauge and listen carefully. Note the patient's systolic pressure as the reading on the gauge at which the "taps" or "thumps" of the pulse waves can first be heard clearly. As the pressure in the cuff is progressively reduced, pulse sounds will continue for a time, then suddenly disappear. Note the patient's diastolic pressure as the reading on the

## Skill Drill 10-3 Obtaining Blood Pressure by Auscultation

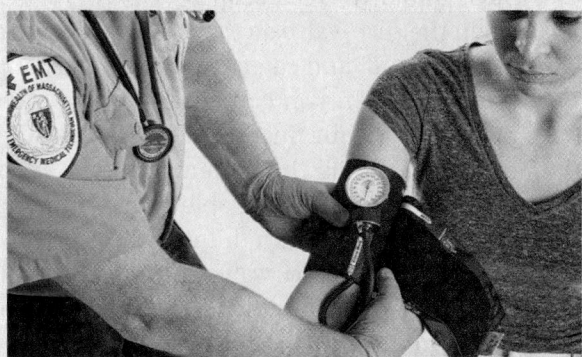

### Step 1

Follow standard precautions. Check for a dialysis fistula, central line, previous mastectomy, and injury to the arm. If any are present, use the brachial artery on the other arm. Apply the cuff snugly. The lower border of the cuff should be about 1 inch (2.5 cm) above the antecubital space.

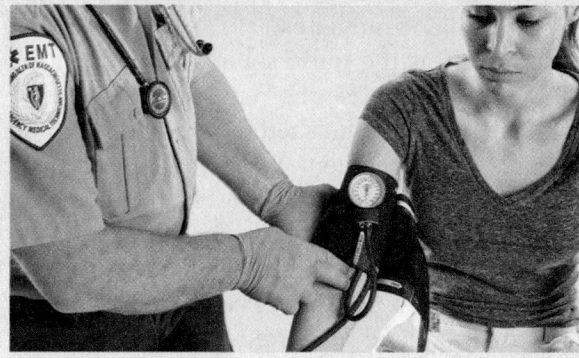

### Step 2

Support the exposed arm at the level of the heart. Palpate the brachial artery.

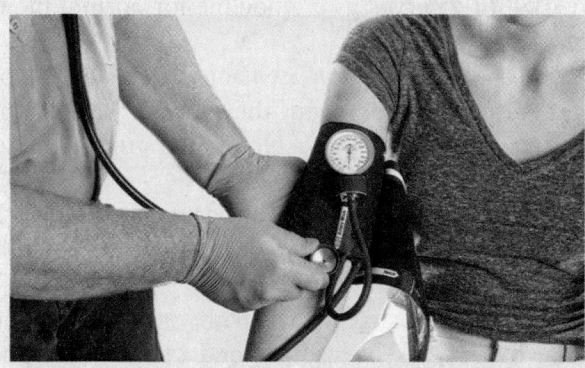

### Step 3

Place the stethoscope over the brachial artery, and grasp the ball-pump and turn-valve.

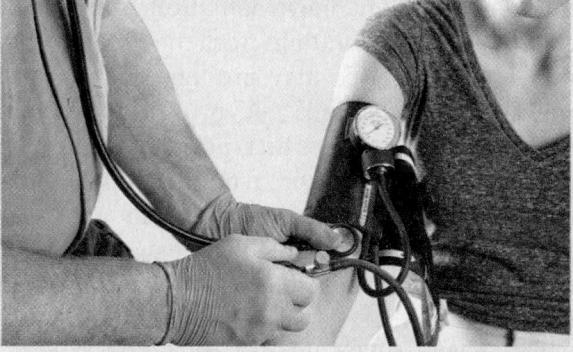

### Step 4

Close the valve, and pump to 30 mm Hg above the point at which you stop hearing pulse sounds. Note the systolic and diastolic pressures as you let air escape slowly.

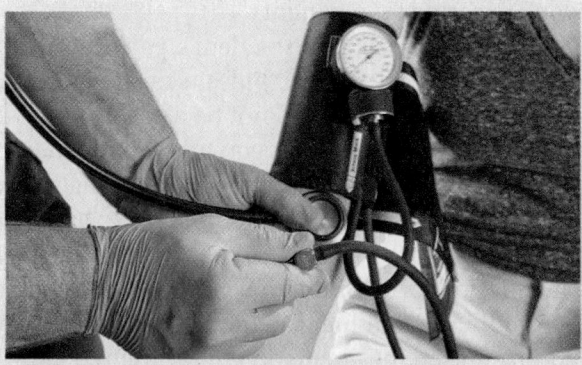

### Step 5

Open the valve, and quickly release remaining air.

gauge at which the sounds stopped (**Step 4**). It is common to see the needle of the sphygmomanometer bounce with the atrial pulsation. Do not mistake these movements as the patient's blood pressure.

6. As soon as the pulse sounds stop, open the valve, and release the remaining air quickly. Once you have finished measuring the blood pressure, document your findings and the time at which the blood pressure was taken. Blood pressure is most often measured by auscultation with the patient in a sitting or semi-Fowler position. Occasionally, when a patient's blood pressure is very low, you will continue to hear pulse sounds from the reading at which they started all the way until the gauge has reached 0. When this occurs, you should record the diastolic pressure as "0" or indicate that it was heard until the gauge read "0" (**Step 5**).

Obtaining a patient's blood pressure accurately by auscultation may be difficult at times. Noisy environments, patient movement from tremors or seizures, external vibrations from the EMS vehicle, and excessive noises may produce sounds that mimic Korotkoff sounds and provide inaccurate readings. Other variables that may make obtaining an accurate blood pressure reading nearly impossible are uncooperative adults, infants and children, and patients who are hypotensive with poor perfusion. In these cases, measure blood pressure by palpation.

The palpation (feeling) method does not depend on your ability to hear sounds and should be used in these cases to obtain a patient's blood pressure. If possible, it is preferable that you first obtain a baseline auscultated blood pressure.

Follow the steps in **SKILL DRILL 10-4** to measure blood pressure by palpation:

1. Secure the appropriate-size cuff around the patient's upper arm in the manner previously described (**Step 1**).
2. With your nondominant hand, palpate the patient's radial pulse on the same arm as the cuff (**Step 2**). Once you have located it, do not move your fingertips until you have completed taking the blood pressure.
3. While holding the ball-pump in your other hand, close the turn-valve and slowly inflate

the cuff until the pulse disappears and then continue to inflate to 200 mm Hg (**Step 3**). As the cuff inflates, you will no longer feel the pulse under your fingertips.

4. Open the turn-valve so that air slowly escapes from the cuff, and carefully observe the gauge (**Step 4**). When you can again feel the radial pulse under your fingertips, note the reading on the gauge as the patient's systolic blood pressure. You will not be able to determine the diastolic pressure with this method.
5. Next, open the turn-valve further, and completely deflate the cuff (**Step 5**). Document your findings, including the time, and note that the pressure was taken by palpation. On your patient care report, record the blood pressure as "120/P" and verbalize it as "120 palpated."

### Normal Blood Pressure

Blood pressure levels vary with age and sex. **TABLE 10-7** serves as a guideline for normal blood pressure ranges.

A patient has **hypotension** when the blood pressure is lower than the normal range and **hypertension** when the blood pressure is higher than the normal range.

Typically, you will see children less frequently than adults; therefore, you might not remember the normal ranges for the various age groups. It is a good idea to carry a chart with you that lists normal blood pressure ranges and other vital signs. Remember, however, that blood pressure will vary somewhat with different patients and how they react to the environment around them. Often, the most important information associated with the blood pressure is not the absolute value at any one point but the trend in the pressure over time while you are caring for a patient.

When assessing the patient's general circulation, the blood pressure, pulse, skin temperature, and capillary refill should not be assessed in an injured limb. However, once you have obtained these vital signs from an uninjured limb, you might want to compare the distal skin temperature, quality of the distal pulse, and/or CRT in the injured limb with those found on the uninjured side. This information is useful in evaluating whether the injury may have compromised the circulation in the injured limb.

## Skill Drill 10-4 Obtaining Blood Pressure by Palpation

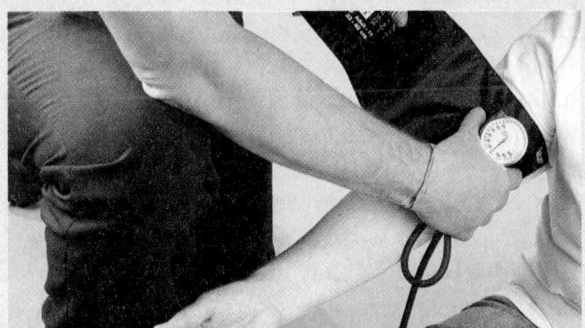

### Step 1

Follow standard precautions. Secure the appropriate-size cuff around the patient's upper arm.

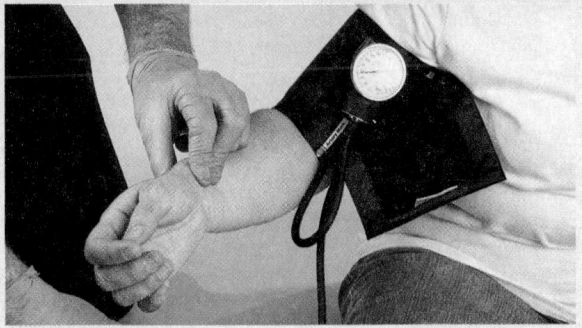

### Step 2

With your nondominant hand, palpate the patient's radial pulse on the same arm as the cuff. Once you have located it, do not move your fingertips until you have completed taking the blood pressure.

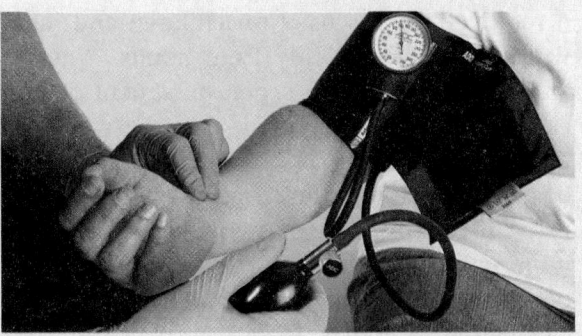

### Step 3

While holding the ball-pump in your other hand, close the turn-valve and slowly inflate the cuff until the pulse disappears and then continue to inflate another 30 mm Hg. As the cuff inflates, you will no longer feel the pulse under your fingertips.

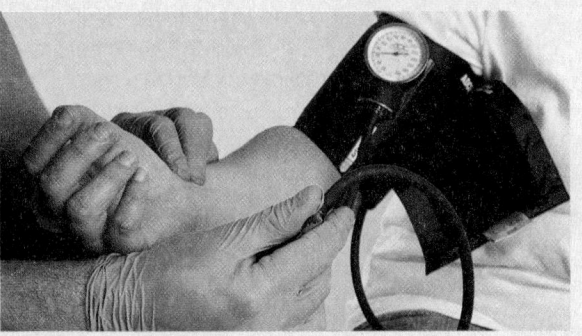

### Step 4

Open the turn-valve so that air slowly escapes from the cuff, and carefully observe the gauge. When you can again feel the radial pulse under your fingertips, note the reading on the gauge as the patient's systolic blood pressure.

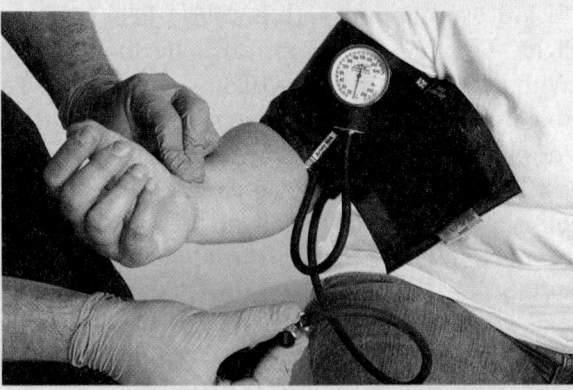

### Step 5

Next, open the turn-valve further, and completely deflate the cuff. Document your findings, including the time, and note that the pressure was taken by palpation.

**TABLE 10-7** Normal Range for Blood Pressure

| Age | Range, mm Hg |
| --- | --- |
| Adults | 90 to 120 (systolic) |
| Adolescent (15 years) | 110 to 131 (systolic) |
| Child (7 years) | 97 to 115 (systolic) |
| Child (2 years) | 86 to 106 (systolic) |
| Infant (1–12 months) | 72 to 104 (systolic) |
| Neonate (96 hours) | 67 to 84 (systolic) |

Data adapted from *Pediatric Advanced Life Support*, 2015, American Heart Association; and National Model EMS Clinical Guidelines, v2.2, 2019, NASEMSO.

## Words of Wisdom

Automated blood pressure machines often display **mean arterial pressure (MAP)** in addition to systolic and diastolic blood pressures. The MAP is a measure of the average arterial pressure through the systolic and diastolic phases of the cardiac cycle. It is increasingly used as a valuable measurement to determine perfusion in conditions such as sepsis. A MAP of greater than 65 is needed to adequately perfuse the vital organs in an adult.

## Neurologic System

Assessment of a patient's neurologic system can be time consuming and detailed. A neurologic assessment should be performed anytime you are confronted with a patient who has changes in mental status, a possible head injury, stupor, dizziness, drowsiness, or syncope. A neurologic assessment begins before you even touch the patient. It can be as simple as talking with the patient, asking questions, and receiving an appropriate reply from the patient during the primary assessment.

Evaluate the LOC and orientation to determine the patient's ability to think. Use the AVPU scale if appropriate to determine the patient's mental status. Is the patient alert, oriented to person, place, time, and events? Is the patient responsive or unresponsive? Does the patient respond to verbal and painful stimuli? If the patient is responsive, evaluate speech for clarity, speed, organization, and logic. What is the patient's activity level? What are the patient's mood and thought content? What do the patient's facial expressions tell you? Is the patient angry, fearful, depressed, anxious, or restless? Does the patient appear uncomfortable? Does the patient make incomprehensible or understandable statements? Is the patient's memory affected? What is the patient's perception or view on what is happening? These are all important considerations when beginning to assess the neurologic system.

Use of the Glasgow Coma Scale (GCS) score can be helpful in providing additional information on patients with changes in mental status. The GCS (discussed further in Chapter 18, *Neurologic Emergencies*) uses parameters that test a patient's eye opening, best verbal response, and best motor response. The scale provides a numeric score that is associated with the relative severity of a patient's brain dysfunction (**TABLE 10-8**). This information provides baseline data on the patient's overall neurologic status and can be used to help determine if that status is changing for better or worse. A modified GCS is used for children and infants, who respond differently from adults. When you are reporting the GCS score, document or report each section (eg, Eye opening: 3, Verbal response: 4, Motor response: 5 = GCS score of 12) to describe baseline function in each area. Similar to blood pressure, the trending of the patient's GCS is often important. The GCS scale can be difficult to remember and you may need to consult a reference when calculating a patient's GCS.

## Pupils

The pupil is the black center portion of the eye. The pupils are normally round, of approximately equal size, and adjust their size depending on the available light. The diameter and reactivity to light of the patient's pupils can reflect the status of the brain's perfusion, oxygenation, and condition. In normal room light, the pupil should appear to be about midsize. With less light, the pupils dilate to allow more light to enter the eye. When a bright light is shined near the eye, the pupils constrict (**FIGURE 10-26A**). When a brighter light is introduced into one eye, both pupils should constrict equally to the appropriate size for the pupil receiving the most light.

In the absence of light, the pupils will become fully relaxed and dilated (**FIGURE 10-26B**). When light is introduced, each eye sends sensory signals to the brain indicating the level of light it is receiving. Pupil size is regulated by a series of continuous motor commands that the brain automatically sends through the

**TABLE 10-8** Glasgow Coma Scale[a]

| Eye Opening | | Best Verbal Response | | Best Motor Response | |
|---|---|---|---|---|---|
| Spontaneous | 4 | Oriented conversation | 5 | Obeys commands | 6 |
| In response to sound | 3 | Confused conversation | 4 | Localizes to pressure | 5 |
| In response to pressure | 2 | Inappropriate words | 3 | Withdraws from pressure | 4 |
| None | 1 | Incomprehensible sounds | 2 | Abnormal flexion | 3 |
| | | None | 1 | Abnormal extension | 2 |
| | | | | None | 1 |

[a]Some systems use a "Not testable (NT)" score for any element that cannot be tested. Eye opening cannot be tested in a patient whose eyes are closed due to a local factor, such as swelling; verbal response cannot be tested in a patient who has a preexisting factor interfering with communication, such as mutism; and motor response cannot be tested in a patient who has preexisting paralysis or other limiting factor.

*Score:* 13–15 may indicate mild dysfunction, although 15 is the score a person without neurologic impairment would receive.

*Score:* 9–12 may indicate moderate dysfunction.

*Score:* 8 or less is indicative of severe dysfunction.

© Jones & Bartlett Learning.

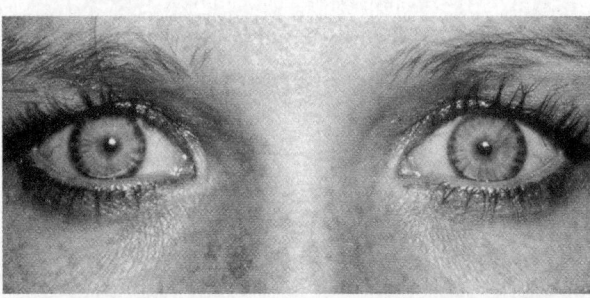
A

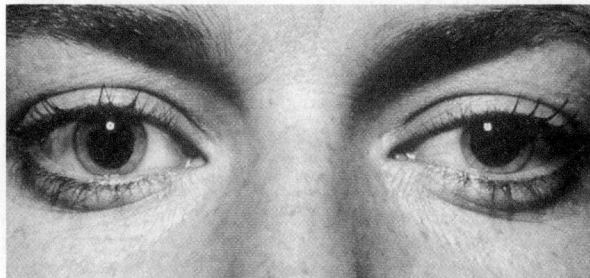
B

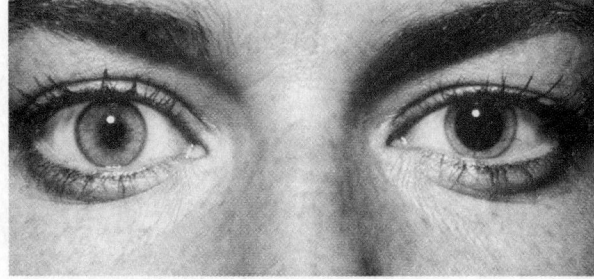
C

**FIGURE 10-26 A.** Constricted pupils. **B.** Dilated pupils. **C.** Unequal pupils.

A., B., C: © American Academy of Orthopaedic Surgeons.

oculomotor nerves to each eye, causing both pupils to constrict to the same appropriate size. Normally, pupil size changes instantly with any change in light level.

Some patients normally have pupils that do not react properly to changes in light as a result of eye surgery or other conditions. A small number of patients exhibit normally unequal pupils (anisocoria) (**FIGURE 10-26C**). If the patient or family member cannot confirm the presence of these conditions, you should presume that abnormal pupillary response indicates altered brain function as a result of central nervous system depression or injury. Specifically, evaluate if the pupils react in any of the following ways:

- Become fixed (either dilated or constricted) with no reaction to changes in light
- Dilate with introduction of a bright light and constrict when the light is removed
- React sluggishly instead of briskly
- Become unequal in size
- Become unequal in size when a bright light is introduced into or removed from one eye

Some of the causes of depressed brain function include the following:

- Injury of the brain or brainstem
- Trauma or stroke
- Brain tumor
- Inadequate oxygenation or perfusion
- Drugs or toxins (central nervous system depressants)

The mnemonic PEARRL is a useful guide in assessing the pupils. The letters stand for the following:

**P** Pupils
**E** Equal
**A** And
**R** Round
**R** Regular in size
**L** React to Light

For patients with normal pupils, you can report "Pupils are Equal And Round, Regular in size, and react properly to Light" or "Pupils = PEARRL." Describe any abnormal findings using the longer form, such as "Pupils are equal and round, the left pupil is fixed and dilated, the right pupil is regular in size and reacts to light."

## Assessing Neurovascular Status

Now perform a hands-on assessment to determine sensory and motor response. How does the patient move? Check for bilateral muscle strength and weaknesses. Complete a thorough sensory assessment. Test for pain, sensations, and position, and compare distal and proximal sensory and motor responses and one side with the other. Remember that a physical examination that deals with a specific chief complaint can be streamlined to assess a specific area of concern.

To assess neurovascular status in a conscious patient, follow the steps in **SKILL DRILL 10-5**:

1. **Pulse.** Palpate the pulse distal to the point of injury. First, palpate the radial pulse in the

## Skill Drill 10-5 Assessing Neurovascular Status

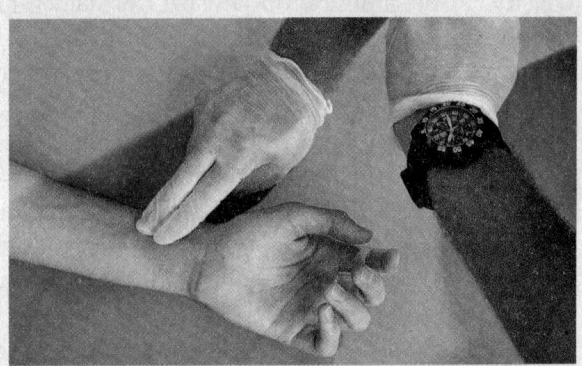

**Step 1**
Palpate the radial pulse in the upper extremity.

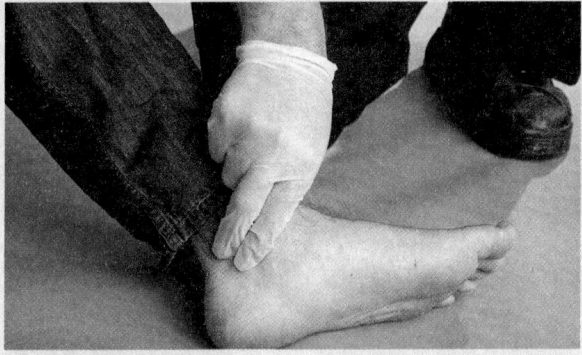

**Step 2**
Palpate the posterior tibial and dorsalis pedis pulses in the lower extremity.

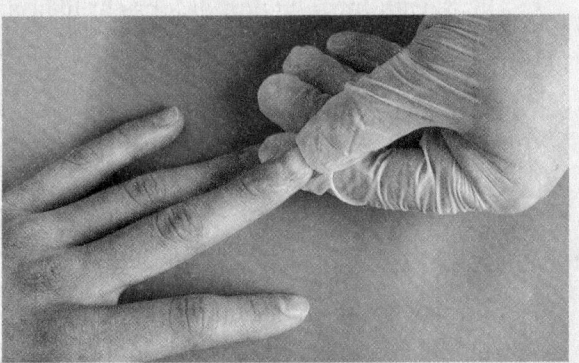

**Step 3**
Assess capillary refill by blanching a fingernail or toenail.

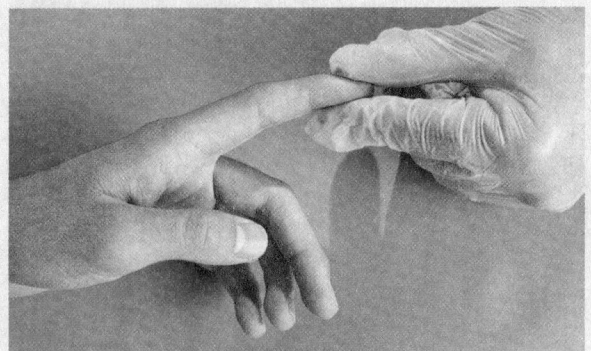

**Step 4**
Assess sensation on the flesh near the tip of the index finger and thumb, as well as the little finger.

# Skill Drill 10-5 Assessing Neurovascular Status (*continued*)

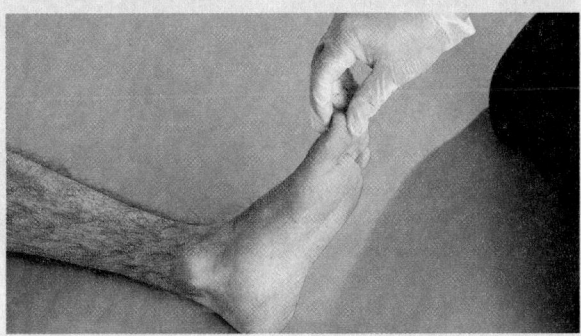

### Step 5

On the foot, first check sensation on the flesh near the tip of the big toe.

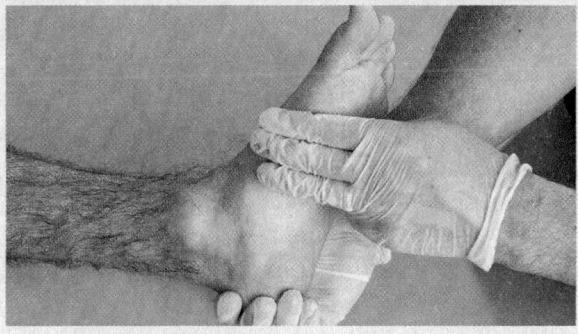

### Step 6

Also check sensation on the side of the foot.

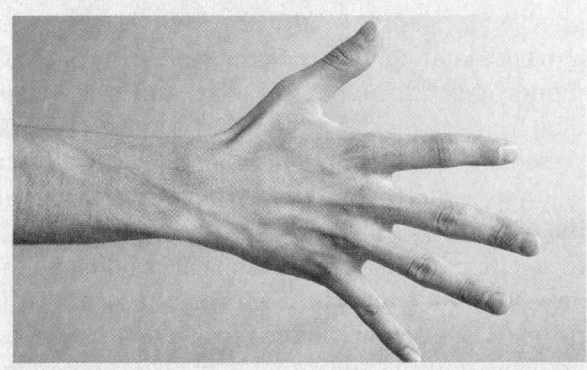

### Step 7

For an upper extremity injury, evaluate motor function by asking the patient to open the hand. (Perform motor tests only if the hand or foot is not injured. Stop a test if it causes pain.)

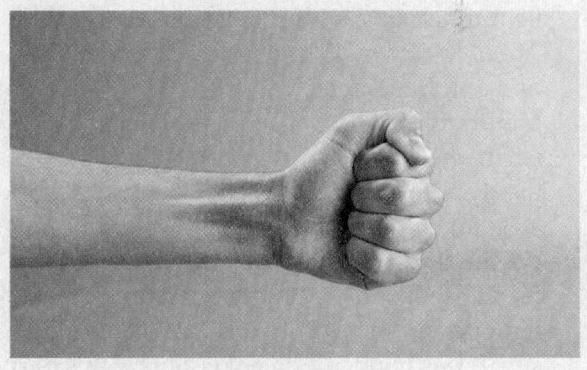

### Step 8

Also ask the patient to make a fist.

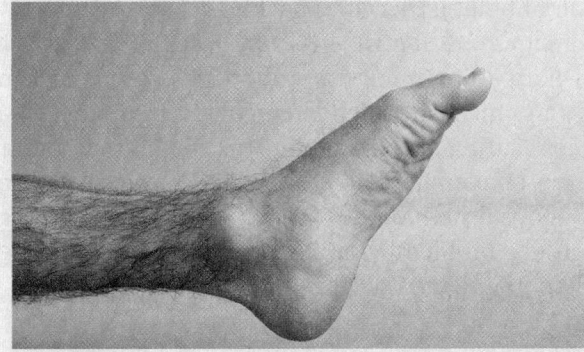

### Step 9

For a lower extremity injury, ask the patient to flex the foot and toes (ask the patient to "push down on the gas").

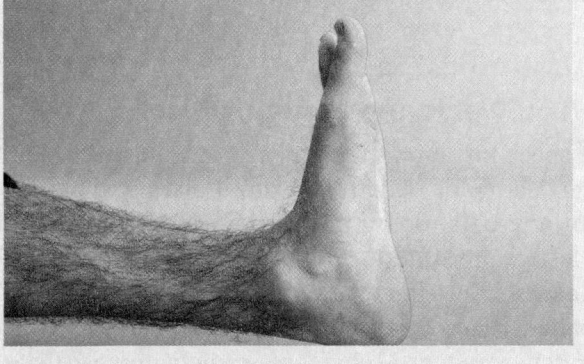

### Step 10

Also have the patient extend the foot and ankle and pull the toes and foot toward the nose.

upper extremity (**Step 1**). Second, in the lower extremity, palpate the posterior tibial and dorsalis pedis pulses (**Step 2**).

2. **Capillary refill.** Note and record the skin color, identifying any pallor or cyanosis. Then apply firm pressure to the tip of the fingernail or toenail, which will cause the skin to blanch (turn white). If normal color does not return within 2 seconds after you release the nail, you can assume that circulation is impaired. This test is typically recommended for use in children, although it can also be used in adults (**Step 3**).

3. **Sensation.** In the hand, check the feeling on the flesh near the tip of the index finger and thumb, as well as the little finger (**Step 4**). In the foot, check the sensation on the flesh of the big toe (**Step 5**) and on the lateral side of the foot (**Step 6**). The patient's ability to sense light touch in the fingers or toes distal to the site of a fracture is a good indication that the nerve supply is intact.

4. **Motor function.** Evaluate muscular activity when the injury is proximal to the patient's hand or foot. Ask the patient to open and close a fist for an upper extremity injury and to wiggle the toes and move the foot up and down for a lower extremity injury. Sometimes, an attempt at motion will produce pain at the injury site. If this happens, do not continue this part of the examination. To avoid causing pain, do not perform this test at all if the injury involves the hand or foot itself (**Steps 7 through 10**).

Because many of the steps require patient cooperation, you will not be able to assess sensory and motor functions in an unconscious patient.

## Anatomic Regions

### Head, Neck, and Cervical Spine

Inspect for abnormalities of the head, neck, and cervical spine. Gently palpate the scalp and skull for any pain, deformity, tenderness, crepitus, and bleeding (**FIGURE 10-27**). Ask a responsive patient if he or she feels any pain or tenderness. Look at the patient's face. Is it symmetrical? Is there evidence of trauma, such as ecchymoses or hematomas? Does the patient have any facial expressions such as a smile or grimace? Check the patient's eyes, and assess pupillary function, shape, and response. Are the pupils equal in size and reactive to light, or are they

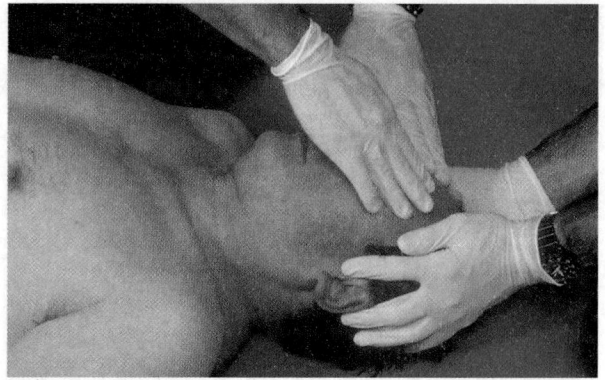

**FIGURE 10-27** Gently palpate the head for any pain, deformity, tenderness, crepitus, and bleeding.
© Jones & Bartlett Learning. Courtesy of MIEMSS.

constricted, dilated, or unequal? Check the color of the sclera. Assess the patient's cheek bones (zygomas) for possible injury. Check the patient's ears and nose for fluid. Next, before opening the patient's mouth, check the upper (maxillae) and lower (mandible) jaw. Once the patient's jaws have been assessed and it has been determined that movement will not create any additional pain or injury, open the patient's mouth, looking for any broken or missing teeth. If blood and secretions have impaired the airway, this should have been corrected during the primary assessment. Before moving on to the neck, note any unusual odors that may be present in the patient's mouth. This may give an indication of what type of emergency you may be dealing with.

Next, check the neck for signs of swelling or bleeding. Palpate the neck for signs of trauma, such as deformities, bumps, swelling, bruising, and bleeding, as well as a crackling sound produced by air bubbles under the skin, known as **subcutaneous emphysema** (**FIGURE 10-28**). Also, in patients in whom spinal injury is not suspected, inspect for pronounced or distended jugular veins with the patient sitting at a 45° angle. This is a normal finding in a person who is lying supine; however, jugular venous distention in a patient who is sitting up suggests a problem with blood returning to the heart. Report and record your findings carefully.

### Chest

When assessing the chest, inspect, visualize, and palpate over the chest area for injury and signs of trauma, including bruising, tenderness, and swelling (**FIGURE 10-29**).

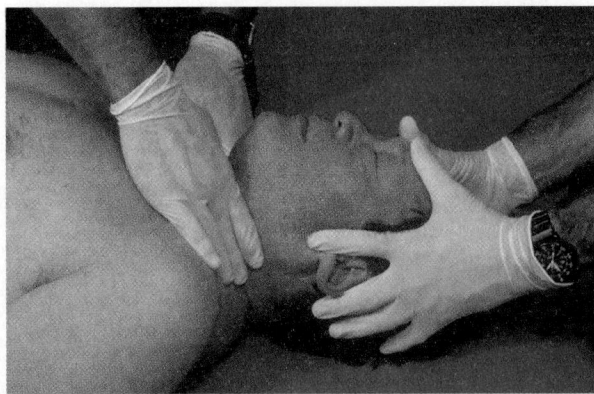

**FIGURE 10-28** Gently palpate the neck.

© Jones & Bartlett Learning. Courtesy of MIEMSS.

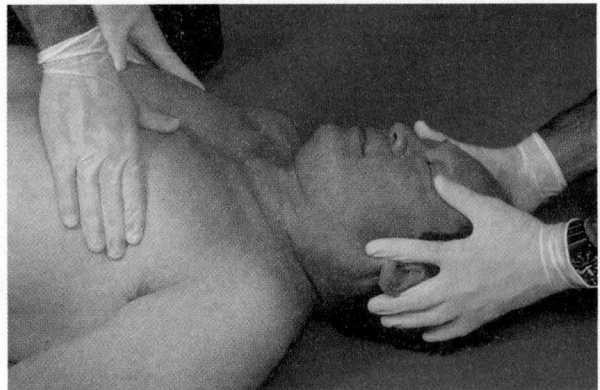

**FIGURE 10-29** Inspect, visualize, and palpate over the chest area for injury and signs of trauma.

© Jones & Bartlett Learning. Courtesy of MIEMSS.

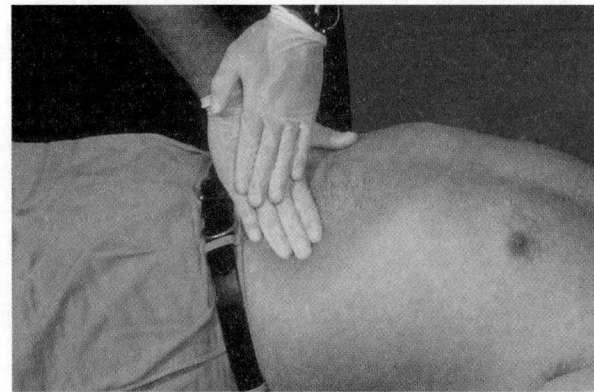

**FIGURE 10-30** Palpate the abdomen, evaluating for tenderness and bleeding.

© Jones & Bartlett Learning. Courtesy of MIEMSS.

When assessing breathing, watch for both sides of the chest to rise and fall together with normal breathing. Observe for abnormal breathing signs, including retractions or **paradoxical motion** (when only one section of the chest rises on inspiration while another area of the chest falls).

Retractions indicate the patient has some condition, usually medical, that is impairing the flow of air into and out of the lungs. Paradoxical motion is associated with a fracture of several ribs (flail), causing a section of the chest to move independently from the rest of the chest wall. Feel for grating of the bones as the patient breathes. Crepitus is often associated with rib fractures. Palpate the chest for subcutaneous emphysema, especially in cases of severe blunt chest trauma, as this could indicate a pneumothorax.

If the patient reports difficulty breathing or has evidence of trauma to the chest, auscultate breath sounds. This helps you to evaluate air movement into and out of the lungs. To auscultate, you need a stethoscope. The position of the patient will determine the way you proceed to check for breathing.

The goal is to hear and document the presence or absence of breath sounds. It is important to compare one side with the other. If you believe the patient's breathing is abnormal, reassess breathing and, if appropriate, assist with ventilations.

### Abdomen

Look for trauma to the abdomen and for distention. Palpate the abdomen for tenderness, rigidity, and patient **guarding** (**FIGURE 10-30**). As you palpate the abdomen, use "firm," "soft," "tender," or "distended" (swollen) to report your findings. If the patient is awake and alert, ask about pain as you perform the examination. The abdomen is divided into four quadrants: left upper quadrant (LUQ), left lower quadrant (LLQ), right upper quadrant (RUQ), and right lower quadrant (RLQ). Always start the palpation of the abdomen in the quadrant that is farthest from the patient's pain. Do not palpate obvious soft-tissue injuries, and be careful not to palpate too firmly. Assess for the presence of rebound tenderness, which is pain created when pressure is released.

### Pelvis

Inspect the pelvis for symmetry and any obvious signs of injury, bleeding, and deformity (**FIGURE 10-31**). If the patient reports no pain, gently press downward and inward on the pelvic bones. Do not rock the

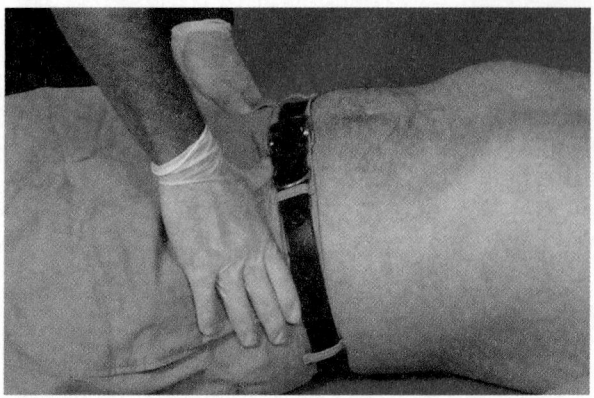

**FIGURE 10-31** Inspect the pelvis for any obvious signs of injury, bleeding, and deformity.

© Jones & Bartlett Learning. Courtesy of MIEMSS.

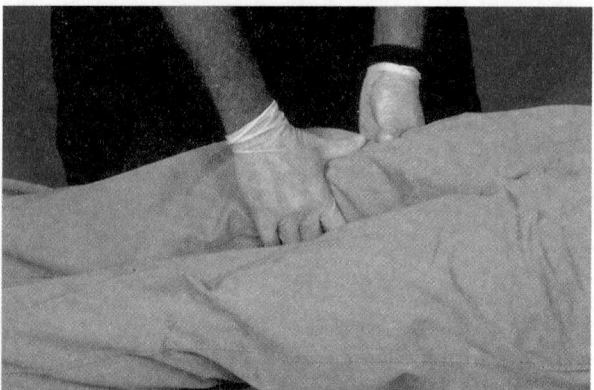

**FIGURE 10-32** Inspect each extremity for cuts, bruises, swelling, obvious injuries, and bleeding.

© Jones & Bartlett Learning. Courtesy of MIEMSS.

pelvis; this action may result in exacerbation of damage to any unstable bones. If you feel any movement or crepitus or the patient reports pain or tenderness, severe injury may be present. Injuries to the pelvis and surrounding abdomen may bleed profusely without any obvious external signs, so continue to monitor the patient's mental status, skin condition, and vital signs.

### Extremities

An assessment of the patient's musculoskeletal system typically is done because of a chief complaint associated with some type of trauma. Do all extremities appear to be properly positioned, and do all extremities appear to be functioning normally? Assess for posture if standing, and look at joints, checking for range of motion. This should be done by asking the patient how much he or she can move the extremity or joint. Never force a painful joint to move. Always compare the right side with the left side, looking for weakness or atrophy, and assess equality of grip strength.

Inspect each extremity for symmetry, cuts, bruises, swelling, obvious injuries, and bleeding (**FIGURE 10-32**). Also palpate along each extremity for deformities. Ask the patient about any tenderness or pain. As you evaluate the extremities, check for pulses, motor function, and sensory function:

- **Pulse.** Check the distal pulses on the foot (dorsalis pedis or posterior tibial) (**FIGURE 10-33** and **FIGURE 10-34**) and wrist. Assess the pulses in the lower extremities for rate, quality, and rhythm. Is the pulse rate fast, slow, or irregular?

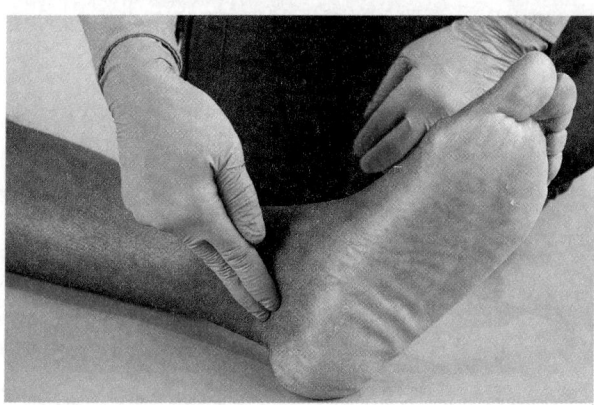

**FIGURE 10-33** Palpation of the posterior tibial pulse.

© Jones & Bartlett Learning.

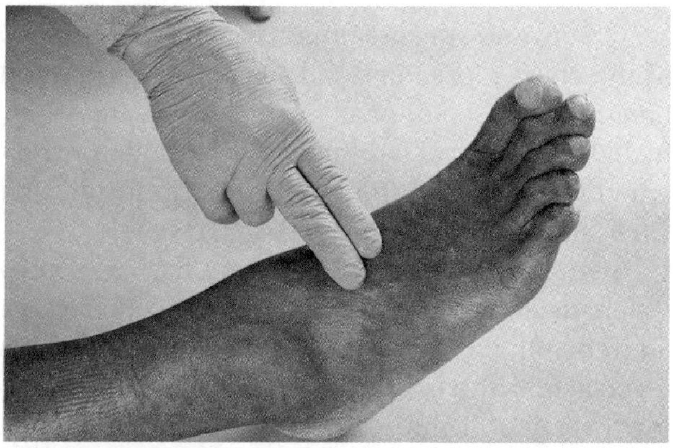

**FIGURE 10-34** Palpation of the dorsalis pedis pulse.

© Jones & Bartlett Learning.

Is the pulse weak, thready, or bounding? Also check circulation. Evaluate the skin color and temperature of the hands and feet. Is it normal? How does it compare with the skin color and temperature of the other extremities? Pale or cyanotic skin may indicate poor circulation in that extremity.

- **Motor function.** Ask the patient to wiggle his or her fingers and toes. An inability to move a single extremity can be the result of a bone, muscle, or nerve injury. An inability to move several extremities may be a sign of a brain abnormality or spinal cord injury. Verify that you are maintaining spinal motion restriction if indicated.

- **Sensory function.** Evaluate sensory function in the extremity by asking the patient to close his or her eyes. Gently squeeze or pinch a finger or toe and ask the patient to identify what you are doing. The inability to feel sensation in the extremity may indicate a local nerve injury. The inability to feel sensation in several extremities may be a sign of a spinal cord injury. Ensure that you are maintaining spinal motion restriction.

### *Posterior Body*

Inspect the back for DCAP-BTLS, symmetry, and open wounds (**FIGURE 10-35**). Carefully palpate the spine from the neck to the pelvis for tenderness and deformity.

## Assess Vital Signs Using the Appropriate Monitoring Device

The use of monitoring equipment in the prehospital setting has continued to expand. EMTs at all levels use a wide variety of devices in the continuous monitoring of patients. It is important to remember that these devices are manufactured and subject to limitations and failures. Such devices should never be used to replace your comprehensive assessment of your patient; think of them as simply adjuncts to the assessment and treatment of your patient. Obtaining and using information from patient monitoring devices includes, but is not limited to, data from pulse oximetry and noninvasive blood pressure monitoring.

### Pulse Oximetry

**Pulse oximetry** is an assessment tool used to evaluate the effectiveness of oxygenation. The pulse oximeter is a photoelectric device that monitors the oxygen saturation of hemoglobin (the iron-containing portion of the red blood cell to which oxygen attaches) in the capillary beds (**FIGURE 10-36**). The parts that make up the pulse oximeter include a monitor and a sensing probe. The sensing probe clips onto a finger or earlobe. The light source must have unobstructed access to a capillary bed, so dark fingernail polish might need to be removed. Results appear as a percentage on the display screen. Normally, pulse oximetry values in ambient air will vary depending on the altitude, with most values falling between 94% and 99%.

The goal of applying oxygen therapy is to increase oxygen saturation to a normal level. This device is a useful assessment tool to determine the effectiveness of oxygen therapy, bronchodilator therapy, and artificial ventilations. However, the pulse oximeter does not take the place of good assessment skills and should not prevent the

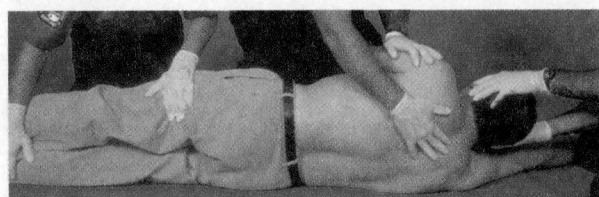

**FIGURE 10-35** Feel the back for tenderness, deformity, and open wounds. Carefully palpate the spine from the neck to the pelvis for tenderness and deformity. Look under the clothing for obvious injuries, including bruising and bleeding.

© Jones & Bartlett Learning. Courtesy of MIEMSS.

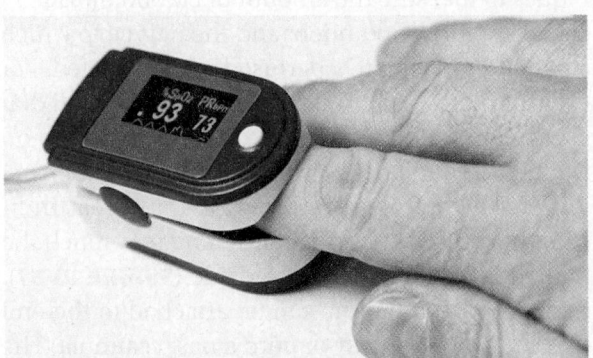

**FIGURE 10-36** The pulse oximeter is a device that measures the saturation of oxygen in the blood as a percentage.

© juanrvelasco/iStock.

application of oxygen to any patient who reports difficulty breathing regardless of the pulse oximetry value seen on the monitor.

Because the device functions properly only with adequate perfusion and numbers of red blood cells, any situation that causes vasoconstriction (such as hypothermia or shock) or loss of red blood cells (such as bleeding or anemia) will result in inaccurate or misleading values. The device also presumes that oxygen is saturating the hemoglobin. Therefore, any chemical that displaces oxygen (such as carbon monoxide) may cause misleading values.

The pulse oximeter is a useful tool as long as you remember that the device is only a tool, not a substitute for a good assessment.

## Capnography

**Metabolism** refers to the chemical reactions that occur in the body or cells to maintain life. To get an idea about the patient's metabolism and adequacy of ventilation, you can measure carbon dioxide ($CO_2$) levels in the air as the patient exhales. Pulse oximetry can measure the amount of oxygen available to the patient's cells for cellular metabolism, but it does not measure how much of that oxygen is being used. **Carbon dioxide** is the by-product of aerobic cellular metabolism and reflects the amount of oxygen being consumed during the process. Think of the oxygen as helping to burn the fuel in metabolism, and the carbon dioxide as the exhaust. You can learn a great deal by measuring this exhaust from a patient.

When you are working with ALS providers, there will be times when they may employ certain techniques to measure the amount of carbon dioxide in exhaled air to help understand the degree to which a patient is adequately perfused and ventilated. For example, **capnography** is a noninvasive method that can quickly and efficiently provide information on a patient's ventilation, circulation, and metabolism. Waveform capnography shows a graph that indicates how easily, how frequently, and how much the patient is exhaling carbon dioxide (**FIGURE 10-37**). Capnography monitors can be attached to the end of an advanced airway or onto a nasal cannula. The continued use of capnography expands the EMT's diagnostic capability. Capnography is used to evaluate the effectiveness of breathing treatments and

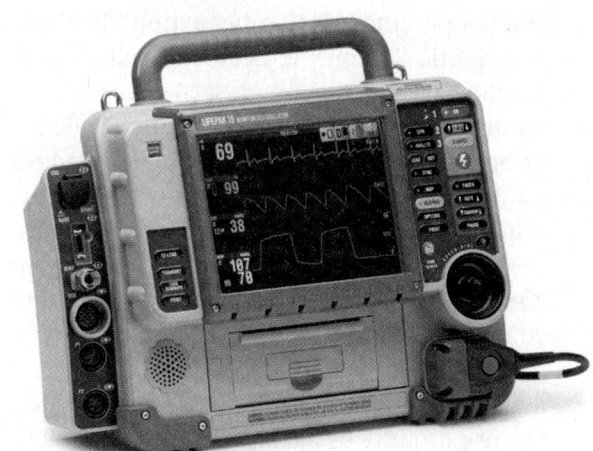

**FIGURE 10-37** This device is capable of monitoring multiple functions simultaneously, including continuous capnography (bottom tracing).

The LIFEPAK 15 defibrillator monitor courtesy of Physio-Control. Used with permission of Physio-Control, Inc., and according to the Material Release Form provided by Physio-Control.

of artificial ventilation and to confirm endotracheal tube placement. It is correlated to lactic acid values in patients with septic shock.

## Blood Glucometry

Measuring the blood glucose level of a patient who has altered mental status can prove invaluable. Blood glucometry measures the level of glucose in the patient's bloodstream. If the glucose level is low, this can help you identify the reason a patient is unresponsive. If the level is high in a patient with nausea, vomiting, abdominal pain, and a change in mental status, it may signal dangerous complications of high blood glucose.

Blood glucose should be assessed in all patients known to have diabetes, all patients who have an altered mental status, and patients with generalized malaise or weakness. In addition, a blood glucose level can be assessed in any patient whom you think has a poor general impression.

To obtain a blood glucose measurement, you will need to use a lancet to obtain a drop of blood. Follow the steps in **SKILL DRILL 10-6** to assess blood glucose level:

1. Take standard precautions. Cleanse the site (finger) with antiseptic and allow it to dry (**Step 1**).
2. Puncture the site with the lancet (**Step 2**).

## Skill Drill 10-6 Assessing Blood Glucose Level

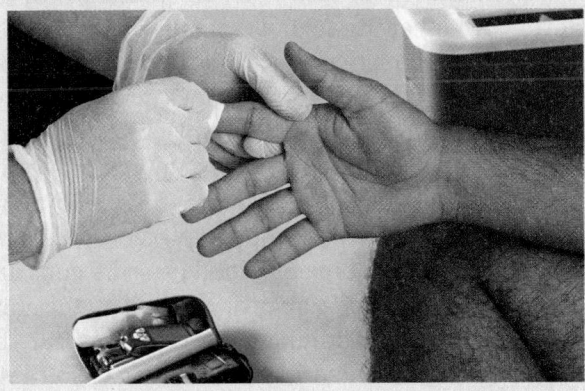

### Step 1

Take standard precautions. Cleanse the site (finger) with antiseptic.

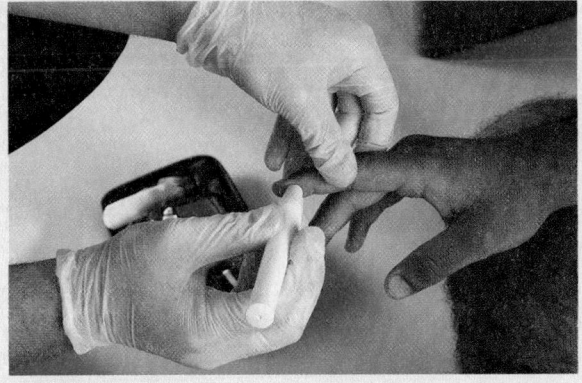

### Step 2

Puncture the site with the lancet.

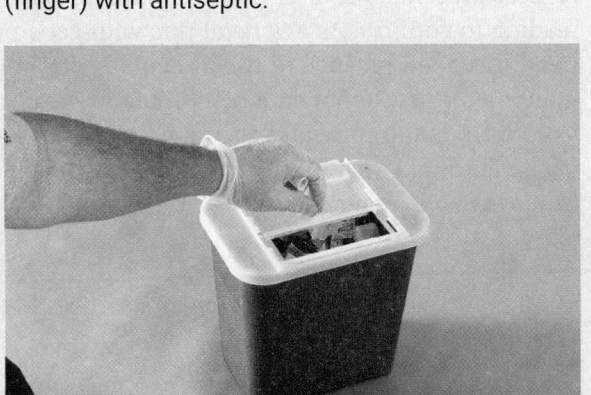

### Step 3

Dispose of the needle in a sharps container.

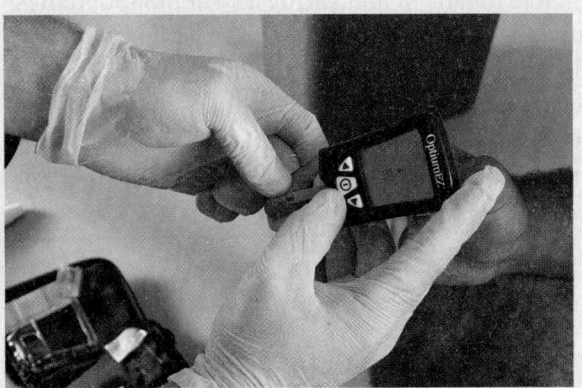

### Step 4

Obtain a drop of blood on the test strip. Insert the test strip into the glucometer and activate the device per the manufacturer's instructions.

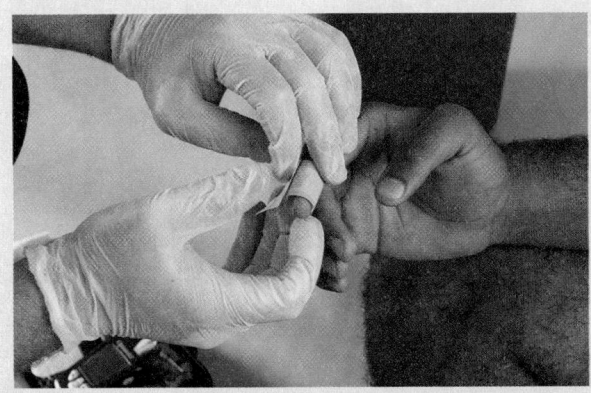

### Step 5

Place a bandage over the puncture site.

3. Immediately dispose of the needle in a sharps container (**Step 3**).
4. Obtain a drop of blood on the test strip. Insert the test strip into the glucometer and activate the device per the manufacturer's instructions (**Step 4**).
5. When finished, place a bandage over the puncture site (**Step 5**).

Most newer glucometers take only a few seconds to provide a reading. Glucometers should be calibrated on a regular basis to maintain accuracy. In addition, you should verify that the test strips match the glucometer you are using and that they have not expired.

## Noninvasive Blood Pressure Measurement

Auscultation with a sphygmomanometer is the most reliable means of measuring a patient's blood pressure. Electronic measurement is another method of obtaining blood pressure readings on patients. An electronic device measures changes in pressure oscillations that occur during cuff inflation or deflation and are related to systolic, mean, and diastolic pressures. Several different types of electronic devices are used in the prehospital setting; the blood pressure cuff deflates differently in each device.

Standard noninvasive blood pressure monitoring, whether through a manual sphygmomanometer or through an electronic, automatic blood pressure cuff, is easy to use and does not involve any advanced or invasive procedures. However, both of these methods are prone to inaccurate readings in moving vehicles, in noisy environments, or if the cuff is not correctly sized or properly placed on the patient. Electronic automated blood pressure cuffs are further subject to inaccuracy depending on the ability of the sensors to accurately ascertain pressure in the blood vessel. The degree of inaccuracy in these devices can vary substantially from patient to patient depending on several factors. When faced with electronic readings that do not correlate with a patient's clinical presentation, it is best to obtain a manual reading to confirm. As a general rule with each patient, it is good practice to use a manual sphygmomanometer first to obtain a blood pressure reading to confirm that it correlates accurately with the electronic automated cuff prior to relying on the electronic measurement.

# Patient Assessment

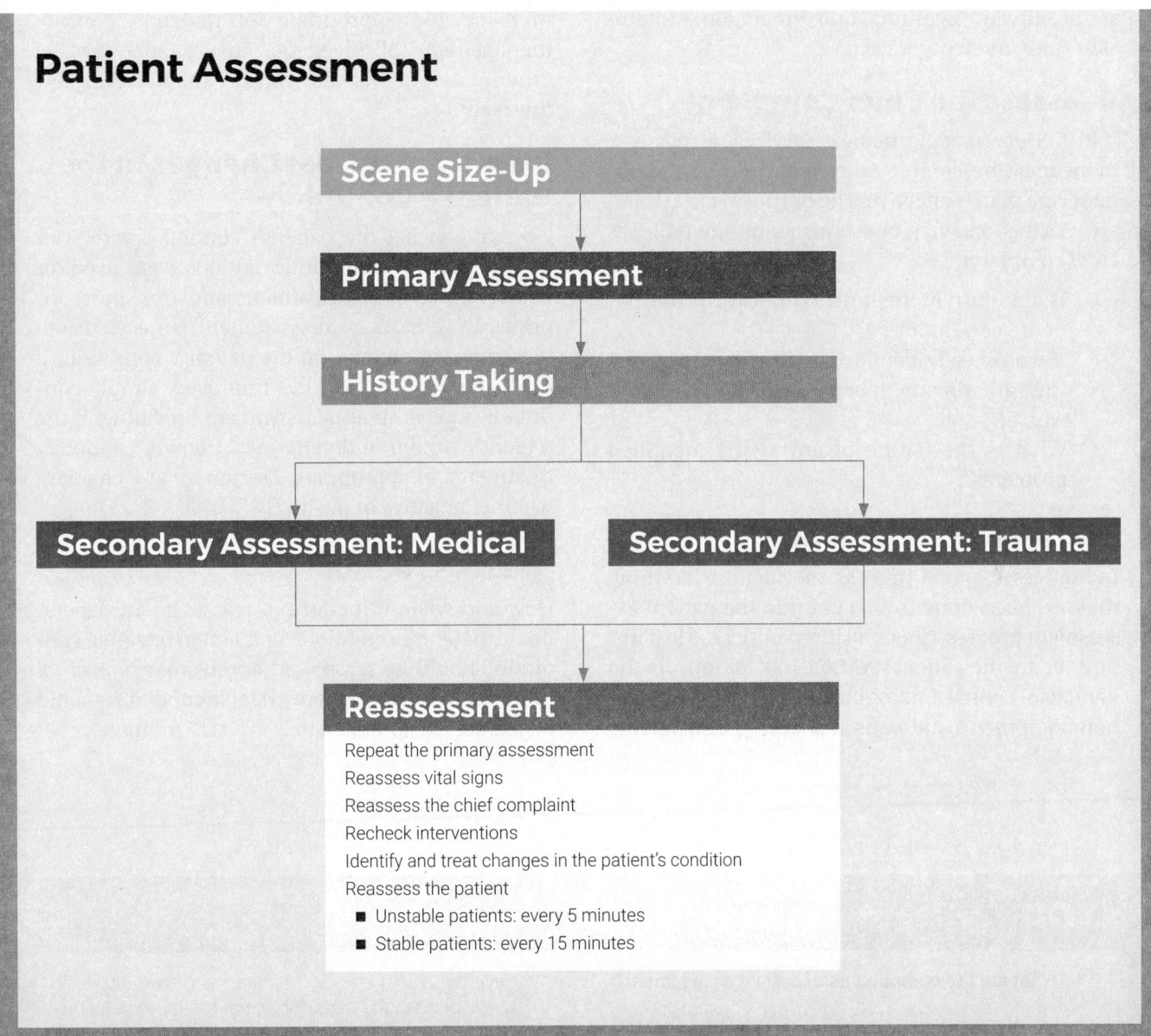

Scene Size-Up

Primary Assessment

History Taking

Secondary Assessment: Medical

Secondary Assessment: Trauma

Reassessment

Repeat the primary assessment
Reassess vital signs
Reassess the chief complaint
Recheck interventions
Identify and treat changes in the patient's condition
Reassess the patient
- Unstable patients: every 5 minutes
- Stable patients: every 15 minutes

## Reassessment

A **reassessment** is performed at regular intervals during the assessment process, and its purpose is to identify and treat changes in a patient's condition.

### Words of Wisdom

**Reassessment should take place:**
- Every 5 minutes for patients in unstable condition
- Every 15 minutes for patients in stable condition

## Repeat the Primary Assessment

The reassessment procedure is to simply repeat the primary assessment (airway, breathing, circulation) to identify and treat any life-threatening changes in the patient's condition.

### Reassess Vital Signs

Reassess and record vital signs. Compare the baseline vital signs obtained during the primary assessment with any and all subsequent vital signs. Look for trends. Have they increased, declined, or stayed the same? If so, how fast? Reassess the mental status, airway, breathing, and circulation. Monitor skin color and temperature.

## Reassess the Chief Complaint

With all emergency medical services, a reassessment must be completed to determine if the patient care plan is effective. The purpose is to ask and answer the following questions about the patient's chief complaint:

- Is the current treatment improving the patient's condition?
- Has an already identified problem gotten better?
- Has an already identified problem gotten worse?
- What is the nature of any newly identified problems?

## Recheck Interventions

In the reassessment process, reevaluate everything that has been done to this point in the patient assessment process. Check all interventions. Most important are the patient's XABCs. In addition, are the bandages, spinal immobilization devices, extrication equipment, and patient-securing instruments in place and appropriate for transport? Ensure management of bleeding. Ensure adequacy of other interventions and consider the need for new interventions.

## Identify and Treat Changes in the Patient's Condition

No matter what the patient's condition was prior to your arrival, which interventions were used, or which decisions on treatment and transport priorities were made, a reassessment is necessary to help monitor changes in the patient's condition. If the patient's condition has improved, simply continue whatever treatments you are providing. If the patient's condition deteriorates, prepare to modify treatments as appropriate. Document any changes, whether negative or positive.

## Reassess Patient

How and when to perform a reassessment depend on the patient's condition. A patient in unstable condition should be reassessed approximately every 5 minutes, whereas a patient in stable condition should be reassessed approximately every 15 minutes.

## YOU are the Provider SUMMARY

**1. What are the components of patient assessment?**

There are five components in the assessment process: scene size-up, primary assessment, history taking, secondary assessment, and reassessment. Each component has an integral role in your overall treatment of the patient. The steps of assessment represent a logical approach to evaluation of a patient, but the order in which they are performed is determined by the patient's condition and the environment in which you are working.

**2. Will your assessment of the patient differ if he or she is injured versus ill? If so, how?**

The same components of patient assessment used to evaluate a medical patient are used to assess a trauma patient. The differences lie in what you find and how you treat it. For example, during the scene size-up of a trauma patient, you will evaluate the MOI to help focus your assessment of the type and severity of injuries your patient may have; you will also consider the need for spinal motion restriction. In medical patients, the NOI is assessed to help determine what category of medical condition you are dealing with (eg, cardiac, respiratory, endocrine), which will help guide your assessment in the appropriate direction.

Whether you are assessing a medical patient or a trauma patient, the key is to remain organized. Furthermore, you should assess the patient for medical conditions *and* injuries, especially if you suspect that the patient's injury was preceded by a medical condition.

**3. Is spinal motion restriction indicated? Why or why not?**

Local protocols for spinal motion restriction vary. If you find that spinal motion restriction is indicated, keep this in mind throughout your assessment process, modifying your assessment as appropriate to ensure that you are not unnecessarily risking additional spinal injury. Remember, however, that any life-threatening injuries *must be addressed immediately*, regardless of your suspicion of a possible spinal injury.

**4. Which of these assessment findings requires your *most* immediate attention?**

The patient's airway, which contains bloody secretions and vomitus, is in *immediate* jeopardy! Immediately use suction to clear his airway. Suction for up to 10 seconds, and then reassess his airway status. If you hear gurgling, think suction!

After ensuring that his airway is clear of secretions and vomitus, insert a simple airway adjunct—while keeping the airway open manually—to further help maintain airway patency.

**5. Does the patient require further treatment at the scene? If so, what?**

At this point, you should continue to support his airway and breathing, monitor his circulatory status (ie, his pulse, which is slow), keep him warm, and be prepared to begin CPR and apply the AED. Apply spinal motion restriction as directed by local protocol and prepare for immediate transport. Remember, there were no witnesses to this event; err on the side of caution and protect the patient's spine.

**6. Should you remain at the scene and wait for the paramedic unit? Why or why not?**

No, do not remain at the scene! Eighteen minutes is too long to remain at the scene with a patient in unstable condition, not to mention one who still needs to be moved from a second-floor apartment. You should advise the paramedic ambulance of the situation, but do so while you are preparing for immediate transport. The longer you remain at the scene, the greater the chance that the patient's condition will further deteriorate.

If the paramedic ambulance arrives before you depart the scene, it would clearly be prudent to transfer care to them.

Consider an intercept with the paramedic unit at a designated location. Your EMS system protocols should have a plan for coordinating a paramedic intercept when transporting a patient in unstable condition or a patient who requires care that is beyond your level of training. You should be aware of the transport time to the nearest definitive care site and weigh this against the time associated with achieving a paramedic intercept or waiting for ALS to arrive on the scene. Your goal is to reach advanced care in the least amount of time possible,

**7. How has your patient's condition changed from the previous assessments?**

Your patient's condition has obviously deteriorated. Compared with earlier assessments, which revealed that he was responsive to pain, he is now unconscious and unresponsive. Furthermore, his oxygen saturation is declining despite assisted ventilation with high-flow oxygen, and cyanosis is developing around his mouth (perioral/circumoral cyanosis).

His heart rate and blood pressure—although still unstable—are essentially unchanged compared with previous assessments. However, they must continue to be closely monitored for further deterioration.

The findings of your reassessment (eg, unresponsive, low $SpO_2$ level, cyanosis) point to a problem with his oxygenation and ventilation status that may be caused by more than one factor. His head may not be properly positioned, the simple airway adjunct may need to be repositioned, his airway may be filling with blood or vomitus, or he is not being adequately ventilated.

**8. What should you do in response to the patient's change in condition?**

Deterioration of a patient's condition should immediately prompt you to repeat the primary assessment, which begins by reassessing airway, breathing, and circulation.

Make sure the patient's head is correctly positioned. Look in his mouth for secretions and remove them with suction, if present. Reassess the position of the simple airway adjunct; is the nasal airway protruding from his nose? If an oral airway is in place, is it protruding from his mouth? Reassess the mask-to-face seal of the bag-mask device; is it adequate, or is there air leaking? Are you ventilating at the appropriate rate (10 to 12 breaths/min in an adult) with the appropriate volume (each breath delivered over 1 second—just enough to cause visible chest rise)?

A rapid, yet careful reassessment of the ABCs will often reveal the cause of the patient's status change, thus allowing you to rapidly correct it.

## YOU are the Provider SUMMARY *continued*

**9. What components of the SAMPLE history, if any, can you obtain when your patient is unresponsive? How would you obtain the information?**

In the absence of any family members, caregivers, or bystanders who know the patient, it may not be possible to obtain a complete and accurate SAMPLE history; however, it may be possible to obtain certain components of the SAMPLE history. Obtaining this information relies on your good assessment skills and thinking outside the box.

Signs and symptoms can be established by simply assessing the patient; although signs and symptoms alone will not tell you what the patient's underlying problem is, they will enable you to direct your initial treatment accordingly.

Look for a medical alert bracelet, a medical alert card, or medical information posted in the patient's home. Are there any prescription medication bottles present? Is there medical equipment present (eg, home oxygen, nebulizer) that indicates an underlying condition? Although an unresponsive patient cannot speak, you can learn something about the patient's conditions based on the medications found at the scene.

**10. Why is reassessing your interventions so important?**

The main purpose of reassessing the interventions you have performed on a patient is to determine their effectiveness. If your intervention has been effective, you should see an improvement in the patient's condition. If your intervention has not been effective, the patient's condition will have remained unchanged or will have deteriorated. Intervention reassessment also enables you to determine if you need to make modifications to existing interventions, cease an intervention, or perform another intervention.

For example, if a conscious patient is receiving oxygen via a nonrebreathing mask, and your reassessment reveals that he is now unresponsive, you may need to ensure that the airway is maintained and clear of secretions, and assess to see if the patient is adequately ventilated. Based on these findings, you may need to take measures to maintain the airway and assist with ventilations.

The mere performance of an intervention does not mean that it will cause your patient's condition to improve, nor does it mean that it will prevent your patient's condition from deteriorating. Reassess, reassess, reassess!

### EMS Patient Care Report (PCR)

| Date: 7-20-20 | Incident No.: 010809 | Nature of Call: Man down | | Location: 3820 121st St. | |
|---|---|---|---|---|---|
| Dispatched: 1815 | En Route: 1816 | At Scene: 1820 | Transport: 1838 | At Hospital: 1904 | In Service: 1923 |

#### Patient Information

| | |
|---|---|
| Age: 25<br>Sex: M<br>Weight (in kg [lb]): 70 kg estimated (155 lb) | Allergies: Unknown<br>Medications: Unknown<br>Past Medical History: Unknown<br>Chief Complaint: Unresponsive; unknown circumstances |

#### Vital Signs

| Time: 1825 | BP: 76/58 | Pulse: 42 | Respirations: 8 | Spo$_2$: 95% |
|---|---|---|---|---|
| Time: 1832 | BP: 78/54 | Pulse: 44 | Respirations: 6 assisted at 10 | Spo$_2$: 88% |
| Time: 1840 | BP: 84/56 | Pulse: 38 | Respirations: 6 assisted at 10 | Spo$_2$: 95% |
| Time: 1851 | BP: 82/64 | Pulse: 40 | Respirations: 6 assisted at 10 | Spo$_2$: 96% |

## YOU are the Provider SUMMARY *continued*

| EMS Treatment (circle all that apply) | | | | |
|---|---|---|---|---|
| Oxygen @ 15 L/min via:<br>NC  NRM  (Bag mask) | | (Assisted Ventilation) | (Airway Adjunct) | CPR |
| Defibrillation | Bleeding Control | Bandaging | Splinting | Other: (Suctioning, spinal precautions, blanket) |

### Narrative

9-1-1 dispatch for a "man down."

Chief Complaint: Unresponsive; unknown circumstances

History: Law enforcement personnel responded and ensured the scene was secure prior to EMS arrival. On arrival at the scene, found the patient, a 25-year-old man, lying prone on the kitchen floor of his second-floor apartment. A neighbor was present but did not know what happened and has no knowledge of the patient's medical history.

Assessment: The patient was responsive to pain.

Treatment (Rx): Manually stabilized the patient's head, and rolled him to a supine position to provide immediate care. Opened his airway with the jaw-thrust maneuver, and noted bloody secretions and vomitus coming from his mouth. Immediately suctioned his oropharynx until clear of debris, and inserted a nasal airway. Assessment of his breathing revealed it to be slow and shallow. Began assisting ventilations with a bag mask device attached to high-flow oxygen. Secondary assessment revealed no obvious signs of trauma, and law enforcement's search of the patient's apartment revealed no medical records, medication bottles, drug paraphernalia, or anything else suspicious. Unable to obtain SAMPLE history. Blood glucose level was assessed and read 108 mg/dL.

Transport: A paramedic unit was available but was 18 minutes away from our location, so decision was made to continue treatment and begin immediate transport. Applied a cervical collar, applied a blanket for warmth, moved the patient down a flight of stairs on a scoop stretcher with the assistance of Engine Company 13, and loaded him into the ambulance. Began transport to hospital; EMT Jones from Engine Company 13 accompanied us with the patient to provide assistance.

Reassessment revealed that the patient was now completely unresponsive, his oxygen saturation had declined, and cyanosis was developing around his mouth. EMS used suction to clear his oropharynx, inserted an oral airway, and continued to assist ventilations. Intervention reassessment revealed improvement in the patient's oxygenation status; however, he remained unresponsive, bradycardic, and hypotensive. Continued to assist patient's ventilations, and reassessed his condition approximately every 5 minutes as treatment would allow. Patient's condition remained unchanged throughout transport. Delivered him to the emergency department staff without incident, and gave verbal report to attending physician. Medic 80 returned to service at 1923.

**End of report**

# Prep Kit

## Ready for Review

- The assessment process begins with the scene size-up, which identifies real or potential hazards. The patient should not be approached until these hazards have been dealt with in a way that eliminates or minimizes risk to the EMTs and the patient or patients.
- The primary assessment is performed on all patients. It includes forming an initial general impression of the patient, including the LOC, and identifies any life-threatening conditions to the XABCs. A primary assessment is performed to assist in prioritizing time and mode of transport. Any life threats identified must be treated before moving on to the next step of the assessment.
- The ABCs are assessed to evaluate the patient's general condition.
- History taking includes an investigation of the patient's chief complaint or history of present illness. A SAMPLE history is generally taken during this step of the assessment process. This information may be obtained from the patient, family, friends, bystanders, caregivers, or medical alert devices or documentation.
- By using the SAMPLE mnemonic, you will be able to determine the patient's signs and symptoms, allergies, medications, pertinent past history, last oral intake, and events leading up to the illness or injury.
- The secondary assessment is a systematic physical examination of the patient. The secondary assessment may be a systematic head-to-toe physical examination or an assessment that focuses on a certain area or region of the body, often determined through the chief complaint. Circumstances will dictate which aspects of the physical examination will be used. The secondary assessment is performed on scene or, more often, in the back of the ambulance en route to the hospital. If the patient has serious life threats, you may not have time to perform a secondary assessment.
- The reassessment is performed on all patients. It gives you an opportunity to reevaluate the chief complaint and to reassess interventions to ensure that they are still being delivered correctly. Information from the reassessment may be used to identify and treat changes in the patient's condition.
- A patient in stable condition should be reassessed every 15 minutes, whereas a patient in unstable condition should be reassessed every 5 minutes.
- The assessment process is systematic and dynamic. Each assessment you perform will be slightly different, depending on the needs of the patient. The result will be a process that will enable you to quickly identify and treat the needs of all patients, both medical and trauma related, in a way that meets their unique needs.

## Vital Vocabulary

**accessory muscles** The secondary muscles of respiration. They include the neck muscles (sternocleidomastoids), the chest pectoralis major muscles, and the abdominal muscles.

**altered mental status** A change in the way a person thinks and behaves that may signal disease in the central nervous system or elsewhere in the body.

**auscultate** To listen to sounds within an organ with a stethoscope.

**AVPU scale** A method of assessing the level of consciousness by determining whether the patient is awake and alert, responsive to verbal stimuli or pain, or unresponsive; used principally early in the assessment process.

**blood pressure** The pressure that the blood exerts against the walls of the arteries as it passes through them.

**bradycardia** A slow heart rate, less than 60 beats/min.

**breath sounds** An indication of air movement in the lungs, usually assessed with a stethoscope.

**capillary refill** A test that evaluates distal circulatory system function by squeezing (blanching) blood from an area such as a nail bed and watching the speed of its return after releasing the pressure.

**capnography** A noninvasive method to quickly and efficiently provide information on a patient's ventilatory status, circulation, and metabolism; effectively measures the concentration of carbon dioxide in expired air over time.

**carbon dioxide** A component of air that typically makes up 0.03% of air at sea level; also a waste product exhaled during expiration by the respiratory system.

**chief complaint** The reason a patient called for help; also, the patient's response to questions such as "What's wrong?" or "What happened?"

**conjunctiva** The delicate membrane that lines the eyelids and covers the exposed surface of the eye.

**crackles** A crackling, rattling breath sound that signals fluid in the air spaces of the lungs.

**crepitus** A grating or grinding sensation caused by fractured bone ends or joints rubbing together.

**cyanosis** A blue skin discoloration that is caused by a reduced level of oxygen in the blood.

**DCAP-BTLS** A mnemonic for assessment in which each area of the body is evaluated for Deformities, Contusions, Abrasions, Punctures/penetrations, Burns, Tenderness, Lacerations, and Swelling.

**diaphoretic** Characterized by light or profuse sweating.

**diastolic pressure** The pressure that remains in the arteries during the relaxing phase of the heart's cycle (diastole) when the left ventricle is at rest.

**distracting injury** Any injury that prevents the patient from noticing other injuries he or she may have, even severe injuries; for example, a painful femur or tibia fracture that prevents the patient from noticing back pain associated with a spinal fracture.

**field impression** The conclusion about the cause of the patient's condition after considering the situation, history, and examination findings.

**focused assessment** A type of physical assessment typically performed on patients who have sustained nonsignificant mechanisms of injury or on responsive medical patients. This type of examination is based on the chief complaint and focuses on one body system or part.

**frostbite** Damage to tissues as the result of exposure to cold; frozen or partially frozen body parts are frostbitten.

**general impression** The overall initial impression that determines the priority for patient care; based on the patient's surroundings, the mechanism of injury, signs and symptoms, and the chief complaint.

**Golden Hour** The time from injury to definitive care, during which treatment of shock and traumatic injuries should occur because survival potential is best; also called the Golden Period.

**guarding** Involuntary muscle contractions (spasm) of the abdominal wall; an effort to protect the inflamed abdomen.

**history taking** A step within the patient assessment process that provides detail about the patient's chief complaint and an account of the patient's signs and symptoms.

**hypertension** Blood pressure that is higher than the normal range.

**hypotension** Blood pressure that is lower than the normal range.

**hypothermia** A condition in which the internal body temperature falls below 95°F (35°C).

**incident command system** A system implemented to manage disasters and mass- and multiple-casualty incidents in which section chiefs, including finance, logistics, operations, and planning, report to the incident commander.

**jaundice** Yellow skin or sclera that is caused by liver disease or dysfunction.

**labored breathing** Breathing that requires greater than normal effort; may be slower or faster than normal and characterized by grunting, stridor, and use of accessory muscles.

**mean arterial pressure (MAP)** The average pressure in the circulatory system during one cardiac cycle.

**mechanism of injury (MOI)** The forces, or energy transmission, applied to the body that cause injury.

**metabolism** The biochemical processes that result in production of energy from nutrients within the cells.

**nasal flaring** Widening of the nostrils, indicating that there is an airway obstruction.

**nature of illness (NOI)** The general type of illness a patient is experiencing.

**OPQRST** A mnemonic used in evaluating a patient's pain: Onset, Provocation/palliation, Quality, Region/radiation, Severity, and Timing.

**orientation** The mental status of a patient as measured by memory of person (name), place (current location), time (current year, month, and approximate date), and event (what happened).

**palpate** To examine by touch.

**paradoxical motion** The motion of the portion of the chest wall that is detached in a flail chest; the motion—in during inhalation, out during exhalation—is exactly the opposite of normal chest wall motion during breathing.

**perfusion** The flow of blood through body tissues and vessels.

**personal protective equipment (PPE)** Protective equipment that blocks exposure to a pathogen or a hazardous material.

**pertinent negatives** Negative findings that warrant no care or intervention.

**primary assessment** A step within the patient assessment process that identifies and initiates treatment of immediate and potential life threats.

**pulse** The wave of pressure created as the heart contracts and forces blood out the left ventricle and into the major arteries.

**pulse oximetry** An assessment tool that measures oxygen saturation of hemoglobin in the capillary beds.

**reassessment** A step within the patient assessment process performed at regular intervals during the assessment process to identify and treat changes in a patient's condition. A patient in unstable condition should be reassessed every 5 minutes, whereas a patient in stable condition should be reassessed every 15 minutes.

**responsiveness** The way in which a patient responds to external stimuli, including verbal stimuli (sound), tactile stimuli (touch), and painful stimuli.

**retractions** Movements in which the skin pulls in around the ribs during inspiration.

**rhonchi** Coarse, low-pitched breath sounds heard in patients with chronic mucus in the upper airways.

**SAMPLE history** A brief history of a patient's condition to determine signs and symptoms, allergies, medications, pertinent past history, last oral intake, and events leading to the injury or illness.

**scene size-up** A step within the patient assessment process that involves a quick assessment of the scene and the surroundings to provide information about scene safety and the mechanism of injury or nature of illness before you enter and begin patient care.

**sclera** The tough, fibrous, white portion of the eye that protects the more delicate inner structures.

**secondary assessment** A step within the patient assessment process in which a systematic physical examination of the patient is performed. The examination may be a systematic exam or an assessment that focuses on a certain area or region of the body, often determined through the chief complaint.

**shallow respirations** Respirations characterized by little movement of the chest wall (reduced tidal volume) or poor chest excursion.

**sign** Objective finding that can be seen, heard, felt, smelled, or measured.

**situational awareness** Knowledge and understanding of one's surroundings and the ability to recognize potential risks to the safety of the patient or EMS team.

**sniffing position** An upright position in which the patient's head and chin are thrust slightly forward to keep the airway open.

**spontaneous respirations** Breathing that occurs without assistance.

**standard precautions** Protective measures that have traditionally been developed by the Centers for Disease Control and Prevention (CDC) for use in dealing with objects, blood, body fluids, and other potential exposure risks of communicable disease.

**stridor** A harsh, high-pitched, respiratory sound, generally heard during inspiration, that is caused by partial blockage or narrowing of the upper airway; may be audible without a stethoscope.

**subcutaneous emphysema** A characteristic crackling sensation felt on palpation of the skin, caused by the presence of air in soft tissues.

**symptom** Subjective findings that the patient feels but that can be identified only by the patient.

**systolic pressure** The increased pressure in an artery with each contraction of the ventricles (systole).

**tachycardia** A rapid heart rate, more than 100 beats/min.

**tidal volume** The amount of air (in milliliters) that is moved into or out of the lungs during one breath.

**triage** The process of establishing treatment and transportation priorities according to severity of injury and medical need.

**tripod position** An upright position in which the patient leans forward onto two arms stretched forward and thrusts the head and chin forward.

**two- to three-word dyspnea** A severe breathing problem in which a patient can speak only two to three words at a time without pausing to take a breath.

**vasoconstriction** Narrowing of a blood vessel.

**vital signs** The key signs that are used to evaluate the patient's overall condition, including respirations, pulse, blood pressure, level of consciousness, and skin characteristics.

**wheezing** A high-pitched, whistling breath sound that is most prominent on expiration, and which suggests an obstruction or narrowing of the lower airways; occurs in asthma and bronchiolitis.

# References

1. Alpert BS. Validation of the Welch Allyn Sure BP (inflation) and Step BP (deflation) algorithms by AAMI standard testing and BHS data analysis. *Blood Press Monit* 2011;16(2):96–98.

2. Alpin G. Once is sometimes too much: cultural competence can reduce medical errors, increase patient satisfaction. *MGMA Connexion* 2007;7(1):21–22.

3. American Academy of Orthopaedic Surgeons. *Advanced Emergency Care and Transportation of the Sick and Injured.* 2nd ed. Burlington, MA: Jones & Bartlett Learning and American Academy of Orthopaedic Surgeons; 2012.

4. American Academy of Orthopaedic Surgeons. *Nancy Caroline's Emergency Care in the Streets.* 7th ed. Burlington, MA: Jones & Bartlett Learning and American Academy of Orthopaedic Surgeons; 2013.

5. Berg MD, Schexnayder SM, Chameides L, et al. Part 13: Pediatric basic life support: 2010 American Heart Association guidelines for cardiopulmonary resuscitation and emergency cardiovascular care. *Circulation* 2010;122(Suppl 3):S862–S875.

6. Brisbin T, McKenna KD, Kim CS, et al. Does paramedic student ethnicity impact the likelihood of providing ALS interventions to Caucasian versus non-Caucasian patients? [abstract]. *Prehosp Emerg Care* 2009;13(1).

7. Chameides L, Samson RA, Schexnayder SM, et al. *Pediatric Advanced Life Support Provider Manual.* Dallas, TX: American Heart Association; 2015.

8. Croskerry P. Diagnostic failure: a cognitive and affective approach. In: Henriksen K, Battles JB, Marks ES, Lewin DI, eds. *Advances in Patient Safety: From Research to Implementation (Vol. 2: Concepts and Methodology).* Rockville, MD: Agency for Healthcare Research and Quality; 2005.

9. Highlights of the 2015 American Heart Association Guidelines Update for CPR and ECC. American Heart Association website. https://eccguidelines.heart.org/index.php/circulation/cpr-ecc-guidelines-2/. Published 2015. Accessed July 4, 2020.

10. McKenna KD. Teaching intercultural competence in emergency medical services. *Educator Update.* Spring 2014:14. http://connection.ebscohost.com/c/articles/99502258/teaching-intercultural-competence-emergency-medical-services. Accessed June 9, 2015.

11. National Association of Emergency Medical Technicians. *PHTLS: Prehospital Trauma Life Support.* 9th ed. Burlington, MA: Jones & Bartlett Learning; 2020.

12. *National Emergency Medical Services Education Standards.* U.S. Department of Transportation. National Highway Traffic Safety Administration. DOT HS 811

077A. January 2009. www.ems.gov/pdf/811077a.pdf. Accessed June 14, 2014.

13. *National Emergency Medical Services Education Standards. Emergency Medical Technician Instructional Guidelines.* U.S. Department of Transportation. National Highway Traffic Safety Administration. DOT HS 811 077C. January 2009. www.ems.gov/pdf/811077c.pdf. Accessed June 14, 2014.

14. National Model EMS Clinical Guidelines. National Association of State EMS Officials website. https://www .nasemso.org/Projects/ModelEMSClinicalGuidelines /index.asp. Accessed October 23, 2014.

15. National Registry of Emergency Medical Technicians. *2015 Paramedic Psychomotor Competency Portfolio (PPCP).* Columbus, OH: NREMT; 2015.

16. National Registry of Emergency Medical Technicians. *Emergency Medical Technician Psychomotor Examination.* Columbus, OH: NREMT. https://www.nremt.org /nremt/about/psychomotor_exam_emt.asp. Accessed June 18, 2014.

17. Oliva NL. When language intervenes: improving care for patients with limited English proficiency. *Am J Nurs* 2008;108(3):73–75.

18. Smedley BD, Stith AY, Nelson AR, eds. *Unequal Treatment: Confronting Racial and Ethnic Disparities in Health Care.* Washington, DC: National Academies Press; 2003.

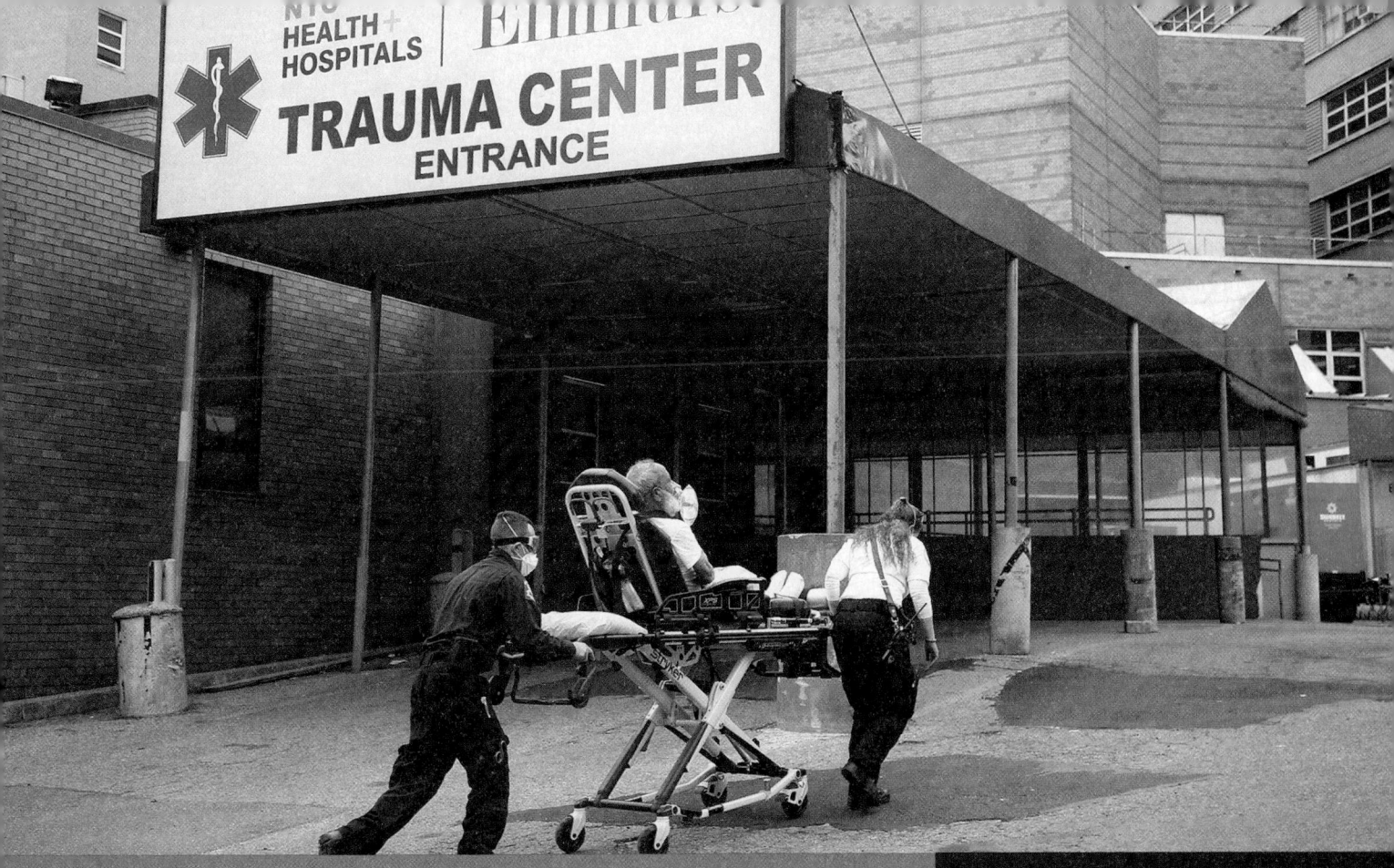

# Airway

**11** Airway Management

SECTION

3

# Chapter 11

# Airway Management

## NATIONAL EMS EDUCATION STANDARD COMPETENCIES

### Airway Management, Respiration, and Artificial Ventilation

Applies knowledge of general anatomy and physiology to patient assessment and management in order to assure a patent airway, adequate mechanical ventilation, and respiration for patients of all ages.

### Airway Management

- Airway anatomy (pp 418–423)
- Airway assessment (pp 431–439)
- Techniques of assuring a patent airway (pp 439–446)

### Respiration

- Anatomy of the respiratory system (pp 418–423)
- Physiology and pathophysiology of respiration
  - Pulmonary ventilation (pp 424–427)
  - Oxygenation (p 427)
  - Respiration (pp 427–429)
    - External (pp 427–428)
    - Internal (p 428)
    - Cellular (pp 428–429)
- Assessment and management of adequate and inadequate ventilation (pp 434–439)
- Supplemental oxygen therapy (pp 451–457)

### Artificial Ventilation

- Assessment and management of adequate and inadequate ventilation (pp 460–469)
- Artificial ventilation (pp 461–469)
- Minute ventilation (pp 424–425)
- Alveolar ventilation (pp 424–425)
- Effect of artificial ventilation on cardiac output (pp 461–462)

### Pathophysiology

Applies fundamental knowledge of the pathophysiology of respiration and perfusion to patient assessment and management.

## KNOWLEDGE OBJECTIVES

1. Describe the major structures of the respiratory system. (pp 418–423)
2. Discuss the physiology of breathing. (pp 423–428)
3. Give the signs of adequate breathing. (p 432)
4. Give the signs of inadequate breathing. (pp 432–434)
5. Describe the assessment and care of a patient with apnea. (p 434)
6. Explain how to assess for adequate and inadequate respiration, including the use of pulse oximetry. (pp 434–439)
7. Explain how to assess for a patent airway. (pp 439–440)
8. Describe how to perform the head tilt–chin lift maneuver. (pp 440–441)
9. Describe how to perform the jaw-thrust maneuver. (pp 441–442)
10. Explain the importance of and techniques for suctioning. (pp 442–446)
11. Explain how to measure and insert an oropharyngeal (oral) airway. (pp 446–448)
12. Describe how to measure and insert a nasopharyngeal (nasal) airway. (p 449)

13. Explain the use of the recovery position to maintain a clear airway. (pp 449–451)

14. Describe the importance of giving supplemental oxygen to patients who are hypoxic. (p 451)

15. Discuss the basics of how oxygen is stored and the various hazards associated with its use. (pp 451–457)

16. Explain the use of a nonrebreathing mask and the oxygen flow requirements for its use. (p 458)

17. Describe the indications for using a nasal cannula rather than a nonrebreathing face mask. (p 458)

18. Describe the indications for using a humidifier during supplemental oxygen therapy. (p 460)

19. Describe how to perform mouth-to-mouth or mouth-to-mask ventilation. (pp 462–463)

20. Describe the use of a one- or two-person bag-mask device. (pp 463–467)

21. Describe the signs associated with adequate and inadequate artificial ventilation. (p 468)

22. Describe the use of continuous positive airway pressure (CPAP). (pp 469–474)

23. Explain how to recognize and care for a foreign body airway obstruction. (pp 474–477)

24. Describe the four-step process of assisting with advanced life support (ALS) skills. (pp 477–482)

25. Discuss the importance of preoxygenation when performing endotracheal (ET) intubation. (p 477)

26. Describe the six steps of the BE MAGIC intubation procedure. (pp 478–481)

27. Describe the signs that indicate a complication with an intubated patient. (pp 481–482)

## SKILLS OBJECTIVES

1. Demonstrate use of pulse oximetry. (pp 435–436, Skill Drill 11-1)

2. Demonstrate how to position the unconscious patient. (pp 439–440, Skill Drill 11-2)

3. Demonstrate how to perform the head tilt–chin lift maneuver. (pp 440–441)

4. Demonstrate how to perform the jaw-thrust maneuver. (pp 441–442)

5. Demonstrate how to operate a suction unit. (pp 442–446)

6. Demonstrate how to suction a patient's airway. (pp 444–446, Skill Drill 11-3)

7. Demonstrate the insertion of an oral airway. (pp 446–447, Skill Drill 11-4)

8. Demonstrate the insertion of an oral airway with a 90° rotation. (p 448, Skill Drill 11-5)

9. Demonstrate the insertion of a nasal airway. (p 449, Skill Drill 11-6)

10. Demonstrate how to place a patient in the recovery position. (p 449)

11. Demonstrate how to place an oxygen cylinder into service. (pp 455–457, Skill Drill 11-7)

12. Demonstrate the use of a partial rebreathing mask in providing supplemental oxygen therapy to patients. (p 459)

13. Demonstrate the use of a Venturi mask in providing supplemental oxygen therapy to patients. (p 459)

14. Demonstrate the use of a humidifier in providing supplemental oxygen therapy to patients. (p 460)

15. Demonstrate how to assist a patient with ventilations using the bag-mask device. (pp 464–467, Skill Drill 11-9)

16. Demonstrate the use of an automatic transport ventilator to assist in delivering artificial ventilation to the patient. (pp 468–469)

17. Demonstrate the use of CPAP. (pp 469–474, Skill Drill 11-10)

# Introduction

The single most important step in caring for patients is to make sure that life threats are rapidly identified and addressed. A primary component of that step is to ensure that patients can breathe adequately. When the ability to breathe is disrupted, oxygen delivery to the body tissues and cells is compromised. Cells require a constant supply of oxygen to survive. Within seconds of being deprived of oxygen, vital organs such as the heart and brain may not function normally. Therefore, it is imperative that you recognize airway and breathing inadequacies and correct them immediately. Brain tissue will begin to die within 4 to 6 minutes without oxygen.

Oxygen reaches body tissues and cells through two separate but related processes: breathing and circulation. During inhalation, oxygen moves from the atmosphere into the lungs, crosses the alveolar membrane, and attaches to hemoglobin by a process called **diffusion**. Diffusion is a process in which molecules move from an area of higher concentration to an area of lower concentration. Next, red blood cells carry the hemoglobin, with the bound oxygen, through the body, ultimately delivering it to the capillaries to oxygenate the body's cells. At the same time, carbon dioxide, the by-product of normal cellular metabolism, moves from the cells into the blood and is carried back to the lungs where it moves into the alveoli by diffusion. The blood, enriched with oxygen, travels through the body by the pumping action of the heart. The carbon dioxide then leaves the body during exhalation.

As an EMT, you must be able to identify the anatomic structures of the respiratory system, understand how the system works, and be able to recognize which patients are breathing adequately and which patients are breathing inadequately. This knowledge will enable you to determine how best to treat your patients. You also play a pivotal role by bringing emergency medicine into patients' homes, assisting with advanced patient care skills, and ensuring the effective transfer of patient care to emergency department (ED) staff when you arrive at the hospital.

This chapter reviews the anatomy, physiology, and pathophysiology of the respiratory system. It describes how to assess patients quickly and to carefully determine their airway and ventilation status. The equipment, procedures, and guidelines that you will need to manage a patient's airway and breathing are described in detail. You will learn several ways to open a patient's airway and specific techniques for removing foreign objects or fluids

that may be compromising the airway. Because airway management equipment can be dangerous if used improperly, the chapter thoroughly discusses airway adjuncts, oxygen therapy devices, and artificial ventilation methods.

# Anatomy of the Respiratory System

The respiratory system consists of all the structures in the body that make up the **airway** and help us breathe, or ventilate (**FIGURE 11-1**). The airway is divided into the upper and the lower airways. Structures that help us breathe include the diaphragm, the intercostal muscles (muscles in between the ribs), and the nerves from the brain and spinal cord that innervate those muscles. In times of increased distress, muscles that are ordinarily not used during normal breathing, called accessory muscles, can be employed. Ventilation is the simple act of moving air into and out of the lungs. The diaphragm and intercostal muscles are responsible for the regular rise and fall of the chest that accompany normal breathing.

## Anatomy of the Upper Airway

The upper airway consists of all anatomic airway structures above the level of the vocal cords. These include the nose, mouth, jaw, oral cavity, pharynx, and larynx. Its major functions are to warm, filter, and humidify air as it enters the body through the nose and mouth. The pharynx (throat) is a muscular tube that extends from the nose and mouth to the level of the esophagus and trachea. The pharynx is composed of the nasopharynx, oropharynx, and

## YOU are the Provider

You and your partner are dispatched to a residence for a 49-year-old woman with respiratory distress. The patient's husband, who called 9-1-1, told the dispatcher that his wife is "turning blue" and is not acting normally. The time is 1930 hours, the temperature outside is 70°F (21°C), and the weather is clear.

1. From the dispatch information, can you determine if this is a problem with the airway, ventilation, or oxygenation? Why or why not?

2. How does ventilation differ from oxygenation?

3. Is it possible for a patient to ventilate but not oxygenate? Why or why not? What should your concerns be about PPE?

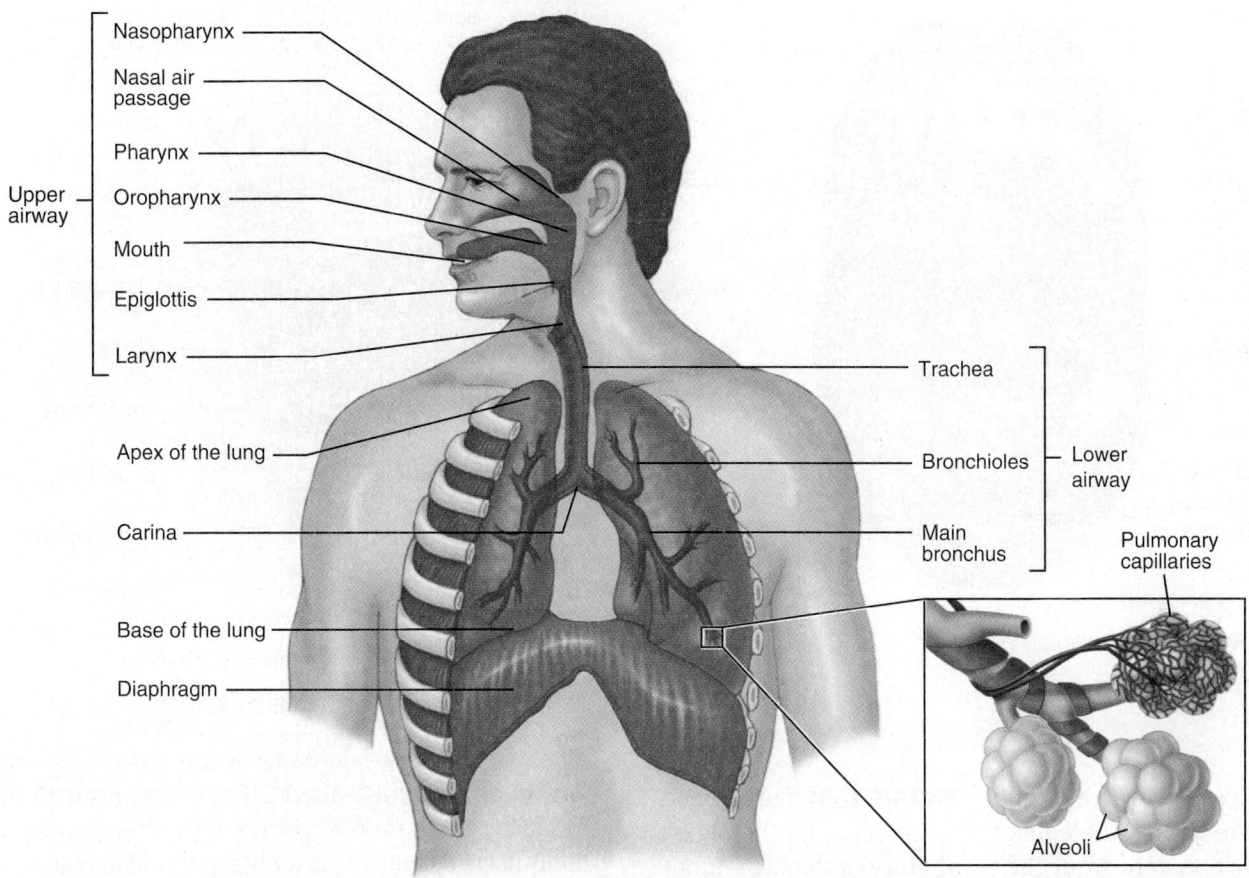

**FIGURE 11-1** The upper and lower airways contain the structures in the body that help us breathe.

© Jones & Bartlett Learning.

the laryngopharynx (also called the hypopharynx) (**FIGURE 11-2**). The laryngopharynx is the lowest portion of the pharynx. At the base, it splits into two lumens, the larynx (and ultimately, the trachea) anteriorly and the esophagus posteriorly.

## Nasopharynx

During inhalation, air typically enters the body through the nose and passes into the **nasopharynx**. The nasopharynx is lined with a ciliated mucous membrane that keeps contaminants such as dust and other small particles out of the respiratory tract. In addition, the mucous membranes warm and humidify air as it enters the body.

## Oropharynx

The **oropharynx** forms the posterior portion of the oral cavity, which is bordered superiorly by the hard and soft palates, laterally by the cheeks, and

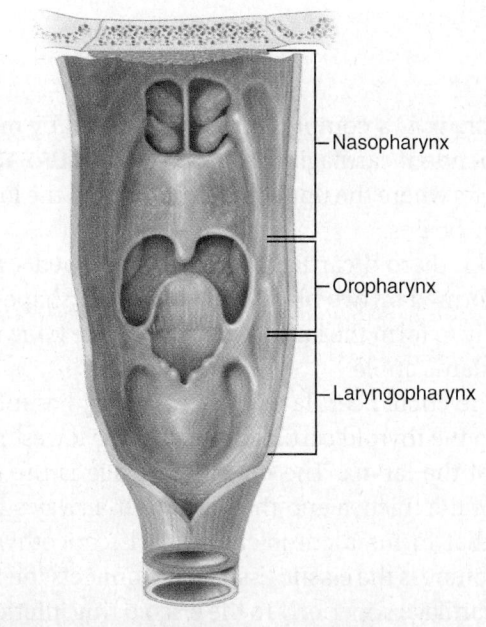

**FIGURE 11-2** The pharynx.

© Jones & Bartlett Learning.

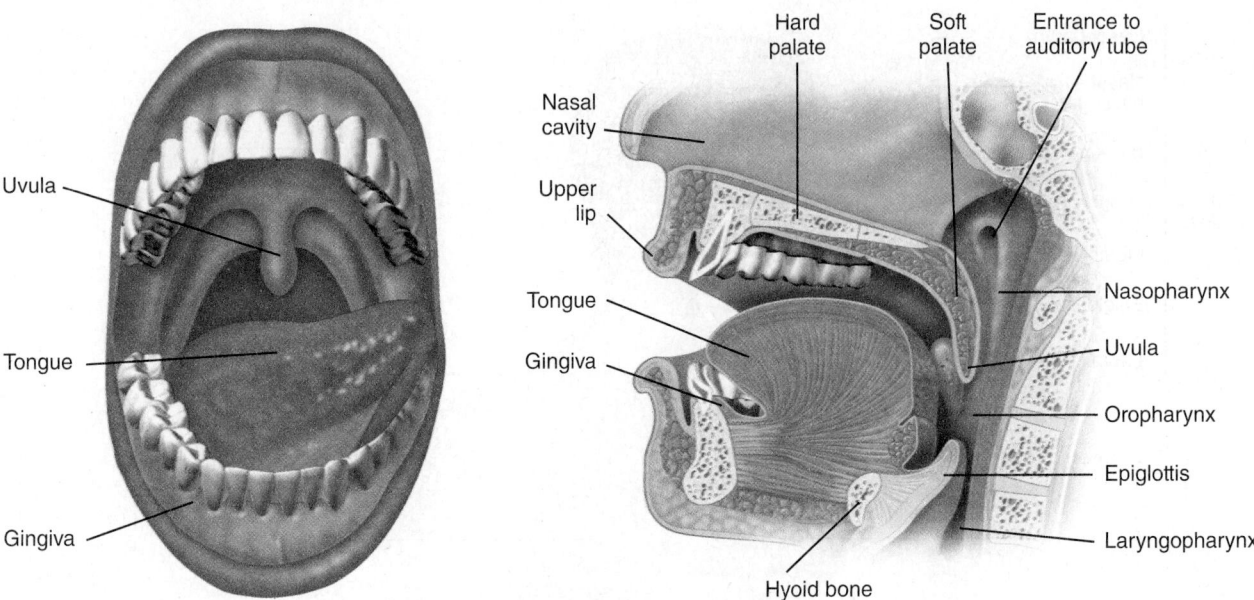

**FIGURE 11-3** The oral cavity.

© Jones & Bartlett Learning.

inferiorly by the tongue (**FIGURE 11-3**). Superior to the larynx, the epiglottis helps separate the digestive system from the respiratory system. Its function is to prevent food and liquid from entering the larynx during swallowing. When swallowing occurs, the larynx is elevated and the epiglottis folds over the glottis to prevent **aspiration** of contents into the trachea.

## Larynx

The **larynx** is a complex structure formed by many independent cartilaginous structures (**FIGURE 11-6**). It marks where the upper airway ends and the lower airway begins.

The thyroid cartilage is a shield-shaped structure formed by two plates that join in a V shape anteriorly to form the laryngeal prominence known as the Adam's apple.

The cricoid cartilage, or cricoid ring, lies inferiorly to the thyroid cartilage; it forms the lowest portion of the larynx. The cricoid cartilage is the first ring of the trachea and the only lower airway structure that forms a complete ring. The cricothyroid membrane is the elastic tissue that connects the thyroid cartilage superiorly to the cricoid ring inferiorly.

The **glottis**, also called the glottic opening, is the space between the vocal cords and the narrowest portion of the adult's airway. The lateral borders of the glottis are the **vocal cords**. These white bands of thin muscle tissue are partially separated at rest and serve as the primary center for speech production. In addition, the vocal cords contain defense reflexes that protect the lower airway, causing a spasmodic closure to the lower airway to prevent substances from entering the trachea (eg, water, vomitus).

## Anatomy of the Lower Airway

The function of the lower airway is to deliver oxygen to the alveoli. Its external boundaries are the fourth cervical vertebra and the xiphoid process, which is the narrow, cartilaginous, lower tip of the sternum. Internally, the lower airway spans the glottis to the pulmonary capillary membrane.

The trachea, or windpipe, is the conduit for air entry into the lungs. This tubular structure is approximately 4 to 5 inches (10 to 12 cm) in length and consists of C-shaped cartilaginous rings. The trachea begins directly below the cricoid cartilage and descends anteriorly down the midline of the neck into the thoracic cavity. Once in the thoracic cavity, the trachea divides at the level of the **carina** into the two main stem bronchi (right and left). The hollow bronchi are supported by cartilage and distribute air into the right and left lungs.

## Special Populations

Generally, the maneuvers, techniques, and indications for airway management are the same in children as they are in adults. However, several anatomic differences in the child require modification of certain techniques.

Infants and small children have a proportionately larger occiput (posterior portion of the cranium), which causes the neck to flex, moving the head forward and backward, when the child lies supine; this position itself can cause an airway obstruction. When positioning the airway of an infant or child, place a folded towel under the child's shoulders to maintain a neutral position of the head.

Compared with adults, children have a proportionately smaller mandible and a proportionately larger tongue (**FIGURE 11-4**). Both factors increase the incidence of airway obstruction in children.

The child's epiglottis is more floppy and omega-shaped than an adult's (**FIGURE 11-5**).

In general, the infant's and the child's airway is smaller and narrower at all levels. The larynx lies more superior and anterior than that of an adult. The larynx is also funnel-shaped due to the narrow, underdeveloped cricoid cartilage. In children younger than 8 years, the narrowest portion of the airway is at the cricoid ring. Further narrowing of the child's inherently narrow airway, such as that caused by soft-tissue swelling or foreign body aspiration, can significantly increase airway resistance and cause breathing inadequacy.

Children do not have well-developed chest musculature, and their ribs and cartilage are softer and more pliable than those of an adult. As a result, the thoracic cavity cannot optimally contribute to lung expansion. Children rely heavily on their diaphragm for breathing, which moves their abdomen in and out. For this reason, infants and small children are commonly referred to as belly breathers.

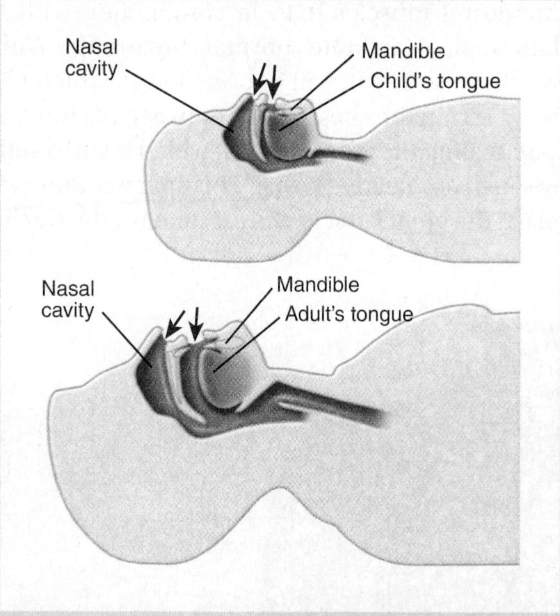

**FIGURE 11-4** In children, the mandible is proportionately smaller and the tongue is proportionately larger than in an adult.
© Jones & Bartlett Learning.

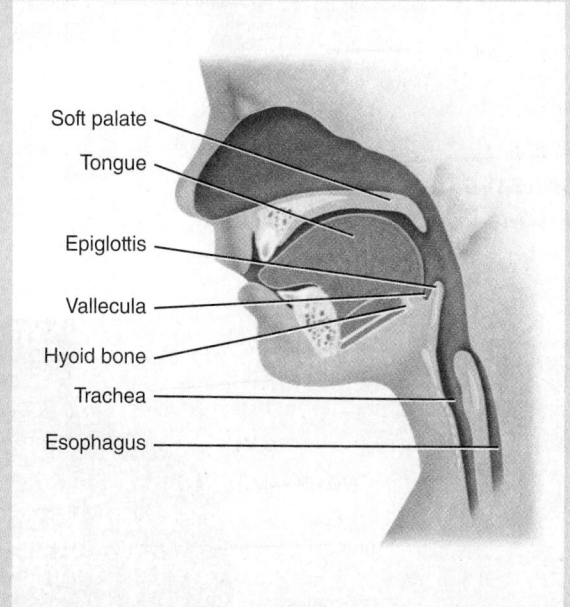

**FIGURE 11-5** The child's epiglottis and surrounding structures.
© Jones & Bartlett Learning.

The lungs consist of the entire mass of tissue that includes the smaller bronchi, bronchioles, and alveoli (**FIGURE 11-7**). The pleurae are thin serous membranes that cover the lungs and line the thoracic cavity. The **visceral pleura** covers the outer surface of the lung tissue, and the **parietal pleura** lines the inside of the thoracic cavity. A small amount of fluid is found between these two pleural layers and serves as a lubricant to prevent friction during breathing.

On entering the lungs, each bronchus divides into increasingly smaller bronchi, which in turn subdivide into bronchioles. The **bronchioles** are thin, hollow tubes made of smooth muscle. The tone of these smooth muscles allows the bronchioles to dilate or constrict in response to various stimuli. The smaller bronchioles branch into alveolar ducts that end at the alveolar sacs.

The alveoli, located at the end of the airway, are millions of thin-walled, balloonlike sacs that serve as the functional site for the exchange of oxygen and carbon dioxide. Surrounding each of these sacs is an intricate bed of blood vessels, known as pulmonary capillaries. Oxygen diffuses through the lining of the alveoli into the pulmonary capillaries where, depending on adequate blood volume and pressure, it is carried back to the heart for distribution to the rest of the body. At the same time, carbon dioxide (waste) diffuses from the pulmonary capillaries into the alveoli, where it is exhaled and removed from the body.

The chest cage (thoracic cavity) contains the lungs, one on each side (**FIGURE 11-8**). The boundaries of the thorax are the rib cage anteriorly, superiorly, and posteriorly and the diaphragm inferiorly. Each individual rib plays a part in the overall protection of the thorax. In between each rib are intercostal muscles that, in conjunction with the diaphragm, facilitate normal breathing. Within the chest cage, you will find the lungs, which hang freely within the chest cavity. Between the lungs is a space called the **mediastinum**, which is surrounded by tough connective tissue. This space contains the heart, the great vessels, the esophagus, the trachea,

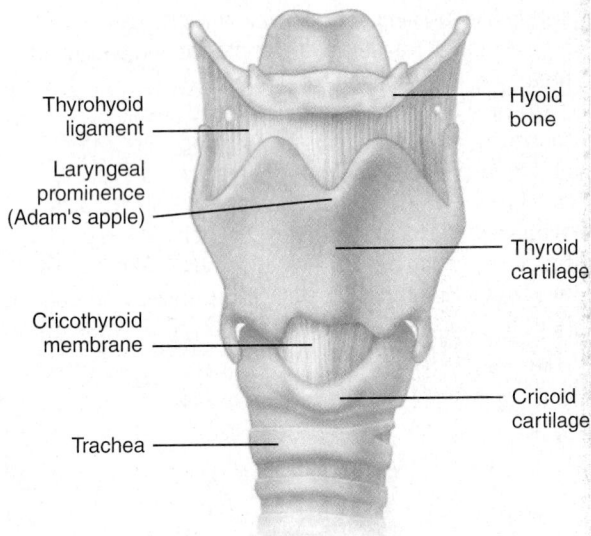

**FIGURE 11-6** The larynx.

© Jones & Bartlett Learning.

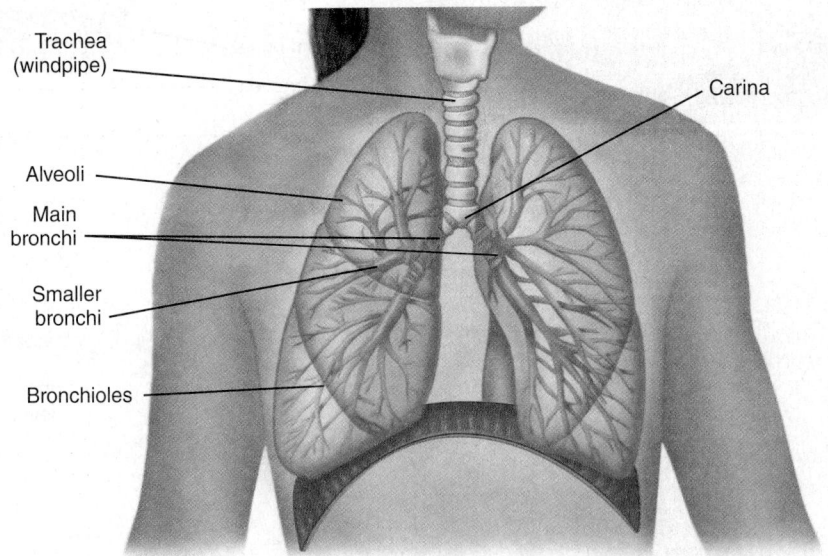

**FIGURE 11-7** The trachea and the lungs are lower airway structures.

© Jones & Bartlett Learning.

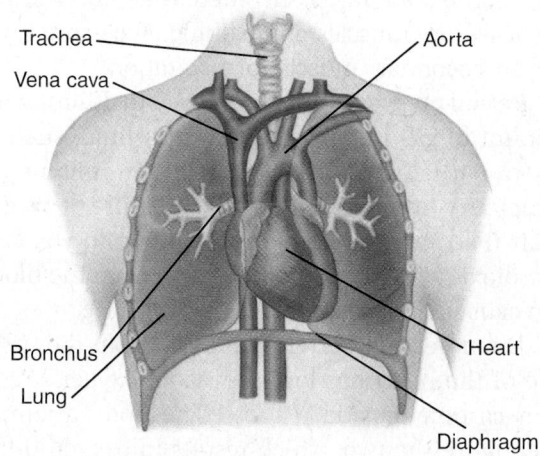

Trachea
Aorta
Vena cava
Bronchus
Heart
Lung
Diaphragm

**FIGURE 11-8** The thoracic cavity contains important anatomic structures for ventilation, oxygenation, and respiration, including the lungs and bronchi, heart, great vessels (the vena cavae and aorta), and trachea.

© Jones & Bartlett Learning.

the major bronchi, and many nerves. The mediastinum effectively separates the right lung space from the left lung space. In addition to the respiratory and circulatory structures found in the thoracic cavity, important structures of the nervous system are also found in the thorax—the **phrenic nerves**. The phrenic nerves, which originate from the third, fourth, and fifth cervical nerves, innervate the diaphragm muscle, allowing it to contract. Contraction of the diaphragm occurs in a downward direction and is necessary for adequate breathing to occur.

## Physiology of Breathing

The respiratory and cardiovascular systems work together to ensure that a constant supply of oxygen and nutrients is delivered to every cell in the body and that carbon dioxide and waste products are removed from every cell. The following sections will describe the process of ventilation, oxygenation, and respiration; however, you first need to understand how the processes of breathing and circulation are connected.

As described earlier, air enters the body through the oral and nasal cavities and travels into the lungs. This occurs because a negative pressure is created in the chest when the thoracic cavity enlarges due

to contraction of the diaphragm and intercostal muscles. Eventually the air reaches the alveolar sacs, where oxygen diffuses across the alveolar membrane and binds to hemoglobin in the bloodstream. At the same time, carbon dioxide diffuses from the bloodstream into the alveoli. The carbon dioxide is exhaled from the lungs, and the oxygen is transported back to the heart, where it is distributed to the rest of the body.

The heart pumps blood to the tissues of the body through a series of arteries and veins. Arteries carry blood away from the heart and eventually branch into capillaries. In the capillaries, the exchange of nutrients and waste products takes place. Oxygen and nutrients leave the capillaries and enter the cells. At the same time, waste products, such as carbon dioxide, diffuse from the cells back into the blood of the capillaries. From here, the deoxygenated blood travels back to the heart. The deoxygenated blood enters the right side of the heart through the right atrium. The right ventricle pumps the blood to the lungs for oxygenation and removal of carbon dioxide. The oxygenated blood then travels back to the heart and into the left atrium. The left ventricle then pumps the oxygenated blood to the rest of the body. Refer back to Chapter 6, *The Human Body*, for an illustration of this process.

It is important to understand that the respiratory and circulatory systems work together to facilitate oxygen delivery to the tissues of the body and removal of waste products from the body (**TABLE 11-1**).

| TABLE 11-1 Ventilation, Oxygenation, and Respiration | |
|---|---|
| **Function** | **Definition** |
| Ventilation | The physical act of moving air into and out of the lungs. |
| Oxygenation | The process of loading oxygen molecules onto hemoglobin molecules in the bloodstream. |
| Respiration | The actual exchange of oxygen and carbon dioxide in the alveoli as well as the tissues of the body. |

© Jones & Bartlett Learning.

When one of these systems is compromised, oxygen delivery is not effective, waste products cannot be removed, and cellular death can result.

## Ventilation

Pulmonary ventilation, the process of moving air into and out of the lungs, is necessary for oxygenation and respiration to occur. Adequate, continuous ventilation is essential for life and therefore is one of the highest priorities in treating any patient. If a patient is not breathing or is breathing inadequately, you must immediately intervene to ensure adequate ventilation.

## Inhalation

The active, muscular part of breathing is called inhalation. When a person inhales, the diaphragm and intercostal muscles contract, allowing air to enter the body and travel to the lungs. When it contracts, the diaphragm moves down slightly, enlarging the thoracic cage from top to bottom. When the intercostal muscles contract, they lift the ribs up and out. The combined actions of these structures enlarge the thorax in all directions. Take a deep breath to see how your chest expands.

The lungs have no muscle tissue; therefore, they cannot move on their own. They need the help of other structures to be able to expand and contract during inhalation and exhalation. Therefore, the ability of the lungs to function properly is dependent on the movement of the chest and supporting structures. These structures include the thorax, the thoracic cage (chest), the diaphragm, the intercostal muscles, and the accessory muscles of breathing. Accessory muscles are secondary muscles of respiration.

Partial pressure is the term used to describe the amount of gas in air or dissolved in fluid, such as blood. Partial pressure is measured in millimeters of mercury (mm Hg). The partial pressure of oxygen in air ($Pao_2$) within the alveoli is 104 mm Hg. Carbon dioxide ($CO_2$) enters the alveoli from the blood and causes a partial pressure of 40 mm Hg.

Deoxygenated arterial blood from the right side of the heart has lower levels of oxygen ($Pao_2$) than carbon dioxide ($Paco_2$). The body attempts to equalize the two, which results in oxygen diffusion across the membrane into the blood and carbon dioxide diffusion in the opposite direction. The carbon dioxide is then eliminated from the lungs as waste during exhalation. This process occurs in reverse when the arterial blood reaches the tissues. Oxygen diffuses into the tissue fluid and then into the cells, and carbon dioxide diffuses out of the cells and then into the tissue fluid and blood.

The air pressure outside the body, called the atmospheric pressure, is normally higher than the air pressure within the thorax. During inhalation, the thoracic cage expands and the air pressure within the thorax decreases, creating a slight vacuum. This pulls air in through the trachea, causing the lungs to fill—a process called negative pressure ventilation. When the air pressure outside equals the air pressure inside, air stops moving. Gases, such as oxygen, will move from an area of higher pressure to an area of lower pressure until the pressures are equal. At this point, the air stops moving, and inhalation stops.

It may help you to understand this if you think of the thoracic cage as a bell jar in which balloons are suspended. In this example, the balloons are the lungs. The base of the jar is the diaphragm, which moves up and down slightly with each breath. The ribs, which are the sides of the jar, maintain the shape of the chest. The only opening into the jar is a small tube at the top, similar to the trachea. During inhalation, the bottom of the jar moves down slightly, causing a decrease in pressure in the jar and creating a slight vacuum. As a result, the balloons fill with air (**FIGURE 11-9**).

The entire process of inspiration is focused on delivering oxygen to the alveoli. However, not all of the air you breathe actually reaches the alveoli. **TABLE 11-2** reviews terminology as it relates to the

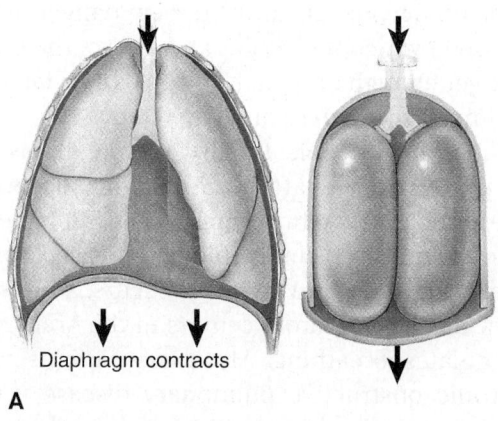 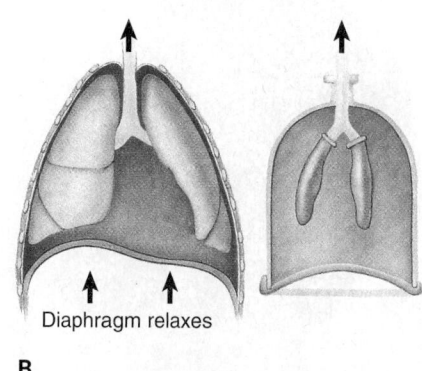

**FIGURE 11-9** The mechanism of ventilation can be illustrated by using a bell jar. **A.** Inhalation and chest expansion, anatomic (left) and bell jar (right). **B.** Exhalation and chest contraction, anatomic (left) and bell jar (right).

A, B: © Jones & Bartlett Learning.

| **TABLE 11-2** Ventilation Terminology | |
|---|---|
| **Term** | **Definition** |
| Tidal volume | The amount of air (in mL) that is moved into or out of the lungs during one breath. |
| Residual volume | The air that remains in the lungs after maximal expiration. |
| Alveolar ventilation | The volume of air that reaches the alveoli; calculated by subtracting the amount of dead space air from the tidal volume. |
| Minute volume | The volume of air moved through the lungs in 1 minute; calculated by multiplying tidal volume and respiratory rate. |
| Alveolar minute volume | The volume of air moved through the lungs in 1 minute minus the dead space; calculated by multiplying tidal volume (minus dead space) and respiratory rate. |
| Vital capacity | The amount of air that can be forcibly expelled from the lungs after breathing in as deeply as possible. |
| Dead space | The portion of the tidal volume that does not reach alveoli and thus does not participate in gas exchange. |

© Jones & Bartlett Learning.

processes of inspiration and expiration. (These processes are discussed further in Chapter 6, *The Human Body*). The average tidal volume, the amount of air in milliliters (mL) moved into or out of the lung during a single breath, for an average adult man is approximately 500 mL. Breathing becomes deeper as the tidal volume responds to the increased metabolic demand for oxygen. However, as noted previously, not all inspired air reaches the alveoli for gas exchange. Dead space is described as the portion of inspired air that fails to reach the alveoli and deliver oxygen.

## Exhalation

Unlike inhalation, **exhalation** does not normally require muscular effort; therefore, it is a passive process. During exhalation, the diaphragm and the intercostal muscles relax. In response, the thorax decreases in size, and the ribs and muscles assume a normal resting position. When the size of the thoracic cage decreases, air in the lungs is compressed into a smaller space. The air pressure within the thorax then becomes higher than the outside pressure, and the air is pushed out through the trachea.

Remember that air will reach the lungs only if it travels through the trachea. This is why clearing and maintaining an open airway is so important. Clearing the airway means removing obstructing material, tissue, or fluids from the nose, mouth, and throat. Maintaining the airway means keeping the airway **patent** so that air can enter and leave the lungs freely (**FIGURE 11-10**).

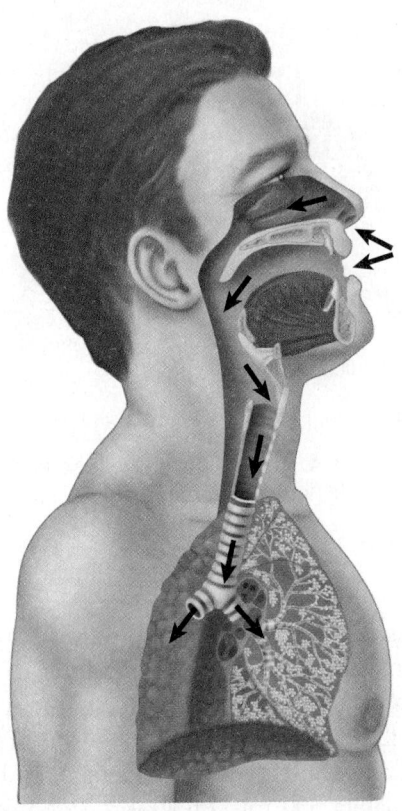

**FIGURE 11-10** Air reaches the lungs only if it travels through the trachea. Maintaining the airway means keeping the trachea and the entirety of the airway patent so that air can enter and leave the lungs freely.

© Jones & Bartlett Learning.

Air may also pass into the chest cavity through an abnormal opening in the throat or chest wall as a result of trauma, remaining outside the bronchi and never reaching the alveoli. In later chapters, you will learn how to recognize and manage these potentially life-threatening conditions.

## Regulation of Ventilation

The body's need for oxygen is constantly changing. The respiratory system must be able to accommodate the changes in oxygen demand by altering the rate and depth of ventilation. The regulation of ventilation involves a complex series of receptors and feedback loops that sense gas concentrations in the body fluids and send messages to the respiratory centers in the brain to adjust the rate and depth of ventilation accordingly. Failure to meet the body's needs for oxygen may result in

hypoxia. Hypoxia is an extremely dangerous condition in which the tissues and cells of the body do not get enough oxygen. Hypoxia can be fatal if not promptly recognized and corrected.

For most people, the drive to breathe is based on pH changes (related to carbon dioxide levels) in the blood and cerebrospinal fluid (CSF). When carbon dioxide levels in the blood increase, the pH of the CSF decreases. When this occurs, a message is sent to the respiratory centers in the brain, which stimulates breathing. However, patients with a chronic obstructive pulmonary disease (COPD), such as emphysema or chronic bronchitis, have difficulty eliminating carbon dioxide through exhalation; thus, they always have higher levels of carbon dioxide. This condition potentially alters their respiratory drive. The theory is that the respiratory centers in the brain gradually adjust to accommodate high levels of carbon dioxide. In patients with COPD, the body uses a backup system to control breathing. This theory of secondary control of breathing, called **hypoxic drive**, is based on levels of oxygen dissolved in plasma. This method is different from the primary control of breathing that uses carbon dioxide as the driving force. Hypoxic drive is typically found in end-stage COPD. Providing high concentrations of oxygen over time will increase the amount of oxygen dissolved in plasma. Some believe this could potentially negatively affect the body's drive to breathe. It is important to remember that high concentrations of oxygen should *never* be withheld from any patient who needs it. Patients with severe respiratory and/or circulatory compromise should receive high concentrations of oxygen regardless of their underlying medical conditions.

Patients who are breathing inadequately will show varying signs and symptoms of hypoxia. The onset and degree of tissue damage caused by hypoxia often depend on the quality of ventilations. Early signs of hypoxia include restlessness, irritability, apprehension, fast heart rate (tachycardia), and anxiety. Late signs of hypoxia include mental status changes, a weak (thready) pulse, and cyanosis. Conscious patients will complain of shortness of breath (**dyspnea**) and may not be able to talk in complete sentences. The best time to give a patient oxygen is before signs and symptoms of hypoxia appear.

## Oxygenation

Oxygenation is the process of loading oxygen molecules onto hemoglobin molecules in the bloodstream. Adequate oxygenation is required for internal respiration to occur; however, it does not guarantee internal respiration is taking place. Oxygenation requires that the air used for ventilation contains an adequate percentage of oxygen. Ventilation without oxygenation can occur in places where oxygen levels in the breathing air have been depleted, such as in mines and confined spaces. Ventilation without adequate oxygenation also occurs in climbers who ascend too quickly to an altitude of lower atmospheric pressure. At high altitudes, the percentage of oxygen remains the same, but the lower atmospheric pressure makes it difficult to adequately bring sufficient amounts of oxygen into the body.

## Respiration

All living cells perform a specific function and need energy to survive. Cells take energy from nutrients through a series of chemical processes. The name given to these processes is metabolism, or cellular respiration. During metabolism, each cell combines nutrients (such as sugar) and oxygen and produces energy (in the form of adenosine triphosphate) and waste products, primarily water and carbon dioxide. Each cell in the body requires a continuous supply of oxygen and a regular means of disposing of waste (carbon dioxide). The body provides for these requirements through respiration.

Respiration is the process of exchanging oxygen and carbon dioxide. This exchange occurs by diffusion, a process in which a gas moves from an area of greater concentration to an area of lower concentration. In the body, gases diffuse rapidly across a distance of micrometers.

## External Respiration

External respiration (pulmonary respiration) is the process of breathing fresh air into the respiratory system and exchanging oxygen and carbon dioxide between the alveoli and the blood in the pulmonary capillaries (**FIGURE 11-11**).

Fresh air that is inspired into the lungs contains approximately 21% oxygen, 78% nitrogen, and 0.3% carbon dioxide. As this air reaches the alveoli, it comes in contact with a fluid called surfactant. Surfactant reduces surface tension within the alveoli and keeps them expanded, making it easier for the gas exchange between oxygen and carbon dioxide to occur. It is important to remember that although adequate ventilation is necessary for external respiration to occur, it does not guarantee that external respiration is being achieved.

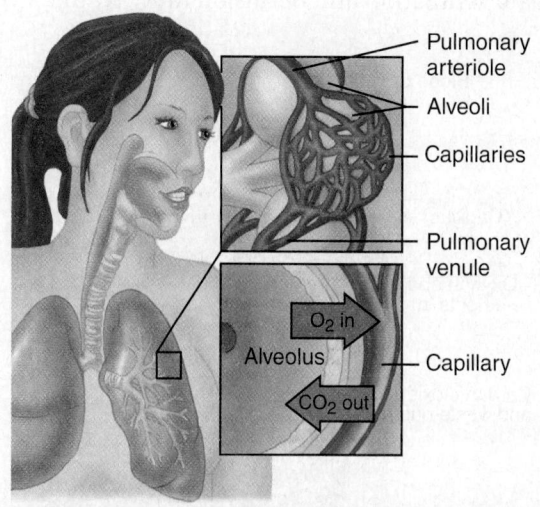

**FIGURE 11-11** External respiration.
© Jones & Bartlett Learning.

Once the oxygen crosses the alveolar membrane, it binds to hemoglobin, an iron-containing molecule that has a great affinity for oxygen molecules. Found in red blood cells, hemoglobin molecules that are low in oxygen concentration are pumped from the right side of the heart through the pulmonary circulation, which ends in the capillaries in the lungs. The capillaries surround alveoli containing high concentrations of oxygen (from inspired air). The hemoglobin molecules bind to oxygen as it crosses the alveolar membrane and transport it back to the left side of the heart, where it is pumped out to the rest of the body. Under normal conditions, 96% to 100% of the hemoglobin receptor sites contain oxygen.

## Internal Respiration

The exchange of oxygen and carbon dioxide between the systemic circulatory system and the cells of the body is called **internal respiration**. As blood travels through the body, it supplies oxygen and nutrients to tissues and cells. Oxygen passes from the blood in the capillaries to the cells in the body's tissues. At the same time, carbon dioxide and cell waste pass from the cells into the capillaries, where they are transported in the venous system back to the lungs (**FIGURE 11-12**).

Every cell in the body needs a constant supply of oxygen to survive. Whereas some tissues are more resilient than others, eventually all cells will die if deprived of oxygen (**FIGURE 11-13**). To deliver sufficient oxygen to the tissues of the body, adequate ventilation and perfusion must occur.

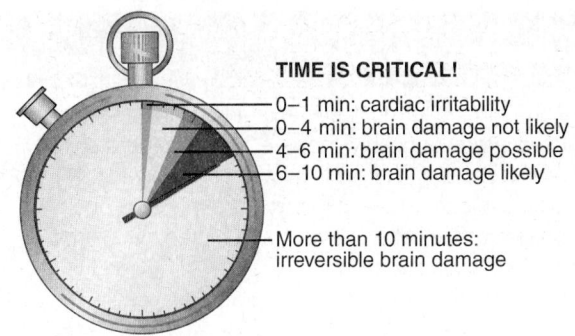

**TIME IS CRITICAL!**

- 0–1 min: cardiac irritability
- 0–4 min: brain damage not likely
- 4–6 min: brain damage possible
- 6–10 min: brain damage likely
- More than 10 minutes: irreversible brain damage

**FIGURE 11-13** Cells need a constant supply of oxygen to survive. Some cells may be severely or permanently damaged after 4 to 6 minutes without oxygen.

© Jones & Bartlett Learning.

In the presence of oxygen, cells convert glucose into energy through a process known as **aerobic metabolism**. Energy is produced through a series of biochemical reactions. Without adequate oxygen, the cells do not completely convert glucose into energy, and lactic acid and other toxins accumulate in the cell. This process, **anaerobic metabolism**, cannot meet the metabolic demands of the cell. If this process is not corrected, the cells will eventually die. Therefore, adequate perfusion (circulation of blood within an organ or tissue) and ventilation must be present for aerobic metabolism to occur. However, although these elements are necessary for aerobic metabolism, they do not guarantee that aerobic metabolism will occur.

When cells use oxygen to convert glucose to energy, carbon dioxide—the main waste product—accumulates in the cell. Carbon dioxide is then transported through the circulatory system and back to the lungs for exhalation.

It is important to understand the processes of ventilation, oxygenation, and respiration. The overall goal of these mechanisms is to deliver an adequate supply of oxygen to the cells of the body. When one of these processes fails or becomes disrupted, cells die. By recognizing the signs and symptoms of inadequate tissue perfusion and oxygenation, you can immediately intervene and correct a potentially life-threatening condition.

## Pathophysiology of Respiration

Multiple conditions inhibit the body's ability to effectively deliver oxygen to the cells. Disruption of pulmonary ventilation, oxygenation, and

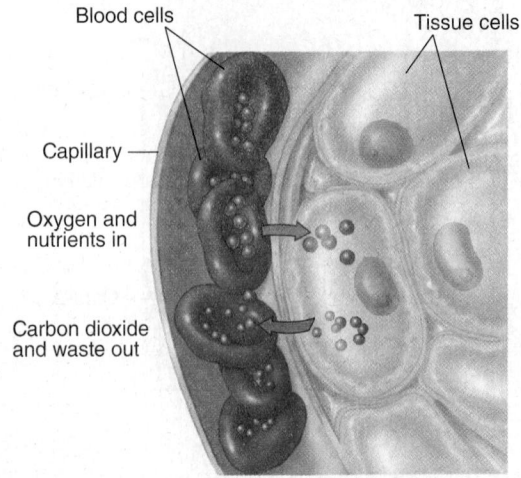

Blood cells

Tissue cells

Capillary

Oxygen and nutrients in

Carbon dioxide and waste out

**FIGURE 11-12** Internal respiration.

© Jones & Bartlett Learning.

respiration will cause immediate effects on the body. As an EMT, you need to recognize these conditions and correct them immediately.

## Factors in the Nervous System

Chemical factors are commonly involved in respiratory control issues because of the level of complexity of the human body. A complex series of chemical reactions are constantly taking place. For example, chemoreceptors monitor the levels of oxygen, carbon dioxide, hydrogen ion concentration, and the pH of the CSF and then provide feedback to the respiratory centers to modify the rate and depth of breathing based on the body's needs at any given time. Central chemoreceptors in the medulla respond quickly to slight elevations in carbon dioxide level or a decrease in the pH of the CSF. The peripheral chemoreceptors, located in the carotid arteries and the aortic arch, are sensitive to decreased levels of oxygen in arterial blood as well as to low pH levels.

When serum carbon dioxide or hydrogen ion levels increase because of medical or traumatic conditions involving the respiratory system, chemoreceptors stimulate the medulla to increase the respiratory rate, thus removing more carbon dioxide or acid from the body. One area in the medulla is responsible for initiating inspiration based on the information received from the chemoreceptors. Another area in the medulla is primarily responsible for motor control of the inspiratory and expiratory muscles.

In addition, stimulation from the pons affects the rate and depth of respirations. If one item in this process is disrupted, then the respiratory process will be affected.

## Ventilation/Perfusion Ratio and Mismatch

The lung has a functional role of placing ambient air in proximity to circulating blood to permit gas exchange by simple diffusion. To accomplish this action, air and blood flow must be directed to the same place at the same time. In other words, ventilation (air flow, $\dot{V}$) and perfusion (blood flow, $\dot{Q}$) must be matched. A failure to match ventilation and perfusion lies behind most abnormalities in oxygen and carbon dioxide exchange.

When ventilation is compromised but perfusion continues, blood passes over some alveolar membranes without gas exchange taking place. This results in a lack of oxygen diffusing across the membrane and into the bloodstream. Carbon dioxide is also not able to diffuse across the membrane into the lungs and is therefore recirculated within the bloodstream. This condition could lead to severe hypoxemia—and eventually hypoxia—if not recognized and treated. It also results in the accumulation of excess carbon dioxide within the circulating bloodstream that leads to a separate set of adverse consequences.

Similar problems can occur when perfusion across the alveolar membrane is disrupted. Although the alveoli are filled with oxygen, disruption in blood flow does not allow for optimal exchange of gases across the membrane. This condition results in less oxygen absorption in the bloodstream and less carbon dioxide removal. It can also lead to hypoxemia, and you need to provide immediate intervention to prevent cellular damage or death.

An example of a ventilation/perfusion ($\dot{V}/\dot{Q}$) mismatch can also be seen with a pulmonary embolism. When a thrombus (blood clot) lodges in a pulmonary artery, blood flow from the right side of the heart to the lungs is partially or completely obstructed, depending on the size and location of the thrombus. Even though the patient continues to ventilate (that is, move air into and out of the lungs), external respiration will be impaired because of decreased blood flow to the lungs.

## Factors Affecting Pulmonary Ventilation

Maintaining a patent airway is critical to the delivery of oxygen to the tissues of the body. There are many intrinsic and extrinsic factors that cause airway obstructions.

### Intrinsic Factors

Intrinsic conditions such as infections, allergic reactions, and unresponsiveness (tongue obstruction) can cause significant restrictions on the ability to maintain an open airway. Swelling from infections and allergic reactions can be fatal if not aggressively managed with medications and possibly advanced airway techniques.

Some factors affecting pulmonary ventilation are not necessarily directly part of the respiratory system. The central and peripheral nervous systems play key roles in the regulation of breathing. Interruptions to these systems can have a drastic effect on the ability to breathe efficiently. Medications that depress the central nervous system lower the respiratory rate and tidal volume. This lower rate and volume will decrease minute volume as well as alveolar volume. As a result, the amount of oxygen in the blood decreases and the amount of carbon dioxide in the bloodstream increases, a condition called **hypercarbia**. Trauma to the head and spinal cord can also interrupt nervous control of ventilation, resulting in decreased respiratory function and even failure. In addition to medications and trauma, conditions such as muscular dystrophy can affect nervous control. This disease causes degeneration of muscle fibers, resulting in a gradual weakening of muscles (such as the diaphragm and intercostal muscles), slowing of motor development, and loss of muscle contractility. Curvature of the spine is also likely in patients with muscular dystrophy and can impair pulmonary function.

The tongue is the most common airway obstruction in the unresponsive patient. This airway obstruction, while easily corrected, can result in hypoxia and hinder adequate tissue perfusion. Obstruction of the airway by the tongue is also associated with hypercarbia. Snoring respirations and the position of the head and/or neck are good indicators that the tongue may be obstructing the airway. Prompt correction of this obstruction is necessary for adequate ventilation and oxygenation.

Patients with allergic reactions not only have a potential airway obstruction from swelling, but may also have a decrease in pulmonary ventilation from bronchoconstriction. As the bronchioles constrict, air is forced through smaller lumens, resulting in decreased ventilation. This condition is also found in patients with COPD such as emphysema.

## Extrinsic Factors

Extrinsic factors affecting pulmonary ventilation can include trauma or foreign body airway obstruction. Trauma to the airway or chest requires immediate evaluation and intervention. The effect of an injury such as a broken jaw is often overlooked. Patients with a fracture to the mandible, especially unconscious patients, may not be able to maintain an open airway and may require the insertion of an airway adjunct. Blunt or penetrating trauma and burns can disrupt airflow through the trachea and into the lungs, quickly resulting in oxygenation deficiencies. In addition, trauma to the chest wall can result in structural damage to the thorax, leading to inadequate pulmonary ventilation. Swelling, punctures, and bruising can have a tremendous effect on the ability to deliver oxygen to the alveoli and into the bloodstream. Proper airway management and high concentrations of oxygen are crucial to the patient's outcome in these situations.

## Factors Affecting Respiration

External elements in the environment can affect the overall process of respiration. For proper respiration to take place at the cellular level, both oxygenation and perfusion need to function efficiently.

## External Factors

Adequate respiration requires proper ventilation and oxygenation. Here, external factors such as atmospheric pressure and the partial pressure of oxygen in the ambient air play a key role in the overall process of respiration. At high altitudes, the percentage of oxygen remains the same, but the partial pressure decreases because the total atmospheric pressure decreases. The low partial pressure of oxygen can make it difficult (or impossible) to adequately oxygenate tissue, thus interrupting internal respiration. In addition, closed environments, such as mines and trenches, may have decreased levels of ambient oxygen, resulting in poor oxygenation and respiration.

Carbon monoxide, along with other toxic and poisonous gases, displaces oxygen in the environment and makes proper oxygenation and respiration difficult. In particular, carbon monoxide has a much greater affinity for hemoglobin than does oxygen (250 times more), and will occupy all sites on hemoglobin that are normally occupied by oxygen. Loading the hemoglobin with carbon monoxide instead of oxygen prohibits oxygen delivery to the tissues. This results in severe hypoxemia which, if uncorrected, can rapidly lead to death.

## Internal Factors

Conditions that reduce the surface area for gas exchange also decrease the body's oxygen supply, leading to inadequate tissue perfusion. Medical conditions such as pneumonia, pulmonary edema, and COPD/emphysema may also result in a disturbance of cellular metabolism. These conditions decrease the surface area of the alveoli either by damaging the alveoli or by leading to an accumulation of fluid in the lungs.

Nonfunctional alveoli inhibit the diffusion of oxygen and carbon dioxide. As a result, blood entering the lungs from the right side of the heart bypasses the alveoli and returns to the left side of the heart in an unoxygenated state, a condition called **intrapulmonary shunting**. The greater the degree of intrapulmonary shunting, the greater the degree of hypoxemia.

Drowning victims and/or patients with pulmonary edema have fluid in the alveoli. This accumulation of fluid inhibits adequate gas exchange at the alveolar membrane and results in decreased oxygenation and respiration. In addition, exposure to certain environmental conditions such as high altitude or occupational hazards such as epoxy resins can result over time in fluid accumulation or other abnormal conditions, resulting in impaired oxygenation. These conditions can interrupt the process of aerobic respiration at the cellular level, resulting in anaerobic respiration and an increase in lactic acid accumulation.

Other conditions affecting cells of the body include hypoxia, hypoglycemia (low blood glucose), and infection. As oxygen and glucose levels decrease, the body is unable to maintain a homeostatic balance regarding energy production. At this point, the energy production cannot meet the needs of the body, and cellular death is likely if the condition is not corrected. Infection also increases the metabolic needs of the body and disrupts homeostasis. If not corrected, this will also cause the cells to die.

## Circulatory Compromise

For respiration to occur, the circulatory system must function efficiently to deliver oxygen to the tissues of the body. When this system becomes compromised, perfusion is inadequate to meet the metabolic demands of the tissues.

Obstruction of blood flow to individual cells and tissue can be related to traumatic emergencies. These conditions include a **hemothorax** or a **pneumothorax**—whether a simple or **tension** **pneumothorax**, open pneumothorax (sucking chest wound), or hemopneumothorax. Although not directly related to traumatic emergencies, a pulmonary embolism can have the same obstructive effects. All of these conditions limit the ability for gas exchange to occur at the tissue level as a result of their effects on the respiratory and circulatory systems. In addition, conditions such as heart failure and cardiac tamponade inhibit the ability of the heart to effectively pump oxygenated blood to the tissues.

Blood loss and anemia, a deficiency of red blood cells, result in a decreased ability of blood to carry oxygen. Without sufficient circulating red blood cells, there is not enough hemoglobin to carry oxygen to the tissues.

When the body is in a state of shock, oxygen is not delivered to the cells efficiently. Hypovolemic shock is an abnormal decrease in circulating volume that causes inadequate oxygen delivery to the body. In contrast, vasodilatory shock is not determined by the amount of circulating blood, but by the size of the blood vessels. As the diameter of the blood vessels increases, the blood pressure in the circulatory system decreases. As the systemic blood pressure decreases, oxygen is not delivered effectively to the tissues. Both forms of shock result in poor tissue perfusion that leads to anaerobic metabolism. Any patient suspected of being in shock should be treated aggressively to prevent further interruptions in tissue perfusion.

### Street Smarts

It is equally important to know *how* and *why* you are performing a particular airway procedure. If you know how and why, you will also know when to perform and when not to perform the procedure. Without sufficient knowledge of respiratory anatomy, physiology, and pathophysiology, airway management is nothing more than a procedure. Remember, your patients need your knowledge as much as they need your hands.

## Patient Assessment

To ensure your safety during a call that involves a patient with breathing difficulties, wear a mask and protective eyewear that includes eye shields (not glasses) whenever airway management involves suctioning or an **aerosol-generating procedure (AGP)**.

Any airway manipulation that induces the production of aerosols constitutes an AGP, such as CPR, nebulizer treatments, endotracheal intubation. and continuous positive airway pressure. Body fluids can become aerosolized, and exposure to the mucous membranes of your mouth, nose, and eyes can easily occur. In the event of a pandemic or if the patient has a highly contagious disease, an N95 or powered, air-purifying respirator and gown should also be worn (if there is risk of tuberculosis or a pandemic such as SARS-CoV-2).

## Recognizing Adequate Breathing

Breathing is something that all people do every day; yet, most of the time, you are not aware of your own breathing or the breathing of others around you. Breathing should be a smooth flow of air moving into and out of the lungs. In general, unless you are directly assessing the patient's airway, you should not be able to see or hear a patient breathe. Signs of normal (adequate) breathing for adult patients are as follows:

- A normal rate (between 12 and 20 breaths/min)
- A regular pattern of inhalation and exhalation
- Clear and equal lung sounds on both sides of the chest (bilateral)
- Regular and equal chest rise and fall (chest expansion)
- Adequate depth (tidal volume)

## Recognizing Abnormal Breathing

An adult who is awake, alert, and talking to you generally has no *immediate* airway or breathing problems. However, you should always have supplemental oxygen and a bag-mask device or pocket mask close at hand to assist with breathing if necessary. An adult who is breathing normally will have respirations of 12 to 20 breaths/min (**TABLE 11-3**).

Adult patients who are breathing slower (fewer than 12 breaths/min) than normal should be evaluated for inadequate breathing by assessing the depth of respirations. Patients with shallow depth of breathing (reduced tidal volume) may require assisted ventilations, even if the respiratory rate is within normal limits.

A patient with inadequate breathing may appear to be working hard to breathe, which is called labored breathing. It requires effort and, especially among children, may involve the use of accessory

| TABLE 11-3  Normal Respiratory Rate Ranges | |
|---|---|
| Adults | 12 to 20 breaths/min |
| Children | 12 to 40 breaths/min |
| Infants | 30 to 60 breaths/min |

*Note*: These ranges are from the AHA (2015) PALS digital reference card and NASEMSO (2019) National Model EMS clinical Guidelines v2.2. Ranges presented in other courses may vary.

© Jones & Bartlett Learning.

## YOU are the Provider

On arrival at the scene, you find the patient sitting in a recliner. She is drooling, and her face and neck are cyanotic. She does not answer when spoken to. Her breathing is slow, shallow, and labored. As your partner opens the jump kit, you assess the patient.

| Recording Time:  0 Minutes | |
|---|---|
| Appearance | Poor breathing effort; skin is cyanotic |
| Level of consciousness | Eyes are barely open; does not answer when spoken to |
| Airway | Open; secretions draining from the mouth |
| Breathing | Slow, shallow, and labored |
| Circulation | Skin, cyanotic; radial pulse, rapid, and weak |

4. Why is slow, shallow breathing so dangerous?

5. How should you proceed with airway management of this patient?

6. What specifically does pulse oximetry measure?

muscles, including the neck muscles (sternocleido-mastoid), the pectoralis major muscles of the chest, and the abdominal muscles.

Accessory muscles are not used during normal breathing. More information about recognizing labored breathing and respiratory distress in children is found in later chapters. Signs of inadequate breathing in adult patients are as follows:

- Respiratory rate of fewer than 12 breaths/min or more than 20 breaths/min in the presence of shortness of breath (dyspnea)
- Irregular rhythm, such as a patient taking a series of deep breaths followed by periods of apnea
- Diminished, absent, or noisy auscultated breath sounds
- Use of tripod position where patient is sitting upright and leaning forward onto arms and hands to facilitate inspiration and expiration (**FIGURE 11-14**).
- Reduced flow of expired air at the nose and mouth
- Unequal or inadequate chest expansion, resulting in reduced tidal volume
- Increased effort of breathing (use of accessory muscles)
- Shallow depth (reduced tidal volume)
- Skin that is pale, cyanotic (blue), cool, or moist (clammy)
- Skin pulling in around the ribs or above the clavicles during inspiration (**retractions**)

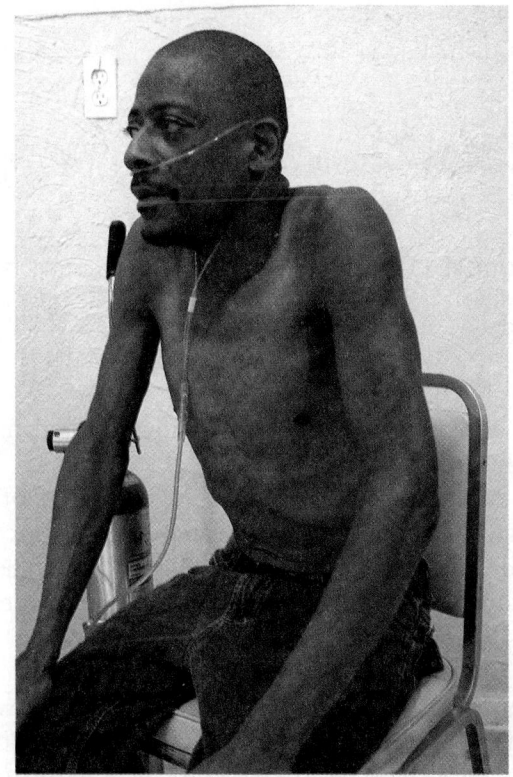

**FIGURE 11-14** The use of the tripod position in which the patient sits or stands with hands on knees or another surface as demonstrated above is commonly seen in patients with labored breathing to facilitate inhalation and exhalation.

© Ray Kemp/Science Source.

When you are assessing a patient with potential airway compromise, pay particular attention to the external environment. Conditions such as high altitude and enclosed spaces alter the partial pressure of oxygen in the environment, making the process of oxygenation difficult for the patient. In addition, poisonous gases, such as carbon monoxide, displace oxygen in the environment and alter the overall metabolism of the patient. The external environment should be considered when deciding on the appropriate treatment.

You should be aware that a patient may appear to be breathing after his or her heart has stopped. These occasional, gasping breaths are called **agonal gasps**. They occur when the respiratory center in the brain continues to send signals to the respiratory muscles. These gasps do not provide adequate oxygen because they are infrequent, gasping respiratory efforts. In patients with agonal gasps, you

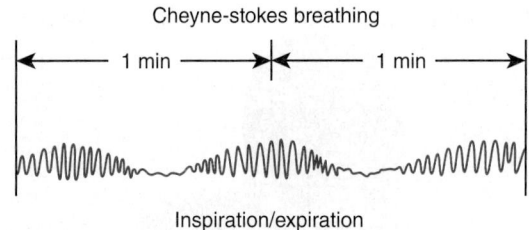

**FIGURE 11-15** Cheyne-Stokes breathing shows irregular respirations followed by a period of apnea.

© Jones & Bartlett Learning.

will need to provide artificial ventilations and, most likely, chest compressions.

Some patients may have irregular respiratory breathing patterns that are related to a specific condition. For example, **Cheyne-Stokes respirations** are often seen in patients with stroke and patients with serious head injuries (**FIGURE 11-15**).

Cheyne-Stokes respirations are an irregular respiratory pattern in which the patient breathes with an increasing rate and depth of respirations that is followed by a period of **apnea**, or lack of spontaneous breathing, followed again by a pattern of increasing rate and depth of respiration. Serious head injuries may also cause changes in the normal respiratory rate and pattern of breathing. The result may be irregular, ineffective respirations that may or may not have an identifiable pattern (**ataxic respirations**). Patients experiencing a metabolic or toxic disorder may display other abnormal respiratory patterns such as Kussmaul respirations. Kussmaul respirations are characterized as deep, rapid respirations commonly seen in patients with metabolic acidosis.

Whereas rapid breathing is a compensatory mechanism to help patients in respiratory distress, some patients are so ill that their bodies are unable to compensate for their respiratory distress. You need to be vigilant when monitoring patients in respiratory distress because their condition may decline rapidly.

Patients with inadequate breathing have inadequate minute volume and need to be treated immediately. If a patient can speak using only minimal words while at rest, he or she is attempting to preserve residual volume in the lungs; this is a sign of inadequate ventilation. Likewise, a slow or fast respiratory rate may result in a reduction in tidal volume and decreased ventilation adequacy. Emergency medical care includes airway management, supplemental oxygen, and ventilatory support.

## Assessment of Respiration

Even though a patient may be ventilating adequately, the actual exchange of oxygen and carbon dioxide at the tissue level may be compromised. You must assess for signs of adequate and inadequate respiration in all patients.

As stated earlier, external factors may disrupt the process of respiration. Be aware of the patient's environment and assess the quality of ambient air when approaching the patient. High altitudes and poisonous gases should always be considered when assessing respiration. Environmental factors can dramatically affect respiration and alter metabolism in your patient. If there is more than one patient with similar symptoms, consider the presence of poisonous or toxic gases or an infectious cause such as pneumonia affecting the community. If your EMS unit carries a handheld carbon monoxide detector, assess ambient air before entering the location. However, if you enter a space and suspect the quality of the ambient air is not safe, remove yourself and the patient (if possible) from the scene immediately and contact the appropriate resources.

A patient's level of consciousness and skin color and condition are excellent indicators of respiration. During normal respiration, oxygen and carbon dioxide diffuse into and out of tissues. When you are assessing mental status and skin color and condition, it will be apparent if the patient has adequate oxygen levels reaching these areas. A patient with an altered level of consciousness may not have adequate oxygen levels reaching the brain. This lack of oxygen can cause rapid changes in the patient's mental status. Therefore, when treating patients with an altered mental status, always consider the possibility that these patients may not be getting adequate oxygen levels to their brain and that you need to consider the possible underlying causes. Be sure to determine the patient's baseline mental status, considering that the baseline mental status may be abnormal because of a preexisting medical condition (eg, previous stroke, traumatic brain injury). Ask family members to describe the patient's normal mental status.

Poor skin color can indicate inadequate respiration, just as an altered level of consciousness does.

As oxygen fails to reach the skin tissue of the body, either from a lack of perfusion or poor oxygenation, the color of the skin changes to reflect the low level of oxygenation. Pale skin and mucous membranes, commonly referred to as pallor, are typically associated with poor perfusion caused by illness or shock. As this condition worsens, cyanosis becomes noticeable first peripherally, in the fingertips, and then centrally, in the mucous membranes and around the lips. Eventually, if the poor perfusion or oxygenation is not corrected, anaerobic metabolism will occur. This could cause the skin to become marked with blotches of different colors, commonly referred to as mottling.

Several methods can be used to assess proper oxygenation, including the use of **pulse oximetry**. The oxygen saturation ($SpO_2$) level measures the percentage of hemoglobin molecules that are bound in arterial blood. Because hemoglobin delivers 97% of the oxygen delivered to the body's tissues, oxygen saturation is an excellent indication of the amount of oxygen available to the end organs. Oxygen dissolved in plasma (the partial pressure of oxygen [$PaO_2$]) delivers the other 3% to the body's tissues.

Assessment of oxygen saturation is the standard of care in the management of patients with respiratory or circulatory problems (**FIGURE 11-16**). The pulse oximeter provides a rapid, reliable, noninvasive measurement of a patient's oxygenation status; however, a pulse oximetry reading should not be the sole determinant of a patient's overall respiratory status. This value should be interpreted together with a full clinical assessment of the patient. This device can be used to assess the adequacy of oxygenation during positive-pressure ventilation and assess the overall effect of interventions on your patient.

A pulse oximeter measures the percentage of hemoglobin saturation. Under normal conditions, the $SpO_2$ should be 94% or greater while breathing room air. Although no definitive threshold exists for normal values, an $SpO_2$ of less than 94% in a nonsmoker may indicate hypoxemia. An $SpO_2$ of 94% or lower generally requires treatment unless the patient has a chronic condition causing perpetually low oxygen saturation levels. In conditions such as stroke or heart attack, oxygen is applied when the $SpO_2$ drops below 94%. Pulse oximeters are highly accurate for $SpO_2$ readings higher than 85%; however, readings below that are less reliable but can certainly indicate profound hypoxemia. Pulse oximeters can take as long as 60 seconds to reflect changes in a patient's oxygenation status. Essentially, a pulse oximeter placed on a patient's finger typically reflects a patient's oxygenation status approximately 1 minute ago. This time delay is important to understand because respiratory insufficiency can develop in a patient well before the pulse oximetry values begin to decline. It is critical to monitor the patient and supplement your assessment with the information from the pulse oximeter.

> ## Words of Wisdom
>
> When caring for patients who live at high altitudes, remember that their normal pulse oximetry reading may be lower than normal. When living at altitude, the body adapts to the decreased pressure of oxygen, resulting in a lower normal $SaO_2$ reading. Your medical assessment must take this adaptation into account.

Pulse oximetry is considered a routine vital sign and can be used as part of any patient assessment. Whereas there are no true contraindications to using pulse oximetry, you must be aware of the limitations associated with this device. To function properly, the pulse oximeter must find a pulsation in the selected tissue. The most commonly used

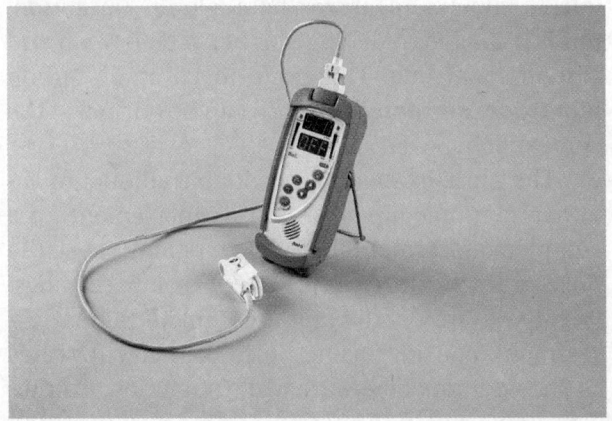

**FIGURE 11-16** A pulse oximeter.

© Jones & Bartlett Learning.

## Skill Drill 11-1 Performing Pulse Oximetry

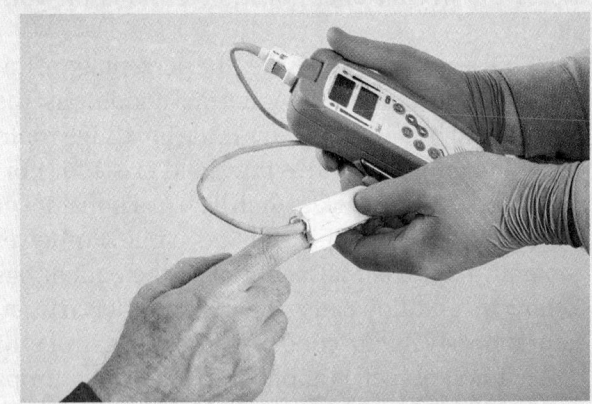

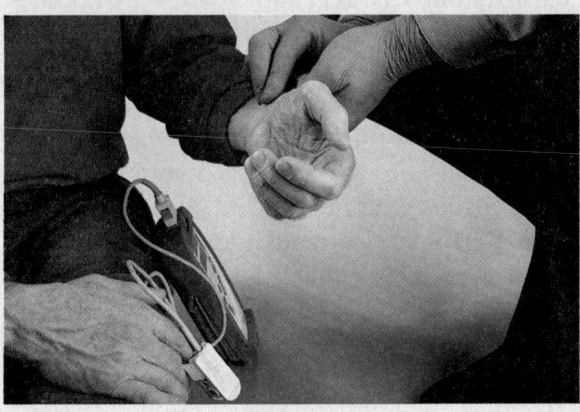

**Step 1**

Clean the patient's finger and place the index or middle finger into the pulse oximeter probe. Turn on the pulse oximeter and note the LED reading of the Spo$_2$.

**Step 2**

Palpate the radial pulse to ensure that it correlates with the LED display on the pulse oximeter.

© Jones & Bartlett Learning.

site is a finger. Follow the steps in **SKILL DRILL 11-1** to measure pulse oximetry:

1. Clean the patient's finger and remove nail polish as needed. Place the index or middle finger into the pulse oximeter probe. Turn on the pulse oximeter and note the LED reading of the Spo$_2$ (**Step 1**).
2. Palpate the radial pulse to ensure that it correlates with the LED display on the pulse oximeter (**Step 2**).

In patients with significant vasoconstriction or very low perfusion (including decompensated shock and cardiac arrest), there may not be enough peripheral perfusion to be detected by the sensor. In these cases, move the sensor to a more central location (bridge of the nose or earlobe). Always consult the manufacturer's guidelines for proper placement and troubleshooting of these devices. An inaccurate pulse oximetry reading may be caused by the following:

- Hypovolemia
- Anemia (decreased level of circulating red blood cells and therefore hemoglobin)

- Severe peripheral vasoconstriction (chronic hypoxia, smoking, or hypothermia)
- Time delay in detecting respiratory insufficiency
- Dark or metallic nail polish
- Dirty fingers
- Carbon monoxide poisoning

When carbon monoxide is present in the inspired gas, it displaces oxygen from the hemoglobin. Pulse oximetry measures hemoglobin saturation, but it is unable to distinguish between oxygen and carbon monoxide. Therefore, in cases of carbon monoxide poisoning, the Spo$_2$ can be normal in the context of hypoxia.

The pulse oximeter is a valuable adjunct to aid in decision making, but is not a replacement for a complete assessment. Many factors may cause the pulse oximeter to give false high or low readings. When you are conducting a complete patient assessment, consider using pulse oximetry readings as one additional measure while obtaining all other comprehensive information you need. Assess the patient for signs and symptoms of adequate oxygenation. If a patient has signs such as cyanosis or pale or clammy skin, or symptoms such as shortness of breath and a normal $SpO_2$, treat the patient's condition, not the device. Bear in mind that otherwise healthy patients may maintain a normal $SpO_2$ for several minutes, even in the face of acute respiratory compromise.

Pulse oximetry cannot measure the effectiveness of ventilation or provide information about cellular metabolism. To assess ventilation, you will need to measure exhaled carbon dioxide levels. Carbon dioxide can be described as the smoke of metabolism. The body uses oxygen as its fuel and makes carbon dioxide as its by-product. As long as oxygen is delivered to the cells and tissues, carbon dioxide production continues. A helpful analogy is a motor vehicle engine. As long as gasoline continues to burn, exhaust is produced. In the human body, carbon dioxide is the exhaust.

**End-tidal $co_2$** is the measure of the maximal concentration of $CO_2$ at the end of an exhaled breath. A low $CO_2$ level could indicate a number of conditions. If the patient is hyperventilating, he or she is eliminating carbon dioxide faster than the body is making it; this would cause a low $CO_2$ level. A low $CO_2$ level could also indicate decreased $CO_2$ return to the lungs because of reduced $CO_2$ production at the cellular level secondary to conditions such as shock and cardiac arrest. When cardiac output increases, end-tidal $CO_2$ levels generally increase—a reflection of improved oxygen delivery. By contrast, a high $CO_2$ level may indicate that the patient is retaining $CO_2$ secondary to ventilation inadequacy. An absence of $CO_2$ can indicate that the patient is not breathing at all.

End-tidal $CO_2$ is measured by using capnometry and capnography devices. **Capnometry** typically refers to use of a device that provides a digital numeric reading of the end-tidal $CO_2$ level. **Capnography** provides both a numeric reading and a graph, or real-time image, of the end-tidal $CO_2$ levels from breath to breath. The digital display of end-tidal $CO_2$ is expressed in millimeters of mercury (mm Hg) (**FIGURE 11-17**). The normal range is 35 to 45 mm Hg. Although end-tidal $CO_2$ monitoring was previously used as the primary method to assess proper advanced airway placement, it is now used routinely on many respiratory distress calls. Paramedic or other advanced life support (ALS) providers use these devices to determine proper placement of an advanced airway, assess a patient's ventilatory status, and avoid inadvertent hyperventilation of

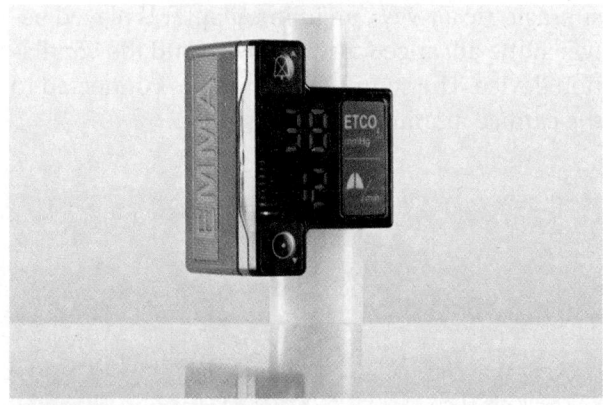

**FIGURE 11-17** A capnometer.

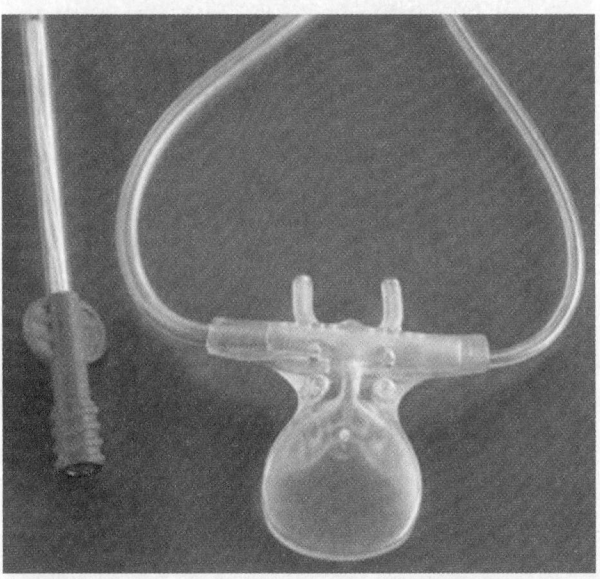

**FIGURE 11-18** Nasal cannula device for monitoring end-tidal carbon dioxide in a spontaneously breathing patient.

patients with head injuries, which has been linked to poor outcomes. Additionally, waveform capnography provides data that can be used to determine changes in cardiac output. It also provides the first indication of return of spontaneous circulation (ROSC) after cardiac arrest.

Waveform capnography can be monitored in spontaneously breathing patients with an adequate airway by applying a special nasal cannula device to the patient and connecting the sampling line to the cardiac monitor (**FIGURE 11-18**). If an advanced airway device is in place (ie, endotracheal tube, supraglottic airway), an inline adapter is placed between the advanced airway device and the ventilation device. The sampling line is then connected to the cardiac monitor (**FIGURE 11-19**).

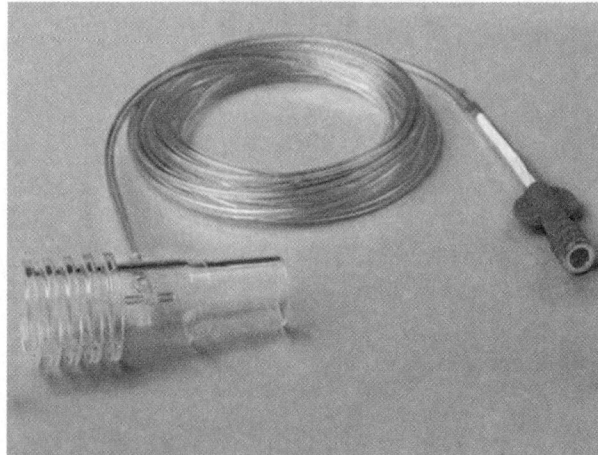

**FIGURE 11-19** Inline end-tidal carbon dioxide device for use in the patient with advanced airway in place.

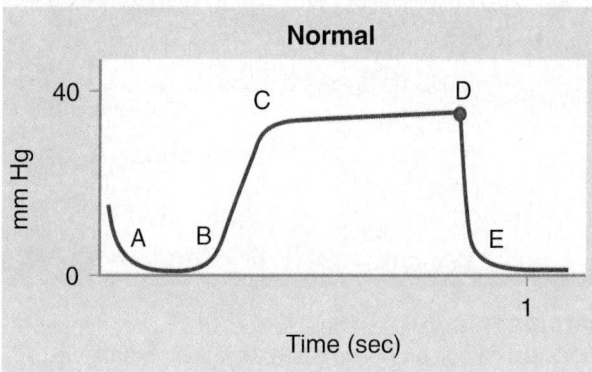

**FIGURE 11-20** Normal capnographic waveform with points A through E shown.

A normal capnographic waveform has four distinct phases (**FIGURE 11-20**). Phase I (**A–B**), also known as the respiratory baseline, is the initial stage of exhalation; the gas sample is dead space gas, free of carbon dioxide (which explains why phase I is flat). Phase II (**B–C**) is called the expiratory upslope. At point B, alveolar gas, which contains a high level of carbon dioxide, mixes with dead space gas, resulting in an abrupt rise in exhaled carbon dioxide (which explains why phase II abruptly rises from the baseline). The alveolar plateau is represented by phase III (**C–D**), and the gas sampled is all alveolar. Point D is the maximal end-tidal $CO_2$ level—the best reflection of the alveolar carbon dioxide level. The height of the waveform at point D correlates with the numeric value of exhaled carbon dioxide that is displayed on the cardiac monitor. Phase IV, called the inspiratory downstroke, occurs when the patient inhales and fresh gas is breathed into the lungs. During inhalation, carbon dioxide is displaced, causing the waveform to return to the baseline level of carbon dioxide—approximately 0 mm Hg. The duration (width) of each waveform corresponds to the duration of ventilation, and the space between waveforms corresponds to the patient's respiratory rate.

The EMT can recognize abnormalities in carbon dioxide levels by noting the height of the capnographic waveform. If the patient is hypoventilating, such as may be seen in cases of opioid overdose, he or she is retaining too much carbon dioxide; therefore, one would expect a tall capnographic waveform (**FIGURE 11-21**). By contrast, if the patient is hyperventilating and eliminating too much carbon dioxide, or if carbon dioxide return to the lungs is decreased (ie, shock, cardiac arrest), the capnographic waveform would be correspondingly smaller (**FIGURE 11-22**).

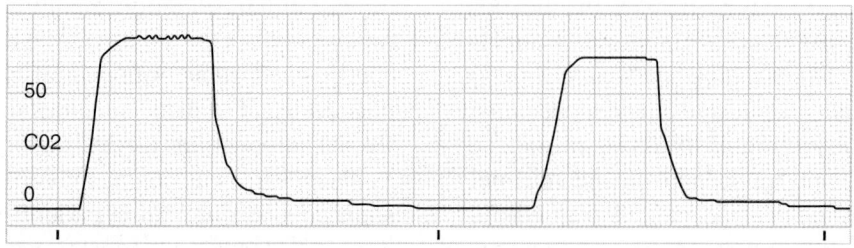

**FIGURE 11-21** Capnographic waveform caused by hypoventilation.

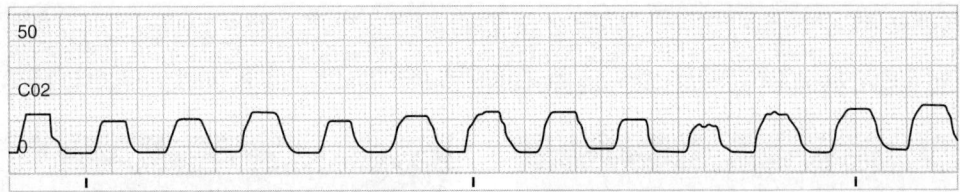

**FIGURE 11-22** Capnographic waveform caused by hyperventilation, or reduced carbon dioxide return to the lungs.

© Jones & Bartlett Learning.

---

**Street Smarts**

Effective airway management is accomplished by a team—not an individual. Never leave an EMT to struggle, attempting to establish a patent airway and adequate ventilation alone! When practicing airway skills (which should be frequently), practice as a team. Plan how you will manage the next airway problem before you receive the call. Remember, practice like you play.

---

## Opening the Airway

Emergency medical care begins with ensuring an open airway. If you cannot immediately open and maintain a patent airway, you cannot ensure adequate oxygenation, ventilation, and respiration. Regardless of the patient's condition, the airway must remain patent at all times.

When you respond to a call and find an unconscious patient, you need to quickly assess for a pulse and breathing; if the patient has a pulse, you need to determine whether breathing is adequate. Remember that airway and breathing are two separate components that are closely related to each other. However, you must understand that adequate breathing does not always equate to an adequate airway. To most effectively open the airway and assess breathing, the unresponsive patient should be in the supine position. However, if your patient is in a situation that delays placement in a supine position (for example, entrapped in a vehicle), the patient's airway must be opened and assessed in the position in which you find the patient. If your patient is found in the prone position (lying facedown), he or she must be repositioned to allow for assessment of airway and breathing and

to begin CPR, should it become necessary. Currently, health care workers are taught to begin CPR with high-quality compressions if cardiac arrest is suspected. The patient should be log rolled as a unit so the head, neck, and spine all move together without twisting. Although care should be taken to avoid injury, remember that airway management almost always takes priority and should not be delayed when caring for patients with life-threatening conditions. Unconscious patients, especially when there are no witnesses who can rule out trauma, should be moved as a unit because of the potential for spinal injury. To position the unconscious patient to open the airway, follow the steps in **SKILL DRILL 11-2**:

1. Kneel beside the patient. Make sure you kneel far enough away so that the patient, when rolled toward you, does not come to rest in your lap. Place your hands behind the patient's head and neck to support the cervical spine as your partner straightens the patient's legs (**Step 1**).
2. Have your partner place his or her hands on the patient's far shoulder and hip (**Step 2**).
3. As you call the count to control movement, have your partner turn the patient toward you by pulling on the far shoulder and hip. Control the head and neck so that they move as a unit with the rest of the torso. In this way, the head and neck stay in the same vertical plane as the back. This single motion will minimize aggravation of any potential spine injury. Place the patient's arms at his or her side (**Step 3**).
4. Once the patient is positioned, maintain an open airway and check for breathing (**Step 4**).

In an unconscious patient, the most common airway obstruction is the patient's tongue, which

## Skill Drill 11-2 Positioning the Unconscious Patient

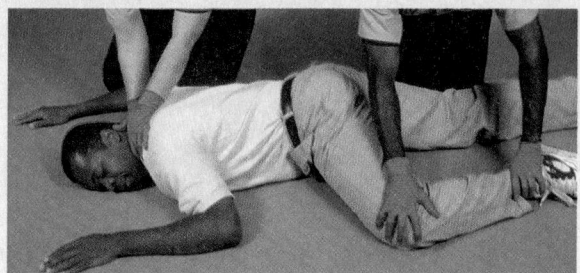

### Step 1

Support the head while your partner straightens the patient's legs.

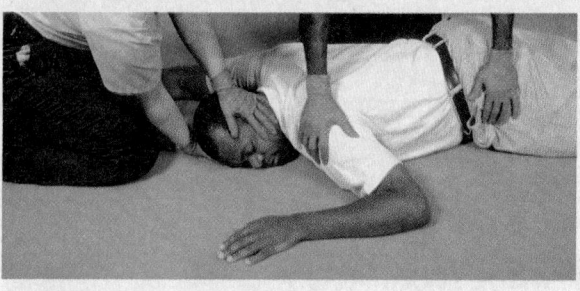

### Step 2

Have your partner place his or her hand on the patient's far shoulder and hip.

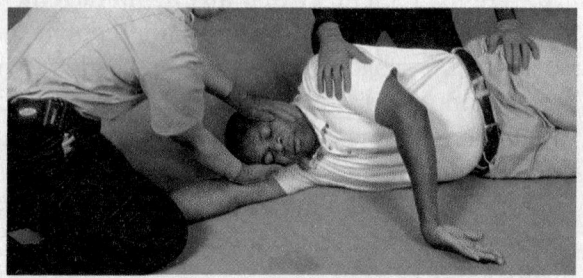

### Step 3

Roll the patient as a unit with the EMT at the patient's head calling the count to begin the move.

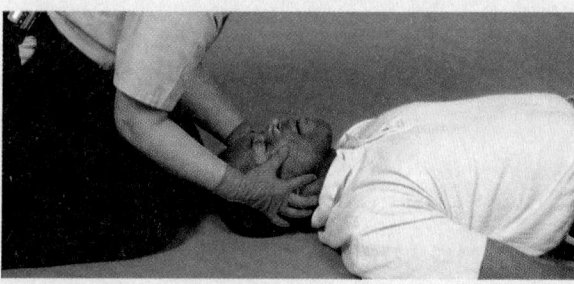

### Step 4

Open and assess the patient's airway and breathing status.

© Jones & Bartlett Learning. Courtesy of MIEMSS.

falls back into the throat when the muscles of the throat and tongue relax (**FIGURE 11-23**). Dentures (false teeth), blood, vomitus, mucus, food, and other foreign objects may also compromise the airway. Therefore, always be prepared to help clear and maintain a patent airway with the use of suction and placement of an airway adjunct, such as an oral or nasal airway.

## Head Tilt–Chin Lift Maneuver

Opening the airway to relieve an obstruction can often be done quickly and easily by simply tilting the patient's head back and lifting the chin in what is known as the **head tilt–chin lift maneuver**.

For patients who have not sustained or are not suspected of having sustained spinal trauma, this simple maneuver is sometimes all that is needed for the patient to resume breathing.

To perform the head tilt–chin lift maneuver, follow these steps:

1. With the patient in a supine position, position yourself beside the patient's head.
2. Place the heel of one hand on the patient's forehead, and apply firm backward pressure with your palm to tilt the patient's head back. This extension of the neck will move the tongue forward, away from the back of the throat, and clear the airway if the tongue is blocking it.

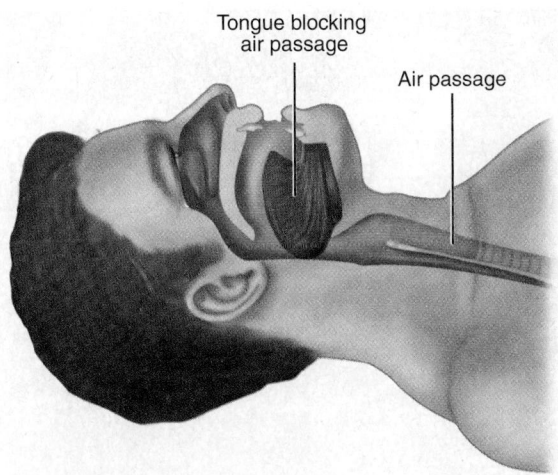

**FIGURE 11-23** The most common airway obstruction is the patient's own tongue, which falls back into the throat when the muscles of the throat and tongue relax.

© Jones & Bartlett Learning.

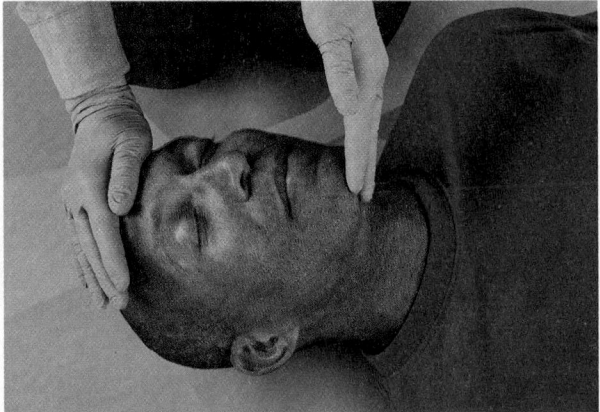

**FIGURE 11-24** The head tilt–chin lift maneuver is a simple technique for opening the airway in a patient without a suspected cervical spine injury.

© Jones & Bartlett Learning.

3. Place the fingertips of your other hand under the lower jaw near the bony part of the chin. Do not compress the soft tissue under the chin, as this may block the airway.

4. Lift the chin upward, bringing the entire lower jaw with it, helping to tilt the head back. Do not use your thumb to lift the chin. Lift so that the teeth are nearly brought together, but avoid closing the mouth completely. Continue to hold the forehead to maintain the backward tilt of the head (**FIGURE 11-24**).

### Words of Wisdom

Causes of airway obstruction include the following:
- Relaxation of the tongue in an unresponsive patient
- Foreign objects (food, small toys, dentures)
- Blood clots, broken teeth, or damaged oral tissue following trauma
- Airway tissue swelling (infection, allergic reaction)
- Aspirated vomitus (stomach contents)

## Jaw-Thrust Maneuver

The head tilt–chin lift maneuver will open the airway in most patients. However, if you suspect a cervical spine injury, use the jaw-thrust maneuver.

The **jaw-thrust maneuver** is a technique to open the airway by placing the fingers behind the angle of the jaw and lifting the jaw upward. You can easily seal a mask around the mouth while doing the jaw-thrust maneuver. Refer to Chapter 29, *Head and Spine Injuries,* for a more detailed discussion of these types of injuries.

Perform the jaw-thrust maneuver in an adult using the following steps (**FIGURE 11-25**):

1. Kneel above the patient's head. Place your fingers behind the angles of the lower jaw, and move the jaw upward. Use your thumbs to help position the lower jaw to allow breathing through the mouth and nose.

2. The completed maneuver should open the airway with the mouth slightly open and the jaw jutting forward.

### Special Populations

Patients with a history of rheumatoid arthritis or Down syndrome are predisposed to instability of the cervical spine, specifically at the first and second cervical vertebrae. The head tilt–chin lift maneuver should be avoided on these patients. Excessive force or hyperextension of the neck can cause partial dislocation of the cervical spine, which can potentially lead to paralysis. It is often better to open the airway of these patients using a jaw-thrust maneuver.

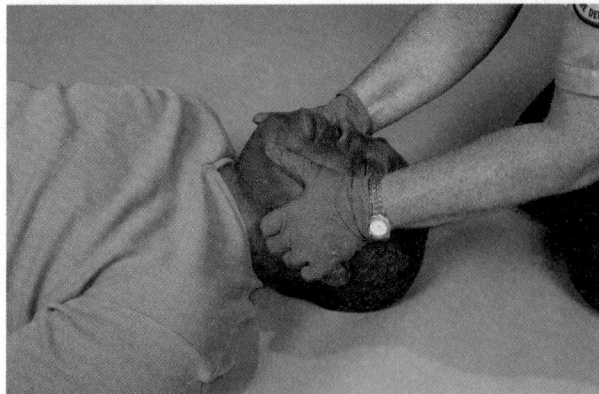

**A**

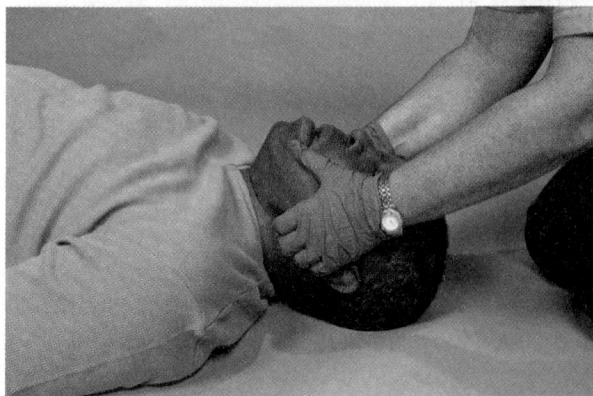

**B**

**FIGURE 11-25** Performing the jaw-thrust maneuver.
**A.** Kneeling above the patient's head, place your fingers behind the angles of the lower jaw, and move the jaw upward. Use your thumbs to help position the lower jaw.
**B.** The completed maneuver should look like this.

A, B: © Jones & Bartlett Learning. Courtesy of MIEMSS.

Patients who have a pulse may start to breathe on their own once the airway has been opened. Assess whether breathing has returned by quickly looking at the chest and observing for obvious movement (**FIGURE 11-26**).

With complete airway obstruction, there will be no movement of air. However, you may see the chest and abdomen rise and fall considerably with the patient's frantic attempts to breathe. This is why the presence of chest wall movement alone does not indicate if adequate breathing is present. Regular chest wall movement indicates a respiratory effort is present. Observing chest and abdominal movement is often difficult with a fully clothed patient. You may see little, if any, chest movement, even with normal breathing. This is particularly true in some patients with chronic

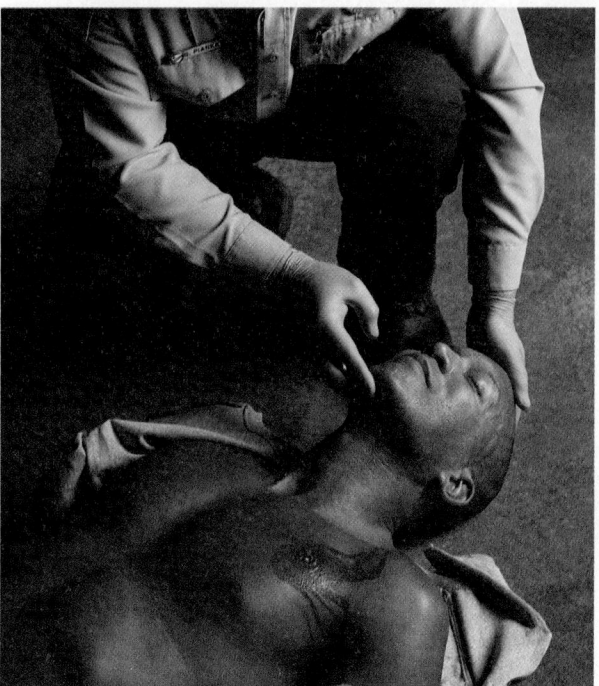

**FIGURE 11-26** Looking at the chest and observing for obvious movement can be used to assess whether breathing has spontaneously returned.

© Jones & Bartlett Learning.

lung disease if you discover that there is no movement of air.

## Opening the Mouth

Even though you may have opened the airway with a head tilt–chin lift or jaw-thrust maneuver, the patient's mouth may still be closed. To open the mouth, place the tips of your index finger and thumb on the patient's teeth. Then, open the mouth by pushing your thumb on the lower teeth and index finger on the upper teeth. This pushing motion will cause the index finger and thumb to cross over each other, which is why this is called the cross-finger technique.

## Suctioning

You must keep the airway clear so that you can ventilate the patient properly. If the airway is not clear, you will force the fluids and secretions into the lungs, resulting in aspiration. If aspiration occurs, mortality increases significantly. Therefore, suctioning is your next priority. If you have any doubt about the situation, remember this rule: If you hear gurgling, the patient needs suctioning!

## Suctioning Equipment

Portable, hand-operated, and fixed (mounted) suctioning equipment is essential for resuscitation (**FIGURE 11-27**).

A portable suctioning unit must provide enough vacuum pressure and flow to allow you to suction the mouth and nose effectively. Hand-operated suctioning units with disposable chambers are reliable, effective, and relatively inexpensive. A fixed suctioning unit should generate a vacuum of more than 300 mm Hg when the tubing is clamped.

A portable or fixed suctioning unit should be fitted with the following:

- Wide-bore, thick-walled, nonkinking tubing
- Plastic, rigid pharyngeal suction tips, called **tonsil tips** (Yankauer tips or DuCanto catheter)
- Nonrigid plastic catheters, called French or whistle-tip catheters
- A nonbreakable, disposable collection bottle
- Water for rinsing the tips

A **suction catheter** is a hollow, cylindrical device that is used to remove fluids from the patient's airway. A tonsil-tip catheter is the best type of catheter for infants and children. The plastic tips have a large diameter and are rigid, so they do not collapse. Another type of suctioning device is designed for routine and emergency airway management (**FIGURE 11-28**).

Tips with a curved contour allow for easy, rapid placement in the oropharynx. Nonrigid plastic catheters, sometimes called French or whistle-tip catheters, are used to suction the nose and thin secretions in the back of the mouth and in situations in which you cannot use a rigid catheter, such as for a patient with a **stoma** (**FIGURE 11-29**). A stoma is an opening through the skin that goes into an organ or other structure.

For example, a rigid catheter could break off a patient's tooth, whereas a flexible catheter may be inserted along the cheeks without injury. Before you insert any catheter, make sure to measure for the proper size. Use the same technique you would use when measuring for an oropharyngeal airway. Be careful not to touch the back of the airway with a suction catheter. This can stimulate the gag reflex, causing vomiting, and increase the possibility of aspiration. Aggressive suctioning can also stimulate the vagus nerve and cause bradycardia, especially in infants and small children.

### Words of Wisdom

Any time there are fluids in the airway, the risk of aspiration increases. Aspiration may increase the risk of mortality by 30% to 70%.

## YOU are the Provider

After suctioning the patient's mouth, you attempt to insert an oropharyngeal airway. However, the patient gags, so instead, you place a nasopharyngeal airway and then begin bag-mask ventilation with high-flow oxygen. Your partner assesses her vital signs.

| Recording Time:  2 Minutes | |
|---|---|
| **Respirations** | 4 breaths/min, labored and shallow (12 breaths assisted) |
| **Pulse** | 130 beats/min, weak |
| **Skin** | Cool and dry; cyanosis to the face and neck |
| **Blood pressure** | 98/64 mm Hg |
| **Oxygen saturation (Spo$_2$)** | 72% (on oxygen) |

**7.** Based on your findings, what adjustments, if any, should be made to the current treatment plan?

**8.** How does negative-pressure ventilation differ from positive-pressure ventilation?

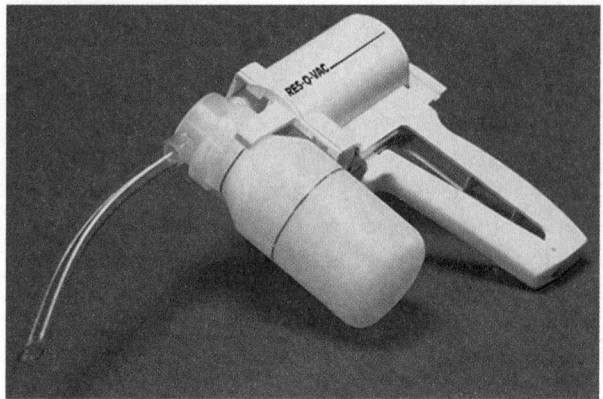

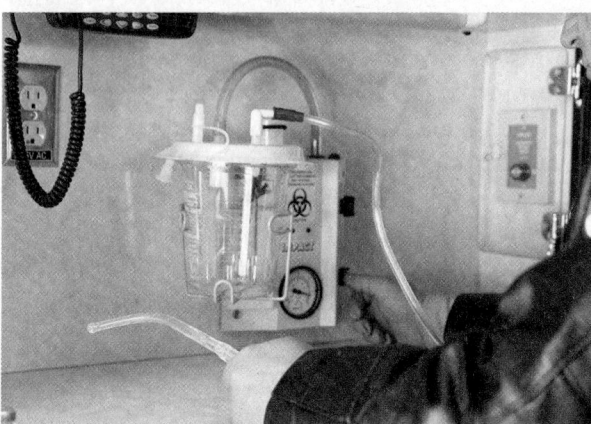

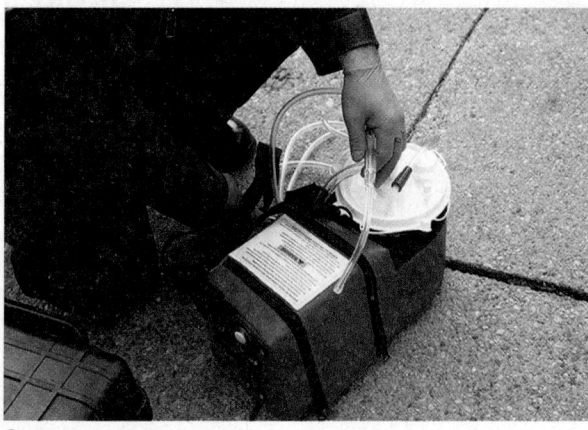

**FIGURE 11-27** Suctioning equipment is essential for resuscitation. **A.** Hand-operated unit. **B.** Fixed unit. **C.** Portable unit.

A, C: © Jones & Bartlett Learning. Courtesy of MIEMSS. **B:** © Jones & Bartlett Learning.

## Techniques of Suctioning

Inspect your suctioning equipment regularly to make sure it is in proper working condition. Turn on the suction, clamp the tubing, and make sure that the unit generates a vacuum of more than 300 mm Hg. Check that a battery-charged unit has charged

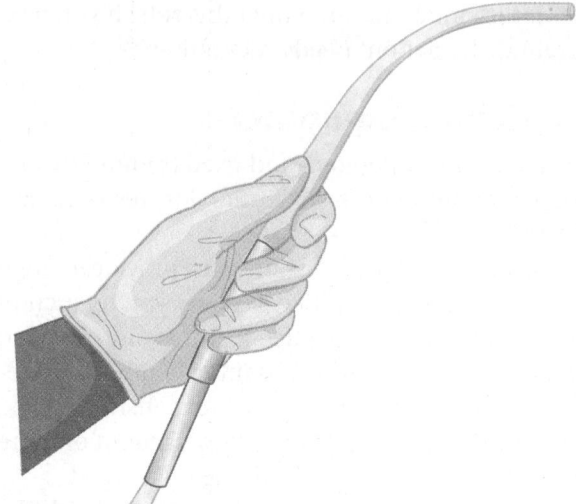

**FIGURE 11-28** A suctioning device used for routine and emergency airway management.

© Jones & Bartlett Learning.

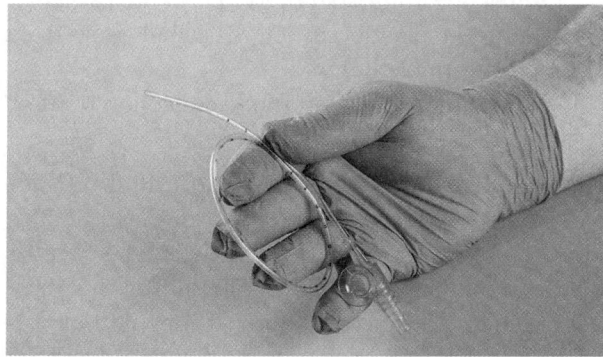

**FIGURE 11-29** French, or whistle-tip, catheters are used in situations in which rigid catheters cannot be used, such as with a patient who has a stoma, patients whose teeth are clenched, or if suctioning the nose is necessary.

© Jones & Bartlett Learning.

batteries. Ensure that your suctioning equipment is placed at the patient's head and is easily accessible. Follow these general steps to operate the suction unit:

1. Check the unit for proper assembly of all its parts.
2. Turn on the suctioning unit and test it to ensure a vacuum pressure of more than 300 mm Hg.
3. Select and attach the appropriate suction catheter to the tubing.

Because mortality increases significantly if a patient aspirates, it is important to suction the airway until it is clear of liquids or other debris. Ventilating a patient whose airway is full of blood, vomitus, or other secretions virtually guarantees aspiration. Repeat suctioning as needed to keep the airway clear, ensuring that the patient remains adequately ventilated and oxygenated. Between suction attempts, rinse the catheter and tubing with water to prevent clogging of the tube with dried vomitus or other secretions.

Use extreme caution when suctioning a conscious or semiconscious patient. Put the tip of the suction catheter in only as far as you can visualize. Be aware that suctioning may induce vomiting.

To properly suction a patient, follow the steps in **SKILL DRILL 11-3**:

1. Turn on the assembled suction unit. To test the suction, clamp the tubing, and make sure that the unit generates a vacuum of more than 300 mm Hg (**Step 1**).
2. Measure the catheter to the correct depth by measuring the catheter from the corner of the

## Skill Drill 11-3 Suctioning a Patient's Airway

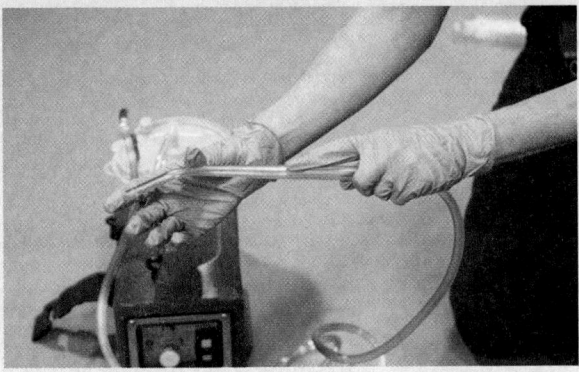

### Step 1

Make sure the suctioning unit is properly assembled and turn it on. Clamp the tubing, and make sure that the unit generates a vacuum of more than 300 mm Hg.

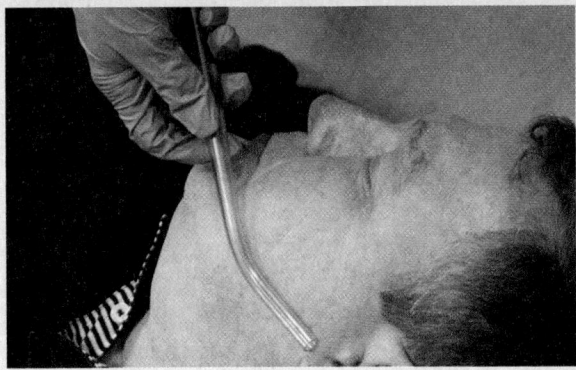

### Step 2

Measure the catheter from the corner of the mouth to the earlobe or angle of the jaw.

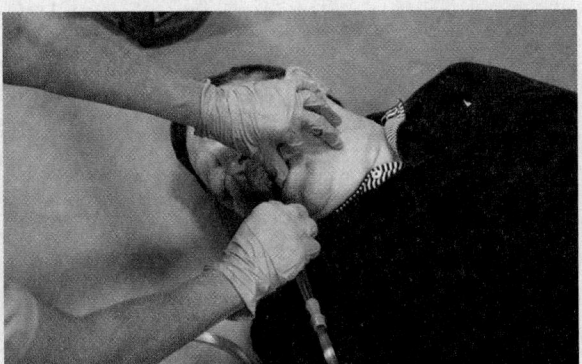

### Step 3

Turn the patient's head to the side (unless you suspect cervical spine injury), open the mouth using the cross-finger technique or tongue-jaw lift, and insert the catheter to the predetermined depth without suctioning.

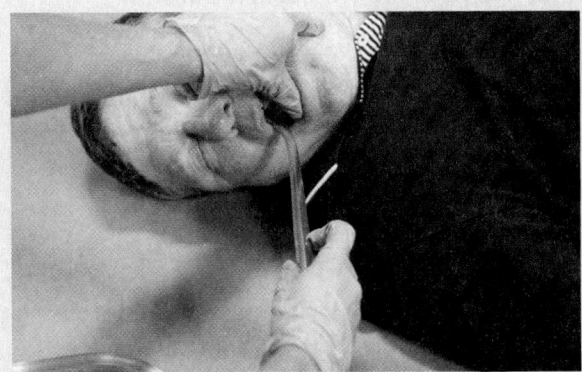

### Step 4

Apply suction in a circular motion as you withdraw the catheter.

patient's mouth to the edge of the earlobe or angle of the jaw (**Step 2**).

3. Before applying suction, turn the patient's head to the side (unless you suspect cervical spine injury). Open the patient's mouth using the cross-finger technique or tongue-jaw lift, and insert the tip of the catheter to the depth measured. Do not suction while inserting the catheter (**Step 3**).

4. Insert the catheter to the premeasured depth and apply suction in a circular motion as you withdraw the catheter (**Step 4**).

At times, a patient may have secretions or vomitus that cannot be suctioned quickly and easily, and some suction units cannot effectively remove solid objects such as teeth, foreign bodies, and food. In these cases, you should remove the catheter from the patient's mouth, log roll the patient to the side, and then clear the mouth carefully with your gloved finger. Only attempt to remove an object if it is visible during examination of the open mouth; blind sweeps of the back of the oropharynx may push an object farther down in the airway, making the obstruction worse. A patient who requires assisted ventilations may also produce frothy secretions as quickly as you can suction them from the airway. In this situation, alternate suctioning with ventilations, ensuring that the airway remains as clear of secretions as possible. Continuous ventilation is not appropriate if vomitus or other particles are present in the airway.

Clean and decontaminate your suctioning equipment after each use according to the manufacturer's guidelines. Place all disposable components (such as catheter, suction tubing) in a biohazard bag.

## Basic Airway Adjuncts

The primary function of an airway adjunct is to prevent obstruction of the upper airway by the tongue and allow the passage of air and oxygen to the lungs.

### Oropharyngeal Airways

An **oropharyngeal (oral) airway** has two principal purposes. The first is to keep the tongue from blocking the upper airway. The second is to make it easier to suction the oropharynx if necessary. Suctioning

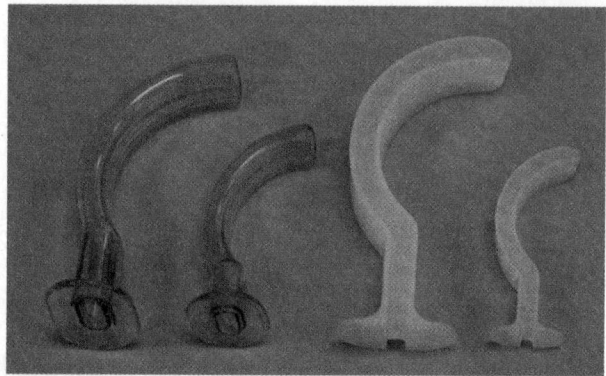

**FIGURE 11-30** An oral airway is used for unconscious patients who have no gag reflex. It keeps the tongue from blocking the airway and makes suctioning the airway easier.

© Jones & Bartlett Learning. Courtesy of MIEMSS.

is possible through an opening down the center or along either side of the oropharyngeal airway (**FIGURE 11-30**).

Indications for the oral airway include the following:

- Unresponsive patients without a gag reflex (breathing or apneic)
- Any apneic patient being ventilated with a bag-mask device

Contraindications for the oral airway include the following:

- Conscious patients
- Any patient (conscious or unconscious) who has an intact gag reflex

The **gag reflex** is a protective reflex mechanism that prevents food and other particles from entering the airway. If you try to insert an oral airway in a patient with an intact gag reflex, the result may be vomiting or a spasm of the vocal cords (laryngospasm). If the patient gags while you are attempting to insert an oral airway, immediately remove the adjunct and prepare to log roll the patient and suction the oropharynx, should vomiting occur. An oral airway is also a safe, effective way to help maintain the airway of a patient with a possible spinal injury. The use of an oral airway may make manual airway maneuvers such as the head tilt–chin lift and the jaw thrust easier to maintain; however, manual maneuvers are often still needed to ensure that the airway remains open.

You must clearly understand when and how this device is used. If the oropharyngeal airway is too large, it could actually push the tongue back into the pharynx, blocking the airway. Conversely, an oral airway that is too small could block the airway directly, just like any foreign body obstruction. The following steps should be used when inserting an oropharyngeal airway (**SKILL DRILL 11-4**):

1. To select the proper size, measure from the patient's earlobe or angle of the jaw to the corner of the mouth (**Step 1**).
2. Open the patient's mouth with the cross-finger technique. Hold the airway upside down with your other hand. Insert the airway with the tip facing the roof of the mouth (**Step 2**).
3. Rotate the airway 180°. When inserted properly, the airway will rest in the mouth with the

curvature of the airway following the contour of the anatomy. The flange should rest against the lips or teeth, with the other end opening into the pharynx (**Step 3**).

### Special Populations

In children, the only acceptable method of inserting an oral airway is to use a tongue blade to hold the tongue down while inserting the airway. Because the airways of children are undeveloped, rotating an oropharyngeal airway in the posterior pharynx may cause damage. For more discussion on pediatric airways, see Chapter 35, *Pediatric Emergencies*.

## Skill Drill 11-4 Inserting an Oral Airway

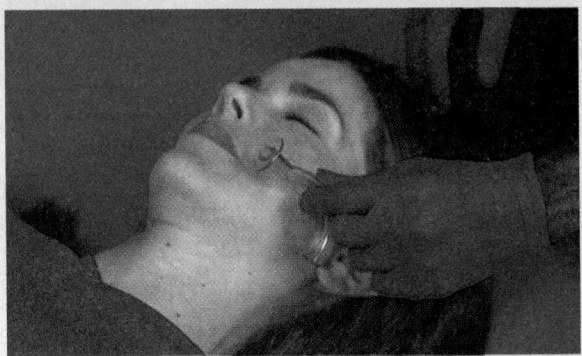

### Step 1

Size the airway by measuring from the patient's earlobe to the corner of the mouth.

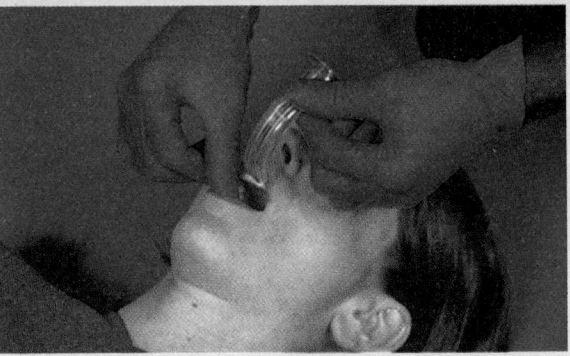

### Step 2

Open the patient's mouth with the cross-finger technique. Hold the airway upside down with your other hand. Insert the airway with the tip facing the roof of the mouth.

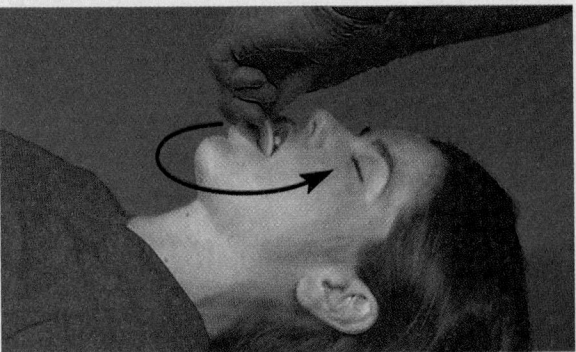

### Step 3

Rotate the airway 180°. Insert the airway until the flange rests on the patient's lips and teeth. In this position, the airway will hold the tongue forward.

Take care to avoid injuring the hard palate (roof of the mouth) as you insert the airway. Roughness can cause bleeding that may aggravate airway problems or even cause vomiting.

If you encounter difficulty while inserting the oral airway, insert the airway with a 90° rotation (**SKILL DRILL 11-5**):

1. Use a tongue depressor or bite stick to depress the tongue, ensuring the tongue remains forward (**Step 1**).
2. Insert the oral airway sideways from the corner of the mouth, until the flange reaches the teeth (**Step 2**).

3. Rotate the oral airway 90°, removing the depressor or bite stick as you exert gentle backward pressure on the oral airway until it rests securely in place against the lips and teeth (**Step 3**).

In some cases, a patient may become responsive and regain the gag reflex after you have inserted an oral airway. If this occurs, gently remove the airway by pulling it out, following the normal curvature of the mouth and throat. Be prepared for the patient to vomit. Have suction available, and log roll the patient onto his or her side and allow any fluids to drain out.

## Skill Drill 11-5 Inserting an Oral Airway With a 90° Rotation

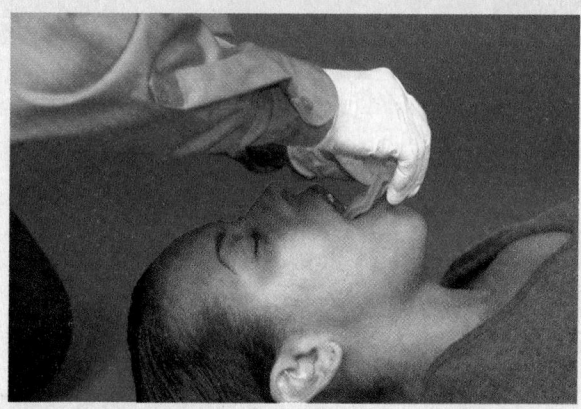

### Step 1

Depress the tongue so that it remains forward.

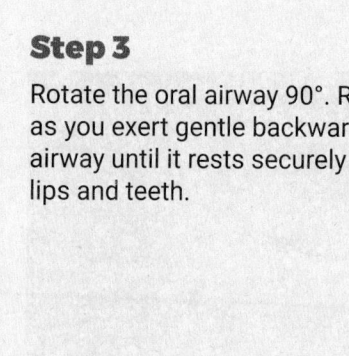

### Step 2

Insert the oral airway sideways from the corner of the mouth, until the flange reaches the teeth.

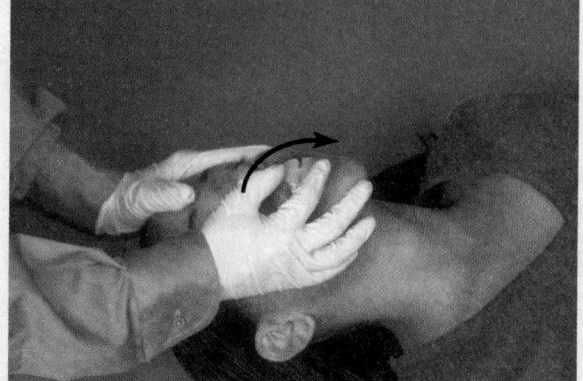

### Step 3

Rotate the oral airway 90°. Remove the bite stick as you exert gentle backward pressure on the oral airway until it rests securely in place against the lips and teeth.

## Nasopharyngeal Airways

A **nasopharyngeal (nasal) airway** is usually used with an unresponsive patient or a patient with an altered level of consciousness who has an intact gag reflex and is not able to maintain his or her airway spontaneously (**FIGURE 11-31**).

Patients with an altered mental status or who have just had a seizure may also benefit from this type of airway. If a patient has sustained severe trauma to the head or face, use extreme caution when inserting a nasopharyngeal airway. If the nasal airway is accidentally pushed through a hole caused by a fracture of the base of the skull, it may enter the cranial vault. Although this is rare, it is possible.

This type of airway is usually better tolerated than an oropharyngeal airway by patients who have an intact gag reflex. It is not as likely to cause vomiting. Coat the airway well with a water-soluble lubricant before inserting it. Be aware that slight bleeding may occur even when the airway is inserted properly. However, never force the airway into place.

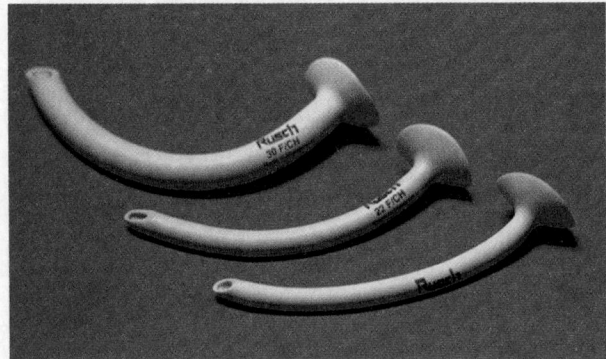

**FIGURE 11-31** A nasal airway is better tolerated than an oral airway by patients who have an intact gag reflex.

© Jones & Bartlett Learning. Courtesy of MIEMSS.

Indications for the nasopharyngeal airway include the following:

- Semiconscious or unconscious patients with an intact gag reflex
- Patients who otherwise will not tolerate an oropharyngeal airway

Contraindications for the nasopharyngeal airway include the following:

- Severe head injury with blood draining from the nose
- History of fractured nasal bone

Follow these steps to ensure correct placement of the nasopharyngeal airway (**SKILL DRILL 11-6**):

1. Before inserting the airway, be sure you have selected the proper size. Measure from the tip of the patient's nose to the earlobe. In almost all patients, one nostril is larger than the other (**Step 1**).
2. The airway should be placed in the larger nostril, with the curvature of the device following the curve of the floor of the nose. If using the right nare, the bevel should face the septum (**Step 2**). If using the left nare, insert the airway with the tip of the airway pointing upward, which will allow the bevel to face the septum.
3. Advance the airway gently (**Step 3**). If using the left nare, insert the nasal airway until resistance is met. Then rotate the nasal airway 180° into position. This rotation is not required if using the right nostril.
4. When completely inserted, the flange rests against the nostril. The other end of the airway opens into the posterior pharynx (**Step 4**). If the patient becomes intolerant of the nasal airway, you may have to remove it. Gently withdraw the airway from the nasal passage. Precautions similar to those used when removing an oral airway should be followed.

## Maintaining the Airway

The **recovery position** is used to help maintain a clear airway in an unconscious patient who is not injured and is breathing on his or her own with a normal respiratory rate and adequate tidal volume (depth of breathing) (**FIGURE 11-32**).

## Skill Drill 11-6 Inserting a Nasal Airway

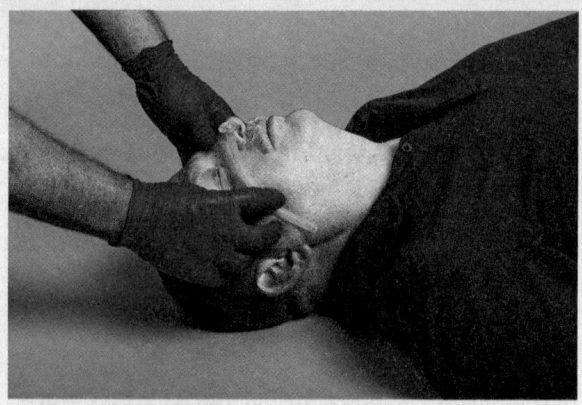

### Step 1

Size the airway by measuring from the tip of the nose to the patient's earlobe. Coat the tip with a water-soluble lubricant.

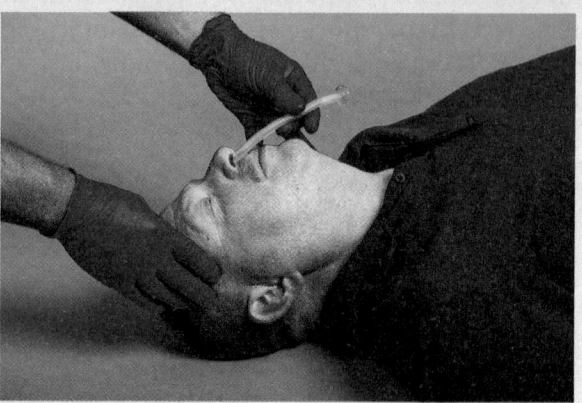

### Step 2

Insert the lubricated airway into the larger nostril with the curvature following the floor of the nose. If using the right nare, the bevel should face the septum. If using the left nare, insert the airway with the tip of the airway pointing upward, which will allow the bevel to face the septum.

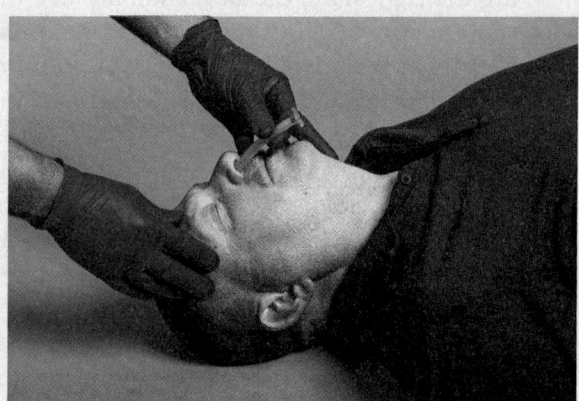

### Step 3

Gently advance the airway. If using the left nare, insert the nasopharyngeal airway until resistance is met. Then rotate the nasopharyngeal airway 180° into position. This rotation is not required if using the right nostril.

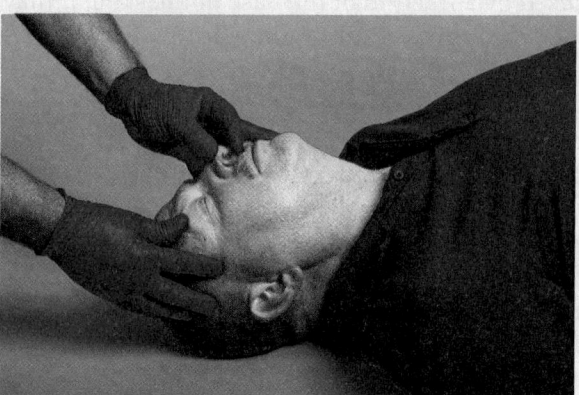

### Step 4

Continue until the flange rests against the nostril. If you feel any resistance or obstruction, remove the airway and insert it into the other nostril.

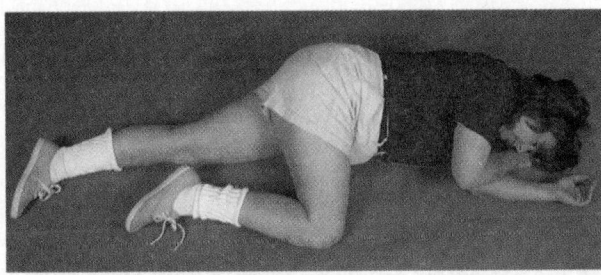

**FIGURE 11-32** In the recovery position, the patient is rolled onto his or her left or right side.

© Jones & Bartlett Learning. Courtesy of MIEMSS.

Take the following steps to put the patient in the recovery position:

1. Roll the patient onto either side so that the head, shoulders, and torso move at the same time without twisting.
2. Extend the patient's lower arm and place the upper hand under his or her cheek.

For patients who have resumed spontaneous breathing after being resuscitated, the recovery position will prevent the aspiration of vomitus. However, this position is not appropriate for patients with suspected spinal, hip, or pelvic injuries or for patients who are unconscious and require ventilatory assistance. Reposition such patients to provide adequate access to the airway while maintaining appropriate spinal stabilization.

## Supplemental Oxygen

Always give supplemental oxygen to patients who are hypoxic because not enough oxygen is being supplied to the tissues and cells of the body. Some tissues and organs, such as the heart, central nervous system, lungs, kidneys, and liver, need a constant supply of oxygen to function normally. *Never withhold oxygen from any patient who might benefit from it, especially if you must assist ventilations.* When ventilating any patient in cardiac or respiratory arrest, use high-concentration supplemental oxygen.

## Supplemental Oxygen Equipment

In addition to knowing when and how to give supplemental oxygen, you must understand how oxygen is stored and the various hazards associated with its use.

## Oxygen Cylinders

The oxygen that you will give to patients is usually supplied as a compressed gas in green, seamless, steel or aluminum cylinders. Some cylinders may be silver or chrome with a green area around the valve stem on top. Newer cylinders are often made of lightweight aluminum or spun steel; older cylinders are much heavier.

Check to make sure that the cylinder is labeled for medical oxygen. Look for letters and numbers stamped into the metal on the collar of the cylinder (**FIGURE 11-33**). The month and year stamps are particularly important because they indicate when the cylinder was last tested. Generally, aluminum cylinders are tested every 5 years; composite cylinders are tested every 3 years.

Oxygen cylinders are available in several sizes. The two sizes that you will most often use are the D (or jumbo D) and M cylinders (**FIGURE 11-34**). The D (or jumbo D) cylinder can be carried from your unit to the patient. The M tank remains on board your unit as a main supply tank. Other sizes that you will see are A, E, G, H, and K (**TABLE 11-4**). Another naming system for identifying the size of the oxygen cylinder has been introduced. Per this naming convention, cylinders are labeled with M (for medical), followed by a number.

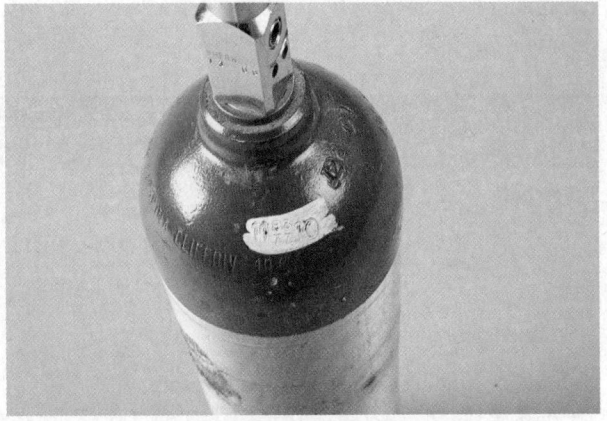

**FIGURE 11-33** Oxygen tanks for medical use have a series of letters and numbers stamped into the metal on the collar of the cylinder.

© Jones & Bartlett Learning.

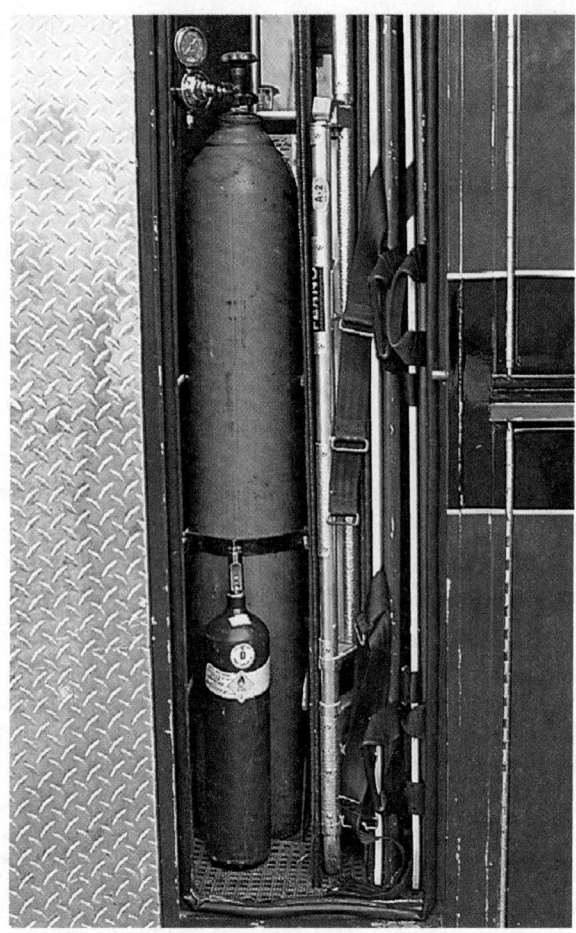

**FIGURE 11-34** The cylinders that are most commonly found on an ambulance are the D (or jumbo D) and M size cylinders. D, jumbo D, and E sizes are typically portable tank systems while the M, G, H, A, and K sizes are mounted inside the ambulance.

© Jones & Bartlett Learning. Courtesy of MIEMSS.

The length of time you can use an oxygen cylinder depends on the pressure in the cylinder and the flow rate. A method of calculating cylinder duration is shown in **TABLE 11-5**.

### Words of Wisdom

Some patients require oxygen continually. Many of these patients have liquid oxygen at home.

Liquid oxygen containers hold a large volume of oxygen and do not need to be filled as often. Liquid oxygen tanks generally need to be kept upright and have special requirements for filling, large-volume storage, and cylinder transfer.

**TABLE 11-4** Oxygen Cylinder Sizes Carried on the Ambulance

| Size | Volume, Liters |
| --- | --- |
| D | 350 |
| Jumbo D | 500 |
| E | 625 |
| M (MM) | 3,000 |
| G | 5,300 |
| H, A (M4), K | 6,900 |

© Jones & Bartlett Learning.

**TABLE 11-5** Oxygen Cylinders: Duration of Flow

**Formula**

$$\frac{(\text{Guage pressure in psi} - \text{Safe residual pressure}) \times \text{Cylinder constant}}{\text{Flow rate in L/min}} \times \text{Duration of flow in minutes}$$

Safe residual pressure = 200 psi

Cylinder constant for a given cylinder size:
A = 3.14   G = 2.41   D = 0.16   H = 3.14   E = 0.28   K = 3.14   M = 1.56

Determine the life of an M cylinder that has a pressure of 2,000 psi and a flow rate of 10 L/min.

$$\frac{(2{,}000 - 200) \times 1.56}{10} = \frac{2{,}808}{10} = 281 \text{ min, or 4 h 41 min}$$

psi = pounds per square inch.

© Jones & Bartlett Learning.

## Safety Considerations

Handle compressed gas cylinders carefully because their contents are under pressure. Cylinders are fitted with pressure regulators to make sure that patients receive the right amount and type of gas. Make sure that the correct pressure regulator is firmly attached before you transport the cylinders. A puncture or hole in the tank can cause the cylinder to become a deadly missile. Do not handle a cylinder by the neck assembly alone. Secure cylinders with mounting brackets when they are stored on the ambulance. Oxygen cylinders that are in use during transport should be positioned and secured to prevent the tank from falling, damaging the valve-gauge assembly, or becoming a dangerous projectile during a collision.

## Pin-Indexing System

The compressed gas industry has established a **pin-indexing system** for portable cylinders to prevent an oxygen regulator from being connected to a carbon dioxide cylinder, a carbon dioxide regulator from being connected to an oxygen cylinder, and so on. In preparing to administer oxygen, always check to be sure that the pinholes on the cylinder *exactly* match the corresponding pins on the regulator.

The pin-indexing system features a series of pins on a yoke that must be matched with the holes on the valve stem of the gas cylinder. The arrangement of the pins and holes varies for different gases according to accepted national standards (**FIGURE 11-35**). Other gases that are supplied in portable cylinders, such as acetylene, carbon dioxide, and nitrogen, use regulators and flowmeters that are similar to those used with oxygen. Each cylinder of a specific gas type has a given pattern and a given number of pins. These safety measures make it impossible for you to attach a cylinder of nitrous oxide to an oxygen regulator. The oxygen regulator will not fit.

The outlet valves on portable oxygen cylinders are designed to accept yoke-type pressure-reducing gauges, which conform to the pin-indexing system (**FIGURE 11-36**).

The safety system for the large cylinders is known as the **American Standard Safety System**. In this system, oxygen cylinders are equipped with threaded gas outlet valves. The inside and outside thread sizes of these outlets vary depending on the

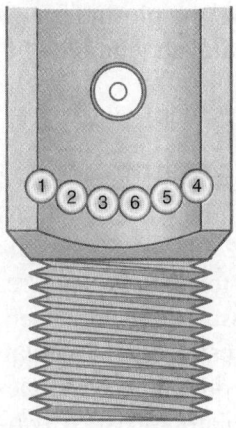

**FIGURE 11-35** The locations of the pin-indexing safety system holes in a cylinder valve face. Each cylinder of a specific gas has a given pattern and a given number of pins.

© Jones & Bartlett Learning.

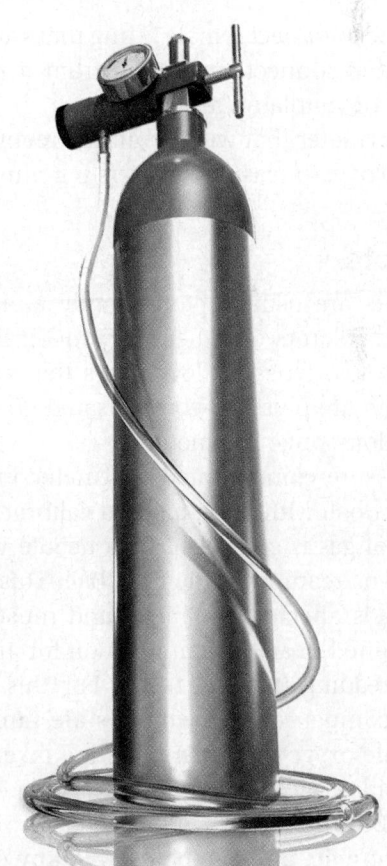

**FIGURE 11-36** A yoke-type pressure-reducing gauge is used with a portable oxygen cylinder.

© dream designs/ShutterStock.

gas in the cylinder. The cylinder will not accept a regulator valve unless it is properly threaded to fit that regulator. The purpose of these safety devices is the same as in the pin-indexing system—to prevent the accidental attachment of a regulator to the wrong cylinder.

## Pressure Regulators

The pressure of the gas in a full oxygen cylinder is approximately 2,000 psi. This is far too much pressure to be safe for patient use. Pressure regulators reduce the pressure to a more useful range, usually 40 to 70 psi. Most pressure regulators currently in use reduce the pressure in a single stage, although multistage regulators exist. A two-stage regulator will reduce the pressure first to 700 psi and then to 40 to 70 psi.

After the pressure is reduced to a workable level, the final attachment for delivering the gas to the patient is usually one of the following:

- A quick-connect female fitting that will accept a quick-connect male plug from a pressure hose or ventilator/resuscitator
- A flowmeter that will permit the regulated release of gas measured in liters per minute

## Flowmeters

Flowmeters are usually permanently attached to pressure regulators on emergency medical equipment. The two types of flowmeters that are commonly used are pressure-compensated flowmeters and Bourdon-gauge flowmeters.

A pressure-compensated flowmeter incorporates a float ball within the tapered calibrated tube. The flow of gas is controlled by a needle valve located downstream from the float ball. This type of flowmeter is affected by gravity and must always be maintained in an upright position for an accurate flow reading (**FIGURE 11-37**). For this reason, pressure-compensated flowmeters are rarely used on portable oxygen cylinders that are taken to the patient's side.

The Bourdon-gauge flowmeter is not affected by gravity and can be used in any position (**FIGURE 11-38**). It is a pressure gauge that is calibrated to record flow rate. This type of flowmeter, however, is now generally considered outdated. Newer flowmeters incorporate a fixable setting with either a dial or a knob that sets the flow. With these regulators, a Bourdon gauge is not necessary.

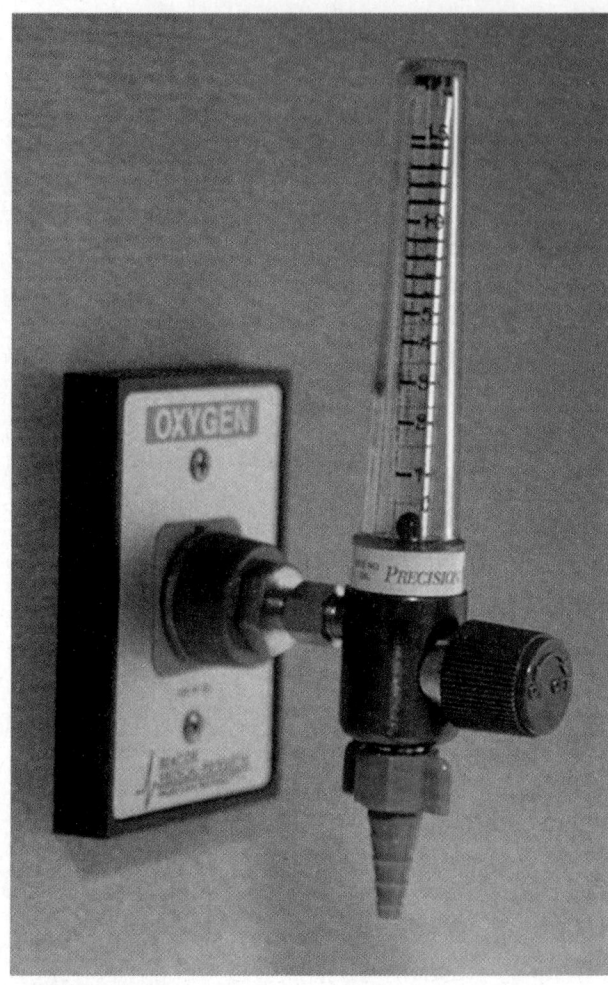

**FIGURE 11-37** A pressure-compensated flowmeter contains a float ball that rises or falls according to the gas flow within the tube. It must be maintained in an upright position for an accurate reading.

© Jones & Bartlett Learning.

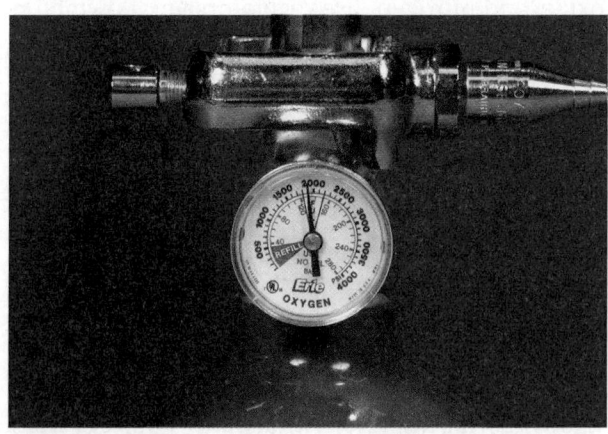

**FIGURE 11-38** The Bourdon-gauge flowmeter is not affected by gravity and can be used in any position.

© Jones & Bartlett Learning.

## Procedures for Operating and Administering Oxygen

To place an oxygen cylinder into service and administer medical oxygen to a patient, follow the steps in **SKILL DRILL 11-7**:

1. Inspect the cylinder and its markings. If the cylinder was commercially filled, it will have a plastic seal around the valve stem covering the opening in the stem. Remove the seal, and inspect the opening to make sure that it is free of dirt and other debris. The valve stem should not be sealed or covered with adhesive tape or any petroleum-based substances. These can contaminate the oxygen and can contribute to combustion when mixed with pressurized oxygen.

## Skill Drill 11-7 Placing an Oxygen Cylinder Into Service

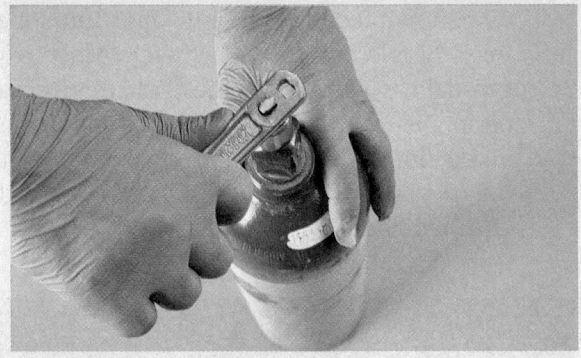

**Step 1**

Using an oxygen wrench, turn the valve counterclockwise to slowly "crack" the cylinder. Genty retighten the valve to stop the oxygen flow to allow the regulator to be attached.

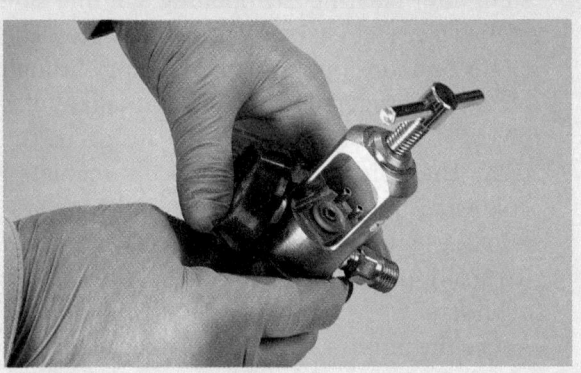

**Step 2**

Attach the regulator/flowmeter to the valve stem using the two pin-indexing holes and make sure that the washer is in place over the larger hole.

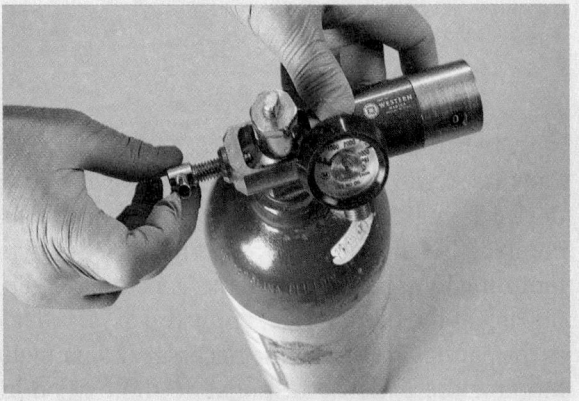

**Step 3**

Align the regulator so that the pins fit snugly into the correct holes on the valve stem, and hand tighten the regulator.

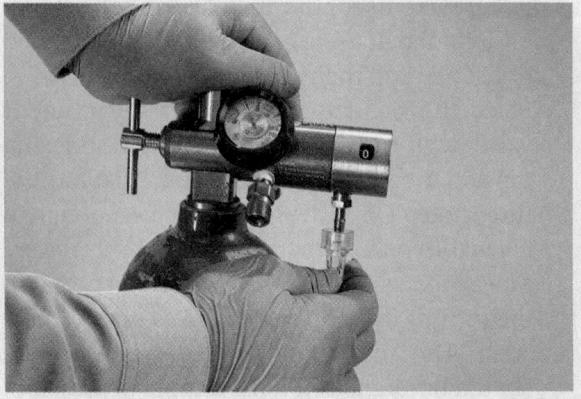

**Step 4**

Attach the oxygen connective tubing to the flowmeter. Use the wrench to fully open the tank.

2. "Crack" the cylinder by slowly opening and then reclosing the valve to help make sure that dirt particles and other possible contaminants do not enter the oxygen flow. Never face the tank toward yourself or others when cracking the cylinder. Open the tank by attaching a tank key (wrench) to the valve and rotating the valve counterclockwise. You should be able to clearly hear the rush of oxygen coming from the tank. Close the tank by rotating the valve clockwise (**Step 1**).

3. Attach the regulator/flowmeter to the valve stem after clearing the opening. On one side of the valve stem, you will find three holes. The larger one, on top, is a true opening through which the oxygen flows. The two smaller holes below it do not extend to the inside of the tank. They provide stability to the regulator. Following the design of the pin-indexing system, these two holes are very precisely located in positions that are unique to the oxygen cylinders.

4. Above the pins on the inside of the collar is the actual port through which oxygen flows from the cylinder to the regulator. A metal-bound elastomeric sealing washer (also called a gasket) is placed around the oxygen port to optimize the airtight seal between the collar of the regulator and the valve stem (**Step 2**). In the past, crush gaskets made of plastic and nylon were used, but they are no longer recommended. If used, crush gaskets can be used only once and then they must be replaced.

5. Place the regulator collar over the cylinder valve, with the oxygen port and pin-indexing pins on the side of the valve stem that has the three holes. Open the screw bolt just enough to allow the collar to fit freely over the valve stem. Move the regulator so that the oxygen port and the pins fit into the correct holes on the valve stem. The screw bolt on the opposite side should be aligned with the dimple depression. As you hold the regulator securely against the valve stem, hand tighten the screw bolt until the regulator is firmly attached to the cylinder. At this point, you should not see any open spaces between the sides of the valve stem and the interior walls of the collar (**Step 3**).

6. With the regulator firmly attached, open the cylinder completely, check for air leaking from the regulator–oxygen cylinder connection, and read the pressure level on the regulator gauge. Most portable cylinders have a maximum pressure of approximately 2,000 psi. Most EMS systems consider a cylinder with less than 500 to 1,000 psi to be too low to keep in service. Learn your department's policies in this regard and follow them.

7. The flowmeter will have a second gauge or a selector dial that indicates the oxygen flow rate. Several popular types of devices are widely used. Attach the selected oxygen device to the flowmeter by connecting the universal oxygen connecting tubing to the "Christmas tree" nipple on the flowmeter. Most oxygen-delivery devices come with this tubing permanently attached; however, some oxygen masks do not. You must attach this tubing to the oxygen-delivery device if it is not already attached (**Step 4**).

## Safety Tips

Slowly open the oxygen tank after attaching the regulator and check for leaks. Remember that although oxygen itself is not combustible, it supports combustion, and any ignition source may cause fire or an explosion in an oxygen-rich environment—especially if oxygen is being released too quickly from the cylinder at the time or if the seal between the regulator and oxygen cylinder is not secure.

Open the flowmeter to the desired flow rate. Flow rates will vary based on the oxygen-delivery device being used. Remember that you must be completely familiar with the equipment before attempting to use it on a patient. Once the oxygen is flowing at the desired rate, apply the oxygen device to the patient and make any necessary adjustments. Monitor the patient's response to the oxygen and to the oxygen device, and periodically recheck the regulator gauge to make sure there is sufficient oxygen in the cylinder. Disconnect the tubing from the flowmeter nipple and turn off the cylinder valve when oxygen therapy is complete or when the patient has been transferred to the hospital and is using the hospital's oxygen system. In a few seconds, the sound of oxygen flowing from the nipple will cease. This indicates that all the pressurized oxygen has been removed from the flowmeter. Turn off the flowmeter. The gauge on the regulator should read zero with the tank valve closed. This reading confirms that there is no pressure left above the valve stem. As long as there is a pressure reading on the regulator gauge, it is not safe to remove the regulator from the valve stem.

## Hazards of Supplemental Oxygen

### Combustion

Oxygen does not burn or explode. However, it does support combustion. The more oxygen present, the faster the combustion process. A small spark, even a glowing cigarette, can become a flame in an oxygen-rich atmosphere. Therefore, you must keep any possible source of fire away from the area while oxygen is in use. Make sure the area is adequately ventilated, especially in industrial settings where hazardous materials may be present and where sparks are easily generated. Be extremely cautious in any enclosed environment in which oxygen is being administered, as an oxygen-rich environment increases the chance of fire if a spark or flame is introduced. A bystander who is smoking or sparks generated during vehicle extrication are possible sources of ignition. Never leave an oxygen cylinder standing unattended. The cylinder can be knocked over, injuring the patient or damaging the equipment.

### Oxygen Toxicity

The administration of oxygen to patients is a common practice. Although many patients in the prehospital environment require high concentrations of oxygen, not all patients do. Excessive supplemental oxygen can have a detrimental effect on patients with certain illnesses (ie, COPD, cerebral vascular accidents, and myocardial infarction).

Recent research has shown that although the administration of oxygen benefits many patients and is rarely problematic, high concentrations of oxygen are potentially harmful for a select population. Oxygen toxicity refers to damage to cellular tissue due to excessive oxygen levels in the blood. Years ago, high concentrations of oxygen were thought to benefit all patients in the prehospital environment. However, current evidence suggests that increased cellular oxygen levels contribute to the production of oxygen free radicals. These free

radicals may lead to tissue damage and cellular death in some patients.

The International Liaison Committee on Resuscitation guidelines published by the American Heart Association recognize there may be negative effects of oxygen toxicity and recommend that oxygen be administered to patients experiencing signs of a myocardial infarction when they have signs of heart failure, are short of breath, or have a room air oxygen saturation less than 94%. In addition, patients experiencing signs of shock should be placed on oxygen. Understand that hypoxemia is immediately life-threatening, whereas oxygen toxicity is not; when in doubt, or if unable to measure oxygen saturation reliably, supplemental oxygen should be administered.

Pulse oximetry is not always available to the EMT. When pulse oximetry is available, tailor oxygen therapy to the patient's needs, and administer the minimum amount of oxygen necessary to maintain oxygen saturation at or above 94%. Exceptions to these minimums include patients who have been exposed to carbon monoxide, patients with potential anemia, or patients with shock.

## Oxygen-Delivery Equipment

In general, the oxygen delivery equipment used in the field should be limited to nonrebreathing masks, bag-mask devices, and nasal cannulas, depending on local protocol. However, you may encounter other devices during transports between medical facilities.

### Words of Wisdom

#### Oxygen-Delivery Devices

| Device | Flow Rate | Oxygen Delivered |
|---|---|---|
| Nasal cannula | 1 to 6 L/min | 24% to 44% |
| Nonrebreathing mask with reservoir | 10 to 15 L/min | Up to 90% |
| Bag-mask device with reservoir | 15 L/min | Nearly 100% |

## Nonrebreathing Masks

The nonrebreathing mask is used to administer high concentrations of oxygen to significantly hypoxemic patients who are otherwise breathing adequately. With a good mask-to-face seal and a flow rate of 15 L/min, the nonrebreathing mask is capable of providing up to 90% inspired oxygen.

The nonrebreathing mask is a combination mask and reservoir bag system. Oxygen fills a reservoir bag that is attached to the mask by a one-way valve. The system is called a nonrebreathing mask because the exhaled gas escapes through flapper valve ports at the cheek areas of the mask (**FIGURE 11-39**). These valves prevent the patient from rebreathing exhaled gases, namely carbon dioxide.

When using this system, you must be sure that the reservoir bag is full before the mask is placed on the patient. Adjust the flow rate so that the bag does not fully collapse when the patient inhales, to about two-thirds of the bag volume, or 10 to 15 L/min. Make sure the bag stays inflated. Should the bag collapse when the patient inhales, increase the flow rate of oxygen. In addition, if oxygen therapy is discontinued, remove the mask from the patient's face. Leaving the mask in place while oxygen is not flowing allows the patient to rebreathe exhaled carbon dioxide. Use a pediatric nonrebreathing mask, which has a smaller reservoir bag, with infants and children, as they will inhale a smaller volume.

## Nasal Cannulas

A nasal cannula delivers oxygen through two small, tubelike prongs that fit into the patient's nostrils (**FIGURE 11-40**). This device can provide 24% to 44% inspired oxygen when the flowmeter is set at 1 to 6 L/min. For the comfort of your patient, flow rates above 6 L/min are not recommended with the nasal cannula. Typically, the nasal cannula is used in patients with mild hypoxemia.

The nasal cannula delivers dry oxygen directly into the nostrils, which, over prolonged periods, can cause dryness or irritate the mucous membrane lining of the nose. Therefore, when you anticipate a long transport time, consider the use of humidification. Remember that humidification may be associated with an increased generation of aerosolized droplets of fluid that may increase the degree to which the patient can transmit disease to other people in the same ambulance compartment. This fact is particularly relevant during pandemics of diseases that are transmitted through respiratory droplets.

The nasal cannula does have some limitations. For example, a patient who breathes through the mouth or who has a nasal obstruction will likely get little or no benefit from a nasal cannula. Use a nonrebreathing mask if the patient is significantly hypoxemic, coaching the patient if necessary. If the patient will not tolerate a nonrebreathing mask, you will have to use a nasal cannula, which some patients find more comfortable. As always, a good assessment of your patient will guide your decision.

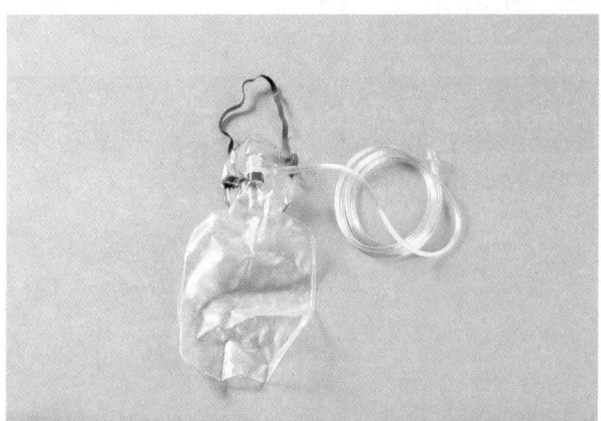

**FIGURE 11-39** The nonrebreathing mask contains flapper valve ports at the cheek areas of the mask to prevent the patient from rebreathing exhaled gases.

© Jones & Bartlett Learning

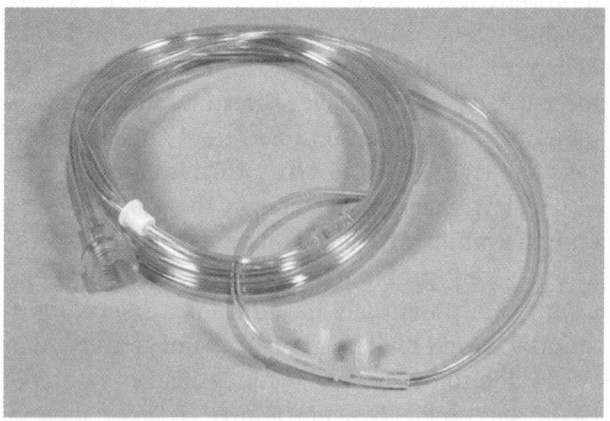

**FIGURE 11-40** The nasal cannula delivers oxygen directly through the nostrils.

© Jones & Bartlett Learning. Courtesy of MIEMSS.

## Partial Rebreathing Masks

The partial rebreathing mask is similar to a nonrebreathing mask except that there is no one-way valve between the mask and the reservoir. Consequently, patients rebreathe a small amount of their exhaled air. This has some benefit when you want to increase the patient's $Paco_2$, which makes this the ideal mask for patients whom you think are experiencing hyperventilation syndrome. The oxygen enriches the air mixture and delivers a gas mix of approximately 80% to 90% oxygen. You can easily convert a nonrebreathing mask to a partial rebreathing mask by removing the one-way valve between the mask and the reservoir bag.

## Venturi Masks

A Venturi mask has a number of attachments that enable you to vary the percentage of oxygen delivered to the patient while a constant flow is maintained from the regulator (**FIGURE 11-41**). This is accomplished by the Venturi principle, which causes air to be drawn into the flow of oxygen as it passes a hole in the line. The Venturi mask is a medium-flow device that delivers 24% to 40% oxygen, depending on the manufacturer.

The main advantage of the Venturi mask is the use of its fine adjustment capabilities in the

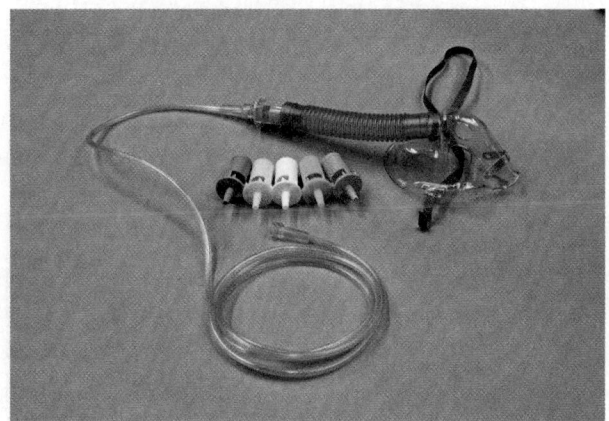

**FIGURE 11-41** The Venturi mask.
© Jones & Bartlett Learning. Courtesy of MIEMSS.

long-term management of physiologically stable patients. However, in the emergency setting, such fine adjustments are not necessary. When you need to adjust the oxygen concentration in an emergency, it is typically done by adjusting the flow rate or changing the delivery device.

## Tracheostomy Masks

Patients with tracheostomies do not breathe through their mouth and nose. A face mask or nasal cannula therefore cannot be used to treat them.

## YOU are the Provider

A fire engine company arrives at the scene to assist you and your partner. You are unable to find any underlying problems that would explain the patient's current condition. During reassessment, you note a change in her clinical status and tell the firefighter to slow his rate of ventilation. Dispatch advises there is no ALS unit available so you ask the officer on the engine to have someone prepare the ambulance stretcher for transport.

**Recording Time: 6 Minutes**

| | |
|---|---|
| Level of consciousness | Unresponsive |
| Respirations | 4 breaths/min (baseline); 12 breaths/min (assisted) |
| Pulse | 148 beats/min, weak |
| Skin | Cool and dry; cyanotic |
| Blood pressure | 86/54 mm Hg |
| $Spo_2$ | 70% (with oxygen and assisted ventilation) |

**9.** How can positive-pressure ventilation affect cardiac output?

**10.** Based on the patient's deteriorating clinical status, what corrective action should be taken?

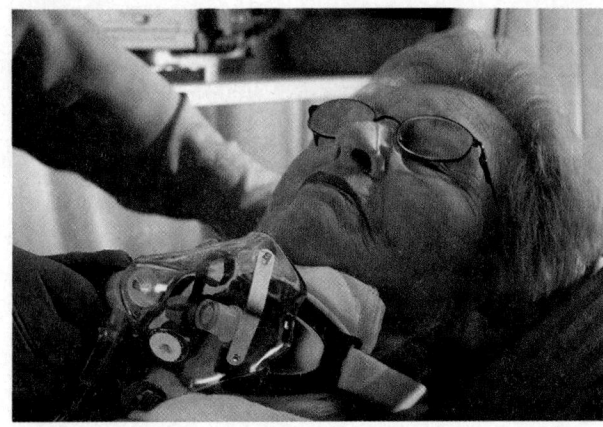

**FIGURE 11-42** For a patient with a tracheostomy, if you do not have a tracheostomy mask, use a face mask instead.

© Jones & Bartlett Learning.

Masks designed specifically for these patients cover the tracheostomy hole and have a strap that goes around the neck. These masks are usually available in intensive care units, where many patients have tracheostomies, and may not be available in an emergency setting. If you do not have a tracheostomy mask, you can improvise by placing a face mask over the stoma. Even though the mask is shaped to fit the face, you can usually get an adequate fit over the patient's neck by adjusting the strap (**FIGURE 11-42**).

## Humidification

Some EMS systems provide humidified oxygen to patients during extended transport or for certain conditions such as croup (**FIGURE 11-43**). However, humidified oxygen is usually indicated only for long-term oxygen therapy. Dry oxygen is not considered harmful for short-term use. An oxygen humidifier consists of a small single-patient-use bottle of sterile water through which the oxygen leaving the cylinder becomes moisturized before it reaches the patient. Because the humidifier must be kept in an upright position, however, it is practical only for the fixed oxygen unit in the ambulance.

## Assisted and Artificial Ventilation

A patient who is not breathing needs artificial ventilation and 100% supplemental oxygen. Assisted ventilation and artificial ventilation are critical skills for any EMS provider—regardless of certification

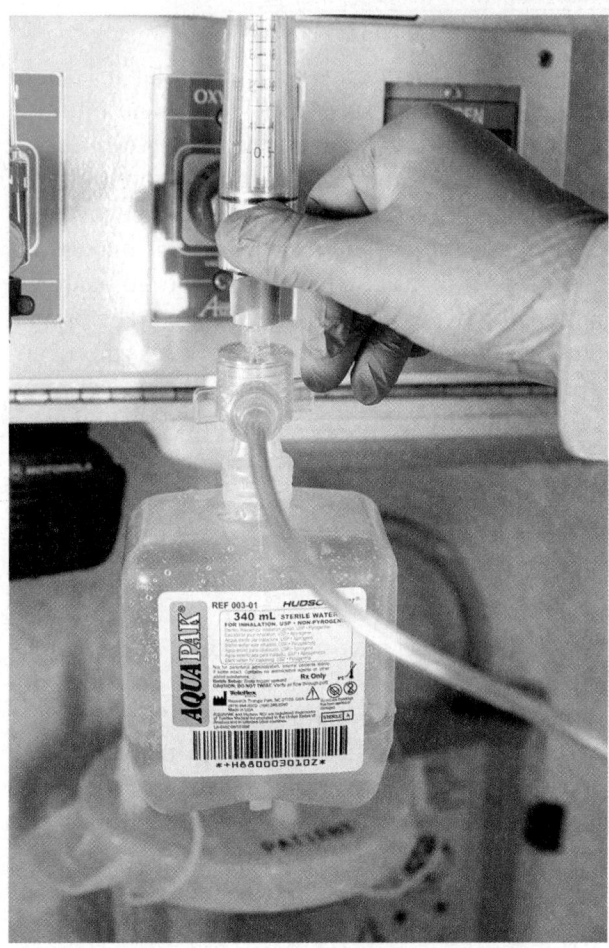

**FIGURE 11-43** Giving humidified oxygen is preferred with long transport times although it increases the aerosolization of droplets and may increase the risk of disease transmission to others in the same ambulance compartment as the patient.

© Jones & Bartlett Learning.

level. Too often emphasis is placed on advanced airway techniques, making the basic airway maneuvers seem ineffective. This cannot be further from the truth. Basic airway and ventilation techniques are extremely effective when administered appropriately. Mastery of these techniques at the EMT level—and continued mastery at the AEMT and paramedic levels—is imperative.

Patients who are breathing inadequately may be unable to speak in complete sentences. An irregular breathing pattern may also require artificial ventilation to assist patients in maintaining adequate minute volume. Keep in mind that fast, shallow breathing can be just as dangerous as very slow breathing. Fast, shallow breathing moves air primarily in the larger airway passages (dead air space) and does not allow for adequate exchange of air and carbon dioxide in the alveoli. Patients with inadequate breathing require assisted ventilations with some form of positive-pressure ventilation. Remember to follow standard precautions as needed when managing the patient's airway.

## Assisting Ventilation in Respiratory Distress/Failure

When a patient is in severe respiratory distress or respiratory failure and not breathing adequately, you must intervene quickly to prevent further deterioration of the patient. Two treatment options are available in these situations: assisted ventilation and continuous positive airway pressure (CPAP). CPAP is discussed later in this chapter; the focus of this section will be on assisted ventilation.

The purpose of assisted ventilations is to improve the overall oxygenation and ventilatory status of the patient. Patients who require assisted ventilations are no longer able to maintain adequate oxygen levels for the body and need assistance to prevent further hypoxia.

You need to be familiar with the signs and symptoms associated with inadequate ventilation. Signs of altered mental status and shallow breathing (reduced tidal volume) are indications for assisted ventilation. In addition, excessive accessory muscle use and fatigue from labored breathing are signs of potential respiratory failure. Patients exhibiting these signs need immediate treatment.

Follow these steps to assist a spontaneously breathing patient's ventilations using a bag-mask device:

1. Explain the procedure to the patient.
2. Place the mask over the patient's nose and mouth.
3. Squeeze the bag each time the patient breathes, maintaining the same rate as the patient.
4. After the initial 5 to 10 breaths, slowly adjust the rate and deliver an appropriate tidal volume.
5. Adjust the rate and tidal volume to maintain an adequate minute volume.

## Artificial Ventilation

Patients who are in respiratory arrest need immediate treatment. Without it, they will die. However, the act of breathing for a patient, or artificial ventilation, is not a skill you should take lightly. Once you determine that a patient is not breathing, begin artificial ventilation immediately. The methods that you may use to provide artificial ventilation include the mouth-to-mask technique (used only in non-work situations when a bag mask is not available) and the one- or two-person bag-mask device technique.

### Normal Ventilation Versus Positive-Pressure Ventilation

It is important to understand that although artificial ventilations are necessary to sustain life, they are not the same as normal breathing. As discussed earlier, the act of air moving into and out of the lungs is based on pressure changes within the thoracic cavity. During normal ventilation, the diaphragm contracts and negative pressure is generated in the chest cavity. This essentially sucks air into the chest from the trachea to equalize the pressure in the chest with the atmospheric pressure. The same vacuum that sucks air into the chest also pulls blood back to the right side of the heart. However, positive-pressure ventilation generated by a device, such as a bag-mask device, forces air into the chest cavity from the external environment, rather than using pressure changes. This difference between normal ventilation and positive-pressure ventilation can create some challenges (**TABLE 11-6**).

The physical act of the chest wall expanding and retracting during breathing helps the circulatory system return blood to the heart. During normal ventilation, the chest wall movement works similarly to a pump. The pressure changes in the thoracic cavity help draw venous blood back to the heart. However, when positive-pressure ventilation is initiated, more air is needed to achieve the same oxygenation and ventilatory effects of normal breathing. This increase in airway wall pressure causes the walls of the chest cavity to push out of their normal anatomic shape. As a result, there is an increase in the overall intrathoracic pressure. This pressure increase affects the return of venous blood to the heart. Considering that the left side of the heart receives only what the right side gives it, reduced venous return would result in reduced cardiac output. Therefore, it is imperative that you regulate the rate and volume of artificial ventilations to help prevent this drop in cardiac output. Cardiac

**TABLE 11-6** Normal Ventilation Versus Positive-Pressure Ventilation

|  | Normal Ventilation | Positive-Pressure Ventilation |
|---|---|---|
| **Air movement** | Air is sucked into the lungs due to the negative intrathoracic pressure created when the diaphragm contracts. | Air is forced into the lungs through a means of mechanical ventilation. |
| **Blood movement** | Normal breathing allows blood to naturally be pulled back to the heart. | Intrathoracic pressure is increased as air is driven into the lungs, which can reduce blood return to the heart and therefore reduce the amount of blood pumped by the heart. |
| **Airway wall pressure** | Not affected during normal breathing. | More volume is required to have the same effects as normal breathing. As a result, the walls are pushed out of their normal anatomic shape. |
| **Esophageal opening pressure** | Not affected during normal breathing. | Air may be forced into the stomach, especially with aggressive ventilation, causing gastric distention that could result in vomiting and aspiration. |
| **Overventilation** | Overventilation is not typical of normal breathing. | Too much volume and/or a fast ventilation rate results in increased intrathoracic pressure, gastric distention, and decrease in cardiac output, resulting in hypotension. |

© Jones & Bartlett Learning.

output is a function of stroke volume and heart rate, such that cardiac output = stroke volume × heart rate. Stroke volume is the amount of blood ejected by the ventricle in one cardiac cycle. The heart rate is assessed by taking the pulse for 1 minute. The cardiac output is the amount of blood ejected by the left ventricle in 1 minute.

### Words of Wisdom

**Ventilation Rates[a]**

| Adult | 1 breath every 6 seconds |
|---|---|
| Child | 1 breath every 2 to 3 seconds |
| Infant | 1 breath every 2 to 3 seconds |

[a]For apneic patients with a pulse.

## Mouth-to-Mouth and Mouth-to-Mask Ventilation

As you learned in your CPR course, mouth-to-mouth ventilations are now routinely done with a barrier device, such as a mask or face shield. Barrier devices provide some protection but not from

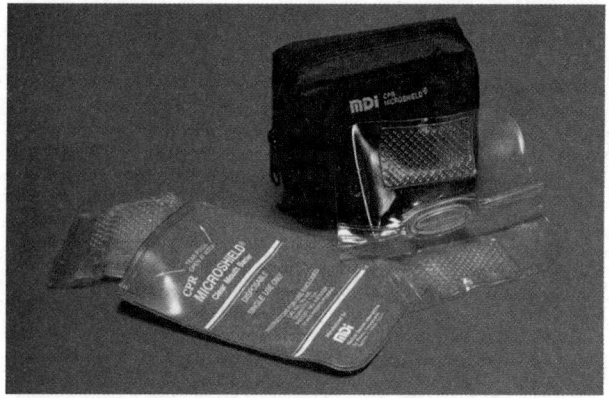

**FIGURE 11-44** Barrier devices, such as a pocket mask with a one-way valve, provide some protection from certain diseases but inadequate protection from SARS-CoV2 or tuberculosis.

© Jones & Bartlett Learning. Courtesy of MIEMSS.

diseases transmitted by airborne pathogens or aerosolized droplets such as SARS-CoV2 or tuberculosis (**FIGURE 11-44**). Mouth-to-mouth ventilations with or without a barrier device should be provided only in extreme situations. Performing mouth-to-mask ventilations with a pocket mask containing a one-way valve with an adequate filter is a safer method to prevent possible disease transmission.

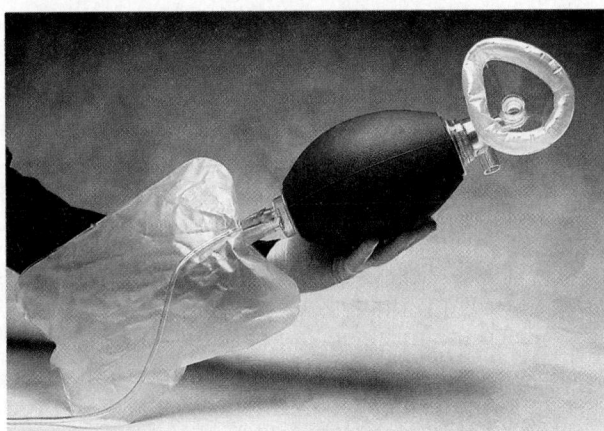

**FIGURE 11-45** A bag-mask device with an oxygen reservoir can deliver nearly 100% oxygen if a good seal between the mouth and mask is achieved and if supplemental oxygen is used.

© American Academy of Orthopaedic Surgeons.

This method is used only when the EMT is off duty in a situation where no bag-mask device is available.

## The Bag-Mask Device

With an oxygen flow rate of 15 L/min and an adequate mask-to-face seal, a bag-mask device with an oxygen reservoir can deliver nearly 100% oxygen (**FIGURE 11-45**). Most bag-mask devices commercially available include reservoirs that permit the delivery of oxygen concentrations approaching 100%; however, the device can deliver only as much volume as you can squeeze out of the bag by hand. The bag-mask device provides less tidal volume than mouth-to-mask ventilation; however, it delivers a higher concentration of oxygen. The bag-mask device is the most common method used to ventilate patients in the field. Although an experienced EMT will be able to supply adequate tidal volume with a bag-mask device, as a new EMT you should develop proficiency at ventilating airway-training manikins before using a bag-mask device on a patient. If you have difficulty adequately ventilating a patient with a bag-mask device, you should immediately switch to an alternative method of ventilation, such as the mouth-to-mask technique.

A bag-mask device should be used when you need to deliver high concentrations of oxygen to patients who are not ventilating adequately. The device is also used for patients in respiratory arrest, cardiopulmonary arrest, and respiratory failure.

The bag-mask device may be used with or without oxygen. However, to ensure the highest concentration of delivered oxygen, you must attach supplemental oxygen and a reservoir. Use an oral or nasal airway adjunct in conjunction with the bag-mask device.

### Bag-Mask Device Components

All adult bag-mask devices should have the following components:

- A disposable self-inflating bag
- No pop-off valve, or if one is present, the capability of disabling the pop-off valve
- An outlet valve that is a true valve for nonrebreathing
- An inline viral filter
- An oxygen reservoir that allows for delivery of high-concentration oxygen
- A one-way, no-jam inlet valve system that provides an oxygen inlet flow at a maximum of 15 L/min with standard 15/22-mm fittings for face mask and endotracheal tube (or other advanced airway adjunct) connection
- A transparent face mask
- Ability to perform under extreme environmental conditions, including extreme heat or cold

The total volume in the bag of an adult bag-mask device is usually 1,200 to 1,600 mL. The pediatric bag volume is 500 to 700 mL, and the infant bag volume is 150 to 240 mL.

The volume of air (and therefore, oxygen) delivered to the patient is based on one key observation—chest rise and fall. Essentially, this is typically the only means of assessing tidal volume in the field. In most situations, you will be using the bag-mask device attached to high-flow oxygen (15 L/min). When using the bag-mask device with high-flow oxygen on an adult patient, you should squeeze the bag enough to cause a noticeable rise of the patient's chest—a volume of about 600 mL (approximately 6 to 7 mL/kg) over 1 second.

By delivering just enough tidal volume to see the chest rise, and not ventilating at a rate that is too fast, the risks of gastric distention (and associated complications of vomiting and aspiration) and cardiac compromise are reduced.

It is not practical for you to accurately measure tidal volume in milliliters per kilogram for each patient ventilated in the field. The key is to watch for good chest rise and fall—let these observations determine the appropriate amount of volume to deliver.

### Bag-Mask Device Technique

Whenever possible, you and your partner should work together to provide bag-mask ventilation. One EMT can maintain a good mask seal by securing the mask to the patient's face with two hands while the other EMT squeezes the bag. Ventilation using a bag-mask device is a challenging skill: it may be very difficult for one EMT to maintain a proper seal between the mask and the face with one hand while squeezing the bag well enough to deliver an adequate volume to the patient. This skill can be difficult to maintain if you do not have many opportunities to practice. Effective one-person bag-mask ventilation requires considerable practice and experience. Also, performance of this skill depends on having enough personnel to carry out other actions that need to be done at the same time, such as chest compressions, putting the stretcher in place, or helping to lift the patient onto the stretcher.

Follow these steps to use the one-person bag-mask device technique (**SKILL DRILL 11-8**):

1. Select the proper size mask and assemble your equipment. Kneel above the patient's head.

Maintain the patient's neck in an extended position unless you suspect a cervical spine injury (**Step 1**). In that case, stabilize the patient's head and neck and use the jaw-thrust maneuver. Have your partner hold the head, or, if you are alone, use your knees to stabilize the head.
2. Open the patient's mouth, and suction as needed. Insert an oral or nasal airway to maintain airway patency (**Step 2**).
3. Place the mask on the patient's face (**Step 3**). Make sure the top is over the bridge of the nose and the bottom is in the groove between the lower lip and the chin. If the mask has a large, round cuff around the ventilation port, center the port over the patient's mouth. Adjust the amount of air in the mask to obtain a better fit and seal to the face if necessary.
4. Create a seal by holding your index finger over the lower part of the mask and your thumb over the upper part of the mask. Then use your remaining fingers to pull the lower jaw into the mask. This is known as the EC-clamp method and will maintain an effective face-to-mask seal.
5. Bring the lower jaw up to the mask with the last three fingers of your hand. This will help to maintain an open airway. Make sure you do not grab the fleshy part of the neck; doing so will push the tongue against the roof of the mouth and block the airway.

## YOU are the Provider

After taking action to correct the patient's previous deterioration, you note improvement in her clinical status. Her level of consciousness has improved; however, she is not resisting your treatment. At this point, she is loaded into the ambulance and transport is initiated. A firefighter/EMT accompanies you in the back to assist with further patient care. You continue your treatment plan en route, monitoring her condition frequently. After reassessing the patient, you call in your report to the ED.

| Recording Time: 10 Minutes | |
|---|---|
| Level of consciousness | Opens her eyes when you speak to her |
| Respirations | 12 breaths/min (assisted with a bag mask) |
| Pulse | 110 beats/min, stronger |
| Skin | Cool and dry; less cyanotic |
| Blood pressure | 104/60 mm Hg |
| SpO$_2$ | 80% (on oxygen with assisted ventilation) |

**11.** How can capnography be used to assess ventilation adequacy?

**12.** What is the clinical significance of cyanosis?

## Skill Drill 11-8 Performing One-Rescuer Bag-Mask Ventilations

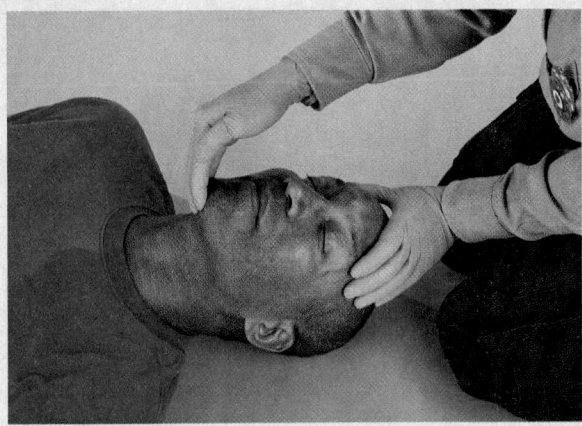

### Step 1

Assemble your equipment and position yourself above the patient's head. Open the airway using the head tilt–chin lift or jaw-thrust maneuver.

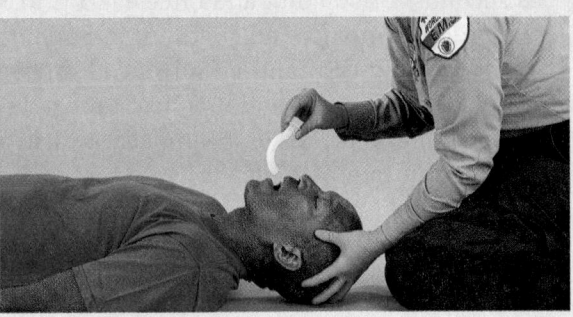

### Step 2

Open the patient's mouth and suction as necessary to clear secretions. Insert an oral or nasal airway.

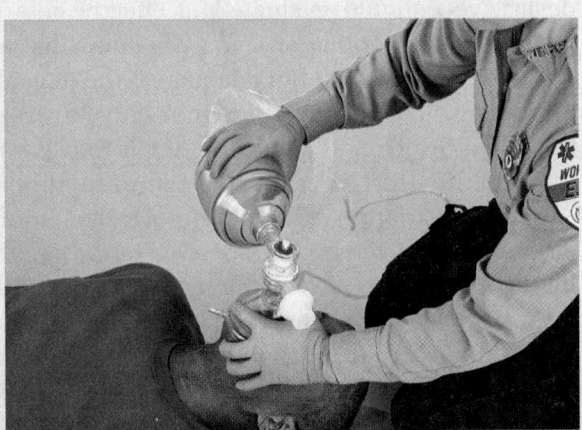

### Step 3

Select the appropriate mask and position it properly on the patient's face. Following the EC-clamp method, make a seal by holding your index finger over the lower part of the mask and your thumb over the upper part of the mask. Then use your remaining fingers to pull the lower jaw into the mask. Bring the lower jaw up to the mask with the last three fingers of your hand. Avoid the fleshy soft tissue of the neck.

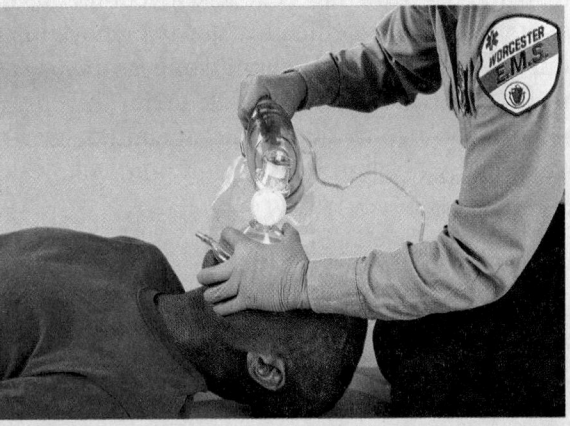

### Step 4

Squeeze the bag with your other hand until you see adequate chest rise. For adults, squeeze once every 6 seconds. For infants and children, squeeze once every 2 to 3 seconds. In patients undergoing CPR and with an advanced airway in place, use a rate of 1 breath every 6 seconds (10 breaths/min).

© Jones & Bartlett Learning.

6. Squeeze the bag with your other hand until you see adequate chest rise (**Step 4**). Perform this in a rhythmic manner once every 6 seconds for an adult and once every 2 to 3 seconds for infants and children. In patients with ongoing CPR and an advanced airway in place, such as an endotracheal tube, a laryngeal mask airway, or a King airway, use a ventilation rate of 1 breath every 6 seconds (10 breaths/min), without pausing chest compressions.

If two EMTs are available to manage the airway, have one EMT hold the mask in position by placing the thumbs over the top part of the mask and the index fingers over the bottom half. Use the last three fingers of the hands to bring the lower jaw up to the mask. This helps to seal the mask to the face and maintain an open airway. The second EMT squeezes the bag with two hands until the chest rises adequately in the same manner as the one-person technique (**FIGURE 11-46**).

When using the device to assist ventilations of a patient who is breathing too slowly (hypoventilation) with reduced tidal volume, squeeze the bag as the patient tries to breathe in. Then, for the next 5 to 10 breaths, slowly adjust the rate and delivered tidal volume until an adequate minute volume is achieved.

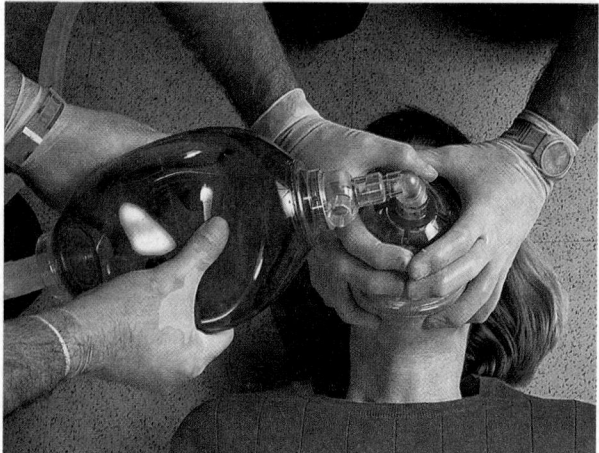

**FIGURE 11-46** With two-person bag-mask ventilation, you hold the mask in place while your partner squeezes the bag with two hands until the patient's chest rises adequately.

© Jones & Bartlett Learning. Courtesy of MIEMSS.

To assist ventilations of a patient who is breathing too fast (hyperventilation) with reduced tidal volume, you must first explain the procedure to the patient if the patient is coherent. Initially assist ventilations at the rate at which the patient has been breathing, squeezing the bag each time the patient inhales. Then, for the next 5 to 10 breaths, slowly adjust the rate and the delivered tidal volume until an adequate minute volume is achieved.

As you are assisting ventilations with a bag-mask device, you should evaluate the effectiveness of your delivered ventilations. You will know that artificial ventilations are not adequate if the patient's chest does not rise and fall with each ventilation, the rate at which you are ventilating is too slow or too fast, the heart rate does not return to normal, or oxygen saturation does not improve. If too much air is escaping from under the mask, reposition the mask for a better seal. If the patient's chest does not rise and fall, you may need to reposition the head or use an airway adjunct. If the patient's chest still does not rise and fall after you have made these corrections, check for an airway obstruction. If an obstruction is not present, attempt ventilations using an alternative method, such as the mouth-to-mask technique.

The bag-mask device may also be used in conjunction with an endotracheal tube or with other advanced airway devices. Advanced airway techniques are beneficial when a good seal is difficult to maintain, the patient has a cervical spine injury, or the patient's condition warrants. These techniques are discussed later in the text.

### Gastric Distention

When using a bag-mask device or any other ventilation device, be alert for **gastric distention**, inflation of the stomach with air. Although gastric distention most commonly affects children, it also affects adults. Gastric distention is most likely to occur when you ventilate the patient too forcefully or too rapidly with a bag-mask device or pocket mask. It may also occur when the airway is obstructed as a result of a foreign body or improper head position. For this reason, give slow, gentle breaths during artificial ventilation over 1 second (enough to see the chest rise) in the adult patient. As compliance decreases, you will notice it becoming increasingly difficult to squeeze the bag-mask device to get air into the lungs. Slight gastric distention is not of concern; however, severe inflation of the stomach is dangerous because it may cause vomiting and increase the risk of aspiration during CPR. Gastric distention can also significantly reduce the lung volume by elevating the diaphragm, especially in infants and children.

To prevent or alleviate distention, do the following: (1) ensure that the patient's airway is appropriately positioned, (2) ventilate the patient at the appropriate rate, and (3) ventilate the patient with the appropriate volume.

If the patient's stomach appears to be distending, recheck and reposition the head, and watch for rise and fall of the chest wall as you perform rescue breathing. Continue slow rescue breathing without attempting to expel the stomach contents. If gastric distention makes it impossible to ventilate the patient and an ALS provider is not available to perform orogastric tube or nasogastric tube decompression, consider positioning the patient onto his or her side and applying manual pressure over the upper abdomen. You should anticipate that vomiting will occur, so have suction immediately available. If necessary, sweep large debris from the mouth with your gloved hand. When the airway is clear, return the patient to a supine position and continue rescue breathing. *Manual decompression should be used only as a last resort and is reserved for extreme circumstances.* Be aware of your local protocols as manual decompression may not be permitted for EMTs in your service or jurisdiction.

## Passive Ventilation

The process of expansion and contraction of the chest creates a pump for air movement in and out of the chest. Normally, the muscles of the chest wall are the driving force behind the expansion and contraction of the chest. However, when a patient is not breathing, the movement of the chest wall depends completely on the EMS providers' ability to provide artificial breathing to the patient—active ventilation.

During cardiac arrest, you are responsible for providing high-quality chest compressions to circulate blood and artificial ventilations to oxygenate the hemoglobin. Because movement of the chest wall has been shown to assist in the ventilation process, patients receiving chest compressions benefit from a process known as **passive ventilation**. This is sometimes also called passive oxygenation or apneic oxygenation. In passive ventilation, air movement into and out of the chest cavity occurs passively as a result of compressing the chest. When the chest is compressed, air is forced out of the thorax. As the chest recoils following compression, a negative pressure is created within the chest, which results in a vacuum. This leads to air being sucked into the chest cavity, similar to what occurs with muscle contraction during active inhalation.

### Words of Wisdom

Prior to and during placement of an endotracheal tube (a procedure performed by ALS providers), consider applying a nasal cannula and setting the flow rate at 15 L/min. This initiates the processes of preoxygenation and denitrogenation. **Denitrogenation** attempts to replace alveolar nitrogen with oxygen; the goal is to increase oxygen reserve in the lungs, thus minimizing the risk of oxygen desaturation during periods of forced apnea that will occur during the intubation attempt.

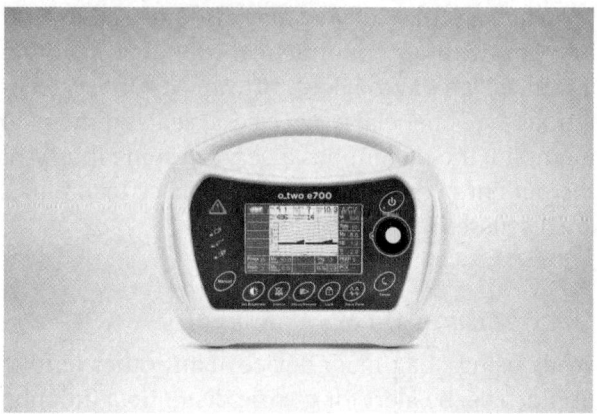

**FIGURE 11-47** Automatic transport ventilator.

Used with permission of O-Two Medical Technologies Inc.

When you are performing chest compressions, passive ventilation can be enhanced by inserting an oropharyngeal airway and providing supplemental oxygen to the patient. You can also improve oxygenation during passive ventilation by applying supplemental oxygen with a nasal cannula or a nonrebreathing mask.

## Automatic Transport Ventilator/Resuscitator

The **automatic transport ventilator (ATV)** is a ventilation device attached to a control box that allows the variables of ventilation to be set (**FIGURE 11-47**). An EMT must be approved and credentialed by the medical director to use these devices. Although some ATVs may not offer the same controls as a hospital ventilator, some are very advanced being very similar to a hospital ventilator but with a simpler interface, with the advantage that it frees you to perform other tasks, such as maintaining

a mask seal or ensuring continued patency of the airway. You can even perform non–airway-related tasks if the patient has an advanced airway in place and is being ventilated with the ATV. As recommended for all ventilators, always have a bag-mask device or a backup ventilator ready in case of malfunction.

Most models have adjustments for respiratory rate and tidal volume; more sophisticated models allow you to regulate the percentage of oxygen delivered to the patient and may offer a pressure cycle. In most cases, the respiratory rate is set at the midpoint or average for the patient's age. Tidal volume is usually estimated using the formula of 6 to 7 mL/kg of ideal body weight because ATVs are oxygen-powered and provide oxygen-enriched breathing gas. The tidal volume can be adjusted based on the patient's chest rise and physiologic response.

The ATV is generally oxygen-powered, although some models may require an external power source. Whereas this device does require oxygen, in some cases it will consume 5 L/min of oxygen run, in other cases the consumed oxygen is the patient only being considered a "zero drive" oxygen consumption, unlike a bag-mask device that uses 15 to 25 L/min. **Compliance** is the ability of the alveoli to expand when air is drawn in during inhalation. Poor lung compliance is the inability of the alveoli to fully expand during inhalation. When ventilating a patient, you would recognize this by noting an increase in resistance when you attempt to ventilate.

Whereas ATVs potentially free you to perform other tasks, constant reassessment of the patient is necessary. Barotrauma can occur in patients being ventilated. In addition, you need to assess for full chest recoil when using an ATV. This step is not only essential with patients in respiratory arrest, but also with patients in cardiac arrest who are also receiving chest compressions.

## Continuous Positive Airway Pressure

Continuous positive airway pressure (CPAP) is a noninvasive means of providing ventilatory support for patients experiencing respiratory distress. Many people in whom obstructive sleep apnea has been diagnosed wear a CPAP unit at night to maintain their airway while they sleep (**FIGURE 11-48**). CPAP in the prehospital environment has proven to be an excellent adjunct in the treatment of respiratory distress associated with COPD, acute pulmonary edema, and acute bronchospasm (such as in asthma). In asthma and COPD it is used in conjunction with bronchodilator medications (eg, albuterol). Typically, many of these patients would be managed with advanced airway techniques,

such as endotracheal intubation. Early intervention with CPAP is an alternative means of providing ventilatory assistance to patients; it helps to decrease overall morbidity and mortality and it can prevent the need to intubate the patient. Because of the simplicity of the device and its great benefit to the patient, CPAP is widely used at the EMT level. Follow your local protocols regarding the use of CPAP in your agency or department.

### Safety Tips

CPAP systems without viral filters may increase the risk of aerosolization of secretions during sleep, which may increase the risk of these patients transmitting certain diseases, such as COVID-19 or tuberculosis, to people around them when they sleep.

### Mechanism

CPAP increases pressure in the lungs, opens collapsed alveoli and prevents further alveolar collapse (atelectasis), pushes more oxygen across the alveolar membrane, and forces interstitial fluid back into the pulmonary circulation. The desired effect of CPAP is to improve pulmonary compliance and make spontaneous ventilation easier for the patient. The therapy is typically delivered through a face mask that is held to the head with a strapping system. A good seal with minimal leakage between the face and mask is essential.

Many CPAP systems use oxygen as the driving force to deliver the positive ventilatory pressure to the patient. Frequently check the oxygen regulator when administering CPAP; depending on the flow and the patient's respiratory rate, some CPAP units can empty a D cylinder in as little as 5 to 10 minutes.

The CPAP device is fitted with a pressure relief valve that determines the amount of pressure the patient must breathe against and overcome, referred to as expiratory positive airway pressure (EPAP). The EPAP setting typically ranges between 5 and 20 cm $H_2O$. As the patient breathes against this pressure, positive pressure is redirected to the lower

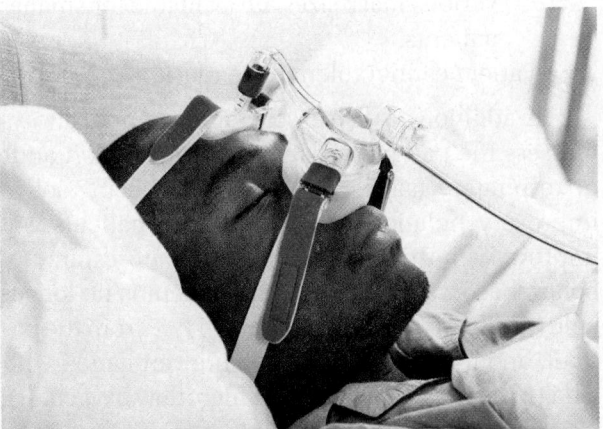

**FIGURE 11-48** Many people in whom obstructive sleep apnea has been diagnosed wear a CPAP unit at night to maintain their airway while they sleep.

© Andrey_Popov/Shutterstock.

airway. Therefore, patients benefit the most from CPAP during exhalation rather than inhalation. The effect of CPAP is similar to hanging your head out the window while driving on the highway. In order to exhale, you must first overcome the high inspiratory flow created by the fast-moving air. Although this may appear to require a great deal of effort on the part of a patient who is already in distress, many patients improve dramatically when CPAP is applied.

Because CPAP increases pressure inside the chest, it reduces the amount of blood flow returning to the heart. As the pressure in the thorax increases, the venous flow of blood returning to the heart meets the resistance of the increased pressure in the chest. The result is a decrease in the workload of the heart and a drop in cardiac output. This is not common with lower levels of CPAP; however, caution should be used when considering CPAP in patients with low blood pressure. Continually monitor blood pressure in patients receiving CPAP treatment.

## Indications

CPAP is indicated for patients experiencing respiratory distress in which their own compensatory mechanisms are not enough to keep up with their oxygen demand. Whereas most patients improve after the application of CPAP, it is important to remember that CPAP is merely treating the symptoms and not necessarily the underlying pathology.

The following are general indications for using CPAP:

- Patient is alert and able to follow commands.
- Patient is displaying obvious signs of moderate to severe respiratory distress (eg, accessory muscle use, tripod position, retractions) from an underlying pathology, such as pulmonary edema or obstructive pulmonary disease (ie, COPD), or bronchospasm.
- Respiratory distress occurs after a submersion incident.
- Patient is breathing so rapidly that it affects overall minute volume.
- Pulse oximetry reading is less than 90%.

Although these guidelines should be considered when assessing the need for CPAP, it is important that you follow your local guidelines and protocols.

## Contraindications

CPAP has proven to be immensely beneficial to patients experiencing respiratory distress from acute pulmonary edema or COPD; however, there are times when CPAP is not appropriate for the patient.

The following are general contraindications for CPAP use:

- Patient is in respiratory arrest or has agonal respirations.
- Patient is hypoventilating (slow respiratory rate and/or reduced tidal volume).
- Patient cannot speak.
- Patient is unresponsive or otherwise unable to follow verbal commands.
- Patient cannot protect his or her own airway.
- Patient has hypotension (systolic blood pressure less than 90 mm Hg).
- Signs and symptoms of a pneumothorax or chest trauma are present.
- Patient has a tracheostomy.
- Active gastrointestinal bleeding, nausea, or vomiting is present.
- Patient has experienced facial trauma.
- Patient is in cardiogenic shock.
- Patient cannot sit upright.
- CPAP system mask and strap cannot be properly fit.
  - Excessive facial hair or dysmorphic facial features can impede your ability to ensure a properly fitting mask.
  - Various mask sizes are available for smaller patients.
- Patient cannot tolerate the mask.

In addition to these contraindications, always reassess the patient for signs of deterioration and/or respiratory failure. CPAP is an excellent tool to improve ventilation; however, not all patients will improve with this device. Once signs of respiratory failure become apparent or the patient is no longer able to follow commands, remove CPAP from the patient, and initiate positive-pressure ventilation with a bag-mask device attached to high-flow oxygen.

## Application

Several varieties of CPAP units are available to EMS providers; however, most follow the same general guidelines for use and setup. CPAP units generally comprise a generator, a mask, a circuit that contains corrugated tubing, a bacteria filter, and a one-way valve. The CPAP generator creates resistance throughout the respiratory cycle. This resistance creates a back pressure into the airways that pushes open the smaller airway structures, such as bronchioles and alveoli, as the patient exhales. The amount of pressure can be determined by adjusting a valve within the system or with a separate valve that can be attached to the CPAP system. A pressure of 7.0 to 10.0 cm $H_2O$ is generally an acceptable therapeutic range for a patient on CPAP. Always consult the operations manual of any CPAP device for proper assembly instructions.

Because most CPAP units are powered by oxygen, it is important to have a full cylinder of oxygen when using CPAP. Some CPAP units use a continuous flow of oxygen, whereas others use oxygen on more of a demand basis. In either situation, continuously monitor the amount of available oxygen in your cylinder. A typical CPAP unit will deplete a full D cylinder of oxygen in 15 to 30 minutes, depending on the fraction of inspired oxygen ($FIO_2$) setting. Therefore, proper planning for oxygen consumption is necessary when considering applying

CPAP. Some newer CPAP devices allow the provider to adjust the $FIO_2$, whereas older CPAP devices are typically set to deliver a fixed $FIO_2$ of 30% to 35%, although some can deliver as high a level as 95%.

In recent years, disposable CPAP devices have become available to the EMS provider. These devices typically have a mask that is secured to the face, similar to standard CPAP devices. However, these devices run entirely off the oxygen system and do not require the adjustment of a valve. Depending on the manufacturer, a valve in either the tubing or the mask creates the pressure needed for the system. Pressure is controlled by changing the oxygen flow. The higher the oxygen flow rate, the higher the pressure. These devices are gaining in popularity because they are lightweight and relatively easy to operate.

Follow the steps in **SKILL DRILL 11-9** to use CPAP:

1.  Take standard precautions. Assess the patient for indications and contraindications of CPAP. Confirm the patient's blood pressure and explain the procedure to the patient. Check your equipment, then connect the circuit to the CPAP generator (**Step 1**).

## Skill Drill 11-9 Using CPAP

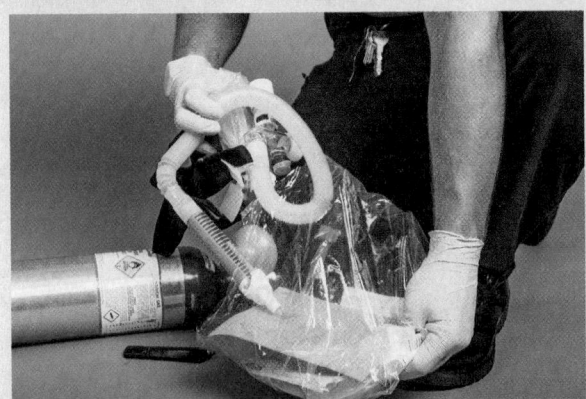

**Step 1**

Take standard precautions. Assess the patient for indications and contraindications of CPAP. Confirm the patient's blood pressure and explain the procedure to the patient. Check your equipment, then connect the circuit to the CPAP generator.

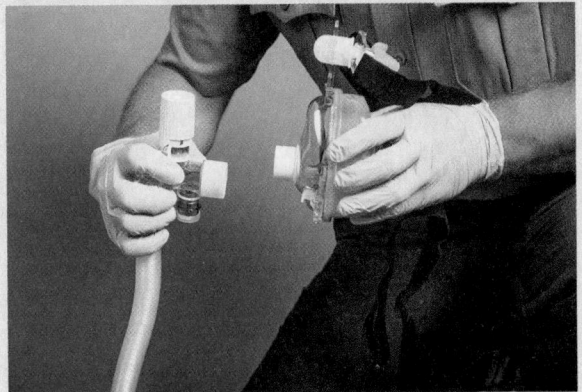

**Step 2**

Connect the face mask to the circuit tubing.

*(continues)*

## Skill Drill 11-9 Using CPAP (continued)

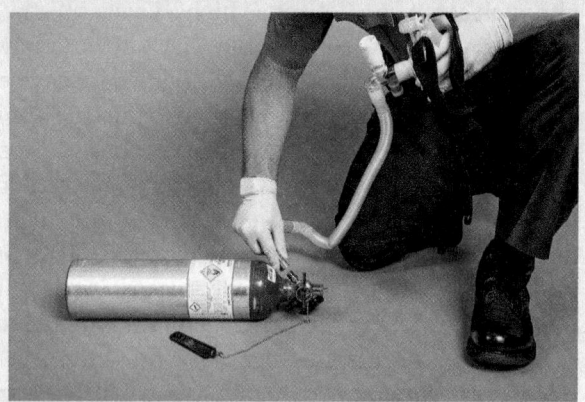

### Step 3

Connect the tubing to the oxygen tank.

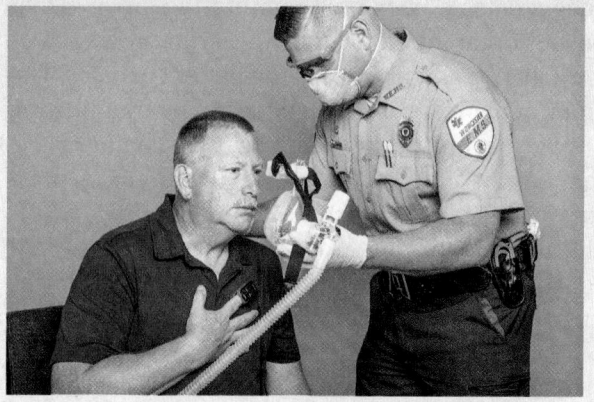

### Step 4

Place the patient in a high Fowler position to facilitate breathing, and coach the patient through the initial application of the mask. Instruct the patient to place the mask over the mouth and nose, creating the most airtight seal possible.

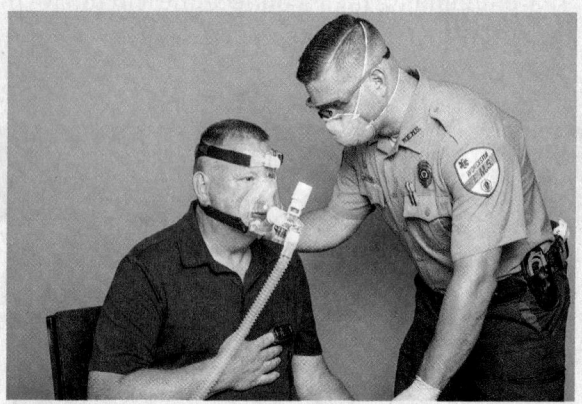

### Step 5

After the mask is placed on the face and the patient adjusts to it, use the strapping mechanism to secure it to the patient's head. Ensure the seal between the mask and face remains intact.

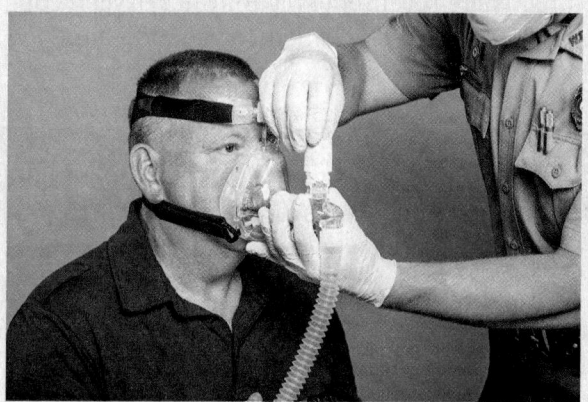

### Step 6

Adjust the PEEP valve and the FIO$_2$ according to the manufacturer's recommendations to maintain adequate oxygenation and ventilation. With CPAP in place, the patient's oxygenation saturation level should improve, the work of breathing should decrease, and the ability to speak should improve. Constantly reassess the patient for signs of clinical deterioration and/or complications (eg, pneumothorax, hypotension).

2. Connect the face mask to the circuit tubing (**Step 2**). Once the system is connected, check to see if there is an on/off button. Some newer models have this feature. Confirm the device is powered on and working before you apply CPAP to the patient.

3. Connect the tubing to the oxygen tank (**Step 3**).

4. Place the patient in a high Fowler position to facilitate breathing, and coach the patient through the initial application of the mask. Instruct the patient to place the mask over the mouth and nose, creating the most airtight seal possible (**Step 4**). Allowing the patient to hold the mask to his or her face initially may help reduce some of the stress and anxiety associated with the application of CPAP; however, some patients may resist application of the mask while in severe respiratory distress.

5. After the mask is placed on the face and the patient adjusts to it, use the strapping mechanism to secure it to the patient's head. Ensure the seal between the mask and face remains intact (**Step 5**). Consult the manufacturer's guidelines for specific strapping instructions.

6. Adjust the positive end-expiratory pressure (PEEP) valve and the $FIO_2$ according to the manufacturer's recommendations to maintain adequate oxygenation and ventilation. With CPAP in place, the patient's oxygenation saturation level should improve, the work of breathing should decrease, and the ability to speak should improve. Constantly reassess the patient for signs of clinical deterioration and/or complications (eg, pneumothorax, hypotension) (**Step 6**).

## Complications

The application and administration of CPAP is a relatively easy process. However, some patients may find CPAP claustrophobic and will resist the application. As patients become more hypoxic, the application of a mask to their face is sometimes perceived as suffocation, rather than helping them breathe. In any event, it is important to explain the application to patients and coach them through the process. Do not force the mask on patients. This will create a higher level of anxiety and increase their oxygen demand. Coach patients through the application of CPAP, allowing them to adjust to the situation. Coaching patients is not always an easy task; it takes practice and a willingness to work closely with your patient during a difficult time.

## YOU are the Provider

Reassessment on delivery at the ED reveals that the patient's condition has continued to improve. Her eyes are open, she responds to verbal stimuli, and she pushes away her bag mask. Her breathing, although still somewhat labored, has improved. Oxygen saturation, however, remains low despite supplemental oxygen via nonrebreathing mask.

| Recording Time: 17 Minutes | |
|---|---|
| Level of consciousness | Eyes open; responsive to verbal stimuli |
| Respirations | 14 breaths/min, slightly labored, adequate depth |
| Pulse | 109 beats/min, strong and regular |
| Skin | Cool and dry |
| Blood pressure | 118/70 mm Hg |
| $SpO_2$ | 86% (on supplemental oxygen) |

You transfer care of the patient to the ED physician, who tells you that she believes the patient is experiencing an acute pulmonary embolism. After further treatment in the ED, the patient is sent for CT scanning of the chest.

**13.** What components of your reassessment are consistent with acute pulmonary embolism?

**14.** What is a ventilation/perfusion mismatch?

Due to the high volume of pressure generated by CPAP, there is the possibility of causing a pneumothorax. Although the medical literature suggests that this is highly unlikely, you should be aware of this risk and continually assess your patients for signs and symptoms of a pneumothorax.

In addition to pneumothorax, high pressure in the chest can lower a patient's blood pressure. As the intrathoracic pressure increases, venous blood returning to the heart meets resistance from the increased pressure in the chest. This can result in a sudden drop in blood pressure. Although this is not common with lower levels of CPAP, continuous monitoring of blood pressure is necessary.

CPAP has consistently shown positive results with patients experiencing moderate and severe respiratory distress; however, there are still cases in which patients deteriorate. It is important that you reassess the patient for signs of deterioration. If the patient is no longer able to follow verbal commands and/or goes into respiratory failure/arrest, you must act quickly to remove CPAP and begin positive-pressure ventilation using a bag-mask device attached to high-flow oxygen.

## Stomas and Tracheostomy Tubes

Bag-mask ventilation may also need to be used for patients who have had a laryngectomy (surgical removal of the larynx). These patients have a permanent tracheal stoma (an opening in the neck that connects the trachea directly to the skin) (**FIGURE 11-49**). This type of stoma, known as the tracheostomy, is an opening at the center front and base of the neck. Many patients who have had a laryngectomy will have other openings in the neck, according to the type of operation performed. You should ignore any opening other than the midline tracheal stoma. The midline opening is the only one that can be used to ventilate the patient.

Neither the head tilt–chin lift nor the jaw-thrust maneuver is required for ventilating a patient with a stoma. If the patient has a tracheostomy tube, ventilate through the tube with a bag-mask device (the standard 15/22-mm adapter on the bag-mask device will fit onto the tube in the tracheal stoma) and 100% oxygen attached directly to the bag-mask device. If the patient has a stoma and no tube is

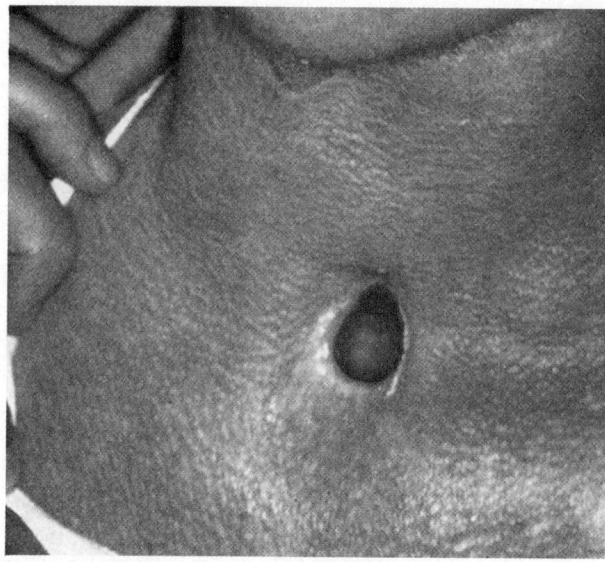

**FIGURE 11-49** A tracheal stoma is typically located in the midline of the neck. The midline opening is the only one that can be used to ventilate the patient.

© American Academy of Orthopaedic Surgeons.

in place, use an infant or child mask with your bag-mask device to make a seal over the stoma. Seal the patient's mouth and nose with one hand to prevent leakage of air through the upper airway when you ventilate through a stoma. Release the seal of the patient's mouth and nose for exhalation. This allows the air to exhale through the upper airway.

If you are unable to ventilate a patient who has a stoma, try suctioning the stoma and the mouth with a French or soft-tip catheter before giving the patient artificial ventilation through the mouth and nose. If you seal the stoma during ventilation via the nose and mouth, the ability to ventilate the patient may be improved, or it may help to clear any obstructions.

## Foreign Body Airway Obstruction

A foreign body that *completely* blocks the airway in a patient is a true emergency that will result in death if not treated immediately. In an adult, sudden foreign body airway obstruction usually occurs during a meal. In a child, it occurs while eating, playing with small toys, or crawling around the house. An otherwise healthy child who has sudden difficulty breathing should be assumed to have a foreign body airway obstruction.

By far, the most common airway obstruction in an unconscious patient is the tongue, which relaxes and falls back into the throat. There are other causes of airway obstruction that do not involve foreign bodies in the airway. These include swelling (from infection or acute allergic reaction) and trauma (tissue damage from injury). With airway obstruction from medical conditions such as infection and acute allergic reactions, repeated attempts to clear the airway as if there were a foreign body will be unsuccessful and potentially dangerous. These patients require specific emergency medical care for their condition; therefore, rapid transport to the hospital is critical.

## Recognition

Early recognition of airway obstruction is crucial for you to be able to provide emergency medical care effectively. Obstruction from a foreign body can result in a **mild airway obstruction** or a **severe airway obstruction**.

Patients with a mild airway obstruction are still able to exchange air but will have varying degrees of respiratory distress. Great care must be taken to prevent a mild airway obstruction from becoming a severe airway obstruction. The patient will usually have noisy breathing and may be coughing. Assess the patient and determine whether the patient has **good air exchange** or **poor air exchange**.

With good air exchange, the patient can cough forcefully, although you may hear **wheezing** (the production of whistling sounds during respiration) between coughs. Wheezing is usually indicative of a mild lower airway obstruction. As long as the patient can breathe, cough forcefully, or talk, you should not interfere with the patient's efforts to expel the foreign object on his or her own. Continue to monitor the patient closely and encourage the patient to continue coughing. Abdominal thrusts are usually not effective for dislodging a partial obstruction. Attempts to remove the object manually could force the object farther down into the airway and cause a severe airway obstruction. Continually reassess the patient's condition and be prepared to provide treatment if the air exchange becomes poor or a mild obstruction becomes a severe obstruction.

With poor air exchange, the patient has a weak, ineffective (not forceful) cough and may have increased difficulty breathing, **stridor** (a high-pitched noise heard primarily on inspiration), and cyanosis. Stridor is an indication of a mild upper airway obstruction. You must quickly recognize this situation and provide immediate care.

For patients with mild airway obstruction with poor air exchange, treat immediately as if there is a severe airway obstruction.

Patients with a severe airway obstruction cannot breathe, talk, or cough. One sure sign of a severe obstruction is the sudden inability to speak or cough during or immediately after eating. The person may clutch or grasp his or her throat (universal distress signal), start to become cyanotic, and have extreme difficulty breathing (**FIGURE 11-50**). There is little or no air movement. Ask the conscious patient, "Are you choking?" If the patient nods "yes," provide immediate treatment. If the obstruction is not cleared quickly, the amount of oxygen in the patient's blood will decrease dramatically. If not treated, the patient will become unconscious and die.

Some patients with a severe airway obstruction will be unconscious as you form your general impression. You may not know that an airway obstruction is the cause of their condition. There are many other causes of unconsciousness and respiratory failure, including stroke, heart attack, trauma, seizures, and drug overdose. A complete and thorough patient assessment by you, therefore, is essential to providing appropriate emergency medical care.

If the patient is found unresponsive, does not appear to be breathing, and does not have a pulse,

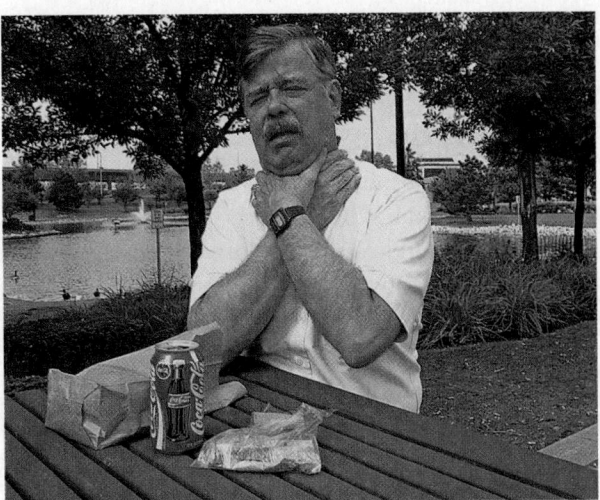

**FIGURE 11-50** The universal sign of choking is a person who grasps his or her throat and has difficulty breathing.

© Jones & Bartlett Learning. Courtesy of MIEMSS.

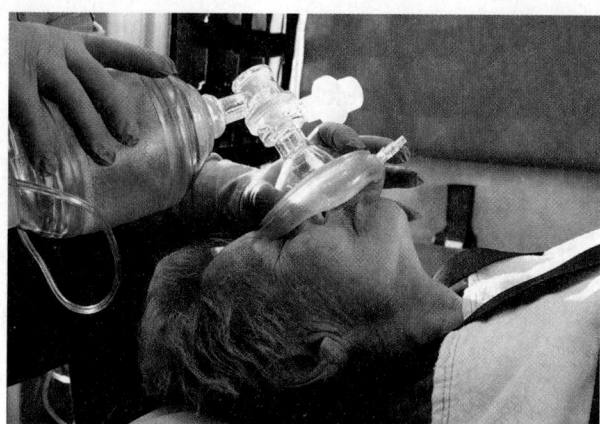

**FIGURE 11-51** When you open the airway and attempt ventilations, it will be obvious to you if the airway is blocked.

© Jones & Bartlett Learning.

begin CPR with high-quality chest compressions. When you open the airway and attempt two ventilations following chest compressions, it will be obvious to you if the airway is blocked (**FIGURE 11-51**). The compressions may have been enough to clear the airway; however, if you are unable to ventilate the patient after several attempts (no chest rise and fall) or you feel resistance while ventilating, consider the possibility of an airway obstruction. Resistance to ventilation can also be due to poor lung compliance. As discussed, compliance is the ability of the alveoli to expand when air is drawn in during inhalation; poor lung compliance is the inability of the alveoli to fully expand during inhalation.

## Emergency Medical Care for Foreign Body Airway Obstruction

Perform the head tilt–chin lift maneuver to clear an obstruction that has been caused by the tongue and throat muscles relaxing back into the airway in any person who is found unconscious. This should be performed on unresponsive patients with adequate or inadequate breathing who are not suspected of having spinal trauma. If spinal trauma is suspected, open the airway with the jaw-thrust maneuver. Large pieces of vomited food, mucus, loose dentures, or blood clots in the mouth should be swept forward and out of the mouth with your gloved index finger. Use suction to clear the airway of thinner secretions.

Abdominal thrusts are the most effective method of dislodging and forcing an object out of the airway of a conscious adult or child. Residual air, which is always present in the lungs, is compressed upward and used to expel the object. Use abdominal thrusts until the object dislodges or the patient becomes unconscious.

For the unresponsive patient with a severe foreign body airway obstruction, reassess to confirm apnea and inability to ventilate. Begin chest compression just as you would for CPR. At the completion of the 30 compressions, perform a tongue-jaw lift by grasping the jaw with your thumb and index finger. Place your thumb onto the tip of the patient's lower teeth and tongue while placing your index finger under the bony portion of the chin. Be careful not to compress the soft tissues under the chin. Pull the jaw/mouth open and look at the back of the oropharynx for any foreign objects. If an object is observed, remove it with a gloved index finger or suction. Attempt to remove an object only if it is visible during examination of the open mouth; blind sweeps of the back of the oropharynx may push an object farther down in the airway, making the obstruction worse. If the object is removed, attempt to ventilate. If no object was seen during the tongue-jaw lift, continue chest compressions.

If you are unable to clear a severe airway obstruction with your initial attempts, begin rapid transport and continue your efforts to relieve the obstruction with abdominal thrusts (chest compressions in the unresponsive patient) on the way to the hospital.

Remember to treat patients with a mild airway obstruction with poor air exchange as if they have a severe airway obstruction.

Patients with a mild airway obstruction and good air exchange should be monitored closely for deterioration of their condition. If the patient is unable to clear the obstruction and remains conscious, support (or let the patient control) the airway position that is most efficient and comfortable. Provide supplemental oxygen, and transport to the hospital.

### Words of Wisdom

If spinal trauma is suspected, open the airway using the jaw-thrust maneuver.

## Dental Appliances

Many dental appliances can cause an airway obstruction. If a dental appliance, such as a crown or bridge, dentures, or even a piece or sections of braces, has become loose, manually remove it before providing ventilations. Simple manual removal may relieve the obstruction and allow the patient to breathe on his or her own.

Providing bag-mask or mouth-to-mask ventilation is usually much easier when dentures can be left in place. Leaving the dentures in place provides more structure to the face and will generally assist you in being able to provide a good face-to-mask seal, thus delivering adequate tidal volume. However, loose dentures make it difficult to perform artificial ventilation by any method and can easily obstruct the airway. Therefore, dentures and dental appliances that do not stay in place should be removed. Dentures and appliances may become loose or be completely out of place following an accident or as you are providing care. Periodically reassess the patient's airway to make sure these devices are firmly in place. If dentures become dislodged, place them in a container and transport with the patient, if possible.

## Facial Bleeding

Airway problems can be especially challenging in patients with serious facial injuries (**FIGURE 11-52**). Because the blood supply to the face is so rich, injuries to the face can result in severe tissue swelling

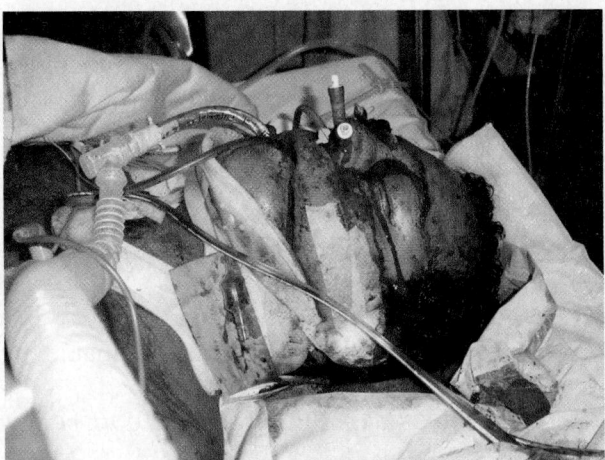

**FIGURE 11-52** Airway problems can be especially challenging in patients with serious facial injuries.

Courtesy of Dr. Ken Harrison, Careflight/NSW Institute of Trauma & Injury Management.

and bleeding into the airway. Control bleeding with direct pressure and suction as necessary.

## Assisting With ALS Airway Procedures

Many EMTs work as a team with a paramedic partner. When a critical patient needs an advanced airway intervention, the paramedic will perform the skill, but the EMT partner will play an essential role in helping set up for the procedure, performing BLS airway and ventilation maneuvers, and helping to monitor the patient.

### Assisting With Placement of Advanced Airways

Endotracheal (ET) intubation is the insertion of a tube into the trachea to maintain and protect the airway. The ET tube can be inserted through the mouth or through the nose. In either case, the ET tube passes directly through the larynx between the vocal cords and then into the trachea. You may also be asked to assist with the placement of other advanced airway devices.

### Patient Preparation

The first step in preparing a patient for ET intubation is oxygenation. Good oxygenation often includes bag-mask ventilation (including the use of an oral or nasal airway) and ensuring a proper seal, ventilation rate, volume of ventilation, and time for patient exhalation. Oxygen enters the bloodstream through the process of diffusion. The more oxygen that is available in the alveoli, the longer the patient can maintain adequate gas exchange in the lungs while the intubation procedure is being performed (**FIGURE 11-53**). This critical phase of the intubation procedure is called preoxygenation.

Maintain a high-flow nasal cannula on the patient during the preoxygenation phase and leave the nasal cannula in place during the intubation attempt, during which bag-mask ventilation and chest rise and fall are not possible. This technique, called apneic oxygenation, allows for continuous oxygen delivery down the airways during all phases of the intubation procedure.

Preoxygenation is a critical step in advanced airway management. Always follow your local protocols regarding the sequence of this procedure.

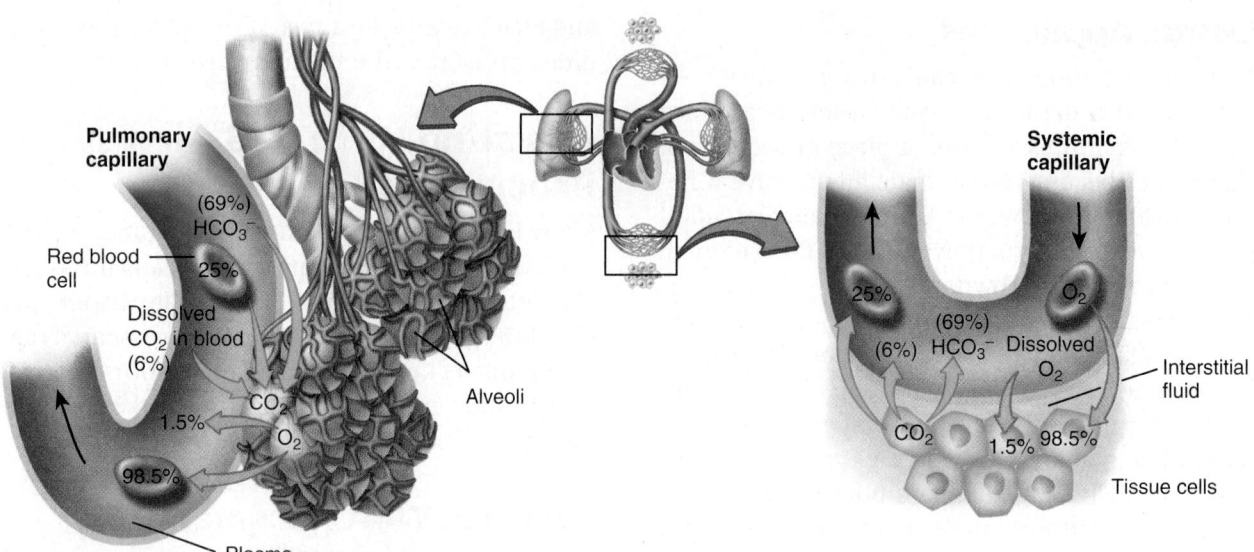

**FIGURE 11-53 A.** Alveolar–capillary exchange. Oxygen-rich air enters the alveoli, where it crosses into the bloodstream. Carbon dioxide leaves the blood and enters the alveoli. **B.** Capillary cellular exchange. Throughout the body, carbon dioxide from the cells enters the capillaries, and oxygen leaves the capillaries and enters the cells. Carbon dioxide is returned to the lungs in red blood cells (25%), in the form of bicarbonate (69%), and dissolved in blood (6%).

**A, B:** © Jones & Bartlett Learning.

## Equipment Setup

Equipment sets vary depending on local protocols, provider preference, and whether **direct laryngoscopy** or **video laryngoscopy** will be used. (Direct laryngoscopy is visualization of the vocal cords with a laryngoscope, while video laryngoscopy is visualization of the vocal cords using a video camera and monitor.) These differences emphasize why it is important for team members to train and practice together. Typically, intubation equipment sets include the following:

- Personal protective equipment, including face mask and eye shield
- Suction unit with rigid, tonsil-tip (Yankauer) and nonrigid, whistle-tip (French) catheters
- Laryngoscope handle and blade (sized for the patient)
- Magill forceps
- ET tube (sized for the patient)
- Stylette or tube introducer (**gum elastic bougie**)
- Water-soluble lubricant
- 10-mL syringe
- Confirmation device or devices, including waveform end-tidal $CO_2$ monitors and/or colorimetric device
- Commercial ET tube securing device
- Alternate airway management devices, such as a supraglottic airway and/or cricothyrotomy kit

### Words of Wisdom

When assembling the intubation equipment, you may have time to take extra steps, such as opening the ET tube package, lubricating the end of the ET tube with the water-soluble lubricant, attaching the 10-mL syringe, testing the cuff and pilot balloon, and checking the laryngoscope's light source.

## Performing the Procedure

While the details of endotracheal intubation may vary depending on available equipment, difficulties encountered, and provider preference, you can remember the six typical steps by using the BE MAGIC mnemonic:

- **B** Perform *Bag-mask* preoxygenation.
- **E** *Evaluate* for airway difficulties.
- **M** *Manipulate* the patient.
- **A** *Attempt* first-pass intubation.
- **GI** Use a supra*Glottic* airway if unable to intubate.
- **C** *Confirm* successful intubation/*Correct* any issues.

### Bag-Mask Device Preoxygenation

As discussed previously, it is crucial that you adequately preoxygenate the patient before the

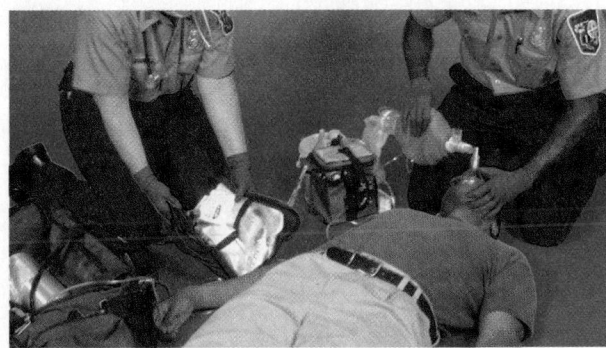

**FIGURE 11-54** One EMT or the paramedic may prepare the intubation equipment while another EMT continues to ventilate and preoxygenate the patient.

© Jones & Bartlett Learning. Courtesy of MIEMSS.

intubation procedure, especially critical patients (**FIGURE 11-54**). Do not hyperventilate the patient during the preoxygenation phase, because this may cause gastric distention and increase the risk of aspiration. Hyperventilation may also cause hypotension. Focus on maintaining a good seal, achieving chest rise and fall, and delivering breaths at a rate appropriate for the patient's age (1 breath every 6 seconds for an adult, and 1 breath every 2 to 3 seconds for an infant or child).

### Evaluate for Airway Difficulties

While you preoxygenate the patient, an ALS provider should evaluate the patient to identify any factors that will present difficulties during the procedure—for example, trauma or anatomic deformities to the airway. It is crucial that difficulties be identified before the procedure begins. You may assist with this process, as well as the preparation of any equipment that will be needed to address the problem or problems.

### Special Populations

It may be difficult for the ALS provider to visualize the vocal cords in bariatric and pediatric patients or patients with suspected cervical spine injuries. Expect to have particularly hands-on involvement with these patients. It is usually necessary to open (undo) a cervical collar to perform intubation. As the cervical collar is opened, you may be asked to maintain cervical spine immobilization while an ALS provider attempts intubation. Good communication and coordination between team members is critical during these advanced procedures.

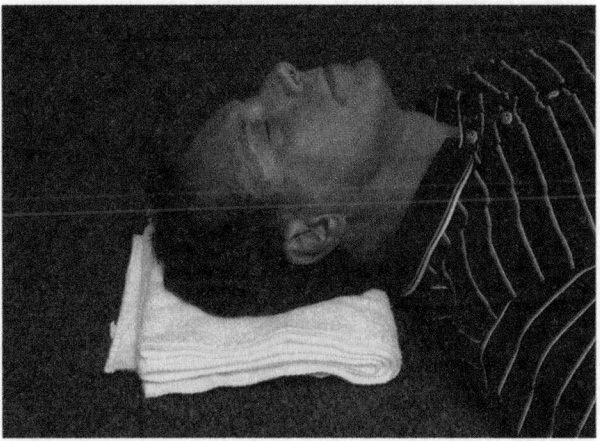

**FIGURE 11-55** The sniffing position: Position the patient so that the ear canal is on the same horizontal plane as the sternal notch.

© Jones & Bartlett Learning. Courtesy of MIEMSS.

### Manipulate the Patient

Before the procedure can begin, position the patient so that the ALS provider can visualize the vocal cords. Use towels, blankets, and pillows to ramp, position, and otherwise manipulate the patient so that the first attempted intubation will be successful. The ideal position is achieved when the patient's ear canal is on the same horizontal plane as his or her sternal notch, known as the sniffing position (**FIGURE 11-55**).

### Attempt Intubation

When the ALS provider is ready to begin the intubation attempt, remove the oral airway and disconnect the mask from the bag in preparation for connecting the bag to the ET tube. Always keep the mask and airway within reach in case the first attempt is unsuccessful and you need to ventilate the patient with the bag-mask device once more. Likewise, keep suction equipment at hand in case you need to suction the patient's airway. The ALS provider will begin by inserting the laryngoscope blade into the patient's mouth and will use it to move structures in the airway, such as the tongue and epiglottis, to gain a view of the vocal cords through which the ET tube will pass (**FIGURE 11-56**).

The ALS provider may ask you for assistance in manipulating the patient's larynx (external laryngeal manipulation) or otherwise positioning the patient for a better view (**FIGURE 11-57**). You may also be asked to hand the ET tube, gum elastic bougie, suction catheter, or other equipment to the ALS provider.

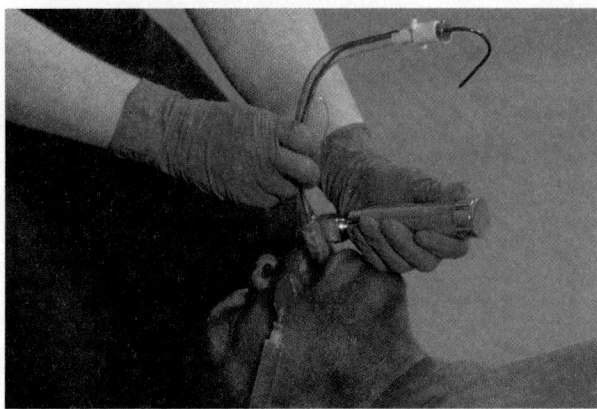

**FIGURE 11-56** The ALS provider will use the laryngoscope blade to visualize the target of the vocal cords through which the ET tube will pass.

© Jones & Bartlett Learning. Courtesy of MIEMSS.

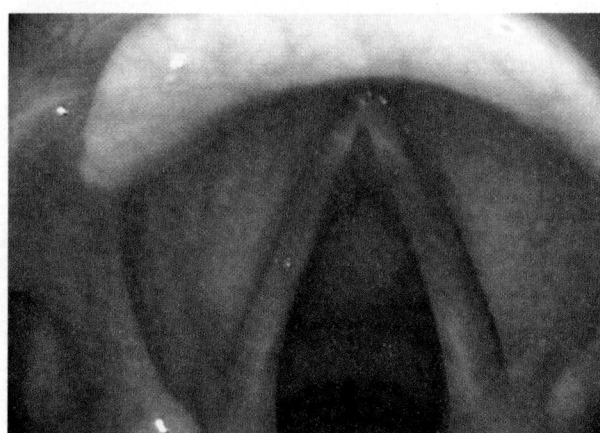

**FIGURE 11-57** The cuff of the ET tube must pass through the vocal cords.

Courtesy of James P. Thomas, M.D. (voicedoctor.net).

## Supraglottic Airway

Should the intubation attempts fail, it may be your responsibility to prepare and hand over the supra-glottic airway device (**FIGURE 11-58**).

### Words of Wisdom

An ALS provider may place an oral airway back into the patient's mouth after a successful intubation attempt to prevent the patient from biting down on the ET tube.

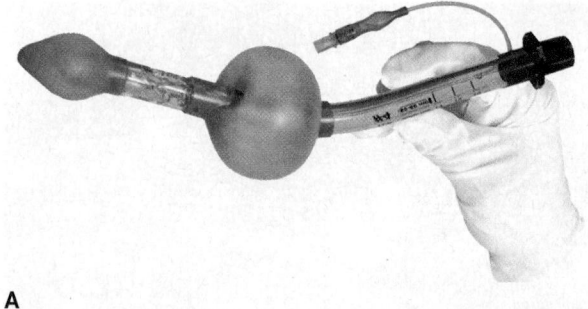

**A**

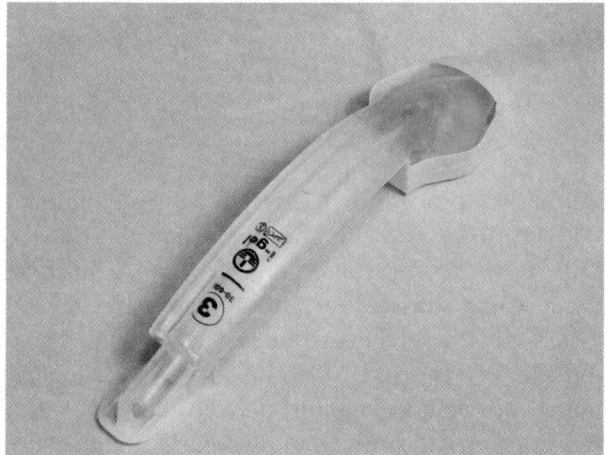

**B**

**FIGURE 11-58** Supraglottic airway devices. **A.** The King LT is a single-lumen supraglottic airway device. **B.** The i-gel airway device.

**A:** Courtesy of King Systems; **B:** © Photo Researchers, Inc/Science Source.

## Confirm Intubation/Correct Issues

If the intubation procedure appears successful, then work with your team to confirm intubation success. You may attach the end-tidal $CO_2$ wave-form detector in line between the ET tube and the bag. You may also either ventilate the patient while another provider checks for positive breath sounds and the absence of gastric sounds, or listen while another team member ventilates (**FIGURE 11-59**). A successfully intubated patient should have an end-tidal $CO_2$ waveform, bilateral breath sounds present, and gastric (or epigastric) sounds absent. Either absence of breath sounds or presence of gastric sounds suggests the ET tube was improp-erly inserted into the esophagus. If the intubation is confirmed as successful, then you may assist in

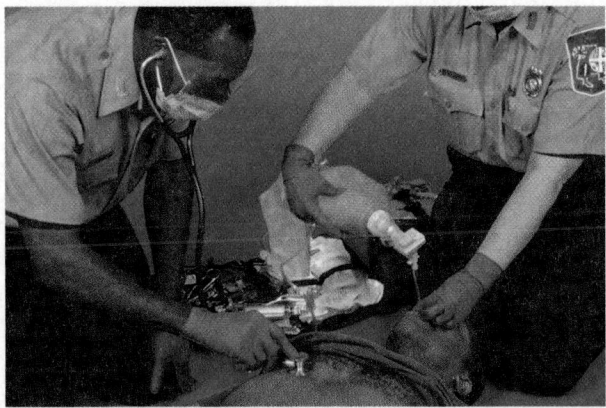

**FIGURE 11-59** Ventilate while listening for breath sounds to confirm successful placement of the ET tube.

© Jones & Bartlett Learning. Courtesy of MIEMSS.

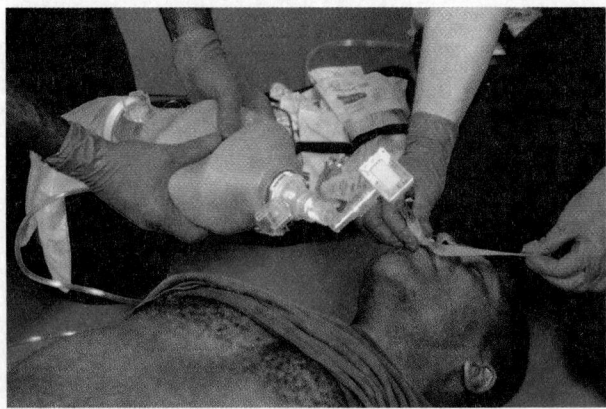

**FIGURE 11-60** Ensure the ET tube does not move while it is being secured or at any point during patient care.

© Jones & Bartlett Learning. Courtesy of MIEMSS.

securing the ET tube (**FIGURE 11-60**). If the intubation cannot be confirmed, or if the ET tube appears to be properly placed but airway or breathing issues remain, then you may assist other team members in correcting these issues.

## Words of Wisdom

The position of the ET tube is unstable before the tube is secured with tape or a mechanical device. Make sure the ET tube is not dislodged by movement at this point in the procedure or at any time during patient care.

## Continuing Care

Once an intubation attempt has been confirmed as successful, the job of airway management is not over for the EMS team. You must continue to observe all of the patient's monitor readings, as well as monitor for signs of potential complications, including the following:

- **Absence of an end-tidal $CO_2$ level.** Alert team members if the end-tidal $CO_2$ waveform suddenly disappears. (This is a sign the ET tube may have shifted out of the proper position.)
- **Decreasing $SpO_2$ level.** Alert team members if the $SpO_2$ level begins to drop, especially below 94%. (This is a sign the ET tube may have shifted out of the proper position.)
- **Increasing resistance when ventilating.** The person assigned the task of ventilation should monitor for increasing resistance when the bag is squeezed for ventilation. When increasing resistance is felt, it could indicate a critical airway or breathing problem that must be addressed, such as the advanced airway device has been mistakenly placed into the esophagus rather than into the trachea, referred to as **esophageal intubation**. When the ET tube is placed in the esophagus, ventilation results in air being pumped into the stomach, which increases the size of the patient's stomach and leads to gastric distention.

## Safety Tips

In the event of a pandemic involving a highly communicable disease, emergency care providers must consider not only the device most appropriate for the patient's emergency condition, but also the safety of using those devices for rescuers. There is a difference in the distance that aerosols are dispersed from various devices. Therefore, some simple modifications may be made for some patients. For example, it may be safer to use a nonrebreathing mask rather than a nasal cannula in these patients.

- **Other physical signs of poor ventilation and perfusion.** Physical signs include pale skin and cyanosis.
- **Improper positioning or dislodgement of the ET tube.** Each time the patient is moved, it is important to reassess the placement of the ET tube. Verify proper ET tube position by ensuring breath sounds are present, gastric sounds are absent, an end-tidal $CO_2$ waveform is visible during ventilation, $SpO_2$ values are stable or rising, and the ET tube is secured at the proper depth marking (**FIGURE 11-61**).

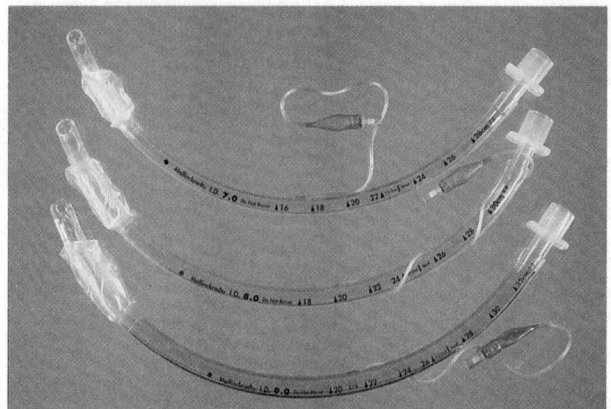

**FIGURE 11-61** Centimeter markings on the ET tube are used to ensure insertion to the appropriate depth.
© American Academy of Orthopaedic Surgeons.

# YOU are the Provider SUMMARY

**1. From the dispatch information, can you determine if this is a problem with the airway, ventilation, or oxygenation? Why or why not?**

Based on the dispatch information, you have no way of knowing the exact origin of the patient's problem. What you do know is that the patient has signs of hypoxia, as evidenced by her "turning blue" and not acting normally. A more detailed assessment will be required to determine if the origin is a problem with the airway, ventilation, or oxygenation. In the interest of the patient, however, you should assume a problem with all three.

**2. How does ventilation differ from oxygenation?**

Ventilation is the physical process of moving air into and out of the lungs. Oxygenation is the process of loading oxygen onto the hemoglobin in the bloodstream. To oxygenate, one must have the ability to breathe oxygen into the lungs during ventilation. Therefore, oxygenation without ventilation is not possible. However, it is possible for a patient to ventilate, but not oxygenate. For example, patients who are trapped in an area devoid of oxygen, such as a structural fire, grain silo, or trench, may continue to ventilate; however, because they are not breathing in oxygen, there is nothing to load onto the hemoglobin.

**3. Is it possible for a patient to ventilate but not oxygenate? Why or why not? What should your concerns be about PPE?**

Recall that ventilation is the simple process of moving air into and out of the lungs. Just because a patient is ventilating, you cannot assume that the patient is oxygenating as well. That determination is made by a careful clinical assessment, including assessment of the patient's surroundings. Prior to loading oxygen onto the hemoglobin (oxygenation), the air breathed in must contain an adequate supply of oxygen. This may not be the case if the patient is breathing in a gas other than oxygen (eg, carbon monoxide). Another example would be a pulmonary embolism. If deoxygenated blood cannot return to the lungs to be reoxygenated, there will not be adequate oxygen to load onto the hemoglobin. The patient may continue to ventilate but is not oxygenating.

Wear a mask and protective eyewear whenever airway management involves aerosol-generating procedures (AGPs) such as CPR, nebulizer treatments, endotracheal intubation, and continuous positive airway pressure.

**4. Why is slow, shallow breathing so dangerous?**

Alveolar minute volume, also called minute alveolar ventilation, is the volume of air that moves into and out of the lungs each minute. It is equal to tidal volume (the volume of air moved into and out of the respiratory tract with each breath) minus the dead space volume (the volume of air that lingers in the upper airway and large bronchi) multiplied by the respiratory rate. Alveolar minute volume depends on an adequate respiratory rate and adequate tidal volume. When tidal volume is reduced, the patient's breathing becomes shallow; this indicates that less air is being drawn into the lungs during inhalation. If the respiratory rate is too slow (or too fast)—especially when tidal volume is reduced—alveolar minute volume will decrease. As a result, oxygenation, and ultimately perfusion, will diminish. Left untreated, the patient will become hypoxic, potentially to the point of respiratory arrest or cardiopulmonary arrest.

**5. How should you proceed with airway management of this patient?**

As evidenced by her depressed level of consciousness and drooling, this patient cannot control her own airway. Therefore, anything that you do to treat her breathing would be ineffective if you do not secure her airway first. You should suction any secretions from her airway to prevent aspiration. To maintain patency of her airway, insert a nasopharyngeal airway. If she still has a gag reflex, an oropharyngeal airway could stimulate vomiting that could potentially lead to aspiration.

**6. What specifically does pulse oximetry measure?**

Pulse oximetry measures the percentage of hemoglobin that is bound to a gas. Despite it being called a pulse oximeter, one must not assume that it is oxygen that is bound to the hemoglobin; this requires a careful clinical assessment, as well as an assessment of the patient's environment. If the patient is not experiencing respiratory difficulty, has a normal rate and depth of breathing, and has normal skin color and condition, then it likely is oxygen that is bound to hemoglobin. However, it is important to remember that the pulse oximeter cannot distinguish oxygen from carbon monoxide, and carbon monoxide will bind to hemoglobin far more readily than oxygen will. Therefore, if the patient was pulled from a burning structure (or any other place that may have a high carbon monoxide content) and is unconscious and cyanotic, you should assume that the reading on the pulse oximeter does not reflect oxygen-hemoglobin binding.

**7. Based on your findings, what adjustments, if any, should be made to the current treatment plan?**

The patient is not ventilating adequately on her own. This is evidenced by numerous findings, including her mental status; cyanosis; slow, shallow breathing; and low oxygen saturation. If the patient cannot breathe in an adequate volume of air, passive oxygenation (such as what is delivered by a nasal cannula or nonrebreathing mask) is of minimal value. The patient requires ventilatory assistance. Use a bag-mask device attached to supplemental oxygen and deliver one breath every 6 seconds (10 breaths/min). If her inadequate breathing effort is not treated, she will become more hypoxic, which could ultimately result in respiratory or cardiopulmonary arrest.

**8. How does negative-pressure ventilation differ from positive-pressure ventilation?**

During the act of normal (unassisted) breathing, the diaphragm and intercostal muscles contract. The combined actions of these muscular contractions enlarge the thoracic cavity. As the thoracic cavity enlarges, intrathoracic pressure falls below that of atmospheric pressure and a vacuum is created in the chest; this pulls air into the lungs and blood back to the right side of the heart. When inhalation stops, exhalation occurs passively. By contrast, positive-pressure ventilation involves pushing air into the lungs, such as occurs during rescue breathing of an apneic patient or assisted ventilation of a patient with inadequate minute volume. When air is pushed into the lungs, intrathoracic pressure increases. If rescue breathing is performed too rapidly and/or with too much volume, the hyperinflated lungs can squeeze the heart, impairing its ability to refill with blood. If venous return is diminished, less blood will be delivered to the left side of the heart; as a result, cardiac output will decrease, and the patient could become hypotensive.

**9. How can positive-pressure ventilation affect cardiac output?**

If positive-pressure ventilation is performed correctly—that is, ventilating with just enough volume to produce visible chest rise and delivering a rate that is appropriate for the patient's age—the effects of positive-pressure ventilation on cardiac output are minimal. Problems arise, however, when the patient is hyperventilated

(ventilated too rapidly and/or with too much volume). Hyperventilation can have lethal consequences for your patient. The high airway pressures created with forceful ventilation can push air into the stomach, increasing the risks of regurgitation and aspiration. Hyperventilation can also increase intrathoracic pressure significantly, which can impair the right heart's ability to refill with blood.

**10. Based on the patient's deteriorating clinical status, what corrective action should be taken?**

First and foremost, the patient is not being adequately ventilated and/or oxygenated, as evidenced by her unresolving cyanosis, decreasing oxygen saturation, and now complete unresponsiveness. Critical to bag-mask ventilation is an adequate mask-to-face seal. Second, the rate of ventilation being used (24 breaths/min) is too fast—in fact, it is twice as fast as it should be. Considering that her blood pressure is continuing to drop without apparent cause, you should suspect that she is being hyperventilated and that her reduced cardiac output (and blood pressure) is secondary to reduced venous return to the right side of the heart. Immediate corrective action is to ensure an adequate mask-to-face seal; it would be optimal to perform two-person bag-mask ventilation. In addition, the patient should be ventilated at a rate of one breath every 6 seconds (10 breaths/min), with just enough volume to cause noticeable chest rise. Anytime a patient is receiving positive-pressure ventilation, it is important to monitor blood pressure and heart rate.

**11. How is capnography used to assess ventilation adequacy?**

Capnography measures the amount of carbon dioxide in exhaled air; it is reported as the end-tidal $CO_2$ and is measured in mm Hg, where the normal range is 35 to 45 mm Hg. $CO_2$ is the primary by-product of aerobic metabolism (metabolism in the presence of oxygen). As the $CO_2$ made at the cellular level returns to the lungs via the circulatory system, it is measured by the capnograph, which reports the information in the form of a numeric value and a waveform (hence the term *quantitative waveform capnography*). Capnography serves as an excellent indicator of ventilation adequacy because adequate ventilation is necessary to eliminate $CO_2$ from the body via the respiratory system. There are several reasons why an abnormal end-tidal $CO_2$ level may be observed. If a

problem with the respiratory system occurs—even if adequate $CO_2$ is being produced at the cellular level—end-tidal $CO_2$ values would increase because $CO_2$ cannot be adequately released from the body. Conversely, if $CO_2$ production at the cellular level is low (eg, during shock or cardiac arrest), or if the patient is eliminating $CO_2$ faster than the body is making it (eg, hyperventilation), end-tidal $CO_2$ levels would be correspondingly low. Another major benefit of capnography is that it provides data in real time, unlike pulse oximetry, which has a 60- to 90-second lag.

**12. What is the clinical significance of cyanosis?**

Cyanosis, a blue-gray discoloration of the skin, indicates that the amount of deoxygenated blood in the body has exceeded the amount of oxygenated blood. Recall that for oxygen to be delivered to the cells, it must first bind to hemoglobin. If minimal (or no) oxygen binds to hemoglobin, there is nothing to deliver to the cells. This is a clinically significant finding because it indicates a severe degree of hypoxia. It is important to note, however, that cyanosis is not an early sign; therefore, its absence should not be used to rule out hypoxia or a significant respiratory problem.

**13. What components of your assessment are consistent with acute pulmonary embolism?**

Although the patient's overall clinical status has improved, there remain a number of abnormalities that could be explained by an acute pulmonary embolism. Throughout the entire patient encounter, you will note that the patient's oxygen saturation never returned to a normal value, despite high-flow oxygen and assisted ventilation. This indicates the presence of ongoing hypoxemia. Initially, the patient was so hypoxic that her mental status was severely depressed, and she was on the verge of respiratory arrest. Although the patient's breathing did improve, it remained labored; although this could be caused by many different problems, labored breathing, hypoxemia that is not corrected with supplemental oxygen, and the initial clinical presentation (sharp chest pain, acute shortness of breath) are highly suspicious for acute pulmonary embolism.

**14. What is a ventilation/perfusion mismatch?**

For respiration to continue, air and blood must reach the same place at the same time; in other words, ventilation and perfusion must be matched. When

## YOU | are the Provider SUMMARY *continued*

this does not occur, a ventilation/perfusion mismatch exists. A pulmonary embolism is a perfect example of a condition that can cause a ventilation/perfusion mismatch. With a pulmonary embolism, air and oxygen reach the alveoli through inhalation. However, due to a thrombus in a pulmonary artery, blood flow does not reach every part of the lungs.

As a result, deoxygenated blood cannot be reoxygenated—a failure of pulmonary respiration. A ventilation/perfusion mismatch could also occur if airflow to the alveoli is reduced, although blood flow to the lungs is not. An example of this condition would be widespread alveolar collapse (atelectasis).

### EMS Patient Care Report (PCR)

| **Date:** 1-15-20 | **Incident No.:** 20014434 | **Nature of Call:** Respiratory | | **Location:** 214 James St. | |
|---|---|---|---|---|---|
| **Dispatched:** 1930 | **En Route:** 1932 | **At Scene:** 1936 | **Transport:** 1945 | **At Hospital:** 1953 | **In Service:** 2010 |

#### Patient Information

| **Age:** 49 <br> **Sex:** F <br> **Weight (in kg [lb]):** 68 kg (150 lb) | **Allergies:** None <br> **Medications:** None <br> **Past Medical History:** None <br> **Chief Complaint:** Respiratory distress |
|---|---|

#### Vital Signs

| **Time:** 1938 | **BP:** 98/64 | **Pulse:** 130 | **Respirations:** 4 | **Spo₂:** 72% |
|---|---|---|---|---|
| **Time:** 1942 | **BP:** 86/54 | **Pulse:** 148 | **Respirations:** 12 assisted | **Spo₂:** 70% |
| **Time:** 1946 | **BP:** 104/60 | **Pulse:** 110 | **Respirations:** 12 assisted | **Spo₂:** 80% |
| **Time:** 1953 | **BP:** 118/70 | **Pulse:** 109 | **Respirations:** 14 | **Spo₂:** 86% |

#### EMS Treatment (circle all that apply)

| **Oxygen @ _15_ L/min via:** <br><br> NC (NRM) Bag mask | **Assisted Ventilation** | **Airway Adjunct** | **CPR** |
|---|---|---|---|
| **Defibrillation** | **Bleeding Control** | **Bandaging** | **Splinting** | **Other** |

## YOU are the Provider SUMMARY *continued*

| Narrative |
| --- |

9-1-1 dispatch for a female patient who is "turning blue."

Chief Complaint: Respiratory distress

History: According to the patient's husband, she experienced acute shortness of breath and sharp chest pain approximately 5 minutes before he called 9-1-1. He further indicated that she started turning blue and deteriorated rapidly. Husband denies any past medical history and states that she takes no medications.

Assessment: Arrived on scene to find the patient, a 49-year-old woman, sitting in a recliner with obvious respiratory compromise. Her eyes were open slightly, and she would not answer when spoken to. Secretions were draining from her mouth. Skin was cool and dry, with cyanosis to the face and neck.

Treatment (Rx): Suctioned the patient's airway and inserted a nasopharyngeal airway for continued airway maintenance. Administered high-flow oxygen via nonrebreathing mask and continued assessment. Vital signs obtained and noted above. Noting poor respiratory effort and further deterioration, began assisting the patient's ventilations with a bag-mask device attached to high-flow oxygen.

Transport: No ALS available so this unit transported to ED and continued treatment en route. Assessment of assisted ventilation revealed that breath sounds were audible bilaterally with a stethoscope and chest rise was visible with each ventilation. En route, the patient's condition improved; assisted ventilation was discontinued, but supplemental oxygen was continued. The patient's breathing remained slightly labored and her oxygen saturation remained at less than 90%. On arrival at the ED, the patient was responsive to verbal stimuli and her cyanosis was resolving. Delivered patient to hospital staff and gave verbal report to attending physician.

**End of report**

# Prep Kit

## Ready for Review

- The upper airway includes the nose, mouth, jaw, oral cavity, pharynx, and larynx. Its function is to warm, filter, and humidify air as it enters the nose and mouth.
- The lower airway includes the trachea and lungs; its function is to exchange oxygen and carbon dioxide.
- Aerosol-generating procedures (AGPs) require enhanced PPE.
- Adequate breathing for an adult features a normal rate of 12 to 20 breaths/min, a regular pattern of inhalation and exhalation, adequate depth, bilaterally clear and equal lung sounds, and regular and equal chest rise and fall.
- Inadequate breathing for an adult features a respiratory rate of fewer than 12 breaths/min or more than 20 breaths/min, shallow depth (reduced tidal volume), an irregular pattern of inhalation and exhalation, and breath sounds that are diminished, absent, or noisy.
- Patients who are breathing inadequately show signs of hypoxia, a dangerous condition in which the body's tissues and cells do not have enough oxygen.
- Patients with inadequate breathing need to be treated immediately. Emergency medical care includes airway management, supplemental oxygen, and ventilatory support.

- Basic techniques for opening the airway include the head tilt–chin lift maneuver or, if trauma is suspected, the jaw-thrust maneuver.
- One basic airway adjunct is the oropharyngeal or oral airway, which keeps the tongue from blocking the airway in unconscious patients with no gag reflex. If the oral airway is not the proper size or is inserted incorrectly, it can cause an obstruction.
- Another basic airway adjunct is the nasopharyngeal or nasal airway, which is typically used with patients who have a gag reflex and is better tolerated than the oral airway.
- Suctioning is the next priority after opening the airway. Rigid tonsil-tip catheters are the best catheters to use when suctioning the pharynx; soft plastic catheters are used to suction the nose and liquid secretions in the back of the mouth.
- The recovery position is used to help maintain the airway in patients without traumatic injuries who are unconscious and breathing adequately.
- You must provide immediate artificial ventilations with supplemental oxygen to patients who are not breathing on their own. Patients with inadequate breathing may also require artificial ventilations to maintain effective tidal volume.
- Excessive supplemental oxygen can have a detrimental effect on patients with certain illnesses when administered for a prolonged time. Patients who require oxygen include (1) patients with signs of dyspnea, (2) patients with signs of shock, and (3) patients experiencing signs of a myocardial infarction with an oxygen saturation level lower than 94%. Use pulse oximetry, when available, to tailor oxygen administration to the patient's needs but do not rely on it exclusively.
- Handle compressed gas cylinders carefully; their contents are under pressure. Always make sure the correct pressure regulator is firmly attached before transporting a cylinder. The pin-indexing safety system features a series of pins on a yoke that must be matched with the holes on the valve stem of the gas cylinder. Pressure regulators reduce the pressure of gas in an oxygen cylinder to between 40 and 70 psi. Pressure-compensated flowmeters and Bourdon-gauge flowmeters permit the regulated release of gas measured in liters per minute.
- When oxygen therapy is complete, disconnect the tubing from the flowmeter nipple and turn off the cylinder valve, then turn off the flowmeter. As long as there is a pressure reading on the regulator gauge, it is not safe to remove the regulator from the valve stem. Keep any possible source of fire away from the area while oxygen is in use.
- Nasal cannulas and nonrebreathing masks are used most often to deliver oxygen in the field. The nonrebreathing mask is the delivery device of choice for providing supplemental oxygen to patients who are breathing adequately but are suspected of having or are showing signs of hypoxia. With a flow rate set at 15 L/min and the reservoir bag preinflated, the nonrebreathing mask can provide more than 90% inspired oxygen. If the patient will not tolerate a nonrebreathing mask, apply a nasal cannula.
- The methods of providing artificial ventilation include mouth-to-mask ventilation, two-person bag-mask ventilation, and one-person bag-mask ventilation. Combined with your own exhaled breath, mouth-to-mask ventilation will give a patient up to 55% oxygen; a bag-mask device with an oxygen reservoir and supplemental oxygen can deliver nearly 100% oxygen.
- CPAP is a noninvasive method of providing ventilatory support for patients in respiratory distress or experiencing sleep apnea.
- When you are providing artificial ventilation, remember that ventilating too forcefully can cause gastric distention. Slow, gentle breaths during artificial ventilation can help to prevent gastric distention. Patients who have a tracheal stoma or a tracheostomy tube need to be ventilated through the tube or the stoma.
- Foreign body airway obstruction usually occurs during a meal in an adult or while a child is

eating, playing with small objects, or crawling about the house. The earlier you recognize an airway obstruction, the better. You must learn to recognize the difference between airway obstruction caused by a foreign object and that caused by a medical condition.

- Foreign body airway obstructions are classified as being mild or severe. Patients with a mild airway obstruction are able to move adequate amounts of air and should be left alone. Patients with a severe airway obstruction cannot move any air at all and require immediate treatment. Perform abdominal thrusts on conscious adults and children with

a severe airway obstruction. If the patient becomes unconscious, open the airway and look in the mouth (do not perform blind finger sweeps), attempt to ventilate the patient, and perform chest compressions if ventilations are unsuccessful.

- Check for loose dental appliances in a patient before assisting ventilations. Loose appliances should be removed to prevent them from obstructing the airway. Tight-fitting appliances should be left in place.
- As an EMT, you may be asked to assist the paramedic in establishing an advanced airway.

## Vital Vocabulary

**aerobic metabolism** Metabolism that can proceed only in the presence of oxygen.

**aerosol-generating procedure** Any airway manipulation that induces the production of aerosols that may present a risk for airborne transmission of pathogens, such as CPR.

**agonal gasps** Abnormal breathing pattern characterized by slow, gasping breaths, sometimes seen in patients in cardiac arrest.

**airway** The upper airway tract or the passage above the larynx, which includes the nose, mouth, and throat.

**alveolar minute volume** The volume of air moved through the lungs in 1 minute minus the dead space; calculated by multiplying tidal volume (minus dead space) and respiratory rate.

**alveolar ventilation** The volume of air that reaches the alveoli. It is determined by subtracting the amount of dead space air from the tidal volume.

**American Standard Safety System** A safety system for large oxygen cylinders, designed to prevent the accidental attachment of a regulator to a cylinder containing the wrong type of gas.

**anaerobic metabolism** The metabolism that takes place in the absence of oxygen; the main by-product is lactic acid.

**apnea** Absence of spontaneous breathing.

**apneic oxygenation** A technique in which oxygen administered via a high-flow nasal cannula is left in place during an intubation attempt, allowing for continuous oxygen delivery into the airways during all phases of the procedure.

**aspiration** In the context of the airway, the introduction of vomitus or other foreign material into the lungs.

**ataxic respirations** Irregular, ineffective respirations that may or may not have an identifiable pattern.

**automatic transport ventilator (ATV)** A ventilation device attached to a control box that allows the variables of ventilation to be set. It frees the EMT to perform other tasks while the patient is being ventilated.

**bag-mask device** A device with a one-way valve and a face mask attached to a ventilation bag; when attached to a reservoir and connected to oxygen, it delivers more than 90% supplemental oxygen.

**barrier device** A protective item, such as a pocket mask with a valve, that limits exposure to a patient's body fluids.

**bilateral** A body part or condition that appears on both sides of the midline.

**bronchioles** Subdivision of the smaller bronchi in the lungs; made of smooth muscle and dilate or constrict in response to various stimuli.

**capnography** A noninvasive method to quickly and efficiently provide information on a patient's ventilatory status, circulation, and metabolism. It effectively measures the concentration of carbon dioxide in expired air over time.

**capnometry** The use of a capnometer, a device that measures the amount of expired carbon dioxide.

**carina** Point at which the trachea bifurcates (divides) into the left and right main stem bronchi.

**chemoreceptors** Monitor the levels of oxygen, carbon dioxide, and pH of the cerebrospinal fluid and then provide feedback to the respiratory centers to modify the rate and depth of breathing based on the body's needs at any given time.

**Cheyne-Stokes respirations** A cyclical pattern of abnormal breathing that increases and then decreases in rate and depth, followed by a period of apnea.

**compliance** The ability of the alveoli to expand when air is drawn in during inhalation.

**continuous positive airway pressure (CPAP)** A method of ventilation used primarily in the treatment of critically ill patients with respiratory distress; can prevent the need for endotracheal intubation.

**dead space** Any portion of the airway that does contain air and cannot participate in gas exchange, such as the trachea and bronchi.

**denitrogenation** The process of replacing nitrogen in the lungs with oxygen to maintain a normal oxygen saturation level during advanced airway management.

**diffusion** Movement of a gas from an area of higher concentration to an area of lower concentration.

**direct laryngoscopy** Visualization of the airway with a laryngoscope.

**dyspnea** Shortness of breath.

**endotracheal (ET) intubation** Insertion of an endotracheal tube directly through the larynx between the vocal cords and into the trachea to maintain and protect an airway.

**end-tidal $CO_2$** The amount of carbon dioxide present at the end of an exhaled breath.

**esophageal intubation** Improper placement of an advanced airway device into the esophagus rather than into the trachea.

**exhalation** The passive part of the breathing process in which the diaphragm and the intercostal muscles relax, forcing air out of the lungs.

**external respiration** The exchange of gases between the lungs and the blood cells in the pulmonary capillaries; also called pulmonary respiration.

**gag reflex** A normal reflex mechanism that causes retching; activated by touching the soft palate or the back of the throat.

**gastric distention** A condition in which air fills the stomach, often as a result of high volume and pressure during artificial ventilation.

**glottis** The space in between the vocal cords that is the narrowest portion of the adult's airway; also called the glottic opening.

**good air exchange** A term used to distinguish the degree of distress in a patient with a mild airway obstruction. With good air exchange, the patient is still conscious and able to cough forcefully, although wheezing may be heard.

**gum elastic bougie** A flexible device that is inserted between the glottis under direct laryngoscopy; the endotracheal tube is threaded over the device, facilitating its entry into the trachea.

**head tilt–chin lift maneuver** A combination of two movements to open the airway by tilting the forehead back and lifting the chin; not used for trauma patients.

**hemothorax** A collection of blood in the pleural cavity.

**hypercarbia** Increased carbon dioxide level in the bloodstream.

**hypoxia** Deficient oxygen concentration in the tissues.

**hypoxic drive** A "backup system" to control respiration; senses drops in the oxygen level in the blood.

**inhalation** The active, muscular part of breathing that draws air into the airway and lungs.

**internal respiration** The exchange of gases between the blood cells and the tissues.

**intrapulmonary shunting** Bypassing of oxygen-poor blood past nonfunctional alveoli to the left side of the heart.

**jaw-thrust maneuver** Technique to open the airway by placing the fingers behind the angle of the jaw and bringing the jaw forward; used for patients who may have a cervical spine injury.

**labored breathing** The use of muscles of the chest, back, and abdomen to assist in expanding the chest; occurs when air movement is impaired.

**larynx** A complex structure formed by many independent cartilaginous structures that all work together; where the upper airway ends and the lower airway begins; also called the voice box.

**mediastinum** Space within the chest that contains the heart, major blood vessels, vagus nerve, trachea, major bronchi, and esophagus; located between the two lungs.

**metabolism** The biochemical processes that result in production of energy from nutrients within the cells; also called cellular respiration.

**mild airway obstruction** Occurs when a foreign body partially obstructs the patient's airway. The patient is able to move adequate amounts of air, but also experiences some degree of respiratory distress.

**minute volume** The volume of air that moves into and out of the lungs per minute; calculated by multiplying the tidal volume and respiratory rate; also called minute ventilation.

**nasal cannula** An oxygen-delivery device in which oxygen flows through two small, tubelike prongs that fit into the patient's nostrils; delivers 24% to 44% supplemental oxygen, depending on the flow rate.

**nasopharyngeal (nasal) airway** Airway adjunct inserted into the nostril of an unresponsive patient or a patient with an altered level of consciousness who is unable to maintain airway patency independently.

**nasopharynx** The part of the pharynx that lies above the level of the roof of the mouth, or palate.

**nonrebreathing mask** A combination mask and reservoir bag system that is the preferred way to give oxygen in the prehospital setting; delivers up to 90% inspired oxygen and prevents inhaling the exhaled gases (carbon dioxide).

**oropharyngeal (oral) airway** Airway adjunct inserted into the mouth of an unresponsive patient to keep the tongue from blocking the upper airway and to facilitate suctioning the airway, if necessary.

**oropharynx** A tubular structure that forms the posterior portion of the oral cavity, which is bordered superiorly by the hard and soft palates, laterally by the cheeks, and inferiorly by the tongue.

**oxygenation** The process of delivering oxygen to the blood by diffusion from the alveoli following inhalation into the lungs.

**oxygen toxicity** A condition of excessive oxygen consumption resulting in cellular and tissue damage.

**parietal pleura** Thin membrane that lines the chest cavity.

**partial pressure** The term used to describe the amount of gas in air or dissolved in fluid, such as blood.

**passive ventilation** The act of air moving into and out of the lungs during chest compressions.

**patent** Open, clear of obstruction.

**phrenic nerves** The two nerves that innervate the diaphragm; necessary for adequate breathing to occur.

**pin-indexing system** A system established for portable cylinders to ensure that a regulator is not connected to a cylinder containing the wrong type of gas.

**pneumothorax** An accumulation of air or gas in the pleural cavity.

**poor air exchange** A term used to describe the degree of distress in a patient with a mild airway obstruction. With poor air exchange, the patient often has a weak, ineffective cough, increased difficulty breathing, or possible cyanosis and may produce a high-pitched noise during inhalation (stridor).

**preoxygenation** The process of providing oxygen, often in combination with ventilation, prior to intubation in order to raise the oxygen levels of body tissues; a critical step in advanced airway management. This extends the time during which an advanced airway can be placed in an apneic patient, because the more oxygen that is available in the alveoli, the longer the patient can maintain adequate gas exchange in the lungs during the procedure.

**pulse oximetry** An assessment tool that measures oxygen saturation of hemoglobin in the capillary beds.

**recovery position** A side-lying position used to maintain a clear airway in unconscious patients without injuries who are breathing adequately.

**residual volume** The air that remains in the lungs after maximal expiration.

**respiration** The process of exchanging oxygen and carbon dioxide.

**retractions** Movements in which the skin pulls in around the ribs during inspiration.

**severe airway obstruction** Occurs when a foreign body completely obstructs the patient's airway. The patient cannot breathe, talk, or cough.

**stoma** An opening through the skin and into an organ or other structure.

**stridor** A harsh, high-pitched respiratory sound, generally heard during inspiration, that is caused by partial blockage or narrowing of the upper airway; may be audible without a stethoscope.

**suction catheter** A hollow, cylindrical device used to remove fluid from the patient's airway.

**surfactant** A liquid protein substance that coats the alveoli in the lungs, decreases alveolar surface tension, and keeps the alveoli expanded; a low level in a premature infant contributes to respiratory distress syndrome.

**tension pneumothorax** An accumulation of air or gas in the pleural cavity that progressively increases pressure in the chest and that interferes with cardiac function, with potentially fatal results.

**tidal volume** The amount of air (in mL) that is moved into or out of the lungs during one breath.

**tonsil tips** Large, semi-rigid suction tips recommended for suctioning the pharynx.

**tracheostomy** A surgical procedure to create an opening (stoma) into the trachea; a stoma in the neck connects the trachea directly to the skin.

**ventilation** The exchange of air between the lungs and the environment; occurs spontaneously by the patient or with assistance from another person, such as an EMT.

**video laryngoscopy** Visualization of the vocal cords, and thereby placement of the endotracheal tube, that is facilitated by use of a video camera and monitor.

**visceral pleura** Thin membrane that covers the lungs.

**vital capacity** The amount of air that can be forcibly expelled from the lungs after breathing in as deeply as possible.

**vocal cords** Thin white bands of tough muscular tissue that are lateral borders of the glottis and serve as the primary center for speech production.

**wheezing** A high-pitched, whistling breath sound that is most prominent on expiration, and which suggests an obstruction or narrowing of the lower airways; occurs in asthma and bronchiolitis.

## References

1. American Heart Association. *Highlights of the 2020 American Heart Association Guidelines Update for CPR and ECC.* https://cpr.heart.org/-/media/cpr-files/cpr-guidelines-files/highlights/hghlghts_2020_ecc_guidelines_english.pdf. Accessed November 6, 2020.

2. American Heart Association. Interim guidance to reduce COVID-19 transmission during resuscitation care. https://newsroom.heart.org/news/interim-guidance-to-reduce-covid-19-transmission-during-resuscitation-care. Published 2020. Accessed May 7, 2020.

3. American Heart Association. Oxygenation and ventilation of COVID-19 patients: Module 2. Airway patients. https://cpr.heart.org/-/media/cpr-files/resources/covid-19-resources-for-cpr-training/oxygenation-and-ventilation-of-covid-19-patients/ovcovid_mod2_airwymgmt_200401_ed.pdf?la=en&hash=F635CB4126F9A8617E

CDA8706E1A8A0D273E36B5. Published 2020. Accessed May 7, 2020.

4. Berg RA, Hemphill R, Abella BS, et al. Part 5: adult basic life support: 2010 American Heart Association guidelines for cardiopulmonary resuscitation and emergency cardiovascular care. *Circulation*. 2010;122(18 Suppl 3): S685-S705.

5. Chameides L, Samson RA, Schexnayder SM, et al. *Pediatric Advanced Life Support Provider Manual*. Dallas, TX: American Heart Association; 2012.

6. Hamber EA, Bailey PL, James SW, et al. Delays in the detection of hypoxemia due to site of pulse oximetry probe placement. *J Clin Anesth*. 1999;11(2):113-118.

7. Hazinski MF. *Highlights of the 2010 American Heart Association Guidelines for CPR and ECC*. Dallas, TX: American Heart Association; 2010. http://www.heart.org /idc/groups/heart-public/@wcm/@ecc/documents /downloadable/ucm_317350.pdf.

8. Hubble MW, Richards ME, Jarvis R, Millikan T, Young D. Effectiveness of prehospital continuous positive airway pressure in the management of acute pulmonary edema. *Prehosp Emerg Care*. 2006;10(4):430-439.

9. Inogen. Types of oxygen tanks and oxygen tank sizes. http://www.inogen.com/resources/oxygen -concentrators/types-of-oxygen-tanks/. Accessed March 26, 2015.

10. National Association of State EMS Officials. *National Model EMS Clinical Guidelines*. https://www.nasemso .org/Projects/ModelEMSClinicalGuidelines/index.asp. Published 2016. Accessed October 23, 2018.

11. National Highway Traffic Safety Administration. *National Emergency Medical Services Education Standards*. DOT HS 811 077A. www.ems.gov/pdf/811077a.pdf. Published January 2009. Accessed June 14, 2014.

12. National Registry of Emergency Medical Technicians. *2015 Paramedic Psychomotor Competency Portfolio* (PPCP). Columbus, OH: National Registry of Emergency Medical Technicians; 2015.

13. National Registry of Emergency Medical Technicians. *Emergency Medical Technician Psychomotor Examination*. https://www.nremt.org/nremt/about/psychomotor_exam _emt.asp. Accessed June 18, 2014.

14. Taylor DM, Bernard SA, Masci K, et al. Prehospital noninvasive ventilation: a viable treatment option in the urban setting. *Prehosp Emerg Care*. 2008;12(1):42-45. Erratum in: *Prehosp Emerg Care*. 2009;13(1):151.

15. Tri-Med, Inc. Cylinder/tank specifications chart. http:// www.tri-medinc.com/page12.htm#cyl-spec. Updated January 1, 2016. Accessed March 26, 2015.

16. US Fire Administration. *Coffee Break Training–Fire Protection Series: Hazardous Materials: Compressed Gas Cylinder Control Valve Safety Systems*. Emmitsburg, MD: US Fire Administration National Fire Academy; 2014. http://www.usfa.fema.gov/downloads/pdf/coffee-break /cb_fp_2014_43.pdf.

17. Warner GS. Evaluation of the effect of prehospital application of continuous positive airway pressure therapy in acute respiratory distress. *Prehosp Disaster Med*. 2010;25(1):87-91.

18. Whittle JS, Pavlov I, Sacchetti AD, Atwood C, Rosenberg MS. Respiratory support for adult patients with COVID-19. *ACEP Open*. 2020;1(2):95-101. doi:10.1002 /emp2.12071. Accessed May 7, 2020.

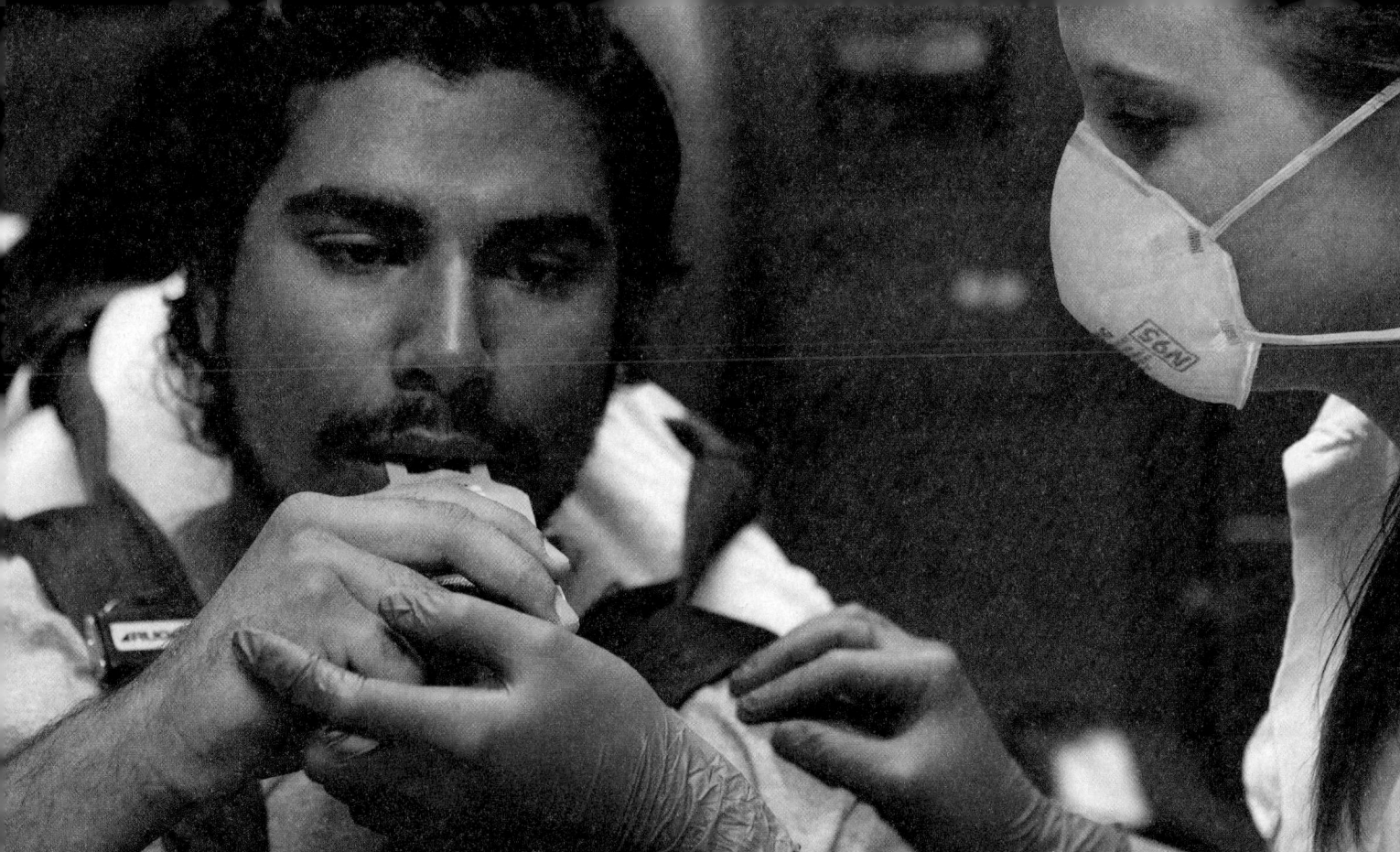

# Pharmacology

| 12 | Principles of Pharmacology |

SECTION

4

# Chapter 12

# Principles of Pharmacology

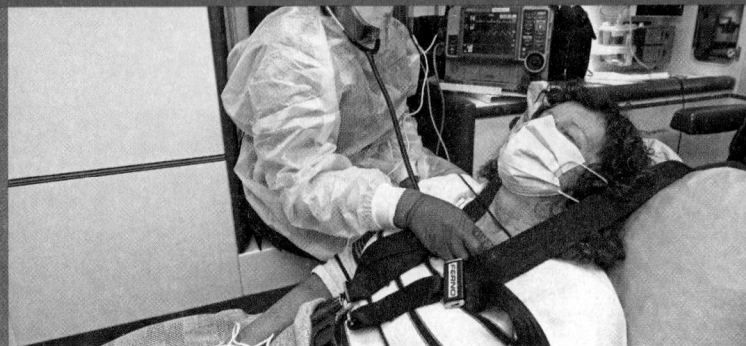

## NATIONAL EMS EDUCATION STANDARD COMPETENCIES

### Pharmacology

Applies fundamental knowledge of the medications that the EMT may administer to a patient during an emergency.

### Principles of Pharmacology

- Medication safety (pp 503–505)
- Kinds of medications used during an emergency (pp 507–518)

### Medication Administration

- Self-administer medication (pp 506–507)
- Peer-administer medication (pp 506–507)
- Assist/administer medications to a patient (pp 506–507)

### Emergency Medications

- Names (pp 497–498)
- Effects (pp 495–497)
- Actions (pp 495–497)
- Indications (p 497)
- Contraindications (p 497)
- Complications (p 497)
- Routes of administration (pp 498–500)
- Adverse effects (p 497)
- Interactions (pp 508–509, 518–519)
- Dosages for the medications administered (pp 496, 504, 508–509)

## KNOWLEDGE OBJECTIVES

1. Define the terms pharmacodynamics, therapeutic effects, indications, adverse effects, pharmacokinetics, onset of action, peak, duration, elimination, unintended effects, and untoward effects. (pp 495–497)
2. Explain medication contraindications; include an example. (p 497)
3. Explain the differences between a generic medication name and a trade medication name; provide an example of each. (p 497)
4. Differentiate enteral and parenteral routes of medication administration. (p 498)
5. Describe rectal, oral, intravenous, intraosseous, subcutaneous, intramuscular, intranasal, inhalation, sublingual, and transcutaneous routes of medication administration; include the rates of absorption. (pp 498–500)
6. Explain the solid, liquid, and gas forms of medication and the routes of administration; provide examples of each. (pp 501–503)
7. List the "rights" of medication administration; include how each one relates to EMS. (pp 503–505)
8. Explain the difference between direct orders (online) and standing orders (off-line) and the role of medical control. (p 506)
9. Discuss the medication administration circumstances involving peer-assisted

medication, patient-assisted medication, and EMT-administered medication. (pp 506–507)

10. Know the generic and trade names, actions, indications, contraindications, routes of administration, adverse effects, interactions, and doses of medications that may be administered by an EMT in an emergency as dictated by state protocols and local medical direction. (pp 497–518)

11. Describe the medication administration considerations related to special populations, including pediatric, geriatric, and pregnant patients. (pp 507, 515, 517)

12. State the steps to follow when administering medications to a patient using an auto-injector. (p 514)

13. Explain why determining what prescription and over-the-counter medications a patient is taking is a critical aspect of patient assessment during an emergency. (pp 518–519)

14. State the steps to take if a medication error occurs. (p 522)

## SKILLS OBJECTIVES

1. Apply the rights of medication administration. (pp 503–505)

2. Perform the medication cross-check procedure prior to administering a medication. (pp 505–506)

3. Demonstrate how to administer oral medication to a patient. (pp 507, 510–511)

4. Demonstrate how to administer aspirin to a patient with chest pain. (p 511)

5. Demonstrate how to administer oral glucose to a patient with hypoglycemia. (pp 507, 510)

6. Demonstrate how to assist a patient with the sublingual administration of a medication. (pp 511–513)

7. Demonstrate how to administer a medication by auto-injector. (p 514)

8. Demonstrate how to administer an intranasal medication. (p 515)

## Introduction

Medications are an important intervention available to you as an EMT. You must understand the medications within your scope of practice, just as paramedics and nurses must understand the medications they administer. Used appropriately, a medication may alleviate pain and improve a patient's condition. Failure to administer medications safely and competently can lead to serious consequences for the patient, including death. Therefore, it is essential that you have the knowledge and skills to administer or assist in administration of these medications.

This chapter describes the various forms of medications, the different ways in which they can be administered, and how they work. It then takes a close look at each of the seven forms of medications you may be asked to administer or help patients to self-administer. It will also explain when it is dangerous to administer these medications.

## How Medications Work

**Pharmacology** is the science of drugs, including their ingredients, preparation, uses, and actions on the body. Although the terms *drugs* and *medications* are often used interchangeably, the term *drugs* may make some people think of narcotics or illegal substances. For this reason, you should use the word *medications*, especially when interviewing patients and families. In general terms, a **medication** is a substance that is used to treat or prevent disease or relieve pain.

> ### Words of Wisdom
>
> It is important for you to become familiar with the "street" names of commonly used and abused drugs. Most users will not tell you they took methylenedioxymethamphetamine; most likely you will hear terms such as ecstasy, XTC, Molly, rolling, or popping. Research these street names using a reliable source, such as the National Institutes of Health (NIH) or the Centers for Disease Control and Prevention (CDC).

**Pharmacodynamics** is the process by which a medication works on the body. Different types of receptors are located throughout the body. Receptors are sites on cells where medications or chemicals produced in the body can bind and produce an effect. When medications are given, they bind to these sites and either stimulate the receptors to produce an effect or block the receptors to prevent other chemicals or medications from binding. Thus, a medication can either increase or decrease a normal function of the body. A medication that causes stimulation of receptors is called an **agonist**. A medication that binds to a receptor and blocks other medications or chemicals from attaching is called an **antagonist**, or blocker.

There are a variety of other ways that medications affect the body. Certain medications may add electrolytes such as potassium to the body. Other medications target the cell walls of invasive organisms. For example, an **antibiotic** targets bacteria, and an **antifungal** medication targets fungi. Finally, medications might change the concentration of substances in certain body compartments, prompting the movement of water molecules and chemicals from one area of the body to another.

The **dose** is the amount of the medication that is given. It often depends on the patient's weight or age. The dose also depends on the desired action of the medication. The **action** is the intended **therapeutic effect** that a medication is expected to have on the body. The therapeutic effect is also referred to as the desired or intended effect. These factors, among others, can help to explain why one dose of medication works quickly and efficiently on one patient and the same dose has little effect on another patient. Doses may need to be decreased for older adults because they cannot process medications as efficiently as younger people.

When administering a medication or treating an overdose, you should also consider how the body absorbs, distributes, changes, or eliminates a particular substance. These actions refer to the **pharmacokinetics** of a medication, or actions of the body upon the medication (or chemical). Pharmacokinetic properties for a medication include the following:

- **Onset of action**. Time from medication administration until clinical effects occur.
- **Duration**. Length of time that clinical effects persist.
- **Elimination**. How medications or chemicals are removed from the body.
- **Peak**. The point or period when the maximum clinical effect is achieved. For EMS providers, these times become particularly important when treating pain with opioid medications or managing an opioid overdose with naloxone (Narcan).

Many medications are transformed by the liver and/or eliminated by the kidneys. Patients with liver or kidney disease will have altered pharmacokinetics of many medications compared to healthy individuals. EMTs should understand both the pharmacodynamics and the pharmacokinetics of a medication when assessing a patient's response to a medication, monitoring for adverse effects, or considering the administration of repeat doses of a medication. These two sets of factors will determine how quickly a medication will begin to work, when its effects will peak, how long it will last, and when additional doses would be safe to administer. The route of administration will often have a

## Street Smarts

Scales in homes, day care centers, schools, and medical offices can be used to obtain an accurate patient weight on scene during EMS responses for infants and children. These devices can offer the most accurate means to calculate weight-based medications.

## YOU are the Provider

You and your partner are dispatched to a residence at 4864 Project Avenue for an older woman with "diabetic problems." The time is 0600 hours, the weather is clear, the traffic is light, and your response time to the scene is approximately 5 minutes.

**1.** What is pharmacology?

**2.** Why is knowledge of pharmacology important to patient care?

significant effect on both the pharmacodynamics and the pharmacokinetics of a particular medication or substance. Shock states, altered vital signs, and medication interactions can profoundly alter both the pharmacodynamics and the pharmacokinetics of medications administered by prehospital providers.

**Indications** are the reasons or conditions for which a particular medication is given. For example, nitroglycerin relaxes the walls of all blood vessels, both veins and arteries. This increases the blood flow and the supply of oxygen to the heart muscle. In this way, nitroglycerin may relieve the discomfort that can occur with the cardiac condition called angina. Therefore, nitroglycerin is indicated for chest pain associated with angina.

There are times when you should not give a medication, even if it usually is indicated for that person's condition. Such situations are called **contraindications**. A medication is contraindicated when it would harm the patient or have no positive effect on the patient's condition. For example, aspirin is an important treatment for patients experiencing a heart attack (acute myocardial infarction [MI]) or when treating pain for fever, yet it would be contraindicated in patients with a suspected head bleed. Some contraindications are absolute, meaning the medication should never be given if the contraindication is present. For example, severe hypotension is an absolute contraindication for nitroglycerin. Some contraindications are relative, meaning the benefits of administering the drug may outweigh the risks. For example, glaucoma (a condition of increased pressure within the eye) is a relative contraindication for many drugs. Consider a patient with anaphylaxis and a history of glaucoma. Glaucoma is a relative contraindication to the use of epinephrine; however, it would likely be more dangerous to withhold epinephrine from this patient than to administer it.

**Adverse effects** are any actions of a medication other than the desired ones. Adverse effects can occur even when medications are administered correctly. There are two types of adverse effects: unintended effects and untoward effects. **Unintended effects** are undesirable but pose little risk to the patient, such as a slight headache after taking nitroglycerin. **Untoward effects** can be harmful to the patient, such as hypotension after taking nitroglycerin.

Consider diphenhydramine (Benadryl). People take this medication for allergic reactions (indication). The medication is supposed to block the effects of histamine (intended effect). Its adverse effects include dry mouth and drowsiness (unintended effect) and it can increase the pressure of the fluid within the eye (untoward effect). Asthma is a relative contraindication for diphenhydramine because it can worsen lower airway constriction.

## Medication Names

Medications usually have two names. The **generic name** (such as ibuprofen) is a simple, clear, nonproprietary name. The generic name is not capitalized. Sometimes a medication is called by its generic name more often than by any of its trade names. For example, you may hear "nitroglycerin" used more often than the trade names Nitromist and Nitrostat. All medications that are licensed for use in the United States are listed by their generic names in the *United States Pharmacopoeia and National Formulary (USP-NF)*. The generic name is approved by the US Food and Drug Administration (FDA) for new drugs. The FDA regulates drug safety and effectiveness in the United States. The Federal Food, Drug, and Cosmetic Act of 1938 gives the FDA authority to enforce drug safety standards.

A **trade name** is the brand name that a manufacturer gives to a medication, such as Tylenol (acetaminophen). As a proper noun, a trade name begins with a capital letter. Trade names are used in every aspect of our daily lives, not just in medications. Well-known examples include Jell-O, Band-Aid, Kleenex, and Coke. A medication may have many different trade names, depending on how many companies manufacture it. Advil, Nuprin, and Motrin all are trade names for the generic medication ibuprofen. A trade name is sometimes designated by use of a raised registered symbol—that is, Advil®.

Medications may be **prescription medications** or **over-the-counter (OTC) medications**. Prescription medications are distributed to patients only by pharmacists according to a physician's order. OTC medications may be purchased directly, without a prescription. In recent years, many medications previously available only by prescription have become available in OTC form, such as Nasacort, Nexium, and Flonase.

You may come in contact with patients who have taken recreational drugs such as heroin or cocaine. Other patients may take herbal remedies, enhancement drugs, vitamin supplements, or alternative medicines. As we have discussed, the body's cells are configured to operate using chemical reactions; they cannot discern between safe and unsafe pharmacologic agents. Any medication that a patient takes can be pharmacologically active and can cause an effect. As an EMT, you need to ask patients about any and all medications they take.

### Street Smarts

Because many herbal medications, supplements, and OTC medications can interact with prescription medicines, it is a good idea to bring them to the hospital so the physician has a full picture of the patient's medication use.

## Routes of Administration

Medications can enter the body through a variety of routes. To simplify this topic, the routes of medication administration are divided into two categories: enteral and parenteral. **Enteral medications** enter the body through the digestive system. Typically, the form of the medication will be a pill or a liquid such as cough medicine. Medications administered via this route tend to absorb slowly. Most emergency medications are not administered orally because the delayed absorption would limit their efficacy when time is crucial. Aspirin and certain **antipyretics** (fever-reducing medications) are common exceptions and may be administered orally by EMS providers in many systems. **Parenteral medications** enter the body by a route other than the digestive tract, the skin, or the mucous membranes. Parenteral medications are often in a liquid form and are generally administered using syringes and needles. These medications are absorbed much more quickly and offer a more predictable and measurable response.

Regardless of the route of administration of a medication, the end goal is to get the medication into the bloodstream. **Absorption** is the process by which medications travel through body tissues until they reach the bloodstream. Often, the rate at which a medication is absorbed into the bloodstream depends on its route of administration (**TABLE 12-1**).

**TABLE 12-1** Routes of Administration and Rates of Absorption

| Route | Rate |
|---|---|
| **Enteral** | |
| Sublingual (SL) | Rapid |
| Per rectum (PR) | Rapid |
| By mouth (PO) | Slow |
| **Parenteral** | |
| Intravenous (IV) | Immediate |
| Intraosseous (IO) | Immediate |
| Inhalation | Rapid |
| Intranasal (IN) | Rapid |
| Intramuscular (IM) | Moderate |
| Subcutaneous | Slow |
| Transcutaneous | Slow |

© Jones & Bartlett Learning.

Common routes of medication administration are described as follows:

- **Per rectum (PR)**. Per rectum literally means through the rectum. This route of delivery is most commonly used with children because of easier administration and more reliable absorption. (Children often regurgitate some or all of a medication.) For similar reasons, many medications that are used for nausea and vomiting come in a rectal suppository form. Some medications to control seizures are administered PR when it is impossible to administer them intravenously. The PR route also is used to give some medications when the patient cannot swallow or is unconscious.
- **Oral**. Many medications are taken by mouth, or **per os (PO)**, and enter the bloodstream through the digestive system. This process often takes as long as 1 hour but may be surprisingly rapid, depending on the substance or form of preparation. One of the advantages of using this route is that it is noninvasive. Patients are often much happier to take a pill than to have a needle stuck in them. It is also often less expensive to use enteral medications than

to use parenteral forms. The main disadvantage of this administration route is the unpredictability of medication absorption. If the patient has vomiting or diarrhea, the amount of medication that is absorbed will be altered. Some medication preparations, referred to as orally disintegrating tablets, are put directly onto the tongue, where they dissolve. This is an alternative administration form for patients who may have difficulty swallowing. Some forms of medications are adversely affected by stomach acids, so dissolving them directly on the tongue avoids breakdown by gastric acids. An example of this type of medication is ondansetron (Zofran), which is used to treat nausea and vomiting.

- **Intravenous (IV) injection.** Intravenous means into the vein. Medications that need to enter the bloodstream immediately may be injected directly into a vein. This is the fastest way to deliver a chemical substance, but the IV route cannot be used for all chemicals. For example, aspirin, albuterol, and oxygen cannot be given by the IV route.
- **Intraosseous (IO) injection.** Intraosseous means into the bone. Medications that are given by this route reach the bloodstream through the bone marrow. Giving a medication by the IO route, into the marrow, requires drilling a needle into the outer layer of the bone. Because this is painful, the IO route is used most often in patients who are unconscious as a result of cardiac arrest or extreme shock. Often, the IO route is used for children who have fewer available (or difficult to access) IV sites. In general, any medication that can be given by the IV route can be given by the IO route. This route may be more desirable in critical patients in whom IV access will take longer.
- **Subcutaneous injection.** Subcutaneous means under the skin. A subcutaneous injection is given into the fatty tissue between the skin and the muscle. Because there is less blood here than in the muscles, medications that are given by this route are generally absorbed more slowly, and their effects last longer. A subcutaneous injection is a useful way to give medications that cannot be taken by mouth, as long as they do not irritate or damage the tissue. Daily insulin injections for patients with

diabetes are given by the subcutaneous route. Some forms of epinephrine can be given by the subcutaneous route.

- **Intramuscular (IM) injection.** Intramuscular means into the muscle. Usually, medications that are administered by IM injection are absorbed quickly because muscles have a lot of blood vessels. However, not all medications can be administered by the IM route. Possible problems with IM injections are damage to muscle tissue and uneven, unreliable absorption, especially in people with decreased tissue perfusion or who are in shock.

  You will typically use the IM route of medication administration with an auto-injector. These devices deliver a predetermined amount of medication into the patient when pressed firmly into the thigh. Examples of this delivery method would be the EpiPen auto-injector, which is used for anaphylactic reactions (see Chapter 21, *Allergy and Anaphylaxis*), and the DuoDote auto-injector and Antidote Treatment-Nerve Agent Auto-Injector (ATNAA), which are used for nerve agent exposure. (See Chapter 41, *Terrorism Response and Disaster Management.*)
- **Inhalation.** Some medications are inhaled into the lungs so that they can be absorbed into the bloodstream more quickly. Others are inhaled because they work in the lungs. Generally, inhalation helps minimize the effects of the medication in other body tissues. Such medications come in the form of aerosols, fine powders, and sprays.
- **Sublingual (SL).** Sublingual means under the tongue. Medications given by the SL route, such as nitroglycerin tablets, enter through the oral mucosa under the tongue and are absorbed into the bloodstream within minutes. This route is faster than the oral route, and it protects medications from chemicals in the digestive system, such as acids that can weaken or inactivate them.
- **Transcutaneous (transdermal).** Transcutaneous means through the skin. Some medications can be absorbed transcutaneously, such as the nicotine in patches used by people who are trying to quit smoking. On occasion, a medication that also comes in another form is administered transcutaneously to achieve a

## Words of Wisdom

Transdermal patches may contain massive quantities of medication that may be released rapidly if the patches are chewed or taken orally through accident or misuse. Children, often toddlers, may face a life-threatening overdose emergency if they chew adult medication patches. Consult a Poison Control Center or online medical control in these situations. Transdermal patches, such as those containing the potent opioid medication fentanyl (Sublimaze), continually release medication and may complicate resuscitation efforts when left in place on critical patients. Consult local protocols or guidelines regarding the removal of transdermal patches during resuscitation or overdose situations.

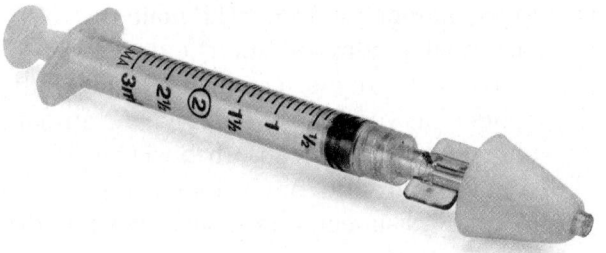

**FIGURE 12-1** Mucosal atomizer device can be used for drugs approved for intranasal use.

within the head and neck are very vascular; therefore, absorption is rather quick with this route.

**TABLE 12-2** lists the words that are used for routes of medication delivery, along with their meanings.

## Safety Tips

Make absolutely certain you follow standard precautions when administering any medication, particularly topical drugs. If the medication can be absorbed into the patient's skin, it can be absorbed into yours as well.

longer-lasting effect. An example is an adhesive patch containing nitroglycerin.

- **Intranasal (IN).** In the intranasal route of medication administration, a liquid medication is pushed through a specialized device called a **mucosal atomizer device (MAD)** (**FIGURE 12-1**). The liquid medication is aerosolized and is administered into a nostril. The mucous membranes lining the sinuses and passageways

### TABLE 12-2 Routes of Administration: Words and Their Meanings

| This Word... | From These Latin Words... | Means |
| --- | --- | --- |
| Inhalation | *inhalatio* (drawing air into the lungs) | inhaling or breathing in |
| Intramuscular (IM) | *intra* (into) and *muscularis* (of the muscles) | into muscle |
| Intraosseous (IO) | *intra* (into) and *osse* (bone) | into bone |
| Intravenous (IV) | *intra* (into) and *venosus* (of the veins) | into vein |
| Per os (PO) | *per* (by) and *os* (mouth) | by mouth |
| Per rectum (PR) | *per* (by) and *rectum* (rectum) | by rectum |
| Subcutaneous | *sub* (under) and *cutis* (skin) | under the skin |
| Sublingual (SL) | *sub* (under) and *lingua* (relating to the tongue) | under the tongue |
| Transcutaneous (transdermal) | *trans* (through) and *cutis* (skin) | through the skin |
| Intranasal | *intra* (into) and *nasal* (nose) | into the nose |

## Medication Forms

The form of a medication usually dictates the route of administration. For example, a tablet or a spray cannot be given through a needle. The manufacturer chooses the form to ensure the proper route of administration, the timing of its release into the bloodstream, and its effects on the target organs or body systems. As an EMT, you should be familiar with the following seven medication forms.

### Tablets and Capsules

Most medications that are given by mouth to adult patients are in tablet or capsule form. Capsules are gelatin shells filled with powdered or liquid medication. If the capsule contains liquid, the shell is sealed and usually soft. If the capsule contains powder, the shell can usually be pulled apart. Tablets often contain other materials that are mixed with the medication.

Some tablets are designed to dissolve quickly in small amounts of liquid so that they can be given sublingually (under the tongue) and absorbed rapidly. An example is the sublingual nitroglycerin tablet used to treat chest pain in patients with cardiac conditions. These medications are especially useful in emergency situations, because medications that must be swallowed and then digested require more time to have an effect. For example, an oral pain medication is less useful than an IV pain medication when pain relief is needed immediately.

### Solutions and Suspensions

A solution is a liquid mixture of one or more substances that cannot be separated by filtering or allowing the mixture to stand. Solutions can be given by almost any route. When given by mouth, solutions may be absorbed from the stomach rather quickly because the medication is already dissolved. Specially prepared solutions can be given as an IV, IM, or subcutaneous injection. If a patient has an anaphylactic reaction, you may help the patient to self-administer a solution of epinephrine using an auto-injector (EpiPen).

Many substances do not dissolve well in liquids. Some of these can be ground into fine particles and evenly distributed throughout a liquid by shaking or stirring. This type of mixture is called a suspension. An example is acetaminophen (Tylenol) suspension, given to infants and children for fever control or pain relief.

## YOU are the Provider

You arrive at the scene and find the patient, a 68-year-old woman, sitting in a recliner in her living room. Her son, who called 9-1-1, tells you that she is not "acting right." He also tells you that she has taken her medications today but is not sure when she last ate. You assess the patient as your partner opens the jump kit and prepares to begin treatment.

| Recording Time: 0 Minutes | |
|---|---|
| Appearance | Confused; diaphoretic; pale |
| Level of consciousness | Conscious but confused |
| Airway | Open; clear of secretions or foreign bodies |
| Breathing | Increased rate; shallow depth |
| Circulation | Radial pulses rapid and weak; skin pale and diaphoretic |

As your partner gives the patient high-flow oxygen via nonrebreathing mask, her son tells you that she has diabetes, heart disease, and depression. Her medication list includes eight different prescription medications, including glimepiride (Amaryl) for her diabetes, nitroglycerin (Nitrostat) for her heart disease, and sertraline (Zoloft) for her depression. You assess her blood glucose level, which reads 36 mg/dL. The patient is disoriented to place and time but able to speak and follow simple commands.

**3.** Other than oxygen, what other medication does this patient require, and why?

**4.** Why is it significant to know the patient took her medications on an empty stomach?

Suspensions separate if they stand or are filtered. It is important that you shake or swirl a suspension before administering it to ensure that the patient receives the right amount of medication.

Suspensions usually are administered by mouth but sometimes are given rectally. Occasionally, suspensions are applied directly to the skin to treat skin problems. You may have used calamine lotion in this way. Injectable suspensions are given via IM or subcutaneous injection only. Certain hormone shots or vaccinations are given this way because of the suspended particles. They cannot be given by IV injection because the suspended particles do not remain dissolved.

## Metered-Dose Inhalers

If liquids or solids are broken into small enough droplets or particles, they can be inhaled. A **metered-dose inhaler (MDI)** is a miniature spray canister used to direct such substances through the mouth and into the lungs (**FIGURE 12-2**) and is often used by a patient with a respiratory illness such as asthma or emphysema. An MDI delivers the same amount of medication each time it is used. Because an inhaled medication usually is suspended in a propellant, the MDI must be shaken vigorously before the medication is administered. Many patients who use MDI medications also self-administer medications with a nebulizer. Use of MDIs and nebulizers will be discussed later in this chapter.

## Topical Medications

Lotions, creams, and ointments are **topical medications**; that is, they are applied to the surface of the skin and affect only that area. Lotions contain the most water, and ointments contain the least. Lotions (such as calamine lotion) are absorbed the most rapidly, and ointments (such as triple antibiotic ointment [Neosporin]) the most slowly. Hydrocortisone cream, to diminish skin itching, is an example of a medical cream that can also be given in ointment form.

## Transcutaneous Medications

Transdermal medications are designed to be absorbed through the skin, or transcutaneously. Medications such as nitroglycerin paste usually have properties or delivery systems that help to dilate the blood vessels in the skin and, thus, speed absorption into the bloodstream. In contrast to most topical medicines, which work directly on the application site, transdermal medications are usually intended for systemic (whole-body) effects. A note of caution: If you touch such a medication with your bare skin while administering it, you will absorb it just as readily as the patient will. This can be very dangerous. For example, if you absorb nitroglycerin paste, your blood pressure may drop and cause you to faint while driving the ambulance to the hospital.

One delivery system for transcutaneous medications is the adhesive patch. Patches attach to the skin and allow even absorption of a medication for many hours (**FIGURE 12-3**). Prescription and OTC

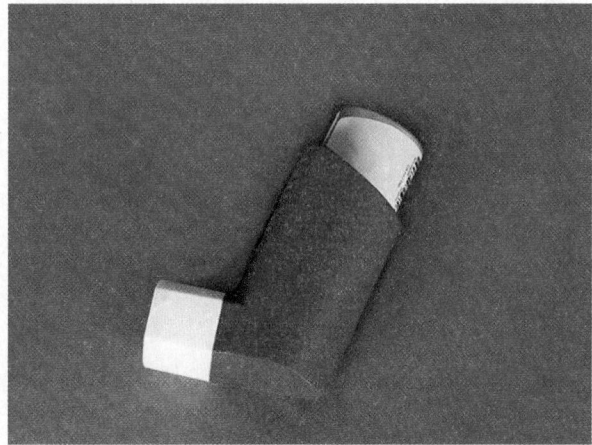

**FIGURE 12-2** Some medications are inhaled into the lungs with a metered-dose inhaler so that they can be absorbed into the bloodstream near the site of desired action more quickly.

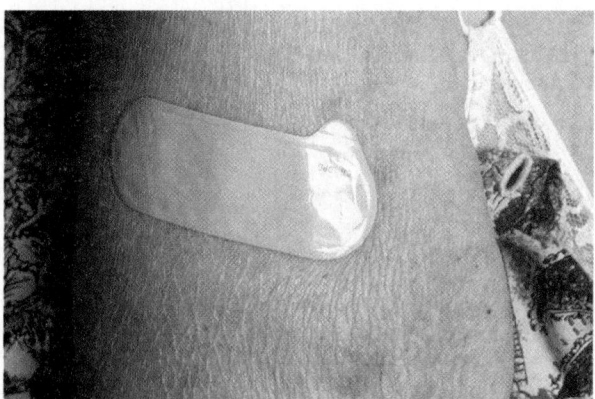

**FIGURE 12-3** Some medications are transcutaneous, or administered through the skin, such as the nitroglycerin patch shown.

medications come in this form. Common examples are nitroglycerin, nicotine, some pain medications, and some oral contraceptives.

## Gels

A **gel** is a semiliquid substance that is administered orally in capsule form or through plastic tubes. Gels usually have the consistency of pastes or creams but are transparent (clear). "Gelatinous" means thick and sticky, like gelatin. Depending on your local medical directives, as an EMT, you may give oral glucose in gel form to a patient with diabetes (**FIGURE 12-4**).

## Gases for Inhalation

Gaseous medications are neither solid nor liquid. The medication most commonly used in gaseous form is oxygen. You might not think of oxygen as a medication; however, in its concentrated form, it is a potent medication that has systemic effects. You will deliver this gas through a nonrebreathing mask,

### Words of Wisdom

When you document the use of oxygen, include the liter flow rate, the time oxygen was delivered (usually recorded in military time), and the type of device used. For example, "0915—Nonrebreathing mask at 15 L/min. Patient states shortness of breath has improved." *Always* remember to document the patient's response to oxygen administration.

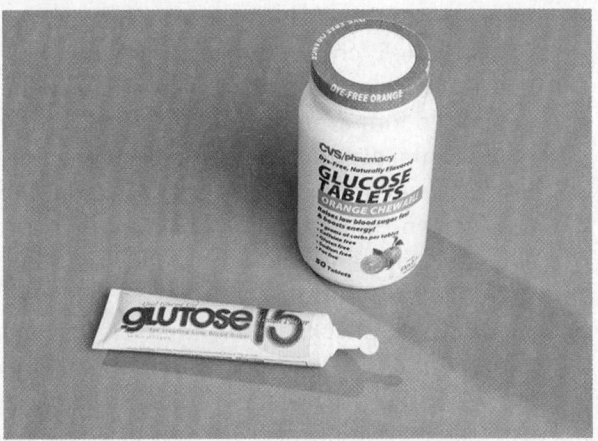

**FIGURE 12-4** Oral glucose, used in diabetic emergencies, is available in gel and tablet forms.
© Jones & Bartlett Learning.

nasal cannula, or bag-mask device. Current guidelines and potential risks of oxygen administration are discussed in Chapter 11, *Airway Management.*

## General Steps in Administering Medication

As an EMT, you may only administer medications for which you have an order from medical control. Medical control may be provided online or offline based on local protocol. You must be familiar with the general steps of administering any medication to a patient. These steps are the "rights" of medication administration (**TABLE 12-3**). Medication errors, which will be discussed later in this chapter, are disturbingly common and almost always result from failure to follow these rights. After the medication has been administered, you will need to reassess the patient to see if it worked. You should look for adverse effects and then be prepared to document your findings and your actions.

When administering or assisting with the administration of patient medications, you must have an order from medical control to do so. If this order is given to you directly through online medical control, it is important that you repeat the order back to the physician. This is referred to as the echo technique, and it is done to ensure that you heard the order correctly.

The following example illustrates the correct way to acknowledge orders for medications. EMT Johnson is talking on the radio to medical control.

**TABLE 12-3** The "Rights" of Medication Administration

| |
|---|
| Right patient |
| Right medication and indication |
| Right dose |
| Right route |
| Right time |
| Right education |
| Right to refuse |
| Right response and evaluation |
| Right documentation |

© Jones & Bartlett Learning.

She has already given the physician all of the patient assessment information and vital signs. She now asks, "Do you have any orders?" Dr. Ortez says, "Yes, please assist the patient with one nitroglycerin tablet. Make sure the tablet is administered sublingually. Reassess the patient's pain and blood pressure and contact me for further orders if needed." EMT Johnson should reply, "Dr. Ortez, I copy one nitroglycerin tablet sublingual, reassess the patient's pain and blood pressure, and contact you again if needed." Dr. Ortez says, "That is correct. ABC Hospital clear."

If at any point while you are receiving an order for a medication you are confused or unclear about what to do, you should tell medical control. It is very important that you understand what the physician wants you to do. With all of the noise on a hectic scene, or in the back of an ambulance, it is important to err on the cautious side. If you are not sure what to do, say so and ask for the order to be clarified. If you believe a medication order may be harmful to the patient, it is your responsibility to address your concerns with the ordering physician.

The other way to receive orders to administer or assist with medications is through indirect or offline medical control. Protocols are documents that contain standing orders for the administration of certain medications in specific circumstances. For example, your system may use a protocol that describes how the medical director wants you to deal with a patient who is having respiratory difficulties. Part of this protocol may direct you to use a nonrebreathing mask to deliver oxygen at 15 L/min. You may do this without calling online medical control if the patient meets the criteria of the protocol.

The "rights" of medication administration are as follows:

1. **Right patient.** For EMS, this safety check may seem unneeded if there is only one patient; however, there will be times when you will be working with more than one patient. Consider the following scenario. You respond to a patient with chest pain and discover that the patient is preparing to self-administer one nitroglycerin tablet sublingually. You check the bottle prior to administration and discover that the medication was actually prescribed for his wife. Depending on local protocols, administering a medication that was prescribed for a different patient may represent a violation.

2. **Right medication and indication.** Verify the proper medication and prescription, if applicable. Once received, confirm the medication order and determine that the patient is still a candidate for the medication. Make sure the patient does not have any contraindications for the medication. It is always a good idea to have your partner confirm the medication before you administer it. Carefully read the label. If it is the patient's own prescription, the bottle may show the trade name or the generic name. If you have any questions, contact online medical control. Make sure that the medication is the patient's own and does not belong to a friend or relative. You should never give a patient a medication that was prescribed for someone else.

3. **Right dose.** Verify the form and dose of the medication. Once you have confirmed the order and verified that the medication is the correct one to give, you must make sure that the form of the medication and the dose are correct. This is where it is important to pay close attention to detail. If you are ordered to give 324 mg of aspirin, you will need to read the bottle to determine how many milligrams are in each tablet. If aspirin is available in 81-mg tablets, how many will you need to give the patient? Again, it is always a good idea to have your partner confirm the dosage before administering it.

4. **Right route.** Verify the route of the medication. You must make sure the route matches the order you received. For example, suppose you are told to give the patient a sublingual nitroglycerin tablet. The patient's nitroglycerin tablet bottle is empty, but he has another bottle of nitroglycerin capsules. These are to be swallowed four times per day. The medication is the same, even the dose may be the same, but the route of delivery is different from the order given. You may not substitute the capsules for the tablets without specific orders from medical control.

5. **Right time.** Check the expiration date and condition of the medication. The last step before administering a medication is to make sure the expiration date has not passed. Prescription and OTC medications have an expiration date. Check the label. If no date can be found, you should examine the medication

with suspicion. If you find discoloration, cloudiness, or particles in a liquid medication, you should not use it. If a patient with asthma gives you an MDI and the expiration date on it is smudged, you should not use it. After the medication is administered, you will need to reassess the patient to see if it has worked. Does the patient still have the same complaint as before you administered the medication? Has it changed? Is the patient experiencing any adverse effects? You should reassess the vital signs, especially heart rate and blood pressure, at least every 5 minutes if the patient's condition changes. If the medication is being administered to help reduce pain, you should ask the patient to rate his or her pain both before and after medication administration. A 0 to 10 scale, or the visual pain scale, is often used to help patients quantify their pain level. In addition, if the physician orders you to repeat the medication, it is important to do so at the right time. For example, if you are advised to repeat administration of nitroglycerin in 10 minutes if the patient's pain is unresolved, you should not wait 15 minutes.

6. **Right education.** Inform the patient of the medication you intend to administer. In this brief discussion, confirm (or reconfirm) whether the patient has any medication allergies or unusual sensitivity to the medication (or medication category). Additionally, inform the patient of any likely adverse effects or unusual sensations he or she may experience as the medication is administered.

7. **Right to refuse.** Patients with decision-making capacity can decline or refuse proposed interventions or medications. If the patient is unresponsive, briefly evaluate whether the patient has an advance directive in place that might preclude the administration of certain medications, particularly during resuscitation situations. When a patient lacks decision-making capacity, a surrogate decision maker has the authority to refuse proposed interventions or medication on a patient's behalf.

8. **Right response and evaluation.** Monitor the patient's vital signs, mental status, signs of perfusion, and respiratory effort after medication administration. Assess for the anticipated response, and observe for any adverse medication effects. Your knowledge of the medication's actions will help guide your reassessment.

9. **Right documentation.** Remember the EMS rule: The work is not done until the paperwork is done. Once the medication has been given, you must document your actions and the patient's response. This includes the time you gave the medication and the name, dose, and route of administration. Did the patient's condition improve, worsen, or not change? Were there any adverse effects? A second EMS rule says, "If you did not write it down, it did not happen." Should your performance ever be questioned, accurate documentation is your best defense.

## Medication Administration Cross-Check Procedure

Merely reviewing the rights of medication administration in your head is often not a sufficient safeguard to prevent a medication error. Using a verbal cross-check procedure that verifies you are giving the right drug to the right patient at the right dose has been found to reduce medication errors. This procedure, initially developed by Sedgwick County EMS in Kansas, should be stated aloud for each medication administration. It uses closed-loop communication and provides a time-out to reflect on whether the proper drug administration is being performed.

To perform the procedure, the person who is prepared to give the medicine alerts his or her partner that an important communication is happening by saying, "Med check." The partner then replies, "Ready." Then the person who will give the medicine says, "I am going to give [medication name, dose, and route] for [indication]." If the teammate thinks this information is correct, he or she responds, "Contraindications?" This is a chance to reflect on whether the patient has allergies or other reasons the medicine should not be given. If there are none, the first team member says, "None." The partner then asks, "Volume?" and shows the partner the medication container and the syringe, tablets, or device that is used to measure the dose. If the partner agrees it is correct, he or she states, "Give it."

This procedure can be done with another EMT, an EMR, or even aloud, alone in the back of the ambulance. The mere act of pausing and consciously verifying these steps aloud may help you catch an error before it is too late.

# Medication Administration and the EMT

There are several medications that may be carried on the EMS unit, including oxygen, oral glucose, aspirin, and epinephrine. When used wisely, each can be a powerful tool. Keep in mind, however, that you may give these medications only according to standing orders in a protocol (offline medical control) or a direct order (online medical control). Along with the several different medications that can be given by EMTs, there are several different routes of administration that will be used to deliver these medications to the patient.

Before specific medications are discussed, the circumstances surrounding the administration of the medications need to be discussed. Over the years, EMTs have been allowed increasing responsibility to work with medications, but this growth has come with some degree of confusion and worry. Many departments throughout the United States have strict controls on when an EMT is allowed to administer a medication. The circumstances are as follows:

- **Peer-assisted medication**
- **Patient-assisted medication**
- **EMT-administered medication**

In peer-assisted medication administration, you are administering medication to yourself or your partner. At times it may be necessary for an EMS crew to receive medications because they were exposed to a toxic nerve agent, such as during a terrorism incident. In this case, you would first treat yourself and then your partner. Typically, nerve agent antidotes are administered via an auto-injector. (See Chapter 41, *Terrorism Response and Disaster Management*, for more information on nerve agent antidotes.)

In patient-assisted medication administration, you are assisting the patient with the administration of his or her own medication, such as an EpiPen, an MDI bronchodilator, or nitroglycerin. Perhaps the patient cannot find his or her medication. Maybe the patient is so upset that he or she cannot open the pill bottle or hold the MDI steady. In this circumstance, the patient is trying to administer the medication, but you need to offer some help so the task can be completed.

The last circumstance is EMT-administered medications. Here you are directly administering the medication to the patient. It can certainly be difficult to find the exact point where assisting a patient ends and actually administering a medication begins. The patient may be severely confused or unable to understand the need for the medication. Common medications that you will administer in this circumstance are oxygen, oral glucose, nitroglycerin, and aspirin.

It is important for you to understand that the medication itself does not necessarily dictate whether you will be assisting or directly administering. Medical control, state guidelines, and local protocols will be the determining factors that define the role of the EMT. The EpiPen is an example of a medication that is both patient-assisted and EMT-administered. Refer to your local standards to obtain a listing of how and when EMTs can administer medications.

## Words of Wisdom

The following is a list of medications that, depending on local protocol, may be administered by EMTs. Keep in mind that this list is ultimately set by the state in which you will be delivering patient care and the medical director of your agency.
- Oxygen
- Oral glucose
- Aspirin
- Epinephrine
- Inhaled beta agonist/bronchodilator and anticholinergic (albuterol/ipratropium)
- MDI medications
- Nitroglycerin
- Naloxone
- Oral OTC analgesics for fever or pain

You may administer or help to administer medications only under the following conditions:
- Medical control gives you a direct order to administer a medication and/or the local medical protocols under which you are working permit you to administer that medication.
- Local medical protocols, developed by a medical physician under whom you are working, include standing orders for the use of a medication in defined situations.

It is imperative that you not give or help patients take any other medications under any other circumstances.

## Special Populations

Pregnant patients are limited in the medications they can take because of the risk to the fetus.

## Special Populations

Doses of medications are usually decreased for infants and children because they have smaller bodies, and in some cases, process the drugs differently. Medications for infants and children are typically ordered based on their weight in kilograms. To safely administer medications to infants and children, EMS providers must be able to accurately determine (or estimate) a patient's weight in kilograms. It might be necessary to convert from pounds to kilograms, by dividing the number of pounds by 2.2. For example, 22 pounds divided by 2.2 equals 10 kg. A length-based resuscitation tape, such as a Broselow tape, is a viable alternative if no scale is available, and the child's caregiver cannot confidently recall a recent measured weight (**FIGURE 12-5**). Visually estimating patient weight is notoriously inaccurate, even by experienced health care providers. Dosing for infants and children is expressed as milligrams (mg) or milliliters (mL) per kg of body weight. For example, an order may state, "Administer acetaminophen 15 mg/kg by mouth."

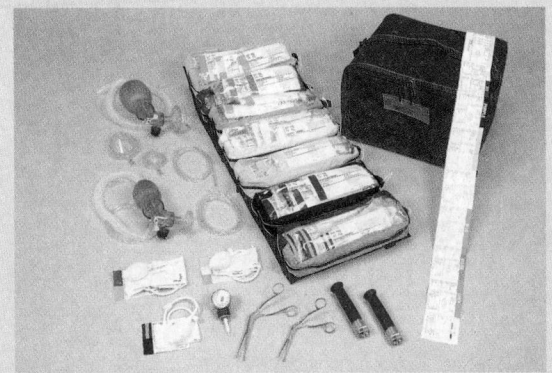

**FIGURE 12-5** Broselow system. The color coding on the Broselow tape helps give accurate medication dosing.
Courtesy of Armstrong Medical Industries.

## Medications Used by EMTs

The following is a discussion of medications that may be administered by EMTs. Again, your state, department, and medical director will ultimately define what medications are carried on your ambulance. **TABLE 12-4** provides an overview of these medications and their actions, indications, contraindications, routes of administration, adverse effects, interactions, and doses.

The 2019 National EMS Scope of Practice Model recognizes that some regions of the country may need EMTs to be involved in the administration of medications beyond oxygen, oral glucose, aspirin for chest pain of ischemic origin, oral OTC analgesics for pain or fever, inhaled beta agonists, naloxone, auto-injectors for chemical/hazardous materials exposures, epinephrine, and nitroglycerin for chest pain (must be the patient's medication). The exact list of medications that you will be allowed to manage is ultimately controlled by the state in which you practice and medical director of your agency.

## Oral Medications

There are several medications you may be asked to administer or to assist with administration. Oral glucose, aspirin, and several OTC medications can be administered by this route. As discussed, the advantages of this route are its ease of access and comfort level for the patient. One of the disadvantages of administering medications orally is that the digestive tract can be easily affected by foods, stress, and illness. The speed of movement of food through the tract dramatically changes the speed of absorption. As with all medications, you need to start with the rights of administration. Follow these steps to perform oral medication administration:

1. Take standard precautions.
2. Confirm the medication is not expired.
3. Obtain medical direction per local protocol.
4. Confirm that the patient has a patent airway and is able to swallow and follow instructions, then instruct the patient to swallow or chew the medication (**FIGURE 12-6**).
5. Monitor the patient's condition and document.

## Oral Glucose

Glucose is a sugar that our cells use as fuel. Although some cells can use other sugars, brain cells must have glucose. If the level of glucose in the blood gets too low, a person can experience a loss of consciousness, have seizures, and ultimately die.

The medical term for an extremely low blood glucose level is **hypoglycemia**. Hypoglycemia can

**TABLE 12-4** EMT Medication Overview

| Generic/Trade | Action | Indications | Contraindications | Routes | Adverse Effects | Interactions | Adult Dose | Administration Concerns |
|---|---|---|---|---|---|---|---|---|
| | | | | Medications EMTs Administer or May Assist in Administering | | | | |
| Aspirin (Bayer) | Anti-inflammatory agent and anti-fever agent; prevents platelets from clumping, thereby decreasing formation of new clots | Relief of mild pain, headache, muscle aches, fever; chest pain of cardiac origin | Hypersensitivity; recent bleeding | PO | Nausea, vomiting, stomach pain, bleeding, allergic reactions | Caution should be used in patients who are taking anticoagulants | 160 to 325 mg; 160- to 325-mg chewable tablets for chest pain | Do not administer for pain caused by trauma or for fevers in children; patients with chest pain must be able to chew tablets |
| Ipratropium [Atrovent], albuterol [Proventil, Ventolin][a] | Stimulates nervous system, causing bronchodilation | Asthma/Difficulty breathing with wheezing | Hypersensitivity; tachycardia (relative); chest pain of cardiac origin | Inhalation | Hypertension, tachycardia, anxiety, restlessness | Increases effects of other nervous system stimulants | 1 to 2 inhalations; wait 5 minutes before repeating dose | Patient must inhale all medication in one breath; coach patient to hold breath for 5 seconds after inhalation |
| Epinephrine (EpiPen) | Stimulates nervous system, causing bronchodilation | Anaphylactic reaction | Chest pain of cardiac origin; hypothermia; hypertension | IM | Hypertension, tachycardia, anxiety, restlessness | Increases effects of other nervous system stimulants | 0.3 mg for adult; 0.15 mg for children | Medication will last approximately 5 minutes; do not repeat dose; ensure ALS is en route for continuing treatment |
| Naloxone (Narcan, EVZIO auto-injector) | Reverses respiratory depression secondary to opioid overdose | Opioid poisoning | Hypersensitivity | IM, IN | Nausea, vomiting | Additional doses may be required for severe opioid overdoses | 2 mg IN or IM auto-injector | Patients may wake up combative |
| Nitroglycerin (Nitrostat, Nitromist) | Dilates blood vessels | Chest pain of cardiac origin | Hypotension; use of sildenafil (Viagra) or another treatment for erectile dysfunction within the previous 24 hours; head injury | SL tablet or spray | Headache, burning under tongue, hypotension, nausea | Increases dilating effects of other blood vessel–dilating medications | 0.3 to 0.4 mg SL; 0.4 mg spray | Ensure ALS is en route |

| Medication | Action | Indications | Contraindications | Route | Side Effects | Interactions/Cautions | Dose | Special Considerations |
|---|---|---|---|---|---|---|---|---|
| Oral glucose (Glutose) | When absorbed, provides glucose for cell use | Low blood glucose (hypoglycemia) | Decreased level of consciousness; nausea; vomiting | PO | Nausea, vomiting | None | 1/2 to 1 tube | Patient must be awake, have control of airway, and be able to follow commands |
| Oxygen (no trade name) | Reverses hypoxia; provides oxygen to be absorbed by lungs | Hypoxia or suspected hypoxia | Very rarely used in patients with COPD; do not use near open flames, as oxygen will support combustion | Inhalation | Decreased respiratory effort in rare cases in patients with COPD | Can support combustion | Use oxygen delivery devices to administer 28% to 100% oxygen | No open flames nearby; do not withhold oxygen from patients in respiratory distress |

### Common Over-the-Counter Medications

| Medication | Action | Indications | Contraindications | Route | Side Effects | Interactions/Cautions | Dose | Special Considerations |
|---|---|---|---|---|---|---|---|---|
| Acetaminophen (Tylenol) | Analgesic and fever reducer | Relief of mild pain or fever, headache, muscle aches | Hypersensitivity | PO | Allergic reaction | Take caution to avoid potential overdosing; many OTC medications contain acetaminophen | 500 to 1,000 mg every 4 hours as needed; dose is weight-based for children | Weight of child is more important than age |
| Diphenhydramine (Benadryl) | Antihistamine (blocks histamine) | Mild allergic reactions | Asthma; glaucoma; pregnancy; hypertension; infants | PO | Sleepiness (although can stimulate children), dry mouth and throat | Do not take with alcohol or MAO inhibitors (a type of psychiatric medication) | 25 to 50 mg | Can use in severe allergic reaction; however, epinephrine is administered first |
| Ibuprofen (Advil, Motrin, Nuprin) | NSAID that reduces inflammation and fever; analgesic | Mild pain or fever, headache, muscle aches | Hypersensitivity | PO | Nausea, vomiting, stomach pain, bleeding, allergic reactions | Do not take with aspirin | 200 to 400 mg every 4 to 6 hours; dose is weight-based in children | Do not take for pain caused by trauma; weight of child is more important than age |

[a] Albuterol and ipratropium are often packed together in the same inhaler or prefilled medication dose for inhalation under the trade name Combivent or DuoNeb.

Abbreviations: COPD, chronic obstructive pulmonary disease; MAO, monoamine oxidase; NSAID, nonsteroidal anti-inflammatory drug; OTC, over the counter; PO, per os

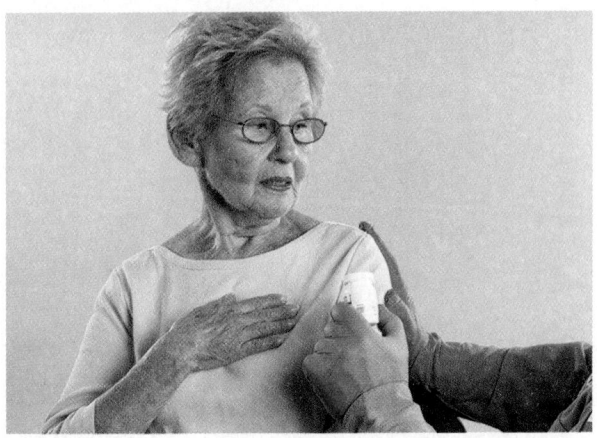

**FIGURE 12-6** Instruct the patient to chew (eg, baby aspirin) or swallow the medication.

© Jones & Bartlett Learning.

be caused by an excess of insulin, which is taken to control blood glucose levels. Patients with diabetes who use insulin regularly usually understand the effects of this medication on the body. The **oral glucose** that is carried in the EMS unit, as well as glucose tablets, can counteract the effects of hypoglycemia in the same way as a caloric beverage such as juice or a non-diet soda, but faster. This is because common table sugar (sucrose) and fruit sugars (fructose) are complex sugars and must be broken down before they can be absorbed. Glucose is a simple sugar that is readily absorbed by the bloodstream.

As an EMT, you can give glucose only by mouth. Hospital personnel and advanced providers (AEMTs and paramedics) can also give a form of glucose (dextrose) intravenously. Glucose is available as a gel designed to be spread on the mucous membranes between the cheek and gum; however, absorption through this route is not as quick as with injection. Because the patient may be conscious one moment and unconscious the next, you must be very careful when administering oral glucose. Never administer oral medications to an unconscious patient or to a patient who is unable to swallow or protect the airway. See Chapter 20, *Endocrine and Hematologic Emergencies*, for more information on the administration of oral glucose.

## Safety Tips

Never attempt to give anything by mouth to a patient with a decreased level of consciousness (LOC). Remember, an altered LOC may be an indication for a medication such as oral glucose; however, a decreased LOC can be a contraindication for oral medications, due to the potential for airway compromise.

## YOU are the Provider

After administering 15 g of oral glucose to the patient, you reassess her and note that her condition has improved. She is conscious and alert and asks you what happened. As you explain what happened to her, your partner takes her vital signs.

| Recording Time: 5 Minutes | |
|---|---|
| **Respirations** | 22 breaths/min; regular and adequate |
| **Pulse** | 112 beats/min; strong and regular |
| **Skin** | Pink; slightly moist |
| **Blood pressure** | 122/72 mm Hg |
| **Oxygen saturation (Spo$_2$)** | 98% (on oxygen) |
| **Blood glucose** | 70 mg/dL |

**5.** What are the "rights" of medication administration, and why are they important?

**6.** What medications are typically carried on an EMT ambulance?

**7.** As an EMT, what medications can you assist the patient to self-administer?

## Aspirin

**Aspirin (acetylsalicylic acid or ASA)** is an antipyretic (reduces fever), analgesic (reduces pain), and anti-inflammatory (reduces inflammation) medication that inhibits platelet aggregation (clumping). This last property makes it one of the most used medications today. Research has shown that the aggregation of platelets in the coronary arteries under certain conditions is one of the direct causes of heart attack. Patients at risk for coronary artery disease are often prescribed one or two "baby" (children's) aspirins per day. During a potential heart attack, aspirin may be life-saving.

Contraindications for aspirin include documented hypersensitivity to aspirin (absolute), pre-existing liver damage (absolute), bleeding disorders (relative), and asthma (relative). Because of the association of aspirin with Reye syndrome (a rare but serious condition that causes swelling in the brain and liver), it should not be given to children.

## Sublingual Medications

The sublingual route of administration has many advantages. Assuming the patient is awake, alert, and able to follow commands, it is easy to talk with the patient and advise him or her to place a pill under the tongue. The membranes that line the mouth and the undersurface of the tongue receive large amounts of blood flow, so absorption rates are relatively quick. Be aware, however, that any medication placed in the mouth requires constant evaluation of the airway. You must also be alert to any signs of choking on the pill. If the patient is uncooperative or unconscious, this route of medication administration should not be used.

## Nitroglycerin

Many patients with cardiac conditions carry some form of fast-acting nitroglycerin to relieve the pain of angina. **Nitroglycerin** has been used medically since the 1800s. Nitroglycerin is typically the only medication that you will help to administer sublingually (**FIGURE 12-7**).

If you have ever run for a prolonged period, you probably remember your muscles developed a painful, heavy, burning sensation. This is because the demand for oxygen by the muscles exceeded the supply. When a similar pain develops in heart muscle, it is called angina pectoris. The cause is the

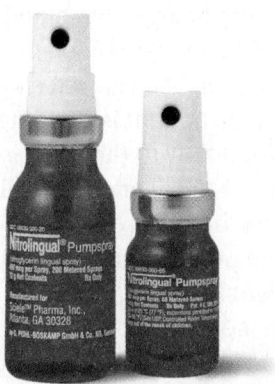

**A**

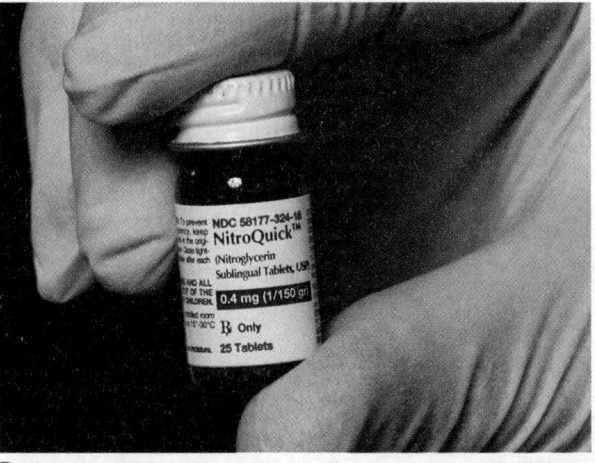

**B**

**FIGURE 12-7** Nitroglycerin, which is prescribed for chest pain, can be given sublingually as a spray (**A**) or tablet (**B**).

A: Courtesy of Shionogi Pharma, Inc.; B: © Jones & Bartlett Learning.

same—not enough oxygen. In this case the pain is due to a blockage or narrowing in the blood vessels that supply the heart. Occasionally, the cause is a spasm in these blood vessels. Unlike a runner with sore legs, the heart muscle cannot stop and rest until the pain goes away.

The purpose of nitroglycerin is to increase blood flow by relieving the spasms or causing the arteries to dilate. It does this by relaxing the muscular walls of the coronary arteries and veins. Nitroglycerin also relaxes veins throughout the body, so less blood is returned to the heart and the heart does not have to work as hard each time it contracts. In short, blood pressure is decreased. Because of this, it is important that you always take the patient's blood pressure before administering nitroglycerin. If the systolic blood pressure is less than 100 mm Hg, the nitroglycerin may have the harmful effect of lowering the blood flow to the heart's own blood vessels. Even a patient who has adequate blood pressure should sit or lie down with the head elevated before taking this medication. If the patient is standing, he or she may faint when blood flow to the brain is reduced as the nitroglycerin starts to work. If a significant decrease in the patient's blood pressure (15 to 20 mm Hg) occurs and the patient suddenly feels dizzy or sick, have the patient lie down.

During a heart attack (myocardial infarction [MI]), a narrowing or blockage in a coronary artery blocks the blood flow to a section of the heart muscle (myocardium). If the blockage is not cleared in time, the section of the heart muscle beyond the clot will die. If nitroglycerin no longer brings relief to a person in whom it has previously worked, the person may be experiencing an MI instead of an angina attack. Therefore, it is important to know how much nitroglycerin a patient has needed in the past to relieve chest pain and how much has been taken during the current emergency, including the use of nitroglycerin patches. Always report this information to medical control. Remember, you cannot administer this medication without clearance from medical control or standing orders.

There are important interactions to consider when administering nitroglycerin. Erectile dysfunction medications, such as sildenafil (Viagra), tadalafil (Cialis), and vardenafil (Levitra), can have potentially fatal interactions with nitroglycerin. When taken together, nitroglycerin and these drugs can cause a dramatic drop in blood pressure. Always ask a patient who has been prescribed nitroglycerin if he or she has used any medication for the treatment of erectile dysfunction within the previous 24 hours. If so, do not administer the nitroglycerin, and report this to medical control. Keep in mind that drugs for erectile dysfunction may be used by both men and women; do not assume women have not taken erectile dysfunction drugs.

Nitroglycerin has the following effects:

- Relaxes the muscular walls of coronary arteries and veins
- Results in less blood returning to the heart
- Decreases blood pressure
- Relaxes arteries throughout the body
- Often causes a mild headache and/or burning under the tongue after administration

## Administering Nitroglycerin by Tablet

Nitroglycerin is usually taken sublingually. The patient places a tiny tablet under the tongue, where it dissolves. The tablet should create a slight tingling or burning sensation under the tongue. Exposure to light, heat, or air may degrade the strength of the medication. If the nitroglycerin does not produce the typical burning sensation, it may have lost potency because of aging or improper storage. If you notice any signs of improper storage, be sure to include that information in the patient's medical history. In addition, be sure to check the expiration date on the bottle.

Sublingual nitroglycerin tablets should be stored in their original glass container with the cap screwed on tightly. Nothing else should be placed in the container, as this can rob nitroglycerin of its power.

### Street Smarts

Do not pour nitroglycerin tablets directly from the bottle into the patient's mouth; doing so may cause you to inadvertently administer multiple tablets. Patients who have an unusually dry mouth might benefit from the metered-dose spray form of nitroglycerin, as the tablets may not dissolve fully in a timely manner.

## Administering Nitroglycerin by Metered-Dose Spray

Some patients who take nitroglycerin use a metered-dose spray, which deposits medication on or under the tongue. Each spray is equivalent to one tablet. To ensure direct, proper dosing on the bottom of the tongue, hold the canister upright when administering, and do not use a spacer with the metered-dose canister when giving nitroglycerin by this method. Do not shake the canister before spraying it.

Whether using the tablets or the metered-dose spray, you should wait 5 minutes for a response before repeating the dose. Closely monitor the patient's vital signs, particularly the blood pressure. Give repeated doses per medical control and/or local protocol. Remember, always wear gloves when handling nitroglycerin tablets or spray, because this medication can be absorbed by your skin.

Next, you must reconfirm that the medication is still indicated for the patient. For example, suppose you have received and verified the order to give one sublingual nitroglycerin tablet to a patient with a cardiac condition. While you were getting the order, however, the patient begins to sweat more and becomes less responsive. Reassessment of the blood pressure reveals a pressure of 80/60 mm Hg. Using your knowledge of nitroglycerin, you recognize the contraindication and decide not to give the medication. Instead, you notify medical control of the changes in the patient's condition and seek new orders.

Knowing and understanding the local protocols under which you will be working are absolutely essential, as is a thorough knowledge of the medications within your scope of practice. Refer to Table 12-4 for a review of all medications and the important information needed for their administration. See Chapter 17, *Cardiovascular Emergencies*, for more information on how to administer nitroglycerin.

---

### Words of Wisdom

#### General Steps in Administering Medication

1. Obtain an order from medical control.
2. Verify the proper medication and prescription.
3. Verify the form, dose, and route of the medication.
4. Check the expiration date and condition of the medication.
5. Complete a cross-check procedure.
6. Reassess the vital signs, especially heart rate and blood pressure, at least every 5 minutes or as the patient's condition changes.
7. Document your actions and the patient's response.

---

## Intramuscular Medications

The intramuscular (IM) route of administration provides quick and easy access to the circulatory system without the need for placing a needle within a vein. Blood flow to the muscles is relatively stable, even during circumstances of severe illness or injury. This advantage makes the IM route an efficient means to deliver some medications. A disadvantage for this route is the use of a needle and the subsequent pain it can cause. Patients may be reluctant for you to use the needle for fear of pain or injury. With proper technique, you can administer medications via the IM route and limit the amount of pain delivered to the patient.

## Epinephrine

**Epinephrine** is the main hormone that controls the body's fight-or-flight response and is the primary medication that you will be administering intramuscularly. Epinephrine is a sympathomimetic. A sympathomimetic mimics the effect of the sympathetic nervous system. The body releases epinephrine when there is sudden stress, such as during exercise or when the patient is suddenly scared. Because epinephrine is secreted by the adrenal glands, it is also known as adrenaline. Epinephrine has different effects on different body tissues and is used as a medication in several forms. Generally, epinephrine will increase the heart rate and blood pressure and dilate passages in the lungs. It can ease breathing problems caused by the bronchial spasms common in asthma and allergic reactions. In a person who is close to anaphylactic shock as a result of an allergic reaction, epinephrine may also help to maintain the patient's blood pressure. However, epinephrine is not indicated for patients who do not show signs of airway obstruction or wheezing due to an allergic reaction. In addition, this medication should not be given to patients with hypertension or hypothermia, or if you believe the patient may be experiencing an MI.

Epinephrine has the following characteristics:

- Secreted naturally by the adrenal glands
- Dilates passages in the lungs
- Constricts blood vessels, causing increased blood pressure
- Increases heart rate and blood pressure

Refer to Chapter 6, *The Human Body*, for more information on epinephrine.

### Administering Epinephrine by Injection

Many states and EMS agencies now authorize the use of epinephrine by EMTs for the treatment of life-threatening anaphylaxis. In certain patients, insect venom or other allergens cause the body to over-release histamine, which lowers blood pressure by relaxing the small blood vessels and allowing them to leak. The over-release of histamine may also cause wheezing from bronchial spasms and swelling of the airway tissues (edema), which make it difficult for the patient to breathe. Epinephrine

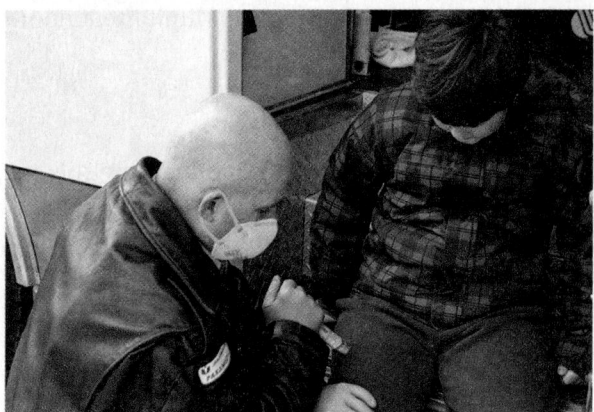

**FIGURE 12-8** An EpiPen auto-injector may be used to administer a preset dose of epinephrine.

© Jones & Bartlett Learning.

acts as a specific antidote to reverse the effects of histamines, countering both of the harmful effects. It constricts the blood vessels, allowing blood pressure to rise and reducing the swelling. In the lungs, it has the opposite effect: It dilates the air passages, so the flow of air is less restricted.

Epinephrine may be dispensed from an auto-injector, which automatically delivers a preset amount of the medication (**FIGURE 12-8**). This is usually 0.3 mg of epinephrine. This is the method that you will most likely use.

Some areas may allow epinephrine to be administered by intramuscular injection using a vial of 1 mg/mL concentration with a needle and syringe. (This is discussed further in Chapter 21, *Allergy and Anaphylaxis.*) Older references or medication labels might refer to epinephrine concentration using "1:1,000" or "1:10,000." This practice has been phased out and replaced by the "mg/mL" concentration language for epinephrine and the other medications that had previously used that same concentration language.

Be sure to familiarize yourself with the procedures for using the auto-injector on your unit. Some manufacturers of auto-injectors include verbal instructions for administration. The general procedure is as follows:

1. Grasp unit with the tip pointing downward.
2. Form a fist around the unit. Do *not* place your thumb over either end of the unit.
3. With the other hand, pull off the activation cap.
4. Hold the tip near the outer part of the patient's thigh.

5. Insert firmly into the outer thigh so that the unit is perpendicular (at a 90-degree angle) to the thigh. Do not allow the unit to bounce.
6. Hold firmly in the thigh for several seconds.
7. Immediately place the unit in an appropriate sharps container after administration.

Epinephrine causes a burning sensation where it is injected, and the patient's heart rate will increase after the injection, so be prepared for these adverse effects. Some services do not permit EMTs to carry epinephrine but do allow them to assist patients in administering their own epinephrine in life-threatening anaphylactic reactions.

### Administering Naloxone by Injection

The US FDA has approved an auto-injector device that delivers an IM or subcutaneous injection of naloxone (Narcan) to reverse the effects of an opioid overdose. This medication can be administered by family members or caregivers to help reverse dangerous adverse effects of opioid overdose, such as life-threatening respiratory depression. One version of auto-injectable naloxone, called EVZIO, provides verbal instructions for administration similar to those provided by AEDs. There are several important considerations for EMTs related to auto-injectable naloxone:

- Consult medical direction to determine if EMTs are allowed to administer naloxone in your region. As always, follow your local protocol. Consider requesting assistance from ALS personnel if available for any suspected opioid overdose. Ensure that another rescuer is ventilating and oxygenating the patient if needed while you prepare the medication.
- Find out if naloxone has been administered by a bystander prior to your arrival.
- Be aware that the effects of naloxone may not last as long as those of opioids. Repeat doses of naloxone may be needed.
- Administration of naloxone to opioid-dependent patients can cause severe withdrawal symptoms, including seizures and cardiac arrest.
- You must consider your safety, as patients may become violent following naloxone administration. Make sure you are wearing proper PPE, including eye protection, mask, and gloves.

Most prefilled naloxone IM preparations are administered in increments of 2 mg, then gradually increase based on the patient response, or lack thereof, to achieve the desired effect of restoring respirations while avoiding withdrawal symptoms and associated complications.

## Intranasal Medications

### Naloxone

Not all EMS departments will use naloxone auto-injectors, due to their expense. The most common technique for naloxone administration is via the intranasal route. Other common routes of administration include intravenous and intramuscular. All of the same considerations described for administering injectable naloxone apply when administering naloxone in any another form.

Follow these steps to administer a medication intranasally:

1. Obtain medical direction per local protocol.
2. Confirm correct medication and expiration date.
3. Attempt to determine if the patient is allergic to any medications.
4. Prepare the medication and attach the atomizer. *Never* use a needle.
5. Place the atomizer in one nostril, pointing up and slightly outward (**FIGURE 12-9**).
6. Administer a half-dose (1 mL maximum) into each nostril.
7. Reassess the patient and document appropriately.

If you do not have naloxone available, note that bag-mask ventilations provide necessary treatment to opioid overdose patients until definitive treatment can be reached.

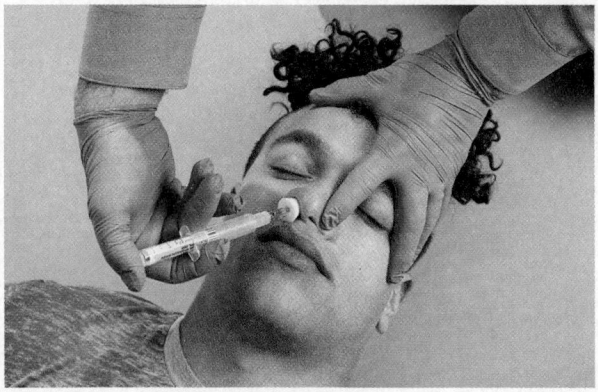

**FIGURE 12-9** Some EMTs may administer naloxone intranasally to treat an opioid overdose.

© Jones & Bartlett Learning.

## Inhalation Medications

### Oxygen

Oxygen is, by far, the most commonly administered medication in the prehospital setting. All cells need **oxygen** to function properly. The heart and brain, especially, cannot function for long if oxygen levels decrease, which is why oxygen is an onboard medication for EMS units. If a patient is not breathing or is having trouble getting air into the lungs, you should administer supplemental oxygen. In general, you will be giving oxygen via either a nonrebreathing mask at 10 to 15 L/min or via nasal cannula at 2 to 6 L/min based on the patient's condition. However, if the patient is not breathing adequately, you must also provide artificial ventilations, so you will need to use a bag-mask device. Oxygen is usually delivered at 15 L/min with this technique.

Outside a hospital, the nonrebreathing mask is the preferred method of giving oxygen to patients who are experiencing significant respiratory difficulties or shock. With a good mask-to-face seal, this mask can provide up to 90% inspired oxygen. With a nasal cannula, oxygen flows through two small, tubelike prongs that fit into the patient's nostrils. This device can provide up to 44% inspired oxygen if the flowmeter is set at 6 L/min.

Remember that, although oxygen itself does not burn, it is a catalyst for combustion. If there is extra oxygen in the air, objects will burn more easily. Ensure there are no open flames, lit cigarettes, or sparks in the area in which you are administering oxygen.

## Words of Wisdom

Oxygen is not helpful, and prolonged use of supplemental oxygen may actually be harmful, in patients who are having a heart attack or stroke when breathing is normal and the oxygen saturation is 94% or greater. Nonetheless, the evidence is very strong that even brief periods of hypoxemia in these patients can be very dangerous. Patients who need supplemental oxygen should receive it promptly. If in doubt, always err on the side of providing supplemental oxygen to patients.

## MDIs and Nebulizers

MDIs and small-volume nebulizers (SVNs) are used to administer liquid medications that have been turned into a fine mist by a flow of air or oxygen (**FIGURE 12-10**). Respiratory illness can be spread through SVNs. When the medication is atomized, it is breathed into the lungs and delivered to the alveoli. Blood flow to the alveoli is very high and absorption rates are close to those found with IV medications. This route is fast and relatively easy to access. MDIs are commonly used because of their convenience and portability. The major

## YOU are the Provider

The patient is placed onto the stretcher and loaded into the ambulance. She remains conscious and alert. Her son tells you that he has to retrieve some items from her house and will follow the ambulance in his car. Shortly before departing the scene, you reassess the patient's vital signs.

| Recording Time:    13 Minutes | |
| --- | --- |
| Level of consciousness | Conscious and alert |
| Respirations | 18 breaths/min; regular and adequate |
| Pulse | 84 beats/min; strong and regular |
| Skin | Pink, warm, and slightly moist |
| Blood pressure | 128/74 mm Hg |
| $SpO_2$ | 99% (on oxygen) |
| Blood glucose | 94 mg/dL |

The patient tells you that she thinks she may have accidentally taken too much of her Amaryl. You reassess her blood glucose level and note that it is 94 mg/dL.

**8.** You are unfamiliar with the medication Amaryl. What should you do?

**9.** If you were unable to obtain a blood glucose reading on this patient, would you still administer oral glucose? Why or why not?

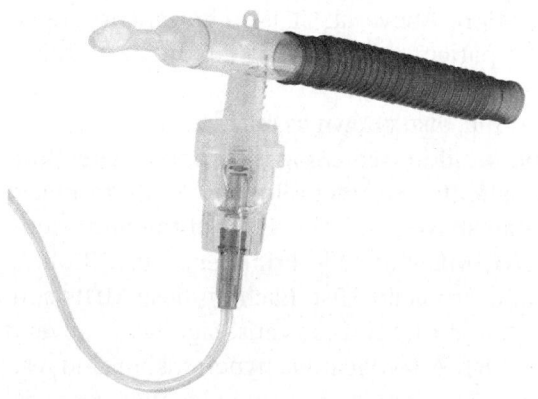

**FIGURE 12-10** Metered-dose inhalers and small-volume nebulizers (shown here) convert liquid medications into a fine mist.

© Charles Brutlag/Shutterstock.

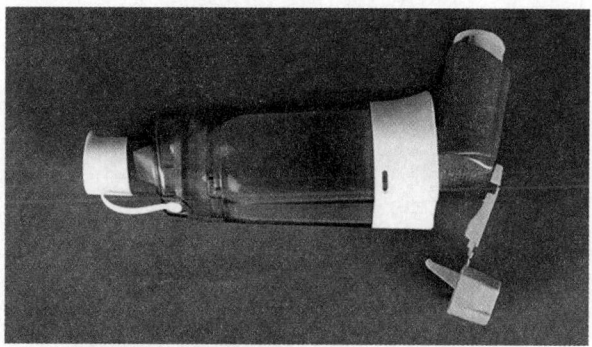

**FIGURE 12-11** Some inhalers have spacer devices to better direct the medication spray.

© Jones & Bartlett Learning.

## Special Populations

Children are not small adults, especially when it comes to the administration of medications. The approach to children differs from that for adults. First, doses of medications are different. Most of the assisted medications will be smaller doses. Children may not have the coordination needed to use an MDI. It will be easier if a spacer device is added to the inhaler to ensure the child receives the full benefit of the medicine. A little more time and effort may be required to explain each procedure. It is also in your best interest to tell the child the truth. It is very important to gain the trust of the child in the short time you have to bond with him or her.

disadvantage of an MDI is that the patient needs to be cooperative and control his or her breathing. If the patient is unconscious, an MDI cannot be used, although you could use a nebulizer. Nebulizers are often used for more severe problems.

## Medications Administered Using an MDI or SVN

Sometimes, a respiratory condition such as asthma is not severe enough to require the use of epinephrine. In such cases, patients may use one of the chemical "cousins" of epinephrine that are more narrowly focused on the lungs. These medications are delivered using an MDI or SVN.

Proper use of an MDI requires some degree of coordination, something that may be difficult to achieve when a person is having trouble breathing. Patients must aim properly and spray just as they start to inhale. If administered improperly, most of the medication ends up on the roof of the patient's mouth. An adapter, called a spacer, fits over the inhaler like a sleeve and can be used to avoid misdirecting the spray (**FIGURE 12-11**). The patient sprays the prescribed dose into the chamber and then breathes in and out of the mouthpiece until the mist is completely inhaled. Spacer devices are especially useful with young children who have difficulty using an MDI.

MDIs contain both the medication and a propellant, a chemical used to help push the medication out of the inhaler. It is possible for the medication to be depleted in the MDI, even though it continues to spray. It may be difficult to determine whether a patient's MDI is still providing needed medicine.

SVNs are much easier to use than MDIs; however, they take longer to deliver the medication and require an external air or oxygen source. An SVN can be more effective than an MDI in moderate to severe respiratory distress. An SVN can also be used while a patient is on continuous positive airway pressure and during bag-mask ventilation. An SVN can easily be adapted to a nonrebreathing mask for patients unable to hold an SVN. This can be especially helpful with children.

Assisting a patient with an SVN involves placing the medication into the nebulizer and then running a flow of oxygen through the device, which will atomize the liquid and allow the patient to breathe in the medication (**FIGURE 12-12**). You will typically use an oxygen tank to deliver an SVN treatment; however, many respiratory patients have a portable SVN machine at home that can also be used. Consult

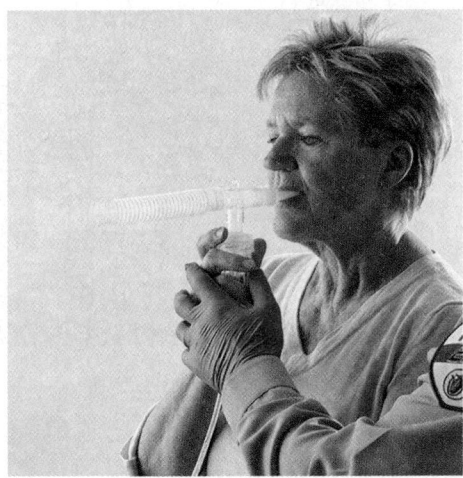

**FIGURE 12-12** With a small-volume nebulizer, liquid medication is atomized by the flow of oxygen. The patient then breathes in the medication.

© Jones & Bartlett Learning.

your local protocol to determine if use of an SVN is within the EMT scope of practice for your agency.

Follow these steps to administer a medication via SVN. See Chapter 16, *Respiratory Emergencies*, for more information on steps for using MDIs and SVNs.

1. Obtain medical direction per local protocol.
2. Confirm correct medication and expiration date.
3. Confirm that the patient is *not* allergic to the medication.
4. Add the appropriate medication and dose to the nebulizer reservoir and assemble according to the manufacturer's instructions.
5. Perform the medication cross-check.
6. Connect to the nebulizer machine (often in the patient's home) or oxygen tank at 6 to 8 L/min.
7. Place the nebulizer in the patient's mouth and instruct the patient to breathe until the medication is gone (usually about 5 minutes).
8. Reassess the patient and document appropriately.

Note: Some nebulizers come preconnected to an oxygen mask for easier administration for patients who are unable to hold the nebulizer.

You can activate the spray by pressing the canister into the adapter just as the patient starts to inhale. If relief is not achieved, wait 3 to 5 minutes and repeat this sequence according to the patient's

prescription. Above all, it is important to ensure that the patient inhales all of the medication in a single-sprayed dose.

Asthma, also known as reactive airway disease, can be a life-threatening condition. Therefore, some patients use rescue inhaler MDIs to relieve bronchial spasms quickly. A few of the more common OTC MDIs include Primatene Mist, Bronitin Mist, and Bronkaid Mist. Each of these MDIs contains epinephrine and can cause significant adverse effects, such as tachycardia, hypertension, and restlessness. Therefore, as mentioned earlier, most patients with asthma use certain chemical cousins of epinephrine that produce fewer adverse effects and act more specifically on the bronchi of the lungs. Common prescription MDIs include albuterol (ProAir, Proventil, and Ventolin), ipratropium bromide (Atrovent), and levalbuterol (Xopenex). Often albuterol and ipratropium are combined in one inhaler (eg, Combivent, DuoNeb). Another type of MDI used by respiratory patients is the maintenance, or controller, inhaler. These MDIs are slow acting and are meant to be used regularly to be effective. Maintenance inhalers are *not* useful for a patient experiencing acute respiratory distress and in need of immediate relief. Common maintenance inhalers include fluticasone propionate (Flovent Diskus), budesonide (Pulmicort), mometasone furoate (Asmanex Twisthaler), beclomethasone dipropionate (Qvar), and ciclesonide (Alvesco).

There are dozens of different MDIs on the market, and often patients may be prescribed several of them at once. The only medications that will be effective during an acute attack of shortness of breath will be the fast-acting rescue inhalers, such as albuterol (Proventil, Ventolin), and levalbuterol (Xopenex). Whether you are assisting the patient with an MDI or an SVN medication, be sure you have the right medication for a patient with acute respiratory distress.

## Patient Medications

Part of your patient assessment includes finding out what medications your patient is currently taking. This information may provide vital clues to your patient's condition that may help guide your treatment or be extremely useful to the ED physician. Often, knowing what medications a patient takes may be the only way you can determine what chronic or underlying conditions your patient may have, such as when a patient is unable to relate his medical history to you. The patient may be unresponsive, confused, not knowledgeable about his or her medical history, uncooperative, or unable to communicate. Discovering what the patient takes and transporting the medications or a list of medications with you to the ED can be crucial in assessing your patient's needs.

## Special Populations

**Polypharmacy** is a term referring to the use of multiple medications by one person. It is not uncommon today to find patients, especially older patients, taking many medications on a regular basis. Often, the prescription regimens can be complex and confusing. The medications may be prescribed by multiple physicians. The person may also be taking nonprescription and herbal medicines. Add to this the possibility of failing memory and confusion, and the potential for overdosing, underdosing, and harmful interactions increases exponentially.

In addition to prescription medications, patients often take nonprescription OTC medications, herbal medications, or other supplements. Many times, they do not consider these substances to be medications and will not report them to you unless you ask about them specifically. Yet, they may be as potent as prescription medications and can have interactions and effects on a patient's health and condition that are just as important. Be sure to ask specifically about these substances.

## Implications for EMS Providers

EMS providers must not underestimate the importance of obtaining a thorough medication history during patient encounters. Medications are frequently not taken as prescribed. Studies show that patients do not fill approximately 20% of new prescriptions, and overall, approximately one-half of

## Street Smarts

When possible, EMS providers should verbally verify which medications are actually being taken, even when presented with a printed medication list.

all prescriptions are not taken correctly. There may be huge gaps between a patient's medication list (or reported history) and what the patient is actually receiving.

A patient may take medications correctly yet still have many opportunities for medication toxicity, adverse medication reactions, or body changes that alter the pharmacodynamics and pharmacokinetics in that individual. Acute illness, dehydration, liver or kidney dysfunction, and a vast array of other variables can alter how a medication affects the body, even if a patient has been stable on that medication for many years. EMS providers should consider a patient's medication in the context of the particular clinical encounter, assessing for cues that the two might be related.

Patient medications may significantly alter the clinical presentation of many acute medical conditions or injuries. Beta adrenergic blocking agents, such as metoprolol (Lopressor) and atenolol (Tenormin), along with calcium channel blocking agents such as amlodipine (Norvasc) and diltiazem (Cardizem), can prevent the patient's heart rate from increasing in sepsis, trauma, hemorrhage, and other conditions that normally would present with tachycardia. Patients who take these medications may demonstrate normal or low heart rate, even when perfusion is impaired and shock is worsening.

Antiplatelet and anticoagulant medications will also complicate EMS assessment and management of many patients. **Antiplatelet** medications, such as aspirin and clopidogrel (Plavix), decrease the ability of blood platelets to aggregate (stick together). **Anticoagulant** medications, such as warfarin (Coumadin), apixaban (Eliquis), and rivaroxaban (Xarelto), interfere with other blood clotting mechanisms in the body. Both groups of medications are prescribed to patients who are susceptible to dysfunctional blood clotting conditions, including acute coronary syndrome, ischemic cerebrovascular accident (stroke), peripheral or pulmonary blood clots, and similar conditions. Patients taking medications from either of these groups are predisposed to bleeding. This bleeding risk becomes more significant when the patient sustains trauma, has an otherwise manageable hemorrhage such as a nosebleed, or a hemorrhage develops that cannot be easily controlled, such as a gastrointestinal bleed. In each instance, hemorrhage control can become quite difficult. EMS providers should

### TABLE 12-5 Common Antiplatelet and Anticoagulant Medications

| Antiplatelet Medications | Anticoagulant Medications |
| --- | --- |
| aspirin | enoxaparin (Lovenox); injectable medication given to patients in their homes |
| clopidogrel (Plavix) | apixaban (Eliquis) |
| prasugrel (Effient) | betrixaban (Bevyxxa) |
| ticagrelor (Brilinta) | dabigatran (Pradaxa) |
| vorapaxar (Zontivity) | edoxaban (Savaysa) |
|  | rivaroxaban (Xarelto) |

Courtesy of Andrew Bartkus.

strongly suspect intracranial hemorrhage in patients who present with altered mental status or other neurologic symptoms. When a complicated hemorrhage is present, EMS providers should consider transport to a health care facility with the capabilities to manage these situations. Some of these medications have approved antidotes, while others require aggressive supportive countermeasures to manage the hemorrhage. **TABLE 12-5** lists common antiplatelet and anticoagulant medications that EMS providers may encounter.

Several of the most commonly prescribed drugs for adults in the United States are used to treat cardiovascular disease and high cholesterol. **TABLE 12-6** lists medications frequently prescribed in the United States and their uses. There are also excellent mobile apps that can help you quickly look up unfamiliar medications.

### TABLE 12-6 Commonly Prescribed Medications in the United States

| Generic Name (Trade Name) | Use |
| --- | --- |
| alprazolam (Xanax) | Treats anxiety disorders |
| amlodipine (Norvasc) | Treats high blood pressure or cardiac conditions |
| amoxicillin (Moxatag) | Treats infection caused by bacteria |
| aripiprazole (Abilify) | Treats psychosis, depression |
| atenolol (Tenormin) | Beta blocker; treats hypertension |
| atorvastatin (Lipitor) | Treats high cholesterol |
| azithromycin (Zithromax) | Treats infection caused by bacteria |
| buprenorphine and naloxone (Suboxone) | Prescribed to prevent opioid withdrawal |
| bupropion (Wellbutrin; Zyban) | Treats depression; also used for smoking cessation |
| celecoxib (Celebrex) | Treats pain |
| citalopram hydrobromide (Celexa) | Treats depression |
| donepezil HCl (Aricept) | Treats dementia |
| duloxetine (Cymbalta) | Treats depression and anxiety disorders |
| escitalopram (Lexapro) | Treats depression and anxiety |
| esomeprazole (Nexium) | Treats gastric reflux, heartburn |

| Generic Name (Trade Name) | Use |
| --- | --- |
| etanercept (Enbrel) | Treats rheumatoid arthritis |
| furosemide (Lasix) | Diuretic; treats hypertension, heart failure |
| gabapentin (Neurontin) | Treats seizures and nerve pain |
| metformin (Glucophage) | Treats diabetes |
| hydrochlorothiazide (Microzide) | Beta blocker; treats hypertension, heart failure |
| hydrocodone (Vicodin) | Narcotic analgesic; pain reliever |
| insulin glargine (Lantus) | Medicine used to treat diabetes that is administered subcutaneously |
| levetiracetam (Keppra) | Treats seizures |
| levothyroxine (Synthroid) | Treats hypothyroidism |
| lisinopril (Zestril) | Angiotensin-converting enzyme (ACE) inhibitor; treats hypertension |
| loratadine (Claritin) | Antihistamine |
| losartan (Cozaar) | Angiotensin receptor blocker; treats hypertension |
| metoprolol (Lopressor) | Beta blocker, treats hypertension, heart failure |
| montelukast (Singulair) | Treats asthma |
| olanzapine (Zyprexa) | Treats schizophrenia and bipolar disorder |
| omeprazole (Prilosec) | Treats gastric reflux, heartburn |
| oxycodone (Oxycontin; also known as Percocet when combined with acetaminophen) | Treats pain (analgesic) |
| pantoprazole (Protonix) | Reduces stomach acid |
| phenytoin (Dilantin) | Treats seizures |
| rosuvastatin (Crestor) | Treats high cholesterol |
| salmeterol (Advair) | Inhaled glucocorticoid and long-acting beta-2 agonist; prevents asthma attacks, COPD |
| sertraline HCl (Zoloft) | Treats depression |
| simvastatin (Zocor) | Treats high cholesterol |
| tamsulosin (Flomax) | Treat urinary disorders related to an enlarged prostate |
| triamcinolone acetonide (Nasacort) | Treats inflammatory conditions |
| valsartan (Diovan) | Treats high blood pressure and congestive heart failure |
| varenicline (Chantix) | Used for smoking cessation |
| zolpidem (Ambien) | Treats insomnia |

Patients are naturally reluctant to tell you about any illegal drugs or medications they may have taken. It is important to ask, and you can assure them that your only interest in asking is to be able to treat them appropriately.

## Medication Errors

As discussed earlier, medication errors are common. A **medication error** is inappropriate use of a medication that could lead to patient harm. For example, this could include incorrect communication of a dose or administration of an incorrect dose. An estimated 1.5 million people in the United States are harmed each year due to medication errors in hospitals, extended care facilities, and outpatient clinics. EMS professionals are not immune to committing medication errors. Medication errors are preventable, so you must be extremely vigilant anytime medications are administered to a patient.

As discussed in Chapter 1, *EMS Systems*, errors can stem from different causes. Administration of a medication that is outside one's scope of practice is a rules-based error. Choosing the wrong medication to administer is a knowledge-based error.

Using incorrect equipment or an incorrect procedure for administering a medication is an example of a skills-based error.

If the circumstances of the errors are understood, it may be possible to minimize them. Ensure that the environment does not contribute to errors—ensure that lighting is sufficient, that equipment is organized, and that distractions are limited as much as possible. Consider using a cheat sheet to help yourself remember all crucial steps to medication administration. Finally, before administering a medication, stop to ask yourself, "Why am I doing this?" Pausing for a moment allows you to sharpen your focus and ensure that you are doing what is correct.

If a medication error does take place, take the following steps. First, rapidly provide any appropriate patient care that is required. Second, notify medical control as quickly as possible. Third, follow your local protocols and document the incident thoroughly, accurately, and honestly. Additionally, talk with your partner, supervisor, or medical director. This is an opportunity for you to learn how to prevent such errors in the future. These discussions can also help identify areas for your agency to target during quality improvement.

## YOU are the Provider

The patient's condition remains stable during transport. You transport in nonemergency mode, reassess her vital signs, and then call in your radio report to the hospital, where you expect to arrive in approximately 8 minutes.

| Recording Time:   19 Minutes | |
| --- | --- |
| Level of consciousness | Conscious and alert |
| Respirations | 18 breaths/min; regular and adequate |
| Pulse | 74 beats/min; strong and regular |
| Skin | Pink, warm, and dry |
| Blood pressure | 126/72 mm Hg |
| $SpO_2$ | 98% (on oxygen) |
| Blood glucose | 94 mg/dL |

You arrive at the hospital and give your verbal report to the charge nurse. The patient's son arrives shortly thereafter and presents the nurse with a plastic bag containing seven medications, including those that you have already noted. After further assessment, treatment, and observation in the ED, the patient is discharged home with modification of her medication regimen and instructions to follow up closely with her primary care provider.

**10.** What does the term "polypharmacy" mean, and why is it important?

**1. What is pharmacology?**

Pharmacology is the study of medications, including their therapeutic uses and actions on the body. Several terms are used when discussing pharmacology. The *dose* is the amount of medication that is given to the patient. The *action* is the therapeutic effect that the medication is expected to have on the body. *Indications* are the reasons or conditions for which a particular medication is given. *Contraindications* are the reasons or conditions for which a particular medication should not be given because it may cause further harm. *Adverse effects* are any actions of a medication other than the desired effects.

**2. Why is knowledge of pharmacology important to patient care?**

Giving a medication to a patient without understanding how it will affect him or her is dangerous. Prior to administering *any* medication—including oxygen—you must understand what effect or effects it will have on the patient. In addition, you must perform a careful and accurate assessment to determine if medication therapy is even indicated.

The patient may have a condition for which a particular drug is indicated; however, various factors that are unique to the patient (eg, known allergy to the drug, unstable vital signs) may otherwise contraindicate its use. Even medications that are normally taken by the patient may be contraindicated at the current time. For example, the nitroglycerin a patient takes for angina should not be administered if the patient's blood pressure is too low. The only way you will be able to determine whether a particular medication should be given is through a careful assessment.

It is easy enough to memorize the indications, contraindications, doses, and adverse effects of the drugs that you may administer as an EMT, but if you do not know how the drug will affect the patient's body, you should not be giving it. *Once you give it, you cannot take it back!*

**3. Other than oxygen, what other medication does this patient require, and why?**

This patient is a candidate for oral glucose. A normal blood glucose level is 80 to 120 mg/dL. This patient's glucose level is 36 mg/dL, which is critically low (hypoglycemia) and would explain the patient's present mental status.

Oral glucose is available as a gel or as tablets. If authorized by medical control, you should administer oral glucose to any patient with a decreased LOC, an ability to protect his or her own airway, and a history of diabetes. The only contraindications to oral glucose are an inability to swallow and decreased level of consciousness, because of the risk of aspiration.

**4. Why is it significant to know the patient took her medications on an empty stomach?**

If a patient with diabetes takes his or her medication but does not eat, either before or right after taking the medication, there is a significant risk of symptomatic hypoglycemia developing. If the blood glucose level becomes too low, a person can experience a loss of consciousness, experience seizures, and ultimately die.

**5. What are the "rights" of medication administration, and why are they important?**

Prior to assisting a patient with his or her prescribed medication or prior to administering a drug from your ambulance, you should review the rights of medication administration, a tool used to promote safe and accurate medication administration, and verify the drugs and dose with your partner using a cross-check procedure, if possible. Most medication errors result from failure to follow the rights.

- **Right patient.** If you are assisting the patient with his or her own medication, look at the medication label to ensure that it reads the same name as your patient.
- **Right medication and indication.** Check the medication label to make sure it is the right medication for the patient's condition.
- **Right dose.** Check the medication label and take note of the dose. The dosing information should be on the medication container. If it is not, contact medical control or follow your local protocols.
- **Right route.** A medication given by the wrong route, even if it is the correct medication, may be ineffective or may even cause harm to the patient.
- **Right time.** Medications that can be repeated must be given at the correct time intervals. After administering the medication, document the time. After the proper time has passed, follow your local protocols or contact medical control again if the drug needs to be readministered.
- **Right education.** Advise the patient of the medication that you intend to give and confirm (or reconfirm) any allergies or other contraindications.
- **Right to refuse.** Remember that patients with decision-making capacity (or their surrogate decision makers) have the right to refuse any proposed interventions.

- **Right response and evaluation.** Monitor the patient for response to the medication, observe for adverse effects, and recheck vital signs at appropriate intervals.
- **Right documentation.** After administering any medication to any patient, you must document the drug, dose, route, time(s) of administration, and reassessment findings after the medication has been given. Proper documentation will ensure that the receiving facility is aware of the medications the patient received in the field and the effects they may have had.

**6. What medications are typically carried on an EMT ambulance?**

There are four medications typically carried on an ambulance that is staffed by EMTs: oxygen, aspirin, oral glucose, and epinephrine. Depending on local protocol, other medications may be carried on the ambulance, including naloxone, nitroglycerin, and MDI or nebulized medications. In particular, naloxone use is rapidly gaining popularity with EMS systems, law enforcement agencies, and other first responders.

It is important to note that, just because these medications are carried on the ambulance, you cannot administer them at will. They may be given only on the direct order of a physician (online medical control) or according to standing orders in your local protocol (offline medical control).

**7. As an EMT, what medications can you assist the patient to self-administer?**

You may be asked to help patients self-administer certain prescription medications, including epinephrine auto-injectors (EpiPens), MDI medications (albuterol [Proventil, Ventolin]), or nitroglycerin (Nitrostat).

First, perform a careful assessment of your patient to determine if medication therapy is indicated. Just because the patient is prescribed a particular medication does not mean that it is indicated. For example, nitroglycerin—a vasodilator drug—is contraindicated if the patient's systolic blood pressure is less than 100 mm Hg. By dilating the patient's blood vessels, nitroglycerin may cause a dangerous drop in his or her blood pressure.

**8. You are unfamiliar with the medication Amaryl. What should you do?**

The simplest and most obvious way of determining the purpose of a medication is to ask the patient. She is conscious and will likely be able to answer your question. If the patient is unsure what it is used for, you should refer to an EMT field guide, drug reference text, or mobile app, or contact medical control. In this case, glimepiride (Amaryl) is an oral medication; commonly used by patients with type 2 diabetes mellitus to help lower their blood glucose level.

As an EMT, you will often encounter patients who take numerous medications. Just because it is not one that you carry on the ambulance or are authorized to assist the patient in taking does not mean that you should not determine its purpose. Much information about a patient's medical history can be obtained by looking at the medications she is taking, especially when the patient is not able to speak and there is no one else who can provide the patient's medical history.

**9. If you were unable to obtain a blood glucose reading on this patient, would you still administer oral glucose? Why or why not?**

Patients with hypoglycemia can experience a rapid loss of consciousness, experience seizures, and even die. Withholding glucose from a patient who needs it is far more dangerous than administering it to a patient who does not. Be sure to follow local protocol regarding administration of any medication.

**10. What does the term "polypharmacy" mean, and why is it important?**

Polypharmacy refers to the use of multiple medications by the same patient. It is not uncommon to find patients, especially older patients, taking multiple prescribed medications, OTC medications, and herbal remedies on a regular basis; this often makes a patient's medication regimen complex and confusing.

The potential for inadvertent underdosing and overdosing and harmful drug interactions increases in patients who take multiple medications. Furthermore, the patient's primary problem may be the result of one or more of the medications he or she is taking. Often older patients see several medical providers for different problems, each of which may prescribe medications without knowing what other medications the patient is taking. In some cases, the prescribed medications may either interfere with other medications or may dangerously increase adverse effects in combination.

You should carry a field guide or similar reference that lists common prescription and nonprescription medications. In cases where the patient is unable to communicate with you and a reliable source (eg, family member, caregiver) is not available to answer your questions, the patient's medications can give you important clues as to his or her medical history.

## YOU are the Provider SUMMARY *continued*

### EMS Patient Care Report (PCR)

| Date: 7-5-20 | Incident No.: 220109 | Nature of Call: Diabetic complications | | Location: 4864 Project Ave. | |
|---|---|---|---|---|---|
| Dispatched: 0600 | En Route: 0601 | At Scene: 0606 | Transport: 0622 | At Hospital: 0630 | In Service: 0636 |

#### Patient Information

**Age:** 68
**Sex:** F
**Weight (in kg [lb]):** 64 kg (140 lb)

**Allergies:** No known drug allergies
**Medications:** Amaryl, Nitrostat, Zoloft
**Past Medical History:** Diabetes, heart disease, depression
**Chief Complaint:** Confused

#### Vital Signs

| Time: 0611 | BP: 122/72 | Pulse: 112 | Respirations: 22 | Spo$_2$: 98% |
|---|---|---|---|---|
| Time: 0619 | BP: 128/74 | Pulse: 84 | Respirations: 18 | Spo$_2$: 99% |
| Time: 0625 | BP: 126/72 | Pulse: 74 | Respirations: 18 | Spo$_2$: 98% |

#### EMS Treatment (circle all that apply)

| Oxygen @ _15_ L/min via:<br><br>NC (NRM) Bag mask | | Assisted Ventilation | Airway Adjunct | CPR |
|---|---|---|---|---|
| Defibrillation | Bleeding Control | Bandaging | Splinting | Other: (Oral glucose) |

#### Narrative

Dispatched to a residence for a 68-year-old woman with "diabetic problems."

Chief Complaint: Confused

History: The patient's son, who called 9-1-1, advised that his mother has type 2 diabetes, and he is not sure when she last ate. Further past medical history includes heart disease and depression.

Assessment: Arrived on scene to find the patient sitting in a recliner in her living room. She was conscious, but confused. Her airway was patent and her breathing, although increased in rate, was producing adequate tidal volume. The patient was disoriented to place and time but able to speak and follow simple commands. Further assessment of patient revealed that her skin was cool, clammy, and pale. She was in no obvious respiratory distress and did not appear to be experiencing any pain.

Treatment (Rx): Applied oxygen at 15 L/min via nonrebreathing mask and obtained initial vital signs. Blood glucose level was assessed and read 36 mg/dL. After ensuring that the patient was able to swallow and follow directions, administered one tube (15 g) of oral glucose. Placed patient onto stretcher, loaded her into the ambulance, and reassessed her status. Her level of consciousness had improved and her vital signs were stable.

Transport: Assisted patient to stand, turn, and pivot onto stretcher, loaded her into the ambulance, and reassessed her status. Her level of consciousness had improved and her vital signs were stable. Began transport to the hospital and closely monitored the patient en route. Her airway and breathing remained adequate and her skin color and condition improved. The patient stated that she could not remember when she had eaten last. She further stated that she thinks that she may have accidentally taken too much of her Amaryl. Reassessed her blood glucose level, which read 94 mg/dL. Delivered patient to the emergency department without incident, gave verbal report to the charge nurse, Elgin, RN, and returned to service.

**End of report**

# Prep Kit

## Ready for Review

- Pharmacology is the science of drugs, including their ingredients, preparation, uses, and actions on the body.
- Medications may be administered through the following routes: intravenous, intramuscular, or subcutaneous injection; intranasal; oral; sublingual; intraosseous; transcutaneous; by inhalation; and by rectum.
- These routes of administration often determine the speed with which the medication takes effect.
- Medications come in seven forms: tablets and capsules, solutions and suspensions, MDIs, topical medications, and transdermal medications, gels, and gases.
- The administration of any medication requires approval by medical control, through direct orders given online or standing orders that are part of the local protocols.
- Once an order from medical control has been obtained, follow these steps in administering medications: Verify the patient, verify the proper medication, verify the dose, verify the route, and verify the time. Once the medication has been administered, reassess vital signs and document the patient's history, assessment, treatment, and response findings.
- Four medications are typically carried on an EMT ambulance: oxygen, aspirin, oral glucose, and epinephrine. Depending on local protocol, some EMS units may carry naloxone, nitroglycerin, and MDI medications.
- There are several medications that you may assist the patient to self-administer, including epinephrine auto-injectors (EpiPens), MDI medications (eg, albuterol [Proventil, Ventolin] and nitroglycerin (Nitrostat). Remember, medication assistance permissions may differ depending on local protocol.
- Knowing what medications a patient takes may be the only way you can determine what chronic or underlying conditions your patient may have.
- You must be extremely vigilant when administering medications. If a medication error occurs, provide any appropriate patient care required, notify medical control as soon as possible, and document the incident.

## Vital Vocabulary

**absorption**  The process by which medications travel through body tissues until they reach the bloodstream.

**action**  The therapeutic effect of a medication on the body.

**adverse effects**  Any unwanted clinical results of a medication.

**agonist**  A medication that causes stimulation of receptors.

**antagonist**  A medication that binds to a receptor and blocks other medications.

**antibiotic**  A medication used to treat infections caused by a bacterium.

**anticoagulant**  A medication that impairs the ability of blood to clot.

**antifungal**  A medication used to treat infections caused by a fungus.

**antiplatelet**  A medication that prevents blood platelets from clumping or sticking together.

**antipyretics**  Medications that treat or reduce a fever.

**aspirin (acetylsalicylic acid or ASA)**  A medication that is an antipyretic (reduces fever), analgesic (reduces pain), anti-inflammatory (reduces inflammation), and a potent inhibitor of platelet aggregation (clumping).

**contraindications**  Conditions that make a particular medication or treatment inappropriate because it would not help, or may actually harm, a patient.

**dose** The amount of medication given on the basis of the patient's size and age.

**duration** The amount of time that clinical effects of a medication last.

**elimination** The process of removing a medication or chemical from within the body.

**EMT-administered medication** Administration of a medication by the EMT directly to the patient.

**enteral medications** Medications that enter the body through the digestive system.

**epinephrine** A medication that increases heart rate and blood pressure but also eases breathing problems by decreasing muscle tone of the bronchiole tree.

**gel** A semiliquid substance that is administered orally in capsule form or through plastic tubes.

**generic name** The original chemical name of a medication (in contrast with one of its proprietary or trade names); the name is not capitalized.

**hypoglycemia** An abnormally low blood glucose level.

**indications** The therapeutic uses for a specific medication.

**inhalation** The active, muscular part of breathing that draws air into the airway and lungs; a medication delivery route.

**intramuscular (IM) injection** An injection into a muscle; a medication delivery route.

**intranasal (IN)** A delivery route in which a medication is pushed through a specialized atomizer device called a mucosal atomizer device (MAD) into the naris.

**intraosseous (IO) injection** An injection into the bone; a medication delivery route.

**intravenous (IV) injection** An injection directly into a vein; a medication delivery route.

**medication** A substance that is used to treat or prevent disease or relieve pain.

**medication error** Inappropriate use of a medication that could lead to patient harm.

**metered-dose inhaler (MDI)** A miniature spray canister used to direct medications through the mouth and into the lungs.

**mucosal atomizer device (MAD)** A device that is used to change a liquid medication into a spray and push it into a nostril.

**nitroglycerin** A medication that increases cardiac perfusion by causing blood vessels to dilate; EMTs may be allowed to assist the patient to self-administer this medication.

**onset of action** The amount of time from the administration of a medication to the onset of clinical effects.

**oral** By mouth; a medication delivery route.

**oral glucose** A simple sugar that is readily absorbed by the bloodstream; it is carried on the EMS unit.

**over-the-counter (OTC) medications** Medications that may be purchased directly by a patient without a prescription.

**oxygen** A gas that all cells need for metabolism; the heart and brain, especially, cannot function without oxygen.

**parenteral medications** Medications that enter the body by a route other than the digestive tract, skin, or mucous membranes.

**patient-assisted medication** When the EMT assists the patient with the administration of his or her own medication.

**peak** The point or period when the maximum clinical effect of a drug is achieved.

**peer-assisted medication** When the EMT administers medication to himself or herself or to a partner.

**per os (PO)** Through the mouth; a medication delivery route; same as oral.

**per rectum (PR)** Through the rectum; a medication delivery route.

**pharmacodynamics** The process by which a medication works on the body.

**pharmacokinetics** The processes that the body performs on a medication, including how it is absorbed, distributed, possibly changed, and eliminated.

**pharmacology** The study of the properties and effects of medications.

**polypharmacy** The use of multiple medications on a regular basis.

**prescription medications** Medications that are distributed to patients only by pharmacists according to a physician's order.

**solution** A liquid mixture that cannot be separated by filtering or allowing the mixture to stand.

**subcutaneous injection** Injection into the fatty tissue between the skin and muscle; a medication delivery route.

**sublingual (SL)** Under the tongue; a medication delivery route.

**suspension** A mixture of ground particles that are distributed evenly throughout a liquid but do not dissolve.

**therapeutic effect** The desired or intended effect a medication is expected to have on the body.

**topical medications** Lotions, creams, and ointments that are applied to the surface of the skin and affect only that area; a medication delivery route.

**trade name** The brand name that a manufacturer gives a medication; the name is capitalized.

**transcutaneous (transdermal)** Through the skin; a medication delivery route.

**unintended effects** Actions that are undesirable but pose little risk to the patient.

**untoward effects** Actions that can be harmful to the patient.

## References

1. Cocchio C. Medication safety win: no more epinephrine ratio expressions. Pharmacy Times website. https://www.pharmacytimes.com/contributor/craig-cocchio-pharmd/2016/01/medication-safety-win-no-more-epinephrine-ratio-expressions. Published January 20, 2016. Accessed April 8, 2020.

2. Darnis S, Fareau N, Corallo CE, Poole S, Dooley MJ, Cheng AC. Estimation of body weight in hospitalized patients. *QJM* 2012;105(8):769–774.

3. da Silva BA, Krishnamurthy M. The alarming reality of medication error: a patient case and review of Pennsylvania and national data. *J Community Hosp Int Med Perspect* 2016;6(4):31758.

4. Guy JS. *Pharmacology for the Prehospital Professional.* 2nd ed. Burlington, MA: Jones & Bartlett Learning; 2020.

5. Misasi P, Keebler JR. Medication safety in emergency medical services: approaching an evidence-based method of verification to reduce errors. *Ther Adv Drug Safety* 2019;10:2042098678821916. doi:10.1177/2042098618821916.

6. National Association of State EMS Officials. *National EMS Scope of Practice Model 2019.* Washington, DC: National Highway Traffic Safety Administration; February 2019. Report No. DOT HS 812-666. https://www.ems.gov/pdf/National_EMS_Scope_of_Practice_Model_2019.pdf. Accessed April 8, 2020.

7. Neiman AB, Ruppar T, Ho M, et al. CDC grand rounds: improving medication adherence for chronic disease management—innovations and opportunities. *Morb Mortal Wkly Rep* 2017;66. http://dx.doi.org/10.15585/mmwr.mm6645a2external icon.

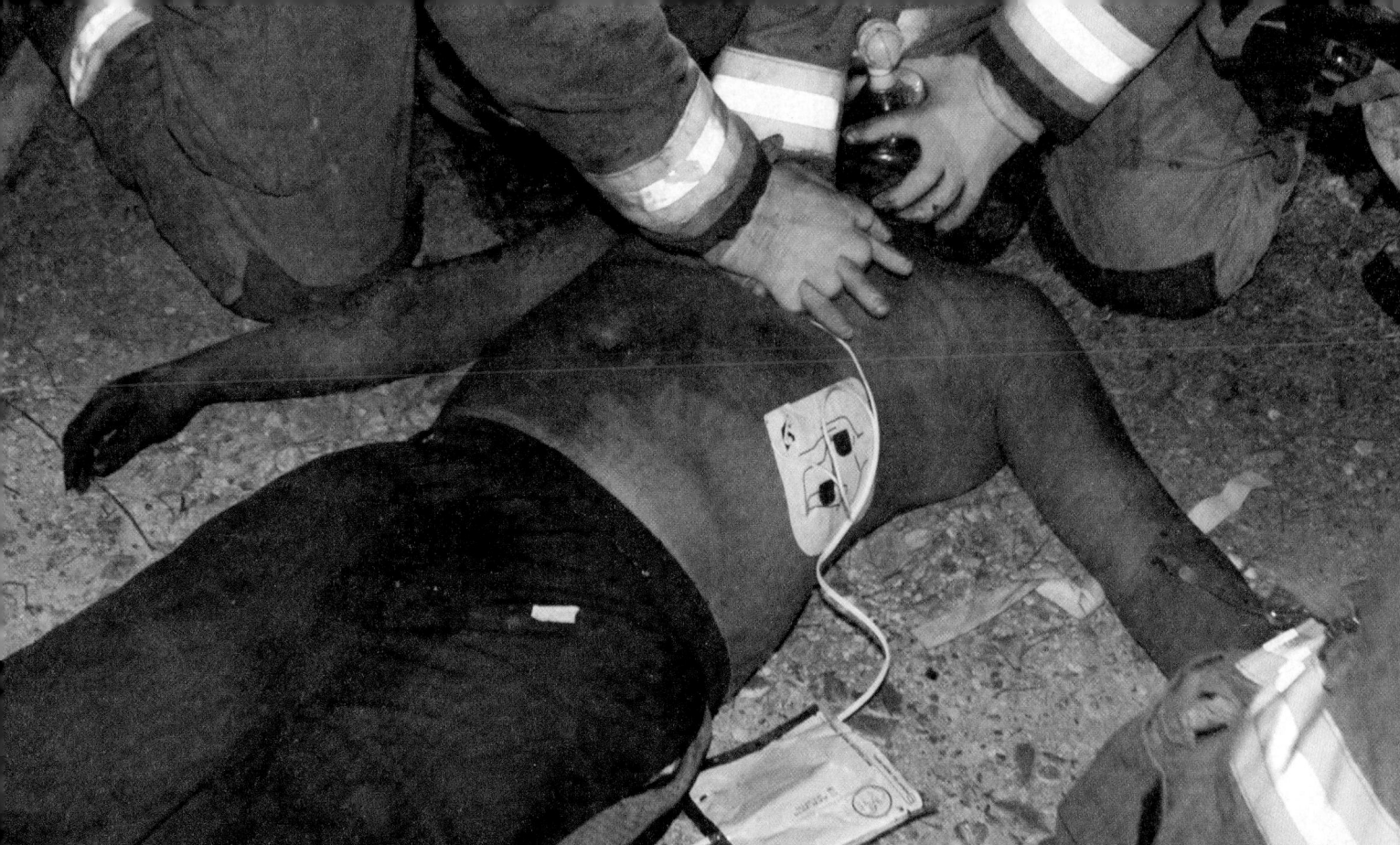

PHOTO: © Glen E. Ellman.

# Shock and Resuscitation

SECTION

# 5

**13** Shock

**14** BLS Resuscitation

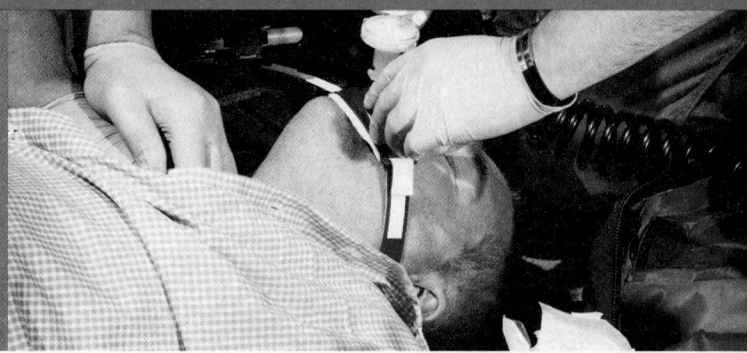

# Chapter 13

# Shock

## NATIONAL EMS EDUCATION STANDARD COMPETENCIES

### Shock and Resuscitation

Applies a fundamental knowledge of the causes, pathophysiology, and management of shock, respiratory failure or arrest, cardiac failure or arrest, and postresuscitation management.

### Pathophysiology

Applies fundamental knowledge of the pathophysiology of respiration and perfusion to patient assessment and management.

## KNOWLEDGE OBJECTIVES

1. Describe the pathophysiology of shock (hypoperfusion). (pp 531–534)
2. Identify the causes of shock. (p 534)
3. Differentiate among the various types of shock. (pp 534–539)
4. Describe the signs and symptoms of shock including compensated and decompensated. (p 540)
5. Discuss key components of patient assessment for shock. (pp 540–542)
6. Describe the steps to follow in the emergency care of the patient with various types of shock. (pp 543–548)

## SKILLS OBJECTIVES

1. Demonstrate how to control shock. (pp 543–548)
2. Demonstrate how to complete an EMS patient care report for a patient with shock. (p 551)

# Introduction

In this chapter, **shock** is defined as inadequate cellular perfusion. Cells require oxygen, water, and glucose to carry out cellular processes to produce energy in the form of adenosine triphosphate. When the cells do not receive these requirements via the bloodstream, the cells cannot create energy and are categorized as hypoperfused. If cells are hypoperfused, tissues and organs are also hypoperfused. In the early stages of shock, the body will attempt to compensate by maintaining **homeostasis** (a balance of all systems of the body); however, as shock progresses from tissues and organs to organ systems and the whole body, blood circulation slows and eventually ceases. This state of inadequate oxygen and nutrient delivery to the cells of the body causes organs and then organ systems to fail. If not treated promptly, shock can be fatal.

Shock can occur because of several medical or traumatic events, such as a heart attack, severe allergic reaction, or bleeding. As an EMT, you will respond to these types of emergencies to provide care and transportation for these patients. Therefore, you must be constantly alert to the signs and symptoms of shock and be able to provide the necessary treatment.

This chapter begins with a close-up look at perfusion. It then examines the physiologic causes of shock, describes each of its major forms, and discusses the emergency treatment of shock. See Chapter 14, *BLS Resuscitation*, for resuscitation techniques.

## Pathophysiology
### Perfusion

**Perfusion** is the circulation of blood to the tissues in adequate amounts to meet the cells' needs. It includes delivery of oxygen and removal of toxic waste products. The circulatory system is a complex arrangement of connected tubes, including the arteries, arterioles, capillaries, venules, and veins, in which blood circulates throughout to the body. There are two circuits in the body: the systemic circulation between the heart and the body and the pulmonary circulation between the heart and the lungs. The systemic circulation carries oxygen-rich blood from the left ventricle through the body and back to the right atrium. In the systemic circulation, as blood passes through the tissues and organs, it delivers oxygen and nutrients. Adequate perfusion is also important for the removal of waste products such as carbon dioxide, a by-product of energy production. The circulatory system carries these waste products for excretion or exhalation.

Organs, tissues, and cells must have adequate oxygenation to survive. Each time you take a breath, the alveoli, which are microscopic, thin-walled air sacs, receive a supply of oxygen-rich air. Oxygen diffuses through the walls of the alveoli into the bloodstream and attaches to hemoglobin, a protein that makes up red blood cells. The red blood cells then circulate the oxygen to the tissues where it can be offloaded.

Oxygen and carbon dioxide pass rapidly across the thin walls of the alveoli by the process of diffusion. Diffusion is a passive process in which molecules move from an area of higher concentration to an area of lower concentration. When the air reaches your alveoli, there is more oxygen in the air than in the bloodstream. Therefore, the oxygen molecules slip between the thin layers of the alveoli into the blood. Carbon dioxide does the same thing in the other direction. When blood is returned to the lungs from the tissues, there is more carbon dioxide in the blood than in the alveoli; thus, it diffuses into the alveoli, where it is exhaled.

Whereas most oxygen is carried to the tissues while attached to hemoglobin, carbon dioxide can be transported in the blood back to the lungs in three ways: dissolved in the plasma, combined with water in the form of bicarbonate, or attached to hemoglobin. Carbon dioxide waste products released from cells can combine with water in the bloodstream to form bicarbonate. Bicarbonate concentrations become higher as more carbon dioxide is produced and blood moves back toward the lungs. Once it reaches the lungs, the bicarbonate breaks down again into carbon dioxide and water and the carbon dioxide is exhaled. In cases of poor perfusion (shock), the transportation of carbon dioxide out of the tissues becomes impaired, resulting in a dangerous buildup of waste products, which may damage cells and tissues.

To protect vital organs from hypoperfusion, the body attempts to compensate by directing blood flow away from organs that are more tolerant of shock (such as the skin and intestines) to organs that cannot tolerate shock (such as the heart, brain, and lungs). If these tissues do not have adequate perfusion restored, they can die, resulting in permanent damage to the tissues and organ.

As described in Chapter 6, *The Human Body*, the cardiovascular system consists of three parts: a pump (the heart), a set of pipes (the blood vessels or arteries that act as the container), and the contents of the container (the blood) (**FIGURE 13-1**). These three parts can be referred to as the perfusion triangle (**FIGURE 13-2**). When a patient is in shock, one or more of the three parts is not working properly.

Blood is the vehicle for carrying oxygen and nutrients through the vessels to the capillary beds and tissue, where they are exchanged for waste products. For this process to happen, the vessels

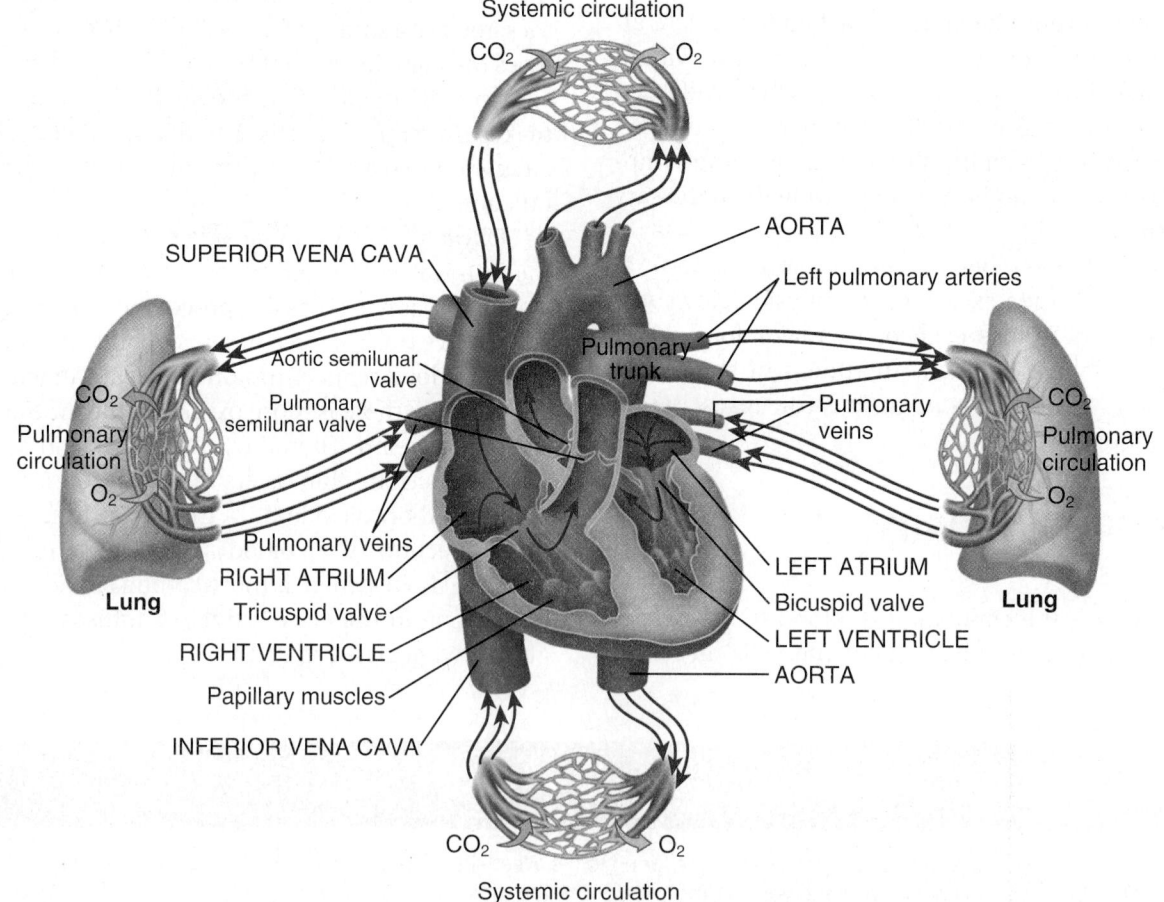

**FIGURE 13-1** The cardiovascular system consists of three parts: the pump (heart), the container (vessels), and the contents (blood). The blood carries oxygen and nutrients through the vessels to the capillary beds, where they diffuse into the tissue; in exchange, waste products diffuse into the bloodstream.

**Perfusion triangle**

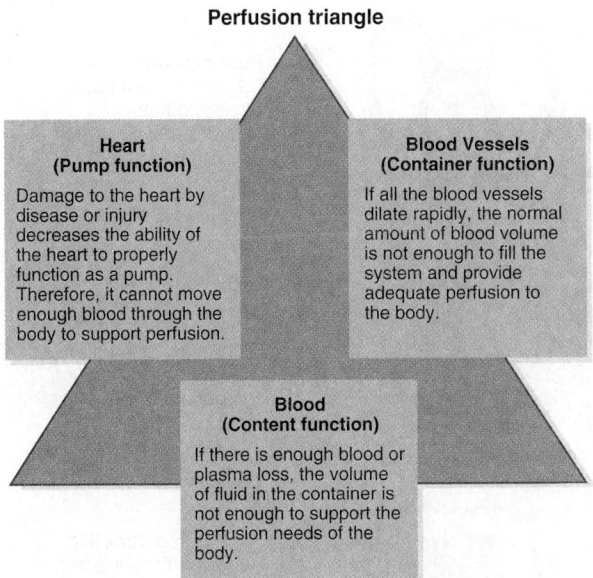

**FIGURE 13-2** The heart, the blood vessels, and the blood represent the three parts of perfusion (the perfusion triangle).

© Jones & Bartlett Learning.

(container) must be intact. Blood is composed of red blood cells, white blood cells, platelets, and a liquid called plasma. As discussed in Chapter 6, *The Human Body*, red blood cells are responsible for transporting oxygen to the cells and transporting carbon dioxide away from the cells to the lungs, where it is exhaled and removed from the body. Each component of blood has an important role in overall health: white blood cells help the body fight infection, platelets assist in forming blood clots, and plasma contains electrolytes and fluid, which are important for cells to function.

These components are all vital to maintain homeostasis. If, at any time, tissue is hypoperfused, the body will attempt to compensate by regulating the blood pressure, or the amount of blood delivered to any given part of the body, thereby preventing shock.

## Words of Wisdom

Capillary hydrostatic pressure (pressure within the capillary bed) tends to force fluids through capillary walls, whereas interstitial fluid hydrostatic pressure (pressure around the capillary bed and between the cells) pushes fluid back into the cells.

Remember, blood pressure is the pressure of blood within the vessels at any moment in time. The *systolic* pressure is the peak arterial pressure, or pressure generated when the heart contracts; the *diastolic* pressure is the pressure maintained within the arteries while the heart is at rest, or between beats. **Pulse pressure** is the difference between the systolic and diastolic pressures (Systolic – Diastolic = Pulse pressure). It signifies the amount of force the heart generates with each contraction.

Blood flow through the capillary beds is regulated by the capillary sphincters, circular muscular walls that constrict and dilate. These **sphincters** are under the control of the **autonomic nervous system**, which regulates involuntary functions such as sweating and digestion. Capillary sphincters also respond to other stimuli such as heat, cold, the need for oxygen, and the need for waste removal. This regulation is important because not all organs require the same amount of blood. Whereas your brain requires a constant amount of blood, your digestive tract requires more blood while digesting food and less when you are not eating.

Thus, regulation of blood flow is determined by cellular need and is accomplished by vessel constriction or dilation and capillary sphincter constriction or dilation. This team effort of the heart, blood, and vessels helps ensure blood gets to the tissues when it is needed.

Perfusion requires more than just having a working cardiovascular system, however. It also requires adequate oxygen exchange in the lungs, adequate nutrients in the form of glucose, and adequate waste removal, primarily through the lungs. Carbon dioxide is one of the primary waste products of cellular work (metabolism) in the body and is removed from the body by the lungs. This is the reason adequate ventilation and oxygenation is one of the EMT's primary concerns. The body has neural and endocrine or hormonal mechanisms in place to help support the respiratory and cardiovascular systems when the need for perfusion of vital organs is increased. These mechanisms include the autonomic nervous system and hormones, which are triggered when the body senses that the pressure in the system is falling. The sympathetic side of the autonomic nervous system, which is responsible for the fight-or-flight response, assumes more control of the body's functions during a state of shock. This response by the autonomic nervous system causes the release of the hormones epinephrine and nor-epinephrine. These hormones cause changes in certain body functions, including an increase in the heart rate and the strength of cardiac contractions. The fight-or-flight response also causes vasoconstriction in nonessential areas, primarily in the skin and gastrointestinal tract. Reducing blood flow to the skin is called peripheral vasoconstriction and helps to shunt blood to the vital organs. Together, these actions help maintain pressure in the system and, as a result, sustain perfusion to the vital organs.

Eventually, a shifting of body fluids to help maintain pressure within the system also occurs by reabsorption of fluid into the bloodstream when it passes through the kidneys. However, the response of the autonomic nervous system and hormones comes within seconds. It is this response that causes the signs and symptoms of shock in a patient.

## Causes of Shock

In all cases of shock, the damage occurs because of insufficient perfusion of organs and tissues. As soon as perfusion becomes impaired, cells and tissues start to die. If the conditions causing shock are not promptly stopped and reversed, death will follow.

> ### Words of Wisdom
>
> Shock is a complex physiologic process that gives subtle signs of its presence before it becomes severe. These early signs relate closely to the events that lead to more severe shock, so it is important for you to know the underlying processes thoroughly. If you understand what causes shock, you will be able to recognize it in many patients before it progresses.

Understanding the basic physiologic causes of shock will better prepare you to treat it (**FIGURE 13-3**). Shock results from three basic causes (**TABLE 13-1**).

## Types of Shock
### Cardiogenic Shock

**Cardiogenic shock** is caused by inadequate function of the heart, or pump failure. Circulation of blood throughout the vascular system requires the constant pumping action of the heart muscle. Many diseases or injuries can cause destruction or

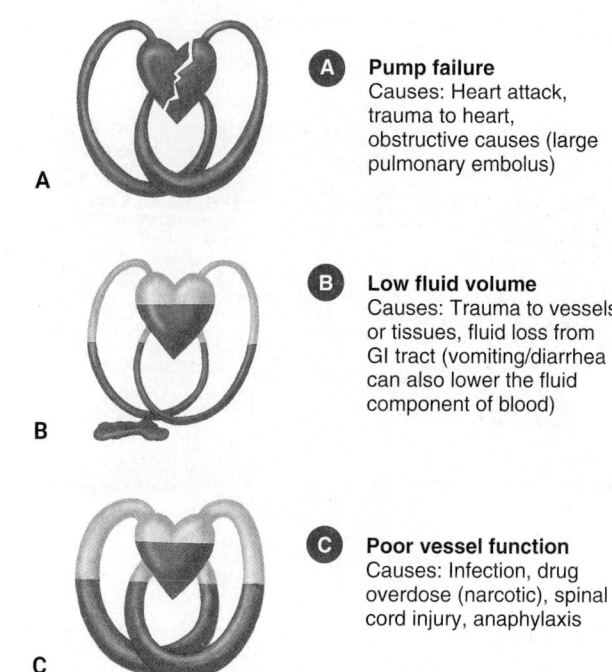

**A** Pump failure
Causes: Heart attack, trauma to heart, obstructive causes (large pulmonary embolus)

**B** Low fluid volume
Causes: Trauma to vessels or tissues, fluid loss from GI tract (vomiting/diarrhea can also lower the fluid component of blood)

**C** Poor vessel function
Causes: Infection, drug overdose (narcotic), spinal cord injury, anaphylaxis

**FIGURE 13-3** There are three basic causes of shock and impaired tissue perfusion. **A.** Pump failure occurs when the heart is damaged by disease or injury, or when an obstruction prevents it from functioning. **B.** Low fluid volume, often a result of bleeding. **C.** The blood vessels can dilate excessively so that the blood within them is inadequate to fill the system.

**A, B, C:** © Jones & Bartlett Learning.

**TABLE 13-1** Causes of Shock

| Cause | Type of Shock |
|---|---|
| Pump failure | Cardiogenic shock<br>Obstructive shock<br>• Tension pneumothorax<br>• Cardiac tamponade<br>• Pulmonary embolism |
| Poor vessel function | Distributive shock<br>• Septic shock<br>• Neurogenic shock<br>• Anaphylactic shock<br>• Psychogenic shock |
| Low fluid volume | Hypovolemic shock<br>• Hemorrhagic shock<br>• Nonhemorrhagic shock |

© Jones & Bartlett Learning.

inflammation of heart muscle. Within certain limits, the heart can adapt. If too much muscular damage occurs, however, as sometimes happens after a heart attack, the heart no longer functions well. A major effect is the backup of blood into the pulmonary vessels. The resulting buildup forces fluid out of the capillary beds that surround the alveoli, leading to pulmonary edema. **Edema** is the presence of abnormally large amounts of fluid between cells in body tissues, causing swelling of the affected area (**FIGURE 13-4**). Red blood cells cannot easily leave the capillaries; however, as blood backs up, the fluid in the vessels is forced out and accumulates in the alveoli. Oxygen cannot diffuse across the fluid-filled alveoli, resulting in tachypnea (rapid respirations) and crackles, or rales, (a rattling sound that may be heard during breathing, typically on inhalation).

The muscular contraction of the heart moves blood through the vessels at distinct pressures. For blood to circulate efficiently throughout the entire system, the amount of pressure must be right and there must be an adequate number of heartbeats.

Cardiogenic shock develops when the heart cannot maintain sufficient output (cardiac output) to meet the demands of the body. Cardiac output is the volume of blood that the heart can pump per minute and depends on several factors. First, the heart must have adequate strength, which is

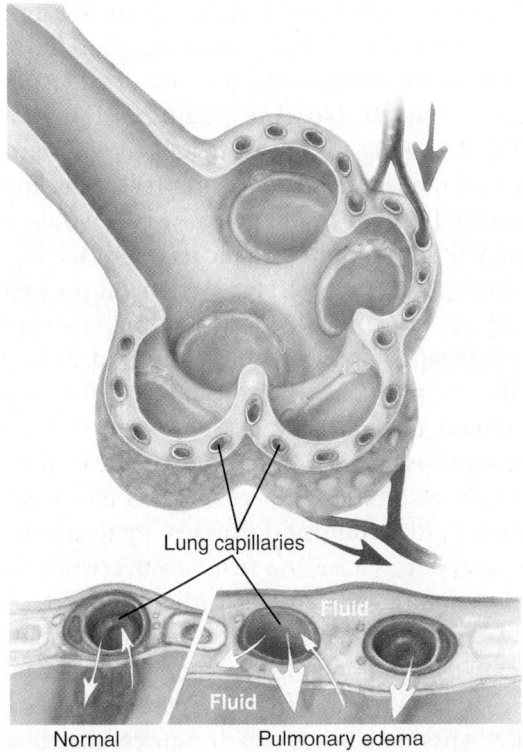

**FIGURE 13-4** Pulmonary edema develops as a result of fluid buildup within the pulmonary tissue. This edema causes swelling and leads to impaired oxygenation.

© Jones & Bartlett Learning.

## YOU are the Provider

You arrive at the clinic and are escorted to the patient by a clinic technician. You find the patient lying supine on an examination table. She is conscious, but restless, and her skin is notably pale and diaphoretic. She has a blanket covering her, and she is receiving oxygen via a nasal cannula at 4 L/min. Several attempts at establishing intravenous (IV) access were unsuccessful. Your assessment of the patient reveals the following:

| Recording Time: 0 Minutes | |
|---|---|
| Appearance | Restless, pale, and diaphoretic |
| Level of consciousness | Conscious and restless |
| Airway | Open and patent |
| Breathing | Increased rate |
| Circulation | Radial pulses weak and rapid; skin cool, pale, and diaphoretic |

The clinic physician tells you that the patient presented approximately 15 minutes ago, reporting abdominal pain and rectal bleeding, which apparently started about 24 hours ago. She has a history of irritable bowel syndrome, she takes lubiprostone (Amitiza) and dicyclomine hydrochloride (Bentyl), and she is allergic to codeine.

**3.** Based on your assessment, what changes, if any, in the patient's current treatment are required?

**4.** How do the patient's signs and symptoms correlate with the body's response to inadequate perfusion?

largely determined by the ability of the heart muscle to contract. This ability to contract is referred to as **myocardial contractility**. Second, the heart must receive adequate blood to pump. As the volume of blood coming to the heart increases, the pressure in the heart builds up. This pressure is known as **preload**. As preload increases, the volume of blood within the ventricles increases, which causes the heart muscle to stretch. When the muscle is stretched, myocardial contractility increases, leading to greater force of contraction and increased cardiac output. Last, the resistance to flow in the peripheral circulation must be appropriate. The force, or resistance against which the heart pumps, is known as **afterload**. In general, as afterload increases, cardiac output decreases. Increased afterload may also cause the heart to overwork while trying to maintain adequate cardiac output. Chronically high afterload is often the reason heart failure develops in patients with hypertension. Cardiogenic shock may result from low cardiac output due to high afterload, low preload, poor contractility, or any combination of the three.

## Obstructive Shock

**Obstructive shock** is caused by an obstruction that prevents an adequate volume of blood from being distributed to the body. Three of the most common examples of obstructive shock are cardiac tamponade, tension pneumothorax, and pulmonary embolism.

A collection of fluid between the pericardial sac and the myocardium is called a **pericardial effusion**. If the effusion becomes large enough, it can prevent the ventricles from filling with blood—a condition called **cardiac tamponade** or pericardial tamponade. This life-threatening condition may also be caused by blunt or penetrating trauma that causes hemorrhage around the heart. Large pericardial effusions leading to cardiac tamponade can also be seen in patients with cancer and autoimmune diseases. Cardiac tamponade occurs when blood leaks into the space between the tough fibrous membrane known as the pericardium and the outer walls of the heart, an area called the pericardial sac. As more blood or fluid accumulates in this confined space, the outer walls of the heart become compressed. Because the pericardium has a limited ability to stretch, the accumulated blood or fluid in the pericardial space

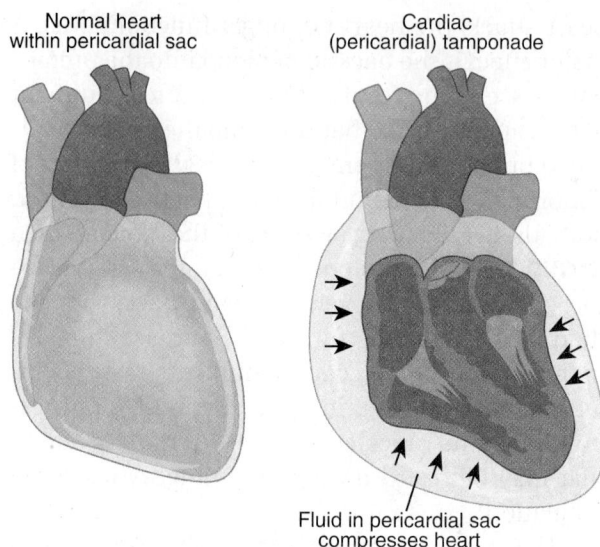

Normal heart within pericardial sac

Cardiac (pericardial) tamponade

Fluid in pericardial sac compresses heart

**FIGURE 13-5** Impaired ventricular filling from a pericardial effusion causes cardiac tamponade.

© Jones & Bartlett Learning.

eventually exerts back pressure on the outer walls of the heart, compressing the walls of the heart and preventing the heart from completely refilling with blood. Continued pressure within the pericardial sac obstructs the flow of blood into the heart, resulting in decreased outflow from the heart (**FIGURE 13-5**). Signs and symptoms of cardiac tamponade are referred to as the Beck triad: the presence of jugular vein distention, muffled heart sounds, and a narrowing pulse pressure, where the systolic and diastolic blood pressures start to merge (systolic pressure decreases and the diastolic pressure increases).

Tension pneumothorax is another obstructive condition (**FIGURE 13-6**). A tension pneumothorax is caused by damage to the lung tissue. This damage allows air normally held within the lung to escape into the chest cavity. The lung eventually collapses, causing a pneumothorax. If a pneumothorax is allowed to progress, air will accumulate within the chest cavity and begin applying pressure to the heart and greater vessels. When the trapped air begins to shift the chest organs toward the uninjured side, a pneumothorax becomes known as a tension pneumothorax, which is a serious, life-threatening condition. As pressure from one side of the chest begins to push the mediastinum toward the other side, the vena cava loses its ability to stay fully expanded. This compression of the vena cava leads to reduced blood return to the right side of the heart and blood pressure drops. As the patient has more difficulty

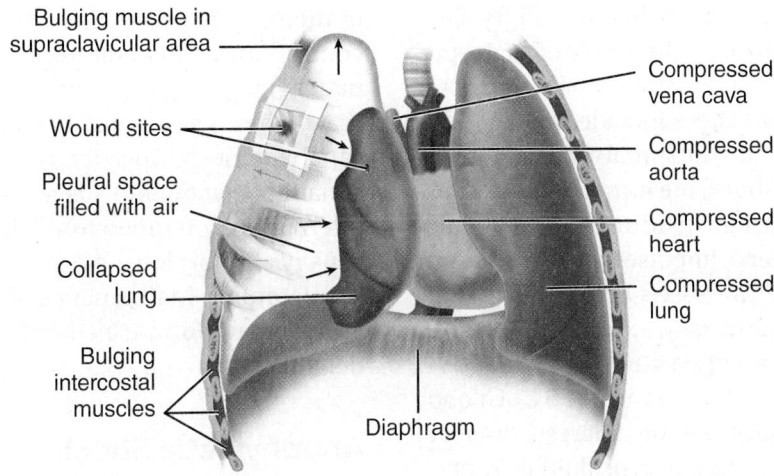

Bulging muscle in supraclavicular area

Wound sites

Pleural space filled with air

Collapsed lung

Bulging intercostal muscles

Compressed vena cava

Compressed aorta

Compressed heart

Compressed lung

Diaphragm

**FIGURE 13-6** A tension pneumothorax is an accumulation of air in the pleural space, which eventually compresses the heart and great vessels.

© Jones & Bartlett Learning.

breathing, the heart also has more difficulty pumping. You may notice difficulty when attempting to ventilate the patient with a bag-mask device. The affected side will have absent lung sounds, and the patient may become cyanotic. Tracheal deviation is a late sign of tension pneumothorax.

A pulmonary embolism can also lead to obstructive shock. A **pulmonary embolism** is a blood clot that occurs in the pulmonary arteries and blocks the flow of blood through the lungs. When a massive pulmonary embolism occurs, it can prevent blood from being pumped from the right side of the heart to the left, resulting in complete backup of blood in the right ventricle and catastrophic obstructive shock.

### Words of Wisdom

Understanding the main differences among the types of shock is as simple as considering the terms themselves.
- **Cardiogenic shock.** Consider the parts of the word *cardiogenic*. *Cardio* suggests the heart, and *genic* means produced by.
- **Obstructive shock.** Think of obstructive shock as an *obstruction* blocking blood flow to an area of the body.
- **Distributive shock.** Think of distributive shock as a problem *distributed* throughout the body.
- **Hypovolemic shock.** Consider the parts of the word *hypovolemic*. *Hypo* means less than normal, and *volemic* suggests volume—specifically, the volume of fluid in the circulatory system.

## Distributive Shock

**Distributive shock** results when there is widespread dilation of the small arterioles, small venules, or both. As a result, the circulating blood volume pools in the expanded vascular beds and tissue perfusion decreases. The four most common types of distributive shock are septic shock, neurogenic shock, anaphylactic shock, and psychogenic shock.

### Septic Shock

**Septic shock** occurs as a result of severe infections, usually bacterial, in which toxins (poisons) are generated by the bacteria. In this condition, the toxins damage the vessel walls, causing increased cellular permeability. The vessel walls leak and are unable to constrict well. Widespread dilation of vessels, in combination with plasma loss through the injured vessel walls, results in shock.

Septic shock is a complex problem. First, there is an insufficient volume of fluid in the container, because much of the plasma has leaked out of the vessels (hypovolemia). Second, the fluid that has leaked out often collects in the alveoli, interfering with respiration. Third, the vasodilation leads to a larger-than-normal vascular volume. This increase in space combined with smaller-than-normal volume of intravascular fluid leads to shock.

### Neurogenic Shock

Damage to the spinal cord, particularly at the upper cervical levels, may cause loss of control to the musculature and vessels below the injury site. **Neurogenic shock** is usually the result of high spinal cord injury. Although not as common, there are medical causes as well. These include brain conditions, tumors, pressure on the spinal cord, and spina bifida. In neurogenic shock, the muscles in the walls of the blood vessels are cut off from the sympathetic nervous system and nerve impulses that cause them to contract. Therefore, all vessels below the level of the spinal injury dilate widely, increasing the size and capacity of the vascular system (**FIGURE 13-7**) and causing blood to pool. The available 6 L of blood in the body can no longer fill the enlarged vascular system. Even if there is no blood or fluid loss, perfusion of organs and tissues becomes inadequate, and shock occurs. In this condition, a change in the size of the vascular system has caused shock. Characteristic signs of this type of shock are the absence of sweating below the level of injury, normal and low heart rate in the presence of hypotension, and normal, warm skin. This is the only type of shock that presents without the characteristic pale, cool skin, because the peripheral vasoconstriction cannot be triggered through the autonomic nervous system.

With neurogenic shock, many other functions that are under the control of the same part of the nervous system are also lost. The most important

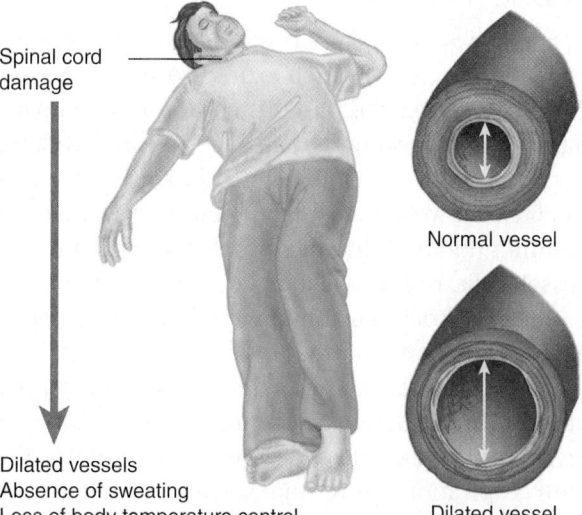

Spinal cord damage

Normal vessel

Dilated vessels
Absence of sweating
Loss of body temperature control

Dilated vessel

**FIGURE 13-7** Damage to the spinal cord can cause significant injury to the part of the nervous system that controls the size and muscle tone of blood vessels. If the muscles in the blood vessels are cut off from their impulses to contract, the vessels dilate widely, increasing the size and capacity of the vascular system. The blood in the body can no longer fill the enlarged vessels, and shock ensues.

© Jones & Bartlett Learning.

of them, in an acute injury setting, is the ability to control body temperature. Body temperature in a patient in neurogenic shock can rapidly fall to match that of the environment. In many situations, significant hypothermia occurs, severely complicating the situation. **Hypothermia** is a condition in which the internal body temperature falls below 95°F (35°C), usually after prolonged exposure to cool or freezing temperatures. Maintenance of body temperature is always an important element of treatment for a patient in shock.

## Anaphylactic Shock

**Anaphylaxis**, or **anaphylactic shock**, occurs when a person reacts quickly to a substance to which he or she has been sensitized. **Sensitization** means becoming sensitive to a substance that did not initially cause a reaction. Do not be misled by a patient who reports no history of allergic reaction to a substance on first or second exposure. Each subsequent exposure after sensitization tends to produce a more severe reaction.

Instances that cause severe allergic reactions commonly fall into the following four categories of exposure:

- Injections (tetanus antitoxin, penicillin)
- Stings (wasps, bees, hornets, ants)
- Ingestion (fish, shellfish, nuts, eggs, medication)
- Inhalation (dust, pollen, mold)

Anaphylactic reactions can develop within minutes after contact with the substance to which the patient is allergic. The signs of such allergic reactions are distinct and not seen with other forms of shock. **TABLE 13-2** lists the signs of anaphylactic shock in the order in which they typically occur. Note that **cyanosis** (blue discoloration of the skin) is a late sign of anaphylactic shock. Although paleness, or a decrease in blood flow, can be difficult to detect in dark-skinned people, it may be observed by examining mucous membranes inside the inner lower eyelid and capillary refill. On general observation, the patient may appear ashen or gray.

In anaphylactic shock, there is no loss of blood or vascular damage. Instead, there is widespread vascular dilation, increased permeability, and bronchoconstriction. The combination of poor oxygenation and poor perfusion in anaphylactic shock may easily prove fatal.

For more information on allergic reactions and anaphylaxis, see Chapter 21, *Allergy and Anaphylaxis*.

**TABLE 13-2** Signs and Symptoms of Anaphylactic Shock

| System | Signs and Symptoms |
|---|---|
| Skin | • Flushed, itchy, or burning, especially over the face and upper part of the chest<br>• Urticaria (hives), which may spread over large areas of the body<br>• Edema, especially of the face, tongue, and lips<br>• Pallor<br>• Cyanosis (a blue cast to the skin resulting from poor oxygenation of circulating blood) about the lips, which in dark-skinned people may be observed by examining mucous membranes inside the inner lower eyelid and capillary refill |
| Circulatory system | • Dilated peripheral blood vessels<br>• Increased vessel permeability<br>• Drop in blood pressure<br>• Weak, barely palpable pulse |
| Respiratory system | • Sneezing or itching in the nasal passages<br>• Stridor<br>• Upper airway obstruction<br>• Tightness in the chest, with a persistent dry cough<br>• Wheezing and dyspnea (difficulty breathing)<br>• Secretions of fluid and mucus into the bronchial passages, alveoli, and lung tissue, causing coughing<br>• Constriction of the bronchi; difficulty drawing air into the lungs<br>• Forced expiration, requiring exertion and accompanied by wheezing<br>• Cessation of breathing |
| Other | • Abdominal cramping<br>• Nausea<br>• Vomiting<br>• Altered mental status<br>• Dizziness<br>• Fainting and coma |

© Jones & Bartlett Learning.

## Psychogenic Shock

A patient in **psychogenic shock** has had a sudden reaction of the nervous system that produces a temporary, generalized vasodilation, resulting in fainting, or **syncope**. The fainting episode is temporary, and

**Words of Wisdom**

Skin findings such as hives without evidence of any other signs and symptoms of anaphylaxis indicate only an allergy, not anaphylaxis. Monitor these patients carefully for development of other findings that suggest anaphylaxis.

the patient rouses soon after. Syncope occurs when blood pools in the dilated vessels, reducing the blood supply to the brain; as a result, the brain temporarily ceases to function normally, and the patient faints.

There are many causes of syncope, and it is important to realize that some are serious. Syncope that is potentially life threatening may be caused by events such as an irregular heartbeat or a brain **aneurysm**. Non–life-threatening events that cause syncope include receiving bad news, experiencing fear, or encountering an unpleasant sight, such as blood. Those experiencing syncope should receive a full assessment.

## Hypovolemic Shock

**Hypovolemic shock** is the result of an inadequate amount of fluid in the circulatory system. There are hemorrhagic and nonhemorrhagic causes of hypovolemic shock. For example, injuries involving bleeding may result in hemorrhagic shock, whereas vomiting and diarrhea may result in nonhemorrhagic hypovolemic shock.

Hypovolemic shock also occurs with severe thermal burns. In this case, intravascular plasma (the colorless part of the blood) loss is caused when fluid leaks from the capillaries into the surrounding tissue. Likewise, crushing injuries may result in the loss of blood and plasma from damaged vessels into injured tissues. These injuries can be thought of as excessive swelling.

**Dehydration**, the loss of water or fluid from body tissues, can cause shock. Fluid loss may be a result of severe vomiting and/or diarrhea. Patients who are very young or old are particularly susceptible to fluid loss and therefore at risk for the development of shock through dehydration. People who exercise in hot weather and are not acclimated to it may experience dehydration if they do not drink enough fluids. In these circumstances, the common factor is an insufficient volume of fluid within the vascular system to provide adequate circulation to the organs of the body.

# The Progression of Shock

The signs and symptoms of shock can become apparent as a patient progresses through them (**TABLE 13-3**). The early stage of shock, while the body can still compensate for blood loss, is called **compensated shock**. The late stage, when blood pressure is falling and the mental status is declining, is called **decompensated shock**. When shock progresses too far, it becomes irreversible; however, there is no way to know when a patient has reached that point. It is therefore important to recognize and treat shock early, before the patient has developed **irreversible shock**, a condition defined by the inability to successfully achieve resuscitation regardless of the methods employed.

## Words of Wisdom

Although skin paleness can suggest a decrease in blood flow, it can be difficult to detect in dark-skinned people. For these patients, you may learn more by examining capillary refill and the mucous membranes inside the inner lower eyelid than by assessing skin color.

| TABLE 13-3 Progression of Shock | |
|---|---|
| **Progression** | **Signs and Symptoms** |
| Compensated shock | • Agitation<br>• Anxiety<br>• Restlessness<br>• Feeling of impending doom<br>• Weak, rapid (thready) pulse<br>• Clammy (pale, cool, moist) skin<br>• Pallor, with cyanosis about the lips<br>• Shallow, rapid breathing<br>• Nausea or vomiting<br>• Capillary refill of longer than 2 seconds in infants and children<br>• Marked thirst<br>• Narrowing pulse pressure |
| Decompensated shock | • Falling blood pressure (systolic blood pressure of 90 mm Hg or lower in an adult)<br>• Declining mental status, altered level of consciousness<br>• Labored or irregular breathing<br>• Ashen, mottled, or cyanotic skin<br>• Thready or absent peripheral pulses<br>• Dull eyes, dilated pupils<br>• Poor urinary output |

Remember that blood pressure may be the last measurable factor to change in shock. As we have seen, the body has several automatic mechanisms to compensate for initial blood loss and to help maintain blood pressure. Thus, by the time you detect a decrease in blood pressure, shock is well developed. This is particularly true in infants and children, who can maintain their blood pressure until they have sustained blood loss equivalent to more than one-half their blood volume. By the time blood pressure drops in infants and children who are in shock, they are close to death.

You should expect shock in many emergency medical situations. For example, you would expect shock to accompany massive external or internal bleeding. You should also expect shock if a patient has any one of the following conditions:

- Multiple severe fractures
- Abdominal or chest injury
- Spinal injury
- Severe infection
- Major heart attack
- Anaphylaxis

## Words of Wisdom

Frequently taking and recording vital signs—and observing perfusion indicators such as skin condition and mental status—will give you a window into the progression of shock. Monitoring vital signs every 5 minutes may reveal a pattern that will alert you to the presence of evolving shock. If suspected, expedite transport and begin treatments for shock immediately.

# Patient Assessment for Shock

## Scene Size-Up

As you approach the scene, be alert to potential hazards to your safety. If this is a trauma scene or bleeding is suspected, put on gloves and eye protection, at a minimum.

## Street Smarts

Put several pairs of gloves in your pocket for easy access in case your gloves tear or there are multiple patients with bleeding.

In incidents involving violence, such as assaults or gunshot wounds, make sure that police are on scene. At times, you may need to stage several blocks away until law enforcement personnel have secured the area.

When you first see the patient, observe the scene and patient for clues to determine the nature of the illness or the mechanism of injury. This could help you anticipate the potential for development of shock.

## Primary Assessment

The primary assessment for a patient with suspected shock should include a rapid exam to look for evidence of severe or exsanguinating hemorrhage, determine level of consciousness, identify and manage life-threatening concerns as they are found, and determine priority of the patient and transport. A patient with massive hemorrhage may require a tourniquet or wound packing *before* the airway is opened. If the patient has obvious life-threatening external bleeding, it should be addressed first (even *before* airway and breathing) by controlling it quickly, then the ABCs can be assessed and treated.

When treating a patient in shock, provide high-flow oxygen to assist in perfusion of damaged tissues. If the patient has bled out, saturating the red blood cells they have left will help prevent hypoxia. If the patient has signs of hypoperfusion, treat aggressively and provide rapid transport to the hospital.

Request advanced life support (ALS) as necessary to assist with more aggressive shock management. Do not delay transport of the seriously injured trauma patient to complete non-lifesaving treatments in the field, such as splinting extremity fractures; instead, complete these types of treatments en route to the hospital.

When you first visually inspect your patient, quickly form an initial general impression. This will help you develop an early sense of urgency for care of a patient who appears sick.

Once you are close to the patient, determine the need for manual spinal stabilization, and assess the patient's level of consciousness using the AVPU scale. A patient who has an altered level of consciousness (LOC) may need emergency airway management. If the patient is awake and alert, determine a chief complaint.

Next, quickly assess the airway to ensure it is patent. Be alert to abnormal airway sounds such as gurgling (suction the airway) or stridor, indicating partial airway obstruction. Consider an adjunct such as an oropharyngeal or nasopharyngeal airway for a patient with an altered LOC.

Quickly assess breathing in the patient. Observe the patient for signs of accessory muscle use such as the muscles of the neck, intercostal retractions, or abnormal use of the abdominal muscles. An increased respiratory rate is often an early sign of impending shock and can be overlooked even by experienced providers. Administer high-flow oxygen, or, if needed, assist respirations with a bag-mask device.

## YOU are the Provider

You continue with the treatment initiated by the clinic; however, you remove the nasal cannula and apply high-flow oxygen via a nonrebreathing mask. Your partner takes the patient's vital signs and reports them to you and the clinic physician.

| Recording Time: 4 Minutes | |
| --- | --- |
| **Respirations** | 24 breaths/min; shallow |
| **Pulse** | 120 beats/min; weak |
| **Skin** | Pale, cool, and diaphoretic |
| **Blood pressure** | 108/58 mm Hg |
| **Oxygen saturation (Spo$_2$)** | 94% (on oxygen) |

You bring the stretcher into the room and prepare the patient for immediate transport. The patient remains conscious and alert, but is becoming increasingly restless and tells you that she is becoming dizzy.

**5.** Is the patient in compensated or decompensated shock? How can you tell?

Assessing the patient's circulatory status can reveal important clues regarding the presence of shock. Check for the presence of a distal pulse. If you cannot obtain a distal pulse, assess for a central pulse. Make a rapid determination if the pulse is fast, slow, weak, strong, or altogether absent. A rapid pulse suggests compensated shock. In shock, the skin may be cool, clammy, or ashen. If the patient has no pulse and is not breathing, immediately begin CPR. Assess for and identify any life-threatening bleeding in trauma patients; if serious bleeding is discovered, treat it immediately when you find it. You must also quickly assess skin temperature, condition, and color, and check for capillary refill time.

## Words of Wisdom

If the shock patient's mental status is starting to deteriorate, the brain is no longer receiving adequate blood flow and the patient is progressing from compensated to decompensated shock.

Once you have assessed perfusion, determine whether the patient should be treated as high priority, whether ALS is needed, and the transport destination.

## History Taking

After the life threats have been managed during the primary assessment, determine the chief complaint. Obtain a medical history and be alert for injury-specific signs and symptoms as well as any pertinent negatives such as loss of sensation. Quickly obtain a SAMPLE history from the patient. Anticoagulants can increase bleeding and worsen shock. Blood pressure medicines such as beta blockers can prevent the heart rate from rising to compensate for shock.

## Secondary Assessment

The secondary assessment is a more detailed, comprehensive examination of the patient that is used to uncover injuries that may have been missed during the primary assessment. The secondary assessment begins by repeating the primary assessment followed by a focused assessment. In some instances, such as a critically injured patient or short transport time, you may not have time to conduct a secondary assessment.

If your patient is a trauma patient with a significant mechanism of injury or multiple injuries, if the patient gives you a poor initial general impression, or if you found problems in the primary assessment, perform a secondary assessment of the entire body. If your patient has a medical problem but is not responsive or if problems were noted in the primary assessment, perform a secondary assessment of the entire body. These assessments should be performed quickly but thoroughly to ensure that you do not miss any significant or life-threatening problems or delay needed care.

If your patient has a simple mechanism of injury, such as a twisted ankle, focus your examination on the specific area affected. Whether your examination is of the entire body or of a specific area, if a life-threatening problem is found, treat it immediately.

When time permits and the patient's condition is stable, perform a thorough examination of the patient, which includes a complete neurologic assessment.

Obtain a complete set of baseline vital signs. If the patient's condition is unstable or could become unstable, reassess vital signs every 5 minutes. If the patient is in stable condition, reassess vital signs every 10 to 15 minutes. Baseline vital signs will help you trend changes in your patient.

In addition to hands-on assessment, use monitoring devices to quantify the patient's oxygenation and circulatory status. Use a noninvasive technique to monitor blood pressure and a pulse oximeter to evaluate the effectiveness of oxygenation. It is recommended that you assess the patient's blood pressure with a sphygmomanometer (blood pressure cuff) and stethoscope (manually), before using a noninvasive blood pressure monitor, to establish a baseline blood pressure and to determine the accuracy of the noninvasive blood pressure monitor.

## Reassessment

Reassess the patient's vital signs, interventions, chief complaint, and mental status. You must determine what interventions are needed for your patient based on the assessment findings. Focus on supporting the cardiovascular system. Treat for shock early and aggressively by providing oxygen and keeping the patient warm.

# Emergency Medical Care for Shock

You must begin immediate treatment for shock as soon as you realize that the condition may exist. As with any type of patient care, you should begin by following standard precautions. Control all obvious external bleeding. Place dry, sterile dressings over the bleeding sites, and secure with bandages. If direct pressure is not rapidly successful in the control of bleeding from an extremity, apply a tourniquet proximal to the bleeding site (**FIGURE 13-8**). The use of tourniquets is further described in Chapter 26, *Bleeding*. Make sure the patient has an open airway. Maintain manual in-line stabilization if necessary, and check breathing and pulse.

Comfort, calm, and reassure the patient, while maintaining the patient in the supine position. Never allow patients to eat or drink prior to being evaluated by a physician.

Apply spinal motion restriction if there is a concern about neck or back injuries. Do not delay transport to apply individual splints in the field when shock is present. If time allows, splint individual extremity fractures during transport. Splinting minimizes pain, bleeding, and discomfort, all of which can aggravate shock. It also prevents the broken bone ends from further damaging adjacent soft tissue.

Remember that inadequate ventilation may be a major factor in the development of shock. Always provide oxygen, assist with ventilations, and use airway control adjuncts as needed, and continue to monitor the patient's breathing. To prevent the loss of body heat, place blankets under and over the patient. Do not use external heat sources, such as hot water bottles or heating pads. They may harm a patient in shock by causing vasodilation and decreasing blood pressure even more.

Transport the patient and treat additional injuries en route. Consider ALS rendezvous if possible, and consider aeromedical transport.

Accurately record the patient's vital signs approximately every 5 minutes throughout treatment and transport. It is essential to transport trauma patients to the ED as rapidly as possible for definitive treatment. The critically important period for the early resuscitation and treatment of severely injured trauma patients is often referred to as the Golden Period. This concept underscores the importance of rapid evaluation, stabilization, and transport. The goal of EMS is to limit on-scene time (time on scene until transport to hospital is started) to 10 minutes or less. Remember to speak calmly and reassuringly to a conscious patient throughout assessment, care, and transport.

**TABLE 13-4** lists the general supportive measures for the major types of shock. Not every measure is used for every type of shock.

## Treating Cardiogenic Shock

The patient who is in shock as a result of a heart attack simply cannot generate the necessary contraction to pump blood throughout the circulatory system.

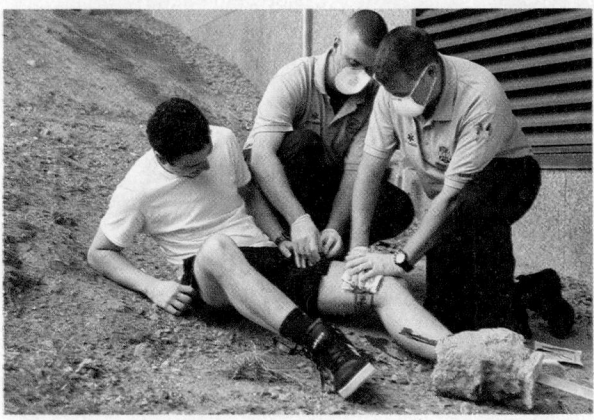

**FIGURE 13-8** If direct pressure does not quickly control bleeding from an extremity, a tourniquet should be applied proximal to the bleeding site.

© Jones & Bartlett Learning.

> ### Words of Wisdom
>
> Keep in mind that chronic lung disease will aggravate cardiogenic shock. If the patient has chronic obstructive pulmonary disease and heart disease, oxygenation of the blood passing through the lungs is impaired. Because fluid is collecting in the lungs, this patient is often able to breathe better in a sitting or semi-sitting position and may tell you so.

Usually, patients with cardiogenic shock do not have an injury, but they may be having chest pain. Such a patient may have taken nitroglycerin before your arrival and may want to take more. Patients in cardiogenic shock should not receive nitroglycerin; by definition, they are hypotensive. In addition to low blood pressure, other signs include a weak,

**TABLE 13-4** Types of Shock

| Type of Shock | Examples of Potential Causes | Signs and Symptoms | Treatment |
|---|---|---|---|
| **Cardiogenic** | Inadequate heart function<br>Disease of muscle tissue<br>Impaired electrical system<br>Disease or injury | Chest pain<br>Irregular pulse<br>Weak pulse<br>Low blood pressure<br>Cyanosis (lips, under nails)<br>Cool, clammy skin<br>Anxiety<br>Crackles (rales)<br>Pulmonary edema | Position comfortably<br>Administer high-flow oxygen<br>Assist ventilations<br>Transport promptly<br>Consider ALS |
| **Obstructive** | Mechanical obstruction of the cardiac muscle causing a decrease in cardiac output<br>1. Tension pneumothorax<br>2. Cardiac tamponade<br>3. Pulmonary embolism | Dependent on cause:<br>• Dyspnea<br>• Rapid, weak pulse<br>• Rapid, shallow breaths<br>• Decreased lung compliance<br>• Unilateral, decreased, or absent breath sounds<br>• Decreased blood pressure<br>• Jugular vein distention<br>• Subcutaneous emphysema<br>• Cyanosis<br>• Tracheal deviation toward unaffected side<br>• Beck triad (cardiac tamponade):<br>　· Jugular vein distention<br>　· Narrowing pulse pressure<br>　· Muffled heart tones | Dependent on cause:<br>• ALS assist and/or rapid transport<br>• Administer high-flow oxygen |
| **Septic** | Severe infection | Warm skin or fever<br>Tachycardia<br>Low blood pressure | Transport promptly<br>Administer high-flow oxygen<br>Assist ventilations<br>Keep patient warm<br>Consider ALS |
| **Neurogenic** | Damaged cervical spine, which causes widespread blood vessel dilation | Bradycardia (slow pulse)<br>Low blood pressure<br>Signs of neck injury | Secure airway<br>Spinal immobilization<br>Assist ventilations<br>Administer high-flow oxygen<br>Preserve body heat<br>Transport promptly<br>Consider ALS |
| **Anaphylactic** | Extreme life-threatening allergic reaction | Can develop within seconds<br>Mild itching or rash<br>Burning skin<br>Vascular dilation<br>Generalized edema<br>Coma<br>Rapid death | Manage the airway<br>Assist ventilations<br>Administer high-flow oxygen<br>Determine cause<br>Assist with administration of epinephrine<br>Transport promptly<br>Consider ALS |

| Type of Shock | Examples of Potential Causes | Signs and Symptoms | Treatment |
|---|---|---|---|
| **Psychogenic (fainting)** | Temporary, generalized vascular dilation Anxiety, bad news, sight of injury or blood, prospect of medical treatment, severe pain, illness, tiredness | Rapid pulse Normal or low blood pressure | Determine duration of unconsciousness Position the patient supine Record initial vital signs and mental status Suspect head injury if patient is confused or slow to regain consciousness Transport promptly |
| **Hypovolemic** | Loss of blood or fluid | Rapid, weak pulse Low blood pressure Change in mental status Cyanosis (lips, under nails) Cool, clammy skin Increased respiratory rate | Secure airway Assist ventilations Administer high-flow oxygen Control external bleeding Keep warm Transport promptly Consider ALS |

ALS, advanced life support

© Jones & Bartlett Learning.

irregular pulse; cyanosis about the lips and underneath the fingernails; anxiety; and nausea.

Treatment of cardiogenic shock should begin by placing the patient in the position in which breathing is easiest as you administer high-flow oxygen. Be ready to assist ventilations as necessary, and have suction nearby in case the patient vomits. Provide prompt transport to the ED. If ALS is not already on the scene, consider a rendezvous en route to the hospital if available. Frequently check for a pulse in an unresponsive patient to identify early whether CPR and an AED are needed.

## Street Smarts

Provide calm reassurance to a patient who has had a suspected heart attack.

## YOU are the Provider

The patient is placed onto the stretcher and loaded into the ambulance. You quickly gather the patient records from the clinic physician and begin transport to a hospital that is only 10 minutes away. En route, you continue with your treatment and reassess the patient's condition.

**Recording Time:   11 Minutes**

| | |
|---|---|
| **Level of consciousness** | Responsive to pain only |
| **Respirations** | 30 breaths/min; shallower |
| **Pulse** | 130 beats/min; absent radial pulses (carotid pulse present) |
| **Skin** | Pale, cool, and diaphoretic |
| **Blood pressure** | 84/44 mm Hg |
| **$SpO_2$** | 89% (on oxygen) |

**6.** How has your patient's condition changed?

**7.** Are adjustments in your current interventions required? If so, what?

## Treating Obstructive Shock

As discussed previously, two of the most common examples of obstructive shock are cardiac tamponade and tension pneumothorax.

Increasing cardiac output should be the priority in treating cardiac tamponade. The preload must be increased because increasing pressure in the pericardium is squeezing the heart. Apply high-flow oxygen. The only definitive treatment for cardiac tamponade is surgery. Pericardiocentesis involves penetrating the pericardium with a needle to withdraw the accumulated blood from the pericardial sac. This procedure is an advanced skill, and it is rarely performed in the field.

To treat a tension pneumothorax, administer high-flow oxygen via nonrebreathing mask early to prevent hypoxia. Usually the only action that can prevent eventual death from a tension pneumothorax is decompression of the injured side of the chest, relieving the pressure in the chest and allowing the heart to expand fully again. Chest decompression is an ALS skill. Ask for ALS assistance early in the call if available; however, do not delay transport waiting for the arrival of ALS.

## Treating Septic Shock

The proper treatment of septic shock requires complex hospital management, including expeditious administration of antibiotics. If you suspect that a patient has septic shock, use appropriate standard precautions and transport as promptly as possible, administering high-flow oxygen during transport. Ventilatory support may be necessary to maintain adequate tidal volume. Use blankets to conserve body heat. Sepsis has become an increasingly common illness. Some hospitals have instituted specialized sepsis teams, which, when notified, will meet the patient in the ED. Sepsis teams have protocols that decrease the amount of time spent in identification of the infectious agent and initiation of the appropriate treatment, thereby decreasing the mortality from septic shock. EMS agencies may have sepsis protocols in which EMTs alert the hospital to the potential for sepsis when giving their radio report. Be familiar with your local protocols for sepsis alerts and notifications.

## Treating Neurogenic Shock

Shock that accompanies spinal cord injury is best treated by a combination of all known supportive measures. Emergency treatment must be directed toward obtaining and maintaining a proper airway, providing spinal stabilization, assisting inadequate breathing as needed, conserving body heat, and ensuring the most effective circulation possible.

A patient in neurogenic shock is usually not losing blood; however, the capacity of the blood vessels has become significantly larger than the available volume of the blood inside the vessels. Supplemental oxygen will boost the concentration of oxygen in the blood. If respirations are weak or inadequate, assist ventilations. Because the injury may have disabled the body's normal temperature controls, keep the patient as warm as possible with blankets. Transport the patient promptly to a facility capable of managing spinal injuries.

## Treating Anaphylactic Shock

The most effective emergency treatment of a severe, acute allergic reaction is to administer epinephrine by way of intramuscular injection. For more information on the emergency care for allergic reactions, see Chapter 21, *Allergy and Anaphylaxis*. A patient who is aware of having a specific sensitivity may carry a kit containing epinephrine (**FIGURE 13-9**). If he or she is unable to inject the medication, you may have to do so if you are allowed by local protocol. Some EMT-staffed ambulances carry pre-filled epinephrine injectors on the ambulance to administer during anaphylaxis. If the patient's signs and symptoms recur or the patient's condition deteriorates, consult medical control for authorization to administer a repeat injection, if available.

A patient with anaphylaxis requires immediate transport to the ED after administration of the epinephrine auto-injector. Additional emergency care includes high-flow oxygen. Assist ventilations with a bag-mask device if necessary. If possible, attempt to determine what agent caused the reaction (for example, drug, insect bite or sting, food item) and how it was received (for example, by mouth, by inhalation, or by injection). The severity of allergic reactions can vary greatly, with symptoms ranging from mild itching to profound coma and rapid death. Keep in mind that a mild reaction may worsen suddenly or over time. Because of the potential for airway compromise, consider requesting ALS backup, if available.

## Treating Psychogenic Shock

In an uncomplicated case of fainting, once the patient collapses and becomes supine, circulation to

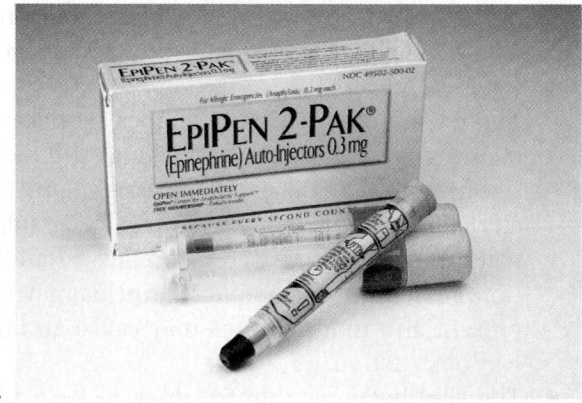

A

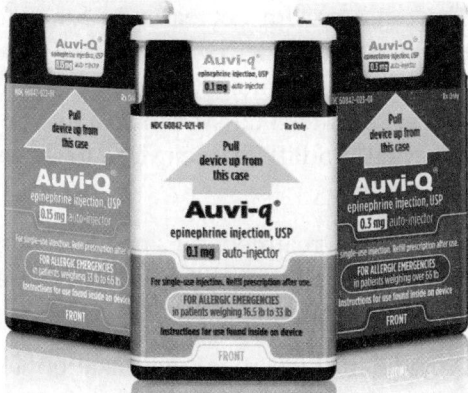

B

**FIGURE 13-9** BLS ambulances or patients may have epinephrine auto-injectors. **A.** An EpiPen. **B.** An Auvi-Q.

A: © Roel Smart/iStockphoto; B: Courtesy of Kaleo, Inc.

the brain is usually restored and with it, a normal state of functioning. Remember that psychogenic shock can significantly worsen other types of shock. If it appears the patient fell as a result of psychogenic shock, check for injuries, especially in older patients. If the patient reports not being able to walk after a fall thought to be related to psychogenic shock, you should suspect another problem, such as head injury. Transport the patient promptly. It is not safe to assume based on EMT assessment that any fainting was caused by psychogenic shock alone. All patients with loss of consciousness, even a brief one, should be transported to the ED for evaluation even if they appear normal once you arrive on scene to evaluate them.

Be sure to record your initial observations of vital signs and level of consciousness. In addition, try to learn from bystanders whether the patient complained of anything before fainting and how long he or she was unconscious.

## Treating Hypovolemic Shock

The emergency treatment of hypovolemic or hemorrhagic shock includes the control of all obvious external bleeding. The best initial method to control external bleeding is direct pressure. To prevent continued bleeding, you must apply sufficient pressure to control obvious external bleeding. If severe extremity bleeding is not controlled with direct

## YOU are the Provider

You ask your partner to call ahead to the hospital because you are busy caring for the patient and cannot free up your hands. The noninvasive automatic vital signs machine records another set of vital signs. With an estimated time of arrival at the hospital of 5 minutes, you reassess the patient.

| Recording Time: 16 Minutes | |
| --- | --- |
| **Level of consciousness** | Responsive to pain only |
| **Respirations** | 30 breaths/min and shallow (baseline); ventilations are being assisted |
| **Pulse** | 128 beats/min; absent radial pulses (carotid pulse present) |
| **Skin** | Pale, cool, and diaphoretic |
| **Blood pressure** | 80/40 mm Hg |
| **Spo$_2$** | 96% (with assisted ventilation; on oxygen) |

You arrive at the hospital and give your report to the charge nurse. Intravenous access is rapidly obtained, the attending physician quickly assesses the patient, and additional treatment is given.

**8.** What part of the patient's perfusion triangle has failed?

**9.** How does shock caused by volume failure differ from shock caused by container failure?

pressure, consider use of a tourniquet. Bleeding control, including application of a tourniquet and wound packing, is discussed in detail in Chapter 26, *Bleeding*. Ensure that you use great care to handle the patient gently and keep the patient warm.

Although you cannot control internal bleeding in the field, it is important to recognize its existence and provide general support and rapid transport. Secure and maintain an airway, and provide respiratory support, including supplemental oxygen and, if needed, assisted ventilations. Start oxygen as soon as you suspect shock and continue it during transport; with too little circulating blood, additional oxygen may be lifesaving. Watch to ensure that the patient does not aspirate blood or vomitus, and transport the patient as rapidly as possible to the ED.

## Treating Shock in Older Patients

Use caution when caring for older patients. As a result of the aging process, older patients generally have more serious complications than younger patients. Although illness is a common complaint among older patients, you must understand that it is not just part of aging. In addition, many older patients take numerous medications that could either mask or mimic signs of shock. Keep in mind the following signs of the normal aging process when managing geriatric patients:

- The central nervous system often has a delayed response; thus, tachypnea and vasoconstriction may be slower to respond to shock.
- The cardiovascular system has a variety of changes that result in a decrease in the efficiency of the system. On assessment, be alert for higher resting heart rates and irregular pulse rates.
- The respiratory system undergoes significant changes as the elasticity of the lungs and their size and strength decrease. On assessment, be alert for higher respiratory rates, lower tidal volume, and a decreased gag reflex. In addition, remember that cervical arthritis may be present and that dentures may cause an airway obstruction.
- The skin becomes thinner, drier, less elastic, and more fragile, thus providing less protection and thermal regulation (cold and hot).
- The renal system decreases in function and may not respond well to unusual demands such as illness or dehydration.
- The gastrointestinal system sustains changes in gastric motility that may lead to slower gastric emptying.

The principles of treatment for a pediatric or geriatric patient in shock are no different than they are for any other shock patient:

1. Provide in-line spinal stabilization if indicated. If spinal immobilization is not indicated, maintain the patient in a position of comfort.
2. Control life-threatening hemorrhage immediately with direct pressure or tourniquet application when appropriate.
3. Suction as necessary and provide high-flow oxygen via a nonrebreathing mask.
4. Maintain body temperature.
5. Provide rapid transportation.

## YOU are the Provider SUMMARY

1. **What additional information should you attempt to gather about the patient while en route to the clinic?**

   The description of "a woman in shock" tells you very little. The patient could have a severe injury with internal bleeding, she could be experiencing a severe allergic reaction, or she may have simply fainted. When you are dispatched to *any* call with minimal information provided, attempt to gather additional information while you are en route. In many cases, the dispatcher will provide additional patient information—without you asking for it—as it becomes available. In other cases, you will need to ask the dispatcher to try to make contact with the caller to obtain a patient update. Many EMS systems use an emergency medical dispatcher (EMD); if this is the case, he or she should be able to provide you with more detailed information, as well as give prearrival instructions to the caller.

**2. What is shock and how does it relate to perfusion?**

Perfusion is the delivery of blood and oxygen and other essential nutrients to the body's cells to keep them alive. While delivering these essential items to the body's cells, waste products such as carbon dioxide are removed from the cell and eliminated from the body. Adequate perfusion is maintained by the perfusion triangle, which consists of three essential components—a functioning pump (the heart), adequate volume (the blood and water), and an intact container (the blood vessels). The respiratory system is also a critical component for adequate perfusion; if oxygen cannot get into the lungs, the heart cannot pump it through the blood vessels and to the cells. Shock is a state of inadequate perfusion (hypoperfusion) and is the result of failure of one or more components of the perfusion triangle or the respiratory system. The type of shock that a patient is experiencing describes the component of the perfusion triangle that has failed. Regardless of the type of shock, the result is the same—inadequate perfusion of the body's tissues and cells, which will lead to death if untreated.

**3. Based on your assessment, what changes, if any, in the patient's current treatment are required?**

The patient clearly has signs of shock—restlessness; tachypnea; tachycardia; weak radial pulses; and cool, pale, diaphoretic skin—and the treatment that has been provided thus far is essentially appropriate. She is being kept warm, and she is receiving oxygen. However, patients with signs of shock need *high-flow* oxygen. She is presently receiving oxygen via a nasal cannula; this should be changed to a nonrebreathing mask with the flow rate set at 15 L/min. Based on this patient's presentation—abdominal pain and rectal bleeding—you should suspect blood loss (bleeding into the intestines) as the cause of her shock. Blood carries oxygen; if the blood volume decreases, so does the ability of oxygen to get to the cells. Providing a high concentration of oxygen will oxygenate the red blood cells that remain in the circulatory system. In addition to receiving high-flow oxygen, the patient needs IV access and volume replacement to help circulate the oxygenated blood. The physician has been unable to obtain IV access, and since IV therapy is beyond

the EMT's scope of practice, you must prepare the patient for immediate transport. If your transport time to the hospital will be prolonged, you should consider an intercept with ALS, because ALS is trained to establish IV access.

**4. How do the patient's signs and symptoms correlate with the body's response to inadequate perfusion?**

During shock, the body mounts a physiologic response aimed at maintaining adequate perfusion, most of which is the result of increased activity of the sympathetic nervous system releasing greater quantities of epinephrine (adrenaline) and norepinephrine. Restlessness, perhaps one of the earliest signs of shock, is caused by a decrease in oxygen to the brain. As a result, the number of signals the brain sends to the respiratory muscles increases, which causes an increase in the patient's respiratory rate (tachypnea). Increased levels of epinephrine cause an increase in heart rate and cardiac contractility, and as a result, blood is pumped faster and with greater force throughout the body to compensate for decreased perfusion. Increased levels of norepinephrine cause the blood vessels to constrict (vasoconstriction), thus maintaining the patient's blood pressure. Early in shock, blood is shunted away from areas of lesser need (ie, the skin and muscles) to areas of greater need (ie, heart, lungs, liver, kidneys) by vasoconstriction. This causes the skin to turn pale (pallor) and become cool to the touch. When the sympathetic nervous system activity increases, sweat gland activity increases as well, resulting in diaphoresis (profuse sweating).

**5. Is the patient in compensated or decompensated shock? How can you tell?**

Signs of compensated shock include restlessness, anxiety, or agitation; tachycardia; rapid, weak (thready) peripheral pulses; tachypnea; and marked thirst. In compensated shock, however, the patient's systolic blood pressure is maintained—usually above 90 mm Hg in adults. Your patient's current blood pressure is 108/58 mm Hg. These signs and symptoms indicate that the patient is in compensated shock. Signs of decompensated shock include systolic blood pressure of 90 mm Hg or lower in an adult; absent peripheral pulses; dilated pupils; ashen, mottled, or cyanotic skin; and a decreasing level of consciousness. It is important to note that the patient's blood pressure is often a very late factor to change in shock. By the time a low blood pressure (hypotension) is detected, shock is well developed. In decompensated shock, the body's compensatory mechanisms are no longer able to maintain adequate perfusion. Survival is less likely—even with rapid transport and aggressive treatment at the hospital.

**6. How has your patient's condition changed?**

Your patient's condition has changed for the worse. Her level of consciousness has decreased (responsive to pain only), her respirations have increased in rate and decreased in depth (reduced tidal volume), her heart rate has increased and her radial pulses are no longer palpable, her blood pressure is below 90 mm Hg (84/44 mm Hg), and her oxygen saturation has fallen—despite the administration of high-flow oxygen. Based on these reassessment findings, your patient is now in decompensated shock with inadequate breathing. As previously discussed, decompensated shock occurs when the body's compensatory mechanisms begin to fail and are no longer able to maintain adequate perfusion. At the clinic, the patient had signs of shock; however, she was still conscious and alert, although restless, and her systolic blood pressure was maintained. Patients can decompensate within a matter of minutes; this fact underscores the criticality of frequent reassessments.

**7. Are adjustments in your current interventions required? If so, what?**

In terms of shock treatment, you are doing everything that you can. The patient is being kept warm with a blanket and she is receiving high-flow oxygen. An intercept with an ALS unit is not practical, because you are too close to the hospital. However, the patient's breathing is no longer adequate (30 breaths/min and shallow) and requires assistance. Because of her decreased level of consciousness, you should insert a nasopharyngeal airway, as she is responsive to pain and likely has an intact gag reflex. Begin assisting her ventilations with a bag-mask device attached to high-flow oxygen and monitor her closely for signs of improvement or further deterioration. Many EMS systems carry noninvasive blood pressure monitoring devices that automatically take the patient's blood pressure and other vital signs. If you have this capability, set the device to reassess the patient's vital signs *at least* every 5 minutes or as deemed appropriate by the patient's condition. You

are the only EMT in the back with the patient; managing her airway and assisting her ventilations clearly has priority over obtaining a manual blood pressure measurement.

**8. What part of the patient's perfusion triangle has failed?**

There are three components to the perfusion triangle, each of which must function well at all times to maintain adequate perfusion: the heart (pump), the blood vessels (container), and the blood (content or volume). Recalling the patient's chief complaint—abdominal pain and rectal bleeding—she is in shock secondary to blood loss (hemorrhagic shock). Therefore, the content function of the perfusion triangle has failed. If there is enough blood or plasma loss, internally or externally, the volume of fluid that remains in the container (blood vessels) will not be able to carry sufficient oxygen to the cells to adequately perfuse them.

**9. How does shock caused by content (volume) failure differ from shock caused by container failure?**

Shock caused by content failure refers to insufficient oxygen delivery to the cells because of inadequate volume and is called hypovolemic shock. Hypovolemia is a generic term that simply means low volume; it could be blood, plasma, water, or a combination. Common causes of hypovolemic shock include blunt or penetrating trauma, burns, and dehydration. Shock that is caused by blood loss specifically is called hemorrhagic shock. The signs of hypovolemic shock include tachycardia; pale, cool, clammy skin; tachypnea; restlessness, agitation, or anxiety; and as a late sign, hypotension. Shock caused by container failure refers to inadequate perfusion because of excessive dilation of the blood vessels, resulting in a decrease in pressure within the circulatory system. Although the volume of blood has not changed, the container that it circulates within has increased; therefore, the normal volume of blood is insufficient to fill the system and provide adequate perfusion. Common causes of shock caused by container failure include anaphylaxis, overdose with drugs that suppress the nervous system (ie, narcotics), and spinal cord injury. The classic signs of hypovolemic shock—specifically, tachycardia, pallor, and diaphoresis—will be absent. Instead, the patient's skin is usually warm and dry, and the heart rate is normal or low.

## YOU are the Provider SUMMARY *continued*

### EMS Patient Care Report (PCR)

| | | | |
|---|---|---|---|
| **Date:** 4-24-20 | **Incident No.:** 011009 | **Nature of Call:** Woman in shock | **Location:** Westlake Urgent Care, 1111 University Avenue |

| | | | | | |
|---|---|---|---|---|---|
| **Dispatched:** 2022 | **En Route:** 2023 | **At Scene:** 2032 | **Transport:** 2043 | **At Hospital:** 2053 | **In Service:** 2105 |

#### Patient Information

**Age:** 39
**Sex:** F
**Weight (in kg [lb]):** 73 kg (160 lb)

**Allergies:** Codeine
**Medications:** Amitiza, Bentyl
**Past Medical History:** Irritable bowel syndrome
**Chief Complaint:** Abdominal pain and rectal bleeding

#### Vital Signs

| Time | BP | Pulse | Respirations | Spo$_2$ |
|---|---|---|---|---|
| 2036 | 108/58 | 120 | 24 | 94% |
| 2043 | 84/44 | 130 | 30 | 89% |
| 2048 | 80/40 | 128 | 30 | 96% |

#### EMS Treatment (circle all that apply)

| Oxygen @ 15 L/min via: NC (NRM) Bag mask | | Assisted Ventilation | Airway Adjunct | CPR |
|---|---|---|---|---|
| **Defibrillation** | **Bleeding Control** | **Bandaging** | **Splinting** | **Other:** (Blanket for warmth) |

#### Narrative

9-1-1 dispatch to Cedar Hills Urgent Care Clinic for a "woman in shock."
Chief Complaint: Abdominal pain and rectal bleeding

History: According to the clinic physician, the patient presented 15 minutes earlier reporting abdominal pain and rectal bleeding, which began approximately 24 hours ago. Prior to EMS arrival, clinic personnel applied oxygen at 4 L/min via nasal cannula and applied a blanket. The physician advised that she attempted to establish IV access several times, but was unsuccessful. The patient denies abdominal trauma and states that she has a history of irritable bowel syndrome.

Assessment: Arrived on scene and found the patient, a 39-year-old female, lying supine on an exam table. She was conscious and alert, but restless. Her airway was patent and her breathing, although increased in rate, was producing adequate tidal volume. Her skin was cool, pale, and diaphoretic. Further assessment revealed that her abdomen was diffusely tender to palpation, and she was actively bleeding from the rectum. Remainder of assessment was unremarkable.

Treatment (Rx): Removed nasal cannula, applied high-flow oxygen via nonrebreathing mask, and obtained vital signs.

Transport: Patient moved from exam table to stretcher using a draw sheet. Departed the scene and continued treatment en route. Reassessment revealed that the patient's mental status had decreased; she was now only responsive to painful stimuli. Her blood pressure had decreased, her radial pulses were absent (carotid pulse was present), her respirations were more rapid and shallow, and her Spo$_2$ had fallen to 89%. Inserted a nasopharyngeal airway and began assisting her ventilations with a bag-mask attached to high-flow oxygen. Partner notified the receiving facility and gave radio report. Continued to assist patient's ventilations and monitor her vital signs. She remained hypotensive and tachycardic; however, her Spo$_2$ increased to 96% with assisted ventilation. Delivered patient to the ED staff without incident and gave verbal report to charge nurse Spergis RN. Medic 4 returned to service at 2105.

**End of report**

# Prep Kit

## Ready to Review

- Perfusion requires an intact cardiovascular system and a functioning respiratory system.
- Remember, most types of shock (hypoperfusion) are caused by dysfunction in one or more parts of the perfusion triangle:
  - The pump (the heart)
  - The pipes, or container (blood vessels)
  - The content, or volume (blood)
- Shock (hypoperfusion) is the collapse and failure of the cardiovascular system, when blood circulation slows and eventually stops.
- Blood is the vehicle for carrying oxygen and nutrients through the vessels to the capillary beds and tissue cells, where these supplies are exchanged for waste products.
- Blood contains red blood cells, white blood cells, platelets, and a liquid called plasma.
- The *systolic* pressure is the peak arterial pressure, or pressure generated every time the heart contracts; the *diastolic* pressure is the pressure maintained within the arteries while the heart rests between heartbeats.
- The various types of shock are cardiogenic, obstructive, septic, neurogenic, anaphylactic, psychogenic, and hypovolemic.
- Signs of compensated shock include anxiety or agitation; tachycardia; pale, cool, moist skin; increased respiratory rate; nausea and vomiting; and increased thirst. If there is any question on your part, treat for shock. Early recognition and rapid treatment are important.
- Signs of decompensated shock include labored or irregular respirations, ashen gray or cyanotic skin color, weak or absent distal pulses, dilated pupils, and profound hypotension (systolic blood pressure of 90 mm Hg or lower in an adult).
- Remember, by the time a decrease in blood pressure is detected, shock is usually in an advanced stage.
- Anticipate shock in patients who have the following conditions:
  - Severe infection
  - Significant blunt force trauma or penetrating trauma
  - Massive external bleeding or index of suspicion for major internal bleeding
  - Spinal cord injury
  - Chest or abdominal injury
  - Major heart attack
  - Anaphylaxis
- Treating a pediatric or geriatric patient in shock is no different from treating any other shock patient.
- Treat all patients suspected to be in shock from any cause as follows and in this order:
  - Open and maintain the airway.
  - Control life-threatening hemorrhage immediately with direct pressure or tourniquet application when appropriate.
  - Provide high-flow oxygen, and as needed, provide bag-mask assisted ventilations.
  - Maintain normal body temperature with blankets.
  - Provide calm reassurance.
  - Provide prompt transport to the appropriate hospital.

## Vital Vocabulary

**afterload** The force or resistance against which the heart pumps.

**anaphylactic shock** Severe shock caused by an allergic reaction.

**anaphylaxis** An extreme, life-threatening, systemic allergic reaction that may include shock and respiratory failure.

**aneurysm** A swelling or enlargement of a part of an artery, resulting from weakening of the arterial wall.

**autonomic nervous system** The part of the nervous system that regulates involuntary activities of the body, such as heart rate, blood pressure, and digestion of food.

**cardiac tamponade** Compression of the heart as the result of buildup of blood or other fluid in the pericardial sac, leading to decreased cardiac output.

**cardiogenic shock** A state in which not enough oxygen is delivered to the tissues of the body, caused by low output of blood from the heart. It can be a severe complication of a large acute myocardial infarction, as well as other conditions.

**compensated shock** The early stage of shock, in which the body can still compensate for blood loss.

**cyanosis** A blue skin discoloration that is caused by a reduced level of oxygen in the blood. Although paleness, or a decrease in blood flow, can be difficult to detect in dark-skinned people, it may be observed by examining mucous membranes inside the inner lower eyelid and capillary refill. On general observation, the patient may appear ashen or gray.

**decompensated shock** The late stage of shock when blood pressure is falling.

**dehydration** Loss of water from the tissues of the body.

**distributive shock** A condition that occurs when there is widespread dilation of the small arterioles, small venules, or both.

**edema** The presence of abnormally large amounts of fluid between cells in body tissues, causing swelling of the affected area.

**homeostasis** A balance of all systems of the body.

**hypothermia** A condition in which the internal body temperature falls below 95°F (35°C).

**hypovolemic shock** A condition in which low blood volume, due to massive internal or external bleeding or extensive loss of body water, results in inadequate perfusion.

**irreversible shock** A condition defined by the inability to successfully achieve resuscitation regardless of the methods employed.

**myocardial contractility** The ability of the heart muscle to contract.

**neurogenic shock** Circulatory failure caused by paralysis of the nerves that control the size of the blood vessels, leading to widespread dilation; seen in patients with spinal cord injuries.

**obstructive shock** Shock that occurs when there is a block to blood flow in the heart or great vessels, causing an insufficient blood supply to the body's tissues.

**perfusion** The flow of blood through body tissues and vessels.

**pericardial effusion** A collection of fluid between the pericardial sac and the myocardium.

**preload** The precontraction pressure in the heart as the volume of blood builds up.

**psychogenic shock** Shock caused by a sudden, temporary reduction in blood supply to the brain that causes fainting (syncope).

**pulmonary embolism** A blood clot that breaks off from a large vein and travels to the blood vessels of the lung, causing obstruction of blood flow.

**pulse pressure** The difference between the systolic and diastolic pressures.

**sensitization** Developing a sensitivity to a substance that initially caused no allergic reaction.

**septic shock** Shock caused by severe infection, usually a bacterial infection.

**shock** A condition in which the circulatory system fails to provide sufficient circulation to maintain normal cellular functions; also called hypoperfusion.

**sphincters** Muscles that encircle and, by contracting, constrict a duct, tube, or opening.

**syncope** A fainting spell or transient loss of consciousness.

# References

1.  National Association of Emergency Medical Technicians. *PHTLS: Prehospital Trauma Life Support*. 9th ed. Burlington, MA: Jones & Bartlett Learning; 2020.

2.  National Association of State EMS Officials. *National Model EMS Clinical Guidelines: Version 2.2*. https://nasemso.org/wp-content/uploads/National-Model-EMS-Clinical-Guidelines-2017-PDF-Version-2.2.pdf. Updated January 5, 2019.Accessed March 10, 2020.

3.  National Highway Traffic Safety Administration. *National Emergency Medical Services Education Standards*. DOT HS 811 077A. www.ems.gov/pdf/811077a.pdf. Published January 2009. Accessed March 10, 2020.

4.  National Highway Traffic Safety Administration. *National Emergency Medical Services Education Standards. Emergency Medical Technician Instructional Guidelines*. DOT HS 811 077C. www.ems.gov/pdf/811077c.pdf. Published January 2009. Accessed March 10, 2020.

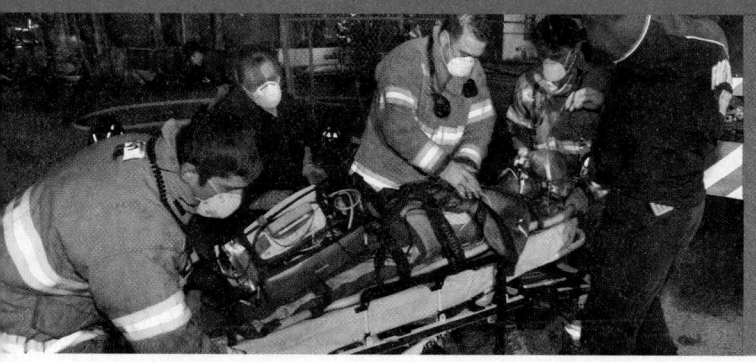

# Chapter 14

# BLS Resuscitation

## NATIONAL EMS EDUCATION STANDARD COMPETENCIES

### Shock and Resuscitation

Applies a fundamental knowledge of the causes, pathophysiology, and management of shock, respiratory failure or arrest, cardiac failure or arrest, and postresuscitation management.

## KNOWLEDGE OBJECTIVES

1. Explain the elements of basic life support (BLS), how it differs from advanced life support (ALS), and why BLS must be applied rapidly. (pp 557–559)
2. Explain the goals of cardiopulmonary resuscitation (CPR) and when it should be performed on a patient. (p 559)
3. Explain the components of CPR, the five links in the American Heart Association (AHA) chain of survival, and how each one relates to maximizing the survival of a patient. (pp 559–560)
4. Discuss guidelines for circumstances that require the use of an automated external defibrillator (AED) on both adult and pediatric patients experiencing cardiac arrest. (pp 561–562)
5. Explain three special situations related to the use of an AED. (p 562)
6. Describe the proper way to position an adult patient to receive BLS care. (pp 562–563)
7. Describe the purpose of external chest compressions. (p 563)
8. Describe the two techniques EMTs may use to open an adult patient's airway and the circumstances that would determine when each technique would be used. (pp 566–567)
9. Describe the recovery position and circumstances that would warrant its use as well as situations in which it would be contraindicated. (pp 567–568)
10. Describe the process of providing artificial ventilations to an adult patient, ways to avoid gastric distention, and modifications required for a patient with a stoma. (pp 568–569)
11. Explain the steps in providing single-rescuer adult CPR. (pp 569–571)
12. Explain the steps in providing two-rescuer adult CPR, including the method for switching positions during the process. (pp 571–573)
13. Describe the different mechanical devices that are available to assist emergency care providers in delivering improved circulatory efforts during CPR. (pp 573, 575–577)
14. Describe the different possible causes of cardiopulmonary arrest in children. (p 577)
15. Explain the four steps of pediatric BLS procedures and how they differ from BLS procedures used in an adult patient. (pp 577–584)
16. Describe the ethical issues related to patient resuscitation, including examples of when not to start CPR on a patient. (pp 584–586)
17. Explain the various factors involved in the decision to stop CPR after it has been started on a patient. (pp 586–587)

18. Explain common causes of foreign body airway obstruction in both children and adults and how to distinguish mild or partial airway obstruction from complete airway obstruction. (pp 587–588)

19. Describe the different methods for removing a foreign body airway obstruction in an infant, child, and adult, including the procedure for a patient with an obstruction who becomes unresponsive. (pp 588–593)

20. Discuss how to provide grief support for a patient's family members and loved ones after resuscitation has ended. (pp 594–595)

21. Discuss the importance of frequent CPR training for EMTs, as well as public education programs that teach compression-only CPR. (p 595)

## SKILLS OBJECTIVES

1. Demonstrate how to position an unresponsive adult for CPR. (pp 562–563)

2. Demonstrate how to check for a pulse at the carotid artery in an unresponsive child or adult. (p 563)

3. Demonstrate how to perform external chest compressions on an adult. (pp 563–565, Skill Drill 14-1)

4. Demonstrate how to perform a head tilt–chin lift maneuver on an adult. (p 566)

5. Demonstrate how to perform a jaw-thrust maneuver on an adult. (pp 566–567)

6. Demonstrate how to place a patient in the recovery position. (pp 567–568)

7. Demonstrate how to perform rescue breathing in an adult. (p 568)

8. Demonstrate how to perform one-rescuer adult CPR. (pp 569–571, Skill Drill 14-2)

9. Demonstrate how to perform two-rescuer adult CPR. (pp 571–573, Skill Drill 14-3)

10. Demonstrate the use of mechanical devices that assist emergency responders in delivering improved circulatory efforts during CPR. (pp 573–577)

11. Demonstrate how to check for a pulse at the brachial artery in an unresponsive infant. (p 579)

12. Demonstrate how to perform external chest compressions on an infant. (pp 579–580, Skill Drill 14-4)

13. Demonstrate how to perform CPR on a child who is between 1 year of age and the onset of puberty. (pp 580–582, Skill Drill 14-5)

14. Demonstrate how to perform a head tilt–chin lift maneuver on a pediatric patient. (p 582)

15. Demonstrate how to perform a jaw-thrust maneuver on a pediatric patient. (pp 582–583)

16. Demonstrate how to perform rescue breathing on a child. (p 583)

17. Demonstrate how to perform rescue breathing on an infant. (p 583)

18. Demonstrate how to remove a foreign body airway obstruction in a responsive adult patient using abdominal thrusts (Heimlich maneuver). (p 588)

19. Demonstrate how to remove a foreign body airway obstruction in a responsive pregnant or obese patient using chest thrusts. (pp 588–591)

20. Demonstrate how to remove a foreign body airway obstruction in a responsive child older than 1 year using abdominal thrusts (Heimlich maneuver). (pp 590–591)

21. Demonstrate how to remove a foreign body airway obstruction in an unresponsive child. (pp 591–592, Skill Drill 14-6)

22. Demonstrate how to remove a foreign body airway obstruction in an infant. (pp 591, 593)

# Introduction

The principles of basic life support (BLS) were introduced in 1960. Since then, the specific techniques for the management of cardiac arrest and the delivery of emergency and cardiac care have been reviewed and revised regularly. The goal is to produce the best recommendations possible given the available scientific evidence and to maximize the chance of successful resuscitation. The updated guidelines are published in peer-reviewed journals: *Circulation* in the United States and *Resuscitation* in Europe. Reviews are conducted and published by the International Liaison Committee on Resuscitation (ILCOR) based on availability of new relevant information. The most recent revision (2020) occurred as a result of a rigorous and systematic review of the newest scientific evidence surrounding the treatment of cardiac arrest and the provision of emergency and cardiac care, using validated, transparent, and scientifically rigorous methodology to produce the best recommendations possible given the available evidence.

This chapter begins with a definition and general discussion of BLS. It then reviews methods for opening and maintaining a patent (open) airway, providing artificial ventilation to a person who is not breathing, providing artificial circulation to a person with no pulse, and removing a foreign body airway obstruction. Each of these topics is followed by a review of the changes in technique that are necessary to treat infants and children. Chapter 2, *Workforce Safety and Wellness*, discusses the methods of preventing the transmission of infectious diseases during cardiopulmonary resuscitation (CPR). Chapter 6, *The Human Body*, discusses the anatomy and physiology of the respiratory and cardiovascular systems. Chapter 9, *The Team Approach to Health Care*, discusses how to work as an effective team in the health care setting. During any emergency, working as a team is critical to giving the patient the best chance for a successful outcome.

## Words of Wisdom

In normal situations, the risk of acquiring an infectious disease while performing CPR is very low. During a pandemic, this risk is escalated dramatically because both CPR and ventilation with a bag-mask device generate aerosol particles that can spread infectious disease. During a pandemic, EMS personnel should wear enhanced PPE that includes goggles, an N95 mask, gloves, and gown. This level of protection makes the physical exertion of CPR more difficult.

## Elements of BLS

**Basic life support (BLS)** is noninvasive emergency life-saving care that is used to treat medical conditions, including airway obstruction, respiratory arrest, and cardiac arrest. BLS follows a specific sequence for adults and for infants and children. This care focuses on the ABCs: airway (obstruction), breathing (respiratory arrest), and circulation (cardiac arrest or severe bleeding). If the patient is in cardiac arrest, then a CAB sequence (compressions, airway, breathing) is used because chest compressions are essential and must be started as quickly as possible (**FIGURE 14-1**). Ideally, only seconds should pass between the time you recognize that a patient needs BLS and the start of treatment. Remember, brain cells die every second they are deprived of oxygen. Permanent brain damage is possible after only 4 to 6 minutes without oxygen (**FIGURE 14-2**).

Check the patient for absent or abnormal breathing and unresponsiveness at the same time. Check for a pulse for no more than 10 seconds, and, if no definite pulse is noted, assume the victim is in cardiac arrest. If a patient has abnormal breathing or breathing is absent, you may be able to restore breathing simply by opening the airway. However, if the patient has no pulse, then you must combine artificial ventilation with artificial circulation (chest compressions). If breathing stops before the heart stops, then the patient may have enough oxygen in the lungs to stay alive for several minutes. When cardiac arrest occurs first, the heart and brain stop receiving oxygen immediately.

**Cardiopulmonary resuscitation (CPR)** is used to re-establish circulation and artificial ventilation in a patient who is not breathing and has no pulse. The steps for CPR include the following:

1. Restore circulation by performing 30 chest compressions at a depth of 2 inches (5 cm) to circulate blood to the vital organs of the body.

## YOU are the Provider

At 1445 hours, you and your partner respond to a local supermarket at 123 Wilshire Avenue where a middle-aged man reportedly collapsed in the parking lot. While you are en route to the scene, dispatch advises you that bystander CPR is in progress. Your response time is less than 5 minutes.

**1.** What should you immediately do on receiving this update from dispatch?

**2.** What should be your initial actions on arriving at this scene?

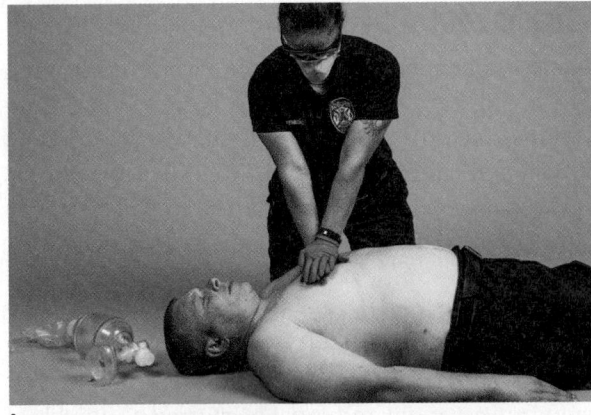

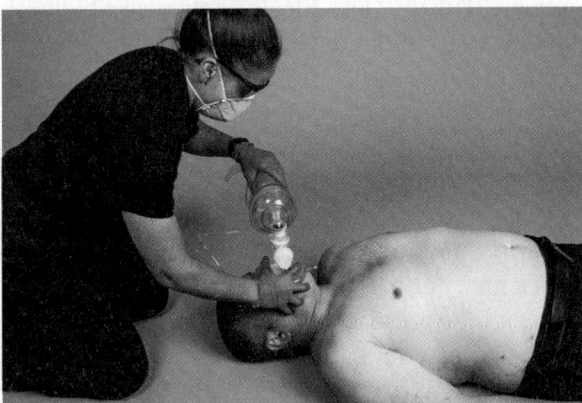

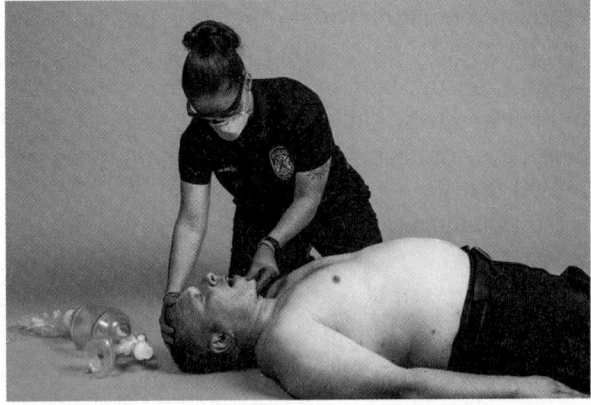

**FIGURE 14-1** CAB: Chest compressions **(A)**, airway **(B)**, and breathing **(C)**.

A, B, C: © Jones & Bartlett Learning.

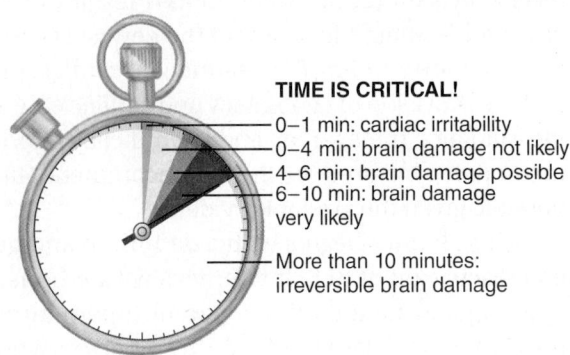

**TIME IS CRITICAL!**
0–1 min: cardiac irritability
0–4 min: brain damage not likely
4–6 min: brain damage possible
6–10 min: brain damage very likely
More than 10 minutes: irreversible brain damage

**FIGURE 14-2** Time is critical for patients who are not breathing. If the brain is deprived of oxygen for 4 to 6 minutes, brain damage is possible.

© Jones & Bartlett Learning.

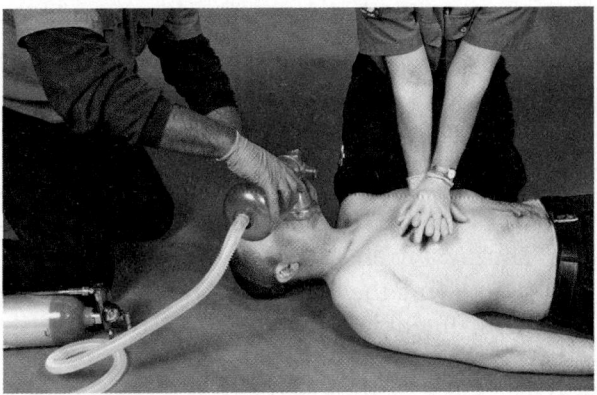

**FIGURE 14-3** You must quickly identify patients in respiratory and/or cardiac arrest so that BLS measures can begin immediately.

© Jones & Bartlett Learning. Courtesy of MIEMSS.

The rate should be at least 100 compressions per minute but no more than 120 per minute.

2. Open the airway with the jaw-thrust or head tilt–chin lift maneuver to restore breathing by providing rescue breaths (via bag-mask device). Administer two breaths, each over 1 second, while visualizing for chest rise. Repeat this sequence.

The goal of CPR is to help restore spontaneous breathing and circulation; however, defibrillation and advanced interventions (ie, medication therapy) are often necessary to achieve this outcome. For CPR to be effective, you must be able to quickly identify a patient who is in respiratory and/or cardiac arrest and immediately begin BLS measures (**FIGURE 14-3**).

BLS differs from **advanced life support (ALS)**, which involves advanced life-saving procedures, such as cardiac monitoring, administration of intravenous (IV) fluids and medications, and the use of advanced airway adjuncts. However, when done correctly, BLS care can maintain life for a short time until ALS measures can be started. In some cases, such as choking, near-drowning, or lightning injuries, early BLS measures may be all that is needed to restore a patient's pulse and breathing. Of course, these patients still require transport to the emergency department (ED) for evaluation.

The BLS measures are only as effective as the person who is performing them. Your skills may be good immediately after training, but as time goes on, skills will deteriorate unless you practice them regularly.

To survive cardiac arrest, effective CPR at an adequate rate and depth with minimal interruptions is essential until defibrillation can be administered. Therefore, the BLS care you provide as an EMT is an extremely critical factor in the patient's chance for survival. In fact, high-quality chest compressions with minimal interruptions and early defibrillation have been proven to be independent predictors of successful resuscitation from cardiac arrest and survival to hospital discharge.

## The Components of CPR

According to the American Heart Association (AHA), 88% of sudden cardiac arrests occur in the home. Few patients who experience cardiac arrest in the prehospital environment survive unless a rapid sequence of events take place. The AHA has determined an ideal sequence of events, termed the chain of survival, that together can improve the chance of successful resuscitation of a patient who experiences sudden cardiac arrest (**FIGURE 14-4**). A successful resuscitation is defined not only by the **return of spontaneous circulation (ROSC)**, but also by the survival of the patient to hospital discharge. The six links in the chain of survival are as follows:

1. **Recognition and activation of the emergency response system.** The first step in the chain of survival requires public education and awareness. Lay people must learn to recognize the early warning signs of a cardiac emergency and immediately activate EMS by calling 9-1-1 and beginning chest compressions during the call. These steps ensure that emergency responders are dispatched to the scene quickly, thus allowing the other links of the chain to be more effective. In modern EMS systems, the 9-1-1 dispatcher can provide prearrival instructions and direct the caller to provide high-quality CPR.

2. **Immediate, high-quality CPR.** The initiation of immediate CPR by a bystander is essential for successful resuscitation of a person in cardiac arrest. CPR will keep blood, and therefore oxygen, flowing to the vital organs to keep the patient alive until the other components of the chain are available. The more people trained in CPR in the community, the better the chances of CPR being administered quickly to a person in cardiac arrest. Immediate, high-quality CPR markedly increases the patient's chance of survival, whereas a delay in CPR leads to poor patient outcomes. The lay public as well as emergency responders should all be trained in CPR. Unfortunately, many bystanders are hesitant to perform CPR on a stranger for fear of contracting a disease from mouth-to-mouth breathing, or out of fear of liability. A perception that bystander CPR involves mouth-to-mouth breathing persists. EMS has a role in educating laypeople in performing compressions-only (hands-only) CPR.

   For chest compressions to be most effective, they must be given hard and fast. The AHA recommends that compressions be started as quickly as possible after onset of cardiac arrest. Compressions should be between 2 and

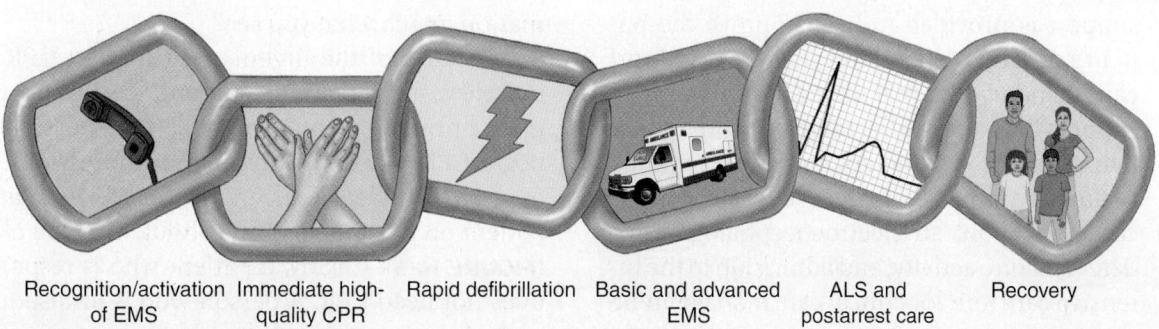

Recognition/activation of EMS     Immediate high-quality CPR     Rapid defibrillation     Basic and advanced EMS     ALS and postarrest care     Recovery

**FIGURE 14-4** The six links of the chain of survival.

2.4 inches in depth (5 to 6 cm) and given at a rate of 100 to 120 per minute. The chest should completely recoil between each compression to maximize blood return to the heart. The rescuer should never lean on the chest between compressions. Interruptions between compressions for any reason should be minimized and no longer than 10 seconds.

3. **Rapid defibrillation.** Provided that immediate, high-quality CPR with minimal interruption is performed, early defibrillation offers the best opportunity to achieve a successful patient outcome. Automated external defibrillators (AEDs) have become readily available in many schools, fitness clubs, airports, concert venues, sports arenas, government buildings, and other mass gathering places. The simple design of the AED makes it easy for emergency medical providers and laypeople to use with little training.

4. **Basic and advanced emergency medical services.** This link in the chain describes care provided by EMTs and ALS providers before the patient arrives at the ED. Such care includes continuing high-quality CPR; basic airway management (ie, oral airway insertion, bag-mask device ventilation); advanced airway management (ie, endotracheal [ET] intubation or use of supraglottic airway devices); manual defibrillation; vascular access; transcutaneous pacing; and administration of medications. In addition to the care provided in the prehospital setting, be familiar with the cardiac resuscitation centers in your service area. Your agency should implement a process to ensure early notification and transport to the appropriate receiving facility.

5. **Advanced life support and postarrest care.** After your team delivers the patient to the ED, further cardiopulmonary and neurologic support is provided to help improve the patient's recovery when indicated. This support can include additional medication therapy to support blood pressure; targeted temperature management (ie, therapeutic hypothermia); maintenance of blood glucose levels; cardiac catheterization; an electroencephalogram to detect seizure activity; and admission to the intensive care unit for critical care management.

6. **Recovery.** Physical and emotional recovery can take a year or longer for people who are eventually resuscitated. After cardiac arrest, survivors can have physical, cognitive, and emotional challenges and may need ongoing therapies and interventions.

If any one of the links in the chain is not maintained, then the patient is more likely to die. For example, fewer patients survive cardiac arrest if CPR is not administered within the first few minutes. Likewise, if the time from cardiac arrest to defibrillation is more than 10 minutes, the chance of survival is decreased. The patient's best chance of survival occurs when all links in the chain are maintained.

## Street Smarts

Cardiac arrest calls are highly emotional. Planning your initial actions and roles en route to the call can avoid confusion and help ensure that the priorities of good-quality CPR and early defibrillation are achieved quickly.

## Assessing the Need for BLS

As always, begin by surveying the scene. Is the scene safe? Is there an environmental hazard or infectious disease that may change your approach? Cardiac arrest calls can be very stressful, particularly on initial arrival. You must be certain that it is safe to proceed with your initial assessment prior to doing so. How many patients are present? What is your initial impression of the patient or patients? Are bystanders present who may have additional information? What is the mechanism of injury or nature of illness? Do you suspect trauma? If you were dispatched to the scene, then does the dispatch information match what you see?

Because of the urgent need to start CPR in a pulseless, nonbreathing patient, you must complete a primary assessment as soon as possible and begin CPR, starting with chest compressions. The first step is to determine unresponsiveness. Tap the patient on the shoulder and shout, "Are you okay?" (**FIGURE 14-5**). Clearly, a patient who is responsive does not need CPR. A person who is unresponsive

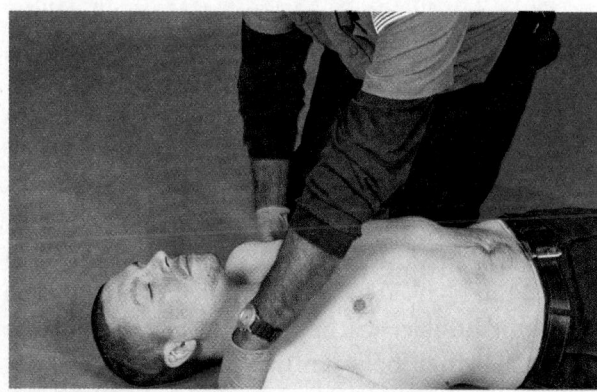

**FIGURE 14-5** Assess an unresponsive patient by first attempting to rouse him or her by tapping on the shoulder.

© Jones & Bartlett Learning. Courtesy of MIEMSS.

may or may not need CPR. Continue your assessment by simultaneously checking for breathing and a pulse; this step should take no more than 10 seconds. If a pulse cannot definitively be felt after 10 seconds, then begin chest compressions immediately. The patient is in cardiac arrest.

In some EMS services, EMTs respond in squad units, before the ambulance. If this is the case in your area, then update the responding crew via radio if possible. In other cases, you may encounter a cardiac arrest patient while off duty. If you are alone and off duty, use your mobile phone to call 9-1-1. You must be familiar with the laws and policies that apply in your service area regarding your duty to act. See Chapter 3, *Medical, Legal, and Ethical Issues*, for more information. If you are alone and do not have a mobile phone, then leave the patient to call 9-1-1 and then return to begin CPR. If you choose to intervene while off duty, then you must continue to provide competent care until an equal or higher medical authority assumes care of the patient.

### Basic Principles of BLS

The basic principles of BLS are the same for infants, children, and adults. For the purposes of BLS, anyone younger than 1 year old is considered an infant. A child is between 1 year of age and approximately 12 to 14 years of age (the onset of puberty), as signified by breast development in girls and underarm, chest, and facial hair in boys. Adulthood is from the onset of puberty and older. Children vary in size. There are two basic differences in providing CPR

for infants, children, and adults. The first is that the emergencies in which infants and children require CPR usually have different underlying causes. The second is that there are anatomic differences in adults, children, and infants, such as smaller airways in infants and children than in adults.

Although cardiac arrest in adults usually occurs before respiratory arrest, the reverse is true in infants and children. In most cases, cardiac arrest in children results from respiratory arrest. If untreated, respiratory arrest will quickly lead to cardiac arrest and death. Respiratory arrest in infants and children has a variety of causes, which are discussed later in this chapter.

## Automated External Defibrillation

Most prehospital cardiac arrests occur as the result of a sudden cardiac rhythm disturbance (dysrhythmia), such as ventricular fibrillation (VF) or pulseless ventricular tachycardia (VT). The normal heart rhythm is known as normal sinus rhythm. VF is the disorganized quivering of the ventricles, resulting in no blood flow and a state of cardiac arrest. VT is a rapid contraction of the ventricles that does not allow for normal filling of the heart. As mentioned previously, according to the AHA, early defibrillation is the link in the chain of survival that is most likely to improve survival rates. The likelihood of survival decreases rapidly over time as long as VF or pulseless VT persists.

When a patient is in cardiac arrest, begin CPR, starting with high-quality chest compressions, and apply an AED as soon as it is available. Defibrillate immediately if indicated. Chapter 17, *Cardiovascular Emergencies*, covers AED use in detail.

### Words of Wisdom

If you witness a patient's cardiac arrest and an AED is available, then deploy the AED immediately and then begin CPR. However, if you did not witness the patient's cardiac arrest or if an AED is unavailable, then perform CPR and apply the AED as soon as it is available. If two or more rescuers are present, one rescuer should begin CPR while the other prepares to defibrillate using the AED.

## AED Usage in Children

AEDs can safely be used in children and infants using the pediatric-size pads and a dose-attenuating system (energy reducer). However, if these items are unavailable, use adult-size AED pads. Apply the AED to infants or children after the first five cycles of CPR have been completed. Recall that cardiac arrest in children is usually the result of respiratory failure; therefore, oxygenation and ventilation are vitally important. After the first five cycles of CPR, use the AED to deliver shocks in the same manner as with an adult patient.

If you use adult-size AED pads on an infant or small child, do not cut the pads to adjust the size. Instead, use the anterior-posterior placement, following the manufacturer's recommendation. More energy through the use of the adult pads is better than no energy.

> ### Words of Wisdom
>
> Remember, if the child is past the onset of puberty, follow the adult CPR sequence, including the use of adult-size AED pads.

## Special AED Situations

It is important to ensure the safety of yourself, others at the scene, and the patient. As such, keep the following factors in mind when using an AED.

### Pacemakers and Implanted Defibrillators

You may encounter a patient who has an automated implanted cardioverter-defibrillator (AICD) or pacemaker that delivers shocks directly to the heart if necessary. These devices are used in patients who are at a high risk for certain cardiac dysrhythmias and cardiac arrest. It is easy to recognize AICDs or pacemakers because they create a hard lump beneath the skin, usually on the upper left side of the chest (just below the clavicle). If the AED pads are placed directly over the device, then the effectiveness of the shock delivered by the AED may be reduced, and the shock could potentially damage the implanted device. Therefore, if you identify an AICD or pacemaker, then you should place the AED pad at least 1 inch (2.5 cm) away from the device.

Occasionally, the implanted device will deliver shocks to the patient. If you observe the patient's muscles twitching as if he or she was just shocked, then continue CPR and wait 30 to 60 seconds before delivering a shock from the AED.

### Wet Patients

Water conducts electricity. Therefore, the AED should not be used in water. If the patient's chest is wet, then the electrical current may move across the skin rather than between the pads to the patient's heart. If the patient is submerged in water, then pull the patient out of the water and quickly dry the skin before attaching the AED pads. Do not delay CPR to dry the patient thoroughly; instead, quickly wipe off as much moisture as possible from the chest. If the patient is lying in a small puddle of water or in the snow, the AED can be used, but again, the patient's chest should be quickly dried as much as possible.

### Transdermal Medication Patches

You may encounter a patient who is receiving medication through a transdermal medication patch, such as nitroglycerin. The medication is absorbed through the skin. The patch could reduce the flow of the electrical current from the AED to the heart and may burn the skin. If the medication patch interferes with AED pad placement, then remove the patch with your gloved hands and wipe the skin to remove any residue prior to attaching the AED pad.

> ### Words of Wisdom
>
> Be familiar with social media platforms and mobile phone dispatch systems used in your service area. For example, free smartphone apps are available that use global positioning system (GPS) technology to alert CPR-trained subscribers that a person nearby is in cardiac arrest. Social media notification systems have not been shown to improve survival from out-of-hospital cardiac arrest. However, the potential benefit of increased bystander-initiated CPR makes it reasonable for you to advocate for the use of such technology.

## Positioning the Patient

For CPR to be effective, the patient must be lying supine on a firm, flat surface, with enough clear space around the patient for two rescuers to perform CPR and use the AED. If the patient is crumpled up or lying facedown (prone), then you will need to move him or her to a supine position. Be mindful that you cannot rule out a spinal injury in an unresponsive patient; therefore, protect the patient's neck and move him or her as a unit, without twisting. If the patient is found in a bed or on a couch, then move him or her to the floor.

## Check for Breathing and a Pulse

After you have determined that the patient is unresponsive, quickly check for breathing and a pulse. These assessments can occur simultaneously and should take no longer than 10 seconds in total.

Visualize the chest for signs of breathing while palpating for a carotid pulse. Feel for the carotid artery by locating the larynx at the front of the neck and then sliding two fingers toward one side (the side closest to you). The pulse is felt in the groove between the larynx and sternocleidomastoid muscle, with the pads of the index and middle fingers held side by side (**FIGURE 14-6**). Light pressure is sufficient to palpate the pulse.

## Provide External Chest Compressions

If the patient is not breathing (or is breathing only slowly or occasionally, known as agonal gasps)

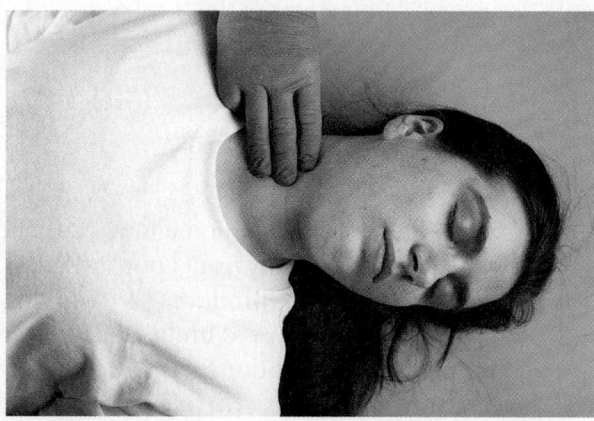

**FIGURE 14-6** Feel for the carotid artery by locating the larynx, then slide your index and middle fingers toward one side. You can feel the pulse in the groove between the larynx and sternocleidomastoid muscle.

© Jones & Bartlett Learning. Courtesy of MIEMSS.

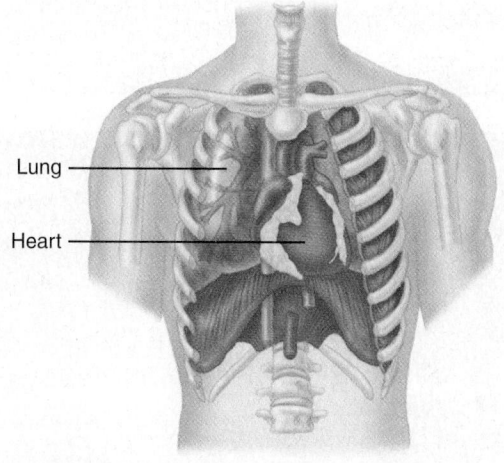

**FIGURE 14-7** The heart lies slightly to the left of the middle of the chest between the sternum and spine.

© Jones & Bartlett Learning.

and does not have a pulse, then begin CPR, starting with chest compressions. It is critical to perform compressions properly. Chest compressions are administered by applying rhythmic pressure and relaxation to the lower half of the sternum. The heart is located slightly to the left of the middle of the chest between the sternum and the spine (**FIGURE 14-7**). Compressions squeeze the heart, thereby acting as a pump to circulate blood. Allow the chest to completely recoil between compressions, which enhances blood return to the heart. Do not lean on the chest between compressions. When artificial ventilation is provided, the blood that is circulated through the lungs during chest compressions is likely to receive adequate oxygen to maintain tissue perfusion. However, even when external chest compressions are performed properly, they circulate only one-third of the blood that is normally pumped by the heart.

## Proper Hand Position and Compression Technique

With the adult patient, correct hand position is established by placing the heel of one hand on the sternum in the center of the chest (lower half of the sternum). Follow the steps in **SKILL DRILL 14-1**:

1. Take standard precautions.
2. Place the heel of one hand on the center of the chest over the lower half of the sternum (**Step 1**).
3. Place the heel of your other hand over the first hand (**Step 2**).

## Skill Drill 14-1 Performing Chest Compressions

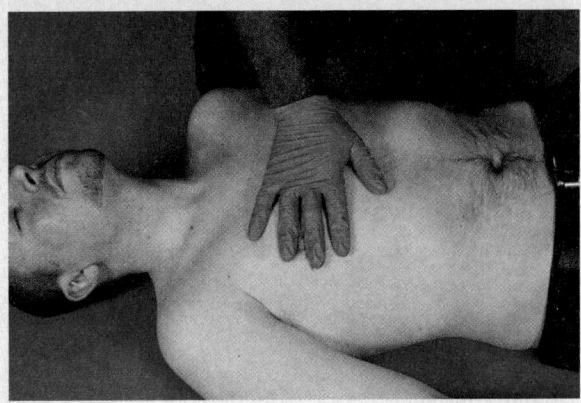

### Step 1

Take standard precautions. Place the heel of one hand on the center of the chest (lower half of the sternum).

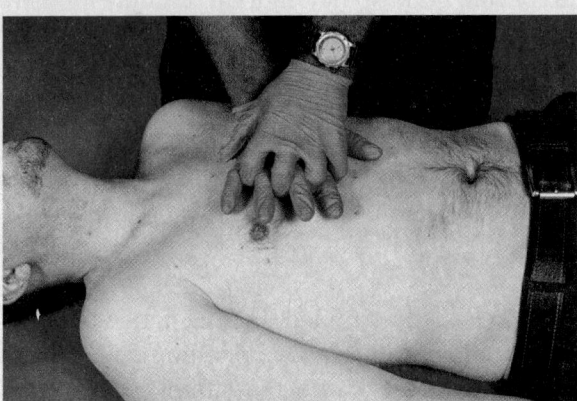

### Step 2

Place the heel of your other hand over the first hand.

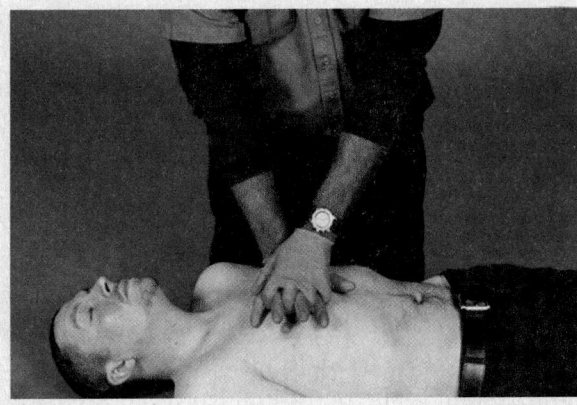

### Step 3

With your arms straight, lock your elbows and position your shoulders directly over your hands. Depress the sternum at a rate of 100 to 120 compressions per minute, and to a depth of 2 to 2.4 inches (5 to 6 cm) using a downward movement. Allow the chest to return to its normal position; do not lean on the chest between compressions. Compression and relaxation should be of equal duration.

© Jones & Bartlett Learning. Courtesy of MIEMSS.

4. With your arms straight, lock your elbows and position your shoulders directly over your hands, so that the thrust of each compression is straight down on the sternum. Your technique may be improved or made more comfortable if you interlock the fingers of your lower hand with the fingers of your upper hand; either way, keep your fingers off the patient's ribs.

5. Depress the sternum to a depth of 2 inches to 2.4 inches (5 cm to 6 cm), using direct downward movement and then rising gently upward (**Step 3**). This motion allows pressure to be delivered vertically from your shoulders. Downward pressure produces a compression that must be followed immediately by an equal period of relaxation. The ratio of time devoted to compression versus relaxation should be 1:1. It is important that you allow the chest to return to its normal position; do not lean on the patient's chest between compressions. Compression and relaxation should be of equal duration.

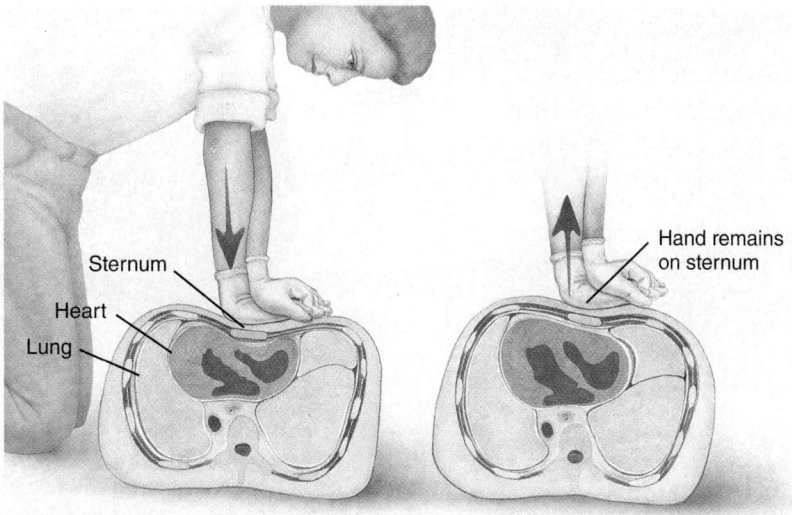

Sternum

Heart

Lung

Hand remains
on sternum

**FIGURE 14-8 A.** Compression and relaxation should be rhythmic and of equal duration (a 1:1 ratio). **B.** Pressure on the sternum must be released so that the sternum can return to its normal resting position between compressions.

A, B: © Jones & Bartlett Learning.

Complications from chest compressions are rare but can include fractured ribs, a lacerated liver, and a fractured sternum. Although these injuries cannot be entirely avoided, you can minimize the chance that they will occur if you use good technique and proper hand placement. Risk of injury to the patient should not delay your initiation of CPR or performance of high-quality CPR.

Your motions must be smooth, rhythmic, and uninterrupted (**FIGURE 14-8A**). Short, jabbing compressions are not effective in producing artificial blood flow. Do not remove the heel of your hand from the patient's chest during relaxation, but make sure that you completely release pressure on the sternum so that it can return to its normal resting position between compressions (**FIGURE 14-8B**).

## Words of Wisdom

When performing chest compressions on an adult, compress the chest to a depth of at least 2 inches (5 cm), but not more than 2.4 inches (6 cm). It is difficult to achieve such a precise depth without the use of a monitoring device that provides immediate feedback (**FIGURE 14-9**). Research continues to support the use of compression feedback devices to improve outcomes in cardiac arrest survivability.

It is more dangerous to compress the chest too lightly than it is to compress too forcefully. Compressing hard can lead to fatigue, and as you become tired, your compressions will become shallower. Therefore, it is critical to push hard and push fast and switch compressors (the person providing chest compressions) every 2 minutes—even if the compressor does not feel tired.

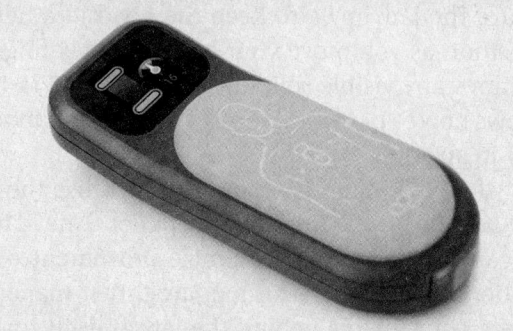

**FIGURE 14-9** CPR feedback devices help ensure a consistent rate and depth of compressions.

Courtesy of Laerdal Medical.

## Words of Wisdom

Chest compressions create blood flow to the heart through filling of the coronary arteries. Every time compressions are stopped, blood flow—and thus, perfusion—to the heart (and brain) drops to zero. It takes 5 to 10 compressions to reestablish effective blood flow to the heart after chest compressions are resumed. Avoid frequent or prolonged interruptions in chest compressions, which lead to poor patient outcomes.

# Opening the Airway and Providing Artificial Ventilation

## Opening the Airway in Adults

Without an open airway, rescue breathing will not be effective. As discussed in Chapter 11, *Airway Management,* the two techniques for opening the airway in adults are the head tilt–chin lift maneuver and the jaw-thrust maneuver. These manual maneuvers are designed to bring the tongue forward and off the throat. The **head tilt–chin lift maneuver** is effective for opening the airway in most patients when there is no indication of a spinal injury (**FIGURE 14-10**).

In patients who have not sustained trauma, this simple maneuver is sometimes all that is required for the patient to resume breathing. If the patient has any foreign material or vomitus in the mouth, then quickly remove it. Remove any liquid materials from the mouth with a suction device; locate the angles of the patient's lower jaw and then move the jaw upward. Keep the head in a neutral position as you move your hooked index finger to remove any visible solid material. **FIGURE 14-11** reviews how to perform the head tilt–chin lift maneuver in an adult.

If spinal injury is suspected, then use the **jaw-thrust maneuver**. Do not tilt the patient's head back, because you want to minimize movement of the patient's neck. To perform a jaw-thrust maneuver, place your fingers behind the jaw and lift upward to open the mouth. If the patient's mouth remains closed, then you can use your thumbs to pull down the patient's lower lip to allow breathing. If the jaw thrust fails to open the airway, then the head tilt–chin lift should be used to open the airway. An

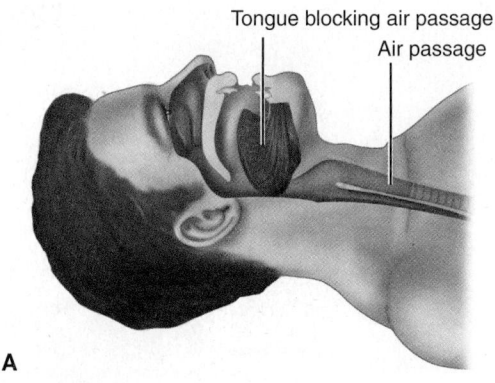

**A**

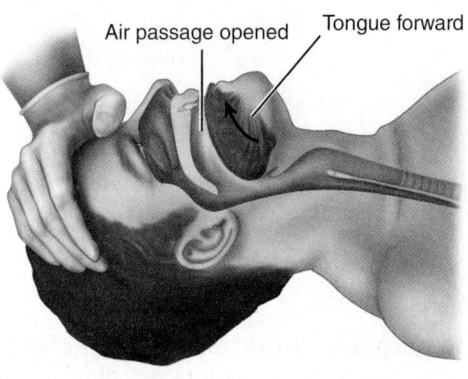

**B**

**FIGURE 14-10 A.** Relaxation of the tongue back into the throat causes airway obstruction. **B.** The head tilt–chin lift maneuver combines two movements of opening the airway; head tilt is shown here.

A, B: © Jones & Bartlett Learning.

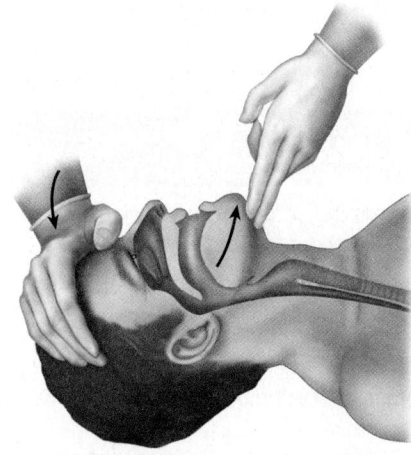

**FIGURE 14-11** To perform the head tilt–chin lift maneuver, place one hand on the patient's forehead and apply firm backward pressure with your palm to tilt the head back. Next, place the tips of the index and middle fingers of your other hand under the lower jaw near the bony part of the chin. Lift the chin upward, bringing the entire lower jaw with it, helping to tilt the head back.

© Jones & Bartlett Learning.

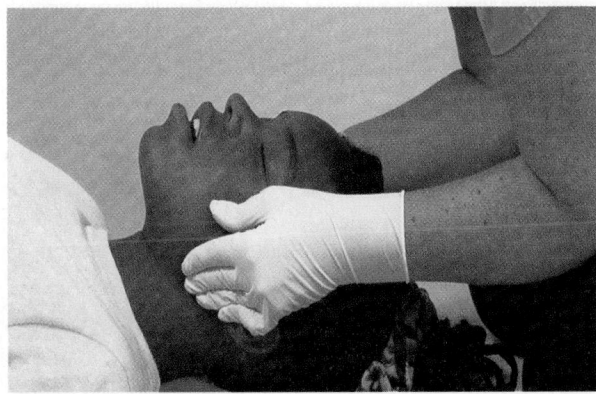

**FIGURE 14-12** To perform the jaw-thrust maneuver, maintain the head in neutral alignment and place your fingers behind the angles of the lower jaw, and move the jaw upward.

© Jones & Bartlett Learning. Courtesy of MIEMSS.

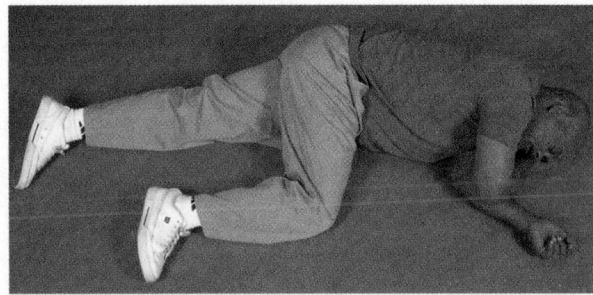

**FIGURE 14-13** The recovery position is used to maintain an open airway in an adequately breathing patient with a decreased level of consciousness who has no spinal injury. It allows vomitus, blood, and any other secretions to drain from the mouth.

© Jones & Bartlett Learning. Courtesy of MIEMSS.

open airway is the primary goal when caring for trauma patients, and you must ensure an open airway to improve survival. **FIGURE 14-12** reviews how to perform the jaw-thrust maneuver in an adult.

## Recovery Position

If the patient is breathing adequately on his or her own and has no signs of injury to the spine, hip,

or pelvis, then place the patient in the **recovery position**. This position helps to maintain a clear airway in a patient with a decreased level of consciousness who has not sustained traumatic injuries and is breathing adequately on his or her own (**FIGURE 14-13**). It also allows vomitus to drain from the mouth. Roll the patient onto his or her side so that the head, shoulders, and torso move as a unit, without twisting. Then place the top hand under the patient's cheek. Avoid placing a patient who has

## YOU are the Provider

You arrive at the scene and find two bystanders performing CPR on the patient, who appears to be in his late 40s. You perform a primary assessment as your partner retrieves the AED.

| Recording Time: | 0 Minutes |
| --- | --- |
| **Appearance** | Motionless; cyanosis of the face |
| **Level of consciousness** | Unresponsive |
| **Airway** | Open; clear of secretions or foreign bodies |
| **Breathing** | Absent |
| **Circulation** | No carotid pulse; skin cool and pale; no gross bleeding |

Your partner takes over ventilations while the bystanders, whose chest compressions are good, continue performing chest compressions, alternating every 2 minutes. One of the bystanders tells you that the patient was about to get into his vehicle when he suddenly grabbed his chest, slumped against the vehicle, and eased himself to the ground. By the time the bystander reached him, he was unresponsive with gasping breaths. The bystander further tells you that he immediately called 9-1-1 and then began CPR.

**3.** What links in the chain of survival have been maintained at this point?

**4.** Why is it so critical to minimize interruptions in CPR?

a suspected head or spinal injury in the recovery position because in this position, the spine is not aligned, spinal stabilization is not possible, and further spinal injury could result.

## Breathing

A lack of oxygen (hypoxia), combined with too much carbon dioxide in the blood (hypercarbia), is lethal. To correct this condition, you must provide slow, deliberate ventilations that last 1 second. This gentle, slow method of ventilating the patient prevents air from being forced into the stomach (discussed later in the chapter).

## Provide Artificial Ventilations

Ventilations can be given by one or two EMS providers. Use a bag-mask device when you administer ventilations in the prehospital environment (**FIGURE 14-14**). Use devices that supply supplemental oxygen when possible. Devices with an oxygen reservoir will provide higher percentages of oxygen to the patient. Regardless of whether you ventilate the patient with or without supplemental oxygen, you should observe the chest for visible rise to assess the effectiveness of your ventilations.

The specific steps of CPR are discussed later in this chapter. Adult BLS procedures are summarized in **TABLE 14-1**. Pediatric BLS procedures are

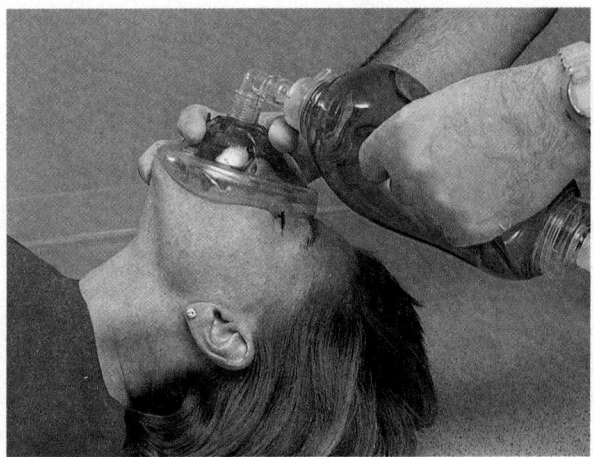

**FIGURE 14-14** When you provide ventilations, use a bag-mask device.

© Jones & Bartlett Learning. Courtesy of MIEMSS.

| TABLE 14-1 Review of Adult BLS Procedures | |
|---|---|
| **Procedure** | |
| **Circulation** | |
| Pulse check | Carotid artery |
| Compression area | In the center of the chest, at the nipple line |
| Compression depth | 2 to 2.4 in. (5 to 6 cm) |
| Compression rate | 100 to 120/min |
| Compression-to-ventilation ratio (until advanced airway is inserted) | 30:2 |
| Foreign body obstruction | Responsive: abdominal thrusts (Heimlich maneuver); chest thrusts if patient is pregnant or has obesity Unresponsive: CPR |
| **Airway** | |
| Airway positioning | Head tilt–chin lift; jaw-thrust maneuver if spinal injury is suspected |
| **Breathing** | |
| Ventilations | 1 breath every 6 seconds (a rate of 10 breaths/min); visible chest rise |
| Ventilations with advanced airway placed | 1 breath every 6 seconds (a rate of 10 breaths/min) |

© Jones & Bartlett Learning.

summarized in Table 14-2 later in this chapter. Resuscitation of a neonate is discussed in Chapter 34, *Obstetrics and Neonatal Care*.

**Hyperventilation** (ventilating too fast or with too much force) may cause increased intrathoracic pressure (pressure inside the chest cavity) by putting pressure on the vena cava, thus reducing the amount of blood that returns to the heart. (Chapter 11, *Airway Management*.) This increased intrathoracic pressure decreases the effectiveness of chest compressions and results in the heart and brain receiving decreased amounts of oxygen.

## Stoma Ventilation

Patients who have undergone a laryngectomy (surgical removal of the larynx) often have a permanent tracheal stoma at the midline in the neck. In this case, a stoma is an opening that connects the trachea directly to the skin (**FIGURE 14-15**). Because it is at the midline, the stoma is the only opening that will move air into the patient's lungs. Patients with a stoma should be ventilated with a bag-mask device placed directly over the stoma.

Not all stomas are disconnected from the nose and mouth. If air leakage through the nose and mouth interferes with ventilation through the stoma, then cover the nose and mouth with your hand to make a seal. Use a pediatric or infant mask to ventilate through the stoma.

## Gastric Distention

Artificial ventilation may result in the stomach becoming filled with air, a condition called **gastric distention**. Although it occurs more easily in children, this condition also happens frequently in adults. Gastric distention is likely to occur if you hyperventilate the patient. If you ventilate too forcefully, or if the patient's airway is not opened adequately, then the excess gas under pressure opens up the collapsible tube (the esophagus) and allows air to enter the stomach. Therefore, it is important for you to give slow, gentle breaths. Such breaths are also more effective in ventilating the lungs. Excessive inflation of the stomach is dangerous because it can cause the patient to vomit during CPR, blocking the airway. It can also reduce lung volume by elevating the diaphragm.

If massive gastric distention occurs, first check for adequate ventilation; if it interferes with adequate ventilation, contact medical control. Check the airway again and reposition the patient, watch for rise and fall of the chest, and avoid giving forceful breaths. Have a suction unit available in case the patient vomits. Remember, mortality increases significantly if aspiration occurs. If an ALS provider is available, then he or she can insert an orogastric or nasogastric tube to decompress the stomach.

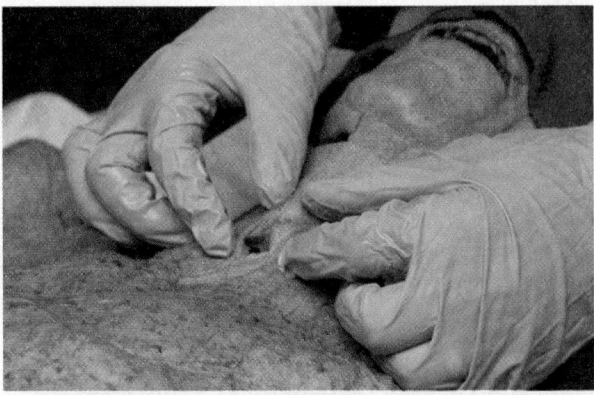

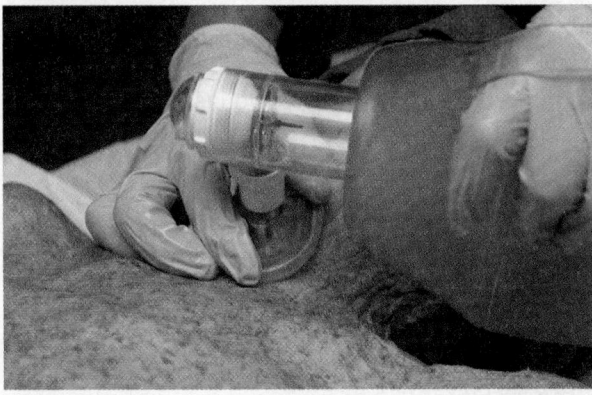

**FIGURE 14-15 A.** This stoma connects the trachea directly to the skin. **B.** Use a bag-mask device to ventilate a patient with a stoma.

A, B: © Jones & Bartlett Learning. Courtesy of MIEMSS.

## One-Rescuer Adult CPR

When you provide CPR alone, you must provide a continuous cycle of 30 chest compressions followed by two artificial ventilations (a ratio of 30:2). To perform one-rescuer adult CPR, follow the steps in **SKILL DRILL 14-2**:

1. Take standard precautions. Establish unresponsiveness and call for additional help (**Step 1**).

## Skill Drill 14-2 Performing One-Rescuer Adult CPR

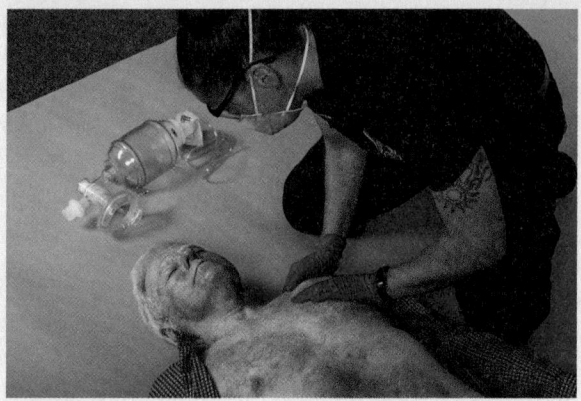

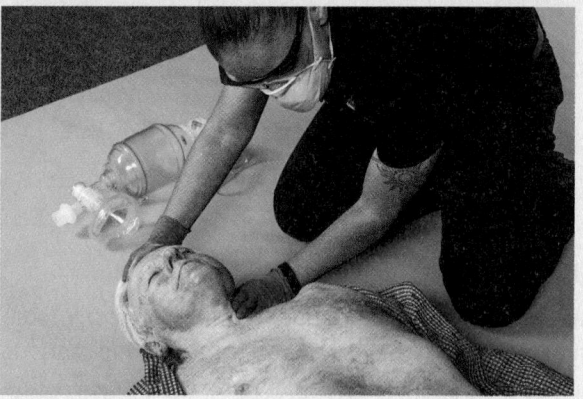

### Step 1

Take standard precautions. Establish unresponsiveness and call for help. Use your mobile phone if needed.

### Step 2

Check for breathing and a carotid pulse for no more than 10 seconds.

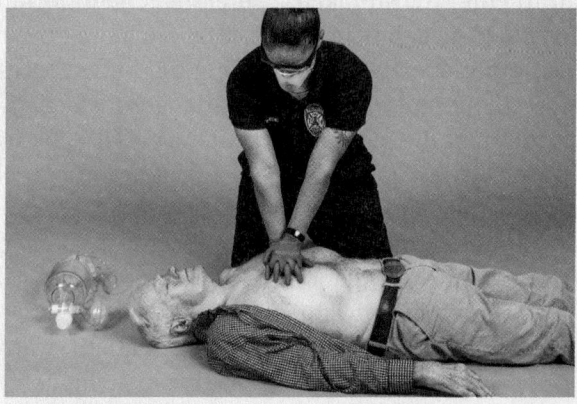

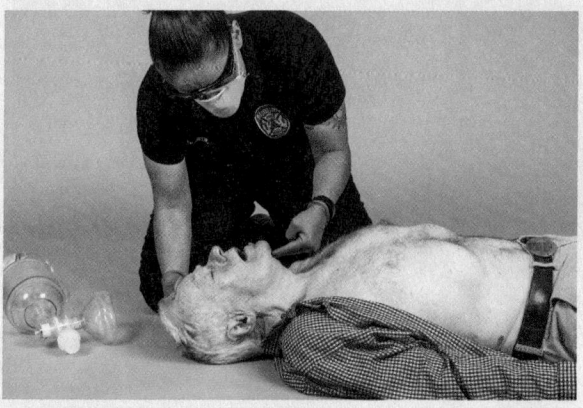

### Step 3

If breathing and pulse are absent, then perform CPR until an AED is available. Give 30 chest compressions at a rate of 100 to 120 per minute.

### Step 4

Open the airway according to your suspicion of spinal injury.

### Step 5

Give two ventilations of 1 second each and observe for visible chest rise. Continue cycles of 30 chest compressions and two ventilations until additional personnel arrive or the patient starts to move.

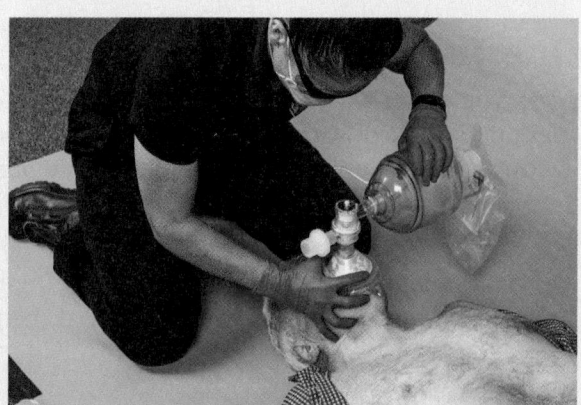

2. Position the patient properly (supine) on a flat surface.

3. Quickly visualize the chest for signs of breathing while simultaneously palpating for a carotid pulse. Take no more than 10 seconds in total to do this (**Step 2**).

4. If pulse and breathing are absent, then perform CPR until an AED is available. Place your hands in the proper position for delivering external chest compressions, as described previously (**Step 3**). Give 30 chest compressions at a rate of 100 to 120 per minute for an adult. Each set of 30 compressions should take about 17 seconds.

5. Open the airway according to your suspicion of spinal injury (**Step 4**).

6. Give two ventilations of 1 second each and observe for visible chest rise (**Step 5**).

7. Continue cycles of 30 chest compressions and two ventilations until additional personnel arrive or the patient starts to move.

## Two-Rescuer Adult CPR

You and your team should be able to perform one-rescuer and two-rescuer CPR with ease. Two-rescuer CPR is always preferable because it is less tiring and it facilitates effective chest compressions. In fact, a team approach to CPR and AED use is far superior to the one-rescuer approach. Once one-rescuer CPR is in progress, additional rescuers can be added to the procedure easily. Before assisting with CPR, a second rescuer should apply airway adjuncts, including a bag-mask device and suction, and insert an oropharyngeal (oral) airway. If CPR is in progress, then the second rescuer should enter the procedure after the AED and then cycle of 30 compressions and two ventilations. To perform two-rescuer adult CPR, follow the steps in **SKILL DRILL 14-3**:

1. Take standard precautions. Establish unresponsiveness while your partner moves to the patient's side to be ready to deliver chest compressions (**Step 1**).

2. If the patient is unresponsive, then simultaneously check for breathing and palpate for a carotid pulse; take no more than 10 seconds to do this (**Step 2**).

3. If the patient is not breathing and has no pulse, then begin CPR, starting with chest compressions. Give 30 chest compressions at a rate of 100 to 120 per minute. If an AED is available, then apply it and follow its voice prompts. Do not interrupt chest compressions to apply the AED pads (**Step 3**).

4. Open the airway according to your suspicion of spinal injury (**Step 4**).

5. Give two ventilations of 1 second each and observe for visible chest rise (**Step 5**).

6. Perform five cycles of 30 compressions and two ventilations (this should take about 2 minutes). After 2 minutes of CPR, the compressor and the ventilator should switch positions. The switch time should take no longer than 5 seconds. Reanalyze the patient's cardiac rhythm with the AED every 2 minutes and deliver a shock if indicated.

7. Continue cycles of 30 chest compressions and two ventilations until ALS providers take over or the patient starts to move.

### Words of Wisdom

When CPR is in progress on a patient who has an advanced airway device in place (ie, ET tube, King LT supraglottic airway, i-gel supraglottic airway), stopping compressions to provide a breath is not necessary. Compressions should be continuous at a rate of 100 to 120 per minute and ventilations should occur at a rate of one breath every 6 seconds (10 breaths/min). Do not attempt to synchronize compressions and ventilations; do not pause between compressions to deliver breaths.

## Switching Positions

It is critical to switch rescuers during CPR to maintain high-quality compressions. After five cycles of CPR (about 2 minutes), the rescuer providing compressions to the patient (the compressor) will begin to tire, and compression quality will decrease. Therefore, compressors should switch positions every 2 minutes. If there are only two rescuers on scene, then the two rescuers will alternate positions. If additional rescuers are available, the compressor should rotate every 2 minutes. During switches, every effort should be made to minimize the time that no compressions are being administered. It should take less than 10 seconds to switch compressors.

## Skill Drill 14-3 Performing Two-Rescuer Adult CPR

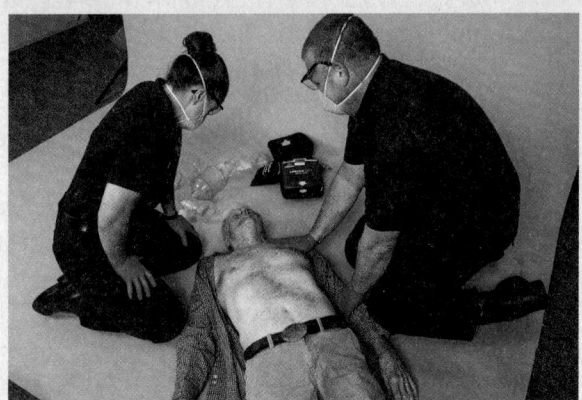

### Step 1

Take standard precautions. Establish unresponsiveness and take positions.

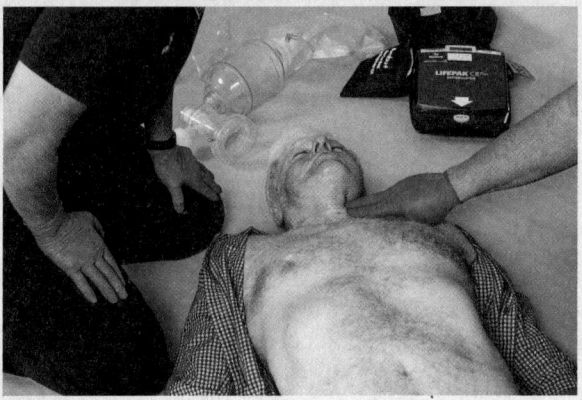

### Step 2

Check for breathing and a carotid pulse.

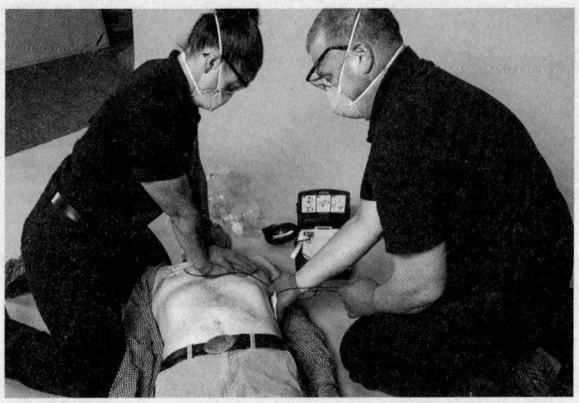

### Step 3

Begin CPR, starting with chest compressions. Give 30 chest compressions at a rate of 100 to 120 per minute. If the AED is available, then apply it and follow the voice prompts.

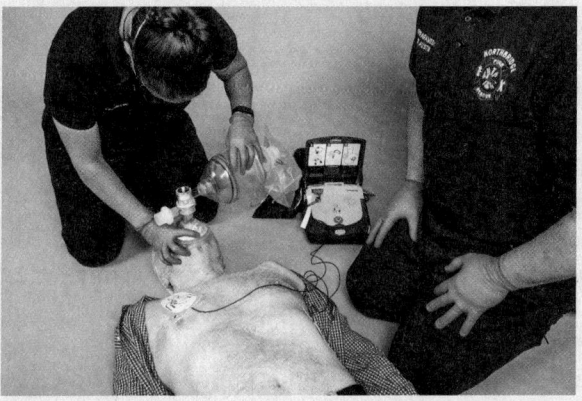

### Step 4

Open the airway according to your suspicion of spinal injury. Give two ventilations of 1 second each and observe for visible chest rise. Continue cycles of 30 chest compressions and two ventilations (switch roles every five cycles [2 minutes]) until ALS providers take over or the patient starts to move. Reanalyze the patient's cardiac rhythm with the AED every 2 minutes and deliver a shock if indicated.

The switch between the two rescuers can be easily accomplished. Rescuer one (the first compressor) should finish the cycle of 30 compressions while the second rescuer moves to the opposite side of the chest and moves into position to begin compressions. Rescuer one should deliver two rescue breaths and then rescuer two should take over compressions by administering 30 chest compressions. Rescuer one will then deliver two ventilations and the CPR cycles will continue as needed until the next 2-minute mark (five cycles) is reached, at which time the process will be repeated.

### Words of Wisdom

Even if the EMT providing compressions does not feel tired after 2 minutes, the compressions being provided are probably less effective. Rotate compressors every 2 minutes, even if you do not feel tired.

A summary of how to manage cardiac arrest in adults is shown in **FIGURE 14-16**.

## Devices and Techniques to Assist Circulation

The effectiveness of CPR depends on the amount of blood circulated throughout the body as a result of chest compressions. Even under ideal conditions, however, manual chest compressions cannot equate to normal cardiac output. In addition, factors such as rescuer fatigue or inaccurate depth or rate of compressions can further impede the resuscitation process. Before you consider the use of mechanical devices to assist circulation, ensure that your manual chest compressions are of consistently high quality. If you decide to use a CPR assist device, the device should be applied quickly with minimal interruptions to CPR. Knowledge about, and frequent training with, the CPR assist device you may use is crucial for best patient outcome.

Several mechanical devices are available to assist emergency responders in maximizing blood flow during CPR. Although improved patient outcomes have not yet been documented, these devices may be considered for use as an adjunct to CPR in select settings when used by properly trained personnel for patients in cardiac arrest in the prehospital or in-hospital setting. These specific settings include instances when limited rescuers are available, when CPR is prolonged, or when CPR is required in a moving ambulance.

### Words of Wisdom

Many EMS systems have implemented a pit crew approach to the management of cardiac arrest. The term originated in motor racing, in which teams of technicians rapidly assess and repair vehicles in a matter of seconds. Following this model, each resuscitation team member is assigned a specific role before beginning care of the cardiac arrest patient. The following provides an example:

- EMT 1 will be the team leader.
- EMT 2 and EMT 3 will perform CPR.
- EMT 4 will operate the AED.

This model clarifies each team member's role and responsibilities and minimizes confusion on the scene. If there are only two EMTs on scene initially—as is the situation in many cases—then a plan should be developed to integrate additional rescuers into the resuscitation effort as they arrive. This preplanned approach allows rescuers to accomplish multiple steps and assessments simultaneously, rather than in the slower, sequential manner used by individual rescuers. Therefore, the pit crew model minimizes the time to first compression. The success of this team approach depends on preplanning, practice, and thorough familiarity with the cardiac arrest algorithm. See Chapter 9, The *Team Approach to Health Care*, for more information.

## Active Compression-Decompression CPR

**Active compression-decompression CPR** is a technique that involves compressing the chest and then actively pulling it back up to its neutral position or beyond (decompression). This technique may increase the amount of blood that returns to the heart, and thus, the amount of blood ejected from the heart during the compression

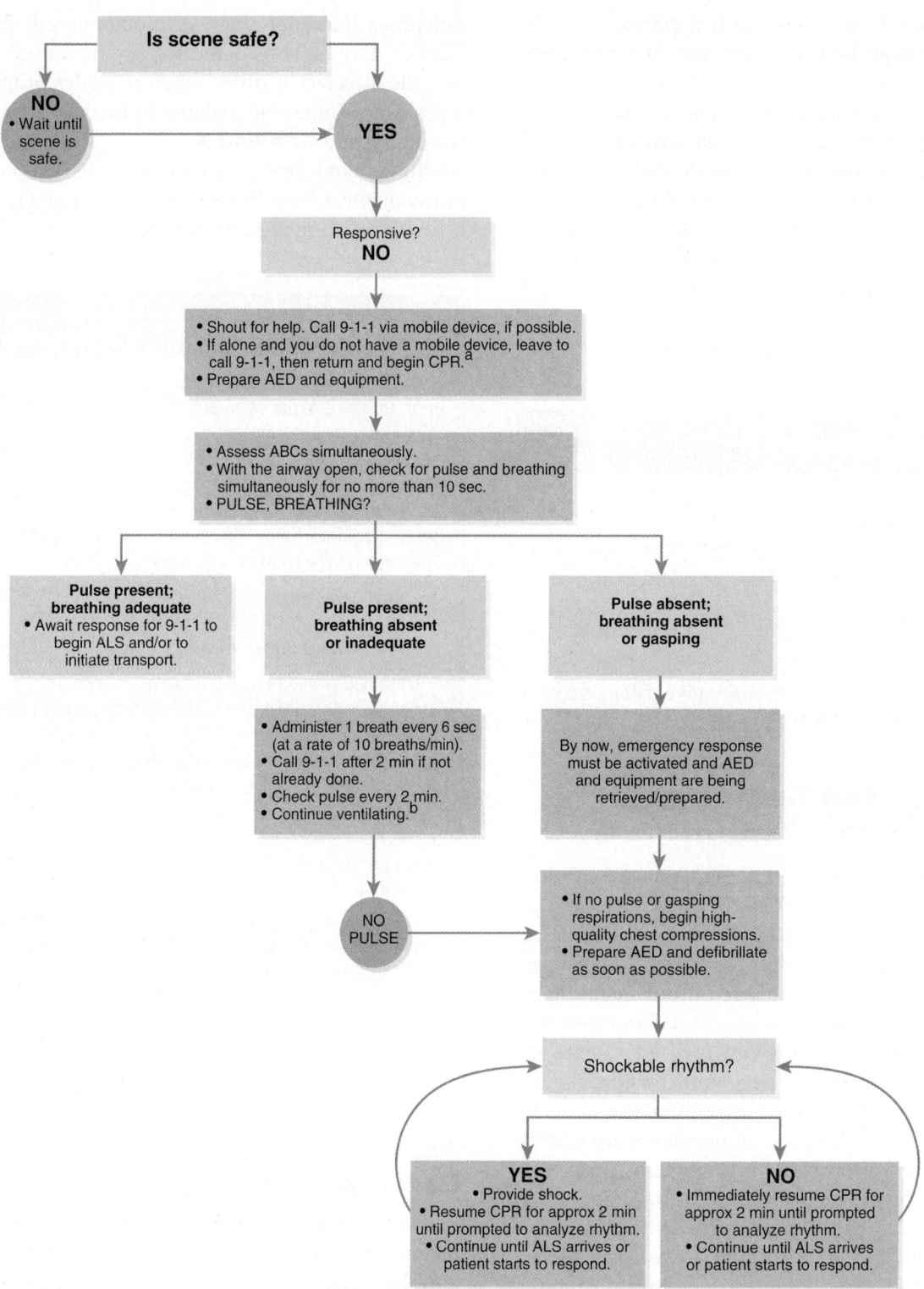

**Is scene safe?**

**NO**
• Wait until scene is safe.

**YES**

Responsive?
**NO**

• Shout for help. Call 9-1-1 via mobile device, if possible.
• If alone and you do not have a mobile device, leave to call 9-1-1, then return and begin CPR.[a]
• Prepare AED and equipment.

• Assess ABCs simultaneously.
• With the airway open, check for pulse and breathing simultaneously for no more than 10 sec.
• PULSE, BREATHING?

**Pulse present; breathing adequate**
• Await response for 9-1-1 to begin ALS and/or to initiate transport.

**Pulse present; breathing absent or inadequate**

**Pulse absent; breathing absent or gasping**

• Administer 1 breath every 6 sec (at a rate of 10 breaths/min).
• Call 9-1-1 after 2 min if not already done.
• Check pulse every 2 min.
• Continue ventilating.[b]

By now, emergency response must be activated and AED and equipment are being retrieved/prepared.

NO PULSE

• If no pulse or gasping respirations, begin high-quality chest compressions.
• Prepare AED and defibrillate as soon as possible.

Shockable rhythm?

**YES**
• Provide shock.
• Resume CPR for approx 2 min until prompted to analyze rhythm.
• Continue until ALS arrives or patient starts to respond.

**NO**
• Immediately resume CPR for approx 2 min until prompted to analyze rhythm.
• Continue until ALS arrives or patient starts to respond.

[a]If the patient is a child or infant, perform 2 minutes of CPR if needed, then call 9-1-1.
[b]If life-threatening opioid overdose is suspected, administer naloxone, if available, per local protocols and see the opioid life-threatening overdose algorithm in Chapter 21, *Toxicology*.

**FIGURE 14-16** Adult cardiac arrest algorithm. Pediatric cardiac arrest follows the same algorithm except for the compression depth and compression-to-ventilation ratio. When performing CPR on pediatric patients, compress to a depth of at least one-third the anterior-posterior diameter of the chest, at a ratio of 30:2 compressions to ventilations (one rescuer) or 15:2 compressions to ventilations (two rescuers).

On occasion, you may encounter a patient who has a left ventricular assist device (LVAD). The LVAD is a mechanical pump that is implanted in the chest and helps pump blood from the left ventricle to the aorta. A tube from the device passes through the skin and is attached to an external power source that the patient wears on their belt or an over-the-shoulder harness. The LVAD is commonly implanted in patients with severe heart failure or in those who are awaiting a heart transplant. If the LVAD is working, then you will hear a humming sound when listening to the chest with a stethoscope. Blood flows continuously through the LVAD, and the more assistance the LVAD is providing to the heart, the weaker the patient's pulse will be. In some patients with an LVAD, you may not feel a pulse at all, even though they are responsive and alert. If the patient is unresponsive with no breathing, poor skin color, and poor or no capillary refill, and the hum of the device is heard, CPR is indicated. If the hum of the device is not heard, check to ensure that all cables are connected and that the power supply is working (batteries have a charge or the device is plugged in to an outlet). When transporting a patient who has an LVAD, be sure to bring all LVAD equipment with you and ensure that the receiving facility is capable of caring for the patient's specific needs.

You should know the location of patients with an LVAD in your service area. If possible, visit with the patient prior to any emergency to determine the patient's specific device and to obtain instructions. Family members are usually knowledgeable about the device; use them as a source of information.

LVAD coordinators are usually available for consult 24 hours per day. These medical professionals typically work at the same facility that placed the device, so they should also be familiar with the patient. Follow your local protocols or contact medical control regarding the treatment of a patient with an LVAD.

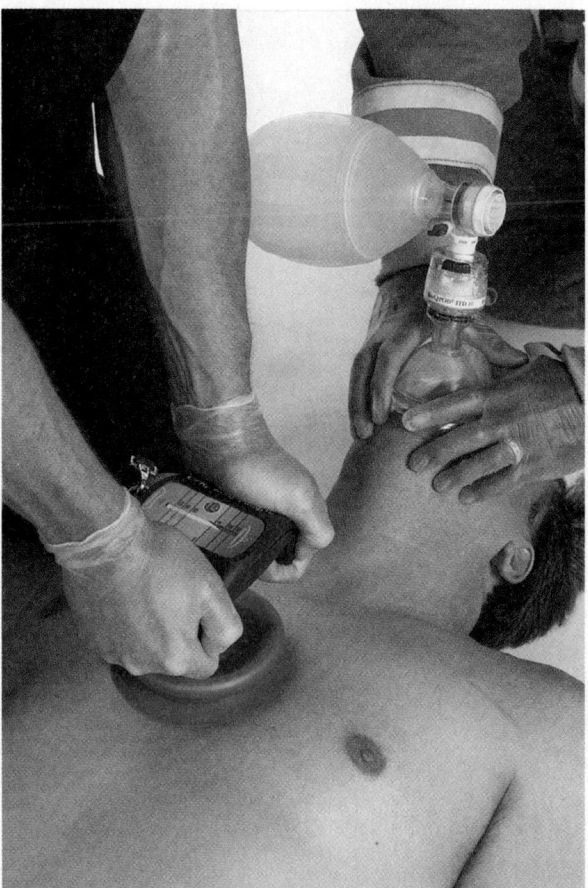

**FIGURE 14-17** An active compression-decompression CPR device.

Provided with permission by ZOLL Medical.

phase. **FIGURE 14-17** shows an active compression-decompression CPR device. It features a suction cup that is placed in the center of the chest. After compressing the chest to the proper depth, the rescuer pulls up on the handle of the device to provide active decompression of the chest, thus ensuring that the chest returns to at least its neutral position or even beyond neutral.

## Impedance Threshold Device

An **impedance threshold device (ITD)** is a valve device placed between the ET tube and a bag-mask device; it may also be placed between the bag and mask if an ET tube is not in place. The ITD is designed to limit the air entering the lungs during the recoil phase between chest compressions (**FIGURE 14-18**). This results in negative intrathoracic pressure that may draw more blood toward the heart, ultimately resulting in improved cardiac filling and circulation during each chest compression. The ITD may be considered when used together with devices that provide active compression-decompression CPR. It is not currently recommended for use with conventional CPR. If ROSC occurs, then the ITD should be removed. You should understand research trends regarding the effectiveness of the ITD.

## Mechanical Piston Device

A **mechanical piston device** is a device that depresses the sternum via a compressed gas-powered or electric-powered plunger mounted on a backboard

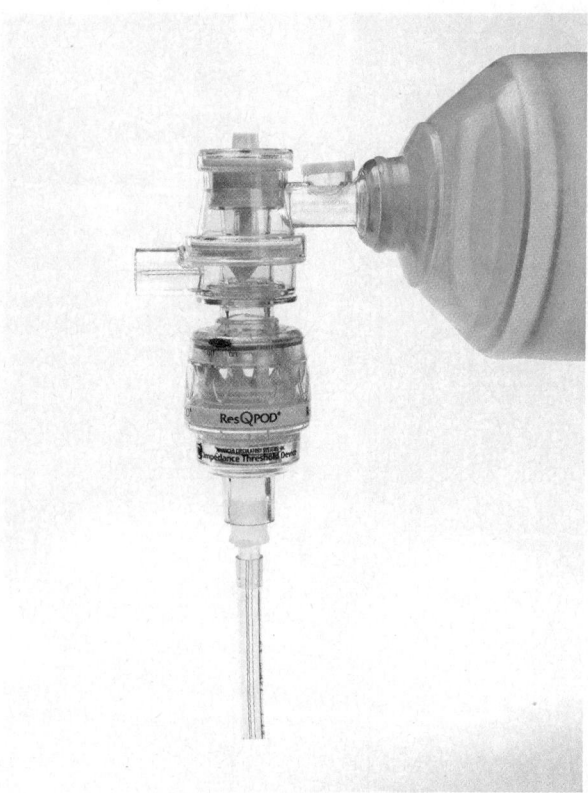

**FIGURE 14-18** An impedance threshold device.

Courtesy of Advanced Circulatory Systems, Inc.

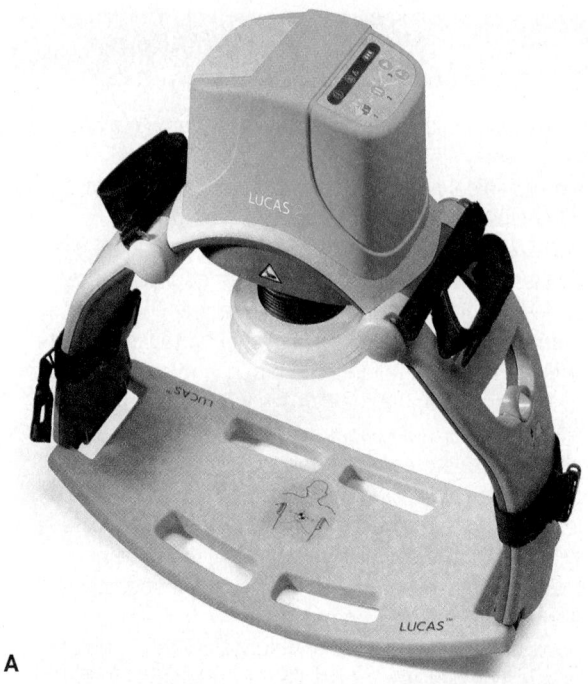

**A**

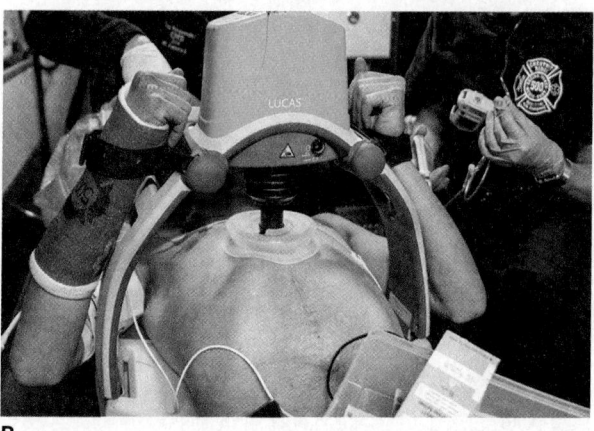

**B**

**FIGURE 14-19 A.** A mechanical piston device. **B.** The device in use.

A: Courtesy of LUCAS CPR (Physio Control Inc.).; B: © Jones & Bartlett Learning.

(**FIGURE 14-19**). The patient is positioned supine on the backboard, with the piston positioned on top of the patient with the plunger centered over the patient's thorax in the same manner as with manual chest compressions. The device is then secured to the backboard.

The mechanical piston device allows rescuers to configure the depth and rate of compressions, resulting in consistent delivery. This frees the rescuer to complete other tasks and eliminates rescuer fatigue that results from continuous delivery of manual chest compressions. These devices have been available for many years. The latest versions of these devices offer you the option of providing compressions using a battery instead of an oxygen tank or a compressed air system, thus eliminating the tanks and hoses.

## Load-Distributing Band CPR or Vest CPR

The **load-distributing band (LDB)** is a circumferential chest compression device composed of a constricting band and backboard (**FIGURE 14-20**). The device is either electrically or pneumatically driven to compress the heart by putting inward pressure on the thorax.

As with the mechanical piston device, use of the LDB frees the rescuer to complete other tasks. The device weighs less than the early-version mechanical piston devices and can be easier to apply.

Although a mechanical CPR device may be a reasonable alternative to conventional CPR in specific settings, manual chest compressions it rapidly. Remember to minimize interruptions to chest compressions while the device is being applied.

## Infant and Child CPR

In most cases, cardiac arrest in infants and children follows respiratory arrest, which triggers hypoxia and **ischemia** (decreased oxygen supply) of the heart. Children consume oxygen two to three times more rapidly than adults, so you must first focus on opening the airway and providing artificial ventilation. Often, this will be enough to allow the child to resume spontaneous breathing and, thus, prevent cardiac arrest. Therefore, airway and breathing are the focus of pediatric BLS (**TABLE 14-2**).

Respiratory issues leading to cardiopulmonary arrest in children can have a number of different causes (as discussed in Chapter 35, *Pediatric Emergencies*). These causes include the following:

- Injury, both blunt and penetrating
- Infections of the respiratory tract or another organ system (croup, epiglottitis)
- Foreign body in the airway
- Submersion (drowning)
- Electrocution
- Poisoning or drug overdose
- Sudden infant death syndrome

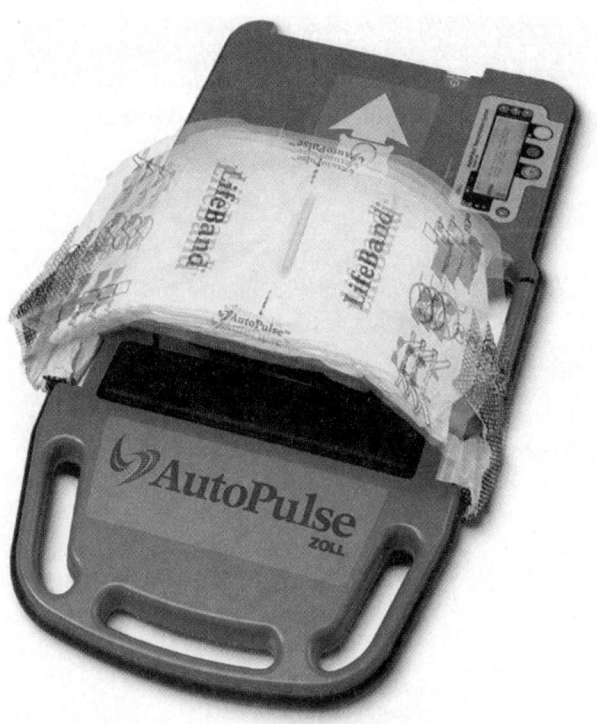

**FIGURE 14-20** A load-distributing band.

Provided with permission by ZOLL Medical.

remain the standard of care. If your EMS service uses a mechanical CPR device, then it is critical to practice frequently to ensure that you can apply

## YOU are the Provider

With CPR ongoing, you open the AED pads and prepare to apply them to the patient's chest. A second EMT unit arrives on the scene to assist with care. You note that the patient has a medication patch on the right upper part of his chest. You also see a bulge with a scar over it on the left upper part of his chest. You apply the AED pads, analyze the patient's cardiac rhythm, and receive a "shock advised" message. After delivering the shock, your partner and another EMT resume CPR.

| Recording Time: 4 Minutes | |
|---|---|
| Level of consciousness | Unresponsive |
| Respirations | Absent (baseline); two breaths are being given after every 30 chest compressions; chest rise is visible with each breath |
| Pulse | Absent (baseline); femoral pulse is palpable with chest compressions |
| Skin | Ashen |
| Blood pressure | Not measurable |
| Oxygen saturation (Spo₂) | Not measurable |

**5.** Should you remove the medication patch or leave it in place? Why or why not?

**6.** What does the bulge and scar over the patient's left chest indicate? How will this affect the way you treat the patient?

**TABLE 14-2** Review of Pediatric BLS Procedures

| Procedure | Infants (between age 1 month and 1 year[a]) | Children (age 1 year to onset of puberty[b]) |
|---|---|---|
| **Circulation** | | |
| Pulse check | Brachial artery | Carotid or femoral artery |
| Compression area | Just below the nipple line | In the center of the chest, in between the nipples |
| Compression width | Two-finger technique or two-thumb-encircling-hands technique | Heel of one or both hands |
| Compression depth | At least one-third anterior-posterior diameter (about 1.5 in. [4 cm]) | At least one-third anterior-posterior diameter (about 2 in. [5 cm]) |
| Compression rate | 100 to 120/min | 100 to 120/min |
| Compression-to-ventilation ratio (until advanced airway is inserted) | 30:2 (one rescuer); 15:2 (two rescuers)[c] | 30:2 (one rescuer); 15:2 (two rescuers)[c] |
| Foreign body obstruction | Responsive: Back slaps and chest thrusts<br>Unresponsive: CPR | Responsive: Abdominal thrusts (Heimlich maneuver)<br>Unresponsive: CPR |
| **Airway** | | |
| | Head tilt–chin lift; jaw-thrust maneuver if spinal injury is suspected | Head tilt–chin lift; jaw-thrust maneuver if spinal injury is suspected |
| **Breathing** | | |
| Ventilations | 1 breath every 2 to 3 seconds (20 to 30 breaths/min); visible chest rise | 1 breath every 2 to 3 seconds (20 to 30 breaths/min); visible chest rise |
| Ventilations with advanced airway placed | 1 breath every 2 to 3 seconds (a rate of 20 to 30 breaths/min) | 1 breath every 2 to 3 seconds (a rate of 20 to 30 breaths/min) |

[a] The AHA defines neonatal patients as birth to age 1 month, and infants as age 1 month to 1 year. Neonatal resuscitation is covered in Chapter 34, *Obstetrics and Neonatal Care*.
[b] Onset of puberty is approximately 12 to 14 years of age, as defined by secondary characteristics (eg, breast development in girls and armpit hair in boys).
[c] Pause compressions to deliver ventilations.

© Jones & Bartlett Learning.

## Determining Responsiveness

Never shake a child to determine whether the child is responsive, especially if the possibility of a neck or back injury exists. Instead, gently tap the child on the shoulder, and say loudly, "Are you okay?" (**FIGURE 14-21**). With an infant, gently tap the soles of the feet. If a child is responsive but struggling to breathe, allow the child to remain in whatever position is most comfortable.

If you find an unresponsive, apneic, and pulseless child while you are alone and off duty, and you did not witness the child's collapse, perform CPR beginning with chest compressions for approximately five cycles (about 2 minutes), and then stop to call 9-1-1 and retrieve an AED. Remember that cardiopulmonary arrest in children is most often the result of respiratory failure, not a primary cardiac event. Therefore, children will require immediate restoration of oxygenation, ventilation,

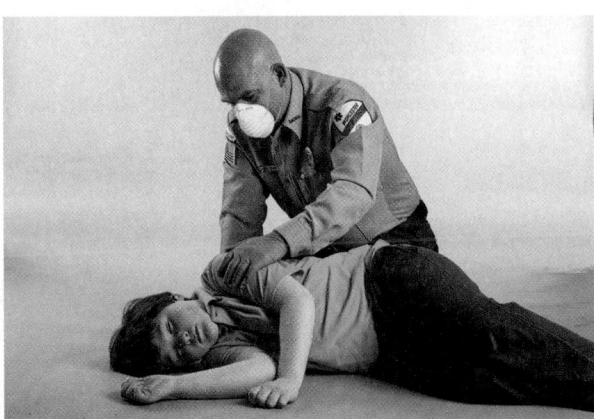

**FIGURE 14-21** Never shake a child to determine responsiveness. Rather, gently tap on the shoulder (child) or tap the soles of the feet (infant), and speak loudly.

© Jones & Bartlett Learning.

and circulation, which can be accomplished by immediately performing five cycles (about 2 minutes) of CPR before activating the EMS system.

## Words of Wisdom

Although uncommon, you may encounter a child whose cardiac arrest was caused by a primary cardiac event rather than a respiratory problem. If an otherwise healthy child without an apparent respiratory condition suddenly collapses and you witness it, first confirm that the child is in cardiac arrest. If you are alone without a mobile phone, then leave the child to call 9-1-1 and get an AED before beginning CPR. If you are not alone, then send someone to call 9-1-1 and get an AED while you begin CPR. The sudden collapse of an otherwise healthy child does not indicate a respiratory problem; instead, it suggests a primary cardiac event that may respond to defibrillation. Therefore, it is critical to get the AED to the child's side as soon as possible.

## Check for Breathing and a Pulse

After you establish responsiveness, you need to assess breathing and circulation. As with an adult, this assessment in a child can occur simultaneously and should take no longer than 10 seconds. Visualize the chest for signs of breathing and palpate for a pulse in a large central artery. In infants, palpate the brachial artery, which is located on the inner side of the arm, midway between the elbow and shoulder. Place your thumb on the outer surface of the arm

between the elbow and shoulder. Then place the tips of your index and middle fingers on the inside of the biceps, and press lightly toward the bone. CPR will be required if the infant or child is not breathing or is not breathing normally (agonal gasps), and a pulse is absent (or less than 60 beats/min).

As with an adult, an infant or child must be lying on a hard, flat surface for effective chest compressions. If you need to carry an infant while providing CPR, then your forearm and hand can serve as the flat surface. Use your palm to support the infant's head. In this way, the infant's shoulders are elevated, and the head is slightly tilted back in a position that will keep the airway open. Ensure that the infant's head is not higher than the rest of the body.

The technique for chest compressions in infants and children differs from that in adults because of several anatomic differences, including the position of the heart, the size of the chest, and the fragile organs of a child. The liver (immediately under the right side of the diaphragm) is relatively large and fragile, especially in infants. The spleen, on the left, is smaller and more fragile in children than in adults. These organs are easily injured if you are not careful in performing chest compressions, so be sure that your hand position is correct before you begin. The chest of an infant is smaller and more pliable than that of an older child or adult; therefore, you should use only two fingers to compress the chest. If two rescuers are performing CPR on an infant, use the two-thumb-encircling-hands technique to deliver chest compressions on the lower half of the sternum, making sure to avoid the xiphoid process (**FIGURE 14-22**). In children, especially those older than 8 years, you can use the heel of one or both hands to compress the chest.

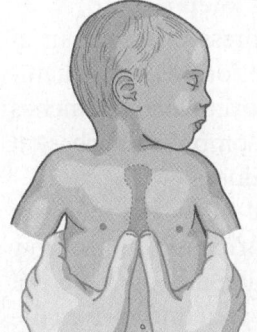

**2-rescuer infant CPR**

- Place both thumbs side by side in center of the chest on the lower half of sternum (thumbs may overlap in small infants)
- Encircle the chest and support the infant's back with the fingers of both hands
- Ratio 15:2, switching roles every 2 minutes

**FIGURE 14-22** Hand positions for 2-rescuer infant CPR.

© Jones & Bartlett Learning.

## Skill Drill 14-4 Performing Infant Chest Compressions

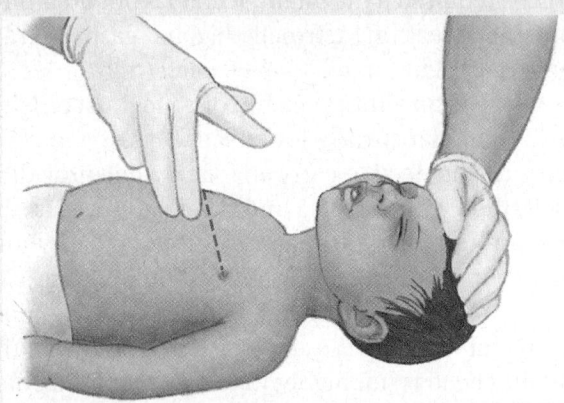

### Step 1

Take standard precautions. Position the infant on a firm surface while maintaining the airway. Place two fingers in the middle of the sternum with one finger just below the nipple line.

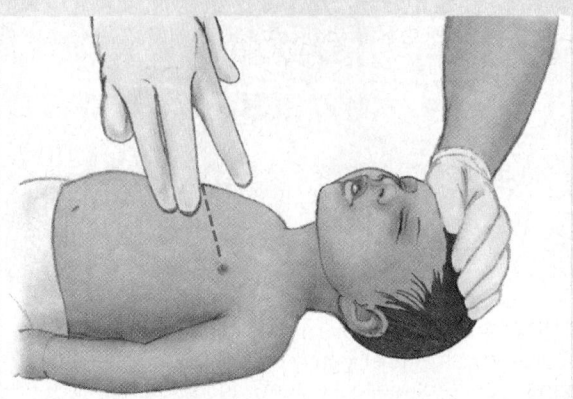

### Step 2

Use two fingers to compress the chest at least one-third its depth at a rate of 100 to 120 per minute. Allow the sternum to return to its normal position between compressions.

© Jones & Bartlett Learning.

Follow the steps in **SKILL DRILL 14-4** to perform infant chest compressions:

1. Take standard precautions. Place the infant on a firm surface, using one hand to keep the head in an open airway position. You can also use a pad or wedge under the shoulders and upper body to keep the head from tilting forward.
2. Imagine a line drawn between the nipples. Place two fingers in the middle of the sternum, just below the nipple line (**Step 1**).
3. Using two fingers, compress the sternum at least one-third the anterior-posterior diameter of the chest (approximately 1.5 inches [4 cm] in most infants). Compress the chest at a rate of 100 to 120 per minute.
4. After each compression, allow the sternum to return briefly to its normal position. Allow equal time for compression and relaxation of the chest. Do not remove your fingers from the sternum, and avoid jerky movements (**Step 2**).

Coordinate compressions and ventilations in a 30:2 ratio if you are working alone, and in a 15:2 ratio if you are working with a trained bystander or another health care provider. Ensure the infant's chest fully recoils in between compressions and that the chest visibly rises with each ventilation. You will find this easier to do if you use your free hand to keep the head in the open airway position. If the chest does not rise, or rises only a little, then use a head tilt–chin lift to open the airway. Reassess the infant for signs of spontaneous breathing or a pulse after five cycles (about 2 minutes) of CPR.

**SKILL DRILL 14-5** shows the steps for performing CPR in children between 1 year of age and the onset of puberty:

1. Take standard precautions. Place the child on a firm surface. Place the heel of one or two hands in the center of the chest, in between the nipples. Avoid compression over the lower tip of the sternum, which is called the xiphoid process (**Step 1**).
2. Compress the chest at least one-third the anterior-posterior diameter of the chest (approximately 2 inches [5 cm] in most children) at a rate of 100 to 120 per minute. With

## Skill Drill 14-5 Performing CPR on a Child

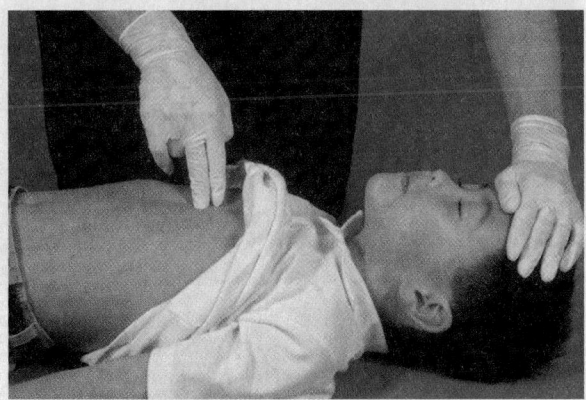

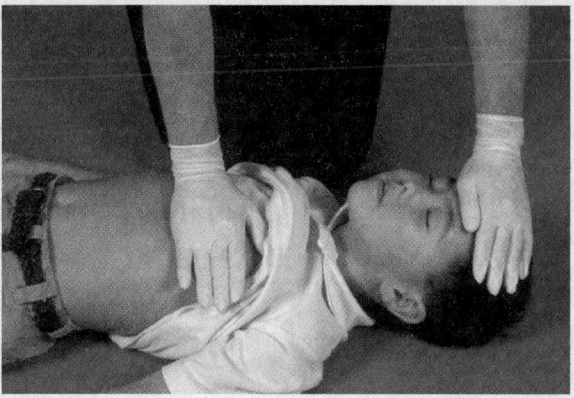

### Step 1

Take standard precautions. Place the child on a firm surface. Identify the location for hand placement, as shown here. Place the heel of one or two hands in the center of the chest, in between the nipples, avoiding the xiphoid process.

### Step 2

Compress the chest at least one-third the anterior-posterior diameter of the chest at a rate of 100 to 120 times/min. Coordinate compressions with ventilations in a 30:2 (one rescuer) or 15:2 (two rescuers) ratio, pausing for two ventilations. Reassess for a pulse after 2 minutes. If there is no pulse and an AED is available, then resume CPR and apply the AED pads.

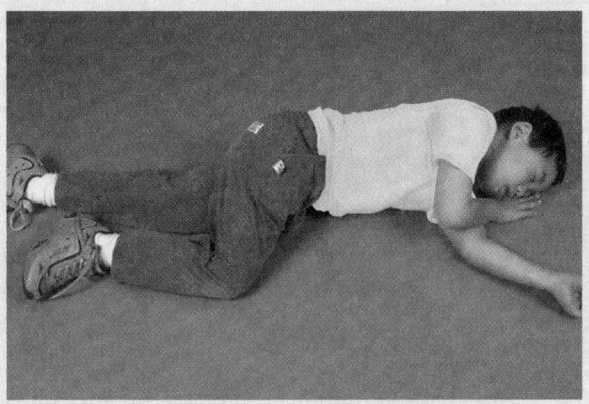

### Step 3

If the child regains a pulse of greater than 60 beats/min and resumes effective breathing, then place the child in a position that allows for frequent reassessment of the airway and vital signs during transport.

pauses for ventilation, the actual number of compressions delivered will be about 80 per minute. In between compressions, allow the chest to fully recoil; do not lean on the chest. Compression and relaxation time should be the same duration. Use smooth movements. Hold your fingers off the child's ribs, and keep the heel of your hand or hands on the sternum.

3. Coordinate compressions and ventilations in a 30:2 ratio for one rescuer and 15:2 for two rescuers, making sure the chest rises with each ventilation. At the end of each cycle, pause for two ventilations (**Step 2**).

4. After five cycles (about 2 minutes) reassess for a pulse. If there is no pulse and you have an AED, continue CPR and apply the AED pads.
5. If the child regains a pulse of greater than 60 beats/min and resumes effective breathing, place the child in a position that allows for frequent reassessment of the airway and vital signs during transport (**Step 3**).

Switching rescuer positions is the same for children as it is for adults, every five cycles (2 minutes) of CPR. Remember, if the child is past the onset of puberty, use the adult CPR sequence, including the use of the AED.

## Airway

Infants and toddlers often put toys and other objects, as well as food, in their mouths; therefore, foreign body obstruction of the upper airway is common. You must make sure that the upper airway is open when managing pediatric respiratory emergencies or cardiopulmonary arrest. If the child is unresponsive and lying in a supine position, then the airway may become obstructed when the tongue and throat muscles relax and the tongue falls backward.

If the child is unresponsive but breathing adequately, then place him or her in the recovery position to maintain an open airway and allow drainage of saliva, vomitus, or other secretions from the mouth. Do not use this position if you suspect injury to the spine, hips, or pelvis unless you can secure the child to a backboard that can be tilted to the side. If the child is responsive and breathing, but in a labored fashion, then provide supplemental oxygen and prompt transport to the closest appropriate hospital.

Opening the airway in an infant or child is done by using the same techniques as used for an adult. However, because a child's neck is so flexible, the techniques should be slightly modified. The jaw-thrust maneuver is the best method to use if you suspect a spinal injury in a child. If a second rescuer is present, he or she should immobilize the child's cervical spine. If spinal injury is not suspected, then use the head tilt–chin lift maneuver but modified so that, as you tilt the head back, you are moving it only into the neutral position or a slightly extended position (**FIGURE 14-23**).

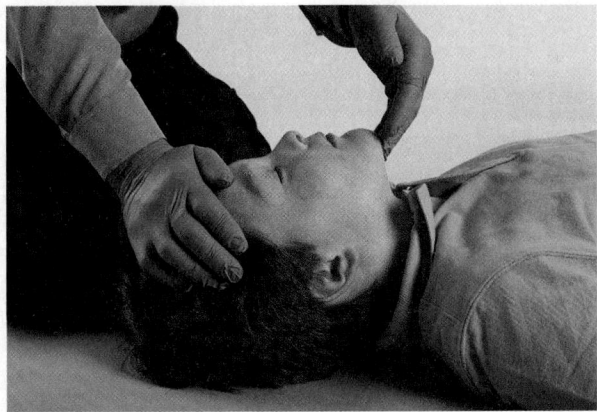

**FIGURE 14-23** Use the head tilt–chin lift maneuver to open the airway in a child who has not sustained a traumatic injury. Do not overextend the neck.

© Jones & Bartlett Learning.

### Head Tilt–Chin Lift Maneuver

Perform the head tilt–chin lift maneuver in a child in the following manner:

1. Place one hand on the child's forehead, and tilt the head back gently, with the neck slightly extended.
2. Place two or three fingers (not the thumb) of your other hand under the child's chin, and lift the jaw upward and outward. Do not close the mouth or push under the chin; either move may obstruct rather than open the airway.
3. Remove any visible foreign body or vomitus.

### Jaw-Thrust Maneuver

Perform the jaw-thrust maneuver in a child in the following manner:

1. Place two or three fingers under each side of the angle of the lower jaw; lift the jaw upward and outward.
2. If the jaw thrust alone does not open the airway and cervical spine injury is not a consideration, then tilt the head slightly. If cervical spine injury is suspected, then use a second rescuer to immobilize the cervical spine.

Remember that the head of an infant or young child is disproportionately large in comparison with the chest and shoulders. As a result, when a child is lying flat on his or her back, especially on a backboard, the head will bend forward (hyperflexion)

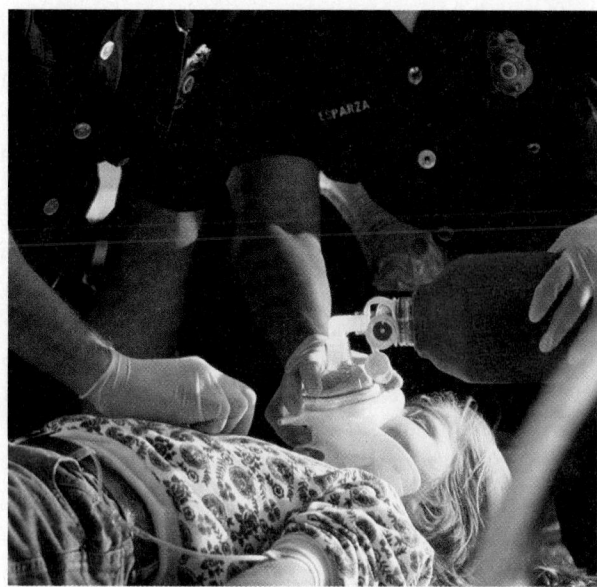

**FIGURE 14-24** Open the child's airway and provide rescue breathing.

© Bruce Ayres/The Image Bank/ Getty Images Plus/Getty Images.

onto the upper chest. This position can partially or completely obstruct the upper airway. To avoid this possibility, place a wedge of padding under the child's upper back and shoulders (torso).

## Provide Rescue Breathing

If the child is not breathing but has a pulse, then open the airway and deliver one breath every 2 to 3 seconds (20 to 30 breaths/min) (**FIGURE 14-24**). If the child is not breathing and does not have a pulse, then deliver two rescue breaths after every 30 chest compressions (15 chest compressions if two rescuers are present). Each ventilation should last about 1 second and should produce visible chest rise. Use the proper-size mask and ensure an adequate mask-to-face seal.

If an infant or small child is breathing, then provide prompt transport. Again, a child who is in respiratory distress should be allowed to stay in whatever position is most comfortable. Children who are unresponsive but breathing with difficulty should be kept in a position that allows you to manage the airway and provide ventilatory support, if needed.

In a child with a tracheostomy tube in the neck, remove the mask from the bag-mask device and connect it directly to the tracheostomy tube to ventilate the child. If a bag-mask device is unavailable, a face mask with one-way valve or other barrier device over the tracheostomy site can be used. Place your hand firmly over the child's mouth and nose to prevent the artificial breaths from leaking out of the upper airway.

### Words of Wisdom

An injured child with a serious airway or breathing problem is likely to need full-time attention from two EMTs. Therefore, it is important for you to arrange for backup from another unit as soon as possible—perhaps even before you arrive at the scene. In such cases, you will need a driver and often additional help with patient care.

## Interrupting CPR

CPR is a crucial, life-saving procedure that provides minimal circulation and ventilation until the patient can receive defibrillation, ALS treatment, and definitive care in the ED. No matter how well CPR is performed, however, it is rarely enough to save a patient's life. If ALS care is unavailable at the scene, you must provide transport based on your local protocols and continue CPR on the way. En route to the ED, consider requesting a rendezvous with ALS providers, if available. This will provide ALS care to the patient sooner, improving the patient's chance

### Special Populations

Children in respiratory distress are often struggling to breathe. As a result, they usually position themselves in a way that keeps the airway open enough for air to move. Let the child stay in that position as long as his or her breathing remains adequate. If you and your partner arrive at the scene and find that the infant or child is not breathing or has cyanosis, then immediate management (including rescue breathing and supplemental oxygen) is essential. Consider requesting additional assistance, if available.

If air enters freely with your initial breaths and the chest rises, then the airway is clear. If air does not enter freely, then check the airway for obstruction. Reposition the patient to open the airway, and attempt to give another breath. If air still does not enter freely, then you must take steps to relieve the obstruction.

for survival. However, not all EMS systems have ALS support available to them, especially in rural settings.

Try not to interrupt CPR for more than 10 seconds, except when it is absolutely necessary. For example, if you have to move a patient up or down stairs, you should continue CPR until you arrive at the head or foot of the stairs, interrupt CPR at a mutually agreed-on signal, and move quickly to the next level where you can resume CPR. Do not move the patient until all transport arrangements are made so that interruptions to CPR can be kept to a minimum. See Chapter 8, *Lifting and Moving Patients*, to review patient lifting and moving techniques.

**Chest compression fraction** is the total percentage of time during a high-quality CPR resuscitation attempt in which chest compressions are being performed. Make every effort to maintain a chest compression fraction greater than 60% (the higher the better, with 80% or higher being a common goal for high-performing EMS systems). The more frequent the interruptions in chest compressions, the lower the compression fraction will be. Low compression fractions lead to worse patient outcomes. Most modern cardiac monitors will provide information about chest compression fraction that you can review after a cardiac arrest. If possible, routinely review this information after every arrest so that you can learn ways to improve the chest compression fraction and improve on other key performance indicators.

## When Not to Start CPR

As an EMT, it is your responsibility to start CPR on virtually all patients you encounter who are in cardiac arrest. There are only three general exceptions to the rule.

First, do not start CPR if the scene is unsafe. The concept of ensuring scene safety applies in cardiac arrest situations, just as it does on any other call.

Second, do not start CPR if the patient has obvious signs of death. These signs are described further in Chapter 3, *Medical, Legal, and Ethical Issues*. Obvious signs of death include an absence of a pulse and breathing, along with any one of the following findings:

- **Rigor mortis**, or stiffening of the body after death
- **Dependent lividity** (livor mortis), a discoloration of the skin caused by pooling of blood (**FIGURE 14-25**)
- Putrefaction (decomposition of the body tissues)
- Evidence of nonsurvivable injury, such as decapitation, dismemberment, or being burned beyond recognition.

Rigor mortis and dependent lividity develop after a patient has been dead for a long period.

## YOU are the Provider

After 2 minutes of CPR, you reanalyze the patient's cardiac rhythm and receive a "no shock advised" message. Your partner and the other EMT immediately resume CPR. During CPR, your partner ventilates the patient with a bag-mask device and high-flow oxygen. As she attempts to insert an oral airway, the patient starts to gag. You quickly reassess him.

| Recording Time:  7 Minutes | |
|---|---|
| **Level of consciousness** | Unresponsive |
| **Respirations** | Occasional agonal gasps; 4 breaths/min |
| **Pulse** | 100 beats/min; strong carotid pulse; absent radial pulses |
| **Skin** | Skin color is improving |
| **Blood pressure** | 70/40 mm Hg |
| **Spo$_2$** | 82% (on oxygen) |

**7.** How should you continue to treat this patient?

**8.** Because the patient is no longer in cardiac arrest, should you remove the AED pads? Why or why not?

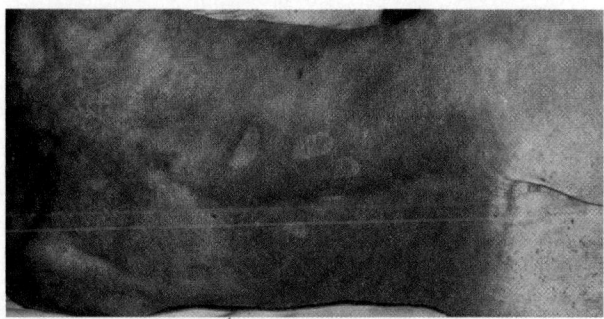

**FIGURE 14-25** Dependent lividity is an obvious sign of death, caused by blood settling to the areas of the body not in firm contact with the ground. The lividity in this figure is seen as purple discoloration of the back, except in areas that are in firm contact with the ground (scapula and buttock).

© American Academy of Orthopaedic Surgeons.

Third, do not start CPR if the patient and the patient's physician have previously agreed on a do not resuscitate (DNR) order or no-CPR order (**FIGURE 14-26**). DNR orders give you permission not to attempt resuscitation. This may apply only to situations in which the patient is known to be in the terminal stage of an incurable disease. In this situation, CPR would only prolong the patient's death. However, end-of-life issues can be complicated. Advance directives, such as living wills, may express the patient's wishes; however, these documents may not be readily producible by the patient's family or caregiver. In such cases, the safest course is to begin CPR under the rule of implied consent and then contact medical control for further guidance.

Figure: 25 TAC §157.25 (h)(2)

# OUT-OF-HOSPITAL DO-NOT-RESUSCITATE (OOH-DNR) ORDER
## TEXAS DEPARTMENT OF STATE HEALTH SERVICES

**STOP DO NOT RESUSCITATE**

This document becomes effective immediately on the date of execution for health care professionals acting in out-of-hospital settings. It remains in effect until the person is pronounced dead by authorized medical or legal authority or the document is revoked. Comfort care will be given as needed.

Person's full legal name _____ Date of birth _____ ☐ Male ☐ Female

**A. Declaration of the adult person:** I am competent and at least 18 years of age. **I direct that none of the following resuscitation measures be initiated or continued for me:** cardiopulmonary resuscitation (CPR), transcutaneous cardiac pacing, defibrillation, advanced airway management, artificial ventilation.

Person's signature _____ Date _____ Printed name _____

**B. Declaration by legal guardian, agent or proxy on behalf of the adult person who is incompetent or otherwise incapable of communication:**

I am the: ☐ legal guardian; ☐ agent in a Medical Power of Attorney; OR ☐ proxy in a directive to physicians of the above-noted person who is incompetent or otherwise mentally or physically incapable of communication.

Based upon the known desires of the person, or a determination of the best interest of the person, **I direct that none of the following resuscitation measures be initiated or continued for the person: cardiopulmonary resuscitation (CPR), transcutaneous cardiac pacing, defibrillation, advanced airway management, artificial ventilation.**

Signature _____ Date _____ Printed name _____

**C. Declaration by a qualified relative of the adult person who is incompetent or otherwise incapable of communication:** I am the above-noted person's:

☐ spouse, ☐ adult child, ☐ parent, OR ☐ nearest living relative, and I am qualified to make this treatment decision under Health and Safety Code §166.088.

To my knowledge the adult person is incompetent or otherwise mentally or physically incapable of communication and is without a legal guardian, agent or proxy. Based upon the known desires of the person or a determination of the best interests of the person, **I direct that none of the following resuscitation measures be initiated or continued for the person: cardiopulmonary resuscitation (CPR), transcutaneous cardiac pacing, defibrillation, advanced airway management, artificial ventilation.**

Signature _____ Date _____ Printed name _____

**D. Declaration by physician based on directive to physicians by a person now incompetent or nonwritten communication to the physician by a competent person:** I am the above-noted person's attending physician and have:

☐ seen evidence of his/her previously issued directive to physicians by the adult, now incompetent; OR ☐ observed his/her issuance before two witnesses of an OOH-DNR in a nonwritten manner.
**I direct that none of the following resuscitation measures be initiated or continued for the person: cardiopulmonary resuscitation (CPR), transcutaneous cardiac pacing, defibrillation, advanced airway management, artificial ventilation.**

Attending physician's signature _____ Date _____ Printed name _____ Lic# _____

**E. Declaration on behalf of the minor person:** I am the minor's: ☐ parent; ☐ legal guardian; OR ☐ managing conservator.

A physician has diagnosed the minor as suffering from a terminal or irreversible condition. **I direct that none of the following resuscitation measures be initiated or continued for the person: cardiopulmonary resuscitation (CPR), transcutaneous cardiac pacing, defibrillation, advanced airway management, artificial ventilation.**

Signature _____ Date _____

Printed name _____

**TWO WITNESSES:** (See qualifications on backside.) We have witnessed the above-noted competent adult person or authorized declarant making his/her signature above and, if applicable, the above-noted adult person making an OOH-DNR by nonwritten communication to the attending physician.

Witness 1 signature _____ Date _____ Printed name _____

Witness 2 signature _____ Date _____ Printed name _____

**Notary in the State of Texas and County of** _____ . The above noted person personally appeared before me and signed the above noted declaration on this date: _____

**FIGURE 14-26** Do not start CPR if the patient and the patient's physician have previously agreed on DNR or no-CPR orders. Learn your local protocols for treating terminally ill patients.

Courtesy of Texas Department of State Health Services.

However, if a valid DNR document or living will is produced, resuscitative efforts may be withheld. Learn your local protocols and the standards in your EMS system for treating terminally ill patients. Some EMS systems have electronic notes on patients who are preregistered with the system. These notes usually specify the amount and extent of treatment that is desired. Other states have specific DNR forms that allow EMS providers to withhold care when the patient, family, and physician have agreed in advance that such a course is most appropriate. It is essential that you understand your local protocols and are aware of the specific restrictions these advance directives imply.

You may also encounter Physician Orders for Life-Sustaining Treatment (POLST) or Medical Orders for Life-Sustaining Treatment (MOLST) forms. These legal documents describe acceptable interventions for the patient in the form of medical orders and must be signed by an authorized medical provider to be valid. Be familiar with POLST or MOLST forms, and learn your local protocols and state laws with regard to withholding end-of-life medical interventions. If you are presented with a POLST or MOLST form, then contact medical control for guidance.

In all other cases, begin CPR on anyone who is in cardiac arrest. It is usually impossible to know how long the patient's brain and vital organs have gone without oxygen. Factors such as air temperature and the basic health of the patient's tissues and organs can affect his or her ability to survive. Therefore, most legal advisers recommend that, when in doubt, always give too much care rather than too little care. Therefore, always start CPR if any doubt exists.

## When to Stop CPR

As an EMT, you are generally not responsible for making the decision to stop CPR. After you begin CPR in the field, you must continue until one of the following events occurs (the STOP mnemonic):

- **S** The patient Starts breathing and has a pulse.
- **T** The patient's care is Transferred to another provider of equal or higher-level training.
- **O** You are Out of strength or too tired to continue CPR.
- **P** A Physician who is present or providing online medical direction assumes responsibility for the patient and directs you to discontinue CPR.

*Out of strength* does not mean merely weary; rather, it means that you are no longer physically able to perform CPR. In short, always continue CPR until the patient's care is transferred to a physician or higher medical authority in the field. In some cases, your medical director or a designated medical control physician may order you to stop CPR on the basis of the patient's condition. ALS providers under Termination of Resuscitation (TOR) protocols may cease resuscitation efforts without online medical direction under specific situations.

### Words of Wisdom

**Termination of Resuscitation (TOR) Protocols**

The BLS criteria for TOR differ from the ALS criteria. BLS criteria include the following three rules:

- Unwitnessed by EMS
- No AED or shock delivered
- No ROSC

ALS criteria include the three BLS rules plus the following additional two rules:

- Unwitnessed by bystander
- No bystander CPR

### Words of Wisdom

Patients who do not achieve ROSC may be potential organ donors in select situations (ie, short transport times, rapid access to an organ recovery program). Follow your local protocols regarding the care of potential organ donors.

### Words of Wisdom

If you choose not to start CPR on a patient in cardiac arrest, then always comply with your local protocols and provide detailed documentation. In particular, record the physical examination signs that led to your decision and reference the protocol that states these signs are a reason not to start CPR. If special circumstances physically prevent you from making resuscitation attempts (for example, if the patient is entrapped in a vehicle), then document the scene conditions thoroughly. These decisions occasionally raise questions that can be put to rest immediately with reference to a well-written report. See Chapter 4, *Communications and Documentation*, for more information.

Every EMS system should have clear standing orders or protocols that provide guidelines for starting and stopping CPR. Your medical director and your system's legal adviser should agree on these protocols, which should be closely administered and reviewed by your medical director.

## Foreign Body Airway Obstruction in Adults

Occasionally, a large foreign body will be aspirated and block the upper airway. An airway obstruction may be caused by various factors, including relaxation of the throat muscles in an unresponsive patient, vomited or regurgitated stomach contents, blood, damaged tissue after an injury, dentures, or foreign bodies such as food or small objects.

Large objects that are visible but cannot be removed from the airway with suction, such as loose dentures, large pieces of food, or blood clots, should be swept forward and out with your gloved index finger. Suctioning can then be used as needed to keep the airway clear of thinner secretions such as blood, vomitus, and mucus.

### Recognizing Foreign Body Airway Obstruction

An airway obstruction by a foreign body in an adult usually occurs during a meal. In children, it usually occurs during mealtime or at play. If the foreign body is not removed quickly, then the lungs will use up their oxygen supply, and unconsciousness and death will follow. Management is based on the severity of the airway obstruction.

### Mild Airway Obstruction

Patients with a mild (partial) airway obstruction are able to exchange adequate amounts of air, but still have signs of respiratory distress. Breathing may be noisy; however, the patient usually has a strong, effective cough. Encourage the patient to continue coughing. Your main concern is to prevent a mild airway obstruction from becoming a severe (complete) airway obstruction. Abdominal thrusts are *not* indicated for patients with a mild airway obstruction.

For the patient with a mild airway obstruction, first encourage the patient to cough or to continue coughing if they are already doing so. Do not interfere with the patient's own attempts to expel the foreign body. Instead, give supplemental oxygen if needed and provide prompt transport to the ED. Closely monitor the patient and observe for signs of a severe airway obstruction (weak or absent cough, decreasing level of consciousness, cyanosis).

### Responsive Patients

A sudden, severe airway obstruction is usually easy to recognize in someone who is eating or has just finished eating. The person is suddenly unable to speak or cough, grasps his or her throat, becomes cyanotic, and makes exaggerated efforts to breathe. Either air is not moving into and out of the airway, or the air movement is so slight that it is not detectable. At first, the patient will be responsive and able to clearly indicate the problem. Ask the patient, "Are you choking?" The patient will usually answer by nodding yes. Alternatively, he or she may use the universal sign to indicate airway blockage (**FIGURE 14-27**).

If there is a minimal amount of air movement, then you may hear a high-pitched sound on inspiration called **stridor**. This occurs when the object is not fully blocking the airway, but the small amount of air entering the lungs is not enough to sustain life and the patient will eventually become unconscious if the obstruction is not relieved.

### Unresponsive Patients

When you discover an unresponsive patient, your first step is to determine whether he or she is

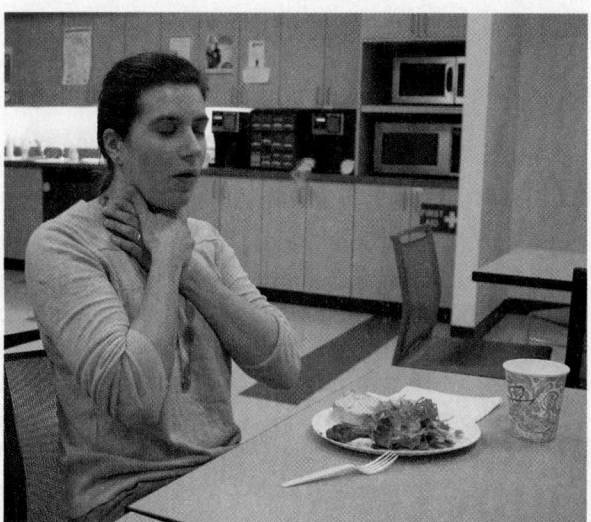

**FIGURE 14-27** Placing the hands at the throat is the universal sign to indicate choking.

breathing and has a pulse. The unconsciousness may be caused by airway obstruction, cardiac arrest, or a number of other conditions. If the patient has a pulse, but is not breathing, then you must make sure that the airway is open and unobstructed.

You should suspect an airway obstruction if the standard maneuvers to open the airway and ventilate the lungs are ineffective. If you feel resistance when attempting to ventilate, the patient probably has some type of obstruction.

## Removing a Foreign Body Airway Obstruction in an Adult

The manual maneuver recommended for removing severe airway obstructions in responsive adults and children older than 1 year is the **abdominal thrust maneuver** (also called the Heimlich maneuver). This technique creates an artificial cough by causing a sudden increase in intrathoracic pressure when thrusts are applied to the subdiaphragmatic region; it is a very effective method for removing a foreign body obstruction from the airway. If the patient with a severe airway obstruction is unresponsive, then perform chest compressions.

### Responsive Patients

#### Abdominal Thrust Maneuver

The goal of the abdominal-thrust maneuver is to compress the lungs upward and force residual air from the lungs to flow upward and expel the object. In responsive patients with a severe airway obstruction, repeat abdominal thrusts until the foreign body is expelled or the patient becomes unresponsive. Each thrust should be deliberate, with the intent of relieving the obstruction.

To perform abdominal thrusts on a responsive adult (**FIGURE 14-28**), use the following technique:

1. Stand behind the patient, and wrap your arms around his or her abdomen. Straddle your legs outside the patient's legs. This will allow you to easily slide the patient to the ground if he or she becomes unresponsive.
2. Make a fist with one hand; grasp the fist with the other hand. Place the thumb side of the fist against the patient's abdomen just above the umbilicus and well below the xiphoid process.

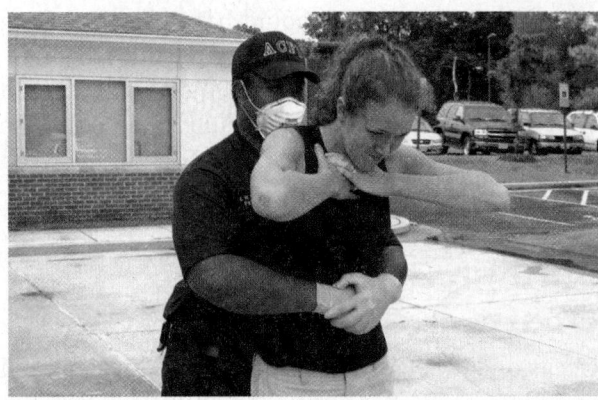

**FIGURE 14-28** The abdominal thrust maneuver in a responsive adult. Stand behind the patient and wrap your arms around the patient's abdomen. Place the thumb side of one fist against the patient's abdomen while holding your fist with your other hand. Press your fists into the patient's abdomen, using inward and upward thrusts.

© Jones & Bartlett Learning. Courtesy of MIEMSS.

3. Press your fist into the patient's abdomen with a quick inward and upward thrust.
4. Continue abdominal thrusts until the object is expelled from the airway or the patient becomes unresponsive.

#### Chest Thrusts

You can perform the abdominal thrust maneuver safely on all adults and children. However, for women in advanced stages of pregnancy and patients who have obesity, use chest thrusts instead.

To perform chest thrusts on the responsive adult, use the following technique (**FIGURE 14-29**):

1. Stand behind the patient with your arms directly under the patient's armpits and wrap your arms around the patient's chest.
2. Make a fist with one hand; grasp the fist with the other hand. Place the thumb side of the fist against the patient's sternum, avoiding the xiphoid process and the edges of the rib cage.
3. Press your fist into the patient's chest with backward thrusts until the object is expelled or the patient becomes unresponsive.
4. If the patient becomes unresponsive, then begin CPR, starting with chest compressions (**FIGURE 14-30**).

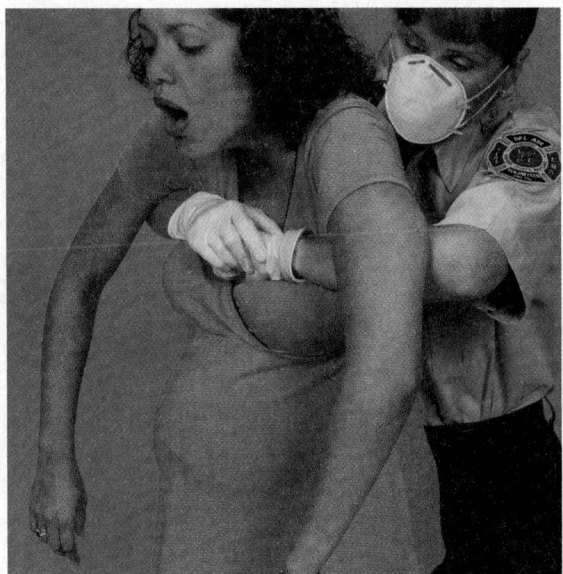

**FIGURE 14-29** Removal of a foreign body obstruction in a responsive adult using chest thrusts. Stand behind the patient and wrap your arms around the patient's chest. Place the thumb side of one fist against the chest while holding your fist with your other hand. Press your fists into the patient's chest with backward thrusts.

© Jones & Bartlett Learning. Courtesy of MIEMSS.

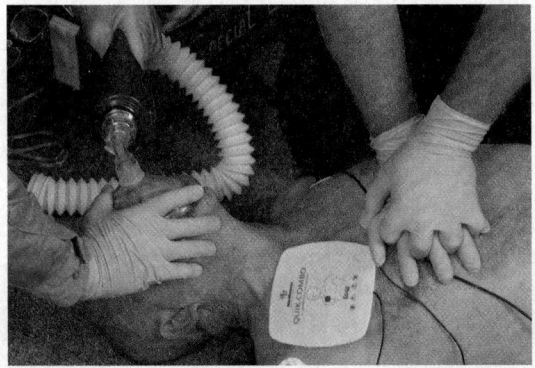

**FIGURE 14-30** An unresponsive patient with an airway obstruction requires CPR.

© Jones & Bartlett Learning.

## Words of Wisdom

If a responsive choking patient is found lying on the floor, then administer abdominal thrusts by straddling the patient's legs, placing your hands just above the umbilicus, and giving rapid thrusts inward and upward under the rib cage, using the heel of your hand with your other hand on top of it.

## Responsive Patients Who Become Unresponsive

A patient with an airway obstruction may become unresponsive while you are attempting to remove the obstruction. In this case, begin CPR, starting with chest compressions. Use the following steps to manage the patient's airway obstruction:

1. Carefully support the patient to the ground and immediately call for help (or send someone to call for help).
2. Perform 30 chest compressions, using the same landmark as you would for CPR (center of the chest, between the nipples). Do not check for a pulse before performing chest compressions.
3. Open the airway and look in the mouth. If you see an object that can easily be removed, then remove it with your fingers and attempt to ventilate. If you do not see an object, then resume chest compressions.
4. Repeat steps 2 and 3 until the obstruction is relieved or ALS providers take over.

If you are able to remove an object from the mouth, then attempt to ventilate. If ventilation produces chest rise, then continue to ventilate and check for a pulse. If a pulse is present but the patient is not breathing, then continue rescue breathing and monitor the pulse. If a pulse is absent, then continue CPR (compressions and ventilations) and apply the AED as soon as it is available.

## Unresponsive Patients

When a patient is found unresponsive, it is unlikely you will know what caused the problem. Begin CPR by determining unresponsiveness and checking for breathing and a pulse simultaneously. If a pulse is present but breathing is absent, then open the airway and attempt to ventilate. If the first ventilation does not produce visible chest rise, then reposition the airway and reattempt to ventilate. If both ventilation attempts do not produce visible chest rise, then perform 30 chest compressions, and then open the airway and look in the mouth. If an object is visible and can easily be removed, then remove it with your fingers and attempt to ventilate. Never perform blind finger sweeps on any patient; doing so may push the obstruction farther into the airway. If an object is not visible or cannot easily be removed, then resume chest compressions. Continue the sequence of chest compressions, opening the airway, and looking inside the mouth until the airway is clear or ALS providers arrive.

# Foreign Body Airway Obstruction in Infants and Children

As mentioned previously, airway obstruction is a common problem in infants and children, usually caused by a foreign body (such as food or a toy) or by an infection, resulting in swelling and narrowing of the airway. Try to identify the cause of the obstruction as soon as possible. In patients who have signs and symptoms of an airway infection, do not waste time trying to dislodge a foreign body. Administer supplemental oxygen if needed and immediately transport the child to the ED.

A previously healthy child who is eating or playing with small toys or an infant who is crawling about the house and who suddenly has difficulty breathing has probably aspirated a foreign body. As in adults, foreign bodies may cause a mild or a severe airway obstruction.

With a mild airway obstruction, the child can cough forcefully, although he or she may wheeze between coughs. As long as the patient can breathe, cough, or talk, do not interfere with his or her attempts to expel the foreign body. As with an adult, encourage the child to continue coughing. Administer supplemental oxygen if needed (and tolerated) and provide transport to the ED.

You should intervene only if signs of a severe airway obstruction develop, such as a weak, ineffective cough; cyanosis; stridor; absent air movement; or a decreasing level of consciousness.

## Removing a Foreign Body Airway Obstruction in a Child
### Responsive Child

If you determine a child older than 1 year has an airway obstruction, then stand or kneel behind the child and provide abdominal thrusts in the same manner as an adult, but use less force, until the object is expelled or the child becomes unresponsive. If the child becomes unresponsive, then follow the same steps as for the unresponsive adult.

To perform the abdominal-thrust maneuver in a responsive child who is in a standing or sitting position, follow these steps (**FIGURE 14-31**):

1. Kneel on one knee behind the child, and circle both of your arms around the child's body. Prepare to give abdominal thrusts by placing your fist just above the patient's umbilicus and well

## YOU are the Provider

You and your partner secure the patient to the cot, load him into the ambulance, and begin transport to a hospital located 5 miles away with one of the other EMTs to assist you. En route, you reassess the patient and then call your radio report to the receiving hospital.

| Recording Time: 12 Minutes | |
|---|---|
| Level of consciousness | Unresponsive |
| Respirations | 8 breaths/min; shallow depth |
| Pulse | 94 beats/min; strong carotid pulse, weak radial pulses |
| Skin | Circulation assessed as adequate by examination of mucous membranes inside the inner lower eyelid and capillary refill with skin cool and dry |
| Blood pressure | 86/66 mm Hg |
| Spo₂ | 95% (on oxygen) |

**9.** Would an ITD benefit your patient at this point?

**10.** What further treatment, if any, is indicated for this patient?

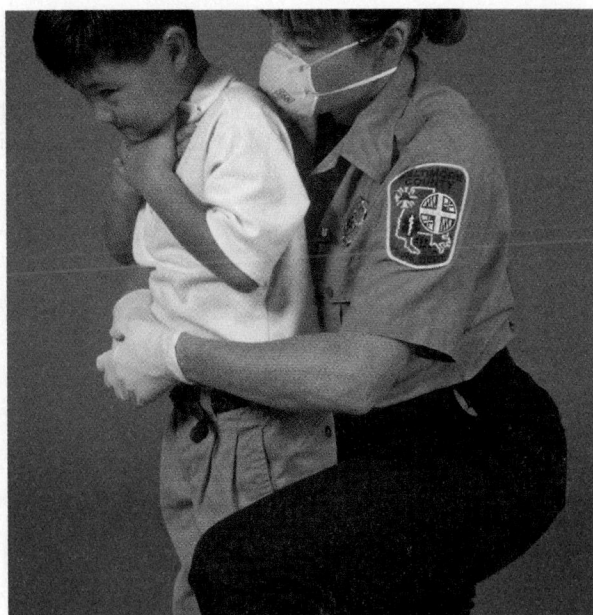

**FIGURE 14-31** To perform the abdominal thrust maneuver on a child, kneel behind the child on one knee, wrap your arms around the child's body, and place your fist just above the umbilicus and well below the lower tip of the sternum.

© Jones & Bartlett Learning. Courtesy of MIEMSS.

below the xiphoid process. Place your other hand over that fist.

2. Give the child abdominal thrusts in an upward direction. Avoid applying force to the lower rib cage or sternum.

3. Repeat this technique until the child expels the foreign body or becomes unresponsive.

4. If the child becomes unresponsive, position the child on a hard surface and immediately call for help (or send someone to call for help).

5. Perform 30 chest compressions (15 compressions if two rescuers are present), using the same landmark as you would for CPR. Do not check for a pulse before performing chest compressions.

6. Open the airway and look inside the mouth. If you see an object that can easily be removed, then remove it with your fingers and attempt to ventilate. If you do not see an object, then resume chest compressions.

7. Repeat steps 5 and 6 until the obstruction is relieved or ALS providers take over.

If you manage to clear the airway obstruction in an unresponsive child but he or she still has no spontaneous breathing or circulation, then perform

CPR (compressions and ventilations) and apply the AED as soon as it is available.

## Unresponsive Child

If a child older than 1 year with an airway obstruction becomes unresponsive, he or she is managed in the same manner as an adult. **SKILL DRILL 14-6** demonstrates the steps for removing a foreign body airway obstruction in an unresponsive child:

1. Take standard precautions. Carefully place the child in a supine position on a firm, flat surface (**Step 1**).

2. Perform 30 chest compressions (15 compressions if two rescuers are present), using the same landmark as you would for CPR (lower half of the sternum). Do not check for a pulse before performing chest compressions (**Step 2**).

3. Open the airway and look in the mouth (**Step 3**).

4. If you see an object that can easily be removed, then remove it with your fingers and attempt to ventilate (**Step 4**).

5. If you do not see an object, then resume chest compressions.

6. Repeat the sequence of chest compressions, opening the airway, and looking inside the mouth until the obstruction is relieved or ALS providers take over (**Step 5**).

## Removing a Foreign Body Airway Obstruction in Infants
### Responsive Infants

Do not use abdominal thrusts on a responsive infant with an airway obstruction because of the risk of injury to the immature organs of the abdomen. Instead, perform back slaps and chest thrusts to try to clear a severe airway obstruction in a responsive infant, as follows (**FIGURE 14-32**):

1. Hold the infant facedown, with the body resting on your forearm. Support the infant's jaw and face with your hand and keep the head lower than the rest of the body.

2. Deliver five back blows between the shoulder blades, using the heel of your hand.

3. Place your free hand behind the infant's head and back and turn the infant faceup on your

## Skill Drill 14-6 Removing a Foreign Body Airway Obstruction in an Unresponsive Child

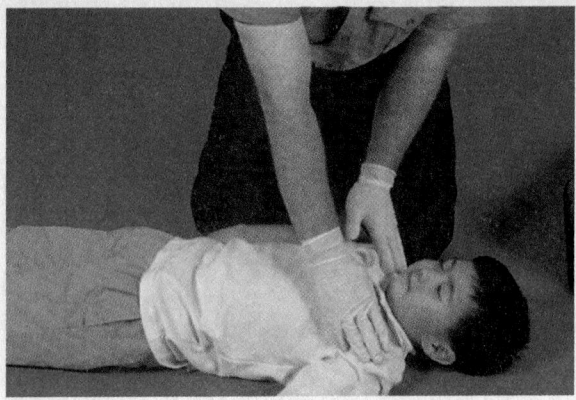

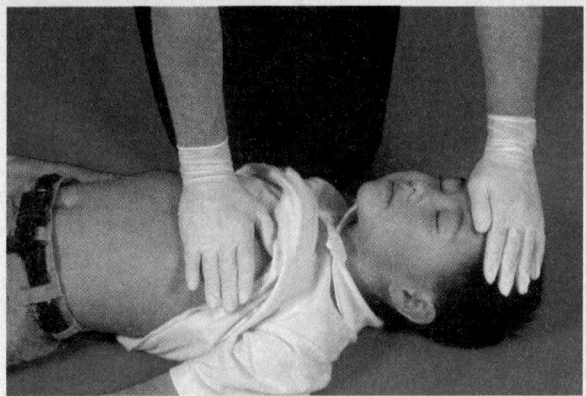

**Step 1**

Take standard precautions. Position the child on a firm, flat surface.

**Step 2**

Perform chest compressions using the same landmark as you would for CPR.

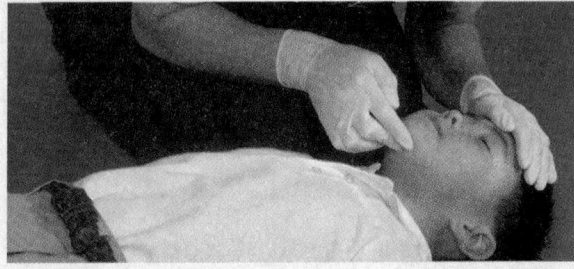

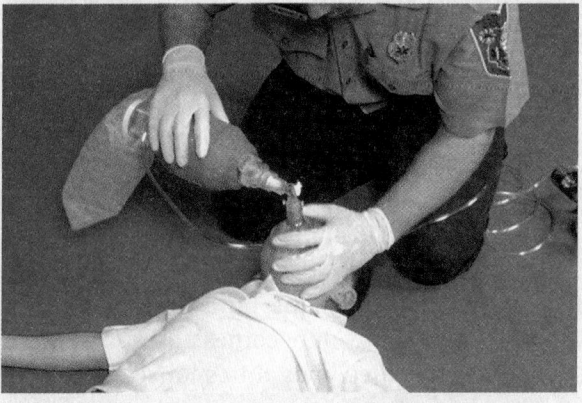

**Step 3**

Open the airway and look inside the mouth.

**Step 4**

If an object is visible and can easily be removed, then remove it with your fingers and attempt rescue breathing.

**Step 5**

If you do not see an object in the mouth, then resume chest compressions. Continue the sequence of chest compressions, opening the airway, and looking inside the mouth until the obstruction is relieved or ALS providers take over.

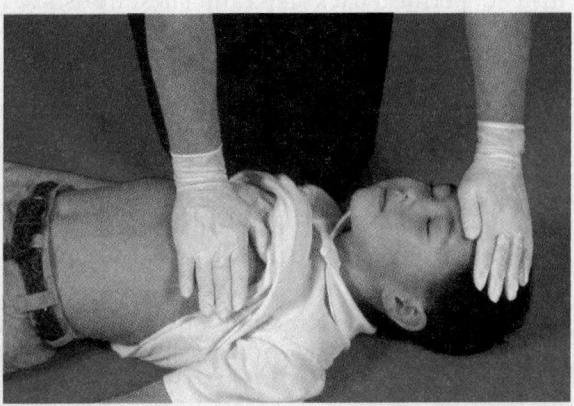

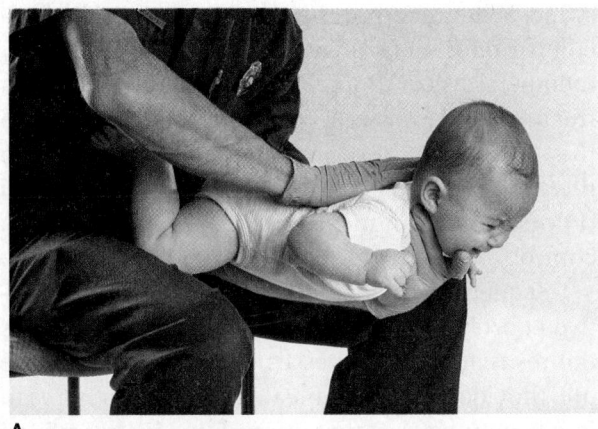
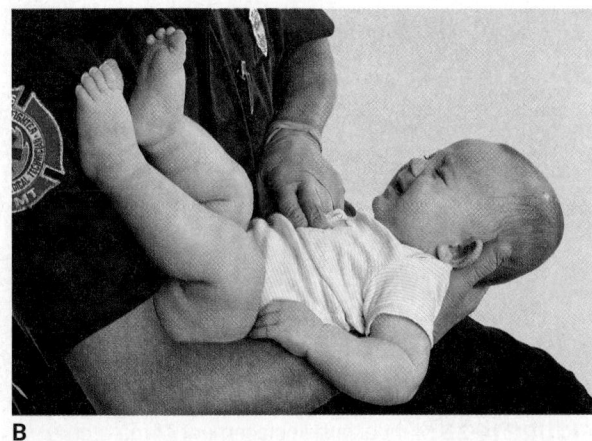

A                                                                          B

**FIGURE 14-32 A.** Hold the infant facedown with the body resting on your forearm. Support the jaw and face with your hand and keep the head lower than the rest of the body. Give the infant five back blows between the shoulder blades, using the heel of your hand. **B.** Give the infant five quick chest thrusts, using two fingers placed on the lower half of the sternum.

A, B: © Jones & Bartlett Learning.

other forearm and thigh, sandwiching the infant's body between your two hands and arms. The infant's head should remain below the level of the body.

4. Give five quick chest thrusts in the same location and manner as chest compressions, using two fingers placed on the lower half of the sternum. For larger infants, or if you have small hands, you can perform this step by placing the infant in your lap and turning the infant's whole body as a unit between back slaps and chest thrusts.

5. Check the airway. If you can see the foreign body, then remove it. If not, then repeat the cycle as often as necessary.

6. If the infant becomes unresponsive, then begin CPR and follow the same sequence as for a child and adult.

### Unresponsive Infants

If the infant becomes unresponsive during your attempts to relieve an airway obstruction, then perform CPR starting with chest compressions. Do not check for a pulse before starting compressions. Open the airway and look in the mouth. If you see an object that can easily be removed, then remove it with your finger and attempt to ventilate; if you do not see an object, then resume chest compressions. Continue the sequence of chest compressions, opening the airway, and looking inside the

mouth until the obstruction is relieved or ALS providers take over.

## Special Resuscitation Circumstances

### Opioid Overdose

An opioid is a narcotic drug that, when taken in excess, depresses the central nervous system and causes respiratory arrest followed by cardiac arrest. Examples of opioids include heroin and oxycodone. Opioids are discussed further in Chapter 22, *Toxicology*.

### Cardiac Arrest in Pregnancy

If you encounter a pregnant patient who is in cardiac arrest, then your priorities are to provide high-quality CPR and relieve pressure from the aorta and vena cava. When the patient lies supine, the pregnant uterus can compress the aorta and vena cava (aortocaval compression). Compression of the vena cava causes a significant decrease in blood return to the heart and, secondarily, in the forward flow of blood to the vital organs.

If the pregnant patient is not in cardiac arrest, then position her on her left side to relieve pressure on the great vessels. However, if she is in cardiac arrest, then this approach is impractical, because she must remain in a supine position to maximize the effectiveness of compressions. Therefore, if the

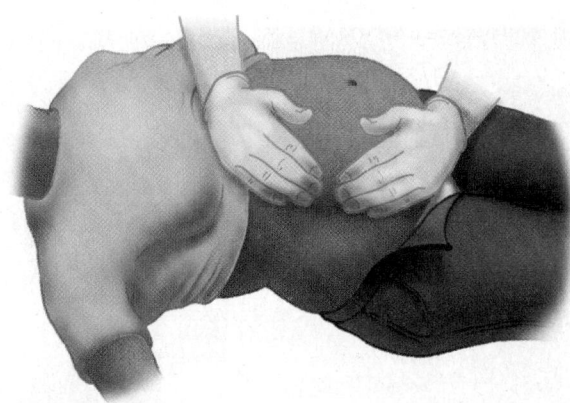

**FIGURE 14-33** Manual left displacement of the uterus. The two-handed technique is shown. Alternatively, one hand can be used.

© Jones & Bartlett Learning.

top of the patient's uterus (fundus) can be felt at or above the level of the umbilicus, perform manual displacement of the uterus to the patient's left to relieve aortocaval compression while CPR is being performed. This step will improve the effectiveness of compressions (**FIGURE 14-33**).

## Grief Support for Family Members and Loved Ones

Whenever you assist a patient, remember that the patient's loved ones will also be affected by the emergency. Serious illness, injury, and pediatric patients create an especially high level of anxiety for family members. A health emergency is often hard for family members to understand. In some cases, family members may experience a psychological crisis that turns into a medical crisis, and may become patients themselves.

Whereas a cardiac arrest may be one of many similar calls in your career, family members and loved ones will remember this event in detail for the rest of their lives. Your reaction to them will form a lasting impression. Conversely, a mismanaged death notification or poor interaction could leave the family feeling disrespected or ignored. A compassionate and sensitive approach will leave a positive impression of you and your agency. Most important, appropriate and supportive care at the onset of grief may positively affect the family's grieving process.

Families do not typically expect EMS providers to stop resuscitation and leave their loved one on scene. When death appears imminent and resuscitative efforts are unsuccessful, make the family members aware the patient is not responding to treatment. Discuss with them what is happening so they may be better prepared for the inevitable. Keep the family informed throughout the resuscitation process because it may also help them feel more in control.

Sequential notification starts during resuscitative efforts; family members should be updated as the resuscitation progresses, if possible. Designate one provider to communicate the patient's status to family members, so that information is streamlined from one source rather than from multiple providers. Be concise and clear. For example, say, "Your husband is not breathing and his heart has stopped. We are attempting to restart his heart with the AED." After resuscitation efforts have stopped, it is appropriate to tell them, "As you know, when we arrived, your husband wasn't breathing and did not have a pulse. He has not responded to any of our treatments. I'm sorry, but he has died." Avoid euphemisms such as "passed away" or "passed on," because these expressions may be confusing or misinterpreted. Law enforcement personnel may be involved in the official death declaration and will likely be responsible for what happens next, such as determining whether the medical examiner should be notified.

### Street Smarts

Allowing family members to watch the resuscitation may be beneficial to their emotional healing. Have a provider sit or stand with the person and verbally walk him or her through the process. If it does not interfere with resuscitation attempts and the bystander wishes, he or she may be allowed to hold the loved one's hand or tell the person goodbye before termination of resuscitation efforts.

After resuscitation has stopped, these other measures can be helpful:

- Take the family to a quiet, private place.
- Introduce yourself and anyone with you.
- Use clear language and speak in a warm, sensitive, and caring manner.
- Try to exhibit calm, reassuring authority.
- Use the patient's name.
- Use eye contact and appropriate touch.

- Expect that family members will show emotion as they begin the grieving process. Be prepared for different reactions, including anger.
- Silence is okay.
- While you are still on scene, be supportive but do not hover.
- Ask if a friend or family member can be called to come and help support them.
- When you need to leave, turn the family over to someone else—for example, a police officer.

Some family members will want to see the deceased. Being able to touch or talk to their loved one may be helpful to them. This may not be advisable in a medical examiner's case. Law enforcement personnel will need to make that determination. It is appropriate to make the body presentable, but follow local protocols regarding movement of the patient or removal of resuscitation equipment.

Another consideration is to ensure that children are not ignored. They may not understand death. Preschool-age children may be less affected, whereas older children understand death but do not expect it to happen to someone they know. Younger children tend to blame themselves. Teenagers may be highly affected but may mask their feelings.

In a situation where ROSC occurs prior to transport, family members may wish to interact with the patient. This can give them comfort, especially if the patient ultimately does not survive.

It is never easy to be the bearer of bad news, but it can help to know you did your best for the family during a difficult situation. Last, consider your own feelings in this stressful situation and make sure you seek assistance if needed. See Chapter 2, *Workforce Safety and Wellness,* for a discussion of the emotional aspects of emergency care and stress management.

## Education and Training for the EMT

You may go weeks or months without performing CPR on a human, depending on how busy your EMS system is. Like any skill, CPR skills can deteriorate over time. You must practice them often using manikin-based training—ideally more frequently than the standard retraining that occurs every 2 years.

The use of high-fidelity manikins for CPR training is encouraged, if your system's budget allows. If this is not an option, then CPR devices that provide corrective feedback are preferred over devices that only provide voice prompts (ie, a metronome).

CPR self-instruction through video and/or computer-based modules with hands-on practice may be a reasonable alternative to instructor-led courses, because it may facilitate frequent retraining.

## Education and Training for the Public

As an EMT, you are a patient advocate. Not only are you responsible for providing the best possible care for your patient, but you must also do your part to facilitate the training of laypeople in the critical skills of CPR and AED operation. Training in CPR and AED usage should not be limited to health care providers. Not enough laypeople are trained to perform these life-saving skills.

As discussed previously, many laypeople assume CPR requires both mouth-to-mouth rescue breathing and chest compressions. As long as this misconception remains, fewer people will be willing to help during an emergency, which means that fewer lives will be saved. If you are asked to train members of your community how to perform compression-only CPR, then you should consider it your professional responsibility and be willing to assist.

It is likely that some citizens in your service area are at increased risk for cardiac arrest. Your agency should make an effort to identify these potential patients and educate their families to recognize cardiac arrest and to train them to perform compression-only CPR.

## YOU are the Provider SUMMARY

**1. What should you immediately do on receiving this update from dispatch?**

After you are informed that CPR is in progress, you should immediately request additional assistance. Effective treatment of a patient in cardiac arrest requires adequate personnel at the scene and during transport. As an EMT, you must be familiar with the resources that are available to you and know when it is appropriate to request them. If your system protocols permit, bystanders who are performing high-quality chest compressions can assist until other help arrives so the compressors can alternate every 2 minutes.

The type of backup you receive (ie, BLS versus ALS) will depend on your EMS system and the resources that are available to you. Combined with high-quality CPR and defibrillation, early advanced care increases the patient's chance for survival.

Regardless of the resources available to you, request them as soon as possible—in this case, as soon as you are advised that CPR is in progress. One EMT cannot effectively treat a patient in cardiac arrest during transport; you would have to perform continuous CPR while your partner drives the ambulance (or vice versa), which could result in rescuer fatigue and decreased effectiveness of chest compressions.

**2. What should be your initial actions on arriving at this scene?**

After ensuring your own safety, approach this patient as you would any other patient, by performing a primary assessment. Although the dispatcher has advised you that bystander CPR is in progress, you must still assess the patient to confirm he is indeed apneic and pulseless and requires CPR.

Your primary assessment should take only a few seconds, just long enough to confirm the patient is in cardiac arrest. If he is in cardiac arrest, then begin CPR immediately, apply the AED as soon as it is available, and analyze the patient's cardiac rhythm. To avoid interrupting CPR, you should apply the AED as chest compressions are being performed (do not stop compressions to do this).

If the AED advises you to shock, then deliver the shock as soon as your partner eliminates any contact with the patient and immediately resume CPR, starting with chest compressions. If the AED does not advise you to shock, then immediately resume CPR, starting with chest compressions. During CPR, ask the two bystanders if they witnessed the event and determine whether they know anything about the patient (ie, past medical history, events leading up to the cardiac arrest).

Regardless of how a call is dispatched and whether or not you are assuming patient care from bystanders or other health care providers, it is important for you to always perform a primary assessment of the patient.

**3. What links in the chain of survival have been maintained at this point?**

The following links in the chain of survival have been established or maintained:

- *Recognition and activation of the emergency response system*, because the bystanders quickly recognized the patient was experiencing a cardiac emergency and immediately called 9-1-1.
- *Immediate, high-quality CPR*, because the bystanders began CPR directly after calling 9-1-1.
- *Basic and advanced emergency medical services*, because EMS providers are at the scene providing specialized care to the patient.

The following links in the chain of survival have not been maintained:

- *Rapid defibrillation*, because it has not yet occurred. Of all the links in the chain of survival, early defibrillation has the most profound impact on patient survival. With early access and early CPR, defibrillation may successfully terminate lethal cardiac dysrhythmias in a significant number of patients. For each minute that defibrillation is delayed, the patient's chance for survival decreases by 7% to 10%.
- *Advanced life support and postarrest care*, because advanced care such as intravenous access and medication administration has not been started, ROSC has not been established, and the patient has not arrived at the hospital.
- *Recovery*, because it takes place after all the links have been maintained.

**4. Why is it so critical to minimize interruptions in CPR?**

Even when CPR is performed correctly (that is, at a rate of 100 to 120 compressions per minute at a depth of 2 to 2.4 inches [5 to 6 cm] in the adult), chest compressions only deliver about one-third of a person's normal cardiac output. When CPR is performed properly and with minimal interruption, it is often enough to keep the patient's vital organs viable until defibrillation and more advanced care can be provided at the scene or at the ED. Of course, this assumes that defibrillation and advanced care are provided within a short period of time.

Within a few seconds of stopping chest compressions, the pressure generated in the arteries drops to near zero; therefore, frequent or prolonged interruptions in chest compressions will not even provide the minimum perfusion needed to keep the vital organs viable. This has been clearly linked to low survival rates from cardiac arrest. Remember to maintain a chest compression fraction of 80% or greater.

As soon as cardiac arrest has been confirmed, it is crucial to begin CPR immediately and apply the AED as soon as it is available. Even when the AED pads are being applied, your partner should continue chest compressions.

**5. Should you remove the medication patch or leave it in place? Why or why not?**

The patch is located on the patient's right upper chest, which is where you will place one of the AED pads. Because of its location, the patch could interfere with the electrical current to the heart and may cause burns to the patient's skin. To prevent this complication, remove the patch, wipe any residue from the skin, and then apply the AED pads. Remember to take standard precautions!

**6. What does the bulge and scar over the patient's left chest indicate? How will this affect the way you treat the patient?**

A hard lump or bulge on the patient's chest, usually with a corresponding scar, indicates an AICD, or pacemaker. These devices are used in patients who are at high risk for certain cardiac dysrhythmias and cardiac arrest. The AICD will deliver shocks directly to the heart if it detects a lethal cardiac dysrhythmia. Implanted pacemakers are used to increase the patient's heart rate if it falls below a given value. Sometimes the implanted device may have both capabilities.

If the AED pads are placed directly over the device, then shocks delivered by the AED may be less effective. In addition, AED or manual defibrillator shocks given by ALS providers may damage the device. Therefore, if you identify an AICD or pacemaker, place the AED pad at least 1 inch (2.5 cm) away from the device. Because most of these devices are implanted in the upper left chest, this should not be an issue. The pads are placed to the right of the upper sternum and to the lower left chest, just below the nipple, so they should be well beyond 1 inch (2.5 cm)

from the device. Follow your local protocols regarding patients with AICDs or implanted pacemakers.

**7. How should you continue to treat this patient?**

You have restored a pulse in your patient; however, his breathing is not adequate. Agonal gasps are ineffective and do not produce adequate minute volume.

Some patients may have an intact gag reflex, despite being unresponsive; in these cases, an oropharyngeal airway is contraindicated. Insert a nasopharyngeal (nasal) airway and continue to provide rescue breathing. Deliver one breath every 5 to 6 seconds (10 to 12 breaths/min); each breath should be delivered over 1 second (just enough to produce visible chest rise). Closely and carefully monitor the patient's pulse and be prepared to resume CPR if necessary.

Assume the patient has a full stomach and have a suction unit ready in case he regurgitates. Remember that mortality increases significantly if aspiration occurs. It is also important to avoid hyperventilating the patient.

**8. Because the patient is no longer in cardiac arrest, should you remove the AED pads? Why or why not?**

Although the patient is not in cardiac arrest, he is still at high risk for recurrence of cardiac arrest. Therefore, do not remove the AED pads; simply turn the AED off, continue rescue breathing, and prepare the patient for prompt transport.

**9. Would an ITD benefit your patient at this point?**

An ITD is a valve device used in some systems that is placed between the ET tube and resuscitation bag; it can also be placed in between the resuscitation bag and mask if the patient is not intubated. It is only used for patients who are apneic and pulseless. At this point, your patient has a pulse and is breathing (albeit slowly and shallowly); therefore, the ITD is not indicated. Use of an ITD is not advised in traditional CPR, but is acceptable when used during active compression-decompression CPR. If ROSC occurs in active compression-decompression CPR, the ITD must be removed.

**10. What further treatment, if any, is indicated for this patient?**

Further treatment of your patient should consist of careful monitoring because he remains at high risk

## YOU are the Provider SUMMARY continued

for recurrence of cardiac arrest. In patients who are responsive and alert, the presence of a pulse is obvious; however, when a patient is unresponsive, you must frequently reassess for a pulse.

Unresponsive patients are at increased risk for regurgitation, which could lead to aspiration and increased mortality. Vigilantly monitor the patient's airway status and be prepared to turn his head to the side if he regurgitates. Maintain his airway with manual positioning and a basic airway adjunct—in this case, a nasal airway.

Although the patient is breathing, his breaths are slow and shallow. Slow, shallow (reduced tidal volume) respirations will not produce adequate minute volume; therefore, continue to assist the patient's

ventilations with a bag-mask device, but do not hyperventilate him. Deliver each breath over 1 second while observing for visible chest rise. Start at 10 breaths per minute (1 every 6 seconds and then monitor his oxygen saturation ($Spo_2$) level and heart rate to help you determine if your assisted ventilations are adequate.

As mentioned earlier, do not remove the AED pads. Turn the AED off, but be prepared to stop the ambulance if cardiac arrest redevelops to safely defibrillate the patient.

The patient's blood pressure (86/66 mm Hg) is still low. Follow your local protocols regarding positioning of the patient to improve his blood pressure.

### EMS Patient Care Report (PCR)

| Date: 12-29-20 | Incident No.: 011109 | Nature of Call: Cardiac arrest | | Location: 123 Wilshire Ave. | |
|---|---|---|---|---|---|
| Dispatched: 1445 | En Route: 1447 | At Scene: 1454 | Transport: 1508 | At Hospital: 1518 | In Service: 1528 |

#### Patient Information

**Age:** 48
**Sex:** M
**Weight (in kg [lb]):** 77 kg (170 lb)

**Allergies:** Unknown
**Medications:** Unknown
**Past Medical History:** Unknown
**Chief Complaint:** Cardiac arrest

#### Vital Signs

| Time: 1454 | BP: N/A | Pulse: 0 | Respirations: 0 | $Spo_2$: N/A |
|---|---|---|---|---|
| Time: 1458 | BP: N/A | Pulse: 0 | Respirations: 0 | $Spo_2$: N/A |
| Time: 1501 | BP: 70/40 | Pulse: 100 | Respirations: 4 | $Spo_2$: 82% |
| Time: 1506 | BP: 86/66 | Pulse: 94 | Respirations: 8 | $Spo_2$: 95% |

#### EMS Treatment (circle all that apply)

| Oxygen @ 15 L/min via:<br><br>NC   NRM   (Bag mask) | (Assisted Ventilation) | (Airway Adjunct) | | (CPR) |
|---|---|---|---|---|
| (Defibrillation) | Bleeding Control | Bandaging | Splinting | Other |

## YOU are the Provider **SUMMARY** *continued*

| Narrative |
| --- |

Medic 51 dispatched to grocery store parking lot for "CPR in progress."

Chief Complaint: Cardiac arrest

History: Per one of the bystanders, the patient was about to get to his vehicle when he suddenly grabbed his chest, slumped against the vehicle, and eased himself to the ground. There was no trauma involved. The bystander further stated that by the time he got to the patient, he was unresponsive and without pulse or breathing. The patient's past medical history was unknown, although he had an AICD and was wearing a medication patch, which was removed.

Assessment: On arrival at the scene, found two bystanders performing CPR on the patient, a 48-year-old male. BLS Medic 48 was dispatched to the scene to assist. ALS was unavailable. Primary assessment revealed that the patient was apneic and pulseless.

Treatment (Rx): Continued CPR for 2 minutes while the AED was being prepared. After 2 minutes of CPR, EMS analyzed patient's cardiac rhythm with the AED and received a shock advised message. Delivered single shock and immediately resumed CPR. Medic 48 arrived at scene and assisted with CPR and airway management. Continued CPR for 2 minutes, reanalyzed the patient's cardiac rhythm, and received a no shock advised message. Continued CPR and attempted to insert an oral airway; however, the patient began to gag. Immediate reassessment revealed that he had a strong carotid pulse, but was not breathing adequately. Inserted a nasal airway, continued ventilations at 10 breaths/min, packaged the patient, and loaded him into the ambulance.

Transport: EMT Jimenez from Medic 48 assisted with patient care en route to the hospital. En route, reassessed patient and found that he remained unresponsive; his respiratory rate increased, but the depth of his breathing remained shallow. Continued assisted ventilation and called in radio report to the receiving facility. Monitored the patient's pulse, provided additional supportive care, and delivered him to the ED without incident. Gave verbal report to attending physician Washburn. Medic 51 cleared the hospital and returned to service at 1528.

\*\*End of report\*\*

# Prep Kit

## Ready for Review

- BLS is noninvasive emergency life-saving care that is used to treat medical conditions, including airway obstruction, respiratory arrest, and cardiac arrest.
- BLS care focuses on the ABCs: airway (obstruction), breathing (respiratory arrest), and circulation (cardiac arrest or severe bleeding). If the patient is in cardiac arrest, a CAB sequence (compressions, airway, breathing) should be used.
- CPR is used to establish artificial ventilation and circulation in a patient who is not breathing and has no pulse.
- The goal of CPR is to help restore spontaneous breathing and circulation; however, advanced procedures such as medications and defibrillation are often necessary for this to occur.
- ALS involves advanced life-saving procedures, such as cardiac monitoring, administration of IV fluids and medications, and use of advanced airway adjuncts.
- The six links in the chain of survival are (1) recognition and activation of the emergency response system; (2) immediate, high-quality CPR; (3) rapid defibrillation; (4) basic and advanced emergency medical services; (5) ALS and postarrest care; and (6) Recovery.
- The AED should be applied as soon as it is available to any patient experiencing cardiac arrest.

- When using an AED on a child between ages 1 and 8 years, use pediatric-size pads and a dose-attenuating system (energy reducer). If these items are unavailable, then use adult-size AED pads. If a manual defibrillator is unavailable, then use an AED equipped with pediatric-size pads and a dose attenuator. If neither option is available, then use adult-size AED pads.
- As an EMT, it is your responsibility to start CPR in virtually all patients who are in cardiac arrest. The three general exceptions to the rule are as follows: (1) you should not start CPR if the scene is unsafe, (2) you should not start CPR if the patient has obvious signs of death, and (3) you should not start CPR if the patient and his or her physician have a previously agreed-on DNR or no-CPR order.
- As an EMT, you are generally not responsible for making the decision to stop CPR. After you begin CPR in the field, you must continue until one of the following events occurs (the STOP mnemonic):
  - S, the patient *Starts* breathing and has a pulse.
  - T, the patient's care is *Transferred* to another provider of equal or higher-level training.
  - O, you are *Out* of strength or too tired to continue.
  - P, a *Physician* who is present or providing online medical direction assumes responsibility for the patient and gives direction to discontinue CPR.
- An airway obstruction may have various causes, including relaxation of the throat muscles in an unresponsive patient, vomited or regurgitated stomach contents, blood, damaged tissue after an injury, dentures, or foreign bodies such as food or small objects.
- The manual maneuver recommended for removing severe airway obstructions in the responsive adult and child is the abdominal thrust maneuver (the Heimlich maneuver). Use back slaps and chest thrusts to treat a responsive infant with a severe airway obstruction.
- If the adult, child, or infant with a severe airway obstruction is unresponsive, then perform CPR, starting with chest compressions.
- As an EMT, you will encounter situations in which grief support for family and loved ones will be part of your role. After resuscitation has stopped, turn your attention to the family and loved ones, and provide clear communication and emotional support.

## Vital Vocabulary

**abdominal thrust maneuver** The preferred method to dislodge a severe airway obstruction in adults and children; also called the Heimlich maneuver.

**active compression-decompression CPR** A technique that involves compressing the chest and then actively pulling it back up to its neutral position or beyond (decompression); may increase the amount of blood that returns to the heart and, thus, the amount of blood ejected from the heart during the compression phase.

**advanced life support (ALS)** Advanced life-saving procedures, some of which are now being provided by the EMT.

**basic life support (BLS)** Noninvasive emergency life-saving care that is used to treat medical conditions, including airway obstruction, respiratory arrest, and cardiac arrest.

**cardiopulmonary resuscitation (CPR)** The combination of chest compressions and rescue breathing used to establish adequate ventilation and circulation in a patient who is not breathing and has no pulse.

**chest compression fraction** The total percentage of time during a resuscitation attempt in which active chest compressions are being performed.

**dependent lividity** Blood settling to the lowest point of the body, causing discoloration of the skin; a definitive sign of death.

**gastric distention** A condition in which air fills the stomach, often as a result of high volume and pressure during artificial ventilation.

**head tilt–chin lift maneuver** A combination of two movements to open the airway by tilting the forehead back and lifting the chin; not used for trauma patients.

**hyperventilation** Rapid or deep breathing that lowers the blood carbon dioxide level below normal; may lead to increased intrathoracic pressure, decreased venous return, and hypotension when associated with bag-mask device use.

**impedance threshold device (ITD)** A valve device placed between the endotracheal tube and a bag-mask device that limits the amount of air entering the lungs during the recoil phase between chest compressions.

**ischemia** A lack of oxygen that deprives tissues of necessary nutrients, resulting from partial or complete blockage of blood flow; potentially reversible because permanent injury has not yet occurred.

**jaw-thrust maneuver** Technique to open the airway by placing the fingers behind the angle of the jaw and bringing the jaw forward; used for patients who may have a cervical spine injury.

**load-distributing band (LDB)** A circumferential chest compression device composed of a constricting band and backboard that is either electrically or pneumatically driven to compress the heart by putting inward pressure on the thorax.

**mechanical piston device** A device that depresses the sternum via a compressed gas-powered or electric-powered plunger mounted on a backboard.

**recovery position** A side-lying position used to maintain a clear airway in unresponsive patients who are breathing adequately and do not have suspected injuries to the spine, hips, or pelvis.

**return of spontaneous circulation (ROSC)** The return of a pulse and effective blood flow to the body in a patient who previously was in cardiac arrest.

**rigor mortis** Stiffening of the body muscles; a definitive sign of death.

**stridor** A harsh, high-pitched respiratory sound, generally heard during inspiration, that is caused by partial blockage or narrowing of the upper airway; may be audible without a stethoscope.

**ventilation** The exchange of air between the lungs and the environment, spontaneously by the patient or with assistance from another person, such as an EMT.

# References

1. Atkins DL, Berger S, Duff JP. Part 11: pediatric basic life support and cardiopulmonary resuscitation quality. *Circulation* 2015;132(Suppl 2):S519–S525.
2. Brooks SC, Anderson ML, Bruder E, et al. Part 6: alternative techniques and ancillary devices for cardiopulmonary resuscitation. *Circulation*. 2015;132(Suppl 2):S436–S443.
3. Callaway CW, Donnino MW, Fink EL, et al. Part 8: post-cardiac arrest care. *Circulation* 2015;132(Suppl 1):S465–S482.
4. CPR statistics. American Heart Association website. https://cprblog.heart.org/cpr-statistics/. Accessed March 24, 2020.
5. Highlights of the 2020 American Heart Association guidelines update for CPR and ECC. https://cpr.heart.org/-/media/cpr-files/cpr-guidelines-files/highlights/hghlghts_2020_ecc_guidelines_english.pdf. Accessed November 6, 2020.
6. Kleinman ME, Brennan EE, Goldberger ZD, et al. Part 5: Adult basic life support and cardiopulmonary resuscitation quality. *Circulation* 2015;132:S414–S435.
7. Lavonas EJ, Drennan IR, Gabrielli A, et al. Part 10: Special circumstances of resuscitation. *Circulation* 2015;132(Suppl 2):S501–S518.
8. Lulla A, Svancarek. Time to stop beating a dead horse: termination of resuscitation in the field. http://www.naemsp-blog.com/emsmed/2016/12/26/title-time-to-stop-beating-a-dead-horse-termination-of-resuscitation-in-the-field. Accessed June 11, 2020.
9. *National Emergency Medical Services Education Standards.* U.S. Department of Transportation, National Highway Traffic Safety Administration. DOT HS 811 077A. January 2009. www.ems.gov/pdf/811077a.pdf. Accessed June 14, 2014.
10. *National Emergency Medical Services Education Standards. Emergency Medical Technician Instructional*

*Guidelines*. U.S. Department of Transportation, National Highway Traffic Safety Administration. DOT HS 811 077C. January 2009. www.ems.gov/pdf/811077c.pdf. Accessed June 14, 2014.

11. *National Model EMS Clinical Guidelines*. National Association of State EMS Officials website. https://www.nasemso.org/Projects/ModelEMSClinicalGuidelines/index.asp. Accessed October 23, 2014.

12. Peberdy MA, Gluck JA, Ornato JP, et al. Cardiopulmonary resuscitation in adults and children with mechanical circulatory support: a scientific statement from the American Heart Association. *Circulation*. 2017;135: e1115-e1134. doi:10.1161/CIR.0000000000000504. Accessed July 23, 2020.

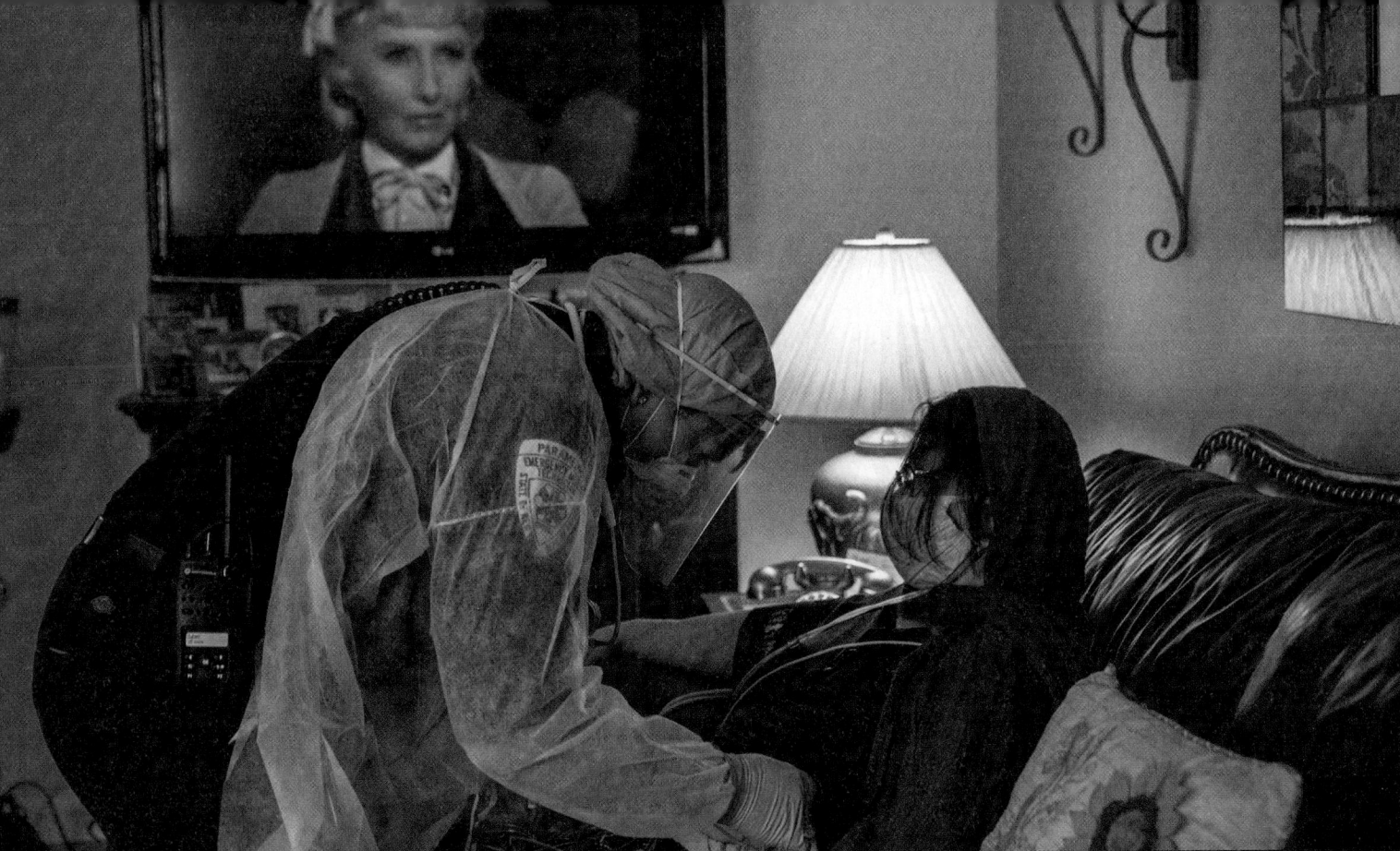

# SECTION 6

# Medical

**15**  Medical Overview

**16**  Respiratory Emergencies

**17**  Cardiovascular Emergencies

**18**  Neurologic Emergencies

**19**  Gastrointestinal and Urologic Emergencies

**20**  Endocrine and Hematologic Emergencies

**21**  Allergy and Anaphylaxis

**22**  Toxicology

**23**  Behavioral Health Emergencies

**24**  Gynecologic Emergencies

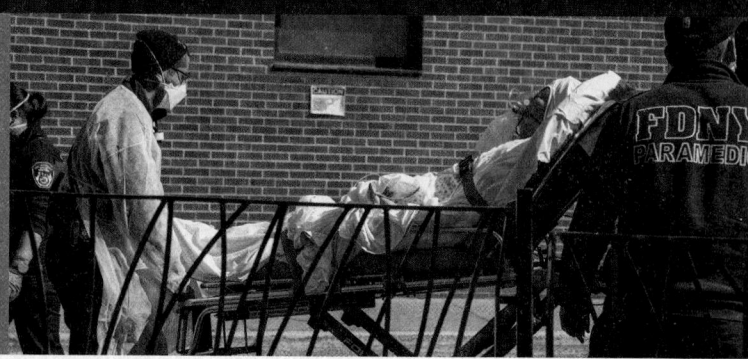

# Chapter 15

# Medical Overview

## NATIONAL EMS EDUCATION STANDARD COMPETENCIES

### Medicine

Applies fundamental knowledge to provide basic emergency care and transportation based on assessment findings for an acutely ill patient.

### Medical Overview

Assessment and management of a
• Medical complaint (pp 605–613)

Pathophysiology, assessment, and management of medical complaints to include

• Transport mode (pp 611–613)
• Destination decisions (p 613)

### Infectious Diseases

Awareness of
• A patient who may have an infectious disease (pp 613–621)

Assessment and management of
• A patient who may have an infectious disease (pp 613–621)

## KNOWLEDGE OBJECTIVES

1. Differentiate between medical emergencies and trauma emergencies, remembering that some patients may have both. (p 605)
2. Name the various categories of common medical emergencies and provide examples. (pp 605–606)
3. Describe the evaluation of the nature of illness (NOI). (p 606)
4. Discuss the assessment of a patient with a medical emergency. (pp 605–611)
5. Explain the importance of transport time and destination selection for a medical patient. (pp 611–613)

6. Define *infectious disease* and *communicable disease*. (p 613)
7. Discuss diseases of special concern and their routes of transmission, including influenza, herpes simplex, human immunodeficiency virus (HIV)/acquired immunodeficiency syndrome (AIDS), hepatitis, meningitis, tuberculosis, whooping cough, methicillin-resistant *Staphylococcus aureus* (MRSA), Middle East respiratory syndrome coronavirus (MERS-CoV), 2019 novel coronavirus (2019-nCoV), and Ebola. (pp 614–620)

## SKILLS OBJECTIVES

There are no skills objectives for this chapter.

# Introduction

Patients who need EMS assistance generally have experienced either a medical emergency or trauma emergency; in some cases both have occurred. **Trauma emergencies** involve injuries resulting from physical forces applied to the body. **Medical emergencies** involve illnesses or conditions caused by disease. Although it is important for you to be able to distinguish between medical and trauma patients, it is equally important for you to remember that patients may have a combination of medical and trauma conditions affecting their health. For example, a person who experiences a heart attack while driving may be involved in a crash, or a patient with diabetes whose blood glucose level is too low may fall and be injured. This chapter discusses medical emergencies. Chapter 25, *Trauma Overview*, discusses trauma emergencies.

# Types of Medical Emergencies

There are many types of medical emergencies (**TABLE 15-1**). Respiratory emergencies occur when patients have trouble breathing or when the amount of oxygen supplied to the tissues is inadequate. Diseases that can lead to respiratory emergencies include asthma, emphysema, and chronic bronchitis. Cardiovascular emergencies are caused by conditions affecting the circulatory system. The most common examples that require EMS intervention include heart attacks (myocardial infarction) and congestive heart failure. Neurologic emergencies involve the brain and may be caused by a seizure, stroke, or fainting (syncope). Many gastrointestinal conditions can result in a call to EMS for help. A well-known gastrointestinal condition is appendicitis, although there are many others, including diverticulitis and pancreatitis. A urologic emergency can involve kidney stones or a bladder infection. The most common endocrine emergencies are caused by complications of diabetes mellitus. Hematologic (blood) emergencies may be the result of sickle cell disease or various types of blood clotting disorders such as hemophilia. Immunologic emergencies involve the body's response to foreign substances. When the body overreacts to a foreign substance, it is commonly referred to as an allergic reaction. Allergic reactions are a type of immunologic medical emergency that can range from fairly

**TABLE 15-1** Common Medical Emergencies

| Type of Medical Emergency | Related Conditions |
| --- | --- |
| Respiratory | Asthma, emphysema, chronic bronchitis |
| Cardiovascular | Heart attack (myocardial infarction), congestive heart failure |
| Neurologic | Seizure, stroke, syncope |
| Gastrointestinal | Appendicitis, diverticulitis, pancreatitis |
| Urologic | Kidney stones, bladder infection |
| Endocrine | Diabetes mellitus |
| Hematologic | Sickle cell disease, hemophilia |
| Immunologic | Anaphylactic reaction (severe allergy to bee stings, food, or other substances) |
| Toxicologic | Substance abuse; food, plant, or chemical poisoning |
| Behavioral | Alzheimer disease, schizophrenia, depression, suicide |
| Gynecologic | Vaginal bleeding, sexually transmitted disease, pelvic inflammatory disease, ectopic pregnancy |

© Jones & Bartlett Learning.

minor to life threatening. Toxicologic emergencies, including poisoning and substance abuse, result in other types of medical emergencies with various presentations. Some medical emergencies are caused by psychological or behavioral problems. Behavioral emergencies may be especially difficult to manage because patients often do not present with typical signs and symptoms. Gynecologic conditions are a special category of medical emergencies that involve the female reproductive organs. The chapters in this section discuss each of these medical emergencies.

# Patient Assessment

Assessment of a medical patient is similar to the assessment of a trauma patient but with a different focus. Whereas trauma assessments focus on the mechanism of injury or physical injuries, some of which can be detected on a physical examination, medical patient assessment focuses on the **nature of illness (NOI)**, symptoms, and the patient's chief complaint. When you are assessing a patient, establish an accurate medical history. Information received from dispatch can help you anticipate what you might find when you arrive on scene, but it is conceivable that what appears to be a traumatic emergency may in fact be a medical emergency, or vice versa. Use the dispatch information to guide your initial response, but do not get locked into a preconceived idea of the patient's condition strictly from what the dispatcher tells you. During assessment, be aware of several challenges. It is possible that a patient has sustained an injury that distracts you from an underlying medical condition. For example, a patient may have a medical condition that resulted in a motor vehicle crash, or the patient may have sustained a large laceration and you fail to recognize that the patient has had a hypoglycemic event that caused him to fall and sustain the injury. Tunnel vision occurs when you become focused on one aspect of the patient's condition and exclude all others, which may cause you to miss an important injury or illness.

Patients may sometimes be uncooperative or even hostile toward those who respond to care for them. Patients may be fearful, angry, and confused and may take out their frustrations on you. It is important that you maintain a professional, calm, and nonjudgmental demeanor at all times.

You are obligated as a medical professional to refrain from labeling patients and displaying personal biases. Never assume that you know what the problem is, even when you are treating patients who frequently call for EMS. This attitude could result in missing a serious condition. For example, an intoxicated patient may call 9-1-1 regularly and then call at another time after a fall resulting in a serious head injury. The head injury may be overlooked if you assume the call is a response only to intoxication. Labeling a patient is dangerous, demeaning, and detrimental to you and the patient. Personal biases should never affect your management of a patient. Any biases you may have need to be resolved before you respond to calls. Patient assessment is discussed in further detail in Chapter 10, *Patient Assessment*. The major components of patient assessment include the following:

- Scene size-up
- Primary assessment
- History taking
- Secondary assessment
- Reassessment

## Scene Size-up

You must complete a scene size-up. The most important aspect of this step is to make sure the scene is safe. Hazards may not be as obvious with medical emergencies as with trauma situations, but they still exist and must be considered. Therefore, remain conscious of your safety and the safety of your crew and patient before you enter a scene and throughout the call.

It is also important that you use standard precautions when you respond to an emergency, including wearing gloves and other personal protective equipment (PPE). As soon as possible after your arrival, determine the number of patients who need assistance. In most medical cases, there will be only one patient, but anticipate the possibility of more patients, and be prepared. Finally, consider whether you need additional help. If you anticipate needing air transport, an advanced life support (ALS) unit, or police assistance, call for them immediately if you have not already done so, so that they will arrive as soon as possible.

Determine the NOI. What signs and symptoms is the patient experiencing? Evaluation of the NOI

## YOU are the Provider

Your unit is dispatched to 125 Green Hills Drive for a 36-year-old man with a fever, diarrhea, and vomiting. The time is 1325 hours, there is a fine mist falling, the temperature is 72°F (22.2°C), and the traffic is moderate. You and your partner respond; the scene is located approximately 10 minutes away.

**1.** What observations should you make when you arrive at the scene before making physical contact with the patient?

for a medical patient will provide you with an **index of suspicion** for different types of serious and/or life-threatening underlying illnesses. The index of suspicion is your awareness and concern for potentially serious underlying and unseen injuries or illnesses. Initiate spinal stabilization if indicated.

## Words of Wisdom

On entering the residence, your general impression will tell you if the patient is "sick or not sick." This determination will guide the speed and detail of your on-scene assessment.

## Primary Assessment

As you approach a medical patient, you should develop a general impression of his or her condition. Perform a rapid examination of the patient to identify life threats. Visual clues include apparent unconsciousness, obvious severe bleeding, or extreme difficulty breathing.

Quickly determine the patient's level of consciousness using the AVPU scale. If the patient is alert on your approach, you can infer several things about his or her condition, such as the existence of a pulse and breathing, but you must always complete a full primary assessment. If the patient is unconscious as you approach, try to see if you can get a response to verbal stimuli by speaking to the patient while using a gentle touch. If the patient does not respond to your verbal stimulation, provide pressure to the nailbed or use the trapezius squeeze test (a pinch on the muscle that runs along the side of the neck to the shoulders) to see whether the patient responds. If there is no response to verbal or painful stimuli, consider the patient unresponsive and quickly continue the assessment.

## Words of Wisdom

Do not let a relatively normal impression lull you into complacency. The conditions of many dangerously ill medical patients may not appear serious at first.

In conscious patients, ensure the airway is open and they are breathing adequately. Check the respiratory rate, depth, and quality. Consider applying oxygen at this time if there is any indication that breathing has been affected. For unconscious patients, make

## YOU are the Provider

You arrive at the residence and knock on the patient's door. His wife answers and escorts you to the bedroom, where you find the patient in a semisitting position in his bed. He is conscious and alert, is covered with several blankets, and is shivering. The patient tells you that he began feeling ill the day before but then started running a fever last night. Other than diarrhea and vomiting, he denies any other symptoms. He took 400 mg of ibuprofen approximately 20 minutes ago, and his wife took his temperature shortly before your arrival; it read 100.6°F (38.1°C). She also tells you her husband is a diabetic and she is worried because he has not been able to keep anything down including the pills he takes for his diabetes.

Your primary assessment reveals the following information:

| Recording Time: 0 Minutes | |
| --- | --- |
| Appearance | Flushed skin |
| Level of consciousness | Conscious and alert |
| Airway | Open; clear of secretions and foreign bodies |
| Breathing | Adequate rate and depth; no accessory muscle use |
| Circulation | Radial pulses, rapid strong; skin, flushed and warm to the touch |

**2.** On the basis of your general impression and primary assessment findings, does this patient require immediate transport?

**3.** How should you proceed with your care of the patient?

sure to open the airway using the proper technique for their condition, and take several seconds to evaluate their breathing. Apply oxygen to patients in shock, with difficulty breathing, and when low oxygen saturation measurements are obtained ($SpO_2$ less than 94%). Consider having your partner administer oxygen as you continue your assessment. Unconscious patients may need airway adjuncts and ventilatory assistance with a bag-mask device.

Quickly assess the circulation in a conscious patient by checking the radial pulse and observing the patient's skin color, temperature, and condition (**FIGURE 15-1**). Because pale skin can be difficult to detect in patients with dark skin, check for pale mucous membranes inside the inner lower eyelid or slow capillary refill. On general observation, the patient may appear ashen or gray. For unconscious patients, assess the circulation at the carotid artery because generally this is the site of the strongest pulse, and it is relatively easy to palpate on a supine person. Also quickly glance around the patient to identify any life threats such as severe bleeding or injury to the chest that affects the breathing. If any life threats are found, address them immediately.

Once you have completed the primary assessment, you should have enough information to make a preliminary transport decision. The following patients should be considered in serious condition and in need of rapid transport: patients who are unconscious or who have an altered mental status, patients with airway or breathing problems, and patients with obvious circulation problems

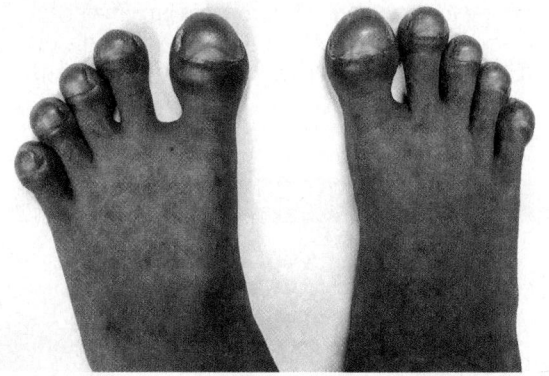

**FIGURE 15-1** Skin color can provide an early and fast indication of several disease processes. Cyanosis presents as blue skin. This photo also shows nail clubbing, associated with chronic hypoxemia seen in various lung and heart diseases.

© Chalie Chulapornsiri/Shutterstock.

such as severe bleeding or signs of shock. Patients identified as needing rapid transport still require additional assessment and care.

If the patient does not meet the criteria for rapid transport at this time, continue your assessment on scene and prepare for transport after you have completed the assessment and treatment. If you find that your patient's condition deteriorates during the primary assessment, prepare the patient for immediate transport and complete the assessment en route to the emergency department (ED).

## History Taking

With a medical patient, history taking may be the only way to determine what the problem is or what may be causing the problem. It is imperative to gather a thorough history from the patient and/or any family, friends, or bystanders who may have pertinent information. Family members may be the only people aware that an older patient sustained a head injury the previous week or that a patient has a history of drug abuse. Bystanders may have seen clues prior to the 9-1-1 call that will lead you and the hospital staff to identify the cause of a patient's condition. Investigate the NOI by inquiring about the chief complaint. Identifying signs and symptoms associated with the chief complaint will often help you determine the nature of the condition. Ask about the history of the present illness and ask follow-up questions such as, "Has anything like this ever happened before?" If the patient answers yes, then ask, "What was done at that time?" and "How does this episode compare with previous episodes?"

If a patient is unconscious, survey the scene for evidence of traumatic events, medication containers, or medical devices the patient may have been using. Try to obtain as much of the patient's medical history as possible from family members, friends, and bystanders or from the scene itself. Family members or friends may know the patient's allergies, medications, or medical conditions. Ask whether the patient reported any symptoms before he or she lost consciousness. If possible, have a family member accompany you to the hospital to answer questions there as well.

As you continue to gather information, remember to obtain a SAMPLE history and to ask questions about the patient's chief complaint using the OPQRST mnemonic. Ask patients to identify all the symptoms they are experiencing. Make sure you record any allergies, medical conditions, and medications they take (**FIGURE 15-2**). Ask about prescriptions, over-the-counter medications, and herbal medications.

Sometimes older patients will report taking numerous medications, both prescription and over the counter. In those situations, it is best to take the medications with you to the hospital, and list them in your report. Ask patients about their medical history to help determine the current problem and identify any other conditions that might cause complications. To obtain a complete history, ask about specific conditions such as heart problems, breathing problems, and blood sugar (glucose) problems. Determine if the patient is taking any medications for these conditions and whether he or she is compliant with the drug regimen. The purpose of these questions is to obtain the most complete medical history possible. In addition, look around the scene for clues, such as prescription pill bottles or home medical equipment, that may help you piece together the patient's medical history and better understand the circumstances surrounding the current medical emergency.

## Secondary Assessment

In some cases in which the patient is critically ill or injured or the transport time is short, you may not have time to conduct a secondary assessment. In other cases, the secondary assessment may occur on scene or en route to the ED.

Conscious medical patients seldom need a secondary assessment of the entire body or a head-to-toe examination, but all conscious patients should undergo a limited or detailed physical examination based on their chief complaint. For example, you should check for pulse, motion, and sensation in all of the patient's extremities and check the patient's pupillary reaction if you suspect a neurologic problem. Unconscious patients are unable to tell you what is wrong, so you should always perform a secondary assessment of the entire body or a head-to-toe examination. A full body assessment should help you obtain clues to assess the problem, but this assessment should be performed quickly so it does not delay transport to the hospital.

### Words of Wisdom

Medical alert jewelry may provide you with valuable information about why the patient is unconscious.

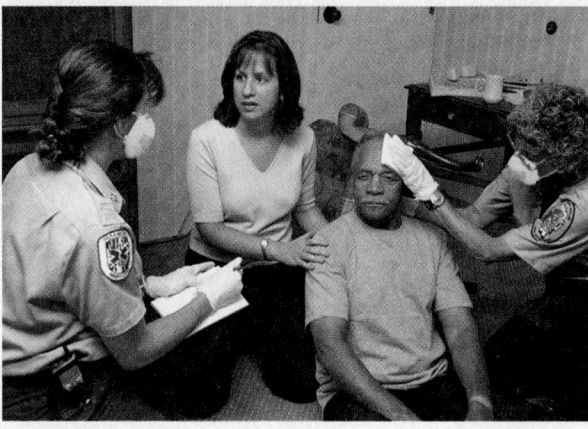

**FIGURE 15-2** History taking is an important part of the patient assessment process.

© Jones & Bartlett Learning. Courtesy of MIEMSS.

If the patient's condition warrants the secondary assessment, begin by carefully examining the head, scalp, and face. Look for evidence of possible trauma, and monitor the patient for any signs of pain with palpation throughout the assessment. Examine the head and face for symmetry, making sure to check the pupils for equality and reactivity to light. Look at the conjunctiva of the eyes for moisture and the ears and nose for any drainage. Look for nasal flaring, and examine the mouth for foreign bodies (including loose teeth or dentures) and pink, moist mucosa.

Examine the neck closely for any evidence of accessory muscle use with respirations. Check for jugular vein distention and tracheal deviation, which can be indicators of respiratory or cardiac problems. While you are examining the neck, make sure to move any clothing so that you can check for a tracheostomy or stoma.

Next, assess the chest and abdomen. At the chest, make sure to check breath sounds and ensure that the patient is breathing adequately with equal chest rise and fall on each side. Carefully inspect and palpate the chest and abdomen to identify any areas of tenderness or swelling. Look for medication patches on the chest or abdomen and any implanted medical devices, which usually can be palpated just under the skin. Check for rigidity and distention in the abdomen, and look for scars on the chest or abdomen that might indicate previous surgeries, including scars from laparoscopic surgery that may be difficult to notice. Finally, check the pelvis and genital area, asking about pain and looking for signs of incontinence or bleeding.

Palpate the legs and arms for swelling and other abnormalities, making sure to check for distal motion, sensation, and circulation. Note any scars or track marks along the veins, which are indicators of intravenous (IV) drug use. Look for medical alert jewelry at the wrists as well. Finally, examine the patient's back to note any irregularities, pain, or scars. At this point, your full assessment of the patient should

be complete, and treatment of non–life-threatening conditions should be instituted. Treatment will depend on each condition and your local protocols.

### Words of Wisdom

Although the use of an automatic blood pressure cuff is convenient, you should always attempt to obtain at least one manual blood pressure reading to be sure it correlates with the automatic reading.

Obtaining a good set of vital signs is critical. Often your partner can begin this process while you are asking about the medical history. Assess the pulse for rate, quality, and regularity at the most appropriate site, either at the radial artery if the patient is conscious, or at the carotid artery if the patient is unconscious. Assess respirations as you assess the pulse to prevent the patient from modifying his or her respirations in response to your observation. Identify the rate, quality, and regularity of the respirations and any difficulties that may be apparent. Finally, obtain an initial blood pressure reading, measuring both systolic and diastolic pressures.

Consider using the automatic blood pressure cuff for future assessments at regular intervals. Depending on your local protocol, other important information to consider obtaining includes a blood glucose level and a pulse oximetry reading.

## YOU are the Provider

Your partner obtains the patient's vital signs. He also obtains a blood glucose level of 242 mg/dL and notes that the patient seems to be showing some signs of dehydration, such as dry mucous membranes. Palpation of the patient's abdomen showed it to be soft and nontender. The patient agrees to transport and asks you to take him to a hospital that he has been to before, which is located 25 miles away. There is another hospital located only 10 miles away.

| Recording Time: 5 Minutes | |
|---|---|
| Respiration | 18 breaths/min; regular and adequate |
| Pulse | 110 beats/min; strong and regular |
| Skin | Flushed and dry; warm to the touch |
| Blood pressure | 124/70 mm Hg |
| Oxygen saturation (Spo$_2$) | 99% |

**4.** Is it appropriate to transport the patient to the hospital he requested, or should you transport him to the closer facility?

## Reassessment

After completing the assessment and treatment, begin reassessment and continue it throughout transport. During the reassessment, repeat the primary assessment and reassess the chief complaint. Look for any changes in the level of consciousness; reassess the airway, breathing, and circulation; and reexamine the transport decision. Consider the need for ALS backup. Obtain another full set of vital signs every 5 minutes for unstable patients or every 15 minutes for stable patients. Reassessment also includes repeating your physical examination to identify and treat changes in the patient's condition.

Finally, the reassessment includes reviewing all treatments that have been performed. Reassess oxygen delivery, any bandages or splints applied, and any other treatment that has been performed.

Document any changes that have developed as a result of the treatments, and, if needed, adjust any of the treatments accordingly. Reassessment is an important step in patient assessment; it allows you to modify care as needed and ensures you have the most current information on the patient's condition when you arrive at the hospital.

## Management, Transport, and Destination

Most medical emergencies require a level of treatment beyond that available in the prehospital setting. Also, the treatments depend on an accurate diagnosis of the exact medical condition, which may require advanced testing that is only available in a hospital. The primary prehospital treatments for medical emergencies address the symptoms more than the actual disease process.

Depending on local protocol, it may be beyond the scope of an EMT to administer medications to a patient. In a few limited circumstances, such as the administration of nitroglycerin to a patient with chest pain or to a patient for whom it has been prescribed, an exception may be made. Another exception may be granted to allow an EMT to assist a patient with a prescribed metered-dose inhaler when it is required because of respiratory difficulty.

Administration of medications that are stored in the ambulance is also limited for EMTs and is dependent on state and local protocols. A few of these protocols include administering aspirin for patients having chest pain, administering oral glucose to a patient with diabetes and a low blood glucose level, and possibly administering albuterol to a patient with respiratory difficulty. The administration of activated charcoal to a patient who has ingested a poison is also allowed when it may be beneficial. Each of these situations and any other administration of medication by an EMT require direct permission from medical control. The process of obtaining permission includes completing a thorough assessment of the patient before calling medical control. After you give a report to the physician and obtain permission, the medication may be administered. Never administer any medication without first obtaining permission from medical control, and always follow your state and local protocols.

You may also use an automated external defibrillator (AED) on a patient who is pulseless and apneic. In some cases of cardiac arrest, immediate treatment with an AED may provide the best option to resuscitate the patient. The AED is discussed in more detail in Chapter 17, *Cardiovascular Emergencies*. Familiarize yourself with the equipment and medications carried on your ambulance, and use them appropriately under a medical director's instruction.

## Scene Time

In many cases, the time on scene may be longer for medical patients than for trauma patients. If the patient is not in critical condition, gather as much information as possible from the scene so that you can transmit that information to the physician at the ED. Briefly check the patient's living conditions—heating, air conditioning, cleanliness of environment, adequate food, and so on. Critical patients include those with altered mental status, airway or breathing difficulties, or any sign of circulatory compromise. In addition, a patient who is very old or very young may be considered critical even if the patient appears to be relatively stable. Critical patients often need expeditious transport. The time on scene should be limited to 10 minutes or less for these patients.

## Type of Transport

Serious consideration should be given to how best to transport a medical patient. If a life-threatening condition exists, the transportation may be meaningfully accelerated by the use of lights and sirens, but if the patient is not critical, or if the degree to which use of lights and sirens would not substantially decrease transport times, consider non-emergency transport. Many patients experiencing a medical emergency can be transported without the use of lights and siren. This is a much safer method of transport and will often result in arrival only a few minutes later than an emergency transport using lights and siren.

Differentiating a high-priority transport from a low-priority transport is a skill developed with experience, but it is a skill that can be learned. A general rule for determining the priority of transport is to consider the results of the patient's primary assessment. Patients with an altered mental status, especially if it is still present at the completion of your assessment and treatment, should be considered a high-priority transport. Patients with circulatory compromise, including signs and symptoms of shock, should also be considered a high-priority transport. Most patients with circulatory problems cannot be stabilized in the prehospital setting and need to undergo treatment at a hospital quickly but safely. Patients with difficulty breathing often require high-priority transport. However, if the patient has responded well to your initial treatment, such as oxygen and albuterol administration, lights and siren may not be necessary. As a rule, if you choose to use lights and siren, you should be able to specifically describe in your report why such emergency transport was medically necessary and why the improved arrival time justified the increased risk to which you exposed the patient and public-at-large (**FIGURE 15-3**).

Modes of transport ultimately come in one of two categories: ground (**FIGURE 15-4**) or air (**FIGURE 15-5**). Ground transportation EMS units are generally staffed by EMTs and paramedics. Air transportation EMS units or critical care transport units are generally staffed by critical care transport professionals such as critical care nurses and paramedics. Although it is not as common to summon an air ambulance for a medical patient, there are instances where it is advisable. In rural areas with long ground transport times, patients who have possibly experienced a heart attack, stroke, or complication of pregnancy could benefit from air transport. Children with serious medical conditions can also benefit from air transport. When you

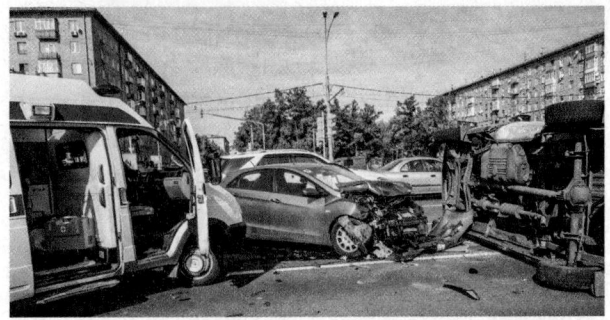

**FIGURE 15-3** Ambulance crash. Additional risk may be posed to the population on the roads by use of lights and sirens.
© Ivanoel/Shutterstock.

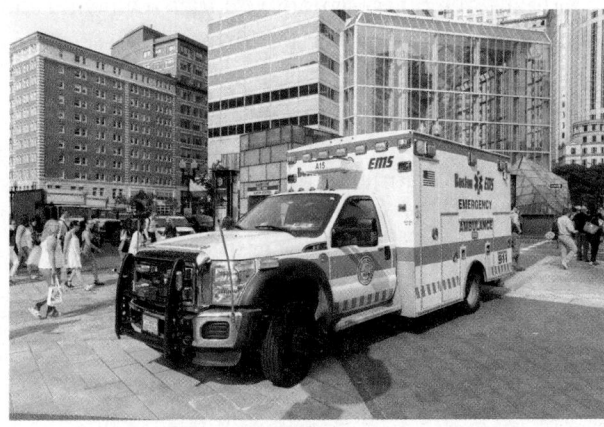

**FIGURE 15-4** Ground transport.
© 2p2play/Shutterstock.

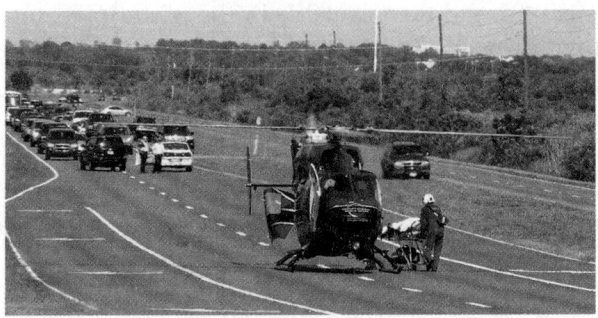

**FIGURE 15-5** Air transport.
LindaCharlton/iStock.

are considering ALS support for a patient, compare the total time for a ground ALS unit to respond and transport to the time required for an ALS helicopter to respond and transport as well as the urgent resources needed by the patient. Follow local protocols and medical direction.

## Destination Selection

It is generally appropriate to select the closest ED as your destination. However, there are times when the closest hospital is not necessarily the most appropriate choice. Patients with chest pain as a result of a heart attack may need a facility that is capable of performing cardiac catheterization, which may not necessarily be available at the closest hospital. If the patient is in cardiac arrest or experiences cardiac arrest during transport, immediately reroute to the closest hospital with emergency facilities. Stroke patients can also benefit from specialized hospital selection. Many hospitals have designated stroke teams and interventional neurology capabilities. Taking a possible stroke patient to a hospital without these resources may result in a delay in definitive treatment and may lead to a worse outcome for the patient.

Some medical patients may benefit from on-scene treatment provided by advanced EMS personnel such as paramedics. It is important to recognize early when paramedics can provide added value on a scene so that, if they are readily available, they can be called to respond in a timely manner.

## Infectious Diseases

An infectious disease is a medical condition caused by the growth and spread of small, harmful organisms within the body. A communicable disease is a disease that can be spread from one person or species to another. Most of these diseases are much harder to be infected with than is commonly believed. In addition, there are many immunizations, protective techniques, and devices that providers can use to minimize their risk of infection. When providers use these protective measures, their risk of contracting a serious infectious disease is substantially decreased.

As an EMT, you will be called on to treat and transport patients with a variety of infectious or communicable diseases. In Chapter 2, *Workforce Safety and Wellness*, the routes of transmission and standard precautions that responders need to take to reduce risk and increase prevention and awareness are described. The assessment and treatment of a patient who may have a communicable or infectious disease are also covered. Chapter 38, *Transport Operations*, discusses decontamination techniques after transport.

## General Assessment Principles

The assessment of a patient suspected of having an infectious disease should be approached much like the assessment of any other medical patient. With most patients who have a potentially infectious disease in the prehospital setting, the next step after scene size-up and primary assessment is to gather patient history using OPQRST to elaborate on the patient's chief complaint. Typical chief complaints include fever, nausea, rash, pleuritic chest pain, difficulty breathing, vomiting, and diarrhea. Obtain a SAMPLE history and a set of baseline vital signs, paying particular attention to medications the patient is currently taking and the events leading up to today's problem. Also ask whether the patient has recently traveled or has come in contact with someone who has traveled. Always show respect for the feelings of the patient, family members, and others at the scene.

## General Management Principles

The general management of the patient with a suspected infectious disease first focuses on any life-threatening conditions that were identified in the primary assessment (airway management, oxygen and ventilatory assistance, and circulatory support). Remember to be empathetic. Because most of these patients will have a fever or mild breathing problems, place the patient in a position of comfort on the stretcher and keep him or her warm. Remember to use appropriate personal protective equipment based on the nature of the call. Always follow your agency's exposure control plan regarding cleaning equipment, properly discarding of any disposable supplies, and washing linens.

## Epidemic and Pandemic Considerations

An epidemic occurs when new cases of a disease in a human population substantially exceed the number expected based on recent experience. A pandemic is an outbreak that occurs on a global scale. A flu pandemic occurs when a new influenza virus for which people have little or no immunity emerges. The disease can spread easily from person to person, cause serious illness, and be found in multiple countries in a short time. Because it is a new virus, there would be no specific vaccine immediately available.

# Common or Serious Communicable Diseases

## Influenza

Influenza, commonly known as flu, is primarily an animal respiratory disease that has mutated to infect humans. It can affect all people, but those with chronic medical conditions, compromised immune systems, the very young, and the very old are particularly susceptible to complications of the disease. All strains of influenza are transmitted by direct contact with nasal secretions and aerosolized droplets from coughing and sneezing by infected people.

The H1N1 virus, which was initially identified as the swine flu in 2009, is a specific form of influenza. Other viruses of concern include Middle East respiratory syndrome (MERS), severe acute respiratory syndrome (SARS), COVID-19, which are discussed later. The H1N1 virus has been present for years in animals. Many deaths have been caused by the H1N1 virus, although deaths caused by other influenza viruses have also occurred. The most positive effect of the outbreak of the H1N1 virus has been the general public's greater awareness of the routes of transmission of contagious diseases. This increased awareness could result in a reduction of all communicable diseases, not only H1N1.

Many potentially serious diseases can be spread by the respiratory route; therefore, you need to wear PPE, such as gloves, eye protection, and a high-efficiency particulate air (HEPA) respirator or an N95 mask, at a minimum. Viruses can live for several days on surfaces, so frequent handwashing is also important. Maintain your vaccinations and stay up to date on the latest Centers for Disease Control and Prevention (CDC) recommendations. Place a surgical mask on patients with suspected or confirmed respiratory disease. Wear a HEPA respirator or an N95 mask during any aerosol-generating procedures such as suctioning of airway secretions, performing cardiopulmonary resuscitation, or assisting with endotracheal intubation.

An annual influenza immunization is important, especially for EMS personnel, to protect both providers and patients. The influenza virus is constantly changing. Experts adjust vaccines from year to year to provide protection against the strains most likely to affect the population. Vaccination effectively decreases transmission rates and limits (though does not eliminate) the disease incidence. Complications of the vaccine are far less common and severe than complications of the flu, which kills an average of 35,000 people in the United States every year. Research has absolutely proven the theory that immunizations cause autism to be untrue.

## Herpes Simplex

Herpes simplex is a common virus strain carried by humans. Eighty percent of people carrying the virus are asymptomatic, but symptomatic infections cause eruptions of tiny fluid-filled blisters called *vesicles* that often appear on the lips or genitals. Herpes simplex can cause more serious illnesses like pneumonia and meningitis in very young, very old, and immunocompromised patients. The primary mode of infection is through close personal contact, so standard precautions are generally sufficient to prevent spread to or from health care workers.

## HIV Infection

Exposure to the virus that causes acquired immunodeficiency syndrome (AIDS) is a risk that EMTs face on a regular basis. It is this prospect that led to the development of standard precautions. There is no vaccine to protect against human immunodeficiency virus (HIV) infection, and despite great progress in drug treatments, AIDS can still be fatal. However, with treatment, patients can expect a near-normal life span. HIV attacks the body's immune system, making it difficult for the natural defenses to fight disease. If the HIV infection develops into AIDS, minor illnesses can become fatal to the patient.

Fortunately, HIV is not easily transmitted in your work setting. For example, it is far less contagious than hepatitis B, although immunization for hepatitis B is important. HIV infection is a potential hazard only when deposited on mucous membranes or directly into the bloodstream. Transmission can occur via sexual contact or exposure to blood or body fluids, meaning your risk of infection is limited to exposure to an infected patient's blood and body fluids. Exposure can take place in the following ways:

- The patient's blood is splashed or sprayed into your eyes, nose, or mouth or into an open sore or cut, however tiny; even a microscopic opening in the skin is an invitation for infection with a virus.
- You have blood from the infected patient on your hands and then touch your own eyes, nose, mouth, or an open sore or cut.
- A needle used to inject the patient breaks your skin. The risk to you from a single injection, even with a hollow-bore needle, is small, probably less than 1 in 1,000. However, this is by far the most dangerous form of exposure.
- Broken glass at a motor vehicle crash or other incident penetrates your glove (and skin), which may have already been covered with blood from an infected patient.

Many patients who are infected with HIV do not show any symptoms. This is why health care workers should wear gloves any time they are likely to come into contact with secretions or blood from any patient. Always put on gloves before leaving the ambulance to care for a patient. Also, take great care in handling and properly disposing of needles and other sharp objects in a sharps container so that you and others are not inadvertently exposed to them. Finally, cover any open wounds that you have whenever you are on the job.

If you have any reason to think that a patient's blood or secretions may have entered your system, especially through contact with a patient's blood, seek medical advice as soon as possible and notify your infectious disease officer. If you know that the patient is infected with HIV, your physician may suggest immediate treatment to try to prevent you from becoming infected. However, if the patient is an unlikely candidate for HIV infection, your physician may recommend that you and the patient be tested before you undergo therapy. As scientists learn more about HIV infection, testing and treatment recommendations change. It is important that you immediately see your physician (or your program's designated physician) any time you have a significant exposure to a communicable or infectious disease. Know the policy for your system, and take time now to consider what you would do in the event of exposure.

## Hepatitis

The term *hepatitis* refers to an inflammation (and often infection) of the liver. Hepatitis can be caused by a number of different viruses and toxins. Early signs of viral hepatitis include loss of appetite, vomiting, fever, fatigue, sore throat, cough, and muscle

## Words of Wisdom

### Causes of Infectious Disease

| Organism | Description | Example |
|---|---|---|
| Bacteria | Grow and reproduce outside the human cell in the appropriate temperature and with the appropriate nutrients | *Salmonella* |
| Viruses | Smaller than bacteria; multiply only inside a host and die when exposed to the environment | Influenza |
| Fungi | Similar to bacteria in that they require the appropriate nutrients and organic material to grow | Mold |
| Protozoa (parasites) | Single-celled microscopic organisms, some of which cause disease | Amoebas |
| Helminths (parasites) | Invertebrates with long, flexible, rounded, or flattened bodies | Worms |

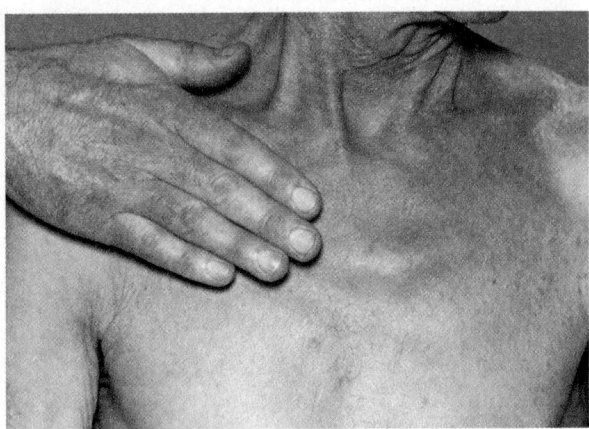

**FIGURE 15-6** Jaundice is a sign of a hepatitis infection. Other causes of jaundice may include hepatitis, alcohol-related liver disease, blocked bile ducts, pancreatic cancer, and certain medications such as acetaminophen, penicillin, birth control pills, and steroids.

© SPL/Science Source.

and joint pain. Several weeks later, jaundice (yellow eyes and skin) and right upper quadrant abdominal pain develop (**FIGURE 15-6**). The severity of toxin-induced hepatitis depends on the amount of agent absorbed and the duration of exposure. Toxin-induced hepatitis is not contagious. There is

no definitive way in the prehospital environment to tell which patients with hepatitis have a contagious form of the disease and which do not. **TABLE 15-2** shows the characteristics of different types of hepatitis, from which you can assess your risk of exposure. Hepatitis A can be transmitted only from a patient who has an acute infection, whereas hepatitis B and hepatitis C can be transmitted from long-term carriers who have no signs of illness. A carrier is a person (or animal) in whom an infectious organism has taken up permanent residence and may or may not cause any active disease. Carriers may never know that they harbor the organism; however, they can infect other people.

Hepatitis A is transmitted orally through oral or fecal contamination. This means that, generally, you must eat or drink something that is contaminated with the virus. Contamination is the presence of an infectious organism on or in an object. The organisms that cause hepatitis B and C are transmitted through vehicles other than food or water. For example, these organisms may enter the body through a transfusion or needlestick with infected blood, which puts health care workers at high risk for contracting hepatitis B, the more contagious and virulent form. **Virulence** is the strength or

**TABLE 15-2** Characteristics of Hepatitis

| Type | Route of Infection | Incubation Period | Chronic Infection | Vaccine and Treatment | Comments |
|---|---|---|---|---|---|
| **Viral Hepatitis** | | | | | |
| Hepatitis A (infectious) | Fecal–oral, infected food or drink | 2–6 wk | Chronic condition does not exist. | Vaccine is available; no specific treatment is available; body will clear the infection on its own. | Mild illness; approximately 2% of patients die; after acute infection, the patient has lifelong immunity. |
| Hepatitis B | Blood, sexual contact, saliva, urine, breast milk | 4–12 wk | Chronic infection affects up to 10% of patients and up to 90% of newborns who have the disease. | Vaccine is available; treatment is minimally effective. | Up to 30% of patients may become chronic carriers; patients are asymptomatic and without signs of liver disease, but they may infect others; approximately 1% to 2% of patients die. |
| Hepatitis C | Blood, sexual contact | 2–10 wk | Chronic infection affects 90% of patients. | No vaccine is available; treatment is costly but effective for many strains of hepatitis C. | Cirrhosis of the liver develops in 50% of patients with chronic hepatitis C; chronic infection increases the risk of cancer of the liver. |
| Hepatitis D | Blood, sexual contact | 4–12 wk | Chronic infection is common. | No vaccine is available; no treatment is available. | Occurs only in patients with active hepatitis B infection; fulminant disease may develop in 20% of patients. |
| **Toxin-Induced Hepatitis** | | | | | |
| Medications, drugs, and alcohol | Inhalation, skin or mucous membrane exposure, oral ingestion, or intravenous administration | Within hours to days following exposure | Some chemicals may initiate an inflammatory response that continues to cause liver damage long after the chemical is out of the body. | No vaccine is available; treatment is to stop exposure; in patients with an overdose of acetaminophen, certain drugs may minimize liver injury if given early enough. | This type of hepatitis is not contagious; patients with toxin-induced hepatitis may have liver damage and jaundice; not every exposure to a toxin will cause liver damage. |

© Jones & Bartlett Learning.

ability of a pathogen to produce disease. Hepatitis B is far more contagious than HIV. For this reason, vaccination with hepatitis B vaccine is highly recommended for EMTs. Unfortunately, not everyone who is vaccinated develops immediate immunity to the virus. Sometimes, but not always, an additional dose will provide immunity. You should be tested after vaccination to determine your immune status.

If you are stuck with a needle or injured in some other way while caring for a patient who might have hepatitis, see your physician immediately.

## Meningitis

**Meningitis** is an inflammation of the meningeal coverings of the brain and spinal cord. Patients with meningitis will have signs and symptoms such as fever, headache, stiff neck, and altered mental status. It is an uncommon but very frightening infectious disease. Meningitis can be caused by viruses or bacteria, most of which are not contagious.

**Meningococcal meningitis**, one form of meningitis, however, is highly contagious. Meningococcal meningitis is an inflammation of the meningeal coverings of the brain and spinal cord. The bacteria that cause meningococcal meningitis can be spread by the exchange of respiratory secretions through coughing and sneezing. The effects are lethal in some cases. Victims who survive can be left with brain damage, hearing loss, or learning disabilities. Patients may present with flulike symptoms, but high fever, severe headache, photophobia (light sensitivity), and a stiff neck in adults are symptoms that are highly suggestive of meningitis. Patients sometimes have an altered level of consciousness and can have red blotches on the skin. Use respiratory protection, provide rapid transportation, and provide early notification to the ED so they can make specific preparations for accepting a highly contagious patient.

Only laboratory tests can sort out the different forms of meningitis; therefore, you should take standard precautions with any patient who is suspected of having meningitis. Wearing gloves and a mask will go a long way to prevent the patient's secretions from getting into your nose and mouth. Again, the risk of infection is small, even if the organism is transmitted. For this reason, vaccines, which are available for most types of meningococcus, are rarely used. Meningitis can be treated at the ED with antibiotics.

After treating a patient with meningitis, contact your employer health representative. Many states consider meningitis reportable and will notify you that one of your patients was diagnosed with meningitis. Prophylactic treatment may be recommended for you.

## Tuberculosis

Most patients who are infected with *Mycobacterium tuberculosis* (the tubercle bacillus) are well most of the time. If the disease involves the brain or kidneys, the patient is only slightly contagious. In the United States, however, **tuberculosis** is a chronic disease that usually strikes the lungs. Disease that occurs shortly after infection is called primary tuberculosis. Except in infants, this infection is not usually serious. After the primary infection, the tubercle bacillus is rendered dormant by the patient's immune system. However, even after decades of lying dormant, this germ can reactivate. Reactive tuberculosis is common and can be much more difficult to treat, especially because an increasing number of tuberculosis strains have grown resistant to most antibiotics.

Although tuberculosis is often hard to distinguish from other diseases, patients who pose the highest risk almost invariably have a cough. Therefore, for your safety, you should consider respiratory tuberculosis to be the only contagious form because it is the only one that is spread by airborne transmission. The droplets produced by coughing are not the real problem. The real problem is the droplet nuclei, which are the remnants of the droplets after the excess water has evaporated. These particles are tiny enough to be invisible and can remain suspended in the air for a long time. In fact, as long as these particles are shielded from ultraviolet light, they can remain alive for decades. Particles that are the size of droplet nuclei are not stopped by routine surgical masks. Inhaled, they are carried directly to the alveoli of the lungs, where the bacteria may begin to grow. N95 or HEPA masks are required to stop droplet nuclei (**FIGURE 15-7**).

Why is tuberculosis not more common than it is? After all, absolute protection from infection with the tubercle bacillus does not exist. Everyone who breathes is at risk. According to the CDC, one-third of the world's population is infected with tuberculosis. The vaccine for tuberculosis, called BCG, is rarely used in the United States. Under normal circumstances, however, the mechanism of

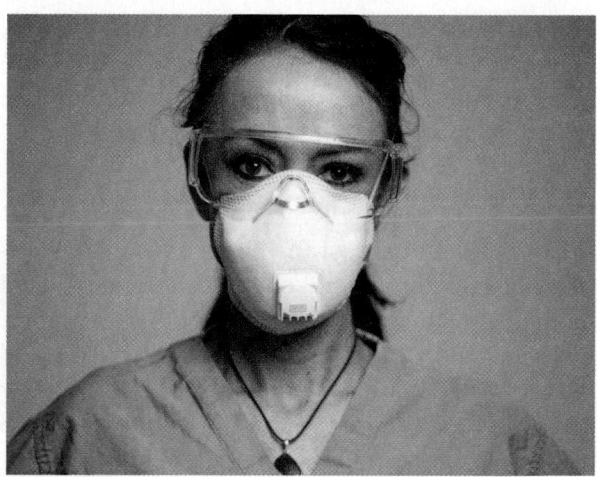

**FIGURE 15-7** Wear an N95 mask when treating a patient whom you suspect has tuberculosis just as you would a patient whom you suspect has COVID-19.

© RichLegg/E+/Getty Images.

## Special Populations

The aging process can pose a threat to the body's natural defense mechanisms against invading microorganisms. As a person ages, his or her physical defenses weaken or are eliminated. The skin's thinning and loss of supportive collagen, along with a reduction in the number of blood vessels, allow bacteria or viruses to enter the body with less resistance. The respiratory system cannot trap and eliminate bacteria and viruses in the airways as efficiently as it once did. Additionally, the gastrointestinal system allows easier entry for bacteria or viruses through the intestines. As the body ages, physical barriers to entry weaken, the immune system deteriorates, and invading organisms are not as easily identified. Infectious agents can take hold in older people much more easily because of reduced defenses.

When transporting an older patient, protect the patient from the environment because extremes in heat or cold can further reduce the body's defenses. If the patient has a cold or the flu, protect yourself. However, remember that your defense system is probably much stronger than that of the patient.

People who are immunosuppressed from chronic illnesses, cancer treatment, or organ transplants may also lack the ability to fight certain infections. Ensure that these patients are not exposed to any additional conditions that could lead to an infection.

transmission used by *M tuberculosis* is not very efficient. Infected air is easily diluted with uninfected air. *M tuberculosis* typically causes no illness in a new host. In fact, many patients with tuberculosis do not even transmit the infection to family members. However, in crowded environments with poor ventilation, the disease spreads more easily.

If you are exposed to a patient who is found to have pulmonary tuberculosis, you will be given a tuberculin skin test. This simple skin test determines whether a person has been infected with *M tuberculosis*. A positive result means that exposure has occurred; it does not mean that the person has active tuberculosis. It takes at least 6 weeks for the bacteria to show up in the laboratory test. So if you are tested for the disease within a few weeks of the exposure and your results are positive, this means that you were exposed to tuberculosis at an earlier time from somebody else. You will probably never identify the source. Most transmissions occur silently, so it is necessary that you have tuberculin skin tests regularly. If the infection is found before you become ill, preventive therapy is almost 100% effective. Usually, a daily dose of the medication isoniazid will prevent the development of active infection.

## Whooping Cough

Whooping cough, also called pertussis, is an airborne disease caused by bacteria that mostly affects children younger than 6 years. Signs and symptoms include fever and a "whoop" sound that occurs when the patient tries to inhale after a coughing attack.

The best way to prevent infection from whooping cough is to be vaccinated with a diphtheria, tetanus, and pertussis vaccine (DTaP). Providers who have previously had this vaccine should make sure they are up-to-date with a booster. For added protection, place a mask on the patient and on yourself.

## Methicillin-Resistant *Staphylococcus aureus*

Methicillin-resistant *Staphylococcus aureus* (MRSA) is a bacterium that causes infections and is resistant to many antibiotics. In health care settings, MRSA is believed to be transmitted from patient to patient via unwashed hands of health care providers. Studies have shown that 5% to 15% of health care providers carry MRSA in their nares. Up to 65% of people presenting with hand infections from the community have MRSA. In addition, children with no health care exposure present with MRSA. The pathogen can subsequently be transferred to skin and other areas of the body through a break in the skin. Surfaces contaminated with MRSA do not seem to be important in transmission. Factors that increase the risk for developing MRSA include antibiotic therapy, prolonged hospital stays, a stay in an intensive care or burn unit, and exposure to an infected patient.

The incubation period for MRSA appears to be between 5 and 45 days. The communicable period varies, as patients who have active infection may carry MRSA for months. MRSA results in soft-tissue infections. Its signs and symptoms may involve localized skin abscesses, and sepsis may be found in older patients with the infection.

## Global Health Issues

### 2019 Novel Coronavirus

Coronaviruses are typically responsible for minor respiratory illnesses such as the common cold, which in most people is not a lethal illness. Past outbreaks of novel (new) strains of coronavirus such as SARS in 2002–2003 and the MERS in 2012 introduced the world to more lethal types of this illness.

In December 2019, a novel coronavirus (COVID-19) originated in Wuhan, Hubei Province, China, and quickly spread, infecting tens of millions and killing over a million. Attempts to control the spread of the virus included social distancing that resulted in massive economic downturns globally. Although much is still unknown at the time of this writing, COVID-19 is spreading worldwide. Signs and symptoms of the disease include fever, cough, and shortness of breath that seem to appear between 2 and 14 days after exposure to an infected person. Asymptomatic infected persons have transmitted infection with COVID-19. For current updates about COVID-19, use the CDC website www.cdc.gov.

### MERS-CoV

MERS coronavirus (MERS-CoV) is a virus most commonly found in bats and camels living in the Middle East. The first human case of MERS-CoV was discovered in 2012 in Saudi Arabia. Although most clusters of human infections are found in the Middle East, reported cases of MERS-CoV have been found in Europe and the United States. Common patient symptoms include high fever, cough, muscle aches, vomiting, and diarrhea. In some cases, renal failure, respiratory failure, and death have been reported.

There is currently no cure or vaccine for this virus. If you suspect your patient might have MERS-CoV, place a surgical mask on him or her, and notify the receiving facility.

### Ebola

In 2014, an outbreak of the Ebola virus in West Africa caused international concern. Several infected people with the virus traveled to other countries, including the United States, motivating EMS and health care facilities to prepare for further outbreaks. The incubation period is approximately 6 to 12 days after exposure; however, symptoms may not begin to appear for as long as 21 days after infection. Symptoms include watery diarrhea, vomiting, fever, body aches, and bleeding. The fatality rate can be as high as 70% if effective supportive treatment in an intensive care unit is not initiated promptly. If you suspect your patient may have this condition, place a surgical mask on him or her and follow PPE precautions as outlined by local protocols and the CDC. Immediately notify the receiving facility that your patient may have or may have been exposed to the Ebola virus.

## Travel Medicine

Every day, thousands of people travel to various countries. Although humans share many common germs, some are confined to certain areas of the world. As an EMS provider, you must be aware of this when assessing a patient who recently traveled outside the United States.

Patients who acquire an illness from another country can present with a variety of symptoms depending on the illness. They may have a fever, cough, vomiting, bloody diarrhea, body aches, and rashes. In many cases, the patient experiences mild symptoms and does not require EMS. However, some patients become extremely ill, requiring urgent evaluation and treatment. When you encounter an ill patient with a recent travel history, place a mask on the patient and gather as much information as possible. Important questions to ask the patient include:

- Where did you recently travel?
- Did you receive any vaccinations before your trip?
- Were you exposed to any infectious diseases?
- Is there anyone else in your travel party who is sick?

- What types of food did you eat?
- What was your source of drinking water?

## Words of Wisdom

The ability of your EMS system to support you in the event of exposure to a communicable disease depends on your understanding of how an exposure to potentially infectious materials can occur and your immediate reporting of the exposure. Make notes right away to ensure that you remember all pertinent information, and report the possible exposure immediately after the response, following your service's guidelines.

If you suspect the patient has a communicable illness, follow appropriate PPE precautions and notify the receiving facility. Although treatment for many travel-related illnesses is primarily supportive in the prehospital environment, always be prepared to manage life-threatening conditions should the patient become unstable.

## Conclusion

Although trauma patients often present with dramatic signs and symptoms, the assessment and treatment you provide for them are fairly straightforward. The assessment and treatment of medical patients, in comparison, can be challenging and interesting because of the highly variable nature of medical conditions. The condition of a medical patient may not be as apparent as that of a trauma patient, and, therefore, treatment may not be as straightforward. You must remember that delays of any kind in an attempt to diagnose a condition can be harmful to the patient and thus are not recommended. Your best approach is to keep calm, use your patient assessment skills, treat the patient's symptoms, report to medical control, and transport the patient safely to the ED. Finally, keep in mind that patients sometimes have more than one problem, so you must be prepared to handle any combination of conditions, including conditions of medical patients who have been involved in traumatic situations.

## YOU are the Provider

With an estimated time of arrival at the hospital of 5 minutes, you reassess the patient and call in your radio report. The hospital acknowledges your report and is awaiting your arrival. The patient tells you that he feels better but is very thirsty. The patient is delivered to the hospital without incident, and you give your verbal report to a staff nurse, who assumes care of the patient. The receiving nurse reassesses the patient's temperature and notes a reading of 99.8°F (37.7°C). After cleaning the ambulance, you return to service.

| Recording Time: 21 Minutes | |
| --- | --- |
| Level of consciousness | Conscious and alert |
| Respiration | 18 breaths/min; regular and adequate |
| Pulse | 102 beats/min; strong and regular |
| Skin | Warm, dry; flushed |
| Blood pressure | 120/72 mm Hg |
| Spo$_2$ | 98% |

**7.** Do the patient's vital signs differ from your initial readings? If so, why might there be a difference?

## YOU are the Provider SUMMARY

**1. What observations should you make when you arrive at the scene before making physical contact with the patient?**

When arriving at any scene, your first priority is to assess for any actual or potential hazards that could pose a safety risk to you or your partners. Remember to use standard precautions before making contact with the patient! Additional precautions or protective equipment may be added based on the dispatch information or findings at the scene. Next, assess the environment in which the patient is found. As you approach the patient, form a general impression that will help you rapidly recognize life-threatening conditions even before making physical contact with the patient. Apparent unconsciousness, obvious external bleeding, and severe difficulty breathing are only a few of the visual clues that you may recognize during the initial general impression. After visually assessing the scene, the patient's environment, and the patient, proceed with the primary assessment.

**2. On the basis of your general impression and primary assessment findings, does this patient require immediate transport?**

Your patient is clearly sick; he has a fever and reports weakness. However, he is conscious and alert and does not have any airway, breathing, or circulation problems. His heart rate and respiratory rate are both increased; however, his heart rate is strong and palpable at the radial artery, and his breathing is producing adequate tidal volume. Tachypnea and tachycardia are common physiologic responses to fever. At the present time, there are no signs indicating the need for immediate transport, although his history of diabetes is an added reason for having him evaluated at the hospital.

**3. How should you proceed with your care of the patient?**

You have already determined the patient's chief complaint and have begun initial treatment. Because his condition is stable, immediate transport is not indicated; therefore, proceed by inquiring about the history of his present illness, taking his vital signs, obtaining a SAMPLE history, and performing a secondary assessment. The secondary assessment of a medical patient should primarily focus on his or her chief complaint and presenting signs and symptoms. A baseline set of vital signs—including pulse oximetry, and if indicated, a blood glucose level—may be obtained by your partner while you are assessing the patient. The baseline vital signs can then be compared with future readings (trending) to determine if the patient's condition is unchanged, has improved, or has worsened.

**4. Is it appropriate to transport the patient to the hospital he requested, or should you transport him to the closer facility?**

Generally, patients should be transported to the hospital of their choice when at all possible, especially if they have been there previously. Ultimately, however, the destination facility should be dictated by the patient's condition as well as local protocols and medical direction. Your patient is in stable condition—that is, he currently has no airway, breathing, or circulation problems. Therefore, it is not unreasonable to comply with his request and transport him to the hospital of his choice. However, you should inform him that that condition worsens, it may be necessary to divert to a closer facility. If his wife will be following you in her personal vehicle, ask for her mobile phone number, if she has one, so you can contact her should diversion to a closer facility become necessary. Documenting the reason for your transport destination choice can influence payment from insurers.

**5. Should you reassess his vital signs at shorter intervals? Why or why not?**

On the basis of your patient's stable condition, reassessing his vital signs every 15 minutes is appropriate at this time. If his condition worsens, you can always record his vital signs at shorter intervals. Vital signs are only one component of reassessment. You should also monitor the patient's level of consciousness and other parameters (eg, skin condition and temperature, breathing status, and pulse regularity and strength) en route. In many cases, these parameters change when a patient's condition is deteriorating even before the vital signs change.

**6. On the basis of the patient's chief complaint, what additional information can you obtain by using the OPQRST mnemonic?**

Not every component of the OPQRST mnemonic will apply to every patient; however, there are some components that will. Your patient's chief complaint was fever, diarrhea, and vomiting with weakness. An acute onset of fever versus fever that developed slowly is important to note and can aid the ED physician in his or her diagnosis, as well as

## YOU are the Provider SUMMARY *continued*

anything leading up to the event. The presence of provoking or palliating factors can also be established. In a patient with a fever, ask him or her if any antipyretics (fever-reducing medications), such as ibuprofen or acetaminophen, were taken and if they seemed to help. Ask if there is a particular position that improves or worsens his symptoms. In this case, the patient had taken ibuprofen, but there is no information on what the fever was prior to taking it, so its effectiveness is not as easy to determine. Although the patient did not report pain initially, you can ask if there is discomfort during vomiting or diarrhea episodes and what that feels like (quality). Radiating or referred pain would be less likely in this patient by history but may be discovered during palpation of the abdomen in the secondary exam. If the patient does have any pain or discomfort, ask the patient to assign it a number initially (severity) and then ask again at regular intervals. In this case, the patient did report some discomfort he rated as 2 out of 10 before he vomited, and it disappeared after the vomiting. When establishing the time of onset, you are asking for a specific time that the symptoms began (eg, yesterday around 1500 hours). If he is unable to give a specific time, he may be able to give a duration (eg, 8 hours) that he has been feeling ill.

**7. How and why do the patient's vital signs differ from your initial readings?**

The patient's blood pressure has remained consistent throughout your encounter with him. This is important as the patient is showing some signs of dehydration (thirst, dry mucus membranes). If there had been a large amount of vomiting, the blood pressure may have decreased and the pulse rate would have likely increased.

Fever can cause shivering, which causes the patient to expend a lot of energy and can make him or her feel weak. Fever also increases a person's metabolic rate, resulting in the production of more heat energy. Physiologically, the body responds to an increased metabolic rate by increasing its vital functions—namely, respirations and heart rate. Additionally, the heart rate and respirations may increase with vomiting episodes. As the temperature decreases after administration of an antipyretic, the heart rate and respiratory rate may decrease.

When a person is actively "running a fever," the skin is typically flushed (red), abnormally warm or hot, and dry. However, as the fever begins to subside, sweating usually occurs, which is the body's way of removing heat through evaporation. However, if as in this case, a person is dehydrated, perspiration cannot increase to cool the body.

### EMS Patient Care Report (PCR)

| Date: 7-29-20 | Incident No.: 011109 | Nature of Call: Sick person | | Location: 125 Green Hills Dr | |
|---|---|---|---|---|---|
| Dispatched: 1325 | En Route: 1325 | At Scene: 1335 | Transport: 1348 | At Hospital: 1402 | In Service: 1413 |

#### Patient Information

| | |
|---|---|
| **Age:** 36<br>**Sex:** M<br>**Weight (in kg [lb]):** 79 kg (175 lb) | **Allergies:** No known allergies<br>**Medications:** Ibuprofen, metformin (oral diabetic medication)<br>**Past Medical History:** Type 2 diabetes<br>**Chief Complaint:** Fever, diarrhea, and vomiting with weakness |

#### Vital Signs

| Time: 1340 | BP: 124/70 | Pulse: 110 | Respirations: 18 | Spo$_2$: 99% |
|---|---|---|---|---|
| Time: 1347 | BP: 122/68 | Pulse: 104 | Respirations: 22 | Spo$_2$: 98% |
| Time: 1356 | BP: 120/72 | Pulse: 102 | Respirations: 18 | Spo$_2$: 98% |

## YOU are the Provider SUMMARY continued

| EMS Treatment (circle all that apply) | | | | |
|---|---|---|---|---|
| Oxygen @ ___ L/min via:<br><br>NC   NRM   Bag mask | | Assisted Ventilation | Airway Adjunct | CPR |
| Defibrillation | Bleeding Control | Bandaging | Splinting | **Other:** Position of comfort |

| Narrative |
|---|

9-1-1 dispatch for a 36-year-old man with fever with diarrhea and vomiting.

Chief Complaint: Fever, diarrhea, vomiting, feeling weak

History: Patient stated that he began feeling bad the day before and began running a fever last night. He also reported diarrhea and vomiting all night and now feels a bit weak, but denied any other symptoms. Approximately 20 minutes prior to EMS arrival, patient took 400 mg of ibuprofen. His wife took his temperature just prior to EMS arrival and noted a reading of 100.6°F (38.1°C).

Assessment: On arrival at the scene, found the patient in a semisitting position in his bed. He was conscious and alert, his airway was patent, and his breathing was adequate. Obtained vital signs and performed additional assessment. Patient's skin was noted to be flushed, warm to touch and dry. His breath sounds were clear to auscultation bilaterally and he denied a cough. His abdomen was soft and nontender on palpation. He further denied any significant past medical history other than diabetes, for which he takes an oral diabetic medication. He stated he has no allergies to medications. A blood glucose reading of 242 mg/dL was obtained.

Treatment (Rx): None administered.

Transport: Patient took two steps with assistance from crew to the stretcher. Began transport to the hospital of patient's choice with the patient in position of comfort. En route, continued to monitor patient's condition and vital signs as indicated. He remained conscious and alert with little change in vital signs. Patient stated that he felt better but was very thirsty. He had one episode of vomiting which consisted of a small amount of clear yellow liquid. Remainder of transport was uneventful. Delivered patient to ED without incident and gave verbal report to staff nurse, Jimenez. Upon arrival, receiving nurse reassessed his temperature; a reading of 99.8°F (37.7°C) was noted. Medic 14 returned to service at 1413.

**End of report**

# Prep Kit

## Ready for Review

- Trauma emergencies are injuries that are the result of physical forces applied to the body. Medical emergencies require EMS attention because of illnesses or conditions not caused by an outside force.
- The assessment of a medical patient is similar to the assessment of a trauma patient but with a different focus. Whereas a trauma assessment focuses on physical injuries, some of which may be detectable by physical examination, medical patient assessment is usually more focused on symptoms and depends more on establishing an accurate medical history.
- Many seriously ill medical patients may not appear to be in critical condition at first glance.
- For conscious medical patients, obtaining a thorough patient history can be one of the most beneficial aspects of the patient assessment. Try to determine the NOI by asking questions about the patient's chief complaint.
- Conscious medical patients seldom need a secondary assessment of the entire body, but all should get a detailed physical examination based on their chief complaint. However, you should always perform a secondary assessment

of the entire body on unconscious patients; this head-to-toe assessment may give you clues to help identify the problem. Your secondary assessment of an unconscious or unstable patient should never delay transport.

- Most medical emergencies require a level of treatment beyond what is available in the pre-hospital setting. Also, the treatments depend on an accurate diagnosis of the exact medical condition; therefore, advanced testing in the hospital may be required.
- If the patient is not in critical condition, you should gather as much important information as possible from the scene so that you can transmit that information to the physician at the ED.
- Many medical emergency patients do not have immediately life-threatening conditions. If a life-threatening condition exists, transportation might be meaningfully expedited by the use of lights and siren, but if that is not the case, careful consideration should be given to nonemergency transport.
- Modes of transport ultimately come in one of two categories: ground or air.
- Many medical patients will benefit from being transported to a specific hospital capable of handling their particular condition.

- Because it is often impossible to tell which patients have infectious diseases, you should avoid direct contact with the blood and body fluids of all patients.
- If you think you may have been exposed to an infectious disease, see your physician (or your employer's designated physician) immediately.
- Seven infectious diseases of special concern are:
  - Influenza
  - HIV infection
  - Hepatitis
  - Meningitis
  - Tuberculosis
  - MERS-CoV
  - COVID-19
  - Ebola
- Infection control should be an important part of your daily routine. Be sure to follow the proper steps when dealing with potential exposure situations.
- Patients who recently traveled outside of the United States should be screened for possible infectious illnesses. If you suspect the patient has a travel-related illness, place a mask on him or her, follow appropriate PPE, and gather as much information as possible.

## Vital Vocabulary

**communicable disease** A disease that can be spread from one person or species to another.

**epidemic** Occurs when new cases of a disease in a human population substantially exceed the number expected based on recent experience.

**herpes simplex** A common virus that is asymptomatic in 80% of people carrying it, but characterized by small blisters on the lips or genitals in symptomatic infections.

**index of suspicion** Awareness that unseen life-threatening injuries or illness may exist.

**infectious disease** A medical condition caused by the growth and spread of small, harmful organisms within the body.

**influenza** A virus that has crossed the animal/human barrier and infected humans and that kills thousands of people every year.

**medical emergencies** Emergencies that are not caused by an outside force; illnesses or conditions.

**meningitis** An inflammation of the meningeal coverings of the brain and spinal cord; it is usually caused by a virus or a bacterium.

**meningococcal meningitis** An inflammation of the meningeal coverings of the brain and spinal cord; can be highly contagious.

**methicillin-resistant *Staphylococcus aureus* (MRSA)** A bacterium that can cause infections in different parts of the body and is often resistant to commonly used antibiotics; it is transmitted by different routes, including the respiratory route, and can be found on the skin, in surgical wounds, in the bloodstream, lungs, and urinary tract.

**nature of illness (NOI)**  The general type of illness a patient is experiencing.

**pandemic**  An outbreak that occurs on a global scale.

**trauma emergencies**  Emergencies that are the result of physical forces applied to the body; injuries.

**tuberculosis**  A chronic bacterial disease, caused by *Mycobacterium tuberculosis*, that usually affects the lungs but can also affect other organs such as the brain and kidneys; it is spread by cough and can lie dormant in a person's lungs for decades and then reactivate.

**virulence**  The strength or ability of a pathogen to produce disease.

# References

1. Bisaga A, Paquette K, Sabatini L, Lovell EO. A prevalence study of methicillin-resistant *Staphylococcus aureus* colonization in emergency department health care workers. *Ann Emerg Med*. 2008;52(5):525-528.

2. Carleton HA, Diep BA, Charlebois ED, Perdreau-Remington S, Perdeau-Remington F. Community-adapted methicillin-resistant *Staphylococcus aureus* (MRSA): population dynamics of an expanding community reservoir of MRSA. *J Infect Dis*. 2004;190(10):1730-1738.

3. Centers for Disease Control and Prevention. 2019 novel coronavirus. https://cdc.gov/coronavirus/2019-ncov/hcp/clinical-criterial.html? Accessed February 12, 2020.

4. Centers for Disease Control and Prevention. Disease burden of influenza. https://www.cdc.gov/flu/about/burden/index.html#:~:text=While%20the%20impact%20of%20flu,61%2C000%20deaths%20annually%20since%202010. Accessed March 5, 2020.

5. Centers for Disease Control and Prevention. What is sepsis? https://www.cdc.gov/sepsis/what-is-sepsis.html. Reviewed August 27, 2019. Accessed February 4, 2020.

6. Ellison RT. MRSA in healthcare workers. *NEJM Journal Watch*. http://www.jwatch.org/id200806250000001/2008/06/25/mrsa-healthcare-workers#sthash.yxYmywlv.dpuf. Published April 25, 2008. Accessed February 4, 2020.

7. MedlinePlus, United States National Library of Medicine. Malaise. https://medlineplus.gov/ency/article/003089.htm. Updated January 6, 2020. Accessed February 4, 2020.

8. National Highway Traffic Safety Administration. *National Emergency Medical Services Education Standards*. DOT HS 811 077A. ems.gov. www.ems.gov/pdf/811077a.pdf. Published January 2009. Accessed February 4, 2020.

9. National Highway Traffic Safety Administration. *National Emergency Medical Services Education Standards. Emergency Medical Technician Instructional Guidelines*. DOT HS 811 077C. ems.gov. www.ems.gov/pdf/811077c.pdf. Published January 2009. Accessed February 4, 2020.

10. Sepsis Alliance. What is sepsis? https://www.sepsis.org/sepsis-basics/what-is-sepsis/. Accessed February 4, 2020.

11. Suffoletto BP, Cannon EH, Ilkhanipour K, Yealy DM. Prevalence of *Staphylococcus aureus* nasal colonization in emergency department personnel. *Ann Emerg Med* 2008;52(5):529-533.

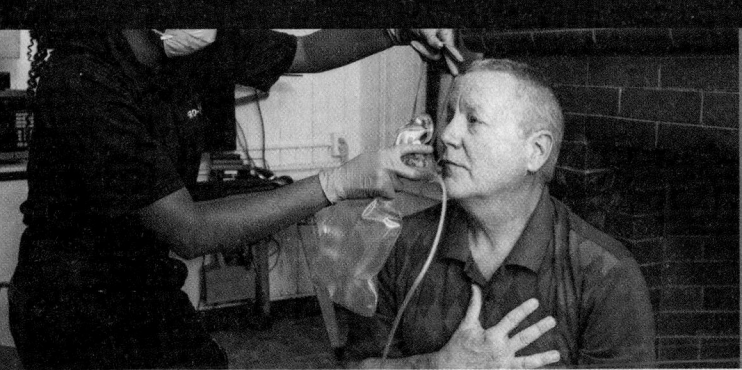

# Chapter 16

# Respiratory Emergencies

## EMS EDUCATION STANDARD COMPETENCIES

### Medicine
Applies fundamental knowledge to provide basic emergency care and transportation based on assessment findings for an acutely ill patient.

### Respiratory
Anatomy, signs, symptoms, and management of respiratory emergencies including those that affect the
- Upper airway (pp 628–638, 656–662)
- Lower airway (pp 628–638, 656–662)

Anatomy, physiology, pathophysiology, assessment, and management of
- Epiglottitis (pp 635, 648–656, 662)
- Spontaneous pneumothorax (pp 644, 648–656, 664)

- Pulmonary edema (pp 638–639, 648–656, 662–663)
- Asthma (pp 642–643, 648–656, 663–664)
- Chronic obstructive pulmonary disease (pp 639–641, 648–656, 663)
- Environmental/industrial exposure (pp 647–656, 665)
- Toxic gas (pp 647–656, 665)
- Pertussis (pp 636–637, 648–656)
- Cystic fibrosis (pp 648–656, 666–667)
- Pulmonary embolism (pp 645–646, 664)
- Pneumonia (pp 636, 648–656, 662)
- Viral respiratory infections (pp 634–637, 648–656, 662)

## KNOWLEDGE OBJECTIVES

1. List the structures and functions of the upper and lower airways, lungs, and accessory structures of the respiratory system. (pp 628–629)
2. Explain the physiology of respiration; include the signs of normal breathing. (pp 629–631)
3. Discuss the pathophysiology of respiration, including examples of the common signs and symptoms a patient with inadequate breathing may present with in an emergency situation. (pp 631–633)
4. Explain the special patient assessment and care considerations that are required for geriatric patients who are experiencing respiratory distress. (pp 633, 636–637, 665–667)

5. Describe different respiratory conditions that cause dyspnea, including their causes, assessment findings and symptoms, complications, and specific prehospital management and transport decisions. (pp 633–634, 656–667)
6. List the characteristics of infectious diseases that are frequently associated with dyspnea. (pp 634–638)
7. Discuss some pandemic considerations related to the spread of influenza type A and coronavirus and strategies EMTs should employ to protect themselves from infection during a possible crisis situation. (pp 634, 637)
8. Explain the special patient assessment and care considerations that are required for pediatric patients who are experiencing respiratory distress. (pp 634–638, 642, 662–667)

9. Describe the assessment of a patient who is in respiratory distress and the relationship of the assessment findings to patient management and transport decisions. (pp 648–655)

10. Describe the primary emergency medical care of a person who is in respiratory distress. (pp 648–651, 656–662)

11. List five different types of adventitious breath sounds, their signs and symptoms, and the disease process associated with each one. (p 651)

12. State the generic name, medication forms, dose, administration, indications, actions, and contraindications for medications that are administered via metered-dose inhalers (MDIs) and small-volume nebulizers. (pp 656–662)

## SKILLS OBJECTIVES

1. Demonstrate the process of history taking to obtain more information related to a patient's chief complaint based on a case scenario. (pp 651–653)

2. Demonstrate how to use the OPQRST assessment to obtain more specific information about a patient's breathing problem. (p 653)

3. Demonstrate how to use the PASTE assessment to obtain more specific information about a patient's breathing problem. (p 653)

4. Demonstrate how to assist a patient with the administration of a metered-dose inhaler. (pp 659–660, Skill Drill 16-1)

5. Demonstrate how to assist a patient with the administration of a small-volume nebulizer. (pp 659–662, Skill Drill 16-2)

# Introduction

As an EMT, you will often encounter the patient complaint of dyspnea, when a patient reports shortness of breath or has difficulty breathing. It is a symptom of many different conditions, from the common cold or asthma to heart failure or pulmonary embolism. You may not be able to determine what is causing dyspnea in a particular patient; this can be difficult even for physicians. Also, several different problems may be contributing to a patient's dyspnea at the same time, including some that are life threatening. Even without making a definitive diagnosis, you will often be able to improve the patient's symptoms or save the patient's life.

This chapter begins with a basic review of respiratory anatomy and physiology. The anatomy and physiology of the respiratory system are defined more thoroughly in Chapter 11, *Airway Management*. The chapter then looks at common medical problems that can impair normal respiratory functioning and cause dyspnea. Next, it explains specific strategies you can use to assess a patient who has difficulty breathing, using the patient assessment template and organized approach (established in Chapter 10, *Patient Assessment*. You will learn the signs and symptoms of each condition and cover topics such as foreign body and anatomic airway obstruction, lung infections, and chronic airway disease. You should keep all these medical possibilities in mind as you obtain the patient's history and perform a physical assessment; these processes will be described in detail in this chapter. The information you collect will help you to decide on the proper treatment, which can differ according to the probable cause of the dyspnea.

Remember, the sensation of not getting enough air can be terrifying, regardless of its cause. As an EMT, you should be prepared to fully treat your patient, addressing not just the symptom and the underlying problem, but also the anxiety it produces.

# Anatomy of the Respiratory System

The respiratory system consists of the structures of the body that contribute to the breathing process (**FIGURE 16-1**). These structures include the diaphragm, the muscles of the chest wall, the accessory muscles of breathing, and the nerves from the brain and spinal cord to those muscles.

The upper airway consists of all anatomic airway structures above the level of the vocal cords. These include the nose, mouth, jaw, oral cavity, pharynx, and larynx. Air enters the upper airway through the nose and mouth, and it is here that the

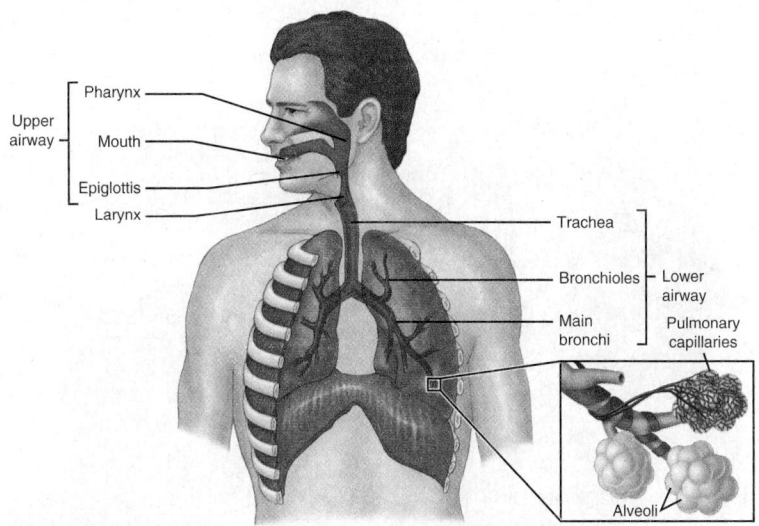

**FIGURE 16-1** The upper airway includes the nose, mouth, jaw, oral cavity, pharynx, and larynx. The lower airway includes the trachea, bronchi, bronchioles, and alveoli surrounded by the pulmonary capillaries.

© Jones & Bartlett Learning.

air is filtered, warmed, and humidified. The upper airway ends at the larynx, which is protected by the epiglottis. This leaf-shaped valve folds over the larynx during swallowing and diverts food and fluid into the esophagus. During normal breathing, the epiglottis returns to an upright position, allowing air to flow freely between the vocal cords into and out of the trachea. Air moves through the trachea into and out of the lungs.

The principal function of the lungs is **respiration**, which is the exchange of oxygen and carbon dioxide. To reach the lower airways, air travels through the trachea into each lung, first passing through the left and right main stem bronchus (larger airways), then on to the bronchioles (smaller airways), and finally into the alveoli. The alveoli are microscopic, thin-walled air sacs where the actual exchange of oxygen and carbon dioxide occurs.

## Physiology of Respiration

As discussed in Chapter 11, *Airway Management*, the two processes that occur during respiration are inspiration, the act of breathing in (inhaling), and expiration, the act of breathing out (exhaling). During respiration, oxygen is provided to the blood, and carbon dioxide is removed from it. In healthy lungs, this exchange of gases takes place rapidly at the level of the alveoli (**FIGURE 16-2**). The alveoli lie against the pulmonary capillary vessels, and as oxygen enters the alveoli from inhalation, it passes freely through tiny passages in the alveolar wall into these capillaries through the process of diffusion. The oxygen bonds to the hemoglobin in the red blood cells and is carried to the heart, which then pumps the oxygen-rich blood around the body. Carbon dioxide produced by the body's

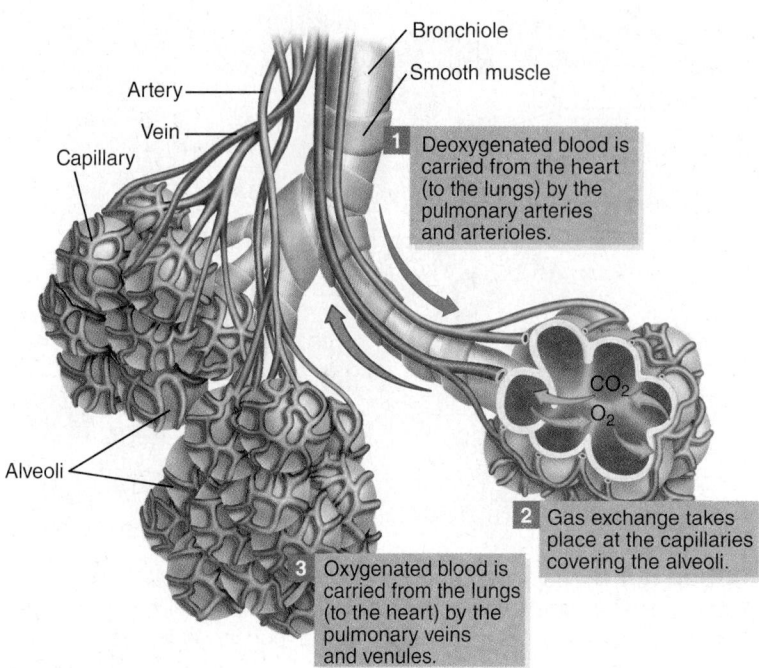

**FIGURE 16-2** An enlarged view of a single alveolus (air sac) showing where the exchange of oxygen and carbon dioxide between air in the sac and blood in the pulmonary capillaries takes place.

© Jones & Bartlett Learning.

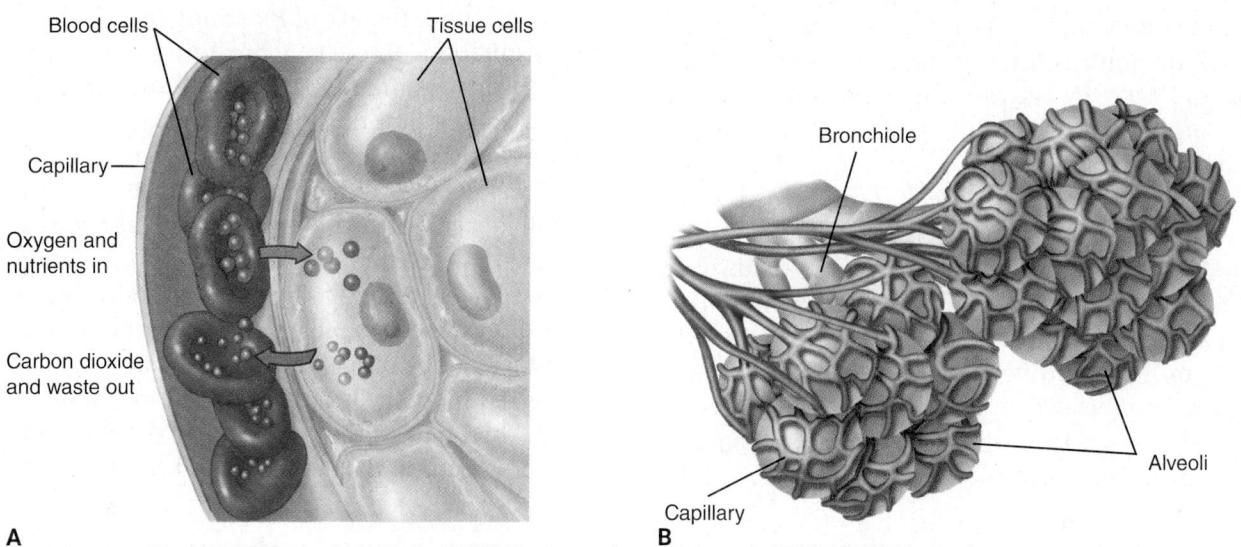

**FIGURE 16-3** The exchange of oxygen and carbon dioxide in the tissues. **A.** Oxygen passes from the blood through capillaries to tissue cells. Carbon dioxide passes from tissue cells through capillaries to the blood. **B.** In the lungs, oxygen is picked up by the blood, and carbon dioxide is given off.

A, B, C: © Jones & Bartlett Learning.

cells returns to the lungs in the blood that circulates through and around the alveolar air spaces. The carbon dioxide diffuses back into the alveoli and travels back up the bronchial tree and out through the upper airways during exhalation (**FIGURE 16-3**). Again, carbon dioxide is exchanged for oxygen, which travels in the opposite direction (during inhalation).

Throughout the whole process of respiration, the brainstem constantly senses the level of carbon dioxide in the arterial blood. The level of carbon dioxide bathing the brainstem stimulates a healthy person to breathe. If the level of carbon dioxide drops too low, the person automatically breathes at a slower rate and less deeply. As a result, less carbon dioxide is expired, allowing carbon dioxide levels in the blood to return to normal. Although considered a waste gas, some level of carbon dioxide in the blood is necessary: In addition to stimulating breathing, it helps balance the pH level. If the level of carbon dioxide in the arterial blood rises above normal, the person breathes more rapidly and more deeply. When more fresh air is brought into the alveoli, more carbon dioxide diffuses out of the bloodstream, thereby lowering the level of carbon dioxide in the blood.

## Pathophysiology

The pathophysiology of respiration refers to conditions under which body processes are not working as they should and, as a result, interfere with normal respiration. Abnormal or pathologic conditions in the anatomy of the airway, disease processes, and traumatic conditions can prevent the proper exchange of oxygen and carbon dioxide. In addition, the pulmonary blood vessels themselves may have abnormalities that interfere with blood flow and thus with the transfer of gases.

Regardless of the reason for breathing difficulty, it is important that you are able to immediately recognize the signs and symptoms of inadequate breathing and know what to do about it. **TABLE 16-1** gives the signs of normal (adequate) breathing, which is measured by rate, rhythm, and quality. **TABLE 16-2** lists the clues that will help you determine if your patient is having difficulty breathing. **TABLE 16-3** provides key signs and symptoms to help you recognize and differentiate between various respiratory-related complaints.

### Carbon Dioxide Retention and Hypoxic Drive

You will sometimes encounter patients who have an elevated level of carbon dioxide in their arterial blood. The level can rise for many reasons. The exhalation process may be impaired by various types of

---

**TABLE 16-1 Signs of Normal Breathing**

- A normal rate (adult: 12 to 20 breaths/min; child: 15 to 30 breaths/min; infant: 30 to 60 breaths/min)
- A regular pattern of inhalation and exhalation
- Clear and equal breath sounds on both sides of the chest
- Regular and equal chest rise (chest expansion) and fall
- Adequate depth (tidal volume)
- Unlabored; without adventitious (abnormal) breath sounds (wheezing, stridor)

*Note:* Respiratory ranges are per the Model EMS Clinical Guidelines and the American Heart Association. Ranges presented in other sources may vary.

© Jones & Bartlett Learning.

---

**TABLE 16-2 Signs and Symptoms of Inadequate Breathing**

- The patient reports difficulty breathing or shortness of breath.
- The patient has an altered mental status associated with shallow or slow breathing.
- The adult patient appears anxious or restless; the pediatric patient appears sleepy or listless.
- The respiratory rate is too fast or too slow (see Table 16-1).
- The breathing rhythm is irregular.
- The skin is pale, cool, clammy, or cyanotic.
- Adventitious breath sounds are heard, including wheezing, gurgling, snoring, crowing, or stridor (harsh, high-pitched, barking sounds).
- Decreased or noisy breath sounds are heard on one or both sides of the chest.
- The patient cannot speak more than a few words between breaths. Ask the patient, "How are you doing?" If the patient cannot speak at all, he or she most likely has a respiratory emergency.
- You observe accessory muscle use, retractions, or labored breathing.
- The patient has unequal or inadequate chest expansion.
- The patient is coughing excessively.
- The patient is sitting up, leaning forward with his or her palms flat on the bed or the arms of the chair. This is called the tripod position because the patient's back and both arms are working together to support the upper body.
- The patient has pursed lips (pursed lip breathing) or nasal flaring.

© Jones & Bartlett Learning.

**TABLE 16-3** Signs and Symptoms Seen in Various Respiratory Conditions

| Condition | Signs and Symptoms | Condition | Signs and Symptoms |
|---|---|---|---|
| Asthma | • Wheezing on inspiration/expiration<br>• Bronchospasm | Epiglottitis | • Dyspnea<br>• High fever<br>• Stridor<br>• Drooling<br>• Difficulty swallowing<br>• Severe sore throat<br>• Tripod or sniffing position<br>• Mostly seen in pediatric patients |
| Anaphylaxis | • Flushed skin or hives (urticaria)<br>• Generalized edema<br>• Decreased blood pressure (hypotension)<br>• Laryngeal edema with dyspnea<br>• Wheezing or stridor | | |
| | | Influenza type A (flu) | • Cough<br>• Fever<br>• Sore throat<br>• Fatigue |
| Bronchiolitis | • Shortness of breath<br>• Wheezing<br>• Coughing<br>• Fever<br>• Dehydration<br>• Tachypnea<br>• Tachycardia | Pertussis (whooping cough) | • Coughing spells<br>• "Whooping" sound<br>• Fever |
| **Bronchitis** | • Chronic cough (with sputum production)<br>• Wheezing<br>• Cyanosis<br>• Tachypnea (increased breathing rate) | Pneumonia | • Dyspnea<br>• Chills, fever<br>• Cough<br>• Green, red, or rust-colored sputum<br>• Localized wheezing or crackles |
| Congestive heart failure | • Dependent (lower extremity) edema<br>• Crackles (pulmonary edema)<br>• **Orthopnea**<br>• **Paroxysmal nocturnal dyspnea** | Pneumothorax | • Sudden chest pain with dyspnea<br>• Decreased breath sounds (affected side)<br>• Subcutaneous emphysema |
| Common cold | • Cough<br>• Runny or stuffy nose<br>• Sore throat | Pulmonary embolus | • Dyspnea<br>• Occasionally will have sharp chest pain<br>• Sudden onset<br>• Tachycardia<br>• Clear breath sounds initially |
| COVID-19 | • Cough<br>• Fever<br>• Dyspnea<br>• Chest pain<br>• Anosmia (inability to smell) | | |
| Croup | • Fever<br>• Barking cough<br>• Stridor<br>• Mostly seen in pediatric patients | Tension pneumothorax | • Severe shortness of breath<br>• Diminished or absent breath sounds on one side<br>• Decreased/altered level of consciousness<br>• Neck vein distention<br>• Tracheal deviation (late sign)<br>• Hypotension; signs of shock |
| **Diphtheria** | • Difficulty breathing and swallowing<br>• Sore throat<br>• Thick, gray buildup in throat or nose<br>• Fever | | |
| | | Respiratory syncytial virus (RSV) | • Cough<br>• Wheezing<br>• Fever<br>• Dehydration |
| Emphysema | • Barrel chest<br>• Pursed lip breathing<br>• Dyspnea on exertion<br>• Cyanosis<br>• Wheezing/decreased breath sounds<br>• Mostly seen in older patients | Tuberculosis (TB) | • Cough<br>• Fever<br>• Fatigue<br>• Productive/bloody sputum |

lung disease. The body may also produce too much carbon dioxide, either temporarily or chronically, depending on the disease or abnormality. If, for a period of years, arterial carbon dioxide levels rise to an abnormally high level and remain there, the respiratory centers in the brain, which sense the carbon dioxide level and control breathing, may work less efficiently.

The failure of these centers to respond normally to a rise in arterial levels of carbon dioxide is due to chronic **carbon dioxide retention**. Normally, the brain senses the levels of carbon dioxide (based on the pH) in the blood and cerebrospinal fluid. (See Chapter 11, *Airway Management*.) When carbon dioxide levels become elevated, the respiratory centers in the brain adjust the rate and depth of **ventilation** accordingly. However, patients with chronic lung diseases have difficulty eliminating carbon dioxide through exhalation; thus, they always have higher levels of carbon dioxide. This condition potentially alters their drive for breathing. The theory is that the brain gradually accommodates high levels of carbon dioxide and then uses a backup system to control breathing based on low levels of oxygen, rather than high levels of carbon dioxide. This condition is called **hypoxic drive**.

Hypoxic drive is frequently found in end-stage chronic obstructive pulmonary disease (COPD). Some experts advocate withholding high concentrations of oxygen, for extended periods of time, from patients with chronic lung diseases for fear that the increased oxygen level in the blood could depress, or completely stop, the patient's respiratory drive. Use caution when providing high concentrations of oxygen on a long-term basis to patients with chronic lung disease, but *never* withhold oxygen therapy from a patient who needs it. Closely monitor patients who are experiencing respiratory distress and be prepared to assist with ventilations if needed.

## Special Populations

As a result of the normal aging process, geriatric patients may have greater difficulties with the exchange of carbon dioxide and oxygen. In respiratory emergencies, begin oxygen therapy early in the assessment and treatment process.

## Words of Wisdom

It is important for you to properly ventilate a patient; both underventilation and overventilation can cause harmful alterations in the level of carbon dioxide in the blood. Avoid hyperventilation when performing bag-mask ventilation during CPR. This is a common pitfall that detracts from the overall quality of CPR and can cause serious alterations in pH, increased intrathoracic pressure, impaired venous return, and hypotension.

## Causes of Dyspnea

Many medical problems may cause dyspnea. Be aware that if the patient's problem is severe and the brain is deprived of oxygen, he or she may not be alert enough to report shortness of breath. Altered mental status may be a sign that the brain is dysfunctional because of severe **hypoxia**, a condition in which the body's cells and tissues do not get enough oxygen.

In addition to the conditions discussed in Table 16-3, patients often have breathing difficulty and/or hypoxia with the following medical conditions:

- Pulmonary edema
- Hay fever
- Pleural effusion
- Obstruction of the airway
- Hyperventilation syndrome
- Environmental/industrial exposure
- Carbon monoxide poisoning
- Drug overdose

As you treat patients with disorders of the lungs, be aware that one or more of the following situations most likely exists:

- Gas exchange between the alveoli and pulmonary circulation is obstructed by fluid in the lung, infection, or collapsed alveoli (**atelectasis**).
- The alveoli are damaged and cannot transport gases properly across their own walls.
- The air passages are obstructed by muscle spasm, mucus, or weakened airway walls.
- Blood flow to the lungs is obstructed by blood clots.
- The pleural space is filled with air or excess fluid, so the lungs cannot properly expand.

All of these conditions prevent the proper exchange of oxygen and carbon dioxide. In addition, the pulmonary blood vessels themselves may have abnormalities that interfere with blood flow and thus with the transfer of gases.

Besides shortness of breath, a patient with dyspnea may report the sensation of chest tightness and air hunger. Air hunger is when a person reports the feeling of "not getting enough air" and has a strong need to breathe. Chest tightness is described as an uncomfortable feeling in the chest, and it is commonly reported by patients with asthma.

Dyspnea is also a common complaint in patients with cardiopulmonary diseases. In some cases, it may be caused by physical exertion that has been made difficult because the patient's heart is damaged. Congestive heart failure is a troublesome cause of breathlessness because the heart is not pumping efficiently and, therefore, the body does not have adequate oxygen. Another condition commonly associated with congestive heart failure is pulmonary edema, in which the alveoli are filled with fluid.

Severe pain can cause a patient to experience rapid, shallow breathing without the presence of a primary pulmonary dysfunction. In some patients, breathing deeply causes pain because it causes expansion of the chest wall.

When you assess your patient for complaints of dyspnea, ask about chest pain; conversely, when you are evaluating your patient for chest pain, ask about dyspnea.

## Upper or Lower Airway Infection

Infectious diseases causing dyspnea may affect all parts of the airway. Some cause mild discomfort; others require aggressive respiratory support. Infections that impair airflow through the airways are problems of respiration. Inadequate oxygen delivery to the tissues is a problem of oxygenation. Infections may cause dyspnea by obstructing airflow in the larger airways due to production of mucus and secretions (colds, diphtheria) or by causing swelling of soft tissues located in the larger, upper airways (epiglottitis, croup). Infections may also impair the exchange of gases between the alveoli and the capillaries (pneumonia). In patients with infectious

diseases, you will be in close contact, so be diligent about your use of appropriate personal protective equipment (PPE), including a mask and face shield. Immunizations, protective techniques, and handwashing can dramatically minimize your risk of contracting an infectious disease. See Chapter 2, *Workforce Safety and Wellness*, for more information on protecting yourself from infection. Follow your local protocols, and stay up to date on the latest Centers for Disease Control and Prevention (CDC) recommendations. A minimum of gloves, eye protection, and a surgical mask or a high-efficiency air particulate (N-95) respirator should be mandatory. Place a surgical mask on patients with suspected or confirmed respiratory disease. Remember to completely disinfect your unit prior to returning to service.

### Street Smarts

Placing a surgical mask on a patient with respiratory disease may make the person feel even more short of breath and uncomfortable. Be sensitive to these feelings, and always ensure the patient is receiving adequate oxygen and ventilations.

The following sections discuss some of the infectious diseases that may be associated with complaints of dyspnea.

## Croup

Croup is caused by inflammation and swelling of the pharynx, larynx, and trachea (**FIGURE 16-4**). This disease is often secondary to an acute viral infection of the upper respiratory tract and is typically seen in children between ages 6 months and 3 years. It is easily passed between children. Peak seasonal outbreaks of this disease occur in the late fall and during the winter.

The disease starts with a cold, cough, and a low-grade fever that develops over a few days. The hallmark signs of croup are stridor and a seal-bark cough, which signal a narrowing of the air passage of the trachea that may progress to significant obstruction.

Croup is rarely seen in adults because their breathing passages are larger and can accommodate

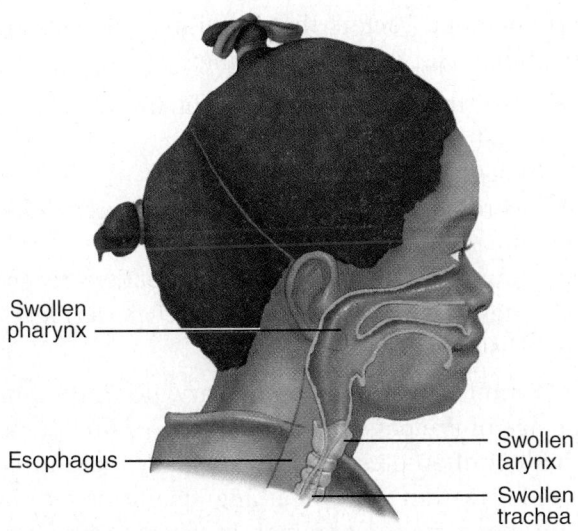

Swollen pharynx

Esophagus

Swollen larynx

Swollen trachea

**FIGURE 16-4** Croup results in swelling of the whole airway: pharynx, larynx, and trachea.

© Jones & Bartlett Learning.

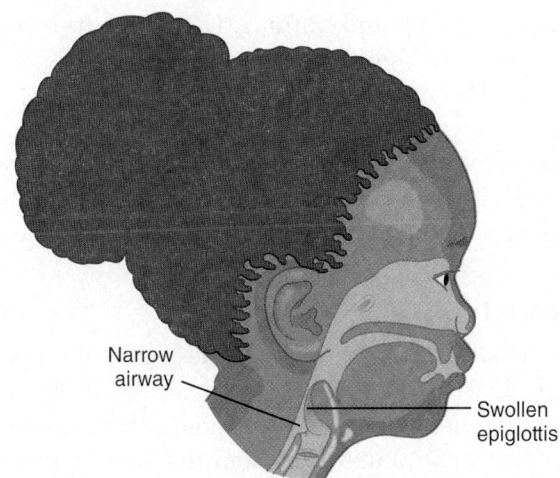

Narrow airway

Swollen epiglottis

**FIGURE 16-5** Acute epiglottitis is caused by a bacterial infection that results in severe swelling of the epiglottis, which could obstruct the airway.

© Jones & Bartlett Learning.

the inflammation and mucus production without producing symptoms. The airways of adults are wider, and the supporting tissue is firmer than in children.

Croup often responds well to the administration of humidified oxygen. Note that bronchodilators are not indicated for croup and can worsen a patient's symptoms.

## Epiglottitis

**Epiglottitis** is a life-threatening inflammatory disease of the epiglottis, the small flap of tissue at the back of the throat that protects the larynx and trachea during swallowing. Bacterial infection is the most common cause (**FIGURE 16-5**). In the past, epiglottitis was most often seen in infants and children. In some cases, it occurs in adults. The development of a childhood vaccine against *Haemophilus influenzae* has dramatically decreased the incidence of this disease.

In preschool and school-age children especially, the epiglottis can swell to two to three times its normal size. This puts the airway at risk of complete obstruction. The condition usually develops in otherwise healthy children, and symptoms are sudden in onset. Children with this infection look ill, report a very sore throat, and have a high fever. They will often be found in the tripod position and

drooling. Stridor is a late sign in the development of airway obstruction.

Treat children with suspected epiglottitis gently and try not to do anything that will cause them to cry. Keep them in a position of comfort, and give them high-flow oxygen. *Do not* put anything in their mouths, as this could trigger a complete airway obstruction.

Deterioration can occur quickly in adults with acute epiglottitis. You should be concerned if your adult patient presents with stridor or any other sign of airway obstruction without an obvious mechanical cause. Focus your patient management on maintaining a patent (adequate) airway, and provide prompt transport to the emergency department (ED).

## Respiratory Syncytial Virus

**Respiratory syncytial virus (RSV)** is a common cause of illness in young children. It causes an infection in the lungs and breathing passages, and can lead to other serious illnesses such as bronchiolitis and pneumonia, as well as serious heart and lung problems in premature infants and in children who have depressed immune systems.

RSV is highly contagious and can be spread through droplets when the patient coughs or sneezes. The virus can also survive on surfaces, including hands and clothing. Therefore, the infection tends to spread rapidly through schools and child care centers.

When you assess a child with suspected RSV, look for signs of dehydration. Infants with RSV often refuse liquids. Treat airway and breathing problems as appropriate. Humidified oxygen is helpful if available.

## Bronchiolitis

Bronchiolitis is a respiratory illness that often occurs due to RSV infection and results in severe inflammation of the bronchioles. Bronchioles, the tiny airways that lead from the larger airways (bronchi) to the alveoli in the lungs, become inflamed, swell, and fill with mucus. This condition occurs most frequently in newborns and toddlers, especially boys, whose airways can easily become blocked. Infections are common during the winter and spring. Young children who require hospitalization for bronchiolitis are at increased risk for developing childhood asthma.

The treatment for a child suffering from bronchiolitis is mainly supportive. Although many of these patients do well, there is still a risk for significant respiratory compromise. You should provide appropriate oxygen therapy and allow the patient to remain in a position of comfort. Suction thick mucus from the nostrils if present. Reassess frequently for signs of worsening respiratory distress. Be prepared to provide airway management and positive-pressure ventilation should the patient develop respiratory failure.

## Pneumonia

According to the World Health Organization, pneumonia is a significant cause of morbidity worldwide. Pneumonia is a general term that refers to an infection of the lungs. The infection collects in the surrounding normal lung tissues, impairing the lung's ability to exchange oxygen and carbon dioxide.

Pneumonia is often a secondary infection, meaning it begins after an upper respiratory tract infection such as a cold or sore throat. It can be caused by a virus or bacterium, or by a chemical injury after an accidental ingestion or a direct lung injury from a submersion incident. Interventions such as intubation and tracheostomy can increase the risk of developing pneumonia. Pneumonia commonly affects people who are chronically and terminally ill. Factors that predispose patients to pneumonia include the following:

- Institutional residence (nursing home or long-term care facilities)
- Recent hospitalization
- Chronic disease processes (such as renal failure requiring dialysis)
- Immune system compromise (patient receiving chemotherapy or diseases such as HIV)
- History of COPD

Symptoms of pneumonia vary, depending on the age of the person and the cause of the illness. Children often present with unusually rapid or labored breathing or breathing characterized by grunting or wheezing sounds. In severe cases where oxygen exchange at the alveoli is markedly impaired, the lips and fingernails may be blue or gray. If the pneumonia is in the lower part of the lungs near the abdomen, there may be fever, abdominal pain, and vomiting rather than dyspnea.

Bacterial pneumonia results in severe symptoms more quickly, including high fevers, which put the child at risk for febrile seizures. A viral pneumonia presents more gradually and is less severe.

Other signs and symptoms include dry skin, decreased skin turgor, exertional dyspnea, a productive cough, chest discomfort or pain that varies with inspiration and expiration, headache, nausea and vomiting, musculoskeletal pain, weight loss, and confusion. The patient may be febrile, tachycardic, or even hypotensive. Assessment of the lungs may reveal diminished breath sounds, along with the presence of wheezing, crackles, or rhonchi. You will need to evaluate the patient's history for possible risk factors. If possible, assess temperature to determine the presence of fever. Pulse oximetry readings, if available, may be low.

Regardless of the cause, treatment includes airway support and providing supplemental oxygen. Use oxygen with appropriate adjuncts, and provide supportive measures if needed. Evaluate patient treatment through reassessment, and prepare for possible deterioration in the patient's condition.

## Pertussis

Pertussis (whooping cough) is an airborne bacterial infection that primarily affects children younger than 6 years. It is highly contagious and is passed through droplet infection.

A patient with pertussis will be feverish and exhibit a "whoop" sound on inspiration after a coughing attack. Symptoms are generally similar to colds, but coughing spells can last for more than 1 minute, during which the child may turn red or purple. This may frighten the parents or caregivers into calling 9-1-1.

Some infants and younger children with pertussis should be treated in a hospital because they are at greater risk for complications such as pneumonia, which occurs mostly in children younger than 1 year. In infants younger than 6 months, pertussis can be life threatening.

Children with pertussis may vomit or not want to eat or drink. Watch for signs of dehydration. You may have to suction thick secretions to clear the airway. Give oxygen by the most appropriate means.

Pertussis can also occur in adults either because they were not vaccinated as children, or more commonly because the vaccine did not confer life-long immunity. When it does occur, it can cause a severe upper respiratory infection, which can lead to pneumonia in geriatric patients or people with compromised immune systems. The infection can cause coughing spells that last for weeks and can be so severe that patients find it hard to breathe, eat, or sleep. In the worst cases of infection, particularly in geriatric patients, coughing can lead to cracked ribs. For patients who are already weak from other chronic conditions, pertussis can lead to hospitalization. According to the CDC, the disease has become a serious issue and physicians are becoming more aggressive about immunizing adults with the pertussis vaccine.

## Influenza Type A

**Influenza type A** is an animal respiratory disease that has mutated to infect humans. In 2009, the H1N1 strain of influenza type A became **pandemic** (an outbreak that occurred on a global scale). Like seasonal flu, it may make chronic medical conditions worse. All strains of influenza type A are transmitted by direct contact with nasal secretions and aerosolized droplets from coughing and sneezing by infected people. Influenza type A viruses cause fever, cough, sore throat, muscle aches, headache, and fatigue and may lead to pneumonia or dehydration.

## COVID-19 (SARS-CoV-2)

**COVID-19** is a respiratory disease caused by the virus SARS-CoV-2. The virus is a coronavirus, similar to the one that causes the common cold. It is believed to have initially been native to bats and transferred to humans by contact in an open-livestock meat market in Wuhan, China, in 2019. Because the virus is extremely contagious, it spread rapidly across the entire world, creating a severe pandemic that resulted in hundreds of thousands of deaths worldwide. The virus preferentially affects the elderly, patients living in close quarters with one another, and those with weakened immune systems, but it has also sickened and even killed many people who were otherwise young and healthy.

COVID-19 is transmitted by aerosol droplets, through airborne particles generated by sneezing or coughing, and by direct contact. The virus can survive on surfaces for several days. Symptoms include high fever, cough, chest pain during inspiration, vomiting and diarrhea, and anosmia (inability to smell). Respiratory deterioration in these patients can be dramatic and rapid.

## Tuberculosis

**Tuberculosis (TB)** is a bacterial infection caused by *Mycobacterium tuberculosis*. TB spreads by cough and is dangerous because many strains are resistant to antibiotics. TB most commonly affects the lungs but can also be found in almost any organ of the body, particularly the kidneys, spine, and lining of the brain and spinal cord (meninges). In some cases, TB can remain dormant (inactive) for years without causing symptoms or being infectious to other people. However, when the person is in a state of weakened immunity, TB can become active again. The patient may not even be aware he or she has the disease.

Patients with active TB involving the lungs will report fever, coughing, fatigue, night sweats, and weight loss. If the lung infection becomes severe, the patient will experience shortness of breath, coughing, productive sputum, bloody sputum, and chest pain.

TB has a higher prevalence among people who live in close contact, such as prison inmates, nursing home residents, and people in homeless shelters. TB is also found in people who abuse intravenous drugs or alcohol and people whose immune systems are compromised by an infection such as HIV. Anyone who comes into close contact with people who have active TB or is in contact with people from countries that have a high prevalence of TB is at risk for contracting the disease. As an EMT, you are also at risk.

If you suspect your patient may have active TB, you need to wear (at a minimum) your gloves, eye protection, and an N-95 respirator. These respirators are fit-tested to the individual to ensure no contaminated air can pass through. Also place a surgical mask or oxygen mask on the patient.

## Acute Pulmonary Edema

Sometimes, the heart muscle is so injured after a heart attack or other illness that it cannot circulate blood properly. In these cases, the left side of the heart cannot remove blood from the lung as fast as the right side delivers it. As a result, fluid builds up within the alveoli and in the lung tissue between the alveoli and the pulmonary capillaries. This accumulation of fluid is referred to as **pulmonary edema**, and it is usually a result of congestive heart failure. By physically separating the alveoli from the pulmonary capillary vessels, the edema interferes with the exchange of carbon dioxide and oxygen (**FIGURE 16-6**). High blood pressure and low cardiac output often trigger this flash (sudden) pulmonary edema. These patients are among the most sick, frightened, and worrisome patients you will encounter. They are literally drowning in their own fluid. The patient usually experiences dyspnea with rapid, shallow respirations. In the most severe cases, you will see frothy pink sputum at the nose and mouth.

Patient risk factors for congestive heart failure include hypertension and a history of coronary artery

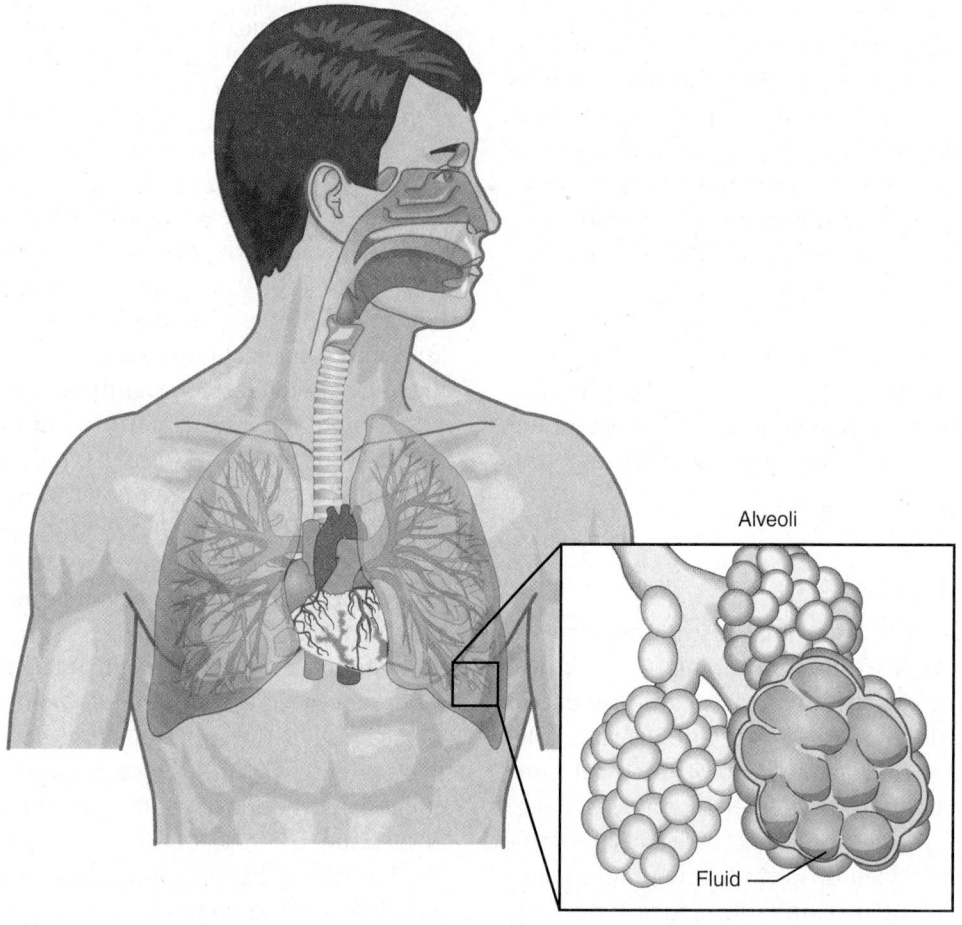

Alveoli

Fluid

**FIGURE 16-6** In pulmonary edema, fluid fills the alveoli and separates the capillaries from the alveolar wall, interfering with the exchange of oxygen and carbon dioxide.

disease and/or atrial fibrillation, a condition in which the atria no longer contract, but instead quiver.

Congestive heart failure (which can lead to pulmonary edema) is often cited as one of the most common causes of hospital admission in the United States. It is not uncommon for a patient to have repeated bouts. In most cases, patients have a long-standing history of chronic congestive heart failure that can be kept under control with medication. However, an acute onset may occur if the patient stops taking the medication, eats food that is too salty, or has a stressful illness, a new heart attack, or an abnormal heart rhythm.

However, not all patients with pulmonary edema have heart disease. Poisonings from inhaling large amounts of smoke or toxic chemical fumes can produce pulmonary edema, as can traumatic injuries of the chest and exposure to high altitudes. In these cases, fluid collects in the alveoli and lung tissue in response to damage to the tissues of the lung or the bronchi.

Signs and symptoms of congestive heart failure include difficulty breathing with exertion because the heart cannot keep up with the body's need for oxygen. Patients may also report a sudden attack of respiratory distress that wakes them at night when they are in a reclining position. This is caused by fluid accumulation in the lungs. Patients also report coughing, feeling suffocated, cold sweats, and tachycardia.

In your primary assessment, you might find the patient has cool, diaphoretic, cyanotic skin and you will hear adventitious breath sounds such as crackles or wheezing. The patient's pulse will be tachycardic. The patient may have hypertension early, followed by deterioration to hypotension as a late finding.

## Chronic Obstructive Pulmonary Disease

Chronic obstructive pulmonary disease (COPD), according to the World Health Organization, is a lung disease characterized by chronic obstruction of lung airflow that interferes with normal breathing and is not fully reversible. According to the US Department of Health and Human Services, COPD has been diagnosed in approximately 16 million people, and millions more people have COPD and do not know it. According to the CDC, it is the fourth leading cause of death in the United States.

COPD is an umbrella term used to describe several lung diseases, including emphysema and chronic bronchitis, an ongoing irritation of the trachea and bronchi.

COPD may be a result of direct lung and airway damage from repeated infections or inhalation of toxic gases and particles, but most often it results from cigarette smoking. Although it is well known that cigarettes are a direct cause of lung cancer, their role in the development of COPD is far more significant and less publicized.

Tobacco smoke is a bronchial irritant and can create chronic bronchitis. With bronchitis, excess mucus is constantly produced, obstructing small airways and alveoli. Protective cells and lung mechanisms that remove foreign particles are destroyed, further weakening the airways. Chronic oxygenation problems can also lead to right-side heart failure and fluid retention, such as edema in the legs.

Pneumonia develops easily when the air passages are persistently obstructed. Ultimately, repeated episodes of irritation and pneumonia cause scarring in the lungs and some dilation of the obstructed alveoli, leading to COPD (**FIGURE 16-7**).

The most common form of COPD is emphysema. Emphysema is a loss of the elastic material in the lungs that occurs when the alveolar air spaces are chronically stretched due to inflamed airways and obstruction of airflow out of the lungs. Smoking can also directly destroy the elasticity of the lung tissue. Normally, the lungs act like spongy balloons that are inflated; once they are inflated, they will naturally recoil because of their elastic nature, expelling gas rapidly. However, when they are constantly obstructed or when the elasticity is diminished, air is no longer expelled rapidly, and the walls of the alveoli eventually fall apart, leaving large holes in the lung that resemble large air pockets or cavities.

Most patients with COPD have elements of both chronic bronchitis and emphysema. Some patients will have more elements of one condition than the other; few patients will have only emphysema or bronchitis. Therefore, most patients with COPD will chronically produce sputum, have a chronic cough, and have difficulty expelling air from their lungs, with long expiration phases and wheezing. Patients may present with adventitious breath sounds such as crackles, rhonchi, and wheezes, or may have severely diminished breath sounds due to poor air movement.

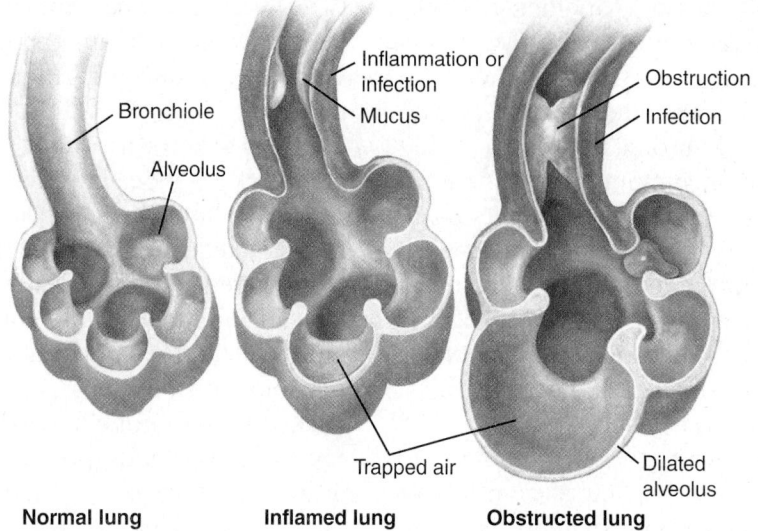

**FIGURE 16-7** Repeated episodes of irritation and inflammation in the alveoli result in the obstruction, scarring, and some dilation of the alveolar sac characteristic of COPD.

© Jones & Bartlett Learning.

## Wet Lungs Versus Dry Lungs and Cardiac Asthma

Be aware that the signs and symptoms of COPD and congestive heart failure significantly overlap. Many patients suffer from both diseases, and it is often difficult to determine which disease is causing the patient's shortness of breath; often these patients are treated for both diseases after arrival to the hospital. Lung sounds (discussed later in the chapter) are one way to help you tell the difference. Patients with pulmonary edema caused most often by congestive heart failure will often have wet lung sounds (crackles), and patients with COPD will often have dry lung sounds (wheezes). However, do not assume *all* patients with COPD have wheezes and *all* congestive heart failure patients have crackles. **TABLE 16-4** compares COPD and congestive heart failure.

Suppose you are called to assist an 80-year-old man who has experienced shortness of breath for 45 minutes. Physical examination reveals that his pulse and respirations are elevated, and you observe pedal edema (swollen legs and feet) and jugular vein distention. His lung sound check reveals wheezing. He has a history of hypertension, congestive heart failure, and myocardial infarction; however, he has no history of smoking, asthma, or COPD. What is your initial general impression?

This patient's elevated blood pressure, pedal edema, jugular vein distention, and history of congestive heart failure should lead you in the direction of congestive heart failure. Unlike a typical patient with COPD, he has no history of smoking and takes diuretics and medication for hypertension. In this case, the alveoli are so full of fluid that bubbles (the condition that gives the sound of crackles) cannot form. The bronchi also become constricted, which produces wheezing. The wheezing this patient is experiencing is called cardiac asthma, which is not a form of asthma, but rather a type of coughing or wheezing that occurs with left-side heart failure.

Patients with COPD wheeze because of bronchial constriction and present with shortness of breath. Their breathing gets progressively worse, and they have the most trouble breathing on exertion. Patients with COPD have chronic coughing and thick sputum. They are usually long-term smokers with a thin, barrel chest appearance. Their medications would include home oxygen, bronchodilators, and corticosteroids.

Patients with COPD often have a slower onset of symptoms because their disease is worsened by infection and other stressors. Patients with congestive heart failure experience a fluid overload in the lung, which may develop quickly from a failing pump.

As you try to discern between COPD and congestive heart failure, keep an open mind so that you do not miss important differences. The best advice is to treat the patient, not the lung sounds.

**TABLE 16-4** Comparison of COPD and Congestive Heart Failure

| | COPD | Congestive Heart Failure |
|---|---|---|
| Description | • A slow process of dilation and disruption of the airways and alveoli caused by chronic bronchial obstruction<br>• Usually in long-term smokers | • A disease of the heart characterized by shortness of breath, edema, and weakness<br>• Patient may or may not smoke |
| Pathophysiology | Emphysema:<br>• Destruction of the airways distal to the bronchiole<br>• Destruction of the pulmonary capillary bed<br>• Decreased ability to oxygenate the blood<br>• Lower cardiac output and hyperventilation<br>• Development of muscle wasting and weight loss<br>Chronic bronchitis:<br>• Excessive mucus production with airway obstruction<br>• Pulmonary capillary bed undamaged<br>• Compensation by decreasing ventilation and increasing cardiac output<br>• Poorly ventilated lungs, leading to hypoxemia<br>• Increased carbon dioxide retention | • Damaged ventricles and failure of heart as a pump<br>• Attempt by heart to compensate with increased rate<br>• Enlarged left ventricle<br>• Backup of fluid into the lungs and body as the heart fails to pump adequately |
| Signs/symptoms | • Use of accessory muscles<br>Emphysema:<br>• Thin appearance with barrel chest<br>• "Puffing" (pursed lip) style of breathing<br>• Tripod position<br>Chronic bronchitis:<br>• May be obese<br>• Difficulty with expiration | • Abdominal distention<br>• Dependent edema (sacral or pedal)<br>• Tachycardia<br>• Increased respiratory rate<br>• Anxiety<br>• Inability to lie flat<br>• Ashen or cyanotic |
| Level of consciousness | Normal or altered | Confusion |
| Neck veins | • Flat<br>• Distended when heart failure also present | Distended |
| Skin color | • In emphysema, pink<br>• In chronic bronchitis, blue, often cyanotic | Blue |
| Lung condition | • In emphysema, dry<br>• In chronic bronchitis, wet when heart failure also present | Wet |
| Breathing | • Shortness of breath (mostly on exertion)<br>• Breathing worsens over time (progressive) | • Shortness of breath all the time<br>• Sudden onset of shortness of breath |
| Breath sounds | Rhonchi, wheezing | Crackles, wheezing |
| Circulation | No dependent edema | Dependent edema |
| Cough | • In emphysema, little or none<br>• In chronic bronchitis, frequent or chronic cough | Coughing may be present; increases when supine |
| Sputum | • In emphysema, no mucus<br>• In chronic bronchitis, excessive, thick mucus | Pink, frothy sputum |
| Medications | Home oxygen, bronchodilators, and steroids help open the airways | Diuretics and antihypertensives help promote cardiac function and reduce fluid loads on the heart |

## Asthma, Hay Fever, and Anaphylaxis

Asthma, hay fever, and anaphylaxis are the result of an allergic reaction to an inhaled, ingested, or injected substance. The substance itself (allergen) is not the cause of the allergic reaction; rather, it is an exaggerated response of the body's immune system to the substance that causes it. In some cases, however, there is no identifiable allergen that triggers the body's immune system.

## Asthma

Asthma is an acute spasm of the bronchioles associated with excessive mucus production and with swelling of the mucous lining of the respiratory passages (**FIGURE 16-8**). According to the CDC, approximately 25 million Americans have asthma. Asthma affects people of all ages, but the highest prevalence rate is seen in children ages 5 to 17 years.

Asthma produces a characteristic wheezing as the patient attempts to exhale through partially obstructed air passages; wheezing is indicative of a partial lower airway obstruction. These same air passages open easily during inspiration. The wheezing may be so loud that you can hear it without a stethoscope. In other cases, the airways are so blocked that no air movement is heard. In severe cases, the actual work of exhaling is tiring, and cyanosis and/or

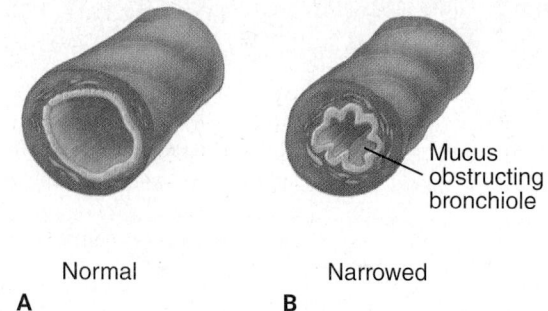

Normal
**A**

Narrowed
**B**

Mucus obstructing bronchiole

**FIGURE 16-8** Asthma is an inflammation of the lungs associated with excessive mucus production and swelling of the bronchioles. **A.** Cross section of a normal bronchiole. **B.** The bronchiole in spasm; a mucus plug has formed and partially obstructed the bronchiole.

A, B: © Jones & Bartlett Learning.

respiratory arrest may quickly develop. Cyanosis is the result of poor oxygenation of the blood as it passes through the capillaries around the alveoli. It can be seen first in the lips and mucous membranes.

An acute asthma attack may be caused by an allergic response to specific foods or some other allergen. Between attacks, patients may breathe normally. Asthma attacks may also be triggered by severe emotional stress, exercise, and respiratory infections. In its most severe form, an allergic reaction can produce anaphylaxis. This, in turn, may cause respiratory distress that is severe enough to result in coma and death.

## YOU are the Provider

After arriving at the scene and entering the patient's house, you smell cigarette smoke. There are numerous full ashtrays in the living room. The patient is sitting on the edge of her couch; she is wearing a nasal cannula attached to home oxygen, is smoking a cigarette, and is experiencing obvious breathing difficulty. She tells you, in two-word sentences, that her shortness of breath has worsened. You perform a primary assessment as your partner prepares to begin treatment.

| Recording Time: 0 Minutes | |
|---|---|
| **Appearance** | Obvious breathing difficulty; breathing through pursed lips |
| **Level of consciousness** | Conscious and alert |
| **Airway** | Open; no secretions or foreign bodies |
| **Breathing** | Rapid and labored |
| **Circulation** | Radial pulse rapid and weak; skin pink, warm, and dry |

**3.** What should be your *most* immediate action?

**4.** How does emphysema differ from chronic bronchitis?

Most patients with asthma are familiar with their symptoms and know when an attack is imminent. Typically, they will have appropriate medication with them. Depending on your local protocols, you may be allowed to assist an asthma patient with an inhaler or nebulizer. Listen carefully to what a patient with asthma tells you; they often know exactly what they need.

## Hay Fever (Allergic Rhinitis)

**Hay fever**, or allergic rhinitis, causes coldlike symptoms, including a runny nose, sneezing, congestion, and sinus pressure. The symptoms are caused by an allergic response, usually to outdoor airborne allergens such as pollen or sometimes indoor allergens such as dust mites and pet dander. For many people, hay fever is at its worst in the spring and summer, but others may have hay fever symptoms year-round. People do not generally call 9-1-1 or request an ambulance for simple hay fever symptoms, but hay fever is included in this discussion of allergic conditions because it affects so many people. People with hay fever tend to be atopic, meaning that they are more likely to have other allergies, and they may also have a higher incidence of severe reactions, including anaphylaxis.

## Anaphylactic Reactions

**Anaphylaxis**, or anaphylactic shock, is a severe allergic reaction characterized by airway swelling and dilation of blood vessels all over the body, which may significantly lower blood pressure (**FIGURE 16-9**). Anaphylaxis may be associated with widespread hives (urticaria), itching, signs of shock, and signs and symptoms similar to asthma. The airway may swell so much that breathing problems can progress to total airway obstruction in a matter of minutes. Most anaphylactic reactions occur within

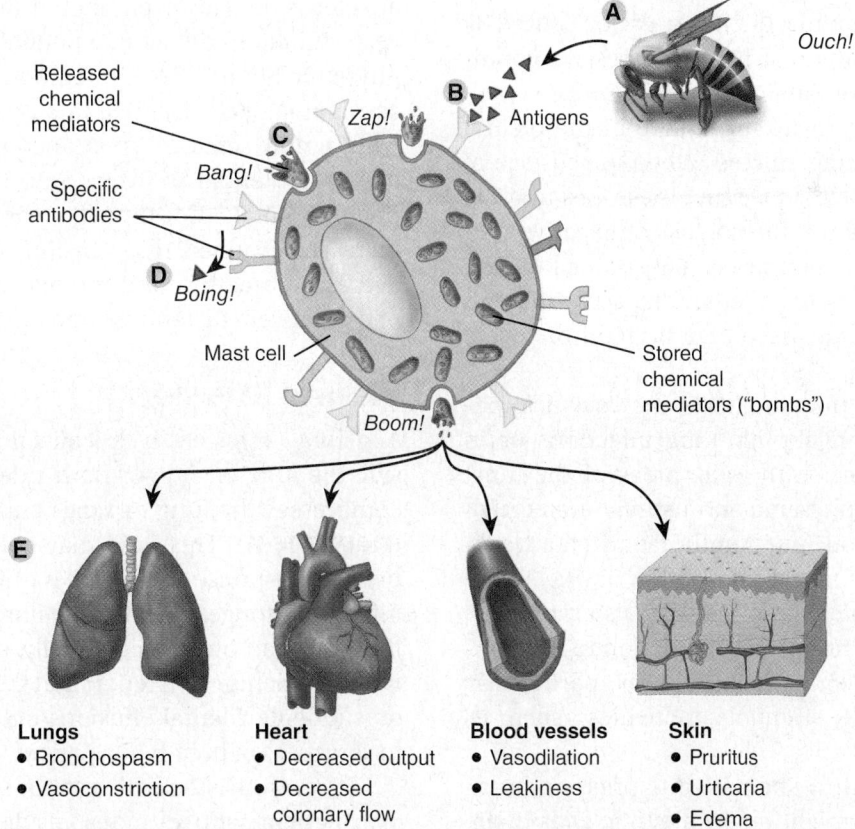

**FIGURE 16-9** The sequence of events in anaphylaxis. **A.** The antigen is introduced into the body. **B.** The antigen–antibody reaction at the surface of a mast cell. **C.** The release of mast cell chemical mediators. **D.** Specific antibody reacts with its corresponding antigen. **E.** Chemical mediators exert their effects on end organs.

**A–E:** © Jones & Bartlett Learning.

30 minutes of exposure to the allergen, which can be anything from food (such as peanuts) to medication (such as penicillin). For some patients, the episode of anaphylaxis may be their first; therefore, they may not know what caused the reaction. In other cases, the patient may be aware of what substance he or she is sensitive to but is unaware that an exposure has occurred, such as eating food that was not supposed to contain nuts. In most cases, epinephrine (adrenalin) is the treatment of choice. Patients may have their own prescribed automatic epinephrine injector, or EpiPen. Oxygen and antihistamines are also useful. As always, medical direction should guide appropriate therapy. For more information about anaphylaxis and the EpiPen, see Chapter 21, *Allergy and Anaphylaxis*.

## Spontaneous Pneumothorax

**Pneumothorax** is a partial or complete accumulation of air in the pleural space. Pneumothorax is most often caused by trauma, but it can also be caused by some medical conditions. In these cases, the condition is called a spontaneous pneumothorax.

Normally, the vacuum pressure in the pleural space keeps the lung inflated. When the surface of the lung is disrupted, however, air escapes into the pleural cavity and results in a loss of negative vacuum pressure. The natural elasticity of the lung tissue causes the lung to collapse. The accumulation of air in the pleural space may be mild or severe (**FIGURE 16-10**).

Spontaneous pneumothorax may occur in patients with certain chronic lung infections or in young people born with weak areas of the lung. Patients with emphysema and asthma are at high risk for spontaneous pneumothorax when a weakened portion of lung ruptures, often during severe coughing. Tall, thin young men are also more susceptible than the rest of the population to development of spontaneous pneumothorax, particularly while performing strenuous activities, such as heavy lifting.

A patient with a spontaneous pneumothorax has dyspnea and might report **pleuritic chest pain**, a sharp, stabbing pain on one side that is worse during inspiration and expiration or with certain movement of the chest wall. By listening to the chest with a stethoscope, you can sometimes detect that breath sounds are absent or decreased on the

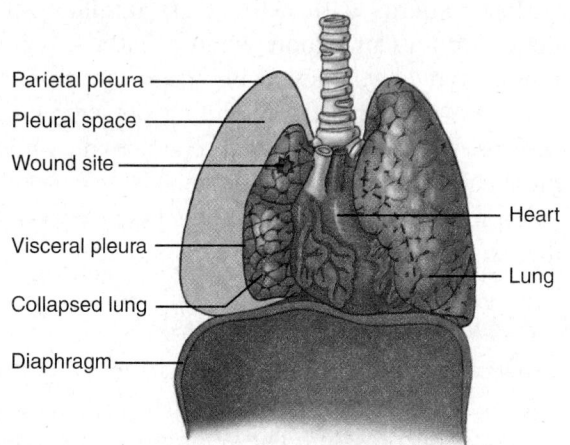

**FIGURE 16-10** A pneumothorax occurs when air leaks into the pleural space from an opening in the chest wall or the surface of the lung. The lung collapses as air fills the pleural space and the two pleural surfaces are no longer in contact.

© Jones & Bartlett Learning.

affected side. However, altered breath sounds are very difficult to detect in a patient with severe emphysema. Spontaneous pneumothorax may be the cause of sudden dyspnea in a patient with underlying emphysema. A spontaneous pneumothorax has the potential to evolve into a life-threatening pneumothorax. Continually reassess for anxiety, increased dyspnea, hypotension, absent or severely decreased breath sounds on one side, the presence of jugular vein distention, and cyanosis.

## Pleural Effusion

A **pleural effusion** is a collection of fluid outside the lung on one or both sides of the chest. It compresses the lung or lungs and causes dyspnea (**FIGURE 16-11**). This fluid may collect in large volumes in response to any form of irritation such as infection, congestive heart failure, or cancer. Although it can build up gradually, over days or even weeks, patients often report that their dyspnea came on suddenly. Pleural effusions may also contribute to shortness of breath in a patient with lung cancer.

When you listen with a stethoscope to the chest of a patient with dyspnea resulting from pleural effusion, you will hear decreased breath sounds over the region of the chest where fluid has moved the lung away from the chest wall. These patients frequently feel better if they are sitting upright. Nothing will completely relieve their symptoms,

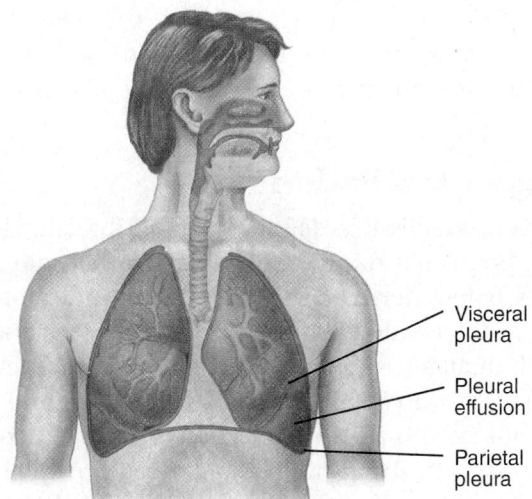

**FIGURE 16-11** With a pleural effusion, fluid may accumulate in large volumes on one or both sides, compressing the lungs and causing dyspnea.

© Jones and Bartlett Learning.

however, except removal of the fluid, which must be done by a physician in the hospital.

## Obstruction of the Airway

As an EMT, you must always be aware of the possibility that a patient with dyspnea may have a mechanical obstruction of the airway and be prepared to treat it quickly. In semiconscious and unconscious patients, the obstruction may be the result of aspiration of vomitus or a foreign object (**FIGURE 16-12A**) or improper positioning of the head so that the tongue is blocking the airway (**FIGURE 16-12B**).

Always consider upper airway obstruction from a foreign body first in patients who were eating just before becoming short of breath.

## Pulmonary Embolism

An embolus is anything in the circulatory system that moves from its point of origin to a distant site and lodges there, obstructing subsequent blood flow in that area. Beyond the point of obstruction, circulation can be significantly decreased or completely blocked, which can result in a life-threatening condition. Emboli can be fragments of blood clots in an artery or vein that break off and travel through the bloodstream, or foreign bodies that enter the circulation, such as a bubble of air.

A pulmonary embolism is a blood clot formed in a vein, usually in the legs or pelvis, that breaks off

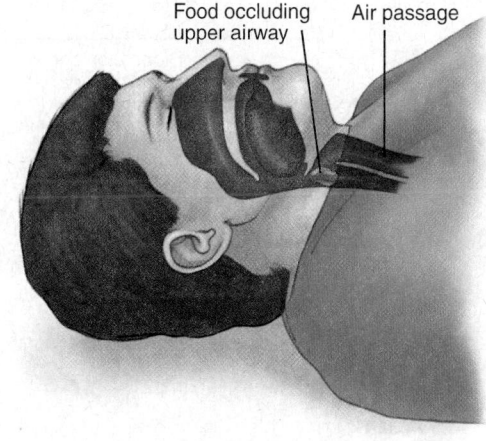

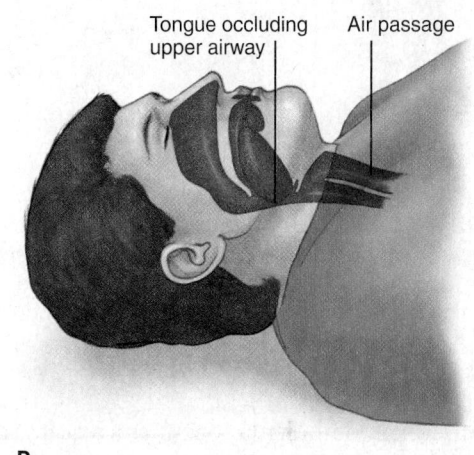

**FIGURE 16-12 A.** Foreign body obstruction occurs when an object, such as food, is lodged in the airway. **B.** Mechanical obstruction also occurs when the head is not properly positioned, causing the tongue to fall back into the throat.

A, B: © Jones & Bartlett Learning.

and circulates through the venous system. The embolus can also come from the right atrium in a patient with atrial fibrillation. The clot moves through the right side of the heart and into the pulmonary artery, where it becomes lodged, significantly decreasing or blocking blood flow (**FIGURE 16-13**). Even though the lung itself can continue the process of inhalation and exhalation, no exchange of oxygen or carbon dioxide takes place in the areas of blocked blood flow because there is no effective circulation. In this circumstance, oxygen levels in the bloodstream may drop enough to cause cyanosis. The severity of cyanosis and dyspnea is directly related to the size of the embolism and the amount of tissue affected.

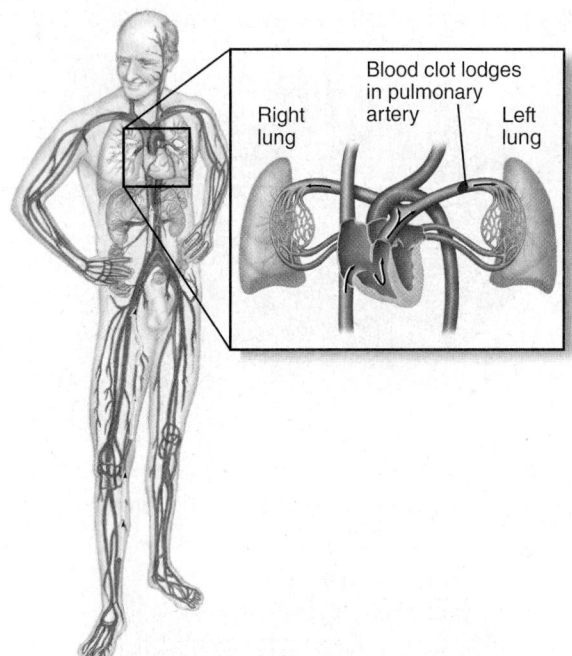

**FIGURE 16-13** A pulmonary embolus is a blood clot from a vein that breaks off, circulates through the venous system, and moves through the right side of the heart into the pulmonary artery. Here, it can become lodged and significantly obstruct blood flow.

© Jones & Bartlett Learning.

Pulmonary emboli may occur as a result of damage to the lining of vessels, a tendency for blood to clot unusually fast, or, most often, slow blood flow in a lower extremity. Slow blood flow in the legs is usually caused by long-term bed rest, which can lead to the collapse of veins. Pregnancy, active cancer, and bed rest are other risk factors. Recent surgery in the legs or pelvis of any type increases the risk of pulmonary embolus. Although uncommon, pulmonary emboli may also occur in active, healthy people in the absence of any other known risk factors.

Although they are fairly common, pulmonary emboli are difficult to diagnose. According to the US Department of Health and Human Services, 100,000 cases of pulmonary embolism occur each year in the United States. Symptoms and signs of pulmonary emboli include the following:

- Dyspnea (often sudden onset)
- Tachycardia
- Tachypnea
- Varying degrees of hypoxia
- Cyanosis
- Acute chest pain
- Hemoptysis (coughing up blood)

With a large enough embolus, complete, sudden obstruction of the output of blood flow from the right side of the heart can result in sudden death.

## Hyperventilation

**Hyperventilation** is defined as rapid breathing to the point that the level of arterial carbon dioxide falls below normal. This may be an indicator of a life-threatening illness. For example, a patient with diabetes who has a high blood glucose level, a patient who has taken an overdose of aspirin, or a patient with a severe infection is likely to hyperventilate. In these cases, rapid, deep breathing is the body's attempt to stay alive. The body is trying to compensate for **acidosis**, the buildup of excess acid in the blood or body tissues that results from the primary illness. Because carbon dioxide, mixed with water in the bloodstream, can add to the blood's acidity, lowering the level of carbon dioxide helps to compensate for the other acids.

Similarly, in an otherwise healthy person, blood acidity can be diminished by excessive breathing because it blows off too much carbon dioxide. The result is a relative lack of acids. The resulting condition, **alkalosis**, is the buildup of excess base (lack of acids) in the body fluids.

Alkalosis is the cause of many of the symptoms associated with **hyperventilation syndrome**, including anxiety, dizziness, numbness, tingling of the hands and feet, and painful spasms of the hands and/or feet (carpopedal spasms). Patients often feel as if they cannot catch their breath despite the rapid breathing. Although hyperventilation can be a response to illness and a buildup of acids, hyperventilation syndrome is not caused by these conditions. Instead, this syndrome occurs in the absence of other physical problems. It commonly occurs when a person is experiencing psychological stress and affects some 10% of the population at one time or another. The respirations of an individual who is experiencing hyperventilation syndrome may be as high as 40 shallow breaths/min or as low as 20 deep breaths/min.

The decision whether hyperventilation is being caused by a life-threatening illness or a panic attack should not be made outside the hospital. Initially, you can verbally instruct the patient to slow his or her breathing; however, if that does not work, give supplemental oxygen and provide transport to the hospital where physicians will determine the cause of the hyperventilation.

## Environmental/Industrial Exposure

Many accidental exposures that cause inhalation injury and dyspnea occur at industrial sites. Pesticides, cleaning solutions, chemicals, chlorine, and other gases can be accidentally released and inhaled by employees. Sometimes chemicals such as ammonia and chlorine bleach are mixed and create a hazardous by-product.

In many cases, industrial sites have their own medical, fire, and/or hazardous materials teams that are familiar with all the chemicals used at their site and know what to do in case of an exposure. They will begin immediate decontamination and medical care. In these cases, the patient needs to be decontaminated by trained responders before you take responsibility.

Once the patient is decontaminated, gather information from the first responders about the substance and the cause of dyspnea. Assess the patient, paying special attention to breath sounds. Inhalation injuries can cause aspiration pneumonia that can result in eventual pulmonary edema. The inhaled substance can also cause lung damage. Blood coming from the airway is an ominous sign. Chapter 40, *Incident Management*, discusses hazardous materials in more detail.

## Carbon Monoxide Poisoning

Toxic gases can also affect people outside the industrial setting. One common type of exposure is carbon monoxide, a colorless, odorless, tasteless, and highly poisonous gas known as "the silent killer." Carbon monoxide is the leading cause of nondrug accidental poisoning deaths in the United States, according to the CDC. People who survive carbon monoxide poisoning can have permanent brain damage.

Carbon monoxide is produced by fuel-burning household appliances such as gas water heaters, space heaters, grills, and generators; it is also present in smoke from fire or cigarettes. The onset of cold weather commonly leads to an increase in carbon monoxide poisonings as people turn on heaters for the first time. The combined effects of incomplete combustion and a poorly ventilated building

can cause a buildup of carbon monoxide. Another common source of carbon monoxide poisoning is motor vehicle exhaust. Some people will attempt suicide by running the engine inside a closed garage and inhaling the fumes.

People who are exposed to carbon monoxide may think they have the flu. They initially report headache, dizziness, fatigue, and nausea and vomiting. They may report dyspnea on exertion and chest pain and display nervous system symptoms such as impaired judgment, confusion, or even hallucinations. The worst exposures may result in syncope or seizure. Carbon monoxide has a much stronger bond with hemoglobin than does oxygen; therefore, oxygen is not being delivered to the tissues of the body. This can lead to cellular death and organ failure if uncorrected.

When you assess the scene, do not put yourself at risk of exposure (**FIGURE 16-14**). Consider toxic gas exposure if more than one patient in the same environment is experiencing the same signs and symptoms. The symptoms of patients will start to improve as soon as they are removed from the toxic environment. High-flow oxygen by nonrebreathing

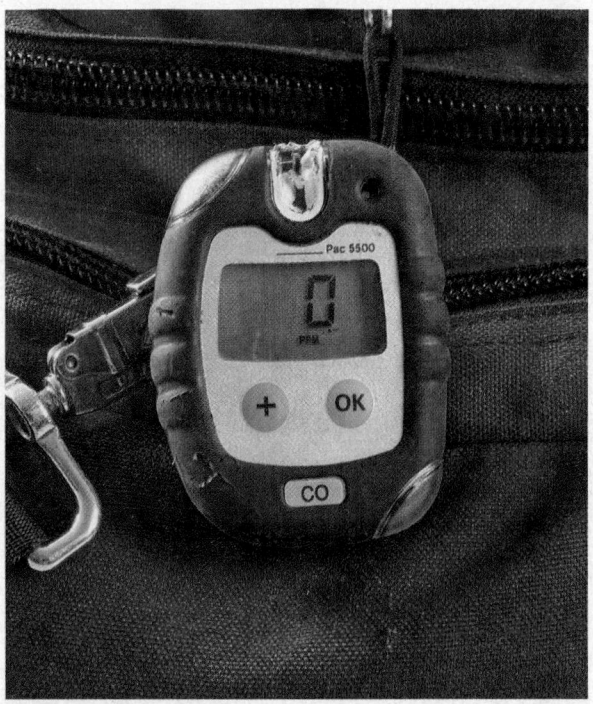

**FIGURE 16-14** A portable carbon monoxide alarm can be attached to your medical bag to alert you to its presence at potential toxic scenes.

mask is the best treatment for conscious patients. Patients who are unconscious or have an altered level of consciousness may need full airway control with insertion of an airway adjunct and ventilation using a bag-mask device. In the worst cases, patients may be treated with hyperbaric or pressurized oxygen therapy.

## Patient Assessment

Your assessment of patients in respiratory distress should be a calm and systematic process. These patients are usually anxious, and they may be some of the most ill and challenging patients you will encounter.

## Scene Size-up

As always, first consider standard precautions and use of PPE. The patient may have a respiratory infection that could be passed to you through sputum and/or airborne droplets. Follow local protocols.

Next, consider whether the respiratory emergency may have been caused by a toxic substance that was inhaled, absorbed, or ingested.

Once you have determined the scene is safe, determine how many patients there are and whether you need additional or specialized resources. If there are multiple people with dyspnea, consider the possibility of an airborne hazardous material release.

If the nature of illness (NOI) is in question, ask why 9-1-1 was activated. By questioning the patient, family, and/or bystanders, you should be able to determine the NOI.

### Words of Wisdom

If there are several patients presenting with the same complaints, there is a good chance the scene is not safe and there is something in the air causing the illness. Do not place yourself in danger. Remember that not all scene safety concerns are visible.

## Primary Assessment

Perform a rapid examination to identify immediate life threats, which includes problems with the ABCs: airway, breathing, and circulation (discussed next). If any major problem is identified, treat it immediately. If you find life-threatening issues, provide rapid transport.

Note your general impression of the patient. What is the patient's age and position? A patient in significant respiratory distress will want to sit up. In a worst-case scenario, you will arrive to see the patient in the tripod position.

Does the patient appear calm? Is the patient anxious and restless, or listless and tired? How severe is the patient's breathing complaint? This initial impression will help you decide whether the patient's condition is stable or unstable.

Use the AVPU scale to check for responsiveness. If the patient is alert or responding to verbal stimuli, you know that the brain is still receiving oxygen. Ask the patient about his or her chief complaint. If the patient is responsive only to painful stimuli or unresponsive, the brain may not be oxygenating well and the potential for an airway or breathing problem is more likely. If there is no gag or cough reflex, you need to immediately assess the patient's airway status. Within seconds you will be able to determine if there are any immediate threats to life.

### Assessing ABCs in Respiratory Patients

Assess the airway; air must flow in and out of the chest easily for the airway to be considered patent. If there is any question about airway patency, immediately open the airway using the head tilt–chin lift maneuver in nontrauma patients and the jaw-thrust maneuver in patients with suspected spinal trauma.

If the airway is patent, next evaluate whether the patient's breathing is adequate. What are the rate, rhythm, and quality of the respirations? Is the rate within normal limits for the patient's age? Is the patient using accessory muscles to assist the respiratory effort, and can you see retractions? Is there abdominal breathing? What is the depth of breathing, and is the tidal volume adequate? Is there adequate rise and fall of the chest? What are the color, temperature, and moisture conditions of the patient's skin? Although cyanosis resulting from low oxygen in the blood can be difficult to detect in dark-skinned people, it may be observed by examining the palms or the mucous membranes of the lips, which may appear pale, ashen, or gray.

Are the patient's respirations labored? If the patient can speak only one or two words at a time before gasping for a breath, ventilations are considered labored. If the respiratory effort is inadequate, you must provide the necessary intervention. If the patient is in respiratory distress, place him or her in a position that best facilitates breathing (generally sitting upright in a full or semi-Fowler position) and begin administering oxygen at 15 L/min via non-rebreathing mask. If the patient's breathing has inadequate depth or the rate is too slow, ventilations may need to be assisted with a bag-mask device.

Ask yourself the following questions:

1. Is air going in and out?
2. Does the chest rise and fall with each breath?
3. Is the rate appropriate for the age of the patient?

If the answer to any of these questions is "no," something is wrong. If the patient is unconscious, try to reposition the patient's head and insert an oral airway to keep the tongue from blocking the airway. Refer to Chapter 11, *Airway Management*, for a review of airway management and ventilation techniques. Continue to monitor the airway for fluid, secretions, and other problems as you move on to assess the adequacy of your patient's breathing.

The next step in assessing breathing in a patient with a respiratory emergency is to assess breath sounds. Techniques for this assessment are described at the end of this section.

After assessing breath sounds, assess circulation—the pulse rate, quality, and rhythm. If the pulse rate is too fast or too slow, the patient may not be getting enough oxygen. Determine the quality of the pulse. Is it strong, bounding, or weak? Also determine whether the rhythm is regular or irregular. Irregular beats could indicate a cardiac problem.

Assessing a patient's circulation includes an evaluation for the presence of shock and bleeding. Respiratory distress in a patient could be caused by an insufficient number of red blood cells to transport the oxygen. Assess capillary refill in infants and children. Normal capillary refill is less than 2 seconds; abnormal capillary refill is greater than 2 seconds. Capillary refill is not considered a reliable assessment tool in the adult patient.

Note that a patient with a severe chest injury, such as flail chest, or obstruction of the airway may be unable to breathe in an adequate amount of oxygen. This affects the ventilation process of respiration because not enough oxygen can be inspired to meet the metabolic demand.

An insufficient concentration of oxygen in the blood can produce a life-threatening situation as rapidly as vascular causes of shock, even if the volume of blood, the volume of the vessels, and the

## YOU are the Provider

Your partner obtains the patient's vital signs as you continue your assessment. You notice she is breathing through pursed lips and has a prolonged exhalation phase, and cyanosis is present in her fingernail beds. You auscultate her breath sounds and hear scattered wheezing in all lung fields. When you talk to her, you note she is now confused, is slow to answer your questions, and appears fatigued.

**Recording Time: 3 Minutes**

| | |
|---|---|
| **Respirations** | 28 breaths/min, labored; prolonged exhalation phase |
| **Pulse** | 110 beats/min; weak |
| **Skin** | Cyanotic, cool, clammy |
| **Blood pressure** | 116/54 mm Hg |
| **Oxygen saturation (SpO$_2$)** | 88% (on 4 L/min oxygen by nasal cannula) |

5. Why do patients with emphysema breathe through pursed lips?
6. What does a prolonged exhalation phase indicate in patients with obstructive lung disease?
7. What treatment is indicated for the patient at this point?

action of the heart are all normal. Without oxygen, the organs in the body cannot survive, and their cells promptly start to deteriorate.

Assess the patient's perfusion by evaluating skin color, temperature, and condition. A loss of perfusion may be caused by chronic anemia, a wound, internal bleeding, or simply shock overwhelming the body's ability to compensate for the illness.

You now know enough to be able to identify any life threats in your patient. They would include any of the following signs or symptoms:

- Problems with the ABCs
- Poor initial general impression
- Unresponsiveness
- Potential hypoperfusion or shock
- Chest pain associated with a low blood pressure
- Severe pain anywhere
- Excessive bleeding

If the patient's condition is unstable and there is a possible life threat, address the life threat and proceed with rapid transport. This means you will keep your scene time short, providing only life-saving interventions. Perform a secondary assessment en route to the hospital. If the patient's condition is stable and there are no life threats, you may decide to perform a thorough secondary assessment on scene, after obtaining the patient history.

## Assessing Breath Sounds

Obtaining breath sounds, or lung sounds, is an important step when you assess a patient who is experiencing respiratory distress. Listen over the bare chest. Trying to listen over clothing or chest hair may give you inaccurate information. The diaphragm of the stethoscope must be in firm contact with the skin. If your patient is lying down, bring him or her to a sitting position, which is a better position for assessing breath sounds.

You need to determine whether your patient's breath sounds are normal (**vesicular breath sounds**, **bronchial breath sounds**) or decreased, absent, or abnormal (**adventitious breath sounds**). With your stethoscope, check breath sounds on the right and left sides of the chest, and compare each side (**FIGURE 16-15**). When listening on the patient's back, place the stethoscope head between and below the scapulae, not over them, or you will have an inaccurate assessment.

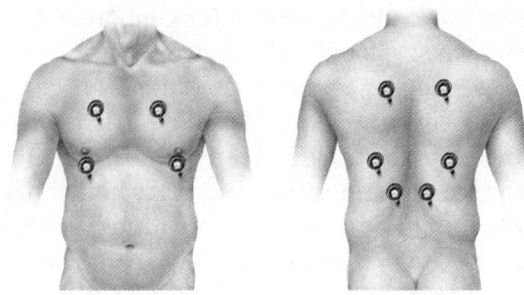

**FIGURE 16-15** Locations of the stethoscope bell for auscultation of breath sounds.
© Jones & Bartlett Learning.

Make sure you listen for a full respiratory cycle at each location on the chest so you can detect the adventitious sounds that may be heard at the end of the inspiratory or expiratory phase. When you assess for fluid collection, pay special attention to the lower lung fields. Start from the bottom up and determine at which level you start hearing clear breath sounds.

You want to hear clear flow of air in both lungs. Not hearing the flow of air is considered an absent lung sound. The lack of air movement in the lung is a significant finding. Listen carefully and do not confuse absent breath sounds with clear breath sounds. See **TABLE 16-5** for examples of breath sounds, the diseases that may be associated with them, and important signs and symptoms.

### Street Smarts

When auscultating lung sounds, providers commonly ask patients to breathe in and out. Do not place the patient in further respiratory distress by asking him or her to breathe too quickly or too slowly just so you can hear lung sounds.

Snoring sounds are indicative of a partial upper airway obstruction, usually in the oropharynx. **Wheezing** indicates constriction and/or inflammation in the bronchus. Wheezing is generally heard on exhalation as a high-pitched, almost musical or whistling sound. This sound is commonly heard in patients with asthma and sometimes in patients with COPD.

**Crackles** (formerly called rales) are the sounds of air trying to pass through fluid in the alveoli. It is a crackling or bubbling sound typically heard on inspiration. High-pitched sounds are called fine

**TABLE 16-5** Signs, Symptoms, and Adventitious Breath Sounds Associated With Specific Respiratory Diseases

| Breath Sounds | Disease | Signs and Symptoms |
|---|---|---|
| Wheezes | Asthma<br>COPD<br>Congestive heart failure/pulmonary edema<br>Pneumonia<br>Bronchitis<br>Anaphylaxis | Dyspnea<br>Productive or nonproductive cough<br>Dependent edema, pink frothy sputum<br>Fever, pleuritic chest pain<br>Clear or white sputum<br>Hives, facial swelling, stridor, nonproductive cough |
| Rhonchi | COPD<br>Pneumonia<br>Bronchitis | Productive cough<br>Fever, pleuritic chest pain<br>Clear or white sputum |
| Crackles | Congestive heart failure/pulmonary edema<br>Pneumonia | Dependent edema, pink frothy sputum<br>Fever, pleuritic chest pain |
| Stridor | Croup<br>Epiglottitis | Fever, barking cough<br>Fever, sore throat, drooling |
| Decreased or absent breath sounds | Asthma<br>COPD<br>Pneumonia<br>Hemothorax<br>Pneumothorax<br>Atelectasis | Nonproductive cough, dyspnea<br>Productive cough<br>Fever, pleuritic chest pain<br>Shock, respiratory distress<br>Dyspnea, pleuritic chest pain<br>Fever, decreased oxygen saturation |

Abbreviation: COPD, chronic obstructive pulmonary disease

© Jones & Bartlett Learning.

crackles, and low-pitched sounds are called coarse crackles. These sounds are often a result of congestive heart failure or pulmonary edema.

**Rhonchi** are low-pitched rattling sounds caused by secretions or mucus in the larger airway. Rhonchi are sometimes referred to as junky lung sounds and can be heard with infections such as pneumonia and bronchitis or in cases of aspiration.

## Words of Wisdom

Adventitious breath sounds are sounds heard by auscultation of abnormal lungs. These sounds can include wheezing, crackles, rhonchi, gurgling, snoring, crowing, and stridor. The ability to hear and distinguish different kinds of breath sounds can give you important clues as to what is wrong with your patient. The only way to develop your ability to identify breath sounds is through practice. Ask your instructor if you can accompany a physician, nurse, or respiratory therapist in the hospital to help you develop this ability.

**Stridor** is the high-pitched sound heard on inspiration as air tries to pass through an obstruction in the upper airway. This sound indicates a partial obstruction of the trachea and occurs in patients with anatomic or foreign body airway obstruction.

## History Taking

The next step of your assessment will provide more information specific to the patient's chief complaint (history of present illness) through history taking. The information you obtain during history taking will be subjective (what the patient expresses, or symptoms) and objective (what you observe, or signs). Both sets of information are important in building a general assessment. Rule out any findings that warrant no care or intervention. Report pertinent negatives to health care providers or ED staff members. Recall that a pertinent negative is any sign or symptom that commonly accompanies a particular condition, but is absent. Examples of pertinent negatives would be a patient in respiratory distress who denies chest pain, or a patient with severe chest pain who denies shortness of breath.

Find out what the patient has done for the breathing problem. Does the patient have home oxygen? Does the patient use a prescribed inhaler or a small-volume nebulizer? If so, when was it used last? How many doses have been taken? Does the patient use more than one inhaler or treatment? Be sure to record the name of each device and when it was used.

## Street Smarts

Although it is easy to assume that patients with a history of a respiratory illness (such as asthma) are having an exacerbation of their condition when they present with dyspnea, it may lead to misdiagnosis and delayed or incorrect treatment. It is critical to keep an open mind and consider all the signs and symptoms in addition to the history before deciding on a treatment plan. A person with asthma may have an anaphylactic reaction, or a patient with COPD may have an acute onset of pulmonary edema caused by congestive heart failure. It is important to get as much information as possible and consider all possibilities before developing a treatment plan.

## Chronic Respiratory Conditions

Different respiratory complaints offer different clues and different challenges. Patients with chronic conditions may have long periods in which they are able to live relatively normal lives but then sometimes experience acute worsening of their conditions. That is when you are called, and it is important for you to be able to determine your patient's baseline status—in other words, his or her normal condition (and what is different this time that made the patient call you). For example, patients with COPD do not cope well with pulmonary infections because the existing airway damage makes them unable to cough up the mucus or sputum produced by the infection. The chronic lower airway obstruction makes it difficult for the patient to breathe deeply enough to clear the lungs. Gradually, the arterial oxygen level falls, and the carbon dioxide level rises. If a new infection of the lung occurs in a patient with COPD, the arterial oxygen level may fall rapidly. In a few patients, the carbon dioxide level may become high enough to cause sleepiness. In these cases,

patients require respiratory support and careful administration of oxygen.

Recall that the patient with COPD usually has a long history of dyspnea with a sudden increase in shortness of breath. There is rarely a history of chest pain. More often, the patient will remember having had a recent "chest cold" with fever and either an inability to cough up mucus or a sudden increase in thick green or yellow sputum. The blood pressure of patients with COPD is often normal; however, the pulse may be rapid and occasionally irregular. Pay particular attention to the respirations. They may be rapid, or they may be very slow.

Patients with asthma may have different triggers, including allergens, cold, exercise, stress, infection, and noncompliance with medication prescriptions. It is important to try to determine what may have triggered the attack so that it can be treated appropriately. For example, an asthma attack that occurred while your patient was jogging in the cold will probably not respond to antihistamines, whereas one brought on by a reaction to pollen might.

Patients with congestive heart failure often walk a fine line between compensating for their diminished cardiac capacity and decompensating. Many take several medications, most often including diuretics (also called water pills) and blood pressure medications. Obtain a list of all medications and ask about the events leading up to the present problem.

## Questioning a Patient With Difficulty Breathing

With patients in respiratory distress, many of the SAMPLE questions can be answered by the family or bystanders if they are present. Limit the number of questions directed to the patient by asking only pertinent ones; a patient who is in respiratory distress does not need to use any additional air to answer questions.

Ask the following questions about a patient in respiratory distress:

- What is the patient's general state of health?
- Has the patient had any childhood or adult diseases?
- Have there been any recent surgical procedures or hospitalizations?
- Have there been any traumatic injuries?

To help determine the cause of your patient's problem, be a detective. Look for medications, medical alert bracelets, environmental conditions, and other clues to what may be causing the problem. Each part of the SAMPLE history may give you clues, so be thorough. For example, you forget to ask about allergies, only to find out later that your patient has a severe allergy to cat dander and that her 8-year-old son had been playing with a cat shortly before the onset of her problem. You would have missed important and possibly life-saving information.

The OPQRST assessment, generally used for determining the specifics of pain, can also be modified to obtain more specific information about the breathing problem. Begin by asking the patient to describe the problem. Pay close attention to OPQRST and include the following open-ended questions:

- When and how did the breathing problem begin, suddenly or gradually? (Onset)
- What makes the breathing difficulty better or worse? (Provocation or palliation)
- How does the breathing feel? (Quality)
- Does the discomfort move? (Radiation/region)
- How much of a problem is the patient having? (Severity)
- Is the problem continuous or intermittent? If it is intermittent, how frequently does it occur and how long does it last? (Timing)

An additional assessment for a complaint of shortness of breath or difficulty breathing uses the mnemonic PASTE:

**P Progression.** Similar to the O in OPQRST, you want to know if the problem started suddenly or has worsened over time.

**A Associated chest pain.** Dyspnea can be a significant symptom of a cardiac problem.

**S Sputum.** Has the patient been coughing up sputum? Mucuslike sputum could indicate a respiratory infection, pink frothy sputum is indicative of fluid in the lungs, and a problem such as a pulmonary embolus may not result in any sputum at all.

**T Talking tiredness.** This is an indicator of how much distress the patient is having. Ask the patient to repeat a sentence and see how many words he or she can speak without needing to take a breath. The assessment results would be reported as the patient "speaks in full sentences" or, perhaps, "speaks in two-to three-word sentences."

**E Exercise tolerance.** Ask the patient a question about what he or she was able to do before this problem started, such as walk across the room, and then ask if the patient could do it now. If the answer is "no," then it is another indicator that your patient is in distress. Exercise tolerance will decrease as the breathing problem and hypoxia increase.

## Secondary Assessment

During the secondary assessment, further investigate the specific chief complaint (for example, dyspnea) by performing a physical examination and taking vital signs.

In respiratory emergencies, as in all other emergencies, only proceed to history taking and the secondary assessment once all life threats have been identified and treated during the primary assessment. If you are busy treating airway or breathing problems, you may not have the opportunity to proceed to a physical examination prior to arriving at the ED. Never compromise the assessment and treatment of airway and breathing problems to conduct a physical examination.

Sometimes it is not possible to quickly and definitively determine what is causing your patient's respiratory distress. If your patient is a 20-year-old woman at a picnic in whom difficulty breathing and hives rapidly develop after being stung by a bee, you have a clear-cut diagnostic picture. Conversely, if your patient is an older woman in a nursing home who is receiving 12 medications and has a cough and increasing shortness of breath that developed during the past week, this is more perplexing. Keep an open mind, gather as complete a history as possible, and perform a secondary assessment.

Conduct an in-depth assessment when a patient reports shortness of breath. In addition to the signs of air hunger present in all patients with respiratory distress, such as the tripod position, rapid breathing, and use of accessory muscles, restriction of the small lower airways in patients with

### Words of Wisdom

Never delay the assessment and treatment of airway and breathing problems to conduct a physical examination.

asthma often causes wheezing. Patients may have a prolonged expiratory phase of breathing as they attempt to exhale trapped air from the lungs. In severe cases, you may actually not hear wheezing because of insufficient airflow. Remember that the brain needs a constant, adequate supply of oxygen to function normally. As your patient tires from the effort of breathing and oxygen levels drop, the respiratory and heart rates may drop, and you will notice an altered level of consciousness. This may manifest itself as confusion, lack of coordination, bizarre behavior, or even combativeness. Your patient may seem to relax or fall asleep. These findings indicate respiratory failure. A change in affect or level of consciousness is one of the early warning signs of respiratory inadequacy, and you must act immediately.

When you perform a secondary assessment on the respiratory system, look for overall symmetry of the chest, adequate rise and fall of the chest, and evidence of retractions or accessory muscle use. Are the patient's respirations labored or unlabored? Assess breath sounds, and perform additional physical assessment if warranted.

A secondary assessment of the cardiovascular system, especially when there is associated chest pain, should include checking and comparing distal pulses, reassessing the skin condition, and being alert for bradycardia and tachycardia.

Feel for the skin temperature, and look for color changes in the extremities and in the core of the body. Cyanosis is an ominous sign that requires immediate, aggressive intervention.

Blood pressure should be auscultated when possible to obtain the systolic and diastolic numbers. If you are in an environment where you cannot hear well enough to auscultate the blood pressure, then palpation of the blood pressure is an alternative.

It is important to assess the neurologic system because the level of consciousness can change. Check the patient's mental status, and determine if the patient's activity can be described as anxious or restless. If so, that would be an indicator of hypoxia. Does the patient have clear thought processes? Disorientation may be another indicator of hypoxia.

Use monitoring devices if you have them available, including, but not limited to, a pulse oximeter. Pulse oximetry is an effective diagnostic tool when used in conjunction with experience, good assessment skills, and clinical judgment. Pulse oximeters measure the percentage of hemoglobin that is saturated by oxygen. In patients with normal levels of hemoglobin, pulse oximetry can be an important tool in evaluating oxygenation. To use pulse oximetry properly, it is important for you to be able to evaluate the quality of the reading and correlate it with the patient's condition. For example, it is doubtful a patient with congestive heart failure in severe respiratory distress will have a pulse oximetry reading of 98% or that a pulse oximetry reading of 80% is reliable in a conscious, alert, active patient with good skin color.

If you get a good reading consistent with your patient's condition, the pulse oximeter can help you determine the severity of the respiratory component of the patient's problem. In addition, if the reading goes steadily up or down, it can give you an indication of improvement or deterioration of the patient's oxygenation status, often even prior to changes in the patient's appearance or vital signs.

> ### Words of Wisdom
>
> Be aware of conditions that can skew pulse oximetry results. Bright light, darkly pigmented skin, and nail polish can cause errors in the readings. Remember that pulse oximetry measures the percentage of hemoglobin that is saturated, but it does not tell you how much hemoglobin the patient needs; nor does it tell you whether it is oxygen that has bound to the hemoglobin (the typical and desired condition) or carbon monoxide.

## Secondary Assessment of COPD Versus Congestive Heart Failure

Additional pieces to the assessment and treatment puzzle may be revealed during the physical examination. For example, you are treating a patient in acute respiratory distress who is breathing at a rate of 40 breaths/min and has audible wheezing. On the basis of this information, you may be unsure whether the patient is in congestive heart failure or is having an asthma attack. The secondary assessment may provide you with additional clues, such as a consistently elevated blood pressure and swollen legs and feet (pedal edema) that would lead you in the direction of congestive heart failure.

Assume you are assessing a patient with COPD. What would you notice? Patients with COPD are

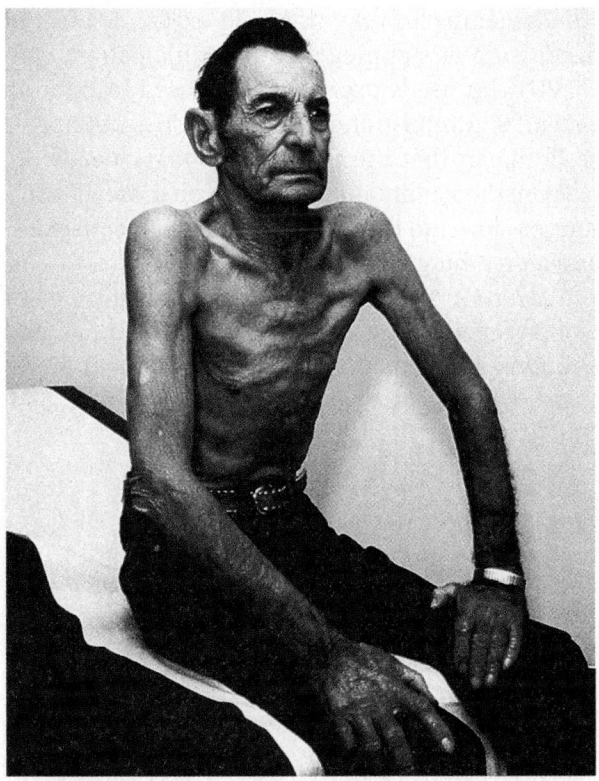

**FIGURE 16-16** Patients with COPD often use accessory muscles and pursed lips for breathing. The increased work of breathing leads to decreased food intake (malnutrition) and muscle wasting. Notice, also, that this patient is sitting in the tripod position.

© American Academy of Orthopaedic Surgeons.

usually older than 50 years. They will often have a history of recurring lung problems and are almost always long-term active or former cigarette smokers. Patients may report tightness in the chest and constant fatigue. Because air has been gradually and continuously trapped in their lungs in increasing amounts, their chests often have a barrellike appearance. Patients with COPD often use accessory muscles to breathe (**FIGURE 16-16**). If you listen to the patient's chest with a stethoscope, you will hear abnormal breath sounds. Patients with COPD will often exhale through pursed lips as a strategy to keep airways open longer. Digital clubbing (abnormal enlargement of the ends of the fingers) is also a sign of COPD.

## Reassessment

Once the assessment and treatment have been completed, you need to reassess the patient and closely watch patients with shortness of breath.

Repeat the primary assessment and maintain an open airway. Monitor the patient's breathing and reassess circulation.

Determine if there have been changes in the patient's condition. Confirm the adequacy of interventions and patient status. Is the current treatment improving the patient's condition? Has an already identified problem improved? Has an already identified problem gotten worse? What is the nature of any newly identified problems?

If the changes you find are improvements, simply continue the treatments; however, if your patient's condition deteriorates, prepare to modify treatments. Be prepared to assist ventilations with a bag-mask device. Monitor the skin color and temperature. Reassess and record vital signs at least every 5 minutes for a patient in unstable condition and/or after the patient uses an inhaler. If the patient's condition is stable and no life threat exists, vital signs should be obtained at least every 15 minutes.

Now that you have completed the secondary assessment and have gathered information about your patient with difficulty breathing, it is time to provide interventions for the problems that are not immediate life threats. Your interventions may be based on standing orders, or you may contact the hospital and ask for specific directions. Remember, interventions for immediate life threats should be been completed during the primary assessment and should not require contacting the hospital first. Interventions for respiratory problems may include the following:

- Providing oxygen via a nonrebreathing mask at 15 L/min
- Providing positive-pressure ventilations using a bag-mask device
- Using airway management techniques such as an oropharyngeal (oral) airway, a nasopharyngeal (nasal) airway, suctioning, or airway positioning
- Providing noninvasive ventilatory support with continuous positive airway pressure (CPAP)
- Positioning the patient in a high Fowler position or a position of choice to facilitate breathing
- Assisting with respiratory medications found in a patient-prescribed metered-dose inhaler or a small-volume nebulizer

Some of these interventions may have been performed in the primary assessment to address life threats. Others are used to support breathing problems until definitive care can be provided at the hospital. Some of your interventions may even correct the problem.

Contact medical control with any change in the patient's level of consciousness or difficulty breathing. Depending on local protocols, contact medical control prior to assisting with any prescribed medications. Be sure to document any changes (and at what time) and any orders given by medical control.

## Emergency Medical Care

Management of respiratory distress involves continuing awareness of scene safety and the use of standard precautions. Management of ABCs and positioning are primary treatments, along with oxygen and suction.

You will usually administer oxygen to patients in respiratory distress. If a patient reports breathing difficulty, administer supplemental oxygen immediately. Adult patients breathing more than 20 breaths/min or fewer than 12 breaths/min should receive high-flow oxygen (defined as 15 L/min). Depending on the level of distress, some patients may benefit from CPAP (discussed later in the chapter). In addition, patients may require ventilatory support with a bag-mask device, particularly if their mental status is declining, if they are in moderate to severe respiratory distress, or if their depth of respiration is inadequate.

Take great care in monitoring the patient's respirations as you provide oxygen. Reevaluate the respirations and the patient's response to oxygen repeatedly, at least every 5 minutes, until you reach the ED. In a person with a chronically high carbon dioxide level (eg, certain patients with COPD), this is critical, because the supplemental oxygen may cause a rapid rise in the arterial oxygen level, which may depress the patient's hypoxic drive.

In patients who have long-standing COPD and probable carbon dioxide retention, administration of low-flow oxygen (2 L/min) is a good place to start, with adjustments to 3 L/min, then 4 L/min, and so on, until symptoms have improved (eg, the patient's breathing becomes easier, or the patient becomes more responsive). Pulse oximetry will help you understand the degree of oxygen deprivation and adjust oxygen therapy accordingly. When in doubt, err on the side of more oxygen, and monitor the patient closely.

Remember, do *not* withhold oxygen for fear of depressing or stopping breathing in a patient with COPD who needs oxygen. A decreased respiratory rate after administration of oxygen does not necessarily mean that the patient no longer needs the oxygen; the patient may need it even more. If respirations slow and the patient becomes unconscious, assist breathing with a bag-mask device.

Always provide emotional support to the patient who is anxious. Always speak with assurance and assume a concerned, professional approach to reassure the patient, who is probably very frightened.

### Words of Wisdom

Some states allow EMTs to administer medication by inhalers or small volume nebulizers or to assist patients in the administration of their own inhalers. With this increased scope of practice comes the responsibility to know the names, doses, indications, contraindications, side effects, and precautions of the numerous medications given by this route. Patients sometimes do not know the difference between their rescue inhalers (immediately effective medication, such as albuterol) and their maintenance inhalers (such as corticosteroids, which have no immediate effect). It is essential, then, that *you* know the difference!

## Metered-Dose Inhaler and Small-Volume Nebulizer

Patients who call for help because of difficulty breathing are likely to have had the same problem before. They probably have prescribed medications to use that are delivered by an inhaler or small-volume nebulizer. If so, you may be able to help them use these devices, depending on local protocols. Some of the most common medications used for shortness of breath are inhaled beta agonists, which dilate breathing passages. Some medications may be administered via a **metered-dose inhaler (MDI)**, which is a miniature spray canister used to direct such substances through the mouth and into the lungs. MDIs are used to administer medications such as albuterol (Proventil, Ventolin), albuterol/ipratropium (Combivent), metaproterenol (Alupent, Metaprel), and terbutaline (Brethine).

The **small-volume nebulizer** works by providing a means for a fine mist of aerosolized medicine to get deep into the patient's lungs and start to work quickly. The patient inhales the mist through a mouthpiece. When the medicine is breathed in correctly, it goes directly into the lungs. Medications typically administered by small-volume nebulizer include, but are not limited to, albuterol, ipratropium, and levalbuterol.

## Medical Control

Consult medical control (online), or follow standing orders (off-line). Remember to report what the medication is, when the patient last self-administered a treatment, how much medication was used at that time, and what the label states regarding dosage. If medical control or standing orders permit, you may assist the patient to self-administer the medication. Be certain that the inhaler belongs to the patient, it contains the correct medication, the expiration date has not passed, and the correct dose is being administered. There may be times when the prescribed dose is not explicitly listed on the inhaler. In this situation, ask the patient how many inhalations of the medication he or she takes. Administer repeated doses of the medication if the maximum dose has not been exceeded and the patient is still experiencing shortness of breath.

Unlike an MDI, a small-volume nebulizer must be assembled prior to use. An oxygen tank, or air compressor, is also required to administer the aerosolized medication. The patient may have a tank available, or you will need to use your own tank.

## Indications and Contraindications

Before helping a patient to self-administer any MDI or small-volume nebulizer medication, make sure that the medication is indicated—that is, the patient has signs and symptoms of shortness of breath. The most common use for an MDI is asthma, and a small-volume nebulizer is used in asthma, bronchiolitis, COPD, and anaphylaxis. Check that there are no contraindications for its use, such as the following:

- The patient is unable to help coordinate inhalation with depression of the trigger on an MDI or is too confused to effectively administer medication through a small-volume nebulizer. These devices will be only minimally effective when patients are in respiratory failure and have only minimal air movement.
- The MDI or small-volume nebulizer is not prescribed for this patient.
- You did not obtain permission from medical control and/or it is not permissible by local protocol.
- The patient has already taken the maximum prescribed dose before your arrival.
- The medication is expired.
- There are other contraindications specific to the medication.

## Actions

Most respiratory inhalation medications relax the muscles that surround the air passages in the lungs,

## YOU are the Provider

After initiating the appropriate treatment, you place the patient onto the stretcher, load her into the ambulance, and begin transport to the hospital. You reassess her and note that her condition has acutely deteriorated.

You insert a nasopharyngeal airway and begin assisting her ventilations with a bag-mask device and high-flow oxygen.

| Recording Time: 9 Minutes | |
|---|---|
| Level of consciousness | Responsive only to pain |
| Respirations | 8 breaths/min; shallow |
| Pulse | 124 beats/min; weak |
| Skin | Cool and dry; cyanosis of the nail beds and around the lips |
| Blood pressure | 108/50 mm Hg |
| Spo$_2$ | 82% (on oxygen) |

**8.** Why is cyanosis a later sign of hypoxemia in patients with emphysema?

**9.** Why does tachycardia develop in patients with hypoxemia?

**TABLE 16-6** Respiratory Medications

| Medication | | | Indications | | | Use: Acute Versus Chronic Disease | |
|---|---|---|---|---|---|---|---|
| Generic Drug Name | Trade Names | Action | Asthma | Bronchitis | COPD | Acute | Chronic |
| Albuterol | Proventil, Ventolin, Volmax | Dilates bronchioles | Yes | Yes | Yes | Yes | No |
| Beclomethasone | Beclovent, Beconase, Qvar, Vanceril | Anti-inflammatory, reduces swelling | Yes | No | No | No | Yes |
| Cromolyn | Intal | Decreases release of histamines | Yes | No | No | No | Yes |
| Fluticasone | Flovent Diskus | Anti-inflammatory, reduces swelling | Yes | No | No | No | Yes |
| Fluticasone, salmeterol | Advair Diskus | Decreases secretions | Yes | No | No | No | Yes |
| Ipratropium bromide | Atrovent | Dilates bronchioles | Yes | Yes | Yes | Yes | No |
| Levalbuterol | Xopenex | Dilates bronchioles | Yes | Yes | Yes | Yes | No |
| Metaproterenol sulfate | Alupent, Metaprel | Dilates bronchioles | Yes | Yes | Yes | Yes | No |
| Montelukast | Singulair, oral tablet | Anti-inflammatory, reduces swelling | Yes | No | Yes | No | Yes |
| Salmeterol | Serevent Diskus | Dilates bronchioles | Yes | Yes | Yes | No | Yes |

© Jones & Bartlett Learning.

leading to enlargement (dilation) of the airways and easier movement of air. See **TABLE 16-6** for a list of respiratory inhalation medications. The medications used for acute symptoms are designed to give the patient rapid relief from symptoms if the condition is reversible. Medications used for chronic symptoms are administered for preventive measures or as maintenance doses. The medications for long-term use will provide little relief of acute symptoms.

## Side Effects

Common side effects of inhalers used for acute shortness of breath include increased pulse rate, nervousness, and muscle tremors. Often, a patient will begin coughing *after* administration of an inhaler as the airways are opened and secretions start to loosen and clear.

If the patient has a prescribed MDI or small-volume nebulizer, read the label carefully to make sure that the medication is to be used for shortness of breath and that it has been prescribed by a physician (**FIGURE 16-17**). When in doubt, consult medical control.

## Dose and Route

Medication from an inhaler is delivered through the respiratory tract to the lung. The dose is one puff for an MDI or continuation of the small-volume nebulizer until all the medication has been administered or the patient's signs and symptoms are resolved.

14. Allow the patient to breathe a few times, then repeat a second dose per direction from medical control or local protocol (**Step 4**).

## Administration of a Small-Volume Nebulizer

To help a patient self-administer medication from a small-volume nebulizer, follow the steps in **SKILL DRILL 16-2**:

1. Follow standard precautions.
2. Obtain an order from medical control or local protocol.
3. Check that you have the right medication, right patient, right dose, and right route, and that the medication is not expired. Ensure there are no issues with contamination, discoloration, or clarity of the medication (**Step 1**).
4. Make sure that the patient is alert enough to use the device.
5. Check whether the patient has already taken any treatments.
6. If assisting to assemble the device, maintain aseptic technique.
7. Open the medication container on the nebulizer and pour the medication (generally the whole volume of the medication) into the container. In some cases, sterile saline may be added (about 3 mL) to achieve the optimal volume of fluid for the nebulized application (**Step 2**).
8. Attach the medication container to the nebulizer mouthpiece and to the oxygen tubing. Attach the oxygen tubing to the oxygen tank.
9. Adjust oxygen flow to 6 L/min to establish a misting effect (**Step 3**).
10. Stop administering supplemental oxygen, and remove the nonrebreathing mask from the patient's face.
11. Ask the patient to put his or her lips around the mouthpiece of the device, inhale the mist, and hold it for 3 to 5 seconds before exhaling (**Step 4**).
12. When the mist dissipates and the container is empty or the patient is no longer experiencing shortness of breath, discontinue use of the device.
13. Place the nonrebreathing mask back on the patient if the patient continues to report shortness of breath.

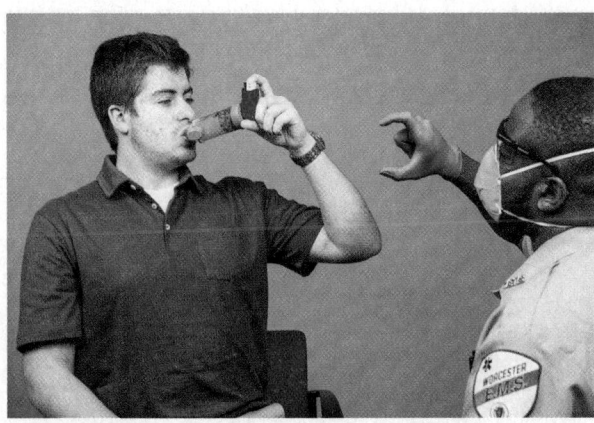

**FIGURE 16-17** Some inhalers have spacer devices to better control the medication delivery to the patient.

© Jones & Bartlett Learning.

## Administration of an MDI

To help a patient self-administer medication from an inhaler, follow the steps in **SKILL DRILL 16-1**:

1. Follow standard precautions.
2. Obtain an order from medical control or local protocol.
3. Check that you have the right medication, right patient, right dose, and right route and that the medication is not expired.
4. Make sure that the patient is alert enough to use the inhaler.
5. Check whether the patient has already taken any doses.
6. Make sure the inhaler is at room temperature or warmer (**Step 1**).
7. Shake the inhaler vigorously several times.
8. Stop administering supplemental oxygen, and remove any mask from the patient's face.
9. Ask the patient to exhale deeply and, before inhaling, to put his or her lips around the opening of the inhaler (**Step 2**).
10. Have the patient depress the hand-held inhaler as he or she begins to inhale deeply.
11. Instruct the patient to hold his or her breath for as long as is comfortable to help the body absorb the medication (**Step 3**).
12. If a spacer is used, the patient may need to take several breaths from the mouthpiece, without depressing the inhaler again, to get the full initial dose of the medication.
13. Continue to administer supplemental oxygen (replace the oxygen mask).

## Skill Drill 16-1 Assisting a Patient With a Metered-Dose Inhaler

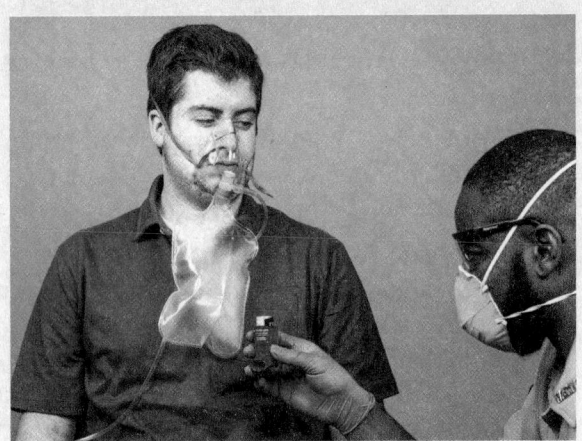

### Step 1

Check that you have the correct medication for the correct patient. Check the expiration date. Ensure the inhaler is at room temperature or warmer. A small-volume nebulizer can be used with a mouthpiece or a mask.

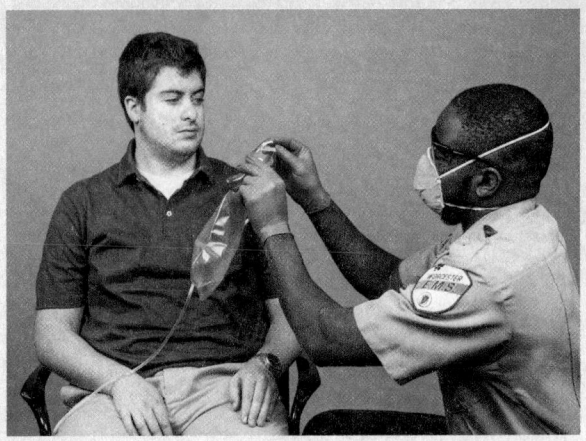

### Step 2

Remove the oxygen mask. Hand the inhaler to the patient. Instruct about breathing and lip seal.

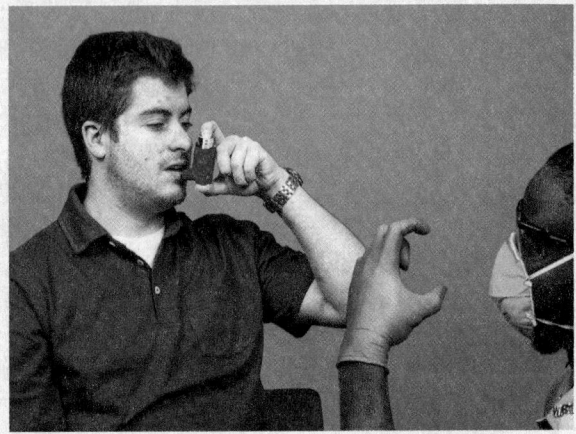

### Step 3

Instruct the patient to press the inhaler and inhale one puff. Instruct about breath holding.

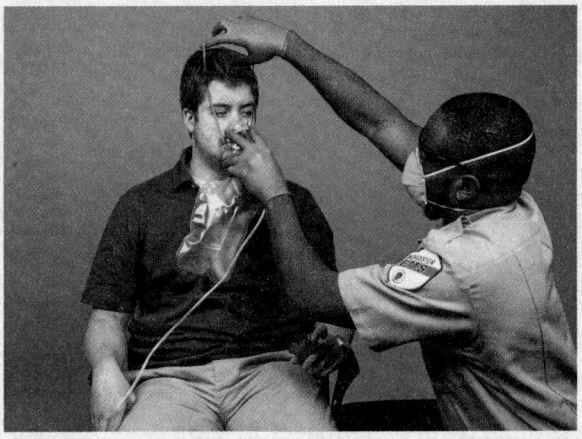

### Step 4

Reapply oxygen. After a few breaths, have the patient repeat the dose if the medical order or protocol allows.

## Skill Drill 16-2 Assisting a Patient With a Small-Volume Nebulizer

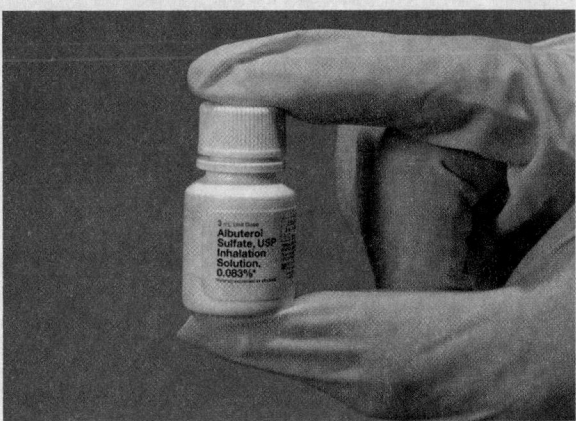

### Step 1

Check that you have the correct medication for the patient. Check the expiration date. Confirm you have the correct patient and the correct dose.

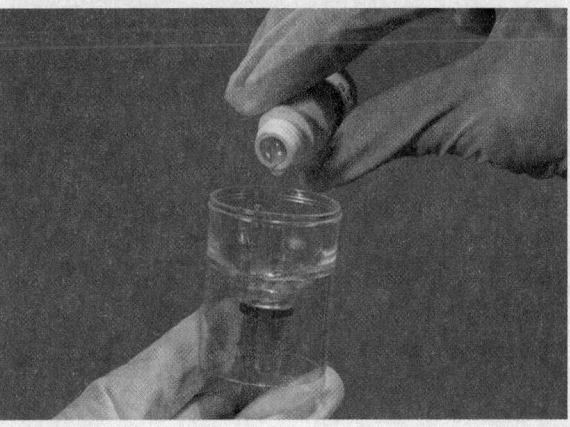

### Step 2

Pour the medication into the container on the nebulizer. In some cases, sterile saline may be added (about 3 mL) to achieve the optimal volume of fluid for the nebulized application.

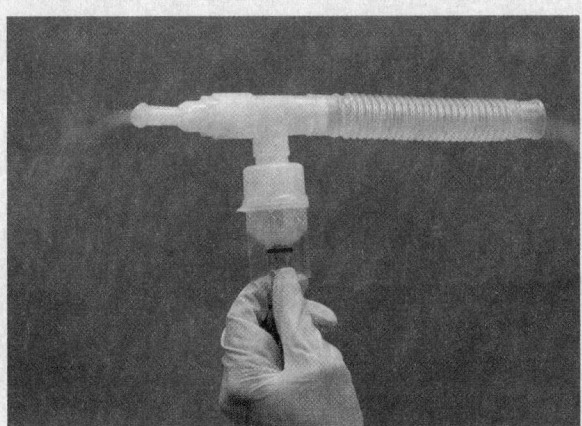

### Step 3

Attach the medication container to the nebulizer, mouthpiece, and tubing. Attach the oxygen tubing to the oxygen tank. Set the flowmeter at 6 L/min.

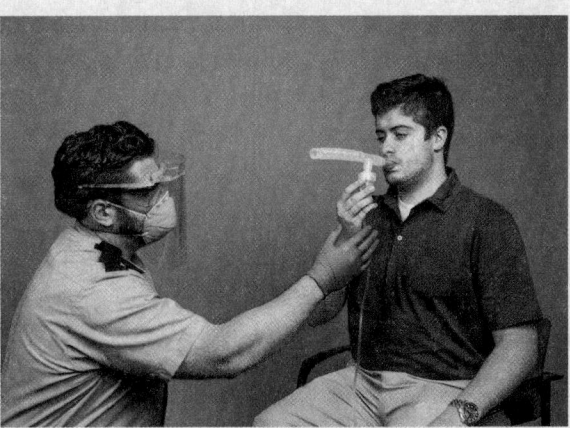

### Step 4

Instruct the patient on how to breathe.

14. Reassess vital signs, and document your actions and the patient's response.

15. Consult with medical control and/or follow local policy if repeated doses are necessary.

## Treatment of Specific Conditions

### Upper or Lower Airway Infection

Dyspnea associated with acute infections is common. In patients with pneumonia, acute bronchitis, or epiglottitis, it can become extremely serious. The acute congestion and stuffiness of a common cold hardly ever require emergency care. Indeed, most people with colds treat themselves with over-the-counter medications. However, people with a common cold who have underlying problems such as asthma or heart failure may experience a worsening of their condition as a result of the additional stress of the infection. In addition, medications for colds may have stressful side effects, such as agitation, increased heart rate, and increased blood pressure. Some people with influenza or another, more serious respiratory viral infection such as COVID-19 may initially mistake their symptoms for those occurring secondary to a common cold. Severe pneumonia with significant respiratory deterioration can rapidly develop in these patients.

For patients with upper airway infections and dyspnea, administer humidified oxygen (if available). Do not attempt to suction the airway or place an oropharyngeal airway in a patient with suspected epiglottitis. These maneuvers may cause a spasm and complete airway obstruction. Transport the patient promptly to the hospital. Allow the patient to sit in the position that is most comfortable. For most patients with respiratory difficulty, this is usually sitting upright and leaning forward in the sniffing position (**FIGURE 16-18**). To force a patient with epiglottitis to lie supine may cause upper airway obstruction that could result in death.

### Acute Pulmonary Edema

Dyspnea caused by acute pulmonary edema may be associated with cardiac disease or direct lung damage. In either case, administer 100% oxygen, and, if necessary, carefully suction any secretions from the airway. The best position for a conscious patient

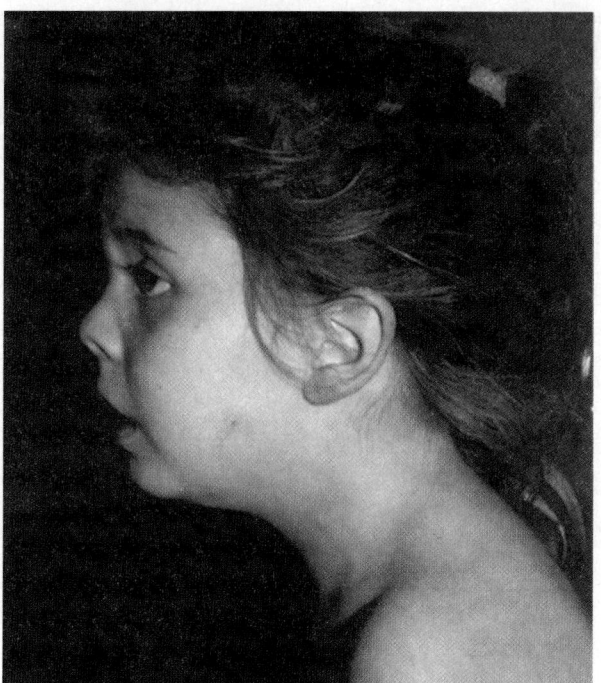

**FIGURE 16-18** A child with epiglottitis may be more comfortable sitting up and leaning forward.
© American Academy of Orthopaedic Surgeons.

who has acute pulmonary edema is the position in which it is easiest to breathe. Usually, this is sitting up. An unconscious patient with acute pulmonary edema may require full ventilatory support, including placement of an airway adjunct, positive-pressure ventilation with a bag-mask device, oxygen, and suctioning.

**Continuous positive airway pressure (CPAP)** is a noninvasive means of providing ventilatory support for patients experiencing respiratory distress associated with obstructive pulmonary disease (such as emphysema) and acute pulmonary edema. CPAP increases pressure in the lungs, opens collapsed alveoli, pushes more oxygen across the alveolar membrane, and forces interstitial fluid back into the pulmonary circulation. See Chapter 11, *Airway Management*, for a complete discussion and Skill Drill 11-10 for instructions on using CPAP. CPAP systems use oxygen to deliver the positive ventilatory pressure to the patient. Many patients show dramatic improvement with the use of CPAP. CPAP can be used for patients who have moderate to severe respiratory distress from an underlying disease, such as pulmonary edema or obstructive pulmonary disease (including emphysema), are alert and able to follow commands, have tachypnea, or have a pulse oximetry reading of less than 90%. One potential contraindication to the use of CPAP is low blood pressure. Because of the increased pressure inside the chest, blood flow returning to the heart is diminished, further decreasing blood pressure. CPAP is also not used in patients in respiratory arrest or who have signs and symptoms of a pneumothorax or chest trauma, a tracheostomy, a decreased level of consciousness, inability to follow commands, or active gastrointestinal bleeding.

If you are authorized to apply CPAP for acute pulmonary edema according to your local protocols, do so. Call for ALS support or provide prompt transport to the nearest appropriate ED. Continue to reassess patients using CPAP for signs of deterioration and/or respiratory failure.

## Chronic Obstructive Pulmonary Disease

Patients with COPD may have an altered level of consciousness or may be unresponsive from hypoxia or carbon dioxide retention. Patients with COPD often find breathing difficult when lying down. Assist with the patient's prescribed inhaler if there is one. Often a patient with COPD will overuse an inhaler, so watch for side effects. If approved by medical direction, the use of CPAP may be helpful for these patients. Promptly transport patients with COPD to the ED, allowing them to sit upright if this is most comfortable.

## Asthma, Hay Fever, and Anaphylaxis

Many lung problems are incorrectly labeled "asthma"; therefore, you must critically assess the patient. Asthma is often a recurring pathologic condition. Confirm whether the patient is able to breathe normally at other times. If possible, ask family members to describe the patient's asthma. Even if they only identify wheezing as a problem, be aware that some forms of heart failure, foreign body aspiration, toxic fumes inhalation, or allergic reactions may cause wheezing.

As you assess the patient's vital signs, note that the pulse rate will be normal or elevated, the blood pressure may be slightly elevated, and respirations will be increased. Ask questions about how and when the symptoms began.

As you care for the patient, be prepared to suction large amounts of mucus from the mouth and to administer oxygen. If you suction, do not withhold oxygen for more than 15 seconds for adult patients, 10 seconds for a child, and 5 seconds for an infant. Allow some time for oxygenation between suction attempts. If the patient is unconscious, you may need to provide airway management.

If the patient has medication, such as an inhaler for an asthma attack, you may help with its administration, as directed by local protocol. Even patients who use their inhaler may continue to get worse. Reassess breathing frequently and be prepared to assist ventilations with a bag-mask device in severe cases. If you must assist ventilations in a patient who is having an asthma attack, use slow, gentle breaths. Remember, the problem in asthma is getting the air out of the lungs, not into them. Resist the temptation to squeeze the bag hard and fast. Always assist with ventilations as a last resort, and then provide only about 10 to 12 shallow breaths/min.

A prolonged asthma attack that is unrelieved may progress into a condition known as *status asthmaticus*. The patient is likely to be frightened, frantically trying to breathe, and using all the accessory muscles. Status asthmaticus is a true emergency. Give oxygen and promptly transport to the ED.

The effort to breathe during an asthma attack is very tiring, and the patient may be exhausted by the time you arrive at the hospital. An exhausted patient may have stopped feeling anxious or even struggling to breathe. This patient is not recovering; the patient is at a critical stage and is likely to stop breathing. Aggressive airway management, oxygen administration, and prompt transport are essential in this situation. Advanced life support (ALS) should be considered. Follow local protocol.

The patient with hay fever is unlikely to need emergency treatment unless the condition has worsened from generalized cold symptoms.

An anaphylactic reaction is a life-threatening emergency. The first step should be to remove the offending agent. For example, if the patient has a stinger from a bee sting still in place, you may need to remove the stinger. Remember to scrape the stinger off because you can inject more venom into the patient if you pinch or squeeze the stinger.

If the patient is still awake, allow him or her to assume a position that does not compromise breathing. Use an appropriate oxygen device for supplemental oxygen administration. Be prepared to assist breathing as needed. Rapid transport and the early administration of epinephrine, should be a priority. Because epinephrine has immediate action, it can rapidly reverse the effects of anaphylaxis.

## Spontaneous Pneumothorax

Patients with spontaneous pneumothorax may have severe respiratory distress, or they may have no distress at all and report only pleuritic chest pain. Provide supplemental oxygen, and provide prompt transport to the hospital. Like most dyspneic patients, those with spontaneous pneumothorax are usually more comfortable sitting up. Monitor the patient carefully, watching for any sudden deterioration in the respiratory status. Be ready to support the airway, assist respirations, and provide CPR if it becomes necessary.

## Pleural Effusion

Treatment of pleural effusion consists of removal of fluid collected outside the lung, which must be done by a physician in a hospital setting. However, you should provide oxygen and other routine support measures to these patients.

## Obstruction of the Airway

If the patient is a small child or someone who was eating just before dyspnea developed, you start by assuming that the problem is an inhaled or aspirated foreign body. If the patient is old enough to talk but cannot make any noise, upper airway obstruction is the likely cause.

Upper airway obstruction may be either partial or complete. If your patient is able to talk and breathe, the wisest course may be to provide supplemental oxygen and transport carefully in a position of comfort to the hospital. As long as the patient is able to obtain sufficient oxygen, avoid doing anything that might turn a partial airway obstruction into a complete airway obstruction.

There is no condition more immediately life threatening than a complete airway obstruction.

The obstructing body must be removed before any other actions will be effective. Clear the patient's upper airway according to basic life support guidelines. The conscious child or adult patient who has an obstructed airway should be given abdominal thrusts and an infant should be given back blows and chest thrust following the American Heart Association guidelines. Opening the airway with the head tilt–chin lift maneuver (or the jaw-thrust maneuver for patients with suspected spinal trauma) may solve the problem. You should perform this maneuver only after you have ruled out a head or neck injury. If simply opening the airway does not correct the breathing problem, you will have to assess the upper airway for the obstruction. Then, whether or not you are successful in clearing the airway, administer supplemental oxygen and transport the patient promptly to the ED.

## Pulmonary Embolism

Because a considerable amount of lung tissue may not be functioning, supplemental oxygen is mandatory in a patient with a pulmonary embolism. Place the patient in a comfortable position, usually sitting, and assist breathing as necessary. Hemoptysis, if present, is usually not severe, but any blood that has been coughed up should be cleared from the airway. The patient may have an unusually rapid and possibly irregular heartbeat. Transport the patient to the ED promptly. Be aware that large pulmonary emboli may cause cardiac arrest.

## Hyperventilation

When you respond to a patient who is hyperventilating, complete a primary assessment and gather a history of the event. Is the patient having chest pain? Is there a history of cardiac problems or diabetes? You must always assume a serious underlying problem even if you suspect that the underlying problem is stress. Do *not* have the patient breathe into a paper bag, even though it was once thought to be the technique for managing hyperventilation syndrome. In theory, breathing into a paper bag causes the patient to rebreathe exhaled carbon dioxide, allowing the level of carbon dioxide in the blood to return to normal. In fact, if the patient is hyperventilating because of a serious medical problem, this maneuver could make things worse. A patient with underlying pulmonary disease who breathes into a bag may become severely hypoxic. Treatment should instead consist of reassuring the patient in a calm, professional manner; supplying supplemental oxygen; and providing prompt transport to the ED. Patients who hyperventilate need to be evaluated in the hospital.

## Environmental/Industrial Exposure

The commonality in these kinds of respiratory problems is the inhalation of a toxic chemical. There are many different types of chemicals, different types of presentations, and certainly different levels of severity. Ensure that all patients are decontaminated prior to treatment. Treat with oxygen, adjuncts, and suction on the basis of the presentation, level of consciousness, and level of distress observed in your patient.

## Foreign Body Aspiration

Upper airway obstruction is common in young children, who put objects in their mouths as a way to learn about them. If you have evidence of a partial or complete airway obstruction in a young child, especially a crawling baby, consider that the child may have swallowed and choked on a small object. Perform the appropriate airway clearing technique specific to the age of the child.

Another scenario to consider is that an object passed through the airway and has been aspirated (inhaled) into the lung. This problem will not be as obvious as an airway obstruction.

Most deaths from foreign body aspiration occur in patients who are younger than 5 years, and most of them are infants. Typical items aspirated include balloons, small balls, and small parts of toys. Toddlers may aspirate pieces of food such as hot dogs or peanuts.

One sign of aspiration in a child may be an abnormality in the voice. The aspirated object will most likely go down the right main stem bronchus. If the bronchus is fully obstructed, the lung could collapse. Aspiration pneumonia may also develop.

Provide oxygen, and transport any child with a suspected aspiration. A radiograph will be needed to confirm the aspiration, its location, and the treatment.

For an older person, the normal process of aging creates conditions that contribute to breathing problems. For example, weakening of the airway musculature can cause decreased breathing capacity. Decreased cough and gag reflexes cause a decreased ability to clear secretions. Difficulty in swallowing means the risk for aspiration is markedly increased. Older people can aspirate food or oral secretions that, in many cases, can develop into a potentially life-threatening aspiration pneumonia.

## Tracheostomy Dysfunction

Children with chronic pulmonary medical conditions may use a home ventilator that is connected by a tracheostomy tube. This tube is placed in an opening in the neck (stoma) and can sometimes become obstructed by secretions, mucus, or foreign bodies. Other tracheostomy tube complications include bleeding, leaking, dislodgement, and infection. Your main goal is to establish a patent airway. Place the patient in a position of comfort and provide suctioning to clear the obstruction. Caregivers, who have been trained to remove the obstructed tracheostomy, are able to replace it with a spare one. If you are unable to clear the airway, request ALS assistance. Once the obstruction is clear, oxygenate the patient and treat based on the patient's presentation.

Geriatric patients may have a tracheostomy tube in place because of airway obstruction, laryngeal cancer, severe infection, trauma, or the inability to manage secretions. As with children, the tube can become obstructed by secretions, foreign bodies, or airway swelling. The stoma itself can become infected. Your immediate goal is to establish airway patency.

## Asthma

Asthma is a common childhood illness. When you assess a pediatric patient, look for retractions of the skin above the sternum and between the ribs. Retractions are typically easier to see in children than in adults. Cyanosis is a late finding in children.

Keep in mind that a cough is not always a symptom of a cold; it could signal pneumonia or asthma. Even if you do not hear much wheezing, the presence of a cough can indicate that some degree of reactive airway disease or an acute asthma attack may be taking place.

The emergency care of a child with shortness of breath is the same as it is for an adult, including the use of supplemental oxygen. However, many small children will not tolerate (or may refuse to wear) a face mask. Rather than fighting with the child, provide blow-by oxygen by holding the oxygen mask in front of the child's face or ask the parent or caregiver to hold the mask (**FIGURE 16-19**).

Many children with asthma also will have prescribed handheld MDIs or small-volume nebulizers. Use these inhalers or nebulizers just as you would with an adult. Pediatric patients and some geriatric patients are more likely to use spacers to assist in inhaler use. Treat as in adult asthma.

Asthma in an older patient causes bronchospasm, swelling of the lining of the airways, and an accumulation of secretions. Attacks are easily triggered by air pollutants, viral infections, allergens, and sometimes something as simple as exposure to cold air. Asthma, like any chronic disease, can become life threatening in older people, especially in patients who have problems with airway control. The condition is made worse by anxiety and dehydration, which is typical in older people. Geriatric

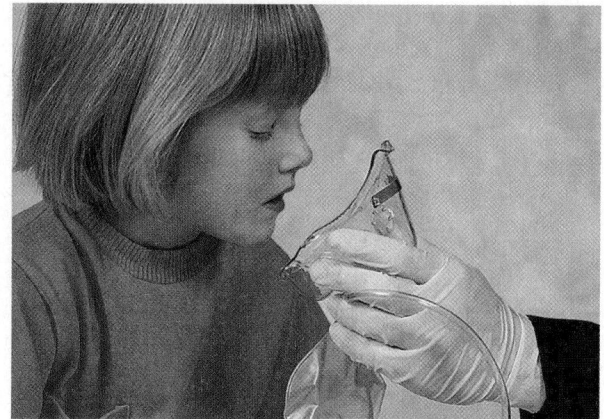

**FIGURE 16-19** Because children may refuse to wear an oxygen mask, you may have to hold the mask in front of the child's face or ask the parents or caregivers for help holding the mask for their child.
© Jones & Bartlett Learning. Courtesy of MIEMSS.

patients with asthma tend to have both inspiratory and expiratory wheezes.

## Cystic Fibrosis

Cystic fibrosis (CF) is a genetic disorder that affects the lungs and digestive system. CF disrupts the normal function of cells that make up the sweat glands

## YOU are the Provider

With an estimated time of arrival at the hospital of 8 minutes, you ask your partner to radio in the patient report. The patient's level of consciousness has not changed; however, the cyanosis around her mouth and in her nail beds has resolved and her oxygen saturation has improved. You complete your reassessment and continue treatment.

| Recording Time: 15 Minutes | |
|---|---|
| **Level of consciousness** | Responsive to pain only |
| **Respirations** | 12 breaths/min assisted |
| **Pulse** | 118 beats/min; weak |
| **Skin** | Cool and dry; cyanosis has resolved |
| **Blood pressure** | 112/70 mm Hg |
| **Spo$_2$** | 90% (with bag-mask device and oxygen) |

You deliver the patient to the ED staff and give your verbal report to the nurse. Because of the patient's decreased level of consciousness and the need for ongoing ventilation assistance, the physician elects to intubate her. She is diagnosed with acute exacerbation of her emphysema and is admitted to the intensive care unit.

**10.** How can positive-pressure ventilation cause a decrease in a patient's blood pressure?

**11.** What does *exacerbation* mean?

**12.** Should oxygen ever be withheld from a patient with COPD?

in the skin and that also line the lungs and the digestive and reproductive systems. The disease predisposes the child to repeated lung infections.

The disease process in CF disrupts the essential balance of salt and water necessary to maintain a normal coating of fluid and mucus inside the lungs and other organs. The end result is that the mucus becomes thick, sticky, and hard to move. The mucus holds germs, causing the lungs to become infected.

In CF, the child's symptoms range from sinus congestion to wheezing and asthmalike complaints. A chronic cough that produces thick, heavy, discolored mucus may develop in the child. As lung function decreases, so does the ability to breathe effectively. The child often has dyspnea; this generally results in the parents or caregivers calling EMS. Treat the child with suction and oxygen using age-appropriate adjuncts.

CF often causes death in childhood because of chronic pneumonia secondary to the thick, pathologic mucus in the airway. It also causes malabsorption of nutrients in the intestines. Because of advances in treatment, the life expectancy for patients with CF becomes better each year. Adults with CF are predisposed to other medical conditions, including arthritis, osteoporosis, diabetes, and liver problems.

## Special Populations

Most geriatric patients take medications, sometimes many, to treat various ailments that are part of the aging process. Some of these medications will blunt the body's normal reactions to stress and the mechanisms the body uses to compensate for respiratory compromise and hypoxia. For example, beta blockers, used for a variety of conditions, prevent heart rate from increasing to compensate for a decrease in blood pressure. Keep this in mind when you evaluate vital signs in geriatric patients.

## YOU are the Provider SUMMARY

**1. What is emphysema? What is the typical cause?**

Emphysema, a form of COPD, is a disease of the respiratory system in which chronic inflammation develops in the airways, and destruction of alveoli and small airways leads to a loss of lung elasticity. As a result, the expiratory phase of respiration becomes difficult and gas exchange in the lungs becomes impaired. Although emphysema is an irreversible condition, its symptoms can be reduced and the disease progression slowed with lifestyle changes (eg, quitting smoking) and certain medications.

The single most common cause of emphysema is heavy, long-term cigarette smoking. Other causes include frequent pulmonary infections and long-term exposure to toxic agents, such as from working in an industrial setting for a long period.

**2. Why is it especially significant that *this* patient called 9-1-1?**

Patients with chronic diseases call 9-1-1 when something is different or has gotten worse. The patient could be experiencing an acute flare-up of her emphysema, a secondary respiratory illness to which she is predisposed (such as pneumonia), or complete respiratory failure. Just because she has refused EMS transport in the past does not mean that she will this time; she has a known respiratory illness, which you should assume has gotten worse, and she should be treated no differently from any other patient with a respiratory emergency.

**3. What should be your *most* immediate action?**

Oxygen and lit cigarettes—or any other source of fire—do not go together! Ask the patient to immediately extinguish her cigarette and then continue your assessment. Although oxygen is not flammable or explosive, it does support the process of combustion. A small spark or lit cigarette can become a flame in an oxygen-rich atmosphere. Oxygen will cause a fire to burn more vigorously, as well as hotter. The patient could literally light her face on fire; you and your partner could be injured as well.

**4. How does emphysema differ from chronic bronchitis?**

Emphysema is a disease in which small airways and the inner walls of alveoli are progressively destroyed, resulting in a loss of lung elasticity. Chronic bronchitis is caused by persistent inflammation in larger airways. With chronic bronchitis, excess mucus is constantly produced, which obstructs the bronchioles and alveoli. As a result, pulmonary gas exchange is less efficient. Many patients with chronic bronchitis have a chronic productive cough. In some patients, however, the cough reflex is weakened; this causes sputum to settle in the lungs and become infected, resulting in pneumonia. Emphysema and chronic bronchitis are both forms of COPD, and both are usually caused by heavy, long-term cigarette smoking.

**5. Why do patients with emphysema breathe through pursed lips?**

With emphysema, the force of exhalation increases intrathoracic pressure and causes premature closure of the small airways, causing air to be trapped in the alveoli. The harder the patient tries to push air out, the more air gets trapped in the alveoli. Chronic air trapping in the lungs explains why many patients with long-term emphysema have a characteristic barrel-shape appearance to their chest. Over time, patients with emphysema learn that if they push air out slowly at a higher residual airway pressure, they can exhale more air than if they try to push it out faster because their airways will remain open for longer. One of the ways they do this is by breathing through pursed lips during exhalation. Pursed lip breathing allows the patient to push air out slowly under controlled pressure.

**6. What does a prolonged exhalation phase indicate in patients with obstructive lung disease?**

A prolonged exhalation phase indicates that the patient is experiencing difficulty exhaling air from the lungs, which, as a result, causes chronic air trapping in the lungs. The inhalation-to-exhalation ratio in healthy people during normal breathing is typically 1:2. In other words, it takes about twice as long to exhale as it does to inhale. Depending on the severity of their disease process, patients with obstructive lung disease may have an inhalation to exhalation ratio of 1:4, 1:5, or longer. Because the patient's bronchioles significantly narrow when he or she exhales, wheezing—a whistling sound—is often heard during the exhalation phase while auscultating the lungs.

**7. What treatment is indicated for the patient at this point?**

Compared with the patient's condition during your initial assessment, it has deteriorated. She is now confused and slow to answer your questions, which indicates decreased oxygen delivery to the brain. Her oxygen saturation level of 88% indicates significant hypoxemia, and the fatigue indicates that she is less able to compensate for her condition. She clearly needs a higher concentration of oxygen than what her nasal cannula is supplying. Apply a nonrebreathing mask, set the flow rate at 12 to 15 L/min, and reassess her condition. CPAP might be helpful, but remember that altered mental status is a contraindication to its use for patients with COPD. If oxygenation does not improve, assisted ventilation with a bag-mask device may be necessary. If you must assist the patient's breathing, however, ensure that you allow *complete* exhalation between positive-pressure breaths. Remember, patients with emphysema have a lot of air trapped in the alveoli.

**8. Why is cyanosis a later sign of hypoxemia in patients with emphysema?**

Patients with emphysema maintain chronically low blood oxygen levels and chronically elevated carbon dioxide levels. Unlike in otherwise healthy people, cyanosis often does not develop in patients with emphysema until significantly more hemoglobin is desaturated (not carrying oxygen). The absence of cyanosis does not rule out hypoxemia in any patient, especially a patient with alveoli who needs a longer period of time to move air out of the lungs.

**9. Why does tachycardia develop in patients with hypoxemia?**

Whenever the body's demand for oxygen increases and its supply decreases (eg, hypoxemia), the nervous system increases the production of epinephrine from the adrenal glands. Epinephrine is a hormone that causes tachycardia (rapid heart rate) and an increase in the strength of cardiac contraction. Tachycardia is a critical physiologic compensatory mechanism that circulates oxygenated blood faster, thus helping to maintain adequate perfusion of the body's vital organs. However, if the underlying cause of the patient's hypoxemia is not corrected, the nervous system, which also requires oxygen, will no longer be able to compensate and the patient's heart rate will begin to fall.

**10. How can positive-pressure ventilation cause a decrease in a patient's blood pressure?**

Recall from Chapter 11, *Airway Management*, that negative-pressure ventilation—the process that occurs with normal breathing—involves contraction of the diaphragm and intercostal muscles and a

## YOU are the Provider SUMMARY *continued*

decrease in intrathoracic pressure; as a result, air is pulled into the lungs. The decreased intrathoracic pressure also increases blood return to the heart by allowing the venae cavae to enlarge. Positive-pressure ventilation involves pushing air into the lungs, as occurs when artificial ventilation is done. It is critical to perform positive-pressure ventilation correctly. Deliver each breath over a period of 1 second, just enough to produce visible chest rise, at a rate that is appropriate for the patient (10 to 12 breaths/min for adults; 12 to 20 breaths/min for infants and children). If positive-pressure ventilation is delivered too fast or with too much force (hyperventilation), the resultant increase in intrathoracic pressure may impair blood return to the right atrium. The reduced blood return to the right side of the heart reduces the amount it can supply to the left side of the heart. If blood supply to the left side of the heart is reduced, less blood is pumped from the left ventricle per contraction (stroke volume). As a result, the patient's blood pressure (and perfusion status) will deteriorate.

### 11. What does *exacerbation* mean?

*Exacerbation* means to intensify or worsen in severity. In acute exacerbation of COPD, sometimes no other condition exists that would clearly explain the patient's sudden deterioration (ie, congestive heart failure, pneumonia). Patients with COPD often experience acute exacerbation of their disease secondary to a change in environmental conditions, such as weather, humidity, or sudden activation of central heating or cooling in the home. Like diseases such as asthma, COPD can also be exacerbated by certain triggers, such as cat dander, dust, and seasonal allergens. In some cases, acute exacerbation is idiopathic (of unknown cause). As the patient's disease progresses, he or she will eventually reach a point at which the lungs simply cannot support oxygenation and ventilation (end-stage COPD). In end-stage COPD, it can be difficult to determine whether the patient is experiencing an exacerbation that can be treated effectively or if he or she has reached the end of the disease process. This will not affect your treatment, however, which involves airway management and ensuring adequate oxygenation and ventilation.

### 12. Should oxygen ever be withheld from a patient with COPD?

Although the brain uses the carbon dioxide level in the blood in regulating respiratory rate, some patients with COPD have a chronically high carbon dioxide level because of the difficulty removing it during exhalation. In those patients, the oxygen level in the blood becomes the stimulus for the respiratory process (hypoxic drive). Some patients who depend on hypoxic drive may decrease their respiratory effort if given increased oxygen. If a patient is hypoxic, however, it is essential that increased oxygen be given. If the respiratory rate and depth start to decrease, the problem can be managed by providing bag-mask ventilation.

### EMS Patient Care Report (PCR)

| Date: 3-12-20 | Incident No.: 130309 | Nature of Call: Respiratory | | Location: 109 East Lawler St. | |
|---|---|---|---|---|---|
| Dispatched: 0430 | En Route: 0432 | At Scene: 0440 | Transport: 0449 | At Hospital: 0510 | In Service: 0519 |

#### Patient Information

| Age: 72 <br> Sex: F <br> Weight (in kg [lb]): 50 kg (110 lb) | Allergies: Sulfa, ibuprofen, aspirin <br> Medications: Oxygen, Combivent, albuterol, lisinopril <br> Past Medical History: Emphysema, hypertension, gout <br> Chief Complaint: Trouble breathing |
|---|---|

#### Vital Signs

| Time: 0443 | BP: 116/54 | Pulse: 110 | Respirations: 28 | $SpO_2$: 88% |
|---|---|---|---|---|
| Time: 0449 | BP: 108/50 | Pulse: 124 | Respirations: 8 | $SpO_2$: 82% |
| Time: 0455 | BP: 112/70 | Pulse: 118 | Respirations: 12 | $SpO_2$: 90% |

## YOU are the Provider SUMMARY *continued*

| EMS Treatment (circle all that apply) | | | | |
|---|---|---|---|---|
| Oxygen @ _15_ L/min via:<br>(NC) NRM (Bag mask) | | Assisted Ventilation | Airway Adjunct:<br>(NPA) | CPR |
| Defibrillation | Bleeding Control | Bandaging | Splinting | Other |

| Narrative |
|---|

Dispatched to the residence of a 72-year-old woman with difficulty breathing.

Chief Complaint: Trouble breathing

History: Past medical history significant for emphysema, hypertension, and gout. The patient states that she is normally short of breath; however, it suddenly worsened today. Patient takes numerous medications and states that she has been compliant with all of them.

Assessment: On arrival at the scene, found the patient sitting on the edge of her couch; she was wearing home oxygen via nasal cannula and was smoking a cigarette. Immediately asked patient to extinguish cigarette and continued with the primary assessment. Patient could only speak in two-word sentences and was experiencing marked respiratory distress. Further assessment revealed pursed lip breathing, prolonged exhalation, and scattered wheezing on auscultation.

Treatment (Rx): Obtained vital signs and applied high-flow oxygen via bag-mask ventilation because of signs of worsened hypoxemia. Placed patient onto stretcher, loaded her into the ambulance, and reassessed her condition. Patient's level of consciousness had markedly decreased (responsive to pain only), her respirations became slow and shallow, her oxygen saturation decreased, and cyanosis developed around her mouth and to her nail beds. Inserted nasal airway and began assisting her ventilations with a bag-mask device and high-flow oxygen.

Transport: Began transport to hospital and continued treatment. En route, noted that patient's oxygen saturation had improved and her cyanosis had resolved; however, her LOC remained unchanged. Continued treatment and reassessment until arrival at the hospital. Transferred patient care to ED staff w/o incident. Verbal report given to staff nurse.

**End of report**

# Prep Kit

## Ready for Review

- Dyspnea is a common complaint that may be caused by numerous medical problems, including infections of the upper or lower airways, acute pulmonary edema, COPD, spontaneous pneumothorax, asthma, allergic reactions, pleural effusion, mechanical obstruction of the airway, pulmonary embolism, and hyperventilation.
- Each of these lung disorders has the capability to interfere with the exchange of oxygen and carbon dioxide that takes place during respiration. This interference may take the form of damage to the alveoli, separation of the alveoli from the pulmonary vessels by fluid or infection, obstruction of the air passages, or air or excess fluid in the pleural space.
- Patients with chronic lung diseases often have high levels of blood carbon dioxide; in some cases, giving too much oxygen to them may depress or stop respirations (hypoxic drive). However, never withhold oxygen from patients with dyspnea.

- Breathing difficulty and/or hypoxia often develop in patients with the following medical conditions: upper or lower airway infection, acute pulmonary edema, COPD, hay fever, asthma, anaphylaxis, spontaneous pneumothorax, and pleural cffusion.
- Infectious diseases associated with dyspnea include epiglottitis, bronchitis, TB, pneumonia, and pertussis.
- Breath sounds (lung sounds) are some of the most important vital signs you should assess when treating a patient in respiratory distress.
- Signs and symptoms of breathing difficulty include adventitious breath sounds (wheezing, stridor, crackles, and rhonchi); nasal flaring; pursed lip breathing; cyanosis; inability to talk; use of accessory muscles to breathe; and sitting in the tripod position, which allows the diaphragm the most room to function.
- Interventions for respiratory problems may include the following:
  - Oxygen via a nonrebreathing mask at 15 L/min, or positive-pressure ventilations using a bag-mask device
  - Airway management techniques such as use of an oropharyngeal (oral) airway, a nasopharyngeal (nasal) airway, suctioning, or airway positioning
  - Providing noninvasive ventilatory support with CPAP
  - Positioning the patient in a high Fowler position or a position of comfort to facilitate breathing
  - Assistance with respiratory medications found in a prescribed MDI or a small-volume nebulizer (Consult medical control to assist with its use or follow standing orders if the orders allow for this.)
- A patient who is breathing rapidly may not be getting enough oxygen as a result of respiratory distress from a variety of problems, including pneumonia or a pulmonary embolism; trying to blow off more carbon dioxide to compensate for acidosis caused by a poison, a severe infection, or a high level of blood glucose; or having a stress reaction.
- In every case, prompt recognition of the problem, administration of oxygen, and prompt transport are essential.

## Vital Vocabulary

**acidosis** The buildup of excess acid in the blood or body tissues that can result from a primary illness.

**adventitious breath sounds** Abnormal breath sounds such as wheezing, stridor, rhonchi, and crackles.

**alkalosis** The buildup of excess base (lack of acids) in the body fluids.

**allergen** A substance that causes an allergic reaction.

**anaphylaxis** An extreme, life-threatening, systemic allergic reaction that may include shock and respiratory failure.

**asthma** An acute spasm of the smaller air passages, called bronchioles, associated with excessive mucus production and with swelling of the mucous lining of the respiratory passages.

**atelectasis** Collapse of the alveolar air spaces of the lungs.

**bronchial breath sounds** Normal breath sounds made by air moving through the bronchi.

**bronchiolitis** Inflammation of the bronchioles that usually occurs in children younger than 2 years and is often caused by the respiratory syncytial virus.

**bronchitis** An acute or chronic inflammation of the lung that may damage lung tissue; usually associated with cough and production of sputum and, depending on its cause, sometimes fever.

**carbon dioxide retention** A condition characterized by a chronically high blood level of carbon dioxide in which the respiratory center no longer responds to high blood levels of carbon dioxide.

**carbon monoxide**  An odorless, colorless, tasteless, and highly poisonous gas that results from incomplete oxidation of carbon in combustion.

**chronic bronchitis**  Irritation of the major lung passageways from long-term exposure to infectious disease or irritants such as smoke.

**chronic obstructive pulmonary disease (COPD)**  A lung disease characterized by chronic obstruction of lung airflow that interferes with normal breathing and is not fully reversible.

**continuous positive airway pressure (CPAP)**  A method of ventilation used primarily in the treatment of critically ill patients with respiratory distress; can prevent the need for endotracheal intubation.

**COVID-19**  A respiratory disease caused by the virus SARS-CoV-2. The virus is a coronavirus, similar to the one that causes the common cold.

**crackles**  Crackling, rattling breath sounds that signal fluid in the air spaces of the lungs.

**croup**  A viral inflammatory disease of the upper respiratory system that may cause a partial airway obstruction and is characterized by a barking cough; usually seen in children.

**diphtheria**  An infectious disease in which a pseudomembrane forms, lining the pharynx; this lining can severely obstruct the passage of air into the larynx.

**dyspnea**  Shortness of breath.

**embolus**  A blood clot or other substance in the circulatory system that travels to a blood vessel where it causes a blockage of blood flow.

**emphysema**  A disease of the lungs in which there is extreme dilation and eventual destruction of the pulmonary alveoli with poor exchange of oxygen and carbon dioxide; it is one form of chronic obstructive pulmonary disease.

**epiglottitis**  A bacterial infection in which the epiglottis becomes inflamed and enlarged and may cause an upper airway obstruction.

**hay fever**  An allergic response, usually to outdoor airborne allergens such as pollen or sometimes indoor allergens such as dust mites or pet dander; also called allergic rhinitis.

**hyperventilation**  Rapid, usually deep, breathing that lowers the blood carbon dioxide level below normal.

**hyperventilation syndrome**  This syndrome occurs in the absence of physical problems. The respirations of a person who is experiencing hyperventilation syndrome may be as high as 40 shallow breaths/min or as low as only 20 very deep breaths/min. This syndrome is often associated with panic attacks.

**hypoxia**  A dangerous condition in which the body tissues and cells do not have enough oxygen.

**hypoxic drive**  A condition in which chronically low levels of oxygen in the blood stimulate the respiratory drive; seen in patients with chronic lung diseases.

**influenza type A**  Virus that has crossed the animal/human barrier and has infected humans, recently reaching a pandemic level with the H1N1 strain.

**metered-dose inhaler (MDI)**  A miniature spray canister used to direct medications through the mouth and into the lungs.

**orthopnea**  Severe dyspnea experienced when lying down and relieved by sitting up.

**oxygenation**  The process of delivering oxygen to the blood by diffusion from the alveoli following inhalation into the lungs.

**pandemic**  An outbreak that occurs on a global scale.

**paroxysmal nocturnal dyspnea**  Severe shortness of breath, especially at night after several hours of reclining; the person is forced to sit up to breathe.

**pertussis (whooping cough)**  An airborne bacterial infection that affects mostly children younger than 6 years. Patients will be feverish and exhibit a "whoop" sound on inspiration after a coughing attack; highly contagious through droplet infection.

**pleural effusion** A collection of fluid between the lung and chest wall that may compress the lung.

**pleuritic chest pain** Sharp, stabbing pain in the chest that is worsened by a deep breath or other chest wall movement; often caused by inflammation or irritation of the pleura.

**pneumonia** An infectious disease of the lung that damages lung tissue.

**pneumothorax** An accumulation of air or gas in the pleural cavity.

**pulmonary edema** A buildup of fluid in the lungs, often as a result of congestive heart failure.

**pulmonary embolism** A blood clot that breaks off from a large vein and travels to the blood vessels of the lung, causing obstruction of blood flow.

**respiration** The process of exchanging oxygen and carbon dioxide.

**respiratory syncytial virus (RSV)** A virus that causes an infection of the lungs and breathing passages; can lead to other serious illnesses that affect the lungs or heart, such as bronchiolitis and pneumonia. RSV is highly contagious and spread through droplets.

**rhonchi** Coarse, low-pitched breath sounds heard in patients with chronic mucus in the upper airways.

**small-volume nebulizer** A respiratory device that holds liquid medicine that is turned into a fine mist. The patient inhales the medication into the airways and lungs as a treatment for conditions such as asthma.

**stridor** A harsh, high-pitched respiratory sound, generally heard during inspiration, that is caused by partial blockage or narrowing of the upper airway; may be audible without a stethoscope.

**tuberculosis (TB)** A contagious disease that attacks the lungs and that can remain dormant in a person's lungs for decades, then reactivate; many strains are resistant to antibiotics. TB is spread by cough.

**ventilation** Exchange of air between the lungs and the environment, spontaneously by the patient or with assistance from another person, such as an EMT.

**vesicular breath sounds** Normal breath sounds made by air moving in and out of the alveoli.

**wheezing** A high-pitched, whistling breath sound that is most prominent on expiration, and which suggests an obstruction or narrowing of the lower airways; occurs in asthma and bronchiolitis.

## References

1. Chameides L, Samson RA, Schexnayder SM, Hazinski MF, eds. *Pediatric Advanced Life Support Provider Manual.* Dallas, TX: American Heart Association; 2012.

2. Jeng MJ, Lee YS, Tsao PC, Yang CF, Soong WJ. A longitudinal study on early hospitalized airway infections and subsequent childhood asthma. *PLoS One* 2015;10(4):e0121906. doi: 10.1371/journal.pone.0121906.

3. Kukla P, McIntyre WF, Koracevic G, et al. Relation of atrial fibrillation and right-sided cardiac thrombus to outcomes in patients with acute pulmonary embolism. *Am J Cardiol* 2015;115(6):825–830.

4. Mankad R. Cardiac asthma: what causes it? Mayo Clinic website. http://www.mayoclinic.org/diseases-conditions /heart-failure/expert-answers/cardiacasthma/FAQ -20058447. Published January 26, 2019. Accessed March 26, 2020.

5. National Association of State EMS Officials. *National EMS Scope of Practice Model 2019.* Washington, DC: National Highway Traffic Safety Administration; February 2019. Report No. DOT HS 812-666.

https://www.ems.gov/pdf/National_EMS_Scope_of _Practice_Model_2019.pdf. Accessed March 26, 2020.

6. National Center for Environmental Health. Asthma data statistics and surveillance. Centers for Disease Control and Prevention website. https://www.cdc.gov/asthma /asthmadata.htm. Reviewed January 28, 2020. Accessed March 26, 2020.

7. National Center for Immunization and Respiratory Diseases. What vaccines are recommended for you. Centers for Disease Control and Prevention website. http://www .cdc.gov/vaccines/adults/rec-vac/index.html. Reviewed November 21, 2019. Accessed March 26, 2020.

8. National Center for Immunization and Respiratory Diseases, Division of Bacterial Diseases. Diphtheria: symptoms. Centers for Disease Control and Prevention website. http://www.cdc.gov/diphtheria/about /symptoms.html. Updated December 17, 2018. Accessed March 26, 2020.

9. National Center for Immunization and Respiratory Diseases, Division of Viral Diseases. Respiratory syncytial

virus infection (RSV): symptoms and care. Centers for Disease Control and Prevention website. http://www.cdc .gov/rsv/about/symptoms.html. Updated June 26, 2018. Accessed March 26, 2020.

10. *National Emergency Medical Services Education Standards.* U.S. Department of Transportation. National Highway Traffic Safety Administration. DOT HS 811 077A. January 2009. www.ems.gov/pdf/811077a.pdf. Accessed March 10, 2020.

11. Poisoning: picture of America report. Centers for Disease Control and Prevention website. https://www.cdc.gov /pictureofamerica/pdfs/Picture_of_America_Poisoning. pdf. Updated 2014. Accessed March 26, 2020.

12. US Department of Health and Human Services. Chronic obstructive pulmonary disease (COPD). National Institutes of Health website. https://archives.nih.gov/asites /report/09-09-2019/report.nih.gov/nihfactsheets /ViewFactSheet7b57.html?csid=77&key=C#C. Updated June 30, 2018. Accessed March 26, 2020.

13. US Department of Health and Human Services. COPD action plan. National Heart, Lung, and Blood Institute website. https://www.nhlbi.nih.gov/health-topics /education-and-awareness/COPD-national-action-plan. Accessed March 26, 2020.

14. US Department of Health and Human Services. What is COPD? National Heart, Lung, and Blood Institute website. http://www.nhlbi.nih.gov/health/health-topics/topics /copd. Accessed March 26, 2020.

15. US Department of Health and Human Services. Who is at risk for pulmonary embolism? National Heart, Lung, and Blood Institute website. http://www.nhlbi.nih.gov /health/health-topics/topics/pe/atrisk. Accessed March 26, 2020.

16. US National Library of Medicine. Epiglottitis. MedlinePlus website. http://www.nlm.nih.gov/medlineplus/ency /article/000605.htm. Updated March 23, 2020. Accessed March 26, 2020.

17. World Health Organization. COPD: definition. https:// www.who.int/respiratory/copd/definition/en/. Accessed March 26, 2020.

18. World Health Organization. Pertussis. https://www.who .int/immunization/diseases/pertussis/en/. Updated May 9, 2018. Accessed March 26, 2020.

19. World Health Organization. Pneumonia. https://www .who.int/news-room/fact-sheets/detail/pneumonia. Updated August 2, 2019. Accessed March 26, 2020.

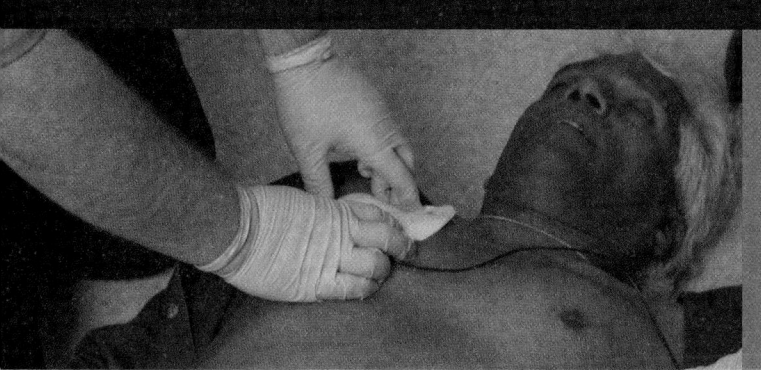

# Chapter 17

# Cardiovascular Emergencies

## NATIONAL EMS EDUCATION STANDARD COMPETENCIES

### Pathophysiology

Applies fundamental knowledge of the pathophysiology of respiration and perfusion to patient assessment and management.

### Medicine

Applies fundamental knowledge to provide basic emergency care and transportation based on assessment findings for an acutely ill patient.

### Cardiovascular

Anatomy, signs, symptoms, and management of
- Chest pain (pp 677–716)
- Cardiac arrest (pp 677–688, 705–716)

Anatomy, physiology, pathophysiology, assessment, and management of
- Acute coronary syndrome (pp 677–688, 692–716)
  - Angina pectoris (pp 677–686, 692–702)
  - Myocardial infarction (pp 677–688, 705–716)
- Aortic aneurysm/dissection (pp 677–684, 692–702)
- Thromboembolism (pp 677–685, 692–702)
- Heart failure (pp 677–684, 688–702)
- Hypertensive emergencies (pp 677–684, 690–702)

## KNOWLEDGE OBJECTIVES

1. Discuss the basic anatomy and physiology of the cardiovascular system. (pp 677–684)
2. Discuss the pathophysiology of the cardiovascular system. (pp 684–692)
3. Describe the anatomy, physiology, pathophysiology, assessment, and management of thromboembolism. (pp 684–688)
4. Describe the anatomy, physiology, pathophysiology, assessment, and management of angina pectoris. (pp 685–686)
5. Describe the anatomy, physiology, pathophysiology, assessment, and management of myocardial infarction. (pp 686–688)
6. Describe the anatomy, signs and symptoms, and management of hypertensive emergencies. (pp 690–692)
7. Describe the anatomy, physiology, pathophysiology, assessment, and management of aortic aneurysm/dissection. (p 691)
8. Explain the assessment for patients with cardiovascular problems. (pp 692–696)
9. Explain the relationship between airway management and the patient with cardiac compromise. (pp 692–693)
10. Give the indications and contraindications for the use of aspirin and nitroglycerin. (pp 697–699)

11. Recognize that many patients will have had cardiac surgery and may have implanted pacemakers or defibrillators. (pp 703–704)
12. Define cardiac arrest. (p 705)
13. Compare the difference between the fully automated and the semiautomated defibrillator. (pp 705–707)
14. Describe the different types of AEDs. (pp 705–707)
15. Explain the use of remote adhesive defibrillator pads. (p 706)
16. Recognize that not all patients in cardiac arrest require an electric shock. (p 707)
17. List the indications and contraindications for use of an AED. (pp 707–708)
18. Discuss the reasons for early defibrillation. (p 707)
19. Explain the circumstances that may result in inappropriate shocks from an AED. (p 708)
20. Explain the reason not to touch the patient, such as by delivering CPR, while the AED is analyzing the heart rhythm and delivering shocks. (pp 708, 710)
21. Describe AED maintenance procedures. (pp 708–710)
22. Explain the relationship of age to energy delivery. (p 708)
23. Explain the role of medical direction in the use of AEDs. (p 710)
24. Discuss the importance of practice and continuing education with the AED. (p 710)
25. Explain the need for a case review of each incident in which an AED is used. (p 710)
26. List quality improvement goals relating to AEDs. (p 710)
27. Discuss the procedures to follow for standard operation of the various types of AEDs. (pp 710–714)
28. Describe the emergency medical care for the patient with cardiac arrest. (pp 710–714)
29. Describe the components of patient care following AED shocks. (p 714)
30. Explain criteria for transport of the patient for advanced life support (ALS) following CPR and defibrillation. (pp 714–715)
31. Discuss the importance of coordinating with ALS personnel. (pp 715–716)

## SKILLS OBJECTIVES

1. Describe the steps to take in the assessment of a patient with chest pain or discomfort. (pp 692–696)
2. Demonstrate how to provide emergency medical care for a patient with chest pain or discomfort. (pp 696–697)
3. Demonstrate how to administer nitroglycerin. (pp 697–699, Skill Drill 17-1)
4. Demonstrate how to attach a cardiac monitor to obtain an ECG. (pp 700–702, Skill Drill 17-2)
5. Demonstrate how to perform maintenance of an AED. (pp 708–710)
6. Demonstrate how to perform CPR. (pp 711, 713–714)
7. Demonstrate the use of an AED. (pp 711–714, Skill Drill 17-3)

# Introduction

The American Heart Association reports that cardiovascular disease claimed 840,768 lives in the United States in 2016. This is 30.6% of all deaths, or approximately 1 in 3 deaths. Although this is a decline from previous years, heart disease has been the leading killer of Americans since 1900.

It is important for EMS providers to understand that many deaths caused by cardiovascular disease occur because of problems that may have been avoided by people living more healthful lifestyles and by access to improved medical technology. The number of deaths can be reduced with better public awareness, early access to medical care, increased numbers of laypeople trained in cardiopulmonary resuscitation (CPR), increased use of evolving technology in dispatch and cardiac arrest response, public access to defibrillation devices, the recognition of the need for advanced life support (ALS) services, and use of cardiac specialty centers when they are available.

This chapter begins with a brief description of the heart and how it works. It then discusses the relationship between chest pain or discomfort and ischemic heart disease. It explains how to recognize and treat acute myocardial infarction (classic heart attack) and its complications—sudden death,

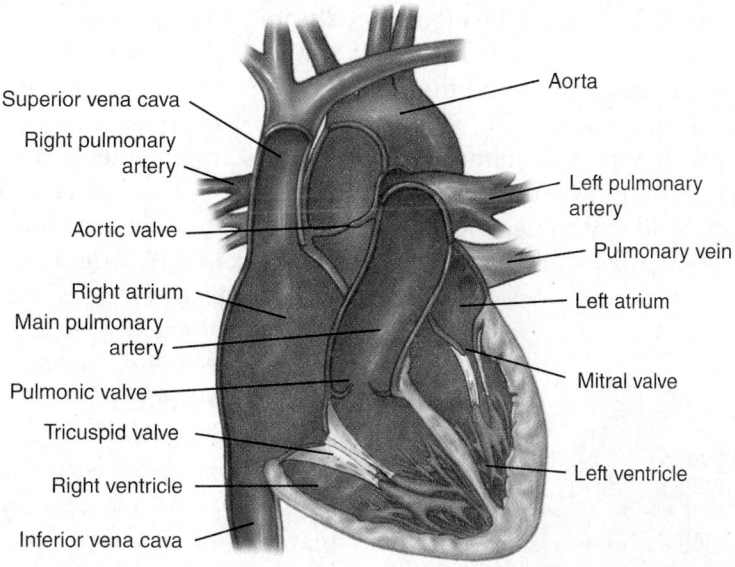

**FIGURE 17-1** The heart is a four-chambered muscle that pumps blood to all parts of the body.

© Jones & Bartlett Learning.

Labels on figure:
- Superior vena cava
- Right pulmonary artery
- Aortic valve
- Right atrium
- Main pulmonary artery
- Pulmonic valve
- Tricuspid valve
- Right ventricle
- Inferior vena cava
- Aorta
- Left pulmonary artery
- Pulmonary vein
- Left atrium
- Mitral valve
- Left ventricle

cardiogenic shock, and congestive heart failure (CHF). The use of nitroglycerin and aspirin are described. The last part of the chapter is devoted to the use and maintenance of the automated external defibrillator (AED).

## Anatomy and Physiology

The heart is a relatively simple organ with a simple job. It pumps blood to supply oxygen-enriched red blood cells to the tissues of the body. The heart is divided down the middle into two sides (left and right) by a wall called the septum. Each side of the heart has an **atrium**, or upper chamber, to receive incoming blood, and a **ventricle**, or lower chamber,

to pump outgoing blood (**FIGURE 17-1**). Blood leaves each of the four chambers of the heart through a one-way valve. These valves keep the blood moving through the circulatory system in the proper direction. The **aorta**, the body's main artery, receives the blood ejected from the left ventricle and delivers it to all the other arteries so they can carry blood to the tissues of the body.

The right side of the heart receives oxygen-poor (deoxygenated) blood from the veins of the body (**FIGURE 17-2A**). Blood from the superior and inferior venae cavae enters the right atrium, which then fills the right ventricle. After contraction of the right ventricle, blood flows into the pulmonary artery and travels through the pulmonary circulation

---

**YOU** are the Provider

You and your partner are returning to your station after completing a call when you are dispatched to 1152 Blanco Road for a 60-year-old woman with chest pain. Dispatch advises you that the patient's son, who called 9-1-1, stated that she has a history of heart problems. You proceed to the scene, which is approximately 5 minutes away. The time is 0942 hours, traffic is light, the weather is clear, and the temperature is 80°F (27°C).

**1.** What is the function of the heart?

**2.** What does the heart require to function effectively?

**3.** What should you include in your primary assessment of a patient with cardiac problems?

in the lungs, where it is reoxygenated. As the blood reaches the lungs, it receives fresh oxygen from the alveoli and carbon dioxide waste is removed from the blood and moved into the alveoli. The blood then returns to the heart through the pulmonary veins. The left side of the heart receives oxygen-rich (oxygenated) blood from the lungs through the pulmonary veins (**FIGURE 17-2B**). Blood enters the left

atrium and then passes into the left ventricle. The left ventricle is more muscular than the right ventricle because it must pump blood into the aorta to supply all the other arteries of the body.

The heart contains more than muscle tissue. The heart's electrical conduction system controls heart rate and enables the atria and ventricles to work together (**FIGURE 17-3**). Normal electrical impulses begin in the sinus node, which is in the upper part of the right atrium and is also known as the sinoatrial (SA) node. The impulses travel across both atria, stimulating them to contract. Between the atria and the ventricles, the impulses cross a bridge of special electrical tissue called the atrioventricular (AV) node. Here, the signal is slowed for about one-to two-tenths of a second to allow blood time to pass from the atria to the ventricles. The impulses then exit the AV node and spread throughout both ventricles via the bundle of His, the right and left bundle branches, and the Purkinje fibers, ultimately causing the muscle cells of the ventricles to contract.

Cardiac muscle cells have a special characteristic called **automaticity** that is not found in any other type of muscle cells. Automaticity allows a cardiac muscle cell to contract spontaneously without a stimulus from a nerve source. Normal impulses in the heart start at the SA node. As long as impulses come from the SA node, the other myocardial cells will contract when the impulse reaches them. However, if no impulse arrives, the other myocardial

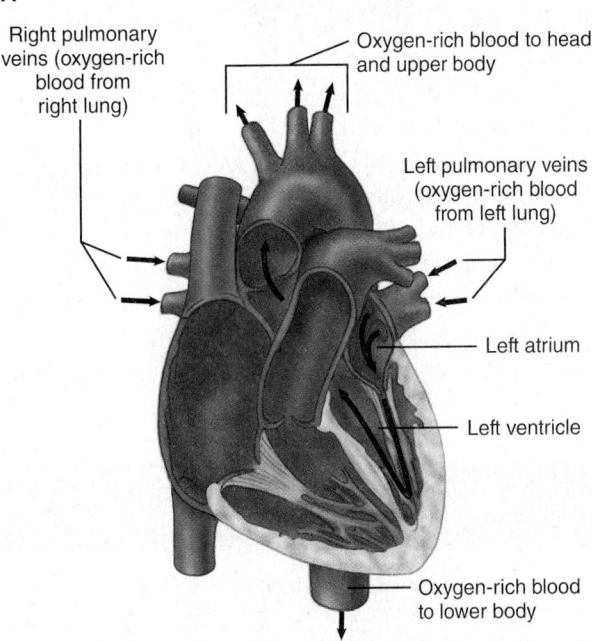

**FIGURE 17-2 A.** The right side of the heart receives oxygen-poor blood from the venous circulation. **B.** The left side of the heart receives oxygen-rich blood from the lungs through the pulmonary veins.

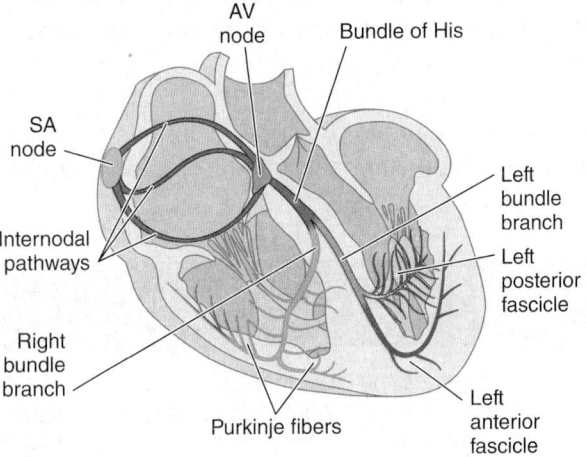

**FIGURE 17-3** The electrical conduction system of the heart controls most aspects of heart rate and enables the four chambers to work together.

AV = atrioventricular; SA = sinoatrial.

cells are capable of creating their own impulses and stimulating a contraction of the heart, although at a generally slower rate.

The stimulus that originates in the SA node is controlled by impulses from the brain, which arrive by way of the autonomic nervous system. The autonomic nervous system is the part of the brain that controls the functions of the body that do not require conscious thought, such as the heartbeat, respirations, dilation and constriction of blood vessels, and digestion of food. The autonomic nervous system has two parts, the sympathetic nervous system and the parasympathetic nervous system. The sympathetic nervous system is also known as the fight-or-flight system and makes adjustments to the body to compensate for increased physical activity. The sympathetic nervous system speeds up the heart rate, increases respiratory rate and depth, dilates blood vessels in the muscles, and constricts blood vessels in the digestive system. The parasympathetic nervous system directly opposes the sympathetic nervous system. The parasympathetic nervous system slows the heart and respiratory rates, constricts blood vessels in the muscles, and dilates blood vessels in the digestive system. Normally, these two systems balance each other, but in times of stress, the sympathetic nervous system gains primary control, whereas in times of relaxation, the parasympathetic system takes control.

## Circulation

To perform the function of pumping blood, the myocardium, or heart muscle, must have a continuous supply of oxygen and nutrients. During periods of physical exertion or stress, the myocardium requires more oxygen. The heart must increase cardiac output to meet the increased metabolic requirements of the body. Cardiac output is increased by increasing the heart rate or stroke volume. In the normal heart, this increased oxygen demand of the myocardium itself is accomplished by increasing the amount of blood flowing (and therefore the amount of oxygen being delivered) to the myocardium by dilation, or widening, of the coronary arteries. The coronary arteries are the blood vessels that supply blood to the heart muscle (**FIGURE 17-4**). They begin at the first part of the aorta, just above the aortic valve. The right coronary artery supplies blood to the right atrium and right ventricle and,

in most people, the bottom part, or inferior wall, of the left ventricle. The left coronary artery supplies blood to the left atrium and left ventricle and divides into two major branches, just a short distance from the aorta.

Two major arteries branching from the upper aorta supply blood to the head and arms (**FIGURE 17-5**). The right and left carotid arteries supply the head and brain with blood. The right and left subclavian arteries (under the clavicles) supply blood to the upper extremities. As the subclavian artery enters each arm, it becomes the brachial artery, the major vessel that supplies blood to each arm. Just below the elbow, the brachial artery divides into two major branches: the radial and ulnar arteries, supplying blood to the lower arms and hands.

At the level of the umbilicus, the descending aorta divides into two main branches called the right and left iliac arteries, which supply blood to the groin, pelvis, and legs. As the iliac arteries enter the legs through the groin, they become the right and left femoral arteries. At the level of the knee, the femoral artery divides into the anterior (front) and posterior (back) tibial arteries and the peroneal artery, supplying blood to the lower legs and feet.

After blood travels through the arteries, it enters smaller and smaller vessels called arterioles and eventually enters the capillaries. Capillaries are tiny blood vessels about one cell thick that connect arterioles to venules. Capillaries, which are found in all parts of the body, allow the exchange of nutrients and waste at the cellular level. As the blood passes through the capillaries, it gives up oxygen to the tissues and picks up carbon dioxide and other waste products to be removed from the body.

Venules are the smallest branches of veins. After traveling through the capillaries, oxygen-poor blood enters the system of veins, starting with the venules, on its way back to the heart. The veins become larger and larger and eventually form the two large venae cavae: the superior vena cava and the inferior vena cava. The superior (upper) vena cava carries blood from the head and arms back to the right atrium. The inferior (lower) vena cava carries blood from the abdomen, pelvis, and legs back to the right atrium. The superior and inferior venae cavae join at the right atrium of the heart, where blood is then returned into the pulmonary circulation for oxygenation.

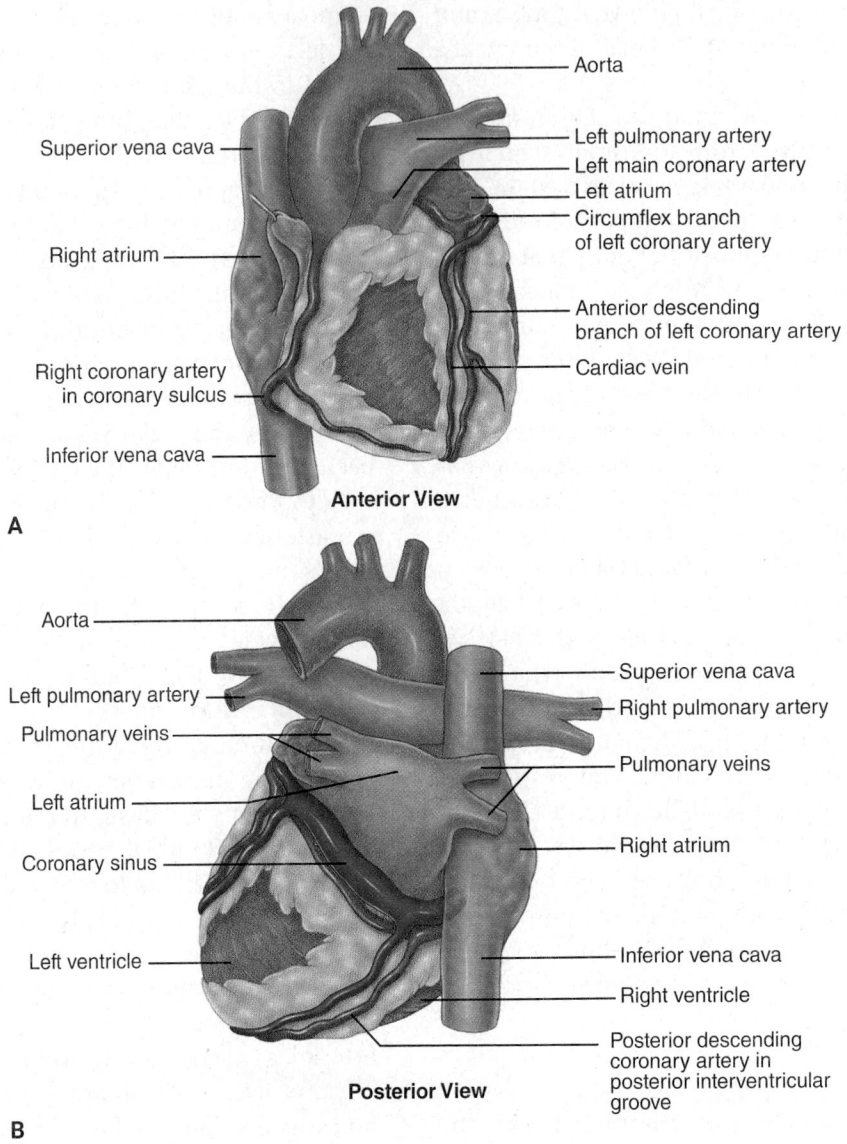

**FIGURE 17-4** Blood flow to the heart. **A.** Coronary arteries (anterior view). **B.** Coronary arteries (posterior view).

**A, B:** © Jones & Bartlett Learning.

Blood consists of fluid and several types of cells (**FIGURE 17-6**). Red blood cells are the most numerous and give the blood its color—bright red when oxygenated and darker red when low on oxygen. Red blood cells carry oxygen to the body's tissues and remove carbon dioxide. Larger white blood cells help to fight infection. Platelets, which help the blood to clot, are much smaller than either red or white blood cells. Plasma is the fluid in which the cells float. It is a mixture of water, salts, nutrients, and proteins.

Blood pressure is the force of circulating blood against the walls of the arteries. Systolic blood pressure is the maximum pressure generated in the arms and legs during the contraction of the left ventricle, during the time period known as systole. As the left ventricle relaxes in the stage known as diastole, the arterial pressure falls. When the left ventricle relaxes, the aortic valve closes and blood flow between the left ventricle and the aorta stops. The diastolic blood pressure is the pressure exerted against the walls of the arteries while the left ventricle is

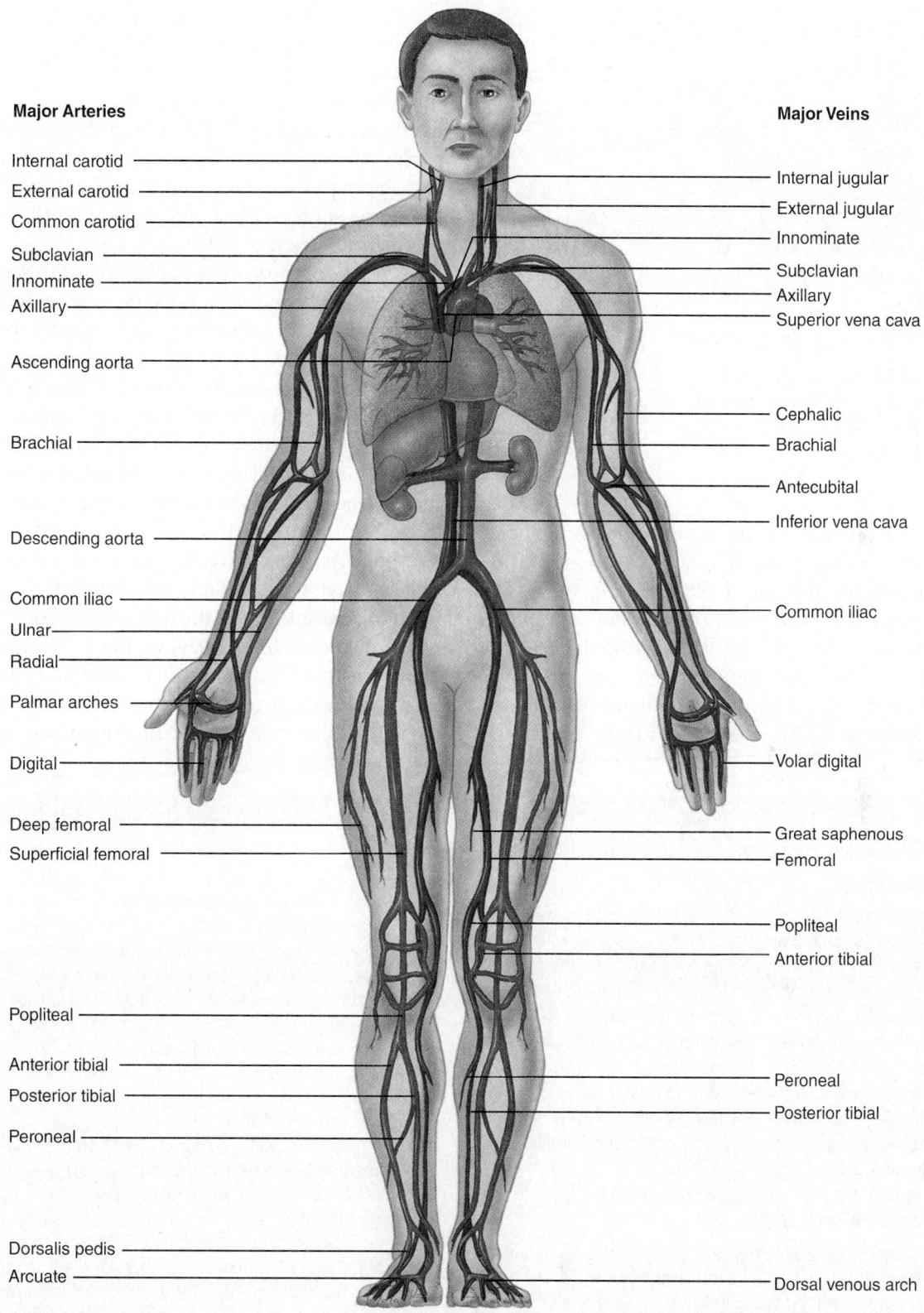

**Major Arteries**

Internal carotid

External carotid

Common carotid

Subclavian

Innominate

Axillary

Ascending aorta

Brachial

Descending aorta

Common iliac

Ulnar

Radial

Palmar arches

Digital

Deep femoral

Superficial femoral

Popliteal

Anterior tibial

Posterior tibial

Peroneal

Dorsalis pedis

Arcuate

**Major Veins**

Internal jugular

External jugular

Innominate

Subclavian

Axillary

Superior vena cava

Cephalic

Brachial

Antecubital

Inferior vena cava

Common iliac

Volar digital

Great saphenous

Femoral

Popliteal

Anterior tibial

Peroneal

Posterior tibial

Dorsal venous arch

**FIGURE 17-5** The major arteries of the body carry oxygen-rich blood to all parts of the body. The major veins of the body carry deoxygenated blood back to the heart.

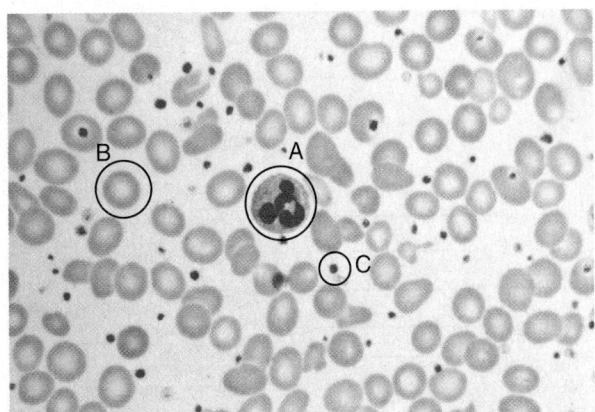

**FIGURE 17-6** Blood consists of fluid and several types of cells, including white blood cells (**A**), red blood cells (**B**), and platelets (**C**).

© Jarun Ontakrai/Shutterstock.

at rest. Remember that the top number in a blood pressure reading is the systolic pressure, and the bottom number is the diastolic, or resting, pressure. The cardiac cycle consists of one systolic and one diastolic time period. The mean arterial pressure (MAP) measures the average blood pressure and is displayed when a noninvasive blood pressure is measured. The MAP is a good measure of perfusion.

As the blood passes through an artery during systole, a pulse is generated. This pulse can be felt by placing a finger on the skin over the artery at a point where the artery lies near the skin surface and gently compressing. Pulses felt in the extremities, such as the radial and the posterior tibial, are called peripheral pulses, whereas pulses near the trunk of the body, such as the femoral and carotid pulses, are known as central pulses.

The rate of cardiac contractions can be increased or decreased by the autonomic nervous system. The heart also has the capability to increase or decrease the volume of blood it pumps with each contraction based on the autonomic nervous system response. To obtain an accurate measure of the efficiency of the heart, the volume of blood pumped and the heart rate are measured. This is determined by calculating the cardiac output. The **cardiac output** is calculated by multiplying the heart rate by the volume of blood ejected with each contraction, or the stroke volume. This is the volume of blood that passes through the heart in 1 minute and is the best measure of the output of the heart. In the field, we have no way of directly measuring the volume of blood being pumped; therefore, we must rely on the heart rate and the strength of the pulse to estimate the cardiac output.

## Words of Wisdom

### Pulsation

As the left ventricle contracts, it ejects a forceful wave of blood through the arteries. You can feel that wave in areas where the artery lies near the surface of the skin. This wave of blood is called the pulse. The evaluation of a patient's pulse is important in the assessment and treatment of cardiovascular emergencies. EMTs should be skilled at finding multiple pulse points and should compare proximal and distal pulses bilaterally, when applicable, to determine any differences in quality or strength that could indicate the patient's condition is progressing to decompensated shock.

Common places to feel for a pulse include the following (**FIGURE 17-7**):

- The carotid pulse can be felt in the neck by placing two fingertips in the center of the throat on the trachea, and then sliding them toward you into the groove between the trachea and the neck muscle. Do not assess both carotid pulses at the same time as this could greatly reduce blood flow to the brain.

- The femoral pulse can be felt in the groin at the crease dividing the lower abdomen from the leg.
- The brachial pulse can be felt on the anterior aspect of the elbow at the level of the crease. This is the pulse that you listen for when you obtain a blood pressure measurement. Pulsations also can be palpated on the medial side of the arm midway between the elbow and armpit.
- The radial pulse can be felt on the thumb side of the wrist, about one fingerbreadth above the wrist crease.
- The posterior tibial pulse can be felt on the inside of the ankle, just behind the medial malleolus. The medial malleolus is the bony bump at the bottom end of the tibia.
- The dorsalis pedis pulse can be felt at the top of the foot. To find the pulse, place your hand across the top of the foot just below the ankle crease. Once you feel something that might be a pulse, use your fingertips to confirm that finding.

Practice feeling for these pulses on yourself and on friends and family members.

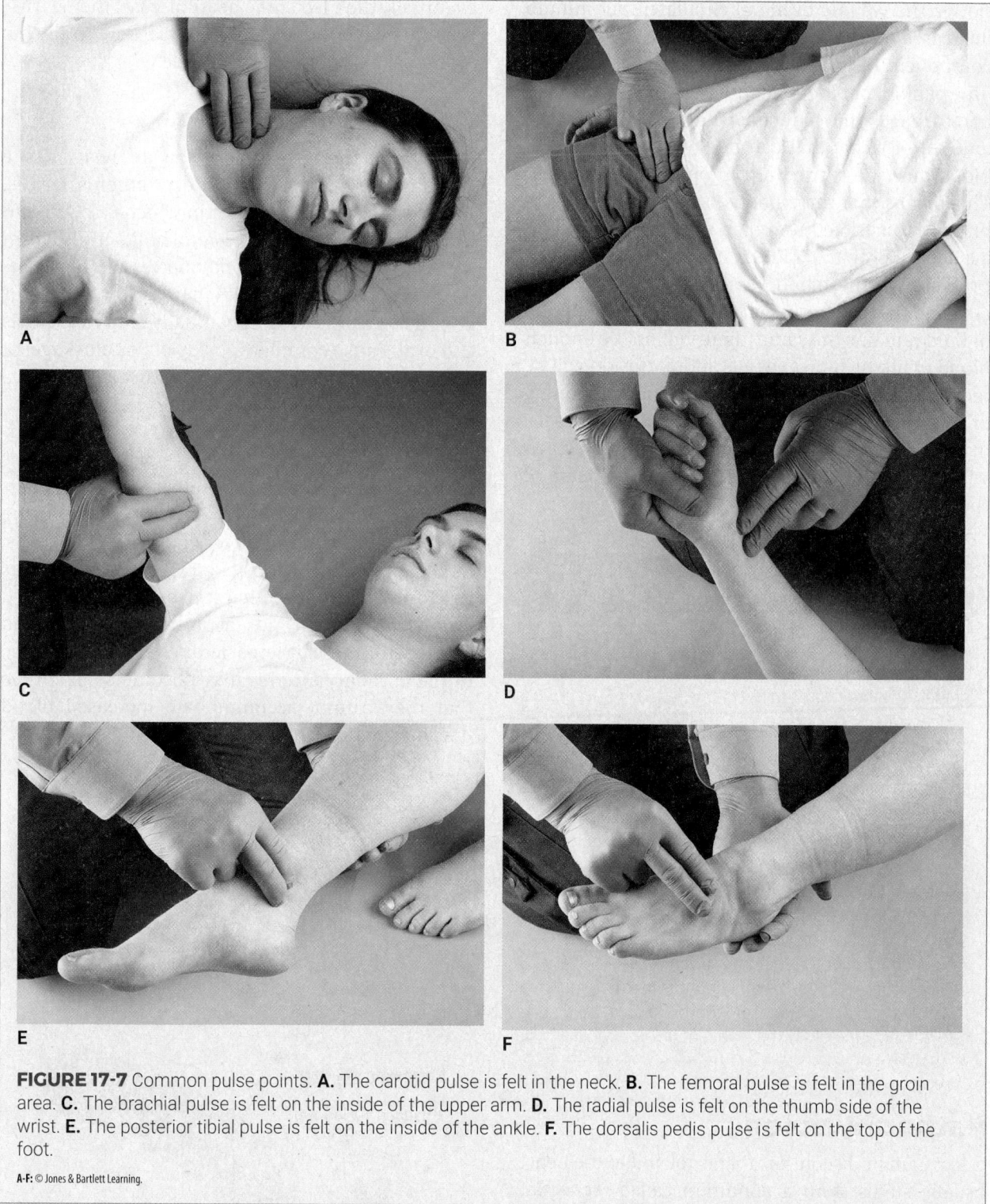

**FIGURE 17-7** Common pulse points. **A.** The carotid pulse is felt in the neck. **B.** The femoral pulse is felt in the groin area. **C.** The brachial pulse is felt on the inside of the upper arm. **D.** The radial pulse is felt on the thumb side of the wrist. **E.** The posterior tibial pulse is felt on the inside of the ankle. **F.** The dorsalis pedis pulse is felt on the top of the foot.

**A-F:** © Jones & Bartlett Learning.

The constant flow of oxygenated blood to the tissues is known as **perfusion**. Good perfusion requires three primary components. The first is a well-functioning heart, or pump. The heart must operate at an appropriate rate because a rate that is too slow or too fast will reduce the volume of blood circulated and, thus, reduce the cardiac output. When the heart beats too rapidly, there is not enough time between contractions for the heart to refill completely, and when the heart beats too slowly, the volume of blood circulated per minute decreases due to the slow pulse rate. The second component of good perfusion is an adequate volume of fluid, or blood. If there is blood loss through hemorrhage, the reduced volume will limit the amount of tissue that can be perfused. Third, the blood must be carried in a proper-size container. This means that the blood vessels must be appropriately constricted to match the volume of blood available so that circulation can occur without problems. If the blood vessels dilate, thereby increasing the size of the container, and the volume of fluid remains the same, there will not be enough blood to fill the blood vessels and perfusion will be reduced. If there is a problem with the functioning of the heart, the functioning of the blood vessels, or the volume of blood, perfusion will fall, which will lead to cellular death and, eventually, death of the patient.

---

### Words of Wisdom

Cardiac output = Heart rate × Stroke volume

Cardiac output is the amount of blood pumped out of the left ventricle in 1 minute.

Heart rate is the number of times the heart contracts in 1 minute.

Stroke volume is the volume of blood pumped out by the left ventricle in one contraction.

Stroke volume is affected by preload, afterload, and contractility. Preload is related to the amount of blood returning to the right ventricle and therefore ultimately to the left ventricle. Afterload is the pressure that the left ventricle pumps against, and it is associated with systemic vascular resistance, which is a function of the constriction of the systemic blood vessels. As the blood vessels constrict, it becomes harder for the ventricle to push the blood into them. Contractility refers to how forcefully the myocardium contracts.

---

## Pathophysiology

Chest pain or discomfort that is related to the heart usually stems from a condition called ischemia, which is decreased blood flow, in this case, to the myocardium. A partial or complete blockage of blood flow through the coronary arteries can cause a portion of the myocardium to be deprived of enough oxygen and nutrients. The tissue soon begins to starve and, if blood flow is not restored,

eventually dies. Ischemic heart disease, then, is disease involving a decrease in blood flow to one or more portions of the heart muscle.

## Atherosclerosis

Most often, the low blood flow to heart tissue is caused by coronary artery atherosclerosis. Atherosclerosis is a disorder in which calcium and a fatty material called cholesterol build up and form a plaque inside the walls of blood vessels, obstructing flow and interfering with their ability to dilate or contract (**FIGURE 17-8**). Eventually, atherosclerosis can even cause complete occlusion, or blockage, of a coronary artery. Atherosclerosis usually involves other arteries of the body as well.

The problem begins when the first trace of cholesterol is deposited on the inside of an artery. This may happen as early as the teenage years. As a person ages, more of this fatty material is deposited; the lumen, or the inside diameter of the artery, narrows. As the cholesterol deposits grow, calcium deposits can form as well. The inner wall of the artery, which is normally smooth and elastic, becomes rough and brittle with these atherosclerotic plaques. Damage to the coronary arteries may become so extensive that they cannot accommodate increased blood flow during times of maximum stress.

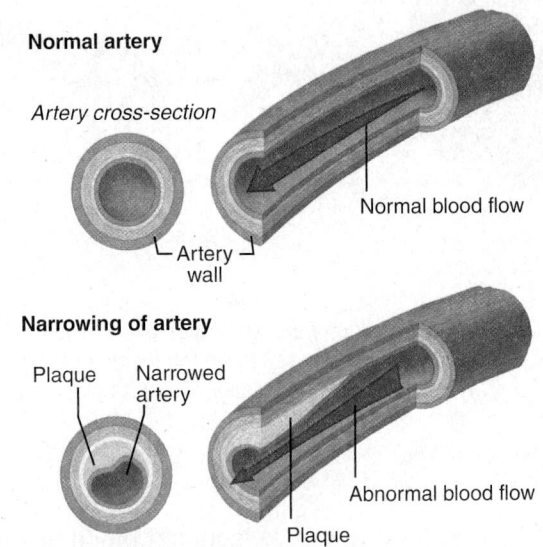

**Normal artery**

*Artery cross-section*

Normal blood flow

Artery wall

**Narrowing of artery**

Plaque    Narrowed artery

Abnormal blood flow

Plaque

**FIGURE 17-8** In atherosclerosis, calcium and cholesterol build up inside the walls of the coronary blood vessels, causing an obstruction in blood flow to the heart.

© Jones & Bartlett Learning.

For reasons that are still not completely understood, a brittle plaque will sometimes develop a crack, exposing the inside of the atherosclerotic wall. Acting like a torn blood vessel, the ragged edge of the crack activates the blood-clotting system, just as when an injury has caused bleeding. In this situation, however, the resulting blood clot will partially or completely block the lumen of the artery. If it does not occlude the artery at that location, the blood clot may break loose and begin floating in the blood, becoming what is known as a thromboembolism. A **thromboembolism** is a blood clot that is floating through blood vessels until it reaches an area too narrow for it to pass, causing it to stop and block the blood flow at that point. Tissues downstream from the blood clot will experience a lack of oxygen (hypoxia). If blood flow is restored in a short time, the hypoxic tissues will recover. However, if too much time goes by before blood flow returns, the hypoxic tissues will die. If a blockage occurs in a coronary artery, the condition results in an **acute myocardial infarction (AMI)**, a heart attack (**FIGURE 17-9**). **Infarction** means the death of tissue. The same sequence may also cause the death of cells in other organs, such as the brain. The death of heart muscle decreases the heart's ability to pump and can also cause it to stop pumping completely (**cardiac arrest**).

In the United States, coronary artery disease is the number one cause of death for men and women. The peak incidence of heart disease is between the ages of 45 and 64 years, but it can also strike teens and people in their 90s. You must be alert to the possibility that, although less likely, a 26-year-old with chest pain could be having an AMI, especially if he or she has a higher than usual risk.

Factors that place a person at higher risk for an AMI are called risk factors. The major controllable factors are cigarette smoking, high blood pressure, elevated cholesterol level, elevated blood glucose level (diabetes), lack of exercise, and obesity. The major risk factors that cannot be controlled are older age, family history of atherosclerotic coronary artery disease, race, ethnicity, and male sex. Other factors that play a role in heart disease are stress, excessive alcohol, and poor diet.

## Acute Coronary Syndrome

Many patients who call for EMS assistance because of chest pain have acute coronary syndrome. **Acute coronary syndrome (ACS)** is a term used to describe a group of symptoms caused by myocardial ischemia. As discussed earlier, myocardial ischemia is a decrease in blood flow to the heart, which leads to chest pain through reduced supply of oxygen and nutrients to the tissues of the heart. This can be a temporary situation known as angina pectoris, or a more serious condition, an AMI. Because the signs and symptoms of these two conditions are very similar, they are treated the same under the designation of ACS. To understand them better, we will examine each one separately.

## Angina Pectoris

Chest pain does not always mean that a person is having an AMI. When, for a brief time, heart tissues are not getting enough oxygen, the pain is called **angina pectoris**, or angina. Although angina can result from a spasm of an artery, it is most often a symptom of atherosclerotic coronary artery disease. Angina occurs when the heart's need for oxygen exceeds its supply, usually during periods of physical or emotional stress when the heart is working hard. A large meal or sudden fear may also trigger an attack. When the increased oxygen demand goes away (eg, the person stops exercising), the pain typically goes away.

Anginal pain is commonly described as crushing, squeezing, or "like somebody standing on my chest." It is usually felt in the midportion of the

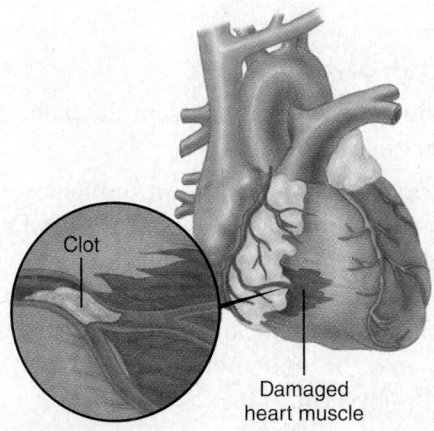

**FIGURE 17-9** An acute myocardial infarction (heart attack) occurs when a blood clot prevents blood flow to an area of the heart muscle. If left untreated, death of myocardium can result.

© Jones & Bartlett Learning.

chest, under the sternum. However, it can radiate to the jaw, the arms (frequently the left arm), the midportion of the back, or the epigastrium (the upper-middle region of the abdomen). The pain usually lasts from 3 to 8 minutes, rarely longer than 15 minutes. It may be associated with shortness of breath, nausea, or sweating. It usually disappears promptly with rest, supplemental oxygen, or nitroglycerin (NTG), all of which decrease the need for or increase the supply of oxygen to the heart. Although angina pectoris is frightening, it does not mean that heart cells are dying, nor does it usually lead to death or permanent heart damage. It is, however, a warning that you and the patient should take seriously. With angina, the electrical system can be compromised because the oxygen supply to the heart is diminished, and the person is at risk for problems with cardiac rhythm.

Angina can be further differentiated into stable and unstable angina. Unstable angina is characterized by pain or discomfort in the chest of coronary origin that occurs in the absence of a significant increase in myocardial oxygen demand. If untreated, it is associated with a very high risk of spontaneous AMI. Stable angina is characterized by pain in the chest of coronary origin that occurs in response to exercise or some activity that increases the demand on the heart muscle beyond the heart's capacity to increase its own blood flow. EMS often becomes involved when stable angina becomes unstable, such as when a patient whose pain is normally relieved by sitting down and taking one nitroglycerin tablet has taken three tablets with no relief. Keep in mind that it can be difficult, even for physicians in hospitals, to distinguish between the pain of angina and the pain of an AMI. Patients experiencing chest pain or discomfort, therefore, should always be treated initially as if they are having an AMI.

## Acute Myocardial Infarction

The pain of an AMI signals the actual death of cells in the area of the heart muscle where blood flow is obstructed. Once dead, the cells cannot be revived. Instead, they will eventually turn to scar tissue and become a burden to the beating heart. Therefore, fast action is critical in treating a heart attack. The sooner the arterial blockage can be cleared, the fewer the cells that may die. About 30 minutes after blood flow is cut off, some heart muscle cells begin to die. After about 2 hours, as many as one-half of the cells in the area can be dead; in most cases, after 4 to 6 hours, more than 90% will be dead. In many cases, however, opening the coronary artery with clot-busting (thrombolytic) medications or angioplasty (mechanical clearing of the artery) can prevent permanent damage to the heart muscle if done within the first few hours after the onset of symptoms. Therefore, immediate prehospital treatment and transport to the emergency department (ED) are essential.

An AMI is more likely to occur in the larger, thick-walled left ventricle, which needs more blood and oxygen than the right ventricle.

### Signs and Symptoms of AMI

A patient with an AMI may show any of the following signs and symptoms:

- Sudden onset of weakness, nausea, and sweating without an obvious cause
- Chest pain, discomfort, or pressure that is often crushing or squeezing and that does not change with each breath
- Pain, discomfort, or pressure in the lower jaw, arms, back, abdomen, or neck
- Irregular heartbeat and **syncope** (fainting)
- Shortness of breath, or dyspnea
- Nausea/vomiting
- Pink, frothy sputum (indicating possible pulmonary edema)
- Sudden death

### The Pain of AMI

The pain of an AMI differs from the pain of angina in three ways:

- It may or may not be caused by exertion but can occur at any time, sometimes when a person is sitting quietly or even sleeping.
- It does not resolve in a few minutes; rather, it can last between 30 minutes and several hours.
- It may or may not be relieved by rest or nitroglycerin.

Not all patients who are having an AMI experience pain or recognize it when it occurs. Approximately one-third of patients never seek medical attention. This can be attributed, in part, to the fact that people are afraid of dying and do not want to face the possibility that their symptoms may be serious (cardiac denial). Middle-aged men, in particular, are likely to minimize their symptoms. However, some patients, particularly older people, women, and people with diabetes, may not experience any pain during an AMI but may have other common complaints associated with ischemia discussed earlier. Others may feel only mild discomfort and call it indigestion. It is not uncommon for the only complaint, especially in older patients and women, to be fatigue. AMI without the classic chest pain is often referred to as a silent myocardial infarction. Heart disease is the number one killer of women in the United States, and EMTs should consider AMI even when the classic symptom of chest pain is not present. This is also true for older people and people with diabetes.

Therefore, when you are called to a scene where the chief complaint is chest pain, complete a thorough assessment, no matter what the patient says. Patients with cardiac risk factors should also be carefully assessed if they have any of the associated symptoms, even if no chest pain is present. Any complaint of chest discomfort is a serious matter. The best thing you can do is to assume the worst.

### Street Smarts

If it appears a patient is having a heart attack, be sure the AED is close by. That way, if it is needed, the delay to the first shock will be minimized.

### Physical Findings of AMI and Cardiac Compromise

The physical findings of AMI vary, depending on the extent and severity of heart muscle damage. The following are common:

- **General appearance.** The patient often appears frightened. There may be nausea, vomiting, and a cold sweat. The skin is often pale or ashen gray because of poor cardiac output and the loss of perfusion, or blood flow through the tissue. Occasionally, the skin will have a blue tint, called cyanosis; this is the result of poor oxygenation of the circulating blood.
- **Pulse.** Generally, the pulse rate increases as a normal response to pain, stress, fear, or actual injury to the myocardium. Because

dysrhythmias are common in an AMI, you may feel an irregularity or even a slowing of the pulse. The pulse may also be dependent on the area of the heart that has been affected by the AMI. Damage to the inferior area of the heart often presents with bradycardia.

- **Blood pressure.** Blood pressure may fall as a result of diminished cardiac output and diminished capability of the left ventricle to pump. However, most patients with an AMI will have a normal or possibly even elevated blood pressure.
- **Respiration.** The respiratory rate is usually normal unless the patient has CHF. In that case, respirations may become rapid and labored with a higher likelihood of cyanosis and possibly frothy sputum. A complaint of difficulty breathing is common with cardiac compromise, so even if the rate seems normal, look at the work of breathing, and treat the patient as if respiratory compromise were present.
- **Mental status.** Patients with AMIs often experience confusion or agitation and sometimes experience an almost overwhelming feeling of impending doom. If a patient tells you, "I feel like I'm going to die," pay attention.

### Words of Wisdom

Documenting exactly how a patient describes chest discomfort, in the patient's own words, is a valuable source of information for hospital staff. Remember OPQRST (Onset, Provocation/Palliation, Quality, Radiation, Severity, Time of onset).

### Consequences of AMI

An AMI can have three serious consequences:

- Sudden death
- Cardiogenic shock
- Congestive heart failure

### Sudden Death

Sudden death is usually the result of cardiac arrest, in which the heart fails to generate effective blood flow. Although you cannot feel a pulse in someone experiencing cardiac arrest, the heart may still be twitching, though erratically. The heart is using up energy without pumping any blood. Such an abnormality of heart rhythm is a ventricular **dysrhythmia**, known as ventricular fibrillation (VF).

A variety of other lethal and nonlethal dysrhythmias may follow an AMI, usually within the first hour. In most cases, premature ventricular contractions, or extra beats in the damaged ventricle, occur. Premature ventricular contractions by themselves may be harmless and are common among healthy people, as well as sick people. Other dysrhythmias include the following:

- **Tachycardia.** Rapid beating of the heart, 100 beats/min or more.
- **Bradycardia.** Unusually slow beating of the heart, 60 beats/min or less.
- **Ventricular tachycardia.** Rapid heart rhythm, usually at a rate of 150 to 200 beats/min. The electrical activity starts in the ventricle instead of the atrium. This rhythm usually does not allow adequate time between beats for the left ventricle to fill with blood. Therefore, the heart pumps less volume and the patient's blood pressure may fall, or the pulse may be lost altogether. The patient may also feel weak or lightheaded or may even become unresponsive. In some cases, existing chest pain may worsen or chest pain that was not there before onset of the dysrhythmia may develop. Most cases of ventricular tachycardia (VT) will be sustained but may deteriorate into VF.
- **Ventricular fibrillation.** Disorganized, ineffective quivering of the ventricles. No blood is pumped through the body, and the patient becomes unconscious within seconds. The only way to convert this dysrhythmia is to defibrillate the heart. To **defibrillate** means to shock the heart with a specialized electric current in an attempt to stop the chaotic, disorganized contraction of the myocardial cells and allow them to start again in a synchronized manner to restore a normal rhythmic beat. Defibrillation is most likely to be successful in terms of saving a life if delivered within the first few minutes of sudden death. If a defibrillator is not immediately available, CPR must be initiated until the defibrillator arrives. Even if CPR is begun at the time of collapse, chances of survival diminish approximately 7% to 10% each minute until defibrillation is accomplished.

If uncorrected, unstable VT or VF will eventually lead to **asystole**, the absence of all heart electrical activity. Without CPR, asystole may occur within minutes. Asystole usually reflects a long period of ischemia, and nearly all patients you find in asystole will die.

## Cardiogenic Shock

Shock is a simple concept but one that few people without medical training really understand. For that reason, Chapter 13 is devoted to a discussion of shock. The discussion of shock in this chapter is limited to that associated with cardiac problems; however, many other medical problems may cause shock as well (**TABLE 17-1**).

Shock is present when body tissues do not get enough oxygen, causing body organs to malfunction. In **cardiogenic shock**, often caused by a heart attack, the problem is that the heart lacks enough power to force the proper volume of blood through the circulatory system. Cardiogenic shock is more commonly found after an AMI that affects the inferior and posterior regions of the left ventricle of the heart because this ventricle provides circulation to the majority of the body. Cardiogenic shock can develop immediately or sometime after an AMI. The various signs and symptoms of cardiogenic shock are produced by the improper functioning of the body's organs. The challenge for you is to recognize shock in its early stages, when treatment is much more likely to be successful.

## Congestive Heart Failure

Failure of the heart occurs when the ventricular myocardium is so profoundly damaged that it can no longer keep up with the return flow of blood from the atria. **Congestive heart failure (CHF)** can occur at any time after a myocardial infarction, in the setting of heart valve damage, or as a consequence of long-standing high blood pressure. Any condition that weakens the pumping strength of the heart may cause CHF, and this often happens after a heart attack.

Just as the pumping function of the left ventricle can be damaged by coronary artery disease, it can also be damaged by diseased heart valves or chronic hypertension. In any of these cases, when the muscle can no longer contract effectively, the

**TABLE 17-1** Cardiogenic Shock and Congestive Heart Failure Facts

| Cardiogenic Shock | Congestive Heart Failure |
|---|---|
| **Signs and Symptoms** | **Signs and Symptoms** |
| • One of the first signs of shock is anxiety or restlessness as the brain becomes relatively starved for oxygen. The patient may report "air hunger." Think of the possibility of shock when the patient is saying that he or she cannot breathe. Obviously, the patient can breathe, because he or she can talk. However, the patient's brain is sensing that it is not getting enough oxygen.<br><br>• As the shock continues, the body tries to send blood to the most important organs, such as the brain and heart, and away from less important organs, such as the skin. Therefore, you may see pale, cool, clammy skin in patients with shock.<br><br>• As the shock gets worse, the body will attempt to compensate by increasing the amount of blood pumped through the heart. Therefore, the pulse rate will be higher than normal. In severe shock, the heart rate usually, but not always, is greater than 120 beats/min. As the shock progresses, the pulses may become irregular and weak.<br><br>• Shock can also present with rapid and shallow breathing, nausea and vomiting, and a decrease in body temperature.<br><br>• Finally, as the heart and other organs begin to malfunction, the blood pressure will fall below normal. A systolic blood pressure less than 90 mm Hg is easy to recognize, but it is a late finding that indicates decompensated shock. It is important not to assume that shock is not present just because the blood pressure is normal (compensated shock). | • This patient usually finds it easier to breathe when sitting up. When the patient is lying down, more blood is returned to the right ventricle and lungs, causing further pulmonary congestion.<br><br>• The patient is often agitated.<br><br>• Chest pain may or may not be present.<br><br>• The patient often has distended neck veins that do not collapse even when the patient is sitting.<br><br>• The patient may have swollen ankles from dependent edema (backup of fluid).<br><br>• The patient generally will have high blood pressure, a rapid heart rate, and rapid respirations.<br><br>• The patient will usually be using accessory breathing muscles of the neck and ribs, reflecting the additional hard work of breathing.<br><br>• Skin is usually pale or cyanotic and sweaty.<br><br>• The fluid surrounding small airways may produce crackles (formerly known as rales), best heard by listening to either side of the patient's chest, about midway down the back. In severe CHF, these soft sounds can be heard even at the top of the lung.<br><br>Once CHF develops, it can be treated but not cured. Regular use of medications may alleviate the symptoms. However, patients with CHF often become ill again and are frequently hospitalized. Approximately one-half will die within 5 years of the onset of symptoms. |
| **Treatment of Cardiogenic Shock**<br>Take the following steps when treating patients with signs and symptoms of cardiogenic shock:<br><br>1. Position the patient comfortably. Some patients will be more comfortable in a semi-Fowler position (head and knees slightly elevated); however, patients with low blood pressure may not tolerate a semi-upright position and may be more comfortable and more alert in a supine position.<br>2. Administer oxygen at a rate to keep the oxygen saturation between 95% and 99%.<br>3. Assist ventilations as necessary.<br>4. Cover the patient with sheets or blankets as necessary to preserve body heat. Be sure to cover the top of the patient's head in very cold weather, as this is where much heat is lost.<br>5. Provide prompt transport to the ED. | **Treatment of CHF**<br>Treat a patient with CHF and pulmonary edema urgently. Call for ALS back-up.<br><br>1. Take the vital signs, and give oxygen by continuous positive airway pressure (CPAP) to move some of the fluid out of the lungs and improve oxygenation. If CPAP is not available or not tolerated by the patient, you may give oxygen by mask or cannula to maintain the oxygen saturation between 95% and 99%.<br>2. Allow the patient to remain sitting in an upright position with the legs down.<br>3. Be reassuring; many patients with CHF are quite anxious because they feel as if they cannot breathe.<br>4. Patients who have had problems with CHF before will usually have specific medications for its treatment. Gather these medications and take them along with you to the hospital.<br>5. Nitroglycerin may be of value in reducing pulmonary edema if the patient's systolic blood pressure is more than 100 mm Hg. If medical control or standing orders advise you to do so, administer nitroglycerin sublingually.<br>6. Prompt transport to the ED is essential. |

heart tries other ways to maintain an adequate cardiac output. Two specific changes in heart function occur: The heart rate increases, and the left ventricle enlarges to increase the amount of blood pumped each minute.

When these adaptations can no longer make up for the decreased heart function, CHF eventually develops. With left-sided heart failure, the lungs become congested with fluid because the left side of the heart fails to pump the blood effectively. Blood tends to back up in the pulmonary veins, increasing the pressure in the capillaries of the lungs. When the pressure in the capillaries exceeds a certain level, fluid (mostly water) passes through the walls of the capillary vessels and into the alveoli. This condition is called pulmonary edema. It may occur suddenly, as in an AMI, or slowly over months, as in chronic CHF. Sometimes, in patients with an acute onset of CHF, severe pulmonary edema will develop, in which the patient has pink, frothy sputum and severe dyspnea. With right-sided heart failure, blood backs up in the venae cavae, resulting in edema in the lower extremities or distention of the veins in the neck.

If the right side of the heart is damaged, fluid collects in the body, often showing up as swelling in the feet and legs. The collection of fluid in the part of the body that is closest to the ground is called **dependent edema**. The swelling causes relatively few symptoms other than discomfort. However, chronic dependent edema may indicate underlying heart disease even in the absence of pain or other symptoms. Because the right side of the heart supplies the preload for the left side of the heart, right heart failure can result in an inadequate supply of blood to the left ventricle, resulting in a drop in the systemic blood pressure. It is important to realize that some patients may present with signs of both left- and right-side heart failure because left-side failure often leads to right-side failure.

## Hypertensive Emergencies

Hypertension is defined as any systolic blood pressure greater than 130 mm Hg or a diastolic blood pressure greater than 80 mm Hg. Another cardiac-related condition is a hypertensive emergency. A **hypertensive emergency** is defined as a

## YOU are the Provider

You arrive at the scene and are escorted by the patient's son to her bedroom. She is sitting up in bed with her fist clutched against her chest. She is conscious and alert, but is notably anxious. Her skin is pale and diaphoretic. Your partner opens the jump kit as you assess the patient.

| Recording Time:   0 Minutes | |
|---|---|
| Appearance | Anxious, pale, and diaphoretic |
| Level of consciousness | Conscious and alert |
| Airway | Open; clear of secretions and foreign bodies |
| Breathing | Increased respiratory rate; adequate depth |
| Circulation | Radial pulse rapid and irregular; skin pale and diaphoretic |

After confirming that she has not taken any medication and that she is not allergic to any medications, you give the patient four 81-mg aspirin tablets to chew and swallow according to your protocols. As you continue your assessment and further inquire about her medical history, your partner applies the pulse oximeter, which shows that the patient's oxygen saturation is 91%. Based on this he applies oxygen via nasal cannula at 4 L/min and prepares to take her vital signs. She tells you that she had a heart attack 3 years ago; has high blood pressure; and takes enalapril (Vasotec), nitroglycerin, and one aspirin per day.

**4.** Why is aspirin given to patients with an acute cardiac event?

**5.** What type of medication is nitroglycerin? How may it help relieve chest pain, pressure, or discomfort?

**6.** When is nitroglycerin indicated for a patient? What is the typical dose?

systolic pressure greater than 180 mm Hg in the presence of impending or progressive organ damage. Because patients do not feel their blood pressure, the signs and symptoms of hypertensive emergency are related to the effects of the hypertension. Some patients with chronic hypertension may not experience signs or symptoms until their systolic pressure is significantly higher than this value. One of the most common signs is a sudden severe headache. If described as "the worst headache I have ever felt," this may also be a sign of cerebral hemorrhage. Other signs and symptoms include strong bounding pulse, ringing in the ears, nausea and vomiting, dizziness, warm skin (dry or moist), nosebleed, altered mental status, and even the sudden development of pulmonary edema. Untreated hypertensive emergencies can lead to a stroke or a dissecting aortic aneurysm.

If you suspect your patient is experiencing a hypertensive emergency, attempt to make him or her comfortable and monitor the blood pressure regularly. Position the patient with the head elevated, and transport rapidly to the ED. Depending on the distance and time involved in transport, you should consider ALS assistance for the patient. Paramedics may be able to administer medications to lower the blood pressure to a safer level. If ALS personnel can be on the scene quickly, contact them early and allow them to transport the patient from the scene. If the transport distance is long, consider asking for an ALS unit to meet you along the way and take over patient care and transportation from that point. Remember that getting the patient with

a hypertensive emergency to the hospital as quickly and safely as possible is the best prehospital treatment you can provide.

An **aortic aneurysm** is a weakness in the wall of the aorta. The aorta dilates at the weakened area, which makes it susceptible to rupture. A **dissecting aneurysm** occurs when the inner layers of the aorta become separated, allowing blood (at high pressures) to flow between the layers. Uncontrolled hypertension is the primary cause of dissecting aortic aneurysms. This separation of layers weakens the wall of the aorta significantly, making it more likely to be ruptured under conditions of continued high blood pressure. If the aorta ruptures, the amount of internal blood loss will be so large that the patient will die almost immediately. The signs and symptoms of a dissecting aortic aneurysm include very sudden chest pain located in the anterior part of the chest or in the back between the shoulder blades. It may be difficult to differentiate the chest pain of a dissecting aortic aneurysm from that of an AMI, but several distinctive features may help. The pain from an AMI is often preceded by other symptoms—nausea, indigestion, weakness, and sweating—and tends to come on gradually, getting more severe with time and often described as "pressure" rather than "stabbing." By contrast, the pain of a dissecting aortic aneurysm usually comes on full force from one minute to the next (**TABLE 17-2**). A patient with a dissecting aortic aneurysm also may exhibit a difference in blood pressure between arms or diminished pulses in the lower extremities. Aortic aneurysms are often difficult to diagnose in the

**TABLE 17-2** AMI Versus Dissecting Aortic Aneurysm

|  | AMI | Dissecting Aneurysm |
| --- | --- | --- |
| Onset of pain | Gradual, with additional symptoms | Abrupt, without additional symptoms |
| Quality of pain | Tightness or pressure | Sharp or tearing |
| Severity of pain | Increases with time | Maximal from onset |
| Timing of pain | May wax and wane | Does not abate once it has started |
| Region/radiation | Substernal; back is rarely involved | Back possibly involved, between the shoulder blades |
| Clinical signs | Peripheral pulses equal | Blood pressure discrepancy between arms or decrease in a femoral or carotid pulse |

prehospital setting, but you must consider them a possibility in any patient with chest and abdominal pain and significant hypertension. Transport the patient without delay.

## Patient Assessment

While en route to the scene, consider the standard precautions that will be needed. The precautions can be as simple as gloves for a patient with chest pain or full precautions for a patient in cardiac arrest. Remember, the patient's condition can change rapidly between the time you are dispatched and your arrival.

## Scene Size-up

Do not let your guard down on medical calls. Always ensure that the scene is safe for all. As you approach the scene, look for and address any hazards. Determine the necessary standard precautions and whether you will need additional resources.

Identification of the nature of illness is important to start your patient assessment in the right direction. Use the information you get from the dispatcher, clues at the scene, and comments of bystanders or family members to begin to develop an idea about the type of problem your patient might be experiencing. For patients with cardiac problems, the clues often include a report of chest pain, difficulty breathing, or sudden loss of consciousness. Once you establish a preliminary nature of illness, you will be able to guide your assessment to find the important information much more effectively. Just remember not to become fixated on a specific condition at this early point in the assessment; sometimes the situation turns out to be very different from how it initially appeared.

## Primary Assessment

As you approach the patient, form a general impression of his or her condition to recognize and address life threats. You will likely begin by determining whether the patient is responsive. Perform a primary assessment of the patient. If the patient is unresponsive and pulseless, begin CPR, starting with chest compressions, and call for an AED. Use of the AED is discussed in the section on cardiac arrest later in this chapter. Generally, an AED should be applied if the patient is pulseless, not breathing (apneic), and unresponsive. Consider calling for ALS backup if possible.

Once you have formed a general impression, the next step in the primary assessment of a conscious patient is to assess airway and breathing. Unless the patient is unresponsive, the airway will most likely be patent. Responsive patients should be able to maintain their own airway. Some episodes of cardiac compromise may produce dizziness or even fainting spells (syncope). If dizziness or fainting has occurred, consider the possibility of a spinal injury from a fall. Assess and treat the patient as appropriate.

Assess the patient's breathing to determine if it is adequate to provide enough oxygen to an ailing heart. If the rate is too fast or too slow, the depth of respiration seems to be too shallow, or if the patient is struggling to breathe, respirations are inadequate. Listen for abnormal breath sounds at this time because these can also be important indicators of respiratory distress. Some patients feel shortness of breath even though there are no obvious signs of respiratory distress. Pulse oximetry is a valuable tool in treatment of cardiac disease and should be applied at this time. If the patient is having any difficulty breathing or if his or her oxygen saturation is less than 94%, administer oxygen at 4 L/min via a nasal cannula. If the saturation does not improve quickly, increase the oxygen concentration. If you cannot get a pulse oximetry reading, apply a nonrebreathing mask at 15 L/min. In general, the goal is to maintain the oxygen saturation level between 95% and 99%. If the patient is not breathing or has inadequate breathing, ensure adequate ventilations with a bag-mask device and 100% oxygen.

Patients experiencing pulmonary edema may require positive-pressure ventilation with a bag-mask device or CPAP. CPAP is the most effective way to assist a person with CHF to breathe effectively and prevent the need to use an invasive airway management technique. Be aware of the indications and contraindications of CPAP and be competent in utilizing this equipment.

After assessing airway and breathing, assess the patient's circulation. Determine the rate and quality of the patient's pulse. Is the pulse rhythm regular or irregular? Is the pulse too fast or too slow? If you find abnormalities in the pulse, you should be more suspicious. Assess the patient's skin condition, color, moisture, and temperature, as well as the capillary refill time. Although paleness, or a decrease in blood flow, can be difficult to detect in dark-skinned people, it may be observed by examining mucous membranes inside the inner lower eyelid, lips, and nail beds and capillary refill. On general observation, the patient may appear ashen or gray. Changes in perfusion may indicate more serious cardiac compromise. Consider treatment for cardiogenic shock early to reduce the workload of the heart. Place the patient in a comfortable position, usually sitting up and well supported. Provide reassurance that appropriate treatment is being given for the condition to reduce the patient's anxiety.

Make a preliminary transport decision based on whether you were able to stabilize life threats during the primary assessment. If the decision is immediate transport, the remainder of the assessment can be initiated en route. In general, most patients with chest pain should be transported immediately. Whether to transport using the lights and siren is determined for each specific patient and may be partially based on the estimated transport time, road conditions, and traffic. As a general rule, however, patients with cardiac problems should be transported in the most gentle, stress-relieving manner possible. You will save little time using the lights and siren, but you can do a lot to calm your patient and reduce the release of heart-damaging adrenaline through your reassurance and by creating a ride to the hospital that is as pleasant as possible. Try not to allow the patient to exert himself or herself, strain, or walk. By default, these patients should not walk to the stretcher or to the ambulance but instead should be carried gently.

Your decision as to where to transport the patient will depend on your local protocol. Patients are generally transported to the closest appropriate facility. If your service is served by only one hospital, the transport decision is easy. In larger urban areas, there may be several hospitals within the service areas. Some medical directors have written protocols requiring patients with suspected cardiac emergencies to be transported to cardiac specialty centers with certain capabilities, such as cardiac catheterization or targeted temperature management after resuscitation from cardiac arrest. Others require the patient to be transported to the nearest facility for stabilization before transporting to a specialty hospital. Be sure you know your local protocol.

## Words of Wisdom

Athletes may have a slower (bradycardic; <60 beats/min) heart rate as a result of normal physiologic changes related to physical conditioning. Tachycardia (>100 beats/min) is a normal physiologic response to exercise to ensure adequate tissue perfusion. Pain, fear, and excitement may also cause a person to be tachycardic. It is important that you assess the patient to determine whether a bradycardic or tachycardic response is appropriate or a sign of something more ominous.

## History Taking

Once you have stabilized life threats, you will want to determine and investigate the chief complaint and discover more about the history of the present illness. For a conscious medical patient, begin with obtaining a brief past medical history, identifying associated signs and symptoms, and identifying pertinent negatives. Friends or family members who are present may also have helpful information.

Remember that not all patients experiencing an AMI have the same signs and symptoms. A chief complaint of chest pain or discomfort, shortness of breath, or dizziness should be taken seriously. Many patients who suspect that something is wrong experience restlessness, appear anxious, and perhaps have a sense of impending doom. Act professionally; be calm. Speak to the patient in a normal voice that is neither too loud nor too soft. Let the patient know that trained responders, including you, are present to provide care and that he or she will soon be taken to the hospital. Remember, some patients may act less concerned, whereas others may be demanding. Most patients, however, are frightened. Your professional attitude may be the single most important factor in winning the patient's cooperation and helping the patient through this event. Patients often have a good idea about what is happening, so do not lie or offer false reassurance. If asked, "Am I having a heart attack?" you can say, "I do not know for sure, but in case you are, we are taking care of you. We are going to help you now, and we will be taking you to the hospital. You are in good hands."

Begin by asking questions about the current situation. Determine whether the patient is experiencing chest pain or discomfort and whether there are any other signs and symptoms. Determine whether the patient is having respiratory difficulty, because this is common among patients with chest pain. If the patient is experiencing dyspnea, find out whether it is related to exertion or whether it is related to the patient's position. Often, patients with chest pain experience worse difficulty breathing when they are lying down. Also determine whether the dyspnea is continuous or if it changes, especially with deep breathing. Note whether the patient has a cough and whether the cough produces sputum. Ask about other signs and symptoms that are commonly found, such as nausea and vomiting, fatigue, headache, and palpitations (a feeling of the heart skipping a beat or racing). Make sure to ask about any trauma the patient might have experienced during the past few days. Be sure to record your findings, including those that are negative (known as pertinent negatives).

If the patient is responsive, obtain the SAMPLE history, and ask the following questions specific to a cardiovascular emergency:

- Have you ever had a heart attack?
- Have you been told that you have heart problems?
  - Have you ever been diagnosed with angina, heart failure, or heart valve disease?
  - Have you ever had high blood pressure?
  - Have you ever been diagnosed with an aneurysm?
  - Do you have any respiratory diseases such as emphysema or chronic bronchitis?

- Do you have diabetes or have you ever had any problems with your blood sugar?
  - Have you ever had kidney disease?
- Do you have any risk factors for coronary artery disease, such as smoking, high blood pressure, or high cholesterol?
  - Is there a family history of heart disease?
  - Do you currently take any medications?

The SAMPLE history provides basic information on the patient's overall medical history. You will want to determine as many signs and symptoms as you can. For example, you may determine that the patient has chest pain at rest or absence of chest pain with respirations or movement. The more signs and symptoms a patient has, the easier it is to identify a particular problem. In addition, ask whether the patient has had the same pain before. If so, ask "Do you take any medications for the pain?" and "Do you have any of the medication with you?" If the patient has had a heart attack or angina before, ask whether the pain is similar.

Make sure to ask about allergies because the patient will likely be given medication in the hospital. If the patient is taking medications, determine whether they are prescribed, over the counter, and/or recreational drugs. Even when a patient may not be able to articulate his or her exact medical condition, knowing the patient's medications may give you important clues. For example, a patient may say he has "heart problems." You see that he is taking furosemide (Lasix), digoxin, and metoprolol (Toprol). Furosemide is a diuretic, digoxin increases

## YOU are the Provider

The patient took two of her prescribed nitroglycerin tablets before her son called 9-1-1; however, she is still experiencing chest pain, which she rates as a 7 on a scale of 0 to 10. Your partner takes her vital signs as you perform a more focused examination, inquire about her past medical history, and prepare for further treatment.

| Recording Time: 2 Minutes | |
| --- | --- |
| **Respirations** | 20 breaths/min; adequate depth |
| **Pulse** | 118 beats/min; strong and irregular |
| **Skin** | Pale, cool, and diaphoretic |
| **Blood pressure** | 150/90 mm Hg |
| **Oxygen saturation (SpO$_2$)** | 98% (on 4 L/min oxygen) |

**7.** What is significant about the patient's vital signs?

**8.** Should you give her additional nitroglycerin? Why or why not?

the strength of heart contractions, and metoprolol lowers blood pressure. These medications are often prescribed together for patients with CHF and may alert you to carefully evaluate the lungs for the presence of crackles, which indicate fluid in the lungs and a need to increase the amount of oxygen being delivered or consider CPAP. When you ask about medical conditions, be sure to ask whether the patient takes medications for any other condition. Also, if the patient tells you that he or she takes prescription medications, ask what condition these are taken to treat. Asking about the last oral intake may seem unnecessary, but this information can be important; it is always better to have too much information rather than not enough. Also remember to ask about any home remedies the patient might have used, because this information can be important, too.

Be sure to include the OPQRST questions when you are obtaining the symptoms as part of the SAMPLE history. Using OPQRST helps you to understand the details of specific complaints, such as chest pain (**TABLE 17-3**).

## Secondary Assessment

Circumstances will determine which aspects of the physical examination will be performed. The secondary assessment of a conscious patient with chest pain or discomfort would likely focus on the patient's cardiac and respiratory systems.

The physical examination of a patient with chest pain begins with the cardiovascular system. Evaluate the patient's circulation by assessing pulses at various locations, and assessing skin color, temperature, and condition. Is the skin cool or moist? How do the mucous membranes look? Are they pink, ashen, or cyanotic? Are the pulses of equal strength bilaterally? Does the patient have any edema in the extremities, especially the lower extremities? All of these physical findings can help identify poor circulation, which may be caused by a failure of the cardiovascular system.

In addition to the cardiovascular system, examine the respiratory system for signs of inadequate ventilation. These two systems are closely related, and cardiovascular issues can cause problems with the respiratory system. Are the lung sounds clear? Wet-sounding lungs indicate fluid is being moved into the lungs from the circulatory system, possibly because of a problem with the heart. Are the breath sounds equal? Are the neck veins distended? Is the trachea deviated, or is it midline? The answers to these questions can help determine whether a problem exists with the lungs or with the heart. Although the physical examination is not usually as

### TABLE 17-3 OPQRST Mnemonic for Assessing Pain

| | |
|---|---|
| Onset | When did the problem begin, and what does the patient think may have caused it? |
| Provocation/palliation | Ask what makes the pain or discomfort better or worse. Is it positional? Does a deep breath or palpation of the chest make it worse? Did you take anything for it (including anything nonprescribed)? |
| Quality | Ask the patient to describe his or her pain. Let the patient use his or her own words to describe what is happening. If the patient is unable to describe the pain, try to avoid supplying only one option. Do not ask, "Does it feel like an elephant is sitting on your chest?" Instead, say, "Tell me what the pain feels like." If the patient cannot answer an open-ended question, then provide a list of alternatives: "There are lots of different kinds of pain. Is your pain more like heaviness, pressure, burning, tearing, dull ache, stabbing, or needlelike?" |
| Region/radiation | Ask where the pain is located and whether the pain has spread to another part of the body. |
| Severity | Ask the patient to rate the pain on a simple scale. Often, a scale ranging from 0 to 10 is used; a 10 represents the worst pain imaginable. Do not use the patient's answer to determine whether the pain has a serious cause. Instead, use it to check whether the pain is getting better or worse. After a few minutes of oxygen or administration of nitroglycerin, ask the patient to rate the pain again. |
| Timing | Find out how long the pain lasts when it is present and whether it has been intermittent or continuous. |

important as the history in a patient with a possible cardiac problem, it may produce important clues to the patient's condition.

Measure and record the patient's vital signs, including pulse, respirations, and blood pressure. You must obtain readings for systolic and diastolic blood pressures. Measure blood pressure on both arms if time allows. Use pulse oximetry to measure the oxygen saturation of the blood and use the pulse rate reading only to confirm your manually obtained pulse rate. Pulse oximetry may not give an accurate measurement if the patient has poor circulation, has been exposed to a toxic chemical, or is in cardiac arrest, but it should be used and the readings noted for all patients with possible cardiac problems.

Be sure to engage in continuous blood pressure monitoring if you have access to it, ensuring that you obtain an accurate manual blood pressure first. Obtain repeat vital signs at appropriate intervals and use the settings on the automatic blood pressure monitoring machine to remind you when it is time to recheck and record the vital signs. Note the time that each set of vital signs is taken.

In patients with chest pain, it is valuable to have a 12-lead ECG tracing from as early as possible after the onset of the pain. EMTs may assist with placing electrodes. This is discussed later in this chapter.

## Reassessment

Repeat the primary assessment by checking to see whether the patient's chief complaint and condition have improved or are deteriorating. Vital signs should be reassessed at least every 5 minutes or anytime significant changes in the patient's condition occur. It is essential to closely monitor the patient with a suspected AMI because sudden cardiac arrest is always a risk. If cardiac arrest occurs, you must be ready to begin automated defibrillation or

### Street Smarts

In some cases, patients who experience sudden cardiac arrest will have what appears to be brief seizure activity as they lose consciousness. This is related to the sudden loss of oxygenation to the brain. An experienced EMT recognizes this situation, checks for a pulse, and if there is none begins chest compressions until the AED can be used.

chest compressions immediately. If an AED is immediately available, use it; if not, perform CPR until the AED is available, as discussed in the later section on cardiac arrest. Reassess your interventions to see whether they are helping and whether the patient's condition is improving. Reassessment will also determine whether further interventions are indicated or contraindicated.

Transport the patient. Early, prompt transport to the ED or specialty center is critical so that treatments such as clot-busting medications or angioplasty can be initiated. To be most effective, these treatments must be started as soon as possible after the onset of the attack. If the patient does not have prescribed nitroglycerin and you do not have permission from medical control to administer nitroglycerin, complete your patient assessment and prepare to transport. Be sure that this process does not consume too much time. Do not delay transport to administer nitroglycerin. The drug can be given en route.

Alert the ED staff about the status of your patient's condition and your estimated time of arrival. Follow the instructions of medical control. Describe the patient's condition to the ED staff on arrival.

It is important to document your assessment and treatment of the patient. All interventions should be initiated according to protocol. If the intervention required an order from medical control, document the intervention and/or medication requested and that prior approval was granted. It must be clear in your documentation that the patient was reassessed appropriately following any intervention. The patient's response to the intervention and the time of each intervention must also be recorded. On completing your documentation, obtain the medical control physician's signature (if required by local protocol) showing approval of medication administration.

## Emergency Medical Care for Chest Pain or Discomfort

Your treatment of the patient begins with proper positioning. As mentioned before, some patients will not tolerate being positioned supine, so they should be allowed to sit up (leaning back on the stretcher). Also loosen tight clothing, trying to make the patient as comfortable as possible.

If it is indicated, you should be giving the patient oxygen by this time, but continually reassess the oxygen saturation and the patient's respiratory status. For patients with mild dyspnea, a nasal cannula may be all that is needed, whereas patients with more serious respiratory difficulty may require a nonrebreathing mask. If signs of pulmonary edema are present, CPAP may be indicated. Remember to titrate the oxygen to obtain an oxygen saturation between 95% and 99% unless ongoing difficulty breathing suggests that respiratory distress is present despite a high pulse oximetry reading. A patient who is unconscious or in obvious respiratory distress may need assistance with breathing. Use a bag-mask device. Be aware that ALS may be valuable to support the use of positive end-expiratory pressure, CPAP, bilevel positive airway pressure, and transport ventilators.

Depending on local protocol, prepare to administer low-dose chewable aspirin and nitroglycerin. Aspirin (acetylsalicylic acid) prevents new clots from forming or existing clots from getting bigger. Administer low-dose aspirin according to local protocol. Low-dose aspirin comes in 81-mg chewable tablets. The recommended dose is 162 mg (two tablets) to 324 mg (four tablets). Be sure you have verified that the patient is not allergic to aspirin before you give it. Also, ask the patient if he or she has any history of internal bleeding such as stomach ulcers, and, if so, contact medical control before giving the patient aspirin.

Nitroglycerin may help to relieve the pain of angina. Nitroglycerin comes in several forms: as a small white tablet, placed sublingually (under the tongue); as a spray, also administered sublingually; and as a skin patch applied to the chest. In any form, the effect is the same. Nitroglycerin relaxes the muscle of blood vessel walls, dilates coronary arteries, increases blood flow and the supply of oxygen to the heart muscle, and decreases the workload of the heart. Nitroglycerin also dilates blood vessels in other parts of the body and can cause a decrease in blood pressure and a severe headache. Other side effects include changes in the patient's pulse rate, including tachycardia or bradycardia. Therefore, you should obtain the patient's blood pressure within 5 minutes after each dose. If the systolic blood pressure is less than 100 mm Hg, do not give nitroglycerin. Other contraindications include the presence of a head injury, use of erectile dysfunction drugs within the previous 24 to 48 hours, and the maximum prescribed dose of

nitroglycerin has already been given (usually three doses). Drugs used for erectile dysfunction include sildenafil (Viagra), tadalafil (Cialis), avanafil (Stendra), and vardenafil (Levitra, Staxyn).

## Administering Nitroglycerin

Check the condition of the medication and its expiration date, and do not administer contaminated or expired medications. Always make sure the medication is prescribed for your patient. Occasionally, patients will try to take medications prescribed for their spouse or a friend if they think it will help them. Be sure to wear gloves when handling nitroglycerin tablets or spray because it is easily absorbed through the skin. If you handle tablets with bare fingers or get the spray on your fingers, it may be absorbed into your body, causing you to experience a very painful headache. If the patient is hypotensive or in cardiac arrest and has a nitroglycerin patch on when you arrive, be sure to carefully remove it before using the AED.

After you obtain permission from medical control, administer the nitroglycerin if required. Nitroglycerin works in most patients within 5 minutes. Most patients who have been prescribed nitroglycerin carry a supply with them. Nitrostat is one trade name for nitroglycerin. Patients are instructed to take one dose of nitroglycerin under the tongue whenever they have an episode of angina that does not immediately go away with rest. If the pain is still present after 5 minutes, patients are typically instructed by their physicians to take a second dose. If the second dose does not work, most patients are told to take a third dose and then call for EMS. If the patient has not taken all three doses, you can administer the medication, if you are allowed to do so by local protocol.

Be aware that nitroglycerin will lose its potency over time, especially if exposed to light and/or heat. Patients who take it only rarely may keep a bottle in their pocket for months. It may lose its potency even before its expiration date. When the nitroglycerin tablet loses its potency, patients may not feel the fizzing sensation when the tablet is placed under their tongue, and they may not experience the normal burning sensation and headache that often accompany nitroglycerin administration. Note that the fizzing only occurs with a potent tablet, not with the spray form. To safely assist the patient with nitroglycerin, follow the steps listed in **SKILL DRILL 17-1**:

1. Obtain an order from medical control—online or through offline protocol.

2. Take the patient's blood pressure. Administer nitroglycerin only if the systolic blood pressure is greater than 100 mm Hg (**Step 1**).

3. Check that you have the right medication, the right patient, the right dose, and the right

## Skill Drill 17-1 Administering Nitroglycerin

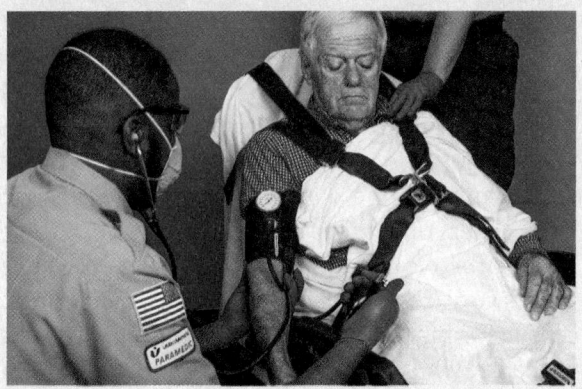

### Step 1

Obtain an order from medical control. Take the patient's blood pressure. Administer nitroglycerin only if the systolic blood pressure is greater than 100 mm Hg.

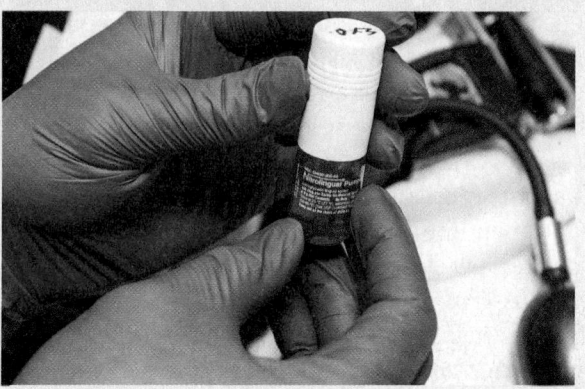

### Step 2

Check the medication and expiration date. Ask the patient about the last dose he or she took and its effects. Make sure that the patient understands the route of administration. Prepare to have the patient lie down to prevent fainting.

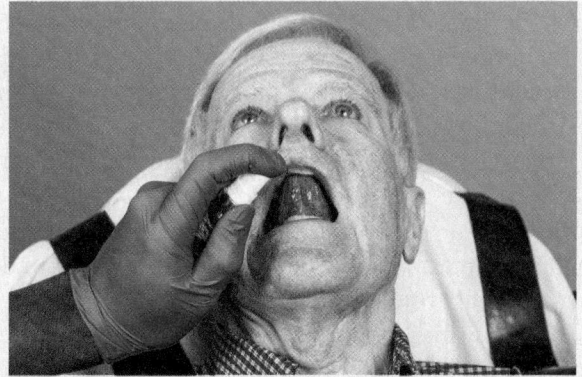

### Step 3

Ask the patient to lift his or her tongue. Place the tablet or spray the dose under the tongue (while wearing gloves), or have the patient do so. Have the patient keep his or her mouth closed with the tablet or spray under the tongue until it is dissolved and absorbed. Caution the patient against chewing or swallowing the tablet.

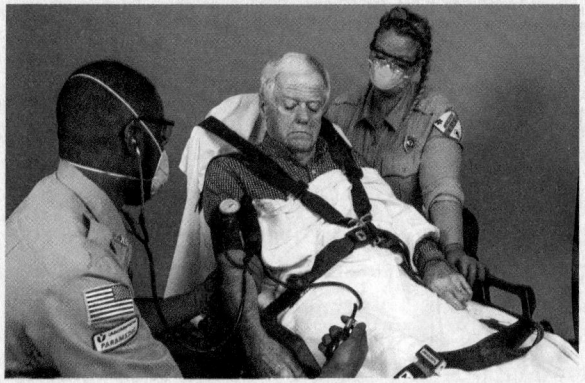

### Step 4

Recheck the blood pressure within 5 minutes. Record each medication and the time of administration. Reevaluate the chest pain and blood pressure, and repeat treatment if necessary.

delivery route. Check the expiration date. Make sure the patient has no contraindications, such as having taken medication for erectile dysfunction in the past 24 hours.

4. Ask the patient about the last dose he or she took and its effects. Make sure that the patient understands the route of administration. Be prepared to have the patient lie down to prevent fainting if the nitroglycerin substantially lowers the patient's blood pressure (the patient gets dizzy or feels faint) (**Step 2**).

5. Ask the patient to lift his or her tongue. Place the tablet or spray the dose under the tongue (while wearing gloves). Have the patient lower the tongue and keep his or her mouth closed with the tablet or spray under the tongue until it is dissolved and absorbed. Caution the patient against chewing or swallowing the tablet (**Step 3**).

6. Recheck the blood pressure within 5 minutes. Record the name and dose of medication given and the time of administration. Reevaluate the chest pain and note the response to the medication. If the chest pain persists and the patient still has a systolic blood pressure greater than 100 mm Hg, repeat the dose every 5 minutes as authorized by medical control. In general, a maximum of three doses of nitroglycerin is given for any one episode of chest pain (**Step 4**).

## Cardiac Monitoring

Some EMS systems will allow EMTs to place electrodes, attach the leads, and obtain and transmit an electrocardiogram (ECG) tracing prior to transport. If your service allows you to perform this skill, the following information will guide you. The goal is to obtain the ECG within less than 10 minutes of your first contact with the patient. Be sure to familiarize yourself with the operation of the monitor that your service uses, including how to obtain and transmit ECG tracings before using it on a call.

## Placing the Electrodes

For an ECG to be reliable and useful, the electrodes must be placed in consistent positions on each patient. **FIGURE 17-10** shows placement of limb lead electrodes, which are used to obtain a 3-lead ECG. **FIGURE 17-11** shows placement of limb lead electrodes and 12-lead ECG electrodes, both of which are used when obtaining a 12-lead ECG.

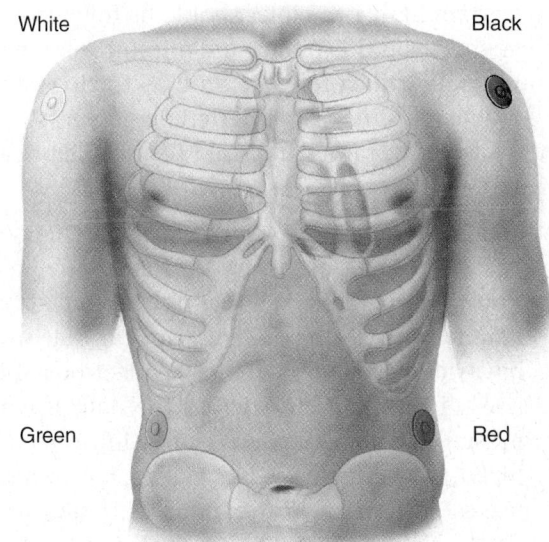

**FIGURE 17-10** Limb electrode placement for cardiac monitoring.

© Jones & Bartlett Learning.

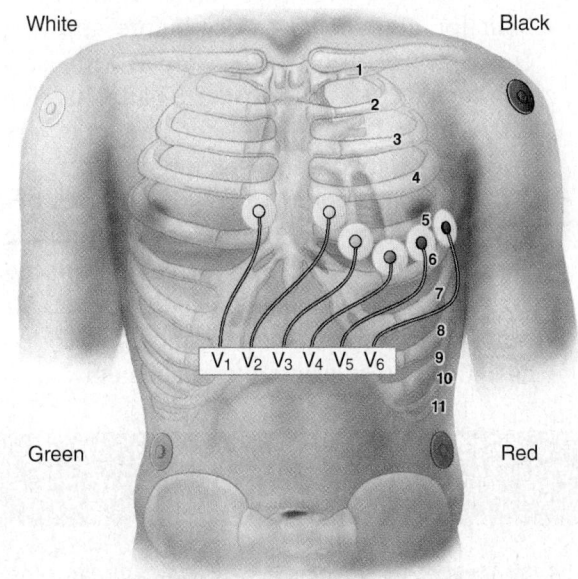

| Lead | Location | View |
|------|----------|------|
| V₁ | 4th intercostal space, right sternal border | Ventricular septum |
| V₂ | 4th intercostal space, left sternal border | Ventricular septum |
| V₃ | Between V₂ and V₄ | Anterior wall of left ventricle |
| V₄ | 5th intercostal space, midclavicular line | Anterior wall of left ventricle |
| V₅ | Lateral to V₄ at the anterior axillary line | Lateral wall of left ventricle |
| V₆ | Lateral to V₅ at the midaxillary line | Lateral wall of left ventricle |

**FIGURE 17-11** 12-lead ECG electrode placement.

© Jones & Bartlett Learning.

To maintain consistency in monitoring and obtaining a useful ECG, there are predetermined locations for each electrode. Electrodes used in the prehospital setting are generally adhesive and have a gel center to aid in skin contact. Whichever type is used, certain basic principles should be followed to achieve the best skin contact and minimize **artifact** in the signal. Artifact refers to an ECG tracing with waves that are the result of interference, such as patient movement, rather than the heart's electrical activity. Guiding principles are as follows:

- To maintain the correct lead placement, it may occasionally be necessary to shave body hair from the electrode site. Do not be fooled by a hairy chest. It may initially appear that you have good skin contact, but the electrode will rise off the skin and stick to the hair. If you must shave the site, be very careful to avoid nicking the skin. If one is available, it is best to use an electric razor to remove hair, because single-blade manual razors irritate the skin and can easily cut a patient.
- To remove oils and dead tissues from the surface of the skin, rub the electrode site briskly with an alcohol swab before application. Wait for the alcohol to dry before applying electrodes or dry it with a quick wipe of a 4 × 4–inch (10 × 10–cm) gauze pad. This step may have to be repeated if the patient is very sweaty, as many cardiac patients are.
- Attach the electrodes to the ECG cables before placement. Confirm that the appropriate electrode now attached to the cable is placed at the correct location on the patient's chest or limbs (each cable is marked and color coded as to the correct location for placement).

## Performing Cardiac Monitoring

Once all electrodes are in place, switch on the monitor, and print a sample rhythm strip. If the strip shows any interference (artifact), verify that the electrodes are firmly applied to the skin and the monitor cable is plugged in correctly. Artifact on the monitor can be tricky. Patient movement, including deep breathing or muscle tremor, may cause a wavy baseline or small up-and-down squiggles on the baseline. These will prevent the ECG from being usable. Make sure that the patient is supine if possible or in the semi-Fowler position if the patient is having difficulty breathing when supine. Also make sure the patient's arms are relaxed by his or her side and feet are uncrossed.

**SKILL DRILL 17-2** shows the steps for performing cardiac monitoring:

1. Take standard precautions (**Step 1**).
2. Explain the procedure to the patient. Prepare the skin for electrode placement (**Step 2**).
3. Attach the electrodes to the leads before placing them on the patient (**Step 3**).
4. Position the limb electrodes on the patient's limbs if you will be acquiring a 12-lead ECG. These electrodes may be placed on the torso only if performing continuous monitoring and a 12-lead ECG will not be required. The RA electrode goes on the right arm distal to the shoulder or on the wrist (avoid placing electrodes directly over a bone). The LA electrode

## Skill Drill 17-2 Performing Cardiac Monitoring

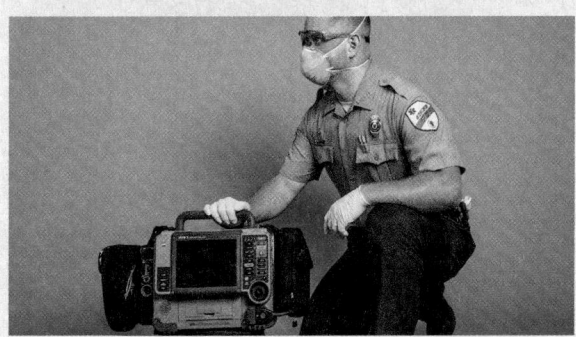

**Step 1**
Take standard precautions.

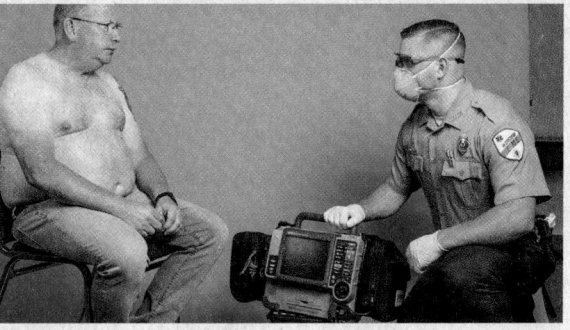

**Step 2**
Explain the procedure to the patient. Prepare the skin for electrode placement.

## Skill Drill 17-2 Performing Cardiac Monitoring (*continued*)

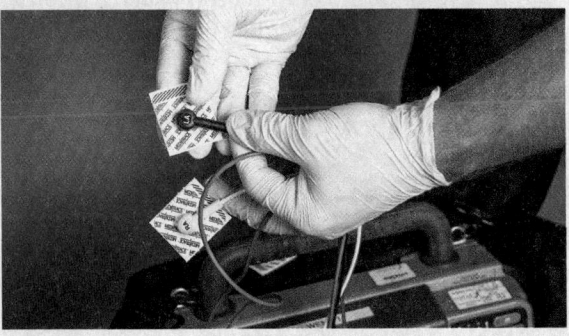

### Step 3

Attach the electrodes to the leads before placing them on the patient.

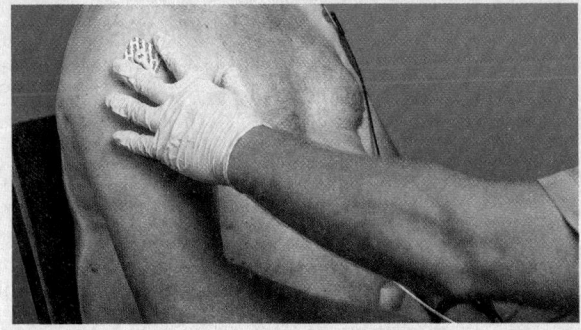

### Step 4

Position the limb electrodes on the patient. Place the leads on the torso if performing continuous monitoring, and on the limbs if you will be acquiring a 12-lead ECG.

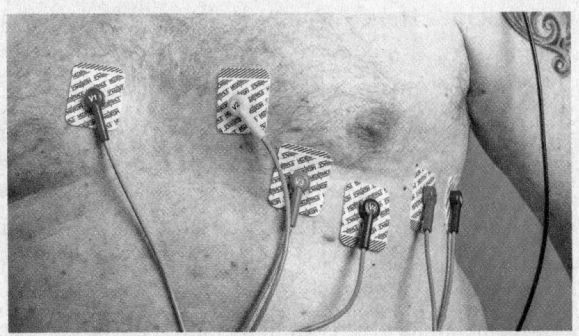

### Step 5

If you plan to obtain a 12-lead ECG tracing, place the chest leads on the chest.

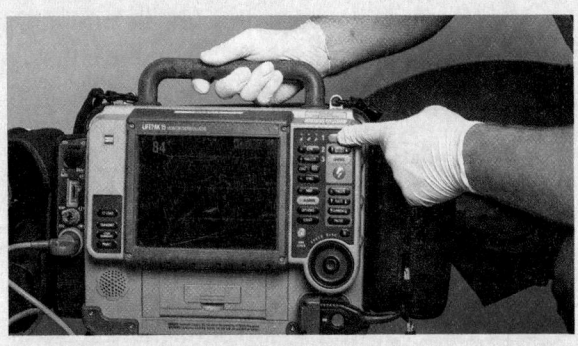

### Step 6

Turn on the monitor.

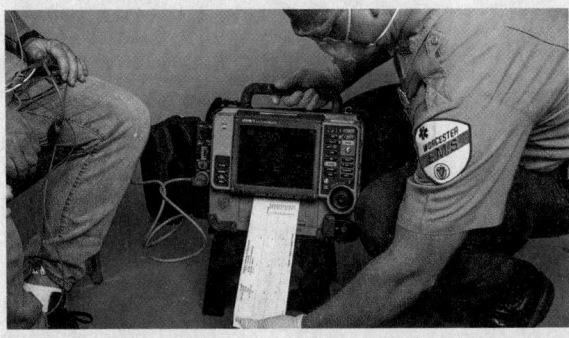

### Step 7

Record tracings.

goes on the left arm at the same location as you placed the RA electrode on the right arm. The LL electrode is placed on the left leg on the thigh or ankle, although if you do not plan to obtain a 12-lead ECG tracing, this electrode may be placed on the lower left side of the abdomen (slightly lower than an AED pad would be placed). Place the RL electrode at the same location on the right side of the body as the LL electrode on the left. Each electrode should be approximately an equal distance from the heart (or the bottom of the sternum) (**Step 4**).

5. If you plan to obtain a 12-lead ECG tracing, place the chest leads on the chest as shown. The $V_1$ electrode is placed on the right side of the sternum between the fourth and fifth ribs. To find this location, place your finger on the angle of Louis (where the manubrium meets the body of the sternum) and slide it to the right. Your finger should now be on the second rib. You can move it down to the third and then fourth rib and place the electrode below this location, between the fourth and fifth ribs. The $V_2$ electrode is placed on the left side of the sternum directly across from $V_1$. The $V_4$ electrode is placed next, between the fifth and sixth ribs in a straight line down from the middle of the clavicle. The $V_3$ electrode is then placed halfway between $V_2$ and $V_4$ in between the fifth and sixth ribs (not on top of a rib). The $V_6$ electrode is placed next and is located horizontally even with $V_4$ in a straight line down from the middle of the armpit. Finally, the $V_5$ electrode is placed halfway between $V_4$ and $V_6$ (**Step 5**).

6. Turn on the monitor (**Step 6**).

7. Record tracings. As soon as a rhythm is visible on the screen, press the print button on the monitor and print a strip while counting slowly to six or seven. Then press the print button again to stop the printout. If the time is not printed correctly on the strip, write it on the edge of the strip. If you are obtaining a 12-lead ECG tracing, ask the patient to hold his or her breath or to take very shallow breaths. Press the 12-lead button and wait for the machine to acquire, analyze, and print or transmit the 12-lead ECG tracing. Gently tear off the tracing when the printer automatically stops (**Step 7**).

8. Label each strip (**Step 8**).

9. Transmit the tracing to the facility where you are transporting the patient. This may be performed electronically on the monitor, or it might require you to scan (or take a photo of) the printout and send it the way a fax or a text or email attachment would be sent. Whichever method your service uses, make sure you are familiar with it and have practiced it.

## Reviewing the ECG Tracing

After obtaining an ECG tracing, it is important to make sure you have a high-quality printout. You should be able to see the QRS complexes (the largest, usually narrow, deflections on the ECG) clearly without interference from artifact. Each QRS complex represents one contraction of the ventricles, so the closer together they are, the faster the heartbeat. The horizontal distance between each wave on the ECG represents time passing. Each small (1-mm) box on the printout represents 0.04 second, and each of the larger (5-mm) boxes represents 0.20 second. The QRS complex should be less than 3 mm wide from where it starts to leave the baseline to where it returns. QRS complexes that are wider than 3 mm are usually signs of dangerous rhythms.

If two QRS complexes are less than 15 mm apart (three large boxes), the heart rate is over 100 and the rhythm is a tachycardia. If the QRS complexes are more than 25 mm apart (five large boxes), the rate is less than 60 beats per minute and the rhythm is a bradycardia. Rhythms such as tachycardia and bradycardia may cause a patient to have altered mental status or a low blood pressure.

You may also see a small rounded wave before the QRS called a P wave, which represents the contraction of the atria. After each QRS complex, you should see a T wave that represents the repolarization (or recharging) of the ventricles. The horizontal line between all of the waves is called the baseline and segments of the baseline are often identified by the waves they connect. For example, the ST segment connects the end of the QRS complex and the beginning of the T wave. Elevation of this ST segment above the baseline in a 12-lead ECG can be an indication of a myocardial infarction in progress.

Identification of cardiac rhythms is a paramedic-level skill, but as an EMT you will likely become familiar with some of the common rhythms.

# Heart Surgeries and Cardiac Assistive Devices

During the past 40 years, hundreds of thousands of open-heart surgeries have been performed to bypass damaged segments of coronary arteries in the heart. In a coronary artery bypass graft, a blood vessel from the chest or leg is sewn directly from the aorta to a coronary artery beyond the point of the obstruction. Another procedure is percutaneous transluminal coronary angioplasty, which aims to dilate, rather than bypass, the coronary artery. In this procedure, which is usually called angioplasty or balloon angioplasty, a tiny balloon is attached to the end of a long, thin tube. The tube is introduced through the skin into a large artery, usually in the groin or wrist, and then threaded under x-ray control into the narrowed coronary artery. Once the balloon is in position inside the coronary artery, it is inflated. The balloon is then deflated, and the tube is removed from the body. Sometimes, a metal mesh cylinder called a stent is placed inside the artery instead of or after the balloon. The stent is left in place permanently to help keep the artery from narrowing again.

A patient who has had an AMI or angina in the past will possibly have had one of these procedures. Patients who have had a bypass graft will have a long surgical scar on the chest from the operation. Patients who have had an angioplasty or a coronary artery stent usually will not. However, newer "keyhole" surgical techniques for bypass surgery may not produce a large scar. You should not assume that a patient who has a small scar has not had bypass surgery because newer minimally invasive procedures have smaller scars that may not be located over the sternum. Chest pain in a patient who has had any of these procedures should be treated in the same manner as chest pain in patients who have not had any heart surgery. Perform all the described tasks, and transport the patient promptly to the ED. If CPR is required, perform it in the usual way, regardless of the scar on the patient's chest. Likewise, if indicated, an AED should be used.

In the United States, many people with heart disease have cardiac pacemakers to maintain a regular cardiac rhythm and rate. Pacemakers are inserted when the electrical control system of the heart no longer functions properly. These battery-powered devices deliver an electrical impulse through wires

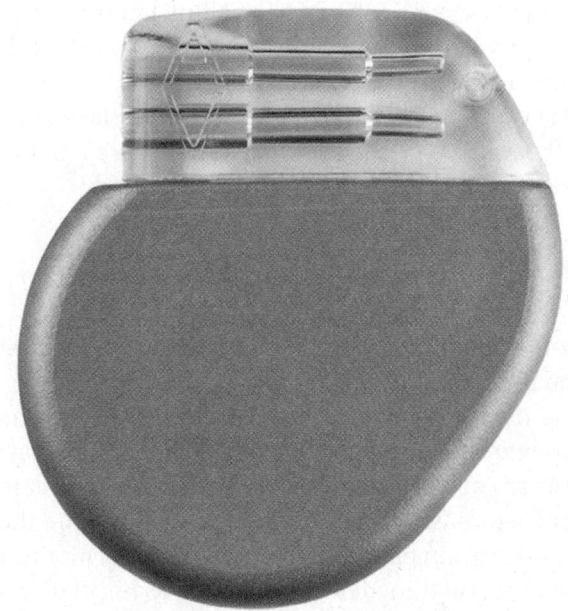

**FIGURE 17-12** A pacemaker, which is typically inserted under the skin in the left upper portion of the chest, delivers an electrical impulse to regulate the heartbeat.
© Carolina K. Smith, MD/ShutterStock.

that are in direct contact with the myocardium. The generating unit is generally placed under a heavy muscle or a fold of skin. It typically resembles a small silver dollar under the skin in the left upper portion of the chest (**FIGURE 17-12**).

Normally, you do not need to be concerned about problems with pacemakers. Thanks to modern technology, an implanted unit will not require replacement for years. Wires are well protected and rarely broken. In the past, pacemakers sometimes malfunctioned when a patient got too close to an electrical radiation source, such as a microwave oven. This is no longer the case; however, patients with pacemakers should avoid exposure to strong magnets. Every patient with a pacemaker should be aware of the precautions, if any, that must be taken to maintain its proper functioning.

If a pacemaker does not function properly, as when the battery wears out, the patient may experience syncope, dizziness, or weakness because of an excessively slow heart rate. The pulse ordinarily will be less than 60 beats/min because the heart is beating without the stimulus of the pacemaker and without the regulation of its own electrical system, which may be damaged. In these circumstances, the heart tends to assume a fixed slow rate that is not fast enough to allow the patient to function normally. A patient with a malfunctioning pacemaker should be promptly transported to the ED; repair of the problem may require surgery. When an AED is used, the patches should not be placed directly over the pacemaker. This will ensure a better flow of electricity through the patient's body.

## Automatic Implantable Cardiac Defibrillators

More and more patients who survive cardiac arrest due to VF have a small automatic implantable cardiac defibrillator implanted (**FIGURE 17-13**). Some patients who are at particularly high risk for a cardiac arrest have them as well. These devices are attached directly to the heart and can prolong the lives of certain patients. They continuously monitor the heart rhythm, delivering shocks as needed. Regardless of whether a patient having an AMI has an automatic implantable cardiac defibrillator, he or she should be treated like all other patients having an AMI. Treatment should include performing CPR and using an AED if the patient goes into cardiac arrest. Generally, the electricity from an automatic implantable cardiac defibrillator is so low that it will not have an effect on rescuers and, therefore, should not be of concern to you.

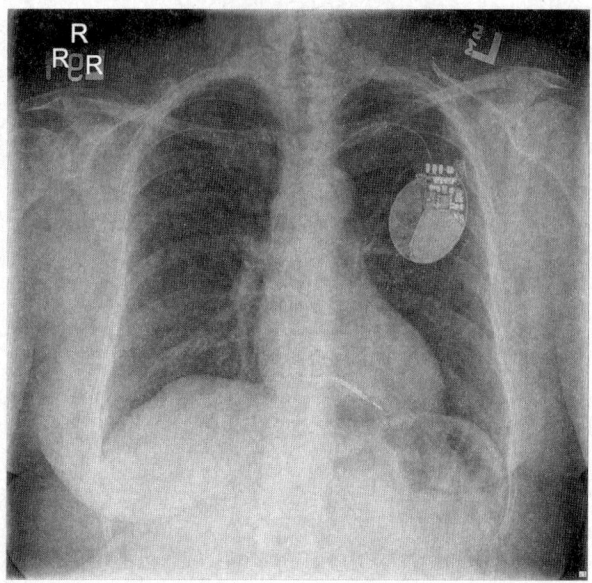

**FIGURE 17-13** An automatic implantable cardiac defibrillator is attached directly to the heart and continuously monitors heart rhythm, delivering shocks as needed. The electricity from the defibrillator is so low that it has no effect on rescuers.

© Andrew Pollak, MD. Used with permission.

## External Defibrillator Vest

A temporary alternative to the implantable cardiac defibrillator is the external defibrillator vest. This device is a vest with built-in monitoring electrodes and defibrillation pads, which is worn by the patient under his or her clothing. The vest is attached to a monitor worn on a belt or hung from a shoulder strap. The monitor provides alerts and voice prompts when it recognizes a dangerous rhythm and before a shock is delivered. It takes 25 to 60 seconds from detection of the rhythm problem to delivery of the shock. Unlike the implantable defibrillator, this device uses high-energy shocks similar to an AED, so you should avoid contact with the patient if the device warns that it is about to deliver a shock. An audible warning alerting rescuers to stay clear will state, "Bystanders, do not interfere," before the shock is delivered. Blue gel under the large defibrillation pads indicates that the device has already delivered at least one shock.

If the patient is in cardiac arrest, the vest should remain in place while CPR is being performed unless it interferes with compressions. If it is necessary to remove the vest, simply remove the battery from the monitor and then remove the vest. You can then use your own AED on the patient. Any patient who is wearing a device that has already delivered a shock should be transported to the hospital for further evaluation.

## Left Ventricular Assist Devices

Left ventricular assist devices (LVADs) are used to enhance the pumping function of the left ventricle in patients with severe heart failure or in patients who need a temporary boost due to a myocardial infarction (**FIGURE 17-14**). There are several types of LVADs; the most common ones have an internal pump unit and an external battery pack. These pumps are almost all continuous, so most of these patients will not have any palpable pulses. If you encounter a patient with an LVAD, he or she (or his or her family members) may be able to tell you about the unit. Unless it malfunctions, you should not need to deal with it. If you are unsure of what to do, contact medical control for assistance. Also, LVADs provide a number to call for assistance. Transport all LVAD supplies and battery packs to the hospital with the patient.

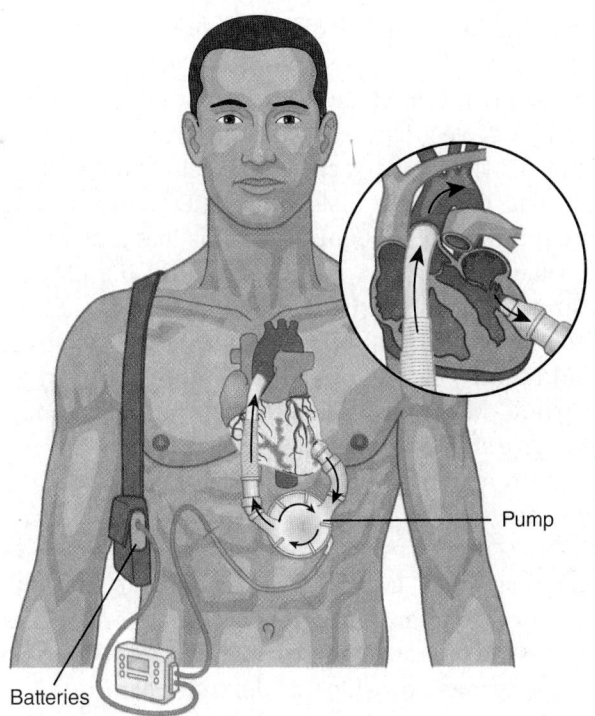

**FIGURE 17-14** Left ventricular assist device.

© Jones & Bartlett Learning.

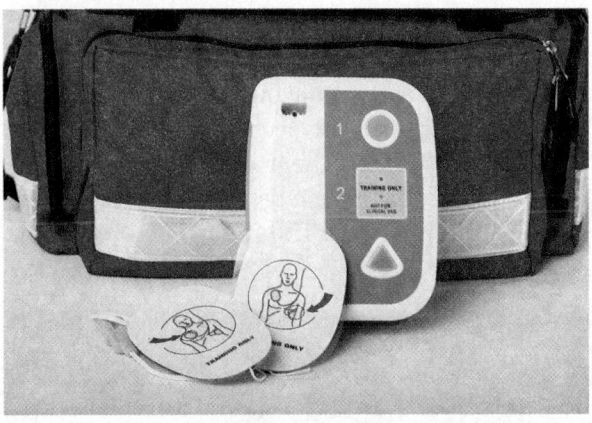

**A**

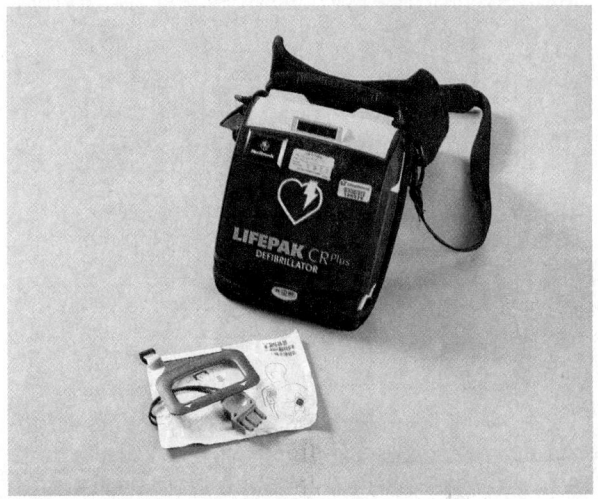

**B**

**FIGURE 17-15** Automated external defibrillators vary in their design, features, and operation. Two types (**A**) and (**B**) of defibrillators.

**A:** Photographee.eu/Shutterstock; **B:** Jones & Bartlett Learning.

## Cardiac Arrest

Cardiac arrest is the complete cessation of cardiac activity. It is indicated in the field by the absence of a carotid pulse. Until the advent of CPR and external defibrillation in the 1960s, cardiac arrest was almost always a terminal event. With good initial CPR, early defibrillation, and access to advanced care, it is now possible for some patients to survive a cardiac arrest without neurologic damage.

When you arrive to find a patient who appears to be in cardiac arrest, you should automatically follow your CPR training. CPR is covered in Chapter 14, *BLS Resuscitation*.

## Automated External Defibrillation

In the late 1970s and early 1980s, scientists developed a small computer that could analyze electrical signals from the heart and determine when VF was taking place. This development, along with improved battery technology, made the automated portable defibrillator—a device that can automatically administer an electrical shock to the heart when needed—possible.

AED machines come in different models with different features (**FIGURE 17-15**). All of them require a certain degree of operator interaction, beginning with turning on the machine and applying the pads. The operator also has to push a button to deliver an electrical shock, regardless of the model. Many AEDs use a computer voice synthesizer to advise the operator which steps to take on the basis of the AED's analysis. Some have a button that tells the computer to analyze the heart's electrical rhythm; other models start doing this as soon as they are turned on. Even though most defibrillators are now semiautomated, we still use the term AED to describe all of these machines. There are few fully automatic AEDs (which would deliver a shock without the operator pressing a button) left. All manufacturers are now producing only semiautomated external defibrillators.

AEDs deliver electrical energy from one pad to the other (and then back to the first pad) to electrically stun the heart and allow it to resume normal function. The amount of electricity delivered by the machine varies among the manufacturers, but each one has shown that the energy delivered is adequate to defibrillate the heart. The factors involved in the defibrillation include voltage, current, and impedance. Most AEDs are set up to adjust the voltage based on the impedance (or resistance of the body to the flow of electricity) to deliver the proper amount of current, which is what causes the cells to defibrillate.

The computer inside the AED is specifically programmed to recognize rhythms that require defibrillation to correct, most commonly VF. AEDs are extremely accurate. It would be rare for an AED to recommend a shock when a shock is not required, and an AED rarely fails to recommend one when it would be helpful. Therefore, if the AED recommends a shock, you can believe that it is indicated.

Automated external defibrillation has several advantages. First, the machine is fast, and it delivers the most important treatment for a patient in VF: an electrical shock. It can be delivered within 1 minute of your arrival at the patient's side. Second, AEDs are easy to operate. ALS providers do not have to be on the scene to provide this definitive care.

Current AEDs offer two other advantages. The shock can be given through remote, adhesive defibrillator pads, which are safe to use. Also, the pad area is larger than manual paddles, which means that the transmission of electricity is more efficient. Usually, there are pictures on the pads to remind you where they go on the patient's chest. As a safety measure, make sure the patient is not lying on wet ground or touching metal objects when he or she is being shocked.

## Special Populations

A pediatric patient with chest pain is not a common call. It is usually associated with a noncardiac condition or with a child who has a preexisting heart condition, which is usually congenital (present since birth). In pediatric situations, it is vital to see family members or caregivers as a valuable source of information.

Cardiac arrest in infants and children is usually the result of respiratory failure and not a primary cardiac event. However, the American Heart Association has determined that AEDs are safe to use in infants and children. If the patient is 8 years old or younger, pediatric-size pads and a dose-attenuating system (energy reducer) are preferred. However, if these are unavailable, a regular adult AED can be used. If the child is between 1 month and 1 year of age (an infant), a manual defibrillator is preferred to an AED. If a manual defibrillator is not available, an AED equipped with a pediatric dose attenuator is preferred. If neither is available, an AED without a pediatric dose attenuator may be used.

## YOU are the Provider

After completing the remainder of your assessment and initial treatment, you place the patient onto the stretcher, load her into the ambulance, and proceed to a hospital located 20 miles away. You ask your partner to notify the hospital to alert the staff as you reassess the patient.

| Recording Time: 10 Minutes | |
|---|---|
| **Level of consciousness** | Conscious and alert; still anxious |
| **Respirations** | 18 breaths/min; adequate depth |
| **Pulse** | 84 beats/min; strong and irregular |
| **Skin** | Pale and cool; less diaphoretic |
| **Blood pressure** | 136/84 mm Hg |
| **SpO$_2$** | 96% (on oxygen) |

**9.** Why is early notification of the receiving facility so important for patients with an acute coronary event?

**10.** Should you apply the AED to determine if this patient is experiencing a cardiac dysrhythmia? Why or why not?

Not all patients in cardiac arrest require an electrical shock. Although the cardiac rhythm of all patients in cardiac arrest should be analyzed with an AED, some do not have shockable rhythms (eg, pulseless electrical activity and asystole). Asystole (flatline) indicates that no electrical activity remains and therefore defibrillation will not help. Pulseless electrical activity refers to a state of cardiac arrest that exists despite an organized electrical complex; defibrillation could possibly make this situation worse. In both cases, CPR should be initiated as soon as possible, beginning with chest compressions.

## Rationale for Early Defibrillation

Few patients who experience sudden cardiac arrest outside a hospital survive unless a rapid sequence of events takes place. The chain of survival is a way of describing the ideal sequence of events that can take place when such an arrest occurs.

The six links in the chain of survival are as follows (**FIGURE 17-16**):

- Recognition of early warning signs and immediate activation of EMS
- Immediate CPR with emphasis on high-quality chest compressions
- Rapid defibrillation
- Basic and advanced EMS
- ALS and postarrest care
- Recovery

If any one of the links in the chain is absent, the patient is less likely to be resuscitated. For example, few patients benefit from defibrillation when more than 10 minutes elapses before administration of the first shock or if CPR is not started within the first 2 to 3 minutes. If all links in the chain are strong, the patient has the best possible chance of survival. The link that is the most common determinant for survival is the third link: rapid defibrillation. This link and those for immediate high-quality CPR and basic and advanced EMS are where EMTs are most involved.

CPR helps patients in cardiac arrest because it prolongs the period during which defibrillation can be effective. Rapid defibrillation has successfully resuscitated many patients with cardiac arrest due to VF. However, defibrillation works best if it takes place within 2 minutes of the onset of the cardiac arrest. Remember, seconds really matter when a patient is in cardiac arrest. The fourth link in the chain of survival is basic and advanced emergency medical services.

The fifth link in the chain of survival is ALS and post–cardiac arrest care. This refers to continuing ventilation at 10 breaths/min; maintaining oxygen saturation between 94% and 99%; ensuring systolic blood pressure is above 90 mm Hg; and using targeted temperature management when the patient arrives at the hospital. It also includes cardiopulmonary and neurologic support at the hospital as well as other advanced assessment techniques and interventions when indicated. The final step in the chain of survival, recovery can take a year or longer for many of the 10% of victims of out-of-hospital cardiac arrest who are fortunate enough to survive.

## Integrating the AED and CPR

Because most cardiac arrests occur in the home, a bystander at the scene may already have started CPR before you arrive. For this reason, you must know how to work the AED into the CPR sequence. Remember that the AED is not very complex, but

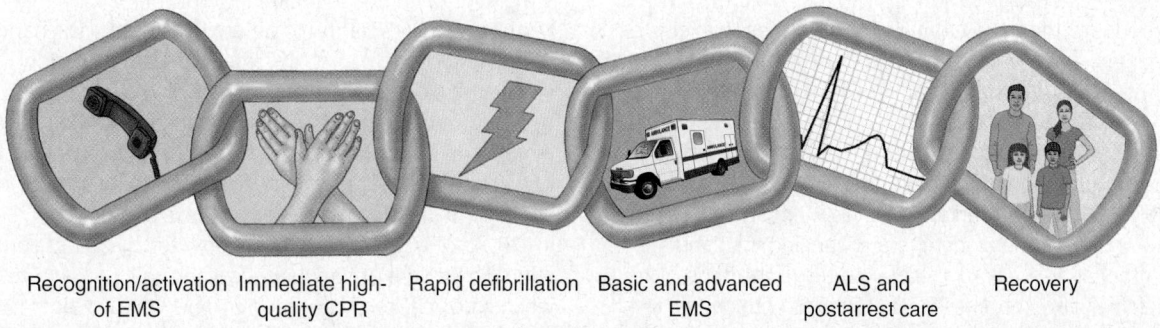

| Recognition/activation of EMS | Immediate high-quality CPR | Rapid defibrillation | Basic and advanced EMS | ALS and postarrest care | Recovery |

**FIGURE 17-16** The six links of the chain of survival.

it may not be able to distinguish other movements from VF. To avoid this problem, apply the AED only to pulseless, unresponsive patients and stay clear of the patient (do not touch the patient) while the AED is analyzing the heart rhythm and delivering shocks. You may perform chest compressions after the "shock advised" message while the AED is charging. Just remember to stop compressions and stay clear of the patient before pressing the button to deliver the shock.

## AED Maintenance

One of your primary missions as an EMT is to deliver an electrical shock to a patient in VF. To accomplish this mission, you need to have a functioning AED. You must become familiar with the maintenance procedures required for the brand of AED your system uses. Read the operator's manual. If your defibrillator does not work on the scene, someone will want to know what went wrong. That person may be your system's administrator, your medical director, the local newspaper reporter, or the family's attorney. You will be asked to show proof that you maintained the defibrillator properly and attended any mandatory in-service sessions.

The main legal risk in using the AED is failing to deliver a shock when one was needed. The three most common errors in using certain AEDs are failure of the machine to shock fine VF; applying the AED to a patient who is moving, squirming, or being transported; and turning off the AED before analysis or shock is complete. Operator errors include failing to apply the AED to a patient in cardiac arrest, not pushing the analyze or shock buttons when the machine advises you to do so, or pushing the power button instead of pushing the shock button when a shock is advised. Like any other manufactured item, the AED can fail, although this is rare. Ideally, you will encounter any such failure while doing routine maintenance, not while caring for a patient in cardiac arrest.

Another risk is failure to deliver a shock due to a battery that did not work, usually because it was not properly maintained. Check your equipment, including your AED, daily at the beginning of each shift and maintain the battery as often as the manufacturer recommends. Ask the manufacturer for a checklist of items that should be checked daily, weekly, or less often (**FIGURE 17-17**).

An error can also occur when the AED is applied to a responsive patient with a rapid heart rate. Most

## Special Populations

Like the other body systems, the cardiovascular system undergoes changes during the aging process. The heart, like other major organs, will show the effects of aging. As the heart's muscle mass and tone decrease, the amount of blood pumped out of the heart per beat decreases. The residual (reserve) capacity of the heart is also reduced; therefore, when the vital organs of the body need additional blood flow, the heart cannot meet the need. When blood flow to the tissues is decreased, the organs suffer. If blood flow to the brain is inadequate, the patient may report weakness, fatigue, or dizziness and may experience syncope (fainting).

The heart muscle is stimulated by electricity and has its own electrical system. Under normal conditions, electrical impulses travel throughout the heart, resulting in the contraction of the heart muscle and the pumping of blood from the heart's chambers. With aging, the electrical system can deteriorate, causing the heart's contraction to weaken or, if blood flow to the heart muscle is affected, extra beats to form. With decreased strength of contraction, the heartbeat is weaker and blood flow to the tissues is reduced. If extra beats are produced, the patient's heart rhythm will be irregular. Although some irregular heart rhythms are not harmful, others can be lethal.

The arteries are also affected by aging. Arteriosclerosis (hardening of the arteries) can develop, reducing perfusion of the tissues. There is an increased chance of heart attack or stroke due to decreased blood flow or plaque formation (atherosclerosis) in the narrowed arteries.

Patients with diabetes can experience reduced circulation to the hands and feet, which makes peripheral pulses harder to detect. It also puts the hands and feet at particular risk for infection and ulceration.

In some older patients with angina or AMI, particularly people with diabetes, chest pain is absent, and the clinical picture can be confused with other, noncardiac conditions. These patients may present with a chief complaint of syncope (fainting), fatigue, or shortness of breath.

The cardiovascular system is affected by aging. You should be aware of the changes, seeking to determine what is normal versus what is chronic versus what is an acute condition for the individual patient.

**AUTOMATED EXTERNAL DEFIBRILLATOR**
Inspection Checklist

Serial # _____ Date _____ Time _____

Model # _____ Inspected by _____

| Item | Pass | Fail |
|------|------|------|
| **Exterior/Cables** | | |
| Nothing stored on top of unit | | |
| Carry case intact and clean | | |
| Exterior/LCD/cables connectors clean and undamaged | | |
| Cables securely attached to unit | | |
| | | |
| **Batteries** | | |
| All chargers plugged in and operational (if applicable) | | |
| All batteries fully charged (battery in unit, spare battery) | | |
| Valid expiration date on both batteries | | |
| | | |
| **Supplies** | | |
| Two sets of electrodes in sealed packages with valid expiration dates | | |
| Razor | | |
| Hand towel | | |
| Alcohol wipes | | |
| Memory/voice recording device—module, card, microcassette | | |
| Manual override—module, key (if applicable) | | |
| Printer paper (if applicable) | | |
| | | |
| **Operation** | | |
| Unit self-test per manufacturer's recommendation/instructions | | |
|     Display (if applicable) | | |
|     Visual indicators | | |
|     Verbal prompts | | |
|     Printer (if applicable) | | |
| Attach AED to simulator/tester | | |
|     Recognizes shockable rhythm | | |
|     Charges to correct energy level within manufacturer's specifications | | |
|     Delivers charge | | |
|     Recognizes nonshockable rhythm | | |
|     Manual override system in working order (if applicable) | | |

Signature:

**FIGURE 17-17** A sample checklist for the automated external defibrillator (AED).

AEDs identify a regular rhythm faster than 150 or 180 beats/min as VT, which should be shocked if the patient is pulseless. However, shocking VT in a patient with a pulse may result in the patient losing his or her pulse and going into cardiac arrest. To avoid this problem, you should apply the AED only to unresponsive *pulseless* patients.

If the AED fails while you are caring for a patient, you must report the problem to the manufacturer and the US Food and Drug Administration. Be sure to follow the appropriate EMS procedures for notifying these organizations.

## Medical Direction

Defibrillation of the heart is a medical procedure. Although AEDs have made the process of delivering electricity much simpler, there is still a benefit in having a physician's involvement. The medical director of your service should approve the written protocol that you will follow in caring for patients in cardiac arrest.

There should be a review of each incident in which the AED is used. After returning from the hospital or the scene, discuss with the rest of the team what happened. This discussion will help all members of the team learn from the incident. Review such events by using the written report and the device's recordings, if applicable.

There should also be a review of the incident by your service's medical director or quality improvement officer. Quality improvement involves meetings between EMTs using AEDs and their EMS system managers or supervisors. This review should focus on speed of defibrillation—that is, the time from the first contact with the patient to the time that the first shock is delivered and, when the monitor can record it, the quality of CPR (to include timing of pauses). Few systems will achieve the ultimate goal: shocking 100% of patients within 1 minute of initial patient contact. However, all systems continuously work on improving patient care. Mandatory continuing education with skill competency review should be required for all EMS providers.

## Emergency Medical Care for Cardiac Arrest

### Preparation

When dispatch reports an unresponsive patient with CPR being performed, the AED is probably one of the first pieces of equipment you will obtain from the ambulance. As the operator of the AED, you are responsible for making sure the electricity does not injure anyone, including yourself. Remote defibrillation using pads allows you to distance yourself safely from the patient. As long as you place the pads in the correct position and make sure no one is touching the patient, you should be safe. Do not defibrillate a patient who is in pooled water. Although there is some danger to you if you are also in the water, there is another problem. Electricity follows the path of least resistance; instead of traveling between the pads and through the patient's heart, it will flow into the water. Therefore, the heart will not receive enough electricity to cause defibrillation. You can defibrillate a soaking wet patient but try first to dry the patient's chest. Do not defibrillate someone who is touching metal that others are touching, and carefully remove a nitroglycerin

### Street Smarts

Very few things we do in EMS have the potential to be as chaotic as treating a patients in cardiac arrest. Adapting the American Heart Association focus on team dynamics, many EMS systems have developed a "pit crew" strategy for handling these scenes. The term derives from the pit crew in Formula One automobile racing, which services a racecar in the middle of a race by changing tires and adding fuel. On a pit crew, each person has a specific job to do, so one person changes the rear tires while another changes the front tires. In the pit crew concept of managing a cardiac arrest, each person also has a specific assignment, which is determined prior to or at the beginning of the scene.

For example, one person will be assigned to start chest compressions and another will perform ventilations with the bag-mask device. Another person should be running the code, or "calling the shots," and another is keeping a record of all that is being done, and still another can be applying and operating the AED. When each person has a specific job to do and can focus on that job, the chaos that often accompanies this type of call can be greatly reduced.

The pit crew concept is also driven by improvement. In many pit crew protocols, many aspects of the cardiac arrest, such as compression depth, rate, and pre- and post-shock pauses, are measured and analyzed to try to meet certain benchmarks. Many systems that have implemented the pit crew approach have significantly improved cardiac arrest survival rates.

patch from a patient's chest and wipe the area with a dry towel before defibrillation to prevent ignition of the patch. It is often helpful to shave the hairy chest of a patient before pad placement to increase conductivity. Be sure to consult local protocols for issues such as pad placement and preparation of the pad site.

Determine the nature of illness and/or mechanism of injury. If the incident involves trauma, consider spinal motion restriction as you begin the primary assessment. Is there only one patient? If you are in a tiered system and the patient is in cardiac arrest, call for ALS assistance. If you suspect that the patient may be in cardiac arrest, discuss who will perform which resuscitation responsibilities prior to arrival on the scene. Preparation tasks should be done concurrently, so that time to defibrillation is minimized. For example, one provider begins compressions while another prepares for ventilation and another prepares the AED. Working as a well-organized team will improve the chances for a successful resuscitation.

## Performing Defibrillation

If you witness a patient's cardiac arrest, begin CPR starting with chest compressions and attach the AED as soon as it is available. As soon as the AED is turned on and attached, follow the instructions to analyze and deliver shocks to the patient. Make sure to minimize the time when you are not performing chest compressions; research has shown the best survival rates for patients in whom compressions were interrupted for the least amount of time. At each defibrillation, the person performing compressions should switch places with the person providing ventilations so that neither gets overtired. Immediately after each defibrillation, resume CPR with compressions first. The steps for using the AED are listed here and shown in **SKILL DRILL 17-3**:

1. If bystander CPR is in progress, assess the effectiveness of chest compressions by palpating for a carotid or femoral pulse. If compressions are effective, you should be able to feel a pulse. If you do, leave your fingers in that position and stop compressions (**Step 1**). If you lose the pulse when compressions stop, immediately resume compressions. It is important to limit the amount of time compressions are interrupted. If the patient is responsive, do not apply the AED.

2. If the patient is unresponsive and CPR has not been started yet, begin providing chest compressions and rescue breaths at a ratio of 30 compressions to two breaths and a rate of 100 to 120 compressions per minute, continuing until an AED arrives and is ready for use. It is important to start chest compressions and use the AED as soon as possible. Compressions provide vital blood flow to the heart and brain, improving the patient's chance of survival. High-quality compressions (ie, performed at the appropriate rate and depth, with no

## Skill Drill 17-3 Using an AED

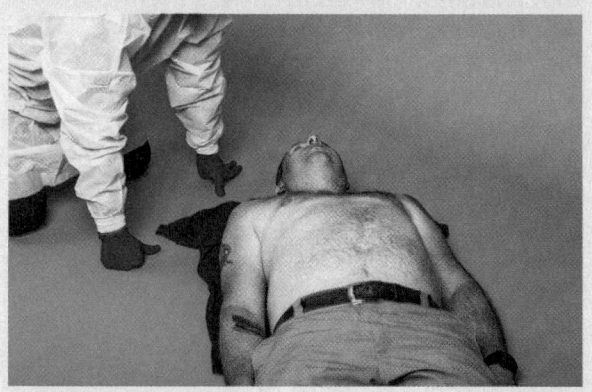

### Step 1

Take standard precautions. Determine scene safety. Question bystanders. Determine responsiveness. Assess compression effectiveness if CPR is already in progress. If the patient is unresponsive and CPR has not been started yet, begin providing chest compressions and rescue breaths at a ratio of 30 compressions to two breaths and a rate of 100 to 120 compressions per minute, continuing until an AED arrives and is ready for use.

*(continues)*

## Skill Drill 17-3 Using an AED (*continued*)

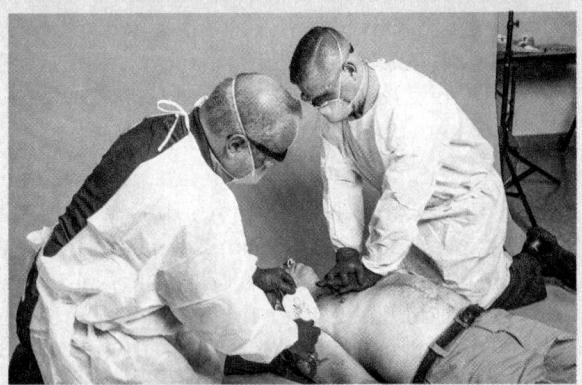

### Step 2

Turn on the AED. Apply the AED pads to the chest and attach the pads to the AED.

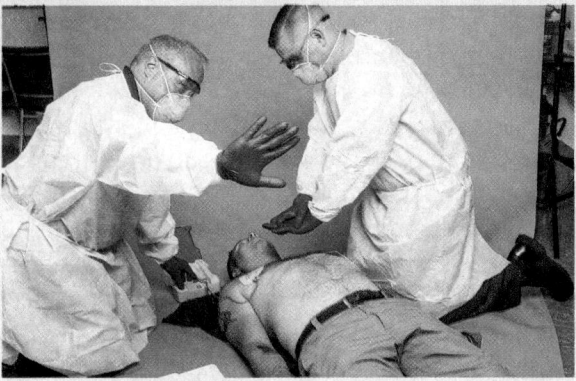

### Step 3

Push the Analyze button, if there is one, and wait for the AED to determine whether a shockable rhythm is present. Stop CPR when the AED instructs you to.

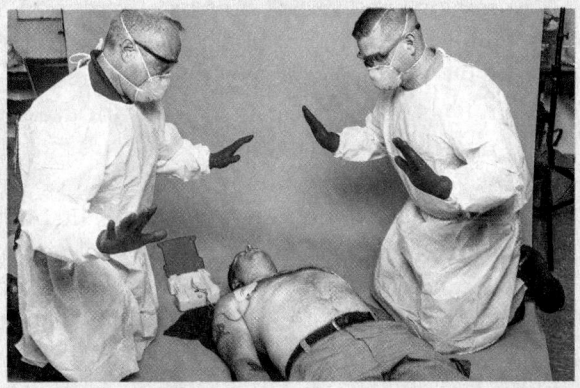

### Step 4

If a shock is advised, state aloud, "Clear the patient," and ensure that no one is touching the patient. Reconfirm that no one is touching the patient and push the Shock button. Continue CPR for five cycles (2 minutes) after the shock is delivered WITHOUT STOPPING to check for a pulse after the shock has been delivered! If no shock is advised, resume CPR immediately.

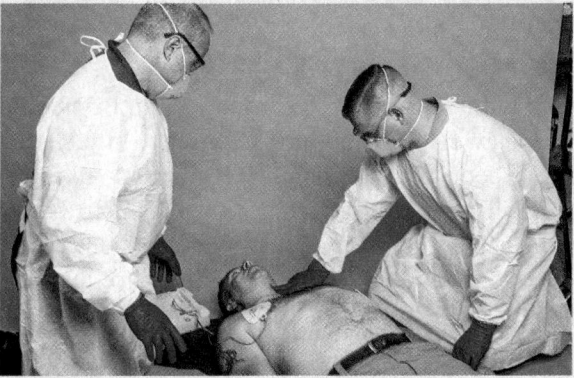

### Step 5

AFTER FIVE CYCLES (or 2 minutes), pause CPR and allow the AED to analyze the rhythm. If a shock is advised, clear the patient, push the Shock button, and immediately resume CPR compressions. If no shock is advised, immediately resume CPR compressions and be sure to switch rescuers. Repeat the cycle of five cycles (2 minutes) of CPR, one shock (if indicated), and 2 minutes of CPR. Transport, and contact medical control as needed.

leaning on the chest during recoil, and interruptions minimized) provide the best cardiac output.

3. Turn on the AED. Remove clothing from the patient's chest area. Apply the pads to the chest: one just to the right of the breastbone (sternum) just below the collarbone (clavicle), the other on the left lower chest area with the top of the pad 2 to 3 inches below the armpit (**Step 2**). Do not place the pads on top of breast tissue in women. If necessary, move the breast out of the way with the back of your hand and place the pad underneath. Ensure that the pads are attached to the patient cables (and that they are attached to the AED in some models). Plug in the pads' connectors to the AED.

4. Push the Analyze button, if there is one, and wait for the AED to determine whether a shockable rhythm is present. Stop CPR when the AED instructs you to (**Step 3**). If a shock is advised, consider performing chest compressions while the AED is charging.

5. If a shock is advised, state aloud, "Clear the patient," and ensure that no one is touching the patient. Reconfirm that no one is touching the patient and push the Shock button (**Step 4**). Immediately resume CPR.

6. If a shock is not advised, perform five cycles (about 2 minutes) of CPR, beginning with chest compressions, and then reanalyze the cardiac rhythm. If at any time the AED advises to check the patient, quickly assess for a carotid or femoral pulse. This should not take longer than 10 seconds. If you feel a pulse, the patient has experienced **return of spontaneous circulation (ROSC)**. ROSC is defined as the return of a pulse and effective blood flow to the body in a patient who previously was in cardiac arrest. Continue to monitor the patient.

7. After any shock is delivered, immediately resume CPR, beginning with chest compressions. Remember to change to a different person for chest compressions each time CPR is paused to prevent rescuer fatigue.

8. After five cycles (about 2 minutes) of CPR, reanalyze the patient's cardiac rhythm (**Step 5**). Do not interrupt chest compressions for more than 10 seconds.

9. Gather additional information about the arrest event.

10. Repeat the cycle of 2 minutes of CPR, one shock (if indicated), and 2 minutes of CPR.

11. Transport, and contact medical control as needed.

## YOU are the Provider

The patient is still conscious and alert and appears less anxious. She tells you that her chest pain has decreased in severity and is now a 3 on a 0 to 10 scale. After reassessing her, you contact the receiving facility and give the staff a patient update.

| Recording Time: 17 Minutes | |
| --- | --- |
| Level of consciousness | Conscious and alert; less anxious |
| Respirations | 16 breaths/min; adequate depth |
| Pulse | 80 beats/min; strong and irregular |
| Skin | Pink, cool, and dry |
| Blood pressure | 128/78 mm Hg |
| SpO$_2$ | 98% (on oxygen) |

You deliver the patient to the ED, where the cardiac team greets you and assumes care of the patient. The physician obtains a 12-lead ECG and determines that she is experiencing an AMI. Within 15 minutes, she is taken to the cardiac catheterization laboratory, where two coronary stents are successfully placed.

**11.** What is the difference between angina pectoris and an AMI?

**12.** As an EMT, how can you distinguish angina pectoris from an AMI?

If the AED advises no shock and the patient has a pulse, check the patient's breathing. If the patient is breathing adequately, give oxygen via nonrebreathing mask, adjusting the flow as soon as pulse oximetry gives a reading, and transport. If the patient is not breathing adequately, provide artificial ventilation with a bag-mask device or pocket mask device attached to 100% oxygen and transport. Ensure that proper airway techniques are used at all times.

If the patient has no pulse, perform five cycles (approximately 2 minutes) of CPR beginning with chest compressions. After 2 minutes of CPR, reanalyze the patient's cardiac rhythm. If the AED advises to shock, deliver one shock, followed immediately by CPR, beginning with chest compressions. Repeat these steps if needed.

If the patient has no pulse and the AED advises no shock, perform five cycles (approximately 2 minutes) of CPR, beginning with chest compressions. After five cycles (2 minutes) of CPR, reanalyze the patient's cardiac rhythm. If no shock is advised, continue CPR. Transport the patient and contact medical control as needed.

## After Automated External Device Shocks

The care of the patient after the AED delivers a shock depends on your location and EMS system; therefore, you should follow your local protocols. After the AED protocol is completed, one of the following outcomes is likely:

- Pulse is regained (ROSC).
- No pulse, and the AED indicates that no shock is advised.
- No pulse, and the AED indicates that a shock is advised.

Patients who do not regain a pulse on the scene of the cardiac arrest usually do not survive. What you do with these patients, again, depends on your EMS system. Whether you should transport the patient or wait for ALS to arrive should be in the local protocols established by medical control. If paramedics or another ALS service is responding to the scene, the best option usually is to stay where you are and continue the sequence of shocks and CPR. The best chance for patient survival occurs when the patient is resuscitated where found, unless the location is unsafe. Administering CPR while patients are being moved or transported is usually not very effective. If moving the patient is necessary with CPR in progress, consider the use of a mechanical chest compression device if one is available and you are trained to use it.

If an ALS service is not responding to the scene and your local protocols agree, you should begin transport when one of the following occurs:

- The patient regains a pulse.
- Six to nine shocks have been delivered (or as directed by local protocol).
- The AED gives three consecutive messages (separated by 2 minutes of CPR) that no shock is advised on a pulseless patient (or as directed by local protocol).

If you transport a patient while performing CPR, you need a plan for managing the patient in the ambulance. Transport is greatly facilitated by the use of a mechanical chest compression device. Performing compressions in a moving vehicle is dangerous to the provider and should be avoided if possible. A mechanical chest compression device makes this possible, as discussed in detail in Chapter 14, *BLS Resuscitation*.

Ideally, you will have two EMTs in the patient compartment while a third EMT drives. You may deliver additional shocks at the scene or en route with the approval of medical control. Keep in mind that AEDs cannot analyze the rhythm as well while the vehicle is in motion; nor is it as safe to defibrillate in a moving ambulance. Therefore, you should consider coming to a complete stop if more shocks are needed. Be sure to memorize the protocol of your EMS system (**FIGURE 17-18**).

## Cardiac Arrest During Transport

If you are traveling to the hospital with an unconscious patient, check the pulse at least every 30 seconds. If a pulse is not present, take the following steps:

1. Stop the vehicle.
2. If the AED is not immediately ready, perform CPR, beginning with chest compressions, until it is available.
3. Call for help in the form of ALS support or any other available resources as appropriate based on circumstances and local protocol.
4. Analyze the rhythm.
5. Deliver one shock, if indicated, and immediately resume CPR.

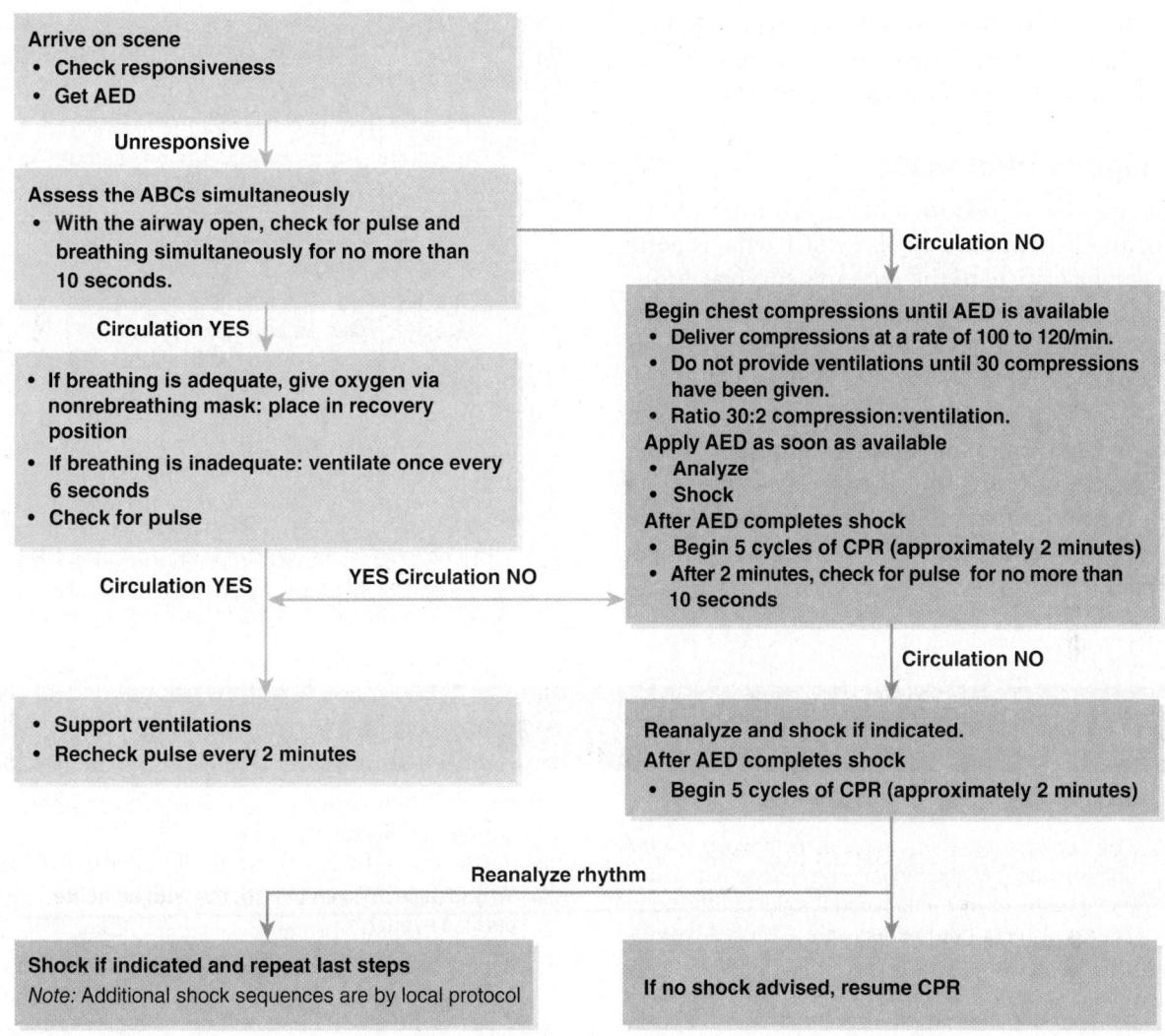

**Arrive on scene**
• Check responsiveness
• Get AED

↓ Unresponsive

**Assess the ABCs simultaneously**
• With the airway open, check for pulse and breathing simultaneously for no more than 10 seconds.

Circulation NO →

↓ Circulation YES

• If breathing is adequate, give oxygen via nonrebreathing mask: place in recovery position
• If breathing is inadequate: ventilate once every 6 seconds
• Check for pulse

**Begin chest compressions until AED is available**
• Deliver compressions at a rate of 100 to 120/min.
• Do not provide ventilations until 30 compressions have been given.
• Ratio 30:2 compression:ventilation.
**Apply AED as soon as available**
• Analyze
• Shock
**After AED completes shock**
• Begin 5 cycles of CPR (approximately 2 minutes)
• After 2 minutes, check for pulse for no more than 10 seconds

Circulation YES ← YES Circulation NO →

↓ Circulation YES                    ↓ Circulation NO

• Support ventilations
• Recheck pulse every 2 minutes

**Reanalyze and shock if indicated.**
**After AED completes shock**
• Begin 5 cycles of CPR (approximately 2 minutes)

Reanalyze rhythm

**Shock if indicated and repeat last steps**
*Note:* Additional shock sequences are by local protocol

**If no shock advised, resume CPR**

**FIGURE 17-18** Automated external defibrillator (AED) algorithm. CPR indicates cardiopulmonary resuscitation.

© Jones & Bartlett Learning.

6. Continue resuscitation according to your local protocol.

If you are en route with a conscious adult patient who is having chest pain and becomes unconscious, take the following steps:

1. Check for a pulse.
2. Stop the vehicle.
3. If the AED is not immediately ready, perform CPR, beginning with chest compressions, until it is ready.
4. Analyze the rhythm.
5. Deliver one shock, if indicated, and immediately resume CPR.
6. Begin compressions, and continue resuscitation according to your local protocol, including transporting the patient.

## Coordination With ALS Personnel

The time to defibrillation is critical to survival after cardiac arrest. As an EMT equipped with an AED, you have the one tool that a dying patient in VF needs most. Furthermore, it is impossible to hurt someone in cardiac arrest with an AED. Therefore, if you have an AED available, do not wait for the paramedics to arrive to administer a shock to a patient in VF. Waiting might seem like a good idea, but it is not. It is throwing away the patient's best chance for survival.

If the patient is unresponsive and does not have a pulse, apply the AED, and push the Analyze button (if there is one) as quickly as you can. Notify the ALS personnel as soon as possible after you recognize a cardiac arrest, but do not delay defibrillation.

After the paramedics arrive at the scene, inform them of your actions to that point and then interact with them according to your local protocols.

## Management of ROSC

If you are able to restore a heartbeat through the use of an AED (also known as ROSC), what is done next can be critical to the patient's survival. Monitor for spontaneous respirations, provide oxygen via bag-mask device at 10 breaths/min, and maintain an oxygen saturation between 95% and 99%. Assess the patient's blood pressure, and see if he or she can follow simple commands such as "Squeeze my fingers." If ALS is not on scene or en route, immediately begin transport to the closest appropriate hospital depending on local protocol.

### Safety Tips

When using an AED, there are several safety items to review.

1. Be aware of the surface on which the patient is lying. Wet and metal surfaces may conduct electricity, making defibrillation of the patient dangerous to EMTs.
2. What is the age of the patient? Use pediatric AED pads when appropriate.
3. Does the patient have a medication patch in the area the AED pads will be placed? If so, remove the medication patch, wipe the area clean, and then attach the AED pad.
4. Does the patient have an implanted pacemaker or internal defibrillator in the same area the AED pads will be placed? If so, place the AED pad below the pacemaker or defibrillator, or place the pads in anterior and posterior positions.

## YOU are the Provider SUMMARY

**1. What is the function of the heart?**

The heart receives deoxygenated blood from the body, sends it to the lungs to be reoxygenated, and then pumps oxygenated blood throughout the body. The heart must pump effectively to ensure that the body's tissues and cells receive an uninterrupted supply of oxygen and that metabolic waste (eg, carbon dioxide) is removed from the tissues and cells and returned, through the heart, for elimination from the body by the respiratory system.

**2. What does the heart require to function effectively?**

Like any other critical organ or muscle, the heart requires a constant supply of oxygen, which it receives from the coronary arteries. It also relies on electricity to stimulate the contraction of the muscular layer of the heart (myocardium). Adequate blood volume is also required for effective cardiac function. As blood returns to the heart, it enters the chambers, stretches their walls, and causes them to contract with greater force. If blood volume is low, the heart will stretch less, and its contractile force will decrease.

**3. What should you include in your primary assessment of a patient with cardiac problems?**

Your primary assessment of a patient with cardiac problems should be no different from your primary assessment of any other patient: To find and immediately correct problems with airway, breathing, and circulation. Look for signs of impaired cardiac function, such as an irregular heartbeat, a fast or slow heart

rate, a weak (thready) pulse, and poor skin condition (eg, pallor, diaphoresis).

**4. Why is aspirin given to patients with an acute cardiac event?**

Aspirin has clearly been shown to reduce mortality from AMI. Unless the patient is allergic to aspirin, it should be given as soon as possible if an acute cardiac event is suspected. An AMI occurs when an atherosclerotic plaque ruptures and occludes a coronary artery. When this occurs, platelets rush to the area and aggregate (clump together), which further occludes the coronary artery. Aspirin makes the platelets less "sticky," which makes them less likely to aggregate. Although aspirin will not dissolve the existing clot that is occluding the coronary artery, it may help prevent it from getting larger by reducing the amount of platelet aggregation.

**5. What type of medication is nitroglycerin? How may it help relieve chest pain, pressure, or discomfort?**

Nitroglycerin is a vasodilator. It works by relaxing the smooth muscle that regulates the diameter of the blood vessels, causing them to dilate (open). Nitroglycerin is used by patients with coronary artery disease who are experiencing chest pain, pressure, or discomfort. It dilates the coronary arteries and increases blood flow to the heart. As a result, the myocardial oxygen supply and demand are rebalanced, and the pain subsides or resolves completely. In some cases, however, nitroglycerin does not relieve the patient's chest pain. In a patient with a cardiac history, this should make you more suspicious that he or she is experiencing an AMI.

**6. When is nitroglycerin indicated for a patient? What is the typical dose?**

Nitroglycerin is indicated for patients with coronary artery disease who experience chest pain, pressure, or discomfort. Many patients with coronary artery disease have prescribed nitroglycerin, which they self-administer. If the patient has not taken any of his or her prescribed nitroglycerin, you may administer it after ensuring that the patient's systolic blood pressure is at least 100 mm Hg and that approval from medical control has been obtained. Because nitroglycerin is a vasodilator, it can cause hypotension. Therefore, it is important to reassess the patient's blood pressure within a few minutes after administering nitroglycerin to ensure that it is at least 100 mm Hg. Nitroglycerin is contraindicated in patients with a systolic blood pressure of less than 100 mm Hg and in patients who have taken drugs for erectile dysfunction (eg, sildenafil [Viagra], tadalafil [Cialis], avanafil [Stendra], and vardenafil [Levitra, Staxyn]) within the past 24 to 36 hours. Drugs for erectile dysfunction are also vasodilators; if given together with nitroglycerin, significant hypotension may occur.

**7. What is significant about the patient's vital signs?**

Pale, cool, clammy (diaphoretic) skin is not exclusive to a cardiac problem. However, in the context of the patient's chief complaint and history of heart problems, it is highly suggestive that her chest pain is of a cardiac origin. An irregular heartbeat indicates a disturbance in the cardiac electrical conduction system (dysrhythmia). Again, in the context of her chief complaint and cardiac history, this should further increase your index of suspicion that she is experiencing a cardiac event. An irregular heartbeat in a patient with a cardiac problem could indicate an impending life-threatening dysrhythmia. The patient's rapid heart rate (tachycardia) and relatively elevated blood pressure (150/90 mm Hg) are also clinically significant; they indicate that her heart is working harder than normal. As the heart rate and blood pressure increase, the heart consumes and requires more oxygen. If the heart is already deprived of oxygen, the patient's condition could worsen.

**8. Should you give her additional nitroglycerin? Why or why not?**

Despite taking two of her prescribed nitroglycerin doses before your arrival, the patient is still experiencing significant chest pain (7 on a scale of 0 to 10). Because her systolic blood pressure is well above 100 mm Hg, you should contact medical control and request permission to assist her with one

more nitroglycerin dose. Remember to reassess her blood pressure within a few minutes after administering the medication.

**9. Why is early notification of the receiving facility so important for patients with an acute coronary event?**

The longer it takes to reestablish blood flow distal to an occluded artery, the greater the amount of cardiac muscle damage (hence the phrase, "time is muscle"). Early reperfusion—with fibrinolytic medications (clot busters) or cardiac catheterization and stent placement—has clearly been shown to minimize the amount of cardiac damage and improve the patient's outcome. The earlier you notify the receiving facility that you are transporting a patient with a possible AMI, the more time the staff will have to allocate the resources needed to facilitate rapid cardiac reperfusion. The physician determines the reperfusion strategy. Your job is to recognize that the patient may be experiencing an AMI, provide immediate life-saving care, promptly notify the appropriate receiving facility, and transport without delay.

**10. Should you apply the AED to determine if this patient is experiencing a cardiac dysrhythmia? Why or why not?**

No. The AED is applied *only* to patients who are apneic and pulseless (eg, in cardiac arrest). Currently, your patient is breathing and has a pulse. Even if you did apply the AED, it would not analyze her cardiac rhythm. An AED will not analyze the cardiac rhythm if it detects patient movement. You should have the AED readily available in case she experiences cardiac arrest, but its application is not indicated at this point.

**11. What is the difference between angina pectoris and an AMI?**

Angina pectoris occurs when the heart's demand for oxygen temporarily exceeds its available supply (ischemia), resulting in chest pain or discomfort. Angina is typically triggered by exertion, which increases myocardial oxygen consumption and demand. When the patient ceases exertion, oxygen supply and demand are rebalanced and the pain resolves, usually in less than 15 minutes. In more severe cases, a combination of rest and nitroglycerin are required for resolution of the patient's chest pain or discomfort.

An AMI occurs when a portion of the heart muscle is completely deprived of oxygen because of complete occlusion of one or more coronary arteries. Unlike angina, the chest pain, pressure, or discomfort associated with an AMI typically does not resolve with rest or nitroglycerin and persists for greater than 15 minutes. The patient experiencing an AMI needs prompt treatment in the hospital, which

## YOU are the Provider SUMMARY continued

is aimed at removing the clot in the coronary artery and reestablishing distal blood flow.

**12. As an EMT, how can you distinguish angina pectoris from an AMI?**

The signs and symptoms of angina and an AMI are essentially the same and usually cannot be distinguished without advanced diagnostic procedures. In both conditions, the chest pain or discomfort may be described as a feeling of pressure or heaviness. The patient requires physician evaluation, blood analysis, and other tests to diagnose an AMI. You should assume that any patient with nontraumatic chest pain or discomfort is experiencing an AMI until ruled out by a physician.

### EMS Patient Care Report (PCR)

| **Date:** 3-10-20 | **Incident No.:** 130209 | **Nature of Call:** Cardiac | | **Location:** 1152 Blanco Road | |
|---|---|---|---|---|---|
| **Dispatched:** 0942 | **En Route:** 0942 | **At Scene:** 0950 | **Transport:** 1000 | **At Hospital:** 1028 | **In Service:** 1041 |

#### Patient Information

**Age:** 60
**Sex:** F
**Weight (in kg [lb]):** 55 kg (121 lb)

**Allergies:** No known drug allergies
**Medications:** Vasotec, aspirin (ASA), nitroglycerin (NTG)
**Past Medical History:** Heart attack, hypertension
**Chief Complaint:** Chest pain

#### Vital Signs

| **Time:** 0952 | **BP:** 150/90 | **Pulse:** 118 | **Respirations:** 20 | **Spo$_2$:** 98% |
|---|---|---|---|---|
| **Time:** 1000 | **BP:** 136/84 | **Pulse:** 84 | **Respirations:** 18 | **Spo$_2$:** 96% |
| **Time:** 1007 | **BP:** 128/78 | **Pulse:** 80 | **Respirations:** 16 | **Spo$_2$:** 98% |

#### EMS Treatment (circle all that apply)

| Oxygen @ _4_ L/min via: (NC) NRM  Bag mask | Assisted Ventilation | Airway Adjunct | CPR |
|---|---|---|---|
| Defibrillation | Bleeding Control | Bandaging | Splinting | Other: (324 mg ASA) |

#### Narrative

Dispatched for a 60-year-old woman with chest pain.

Chief Complaint: Chest pain

History: Patient states that she had a heart attack 3 years ago and has hypertension. She is presently taking Vasotec, NTG, and one (1) ASA per day and states that she has been compliant with her medications. Patient took two doses of her prescribed NTG before EMS arrival; however, she states that the medication had no effect; she presently describes her pain as a 7 on a scale of 0 to 10.

Assessment: On arrival at the scene, found the patient sitting up in her bed with her fist clenched against her chest. She was conscious and alert, although anxious. Her airway was patent, and her breathing was adequate. She was markedly diaphoretic; had pale, cool skin; and had a rapid, irregular pulse.

Treatment (Rx): Administered 324 mg ASA (patient stated she had no known drug allergies), applied oxygen at 4 L/min via nasal cannula to raise the oxygen saturation from 91% to just above 95%, and obtained vital signs. Contacted medical control, who authorized the administration of one more NTG dose. NTG was administered per medical control orders.

Transport: The patient was placed onto the stretcher, loaded into the ambulance, and transported to the hospital. Contacted hospital shortly after departing the scene and advised that we were transporting patient with possible AMI. En route to the hospital, allowed patient to assume position of comfort and reassessed her vital signs. She was still reporting chest pain (3/10); however, her pulse rate, although still irregular, was notably slower. Reassessment of her skin revealed that it was pink, cool, and dry, and she was noted to be less anxious. Continued to monitor patient's condition throughout transport; there was no gross evidence of deterioration, and she remained conscious and alert. Delivered her to emergency department staff w/o incident. On arrival at the hospital, we were greeted by the cardiac team, who assumed patient care. Gave verbal report to charge nurse and returned to service.

**End of report**

# Prep Kit

## Ready for Review

- The heart is divided down the middle into two sides, right and left, each with an upper chamber called the atrium and a lower chamber called the ventricle.
- The heart valve that keeps blood moving through the circulatory system in the proper direction is the aortic valve, which lies between the left ventricle and the aorta, the body's main artery.
- The heart's electrical system controls the heart rate and helps the atria and ventricles work together to pump the blood.
- During periods of exertion or stress, the myocardium requires more oxygen. The oxygen is supplied by dilation of the coronary arteries, which increases blood flow.
- Common places to feel for a pulse include the carotid, femoral, brachial, radial, posterior tibial, and dorsalis pedis arteries.
- Low blood flow to the heart is usually caused by coronary artery atherosclerosis, a disease in which cholesterol plaques build up inside blood vessels, eventually occluding them.
- Occasionally a brittle plaque in an artery will crack, causing a blood clot to form. Heart tissue downstream suffers from a lack of oxygen and, within 30 minutes, will begin to die. This condition is called an AMI, or heart attack.
- Heart tissues that are not getting enough oxygen but are not yet dying can cause pain called angina. The pain of an AMI is different from the pain of angina in that it can come at any time, not just with exertion; it lasts up to several hours, rather than just a few moments; and it is not relieved by rest or nitroglycerin.
- In addition to crushing chest pain, signs of AMI include sudden onset of weakness, nausea, and sweating; sudden dysrhythmia; pulmonary edema; and even sudden death.
- Heart attacks can cause sudden death, usually the result of cardiac arrest caused by abnormal heart rhythms called dysrhythmias. These include tachycardia, bradycardia, VT, and, most commonly, VF.

- A second consequence of an AMI is cardiogenic shock. Symptoms include restlessness; anxiety; pale, clammy skin; pulse rate higher than normal; and blood pressure lower than normal. Patients with these symptoms should receive oxygen, assisted ventilations as needed, and immediate transport.
- A third consequence of an AMI is CHF, in which damaged heart muscle can no longer contract effectively enough to pump blood through the system. The lungs become congested with fluid, breathing becomes difficult, the heart rate increases, and the left ventricle enlarges.
- Signs of CHF include swollen ankles from dependent edema, rapid heart rate and respirations, crackles, and, sometimes, the pink sputum and dyspnea of pulmonary edema.
- Treat a patient with CHF similar to how as you would a patient with chest pain. Monitor the patient's vital signs. Apply CPAP if it is available and you are authorized to use it. Give the patient oxygen via a nonrebreathing mask if he or she will not tolerate CPAP or it is not available. Allow the patient to remain sitting up.
- When treating patients with chest pain or discomfort, obtain a SAMPLE history, following the OPQRST mnemonic to assess the pain; measure and record vital signs; ensure the patient is in a comfortable position, usually semireclining or half sitting up; administer aspirin, prescribed nitroglycerin and oxygen; and transport the patient, reporting to medical control as you do.
- If a patient is not responsive, is not breathing, and does not have a pulse, you may perform the following, depending on the patient's age and your local protocol:
  - With an unresponsive adult or child older than 8 years, perform automated external defibrillation.
  - With an unresponsive child younger than 8 years, perform automated external defibrillation with pediatric pads and dose attenuator;

if neither is available, an adult AED may be used.

- An unresponsive infant between the ages of 1 month and 1 year should be manually defibrillated (an ALS skill). If ALS is not available, use an AED equipped with pediatric pads and a dose attenuator. If neither is available, adult AED pads may be used.

- The AED requires the operator to apply the pads, power on the unit, follow the AED prompts, and press the shock button as indicated. The computer inside the AED recognizes rhythms that require shocking and will not mislead you.

- The three most common errors in using certain AEDs are failure of the machine to shock fine VF; applying the AED to a patient who is moving, squirming, or being transported; and turning off the AED before analysis or shock is complete.

- Do not touch the patient while the AED is analyzing the heart rhythm or delivering shocks.

- Effective CPR and early defibrillation with an AED are critical interventions for the survival of a patient in cardiac arrest. Begin CPR starting with high-quality chest compressions and apply the AED as soon as it is available.

- If an ALS service is responding to the scene, stay where you are and continue CPR and defibrillation as needed. If ALS is not responding, begin transport if the patient regains a pulse, if you have delivered six to nine shocks, or if the AED gives three consecutive messages (separated by 2 minutes of CPR) that no shock is advised. Follow your local protocols regarding when it is appropriate to transport the patient.

- If an unconscious patient becomes pulseless during transport, stop the vehicle, reanalyze the rhythm, and defibrillate again or begin CPR, as appropriate.

- The chain of survival, which is the sequence of events that must happen for a patient with cardiac arrest to have the best chance of survival and recovery, includes recognition of early warning signs and immediate activation of EMS, immediate high-quality CPR, rapid defibrillation, basic advanced EMS, ALS and postarrest care, and a recovery plan.

## Vital Vocabulary

**acute coronary syndrome (ACS)** A group of symptoms caused by myocardial ischemia; includes angina and myocardial infarction.

**acute myocardial infarction (AMI)** A heart attack; death of heart muscle following obstruction of blood flow to it. "Acute" in this context means "new" or "happening right now."

**angina pectoris** Transient (short-lived) chest discomfort caused by partial or temporary blockage of blood flow to the heart muscle; also called angina.

**anterior** The front surface of the body; the side facing you in the standard anatomic position.

**aorta** The main artery, which receives blood from the left ventricle and delivers it to all the other arteries that carry blood to the tissues of the body.

**aortic aneurysm** A weakness in the wall of the aorta that makes it susceptible to rupture.

**aortic valve** The one-way valve that lies between the left ventricle and the aorta and keeps blood from flowing back into the left ventricle after the left ventricle ejects its blood into the aorta; one of four heart valves.

**artifact** A tracing on an ECG that is the result of interference, such as patient movement, rather than the heart's electrical activity.

**asystole** The complete absence of all heart electrical activity.

**atherosclerosis** A disorder in which cholesterol and calcium build up inside the walls of blood vessels, eventually leading to partial or complete blockage of blood flow.

**atrium** One of the two upper chambers of the heart.

**automaticity** The ability of cardiac muscle cells to contract without stimulation from the nervous system.

**autonomic nervous system** The part of the nervous system that controls the involuntary activities of the body such as the heart rate, blood pressure, and digestion of food.

**bradycardia** A slow heart rate, less than 60 beats/min.

**cardiac arrest** When the heart fails to generate effective and detectable blood flow; pulses are not palpable in cardiac arrest, even if muscular and electrical activity continues in the heart.

**cardiac output** A measure of the volume of blood circulated by the heart in 1 minute, calculated by multiplying the stroke volume by the heart rate.

**cardiogenic shock** A state in which not enough oxygen is delivered to the tissues of the body, caused by low output of blood from the heart. It can be a severe complication of a large acute myocardial infarction, as well as other conditions.

**congestive heart failure (CHF)** A disorder in which the heart loses part of its ability to effectively pump blood, usually as a result of damage to the heart muscle and usually resulting in a backup of fluid into the lungs.

**coronary arteries** The blood vessels that carry blood and nutrients to the heart muscle.

**defibrillate** To shock a fibrillating (chaotically shaking) heart with specialized electric current in an attempt to restore a normal, rhythmic beat.

**dependent edema** Swelling in the part of the body closest to the ground, caused by collection of fluid in the tissues; a possible sign of congestive heart failure.

**dilation** Widening of a tubular structure such as a coronary artery.

**dissecting aneurysm** A condition in which the inner layers of an artery, such as the aorta, become separated, allowing blood (at high pressures) to flow between the layers.

**dysrhythmia** An irregular or abnormal heart rhythm.

**hypertensive emergency** An emergency situation created by excessively high blood pressure, which can lead to serious complications such as stroke or aneurysm.

**infarction** Death of a body tissue, usually caused by interruption of its blood supply.

**inferior** Below a body part or nearer to the feet.

**ischemia** A lack of oxygen that deprives tissues of necessary nutrients, resulting from partial or complete blockage of blood flow; potentially reversible because permanent injury has not yet occurred.

**lumen** The inside diameter of an artery or other hollow structure.

**myocardium** The heart muscle.

**occlusion** A blockage, usually of a tubular structure such as a blood vessel.

**parasympathetic nervous system** The part of the autonomic nervous system that controls vegetative functions such as digestion of food and relaxation.

**perfusion** The circulation of oxygenated blood within an organ or tissue in adequate amounts to meet the cells' current needs.

**posterior** The back surface of the body; the side away from you in the standard anatomic position.

**return of spontaneous circulation (ROSC)** The return of a pulse and effective blood flow to the body in a patient who previously was in cardiac arrest.

**stroke volume** The volume of blood ejected with each ventricular contraction.

**superior** Above a body part or nearer to the head.

**sympathetic nervous system** The part of the autonomic nervous system that controls active functions such as responding to fear (also known as the fight-or-flight system).

**syncope** A fainting spell or transient loss of consciousness.

**tachycardia** A rapid heart rate, more than 100 beats/min.

**thromboembolism** A blood clot that has formed within a blood vessel and is floating within the bloodstream.

**ventricle** One of the two lower chambers of the heart.

**ventricular fibrillation** Disorganized, ineffective quivering of the ventricles, resulting in no blood flow and a state of cardiac arrest.

**ventricular tachycardia** A rapid heart rhythm in which the electrical impulse begins in the ventricle (instead of the atria), which may result in inadequate blood flow and eventually deteriorate into cardiac arrest.

# References

1. American Academy of Orthopaedic Surgeons. *Nancy Caroline's Emergency Care in the Streets*. 8th ed. Burlington, MA: Jones & Bartlett Learning and American Academy of Orthopaedic Surgeons; 2018.

2. American Heart Association. *Highlights of the 2020 American Heart Association Guidelines Update for CPR and ECC*. Dallas, TX: American Heart Association; https://cpr.heart.org/-/media/cpr-files/cpr-guidelines-files/highlights/hghlghts_2020_ecc_guidelines_english.pdf. Accessed November 6, 2020.

3. Benjamin EJ, Muntner P, Alonso A, et al. Heart disease and stroke statistics—2019 update: a report from the American Heart Association. *Circulation* 2019;139(10):e56–e528. doi:10.1161/CIR.0000000000000659.

4. Callaway CW, Donnino MW, Fink EL, et al. Part 8: post-cardiac arrest care. *Circulation* 2015;132(Suppl 1):S465–S482.

5. Chopra HK, Ram VS. Recent guidelines for hypertension: a clarion call for blood pressure control in India. *Circulation Res.* 2019;124:984–986.

6. Hopkins CL, Burk C, Moser S, et al. Implementation of pit crew approach and cardiopulmonary resuscitation metrics for out-of-hospital cardiac arrest improves patient survival and neurological outcome. *JAHA.* 2016;5(1). https://doi.org/10.1161/JAHA.115.002892.

7. Hypertensive crisis. American Heart Association website. http://www.heart.org/HEARTORG/Conditions/HighBloodPressure/AboutHighBloodPres sure/Hypertensive-Crisis_UCM_301782_Article.jsp. Reviewed November 30, 2017. Accessed March 27, 2020.

8. Kleinman ME, Brennan EE, Goldberger ZD, et al. Part 5: adult basic life support and cardiopulmonary resuscitation quality. *Circulation* 2015;132:S414–S435.

9. MacDonald RD, Swanson JM, Mottley JL, Weinstein C. Performance and error analysis of automated external defibrillator use in the out-of-hospital setting. *Ann Emerg Med* 2001;38(3):262–267.

10. Mozaffarian D, Benjamin EJ, Go AS, et al. Heart disease and stroke statistics—2015 update: a report from the American Heart Association. *Circulation*. 2015;131:e29–e322. doi:10.1161/CIR.0000000000000152.

11. National Association of State EMS Officials. *National EMS Scope of Practice Model 2019.* Washington, DC: National Highway Traffic Safety Administration; February 2019. Report No. DOT HS 812-666. https://www.ems.gov/pdf/National_EMS_Scope_of_Practice_Model_2019.pdf. Accessed March 27, 2020.

12. *National Emergency Medical Services Education Standards. Emergency Medical Technician Instructional Guidelines.* US Department of Transportation. National Highway Traffic Safety Administration. DOT HS 811 077C. January 2009. www.ems.gov/pdf/811077c.pdf. Accessed March 27, 2020.

13. National Registry of Emergency Medical Technicians. *2015 Paramedic Psychomotor Competency Portfolio (PPCP).* Columbus, OH: National Registry of Emergency Medical Technicians; 2015. https://content.nremt.org/static/documents/Paramedic_Psychomotor_Competency_Portfolio_Manual_v4.pdf. Accessed March 27, 2020.

14. O'Connor RE, Al Ali AS, Brady WJ, et al. Part 9: acute coronary syndromes. 2015 American Heart Association guidelines update for cardiopulmonary resuscitation and emergency cardiovascular care. *Circulation* 2015;132:S483–S500.

15. Psychomotor exams. National Registry of Emergency Medical Technicians website. https://www.nremt.org/nremt/about/psychomotor_exam_emt.asp. Accessed March 27, 2020.

16. Wacht O, Kohn J, Strugo R. Mechanical CPR devices: where is the science? *JEMS* website. https://www.jems.com/2019/11/12/mechanical-cpr-devices-where-is-the-science/. Published November 12, 2019. Accessed March 27, 2020.

17. What is the LifeVest wearable defibrillator? ZOLL LifeVest website. http://lifevest.zoll.com/medical-professionals. Accessed March 27, 2020.

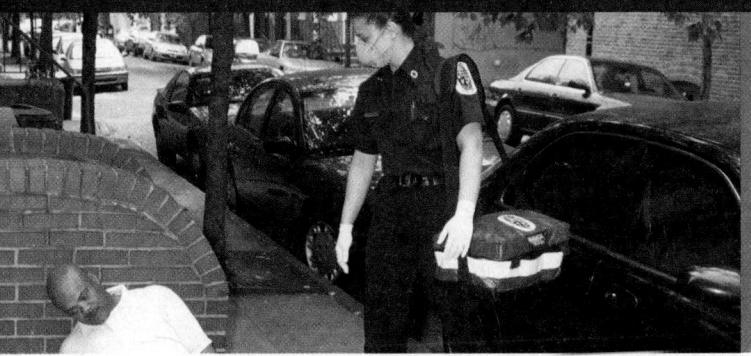

# Chapter 18

# Neurologic Emergencies

## NATIONAL EMS EDUCATION STANDARD COMPETENCIES

### Medicine

Applies fundamental knowledge to provide basic emergency care and transportation based on assessment findings for an acutely ill patient.

### Neurology

Anatomy, presentations, and management of
- Decreased level of responsiveness (pp 724–725, 735–737, 749)
- Seizure (pp 724–725, 732–735, 748–749)
- Stroke (pp 724–725, 727–731, 747–748)

Anatomy, physiology, pathophysiology, assessment, and management of
- Stroke/transient ischemic attack (pp 724–731, 737–748)
- Seizure (pp 724–725, 737–744, 748–749)
- Status epilepticus (pp 724–725, 737–745, 744–749)
- Headache (pp 724–727, 737–741, 744–747)

## KNOWLEDGE OBJECTIVES

1. Describe the anatomy, physiology, and functions of the brain and spinal cord. (pp 724–726)
2. Discuss the different types of headaches, the possible causes of each, and how to distinguish a harmless headache from a potentially life-threatening condition. (pp 726–727)
3. Explain the various ways blood flow to the brain may be interrupted and cause a cerebrovascular accident. (pp 727–728)
4. Discuss the causes, similarities, and differences of an ischemic stroke, hemorrhagic stroke, and transient ischemic attack. (pp 728–730)
5. List the general signs and symptoms of stroke and how those symptoms manifest if the left hemisphere of the brain is affected and if the right hemisphere of the brain is affected. (pp 730–731)
6. List three conditions with symptoms that mimic stroke and the assessment techniques EMTs may use to identify them. (p 731)

7. Define a general seizure, focal-onset seizure, and status epilepticus; include how they differ from each other and their effects on patients. (pp 732–733)
8. Describe how the different stages of a seizure are characterized. (p 733)
9. Discuss the importance for EMTs to recognize when a seizure is occurring or whether one has already occurred in a patient. (pp 734–735)
10. Explain the postictal state and the specific patient care interventions that may be necessary. (p 735)
11. Define altered mental status; include possible causes and the patient assessment considerations that apply to each. (pp 735–737, 749)
12. Discuss scene safety considerations when responding to a patient with a neurologic emergency. (pp 737–738)
13. Explain the special considerations required for pediatric patients who exhibit altered mental status. (p 737)

14. Explain the primary assessment of a patient who is experiencing a neurologic emergency and the necessary interventions that may be required to address all life threats. (pp 738–739)

15. Describe the process of history taking for a patient who is experiencing a neurologic emergency and how this process varies depending on the nature of the patient's illness. (pp 739–741)

16. Explain the secondary assessment of a patient who is experiencing a neurologic emergency. (pp 741–744)

17. Explain how to use stroke assessment tools to rapidly identify a stroke patient; include two commonly used tools. (pp 741–744)

18. Explain the concept of a stroke alert and the important time frame for the most successful treatment outcome for a patient who is suspected of having a stroke. (pp 745–746)

19. List the key information EMTs must obtain and document for a stroke patient during assessment and reassessment. (pp 741–745)

20. Explain the care, treatment, and transport of patients who are experiencing headaches, stroke, seizure, and altered mental status. (pp 745–749)

21. Explain the special considerations required for geriatric patients who are experiencing a neurologic emergency. (p 747)

## SKILLS OBJECTIVE

1. Demonstrate how to use a stroke assessment tool such as the Cincinnati Prehospital Stroke Scale, 3-Item Stroke Severity Scale (LAG), or BE-FAST mnemonic to test a patient for aphasia, facial weakness, and motor weakness. (pp 741–745)

# Introduction

Stroke is the fifth leading cause of death and a leading cause of disability in the United States, according to the American Stroke Association. Although stroke is common in geriatric patients, it may happen to anyone. Contributing factors for stroke include family history and race and ethnicity; African Americans, Hispanics, and Asians have an increased risk of stroke. Fortunately, treatments are available for stroke, and many hospitals are certified stroke centers. Some patients can avoid the devastating consequences of an acute stroke if they reach a hospital in time for treatment.

Seizures and altered mental status may occur in patients with brain disorders. Seizures may occur as a result of a recent or a prior head injury, a brain tumor, a metabolic disease, fever, or a genetic disposition. Your ability to recognize when a seizure has occurred or is occurring is a critical step because you can then provide the appropriate management.

Altered mental status is common in patients with a wide variety of medical conditions. However, avoid making assumptions about the cause of a patient's altered mental status. Many causes are possible, some obvious, some not: intoxication, head injury, hypoxia, stroke, metabolic disturbances, and many more. Treatment also varies based on what causes the altered mental status. Patients with altered mental status can be challenging in that they may be difficult to handle and frustrating to treat. This chapter will help you better understand, communicate with, and care for patients experiencing neurologic emergencies. Remember, your professionalism is paramount in these situations.

This chapter describes the structure and function of the brain and reviews the most common causes of brain disorders, including stroke, transient ischemic attacks (TIAs), seizures, headaches, and altered mental status. The signs and symptoms of each condition are explained as well as how to approach and assess a patient with a neurologic emergency and why prompt transport to an appropriate medical facility is so important.

## Anatomy and Physiology

The brain is the body's computer. It controls breathing, speech, and all other body functions. All thoughts, memories, needs, and desires reside in the brain. Different parts of the brain perform different functions. For example, some parts of the brain receive input from the senses, including sight, hearing, taste, smell, and touch; some control the

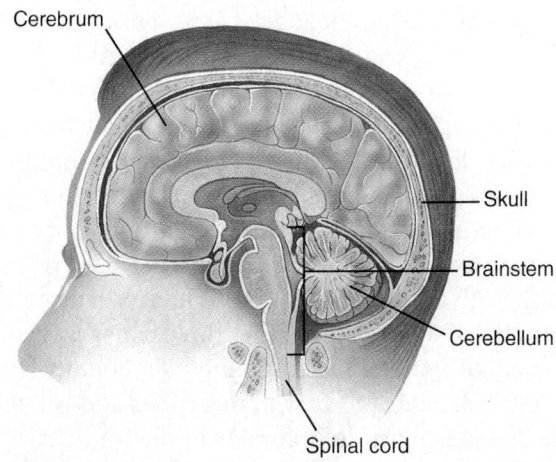

**FIGURE 18-1** The brain is well protected within the skull. The brain's major parts are the cerebrum, the cerebellum, and the brainstem.

© Jones & Bartlett Learning.

muscles and movement; and some control the formation of speech.

The brain is divided into three major parts: the brainstem, the cerebellum, and the cerebrum, which is the largest part (**FIGURE 18-1**). The brainstem controls the most basic functions of the body, such as breathing, blood pressure, swallowing, and pupil constriction. Located just behind the brainstem is the cerebellum, which controls muscle and body coordination. The cerebellum is responsible for coordinating complex tasks that involve many muscles, such as standing on one foot without falling, walking, writing, picking up a coin, and playing the piano.

The cerebrum, located above the cerebellum, is divided down the middle into the right and left cerebral hemispheres. Each hemisphere controls activities on the opposite side of the body. The front part of the cerebrum controls emotion and thought, and the middle part controls sensation and movement. The back part of the cerebrum processes sight. In most people, speech is controlled on the left side of the brain, near the middle of the cerebrum.

Messages sent to and from the brain travel through nerves. Twelve pairs of cranial nerves run directly from the brain to various parts of the body, especially in the head, such as the eyes, ears, nose, and face. The remaining nerves join in the spinal cord and exit the brain through a large opening in the base of the skull called the foramen magnum (**FIGURE 18-2**). At each vertebra in the neck and back, two nerves, called spinal nerves, branch out from the spinal cord, one on each side, and carry signals to and from the body.

## Pathophysiology

Many different disorders may cause brain dysfunction or other neurologic symptoms and may affect the patient's level of consciousness, speech, and voluntary muscle control. The brain is most sensitive to changes in oxygen, glucose, and temperature levels. A significant change in any one of these three levels will result in a neurologic change. In general, if the problem is caused primarily by disorders in the heart and lungs, the entire brain will be affected. For example, when blood flow is stopped (cardiac arrest), the patient will go into a coma, a state of profound unconsciousness, and permanent brain damage can result within minutes. However, if the primary problem is in the brain, such as a poor blood supply to one side of the brain, the patient may have signs and symptoms affecting only one side of the body. A low oxygen level in the bloodstream will affect the entire brain, often causing

**YOU** **are the Provider**

At 1823 hours, your unit is dispatched to 106 Scottie Drive. The dispatcher states that a 58-year-old woman is reported to be experiencing a seizure. Bystanders report the patient is unresponsive, with shaking of her extremities and torso. You respond to the scene, which is located approximately 4 miles from your station. The weather is cloudy, the traffic is moderate, and the temperature is 87°F (30.6°C). While en route, you and your partner discuss the different types of seizures.

1. On the basis of the dispatch information, what type of seizure is the patient most likely experiencing?

2. What are some common causes of seizures in this patient's age group?

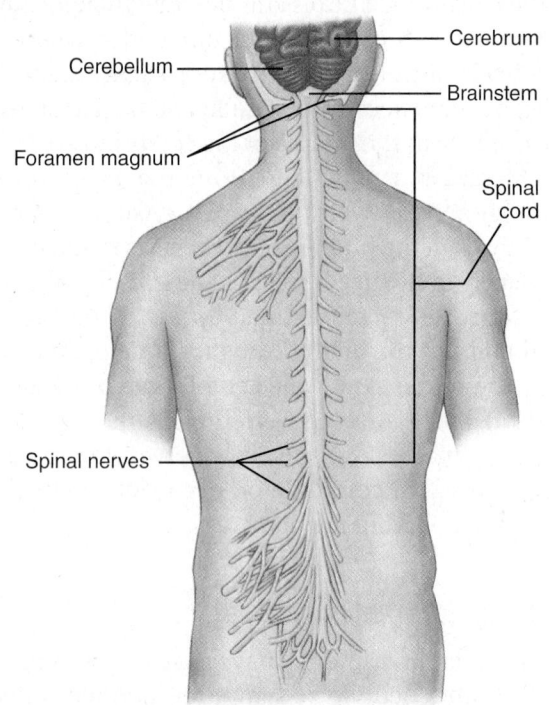

**FIGURE 18-2** The spinal cord is the continuation of the brainstem. It exits the skull at the foramen magnum and extends down to the level of the second lumbar vertebra.

© Jones & Bartlett Learning.

anxiety, restlessness, and confusion. Low blood glucose levels (hypoglycemia) can cause a wide spectrum of symptoms ranging from mild confusion to symptoms that mimic stroke.

## Headache

One of the most common complaints of pain you will hear from your patients is headache. Because a headache is subjective, it may be a symptom of another condition or it may be considered a neurologic condition on its own. Millions of people experience a headache every year, but only a small percentage of these are caused by a serious medical condition. The brain and skull do not actually sense pain because neither contains pain receptors. The pain associated with a headache is felt from the surrounding areas of the face; scalp; meninges (membranes that cover the brain and spinal cord); larger blood vessels; and muscles of the head, neck, and face.

Tension headaches, migraines, and sinus headaches are the most common types of headaches. These types of headaches are not considered life threatening, although they may be debilitating for the patient. Tension headaches are caused by muscle contractions in the head and neck and are attributed to stress. Patients usually describe the pain as squeezing, dull, or an ache. This type of headache typically does not have any associated symptoms and usually does not require medical attention.

Migraine headaches are thought to be caused by changes in blood vessel size in the base of the brain. Both adults and children can experience migraine headaches. Women are three times as likely as men to experience migraines. Frequently, the patient will have a history of migraines and will tell you that this episode is similar to one in the past. Pain from a migraine headache is usually described as pounding, throbbing, or pulsating. Migraines are often associated with nausea and vomiting and may be preceded by visual warning signs such as flashing lights or partial vision loss. These headaches can last for several hours to days.

Sinus headaches are caused by pressure that is the result of fluid accumulation in the sinus cavities. Patients may also have coldlike signs and symptoms of nasal congestion, cough, and fever if they have a sinus infection. Patients may report increased pain when they bend over or when their heads are moved forward. This type of headache is usually self-limiting, and prehospital emergency care is not required.

Although most headaches are not life threatening, some patients with a chief complaint of headache will require medical attention. Hemorrhagic stroke (bleeding in the brain), brain tumor, and meningitis are serious neurologic conditions that may include headache as a symptom. Be concerned if the patient reports a sudden-onset, severe headache or a sudden-onset headache that has associated symptoms. Headaches accompanied by fever, stiff neck, seizures, or altered mental status or following a head trauma are potentially life threatening and require a complete assessment and transport to the hospital (**TABLE 18-1**). A hemorrhagic stroke will often present with a complaint of headache that is described as "the worst headache of my life." If a patient describes a headache this way, you should have a very high index of suspicion and transport expeditiously to the hospital. An incident with multiple patients reporting a headache may indicate carbon monoxide poisoning.

A sudden, severe headache, often described as the worst pain the patient has ever had, could

**TABLE 18-1** Headache Red Flags

A patient who has a headache associated with any of the following should be evaluated for a potentially life-threatening condition:

- Sudden onset of symptoms
- Headache described by the patient as "the worst headache of my life"
- Explosive/thunderclap pain
- Altered mental status
- Age older than 50 years
- Depressed immune system (known to be at higher risk for infection)
- Neurologic deficits
- Neck stiffness/pain
- Fever
- Changes in vision
- One-sided paralysis or weakness

© Jones & Bartlett Learning.

be a sign of a hemorrhagic stroke. The blood from a ruptured blood vessel irritates the tissues of the brain and can cause increased intracranial pressure (ICP), resulting in severe headache pain. This type of pain may initially be localized and then become more diffuse as the irritation in the meninges spreads. You should suspect a hemorrhagic stroke in patients with a severe headache, seizures, and altered mental status. Early signs of increased ICP include headache, vomiting, altered mental status, and seizures. Increasing ICP may also be caused by a hemorrhagic stroke (a blood vessel swells and ruptures), a tumor, or head trauma that may have occurred hours or days before this event. During your patient assessment, ask if the patient has experienced any recent head trauma.

Bacterial meningitis, an inflammation of the meninges caused by a bacterial infection, is a central nervous system infection in which the patient may complain of a headache, stiff neck, fever, and sensitivity to light. This is a serious condition requiring prompt medical attention and is highly contagious. Use standard precautions and provide supportive care of the XABCs. Provide a quiet, darkened environment when possible and avoid using lights and siren.

## Stroke

A **cerebrovascular accident (CVA)**, or **stroke**, is an interruption of blood flow to an area within the brain that results in the loss of brain function. In the context of a total lack of oxygen, brain cells

---

**YOU** are the Provider

You arrive at the scene, where you are greeted by the patient's sister. She tells you they were having a conversation when the patient suddenly grabbed both sides of her head and then began "shaking all over." The patient is lying on the floor in her living room with a pillow under her head. She is conscious but confused and reports a severe headache. You perform an assessment as your partner opens the jump bag.

| Recording Time: 0 Minutes | |
|---|---|
| **Appearance** | Slightly pale; skin is dry |
| **Level of consciousness** | Conscious, but confused |
| **Airway** | Open; clear of secretions and foreign bodies |
| **Breathing** | Rapid rate; adequate depth |
| **Circulation** | Radial pulse rapid and bounding |

Your partner prepares to take the patient's vital signs. The patient's sister tells you her sister has never had a seizure before. The patient is wearing a medical alert bracelet, which identifies her medical history of high blood pressure, heart disease, and type 2 diabetes.

**3.** What additional questions should you ask the patient's sister?

**4.** What prehospital assessments can you perform to determine the possible cause of the patient's seizure?

**5.** What treatment is indicated at this point?

stop functioning and begin to die within minutes. Medical science currently has little to offer in the way of treatment once brain cells are dead. However, when oxygen levels are decreased, but not absent, because an insufficient amount of blood is getting through, brain cells may be damaged more slowly. It may take several hours or more for brain cells to die in this situation. When brain cells die or are injured, severe disability may result. For example, if cells that are responsible for controlling the left arm are starved for oxygen, the patient will not be able to move that arm. The brain cells will develop **ischemia**, a reduction in blood supply that results in inadequate oxygen being supplied to the brain cells. This causes those cells to stop functioning properly. If normal blood flow is restored to that area of the brain in time, the cells will not die and the patient may regain full use and control of the arm.

Unfortunately, many patients experiencing a stroke deny or ignore their symptoms and delay seeking medical attention. The delay in seeking care can result in devastating consequences, because "time is brain."

---

### Words of Wisdom

Stroke patients who receive treatment within the first few hours of the onset of stroke symptoms have a much greater chance of surviving and avoiding long-term brain damage. Patients with ischemic strokes, the most common type of stroke, may be candidates for treatment with medications to lyse or dissolve the clot that is causing the stroke or with treatment to remove the clot under x-ray control, but these treatments must be completed soon after a stroke to have the best chance of reversing the symptoms. Note the time of symptom onset and transport to a stroke center depending on local protocol. Sometimes the gap from last known well time to initiation of effective treatment can be 24 hours or longer, but sooner is better in terms of restoring long-term function.

---

## Types of Stroke

The two main types of stroke are ischemic and hemorrhagic. An ischemic stroke occurs when blood flow through the cerebral arteries is blocked. In hemorrhagic stroke, a blood vessel ruptures and the accumulated blood causes increased pressure in the brain.

## Ischemic Stroke

According to the American Stroke Association, **ischemic stroke** is the most common type of stroke, accounting for 87% of all strokes. When blood flow to a specific part of the brain is stopped by a blockage (blood clot) inside a blood vessel, the result is an ischemic stroke. Patients who experience an ischemic stroke may have dramatic symptoms, including loss of movement on the side of the body opposite the side where the occlusion has occurred.

This blockage may be due to **thrombosis**, where a clot forms at the site of blockage, or an **embolus**, where the blood clot forms in a remote area (such as a diseased heart) and then travels to the site of the blockage. Patients with atrial fibrillation (a heart rhythm where the atria shake rather than squeeze) are prone to ischemic strokes caused by an embolus and often take blood thinners to reduce the risk of these events.

As with coronary artery disease, atherosclerosis in the blood vessels is often the cause of ischemic stroke. **Atherosclerosis** is a disorder in which calcium and cholesterol build up, forming plaque inside the walls of the blood vessels. This plaque may obstruct blood flow and interfere with the vessels' ability to dilate. Eventually, atherosclerosis may cause complete occlusion of an artery (**FIGURE 18-3**). In other cases, an atherosclerotic plaque in the carotid artery in the neck ruptures.

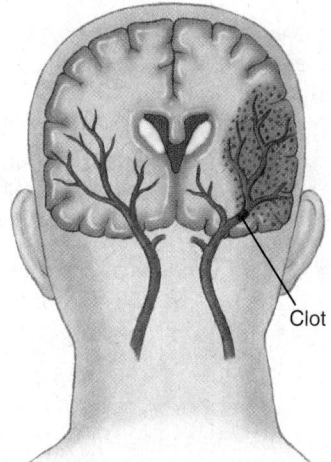

Clot

**FIGURE 18-3** Atherosclerosis can damage the wall of a cerebral artery, producing narrowing and/or a blood clot. When a vessel is narrowed or completely blocked, blood flow to part of the brain may be blocked, causing brain cells to die because of the lack of adequate oxygenation.

© Jones & Bartlett Learning.

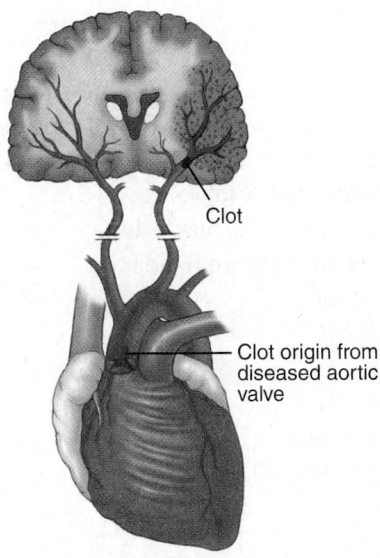

**FIGURE 18-4** An embolus, a blood clot formed elsewhere in the body (for example, on a diseased heart valve), can travel through the body's vascular system, lodge in a cerebral artery, and cause a stroke.

© Jones & Bartlett Learning.

A blood clot forms over the crack in the plaque. Sometimes, it grows large enough to completely block all blood flow through that artery. The parts of the brain supplied by the artery are deprived of oxygen and stop functioning.

Even if the blockage in the carotid artery is not complete, smaller pieces of the blood clot may embolize (break off and be carried by the normal flow of blood) deep into the brain, where they may become lodged in a smaller branch of a blood vessel. This cerebral embolism then blocks blood flow (**FIGURE 18-4**). Depending on the location of the lodged blood clot, the patient's symptoms can vary widely, from nothing at all to complete paralysis or loss of function to the areas or functions of the body controlled by that portion of the brain.

## Hemorrhagic Stroke

**Hemorrhagic stroke** occurs as a result of bleeding inside the brain. According to the American Stroke Association, hemorrhagic strokes account for 13% of all strokes. In hemorrhagic stroke, a blood vessel ruptures and the accumulated blood then forms a blood clot, which compresses the brain tissue next to it. The compression prevents oxygenated blood from getting into the area, and the brain cells begin to die. Cerebral hemorrhages are often massive and rapidly fatal.

Hemorrhagic stroke commonly occurs in people experiencing stress or exertion. The people at highest risk for hemorrhagic stroke are those with extremely high blood pressure or long-term untreated elevated blood pressure. Many years of high blood pressure weaken the blood vessels in the brain. If a vessel ruptures, the bleeding in the brain will increase the pressure inside the cranium. Proper treatment of high blood pressure can help prevent this long-term damage to the blood vessels, decreasing the risk of this devastating complication.

Some people are born with a weakness in the walls of an artery. An **aneurysm**, a swelling or enlargement of the wall of an artery resulting from a defect or weakening of the arterial wall, may then develop. **FIGURE 18-5** is an angiogram showing a cerebral aneurysm. The most notable symptom of a ruptured aneurysm is often a sudden-onset, severe headache, typically described by the patient as the worst headache he or she has ever had. The headache is caused by the irritation of blood on the brain tissue after the artery swells and ruptures. A hemorrhagic stroke in an otherwise healthy young person is often caused by a weakness in a blood vessel called a *berry aneurysm*. This type of aneurysm resembles a tiny balloon (or berry) that juts out from

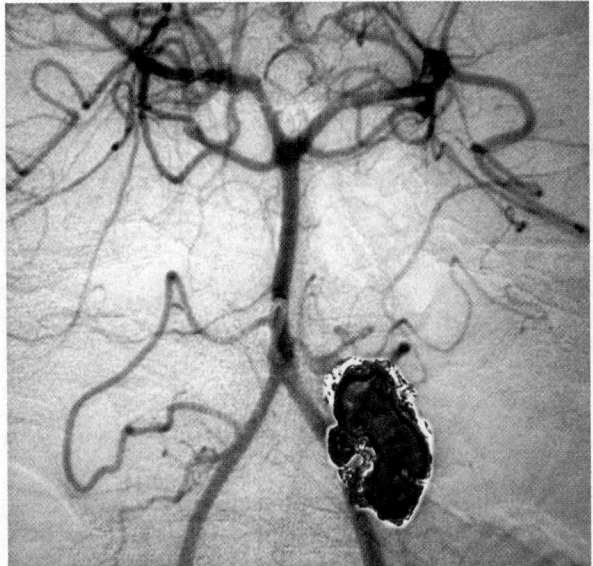

**FIGURE 18-5** An angiogram showing a cerebral aneurysm.

© Living Art Enterprises/Science Source.

the artery. When the aneurysm is overstretched and ruptures, blood spurts into an area between two of the coverings of the brain called the subarachnoid space. These types of strokes are called subarachnoid hemorrhages. If the patient gets to the hospital quickly, surgical repair of the aneurysm may be possible. However, like other brain bleeding and cerebral hemorrhage, this condition is often fatal.

## Transient Ischemic Attack

In a patient with coronary artery disease, blood flow to the heart muscle may be obstructed, causing chest pain (angina), which is considered a warning sign of a potential myocardial infarction. Similarly, when blood flow to the brain is obstructed due to atherosclerosis or a small blood clot, the patient may exhibit signs of a stroke. When these stroke-like symptoms resolve on their own in less than 24 hours, the event is called a **transient ischemic attack (TIA)**. Some people call these *mini strokes*. As with angina, no actual death of tissue (infarction) occurs with a TIA. However, because symptoms of a TIA can last up to 24 hours, you may not be able to differentiate between a stroke and a TIA.

Although most patients with TIAs do well, every TIA is an emergency. It may be a warning sign that a more significant stroke may occur in the future. Approximately one-third of patients who have a TIA will experience a stroke soon after the TIA. For this reason, all patients with a TIA should be evaluated by a physician to determine whether preventive action should be taken.

## Signs and Symptoms of Stroke

The general signs and symptoms of stroke include the following:

- Facial drooping
- Sudden weakness or numbness in the face, arm, leg, or one side of the body
- Decreased or absent movement and sensation on one side of the body
- Lack of muscle coordination (ataxia) or loss of balance
- Sudden vision loss in one eye; blurred or double vision or abnormal eye movements
- Difficulty swallowing (a primary reason for good airway management in a patient with a stroke)

- Decreased level of responsiveness
- Speech disorders
- Aphasia; difficulty expressing thoughts or inability to use the right words (expressive aphasia) or difficulty understanding spoken words (receptive aphasia)
- Slurred speech (**dysarthria**)
- Sudden and severe headache
- Confusion
- Dizziness
- Weakness
- Combativeness
- Restlessness
- Tongue deviation
- Coma

## Left Hemisphere

If the left cerebral hemisphere has been affected by a stroke, the patient may exhibit a speech disorder called **aphasia**, the inability to produce or understand speech. Speech problems can vary widely. Some patients will have trouble understanding speech but will be able to speak clearly. You can detect this problem by asking the patient a question such as "What day is today?" The patient may respond with an inappropriate answer such as "Green." The speech is clear, but it does not make sense. Other patients will be able to understand the question but cannot produce the right sounds to provide an answer. Strokes that affect the left side of the brain can also cause paralysis of the right side of the body.

## Right Hemisphere

If the right cerebral hemisphere of the brain is not getting enough blood, the patient will have trouble moving the muscles on the left side of the body. Usually, the patient will understand language and be able to speak, but the words may be slurred and hard to understand.

Interestingly, patients with right-hemisphere strokes may be completely oblivious to their problems. If you ask these patients to lift their left arms and they cannot, they will lift their right arms instead. Patients will seem to have forgotten that their left arms even exist. This symptom is called neglect. Patients with conditions affecting the back part of the cerebrum may neglect certain parts of their vision. Generally, this is hard to detect in the field because patients compensate without conscious effort. Nevertheless, be aware of the possibility. Sit or stand on the patient's "good" side because he or she may be unable to see things on the "bad" side.

Neglect and lack of pain cause many patients who have had strokes to delay seeking help. A patient may be unaware that he or she has a problem until someone points out that some part of the patient's body is not functioning properly.

## Bleeding in the Brain

Patients with bleeding in the brain (cerebral hemorrhage) may have very high blood pressure. High blood pressure can either cause the bleeding or be a compensatory response to the bleeding. Blood pressure increases as the body attempts to force more oxygen to the area of the brain where the damage is occurring. Remember, the brain is located inside a box (skull) with only a few openings. When bleeding occurs inside the brain, the pressure inside the skull increases. The body must increase the blood pressure to get blood to the brain's tissues, increasing the pressure even further. A trend of increasing blood pressure is an important sign. Blood pressure may then taper off and return to normal. Significant drops in blood pressure may also occur as the patient's condition worsens. Therefore, it is important to monitor the blood pressure for changes in these patients.

## Conditions That May Mimic Stroke

The following conditions may appear to be a stroke:

- Hypoglycemia
- A postictal state (period following a seizure that lasts between 5 and 30 minutes, characterized by labored respirations and some degree of altered mental status)
- Subdural or epidural bleeding (a collection of blood near the skull that presses on the brain)

Because oxygen and glucose are needed for brain metabolism, a patient with hypoglycemia may present in a manner similar to a patient who is experiencing a stroke. Good patient assessment includes finding out whether the patient's medical history includes diabetes. Always check the blood glucose level in patients with altered mental status if allowed by your local protocol.

A patient in a postictal state may look like a patient who is experiencing a stroke. However, in most cases, a patient who has had a seizure will recover rapidly, within several minutes.

Subdural and epidural bleeding usually occur as a result of trauma. The dura is the leathery covering of the brain that lies next to the skull. A fracture near the temples may cause an artery to bleed on top of the dura, resulting in pressure on the brain (**FIGURE 18-6A**). The onset of epidural bleeding is usually very rapid after injury. When the veins just below the dura bleed, this is referred to as subdural bleeding (**FIGURE 18-6B**). Subdural bleeding is slower than epidural bleeding, sometimes occurring over a period of several days.

With subdural and epidural bleeding, the onset of strokelike signs and symptoms may be subtle. The patient or family may not even remember the original injury that is causing the bleeding.

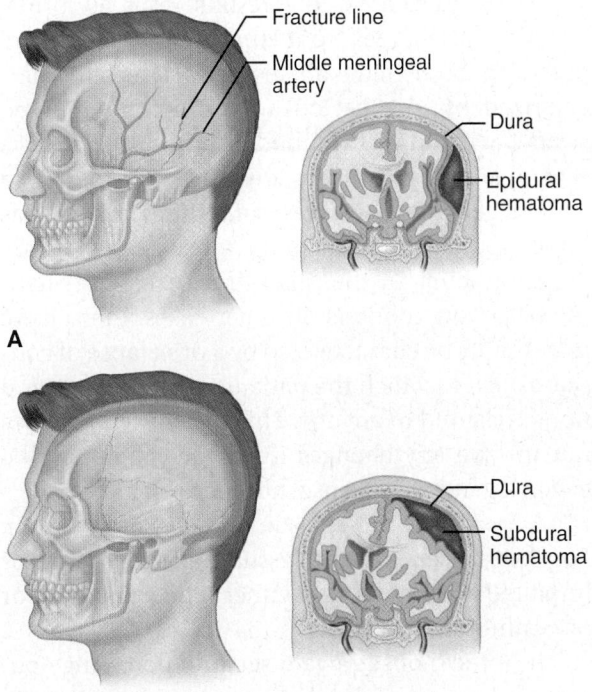

**FIGURE 18-6** Trauma to the head may result in intracranial bleeding. **A.** Bleeding outside the dura and under the skull is called epidural bleeding. **B.** Bleeding beneath the dura but outside the brain is called subdural bleeding.

**A, B:** © Jones & Bartlett Learning.

# Seizures

EMS calls frequently involve seizures. A **seizure** is a neurologic episode caused by a surge of electrical activity in the brain. It can take the form of a convulsion, characterized by generalized, uncoordinated muscle activity, and/or possibly a temporary alteration in consciousness. Nearly 3.5 million people in the United States have **epilepsy**, which is a common cause of seizures. Seizures are classified as either generalized or focal, and their underlying cause can be either known (ie, secondary to a brain tumor or a metabolic disorder) or unknown (idiopathic).

A **generalized seizure** results from abnormal electrical discharges from large areas of the brain, involving both hemispheres. It is typically characterized by unconsciousness and a generalized severe twitching of the body's muscles that lasts several minutes or longer (identified as "motor"). In generalized motor seizures (sometimes classified as tonic-clonic), almost all of the muscles in the body are contracting at the same time, causing twitching or jerking motions. In other cases, the seizure may simply be characterized by a brief lapse of consciousness in which the patient seems to stare and not to respond to anyone. This type of seizure does not involve any changes in motor activity and is called a generalized-onset absence seizure.

A **focal seizure** begins in one part of the brain. Focal-onset seizures are classified as either aware or impaired-awareness, and either type can be motor or nonmotor (absence).

In a focal-onset aware seizure, no change occurs in the patient's level of consciousness. Patients may report numbness, weakness, or dizziness. The senses may also be involved; the patient may report visual changes and unusual smells or tastes. A focal-onset aware (motor) seizure may also cause twitching of the muscles and the extremities that may spread slowly from one part of the body to another, but it is not characterized by the dramatic severe twitching and muscle movements seen in a generalized seizure. The patient may also experience brief paralysis.

In a focal-onset, impaired-awareness seizure, the patient has an altered mental status and does not interact normally with his or her environment. This type of seizure results from abnormal discharges from the temporal lobe of the brain. Other signs may include lip smacking, eye blinking, and isolated convulsions or jerking of the body or one part of the body such as an arm. The patient may experience unpleasant smells and visual hallucinations, exhibit uncontrollable fear, or exhibit repetitive physical behavior such as constant sitting and standing. In impaired-awareness seizures, the patient usually does not remember events occurring during the seizure.

Some focal-onset seizures remain on only one side of the body. Others begin on one side and gradually progress to the entire body. In focal-onset aware seizures, the patient may have no loss of consciousness but still experience body shaking or muscle tremors. Most people with lifelong or chronic seizures tolerate these events reasonably well without complications, but in some patients, seizures may signal life-threatening conditions.

Often, a patient may experience a warning sign prior to the event. This is referred to as an **aura**. An aura can include visual changes (flashing lights or blind spots in the field of vision) or hallucinations (seeing, hearing, or smelling things that are not actually present). People with a history of seizures recognize their auras and usually take steps to minimize injury, such as sitting or lying down, knowing what is about to happen. However, be aware that auras do not occur prior to every seizure, and not all patients with a seizure disorder experience an aura.

A generalized motor seizure may be characterized by sudden loss of consciousness followed by chaotic muscle movement and tone. The patient may experience a tonic phase, usually lasting only seconds, in which there is a period of extreme muscular rigidity. This period is usually followed immediately by a clonic phase, lasting much longer, of constant muscle contraction and trembling, tongue biting, bladder incontinence, or bowel incontinence. During a generalized seizure, the patient typically may exhibit bilateral movement characterized by a cycle of muscle rigidity and relaxation. Throughout a generalized seizure, the patient exhibits tachycardia, hyperventilation, sweating, and intense salivation; however, other responses are also possible.

Generalized motor seizures typically last less than 5 minutes and are followed by a lengthy period (5 to 30 minutes or more) called a postictal state, in which a patient is unresponsive at first and gradually regains consciousness. The postictal state is over when the patient regains a complete return of his or her normal level of consciousness. In most cases, the patient will gradually begin to recover and awaken but appear dazed, confused, and fatigued. In contrast, a generalized nonmotor or absence seizure may last for just seconds, after which the patient fully recovers with only a brief lapse of memory of the event.

Seizures lasting more than 5 minutes are at risk for progressing to **status epilepticus**, which describes seizures that continue every few minutes without the person regaining consciousness or that last longer than 30 minutes.

Recurring or prolonged seizures should be considered immediately life-threatening situations in which patients need emergency medical care. If the patient does not regain consciousness or the seizure continues, protect the patient from self-harm, and call for advanced life support (ALS) backup. These patients need advanced airway management and medication to stop the seizure.

## Causes of Seizures

Some seizure disorders, such as epilepsy, are congenital. Other types of seizures may be caused by high fevers, structural problems in the brain, or metabolic or chemical problems in the body (**TABLE 18-2**). In addition, a percentage of the population will experience a seizure for which the cause cannot be determined (idiopathic). Epileptic seizures can usually be controlled with medications. Medications used most often to treat seizures include the following:

- Levetiracetam (Keppra)
- Phenytoin (Dilantin)
- Phenobarbital
- Carbamazepine (Tegretol)

**TABLE 18-2** Common Causes of Seizures

| Type | Cause |
|------|-------|
| Epileptic | Congenital origin |
| Structural | Tumor (benign or cancerous) <br> Infection (brain abscess) <br> Scar tissue from injury (within the skull) <br> Head trauma <br> Stroke |
| Metabolic | Hypoxia <br> Abnormal blood chemical values <br> Hypoglycemia <br> Poisoning <br> Drug overdose <br> Sudden withdrawal from alcohol or medications |
| Febrile | Sudden high fever (primarily in children) |

© Jones & Bartlett Learning.

- Valproate (Depakote)
- Topiramate (Topamax)
- Clonazepam (Klonopin)

Patients with epilepsy will often have seizures if they stop taking their medications or if they do not take the prescribed dose on a regular basis.

Seizures may also be caused by abnormalities in the brain, such as a benign or cancerous tumor, an infection (brain abscess, meningitis), or scar tissue from some type of injury within the skull. These seizures are said to have a structural cause. Seizures from a metabolic cause may result from abnormal levels of certain blood chemicals (eg, extremely low sodium level), **hypoglycemia** (low blood glucose level), **hyperglycemia** (high blood glucose level), poisons, drug overdoses, or sudden withdrawal from routine heavy alcohol or sedative drug use or even from prescribed medications. Phenytoin, a drug that is used to control seizures, may itself cause seizures if the person takes too much.

Seizures may also result from sudden high fevers, primarily in children. These **febrile seizures** are frightening for parents but are generally well tolerated by the child. Always transport a child who has had a febrile seizure to the hospital, as the seizure may be a sign of a serious medical condition.

## The Importance of Recognizing Seizures

Regardless of the type or the cause of a seizure, it is important for you to recognize when a seizure is occurring or whether one has already occurred. You must also determine whether this episode differs from any previous ones. For example, if the previous seizure occurred on only one side of the body and this seizure occurs over the entire body, an additional or new problem may be involved. In addition to recognizing that seizure activity has occurred and/or that something different may now be occurring, you must recognize the postictal state and the complications of seizures.

Because most seizures involve a vigorous twitching of the muscles, the muscles use a lot of oxygen. This excessive demand consumes oxygen that is needed for the vital functions of the body. As a result, there is a buildup of acids in the bloodstream, and the patient may turn cyanotic (blue lips, tongue, and skin) from the lack of oxygen. Often, the seizures themselves prevent the patient from breathing normally, making the problem worse. In a patient with diabetes, the blood glucose level may decrease because of the excessive muscular contraction of a seizure. If possible, closely monitor the blood glucose level after a patient with diabetes has a seizure.

Recognizing seizure activity also means looking at other problems associated with the seizure. For example, the patient may have fallen during the seizure episode and been injured; head injury is the most serious possibility. Some patients may experience **incontinence** during a generalized seizure, meaning that they may have a loss of bowel or bladder control. Therefore, one clue that unresponsive or confused patients may have had a seizure is to find that they were incontinent. Although incontinence can occur with other medical conditions,

### Words of Wisdom

The physician's examination of a patient who has had a seizure will be aided greatly by information you provide about the seizure pattern and changes in that pattern. Record all pertinent information about the seizure in terms of duration, areas of body movement, and possible triggering factors. This requires effective interviewing of available witnesses, family members, and/or caregivers.

## YOU are the Provider

Your partner reports the patient's vital signs. The patient tells you she is nauseated and her headache, which is still severe, is located on both sides of her head. She further tells you the last thing she remembers was the sudden, severe headache. When she woke up, she was lying on the floor with a pillow under her head. She appears to be having difficulty moving her left side. Her sister tells you she caught the patient before she struck the ground.

| Recording Time: 4 Minutes | |
| --- | --- |
| **Respirations** | 14 breaths/min; adequate depth |
| **Pulse** | 100 beats/min; strong and regular |
| **Skin** | Pink, warm, and moist |
| **Blood pressure** | 200/112 mm Hg |
| **Oxygen saturation (Spo₂)** | 96% (on ambient air) |

The patient's blood glucose level is assessed and noted to be 97 mg/dL. Her sister hands you the patient's medication list, which includes benazepril, hydrochlorothiazide, and metformin. The patient says she is noncompliant with her medication regimen.

**6.** What is your field impression of this patient? Why?

**7.** On the basis of your field impression, you should monitor the patient for which additional signs and symptoms?

sudden incontinence is likely a sign of a seizure. When the patient regains consciousness, he or she is likely to be embarrassed by this temporary loss of control. Minimize the patient's discomfort by covering the patient and assuring him or her that incontinence is part of the loss of control that accompanies a seizure.

## The Postictal State

Once a seizure has stopped, the patient's muscles relax, becoming almost flaccid, or floppy, and the breathing becomes labored (fast and deep) to compensate for the buildup of acids in the bloodstream. By breathing faster and more deeply, the body can balance the acidity in the bloodstream. With normal circulation and liver function, the acids clear away within minutes, and the patient will begin to breathe more normally. The longer and more intense the seizures, the longer it will take for this imbalance to correct itself. Likewise, longer and more severe seizures will result in longer postictal unresponsiveness and confusion. Once the patient regains a normal level of consciousness, the postictal state is over.

> ### Words of Wisdom
>
> Interventions during the postictal state are important. Patients may be unable to maintain an open airway because of their relaxed and exhausted state; therefore, patient positioning, clearing the airway of secretions, and preventing aspiration are critical steps for achieving the best patient outcomes.

In some situations, the postictal state may be characterized by hemiparesis, or weakness on one side of the body, resembling a stroke. However, unlike a stroke, hypoxic hemiparesis soon resolves. Most commonly, the postictal state is characterized by lethargy and confusion to the point that the patient may be combative. Be prepared for these circumstances in your approach to scene control and in your treatment of the patient's symptoms. If the patient's condition does not improve, consider other possible underlying conditions such as hypoglycemia or infection.

> ### Special Populations
>
> Status epilepticus is harmful at any age, but because of physical changes caused by the normal aging process, geriatric patients are at greater risk of hypoxia, hypotension, and/or cardiac dysrhythmias.

## Syncope

Seizures are often mistaken for syncope (fainting); however, fainting typically occurs while the patient is standing, whereas seizures may occur in any position. Fainting is not associated with a postictal state.

## Altered Mental Status

Aside from stroke and seizures, the most common type of neurologic emergency you will encounter is a patient with altered mental status. Simply put, altered mental status means the patient is not thinking clearly or is incapable of being awakened. In some cases, the patient will be unconscious; other times, the patient may be alert but confused (**FIGURE 18-7**). The range of problems is wide and the causes are many, including hypoglycemia, hypoxemia, intoxication, delirium, drug overdose, unrecognized head injury, brain infection, body temperature abnormalities, brain tumors, and overdoses and/or poisonings.

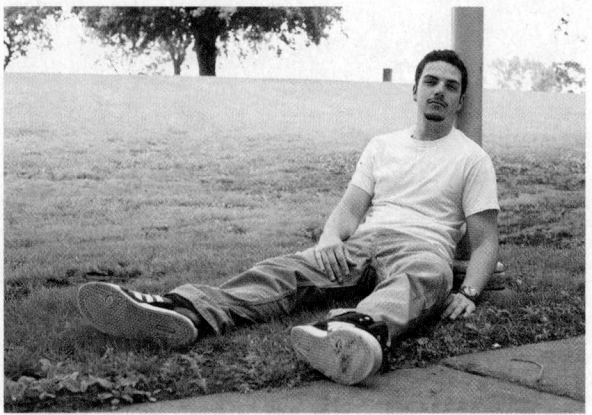

**FIGURE 18-7** Some patients with altered mental status may be unconscious; others may be alert but confused.
© Jones & Bartlett Learning.

## Causes of Altered Mental Status
### Hypoglycemia

The clinical picture of patients with altered mental status caused by hypoglycemia is complex. Because oxygen and glucose are needed for brain function, hypoglycemia can mimic conditions in the brain associated with stroke. In these cases, the patient may have hemiparesis similar to that seen with a stroke. The principal difference is that a patient who has experienced a stroke may be alert and attempting to communicate normally, whereas a patient with hypoglycemia almost always has an altered or decreased level of consciousness (**FIGURE 18-8**).

Patients with hypoglycemia commonly, but not always, take medications that lower their blood glucose level. Thus, if the patient appears to have signs and symptoms of stroke and altered mental status, report your findings to medical control and treat the patient accordingly. Remember, patients with a decreased level of consciousness should not be given anything by mouth.

Patients with hypoglycemia may also experience seizures, and you may arrive at the scene to find a patient in a postictal state: confused and disoriented or unresponsive. The mental status of a patient who has had a typical seizure is likely to improve soon after the seizure stops. In a patient with hypoglycemia, however, mental status is not likely to improve, even after several minutes. Consider the possibility of hypoglycemia in a patient who has had a seizure, especially if the patient has a history of diabetes.

Likewise, consider hypoglycemia in a patient who has altered mental status after an injury such as a motor vehicle crash, even when there is the possibility of an accompanying head injury. As with any other patient, look for medical identification jewelry or medications that might confirm your suspicions.

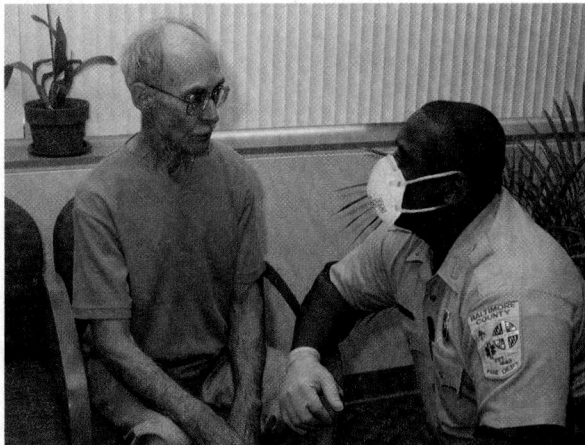

**FIGURE 18-8** During your assessment of a patient with an altered or decreased level of consciousness, consider the possibility of hypoglycemia.

© Jones & Bartlett Learning. Courtesy of MIEMSS.

> ### Words of Wisdom
>
> Always remember that altered mental status is a symptom, not a disease.

> ### Words of Wisdom
>
> A helpful mnemonic to use when reviewing the possible causes of altered mental status is AEIOU TIPS:
>
> A  Alcohol
> E  Epilepsy, endocrine, electrolytes
> I  Insulin
> O  Opiates and other drugs
> U  Uremia (kidney failure)
> T  Trauma, temperature
> I  Infection
> P  Poisoning, psychogenic causes
> S  Shock, stroke, seizure, syncope, space-occupying lesion, subarachnoid hemorrhage

### Delirium

**Delirium** is a symptom, not a disease. It presents as a new complaint, rather than a long-standing alteration in behavior. It is a temporary state that often has a physical or mental cause (eg, infection, changes in medications, hypoxia) and may be reversed with proper treatment.

Signs and symptoms include confusion and disorientation, disorganized thoughts, inattention, memory loss, striking changes in personality and affect, hallucinations, delusions, or a decreased level of consciousness. The patient may experience a rapid alteration between mental states such as lethargy and agitation. Symptoms of delirium may mimic intoxication, drug abuse, or severe psychological disorders such as schizophrenia. Delirium is discussed in detail in Chapter 36, *Geriatric Emergencies*.

## Other Causes of Altered Mental Status

Other causes of altered mental status include unrecognized head injury and severe alcohol intoxication. Considering other possibilities is important because a patient with altered mental status may be combative and may refuse treatment and transport. Be prepared for difficult patient encounters and follow local protocols for dealing with these situations.

In most cases, a patient who appears intoxicated is just that; however, you must consider other causes as well. A person with chronic alcoholism may have decreased liver function, blood clotting, and immune system abnormalities, causing a predisposition to intracranial bleeding, brain and bloodstream infections, and hypoglycemia.

Psychological disorders and medication complications are also possible causes of altered mental status. A person who appears to have a psychological disorder may also have an underlying medical condition.

Infections, particularly those involving the brain or bloodstream, are another possible cause of altered mental status. Infections in the brain and bloodstream are life threatening and require immediate medical attention. Patients may not demonstrate the typical signs of infection, such as fever, particularly if they are very young or very old or have an impaired immune system. Altered mental status may also be caused by a drug overdose or poisoning.

## Patient Assessment

### Scene Size-up

Your dispatcher may obtain a lot of information about your patient or very little. In some calls, the description of the patient's signs and symptoms will give you a fairly good idea of what the problem may be (the patient has slurred speech or one-sided paralysis). In other calls, the description may be vague (the patient has a headache). Dispatchers are frequently given information regarding a seizure by the caller. Even if the caller has never seen a seizure before, on the basis of the caller's description of the convulsions, the dispatcher will be able to convey this information to the responding crew.

Patients with altered mental status may exhibit a wide range of signs and symptoms and behaviors. The most significant difference between a patient

### Special Populations

Children can have altered mental status caused by strokes, seizures, high or low blood glucose levels, infection (eg, meningitis), poisoning, or tumors. Hemorrhagic strokes in children are usually caused by congenital defects in blood vessels, such as berry aneurysms. Ischemic strokes can be caused by disorders such as sickle cell anemia. Children who have sickle cell anemia are at a particularly high risk for ischemic stroke. Treat stroke and altered mental status in children the same way you do in adults.

Remember that in children, seizures can result from sudden high fevers. Also remember that although febrile seizures are generally well tolerated by children, you must provide transport to the hospital to assess for the underlying cause of the seizure. The possibility of a second seizure makes transport mandatory for an evaluation of life-threatening conditions and so that if other problems develop, the child is in the hospital and can receive immediate definitive care.

If you suspect that a patient with altered mental status has hypoglycemia and you are trained and approved to do so, use your glucometer to test the blood glucose level and treat the patient according to local protocols. The patient will require close monitoring, particularly of the airway, en route to the hospital.

with altered mental status and other emergencies is that a patient with altered mental status cannot reliably tell you what is wrong, and there may be more than one cause. Make an early determination whether the call is medical or trauma related because this will help determine the approach of care for the patient.

Do not be distracted by the seriousness of the situation or by frightened family members who want you to rush. Look first for threats to your safety, and follow standard precautions.

Consider the need for spinal motion restriction based on dispatch information and your assessment of the scene as you approach the patient. Many calls involving a neurologic emergency would benefit from ALS assistance if it is available. Call for additional resources early.

Look for clues to help you determine the nature of the illness. Special considerations for a patient with a suspected neurologic emergency include an evaluation of the patient's environment, assessing for any signs of potential trauma (mechanism of injury), indications of a medical condition, such as diabetic supplies, medical alert tags, and evidence of a seizure. Answers to the following questions may help you determine the nature of the illness: Did anyone witness what happened? When was the last time the patient appeared normal? Is the patient's bed or furniture in disarray? Most patients with a neurologic emergency display a change in their level of consciousness and their ability to interact with their environment and others.

## Primary Assessment

Your first priority is to look for and treat any life-threatening conditions. Perform a rapid exam. Patients become unresponsive or have an altered level of consciousness, especially from a neurologic cause, for many reasons. Use a sound approach to assessing whether the patient is bleeding and the patient's airway, breathing, and circulation to have significant effect on how well these systems respond to your care and treatment.

As you approach the patient, gather information from the scene (is this medical or trauma related?) and note the patient's body position and level of consciousness. This initial impression will help you determine the severity of the situation and help set the pace of your call. A patient lying on the ground in an unnatural position is more likely to have a potentially life-threatening condition than one sitting up in bed. In a call that indicates that a seizure is taking place, you should be able to tell whether the patient is still experiencing a seizure. Unless your arrival time is 1 minute or less, most seizures will be over by the time you arrive. If the seizure is still occurring, the potentially life-threatening condition of status epilepticus may be present. If the patient is in a postictal state, he or she may be unresponsive or starting to regain awareness of the surroundings. When you treat any patient with altered mental status, first determine the patient's level of consciousness. To assess the patient's level of consciousness, use the AVPU scale.

As with any other situation, focus on the patient's airway and breathing on arrival. Stroke affects how the body functions in many ways. Patients may have difficulty swallowing and are at risk for choking on their own saliva. Evaluate the airway of an unresponsive patient to make sure it is patent and will remain so (**FIGURE 18-9**). If the patient requires assistance maintaining an airway, consider

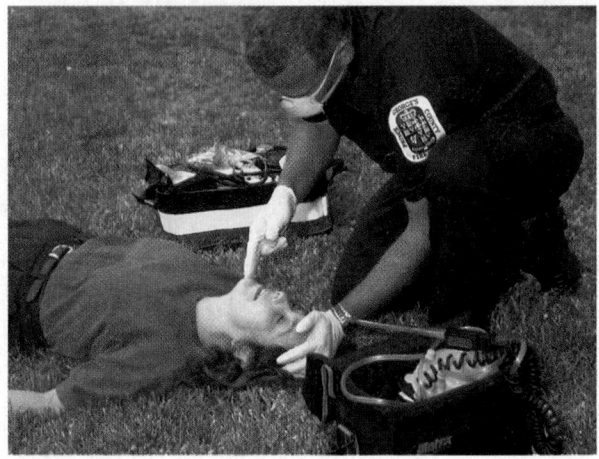

**FIGURE 18-9** Securing and maintaining the airway in a patient who is unconscious is extremely important. Have suction readily available in case the patient vomits.

© Jones & Bartlett Learning. Courtesy of MIEMSS.

an oropharyngeal or nasopharyngeal airway. Be prepared to provide suction, and position the patient to prevent aspiration. If you determine that the patient cannot protect his or her airway, place the patient in the recovery position to help prevent secretions from entering the airway.

A patient who has had or is experiencing a seizure may have been eating or chewing gum at the time of the seizure, so check for foreign body obstruction. Bystanders may have tried to put objects in the patient's mouth to keep the person from "swallowing the tongue," even though this practice is not advised, and swallowing the tongue is not something that is possible.

Assess the patient's breathing. Some causes of altered mental status, such as opioid overdose, can also cause alterations in the patient's breathing and ability to manage his or her own airway. Alternatively, hypoxia can be the cause of an altered mental state, as in the case of unconsciousness from airway obstruction. Seizures cause patients to use oxygen quickly, resulting in hypoxia. Again, in the immediate postictal state following a seizure, you should anticipate rapid, deep respirations and an accompanying fast heart rate as a result of the stress of the severe convulsions. However, the respirations and the heart rate should begin to slow to normal rates after several minutes.

If the patient's breathing is absent or inadequate, it is important to ventilate the patient at the appropriate rate with the proper volume. Deliver each breath over a period of about 1 second (with just enough volume to produce visible chest rise) at a rate of 10 to 12 breaths/min. Do not hyperventilate the patient; doing so may have several negative consequences. Hyperventilation overinflates the lungs, which can impair blood return to the right atrium and cause a decrease in blood pressure and cardiac output. Hyperventilation also increases the risks of regurgitation and aspiration. In addition to the risks already discussed, hyperventilation may cause severe injury in patients with intracerebral bleeding and increased ICP; it causes cerebral vasoconstriction, which shunts blood (and oxygen) away from the brain. This decrease in cerebral perfusion may cause further injury to the brain.

Circulation should be confirmed as normal or treated as necessary. Your assessment of the patient's circulation should begin with checking the pulse if the patient is unresponsive. If no pulse is found, immediately begin CPR, and attach an AED. If a pulse is present, determine whether the pulse is fast or slow, weak or strong. Oxygen administration is helpful for limiting the effects of hypoperfusion of the brain. Evaluate the patient quickly for external bleeding. A patient experiencing a stroke is unlikely to have sustained trauma; it is more likely in a patient who has had a seizure. Consider this possibility and assess appropriately.

Establish your priorities of care based on your assessment of the patient's level of consciousness and the XABCs. How the patient presents will guide you as to whether you stay at the scene for further assessment or proceed to immediate transport. If you suspect the patient is experiencing a stroke, provide rapid transport to an appropriate facility. Prompt treatment is a critical action to minimize the disability caused by an ischemic stroke.

### Street Smarts

When caring for patients with neurologic issues such as stroke or seizures, good interpersonal skills are crucial. Good communication, including active listening with everyone involved, makes potentially difficult calls easier. Compassion and empathy are important in managing these patients. The patient and family may regard the emotional support you provide as more valuable than the physical skills you perform. Your ability to reassure the patient and make him or her comfortable during assessment and transport is always beneficial.

### History Taking

If the patient is unresponsive, you will need to gather any history of the present illness from family or bystanders. If no one is around, quickly look for explanations for the altered mental status (eg, signs of trauma, medical alert tags, track marks resulting from intravenous drug injections, environmental

### YOU are the Provider

An engine crew arrives shortly before you load the patient onto the stretcher. Shortly after loading her into the ambulance, you reassess her and note that her condition has deteriorated. One of the engine crew EMTs accompanies you in the back of the ambulance, and you proceed to the hospital.

**Recording Time: 10 Minutes**

| | |
|---|---|
| **Level of consciousness** | Unconscious and unresponsive |
| **Respirations** | 6 breaths/min; snoring, irregular, and shallow |
| **Pulse** | 60 beats/min; bounding |
| **Skin** | Pink, warm, and dry |
| **Blood pressure** | 198/110 mm Hg |
| **SpO$_2$** | 78% (on ambient air) |

**8.** What should be your most immediate action?

**9.** What additional treatment does this patient require?

clues such as empty alcohol or medication containers).

To determine the chief complaint in a responsive patient, begin by asking the patient what happened. Look for signs and symptoms that may indicate a cause for the patient's altered mental status, such as a stroke (eg, hemiparalysis or one-sided weakness), or any evidence of a seizure (eg, incontinence, bitten tongue). Evaluate the patient's speech. Is the patient making sense? Is his or her speech slurred?

If you know that the patient has had a seizure and is now in a postictal state, you will not be able to obtain a history from the patient. Look for any obvious trauma or explanations as to why the patient may have had a seizure.

If the patient is responsive and breathing, obtain a SAMPLE history. Also speak with family or friends who may be able to explain the events leading up to the altered mental status (**FIGURE 18-10**), remembering that time is critically important in a neurologic emergency. Make a special effort to determine the exact time that the patient last appeared to be healthy. In the case of a patient experiencing a stroke, this information will help physicians decide whether it is safe to begin certain treatments that must be given within the first hours after the onset of stroke symptoms. You may be the only person with the opportunity to speak with bystanders to obtain this critical information. Many times, you will be able to find out only that the patient was healthy when he or she went to sleep the night before. In those cases, the time the

patient was last seen to be healthy was at bedtime, not when the patient awoke with symptoms. Collect or list all medications the patient has taken. When possible, determine allergies and the patient's last oral intake.

Although a patient who has had a stroke may appear to be unconscious and unable to speak, the patient may still be able to hear and understand what is taking place. Therefore, avoid making unnecessary or inappropriate remarks. Communicate with the patient by looking for indications that the patient may understand you, such as a glance, gaze, motion or pressure of the hand, effort to speak, or head nod. Reassure your patient that you understand that communication between the two of you may be difficult at this point but that you will provide him or her with continuous information as to what you and the other team members are doing. Establish effective communication to help you calm the patient and lessen the fear that accompanies an inability to communicate (**FIGURE 18-11**). Keep in mind that the patient has just experienced a potentially life-threatening event and that anxiety, frustration, and embarrassment may inhibit communication with you.

With patients who have had a seizure, your SAMPLE history should reveal if the patient has a history of seizures. If so, it is important to find

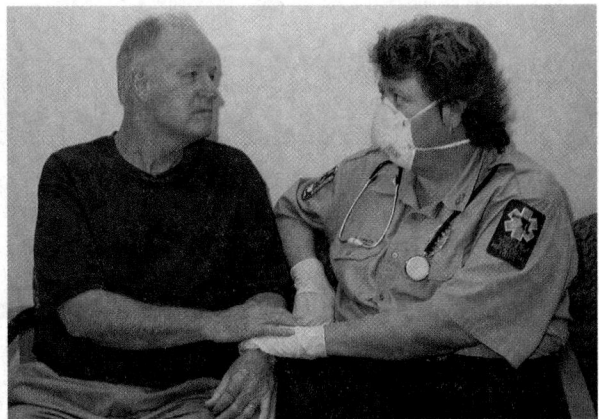

**FIGURE 18-11** Make a special effort to establish communication with a patient who may have had a stroke, seizure, or other neurologic emergency that impairs the patient's ability to communicate. Look for indications that the patient understands you, such as a glance, gaze, squeeze of the hand, efforts to speak, or nodding of the head.

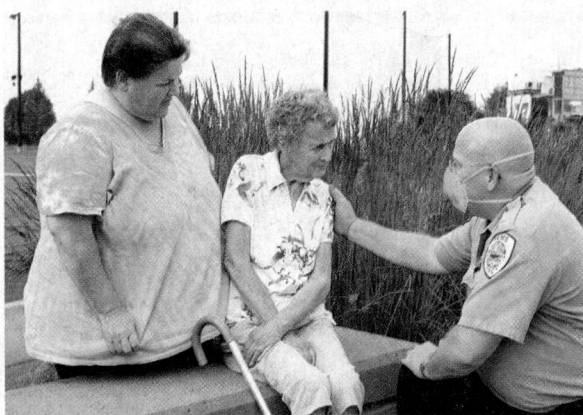

**FIGURE 18-10** Speak with family members or bystanders who may know what happened. They may be able to tell you when the patient last appeared healthy.

out how the patient's seizures typically occur and whether this episode differs in some way from previous episodes. Also, ask what medications the patient has been taking, and note medications used to treat a seizure disorder. You might find that the patient ran out of medication or stopped taking the medication for a time. A patient who has a history of seizures *and* diabetes may use up all the glucose in the body to fuel the seizure.

If a patient with no history of seizures suddenly has a seizure, a serious condition should be suspected, such as a brain tumor, intracranial bleeding, or serious infection. This part of the patient assessment process is the time to determine whether the patient takes medications that lower blood glucose, such as insulin or oral hypoglycemic agents. In other situations, you may want to inquire about illicit drug use or exposure to poisons.

## Words of Wisdom

When assessing a patient who might have had a stroke, it is important to pinpoint when the symptoms first started. Outcomes are best when treatment is initiated as soon after onset of symptoms as possible. In select cases, there may be a possibility of some recovery of neurologic function, with treatment initiated as long as 24 hours after onset of symptoms. During transport, notify the receiving hospital of when the patient's symptoms first began. When appropriate, this will allow hospitals to activate stroke alerts and be ready to immediately start treating these patients as soon as they enter the ED. Follow your local protocols.

## Secondary Assessment

Your assessment of the patient should continue with a secondary assessment of the entire body, paying particular attention to the system involved. If you suspect your patient is experiencing a stroke, then you should direct particular attention to the neurologic assessment. As always, your secondary assessment should include a complete set of vital signs using the monitoring devices you have available.

Patients with significant intracranial bleeding (hemorrhagic stroke) may have a great deal of pressure in the skull that is compressing the brain, thus slowing the pulse and causing respirations to be erratic. Blood pressure is usually high

to compensate for poor perfusion in the brain. Unequal pupil size and reactivity indicate significant bleeding and pressure on the brain. If the patient has altered mental status (regardless of the cause), check the blood glucose level if your local protocol allows. Most commonly, this is done using a portable blood glucose monitor (glucometer), similar to the one your patient may use at home. The portable blood glucose monitor measures the glucose level in whole blood, using capillary or venous samples. Chapter 10, *Patient Assessment*, discusses the use of a glucometer in more detail.

Evaluating vital signs is impossible during most active seizures, and this should not be your priority. In most cases, the vital signs of a patient in a postictal state will be within normal limits. Obtain pulse rate, rhythm, and quality; respiratory rate, rhythm, and quality; blood pressure; skin color, temperature, and condition; oxygen saturation; and pupil size and reactivity. Although paleness, or a decrease in blood flow, can be difficult to detect in dark-skinned people, it may be observed by examining mucous membranes inside the inner lower eyelid, the lips, and the nail beds. On general observation, the patient may appear ashen or gray.

It is recommended that the first blood pressure reading be taken manually, with a sphygmomanometer (blood pressure cuff) and a stethoscope. You may also use automated noninvasive methods to monitor blood pressure if they are available and you are approved to use them.

## Stroke Assessment

A stroke assessment tool should be part of your secondary assessment in patients with a neurologic disorder. Many EMS units use stroke scales to rapidly identify stroke in the field. Stroke scales evaluate balance, eyes, the face, arms, speech, and time of onset, which can be remembered with the mnemonic BE-FAST (**TABLE 18-3**). If the patient does not have a normal response to these evaluations, you should strongly suspect a stroke. Rapid transport to a designated stroke center is indicated.

In the prehospital setting, the most commonly used stroke screening tools are the Cincinnati Prehospital Stroke Scale (**TABLE 18-4**) and the Los Angeles Prehospital Stroke Screen (**TABLE 18-5**). Hospitals most commonly use the National Institutes of Health (NIH) Stroke Scale.

### TABLE 18-3 BE-FAST Stroke Assessment

| | |
|---|---|
| Balance | Did the patient experience a sudden loss of balance or inability to walk? |
| Eyes | Is there a change in vision? Loss of vision, double vision, or no side or top vision? |
| Facial droop (Ask patient to show teeth or smile.) | Does one side of the patient's face droop when he or she smiles? |
| Arm drift (Ask patient to close eyes and hold both arms out with palms up.) | Does the patient demonstrate weakness or the inability to move one of the arms? |
| Speech | Is the patient slurring words or using words that do not make sense? |
| Time | When did the symptoms first appear? Do not delay transport to an appropriate stroke facility. |

© Jones & Bartlett Learning.

### TABLE 18-4 Cincinnati Prehospital Stroke Scale

| Test | Normal Response | Abnormal Response |
|---|---|---|
| Facial droop (Ask patient to show teeth or smile.) | Both sides of face move equally well. | One side of face does not move as well as the other (droops). |
| Arm drift (Ask patient to close eyes and hold both arms out with palms up.) | Both arms move the same, or neither arm moves. (The latter response requires a retest because it may indicate the patient did not understand the instructions.) | One arm does not move, or one arm drifts down compared with the other side. |
| Speech (Ask patient to say, "You can't teach an old dog new tricks.") | Patient uses correct words with no slurring. | Patient slurs words, uses inappropriate words, or is unable to speak. |

© Jones & Bartlett Learning.

## Words of Wisdom

In the hospital, the most commonly used instrument for evaluating a possible stroke is the NIH Stroke Scale. This 11-step numerical grading system provides the hospital with very specific information about the patient's condition. In addition, the NIH evaluation can be repeated throughout the patient's hospital stay to compare numerical values related to any changes in condition. This scale is rarely used in the prehospital setting due to its complexity; however, some components of this evaluation can be assessed by asking the patient to identify common objects in the room and to read a short, written passage.

To test speech, ask the patient to repeat a simple sentence such as "You can't teach an old dog new tricks." If the patient does this correctly, you know the patient understands and can produce speech. If the patient cannot repeat the phrase, the problem may be with either understanding speech or producing it.

To test facial movement, ask the patient to smile, showing his or her teeth (or gums if the patient does not have teeth). Watch whether both sides of the face around the mouth move equally. If only one side is moving well, you know something is wrong with the control of the muscles on the other side.

**TABLE 18-5** Los Angeles Prehospital Stroke Screen

| Criterion | Yes | Unknown | No |
|---|---|---|---|
| **Interpretation: If all criteria 1–6 are marked yes, the probability of a stroke is 97%.** | | | |
| 1. Age older than 45 y | ☐ | ☐ | ☐ |
| 2. History of seizures or epilepsy absent | ☐ | ☐ | ☐ |
| 3. Symptoms <24 h | ☐ | ☐ | ☐ |
| 4. At baseline, patient is not wheelchair-bound or bedridden | ☐ | ☐ | ☐ |
| 5. Blood glucose between 60 and 400 mg/dL | ☐ | ☐ | ☐ |
| 6. Obvious asymmetry (right versus left) in any of the following three exam categories (must be unilateral): | ☐ | ☐ | ☐ |

| | Equal | Right Weak | Left Weak |
|---|---|---|---|
| Facial smile/grimace | ☐ | ☐ Droop | ☐ Droop |
| Grip | ☐ | ☐ Weak grip<br>☐ No grip | ☐ Weak grip<br>☐ No grip |
| Arm strength | ☐ | ☐ Drifts down<br>☐ Falls rapidly | ☐ Drifts down<br>☐ Falls rapidly |

© Jones & Bartlett Learning.

## YOU are the Provider

You continue treatment en route to the hospital. You reassess the patient and note that her condition has deteriorated further. Her pupils are unequal, and she exhibits decorticate posturing (flexion posturing to painful stimulus). You call in your report to the receiving facility, with an estimated time of arrival of 6 minutes.

| Recording Time: 17 Minutes | |
|---|---|
| **Level of consciousness** | Unconscious and unresponsive |
| **Respirations** | 10 breaths/min via bag-mask device |
| **Pulse** | 64 beats/min; bounding |
| **Skin** | Pink, warm, and dry |
| **Blood pressure** | 194/104 mm Hg |
| **Spo$_2$** | 98% (on oxygen via bag-mask device) |

You arrive at the hospital and transfer patient care to the emergency department (ED) staff. After further treatment in the ED, a computed tomography (CT) scan of the patient's brain was performed and revealed massive intracerebral hemorrhage. Despite aggressive treatment in the intensive care unit, the patient died the next day.

**10.** What do unequal pupils indicate?

**11.** On the basis of your last assessment, what is the patient's Glasgow Coma Scale (GCS) score?

To test arm movement, ask the patient to hold both arms in front of his or her body, palms up toward the sky, with eyes closed and without moving. During the next 10 seconds, watch the patient's hands. If you see one side drift down toward the ground, you know that side is affected. If both arms stay up and do not move, you know both sides of the brain are functioning. If both arms fall to the ground, you have not really identified any problems. Perhaps the patient did not understand your instructions. Perform the arm test again, but this time move the patient's arms into position yourself.

In addition, a newer scoring system called the 3-Item Stroke Severity Scale, sometimes called the LAG scale, looks specifically at three items—*l*evel of consciousness, *a*rm drift (motor function), and *g*aze. This system may be used to assess the likelihood your patient is experiencing a stroke. Each item is scored from 0 to 2, with zero (0) being normal and two (2) being a severe abnormality (**TABLE 18-6**). Data show that a score of 5 or 6 indicates a high probability the patient is experiencing a stroke. Become familiar with what is used in your local protocol.

Recently it has been determined that large vessel occlusion (LVO) strokes, which are a subtype of ischemic stroke, can be fairly reliably identified by EMS. These strokes, caused by an occlusion of a large blood vessel in the brain, respond well to fibrinolytics or mechanical thrombectomy but require rapid identification to provide the best results. The Los Angeles Motor Scale (LAMS), which is based on the Los Angeles Prehospital Stroke Screen, was developed to identify LVO strokes faster and more accurately to guide EMS to the best transport destination for the patient. The LAMS gives points for facial droop (absent = 0, present = 1), arm drift (absent = 0, slow drift = 1, rapid fall = 2), and grip strength (normal = 0, weak grip = 1, no grip = 2). A score of 4 or more is a strong indication of an LVO stroke and indicates consideration of transport to a comprehensive stroke center, if available.

You should calculate the GCS score (**TABLE 18-7**) for all patients with altered mental status (stroke, TIA, seizure of unknown cause).

## Reassessment

The reassessment should focus on reassessing the XABCs, vital signs, and interventions provided so far. Patients who are experiencing a stroke may lose their airway, or their breathing may stop without warning. Multiple interventions may be necessary. The effectiveness of airway adjuncts, positive pressure ventilations, and other treatments can be determined only with immediate and continuous observation after providing the intervention. If an intervention is not working, try something else.

You have already established baseline vital signs during your assessment, as well as a GCS score. Now is the time to compare that baseline information with updated information. Any changes may indicate if treatments are effective. Watch carefully for changes in pulse, blood pressure, respirations, and GCS scores.

**TABLE 18-6** 3-Item Stroke Severity Scale (LAG)

| Item | Criteria | Score |
|---|---|---|
| Level of consciousness | Normal | 0 |
| | Mild dysfunction | 1 |
| | Severe dysfunction (unconscious) | 2 |
| Arm drift (hemiparesis) | Normal function | 0 |
| | Mild dysfunction | 1 |
| | Severe dysfunction (flaccid) | 2 |
| Gaze | Normal gaze (follows pen/finger to left and right sides) | 0 |
| | Mild dysfunction | 1 |
| | Severe dysfunction (fixed gaze) | 2 |
| **Score (total)** | | **>4 indicates stroke is likely** |

| TABLE 18-7 Glasgow Coma Scale[a] | | | | | |
|---|---|---|---|---|---|
| **Eye Opening** | | **Best Verbal Response** | | **Best Motor Response** | |
| Spontaneous | 4 | Oriented conversation | 5 | Obeys commands | 6 |
| In response to sound | 3 | Confused conversation | 4 | Localizes pressure | 5 |
| In response to pressure | 2 | Inappropriate words | 3 | Withdraws from pressure | 4 |
| None | 1 | Incomprehensible sounds | 2 | Abnormal flexion | 3 |
| | | None | 1 | Abnormal extension | 2 |
| | | | | None | 1 |

[a]Some systems use a "Not testable (NT)" score for any element that cannot be tested. Eye opening cannot be tested in a patient whose eyes are closed due to a local factor, such as swelling; verbal response cannot be tested in a patient who has a preexisting factor interfering with communication, such as mutism; and motor response cannot be tested in a patient who has preexisting paralysis or other limiting factor.

Score: 13–15 may indicate mild dysfunction, although 15 is the score a person without neurologic disabilities would receive.

Score: 9–12 may indicate moderate dysfunction.

Score: 8 or less indicatives severe dysfunction.

© Jones & Bartlett Learning.

## Words of Wisdom

The following is key information to document for a patient who may have had a stroke:

- Time of onset of the signs and symptoms
- Score on the GCS
- Results of a stroke assessment tool (Cincinnati, Los Angeles, LAG, or BE-FAST)
- Changes noted on reassessment

Establishing the time of onset is critical information because it helps determine whether the patient is a candidate for treatment with blood clot-dissolving drugs or clot-retrieval therapy. If the person who last saw the person well cannot come to the hospital, ask for his or her phone number to give to hospital personnel.

Notify the receiving facility of your patient's chief complaint and your assessment findings. Your local protocol will tell you if the designated stroke centers in your call area want you to call in a stroke alert for patients you have assessed and suspect to be experiencing a stroke. This will alert the stroke team members at the hospital and give them time to assemble their resources to be ready to treat the patient without delay. Report the time the patient last appeared to be healthy, the findings of your neurologic examination, and the time you anticipate arriving at the hospital.

A key piece of information to document is the time of onset of the patient's signs and symptoms. If the diagnosis is an ischemic stroke, time of onset of the signs and symptoms is critical information in determining whether the patient is a candidate for clot-retrieval or for blood clot-dissolving drugs. It is also important to document your findings from your stroke scale and the GCS score, along with any changes you found in your reassessment. Document airway management and interventions performed, including the position in which the patient was placed.

For patients who have had a seizure, give a description of the seizure activity, if known. Include bystanders' comments if they witnessed the seizure. Document the onset and duration of the seizure. Did the patient mention noticing an aura? Record any evidence of trauma and interventions performed. Document whether this is the patient's first seizure or whether the patient has a history of seizures. If the patient has a history of seizure activity, determine how often the seizures occur and if there is any history of status epilepticus. Document your interventions and record the time the intervention was performed, the patient's response to the intervention, and the findings of continued reassessments.

## Emergency Medical Care

A patient experiencing stroke, seizure, hypoglycemia, or hypoxia typically shows relatively easily identifiable signs or symptoms, and treatment options are readily available. With other neurologic emergencies, the cause of the patient's symptoms will not always be obvious, and more time and diagnostic testing may be needed at the hospital to determine the cause. This may make it difficult for you to provide definitive treatment in the field. Most of your interventions will be based on your assessment findings. For example, if the blood glucose level is low, you may give oral glucose according to your local protocol; if a patient is unresponsive, you may need to position him or her in the recovery position to protect the airway. Remember, never give anything orally to a patient with altered mental status or to a patient who is unable to swallow normally, as this may result in aspiration. Your best treatment in these situations is to perform a thorough assessment and maintain the XABCs.

In most patients suspected of experiencing stroke, the physicians in the ED will need to determine whether there is bleeding in the brain. If there is no bleeding, the patient may be a candidate for blood clot-dissolving medication that may help brain cells survive. However, if bleeding is present this medication will increase the bleeding, with disastrous consequences. The only reliable way to tell whether there is bleeding in the brain is with a special type of imaging test called a CT scan of the head. Blood is usually easy for the physician to see on the CT scan.

Some EMS systems designate specific hospitals, typically accredited stroke centers, to receive patients who may be experiencing a stroke. These institutions have CT technicians, radiologists, and neurosurgeons on duty 24 hours per day. Most hospitals that are not accredited stroke centers have only one CT scanner and may not have CT technicians available 24 hours per day. It is important that you recognize the signs and symptoms of a stroke and notify the hospital staff as early as possible if you have a stroke alert patient. If the ED staff knows you are transporting a possible stroke patient, they can call in the technician if needed or may be able to free up the CT scanner so it is immediately available. Keep in mind that most treatments for stroke must be started as soon as possible after the onset of the event (**TABLE 18-8**). A limited number of treatments are available that are effective if started more than 3 hours after the stroke begins. Even if 3 hours has passed, prompt action on your part is essential. It is important to notify the hospital regarding the last time the patient was known to be well (without the current signs and symptoms of stroke).

| **TABLE 18-8** Tips on Patient Care |
| --- |
| • Patients who experience a TIA may exhibit most of the same signs and symptoms as patients who are experiencing a stroke. These signs and symptoms may last from minutes up to 24 hours. Therefore, the signs of stroke that you note on arrival may gradually disappear. Patients who appear to have experienced a TIA should be transported for further evaluation. |
| • Place the patient's affected or paralyzed extremity in a secure and safe position during patient movement and transport. |
| • Some patients who have had a stroke may be unable to communicate, but they can often understand what is being said around them. Be aware of this possibility. |
| • New therapies for stroke are available but must be used as soon as possible after the start of symptoms. Minimize time on the scene, and notify the receiving hospital as soon as possible. |

Abbreviation: TIA, transient ischemic attack

© Jones & Bartlett Learning.

In most situations, patients who have had a seizure require definitive evaluation and treatment in the hospital. Unless the patient has a well-established history of seizures and is completely alert and oriented, supplemental oxygen is strongly advised, to provide extra oxygen.

Seizures are usually short-lived. Most seizures will not require a significant amount of intervention on your part because the seizure will have ended by the time you arrive. For patients who are experiencing a seizure, protect them from harm, maintain a clear airway by suctioning as necessary, and administer oxygen as quickly as possible. If head or neck trauma is suspected, provide spinal motion restriction. In the case of recurrent seizures, protect the

### Words of Wisdom

Use the same process as with all other patients in determining whether an adequate airway is present and whether the patient is able to sufficiently maintain that airway on his or her own. Do not assume that a patient who has had a seizure is in need of an airway adjunct. Conversely, do not assume that a patient who has had a seizure has an airway that is intact. Conduct a thorough assessment, and then decide.

patient from further injury, and manage the airway once the seizure ceases.

For patients who continue to have a seizure, as in status epilepticus, suction the airway, provide positive-pressure ventilations (bag-mask ventilations), and transport quickly to the hospital. If you have the option to rendezvous with ALS, you should do so. ALS providers have medications that can stop a prolonged seizure.

In all cases, show patience and tolerance because many of the patients are likely to be confused and occasionally frightened after a seizure. Many patients who experience seizures are frustrated with their condition and may refuse transport. Kindness and professional behavior are required to help convince the patient that transport is necessary for definitive care.

## Headache

As discussed earlier, most headaches are harmless and do not require emergency medical care. However, be concerned if the patient complains of a sudden-onset, severe headache or a sudden headache that has associated symptoms. Headaches with fever, seizures, or altered mental status, or following head trauma, are potentially life threatening. Complete a thorough patient assessment, and transport the patient to the hospital.

## Migraine

Treatment of a migraine headache is supportive; however, always assess the patient for other signs and symptoms that might indicate a more serious condition. Applying high-flow oxygen, if tolerated, may help ease the patient's condition. When possible, provide a darkened and quiet environment because patients with migraines are sensitive to light and sound. Do not use lights and siren during transport.

## Stroke

Management of a patient experiencing a stroke in the field is based on supporting the XABCs and providing rapid transport to a stroke center. Depending on the location of the stroke in the brain and the signs and symptoms, the patient may require manual airway positioning. Patients may have difficulty swallowing and controlling their own secretions; therefore, use suction as needed. Provide oxygen to maintain an $SpO_2$ level of at least 94%, and monitor the patient's oxygen saturation with a pulse oximeter. Routine use of oxygen therapy in a stroke patient is not recommended if the patient clearly demonstrates no evidence of respiratory distress and has no signs of hypoxia. If there is any doubt, however, err on the side of providing oxygen therapy as the

### Special Populations

The brain gradually deteriorates and shrinks as a part of the normal aging process. These processes increase the risk of brain injury from minor forces because the brain can more readily impact the inside of the skull as a result of the increased space and because the veins that connect the brain to the dura are stretched. A reduced brain mass may also reduce the patient's mental status and capacity. A smaller brain can impair memory function. A geriatric patient with lapses in short-term memory may often ask the same or similar questions repeatedly.

When you are called to care for a geriatric patient with altered mental status, consider the possibility of a stroke or TIA. At the scene of a motor vehicle crash involving an older driver, consider a stroke or TIA as a possible cause in the crash. Be alert for altered mental status and unusual pupil responses (eg, constricted pupils in dim light, unequal pupils).

Take special note of complaints of a headache. Although geriatric patients get tension headaches, they are far less common in the older population. Consider any headache as potentially serious.

As with the general population, older people can experience seizures. Remember, seizures are not necessarily caused by epilepsy. Consider and assess for the possibility of a drug overdose, stroke, head injury, or central nervous system infection. Status epilepticus in a geriatric patient increases the risk of hypoxia, irregular heart rhythm, hypotension, elevated body temperature, low blood glucose level, and, if the patient vomits, aspiration.

Remember, geriatric patients are at a higher risk for central nervous system illnesses and injuries, including brain injury, TIA, stroke, and seizures. Do not be surprised to find a serious head injury from what you might consider a simple bump on the head.

adverse consequences of hypoxemia, even for brief periods of time, are far greater than the potential consequences of excess oxygenation for brief periods. If the patient's extremities are paralyzed, they will require protection from injury because the patient may not be able to feel the extremities or move them out of harm's way as you prepare and move the patient for transport. Continuously talk to the patient and inform him or her of what is going on. Many patients who are experiencing or who have had a stroke understand what is going on, even though they may not be able to communicate with you. The patient may not be able to speak, or when he or she does, inappropriate words may come out. Regardless, the patient will be scared. Reassure the patient and provide emotional support throughout the call.

Fibrinolytic therapy (blood clot-dissolving drugs) and methods to mechanically remove the blood clot may reverse stroke symptoms and even stop the stroke if implemented within 3 hours (drugs) or 6 hours (mechanical methods) of the onset of symptoms. In some very specific situations at centers with advanced capabilities, the window during which mechanical removal of the clot may offer benefit may extend as long as 24 hours after the time at which the patient was last seen to be normal. These therapies may not work for all patients, and they cannot be given to patients with bleeding-type (hemorrhagic) strokes. Comprehensive stroke centers are able to offer advanced stroke care, and in some cases, may be able to provide thrombolytic therapy even well after the 3- to 6-hour window and in some specific cases up to 24 hours after onset of symptoms. Because hospital personnel will ultimately make these treatment decisions, you should proceed under the assumption that the affected area of the brain may be saved. The sooner the treatment is begun, the better the prognosis for the patient.

Spend as little time on scene as possible. Remember, stroke is an emergency and "time is brain." Treatment may be available for the patient at the hospital, and rapid transport is essential to maximize the possibility of recovery. If you have a choice of hospitals, transport the patient to one that is a designated stroke center.

## Seizure

Most patients who have had a seizure will be in a postictal state on your arrival. For those patients who are still experiencing a seizure, continue to assess and treat the XABCs. It may be necessary to maintain the patient's airway with manual airway positioning. Use suction to clear the airway of any excessive secretions or vomitus. Oxygen is rapidly consumed by the body during seizure activity, so you should monitor the patient's oxygen saturation level with a pulse oximeter and apply high-flow oxygen. Administer oxygen even if you are unable to get an accurate pulse oximetry reading because of the patient's seizure activity, shaking, or tremors. Provide emotional support.

It is difficult to safely prepare a patient for transport when he or she is experiencing a seizure. Assess the patient for trauma and restrict movement of the spine if indicated. Protect the patient from his or her surroundings. Never attempt to tightly restrain a patient experiencing a seizure. Injury could result from tonic-clonic movement. Use soft materials for padding, and move any objects out of the way that may harm your patient.

Not every patient who has had a seizure wants to be transported, but it is usually in the best interest of the patient to be evaluated by a physician in the ED after a seizure. Your goal is to encourage the patient to be seen by a physician. Should the patient refuse transport, be prepared to discuss the situation with the hospital staff on the radio before releasing the patient. Ask yourself the following questions if a patient who was in a postictal state now refuses transport:

- Is the patient fully awake and completely oriented after the seizure (GCS score of 15)?
- Does your assessment reveal no indication of trauma or complications from the seizure?
- Has the patient ever had a seizure before?
- Was this seizure the "usual" seizure in every way (length, activity, recovery)?
- Is the patient currently being treated with medications and receiving regular evaluations by a physician?

If the answer to all of these questions is "yes," you can consider agreeing to a patient's refusal for transport if the patient can be released to a responsible person and monitored. If the patient responds "no" to any questions, strongly encourage the patient to be transported and evaluated. In all cases where a patient refuses transport after a seizure, contact online medical direction and ask them to speak directly to the patient to encourage the patient to consent to transport. Follow your local protocols for patients who refuse care and transport.

## Altered Mental Status

The signs and symptoms of altered mental status can vary widely, from simple confusion to coma.

No matter what the cause, consider altered mental status to be an emergency that requires immediate attention, even when it appears that it may be caused by alcohol intoxication or minor head trauma. Determine the cause (mechanism of injury versus nature of illness) and provide spinal motion restriction as indicated, airway and ventilation support, and transport to the appropriate facility.

## YOU are the Provider SUMMARY

**1. On the basis of the dispatch information, what type of seizure is the patient most likely experiencing?**

Given the patient's age (58 years), loss of consciousness, and the fact that the convulsions affect her extremities and torso, the patient is most likely experiencing a generalized seizure.

**2. What are some common causes of seizures in this patient's age group?**

Seizures in adults are typically caused by one of three underlying problems: epilepsy, structural brain problems (eg, brain tumors and abscesses, head trauma, and stroke), or metabolic derangements (eg, cerebral hypoxia, hypoglycemia, hyperglycemia, drug overdose, poisoning, and alcohol withdrawal). Febrile seizures are rare in adults. However, fever may be a sign of brain infection, such as meningitis.

**3. What additional questions should you ask the patient's sister?**

Important questions that need to be answered include: What was the patient doing and what position was she in when the seizure began? Was she sitting or standing? Did she hit her head during the episode? Did the patient describe experiencing an aura? If neither the patient nor her sister mentioned an aura, this does not rule out a seizure.

How long did the seizure last? Was the patient unconscious following the seizure? If so, how long was she unconscious? Does the patient have a history of recent head trauma?

**4. What prehospital assessments can you perform to determine the possible cause of the patient's seizure?**

In most cases, you will not be able to determine the underlying cause of the patient's seizure in the prehospital setting. However, there are a few

assessments you can perform and observations you can make that may increase your index of suspicion. Assess the patient's blood glucose level to rule out hypoglycemia as the cause of her seizure. If the patient is conscious and able to follow commands, test the patient by using a stroke scale, such as the Cincinnati Prehospital Stroke Scale. You should also assess and closely monitor the patient's vital signs and assess her neurologic status using the GCS. In some cases, taking a temperature may help to uncover an underlying illness that may have caused the seizure.

**5. What treatment is indicated at this point?**

Unless the patient was injured during the seizure or you have identified an underlying cause of her seizure that can be treated in the prehospital setting (eg, hypoglycemia), additional treatment is mainly supportive. Maintaining a patent airway and ensuring adequate oxygenation and ventilation are your highest priorities. Provide a calm, quiet environment; reassure and reorient the patient as needed; avoid any loud or bright stimuli, which may cause another seizure; and safely transport her to the hospital. Continuously monitor the patient's XABCs, level of consciousness, and vital signs.

**6. What is your field impression of this patient? Why?**

From the sister's description, it is likely that the patient experienced a seizure. Her present signs and symptoms (confusion; sudden, severe headache; nausea; left-sided weakness) and medical history (poorly controlled hypertension) should make you suspicious that she is experiencing a hemorrhagic stroke, which likely caused the seizure. Signs of increased ICP include changes in level of consciousness, nausea and vomiting, seizures, and high blood pressure, among others; your patient is experiencing all of these signs and symptoms.

**7. On the basis of your field impression, you should monitor the patient for which additional signs and symptoms?**

Your patient's present condition suggests that a cerebral artery may be leaking and blood is slowly accumulating in her brain tissue, which will increase ICP. As the ICP increases, the patient's level of consciousness will deteriorate; therefore, the level of consciousness is the single most important assessment parameter to monitor. Because of the cerebral ischemia caused by the increased ICP, the patient may experience another seizure. As the ICP increases further, the blood pressure often increases and the heart rate commonly decreases. Pressure on the brainstem may cause irregular and ineffective breathing; therefore, assisted ventilation may be necessary. It is important to continuously monitor your patient's condition and be prepared to intervene if her condition deteriorates.

**8. What should be your most immediate action?**

Airway, airway, airway! Snoring respirations indicate partial obstruction of the airway by the tongue. Performing the head tilt–chin lift maneuver is the quickest way to correct the problem. The patient is now unconscious and unresponsive; insert an airway adjunct (eg, oral or nasal airway) to help maintain airway patency. Patients with increased ICP often vomit; remain alert to this possibility and have suction readily available. Regardless of the situation, you must ensure the patient's airway remains patent at all times. No airway, no patient—it's that simple!

**9. What additional treatment does this patient require?**

After establishing a patent airway, your next priority is to assist the patient's breathing. A slow (6 breaths/min), irregular breathing pattern will not support adequate minute volume; therefore, deliver positive pressure ventilation with a bag-mask device. Be sure to attach 100% oxygen to the ventilation device you will be using.

**10. What do unequal pupils indicate?**

In the context of a traumatic brain injury or hemorrhagic stroke, unequal pupil size is an ominous sign. It indicates significantly increased ICP and compression of one of the oculomotor nerves (the nerves that control the pupillary response). The affected pupil is often fully dilated (blown) and does not constrict when a light source is shone into it.

**11. On the basis of your last assessment, what is the patient's GCS score?**

The GCS assesses three parameters: eye opening, verbal response, and motor response. Your last assessment revealed that the patient was unconscious and unresponsive (she did not open her eyes and was unresponsive to all stimuli) and was exhibiting decorticate (abnormal flexion) posturing. Therefore, she would receive a GCS score of 5, based on the following values (the numeric value for each component is in bold):

*Eye opening:*
- Spontaneous: 4
- Responsive to speech: 3
- Responsive to pain: 2
- **None: 1**

*Best verbal response:*
- Oriented conversation: 5
- Confused conversation: 4
- Inappropriate words: 3
- Incomprehensible sounds: 2
- **None: 1**

*Best motor response:*
- Obeys commands: 6
- Localizes pain: 5
- Withdraws from pain: 4
- **Abnormal flexion: 3**
- Abnormal extension: 2
- None: 1

## YOU are the Provider SUMMARY *continued*

### EMS Patient Care Report (PCR)

| Date: 3-16-20 | Incident No.: 140109 | Nature of Call: Seizure | | Location: 106 Scottie Drive | |
|---|---|---|---|---|---|
| Dispatched: 1823 | En Route: 1823 | At Scene: 1827 | Transport: 1839 | At Hospital: 1852 | In Service: 1909 |

### Patient Information

**Age:** 58
**Sex:** F
**Weight (in kg [lb]):** 77 kg (170 lb)

**Allergies:** Penicillin, codeine
**Medications:** Benazepril, hydrochlorothiazide, metformin
**Past Medical History:** Hypertension, heart disease, type 2 diabetes mellitus
**Chief Complaint:** Severe headache and nausea

### Vital Signs

| Time: 1831 | BP: 200/112 | Pulse: 100 | Respirations: 14 | Spo₂: 96% (on ambient air) |
|---|---|---|---|---|
| Time: 1837 | BP: 198/110 | Pulse: 60 | Respirations: 6 | Spo₂: 78% (on ambient air) |
| Time: 1844 | BP: 194/104 | Pulse: 64 | Respirations: 10 | Spo₂: 98% (on oxygen via bag mask) |

### EMS Treatment (circle all that apply)

| Oxygen @ _15_ L/min via:<br><br>NC    NRM    (Bag mask) | Assisted Ventilation | Airway Adjunct:<br>(Oral airway) | CPR |
|---|---|---|---|
| Defibrillation | Bleeding Control | Bandaging | Splinting | Other: (Blood glucose level) |

### Narrative

Dispatched for a 58-year-old woman experiencing a seizure.

Chief Complaint: Severe headache and nausea

History: Per the patient's sister, they were having a conversation when the patient suddenly grabbed both sides of her head and then began "shaking all over." Her sister indicated she caught her sister before the patient fell to the ground. The patient had never experienced a seizure before today. The patient reports nausea and the "worst headache of my life." Past medical history significant for hypertension, heart disease, and type 2 diabetes mellitus. Medications listed above; patient admits to being noncompliant with her prescribed medications.

Assessment: On arrival at the scene, found the patient lying supine on her living room floor with a pillow under her head. She was conscious but confused. She was also having trouble moving her left-sided extremities. There was no trauma noted.

Treatment (Rx): Administered oxygen and obtained vital signs. Blood glucose level was assessed and noted to be 97 mg/dL. Further assessment did not reveal any trauma or urinary incontinence. Engine 60 arrived at the scene to provide assistance. Patient was lifted onto ambulance stretcher using a soft stretcher for movement to the ambulance. As the patient was being loaded into the ambulance, she became unconscious and unresponsive. Reassessment revealed that her respirations were slow, irregular, and shallow. Inserted an oral airway and began assisting the patient's ventilations with a bag-mask device and high-flow oxygen.

Transport: Requested assistance from Engine 60 EMT and began transport to the hospital. Continued to assist the patient's ventilations en route and reassessed her vital signs. Shortly before arriving at the hospital, reassessed the patient and noted her pupils were unequal and she began exhibiting decorticate posturing. Assigned a Glasgow Coma Scale score of 5. Quickly transferred patient to the ED staff and gave verbal report to attending physician, Emerson.

**End of report**

# Prep Kit

## Ready for Review

- The cerebrum, the largest part of the brain, is divided into right and left cerebral hemispheres, each controlling the opposite side of the body.
- Different areas of the brain control different functions. The front part of the cerebrum controls emotion and thought; the middle part controls touch and movement; and the back part of the cerebrum is involved with vision. In most people, speech is controlled on the left side of the brain, near the middle of the cerebrum.
- Many different disorders can cause brain or other neurologic symptoms. In general, if the problem is primarily in the brain, only part of the brain will be affected. If the problem is in the heart or lungs, the whole brain will be affected.
- Stroke is a common brain disorder and is a leading cause of death and disability. The most effective treatment is time dependent. Seizures and altered mental status are also common brain disorders. You must learn to recognize the signs and symptoms of each condition.
- Other causes of neurologic dysfunction include coma, infections, and tumors.
- Strokes occur when part of the blood flow to the brain is suddenly cut off; within minutes, brain cells begin to die.
- Signs and symptoms of stroke include receptive and/or expressive aphasia, slurred speech, muscle weakness or numbness on one side of the body, facial droop, and sometimes high blood pressure.
- Always perform at least three neurologic tests on a patient you suspect of experiencing a stroke: testing speech, facial movement, and arm movement. Also observe the patient's balance and ask about vision changes.
- In a TIA, normal body processes break up the blood clot, restoring blood flow and ending symptoms in less than 24 hours. However, patients experiencing a TIA are at a higher risk for a repeat episode or a more serious stroke.
- Because current treatments for stroke must be administered within 3 hours of the onset of symptoms to be most effective, provide prompt transport.
- Always notify the hospital as soon as possible that you are bringing in a patient with a possible stroke, so staff can prepare to test and treat the patient without delay.
- Generalized seizures are usually characterized by unconsciousness and generalized jerking or twitching of all or part of the body.
- Most generalized seizures last less than 5 minutes and are followed by a postictal state in which the patient may be unresponsive and have labored breathing or hemiparesis. The patient may have a loss of bladder or bowel control as a result of the seizure.
- Recognize the signs and symptoms of seizures so you can provide the ED staff with information as you transport the patient.
- Altered mental status is a common neurologic disorder that you will encounter as an EMT. Signs and symptoms vary widely, as do the causes for this condition.
- Among the most common causes of altered mental status are hypoglycemia, intoxication, drug overdose, and poisoning.
- Do not always assume intoxication when you assess a patient with an altered mental status; hypoglycemia is just as likely a cause. Prompt transport with close monitoring of vital signs en route is indicated.

## Vital Vocabulary

**altered mental status** Any deviation from alert and oriented to person, place, time, and event, or any deviation from a patient's normal baseline mental status.

**aneurysm** A swelling or enlargement of a part of an artery, resulting from weakening of the arterial wall.

**aphasia** The inability to understand and/or produce speech.

**atherosclerosis** A disorder in which cholesterol and calcium build up inside the walls of blood vessels, eventually leading to partial or complete blockage of blood flow.

**aura** A sensation experienced before a seizure; serves as a warning sign that a seizure is about to occur.

**cerebrovascular accident (CVA)** An interruption of blood flow to the brain that results in the loss of brain function; also called a stroke.

**coma** A state of profound unconsciousness from which the patient cannot be roused.

**delirium** A temporary change in mental status characterized by disorganized thoughts, inattention, memory loss, disorientation, striking changes in personality and affect, hallucinations, delusions, or a decreased level of consciousness.

**dysarthria** Slurred speech.

**embolus** A blood clot or other substance in the circulatory system that travels to a blood vessel where it causes a blockage of blood flow.

**epilepsy** A disorder in which abnormal electrical discharges occur in the brain, causing seizures and possible loss of consciousness.

**febrile seizures** Seizures that result from sudden high fevers; most often seen in children.

**focal seizure** A seizure affecting a limited portion of the brain.

**generalized seizure** A seizure characterized by severe twitching of all of the body's muscles that may last several minutes or more; formerly known as a grand mal seizure.

**hemiparesis** Weakness on one side of the body.

**hemorrhagic stroke** A type of stroke that occurs as a result of bleeding inside the brain.

**hyperglycemia** An abnormally high blood glucose level.

**hypoglycemia** An abnormally low blood glucose level.

**incontinence** Loss of bowel and/or bladder control; may be the result of a generalized seizure.

**ischemia** A lack of oxygen that deprives tissues of necessary nutrients, resulting from partial or complete blockage of blood flow; potentially reversible because permanent injury has not yet occurred.

**ischemic stroke** A type of stroke that occurs when blood flow to a particular part of the brain is cut off by a blockage (eg, a blood clot) inside a blood vessel.

**postictal state** The period following a seizure that lasts 5 to 30 minutes; characterized by labored respirations and some degree of altered mental status.

**seizure** A neurologic episode caused by a surge of electrical activity in the brain; can be a convulsion characterized by generalized, uncoordinated muscular activity, and can be associated with loss of consciousness.

**status epilepticus** A condition in which seizures recur every few minutes or last longer than 30 minutes.

**stroke** An interruption of blood flow to the brain that results in the loss of brain function; also called a cerebrovascular accident (CVA).

**syncope** A fainting spell or transient loss of consciousness.

**thrombosis** A blood clot, either in the arterial or venous system. When the clot occurs in a cerebral artery, it may result in the interruption of cerebral blood flow and subsequent stroke.

**transient ischemic attack (TIA)** A disorder of the brain in which brain cells temporarily stop functioning because of insufficient oxygen, causing strokelike symptoms that resolve completely within 24 hours of onset.

# References

1. American Stroke Association. Hemorrhagic strokes (bleeds). American Stroke Association website. http://www.strokeassociation.org/STROKEORG/AboutStroke/TypesofStroke/Hemorrhag icBleeds/Hemorrhagic-Strokes-Bleeds_UCM_310940_Article.jsp. Updated March 28, 2016. Accessed April 13, 2020.

2. American Stroke Association. Stroke treatment. American Stroke Association website. http://www.strokeassociation.org/STROKEORG/AboutStroke/Treatment/StrokeTreatments_UCM_310892_Article.jsp. Updated 2020. Accessed April 13, 2020.

3. American Stroke Association. Types of stroke. American Stroke Association website. http://www.strokeassociation.org/STROKEORG/AboutStroke/TypesofStroke/Types-ofStroke_UCM_308531_SubHomePage.jsp. Accessed April 13, 2020.

4. Aroor S, Singh R, Goldstein LB. BE-FAST (balance, eyes, face, arm, speech, time): reducing the proportion of strokes missed using the FAST mnemonic. *Stroke* 2017;48(2):479–481.

5. Fisher RS, Cross H, D'Souza C, et al.; ILAE Commission for Classification and Terminology. Instruction manual for the ILAE 2017 Operational Classification of Seizure Types. *Epilepsia* 2017;58(4):531–542.

6. National Association of State EMS Officials. *National EMS Scope of Practice Model 2019.* Washington, DC: National Highway Traffic Safety Administration; February 2019. Report No. DOT HS 812-666. https://www.ems.gov/pdf/National_EMS_Scope_of_Practice_Model_2019.pdf.

7. National Center for Chronic Disease Prevention and Health Promotion, Division of Population Health. Epilepsy data and statistics. Centers for Disease Control and Prevention website. https://www.cdc.gov/epilepsy/data/index.html. Reviewed January 25, 2019. Accessed April 13, 2020.

8. *National Emergency Medical Services Education Standards.* U.S. Department of Transportation. National Highway Traffic Safety Administration. DOT HS 811 077A. January 2009. www.ems.gov/pdf/811077a.pdf. Accessed April 13, 2020.

9. *National Emergency Medical Services Education Standards. Emergency Medical Technician Instructional Guidelines.* U.S. Department of Transportation. National Highway Traffic Safety Administration. DOT HS 811 077C. January 2009. www.ems.gov/pdf/811077c.pdf. Accessed April 13, 2020.

10. National Institutes of Health, National Institute of Neurological Disorders and Stroke. NIH stroke scale. Know Stroke website. https://www.stroke.nih.gov/documents/NIH_Stroke_Scale_508C.pdf. Accessed April 13, 2020.

11. On behalf of the American Heart Association Stroke Council: Powers WJ, Rabinstein AA, Ackerson T, et al. 2018 guidelines for the early management of patients with acute ischemic strok: a guideline for healthcare professionals. From the American Heart Association/American Stroke Association. *Stroke.* 2018; 49 (3):e46–e99.

12. Ozkurt B, Cinar O, Cevik E, et al. Efficacy of high-flow oxygen therapy in all types of headache: a prospective, randomized, placebo-controlled trial. *Am J Emerg Med* 2012;30(9):1760–1764.

13. Shafer PO, Sirven JI. Epilepsy statistics. Epilepsy Foundation website. http://www.epilepsy.com/learn/epilepsy-statistics. Published October 2013. Accessed April 13, 2020.

14. Theodore WH, Spencer SS, Wiebe S, et al. Epilepsy in North America: a report prepared under the auspices of the Global Campaign Against Epilepsy, the International Bureau for Epilepsy, the International League Against Epilepsy, and the World Health Organization. *Epilepsia* 2006;47(10):1700–1722.

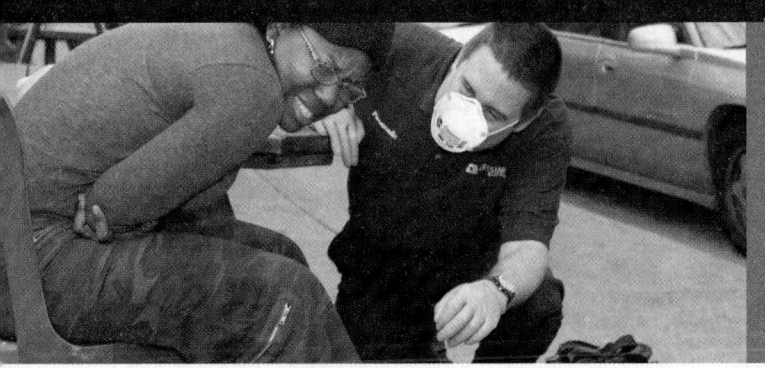

# Chapter 19

# Gastrointestinal and Urologic Emergencies

## NATIONAL EMS EDUCATION STANDARD COMPETENCIES

### Medicine

Applies fundamental knowledge to provide basic emergency care and transportation based on assessment findings for an acutely ill patient.

### Abdominal and Gastrointestinal Disorders

Anatomy, presentations, and management of shock associated with abdominal emergencies

- Gastrointestinal bleeding (pp 756–757, 762, 766–768, 770–772)

Anatomy, physiology, pathophysiology, assessment, and management of

- Acute and chronic gastrointestinal hemorrhage (pp 756–757, 762, 766–770)

- Peritonitis (pp 756–760, 766–771)
- Ulcerative diseases (pp 756–757, 760–761, 766–770)

### Genitourinary/Renal

- Blood pressure assessment in hemodialysis patients (pp 771–772)

Anatomy, physiology, pathophysiology, assessment, and management of

- Complications related to
  - Renal dialysis (pp 764–765, 771–772)
  - Urinary catheter management (not insertion) (p 772)
- Kidney stones (pp 764–765)

## KNOWLEDGE OBJECTIVES

1. Describe the basic anatomy and physiology of the gastrointestinal, genital, and urinary systems. (pp 756–758)

2. Define the term *acute abdomen*. (p 758)

3. Describe pathologic conditions of the gastrointestinal, genital, and urinary systems. (pp 758–766)

4. Explain the concept of referred pain. (p 760)

5. Describe other organ systems that can cause abdominal pain. (pp 759–760, 765–766)

6. Identify the signs and symptoms, and common causes, of an acute abdomen. (pp 760–764)

7. Describe the assessment and management of acute and chronic gastrointestinal hemorrhage, peritonitis, and ulcerative diseases. (pp 758–764, 766–770 )

8. List the most common abdominal emergencies, along with the most common locations of direct and referred pain. (p 760)

9. Describe the assessment of a patient with a gastrointestinal or urologic emergency. (pp 766–770)

10. Describe the procedures to follow in managing the patient with shock associated with abdominal emergencies. (pp 767–768)

11. Describe the emergency medical care of the patient with a gastrointestinal or urologic emergency. (pp 770–772)

12. Explain the principles of kidney dialysis. (pp 771–772)

## SKILLS OBJECTIVE

1. Demonstrate the assessment of a patient's abdomen. (pp 769–770)

# Introduction

Abdominal pain is a common complaint; however, the cause is often difficult to identify, even for a physician. As an EMT, you do not need to determine the exact cause of acute abdominal pain, but it is helpful for you to understand the pathophysiology and the signs and symptoms of common illnesses. You need to be able to recognize a life-threatening problem and act swiftly in response. Remember, the patient is in pain and is probably anxious, requiring your skills of rapid assessment and emotional support.

# Anatomy and Physiology

The abdominal cavity contains solid and hollow organs that make up the gastrointestinal (GI), genital, and urinary systems (**FIGURE 19-1**). Solid organs include the liver, spleen, pancreas, kidneys, and ovaries (in women). Technically, organs such as the kidneys, ovaries, and the pancreas are retroperitoneal (behind the peritoneum). However, because they lie next to the peritoneum, they can cause abdominal pain. An injury to a solid organ can cause shock and bleeding because of the amount of blood vessels contained in the organ.

Hollow organs include the gallbladder, stomach, small intestine, large intestine, and urinary bladder. If there is a perforation of these hollow organs, the contents of the organ will leak and contaminate the abdominal cavity.

## The GI System

The GI system is responsible for the digestion process. Digestion begins when food is put into the mouth and chewed; the salivary glands secrete saliva and begin to break down the food, then it is swallowed. The food travels down the esophagus to

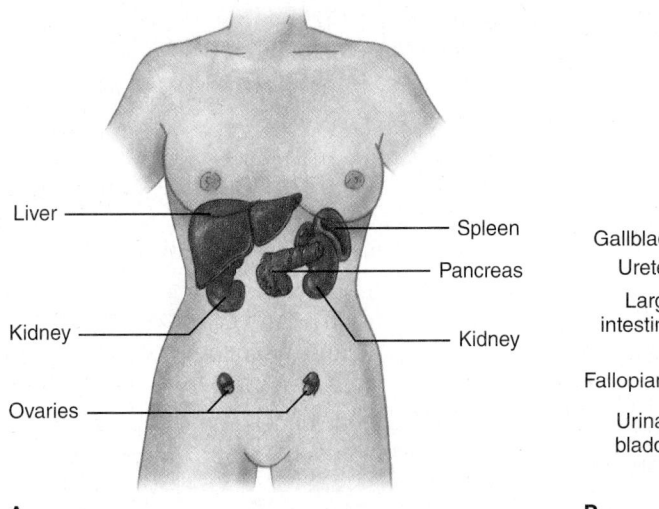

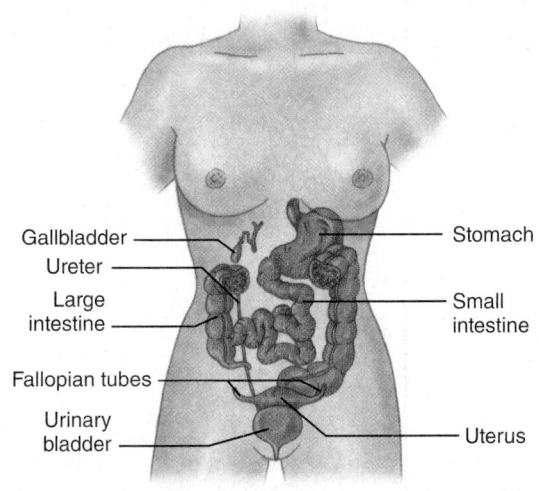

**A**                                                                 **B**

**FIGURE 19-1** The solid and hollow organs of the abdomen. **A.** Solid organs include the liver, spleen, pancreas, kidneys, and ovaries (in women). **B.** Hollow organs include the gallbladder, stomach, small intestine, large intestine, and bladder.

**A, B:** © Jones & Bartlett Learning.

the stomach. The stomach is the main organ of the digestive system. Absorption of nutrients occurs at various places along the digestive tract. Sugars start to be absorbed while in the mouth. Most digestion takes place in the stomach, where gastric juices break down food to a form that can be used by the body.

The liver secretes bile, which aids in the digestion of fats. The liver also filters toxic substances produced by digestion, creates glucose stores, and produces substances necessary for blood clotting and immune function. The gallbladder is a hollow pouch located beneath the liver that acts as a reservoir for bile.

From the stomach, food travels down into the small intestine, which consists of three sections: the duodenum, jejunum, and ileum. The duodenum is where digestive juices from the pancreas and liver mix together. The pancreas secretes juice containing enzymes that help break down starches, fats, and proteins. Amylase, which breaks down starches into sugar, is one enzyme the pancreas secretes. The pancreas also produces bicarbonate, insulin, and glucagon. Bicarbonate neutralizes the stomach acid in the duodenum. Insulin and glucagon help regulate the levels of glucose in the bloodstream.

The jejunum, the next part of the small intestine, plays a major role in the absorption of digestive products. The jejunum comprises a large amount of the surface area of the small intestine and does much of the work. The final part of the small intestine is the ileum, which absorbs the remaining nutrients. It also absorbs bile acids so they can be returned to the liver for future use and vitamin $B_{12}$ for making nerve cells and red blood cells.

The food that was not broken down and used as nutrients then moves into the colon, or large intestine, as waste products. A wavelike contraction of smooth muscle called peristalsis moves the waste matter through the intestines. Water is absorbed and stool is formed. The stool passes through the rectum to the anus, where it is defecated.

## Additional Abdominal Organs

The spleen is also located in the abdomen but has no digestive system function. The spleen is part of the lymphatic system and plays a significant role in relation to red blood cells and the immune system. It assists in the filtration of blood, removes old red blood cells, recycles iron, and serves as a blood reservoir. The spleen also produces antibodies to help the body fight off disease and infection.

## The Genital System

The abdominal space also holds the male and female reproductive organs. The male reproductive system consists of the testicles, epididymis, vasa deferentia, seminal vesicles, prostate gland, and penis. The female reproductive system includes the ovaries, fallopian tubes, uterus, cervix, and vagina.

## The Urinary System

The urinary system controls the discharge of certain waste materials filtered from the blood by the kidneys. In the urinary system, the kidneys are solid organs, and the ureters, bladder, and urethra are hollow organs (**FIGURE 19-2**). Ordinarily, the urinary and genital systems are referred to jointly as the genitourinary system because they share many organs. One system can directly affect the other. For example, if the prostate gland in the male genital system enlarges, then the urethra will narrow, impairing emptying of the bladder, and eventually leading to urinary retention.

## YOU are the Provider

At 0320 hours, you and your partner are dispatched to 1500 East River Road, Apartment 5, for a 79-year-old man with abdominal pain. You proceed to the scene, which is approximately 8 miles from your station. The weather is clear, the temperature is 67°F (19.4°C), and the traffic is light.

**1.** What is the definition of an acute abdomen?

**2.** What is your role as an EMT in treating a patient with abdominal pain?

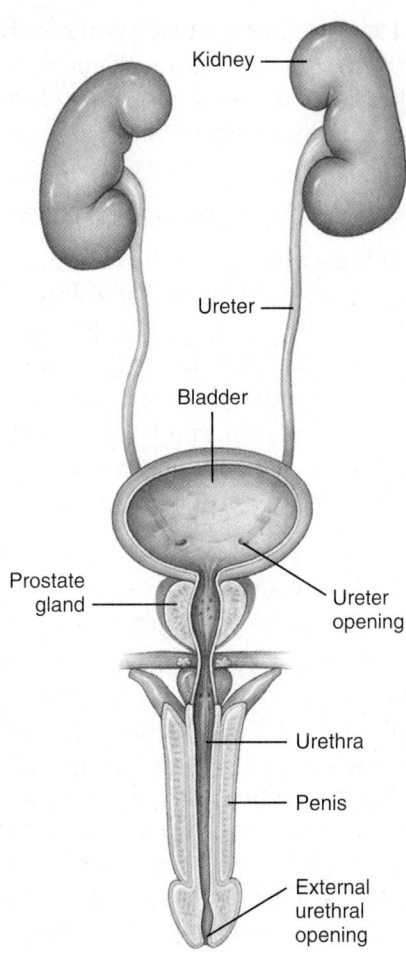

Kidney

Ureter

Bladder

Prostate gland

Ureter opening

Urethra

Penis

External urethral opening

**FIGURE 19-2** The urinary system lies in the retroperitoneal space behind the organs of the digestive system. The urinary system in men and women includes the kidneys, ureters, bladder, and urethra. This diagram shows the male urinary system.

© Jones & Bartlett Learning.

The body contains two kidneys, one on each side, which lie on the posterior muscular wall of the abdomen behind the peritoneum in the retroperitoneal space. The kidneys play an important role in the regulation of the acid–base balance (the body's pH) and blood pressure. Blood pressure regulation is associated with the kidney's ability to remove sodium chloride from the body. Kidney disease is a common cause of secondary hypertension. Most patients with chronic kidney disease also have hypertension. The kidneys also rid the body of toxic wastes and control the body's balance of fluid and electrolytes. Blood flow in the kidneys is high. Nearly 20% of the output of blood from the heart passes through the kidneys each minute. Large

vessels attach the kidneys directly to the aorta and the inferior vena cava. Waste products and water are constantly filtered from the blood to form urine. The kidneys continuously concentrate this filtered urine by reabsorbing the water as it passes through a system of specialized tubes within them. The tubes eventually unite to form the renal pelvis, a cone-shaped collecting area that connects the ureter and the kidney.

A ureter passes from the renal pelvis of each kidney along the surface of the posterior abdominal wall behind the peritoneum to drain into the urinary bladder. The ureters are small (0.2 inch in diameter), hollow, muscular tubes. Peristalsis occurs in these tubes to move the urine to the bladder.

The urinary bladder is located immediately behind the pubic symphysis in the pelvic cavity and is composed of smooth muscle with a specialized lining membrane. The two ureters enter posteriorly at its base on either side. The bladder empties to the outside of the body through the urethra. In the male body, the urethra passes from the anterior base of the bladder through the penis. In the female body, the urethra opens at the front of the vagina. The healthy adult forms 1.5 to 2 liters of urine every day, which is held in the urinary bladder until it is excreted through the urethra.

## Pathophysiology

The abdominal cavity is lined by a membrane called the **peritoneum**. The peritoneum also covers the organs of the abdomen. The parietal peritoneum lines the walls of the abdominal cavity, and the visceral peritoneum covers the organs themselves. The abdominal space normally contains a small amount of peritoneal fluid to bathe and lubricate the organs in the abdominal cavity. Any foreign material, such as blood, pus, bile, pancreatic juice, or amniotic fluid, can cause irritation of the peritoneum, called **peritonitis.**

**Acute abdomen** is a medical term referring to the sudden onset of abdominal pain, often associated with severe, progressive problems that require medical attention. Peritonitis is usually associated with the acute abdomen, which, if not treated, can be fatal.

Peritonitis typically causes **ileus**, or paralysis of the muscular contractions that normally propel material through the intestine. The retained gas and feces, in turn, cause abdominal distention. Distention usually begins after the muscular contractions cease. In the presence of such paralysis, nothing that is eaten can pass normally out of the stomach or through the bowel. In this situation, the only way the stomach can empty itself is by **emesis**, or vomiting. For this reason, peritonitis is frequently associated with nausea and vomiting. These symptoms do not point to a particular cause because they can accompany almost every type of gastrointestinal disease or injury.

Peritonitis can be associated with a loss of body fluid into the abdominal cavity. The loss of fluid usually results from abnormal shifts of fluid from the bloodstream into body tissues. This fluid shift decreases the volume of circulating blood and may lead to decreased blood pressure or even shock. The patient may have normal vital signs or, if the peritonitis has progressed further, the patient may present with tachycardia and hypotension. When peritonitis is accompanied by hemorrhage, the signs of shock are much more apparent.

Fever may or may not be present, depending on the cause of the peritonitis. Patients with **diverticulitis** (inflammation in small pockets at weak areas in the muscle walls of the intestines)

or **cholecystitis** (inflammation of the gallbladder) may have a substantial elevation in body temperature. However, patients with acute appendicitis may have a temperature within normal limits until the appendix ruptures and contaminates the peritoneal cavity.

## Abdominal Pain

Abdominal pain can have different qualities because two different types of nerves supply the peritoneum. The nerves from the spinal cord that supply the skin of the abdomen also supply the parietal peritoneum. Therefore, the parietal peritoneum and the skin of the abdomen can perceive much the same sensations: pain, touch, pressure, heat, and cold. These sensory nerves can easily identify and localize a point of irritation. In contrast, the visceral peritoneum is supplied by the autonomic nervous system. These nerves are far less able to localize sensation. This means that your patient will not be able to describe exactly where the pain is located. The visceral peritoneum is stimulated when distention or contraction of the hollow abdominal organs activates the stretch receptors. Patients sometimes describe it as a deep pain. Other painful sensations

## YOU are the Provider

When you arrive at the scene and enter the patient's residence, you find him lying on the couch on his side in obvious discomfort. He is notably diaphoretic (sweaty) and pale and is in obvious severe discomfort. You introduce yourself and begin your assessment.

### Recording Time: 0 Minutes

| | |
|---|---|
| **Appearance** | Lying on his side, diaphoretic, in obvious pain |
| **Level of consciousness** | Conscious and alert; restless |
| **Airway** | Open; clear of secretions or foreign bodies |
| **Breathing** | Rapid, shallow respirations; Sao$_2$ unobtainable |
| **Circulation** | Radial pulse weak and rapid; skin is pale and diaphoretic |

Your partner administers oxygen at 15 L/min via a nonrebreathing mask as you continue your assessment. The patient tells you that his abdominal pain began suddenly and has been severe from the onset. He describes the pain as like something being pulled apart and indicates that it radiates to his lower back. He denies nausea, vomiting, fever, or any other symptoms. As you examine his abdomen, your partner prepares to take his vital signs.

**3.** What is the proper technique of assessing a patient's abdomen? What should you assess for?

**4.** What is the difference between radiating pain and referred pain?

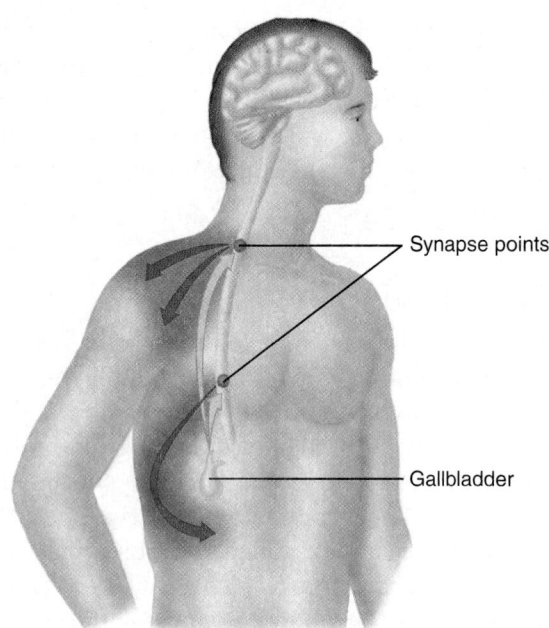

**FIGURE 19-3** Acute cholecystitis causes referred pain in the right shoulder as well as in the abdomen.

© Jones & Bartlett Learning.

**TABLE 19-1** Common Abdominal Conditions

| Condition | Localization of Pain |
|---|---|
| Appendicitis | Right lower quadrant (direct); around navel (referred); rebound tenderness (pain felt on the rebound after palpation) |
| Cholecystitis | Right upper quadrant (direct); right shoulder (referred) |
| Ulcer | Upper midabdomen or upper part of back |
| Diverticulitis | Left lower quadrant |
| Abdominal aortic aneurysm (ruptured or dissecting) | Low part of back and lower quadrants |
| Cystitis (inflammation of the bladder) | Lower midabdomen (retropubic) |
| Kidney infection | Costovertebral angle |
| Kidney stone | Right or left flank, radiating to genitalia |
| Pancreatitis | Upper abdomen (both quadrants); back |
| Hernia | Anywhere in the abdominal area |
| Peritonitis | Diffuse abdominal pain area |

© Jones & Bartlett Learning.

that occur because of an irritated visceral peritoneum may be perceived at a distant point on the surface of the body, such as the back or shoulder. This phenomenon is called **referred pain**.

Referred pain is the result of connections between the body's two separate nervous systems. The nerves connecting the somatic nervous system and autonomic nervous system cause the stimulation of the autonomic nerves to be perceived as stimulation of the spinal sensory nerves. For example, acute cholecystitis may cause pain in the right shoulder because the autonomic nerves serving the gallbladder lie near the spinal cord at the same anatomic level as the spinal sensory nerves that supply the skin of the shoulder (**FIGURE 19-3**).

The most common abdominal emergencies, with the most common locations of direct and referred pain, are listed in **TABLE 19-1**.

## Causes of Acute Abdomen

Almost any problem with an abdominal organ can cause an acute abdomen. Some of the more common causes are discussed here. It is rare for the EMT to determine the exact cause. Because the visceral peritoneum is usually irritated first, early abdominal pain tends to be vague and poorly localized.

As the parietal peritoneum becomes irritated, pain becomes more severe and may be more specifically located.

## Ulcers

The stomach and duodenum are subjected to high levels of acidity. To prevent damage to these organs, protective layers of mucus line both organs. In peptic ulcer disease (PUD), the protective layer is eroded, allowing the acid to eat into the organ itself over the course of weeks, months, or even years.

Most peptic ulcers are the result of infection of the stomach with *Helicobacter pylori* bacteria. Another major cause is chronic use of nonsteroidal anti-inflammatory drugs (NSAIDs), such as aspirin and ibuprofen. Alcohol and smoking can also affect the severity of PUD by increasing gastric acidity.

PUD affects men and women equally, but tends to occur more often in the older population. As people age, the immune system's ability to fight infection decreases, making infection more likely. The geriatric population, in general, also uses NSAIDs more frequently for arthritis and other musculoskeletal conditions.

Patients with PUD experience a classic sequence of burning or gnawing pain in the stomach that subsides or diminishes immediately after eating and then reemerges 2 to 3 hours later. The pain usually presents in the upper abdomen, but sometimes may be found below the sternum. With some patients, the pain occurs immediately after eating. Nausea, vomiting, belching, and heartburn are common symptoms. If the erosion is severe, gastric bleeding can occur, resulting in **hematemesis** (vomiting blood) and **melena** (black, tarry stools containing blood).

Some ulcers will heal without medical intervention, but often complications can occur from bleeding or perforation (a hole through the wall of the stomach). More serious ulcerative conditions can cause severe peritonitis and an acute abdomen.

## Gallstones

The gallbladder is a storage pouch for digestive juices and waste from the liver. Gallstones can form and block the outlet of the gallbladder, causing pain. Sometimes the blockage will pass, but if not, it can lead to severe inflammation of the gallbladder, called cholecystitis. This is a condition in which the wall of the gallbladder becomes inflamed. In severe cases, the gallbladder may rupture, causing inflammation to spread and irritating surrounding structures such as the diaphragm and bowel.

This condition presents as a constant, severe pain in the right upper or midabdominal region and may refer to the right upper back, shoulder area, or flank. The pain may steadily increase for hours or may come and go. Cholecystitis commonly produces symptoms about 30 minutes after a particularly fatty meal and usually at night. Other symptoms include general GI distress such as nausea and vomiting, indigestion, bloating, gas, and belching. People at a higher risk for the development of cholecystitis include women, older adults,

obese people, and people of Scandinavian, Native American, and Hispanic descent. Older adults may present without the normal symptoms described here. Localized tenderness may be the only finding.

## Pancreatitis

The pancreas forms digestive juices and is also the source of insulin and glucagon. Inflammation of the pancreas is called **pancreatitis**. Pancreatitis can be caused by an obstructing gallstone, alcohol abuse, and other diseases. Severe pain may present in the upper left and right quadrants and may often radiate to the back. In addition, the patient may report that the pain is worse after eating. Other signs and symptoms accompanying the pain are nausea and vomiting, abdominal distention, and tenderness. Complications such as sepsis or hemorrhage can occur, in which case assessment may also reveal fever or tachycardia.

## Appendicitis

The appendix is a small recess in the large intestine. Inflammation or infection in the appendix is called **appendicitis**, and it is a frequent cause of acute abdomen. This inflammation can eventually cause the tissues to die and/or rupture, causing an abscess, peritonitis, or shock. Initially, the pain caused by appendicitis is generalized, dull, and diffuse and may center in the umbilical area. The pain later localizes to the right lower quadrant of the abdomen. Appendicitis can also cause referred pain. The patient may also report nausea and vomiting, anorexia (lack of appetite for food), fever, and chills. A classic symptom of appendicitis is rebound tenderness. Rebound tenderness is a result of peritoneal irritation. This can be assessed by pressing down gently and firmly on the abdomen and then quickly releasing the pressure. The patient will feel pain when the pressure is released. Women with appendicitis who are also pregnant may not exhibit this symptom. Because the pain often increases when the patient's legs are straightened, the patient is often more comfortable in the fetal position.

## Gastrointestinal Hemorrhage

Bleeding within the GI tract is a symptom of another disease, not a disease itself. GI hemorrhage can be acute, which may be shorter term and more severe, or chronic, which may be of longer duration and less severe. All complaints of bleeding should be considered serious.

A GI hemorrhage can occur in the upper or lower GI tract. Bleeding in the upper GI tract occurs from the esophagus to the upper small intestine. In the esophagus, problems might include esophagitis, esophageal varices secondary to liver failure, or a Mallory-Weiss tear, which results from excessive retching or vomiting. Hematemesis is frequently seen in patients with upper GI bleeding. The blood is either bright red or has the appearance of coffee grounds, depending on where in the GI tract it originated and how briskly it is occurring. In upper GI bleeding, the bleeding often manifests as melena, or dark tarry stools, as a result of partial digestion of the blood.

Lower GI bleeding occurs between the upper part of the small intestine and the anus. Bowel inflammation, diverticulosis, diverticulitis, cancer, and hemorrhoids are common causes of bleeding in the lower GI tract. When bleeding originates in the lower GI tract, the stools are often bright red or maroon in color.

## Esophagitis

Esophagitis occurs when the lining of the esophagus becomes inflamed by infection or from the acids in the stomach (**gastroesophageal reflux disease [GERD]**). GERD is a condition in which the sphincter between the esophagus and the stomach opens, allowing stomach acid to move up into the esophagus. Also referred to as acid reflux disease, this condition can cause a burning sensation within the chest (heartburn). It is estimated that 60 million people in the United States have GERD. This is approximately 18% of the total population, making GERD extremely common. People diagnosed with

GERD may use antacids, proton pump inhibitors (eg, omeprazole [Prilosec], lansoprazole [Prevacid]), and H$_2$ blockers (eg, nizatidine [Axid], famotidine [Pepcid]) to treat their condition.

The patient with esophagitis may report pain with swallowing and feeling as if an object is stuck in his or her throat. Additional symptoms include heartburn, nausea, vomiting, and sores in the mouth. In the worst cases, bleeding can occur from the small capillary vessels within the esophageal lining or the main blood vessels.

## Esophageal Varices

Esophageal varices occur when the pressure within the blood vessels surrounding the esophagus increases, frequently as a result of liver failure. The esophageal blood vessels eventually drain their blood into the liver. If the liver becomes damaged and blood cannot flow through it easily, blood begins to back up into these portal vessels, dilating the vessels and causing the capillary network of the esophagus to begin leaking. If pressure continues to build, the vessel walls may fail, causing massive upper GI bleeding and, quickly afterward, hematemesis.

In industrialized countries, alcohol is the main cause of liver damage. Long-term alcohol consumption damages the interior of the liver (cirrhosis), leading to slower blood flow. In developing countries, viral hepatitis is the main cause of liver damage.

Presentation of esophageal varices takes two forms. Initially, the patient shows signs of liver disease—fatigue, weight loss, jaundice, anorexia, edema in the abdomen, abdominal pain, nausea, and vomiting. This gradual disease process takes months to years before the patient reaches a state of extreme discomfort.

By contrast, the rupture of the varices is far more sudden. The patient may report sudden-onset discomfort in the epigastric region or sternum. He or she may have severe difficulty swallowing, vomiting of bright red blood, hypotension, and signs of shock. If the bleeding is less dramatic, hematemesis and melena are likely. Regardless of the speed of bleeding, damage to these vessels can be life threatening. Spontaneous rupture is often life threatening and significant blood loss at the scene may be evident. Major ruptures can lead to death in a matter of minutes.

## Mallory-Weiss Tear

A Mallory-Weiss tear is a tear in the junction between the esophagus and the stomach, causing severe bleeding and potentially death. Primary risk factors include alcoholism and eating disorders.

Violent coughing or vomiting is the principal cause. In women, this syndrome may be associated with severe vomiting related to pregnancy. The extent of the bleeding can range from minor bleeding, resulting in little blood loss, to severe bleeding and extreme fluid loss. In extreme cases, patients may experience signs and symptoms of shock, upper abdominal pain, hematemesis, and melena.

## Gastroenteritis

Acute gastroenteritis comprises a family of conditions revolving around a central theme of infection combined with diarrhea, nausea, and vomiting. Bacterial and viral organisms can cause this condition. These organisms typically enter the body through contaminated food or water. Patients may begin to experience an upset stomach and diarrhea as soon as several hours or several days after contact with the contaminated matter. The disease can then run its course in 2 to 3 days or continue for several weeks.

Gastroenteritis may also be caused by noninfectious conditions such as adverse reactions to medications, exposure to certain toxins, or chemotherapy. The symptoms are similar regardless of the underlying cause.

Diarrhea is the principal symptom in both infectious and noninfectious gastroenteritis. Patients may experience large dumping-type diarrhea or frequent small liquid stools. The diarrhea may contain

### Safety Tips

Infection from the bacterium *Clostridium difficile* (commonly referred to as *C diff*) presents with GI symptoms such as diarrhea. You can spread *C difficile* to other patients if proper hand hygiene is not employed and proper decontamination is not performed after each call.

Transmission of *C difficile* occurs in susceptible patients by contact with surfaces contaminated with feces. The bacterium can occasionally be transmitted to patients by contact with the unwashed hands of health care providers. Infections with *C difficile* are generally related to use of antibiotics in patients who are being treated for other infections.

*C difficile* is not inactivated by alcohol-based hand products. Glove use, good handwashing technique, and cleaning of contaminated surfaces with a chlorine-based cleaning agent are important in preventing spread of this bacterium.

### YOU are the Provider

The patient's vital signs are obtained and recorded. Your assessment of his abdomen reveals that it is tender to palpation and that you are able to palpate a pulsatile mass. As your partner retrieves the stretcher from the ambulance, the patient tells you that he has high blood pressure, depression, and had his appendix removed 30 years ago. He says he takes Toprol and Diovan for high blood pressure. You note that he is becoming more restless and is still experiencing intense pain, which he describes as a 10 on a scale of 0 to 10 (10/10).

| Recording Time: 3 Minutes | |
|---|---|
| **Respirations** | 28 breaths/min; shallow |
| **Pulse** | 124 beats/min; regular |
| **Skin** | Pale, cool, and diaphoretic |
| **Blood pressure** | 98/60 mm Hg |
| **Oxygen saturation (Spo₂)** | 96% (on oxygen) |

**5.** What do the patient's vital signs indicate?

**6.** What do you suspect is the cause of the patient's abdominal pain?

blood and/or pus, and it may have a foul odor or be odorless. Abdominal cramping is frequently reported. Nausea, vomiting, fever, and anorexia are also present. If the diarrhea continues, dehydration will result. As the volume of fluid loss increases, the likelihood of shock increases.

## Diverticulitis

As the amount of fiber consumed as part of the diet decreases, the consistency of the normal stool becomes more solid. This hard stool requires more intestinal contractions, subsequently increasing pressure within the colon. In this environment, small defects within the colonic wall that would otherwise never pose a problem now fail, resulting in bulges in the wall. These small outcroppings eventually turn into pouches, called diverticula. Feces may become trapped within these pouches. When bacteria grow there, they cause localized inflammation and infection.

The most common cause of lower GI bleeding in the United States is diverticulosis. Bleeding from diverticulosis is usually bright red (as the blood products do not have time to be digested) and typically painless.

The main symptom of diverticulitis is abdominal pain, which tends to be localized to the left side of the lower abdomen. Classic signs of infection include fever, malaise, body aches, chills, nausea, and vomiting. Bleeding is rare with this condition. Because of the local infections of these pouches, scar tissue forms, causing the tissue to stick together. This narrows the diameter of the colon and results in constipation and bowel obstruction. In severe cases, these infected outcroppings may burst, causing perforation of the affected segment of colon. This may lead to peritonitis, severe infection, and if left untreated, septic shock.

## Hemorrhoids

Hemorrhoids are created by swelling and inflammation of the blood vessels surrounding the rectum. They are a common problem, with almost half the population having at least one hemorrhoid by age 50 years. Hemorrhoids may result from conditions that increase pressure on the rectum or irritation of the rectum. Pregnancy, straining at stool, and chronic constipation cause increased pressure. Diarrhea can cause irritation.

Hemorrhoids may be internal (high in the rectum, usually not visible, often painless, and often associated with bright red, brisk bleeding) or external (low in the rectum, often clearly visible, and painful).

Hemorrhoids present as bright red blood during defecation. This bleeding tends to be minimal and is easily controlled. Additionally, patients may experience itching and a small mass on the rectum. Typically, this mass is a clot formed in response to the mild bleeding.

## Urinary System

Issues in the urinary system can cause acute abdominal pain. Bladder inflammation, called **cystitis**, is common, especially in women. This condition is generally caused by a bacterial infection and can be referred to as a **urinary tract infection (UTI)**. A bladder infection can be painful. Patients with cystitis usually have midline lower abdominal pain. They may also report blood in the urine, an urgency and frequency in urination, and pressure and pain around the bladder. If the infection is severe, the urethra can become inflamed, causing urinary retention. When you are assessing a patient with cystitis, the patient may report tenderness when you are palpating the abdomen over the bladder (just above the pubic bone). Cystitis can become a serious health problem if the infection spreads to the kidneys.

## Kidneys

The kidneys play a major role in maintaining homeostasis, or keeping all body systems in balance. The kidneys preserve this balance by eliminating waste from the blood. When the kidneys fail, the patient loses the ability to excrete waste from the body, leading to a condition called **uremia**. This means that the waste product, urea, which is normally excreted into the urine, remains in the blood.

Chemicals may crystallize in the urine and form **kidney stones** (renal calculi). Kidney stones can grow over time, and if a stone passes into the ureter, it can cause a blockage. Pressure will build up behind the kidney stone and cause swelling in the kidney. Patients with a kidney stone blockage may initially report vague discomfort in the flank, but the pain can become quite intense and typically will radiate to the groin. These patients are often agitated and restless as they try to get into a comfortable position to relieve the pain. They may also report nausea and vomiting. The pain from kidney stones is often caused when the stone moves within the ureter. Stones cause blockage that prevent urine from passing, stretching and dilating the ureter behind the location of the stone, which is the source of the pain. In many cases, the stone will pass on its own, but in other cases it may have to be surgically removed (or broken up). A slight amount of blood in the urine (hematuria) before or after the stone passes may be present because of irritation of the ureter.

Kidney (renal) failure can be acute or chronic. Acute kidney injury (AKI) is a sudden (possibly over a period of days) decrease in function. It occurs from a variety of causes including hemorrhage, dehydration, trauma, shock, sepsis, heart failure, medications, drug abuse, and kidney stones. AKI very often can be reversed with prompt diagnosis and treatment.

Chronic kidney disease (CKD) is irreversible. It is progressive and develops over months and years. It is often caused by diabetes or hypertension. The kidney tissue shrinks and function diminishes. Eventually the patient requires dialysis or a kidney transplant to remove waste products from the bloodstream.

Patients with untreated CKD or patients with CKD who have missed scheduled dialysis may exhibit a wide variety of symptoms ranging from simply not feeling well to an altered level of consciousness. In later stages, seizures and coma are possible. Additional signs and symptoms include lethargy, nausea, headaches, cramps, and edema in the extremities and face because of fluid imbalances. Patients with CKD have a high incidence of heart disease and tend to bleed easily. There is an increased risk of heart failure and cardiac arrest in these patients.

## Female Reproductive Organs

Gynecologic problems are a common cause of acute abdominal pain. Always consider that a woman with lower quadrant abdominal pain and tenderness may have a problem related to her ovaries, fallopian tubes, or uterus. Chapter 24, *Gynecologic Emergencies*, covers gynecologic emergencies in depth.

## Other Organ Systems

The aorta lies immediately behind the peritoneum. In older people, the wall of the aorta sometimes develops weak areas that swell to form an abdominal aortic aneurysm (AAA). A pulsating mass may be felt in the abdomen, although this is a rare sign and is often hard to detect. Use extreme caution when trying to assess or detect this condition. The development of an aneurysm is rarely associated with symptoms because it occurs slowly, but if the aneurysm tears and ruptures, massive hemorrhage may occur, and the patient will present with signs of acute peritoneal irritation and hemorrhagic shock. The patient may also report radiation of severe pain to the back because the peritoneum can be stripped away from the wall of the main abdominal cavity by the hemorrhage. Back pain is a common symptom when an aneurysm has started to expand and the aortic linings begin to tear. Back pain that cannot be easily explained should be investigated closely in patients who are suspected of having an AAA. The patient may describe the pain as tearing, which is different than most other descriptions of abdominal pain. The association of acute abdominal signs and symptoms of shock requires prompt transportation. Because this is a fragile situation with a large, leaking artery, avoid unnecessary or vigorous palpation of the abdomen. If the patient develops signs of shock, avoid any actions that can cause a small tear to expand. At the EMT level, aggressive treatment for shock includes administering oxygen, covering the patient with a blanket, and providing rapid transport. Remember to handle the patient gently during transport.

A hernia is a protrusion of an organ or tissue through a hole or opening into a body cavity where it does not belong. Hernias can occur as a result of the following:

- A congenital defect, as around the umbilicus
- A surgical wound that has failed to heal properly
- A natural weakness in an area, such as in the groin

Hernias do not always produce a mass or lump that the patient will notice. At times, the mass will disappear back into the body cavity in which it belongs. In this case, the hernia is said to be reducible. If the mass cannot be pushed back within the body, it is said to be incarcerated.

A hernia that can gently be pushed back through the abdominal wall is reducible. Reducible hernias pose little risk to the patient; some people

## Special Populations

Geriatric patients are as susceptible to acute abdomen. However, the signs and symptoms in geriatric patients might be different than in younger patients. Because of altered pain sensation, geriatric patients with an acute abdomen may not feel any discomfort or may describe the discomfort as mild, even in severe conditions. Be mindful that older patients may not exhibit rigidity or guarding as would a younger adult.

Because the older patient has decreased body temperature regulation and response, the patient with an acute abdomen, including peritonitis, may have little or no fever at all.

Also keep in mind that abdominal pain can be suggestive of other problems. It is sometimes related to cardiac conditions, and it is frequently caused by bowel impaction or obstruction. Obstructions can be very serious and can lead to bowel ruptures that often are life threatening.

Because of the older patient's response to the acute abdomen, a delay in identifying the condition and seeking medical attention is possible, putting the patient at risk for complications. You should ask about the patient's medical history, especially the history of recent illness, to identify a potential illness. Ask about abdominal discomfort, when the patient last had a bowel movement, and whether she or he was constipated or had diarrhea. Inquire if the patient has had previous bowel obstructions. Inquire as to when the patient last ate, how much fluid he or she has consumed, and whether he or she has vomited. A geriatric patient may think a few cups of coffee a day is adequate fluid intake, but coffee (especially caffeinated) causes vasoconstriction and dehydration within the digestive system.

Quickly determining the severity of the patient's problem can hasten proper treatment and recovery. Provide transport to an appropriate facility that can meet the needs of a geriatric patient.

Any of these signs and symptoms is cause for prompt transport to the emergency department (ED).

## Special Populations

Causes of abdominal pain are difficult enough to determine in adults who can provide a good history, but for children who can only tell you they have a stomachache it is even more problematic. It is hard for a parent or caregiver to provide accurate information when pain is so subjective. Confirm with the parent or caregiver the details of the medical history and whether the current problem could be an exacerbation (worsening) of a chronic problem. Chapter 35, *Pediatric Emergencies*, covers the acute abdomen in pediatric patients in depth.

Abdominal pain could be caused by an infection, be related to something the child ate, or indicate a poisoning. Look for clues that may indicate if the child ingested something poisonous. Consider environmental causes like spider bites (black widow or brown recluse) or metabolic issues like diabetic complications. Confirm the duration and location of the pain and if there has been vomiting.

Assess the child's appearance. Ask if there has been diarrhea or any kind of rash. It is always wise to transport a child with abdominal pain for further assessment.

## Words of Wisdom

An acute abdomen usually indicates peritonitis, in which generalized signs can make it challenging to determine exactly where the problem lies, even for physicians. Knowing abdominal assessment steps well and recording your findings in detail are important early factors in the process that results in diagnosis.

## Patient Assessment

### Scene Size-up

As always, ensure that the scene is safe and follow standard precautions with a minimum of gloves and eye protection. Consider donning a face shield, gown, and covering your shoes with disposable, protective covers because there may be feces and urine on the floor and some patients may have active projectile vomiting.

Determine the number of patients at the scene. If your call involves going to the patient's home and

live with them for years. When a hernia is incarcerated, however, its contents may become seriously compressed by the surrounding tissue, eventually compromising the blood supply. This situation, called strangulation, is a serious medical emergency. Immediate surgery is required to remove any dead tissue and repair the hernia.

The following signs and symptoms indicate a serious hernia problem:

- Reducible mass that is no longer reducible
- Pain at the hernia site
- Tenderness when the hernia is palpated
- Red or blue skin discoloration over the hernia

he or she does not come to the door, the patient may have had a syncopal episode (fainted). Request police assistance to help you gain access to the patient. Consider the need for additional or specialized medical resources and request them early.

Be alert for clues to help you determine the nature of illness (NOI) or the mechanism of injury. Acute abdomen can be the result of violence, such as blunt or penetrating trauma, so always be vigilant. Chapter 31, *Abdominal and Genitourinary Injuries*, discusses traumatic injuries in detail. Clues will help you develop an early index of suspicion for life threats. For example, a pale and sweating patient who reports tearing pain may have an AAA. Observe the scene closely and interview bystanders or family members if the NOI is not obvious. In some cases, your senses can help give you a clue as to the NOI. For example, GI bleeding often has a characteristic odor that you will learn to recognize.

## Primary Assessment

Begin assessing the patient by first looking for and treating any life-threatening conditions. Assess the patient's level of consciousness and ABCs; threats to airway, breathing, or circulation are considered life threatening and must be treated immediately. Rapidly observe the patient and the environment. Note the position of the patient. Commonly the patient will have his or her knees drawn up to help alleviate the pain associated with acute abdomen. Consider necessary treatment and transport options and the need for early advanced life support (ALS) assistance.

If the chief complaint indicates a life-threatening problem, assess and treat it immediately. If the chief complaint is a minor problem, it should wait until you have had a chance to assess for and treat any potential life threats.

Ensure that the patient's airway is clear and that the patient's respirations are adequate. Administer oxygen to the patient when needed. As a result of the abdominal pain, the patient may show shallow or inadequate respirations because deep breaths often intensify the pain.

When you are assessing the patient's circulation, remember to assess for major bleeding. Ask the patient about amount and frequency of blood in the vomit (hematemesis); black, tarry stools (melena); or bright red, bloody stools. The patient's pulse rate and quality, as well as skin condition, may indicate shock. Because skin paleness can be difficult to detect in patients with dark skin, check for pale mucous membranes inside the inner lower eyelid or slow capillary refill. On general observation, the patient may appear ashen or gray. Check the pulses in both feet because a difference in pulse strength may indicate AAA. The abdomen should be inspected for wounds or bruising. Bruising around the umbilicus or on the flanks may indicate internal abdominal bleeding.

Shock may be caused by hypovolemia or may be the result of a severe infection (septic). If evidence

## YOU are the Provider

After providing further assessment, you place the patient onto the stretcher, load him into the ambulance, and proceed to the closest appropriate hospital, which is located 20 miles away. En route, you reassess the patient.

| Recording Time: 12 Minutes | |
|---|---|
| **Level of consciousness** | Conscious and alert; restless |
| **Respirations** | 28 breaths/min; shallow |
| **Pulse** | 130 beats/min; weak and regular |
| **Skin** | Cool, pale, and diaphoretic |
| **Blood pressure** | 100/62 mm Hg |
| **Spo₂** | 98% (on oxygen) |

**7.** Are there any special considerations for this patient? If so, what are they?

of shock (inadequate perfusion) is present, interventions should include high-flow oxygen, placing the patient supine, and keeping the patient warm. Ensure that you provide prompt treatment for life threats and do not delay transport.

Certain patients should be transported quickly. These include patients who have airway, breathing, or circulation problems, including problems with pulse and perfusion, and patients with suspected internal bleeding. Included in the group to call for ALS intercept and to package quickly and transport rapidly are patients who have a poor general impression, especially pediatric and geriatric patients. Pale, cool, diaphoretic skin; tachycardia; hypotension; and altered level of consciousness are all signs of significant illness.

Ensure that the ride during transport is as gentle as possible for the patient. Drive smoothly and steadily. A rough drive can result in increased vehicle movement, potentially aggravating and possibly worsening the patient's abdominal pain.

## History Taking

If the patient is responsive, begin with obtaining the SAMPLE history. When you are obtaining the medication history, ask if the patient has taken antibiotics or pain relievers such as ibuprofen or aspirin recently. Inquire about recent use of alcohol. Ask the following questions specific to the signs and symptoms of a gastrointestinal or urologic emergency:

- **Nausea and vomiting.** Do you feel nauseous? Have you vomited? How many times? Over what period of time? Was there red blood? Did it look like coffee grounds?
- **Changes in bowel habits.** Has there been any change in your bowel habits? Have you been constipated? Did the stool look dark and tarry? Have you had diarrhea? How many times and over what period of time? Was there any red blood in it?
- **Urination.** Have you been urinating more or less often? Is there pain when you urinate? Is the color dark or unusual? Is there an unusual odor?
- **Weight loss.** Have you had unexplained weight loss recently? How many pounds?
- **Belching or flatulence.** Have you experienced belching or flatulence? For how long?

- **Pain.** What does the pain feel like? How long have you had this pain? Is the pain constant or intermittent? Have you had similar pain in the past? Have you done anything to relieve the pain? For any abdominal discomfort, use OPQRST to ask the patient what makes the pain better or worse.
- **Other.** Ask about any other signs or symptoms related to this complaint, such as "Are there any changes you have noted recently that may be contributing to your pain?" "Have you had a fever?"
- **Concurrent chest pain.** If the patient reports chest pain, use OPQRST to ask the patient what makes the pain better or worse.

Continue with the SAMPLE history. If the patient is a woman and of childbearing age, determine the date of her last menstrual period. This will determine if the patient could possibly be pregnant or raise the suspicion of other obstetric emergencies.

Ask the patient about his or her last oral intake. It is important to determine whether the patient has ingested any substance that could be causing the acute abdomen. If eating causes pain, discomfort, vomiting, or diarrhea, the patient will eat less frequently or stop eating altogether. Do not give the patient anything by mouth. Food or fluid may only aggravate many of the symptoms. Also, the presence of food in the stomach increases the risk of aspiration.

### Words of Wisdom

Consider and document pertinent negatives, which are a record of normal findings that warrant no care or intervention. It is important to know and document that the patient denies shortness of breath or radiation of abdominal pain.

Finally, determine the events that led up to the patient's present illness. Question the patient about any recent trauma.

The SAMPLE history may not affect the interventions you perform, but it will help provide needed information for the physician in the ED to aid in determining the cause of the acute abdomen.

## Secondary Assessment

In some situations, patients are comfortable only when lying in one particular position, which tends to relax muscles adjacent to the inflamed organ and thus lessen the pain. Therefore, the position of the patient may provide you with an important clue. For example, a patient with appendicitis may draw up the right knee. A patient with pancreatitis may lie curled up on one side.

Information gathered in the history-taking portion of the patient assessment may be used to focus your physical examination of the abdomen. A normal abdomen is soft and not tender to the touch. Pain and tenderness are the most common symptoms of an acute abdomen. The pain may be sharply localized or diffuse and will vary in its severity. Localized pain gives a clue to the problem organ or area causing it. Tenderness may be minimal or so great that the patient will not allow you to touch the abdomen. In some instances, the muscles of the abdominal wall become rigid in an involuntary effort to protect the abdomen from further irritation. This boardlike muscle spasm, called **guarding**, can be seen with major problems such as a perforated ulcer or pancreatitis.

Remember, the patient with peritonitis usually has abdominal pain, even when lying quietly. The patient may have difficulty breathing and may take rapid, shallow breaths because of the pain. Usually, you will find tenderness on palpation of the abdomen or when the patient moves. The degree of pain and tenderness is usually related directly to the severity of peritoneal inflammation.

Use the following steps to assess the abdomen:

1. Explain to the patient how you will assess the abdomen.
2. Place the patient in a supine position with the legs drawn up and flexed at the knees to relax the abdominal muscles, unless there is any trauma, in which case the patient will remain supine and stabilized. Determine whether the patient is restless or quiet, and whether motion causes pain.
3. Expose the abdomen and visually assess it. Does the abdomen appear distended (enlarged)? Do you see any pulsating masses (indicates an AAA)? Is there bruising to the abdominal wall? Are there any surgical scars?
4. Ask the patient where the pain is most intense. Palpate in a clockwise direction beginning with the quadrant *after* the one the patient indicates is tender or painful; end with the quadrant the patient indicates is tender or painful.

If the most painful area is palpated first, the patient may guard against further examination, making your assessment more difficult and less reliable.

5. Remember to be very gentle when palpating the abdomen. Occasionally, an organ within the abdomen will be enlarged and very fragile. Rough palpation could cause further damage. If you see a pulsating mass, do not touch it; manipulating an aortic aneurysm could cause it to rupture.
6. Palpate the four quadrants of the abdomen gently to determine whether each quadrant is tense (guarded) or soft when palpated (**FIGURE 19-4**).
7. Note whether the pain is localized to a particular quadrant or diffuse (widespread).
8. Palpate and wait for the patient to respond, looking for a facial grimace or a verbal "ouch." Do not ask the patient, "Does it hurt here?" as you palpate.
9. Determine whether the patient exhibits rebound tenderness (may be tender when direct pressure is applied, but very painful when pressure is released). This is an indicator of peritonitis. When you are palpating for rebound tenderness, you should use extreme caution.
10. Determine whether the patient can relax the abdominal wall on command. Guarding or rigidity may be present, which can indicate peritoneal irritation.

Findings of a high respiratory rate with a normal pulse rate and blood pressure may indicate the patient is unable to ventilate properly because deep

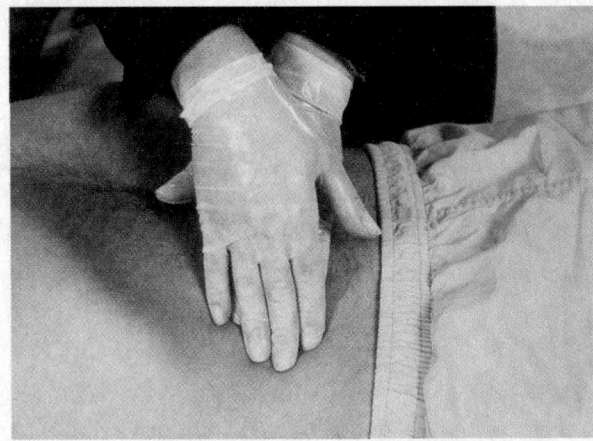

**FIGURE 19-4** Check for tenderness or rigidity by gently palpating the abdomen.

© Jones & Bartlett Learning.

breathing causes pain. A high respiratory rate and pulse rate with signs of shock, such as pallor and diaphoresis (profuse sweating), may indicate septic or hypovolemic shock. When treating a patient who has a dialysis shunt or fistula in his or her arm, it is important not to take a blood pressure in the same arm as the shunt to avoid damaging it.

## Reassessment

Because it is often difficult to determine the cause of an acute abdominal emergency, it is extremely important to reassess your patient frequently to determine whether the patient's condition has changed. Remember, the condition of a patient with an acute abdomen can change rapidly from stable to unstable.

Vital signs must be reassessed and compared with the patient's baseline vital signs. If anything changes en route to the hospital, manage the problem and document any changes or additional treatment.

Reassess the patient and then ask the following questions (where appropriate):

- Has the patient's level of consciousness changed?
- Has the patient become more anxious?
- Has the appearance of the skin changed?
- Has the pain gotten better or worse?
- Has bleeding increased or decreased?
- Is current treatment improving the patient's condition?

- Has an already identified problem gotten better or worse?
- What is the nature of any newly identified problems?

Interventions generally include treatment for shock, providing emotional support, and keeping the patient as comfortable as possible. Administer oxygen if the patient is hypoxemic, cover the patient with a blanket for warmth, and provide gentle transport for the patient without delay. Place the patient in a position of comfort. You will find that patients often want to be supine with their knees drawn up. If the patient wants to lie on his or her side, try to make that possible. Be sure that you can observe and maintain the patient's airway because vomiting is common. If the patient's pain is extreme or he or she is showing significant signs of shock, consider the use of ALS assistance (if available) for intravenous fluids and management of pain, nausea, or vomiting. If transport time is extended and rapid transport is needed, consider air medical transport if available.

## Emergency Medical Care

Although you cannot treat the causes of acute abdomen, you can take steps to provide comfort and lessen the effects of shock by reassuring the patient and making the patient feel at ease. Treat the patient for shock even when obvious signs of shock are not apparent. Position patients who are vomiting to

## YOU are the Provider

With an estimated time of arrival at the hospital of 22 minutes, you reassess the patient and then call in your radio report. The patient remains conscious and alert, but restless, and is still experiencing 10/10 abdominal pain.

| Recording Time: 17 Minutes | |
|---|---|
| Level of consciousness | Conscious and alert; restless |
| Respirations | 28 breaths/min; shallow |
| Pulse | 128 beats/min; weak and regular |
| Skin | Cool, clammy, and diaphoretic |
| Blood pressure | 96/58 mm Hg |
| Spo$_2$ | 97% (on oxygen) |

The patient's condition is unchanged on arrival at the hospital. You give your verbal report to the charge nurse. After further assessment and treatment in the ED, the patient is taken to surgery. You later learn that he had an expanding AAA, which was successfully repaired.

**8.** Could you have done anything definitively for this patient in the field? Why or why not?

maintain a patent airway. Contain the vomitus to prevent the spread of infections (by using a biohazard bag). Airborne bacteria and viruses produced from vomiting can be easily transmitted to others. Ensure you are wearing gloves, eye protection, and a gown to prevent contamination of yourself, and wear a mask to prevent breathing in any infectious organisms. When you have released your patient to the hospital staff, clean the ambulance and any equipment you have used, preferably with an antibacterial cleaner. Do not forget to wash your hands even though you were wearing gloves.

Loosen restrictive clothing and transport the patient gently in a position of comfort. Constantly reassess your patient's condition for signs of deterioration.

## Dialysis Emergencies

Patients with end-stage renal disease (ESRD), also referred to as chronic renal failure, are treated with either peritoneal dialysis (PD) or hemodialysis. In these processes, the patient's blood is filtered and cleansed of the toxins and then returned to the body. The treatment eliminates waste, normalizes the blood chemistry, and reduces excess fluid. If a patient misses a dialysis treatment, weakness and pulmonary edema can be the first in a series of conditions that can become progressively more serious if normal balance is not returned to the patient's body.

In the past, hemodialysis required the patient to make trips to a dialysis center several times a week for treatment. Now, patients and their care partner have the option to receive training and perform hemodialysis in the comfort of their home. This method allows the patient flexibility over his or her dialysis schedule. Unfortunately, complications once encountered in a controlled medical environment will now be seen in private residences, where trained medical staff are not there to assist.

In PD, fluid circulates within the peritoneal cavity. Urea and other toxins diffuse across the peritoneum into the dialysis fluid, which is then drained from the peritoneum, allowing the peritoneum to essentially function as a kidney. Patients on home PD will have a catheter in their abdomen that they use to connect to a PD machine, typically at night.

In hemodialysis, the patient's blood circulates through a dialysis machine that functions in much the same way as the normal kidneys. Most patients undergoing long-term hemodialysis have some sort

### Words of Wisdom

Contact local dialysis centers and inquire about home hemodialysis programs. They may be able to provide training to your department, which will help you care for home dialysis patients more effectively if an emergency arises.

of shunt or fistula, a surgically created connection between a vein and an artery. The patient is connected to the dialysis machine through the shunt or fistula, which allows blood to flow from the body into the dialysis machine and back to the body. The shunt or fistula is usually located in the forearm or upper arm (**FIGURE 19-5**).

In PD, large amounts of specially formulated dialysis fluid are infused into (and back out of) a large catheter in the abdominal cavity (**FIGURE 19-6**). This fluid stays in the cavity for 1 to 2 hours, allowing equilibrium to occur. With proper training, PD can be performed in the home. PD is very effective but carries a very small risk of peritonitis. Peritonitis can occur due to bacteria contaminating the dialysis site. A patient with peritonitis may present with abdominal pain, hypotension, fever, nausea, diarrhea, and cloudy dialysis fluid.

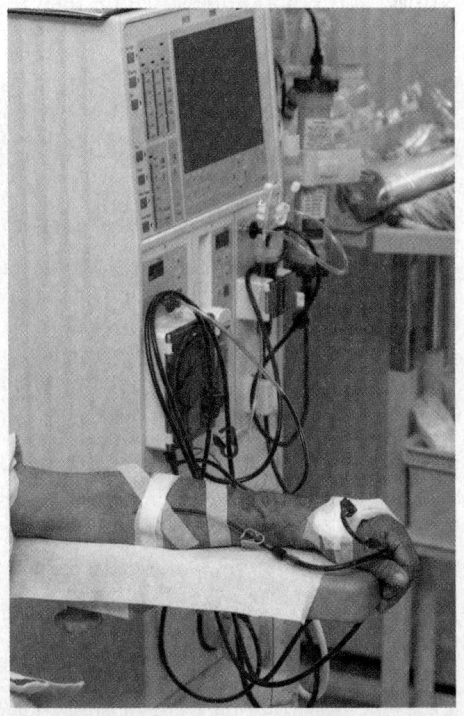

**FIGURE 19-5** Patient connected to a dialysis machine.
© Picsfive/iStock/Getty Images Plus/Getty Images.

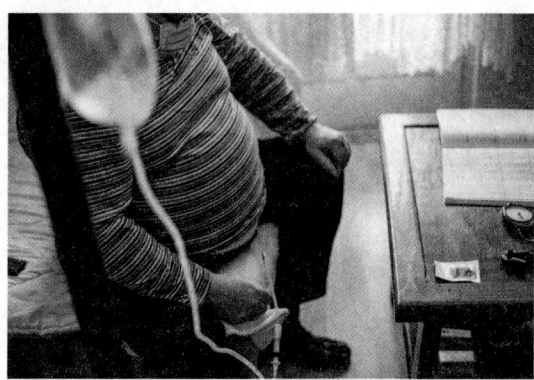

**FIGURE 19-6** Patient receiving peritoneal dialysis.

© Jakovo/iStock/Getty Images Plus/Getty Images.

The adverse effects of dialysis include hypotension, dysrhythmias, chest pain, muscle cramps, nausea and vomiting, altered mental status, electrolyte imbalances, hemorrhage from the access site, and infection at the access site. If your call involves a patient on dialysis, start with the XABCs: control life-threatening hemorrhage (exsanguination), and assess and manage the airway, breathing, and circulation. Provide high-flow oxygen if indicated. Position the patient sitting up in cases of pulmonary edema or supine if the patient is in shock, and transport promptly. Remember, when assessing vital signs in a patient with a dialysis shunt or fistula, do not place a blood pressure cuff over the site.

Doing so may damage the shunt or fistula or cause a blood clot to form. If possible, avoid using the arm with the shunt or fistula for vital signs; instead, use the patient's other arm.

## Words of Wisdom

Bleeding from a fistula that cannot be controlled with pressure after the dialysis needle is removed may be difficult to manage. If bleeding is brisk, firm fingertip pressure should be applied over the bleeding site with one hand while pressure is applied proximal to the bleeding area with the fingers of the other hand for 15 to 30 minutes. Massive bleeding that cannot be controlled in this manner may require application of a tourniquet.

Some dialysis patients also have urinary catheters. The catheter is placed in the bladder so the urine can run into a bag. These catheters can often be a source of infection. The patient may report fever and general malaise (illness) in addition to any symptoms specific to kidney failure. Leave the device in place. Treat any signs and symptoms and transport the patient for further evaluation.

During transport, unless there is a life-threatening event, make all attempts to deliver the patient to a hospital with dialysis capability.

## YOU are the Provider SUMMARY

**1. What is the definition of an acute abdomen?**

Acute abdomen is a term used to describe the sudden (acute) onset of abdominal pain that is not caused by a traumatic injury. It is generally associated with severe, progressive symptoms that require medical attention. Acute abdominal pain can be caused by dysfunction of one or more of the abdominal organs, such as the liver, spleen, gallbladder, stomach, pancreas, kidneys, large or small intestines, or appendix. It can also be due to an irritation or infection of the lining of the abdominal cavity—the peritoneum.

**2. What is your role as an EMT in treating a patient with abdominal pain?**

The underlying cause of a patient's abdominal pain, acute or chronic, is often difficult to identify—even for a physician. As an EMT, it is far more important for you to recognize life-threatening conditions and

provide prompt emergency care than it is to identify the underlying cause of the patient's pain. It is important to watch for signs of shock and treat it quickly. Patients who are in pain, especially when the pain occurs suddenly, are often very anxious and scared; providing emotional support is an important part of your role. Allowing the patient to assume a position of comfort may also help.

**3. What is the proper technique of assessing a patient's abdomen? What should you assess for?**

Although assessment of the abdomen may help localize the source of a patient's pain, it should not be prolonged. During the exam, place the patient supine with the legs drawn up and flexed at the knees; this position will relax the abdominal muscles and may alleviate some of his or her pain. Look at the abdomen first; does it appear distended (enlarged)? Do you see any pulsating masses (suggests an AAA)? Is there bruising of the abdominal wall (suggests internal hemorrhage)? Ask the patient where the pain is most intense and assess that area last. If the most painful area is palpated first, the patient may guard against further examination, making your assessment more difficult and less reliable. Gently palpate the four abdominal quadrants to determine whether each quadrant is rigid or soft or if there is tenderness, and note the presence of any masses. Pay particular attention to the patient's facial expressions when palpating each abdominal quadrant; this may yield valuable information. Note whether the pain is localized to a particular quadrant or diffuse (widespread). Determine whether the patient can relax the abdominal wall on command; if he or she cannot, the abdomen is said to be rigid. Avoid vigorous palpation of the abdomen; doing so will only cause the patient more pain and can worsen his or her condition, especially if one of the abdominal organs is enlarged and fragile.

**4. What is the difference between radiating pain and referred pain?**

Radiating pain moves from its point of origin to other parts of the body, such as the pain from pancreatitis, which may radiate to the back, or the pain from a kidney stone blockage, which may radiate to the groin. With radiating pain, there is pain at point A and point B, with a trail of pain in between the two points.

Referred pain originates in a particular organ but is described or perceived by the patient as pain in a different location or pain at the point of origin and another location. For example, the origin of pain associated with cholecystitis—inflammation of the gallbladder—is usually the right upper quadrant of the abdomen. However, the patient commonly reports pain in the right shoulder. In some cases, the patient reports pain in both the right upper quadrant and the right shoulder. Unlike with radiating pain, there is no pain in between the two points.

**5. What do the patient's vital signs indicate?**

The patient's vital signs indicate shock. His respirations are rapid (tachypnea); he has a rapid heart rate (tachycardia); his skin is cool, pale, and diaphoretic (sweaty); and his blood pressure—considering the fact that he has a history of hypertension—is low. Whether the patient has an intra-abdominal infection (peritonitis) or intra-abdominal bleeding, the end result, if untreated, will be the same—death!

It is more important to recognize life-threatening conditions (eg, shock) than it is to determine the exact cause of a patient's abdominal pain, or any pain for that matter. You must begin immediate treatment aimed at maintaining adequate perfusion, such as applying high-flow oxygen when indicated (your partner has already done this), keeping him warm, and rapidly preparing for transport.

**6. What do you suspect is the cause of the patient's abdominal pain?**

The lack of fever, vomiting, or diarrhea makes an infectious cause less likely in this patient.

Although only a physician can determine the exact cause of the patient's pain, a severe abdominal pain that radiates to the lower back is characteristic of an AAA.

The typical patient with an AAA is a male in his late 60s or older. As long as the aneurysm is not expanding, the patient usually will be asymptomatic. When the aneurysm starts to expand, however, the patient has a sudden onset of abdominal pain, which is classically described as a ripping or searing sensation in the abdomen that radiates to the back. When an AAA starts expanding and producing symptoms, rupture may be imminent. If aortic rupture occurs, the patient often bleeds to death (exsanguination) very quickly. If the aneurysm is leaking, however, blood will accumulate in the retroperitoneal space and cause signs of shock; this is what may be happening to your patient.

**7. Are there any special considerations for this patient? If so, what are they?**

As with any patient exhibiting signs of shock, your priority is to provide transport to an appropriate medical facility with surgical capability without delay. Patients with a suspected aortic aneurysm must be handled carefully; avoid rough driving and unnecessary bumps in the road. Because this is a potentially a fragile situation, with a large, leaking artery, avoid further palpation of the abdomen. Some patients with an abdominal aortic aneurysm have a pulsating mass that can be palpated (and sometimes seen) near the umbilicus. If you see a pulsating mass, do *not* touch it; manipulating an aortic aneurysm could cause it to rupture. However, if you do not see or feel a pulsating mass, it does not necessarily rule out the patient having an abdominal aneurysm, so the same precautions in assessment and treatment should be considered.

Avoid anything that will make the patient more anxious; anxiety causes increases in heart rate and blood pressure. An acute increase in blood pressure, even a slight one, may be all that is needed to cause an aortic rupture. In this particular patient, you should avoid elevating the patient's legs. Elevating the lower extremities may cause a surge of blood back to the heart, resulting in an increase in blood pressure.

**8. Could you have done anything definitively for this patient in the field? Why or why not?**

No. Definitive care (eg, surgically repairing the aneurysm) can only be provided at the hospital. Although paramedics can start intravenous lines and give pain medications, these interventions are simply aimed at controlling pain and partially treating shock, not fixing the aneurysm. Your role as an EMT is to recognize the patient's condition is serious, provide emergency medical treatment, and transport without delay.

## EMS Patient Care Report (PCR)

| **Date:** 3-20-20 | **Incident No.:** 150109 | **Nature of Call:** Abdominal pain | | **Location:** 1500 E. River Rd., Apt. 5 | |
|---|---|---|---|---|---|
| **Dispatched:** 0320 | **En Route:** 0321 | **At Scene:** 0333 | **Transport:** 0345 | **At Hospital:** 0410 | **In Service:** 0420 |

### Patient Information

| | |
|---|---|
| **Age:** 79<br>**Sex:** M<br>**Weight (in kg [lb]):** 86 kg (190 lb) | **Allergies:** None<br>**Medications:** Toprol, Diovan<br>**Past Medical History:** Hypertension, depression, appendectomy<br>**Chief Complaint:** Abdominal pain |

### Vital Signs

| **Time:** 0335 | **BP:** 98/60 | **Pulse:** 124 | **Respirations:** 28 | **Spo$_2$:** 96% |
|---|---|---|---|---|
| **Time:** 0345 | **BP:** 100/62 | **Pulse:** 130 | **Respirations:** 28 | **Spo$_2$:** 98% |
| **Time:** 0350 | **BP:** 96/58 | **Pulse:** 128 | **Respirations:** 28 | **Spo$_2$:** 97% |

### EMS Treatment (circle all that apply)

| **Oxygen @ _15_ L/min via:**<br>NC (NRM) Bag mask | | **Assisted Ventilation** | **Airway Adjunct** | **CPR** |
|---|---|---|---|---|
| **Defibrillation** | **Bleeding Control** | **Bandaging** | **Splinting** | **Other:** Shock management |

### Narrative

Unit 1 dispatched for 79-year-old man who complains of abdominal pain.

Chief Complaint: Abdominal pain

History: History is significant for hypertension, depression, and an appendectomy 30 years ago. The patient states that the pain, which began suddenly, is in his abdomen and is severe and feels like something is being pulled apart. He further states that the pain radiates to his lower back. Pain severity, per patient, is a 10 on a scale of 0 to 10. Patient denies nausea, vomiting, fever, or any other symptoms.

Assessment: On arrival at the scene, found the patient lying in bed in obvious discomfort. He was conscious and alert, but very restless and in severe pain. His skin was cool, pale, and diaphoretic. Vital signs as above. Abdomen was diffusely tender to palpation and guarded. No abdominal distention was noted.

Treatment (Rx): Applied high-flow oxygen via nonrebreathing mask due to signs of shock and unobtainable Sao$_2$ initially, obtained vital signs, and performed further assessment.

Transport: Covered patient with blanket to keep him warm, slid patient from the bed to the stretcher using a soft stretcher, loaded him into the ambulance, and began transport to the hospital. Continued oxygen therapy en route and continuously monitored his condition. He remained conscious and alert, but restless, and stated that his pain was still a 10/10. Called radio report to the hospital; no further orders were given by the attending physician. ALS was not available so transported BLS. Delivered patient to the emergency department without incident. Verbal report was given to charge nurse Jackson.

**End of report**

# Prep Kit

## Ready for Review

- The acute abdomen is a medical emergency, requiring prompt but gentle transport.
- The pain, tenderness, and abdominal distention associated with an acute abdomen may be signs of peritonitis, which may be caused by any condition that allows pus, blood, feces, urine, gastric juice, intestinal contents, bile, pancreatic juice, amniotic fluid, or other foreign material to lie within or adjacent to the peritoneum.
- In addition to abdominal disease or injury, problems in the gastrointestinal, genital, and urinary systems may cause peritonitis.
- Signs and symptoms of acute abdomen include pain, nausea, vomiting, and a tense, distended abdomen.
- Pain is common directly over the inflamed area of the peritoneum, or it may be referred to another part of the body. Referred pain occurs because of the connections between the two different nervous systems supplying the parietal peritoneum and the visceral peritoneum.
- Do not give the patient with an acute abdomen anything by mouth.
- A patient in shock or with any life-threatening condition should be transported without delay. Call for advanced life support assistance if your patient's condition deteriorates during transport.

## Vital Vocabulary

**acute abdomen** A condition of sudden onset of pain within the abdomen, usually indicating peritonitis; immediate medical or surgical treatment is necessary.

**appendicitis** Inflammation or infection of the appendix.

**cholecystitis** Inflammation of the gallbladder.

**cystitis** Inflammation of the bladder.

**diverticulitis** Inflammation in small pockets at weak areas in the muscle walls of the intestines.

**emesis** Vomiting.

**gastroesophageal reflux disease (GERD)** A condition in which the sphincter between the esophagus and the stomach opens, allowing stomach acid to move up into the esophagus, usually resulting in a burning sensation within the chest; also called acid reflux.

**guarding** Involuntary muscle contractions (spasm) of the abdominal wall; an effort to protect the inflamed abdomen.

**hematemesis** Vomiting blood.

**hernia** The protrusion of an organ or tissue through an abnormal body opening.

**ileus** Paralysis of the bowel, arising from any one of several causes; stops contractions that move material through the intestine.

**kidney stones** Solid crystalline masses formed in the kidney, resulting from an excess of insoluble salts or uric acid crystallizing in the urine; may become trapped anywhere along the urinary tract.

**melena** Black, foul-smelling, tarry stool containing digested blood.

**pancreatitis** Inflammation of the pancreas.

**peritoneum** The membrane lining the abdominal cavity (parietal peritoneum) and covering the abdominal organs (visceral peritoneum).

**peritonitis** Inflammation of the peritoneum.

**referred pain** Pain felt in an area of the body other than the area where the cause of pain is located.

**strangulation** Complete obstruction of blood circulation in a given organ as a result of compression or entrapment; an emergency situation causing death of tissue.

**uremia** Severe kidney failure resulting in the buildup of waste products within the blood. Eventually brain functions will be impaired.

**urinary tract infection (UTI)** An infection, usually of the lower urinary tract (urethra and bladder), that occurs when normal flora bacteria enter the urethra and grow.

## References

1. Anand B. Peptic ulcer disease. *Medscape.* https://emedicine.medscape.com/article/181753-overview#a3. Updated August 1, 2019. Accessed November 2, 2019.

2. Antunes C, Curtis S. *Gastroesophageal Reflux Disease.* StatPearls [Internet]. Treasure Island, FL: StatPearls Publishing; 2019. https://www.ncbi.nlm.nih.gov/books/NBK441938/. Accessed November 2, 2019.

3. Bloom A. Cholecystitis clinical presentation. *Medscape.* https://emedicine.medscape.com/article/171886-clinical#b1. Updated March 12, 2019. Accessed November 2, 2019.

4. Burkhart J. Patient education: peritoneal dialysis (beyond the basics). *uptodate.com.* https://www.uptodate.com/contents/peritoneal-dialysis-beyond-the-basics#H15. Updated March 12, 2018. Accessed November 2, 2019.

5. Krause R. Dialysis complications of chronic renal failure. *Medscape.* https://emedicine.medscape.com/article/1918879-overview#a1. Updated September 28, 2015. Accessed November 2, 2019.

6. Mann J. Overview of hypertension in acute and chronic kidney disease. *uptodate.com.* https://www.uptodate.com/contents/overview-of-hypertension-in-acute-and-chronic-kidney-disease. Published December 6, 2018. Accessed November 2, 2019.

7. National Association of State EMS Officials. National Model EMS Clinical Guidelines. https://nasemso.org/wp-content/uploads/National-Model-EMS-Clinical-Guidelines-2017-PDF-Version-2.2.pdf. Published January 2019. Accessed November 2, 2019.

8. National Highway Traffic Safety Administration. *National Emergency Medical Services Education Standards.* DOT HS 811 077A. ems.gov. www.ems.gov/pdf/811077a.pdf. Published January 2009. Accessed November 2, 2019.

9. National Highway Traffic Safety Administration. *National Emergency Medical Services Education Standards. Emergency Medical Technician Instructional Guidelines.* DOT HS 811 077C. ems.gov. www.ems.gov/pdf/811077c.pdf. Published January 2009. Accessed November 2, 2019.

10. National Kidney Foundation. Home dialysis. https://www.kidney.org/atoz/content/homehemo. Accessed November 2, 2019.

11. Rawla P, Devasahayam J. *Mallory Weiss Syndrome.* StatPearls [Internet]. Treasure Island, FL: StatPearls Publishing. https://www.ncbi.nlm.nih.gov/books/NBK538190/. Updated June 26, 2019. Accessed November 2, 2019.

12. Ridao N, Luño J, García de Vinuesa S, et al. Prevalence of hypertension in renal disease. *Nephrol Dial Transplant.* 2001;16(1):70-73.

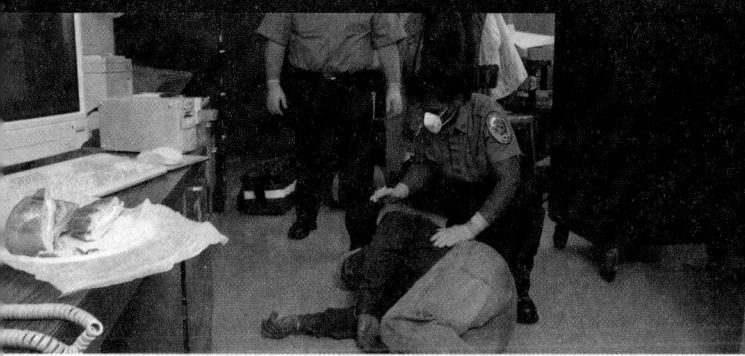

# Chapter 20

# Endocrine and Hematologic Emergencies

## NATIONAL EMS EDUCATION STANDARD COMPETENCIES

### Medicine

Applies fundamental knowledge to provide basic emergency care and transportation based on assessment findings for an acutely ill patient.

### Endocrine Disorders

Awareness that
- Diabetic emergencies cause altered mental status (pp 780–781, 787–789, 790–792)

Anatomy, physiology, pathophysiology, assessment, and management of
- Acute diabetic emergencies (pp 778–793)

### Hematology

Anatomy, physiology, pathophysiology, assessment, and management of
- Sickle cell crisis (pp 793–797)
- Clotting disorders (pp 793–797)

## KNOWLEDGE OBJECTIVES

1. Describe the anatomy and physiology of the endocrine system and its main function in the body. (pp 778–780)
2. Discuss the role of glucose as a major source of energy for the body and its relationship to insulin. (pp 778–780)
3. Define the terms diabetes mellitus, hyperglycemia, and hypoglycemia (pp 780–781)
4. Describe the differences and similarities between hyperglycemic and hypoglycemic diabetic emergencies, including their onset, signs and symptoms, and management considerations. (pp 780–781)
5. Distinguish between the individual types of diabetes and how their onset and presentations are different. (pp 782–784)
6. Describe the interventions for providing emergency medical care to both a conscious

and unconscious patient with an altered mental status and a history of diabetes who is having symptomatic hyperglycemia. (pp 784–785)

7. Describe the interventions for providing emergency medical care to both a conscious and unconscious patient with an altered mental status and a history of diabetes who is having symptomatic hypoglycemia. (pp 785–786)
8. Explain the process for assessing and managing the airway of a patient with an altered mental status, including ways to differentiate a hyperglycemic patient from a hypoglycemic patient. (pp 784–786, 792)
9. Explain some age-related considerations when managing a pediatric patient who is experiencing symptomatic hypoglycemia. (p 786)

10. Discuss the steps the EMT should follow when conducting a primary and secondary assessment of a patient with an altered mental status who is suspected of having diabetes. (pp 786–788)

11. Explain when it is appropriate to obtain medical direction when providing emergency medical care to a patient with diabetes. (pp 788–791)

12. Explain some age-related considerations when managing an older patient who has undiagnosed diabetes. (p 790)

13. Provide the forms, dose, administration, indications, and contraindications for giving oral glucose to a patient with a decreased level of consciousness who has a history of diabetes. (p 791)

14. Discuss the composition and functions of blood. (p 793)

15. Describe the pathophysiology, complications, and management of sickle cell disease. (pp 793–794, 797)

16. Describe two types of blood clotting disorders, and the risk factors, characteristics, and management of each. (pp 794–797)

## SKILLS OBJECTIVES

1. Demonstrate the assessment and care of a patient with hypoglycemia and a decreased level of consciousness. (pp 780–781, 786–793)

## Introduction

The endocrine system directly or indirectly influences almost every cell, organ, and function of the body. Consequently, patients with an endocrine disorder often are seen with a multitude of signs and symptoms that require a thorough assessment and immediate treatment.

This chapter discusses diabetes mellitus types 1 and 2. You will gain an understanding of the role of the pancreas in hormone production and release. The determination of hyperglycemia versus hypoglycemia is explained in detail, because their presentations can be similar with only subtle differences. Further discussion focuses on the signs and symptoms of low and high blood glucose levels as well as the adverse effects of chronically high blood glucose levels.

This chapter also discusses common hematologic emergencies that are often missed in patients. Although hematologic disorders can be difficult to assess and treat in a prehospital setting, your actions may save a patient's life.

## Endocrine Emergencies
### Anatomy and Physiology

The **endocrine system** is a communication system that controls functions inside the body. This system, along with the other systems, maintains the body's homeostasis. **Endocrine glands** secrete messenger **hormones**, which are chemical substances produced by a gland. Hormones travel through the blood to the end organs, tissues, or cells that they are intended to affect. When the hormone arrives,

### YOU are the Provider

A call for service comes in at 1500 hours. The call details from dispatch describe a 23-year-old man with weakness and nausea. You arrive on scene to find a previously healthy man who has had weakness for the past 6 days. He reports recent weight loss, unquenchable thirst, unrelenting hunger, and increased frequency of urination. The patient's other medical history is unremarkable. Your interview reveals that he has two family members with diabetes mellitus.

1. What processes are being described by the patient?
2. What hormone is missing in type 1 diabetes mellitus?

the cell, tissue, or organ receives the message and an action or cellular process takes place.

Endocrine disorders are caused by an internal communication problem. If a gland is not functioning normally, it may produce more hormone (hypersecretion) than is needed or it may not produce enough hormone (hyposecretion). A gland may be functioning correctly, but the receiving organ may not be responding. In these cases, the receiving organ is less responsive to the amount of hormone that it would take to initiate an action or cellular response under normal circumstances.

The brain needs two things to survive: glucose and oxygen. Insulin is necessary for glucose to enter the cells for metabolism. Without the proper balance of hormones (ie, without enough insulin), the cells do not get fed.

The pancreas produces and stores two hormones that play a major role in glucose metabolism: glucagon and insulin. A small portion of the pancreas is filled with the islets of Langerhans. Within these islets are alpha and beta cells. The alpha cells produce glucagon and the beta cells produce insulin.

In a person without diabetes, the pancreas stores and secretes insulin and glucagon in response to the level of glucose in the blood (**FIGURE 20-1**). When a person eats, the level of glucose in his or her blood rises. In response, the pancreas secretes insulin into the blood; this allows the glucose to enter the body's cells and be used for energy. It also allows glucose to be stored in the form of glycogen in the liver and skeletal muscles for use at a later time. As blood glucose levels return to normal, insulin stops being secreted and the body is said to be in a state of being fed.

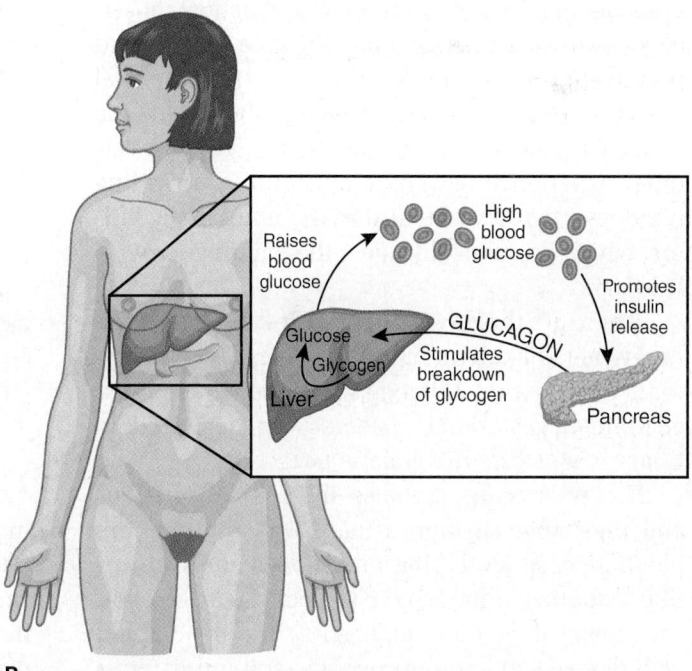

**FIGURE 20-1** Glucose metabolism in a person without diabetes. **A.** Person eats, blood glucose level rises, pancreas secretes insulin into the blood, glucose enters body's cells and is used for energy, glucose is also stored as glycogen in the liver and skeletal muscles for use later, blood glucose levels return to normal, insulin stops being secreted. **B.** Person becomes hungry but does not eat, message is sent to the pancreas to secrete glucagon, glucagon stimulates liver and skeletal muscles to release glycogen, converts glycogen back to glucose for use as cellular fuel.

As time passes, the body will become hungry again. If the hungry individual skips or delays a meal, a message is sent to the pancreas to secrete glucagon. Glucagon then stimulates the liver and the skeletal muscles to release glycogen and converts it back to glucose for use as cellular fuel.

## Pathophysiology

According to the American Diabetes Association, in 2015 diabetes mellitus affected approximately 9.4% of the population. Each year, diabetes is diagnosed in 1.5 million Americans. **Diabetes mellitus** is a disorder of glucose metabolism, such that the body has an impaired ability to get glucose into the cells to be used for energy. The patient with diabetes has either impaired insulin production or not enough functional receptors on the surface of the cells for the insulin to bind to. Glucose cannot get into the cell, the cell goes unfed, and the level of glucose in the blood remains high and continues to rise (**FIGURE 20-2**).

Without treatment, blood glucose levels become too high, which in severe cases may cause life-threatening illness, or coma and death. When diabetes mellitus is properly and effectively managed, a process that involves both the patient and physician, the patient can live a relatively normal life. However, people with diabetes who are unable to achieve good control of their blood glucose levels often experience severe complications, including blindness, cardiovascular disease, and kidney failure, which dramatically affect the length and quality of life.

There are three types of diabetes: diabetes mellitus type 1, diabetes mellitus type 2, and pregnancy-induced gestational diabetes. A more detailed discussion of gestational diabetes can be found in Chapter 34, *Obstetrics and Neonatal Care.*

Treatments for diabetes include medications and injectable hormones that lower the patient's blood glucose level. These hormones and medications, whether administered correctly or incorrectly, can create a medical emergency for the patient with diabetes. If left unrecognized and untreated, a low blood glucose level (hypoglycemia) can be life threatening. You must also recognize the signs and symptoms of a high blood glucose level (hyperglycemia) so you can provide the appropriate treatment and deliver the patient to the next level of care.

**Hyperglycemia** is a state in which the blood glucose level is above normal. **Hypoglycemia** is a state

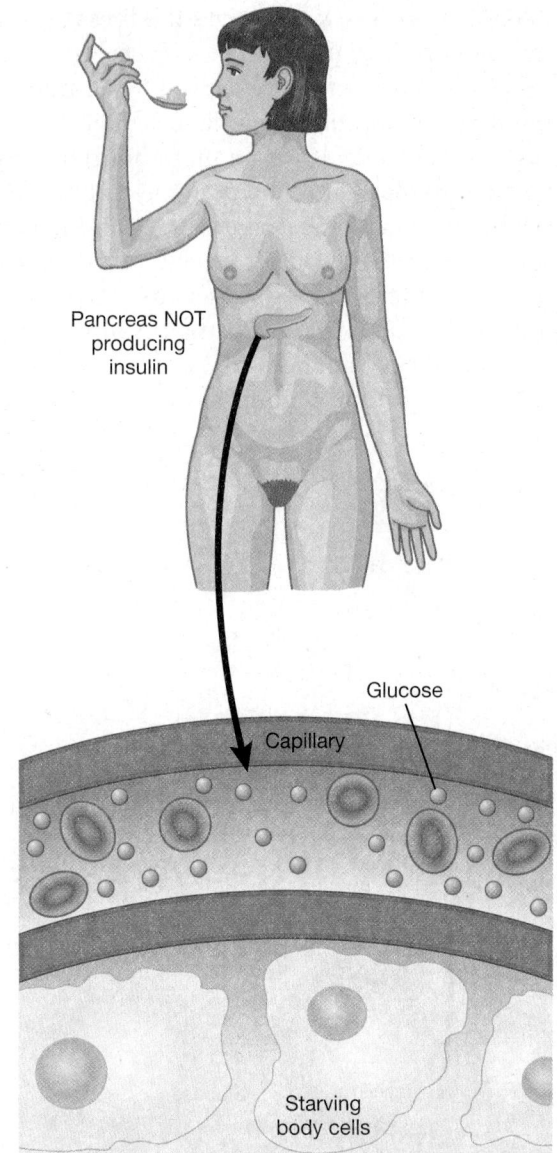

**FIGURE 20-2** Diabetes is defined as the lack of or ineffective action of insulin. Without insulin, cells begin to starve because insulin is needed to allow glucose to enter and nourish the cells.

© Jones & Bartlett Learning.

in which the blood glucose level is below normal (**FIGURE 20-3**). Hyperglycemia and hypoglycemia can occur with both diabetes mellitus types 1 and 2. In the field, you will encounter many patients displaying the signs and symptoms of both high and low blood glucose levels.

Hyperglycemia and hypoglycemia have some similarities in their presentation. As an EMT, you must look for the differences that define one disorder from the other (**TABLE 20-1**). Patients at both extremes, with extremely low and extremely high blood glucose levels, can present with altered

**Blood Glucose Level** (mg/dL)          **Diabetic Emergency**

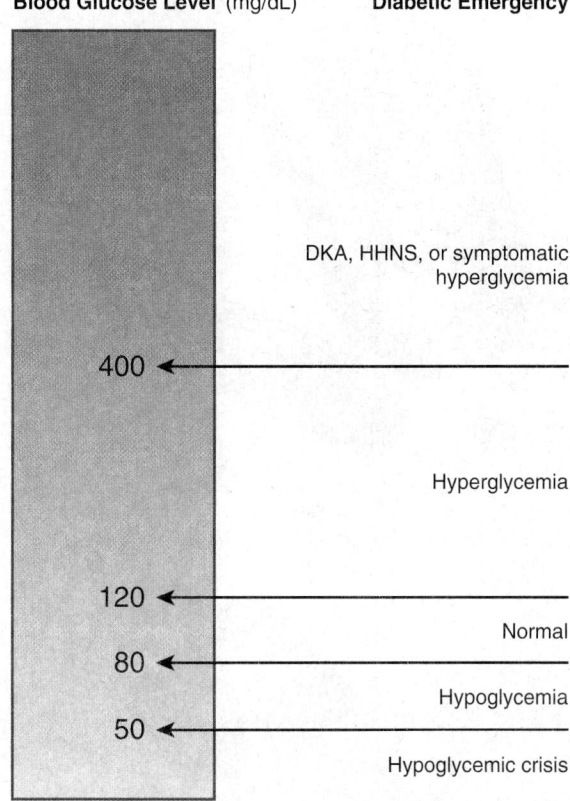

**FIGURE 20-3** The left column illustrates blood glucose levels; the right column illustrates the conditions associated with that particular level of blood glucose. Notice that the normal range is rather small in comparison to the other ranges.

Abbreviations: DKA, diabetic ketoacidosis; HHNS, hyperosmolar hyperglycemic nonketotic syndrome.

© Jones & Bartlett Learning.

mental status. Patients with severe hypoglycemia are more likely to have a depressed level of consciousness than patients with hyperglycemia. Be careful not to incorrectly label patients as being intoxicated. Altered mental status related to diabetic emergencies can often mimic alcohol intoxication, and intoxicated patients often have abnormal glucose levels. Be thorough and check a fingerstick glucose level for all patients with altered mental status.

Hypoglycemia can develop if a person with diabetes takes his or her medications (pills or insulin) as prescribed but fails to eat enough food. Alternatively, a person with diabetes may intentionally or accidentally take too much medication, resulting in low blood glucose levels despite normal dietary intake. All hypoglycemic patients require prompt treatment with oral glucose paste (if alert and able to protect their airway) or injection of glucose (dextrose) or glucagon by an advanced life support (ALS) provider.

**TABLE 20-1** Hyperglycemia Versus Hypoglycemia

| History | Hyperglycemia | Hypoglycemia |
|---|---|---|
| Onset | Gradual (hours to days) | Rapid (within minutes) |
| Skin | Warm and dry | Pale, cool, and moist[a] |
| Infection | Common | Uncommon |
| **Gastrointestinal tract** | | |
| Thirst | Intense | Absent |
| Hunger | Present and increasing | Absent |
| Vomiting/ abdominal pain | Common | Uncommon |
| **Respiratory system** | | |
| Breathing | With DKA there are rapid, deep (Kussmaul) respirations | Normal; may become shallow or ineffective if hypoglycemia is severe and mental status is depressed |
| Odor of breath | With DKA there may be a sweet, fruity odor | Normal |
| **Cardiovascular system** | | |
| Blood pressure | Normal to low | Normal to low |
| Pulse | Rapid, weak, and thready | Rapid, weak |
| **Nervous system** | | |
| Consciousness | Restlessness, possibly progressing to coma; abnormal or slurred speech; unsteady gait | Irritability, confusion, seizure, or coma; unsteady gait |
| **Treatment** | | |
| Response | Gradual, within 6 to 12 hours following medical treatment | Immediate improvement after administration of glucose |

Abbreviation: DKA, diabetic ketoacidosis.

[a]Although paleness, or a decrease in blood flow, can be difficult to detect in dark-skinned people, it may be observed by examining mucous membranes inside the inner lower eyelid and capillary refill. On general observation, the patient may appear ashen or gray.

© Jones and Bartlett Learning.

## Diabetes Mellitus Type 1

**Type 1 diabetes** is an autoimmune disorder in which the individual's immune system produces antibodies against the pancreatic beta cells. Essentially, this disease is about the missing pancreatic hormone insulin. Insulin is the "key" to the "door" of the cell. Without insulin, glucose cannot enter the cell, and the cell cannot produce energy.

The onset of this disorder usually happens from early childhood through the fourth decade of life. The patient's immune system progressively destroys the ability of the pancreas to produce insulin. Without the insulin from the pancreatic beta cells, the patient must obtain insulin from an external source. Patients with type 1 diabetes cannot survive without insulin. Patients who inject insulin often need to check their blood glucose levels up to six times per day or more using a lancet and a small capillary blood sample read by using a glucometer (**FIGURE 20-4**).

Many people with type 1 diabetes have an implanted insulin pump. Some of these devices continuously measure the body's glucose levels and provide an (adjustable) infusion of insulin and correction doses of insulin based on carbohydrate intake at mealtimes (**FIGURE 20-5**). The presence of an insulin pump that automatically measures blood glucose limits the number of times patients have to check their fingerstick glucose level. Some insulin pumps do not measure blood glucose automatically, but rather deliver a continuous baseline dose of insulin that may be supplemented by an additional bolus dose depending on the blood glucose measurement the patient takes at mealtimes. Unfortunately, insulin pumps can malfunction and hyperglycemic or hypoglycemic diabetic emergencies can develop. Always inquire about the presence of an insulin pump—particularly in patients with type 1 diabetes—and ask the patient if it is working properly.

Type 1 diabetes is the most common metabolic disease of childhood. A patient with new-onset type 1 diabetes will have symptoms related to eating and drinking:

- Polyuria
- Polydipsia
- Polyphagia
- Weight loss
- Fatigue

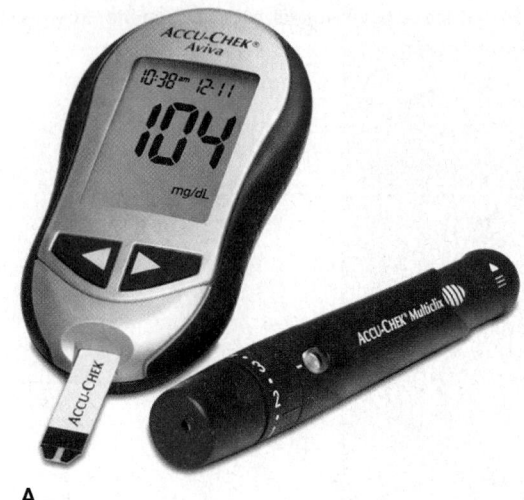

**A**

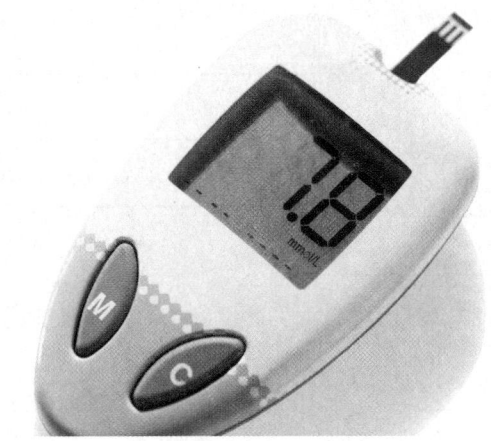

**B**

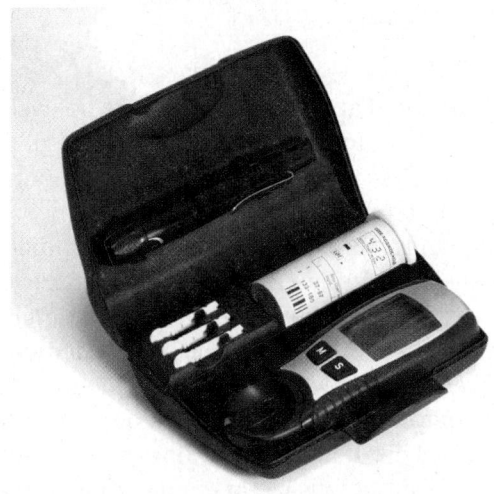

**C**

**FIGURE 20-4** The blood glucose self-monitoring kit with digital meter is a device used by patients at home and by EMTs in the field in many EMS systems. Three types (**A-C**) are shown.

**A:** Accu-Chek® Aviva used with permission of Roche Diagnostics; **B:** © Stockbyte/Thinkstock; **C:** © instamatic/iStock.

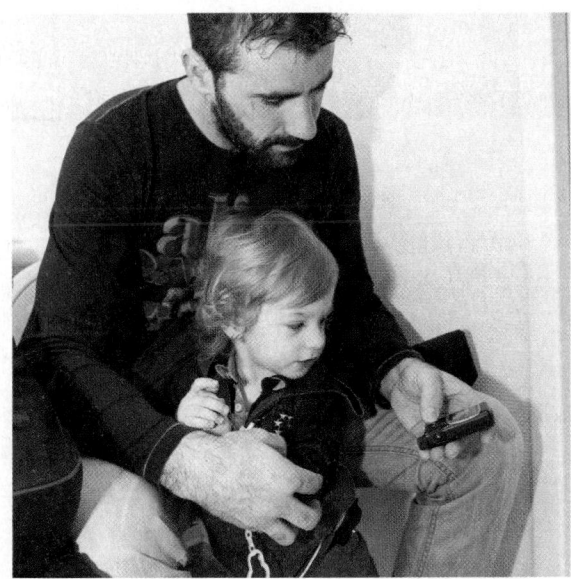

**FIGURE 20-5** An insulin pump.

© BSIP/Contributor/Universal Images Group/Getty Images.

Normal blood glucose level is between 80 and 120 mg/dL. The body's metabolism is sensitive to the levels of particular substances, such as glucose, in the blood. The kidneys filter the blood and thus manage all substances present in the blood. At normal levels, glucose remains in the blood as it is filtered.

When a patient's blood glucose level is above normal, the kidney's filtration system becomes overwhelmed and glucose spills into the urine. The increased amount of glucose in the urine causes more water to be pulled out of the bloodstream into the urine. This results in more frequent urination, or **polyuria**.

Increased urine production and urination also cause dehydration and increased thirst, which can lead to severe electrolyte abnormalities. An increase in fluid consumption, called **polydipsia**, occurs in an attempt to quench this thirst.

In the early phase of diabetes, patients may report severe hunger and increased food intake, a condition known as **polyphagia**. Over time, particularly if diabetes remains undiagnosed or untreated, appetite will decrease and patients often lose weight.

The autoimmune destruction of the pancreatic beta cell takes time to progress. For this reason, initial symptoms are typically subtle and not readily apparent to the patient. As the lack of insulin becomes more profound, the patient will notice increasing fatigue and malaise along with vague symptoms of generalized illness.

When the body's cells do not receive the glucose they require for energy, the body resorts to burning fat for energy. When the body burns fat rather than glucose, acid waste is produced. These acids are called ketones. As ketone levels increase in the blood, the ketones also begin to spill into the urine (as does the excess glucose). When the kidneys become saturated with glucose and ketones, they do not work properly to maintain acid–base balance in the body. The body responds with a backup system and the patient begins to breathe faster and deeper. This respiratory pattern is the body's attempt to reduce the acid level by releasing more carbon dioxide through the lungs. This breathing pattern is known as **Kussmaul respirations**.

If fat metabolism and ketone production continue, a life-threatening illness called **diabetic ketoacidosis (DKA)** can develop in patients with diabetes. DKA may present as:

- Generalized illness, accompanied by:
  - Abdominal pain
  - Body aches
  - Nausea
  - Vomiting
  - Altered mental status or unconsciousness (if severe)

If DKA is not rapidly recognized and treated, it can result in death.

## Street Smarts

Do not attempt to coach the patient to slow his or her breathing if you suspect Kussmaul respirations. This rapid, deep breathing is helping the patient compensate for acidosis. If breathing is slowed, more acids can accumulate and the patient's condition will worsen.

When a patient with DKA has an altered mental status, ask the patient's family and friends about the patient's history and presentation. Obtain a glucose level with a fingerstick using a lancet and a glucometer. (This procedure is covered in Chapter 10, *Patient Assessment.*) The patient with DKA will generally have a fingerstick glucose level higher than 400 mg/dL.

This presentation of the patient with type 1 diabetes in DKA does not only occur when there is an absolute lack of insulin. DKA may also present in cases of a relative lack of insulin, which may occur when there is an acute illness, or an untreated infection or other stressor on the body that leaves the patient with type 1 diabetes in a weakened condition.

## Diabetes Mellitus Type 2

**Type 2 diabetes** is caused by resistance to the effects of insulin at the cellular level. Recall that we described insulin as the key to the door of the cell. Insulin resistance means the lock is unable to accept the key. As a review, in type 1 diabetes, no insulin is produced, so there are no keys. In type 2 diabetes there are typically fewer insulin receptors.

Obesity predisposes patients to type 2 diabetes; there is an association between obesity and increased resistance to the effects of insulin. As the number of obese people continues to rise, so does the number of patients with type 2 diabetes.

When diabetes begins, the individual's pancreas produces more insulin to make up for the increased levels of blood glucose and dysfunction of cellular insulin receptors. Over time this response becomes inefficient. The blood glucose levels continue to rise and do not respond when the pancreas secretes insulin, a process called insulin resistance. In some cases, insulin resistance can be improved by exercise and dietary modification.

In many instances diet and exercise alone cannot control insulin resistance, and oral medications must be started to better control blood glucose levels. Oral medications used to treat type 2 diabetes vary widely. Some of them increase the secretion of insulin and create a high risk of hypoglycemic reaction, whereas others do not (**TABLE 20-2**). Injectable medications and various insulin preparations are also used for type 2 diabetes when oral medications alone will not regulate blood glucose.

Insulin is a hormone that is destroyed when taken by mouth, so it must be injected. Many of the oral medications listed in Table 20-2 either encourage the pancreas to produce more insulin or the cells to stimulate receptors for insulin. Other medications decrease the effects of glucagon, decrease the release of glucose stored in the liver (glycogen), and prevent increased blood glucose levels during sleep or sedentary periods. None of the available medications is the perfect solution for every patient, however.

| **TABLE 20-2** Common Oral Medications Used to Treat Type 2 Diabetes |
| --- |
| Glipizide (Glucotrol, Glucotrol XL)[a] |
| Glyburide (DiaBeta, Glynase, Micronase)[a] |
| Metformin (Glumetza, Glucophage, Glucophage XR) |
| Pioglitazone (Actos), rosiglitazone (Avandia) |
| Exenatide (Byetta, Bydureon), liraglutide (Victoza), semaglutide (Ozempic) |
| Sitagliptin (Januvia) |

[a]These medications increase the risk of hypoglycemia.

© Jones & Bartlett Learning.

Diabetes mellitus type 2 is often diagnosed at a yearly medical examination. In some cases, the patient's physician discovers diabetes mellitus type 2 when treating the patient for a complaint related to high blood glucose levels. Examples of such complaints include recurrent infection, change in vision, or numbness in the feet.

### Words of Wisdom

The patient with diabetes needs to be vigilant about maintaining a proper glucose level through diet, exercise, and often, taking medication. If patients with diabetes have prolonged hyperglycemia or other associated conditions, serious long-term complications may develop. Patients with diabetes take a blood test called the A1C several times a year to estimate their average blood glucose level over time. The A1C level helps patients with diabetes and their physicians know how well they have been managing their blood glucose levels over 2 to 3 months.

## Symptomatic Hyperglycemia

**Symptomatic hyperglycemia** occurs when blood glucose levels are very high. Early signs and symptoms include frequent urination, increased thirst, blurred vision, and fatigue. If the high blood glucose levels go untreated, the patient may present with a fruity odor on his or her breath, nausea and vomiting, shortness of breath, dry mouth, weakness, or altered mental status. The patient is in a state of altered mental status resulting from several combined problems. In type 1 diabetes, hyperglycemia leads to ketoacidosis and dehydration from excessive urination. In type 2 diabetes, hyperglycemia leads to a state of dehydration due to the discharge of fluids from all body systems and eventually out through the kidneys, leading to a much more ominous situation of fluid imbalance known as **hyperosmolar hyperglycemic nonketotic syndrome (HHNS)**. Hyperglycemia does not always result in a crisis event. If an individual has hyperglycemia for a prolonged time, it is not uncommon for the secondary consequences of diabetes to present. These are wounds that do not heal, numbness in the hands and feet, blindness, renal failure, and gastric motility problems, to name a few.

When blood glucose levels are not controlled in diabetes mellitus type 2, HHNS can develop. HHNS can present similarly to the DKA seen in patients with type 1 diabetes. The onset of this disorder is commonly associated with a profound infection or illness.

Key signs and symptoms of HHNS include the following:

- Hyperglycemia
- Altered mental status, drowsiness, lethargy
- Severe dehydration, thirst, dark urine
- Visual or sensory deficits
- Partial paralysis or muscle weakness
- Seizures

Higher glucose levels in the blood cause the excretion of glucose in the urine. Patients respond by increasing their fluid intake precipitously (polydipsia) causing an equally precipitous excretion of fluid (polyuria). In HHNS, however, the patient cannot drink enough fluid to keep up with the exceedingly high glucose levels in the blood. The kidneys become overwhelmed and the patient's blood becomes much more concentrated than normal. As HHNS progresses, the urine becomes rather dark and concentrated. The term *hyperosmolarity* describes very concentrated blood as a result of relative dehydration. As HHNS progresses, the patient may become unconscious or have seizure activity due in part to the severe dehydration that results.

## Symptomatic Hypoglycemia

**Symptomatic hypoglycemia** is an acute emergency in which a patient's blood glucose level drops and must be corrected swiftly. A low blood glucose level can occur in patients who inject insulin or use oral medications that stimulate the pancreas to produce more insulin. When insulin levels remain high, glucose is rapidly taken out of the blood to fuel the cells. If glucose levels fall too low, there may

---

### YOU are the Provider

You perform a primary assessment of the patient. You attempt to obtain more information from the patient, but he is slow to answer your questions and is slightly confused. He can tell you that he has been getting progressively worse over the past 3 to 5 days. The patient's friends and wife tell you he has been experiencing weight loss for the past month but he seems to be eating more and more.

| Recording Time: 0 Minutes | |
|---|---|
| **Appearance** | Weak and confused |
| **Level of consciousness** | Conscious, slow to respond, and confused |
| **Airway** | Open; clear of secretions or foreign bodies |
| **Breathing** | Increased rate and depth |
| **Circulation** | Radial pulses rapid and weak; skin warm and dry with poor turgor |

The patient's wife tells you that he has been urinating frequently and has been drinking large quantities of water, soda, and milk. Your partner assesses his blood glucose level using the glucometer.

**3.** What should you expect the patient's blood glucose level to read? Why?

**4.** What is causing the patient's frequent urination and deep, rapid breathing?

be an insufficient amount to supply the brain. The mental status of the patient declines precipitously and he or she may become aggressive or display unusual behavior. If blood glucose remains low, unconsciousness and permanent brain damage can quickly follow.

Symptomatic hypoglycemia can occur for many different reasons. Some of the more common reasons for a low blood glucose level to develop are because the patient or caregiver administered one of the following:

- A correct dose of insulin with a change in routine (the patient exercised more, consumed a meal later than usual, or skipped the meal)
- More insulin than necessary
- A correct dose of insulin without the patient eating a sufficient amount
- A correct dose of insulin and an acute illness developed in the patient

Hypoglycemia develops much more quickly than hyperglycemia. In some instances, it can occur in a matter of minutes. Hypoglycemia can be associated with the following signs and symptoms:

- Normal to shallow or rapid respirations
- Pale, moist (clammy) skin (in dark-skinned people, paleness is more apparent by examining the mucous membranes inside the lower eyelid)
- Diaphoresis (sweating)
- Dizziness, headache
- Rapid pulse
- Normal to low blood pressure
- Altered mental status (aggressive, confused, lethargic, or unusual behavior)
- Anxious or combative behavior
- Seizure, fainting, or coma
- Weakness on one side of the body (may mimic stroke)
- Rapid changes in mental status

Hyperglycemia is a complex metabolic condition that usually develops over time and involves all the tissues of the body. Correcting this condition may take many hours in a well-controlled hospital setting. Hypoglycemia, however, is an acute condition that can develop rapidly. A patient with diabetes who has taken his or her standard insulin dose and missed lunch may have symptomatic hypoglycemia before dinner. The condition is just as quickly reversed by giving the patient glucose. Without the glucose, however, the patient can sustain permanent brain damage. Minutes count.

## Special Populations

Low blood glucose level events are not uncommon in pediatric patients. Most children adapt well to the routine of managing their diabetes, but during periods of growth, their blood glucose may be more difficult to regulate. Some toxic ingestions and overdose cause hypoglycemia in children. Children cannot store excess glucose as effectively as adults; therefore, the blood glucose level can drop in children even in the absence of diabetes or medication. As an EMT, you must have a high index of suspicion for a low glucose level when you encounter a child who has an altered mental status or depressed level of consciousness.

# Patient Assessment of Diabetes

## Scene Size-up

Evaluate scene safety as you arrive on scene and as you approach the patient. Make sure that all hazards are addressed. Remember that patients with diabetes often use syringes to administer insulin. It is possible you may be stuck by a used needle that was not disposed of properly. Insulin syringes on the nightstand, insulin bottles in the refrigerator, a plate of food, or a glass of orange juice are important clues that may help you decide what is possibly wrong with your patient. Evaluate each situation quickly, and make sure necessary personal protective equipment is readily available. Use standard precautions. As you approach, question bystanders on events leading to your arrival.

Although your report from dispatch may be for a patient with an altered mental status, keep open the possibility that trauma may have occurred because of a medical incident. Determine the mechanism of injury and/or nature of illness. Do not let your guard down, even on what appears to be a routine call.

## Primary Assessment

Perform a primary assessment to form a general impression of the patient. How does the patient look? Does the patient appear anxious, restless, or listless? Is the patient apathetic or irritable? Is the patient interacting appropriately with his or her environment? These initial observations may lead you to suspect high or low blood glucose values. Identify life threats, and provide life-saving interventions, particularly airway management. Determine the patient's level of consciousness using the AVPU scale. If a patient whom you suspect has diabetes is unresponsive, call for ALS immediately. An unconscious patient may have undiagnosed diabetes. In patients with altered mental status, you may be able to determine whether a diabetic emergency exists by assessing the patient's blood glucose level. At the emergency department (ED), diabetes and its complications can be quickly diagnosed.

Remember that even though a person has diabetes, the diabetes may not be causing the current problem; heart attack, stroke, or another medical emergency may be the cause. For this reason, you must always carry out a thorough, careful primary assessment, paying attention to the ABCs.

While you are forming your general impression, assess the patient's airway and breathing. Patients showing signs of inadequate breathing, a pulse oximetry level less than or equal to 94% on room air, or altered mental status should receive high-flow oxygen at 12 to 15 L/min via nonrebreathing mask. A patient who is hyperglycemic may have rapid, deep respirations (Kussmaul respirations) and sweet, fruity breath. A patient who is hypoglycemic will have normal or shallow to rapid respirations. If the patient is not breathing or is having difficulty breathing, open the airway and insert an airway adjunct, administer oxygen, and assist ventilations. Continue to monitor the airway while you provide care.

Once you have assessed the airway and breathing and have performed the necessary life-saving interventions, check the patient's circulatory status. Dry and warm skin indicates hyperglycemia, whereas moist and pale skin indicates hypoglycemia. Because skin paleness can be difficult to detect in patients with dark skin, instead check for pale mucous membranes inside the inner lower eyelid or slow capillary refill. The patient with symptomatic hypoglycemia will have a rapid, weak pulse.

Whether you decide to transport at this stage of the assessment will depend on the patient's level of consciousness and the ability to swallow. Patients with an altered mental status and impaired ability to swallow should be transported promptly.

Patients who have the ability to swallow and are conscious enough to maintain their own airway may be further evaluated on scene and interventions performed if appropriate.

## History Taking

Investigate the chief complaint or the history of the present illness. Responsive patients usually are able to provide their own medical history. If the patient has eaten but has not taken insulin, it is more likely that hyperglycemia is developing. If the patient has taken insulin but has not eaten, the problem is more likely to be hypoglycemia. A patient with diabetes will often know (or strongly suspect) what is wrong. If the patient is not thinking or speaking clearly (or is unconscious), ask a family member or bystander the same questions.

Physical signs such as tremors, abdominal cramps, vomiting, a fruity breath odor, or a dry mouth may guide you in determining whether the patient is hypoglycemic or hyperglycemic.

You will need to obtain a SAMPLE history from your patient or the family or bystanders if the patient is unable to speak. In addition, be sure to ask the following questions of a patient known to have diabetes:

- Do you take insulin or any pills that lower your blood sugar?
- Do you wear an insulin pump? Is it working properly?
- Have you taken your usual dose of insulin (or pills) today?
- Have you eaten normally today?
- Have you had any illness, unusual amount of activity, or stress?

When you are assessing a patient who might have diabetes, check to see whether the patient has an emergency medical identification device—a wallet card, necklace, or bracelet—or ask the patient or a family member. Remember that the environment, bystanders, and medical identification devices may provide important clues about your patient's condition.

## Secondary Assessment

In some instances where the patient is critically ill or injured or the transport time is short, you may not have time to conduct a secondary assessment.

In other instances, the secondary assessment may occur on scene or en route to the ED.

First, assess unresponsive patients from head to toe with a secondary assessment of the entire body, looking for clues to their condition. The patient may have experienced trauma resulting from dizziness or from changes in level of consciousness.

As with every call, you should perform a secondary assessment when time permits. With unconscious patients or patients with an altered mental status, you must assume the role of detective and look for problems or injuries that are not obvious because the patient is unable to communicate these to you. Although an altered mental status may be caused by a blood glucose level that is too high or too low, the patient may have sustained trauma or have another metabolic problem. An altered mental status may also be caused by something else, such as intoxication, poisoning, or a head injury. A systematic examination of the patient may provide you with information essential to proper patient care.

When you suspect a diabetes-related problem, a secondary assessment should focus on the patient's mental status and ability to swallow and protect the airway. Obtain a Glasgow Coma Scale score to track the patient's neurologic status.

Obtain a complete set of vital signs, including a measurement of the patient's blood glucose level using a glucometer. The portable blood glucose monitor measures the glucose level in whole blood using either capillary or venous samples. Advances in technology now allow patients to track their blood glucose in real time using wearable sensors such as Dexcom and FreeStyle that send information via Bluetooth to the patient's phone (**FIGURE 20-6**).

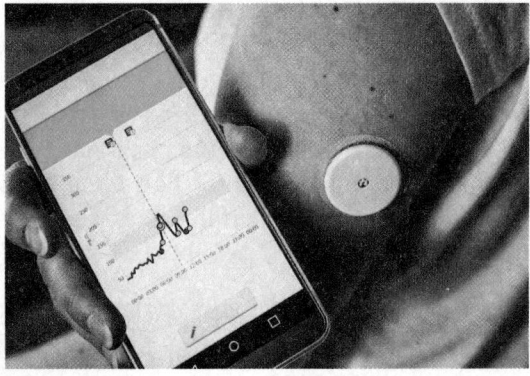

**FIGURE 20-6** Patients can track their blood glucose in real time by wearing a sensor that sends information via Bluetooth to their phone.

© Lukasz Pawel Szczepanski/Shutterstock.

In hypoglycemia, respirations are normal to rapid, pulse is weak and rapid, and skin is typically pale and clammy with a low blood pressure. Although paleness, or a decrease in blood flow, can be difficult to detect in dark-skinned people, it may be observed by examining mucous membranes inside the inner lower eyelid and capillary refill. On general observation, the patient may appear ashen or gray. In hyperglycemia, respirations may be deep and rapid; pulse may be rapid, weak, and thready; and skin may be warm and dry with a normal blood pressure. At times the blood pressure may be low. It should be easier for you to identify abnormal vital signs when you know the blood glucose level is too high or too low. Remember, the patient may have abnormal vital signs and a normal blood glucose value. When this is the case, something else may be causing the patient's altered mental status, vomiting, or other complaints.

It is important to read and understand the operator's manual before using a portable glucometer because the specifications of the device may vary depending on the manufacturer. Some glucometers indicate low ("Lo") when they detect a glucose reading less than 20 mg/dL, whereas others display Lo when they detect a reading less than 30 mg/dL. The same is true with a high ("Hi") reading; some glucometers read Hi at 550 mg/dL and some at 600 mg/dL; therefore, it is important to know both the upper and lower ranges at which your glucometer functions.

The normal range for glucose levels in blood in nonfasting adults and children is 80 to 120 mg/dL; the blood glucose level in neonates should be above 70 mg/dL.

## Reassessment

It is important to reassess the patient with diabetes frequently to assess changes. Is there an improvement in the patient's mental status? Are the ABCs still intact? How is the patient responding to the interventions performed? How must you adjust or change the interventions? In many patients with diabetes, you will note marked improvement with appropriate treatment. Document each assessment, your findings, the time of the interventions, and any changes in the patient's condition. Base your administration of glucose on serial glucometer readings. If a glucometer is not available, a deteriorating level of consciousness indicates that you need to provide more glucose.

If your patient is hypoglycemic, conscious, and able to swallow without the risk of aspiration, encourage him or her to take glucose tablets. If those are not available, household sources of glucose may be used, such as juice or other drinks that contain sugar. Do not be afraid to give too much sugar. Do not give sugar-free drinks that are sweetened with saccharin or other synthetic sweetening compounds, because they will have little or no effect. If you are permitted by local protocol, you may also assist the patient in administering a gel preparation or sugar drink. If your patient with hypoglycemia is unconscious, or if there is any risk of aspiration, the patient will need intravenous (IV) glucose, or intramuscular (IM) or intranasal (IN) glucagon, which most EMTs are not authorized to give. Your responsibility is to provide prompt transport to the hospital, where the proper care can be given. If you are working in a tiered system, AEMTs and paramedics are able to start an IV line and administer IV glucose.

A patient with symptomatic hypoglycemia (rapid onset of altered mental status, hypoglycemia) needs glucose immediately. A patient with symptomatic hyperglycemia (**acidosis**, dehydration, hyperglycemia) needs insulin and IV fluid therapy. These patients need prompt transport to the hospital for appropriate medical care.

When there is any doubt about whether a conscious patient with diabetes is going into symptomatic hypoglycemia or symptomatic hyperglycemia, most protocols will err on the side of giving glucose,

### Words of Wisdom

Intranasal glucagon is now available for use in some areas of the country to treat symptomatic hypoglycemia. This has the advantage of not requiring injection yet still achieving rapid absorption even in patients with markedly decreased levels of consciousness. Be aware of this medication and understand your local protocols regarding its use and indications.

### Safety Tips

Before you give a conscious patient glucose tablets, anything to eat or drink, or instant glucose, you must ensure that there is no danger of aspiration. As a general rule, if patients can lift the cup or squirt the glucose into their own mouths, they are most likely not in danger of aspiration. Watch them carefully!

even though the patient may have hyperglycemia or DKA. Untreated hypoglycemia will result in loss of consciousness and can quickly cause significant brain damage or death. The condition of a patient with symptomatic hypoglycemia is far more critical and far more likely to cause permanent problems than the condition of a patient with hyperglycemia or DKA. Furthermore, the amount of sugar that is typically given to a patient with symptomatic hypoglycemia is unlikely to make a patient with DKA significantly worse. When in doubt, consult medical control.

### YOU are the Provider

Your partner reports that the patient's blood glucose reading on the glucometer is 456 mg/dL. You continue to assess the patient while your partner obtains his vital signs. The patient's wife calls his doctor, who requests that you transport him to the closest hospital. A community hospital is located about 15 miles away.

| Recording Time: 5 Minutes | |
|---|---|
| **Respirations** | 30 breaths/min; deep |
| **Pulse** | 120 beats/min; weak radial pulses |
| **Skin** | Pink, warm, and dry; poor turgor |
| **Blood pressure** | 112/54 mm Hg |
| **Oxygen saturation (SpO$_2$)** | 97% (on room air) |

**5.** What other factors can cause hyperglycemia in patients with diabetes?

**6.** How can you distinguish symptomatic hyperglycemia from symptomatic hypoglycemia?

Determining whether the blood glucose level is too high or too low in a patient in whom diabetes is diagnosed can be difficult when signs and symptoms are confusing and you have no way to test for a blood glucose value. In these situations, perform a thorough assessment and contact the hospital to help sort out the signs and symptoms. The hospital should be a resource for you to help problem-solve situations and provide guidance on how to manage your patient.

## Safety Tips

Managing problems related to diabetes and altered mental status poses minimal risk to you because exposure to body fluids is generally very limited. However, some patients can become confused and even aggressive at times. Follow standard precautions, as you would with any other patient. Always use gloves, a mask, and appropriate eye protection and carefully wash your hands after obtaining and checking a blood sample or coming in contact with any airway secretions.

Communication with hospital staff is important for continuity of care. Hospital personnel need to be informed about the patient's history, the present situation, your assessment findings, and your interventions and their results.

Document your assessment findings clearly, because they represent the basis for your treatment.

## Special Populations

You may encounter an older patient who has undiagnosed diabetes. The patient is likely to report that he or she has not been feeling well for a while but has not seen a physician. A patient with undiagnosed diabetes or one who is in denial or ignores the advice of his or her physician may call 9-1-1 when the signs and symptoms become pronounced. Nonhealing wounds (which can lead to infection), blindness, renal failure, atypical (silent) myocardial infarction presentation, and other complications are associated with longstanding poorly controlled or uncontrolled diabetes. As an EMT, you may be the first to recognize and suggest medical treatment to an older patient. It is important that you recognize the signs and symptoms of diabetes.

## Street Smarts

Just as you are learning about the signs and symptoms of diabetes, your patient may not be aware of the long-term effects of the disease. Take a moment and share information with your patient. Your patient's life may one day depend on it!

Patients who refuse transport because their symptoms improve after taking oral glucose may require even more thorough documentation. Patients who receive treatment in the field for hypoglycemia are

## YOU are the Provider

Because of the patient's signs and symptoms, history, and a glucometer reading that indicates a high blood glucose level, you determine that oral glucose is not indicated. The patient is moved onto the stretcher and loaded into the ambulance. Shortly after departing the scene, you reassess his mental status and vital signs.

| Recording Time: 11 Minutes | |
| --- | --- |
| Level of consciousness | Conscious but confused |
| Respirations | 30 breaths/min; deep |
| Pulse | 124 beats/min; weak radial pulses |
| Skin | Pink, warm, and dry; poor turgor |
| Blood pressure | 108/56 mm Hg |
| Spo$_2$ | 97% (on room air) |

**7.** What additional treatment should you provide to this patient?

at great risk for development of symptomatic hypoglycemia in the near future and should be strongly discouraged from refusing further treatment or transportation to the hospital. Many long-acting forms of insulin and most oral diabetic medications remain in the bloodstream far longer than the glucose used to treat these patients. Follow your local protocols for patients who refuse treatment or transport.

## Emergency Medical Care for Diabetic Emergencies

### Giving Oral Glucose

There are three types of oral glucose preparations available commercially. The most common for EMS providers is a rapidly dissolving gel (**FIGURE 20-7**). The second preparation comes in a large chewable tablet. The third preparation is a liquid formulation. Glucose gel acts to increase a patient's blood glucose levels. If authorized by your system, you should administer glucose gel to any patient with a decreased level of consciousness who has a history of diabetes. The only contraindications to oral glucose are an inability to swallow and unconsciousness, because aspiration (inhalation of the substance) can occur. Oral glucose itself has no side effects if it is administered properly; however, the risk of aspiration in a patient who does not have a gag reflex is substantial. A conscious patient (even if confused) who does not really need glucose will not be harmed by it. Therefore, do not hesitate to give glucose under these circumstances.

Be sure to wear gloves before placing anything into a patient's mouth. After you have confirmed that the patient is conscious and able to swallow and have obtained an online or offline order, open the glucose pouch, and either the EMT or the patient can squeeze the glucose into the mouth either under the tongue or into the buccal space and then swallow.

As an EMT, you know the importance of reassessment. The patient with diabetes experiencing an altered mental status event that you treat with a glucose product is one of the most important patients to reassess frequently. As rapidly as you may see a response to your treatment, you can see a deterioration. Be mindful of the airway when giving an oral medication such as a glucose product—not only from the standpoint of placing something into the mouth but for resultant regurgitation of that product, which can be aspirated. Anytime you change a patient's mental status with a drug, follow-up must be provided. Therefore, it is always best to provide transport to the next level of care.

### Street Smarts

If the patient's mental status, vital signs, and blood glucose level become normal after administering glucose, encourage the patient to eat a meal or snack containing carbohydrates and protein such as eggs or a peanut butter sandwich. Although the oral glucose is essential to quickly raise the patient's blood glucose level, the snack will help to prevent the glucose level from dropping again.

### Words of Wisdom

Diabetes is a systemic disease affecting all tissues of the body, especially the kidneys, eyes, small arteries, and peripheral nerves. Therefore, you are likely to be called to treat patients with a variety of complications of diabetes, such as heart disease, visual disturbances, renal failure, stroke, and ulcers or infections of the feet or toes. Except for heart attack and stroke, most of these will not be acute emergencies. Considering that diabetes is a major risk factor for cardiovascular disease, patients with diabetes should always be suspected of having a potential for heart attack, particularly older patients, even when they do not present with classic symptoms such as chest pain and shortness of breath.

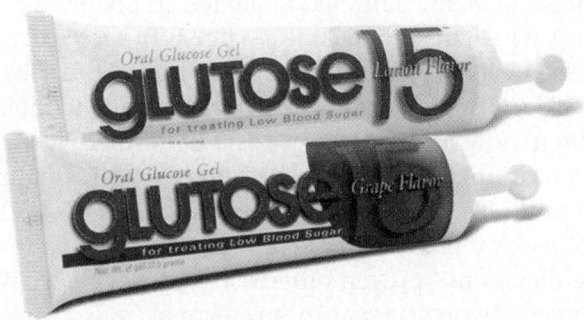

**FIGURE 20-7** Oral glucose is commercially available in gel and tablet form. One tube of gel equals one 15-gram dose.

Courtesy of Paddock Laboratories, Inc.

# The Presentation of Hypoglycemia

Recognition of the patient with hypoglycemia requires an intuitive approach. There are many classic, by-the-book presentations of hypoglycemia. However, each of the altered mental status presentations is identified in much the same way. The discovery comes from a rapid examination utilizing a list of possible conditions to rule out, leading to the ultimate identification of hypoglycemia.

## Seizures

Although seizures are rarely life threatening, you should consider them to be very serious, even in patients with a history of chronic seizures. Seizures, which may be brief or prolonged, are often caused by infections, poisoning, hypoglycemia, trauma, or decreased levels of oxygen, or they may be idiopathic (of unknown cause). In children, they may be caused by fever or epilepsy. Although brief seizures are not harmful, they may indicate a more dangerous and potentially life-threatening underlying condition. Because seizures can be the result of a head injury, consider trauma as a cause. In the patient with diabetes, you should also consider hypoglycemia.

Emergency medical care of seizures includes ensuring that the airway is clear and placing the patient on his or her side. Do not attempt to place anything in the patient's mouth (eg, a bite stick or an oral airway). Be sure to have suctioning equipment ready in case the patient vomits. Provide oxygen or artificial ventilation if the patient is cyanotic or appears to be breathing inadequately, and provide prompt transport.

## Altered Mental Status

Although altered mental status is often caused by complications of diabetes, it may also be caused by a variety of other conditions, including poisoning, infection, head injury, part of the postictal state (period following a seizure), and decreased perfusion to the brain. In diabetes, altered mental status can be caused by hypoglycemia and by ketoacidosis.

The mnemonic AEIOU-TIPS is easily remembered and covers a multitude of conditions that can lead to altered mental status. As such, many of the conditions covered by the mnemonic can be confused, resulting in a misdiagnosis when the patient's blood glucose level is not assessed. AEIOU-TIPS stands for the following conditions:

- Alcohol
- Epilepsy, endocrine, electrolytes
- Insulin
- Opiates and other drugs
- Uremia (kidney failure)
- Trauma, temperature
- Infection
- Poisoning, psychogenic causes
- Shock, stroke, seizure, space-occupying lesion, subarachnoid hemorrhage

Most of the items on the preceding list can be associated with or can cause hypoglycemia. A patient might have a seizure due to hypoglycemia. A patient with an altered mental status after a heroin overdose might also be hypoglycemic. Remember to consider diabetic emergencies in patients who present with any of these emergencies, which can alter or depress mental status. Also remember that patients who present with trauma and are unconscious may have become unconscious as a result of a low blood glucose level and secondarily became injured. Always suspect and check for low blood glucose in a patient with altered mental status.

Begin emergency medical care of altered mental status by ensuring that the airway is clear. Be prepared to provide artificial ventilation and suctioning in case the patient vomits, and provide prompt transport.

## Misdiagnosis of Neurologic Dysfunction

Occasionally, patients with hypoglycemia or hyperglycemia are thought to be intoxicated, especially if their condition has caused a motor vehicle crash or other incident. Confined by police at a police station, a patient with diabetes is at risk. In such situations, an emergency medical identification bracelet, necklace, or card may help to save the patient's life. Often, only a blood glucose test performed at the scene or in the ED will identify the real problem. In many EMS systems, you will be trained and allowed to perform blood glucose testing at the scene. Regardless, until proven otherwise, you must always suspect hypoglycemia in any patient with an altered mental status.

Certainly, diabetes and alcoholism can coexist in a patient. You must be alert to the similarity in symptoms of acute alcohol intoxication and diabetic emergencies. Likewise, hypoglycemia and a head injury can coexist, and you must appreciate the potential for hypoglycemia even when the head injury is obvious.

---

**Street Smarts**

Don't judge a book by its cover. What may appear to be a patient under the influence of alcohol may be a patient with hypoglycemia. Be a patient advocate and check the glucose level before making a judgment.

---

## Relationship to Airway Management

Patients with an altered mental status, particularly those who are difficult to awaken, may not have a gag reflex. When the gag reflex is not working, patients cannot expel foreign materials in their mouths (including vomit), and their tongues will often relax and obstruct the airway. Therefore, you must carefully monitor the airway in patients with hyperglycemia, hypoglycemia, or a complication related to diabetes such as stroke or seizure. Place the patient in a lateral recumbent position, and make sure suction is readily available.

## Hematologic Emergencies

Hematology is the study of blood-related diseases. This section begins by explaining the composition of blood. It then focuses on four disorders that may be seen in a prehospital emergency:

- Sickle cell disease (also called hemoglobin S disease)
- Hemophilia A (also called classic hemophilia or factor VIII deficiency)
- Thrombophilia
- Anemia

## Anatomy and Physiology
### Blood and Its Parts

Blood is made up of four components:

- Erythrocytes (red blood cells)
- Leukocytes (white blood cells)
- Platelets
- Plasma

Each of the components of the blood serves a purpose in maintaining a person's homeostatic balance. Each of the body's other systems provides for and utilizes the blood in a specific way. In turn, the blood transports oxygen and carbon dioxide into and out of tissues to sustain the function of the organ system and tissues.

Red blood cells (RBCs) make up 42% to 47% of a person's total blood volume. RBCs contain an important protein, hemoglobin, which carries 97% of the oxygen in the blood and some of the carbon dioxide.

White blood cells (WBCs) make up 0.1% to 0.2% of a person's blood cell volume. In a healthy person, WBCs collect dead cells and provide for their correct disposal. In times of health, WBC levels are low. When an infection develops, WBCs and all of their complementary defense systems are activated and their numbers grow.

Platelets make up 4% to 7% of a person's blood cell volume and are essential for clot formation. When damage occurs to your skin or to a blood vessel, platelets are sent to the site of injury to assist in forming a blood clot to stop the bleeding. Without this protective response, bleeding from a simple cut could be uncontrollable.

Plasma serves as the transportation medium for all blood components as well as proteins and minerals.

## Pathophysiology
### Sickle Cell Disease

Sickle cell disease, also called hemoglobin S disease, is an inherited blood disorder that affects the RBCs. The name sickle cell comes from the first case report of the disease in 1910, when Dr. James Herrick wrote that the RBCs looked like a sickle (**FIGURE 20-8**). The odd-shaped cells protect the individual from contracting malaria. This protection is useful to people who live in sub-Saharan Africa where malaria is common, but it is not useful to people who do not live in regions endemic for malaria.

There are several variants that make up this genetic disease. It is sufficient to simply understand that the issues of sickle cell can happen with any of the variants. This disease is common among people of African, Caribbean, and South American ancestry. It is present but less common in Mediterranean and

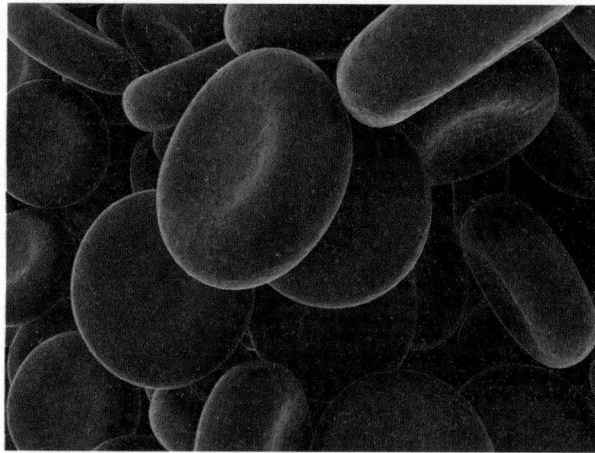

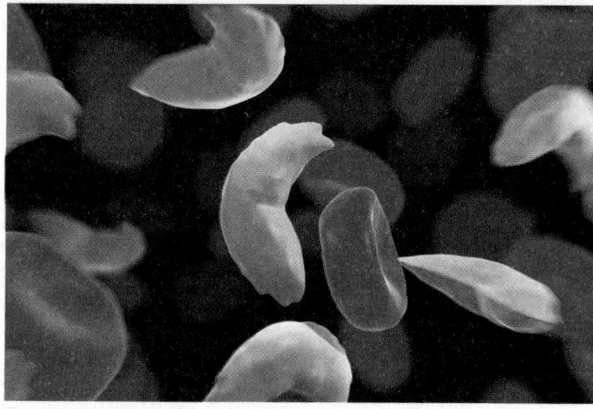

**FIGURE 20-8 A.** Normal red blood cells. **B.** Sickle cells.

A: © Sebastian Kaulitzki/Shutterstock; B: © Science Picture Co/Science Source.

Middle Eastern people. All newborns in the United States are tested for sickle cell disease shortly after birth, regardless of their race or ethnic background.

The sharp and misshapen cells lead to dysfunction in oxygen binding and unintentional clot formation. These unintentional clots may result in a blockage known as **vasoocclusive crisis**.

People with sickle cell disease can experience hypoxia, or a lack of oxygen in the body's cells and tissues. The blockages that result from sickle cell crises or vasoocclusive crises can result in substantial pain and organ damage, which can trigger calls to EMS for help.

The life span of normal RBCs is approximately 110 to 120 days; sickled cells have a much shorter life span. This results in more cellular waste products in the bloodstream, which can contribute to sludging (clumping) of the blood. Maintaining hydration status is important to these patients, as is

maintaining their general health, because insufficient hydration leads to increased clumping of cells.

Complications associated with sickle cell disease include the following:

- Anemia
- Gallstones
- Jaundice
- Splenic dysfunction
- Vascular occlusion with ischemia:
  - Acute chest syndrome (hypoxia, dyspnea, chest discomfort, and fever)
  - Stroke
  - Bone necrosis (avascular necrosis; specifically the head of the femur and the humerus)
  - Pain crises
  - Acute and chronic organ dysfunction/failure
  - Retinal hemorrhages
  - Increased risk of infection

Many of these complications are very painful and potentially life threatening. In the face of these complications the patient with sickle cell anemia is also more susceptible to infections.

## Hemophilia

**Hemophilia** is rare; according to the Hemophilia Federation of America, there are only approximately 20,000 Americans who have the disorder.

Hemophilia A mostly affects males. Males inherit the condition from a mother who is a carrier but does not have the disease; females only inherit the condition if their mother is a carrier and their father has the disease.

People with hemophilia A have a decreased ability to create a clot after an injury. The blood of a healthy individual will clot in as little as 13 seconds after a paper cut and not longer than approximately 7 minutes following a more serious injury that requires direct pressure. Having an extended bleeding time from the inability to clot can be life threatening.

A patient who is otherwise healthy but has hemophilia A can have a serious reaction to a minor trauma, such as a simple ankle sprain while playing soccer. Most people would ignore the sprain and simply continue to play the game. The patient with hemophilia A would begin to experience swelling from uncontrolled bleeding in the region of the injury and continue to do so, making the seemingly minor injury a significant problem.

Acute bleeding from any source may be life threatening, depending on where the bleeding occurs. Patients with hemophilia A can be prescribed medications to replace the missing clotting factors, release the clotting factors that are stored in the patient's body, or prevent the breakdown of blood clots.

Common complications of hemophilia A include the following:

- Long-term joint problems, which may require a joint replacement
- Bleeding in the brain (intracerebral hemorrhage)
- Thrombosis due to treatment

## Thrombophilia

Thrombophilia is a disorder in the body's ability to maintain the viscosity and smooth flow of blood through the venous and arterial systems. In thrombophilia, the concentration of particular elements in the blood creates what amounts to clogging or blockage issues.

Thrombophilia is a general term for many different conditions that result in the blood clotting more easily than normal. This results from either inherited (genetic) disorders, medications, or other factors. Patients with cancer are at increased risk of forming life-threatening blood clots. Whatever the risk factors, the common theme is that clots can spontaneously develop in the blood of the patient.

## Deep Vein Thrombosis

Deep vein thrombosis (DVT) is a common medical problem in sedentary patients and in patients who have had recent injury or surgery. Although several risk factors increase the chance that a DVT will develop, there are several methods to prevent blood clot formation, including blood-thinning medications, compression stockings, and mechanical devices—all of which you may encounter in the field.

DVT is a particularly worrisome risk for patients who have had joint replacement surgery. Be suspicious of this in a patient with a recent history of joint replacement who complains of leg swelling. Travelers, truck and long-distance bus drivers, and bedridden nursing home patients all are at higher risk for DVT because they are sedentary for long periods of time.

If DVT develops in an individual, anticoagulation therapy may be administered. A patient with DVT may be treated in the hospital with IV medications and then transitioned to oral medications or self-administered subcutaneous injectable medications to treat or prevent DVT. Patients who have been prescribed medications such as heparin,

## YOU are the Provider

You reassess the patient and then call your radio report to the receiving hospital. The patient is still conscious, but confused. Your estimated time of arrival at the hospital is 8 minutes.

| Recording Time: 17 Minutes | |
| --- | --- |
| **Level of consciousness** | Conscious, but confused |
| **Respirations** | 28 breaths/min; deep |
| **Pulse** | 118 beats/min; weak radial pulses |
| **Skin** | Pink, warm, and dry; poor turgor |
| **Blood pressure** | 110/58 mm Hg |
| **Spo₂** | 97% (on room air) |

You arrive at the hospital and transfer patient care to the attending physician. After further assessment and treatment in the ED, the patient is admitted to the medical intensive care unit.

**8.** What treatment is provided at the hospital for patients with symptomatic hyperglycemia that cannot be provided in the prehospital setting?

warfarin (Coumadin), dabigatran (Pradaxa), or rivaroxaban (Xarelto) to treat DVT are at increased risk of bleeding complications (ie, gastrointestinal bleeding or stroke), and minor trauma is more likely to produce severe internal or external hemorrhage.

A life threat can develop if the clot from the DVT travels from the patient's lower extremity to the lung, causing a pulmonary embolus. Pulmonary emboli can cause chest pain, difficulty breathing, or, if the clots are large, sudden cardiac arrest. Pulmonary embolism is discussed in Chapter 16, *Respiratory Emergencies*.

## Anemia

Anemia is an abnormally low number of RBCs. RBCs contain hemoglobin, an iron-containing pigment that is responsible for 97% of the transport of oxygen from the lungs to the cells of the body. Each hemoglobin molecule is able to bind to and carry four molecules of oxygen. Anemia may be the result of either chronic or acute bleeding, a deficiency in certain vitamins or minerals, or an underlying disease process. If anemia is present, tissues may become hypoxic because the blood is unable to deliver adequate amounts of oxygen to the tissues, even though the available hemoglobin is fully saturated with oxygen and the lungs are delivering enough oxygen to the blood. In this situation, a pulse oximeter may indicate that there is adequate saturation, even though the tissues are hypoxic. This type of hypoxia is known as hypoxemic hypoxia.

## Patient Assessment of Hematologic Disorders

### Scene Size-up

Although your report from dispatch may be for a patient with an unknown medical problem, most patients presenting with a sickle cell crisis have had a crisis before and will relay that information to the dispatcher. As you approach the scene, ensure your safety by assessing for hazards. Standard precautions should consist of gloves, mask, and eye protection at a minimum.

Determine whether this is your only patient and whether trauma was involved. Decide whether you will need any additional resources. Patients experiencing a vasoocclusive crisis are often in extreme pain and would benefit from ALS providers being able to administer analgesics.

Remember that trauma may have occurred because of a medical incident. Determine the mechanism of injury and/or nature of illness.

### Primary Assessment

An African American patient or any patient of Mediterranean descent who reports severe pain may have undiagnosed sickle cell disease.

Perform a primary assessment to form an initial general impression of the patient. How does the patient look? Does the patient appear anxious, restless, or listless? Is the patient apathetic or irritable? Determine the patient's level of consciousness.

While you are forming your general impression, assess the patient's airway and breathing. Patients showing signs of inadequate breathing or altered mental status should receive high-flow oxygen at 12 to 15 L/min via nonrebreathing mask. A patient who is experiencing a sickle cell crisis may have increased respirations as a result of severe pain or exhibit signs of pneumonia. If the patient is having difficulty breathing, open the airway and insert an airway adjunct, administer oxygen, and assist ventilations. Continue to monitor the airway as you provide care.

Once you have assessed the airway and breathing and have performed the necessary interventions, check the patient's circulatory status. An increased heart rate represents a compensatory mechanism to force the sickled cells through smaller blood vessels.

In patients with suspected hemophilia, be alert for signs of acute blood loss such as pallor, weak pulse, and hypotension. Note any bleeding, such as nosebleeds, bloody sputum, swollen joints, and blood in the urine or stool. Because of blood loss, patients with hemophilia may exhibit signs of hypoxia.

Whether you decide to rapidly transport the patient will depend on the severity of the patient's pain and the patient's wishes. Patients with a history of sickle cell disease, but those who have not had a crisis in some time, may require emotional support and refuse transport. However, transport to an ED should always be recommended to any patient who is experiencing a sickle cell crisis or hemophilia.

### History Taking

If the patient is conscious, what is the chief complaint or history of present illness?

Responsive medical patients are able to provide their own medical history to help you identify a cause for their severe pain. Physical signs, such as swelling of the fingers and toes, priapism, and jaundice, may guide you in determining whether the patient is experiencing a sickle cell crisis. It is also important to ascertain whether the pain is isolated to a single location or if pain is felt throughout the entire body. Is the patient having any visual disturbances? Is the patient experiencing any gastrointestinal problems, such as nausea, vomiting, or abdominal cramping? Is the patient reporting any chest pain or shortness of breath?

In a patient with known sickle cell disease, ask the following questions in addition to obtaining a SAMPLE history:

- Have you had a crisis before?
- When was the last time you had a crisis?
- How did your last crisis resolve?
- Have you had any illness, unusual amount of activity, or stress lately?

## Secondary Assessment

Next, systematically examine the patient, focusing on major joints at which cells congregate. Evaluate and document mental status using the AVPU scale.

Obtain a complete set of vital signs, including a measurement of the patient's oxygen saturation level. In patients experiencing a sickle cell crisis, respirations are normal to rapid, pulse is weak and rapid, and skin is typically pale and clammy with a low blood pressure.

Use pulse oximetry, if available. However, keep in mind that the oxygen saturation reading you obtain may be inaccurate as a result of the patient's anemic state.

## Reassessment

Reassess the patient frequently to determine if there have been changes in the patient's condition. For example, are there changes in the patient's mental status? Are the ABCs still intact? How is the patient responding to the interventions performed? Should you adjust or change the interventions? Document each assessment, your findings, the time of the interventions, and any changes in the patient's condition.

Administer supplemental oxygen via nonrebreathing mask at 12 to 15 L/min to attempt to compensate for decreased cellular oxygenation related to the sickled cells or hemophilia.

At the hospital, care for patients with sickle cell disease can include analgesics for pain, penicillin to treat infection, IV fluid for hydration, and, depending on the severity of the crisis, a blood transfusion.

Distinguishing a true sickle cell crisis from other nonspecific causes of pain can be difficult. Remember to perform a thorough assessment and consult with medical control as soon as feasible.

Hospital care for a patient with hemophilia may include IV therapy to treat hypotension and a transfusion of plasma. Analgesics may also be appropriate.

Communication with hospital staff is important for continuity of care. Inform hospital personnel about the patient's history, the current situation, your assessment findings, and your interventions and their results.

Document your assessment findings clearly, as they represent the basis for your treatment. Follow your local protocols for patients who refuse treatment or transport.

## Emergency Medical Care for Hematologic Disorders

Emergency care for patients with hematologic disorders is mainly supportive and symptomatic. Patients showing signs of inadequate breathing, decreased oxygen saturation, or altered mental status should receive high-flow oxygen at 12 to 15 L/min via nonrebreathing mask and should be placed in a position of comfort and transported rapidly to the hospital.

## YOU are the Provider SUMMARY

**1. What processes are being described by the patient?**

This presentation can be typical of many illnesses until you ask the correct questions. The 3- to 5-day, subtle flulike presentation is often how type 1 diabetes mellitus presents. People must eat to have energy, but the lack of insulin deprives cells of the fuel they need, and therefore no energy is produced.

The onset of type 1 diabetes mellitus takes some time to progress. For this reason, symptoms are initially subtle and are overlooked by the patient. As the lack of insulin becomes more profound, the patient will notice increasing fatigue and malaise along with weight loss.

The patient is also experiencing (1) polydipsia, (2) polyuria, and (3) polyphagia.

Without insulin, glucose accumulates in the blood. Glucose spills into the urine until it reaches the kidney's maximum level to excrete. The glucose in the urine pulls a substantial amount of water with it, resulting in large amounts of urination (*polyuria*), causing dehydration. The patient experiences thirst, causing the patient to drink large amounts of fluid; this is called *polydipsia*. Finally, eating in excess (*polyphagia*) occurs in the face of weight loss. Polyphagia develops because of the starvation of the patient at the cellular level.

Many times the patient does not recognize these symptoms, but family and friends might, especially if they have had previous experience with diabetes.

**2. What hormone is missing in type 1 diabetes mellitus?**

The missing hormone is insulin. Insulin is the key to the door of the cell. Without insulin, nutrition in the form of glucose cannot get into the cell and the cell cannot function normallly.

**3. What should you expect the patient's blood glucose level to read? Why?**

Based on the description of increased food intake with weight loss, increased fluid intake, and increased urination, this patient appears to be hyperglycemic and may be in DKA. In these cases, the blood glucose level will be in the mid 400s to 500s or even higher. This level is much higher than the normal blood glucose level of 80 to 120 mg/dL.

**4. What is causing the patient's frequent urination and deep, rapid breathing?**

The frequent urination is occurring because an increase in his blood glucose level resulted in glucose spilling into the urine. He is excreting large amounts of urine because glucose in the urine pulls water out with it. This secondarily causes him to experience excessive thirst and to drink large amounts of fluid.

Deep, rapid breathing, known as Kussmaul respirations, is caused by the ketones that are accumulating in the blood and are being eliminated from the lungs during exhalation. Kussmaul respirations often have a fruity or sweet odor.

**5. What other factors can cause hyperglycemia in patients with diabetes?**

Changing mealtimes, insulin dosage changes, or a variation in exercise can result in a hyperglycemic or hypoglycemic event. An infection or other major stressors to the body could easily put an otherwise well-regulated patient with type 1 diabetes into DKA. Noncompliance with medication use can also result in hyperglycemic episodes. The patient in this chapter's scenario has new-onset diabetes and is in DKA. Noncompliance with medication use can also result in hyperglycemic episodes.

**6. How can you distinguish symptomatic hyperglycemia from symptomatic hypoglycemia?**

A key to distinguishing a hyperglycemic emergency from a hypoglycemic emergency is the time of symptom onset. Hyperglycemia, ketoacidosis, and dehydration typically progress over hours to days. By contrast, hypoglycemia has an acute onset—often over a period of a few minutes.

Symptomatic hyperglycemia and symptomatic hypoglycemia also present with relatively different signs and symptoms. Signs and symptoms of symptomatic hyperglycemia may include tachycardia; signs of dehydration (warm, dry skin, poor skin turgor, and sunken eyes); deep, rapid breathing (Kussmaul respirations), which indicates the respiratory system is attempting to eliminate ketones from the body; a sweet or fruity (acetone) breath odor; and mental status changes ranging from confusion to coma.

Symptomatic hypoglycemia presents with signs and symptoms similar to hypoxemia and shock that may include rapid, shallow respirations; pale, cool, clammy (diaphoretic) skin; tachycardia; weakness, which may be confined to one side of the body and mimic a stroke; and varying degrees of mental status change, including confusion, irritability, combativeness, seizures, and coma.

**7. What additional treatment should you provide to this patient?**

The patient's signs and symptoms clearly point to symptomatic hyperglycemia, and DKA. Symptomatic

## YOU are the Provider SUMMARY *continued*

hyperglycemia requires definitive care that can only be provided at the hospital. Prehospital treatment at the EMT level is aimed at providing supportive care (ie, maintaining the ABCs) and promptly transporting the patient to the hospital. En route, closely monitor the patient's mental status and breathing adequacy; if his respirations become slow and/or shallow—especially if his mental status deteriorates further—assist his ventilations with a bag-mask device.

Some patients with symptomatic hyperglycemia become so dehydrated that hypovolemic shock develops; therefore, it is important to closely monitor the patient's perfusion status (eg, heart rate, peripheral pulse quality, blood pressure, mental status). If signs of shock are observed, keep the patient warm and in a supine position and administer oxygen if not already applied. Although the patient is extremely thirsty, do not give him anything to drink; doing so increases the risk of aspiration if he vomits.

**8. What treatment is provided at the hospital for patients with symptomatic hyperglycemia that cannot be provided in the prehospital setting?**

Symptomatic hyperglycemia is a complex medical problem that causes numerous complications; it cannot be treated in the prehospital setting, and it cannot be changed quickly. Insulin is needed to restore circulating blood glucose to a normal level, and IV fluids are needed to correct dehydration.

This underscores the importance of performing a rapid assessment, initiating treatment without delay, and promptly transporting the patient to the hospital.

If your transport time will be prolonged, consider an intercept with an ALS unit, if available; AEMTs and paramedics are trained to start IV lines and administer fluids.

### EMS Patient Care Report (PCR)

| **Date:** 09-19-20 | **Incident No.:** 011609 | **Nature of Call:** Weakness, nausea | | **Location:** 445 Landon Way | |
|---|---|---|---|---|---|
| **Dispatched:** 1500 | **En Route:** 1502 | **At Scene:** 1508 | **Transport:** 1529 | **At Hospital:** 1545 | **In Service:** 1558 |

#### Patient Information

| | |
|---|---|
| **Age:** 23<br>**Sex:** M<br>**Weight (in kg [lb]):** 91 kg (200 lb) | **Allergies:** No known drug allergies<br>**Medications:** None<br>**Past Medical History:** None<br>**Chief Complaint:** Weakness and confusion |

#### Vital Signs

| **Time:** 1513 | **BP:** 112/54 | **Pulse:** 120 | **Respirations:** 30 | **Spo$_2$:** 95% |
|---|---|---|---|---|
| **Time:** 1519 | **BP:** 108/56 | **Pulse:** 124 | **Respirations:** 30 | **Spo$_2$:** 96% |
| **Time:** 1525 | **BP:** 110/58 | **Pulse:** 118 | **Respirations:** 28 | **Spo$_2$:** 97% |
| **Time:** 1539 | **BP:** 106/60 | **Pulse:** 116 | **Respirations:** 30 | **Spo$_2$:** 97% |

#### EMS Treatment (circle all that apply)

| **Oxygen @ __ L/min via:**<br><br>NC   NRM   Bag mask | | **Assisted Ventilation** | **Airway Adjunct** | **CPR** |
|---|---|---|---|---|
| **Defibrillation** | **Bleeding Control** | **Bandaging** | **Splinting** | **Other:** Blood glucose level |

# YOU are the Provider SUMMARY *continued*

| Narrative |
|---|

9-1-1 dispatch for a patient with weakness/nausea.

Chief Complaint: Weakness and confusion

History: The patient's wife advised that he has been sick for the past few days. He has been urinating excessively and has been drinking a lot of water.

Assessment: Arrived on scene and found the patient, a 23-year-old man, lying on the couch in his living room. He was conscious but confused. His airway was patent, and his breathing was deep and rapid. Further assessment of the patient revealed that his radial pulse was rapid and weak; his skin was pink, warm, and dry; and he had poor skin turgor. Breath sounds were clear to auscultation bilaterally, pupils were equal and reactive to light, there were no gross signs of trauma, and the patient had a sweet, fruity odor on his breath.

Treatment (Rx): Vital signs were obtained and blood glucose level was assessed and noted to be 456 mg/dL.

Transport: The patient's wife spoke with his physician, who requested EMS transport to the closest appropriate facility. Patient stood and pivoted onto stretcher with assistance and loaded into the ambulance. Mental status and vital signs were reassessed during transport; his mental status and vital signs remained unchanged. Notified receiving facility of our impending arrival; no further medical direction was given. Delivered patient to emergency department; his condition was unchanged. Gave verbal report to attending physician Ehlert, transferred patient care, and returned to service.

**End of report**

# Prep Kit

## Ready for Review

- Diabetes is a disorder of glucose metabolism or difficulty metabolizing carbohydrates, fats, and proteins.
- There are two types of diabetes. Type 1 diabetes typically develops in childhood and requires daily insulin to control blood glucose. Type 2 diabetes typically develops in middle age and often can be controlled with diet, activity, and oral medications.
- Both types of diabetes are serious systemic diseases, especially affecting the kidneys, eyes, small arteries, and peripheral nerves.
- Patients with diabetes have chronic complications that place them at risk for other diseases, such as heart attack, stroke, and infections. Most often, however, you will be called on to treat the acute complications of blood glucose imbalance. These include hyperglycemia (excess blood glucose) and hypoglycemia (insufficient blood glucose).

- Hyperglycemia is typically characterized by excessive urination and resulting thirst, in conjunction with the deterioration of body tissues.
- Hyperglycemia is usually associated with dehydration and ketoacidosis and can result in marked rapid (often deep) respirations; warm, dry skin; a weak pulse; and a fruity breath odor. Hyperglycemia must be treated in the hospital with insulin and IV fluids.
- Symptoms of hypoglycemia classically include confusion; rapid respirations; pale, moist skin; diaphoresis; dizziness; fainting; and even coma and seizures. Although paleness, or a decrease in blood flow, can be difficult to detect in dark-skinned people, it may be observed by examining mucous membranes inside the inner lower eyelid and capillary refill. On general observation, the patient may appear ashen or gray. This condition is rapidly reversible with the administration of glucose or sugar. Without

- treatment, however, permanent brain damage and death can occur.
- Because a blood glucose level that is either too high or too low can result in altered mental status, you must perform a thorough history and patient assessment to determine the nature of the problem. When the problem cannot be determined, it is best to treat the patient for hypoglycemia.
- Be prepared to give oral glucose to a conscious patient who is confused or has a slightly decreased level of consciousness; however, do not give oral glucose to a patient who is unconscious or otherwise unable to swallow properly or protect his or her own airway.
- In all cases, providing emergency medical care and prompt transport is your primary responsibility.

- Sickle cell disease is a blood disorder that affects the shape of RBCs.
- Symptoms of sickle cell disease are pain in the joints, fever, respiratory distress, and abdominal pain.
- Patients with sickle cell disease have chronic complications that place them at risk for other diseases, such as heart attack, stroke, and infection. Most often, however, you will be called on to treat the acute complications of severe pain.
- Patients with hemophilia are not able to control bleeding because clots do not develop as they should.
- Emergency care in the prehospital setting is supportive for patients with sickle cell disease or a clotting disorder such as hemophilia.

## Vital Vocabulary

**acidosis** The buildup of excess acid in the blood or body tissues that can result from a primary illness.

**diabetes mellitus** A metabolic disorder in which the ability to metabolize carbohydrates (sugars) is impaired, usually because of a lack of insulin.

**diabetic ketoacidosis (DKA)** A form of hyperglycemia in uncontrolled diabetes in which certain acids accumulate when insulin is not available.

**endocrine glands** Glands that secrete or release chemicals that are used inside the body.

**endocrine system** The complex message and control system that integrates many body functions, including the release of hormones.

**glucose** One of the basic sugars; it is the primary fuel, in conjunction with oxygen, for cellular metabolism.

**hematology** The study and prevention of blood-related disorders.

**hemophilia** A hereditary condition in which the patient lacks one or more of the blood's normal clotting factors.

**hormones** Substances formed in specialized organs or glands and carried to another organ or group of cells in the same organism; they regulate many body functions, including metabolism, growth, and body temperature.

**hyperglycemia** An abnormally high blood glucose level.

**hyperosmolar hyperglycemic nonketotic syndrome (HHNS)** A life-threatening condition resulting from high blood glucose that typically occurs in older adults and which causes altered mental status, dehydration, and organ damage.

**hypoglycemia** An abnormally low blood glucose level.

**insulin** A hormone produced by the islets of Langerhans (endocrine gland located throughout the pancreas) that enables glucose in the blood to enter cells; used in synthetic form to treat and control diabetes mellitus.

**Kussmaul respirations** Deep, rapid breathing; usually the result of an accumulation of certain acids when insulin is not available in the body.

**polydipsia** Excessive thirst that persists for long periods despite reasonable fluid intake; often the result of excessive urination.

**polyphagia** Excessive eating; in diabetes, the inability to use glucose properly can cause a sense of hunger.

**polyuria** The passage of an unusually large volume of urine in a given period; in diabetes, this can result from the wasting of glucose in the urine.

**sickle cell disease** A hereditary disease that causes normal, round red blood cells to become oblong, or sickle shaped.

**symptomatic hyperglycemia** A state of unconsciousness resulting from several problems, including ketoacidosis, dehydration because of excessive urination, and hyperglycemia.

**symptomatic hypoglycemia** Severe hypoglycemia resulting in changes in mental status.

**thrombophilia** A tendency toward the development of blood clots as a result of an abnormality of the system of coagulation.

**thrombosis** A blood clot, either in the arterial or venous system.

**type 1 diabetes** An autoimmune disorder in which the individual's immune system produces antibodies to the pancreatic beta cells, and therefore the pancreas cannot produce insulin; onset in early childhood is common.

**type 2 diabetes** A condition in which insulin resistance develops in response to increased blood glucose levels; can be managed by exercise and diet modification, but is often managed by medications.

**vasoocclusive crisis** Ischemia and pain caused by sickle-shaped red blood cells that obstruct blood flow to a portion of the body.

# References

1. Dexcom continuous glucose monitoring [Home page]. Dexcom website. https://www.dexcom.com/. Accessed March 31, 2020.

2. Eckel RH, Kahn SE, Ferrannini E, et al. Obesity and type 2 diabetes: what can be unified and what needs to be individualized? *Diabetes Care* 2011;34(6):1424–1430.

3. FreeStyle Libre: patients can get accurate glucose readings without daily calibration. Myfreestyle.com website. https://provider.myfreestyle.com/sensor-technology .html. Accessed March 31, 2020.

4. Hyperglycemia in diabetes: symptoms. Mayo Clinic website. https://www.mayoclinic.org/diseases-conditions /hyperglycemia/symptoms-causes/syc-20373631. Accessed March 31, 2020.

5. National Association of State EMS Officials. *National EMS Scope of Practice Model 2019*. Washington, DC: National Highway Traffic Safety Administration; February 2019. Report No. DOT HS 812-666. https:// www.ems.gov/pdf/National_EMS_Scope_of_Practice _Model_2019.pdf. Accessed March 31, 2020.

6. *National Emergency Medical Services Education Standards*. U.S. Department of Transportation, National Highway Traffic Safety Administration. DOT HS 811 077A. January 2009. www.ems.gov/pdf/811077a.pdf. Accessed March 31, 2020.

7. *National Emergency Medical Services Education Standards. Emergency Medical Technician Instructional Guidelines*. U.S. Department of Transportation, National Highway Traffic Safety Administration. DOT HS 811 077C. January 2009. www.ems.gov/pdf/811077c.pdf. Accessed March 31, 2020.

8. Ogden CL, Carroll MD, Kit BK, Flegal KM. Prevalence of childhood and adult obesity in the United States, 2011–2012. *JAMA* 2014;311(8):806–814.

9. Savitt TL, Goldberg MF. Herrick's 1910 case report of sickle cell anemia: the rest of the story. *JAMA* 1989;261(2):266–271.

10. Statistics about diabetes: overall numbers. American Diabetes Association website. https://www.diabetes.org/ resources/statistics/statistics-about-diabetes. Accessed March 31, 2020.

11. Type 2 diabetes. Mayo Clinic website. https://www .mayoclinic.org/diseases-conditions/type-2-diabetes /diagnosis-treatment/drc-20351199. Accessed March 31, 2020.

12. What is hemophilia? Centers for Disease Control and Prevention website. https://www.cdc.gov/ncbddd /hemophilia/facts.html. Reviewed June 3, 2019. Accessed March 31, 2020.

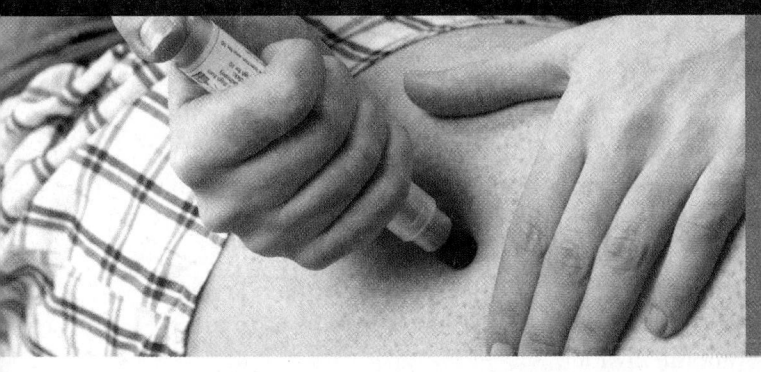

# Chapter 21

# Allergy and Anaphylaxis

## NATIONAL EMS EDUCATION STANDARD COMPETENCIES

### Medicine
Applies fundamental knowledge to provide basic emergency care and transportation based on assessment findings for an acutely ill patient.

### Immunology
Recognition and management of shock and difficulty breathing related to

- Anaphylactic reactions (pp 808–816)

Anatomy, physiology, pathophysiology, assessment, and management of
- Hypersensitivity disorders and/or emergencies (pp 804–816)
- Anaphylactic reactions (pp 804–816)

## KNOWLEDGE OBJECTIVES

1. Define the terms *allergic reaction* and *anaphylaxis*. (p 804)
2. Explain the difference between a local response and a systemic response to allergens. (p 804)
3. List the five categories of stimuli that could cause an allergic reaction or an extreme allergic reaction. (p 806)
4. Differentiate the primary assessment for a patient with a systemic allergic or anaphylactic reaction and with a local reaction. (pp 808–809)
5. Explain the importance of managing the ABCs of a patient who is having an allergic reaction. (p 808)
6. Discuss the steps in the primary assessment that are specific to a patient who is having an allergic reaction. (pp 808–810)

7. Explain the factors involved when making a transport decision for a patient having an allergic reaction. (p 809)
8. Review the process for providing emergency medical care to a patient who is experiencing an allergic reaction. (pp 811–816)
9. Explain the rationale, including communication and documentation considerations, when determining whether to administer epinephrine to a patient who is having an allergic reaction. (pp 813–816)
10. Describe some age-related contraindications to using epinephrine to treat an allergic reaction in a geriatric patient. (p 816)

## SKILLS OBJECTIVES

1. Demonstrate how to remove the stinger from a honeybee sting and proper patient management following its removal. (pp 812–813)

2. Demonstrate how to use an EpiPen auto-injector. (pp 813–815, Skill Drill 21-1)

# Introduction

Approximately 1,500 to 2,000 deaths in the United States per year are attributed to systemic anaphylaxis. The lifetime incidence of systemic anaphylaxis in adults is estimated at 2% to 8%. Half of the anaphylactic reactions in the United States occur at home.

Death as a result of allergic reaction is rare, but it is possible. The fatality rate in the United States is less than 1 per million. Case fatality rates for those reaching the hospital emergency department (ED) in anaphylaxis are slightly higher. As an EMT, you will often respond to calls involving an allergic reaction. When managing allergy-related emergencies, you must be aware of the possibility of acute airway obstruction and cardiovascular collapse and be prepared to treat these life-threatening complications. You must also be able to distinguish between the body's usual response to a sting or bite and an allergic reaction, which may require epinephrine. Your ability to recognize and manage the many signs and symptoms of allergic reactions may be the only thing standing between a patient's life and imminent death.

This chapter describes immunology, the study of the body's immune system, and the five categories of stimuli that may provoke allergic reactions. You will learn what to look for in assessing patients who may be having an allergic reaction and how to care for them, including administration of epinephrine.

# Anatomy and Physiology

The immune system protects the human body from foreign substances and organisms. Without the immune system for protection, life as you know it would not exist. You would be under constant attack from multiple types of invaders, such as bacteria or viruses, that wanted to make your body a home. Fortunately, most people have immune systems that are well equipped to detect unauthorized visits or invading attacks by foreign substances. Once a foreign substance invades the body, the body goes on alert and initiates a series of responses to inactivate the invader.

# Pathophysiology

There are many conditions related to the immune system, but an allergic reaction is the only immunologic emergency you will treat as an EMT. Contrary to what many people think, an allergic reaction, an exaggerated immune response to any substance, is not caused directly by an outside stimulus, such as a bite or sting or ingestion of food or medicine. Rather, it is a reaction by the body's immune system, which releases chemicals to combat the stimulus. Among these chemicals are histamines and leukotrienes, both of which contribute to an allergic reaction. Given the right person and the right circumstances, almost any substance can become an allergen. However, some people do not experience allergic reactions the first time they are exposed to an allergen. First, the person becomes *sensitized* (exposed for the first time) to the substance, and then his or her immune system learns to recognize it. When the patient is exposed to the substance again, an allergic reaction occurs. As a result, some patients may not have any idea what is causing their allergic reaction—they may not realize they are having one at all—so you must be able to recognize the signs and symptoms and maintain a high index of suspicion. An allergic reaction may be mild and local—characterized by itching, redness, or tenderness—or it may be severe and systemic, a condition known as anaphylaxis (**FIGURE 21-1**).

## YOU are the Provider

You and your partner respond to a call involving a 33-year-old man experiencing shortness of breath. On arrival, you observe a conscious patient in obvious respiratory distress, breathing rapidly with audible wheezing. His skin is flushed red and covered in hives. When you attempt to question the patient, you find he can only speak in two- to three-word sentences.

**1.** What, if any, additional resources should you request?

**2.** What intervention or interventions should you perform without delay?

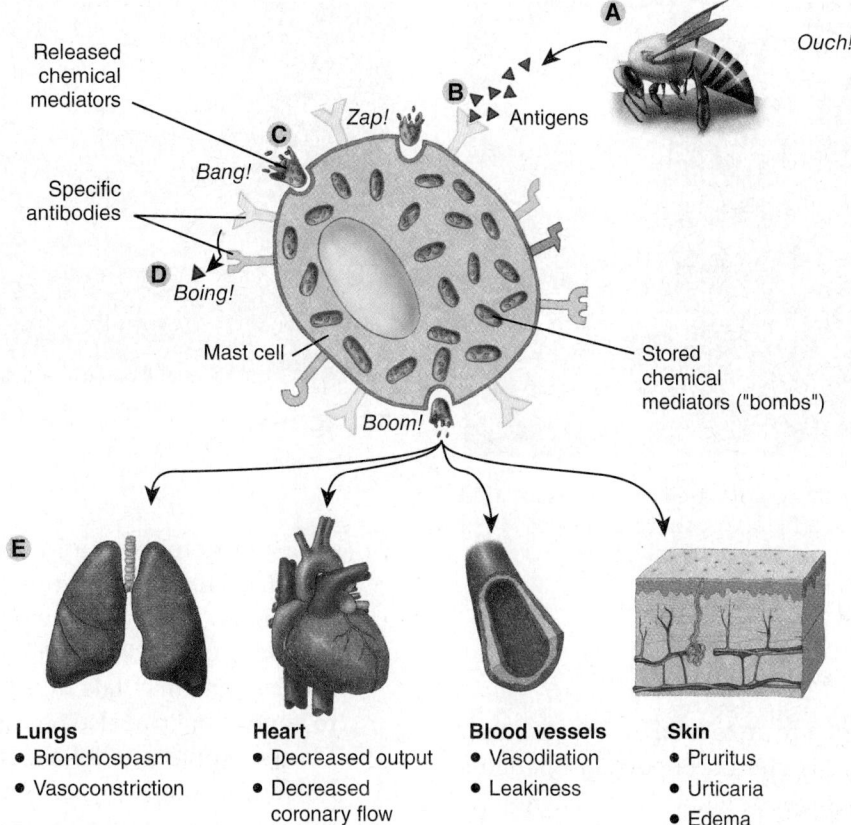

**FIGURE 21-1** The sequence of events in anaphylaxis. **A.** The antigen is introduced into the body. **B.** The antigen–antibody reaction at the surface of a mast cell. **C.** The release of mast cell chemical mediators. **D.** Specific antibody reacts with its corresponding antigen. **E.** Chemical mediators exert their effects on end organs.

© Jones & Bartlett Learning.

Anaphylaxis is an extreme allergic reaction that is life threatening and involves multiple organ systems. In severe cases, anaphylaxis can rapidly result in shock and death. Two of the most common signs of anaphylaxis are widespread urticaria, or hives, small areas of generalized itching or burning that appear as multiple small, raised areas on the skin (**FIGURE 21-2**), and angioedema, areas of localized swelling (**FIGURE 21-3**). Another often-observed sign is wheezing, a high-pitched, whistling breath sound that is typically heard on expiration, usually resulting from bronchospasm/bronchoconstriction and increased mucus production. Signs of possible upper airway narrowing include voice changes and stridor, a high-pitched respiratory sound that is usually heard during inspiration. You may also note hypotension due to vasodilation, as well as increased capillary permeability (causing

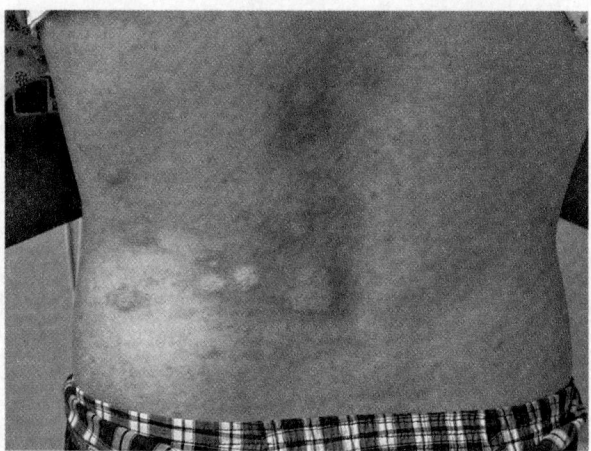

**FIGURE 21-2** Urticaria, or hives, may appear following exposure to an allergen and is characterized by multiple small, raised areas on the skin. Urticaria may be one of the warning signs of an impending anaphylactic reaction.

© Charles Stewart MD, EMDM MPH.

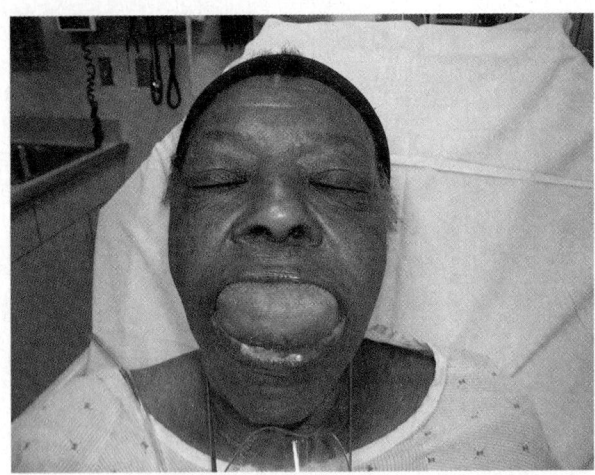

**FIGURE 21-3** Angioedema is localized swelling associated with allergic reactions. If the site of swelling includes the lips, tongue, larynx, or other such structures, airway obstruction may occur.

© E.M. Singletary, MD. Used with permission.

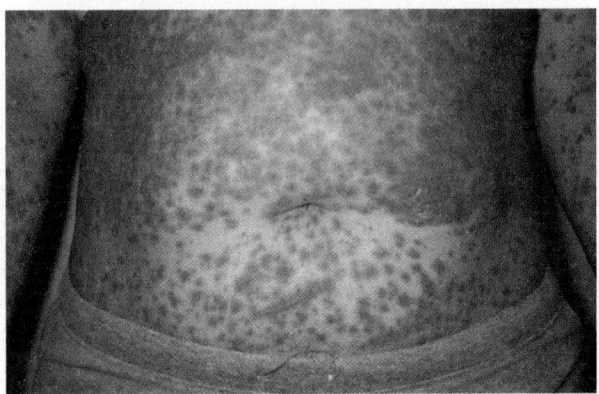

**FIGURE 21-4** A severe allergic reaction to medication.

Courtesy of Carol B. Guerrero.

fluid from the bloodstream to seep into the tissues). One symptom that is often overlooked in patients experiencing an allergic reaction is persistent gastrointestinal dysfunction (eg, nausea, vomiting, and abdominal cramps). Patients can also become confused.

## Common Allergens

The most common allergens fall into one of the following five general categories:

- **Food.** Certain foods, such as shellfish and peanuts, may be the most common trigger of anaphylaxis. These foods account for 30% of deaths from anaphylaxis, most commonly in adolescents and young adults. Symptoms of a food allergy may take more than 30 minutes to appear and may not include the presence of skin signs, such as hives. Abdominal cramping, vomiting, and diarrhea are common, and the reaction can be quite severe and involve the respiratory and/or cardiovascular systems. It is possible for a patient to be unaware of the exposure; for example, a person who is allergic to peanuts may eat something without knowing that one of the ingredients is peanuts.
- **Medication.** The second most common source of anaphylactic reactions is medication, particularly antibiotics (eg, penicillin)

and nonsteroidal anti-inflammatory drugs (NSAIDs). If the medication is injected, the reaction may be immediate (within 30 minutes) and severe (**FIGURE 21-4**). Reactions to oral medications may take more than 30 minutes to appear, but can also be very severe.
- **Plants.** People who inhale dust, pollen, mold, mildew, or other organic materials to which they are sensitive may experience an allergic reaction. Some common plant allergens include ragweed, ryegrass, maple, and oak.
- **Chemicals.** Certain chemicals, makeup, soap, hair dye, latex, and various other substances can cause severe allergic reactions. Latex is of particular concern to health care providers; patients can be sensitive to it, but so can you! Up to 10% of health care providers will become sensitized to latex. For some, simply being in the same room as someone wearing powdered latex gloves can cause a reaction. As a result, almost all EMS agencies use latex alternatives such as nitrile gloves. Follow your local protocol.
- **Insect bites and stings.** When an insect bites or stings, the act of injecting its venom is called envenomation. Envenomation by a honeybee, wasp, ant, yellow jacket, or hornet may cause a localized reaction, causing swelling and itching at the site, or a severe and systemic reaction (ie, anaphylaxis).

## Insect Stings

There are more than 100,000 species of bees, wasps, and hornets in the world. According to the Cleveland

Clinic, approximately 2 million Americans are allergic to the venom of these stinging insects, accounting for at least 62 deaths in the United States per year. Deaths from anaphylactic reactions to stinging insects far outnumber deaths from snake bites. In about one-half of these deaths, the victim had never experienced a reaction to prior stings.

The stinging organ of most bees, wasps, and hornets is a small, hollow spine projecting from the abdomen. Venom can be injected through this spine directly into the skin. The stinger of the honeybee is barbed, so the bee cannot withdraw it (**FIGURE 21-5A**). Therefore, the bee leaves a part of its abdomen embedded with the stinger and dies shortly after flying away. If the stinger is not removed from the skin (discussed later in this chapter), it can continue to inject venom for up to 20 minutes. Wasps and hornets do not have this handicap; they can sting repeatedly (**FIGURE 21-5B**). Because these insects usually fly away after stinging, it is often impossible to identify which species was responsible for the injury.

Some ants, especially the fire ant (**FIGURE 21-6A**), also strike repeatedly, injecting a particularly irritating toxin, or poison, at the bite sites. It is not uncommon for a patient to rapidly sustain multiple ant bites, usually on the feet and legs (**FIGURE 21-6B**).

Signs and symptoms of insect stings and bites include sudden pain, swelling, localized heat, widespread urticaria, and redness in light-skinned people, usually at the site of injury. There may be itching and sometimes a wheal, which is a raised, swollen, well-defined area on the skin (**FIGURE 21-7**). The swelling associated with an insect bite may be dramatic and sometimes frightening to the patient or to you. However, as long as these manifestations remain localized, they are not usually serious.

In more severe (anaphylactic) cases, patients may experience stridor, bronchospasm and wheezing, chest tightness and coughing, dyspnea, anxiety,

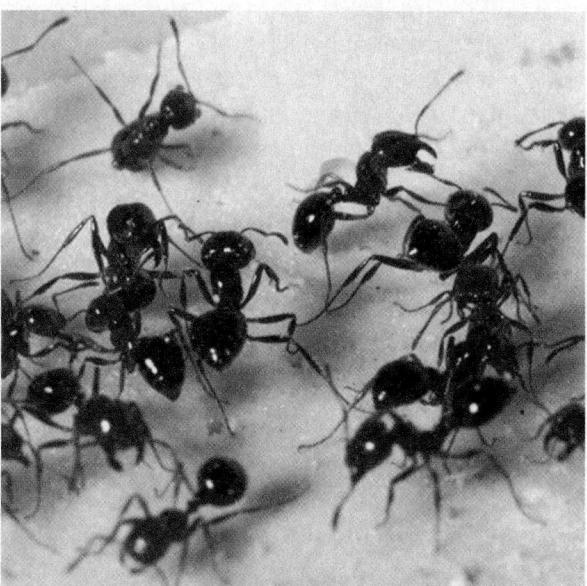
**A**

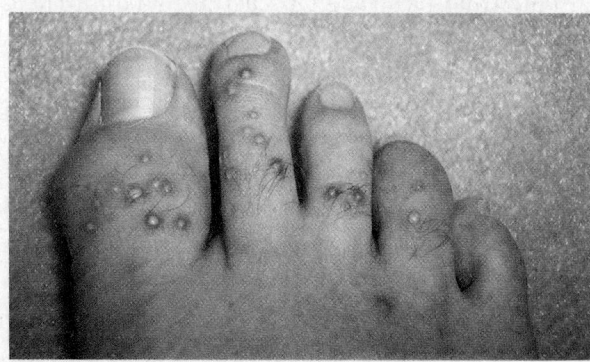
**B**

**FIGURE 21-6 A.** The fire ant. **B.** Fire ants inject an irritating toxin at multiple sites. Bites are generally found on the feet and the legs and appear as multiple small, raised pustules.

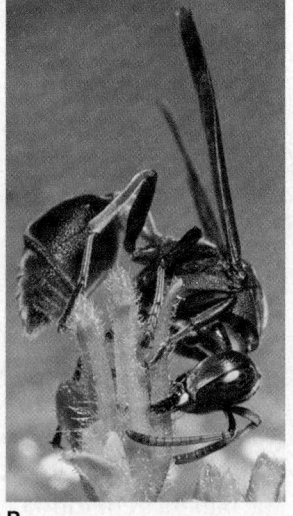
**A**      **B**

**FIGURE 21-5** Most stinging insects inject venom through a small, hollow spine that projects from the abdomen. **A.** The stinger of the honeybee is barbed; the honeybee cannot withdraw its stinger once it has stung someone. **B.** The wasp's stinger is unbarbed, meaning that it can inflict multiple stings.

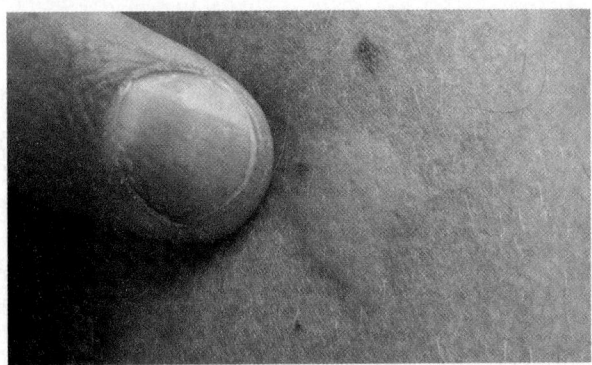

**FIGURE 21-7** A wheal is a whitish, firm elevation of the skin that occurs after an insect sting or bite.

© Simon Krzic/ShutterStock.

gastrointestinal complaints, and hypotension. Occasionally, respiratory failure and confusion occur. If untreated, an anaphylactic reaction can proceed rapidly to death. In fact, more than two-thirds of patients who die of anaphylaxis do so within the first 30 minutes, so rapid treatment and transport is essential.

## Patient Assessment of an Immunologic Emergency

### Scene Size-up

First and foremost, ensure the scene is safe. The patient's environment or recent activity may indicate the source of the reaction, such as a sting or bite from an insect, a food allergy at a restaurant, or a new medication. A respiratory problem reported by dispatch may be an allergic reaction, but until a field impression of allergic reaction is firmly established, be mindful of other potential causes of respiratory distress as well. Do not neglect the possibility that traumatic injury may also be present, secondary to the medical emergency. Follow standard precautions with a minimum of gloves and eye protection. Consider the need for additional resources, such as advanced life support (ALS) personnel, who can provide advanced airway management and additional medications if needed.

### Primary Assessment

When a patient presents with an allergic reaction, you should quickly identify and treat any immediate or potential life threats. It is essential that you pay careful attention to the patient's ABCs, as deterioration can occur at almost any time and with little warning. This is not only paramount during the primary assessment; ABCs should continue to be reassessed repeatedly throughout transport to the ED.

Allergic reactions may present as respiratory distress or as cardiovascular distress in the form of shock. Patients experiencing a severe allergic reaction will often appear very anxious. If your general impression finds the person anxious and in distress, immediately call for ALS backup, if available. Sometimes patients who are known to have severe allergies wear a medical identification tag (eg, necklace or bracelet). Such clues could provide crucial information in situations where the patient is found unresponsive or is otherwise unable to answer questions about his or her medical history.

The most severe form of allergic reaction, anaphylaxis, can cause rapid swelling of the upper airway. You may have only a few minutes to assess the airway and provide life-saving measures; however, not all allergic reactions are anaphylactic reactions. So, work quickly to assess the patient to determine the severity of the symptoms and the number of body systems affected.

Quickly assess for signs of impending airway obstruction, such as swollen lips or tongue, hoarseness, or stridor. Dyspnea may present with increased work of breathing, use of accessory muscles, head bobbing, tripod positioning, nostril flaring, and abnormal breath sounds. Recall that wheezing occurs because of narrowing of the lower air passages, which is mainly the result of contraction of muscles around the bronchioles in reaction to the allergen, and mobilization of mucus in an attempt to push out the allergen. Exhalation, normally the passive, relaxed part of breathing, becomes harder as the patient tries to cough up the secretions or move air past the constricted airways. The fluid in the air passages and the constricted bronchi together produce the wheezing sound. As the patient's condition worsens, breath sounds may diminish to the point of being almost silent. Stridor, a harsh, high-pitched sound heard on inspiration, occurs when swelling in the upper airway (near the vocal cords and throat) begins to close off the airway. It can eventually lead to total obstruction.

As the patient with respiratory failure attempts to compensate by breathing more rapidly, and as respirations become more difficult, the patient may eventually fatigue and may even stop breathing. In the latter case, cardiac arrest will shortly follow respiratory arrest.

Assist the patient into a comfortable position, generally a high Fowler position, in an effort to maximize ventilations. This position may ease respiratory effort. However, if signs of shock emerge, the patient should immediately be placed in the supine position as tolerated.

Quickly listen to the lungs on each side of the chest. Do not hesitate to initiate high-flow oxygen therapy. For a patient in severe respiratory distress, you may have to assist ventilations using a bag-mask device attached to high-concentration oxygen. This can be done in an unresponsive patient or a patient with an altered level of consciousness. The positive-pressure ventilations you provide will force air beyond the swelling in the airway and into the lungs while you await more definitive treatment.

Although respiratory complaints are most common, some patients in anaphylaxis may not present with severe respiratory symptoms but primarily with signs and symptoms of circulatory distress, such as hypotension. Palpating for the presence and quality of a radial pulse will help you quickly identify how the circulatory system is responding to the reaction.

Assess for a rapid pulse rate; pale, cool, cyanotic or red, moist skin; and delayed capillary refill, all of which may indicate hypoperfusion. Because skin paleness can be difficult to detect in patients with dark skin, instead check for pale mucous membranes inside the inner lower eyelid or slow capillary refill. Treatment for shock includes oxygen, proper positioning (ie, recumbent or supine as tolerated), and preventing the loss of body heat. The definitive treatment for shock resulting from anaphylaxis is epinephrine. It should be the treatment priority in these patients.

If anaphylaxis is suspected, or if a relatively mild allergic reaction appears to be worsening, immediate transport is warranted after epinephrine is given. Before leaving the scene, be sure to take along the patient's medications (eg, auto-injectors and inhalers). If the patient is calm and does not exhibit severe signs and symptoms, consider continuing the assessment at the scene. However, if in doubt, always err on the side of urgently initiating transport.

## History Taking

Investigate the patient's chief complaint or history of the present illness. Identify signs and symptoms (**TABLE 21-1**).

If the patient is responsive, begin by obtaining the SAMPLE history (including OPQRST) and the following information specific to allergic reactions:

- **Have any interventions already been completed?** Prior to your arrival, the patient may have begun self-treatment with his or her own medication, such as an epinephrine

## YOU are the Provider

The closest hospital is 15 minutes away, while the closest ALS ambulance is over 1 hour away. You perform a primary assessment of the patient and note the following:

| Recording Time: 0 Minutes | |
| --- | --- |
| Appearance | Anxious; widespread hives |
| Level of consciousness | Conscious and alert, but mildly confused |
| Airway | Open, clear of obstructions or foreign bodies |
| Breathing | Rapid with audible wheezing |
| Circulation | Radial pulse rapid rate and strong; skin flushed and warm, covered with urticaria |

The patient reports dyspnea and states that his entire body is itching. Your partner applies high-concentration oxygen via a nonrebreathing mask.

**3.** Is this patient experiencing a local reaction or anaphylaxis?

**4.** What body system or systems should you focus your secondary assessment on and why?

**TABLE 21-1** Additional Signs and Symptoms of an Allergic Reaction

| Respiratory System | Cardiovascular System | Skin | Other Findings |
|---|---|---|---|
| • Sneezing or an itchy, runny nose (early sign)<br>• Shortness of breath (dyspnea)<br>• Tightness in the chest or throat<br>• Irritating, persistent dry cough<br>• Hoarseness<br>• Rapid, labored, or noisy respirations<br>• Wheezing and/or stridor (which may progress to a silent chest with anaphylaxis; late sign) | • Increase in pulse rate (tachycardia; early sign)<br>• Red, flushed, hot skin (early sign) or pale, cyanotic, cool skin (late sign) as the vascular system fails<br>• Decrease in blood pressure (hypotension) as the blood vessels dilate (late sign) | • Flushing, itching, or burning skin, especially common over the face and upper chest<br>• Urticaria over large areas of the body; may be internal or external<br>• Swelling, especially of the face, neck, hands, feet, and/or tongue, either local (angioedema) or generalized<br>• Cyanosis or pallor around the lips<br>• Warm, tingling feeling in the face, mouth, chest, feet, and hands | • Decreasing mental status (early sign of hypoperfusion), from mild confusion or lethargy to loss of consciousness or coma<br>• Anxiety; a sense of impending doom<br>• Gastrointestinal problems, including nausea, vomiting, or abdominal cramps<br>• Headache<br>• Itchy, watery eyes<br>• Dizziness |

© Jones & Bartlett Learning.

auto-injector, a bronchodilator inhaler, or antihistamines such as chlorpheniramine (Chlor-Trimeton), cetirizine (Zyrtec), or diphenhydramine (Benadryl).

- **Has the patient experienced a severe allergic reaction in the past?** If so, what happened? The patient's answers may indicate how severe the present reaction may become. For example, if the patient was hospitalized or required intubation and prolonged mechanical ventilation due to a previous reaction, you should perceive this as an ominous sign and assume that he or she may have another reaction of equal or even greater severity. In such cases, rapid transport and treatment, as well as ALS care, are among the highest priorities.
- **Be alert for any statements regarding the ingestion of foods that commonly cause allergic reactions.** What was the patient doing, or

what was the patient exposed to, before the onset of symptoms? This information may be the key to effective treatment, regardless of any prior history of allergic reactions.

Inquire about the presence of gastrointestinal complaints such as nausea and vomiting.

## Secondary Assessment

If indicated, perform a rapid full-body scan or conduct a physical examination focused on the area or areas of chief complaint.

If the patient is unconscious or otherwise unable to communicate, remove clothing as necessary, and observe for the presence of bee stingers, signs of contact with chemicals, and other clues suggestive of a reaction. Remember to look for a medical alert tag, which could indicate a severe allergy to a particular substance.

If you have not already done so, auscultate for abnormal breath sounds such as stridor or wheezing, and carefully inspect the skin for swelling, rashes, or urticaria. A rapidly spreading rash can be concerning because it may indicate a systemic reaction. The skin (or mucous membranes) may appear pale or cyanotic and cool; however, red, hot skin is typical in the early stages, suggesting a systemic reaction as the blood vessels lose their ability

## Street Smarts

If the patient self-administered epinephrine before you arrived and does not seem to be responding, check the expiration date. Patients without insurance may not fill their prescriptions because of the high cost of these devices.

to constrict and blood moves outward and closer to the skin. If a systemic reaction continues, the body will have difficulty supplying blood and oxygen to the vital organs. One of the first signs that this has occurred will be altered mental status, as the brain becomes relatively deprived of oxygen and glucose.

Vital signs help determine whether the body is compensating for the stress imposed by the reaction. Assess baseline vital signs, including the pulse and respiratory rate, blood pressure, pupillary response, and oxygen saturation. Remember that skin signs may be unreliable indicators of hypoperfusion, as they may vary widely or be hidden by rashes and swelling.

In a patient experiencing an allergic reaction, pulse oximetry can be a useful method to assess the patient's oxygenation status. However, it is important to remember that pulse oximetry is just another tool in your toolbox. The decision to apply oxygen to a patient experiencing an allergic reaction should be based on a careful assessment of the patient's airway patency, work of breathing, and abnormal lung sounds on auscultation, not solely on the pulse oximetry readings.

## Reassessment

En route to the receiving hospital, repeat the primary assessment. Reassess vital signs, and repeat a focused physical examination of the affected body systems. If the patient is unstable, conduct this reassessment every 5 minutes. If the patient is stable, reassess every 15 minutes. The patient experiencing a suspected allergic reaction should be monitored with vigilance. Deterioration of the patient's condition can be rapid and fatal, so special attention should be given to any signs of airway compromise. The patient's anxiety level and mental status should be monitored as well, as these may provide additional information about the course of the reaction. Monitor for signs of shock, and, if present, treat immediately.

To treat allergic reactions, you must first identify the severity of the reaction. Mild reactions may only require supportive care and monitoring. However, anaphylaxis can produce severe or rapidly progressing signs and symptoms, requiring more aggressive treatment, including epinephrine and ventilatory support. In either situation, the patient

## YOU are the Provider

The patient's wife brings his medications, which include an EpiPen and albuterol inhaler, just before you begin rapid transport to the emergency department (ED). As you move him to the ambulance, you obtain a SAMPLE history and learn that the patient is allergic to peanuts and that he was eating dinner 20 minutes before his symptoms began. Since then, his symptoms have intensified, and he wonders if his meal contained or came into contact with peanuts or peanut oil. He also tells you he has been hospitalized in the past for a severe peanut reaction at which time he was prescribed an EpiPen but he could not get to it in the upstairs bathroom. You reassess his vital signs.

| Recording Time: 5 Minutes | |
|---|---|
| Respirations | 28 breaths/min; labored |
| Pulse | 120 beats/min; weak at the radial artery |
| Skin | Pale and cool; widespread urticaria; angioedema of the lips |
| Blood pressure | 88/60 mm Hg |
| Oxygen saturation (Spo₂) | 88% (on oxygen) |

During the secondary assessment, you note increased swelling of the patient's face and lips. He is having greater difficulty speaking but tries to say he feels like he has a lump in his throat. Auscultation reveals worsening wheezes on exhalation and decreased air movement. As you reach the ambulance your partner removes the nonrebreathing mask and begins assisting the patient's respirations using a bag-mask device attached to high-flow oxygen.

**5.** During the primary assessment, why did the patient first present with warm skin? What is the significance of the changes in his skin color and temperature to pale and cool?

**6.** What are the therapeutic effects of epinephrine if given for anaphylaxis, and would you administer it to this patient?

should be transported to a medical facility for further evaluation.

Recheck your interventions. If you administered epinephrine, what was the effect? Has the patient's condition improved? Does the patient need a second dose? If so, remember to consult medical control before administering any subsequent doses for which you have not already obtained authorization. Also, keep in mind that even if the patient experiences relief following the administration of epinephrine, transport to the ED is still warranted, as the medication's effect will wear off and the symptoms may return.

Your documentation should not only include the signs and symptoms found during your assessment, but should also clearly show *why* you chose the care you provided. Finally, be certain to record the patient's response to your treatment.

## Emergency Medical Care of Immunologic Emergencies

If the patient appears to be having a severe allergic or anaphylactic reaction, you should administer basic life support and provide prompt transport to the hospital. If the allergic reaction was caused by an insect sting and the stinger is still in place, attempt to remove the stinger by scraping the skin with the edge of a sharp, stiff object such as a credit card

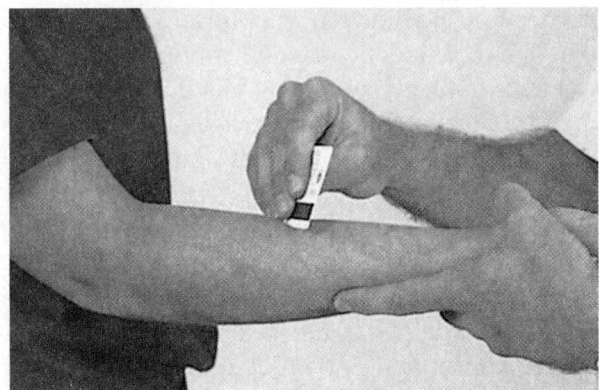

**FIGURE 21-8** To remove the stinger of a honeybee, gently scrape the skin with the edge of a sharp, stiff object such as a credit card.

© Jones & Bartlett Learning.

(**FIGURE 21-8**). Do not use tweezers or forceps to remove the stinger because this may squeeze more venom into the wound. Gently wash the area with soap and water or a mild antiseptic. Try to remove any jewelry from the area before swelling begins. Position the patient with the injection site slightly below the level of the heart, and apply ice or cold packs to the area.

Be alert for signs of airway swelling and other signs of anaphylaxis such as nausea, vomiting, and abdominal cramps, and do not give the patient anything by mouth. Place the patient in the supine position as indicated, and give oxygen if needed. Monitor the patient's vital signs, and be prepared to provide further support as needed.

## Epinephrine

The body normally produces epinephrine (**TABLE 21-2**). Epinephrine is a sympathomimetic hormone. This means it mimics the sympathetic (fight or flight) response. Epinephrine has various properties that cause the blood vessels to constrict, which reverses vasodilation and hypotension; this, in turn, elevates the diastolic pressure and improves coronary blood flow. Other properties of epinephrine increase cardiac contractility and relieve bronchospasm in the lungs. Because epinephrine has immediate action, it can rapidly reverse the effects of anaphylaxis. Epinephrine is prescribed by a physician and comes predosed in an epinephrine auto-injector (EpiPen). In addition to the EpiPen, you may also encounter an Auvi-Q, another type of epinephrine injection, in the home. They are shaped differently than an EpiPen and come in a third dose of 0.1 mg for those patients weighing 17 to 33 lb (7.5 to 15 kg).

In some EMS systems, you may be authorized to carry epinephrine as part of your regular on-board

medications; in others, you may only be permitted to help patients self-administer their own medication. Refer to local protocols or consult online medical control.

## Administering an Epinephrine Auto-injector

All allergic emergency kits should contain a prepared, auto-injectable syringe of epinephrine, ready for intramuscular (IM) injection, along with instructions for its use (**FIGURE 21-9**).

The adult EpiPen system delivers 0.3 mg of epinephrine via a spring-loaded needle and syringe system; the infant–child system (EpiPen Jr) delivers 0.15 mg. The spring-loaded needle automatically injects the epinephrine when the user firmly presses the device into the lateral thigh (thus the term *auto-injector*). If the patient is known to have an allergy, he or she may carry his or her own EpiPen. If the patient is able to use the auto-injector, your role is limited to assisting the patient, if needed.

To use, or help the patient use, the auto-injector, you should first receive a direct order from medical control or follow local protocol. Follow standard precautions, and make sure the medication has been prescribed specifically for that patient. If it has expired or is discolored, do not give the medication. In such an instance, you should inform medical control and continue to provide emergency transport.

| TABLE 21-2 Epinephrine | |
|---|---|
| Indications | Severe allergic reaction causing airway, breathing, or circulatory compromise or an anaphylactic reaction |
| Contraindications | None in a life-threatening emergency; however, consult medical control when the patient has a history of heart disease or acute coronary syndrome |
| Actions | Vasoconstriction and increased cardiac contractility, bronchodilation |
| Side effects | Tachycardia, sweating, pale skin, dizziness, headache, palpitations |
| Typical dose | Adults: 0.3 mg (EpiPen) IM  Children: 0.15 mg (EpiPen Jr) IM |

Abbreviation: IM, intramuscular

© Jones and Bartlett Learning.

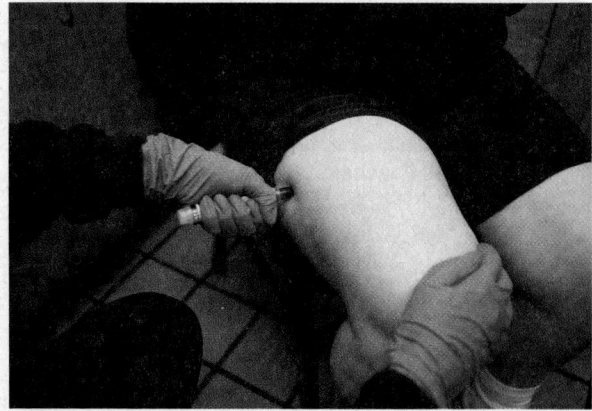

**FIGURE 21-9** Patients who experience severe allergic reactions often carry their own prescription epinephrine, which comes predosed in an auto-injector or a prefilled syringe.

Once you have done these things, follow the steps in **SKILL DRILL 21-1**.

1. Remove the safety cap from the auto-injector, and, if possible, quickly wipe the patient's thigh with alcohol or some other antiseptic (**Step 1**). (Note: Although it is best practice to clean the site, do not delay administration of the drug to do so.) If the patient is displaying signs of life-threatening anaphylaxis, it is possible to administer the auto-injector directly through the patient's clothing.

2. Place the tip of the auto-injector against the lateral part of the patient's thigh, midway between the groin and the knee (**Step 2**).

3. Push the injector firmly against the thigh until a click is heard. This indicates that the injector has activated and medication is being administered. Maintain steady pressure to prevent kickback from the spring in the syringe, and prevent the needle from being pushed out of the injection site too soon. Hold the injector in place until the medication has been injected (3 seconds).

4. Remove the injector from the patient's thigh and dispose of it in the proper biohazard container.

5. Rub the area for 10 seconds (**Step 3**).

6. Record the time and dose of the injection on your patient care report.

7. Reassess and record the patient's vital signs after using the auto-injector.

8. If the patient's signs and symptoms do not improve after 5 minutes and the patient has another auto-injector, consider assisting the patient with the administration of a second (and final) dose of epinephrine.

Other allergy kits may contain oral or IM antihistamines, agents that block the effect of histamine. These work relatively slowly, within several minutes to 1 hour. Because epinephrine can have an effect within 1 minute, it is the primary way to save the life of someone having a severe anaphylactic reaction.

Because epinephrine constricts blood vessels, it may cause the patient's blood pressure to rise significantly. Other side effects include increased pulse rate, anxiety, cardiac dysrhythmias, pallor, dizziness, chest pain, headache, nausea, and vomiting. In a life-threatening situation, the administration of epinephrine outweighs the risk of side effects. Remember that *patients who do not exhibit signs of respiratory compromise or hypotension and do not meet the criteria for a diagnosis of anaphylaxis should not be given epinephrine.*

## YOU are the Provider

Following standing orders, you administer a dose of albuterol from the patient's metered-dose inhaler in order to treat the bronchospasm responsible for his wheezing. A few minutes later, you call the receiving hospital and supply your radio report, including the most recent set of vital signs:

| Recording Time: 20 Minutes | |
| --- | --- |
| Level of consciousness | Conscious and alert |
| Respirations | 18 breaths/min; unlabored; wheezing improved |
| Pulse | 114 beats/min; strong and regular |
| Skin | Pink, warm, and dry; scattered hives |
| Blood pressure | 128/72 mm Hg |
| SpO$_2$ | 97% (on oxygen by nonrebreathing mask; patient no longer requires positive-pressure assistance) |

You deliver the patient to the ED, where the attending physician asks you how much epinephrine the patient has received when you give him your report.

**9.** What is the dose and concentration of epinephrine contained in an adult EpiPen?

## Skill Drill 21-1 Using an EpiPen Auto-injector

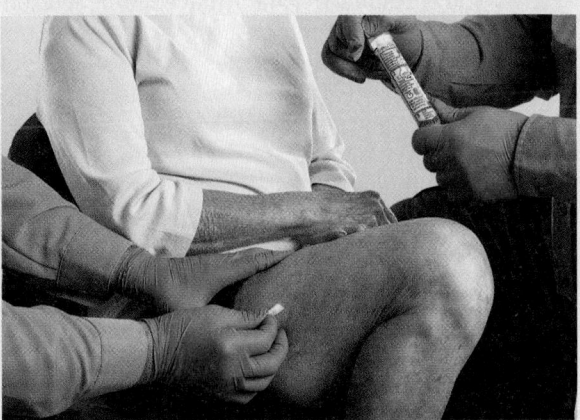

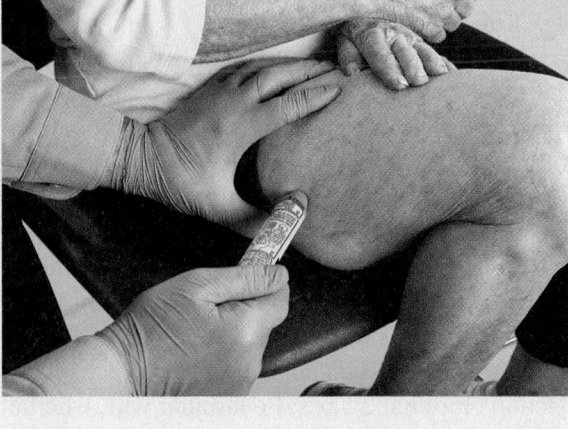

### Step 1

Remove the auto-injector's safety cap, and quickly wipe the thigh with antiseptic, if possible.

### Step 2

Place the tip of the auto-injector against the lateral part of the thigh. Push the auto-injector firmly against the thigh until a click is heard. Hold it in place until all the medication has been injected (3 seconds).

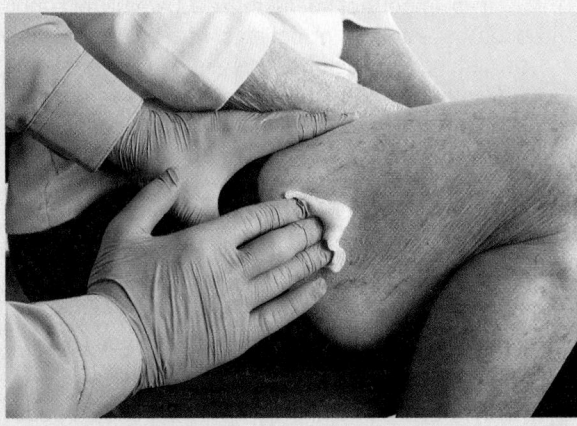

### Step 3

Rub the area for 10 seconds.

All images © Jones & Bartlett Learning.

### Words of Wisdom

Allergic reactions to bites and stings can progress quickly to life threats. With good care, severe signs and symptoms may subside just as quickly. Performing a multisystem examination and documenting your findings are important steps to take before and after treatment. Give particular attention to skin signs and respiratory, circulatory, and mental functioning. If the patient's symptoms seem to resolve and he or she no longer desires to go to the hospital, explain that the effects of epinephrine can wear off before the underlying allergic reaction has fully resolved, and life-threatening symptoms may recur.

## Administering IM Epinephrine

Some areas may allow administration of epinephrine by IM injection, using a vial of 1:1,000 concentration (1 mg/mL) epinephrine along with a needle and syringe. The typical adult dose is 0.3 mg, injected into the midanterolateral thigh. An adult EpiPen can be used for a patient weighing over 66 lb (30 kg). The pediatric dose is weight-based, with the most commonly administered dosage being 0.15 mg in the form of the EpiPen Jr, with a maximum single dose of 0.3 mg. Patients weighing less than 33 lb (15 kg) will have to be dosed individually (0.01 mg/kg IM in the thigh). It is critical to remember that with IM epinephrine injection, the concentration must be 1 mg/mL. Other concentrations are available, but are not used in IM injections for anaphylaxis. Be familiar with whether your protocols allow for epinephrine IM injection.

### Special Populations

When you encounter a geriatric patient experiencing anaphylaxis, obtain a complete and accurate medical history. Because of the potential side effects of epinephrine, such as increased pulse rate, increased myocardial oxygen demand, and increased workload of the heart, you must monitor the patient carefully after epinephrine administration. Do not withhold the administration of a life-saving medication based on a patient's age alone. If the patient is prescribed an EpiPen and has signs and symptoms of anaphylaxis, assist the patient with administration if needed.

## YOU are the Provider SUMMARY

**1. What, if any, additional resources should you request?**

You should consider requesting the response of an ALS unit. Consider the time it will take to reach the nearest hospital versus the time needed to rendezvous with an ALS unit, the feasibility of requesting transport by helicopter, etc. Understand and follow your local protocols. If those resources are not quickly available, transport to the hospital as quickly as is safely possible for more advanced care.

**2. What intervention or interventions should you perform without delay?**

Because the patient's respiratory distress is an immediate life threat, providing high-concentration oxygen is the first action you should take.

**3. Is this patient experiencing a local reaction or anaphylaxis?**

The presence of widespread urticaria (hives) indicates that the patient is experiencing a systemic allergic reaction. Systemic reactions vary in severity and can range from diffuse (widespread) hives and itching to cardiovascular collapse and death.

A local reaction is characterized by tenderness, redness, itching, and swelling at and immediately adjacent to a bite or sting. In many cases, the reaction is not "allergic" in nature—it is simply irritation and inflammation that is caused by the bite or sting itself.

It is important to perform a careful and thorough assessment of patients who are exposed to something to which they have a confirmed allergy. A seemingly local and mild reaction can become systemic and severe within a matter of minutes. Additionally, reaction to something that is eaten may take longer to have its full effects than something that is injected or inhaled, so the route of exposure to a possible allergen can make a difference in the progression of symptoms.

**4. What body system or systems should you focus your secondary assessment on and why?**

Further assessment of the patient should focus on body systems that are commonly affected by an allergic reaction—the respiratory and circulatory systems and the skin. In most cases, a severe allergic reaction occurs within minutes of exposure; however, it may be delayed for up to 1 hour in some patients.

Your primary assessment revealed significant respiratory distress with wheezing. Additionally, the presence of a widespread rash indicates a systemic reaction and warrants a more thorough assessment. As you continue to assess the patient, look for clinical signs that indicate a worsening reaction and be prepared to assist ventilations and treat for shock.

Signs of respiratory system involvement include respirations that become rapid, labored, or noisy;

## YOU are the Provider SUMMARY *continued*

wheezing; stridor; an irritating, persistent dry cough; hoarseness; and tightness in the chest or throat.

Signs of circulatory system involvement include tachycardia (initially), followed by pallor, dizziness, and hypotension. A decreasing level of consciousness indicates a decrease in cerebral blood flow; this is usually secondary to vascular dilation causing hypotension.

The patient already has widespread hives, and his skin is flushed. However, you should further assess the skin by looking for swelling—especially of the face, tongue, neck, hands, and feet. If the patient reports a warm, tingling feeling in the face, mouth, chest, feet, and hands, this should also be cause for concern.

**5. During the primary assessment, why did the patient first present with warm skin? What is the significance of the changes in his skin color and temperature to pale and cool?**

When vasodilation and increased capillary permeability occur in the early stages of an allergic reaction, fluid leaks out of the bloodstream and into the subcutaneous (fatty) layer of the skin. This causes swelling, redness, warmth, and urticaria of the skin. But as the reaction progresses, bronchoconstriction impairs oxygenation and ventilation, producing hypoxemia. Clinical signs of hypoxemia include altered mental status, tachycardia, cyanosis, and a low oxygen saturation ($Spo_2$).

Tachycardia indicates that the body is attempting to compensate for decreased perfusion and hypoxemia by releasing more epinephrine (adrenaline) into the bloodstream to pump more blood to the body's organs, tissues, and cells.

Hypotension occurs because of widespread vasodilation and a decrease in arterial pressure—again, in response to the body's massive release of histamines. As the blood pressure falls, the brain and other vital organs are deprived of oxygen.

**6. What are the therapeutic effects of epinephrine if given for anaphylaxis, and would you administer it to this patient?**

Epinephrine—a hormone that is normally produced by the body—works to rapidly increase the heart rate, dilate the bronchioles in the lungs, and raise the blood pressure by constricting the blood vessels. During anaphylaxis, however, the body may not produce enough epinephrine to enable these actions;

therefore, epinephrine is administered to compensate for the body's inadequate response.

Epinephrine does not stop the allergic reaction itself; it reverses the negative effects of bronchoconstriction and vasodilation, which are caused by the reaction. Therefore, when epinephrine is administered to the patient, it dilates the bronchioles, which improves breathing, and constricts the blood vessels, which increases the blood pressure and improves perfusion.

**7. In addition to the patient's vital signs, what else should you reassess?**

Ask him if he still feels as if he has a lump in his throat; this was likely the result of mild upper airway swelling caused by angioedema and *must* be reassessed. Even though he did not present with obvious external angioedema, you should still reassess his face, lips, tongue, neck, and other parts of his body for swelling.

If bronchoconstriction worsens, the patient may have decreased lung sounds as less air is moved through the narrowed airways. If the epinephrine sufficiently dilates the bronchioles, scattered wheezing may still be heard, even though the patient is not exhibiting any outward signs of respiratory distress.

Reassess his skin to determine if his hives are resolving or if they are still present. In most cases, hives will persist, at least to some degree, following the administration of epinephrine. You will usually notice improvement in the patient's breathing and perfusion status (eg, mental status, blood pressure, peripheral pulse quality) before you see resolution of hives.

**8. How often should you reassess this patient?**

This patient should be considered high priority or critical and, therefore, should be reassessed every 5 minutes en route to the receiving facility.

**9. What is the dose and concentration of epinephrine contained in an adult EpiPen?**

The adult EpiPen contains 0.3 mg of a 1 mg/mL concentration for IM injection. Also sometimes referred to as a 1:1,000 concentration, this contains 1 mg of epinephrine per 1 mL. Therefore, 0.3 mL contains 0.3 mg of epinephrine—all of which is injected into the patient's thigh. Be sure to hold the injector against the thigh for at least 3 seconds to ensure the whole dose has been administered.

## EMS Patient Care Report (PCR)

| **Date:** 01-3-20 | **Incident No.:** 011709 | **Nature of Call:** Shortness of breath | | **Location:** 1444 City Park Drive | |
|---|---|---|---|---|---|
| **Dispatched:** 1310 | **En Route:** 1310 | **At Scene:** 1316 | **Transport:** 1322 | **At Hospital:** 1339 | **In Service:** 1350 |

### Patient Information

| | |
|---|---|
| **Age:** 33<br>**Sex:** M<br>**Weight (in kg [lb]):** 73 kg (160 lb) | **Allergies:** Peanuts; no known drug allergies<br>**Medications:** Prescribed EpiPen and albuterol inhaler<br>**Past Medical History:** Previous allergic reaction to peanuts; required hospitalization<br>**Chief Complaint:** Dyspnea, urticaria, and itching |

### Vital Signs

| **Time:** 1322 | **BP:** 88/60 | **Pulse:** 120 | **Respirations:** 28 | **Spo$_2$:** 88% |
|---|---|---|---|---|
| **Time:** 1327 | **BP:** 104/66 | **Pulse:** 124 | **Respirations:** 22 | **Spo$_2$:** 95% |
| **Time:** 1337 | **BP:** 128/72 | **Pulse:** 112 | **Respirations:** 18 | **Spo$_2$:** 97% |

### EMS Treatment (circle all that apply )

| **Oxygen @ _15_ L/min via:**<br><br>NC (NRM) (Bag mask) | | **Assisted Ventilation** | **Airway Adjunct** | **CPR** |
|---|---|---|---|---|
| **Defibrillation** | **Bleeding Control** | **Bandaging** | **Splinting** | **Other:** Epinephrine 0.3 mg via EpiPen, albuterol inhaler; bag-mask device when NRM not enough |

### Narrative

Medic 85 dispatched to a residence where a 33-year-old man is experiencing shortness of breath.

Chief Complaint: Dyspnea, urticaria, and itching

History: Patient presented with dyspnea, generalized urticaria, and itching approximately 20 minutes after eating his meal. He stated that he was uncertain whether or not his meal had contained peanuts, a food to which he is severely allergic. He further stated that the last time he ingested a product containing peanuts, he had to be hospitalized. Patient denied chest discomfort and other past medical history.

Assessment: On arrival, the patient was conscious and alert; his airway was patent and his breathing was rapid with audible wheezes. Patient's skin was flushed, with urticaria noted on the trunk and extremities. Patient's condition deteriorated en route. He remained conscious, but became confused and he began experiencing increasing respiratory distress, hypotension, and a falling oxygen saturation. Auscultation revealed bilateral expiratory wheezing in all lung fields. The patient's face and lips began to show signs of swelling.

Treatment (Rx): The patient was placed on oxygen via nonrebreathing mask. When his breathing deteriorated his respirations were assisted with a bag mask device attached to 15 L/min of oxygen. The patient was unable to self-administer his EpiPen; therefore, it was given by EMS, following standing orders, in the lateral aspect of his right thigh; dose given was 0.3 mg of 1 mg/mL concentration. Reassessment showed that his symptoms had begun to resolve; his mental status had improved and he stated that it was easier to breathe. Blood pressure and oxygen saturation also improved. Hives were still present, although they appeared to be resolving. However, the wheezing continued; thus, per standing orders, the patient was assisted in the administration of his albuterol inhaler.

Transport: Patient stood and pivoted onto the stretcher, was loaded into the ambulance, and transported BLS to the hospital with lights and siren as ALS was not available.

Continued to monitor patient's condition throughout transport; he continued to improve and was delivered to the ED staff without incident. Gave verbal report to charge nurse and returned to service.

**End of report**

# Prep Kit

## Ready for Review

- An allergic reaction is a response to chemicals the body releases to combat certain stimuli, called allergens.
- Allergic reactions occur most often in response to five categories of stimuli: food, medication, plants, chemicals, and insect bites and stings.
- The reaction may be mild and local, involving itching, redness, and tenderness, or it may be severe and systemic, including shock and respiratory failure.
- Anaphylaxis is a life-threatening allergic reaction mounted by multiple organ systems, which must be treated with epinephrine.
- Wheezing and skin wheals can be signs of anaphylaxis.
- All patients with suspected anaphylaxis require oxygen.
- When assessing a person who may be having an allergic reaction, you should check for flushing, itching, and swelling skin, hives, wheezing and stridor, a persistent cough, a decrease in blood pressure, a weak pulse, dizziness, abdominal cramps, and headache.
- Because epinephrine can have an effect within 1 minute, it is the primary way to save the life of someone having a severe anaphylactic reaction.
- You may help a patient to administer an epinephrine auto-injector (EpiPen) with authorization from medical control.
- Always provide prompt transport to the hospital for any patient who is having an allergic reaction. Remember that signs and symptoms can rapidly become more severe. Carefully monitor the patient's vital signs en route; be especially alert for airway compromise.

## Vital Vocabulary

**allergen** A substance that causes an allergic reaction.

**allergic reaction** The body's exaggerated immune response to an internal or surface agent.

**anaphylaxis** An extreme, life-threatening, systemic allergic reaction that may include shock and respiratory failure.

**angioedema** Localized areas of swelling beneath the skin, often around the eyes and lips, but can also involve other body areas as well.

**envenomation** The act of injecting venom.

**epinephrine** A substance produced by the body (commonly called adrenaline), and a drug produced by pharmaceutical companies that increases pulse rate and blood pressure; the drug of choice for an anaphylactic reaction.

**histamines** Chemical substances released by the immune system in allergic reactions that are responsible for many of the symptoms of anaphylaxis, such as vasodilation.

**immune response** The body's response to a substance perceived by the body as foreign.

**immune system** The body system that includes all of the structures and processes designed to mount a defense against foreign substances and disease-causing agents.

**immunology** The study of the body's immune system.

**leukotrienes** Chemical substances that contribute to anaphylaxis; released by the immune system in allergic reactions.

**stridor** A harsh, high-pitched respiratory sound, generally heard during inspiration, that is caused by partial blockage or narrowing of the upper airway; may be audible without a stethoscope.

**toxin** A harmful substance produced by living cells or organisms.

**urticaria** Small areas of generalized itching and/or burning that appear as multiple raised areas on the skin; hives.

**wheal** A raised, swollen, well-defined area on the skin resulting from an insect bite or allergic reaction.

**wheezing** A high-pitched, whistling breath sound that is most prominent on expiration and which suggests an obstruction or narrowing of the lower airways; occurs in asthma and bronchiolitis.

## References

1. Bock S. Fatal anaphylaxis. uptodate.com. https://www.uptodate.com/contents/fatal-anaphylaxis#H7. Updated October 22, 2019. Accessed November 30, 2019.

2. Cleveland Clinic. Insect sting allergies. https://my.clevelandclinic.org/health/articles/17131-insect-sting-allergies. Accessed February 6, 2020.

3. Freeman T. Bee, yellow jacket, wasp, and other Hymenoptera stings: reaction types and acute management. uptodate.com. https://www.uptodate.com/contents/bee-yellow-jacket-wasp-and-other-hymenoptera-stings-reaction-types-and-acute-management?topicRef=4095&source=see_link. Updated October 1, 2019. Accessed November 30, 2019.

4. Kerr M. Pollen library: plants that cause allergies. healthline.com. https://www.healthline.com/health/allergies/pollen-library#1. Published February 16, 2016. Accessed November 30, 2019.

5. Ma L, Danoff TM, Borish L. Case fatality and population mortality associated with anaphylaxis in the United States. *J Allergy Clin Immunol*. 2014;133(4):1075-1083.

6. Mayo Clinic. Anaphylaxis. https://www.mayoclinic.org/diseases-conditions/anaphylaxis/symptoms-causes/syc-20351468. Accessed November 30, 2019.

7. National Highway Traffic Safety Administration. *National Emergency Medical Services Education Standards*. DOT HS 811 077A. ems.gov. http://www.ems.gov/pdf /811077a.pdf. Published January 2009. Accessed November 2, 2019.

8. National Highway Traffic Safety Administration. *National Emergency Medical Services Education Standards: Emergency Medical Technician Instructional Guidelines*. DOT HS 811 077C. ems.gov. www.ems.gov/pdf/811077a.pdf. Published January 2009. Accessed November 2, 2019.

9. National Vital Statistics System. About underlying cause of death, 1999-2017. https://wonder.cdc.gov/ucd-icd10.html. Accessed March 10, 2020.

10. Turner P, Jerschow E, Umasunthar T, et al. Fatal anaphylaxis: mortality rate and risk factors. *J Allergy Clin Immunol Pract*. 2017;5(5):1169-1178.

11. WebMD. Allergic reactions to insect stings. https://www.webmd.com/skin-problems-and-treatments/insect-stings#1. Updated October 14, 2019. Accessed November 30, 2019.

12. Wesley K, Wesley K. Is epinephrine safe for older patients with anaphylaxis? *J Emerg Med Serv*. 2017;42(6). https://www.jems.com/2017/06/01/is-epinephrine-safe-for-older-patients-with-anaphylaxis/. Accessed February 6, 2020.

13. Wu M, McIntosh J, Liu J. Current prevalence rate of latex allergy: why it remains a problem. *J Occup Health*. 2016;58(2):138-144.

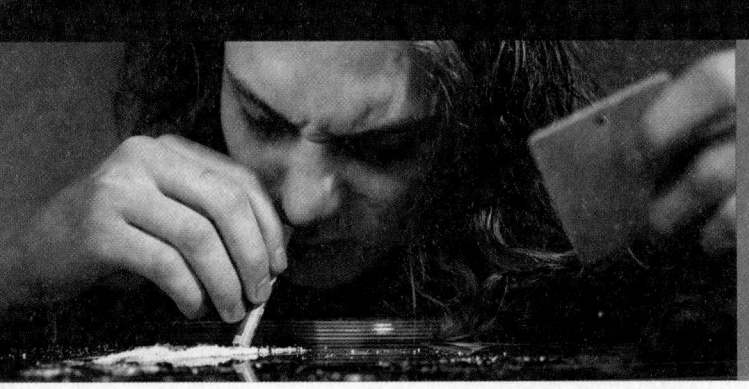

# Chapter 22

# Toxicology

## NATIONAL EMS EDUCATION STANDARD COMPETENCIES

### Medicine
Applies fundamental knowledge to provide basic emergency care and transportation based on assessment findings for an acutely ill patient.

### Toxicology
- Recognition and management of
  - Carbon monoxide poisoning (pp 826–827)
  - Nerve agent poisoning (pp 842–843)

- How and when to contact a poison control center (p 826)
- Anatomy, physiology, pathophysiology, assessment, and management of
  - Inhaled poisons (pp 826–827, 830–833)
  - Ingested poisons (pp 828–829, 830–833)
  - Injected poisons (pp 829–833)
  - Absorbed poisons (pp 827–828, 830–833)
  - Alcohol intoxication and withdrawal (pp 834–836)

## KNOWLEDGE OBJECTIVES

1. Define toxicology, poison, toxin, and overdose. (p 822)
2. Identify the common signs and symptoms of poisoning or toxic exposure. (pp 823–824)
3. Describe how poisons and toxins can enter the body. (pp 824–830)
4. Describe the assessment and treatment of a patient with a suspected poisoning or toxic exposure. (pp 830–846)
5. Describe the assessment and treatment of a patient with a suspected overdose. (pp 830–843)
6. Discuss scene safety considerations for working at a scene with a potentially hazardous material or violent patient. (p 830)
7. Understand the role of airway management in a patient suffering from poisoning or overdose. (pp 830–845)
8. Explain the use of activated charcoal, including indications, contraindications, and the need to

obtain approval from medical control before administration. (pp 829–834)
9. Identify the main types of toxins and poisons and their effects, including alcohol, opiates and opioids, sedative-hypnotic drugs, inhalants, hydrogen sulfide, sympathomimetics, synthetic cathinones, marijuana, hallucinogens, anticholinergic agents, and cholinergic agents. (pp 834–843)
10. Discuss how to manage a patient who has overdosed on an opioid or opiate and who has gone into cardiac or respiratory arrest. (pp 836–837)
11. Describe the assessment and treatment of a patient with suspected food poisoning. (pp 843–845)
12. Describe the assessment and treatment of a patient with suspected plant poisoning. (pp 846–847)

# Introduction

Every day, each of us comes in contact with things that are potentially poisonous. This is not surprising when you consider that almost any substance may be a poison in certain circumstances. Different doses can turn even a remedy into a poison. Consider a common medication such as aspirin. When taken in recommended doses, it is a safe and effective pain reliever (analgesic). However, too much aspirin can result in death.

According to the National Poison Data System, acute poisoning affects over 2 million people each year. Chronic poisoning—often caused by the long-term abuse of medications, tobacco, and alcohol—is more common. Fortunately, deaths caused by acute poisoning are fairly rare. Rates of death as the result of acute poisoning in children have decreased steadily since the late 1960s, when child-resistant caps were introduced for drug bottles and containers. However, deaths caused by chronic poisoning in adults have risen in the past few years, primarily as the result of drug abuse.

In this chapter, the term *poisoning* includes acute and chronic poisonings. As an EMT, you must recognize that patients with either type of condition may have a variety of symptoms. Although you cannot stop chronic substance abuse in a patient, you may be able to prevent death caused by the acute effects of a poison, simply by providing airway management and symptomatic care during transport.

This chapter discusses how to identify a patient who has been poisoned or exposed to a toxin, and how to gather clues about the substance. Also described are the different ways in which a poison or toxin is introduced into the body. The chapter then discusses the signs, symptoms, and treatment of specific poisons. Hazardous materials exposure, food poisoning, and plant poisoning are also discussed.

## Words of Wisdom

Drugs interact with one another. Food, alcohol, vitamins, over-the-counter (OTC) medications, homeopathic agents, and other substances can prevent a drug from working as expected. These interactions can alter the effectiveness of the drug and increase the risk of adverse (harmful) effects.

# Identifying the Patient and the Poison

**Toxicology** is the study of toxic or poisonous substances. A **poison** is any substance whose chemical action can damage body structures or impair body function. A **toxin** is a poisonous substance produced by bacteria, animals, or plants that acts by changing the normal metabolism of cells or by destroying them. Toxins can have acute effects (for example, an injection of heroin may cause respiratory arrest) and chronic effects (for example, years of substance abuse may lead to a weakened immune system). **Substance abuse** is the misuse of any substance to produce a desired effect (for example, heroin—intoxication). A common complication of substance abuse is **overdose**, when a patient takes a toxic or lethal dose of a substance.

Your primary responsibility to the patient who has been poisoned is to recognize that a poisoning has occurred. Your own safety plays a key role here as well; pay attention to your surroundings (**FIGURE 22-1**).

The where, what, and how of the exposure is important. Keep in mind that very small amounts of some poisons or toxins can cause considerable harm or death. Never let your guard down and allow yourself to become exposed to the same substance. If you have even the slightest suspicion that an **ingestion** (swallowing) or exposure to a toxic

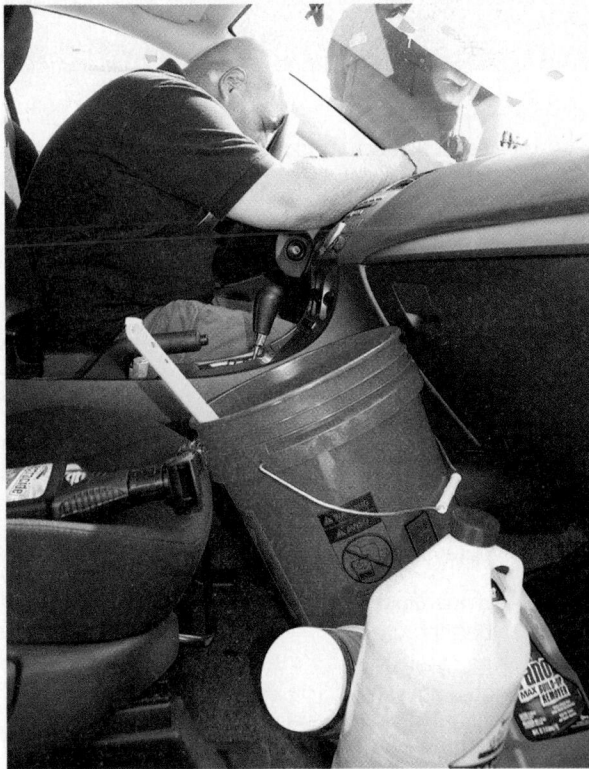

**FIGURE 22-1** Never open a door or approach a scene until you have ascertained that the area is safe to enter. Keep in mind that very small amounts of some poisons or toxins can cause considerable harm or death.

Courtesy of Darin Dowe/*Law and Order Magazine*/Hedon Media Group.

substance has occurred, notify medical control and begin emergency treatment immediately. A discussion of issues relating to suicide is presented in Chapter 23, *Behavioral Health Emergencies*.

Symptoms and signs of poisoning or overdose vary according to the specific agent, as shown in **TABLE 22-1**. Some poisons cause the pulse to speed up, whereas others cause it to slow down; some poisons cause the pupils to dilate, whereas others cause the pupils to constrict. If respiration is depressed or difficult, cyanosis may occur. Some chemical compounds will irritate or burn the skin or mucous membranes, resulting in burning or blistering. The presence of such injuries at the patient's mouth strongly suggests the ingestion of a poison, such as lye. If possible, ask the patient the following questions while you obtain the SAMPLE history (Signs and symptoms; Allergies; Medications; Pertinent past medical history; Last oral intake; Events leading up to the injury or illness):

- What substance did you take?
- When did you take it (or become exposed to it)?
- How much did you ingest?
- Did you have anything to eat or drink before or after you took it?
- Has anyone given you an antidote or any substance orally since you ingested it?
- How much do you weigh?

Be extremely careful in dealing with a child who has ingested a poisonous substance. Although such incidents usually do not lead to death, family members may be distraught, and your calm, professional attitude will help to ease the tension. Remember, however, that a single swallow or single pill of some substances can kill a child.

### Street Smarts

Do not judge the patient for becoming exposed to a poisonous substance, especially if the exposure was an incident of self-harm. Similarly, do not judge a parent or caregiver if the victim was a child. Always treat the patient and others with respect and compassion.

Try to determine the nature of the poison. Look around the immediate area for objects that may provide clues: an overturned bottle, a needle or syringe, scattered pills, chemicals, the remains of food or drink items, or even an overturned or damaged plant. Place any suspicious material in a plastic bag and take it with you to the hospital, along with any containers you find.

Drug containers at the scene can provide critical information. In addition to the name and concentration of the drug, a pill bottle label may list specific ingredients, the number of pills that were originally in the bottle, the name of the manufacturer, and the dose that was prescribed. This information can help emergency department (ED) physicians determine how much has been ingested and what specific treatment may be required. For certain food poisonings, a food container that lists the name and location of the restaurant or vendor may help save the life of the patient and possibly other customers.

If the patient vomits, examine the contents for pill fragments. Wear proper personal protective equipment (PPE) for this activity. Note and document anything unusual that you see.

**TABLE 22-1** Typical Signs and Symptoms of Specific Overdoses

| Agent | Signs and Symptoms |
|---|---|
| Opiates (Examples: morphine, codeine)<br>Opioids (Examples: heroin, fentanyl, methadone, oxycodone) | • Hypoventilation or respiratory arrest<br>• Pinpoint pupils<br>• Sedation or coma<br>• Hypotension |
| Sympathomimetics (Examples: mephedrone, cocaine, methamphetamine) | • Hypertension<br>• Tachycardia<br>• Dilated pupils<br>• Agitation or seizures<br>• Hyperthermia |
| Sedative-hypnotics (Examples: diazepam, secobarbital, temazepam, midazolam) | • Slurred speech<br>• Sedation or coma<br>• Hypoventilation<br>• Hypotension |
| Anticholinergics (Examples: atropine, diphenhydramine, chlorpheniramine, doxylamine, *Datura stramonium* [jimsonweed]) | • Tachycardia<br>• Hyperthermia<br>• Hypertension<br>• Dilated pupils<br>• Dry skin and mucous membranes<br>• Sedation, agitation, seizures, coma, or delirium<br>• Decreased bowel sounds |
| Cholinergics (Examples: organophosphates, pilocarpine, nerve gas) | • Airway compromise<br>• SLUDGEM:<br>  • **S** Salivation, sweating<br>  • **L** Lacrimation (excessive tearing of the eyes)<br>  • **U** Urination<br>  • **D** Defecation, drooling, diarrhea<br>  • **G** Gastric upset and cramps<br>  • **E** Emesis (vomiting)<br>  • **M** Muscle twitching/miosis (pinpoint pupils) |

© Jones & Bartlett Learning.

# How Poisons Enter the Body

Emergency care for a patient who has been poisoned may range from reassuring an anxious parent or caregiver to performing CPR. For these patients, definitive treatment can only be provided at the ED, so transport promptly whenever poisoning is involved. Often, you will not administer a specific antidote (a substance that will counteract the effects of a particular poison) because most poisons do not have one. Depending on local protocols, the antidote most commonly available to EMTs is naloxone (Narcan), which is used to reverse the effects of an opioid overdose. Naloxone is discussed later in the chapter. If you work in a tiered system, advanced life support (ALS) backup may also be appropriate, because these providers can administer additional medications and therapies.

In general, the most important treatment you can perform for a poisoning is to dilute and/or physically remove the poisonous agent. How you do this depends on how the poison entered the patient's body in the first place. The four routes to consider are as follows:

- Inhalation (**FIGURE 22-2A**)
- Absorption (surface contact) (**FIGURE 22-2B**)
- Ingestion (**FIGURE 22-2C**)
- Injection (**FIGURE 22-2D**)

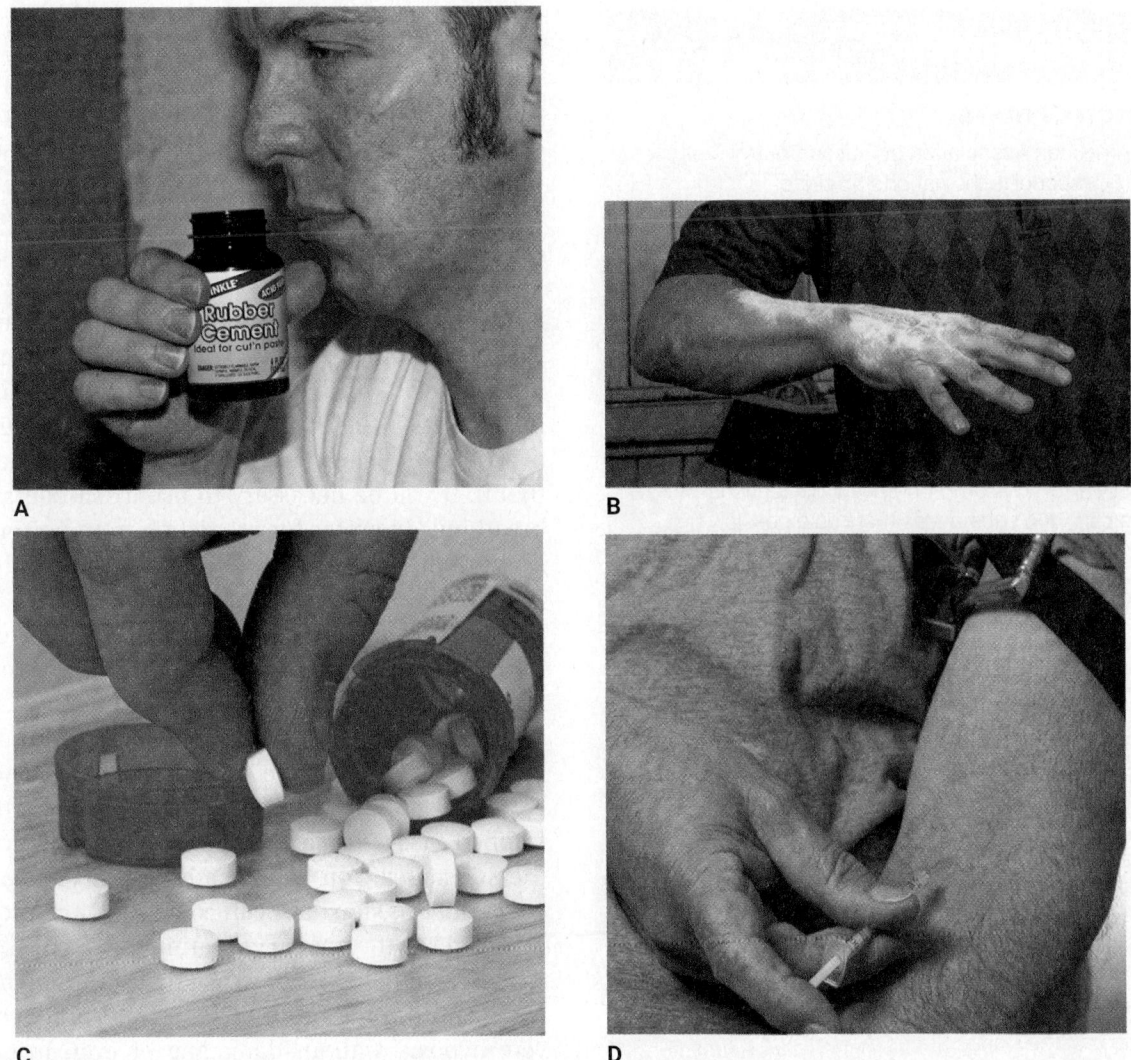

**FIGURE 22-2** There are four routes by which a poison can enter the body. **A.** Inhalation. **B.** Absorption (surface contact). **C.** Ingestion. **D.** Injection.

## YOU are the Provider

It is 0220 hours. Your unit is dispatched to a prominent gated community. A security guard meets you and fire department personnel at the gate and escorts you to 1968 Holly Creek Place. Dispatch advises you the patient is female with acute onset of "flulike symptoms." As you arrive, you notice several police cars on scene as well. You and your EMT partner enter the home and find a 17-year-old girl slouched on the couch. There is a strong odor of vomit on her clothing and she appears sleepy.

The patient's mother is by her side and there is a basin with vomit on the floor beside them. The father reports he was awakened when the teenager and her friends came home from a party and were making a lot of noise. He found his daughter on the front porch and brought her inside.

**1.** In addition to providing immediate life-saving treatment, what else should you do when you arrive at this scene?

**2.** How can knowledge of various signs and symptoms caused by different types of medications improve the care you provide to a patient?

All four routes of poisoning can lead to serious and possibly life-threatening conditions. Take care to treat these patients appropriately and to keep yourself safe from harm. If you are uncertain how to treat a patient who has been poisoned or exposed to a specific substance, find the container if possible, and contact medical control and/or the poison control center before you proceed. Always assess the situation and determine whether the scene is safe before you approach the patient.

## Inhaled Poisons

Patients who have inhaled poison—including natural gas, sewer gas, certain pesticides, carbon monoxide, and chlorine—should be moved to fresh air immediately. Depending on how long the patient was exposed, he or she may require supplemental oxygen (**FIGURE 22-3**). During the scene size-up, if you suspect the presence of a toxic gas, call for specialized resources such as the hazardous materials (hazmat) team. Never approach a contaminated patient unless you have specialized hazmat training and are using the appropriate PPE (not all patients exposed to toxic gases will have contaminants on them). It will be necessary to use a self-contained breathing apparatus for protection from poisonous fumes if they are present. If you are not specifically trained in the use of this apparatus or do not have appropriately fit-tested equipment available, defer to appropriately trained and equipped personnel. Some patients may need to be decontaminated by the hazmat team after they are removed from the toxic environment. The patient's clothing should be removed in this process because it may contain trapped gases that can be released, exposing you to the substance. You cannot administer emergency care until this step has been completed and there is no danger of the poison contaminating you.

Some inhaled poisons, such as carbon monoxide, are colorless and odorless and produce severe hypoxia without damaging or even irritating the lungs. Others, such as chlorine, are very irritating to the tissues and cause airway obstruction and

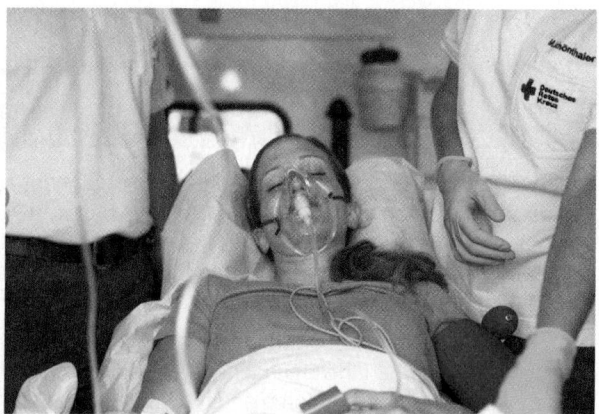

**FIGURE 22-3** Patients who have inhaled poisons may need supplemental oxygen and prompt transport to the emergency department.

pulmonary edema. The patient may have the following signs and symptoms: burning eyes, sore throat, cough, chest pain, hoarseness, wheezing, respiratory distress, dizziness, confusion, headache, or stridor in severe cases. The patient may also have seizures or an altered mental status. Most inhaled toxins can be treated by removing the patient from the exposure and applying oxygen. However, some inhaled agents cause progressive lung damage, even after the patient has been removed from direct exposure; this damage may not be evident for several hours. Meanwhile, it may take 2 or 3 days or more of intensive care to restore normal lung function. Therefore, all patients who have inhaled poison require prompt transport to an ED. Be prepared to use supplemental oxygen via a nonrebreathing mask and/or ventilatory support with a bag-mask device, if necessary. Remember that pulse oximetry readings may be inaccurate with some inhaled poisons. Make sure a suction unit is available in case the patient vomits.

## Words of Wisdom

According to the Centers for Disease Control and Prevention, during the winter months, the increased use of alternative heating systems in poorly ventilated spaces is associated with an increase in carbon monoxide poisonings.

Some patients use inhaled poisons to commit suicide. A common method is for the patient to sit inside a vehicle with the engine running in an enclosed garage. The exhaust fumes from the vehicle contain high levels of carbon monoxide that will cause the patient to become unconscious and eventually stop breathing.

## Words of Wisdom

Anytime there is more than one patient and no evidence of the mechanism of injury (MOI) or nature of illness (NOI), be suspicious. This is especially true when you encounter patients with changes in level of consciousness, especially at an industrial site or in an enclosed space. Toxic fumes may be odorless and colorless or may seem harmless, such as in the case of sewer gas. If the substance is in the atmosphere, it will affect the emergency providers as well as the patients. An EMT who is incapacitated is no help to anyone.

## Absorbed and Surface Contact Poisons

Poisons that come in contact with the surface of the body can affect the patient in many ways. Many corrosive substances will damage the skin, mucous membranes, or eyes, causing chemical burns, rashes, or lesions. Acids, alkalis, and some petroleum (hydrocarbon) products are very destructive. Other substances are absorbed into the bloodstream through the skin and have systemic effects, just like medications or drugs taken via the oral or injectable routes. Other substances, such as poison ivy or poison oak, may cause an itchy rash without being dangerous to the patient's health. It is important, therefore, to distinguish between contact burns and contact absorption.

## Words of Wisdom

Absorption of toxic substances through the skin is a common problem in the agriculture and manufacturing industries. Most solvents, insecticides, herbicides, and pesticides are toxic and can be readily absorbed through the skin.

Signs and symptoms of absorbed poisons include a history of exposure, liquid or powder on a patient's skin, burns, itching, irritation, redness of the skin in light-skinned people, or typical odors of the substance.

Emergency treatment for a typical contact poisoning includes the following two steps:

1. Avoid contaminating yourself or others.
2. While protecting yourself from exposure, remove the irritating or corrosive substance from the patient as rapidly as possible.

Remove all clothing that has been contaminated with poisons or irritating substances. If a dry powder has been spilled, thoroughly brush off the chemical (avoid creating a dust cloud), flush the skin with clean water for 15 to 20 minutes, and then wash the skin with soap and water. If liquid material has been spilled on a patient, flood the affected part for 15 to 20 minutes. If the patient has a chemical agent in the eyes, irrigate them quickly and thoroughly. To avoid contaminating the other eye as you irrigate the affected eye, make sure the fluid runs

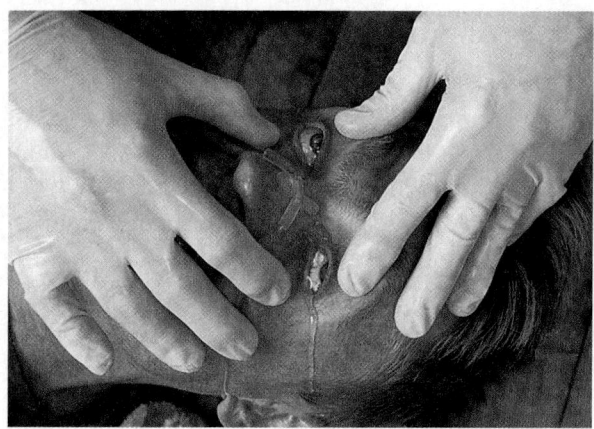

**FIGURE 22-4** If chemical agents are in the patient's eyes, irrigate the eyes quickly and thoroughly, ensuring that the irrigation fluid runs from the bridge of the nose outward. (Use of a nasal cannula is shown.).

© American Academy of Orthopaedic Surgeons.

from the bridge of the nose outward (**FIGURE 22-4**). Initiate this action on the scene and continue it during transport. Keep in mind that you may have to help the patient keep his or her eyes open.

Many chemical burns occur in industrial settings, where safety showers and specific protocols for handling surface burns are available. If you are called to such a scene, a hazmat team should be available to assist you. Always ensure you, your team members, and the exposed patient are thoroughly decontaminated prior to transport. Failure to do so will result in the risk of contaminating the entire ED and staff. After effective decontamination has occurred, promptly transport to the ED for definitive care. Obtain a **material safety data sheet (MSDS)** (or safety data sheet [SDS]) from industrial sites and transport it with the patient. If it is not immediately available, ask the company to send it to the receiving hospital while you are en route. This will help to identify and quickly make available specific interventions and potential antidotes. Chapter 40, *Incident Management*, discusses hazardous materials and decontamination in detail.

## Ingested Poisons

According to the AAPCC, over 80% of all poisonings are by mouth (ingestion). Ingested poisons include liquids, household cleaners, contaminated food, plants, and, in most cases, drugs. Ingested poisoning is usually accidental in children and, except for contaminated food, deliberate in adults. Plant poisonings are common among children, who like to explore and often bite the leaves of various bushes or shrubs.

The signs and symptoms of ingested poisons vary greatly with the type of poison, the age of the patient, and the time that has passed since the ingestion. Small children may respond by crying if the poison is an acid or alkaline, and these types of poisons often cause burns around the mouth. Gastrointestinal pain may be present in some cases, and patients may vomit before or after your

## YOU are the Provider

You approach the patient, and the mother tells you she vomited up some pills. You glance down at the basin of vomit on the floor and note several different colors of pill fragments. You also notice a vomit stain on the patient's shirt is speckled with different colors. As you begin your assessment of the patient, you note her respirations are very slow.

| Recording Time: 0 Minutes | |
| --- | --- |
| **Appearance** | Slouched into the couch with her head down, motionless |
| **Level of consciousness** | Sleepy and not responding without stimulation; constricted pupils |
| **Airway** | Oral secretions; snoring respirations |
| **Breathing** | Slow rate; shallow depth; breath sounds diminished to absent |
| **Circulation** | Radial pulses rapid and weak; skin cool, pale, and wet; no gross bleeding |

**3.** On the basis of your initial assessment, what is the most appropriate treatment for this patient?

**4.** On the basis of the patient's initial presentation, what type of drug should you suspect she overdosed on?

arrival. If the patient has an altered mental status, it is critical that you protect the patient from aspirating if he or she vomits. Other signs and symptoms depend on the substance involved; for example, some poisons may cause cardiac dysrhythmias, whereas others may cause seizures. It is important to treat these signs and symptoms and notify the poison center and medical control of the patient's condition. Consider whether there is unabsorbed poison remaining in the gastrointestinal tract and whether you can safely and effectively prevent its absorption.

### Words of Wisdom

Be aware that some chemicals react with water. Although small amounts can usually be flushed safely with large quantities of water, larger amounts of such chemicals can give off toxic fumes or explode when wet. Be sure to check the relevant warnings and placards, and avoid potential injury to your patient and yourself by calling for additional resources (hazmat team) when in doubt.

When the patient has ingested a toxin, some EMS systems allow EMTs to administer activated charcoal by mouth. Activated charcoal is discussed later in the chapter.

Although every poison will result in a specific set of symptoms and signs, always immediately assess the XABCs of every patient who has been poisoned. Many patients have died as a result of conditions related to the XABCs that might have been managed easily. Be prepared to provide aggressive ventilatory support and CPR, if necessary, to a patient who has ingested an opioid, a sedative, or a barbiturate, each of which can depress the central nervous system (CNS) and slow breathing.

## Injected Poisons

Exposure by injection includes intravenous (IV) drug abuse and envenomation by insects, arachnids, and reptiles. (These injuries are covered in Chapter 21, *Endocrine and Hematologic Emergencies*, and Chapter 33, *Environmental Emergencies*, respectively.) Injected poisons cannot be diluted or removed from the body in the field because they

## YOU are the Provider

The patient's respirations continue to slow and then stop completely. You, your partner, and the fire crew begin to treat the patient. She is placed on the floor supine. One of the firefighters inserts an oropharyngeal airway and begins ventilation with a bag-mask device and oxygen.

| Recording Time: 6 Minutes | |
| --- | --- |
| **Respirations** | Apneic; assisted ventilations |
| **Pulse** | 116 beats/min; weak and regular |
| **Skin** | Cool, pale, and wet |
| **Blood pressure** | 96/50 mm Hg |
| **Oxygen saturation (Spo$_2$)** | 99% (on oxygen) |

As you treat the patient, a law enforcement officer brings inside one of the friends who brought the patient home. He reports they went to a "Skittles party" earlier that night. He explains the teenagers took prescription pills from their parents' medicine cabinets, mixed them up in a bowl, and then took turns selecting pills to get high. They were also drinking beer and liquor.

You check the patient's pupils. You and your partner agree they are pinpoint. Your partner prepares a preloaded syringe of naloxone to be administered nasally to the patient. You hand the syringe to your partner, then check the patient's blood glucose level. The glucometer registers a fingerstick glucose level of 112 mg/dL.

**5.** Would activated charcoal benefit this patient? Why or why not?

**6.** Why is naloxone being given to this patient?

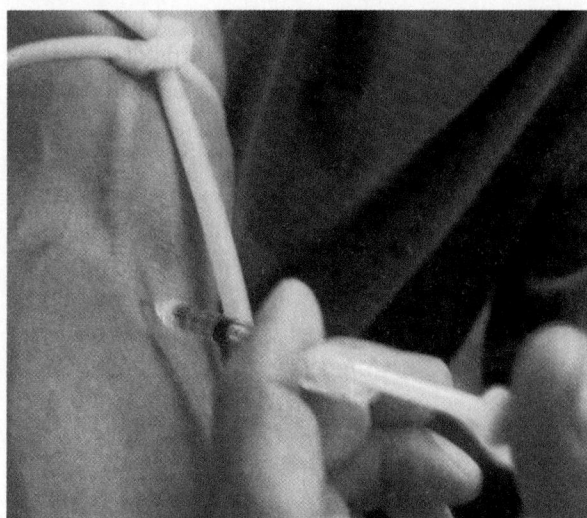

**FIGURE 22-5** Injected poisons are impossible to dilute or remove from the body in the field; therefore, prompt transport to the emergency department is critical.

© Oscar Knott/FogStock/Alamy Stock Photo.

are usually absorbed quickly into the body or cause intense local tissue destruction. When people become ill from an injected poison, their condition can be life threatening and you must act quickly (**FIGURE 22-5**).

### Words of Wisdom

Take time at the scene to make thorough notes about the nature of the poisoning. You can then use this information to state the type and amount of substance and the time and route of exposure in your radio, verbal, and written reports. The busy ED staff will also appreciate clear notes that can quickly be handed over on arrival.

Signs and symptoms of poisoning by injection depend on the toxin that was injected. They include weakness, dizziness, fever, chills, slow breathing, and unresponsiveness, or the patient may be easily excited.

If you suspect that rapid absorption has occurred, monitor the patient's airway, provide high-flow oxygen for any patient with respiratory distress or signs of hypoxia (ie, oxygen saturation level of less than 94%, cyanosis), and be alert for nausea and vomiting. Remove rings, watches, and bracelets from areas around the injection site if swelling occurs. Prompt transport to the ED is

essential. Take all containers, bottles, and labels with the patient to the hospital.

## Patient Assessment

### Scene Size-up

When you have a situation that involves a toxicologic emergency, a well-trained dispatcher can obtain important information pertaining to a poisoning call that will help you anticipate the proper protection needed to ensure your safety. The dispatcher may be able to obtain information pertaining to the MOI/NOI, the number of patients involved, whether additional resources are needed, and whether trauma is involved. If this information has been obtained before your arrival, you must assess the scene nevertheless to ensure your safety and to determine the accuracy of the dispatcher's information.

Because of the risk of possible cross-contamination by poisons that can be inhaled, absorbed, ingested, and injected, you must take appropriate standard precautions. As you approach the scene, think like a detective and look for clues that might indicate the substance involved. Ask yourself the following questions:

- Is there an unpleasant or odd odor in the room? If so, is the scene safe? (This could indicate an inhaled poison.)
- Are there medication bottles near the patient or at the scene? If so, is there medication missing that might indicate an overdose?
- Are there alcoholic beverage containers present?
- Are there syringes or other drug paraphernalia on the scene?
- Is there a suspicious odor and/or drug paraphernalia present that may indicate the presence of an illegal drug laboratory? Drug laboratories can be volatile, so ensure scene safety (**FIGURE 22-6**).

The location of the patient may help contribute to identifying a suspected poisoning, and other clues such as empty pill bottles or open bottles of household cleaners near the patient may provide further information to help you determine what happened. Keep a constant eye on the surroundings, and keep an open mind when questioning the patient or bystanders to avoid mistaken conclusions.

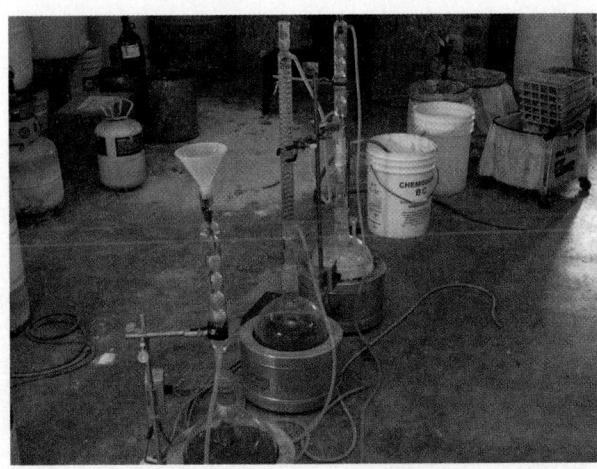

**FIGURE 22-6** An illegal laboratory capable of producing large quantities of methamphetamine.

Courtesy of DEA.

## Primary Assessment

To best determine the severity of the patient's condition, first obtain a general impression of the patient, assess his or her level of consciousness, and determine any life threats. With substance abuse and poisonings, do not assume a conscious, alert, and oriented patient is in stable condition and has no apparent life threats. The patient may have a harmful or even lethal amount of poison in his or her system that has not had time to produce systemic reactions. A primary assessment that reveals a patient with signs of distress and/or altered mental status gives you early confirmation that the poisonous substance is causing systemic reactions.

Quickly ensure that the patient has an open airway and adequate ventilation. If the patient is hypoxic, begin oxygen therapy. In situations where a patient may have an inhalation injury (typically carbon monoxide and/or cyanide poisoning), place the patient on high-flow oxygen regardless of the pulse oximetry reading. If the patient is unresponsive to painful stimuli, consider inserting an airway adjunct to ensure an open airway. Have suction available; these patients are susceptible to vomiting. You may also have to assist a patient's ventilations with a bag-mask device because some substances act as depressants on the body's systems.

Once the airway and breathing have been assessed and appropriate interventions performed, assess the patient's circulatory status. You will find variations in a patient's circulatory status

depending on the substance involved. Assess the pulse and skin condition. Although paleness, or a decrease in blood flow, can be difficult to detect in dark-skinned people, it may be observed by examining mucous membranes inside the inner lower eyelid and capillary refill. On general observation, the patient may appear ashen or gray.

Some poisons are stimulants, and others are depressants. Some poisons will cause vasoconstriction and others vasodilation. Although bleeding may not be obvious, alterations in consciousness may have contributed to trauma and bleeding.

### Street Smarts

Do not rule out the possibility of an overdose or an exposure when assessing a patient who has sustained trauma. Medications that promote vasodilation or bleeding can speed up the development of shock due to hypovolemia. Also, identifying an overdose or exposure can help the medical team prepare for unforeseen complications.

Consider prompt transport for patients with obvious alterations in the XABCs or for patients you have determined have a poor general impression. Some industrial settings may have specific decontamination stations and antidotes available at the site. Remember, everyone who is exposed to the hazardous material must be thoroughly decontaminated by the hazmat team before leaving the scene.

## History Taking

After you have managed the life threats during the primary assessment, investigate the chief complaint or history of present illness. Obtain the patient's medical history. In many situations, you can perform this in the ambulance en route to the hospital. If your patient is responsive and can answer questions, begin with an evaluation of the exposure and the SAMPLE history. If the patient is unresponsive, attempt to obtain the history from coworkers, bystanders, friends, or family members. Medical identification jewelry and wallet cards may also provide information about the patient's medical history.

In these situations, the SAMPLE history guides you in what to focus on as you continue to assess the patient's complaints, and the physical examination and vital signs tell you what is happening to the patient's body. These three assessments give you direction in the interventions your patient might need.

In addition to the SAMPLE history, ask the following questions:

- **What is the substance involved?** If you know the substance involved, you will be better able to access the appropriate resource, such as the poison center, to determine lethal doses, time before adverse effects begin, effects of the substance at toxic levels, and appropriate interventions.

- **When did the patient ingest or become exposed to the substance?** This will let you know if and when the adverse effects will begin. This will also let the emergency physician know what adverse effects can be reversed and which ones cannot because of the length of time the patient has been exposed to the substance.

- **How much did the patient ingest or what was the level of exposure?** With this information, the poison center will be able to inform you whether the patient has had a harmful or lethal dose.

- **Over what period did the patient take or was the patient exposed to the substance?** Did the exposure occur all at once or over minutes or hours?

- **Has the patient or a bystander performed any intervention on the patient? Has the intervention helped?** The patient's or bystander's intervention may cause complications. The emergency physician will need to know this information to be able to adjust interventions accordingly.

- **How much does the patient weigh?** If activated charcoal is indicated and permitted by local protocols, you will need to determine the dose based on the patient's weight. The antidote or neutralizing agent given by the emergency physician may be based on the patient's weight as well.

## Secondary Assessment

In some instances, such as a critically ill patient or a short transport time, you may not have time to conduct a secondary assessment.

Your physical examination should focus on the area of the body involved with the route of exposure

and the particular drug or chemical the patient was exposed to. For example, if you suspect a person has ingested a poison, inspect the mouth for indications of poisoning. Are there burns from caustic chemicals? Are there plant or pill fragments? If the person's skin came in contact with a poison, is there a rash or burns? How large an area is involved? If a respiratory exposure occurred, auscultate the lungs. Is there good air movement in and out of the lungs? Do you hear any wheezing or crackles? Learn about the effects of general classes of drugs and chemicals so that you will be familiar with specific and common poisons.

Your priority is to manage the XABCs during the primary assessment. These interventions take precedence over a thorough physical examination. However, once the XABCs have been addressed and managed, conducting a thorough physical examination will often provide additional information on the exposure the patient experienced. A general review of all body systems may help to identify systemic problems. Perform this review, at a minimum, on patients with extensive chemical burns or other significant trauma and on patients who are unresponsive.

A complete set of baseline vital signs is important. Many poisons have no outward indications of the seriousness of the exposure. Alterations in the level of consciousness, pulse, respirations, blood pressure, and skin are more sensitive indicators that something serious is wrong.

## Reassessment

The condition of patients exposed to poisons may change suddenly and without warning. Continually reassess the adequacy of the patient's XABCs. Repeat the vital signs, and compare them with the baseline set obtained earlier in your assessment. Evaluate the effectiveness of interventions you have provided. If your assessment has provided necessary information about the poisonous substance, you may be able to anticipate changes in the patient's condition. If the patient has consumed a harmful or lethal dose of a poisonous substance, reassess the vital signs at least every 5 minutes. If the patient is in stable condition and there are no life threats, reassess every 15 minutes. If the poison or the level of exposure (eg, the number and type of pills taken) is unknown, careful and frequent reassessment is mandatory.

The treatment you provide for poisoned patients depends a great deal on what they were exposed to, how they were exposed, and other signs and symptoms found in your assessment. Remember, supporting the XABCs is your most important task. Contact your medical control or a poison center to discuss treatment options for particular poisonings. Manage airborne exposures with oxygen if indicated, remove contact exposures with large amounts of water unless contraindicated, and consider activated charcoal for ingested poisons (if permitted by local protocol).

Once you have completed your primary assessment, history taking, and secondary assessment, contact medical control to request necessary interventions. Report to the hospital as much information as you have about the poison or chemical to which the patient was exposed. If a material safety data sheet is immediately available in a work setting, take it with you to the hospital.

## Emergency Medical Care

First, ensure scene safety by following standard precautions and performing external decontamination. Suction tablet or pill fragments from the patient's mouth, and wash or brush dry poison from the patient's skin. Treatment focuses on support. Assess and maintain the patient's XABCs. Provide oxygen to the patient, and assist ventilations if necessary. Keep the patient warm, treat for shock as necessary, and transport promptly to the nearest appropriate hospital.

In certain cases, some EMS systems allow EMTs to give activated charcoal by mouth. Activated charcoal binds to specific toxins—for example, pills that have been ingested—and prevents their absorption by the body. The toxins are then carried out of the body in the stool.

Activated charcoal is not indicated, nor will it be effective, for patients who have ingested alkali poisons, cyanide, ethanol, iron, lithium, methanol, mineral acids, or organic solvents. If the patient has a decreased level of consciousness and cannot protect his or her airway, do not give activated charcoal.

If local protocol permits, your ambulance will likely carry plastic bottles of premixed suspension, each containing up to 50 g of activated charcoal (**FIGURE 22-7**). Some common trade names for the suspension form are InstaChar, Actidose, and

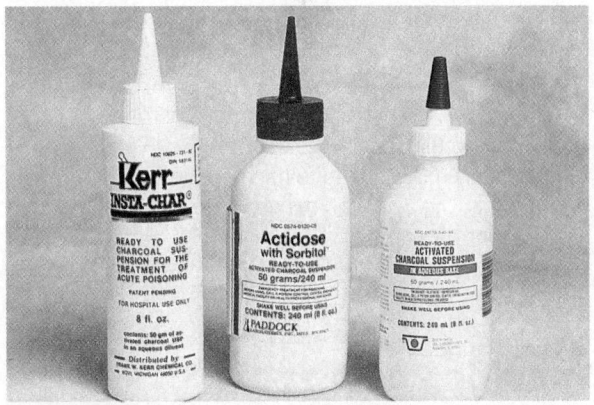

**FIGURE 22-7** Activated charcoal comes as a premixed suspension.
© American Academy of Orthopaedic Surgeons.

LiquiChar. The usual dose for an adult or child is 1 g of activated charcoal per kilogram of body weight (more if food is present). The usual adult dose is 30 to 100 g, and the usual pediatric dose is 15 to 30 g for children younger than age 13 years.

Before you give a patient charcoal, obtain approval from medical control. Consider the amount and type of the toxin and the patient's condition. In most cases, the activated charcoal should be used within 1 hour of ingestion. Next, shake the bottle vigorously to mix the suspension. The medication looks like mud, so it is best to cover the outside of the container so that the fluid is not visible and ask the patient to drink it with a straw. Some patients may not tolerate the medication due to its gritty texture. You might need to convince the patient why this intervention is important, particularly if the patient is a child, but never force the patient. If the patient takes a long time to drink the mixture, you will have to shake the container frequently to keep the medication mixed. Once the patient has finished, discard the container from which the charcoal was administered. Be sure to record the time when you administered the activated charcoal. If the patient refuses the activated charcoal, document the refusal and your attempts to counsel the patient, and transport the patient for further evaluation.

The adverse effects of ingesting activated charcoal include constipation and black stools. If the patient has ingested a poison that causes nausea, he or she may vomit after taking activated charcoal, and the dose will have to be repeated. As you reassess the patient, be prepared for vomiting, nausea, and possible airway conditions.

## Specific Poisons

Over time, a person who routinely misuses a substance may need increasing amounts of it to achieve the same result. This is called developing a **tolerance** to the substance. A person with an **addiction** has an overwhelming desire or need to continue using the substance, at whatever cost, with a tendency to increase the dose. This does not happen only with the classic drugs of abuse, such as cocaine or heroin. Almost any substance can be abused, including laxatives, nasal decongestants, vitamins, and food. You should be familiar with the concepts of tolerance, addiction, and abuse and the differences between the terms.

The importance of safety awareness when caring for drug users cannot be overemphasized. Known drug users have a fairly high incidence of serious and undiagnosed infections, including human immunodeficiency virus and hepatitis. These patients, when intoxicated, may bite, spit, hit, or otherwise injure you, causing you to come in contact with their blood and other body fluids. Always wear appropriate PPE. A calm, professional approach can defuse frightening situations, but keep your safety and that of your team uppermost in mind. Expect the unexpected and remember: The drug user, not the drug, can pose the greatest threat.

## Alcohol

As a new EMT, you will notice that many calls for service have a connection to alcohol use. Alcohol can damage the liver, whether thorough chronic overuse or occasional heavy use (binge drinking). According to the Centers for Disease Control and Prevention, 1 in 10 deaths among working-age adults in the United States can be attributed to excessive alcohol use. Many people dismiss the dangers of drinking and do not understand that binge use can be more damaging than chronic use, depending on the frequency of the binging and the surrounding circumstances. Binge drinking is a serious health concern in the United States. In a 2018 study, more than one in four participants admitted binge drinking within the past month.

Alcohol is a powerful CNS depressant. It is a **sedative**, a substance that decreases activity and excitement, and a **hypnotic**, meaning that it induces sleep. In general, alcohol dulls the sense of awareness, slows reflexes, and decreases reaction time (**FIGURE 22-8**). It may also cause aggressive and inappropriate behavior and lack of coordination. However, a person who appears intoxicated may have other medical conditions as well. Look for signs of head trauma, mental illness, toxic reactions, or uncontrolled diabetes. Severe acute alcohol ingestion may cause hypoglycemia, which may contribute to the symptoms. You should assume that all intoxicated patients are experiencing a drug overdose and require a thorough examination by a physician. In most states, patients who are impaired in any way—whether by mental illness, medical condition, or intoxication—cannot legally refuse transport. Always consult with your supervisor, law enforcement, or medical control in these situations. Chapter 23, *Behavioral Health Emergencies*, covers this topic in more detail.

Alcohol increases the effects of many drugs and is commonly taken with other substances. OTC drugs, including antihistamines and diet medications, can cause serious complications when combined with alcohol.

If a patient exhibits signs of serious CNS depression, provide respiratory support. This may be difficult, however, because depression of the respiratory system can also cause **emesis**, or vomiting. The vomiting may be forceful or even bloody

(**hematemesis**) because large amounts of alcohol irritate the stomach. Internal bleeding should also be considered if the patient appears to be in shock (hypoperfusion) because blood might not clot effectively in a patient who has a prolonged history of alcohol abuse.

## Special Populations

Drug and alcohol abuse among teenagers is one of the most common issues in society. Most teenagers are encouraged to experiment with drugs through peer pressure. Often, older teenagers will encourage younger teenagers to try combinations of drugs. In other cases, an older teenager who has developed a tolerance will give too large of a dose of a drug to a first-time user, resulting in an overdose. Many teenagers will do things they know are not safe just to gain acceptance from their peers. Often teenagers will lie about taking drugs out of fear of being arrested. Reassure them that your intent is only to give them the best treatment possible.

Also be aware that some teenagers use drugs to attempt suicide. According to the American Psychological Association, teen suicide is a growing health concern and the third leading cause of death for young people ages 15 to 24 years.. Do not be judgmental with these teenagers, and treat them as you would any other patient, with empathy and patience.

A patient in alcohol withdrawal may experience frightening hallucinations, or **delirium tremens (DTs)**. Approximately 1 to 7 days after a person stops drinking or when alcohol consumption levels are decreased suddenly, DTs may develop. Alcoholic hallucinations come and go. A patient with an otherwise clear mental state may see fantastic shapes or figures or hear odd voices. Such auditory and visual hallucinations often precede DTs, which are a more severe complication.

Patients may experience one or more of the following signs and symptoms:

- Agitation and restlessness
- Fever
- Sweating
- Tremors
- Confusion and/or disorientation
- Delusions and/or hallucinations
- Seizures

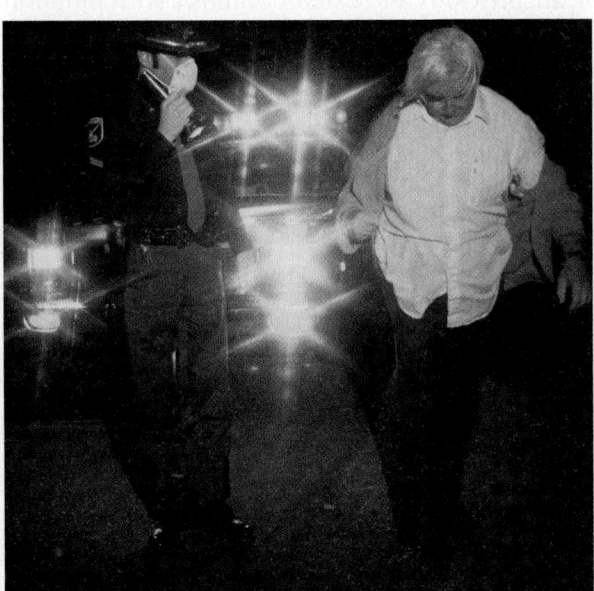

**FIGURE 22-8** Alcohol intoxication causes altered mental status, slowed reflexes, and impaired reaction time.
© David R. Frazier/Science Source.

Provide prompt transport after you have completed your assessment and given necessary care. A person who is experiencing hallucinations or DTs is extremely ill. Should seizures develop, treat them as you would any other seizure. Do not restrain the patient, although you must protect him or her from self-injury. If the patient has difficulty breathing, provide supplemental oxygen and watch carefully for vomiting; have suction ready. Hypovolemia may develop because of sweating, fluid loss, insufficient fluid intake, or vomiting associated with DTs. If you see signs of hypovolemic shock, clear the airway and turn the patient's head to one side to minimize the chance of aspiration during transport. These patients may not respond appropriately to suggestions or conversation; they are often confused and frightened. Therefore, use a calm and relaxed approach. Reassure the patient, and provide emotional support.

## Safety Tips

In situations that involve toxic substances, your safety is paramount. Always be aware of the environment. When dealing with patients who have taken illegal drugs, be cautious and be prepared for unexpected violence. Do not hesitate to call for law enforcement support.

## Opiates and Opioids

A **narcotic** is a drug that produces sleep or altered mental consciousness. An **opioid** is a type of narcotic medication used to relieve pain. An **opiate** is a subset of the opioid family, and refers to natural, nonsynthetic opioids. Opioids are named for the opium in poppy seeds, from which the opiates codeine and morphine are derived. According to the National Institute on Drug Abuse (NIDA), prescription opioid drugs are among the most commonly abused drugs in the United States. Some people become physically dependent on opioids after taking an appropriate medical prescription. These drugs include several synthetic (laboratory-manufactured) opioids, such as hydromorphone, oxycodone, hydrocodone, and methadone (**TABLE 22-2**). According to NIDA, there were over 46,000 deaths in 2018 from opioid overdoses.

## TABLE 22-2 Common Opioids and Opiates

- Butorphanol (Stadol)
- Codeine
- Fentanyl (Sublimaze)
- Heroin
- Hydrocodone (Vicodin)
- Hydromorphone (Dilaudid)
- Morphine
- Methadone (Dolophine)
- Oxycodone hydrochloride (OxyContin)
- Oxymorphone (Opana)

© Jones & Bartlett Learning.

These agents are CNS depressants and can cause severe respiratory depression. However, with IV administration, they produce a characteristic "high" or "kick." Tolerance develops rapidly, so some users may require massive doses to experience the same high. In general, emergency medical conditions related to opioids are caused by respiratory depression, including a decreased volume of inspired air and decreased respirations. This can lead to respiratory and then cardiac arrest if not treated promptly. These drugs often cause nausea and vomiting and may lead to hypotension. Although seizures are uncommon, they can occur and an overdose can result in the patient entering a comatose condition. Patients typically appear sedated or unconscious and exhibit cyanosis with pinpoint pupils. Whereas all of these signs and symptoms may be present with other drugs, the pinpoint pupils is a classic sign of opiate intoxication.

## Words of Wisdom

Some patients who abuse opioids via IV injection are at high risk for hepatitis C and human immunodeficiency virus. Be aware of your surroundings and practice bloodborne precautions. Be alert for improperly disposed needles.

Naloxone (Narcan) is an antidote that reverses the effects of opiate or opioid overdose. This medication can be given intravenously, intramuscularly, or intranasally. Ideally, naloxone is administered intravenously. In many instances, however, IV access is difficult to obtain in the chronic user of illicit IV drugs such as heroin. These patients have venous scarring, called track marks, from repeated use of needles on peripheral veins. Therefore, the intranasal route is becoming a preferred alternative route for the administration of naloxone. It is safer than giving an IM injection because a needle is not required to administer the medication.

EMTs are permitted to administer prefilled naloxone by the intramuscular route or by the intranasal route, in which the antidote is atomized through the nares onto the nasal mucosa. Be aware that this drug can cause harm. This medication should only be used when the patient has agonal respirations or apnea. Place an oropharyngeal (oral) or nasopharyngeal (nasal) airway and ventilate the patient using a bag-mask device prior to administering naloxone. Adequate ventilation while you prepare to administer naloxone decreases the risk of permanent brain damage related to hypoxia. Watch the patient closely; as the level of consciousness rises, the patient will no longer tolerate the oropharyngeal airway and you will have to remove it to prevent aspiration.

In some areas, lay people are permitted to administer naloxone. Be aware that it may have been administered prior to your arrival. Find out from bystanders what has occurred and who was given naloxone.

When a patient goes into cardiac arrest, follow the algorithm shown in **FIGURE 22-9**, including administration of naloxone if it is available. However, providing bag-mask ventilations is a critical treatment for these patients as well. Whether or not naloxone is available, provide ventilations and rapid transport.

## Sedative-Hypnotic Drugs

Barbiturates and benzodiazepines have been a part of legitimate medicine for a long time. They are easy to obtain and relatively cheap. People sometimes solicit prescriptions from several physicians for the same hypnotics or a variety of sedative-hypnotics (**TABLE 22-3**). These drugs are CNS depressants and alter the level of consciousness, with effects similar

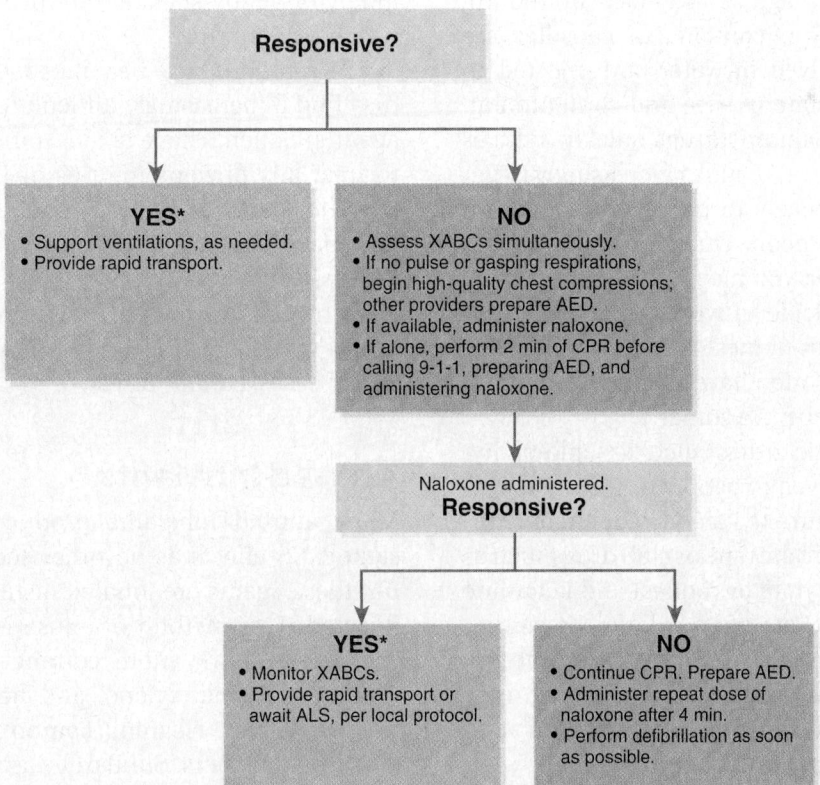

*If at any point the patient loses a pulse or develops agonal breathing, move to "NO" at right.

**FIGURE 22-9** Opioid life-threatening overdose algorithm.

**TABLE 22-3 Examples of Sedative-Hypnotic Drugs**

| Barbiturates | Benzodiazepines | Others |
| --- | --- | --- |
| Amobarbital (Amytal) | Alprazolam (Xanax) | Carisoprodol (Soma) |
| Butabarbital (Butisol) | Chlordiazepoxide (Librium) | Chloral hydrate ("Mickey Finn") |
| Pentobarbital (Nembutal) | Diazepam (Valium) | Cyclobenzaprine (Flexeril) |
| Phenobarbital (Luminal) | Flunitrazepam (Rohypnol) | Eszopiclone (Lunesta) |
| Secobarbital (Seconal) | Lorazepam (Ativan) | Ethchlorvynol (Placidyl) |
| | Oxazepam (Serax) | Ethyl alcohol (drinking alcohol) |
| | Temazepam (Restoril) | Isopropyl alcohol (rubbing alcohol) |
| | | Ketamine (Ketalar) |
| | | Meprobamate (Equagesic) |

© Jones & Bartlett Learning.

to those of alcohol so that the patient may appear drowsy, peaceful, or intoxicated. By themselves, these drugs do not relieve pain, nor do they produce a specific high, although users often take alcohol or an opioid at the same time to boost their effects.

In general, these agents are taken by mouth. Occasionally, however, contents of capsules are suspended or dissolved in water and injected to produce a sudden state of ease and contentment. Use of IV sedative-hypnotic drugs quickly induces tolerance, so the person requires increasingly larger doses. You are less likely to be called to treat an acute overdose in someone who chronically abuses these drugs; however, you may be called to a scene of an attempted suicide in which the patient has taken large quantities of these drugs. In these situations, patients will often have marked respiratory depression and may be in a coma.

Sedative-hypnotic drugs such as chloral hydrate may also be given to people as a "knock-out" drink, or "Mickey Finn," to incapacitate them without their knowledge. Date rape or club drugs such as flunitrazepam (Rohypnol or roofies) and ketamine (Ketalar or Special K) are often colorless, tasteless, and odorless. They cause an unwary person to become sedated and even unconscious, which may facilitate sexual assault or rape. The person later awakens, confused and unable to remember what happened. Chapter 24, *Gynecologic Emergencies*, discusses this topic in more detail.

In general, your treatment of patients who have overdosed with sedative-hypnotics and have

respiratory depression is to ensure the airway is patent, assist ventilations, and give supplemental oxygen when appropriate. Provide prompt transport. and closely monitor the patient's mental status. You may attempt to stimulate the person by speaking loudly or gently shaking him or her; remember to watch for vomiting.

As multidrug use becomes more common, you may find it increasingly difficult to determine what agent(s) patients have taken. Your best approach is to treat any obvious injuries or illnesses, keeping in mind that drug use may complicate the picture and make full life support necessary. Focus on the XABCs, especially the possibility of airway problems (relaxation of the tongue, causing obstruction), vomiting, respiratory depression, and, in severe cases, cardiac arrest.

## Abused Inhalants

Many abused inhalants produce several of the same CNS effects as do other sedative-hypnotics, but these agents are inhaled instead of ingested or injected. This method of abuse is known as huffing. Some of the more common agents include acetone, toluene, xylene, and hexane, which are found in glues, cleaning compounds, paint thinners, and lacquers. Similarly, gasoline and various halogenated hydrocarbons, such as Freon or difluoroethane (used as propellants in aerosol sprays such as compressed air to dust off electronics), are also abused as inhalants. None of these inhalants are medications; rather, these substances briefly displace oxygen in the brain and cause a rush of euphoria. Because these are inexpensive products that can be bought in hardware stores, they are commonly abused by teenagers and curious adults seeking an alcohol-like high. The effective dose and the lethal dose are very close, making these extremely dangerous drugs. Long-term abuse can lead to permanent brain damage.

Take special care in dealing with a patient who may have used inhalants. Effects of inhalants range from mild drowsiness to coma, but unlike most other sedative-hypnotics, these agents often cause seizures. The lack of oxygen to the brain may cause a loss of brain function. Also, halogenated hydrocarbon solvents can make the heart hypersensitive to the patient's own adrenaline, putting the patient at high risk for sudden cardiac death because of ventricular fibrillation; even the action of walking may release enough adrenaline to cause a fatal ventricular dysrhythmia. You must try to keep such patients from struggling with you or exerting themselves. Give supplemental oxygen for patients with respiratory distress or signs of hypoxia, and use a stretcher to move the patient. Prompt transport to the hospital is essential; monitor vital signs en route.

## Hydrogen Sulfide

Hydrogen sulfide is a highly toxic, colorless, and flammable gas with a distinctive rotten-egg odor. Poisoning by hydrogen sulfide usually occurs by inhalation. Hydrogen sulfide affects all organs, but it has the most impact on the lungs and CNS.

Hydrogen sulfide occurs naturally in sewers, swamps, volcanoes, and crude petroleum. Hydrogen sulfide poisoning is also a method used to commit suicide, referred to as chemical or detergent suicide. According to the Chemical Hazards Emergency Medical Management database, this method of self-inflicted exposure to toxic gas originated in Japan and reached the United States via the Internet. The patient may obtain a warning sign to place near the area of the suicide, such as an enclosed vehicle, to warn responders of the deadly gas. If you approach an enclosed vehicle with an unconscious patient inside, be alert for warning signs, as well as containers, buckets, or pots. Remember, do not enter a scene where a toxic gas may be present. Be aware of your surroundings as you approach, and

if you suspect the presence of a toxic gas, wait for a hazmat team to tell you the scene is safe.

Workers in industrial settings may experience low-level exposure to hydrogen sulfide over a long period of time, leading to eye, nose, and throat irritation, as well as headaches and bronchitis. Chronic exposure to this gas may cause an inability to smell the gas. When patients are exposed to high concentrations of the gas, they will experience nausea and vomiting, confusion, dyspnea, and a loss of consciousness. Seizures, shock, coma, and cardiopulmonary arrest may also result.

There is no antidote for hydrogen sulfide poisoning. Therefore, a hazmat team must quickly remove the patient from the contaminated area. Once the patient has been decontaminated, management is largely supportive. Monitor and assist the patient's respiratory and cardiovascular functions and provide rapid transport.

### Street Smarts

Fire departments often carry four-gas meters. Using these meters, fire personnel can check the environment for dangerous levels of oxygen, carbon monoxide, hydrogen sulfide, and combustible gas to ensure it is safe for you to enter.

## Sympathomimetics

Sympathomimetics are CNS stimulants that mimic the effects of the sympathetic (fight-or-flight) nervous system. These stimulants frequently cause hypertension, tachycardia, and dilated pupils. A **stimulant** is an agent that produces an excited state. Examples include amphetamine and methamphetamine (also called meth or ice), which are commonly taken by mouth or smoked. They are also injected by drug abusers in many cases. Sympathomimetic drugs are typically taken to make the user "feel good," improve task performance, suppress appetite, or prevent sleepiness. They may also produce irritability, anxiety, fear, lack of concentration, or seizures. Paranoia and delusions are common symptoms of sympathomimetic abuse. Other examples include phentermine hydrochloride, an appetite suppressant, and amphetamine sulfate (Benzedrine), taken for weight control (short term), narcolepsy, and chronic fatigue syndrome. Caffeine and phenylpropanolamine (a nasal decongestant) are mild sympathomimetics. So-called designer drugs such as 3,4-methylenedioxymethamphetamine (MDMA, known as ecstasy or Molly) are also frequently abused in the United States.

Sympathomimetic drugs are known by various street names that change often (**TABLE 22-4**).

Cocaine, also called crystal, snow, freebase, rock, gold dust, blow, and lady, is one of the most addictive substances known. It may be taken several different ways. Classically, it is inhaled into the nose and absorbed through the nasal mucosa, damaging tissue, causing nosebleeds, and ultimately destroying the nasal septum. It can also be injected intravenously or subcutaneously (skin popping). Cocaine can be absorbed through all mucous membranes and even across the skin. In any form, the immediate effects of a given dose, including excitement and euphoria, last less than 1 hour.

Another method of abusing cocaine is by smoking it. Crack is pure cocaine. It melts at 93°F (33.9°C) and vaporizes at a slightly higher temperature. Therefore, crack is easily smoked. In this form, it reaches the capillary network of the lungs and can be absorbed into the body in seconds. The immediate outflow of blood from the heart speeds the drug to the brain, so its effect is felt at once. Smoked crack produces the most rapid means of absorption and, therefore, the most potent effect.

Acute cocaine overdose is a genuine emergency because patients are at high risk for seizures, cardiac dysrhythmias, and stroke. You may see blood pressure measurements as high as 250/150 mm Hg. Chronic cocaine abuse may cause hallucinations; patients with "cocaine bugs" think that bugs are crawling out of their skin.

Be aware that patients who have been poisoned by a sympathomimetic may be paranoid, putting you and other health care providers in danger. Law enforcement officers should be at the scene to restrain the patient, if necessary. Do not leave the patient unattended and unmonitored during transport.

All of these patients need prompt transport to the ED. Give supplemental oxygen if necessary and be ready to provide suctioning. If the patient is already having a seizure, protect him or her against self-injury.

## Synthetic Cathinones (Bath Salts)

Bath salts, or synthetic cathinones, are an emerging class of drugs similar to MDMA. The drug commonly includes the chemical methylenedioxypyrovalerone (MDPV). Bath salts should not be confused with products such as Epsom salt (magnesium sulfate), although selling it under this umbrella label has allowed its manufacturers and users to escape the legal restrictions imposed on illicit drugs. Brand names include Ivory Wave and Cloud Nine. Many states are working to make it illegal to manufacture or possess this drug.

Bath salts produce euphoria, increased mental clarity, and sexual arousal. Most users of this drug snort or insufflate the powder nasally. The effects reportedly last as long as 48 hours. Adverse effects include teeth grinding, appetite loss, muscle twitching, lip-smacking, confusion, gastrointestinal

**TABLE 22-4** Examples of Street Names for Sympathomimetics

| Street Name | Drug Name |
| --- | --- |
| Adam | 3,4-Methylenedioxymethamphetamine (MDMA) |
| Angel dust | Phencyclidine (PCP) |
| Bennies | Amphetamines |
| Coke | Cocaine |
| Crank | Crack cocaine, heroin, amphetamine, methamphetamine, methcathinone |
| DOM | 4-Methyl-2,5-dimethoxyamphetamine |
| Ecstasy | MDMA |
| Eve | MDMA |
| Golden eagle | 4-Methylthioamphetamine |
| Ice | Cocaine, crack cocaine, smokable methamphetamine, methamphetamine, MDMA, PCP |
| MDA | Methaqualone |
| Meth | Methamphetamine |
| Molly | MDMA |
| Speed | Crack cocaine, amphetamine, methamphetamine |
| Uppers | Amphetamines |

© Jones & Bartlett Learning.

conditions, paranoia, headache, elevated heart rate, and hallucinations.

Keep the patient calm and transport. Consider ALS assistance; some of these patients may require chemical restraint to facilitate safe transport.

## Marijuana

The flowering hemp plant, *Cannabis sativa*, called marijuana, is abused throughout the world. According to the Pew Research Center, almost one-half (49%) of Americans say they have tried marijuana. Tetrahydrocannabinol, or THC, is the chemical in the marijuana plant that produces its high. Inhaling marijuana smoke from a cigarette or pipe produces euphoria, relaxation, and drowsiness. It also impairs short-term memory and the capacity to do complex thinking and work. In some people, the euphoria progresses to depression and confusion. An altered perception of time is common, and anxiety and panic can occur. With very high doses, some patients may experience hallucinations or become very anxious or paranoid. In these cases, keep the patient calm and provide transport. However, be aware that marijuana may be used as a vehicle to get other drugs into the body. For example, it may be laced with crack, fentanyl, or PCP.

Several states have legalized the recreational use of marijuana, and many others allow for the medical use of marijuana and products that contain THC. As the move toward legalization continues and as people become more aware of the health risks associated with smoking, delivery methods have evolved. Many medical users opt against smoking marijuana and instead obtain THC in the form of edibles or baked goods, candies, and other food additives that have been infused with marijuana. These edibles are attractive to children and have led to an increase in emergency visits related to THC ingestion in children. The ingestion of marijuana can also lead to *cannabinoid hyperemesis syndrome*, characterized by chronic marijuana use and extreme nausea and vomiting that is relieved only by a hot shower or bath. Bathing can become compulsive in these patients. The definitive treatment for this condition is to stop using marijuana; however, these users often believe that more marijuana will help the nausea and continue to consume it.

Synthetic marijuana or "spice" refers to a variety of herbal incense or smoking blends that resemble THC and produce a similar high. Synthetic marijuana is often marketed as a "safe" alternative to that drug under brand names such as K2 and Skunk. However, according to NIDA, the chemicals commonly found in spice products have no medical benefit and have a high potential for abuse. Powerful and unpredictable effects may result, ranging from simple euphoria to complete loss of consciousness.

## Hallucinogens

A **hallucinogen** alters a person's sensory perceptions (**TABLE 22-5**). The classic hallucinogen is lysergic acid diethylamide (LSD). Abuse of another hallucinogen, phencyclidine (PCP, or angel dust), is relatively uncommon among young adults. PCP is a dissociative anesthetic that is easily synthesized and highly potent. Its effectiveness by oral, nasal, pulmonary, and IV routes makes it easy to add to other street drugs. It is dangerous because it causes severe behavioral changes in which people often inflict injury on themselves.

All these agents cause visual hallucinations, intensify vision and hearing, and generally separate the user from reality. The user, of course, expects that the altered sensory state will be pleasurable. Often, however, it can be terrifying. At some point, you are bound to encounter patients who are having a "bad trip." They will usually have hypertension, tachycardia, anxiety, and paranoia.

Many hallucinogens have sympathomimetic properties. Your care for a patient who is having a bad reaction to a hallucinogenic agent is the same

| **TABLE 22-5** Commonly Abused Hallucinogens |
| --- |
| • Bufotenine (toad skin) |
| • *Datura stramonium* (jimsonweed) |
| • Dextromethorphan (DXM) |
| • Dimethyltryptamine (DMT) |
| • Ketamine |
| • LSD |
| • Mescaline (peyote) |
| • Morning glory |
| • Nutmeg |
| • PCP |
| • Psilocybin (mushrooms) |
| • Salvia |

© Jones & Bartlett Learning.

as that for a patient who has taken a sympathomimetic. Use a calm, professional manner, and provide emotional support. Do not use restraints unless you or the patient is in danger of injury. Follow the guidelines specified by local authorities. These patients may suddenly experience hallucinations or odd perceptions, so watch them carefully throughout transport. Never leave a patient who has taken a hallucinogen unattended and unmonitored. Request ALS assistance when appropriate.

## Anticholinergic Agents

Anticholinergic agents are medications that block the parasympathetic nerves. The classic picture of a person who has taken too much of an anticholinergic medication is "hot as a hare, blind as a bat, dry as a bone, red as a beet, and mad as a hatter." In other words, the patient will exhibit hyperthermia, dilated pupils, dry skin and mucous membranes, reddened skin, and agitation or delirium. Common drugs with a significant anticholinergic effect include atropine, antihistamines such as diphenhydramine (Benadryl), *Datura stramonium* (jimsonweed), and certain tricyclic antidepressants such as amitriptyline (Elavil). With the exception of jimsonweed, these medications usually are not abused drugs but may be taken as an intentional overdose. It is often difficult to distinguish between an anticholinergic overdose and a sympathomimetic overdose. Both groups of patients may be agitated and have tachycardia and dilated pupils.

In addition to its anticholinergic effects, a tricyclic antidepressant overdose may cause more serious and life-threatening effects because the medication may block the electrical conduction system in the heart, leading to lethal cardiac dysrhythmias. Patients with acute tricyclic antidepressant overdose must be transported immediately to the ED; they may appear "normal," but seizure and death can occur within 30 minutes. The seizures and cardiac dysrhythmias caused by a severe tricyclic antidepressant overdose are best treated in the hospital. If you work in a tiered system, consider calling for ALS backup when you are en route to the scene.

## Cholinergic Agents

Cholinergic agents are medications that overstimulate the normal body functions controlled by the parasympathetic nervous system. These agents have been used for chemical warfare, such as during the sarin gas attack on the Tokyo subway system in 1995. These agents also occur in organophosphate insecticides, which are commonly used for lawn and garden care. A patient who has been poisoned by a cholinergic agent will exhibit excessive salivation or drooling; mucous membrane oversecretion, resulting in a runny nose (rhinorrhea); excessive urination; excessive tearing of the eyes; uncontrolled diarrhea; and an abnormal heart rate. The signs and symptoms of cholinergic drug poisoning are easy to remember using the mnemonic DUMBELS:

**D**    Diarrhea
**U**    Urination
**M**    Miosis (constriction of the pupils), muscle weakness
**B**    Bradycardia, bronchospasm, bronchorrhea (discharge of mucus from the lungs)
**E**    Emesis (vomiting)
**L**    Lacrimation (excessive tearing)
**S**    Seizures, salivation, sweating

Alternatively, you can use the mnemonic SLUDGEM:

**S**    Salivation, sweating
**L**    Lacrimation (excessive tearing)
**U**    Urination
**D**    Defecation, drooling, diarrhea
**G**    Gastric upset and cramps
**E**    Emesis (vomiting)
**M**    Muscle twitching/miosis (pinpoint pupils)

Patients who have been poisoned will have excessive body secretions. In addition, patients may have bradycardia.

The most important consideration in caring for a patient who has been exposed to a cholinergic agent is to avoid exposure yourself. Because these agents may cling to a patient's clothing and skin, decontamination will take priority over prompt transport to the ED. In many jurisdictions, the hazmat team will provide decontamination and contain the exposure chemical.

To care for the exposed patient, hospital staff or paramedics can use the anticholinergic drug atropine to dry up the patient's secretions, followed by the use of pralidoxime to reverse the nerve agent's effect on the patient's nervous system. In the meantime, your priorities after decontamination are to decrease the secretions in the mouth and trachea that threaten to suffocate the patient and provide airway support.

The military has developed antidotes to nerve gas agents that responders can self-administer if the agents are available. In some areas across the country, these kits are issued to emergency medical providers depending on local protocols. The most common kit is the DuoDote Auto-Injector. The Antidote Treatment Nerve Agent Auto-Injector (ATNAA) is the military form of the DuoDote Auto-Injector.

The DuoDote Auto-Injector is a single auto-injector containing 2 mg of atropine and 600 mg of pralidoxime. If a known exposure to nerve agents or organophosphates with manifestation of signs and symptoms has occurred, use the antidote kit only on yourself. If your service carries these antidote kits, you should receive training on their proper use prior to administering them.

## Miscellaneous Drugs

Accidental or intentional overdose with cardiac medications has become common because there are so many patients who have these medications prescribed for them. For example, children may ingest these medications at their grandparent's house, thinking they are candy. Another common scenario is older patients who have forgotten they have already taken their medication and take a second dose. Occasionally people wanting to commit suicide will take an overdose of cardiac medications if that is all they have available. The signs and symptoms of cardiac medication overdose depend on the medication ingested. These drugs may cause bleeding, cardiac dysrhythmias, unconsciousness, and even cardiac arrest. Most of these medications are powerful, so contact the poison center as soon as possible. Depending on local protocol, you may be ordered to administer activated charcoal, but check with the poison center first.

Aspirin poisoning is a potentially lethal condition. Ingesting too many aspirin tablets, acutely or chronically, is an emergency that may result in nausea, vomiting, hyperventilation, and ringing in the ears. Patients with this condition frequently have anxiety, confusion, tachypnea, and hyperthermia, and are in danger of having seizures. Rapidly transport these patients to the hospital.

When consumed in excess, acetaminophen becomes toxic. Overdosing with acetaminophen and combination medications containing acetaminophen is also common. According to the US Food and Drug Administration, acetaminophen is among the top 25 substances with the largest number of fatalities due to poisoning.

It is essential to determine what medications the patient takes or has taken, including OTC medications. Acetaminophen overdose, unintentional or intentional, must be treated promptly and aggressively.

Accidental acetaminophen overdose is as serious as intentional overdose. In fact, its effects can be worse because the patient is unaware of the continuous exposure to the toxin. For example, massive liver failure may not be apparent for a full week. In addition, patients may not provide the information necessary for a correct diagnosis. For this reason, gathering information at the scene is very important. By finding an empty acetaminophen bottle, you may save a patient's life. If a specific antidote is given early enough (before liver failure occurs), liver damage may be prevented.

Some alcohols, including methyl alcohol and ethylene glycol, are even more toxic than ethyl alcohol (drinking alcohol). Methyl alcohol is found in dry gas products and stove kits (Sterno); ethylene glycol is found in some antifreeze products. Both cause a feeling of intoxication. Left untreated, both will also cause severe tachypnea, blindness (methyl alcohol), renal failure (ethylene glycol), and eventually death. Even ethyl alcohol can stop a patient's breathing if taken in too high a dose or too fast, particularly in children. Although methyl alcohol or ethylene glycol may be used as a substitute by a chronic abuser of alcohol who is unable to obtain ethyl alcohol, they are more often taken by someone attempting suicide. In either case, prompt transport to the ED is essential. **TABLE 22-6** lists the most common fatally ingested poisons.

## Food Poisoning

The term *ptomaine poisoning* was coined in 1870 to indicate poisoning by a class of chemicals found in rotting food. It is still used currently in many news accounts of food poisoning. Food poisoning is almost always caused by eating food that is contaminated by bacteria. The food may appear normal, with little or no decay or odor to suggest danger.

There are two main types of food poisoning. In one, the organism itself causes disease; in the other,

### TABLE 22-6 Examples of Fatally Ingested Poisons

- Sedative-hypnotics (alprazolam [Xanax], diazepam [Valium], zolpidem [Ambien])
- Calcium channel blockers (verapamil, nifedipine, diltiazem)
- Stimulants and street drugs
- Opioids (heroin, fentanyl, oxycodone)
- Beta blockers (metoprolol, atenolol)
- Acetaminophen alone or combinations
- Alcohols
- Antidepressants (selective serotonin reuptake inhibitors such as sertraline [Zoloft] and others)
- Hypoglycemic drugs
- Acetylsalicylic acid (aspirin, oil of wintergreen)
- Tricyclic antidepressants (amitriptyline [Elavil], imipramine [Tofranil], nortriptyline [Pamelor])

*Data from American Association of Poison Control Centers, Annual Report, 2018.*

### TABLE 22-7 Common Causes of Food Poisoning

- *Campylobacter*
- *Clostridium botulinum* toxin
- *Clostridium perfringens*
- *Cryptosporidium*
- *Cyclospora*
- *Escherichia coli*
- *Giardia lamblia*
- *Listeria monocytogenes*
- Norovirus
- Rotavirus
- *Salmonella*
- *Shigella*
- *Staphylococcus* toxin
- *Vibrio parahaemolyticus*
- *Yersinia enterocolitica*

© Jones & Bartlett Learning.

the organism produces toxins that cause disease (**TABLE 22-7**).

One organism that produces direct effects of food poisoning is the *Salmonella* bacterium. Salmonellosis is a condition characterized by severe gastrointestinal symptoms within 72 hours of ingestion, including nausea, vomiting, abdominal pain, and diarrhea. In addition, patients with salmonellosis may be systemically ill with fever and generalized weakness. Some people are carriers of certain bacteria; although they may not become ill themselves, they may transmit diseases, particularly if they work in the food services industry. Usually, proper cooking kills bacteria, and proper cleanliness in the kitchen prevents the contamination of uncooked foods.

The more common cause of food poisoning is the ingestion of powerful toxins produced by

## YOU are the Provider

You begin transport to the hospital, which is located a short distance away. You and your partner watch the patient closely because she has been retching and her airway may become compromised if she vomits. You reassess the patient and her vital signs remain normal. You call in your radio report to the hospital. The estimated time of arrival is 6 minutes.

| Recording Time: 17 Minutes | |
| --- | --- |
| Level of consciousness | Conscious, but sleepy |
| Respirations | 14 breaths/min; adequate depth |
| Pulse | 72 beats/min; strong and regular |
| Skin | Pink, warm, and dry |
| Blood pressure | 108/60 mm Hg |
| Spo$_2$ | 100% (on oxygen) |

**9.** What additional treatment is required for this patient?

**10.** What information should you relay to the hospital staff during your verbal report?

bacteria, often in leftovers. The bacterium *Staphylococcus*, a common culprit, is quick to grow and produce toxins in foods that have been prepared in advance and kept too long, even in the refrigerator. Foods left unrefrigerated are a common vehicle for the development of staphylococcal toxins. Usually, staphylococcal food poisoning results in sudden gastrointestinal symptoms, including nausea, vomiting, and diarrhea. Although time frames may vary from person to person, these symptoms usually start within 2 to 3 hours after ingestion or as long as 8 to 12 hours after ingestion.

The most severe form of toxin ingestion is botulism. This often-fatal disease usually results from eating improperly canned food, in which the spores of *Clostridium* bacteria have grown and produced a toxin. The symptoms of botulism are neurologic: blurring of vision, weakness, and difficulty in speaking and breathing. Botulism can also cause muscle paralysis and is typically fatal when it reaches the muscles of respiration. Symptoms of botulism may develop as long as 4 days after ingestion or as early as the first 24 hours.

In general, do not try to determine the specific cause of acute gastrointestinal conditions. After all, severe vomiting may be a sign of food poisoning, a bowel obstruction requiring surgery, or poisoning by substances such as copper, arsenic, zinc, cadmium, scombrotoxin (fish poison), or *Clitocybe* or *Inocybe* mushrooms. Instead, gather as much history as possible from the patient and transport him or her promptly to the hospital. When two or more people in one group have the same illness, take along some of the suspected food to the hospital. In advanced cases of botulism, you may have to assist ventilation and give basic life support.

## Special Populations

Geriatric patients are susceptible to toxicity for several reasons. Consider the case of an accidental overdose or poisoning. The older patient may have forgotten that the medication had been taken and take repeated doses. Alcohol abuse can make a patient more likely to make medication mistakes. Many older patients take multiple prescriptions that may negatively interfere with each other, resulting in increased effects or unwanted drug interactions. The aging process may also impair the older patient's ability to metabolize or excrete the poison. The drug could quickly accumulate to toxic levels and become fatal in lesser doses than in a younger person. Chapter 36, *Geriatric Emergencies*, discusses these risk factors in more detail.

If an older person inhales a poison, even in tiny quantities, lung damage can be severe. Consider the decreased lung capacity and ability to exchange oxygen and carbon dioxide in an older patient's lungs. Pulmonary function could be worsened to potentially fatal levels with the inhalation of minute amounts of poison. For poisons that are absorbed by or injected into the skin, reduced circulation to the skin can decrease or delay absorption into the body. Watch for an increased reaction or irritation at the skin site.

A geriatric patient may also intentionally overdose in an attempt to commit suicide. Be alert for any indication of an intentional overdose or poisoning, even though the patient might deny an attempted suicide.

## Special Populations

Small children or toddlers may experience accidental poisoning due to their natural curiosity. Children at this age commonly put objects in their mouth as a means to learn about them. When they gain access to toxic substances, they will almost always ingest them. Most parents and caregivers are aware of these dangers and properly secure cabinets or store substances out of reach, but often grandparents or older adults without children will store household chemicals in easy-to-reach, lower cabinets without locks. This creates a serious hazard when young children visit. It is fortunate that most accidental poisonings of children are not fatal. Avoid blaming the adults and focus instead on treating the child in the most appropriate manner.

## Street Smarts

Consider initiating a community program to help make homes safer for children. Identifying cleaning agents that resemble children's drinks and placing them out of reach, placing child locks on cabinets, identifying poisonous plants, and educating parents about the potential for accidental poisoning or exposure could save a life.

# Plant Poisoning

According to the National Poison Data System, tens of thousands of cases of poisoning from plants occur each year, some severe. Many household plants are poisonous if ingested; children have been known to nibble on the leaves (**TABLE 22-8**). Some poisonous plants cause local irritation of the skin; others can affect the circulatory system, the gastrointestinal tract, or the CNS. It is impossible for you to memorize every plant and poison, let alone their effects (**FIGURE 22-10**). You can and should do the following:

1. Assess the patient's airway and vital signs.
2. Notify the regional poison center for assistance in identifying the plant.
3. Take the plant to the ED.
4. Provide prompt transport.

Irritation of the skin and/or mucous membranes is a problem with the common houseplant called dieffenbachia, which resembles elephant ears. When chewed, a single leaf may irritate the lining of the upper airway enough to cause difficulty swallowing, breathing, and speaking. For this reason, dieffenbachia has been called "dumb cane." In rare circumstances, the airway may be completely obstructed. Emergency medical treatment of dieffenbachia poisoning includes maintaining an open airway, giving oxygen when necessary, and transporting the patient promptly to the hospital for respiratory support. Assess the patient for airway difficulties throughout transport. If necessary, provide positive pressure ventilation.

**TABLE 22-8** Common Toxic Plants

| Scientific Name | Common Name |
| --- | --- |
| *Abrus precatorius* | Jequirity bean/rosary pea |
| *Cicuta* species | Water hemlock/wild carrot |
| *Colchicum autumnale* | Autumn crocus |
| *Conium maculatum* | Poison hemlock |
| *Convallaria majalis* | Lily of the valley |
| *Datura* species | Jimsonweed/stinkweed |
| *Dieffenbachia* | Dumbcane |
| *Digitalis purpurea* | Foxglove |
| *Nerium oleander* | Oleander or rose laurel |
| *Nicotiana glauca* | Tree tobacco |
| *Phoradendron* | Mistletoe |
| *Phytolacca americana* | Pokeweed |
| *Rheum rhabarbarum* | Rhubarb |
| *Rhododendron* | Rhododendron or azalea |
| *Ricinus communis* | Castor bean |
| *Solarium nigrum* | Nightshade |
| *Zygadenus* species | Death camas |

© Jones & Bartlett Learning.

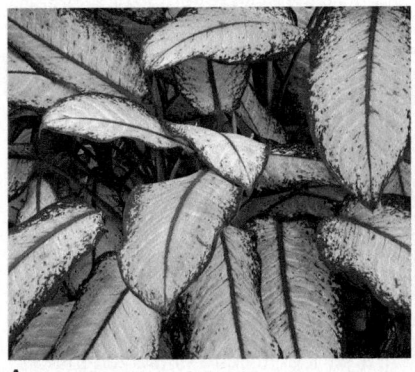
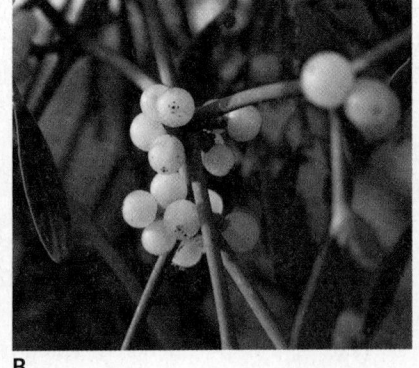
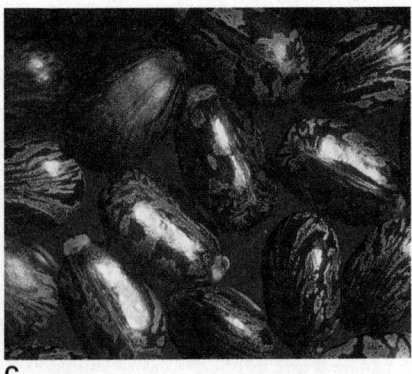

**A** **B** **C**

**FIGURE 22-10** The toxins in these common poisonous plants are often ingested or absorbed through the skin. **A.** Dieffenbachia. **B.** Mistletoe. **C.** Castor bean.

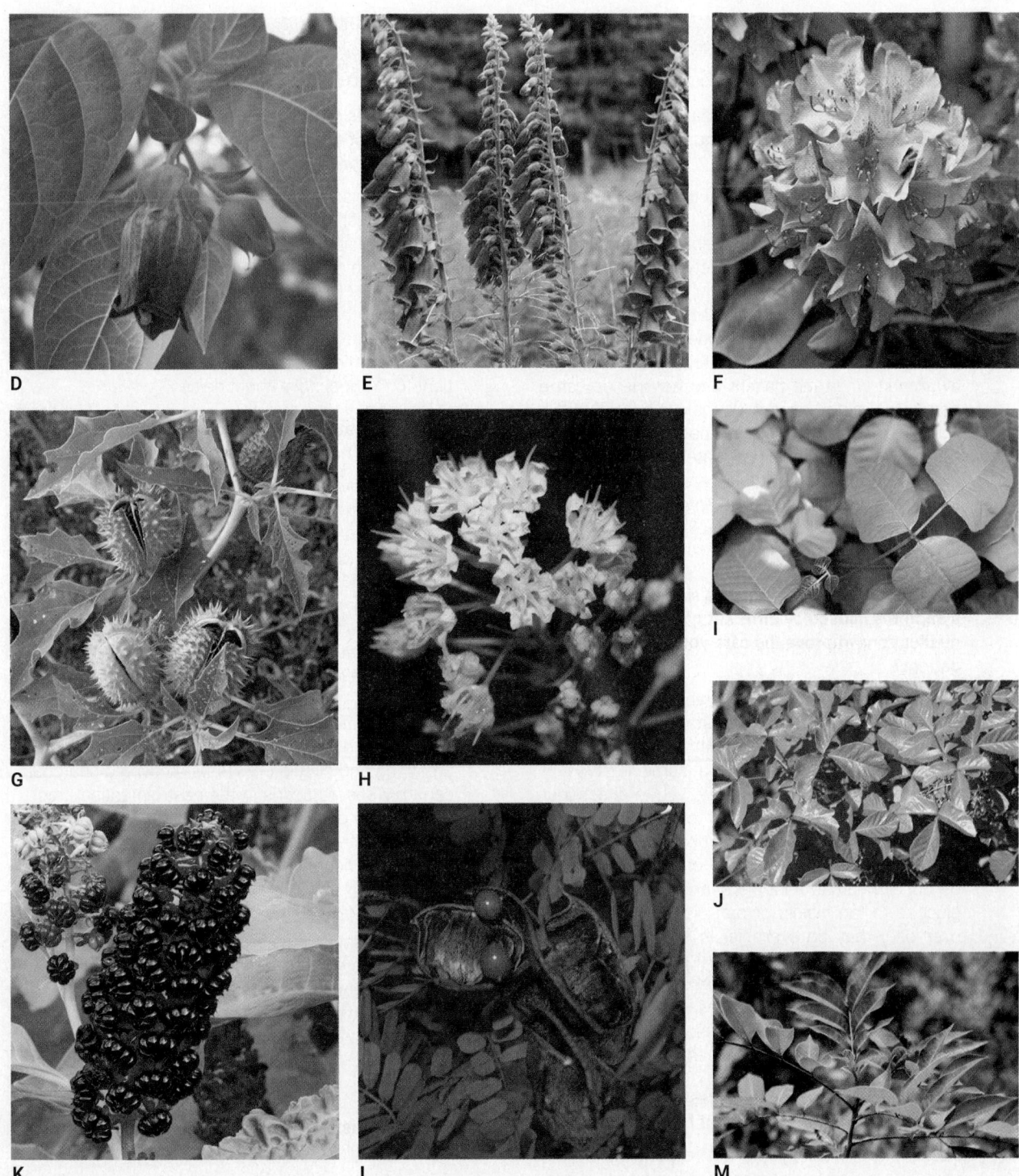

**FIGURE 22-10 D.** Nightshade. **E.** Foxglove. **F.** Rhododendron. **G.** Jimsonweed. **H.** Death camas. **I.** Poison ivy. **J.** Poison oak. **K.** Pokeweed. **L.** Rosary pea. **M.** Poison sumac.

## YOU are the Provider SUMMARY

**1. In addition to providing immediate life-saving treatment, what else should you do when you arrive at this scene?**

Never make assumptions about the scene. Although the home is located in an affluent neighborhood with law enforcement officers available at the scene, always remember that your safety is of the utmost importance. If possible, obtain information from family members or bystanders at the scene. This information is essential to the proper treatment of your patient. In this case, the father reported that he was awakened when the patient and her friends came home from a party and were making a lot of noise. A full secondary assessment may reveal injuries or symptoms that are not immediately apparent. It may also be useful to ask if others are having the same symptoms: Could there be an environmental exposure risk or other group exposure? Because both patients are available, obtain a full SAMPLE history.

**2. How can knowledge of various signs and symptoms caused by different types of medications improve the care you provide to a patient?**

When you assess a patient who has overdosed on a medication or other substance, a careful assessment may help you identify a series of signs and symptoms that indicate a particular type of toxic exposure—thereby allowing you to direct your treatment accordingly. For some toxins (eg, barbiturate-type sedative drug overdose), only supportive treatment such as oxygen or ventilation might be done, whereas for others, an antidote (eg, oral glucose for an insulin or oral diabetes medication overdose) may be available. In some cases, activated charcoal may be useful, if permitted by local protocols. Knowing that a patient has taken or been exposed to certain types of overdoses (eg, stimulant-type drugs) may make you better prepared if agitation, hallucinations, or even seizures develop.

**3. On the basis of your initial assessment, what is the most appropriate treatment for this patient?**

Your patient is sleepy and not responding without stimulation. She has vomited but her airway is currently patent. Her ventilation status is inadequate and requires immediate attention.

With the help of your partner and the members of the fire crew, position the patient supine. Ensure the patient and other providers are not injured in the process. You have assigned a firefighter to manage her airway with a bag-mask device and an airway adjunct as she does not have a gag reflex. Blood glucose level should be determined. This patient requires aggressive treatment and monitoring.

**4. On the basis of the patient's initial presentation, what type of drug should you suspect she overdosed on?**

On the basis of the patient's initial presentation—unconsciousness, hypoventilation, and pinpoint pupils—you should suspect that she has overdosed on an opiate or opioid.

As an EMT, your job is to recognize the signs and symptoms that are associated with these types of drugs, begin immediate treatment to support the XABCs, administer naloxone, and transport the patient to the hospital without delay.

**5. Would activated charcoal benefit this patient? Why or why not?**

There are several reasons why activated charcoal is not indicated for this patient. First, the patient is unconscious, is unable to protect her own airway, and clearly cannot swallow. Pouring anything into her mouth would lead to aspiration, thus substantially increasing her chance of death.

On the basis of the patient's clinical presentation, it is clear that at least some of the medications she ingested are no longer in her stomach. Therefore, it may be too late for charcoal, even if she was alert enough to safely swallow it. She is now experiencing systemic effects that are causing compromise of her breathing and circulatory status. Activated charcoal can only absorb toxins in the gastrointestinal tract, so it has no effect on the drug(s) already absorbed into the system. There are also many drugs/toxins that are not neutralized by charcoal.

**6. Why is naloxone being given to this patient?**

Naloxone blocks opiate receptors in the body and reverses the effects of an opioid overdose. The patient's presentation indicates that one (or many) of the unknown medications she ingested is a narcotic, based on the patient's pinpoint pupils, level of sedation, and decreased ventilation; therefore, naloxone is indicated.

**7. What other issues about this patient should concern you?**

Although the patient's condition has improved following the administration of naloxone, the fact remains that she also ingested an unknown quantity of unknown medications. Because the drugs were taken orally, they may be absorbed or metabolized over a longer period of time and she could have symptoms return. Also, other drugs she may have ingested that take longer to be absorbed and have maximum effect, or that had their effects decreased by the opiates (eg, stimulants), may begin to produce symptoms as time passes. By no means is she out of danger.

# YOU are the Provider SUMMARY *continued*

**8. How would this patient's presentation have differed had she overdosed on a sympathomimetic?**

Unlike CNS depressants, sympathomimetics are CNS stimulants. A sympathomimetic is any substance that mimics the effects of the sympathetic (fight-or-flight) nervous system. When the sympathetic nervous system is stimulated, it releases epinephrine and norepinephrine, resulting in hypertension, tachycardia, and restlessness or agitation.

Had the patient overdosed on a sympathomimetic, her clinical presentation would have been the exact opposite. Her vital functions, such as breathing, heart rate, and blood pressure, would have significantly increased. Furthermore, she would likely have experienced paranoia, delusions, and disorganized behavior. She may even have experienced heart dysrhythmias or seizures.

**9. What additional treatment is required for this patient?**

Further treatment for this patient is mainly supportive; closely monitor her XABCs and be alert for the recurrence of CNS depression (eg, decreased level of consciousness, hypoventilation, hypotension). Monitor her vital signs at regular intervals.

Naloxone is a short-acting reversal agent compared with most opiate/narcotics. Assisted ventilation and additional naloxone may be required if the patient lapses back into CNS depression.

**10. What information should you relay to the hospital staff during your verbal report?**

Your verbal (hand-off) report at the hospital should be more in-depth than what was provided over the radio. Advise the receiving nurse or physician of how you found the patient and the suspected circumstances leading up to the onset of her symptoms, what you initially did to treat her, and how she responded to your treatment.

Inform the hospital staff of the patient's condition en route to the hospital, and advise them of any changes—good or bad—that may have occurred after you gave your radio report.

| EMS Patient Care Report (PCR) | | | | | |
|---|---|---|---|---|---|
| **Date:** 12-04-20 | **Incident No.:** 03188 | **Nature of Call:** "Flulike symptoms" | | **Location:** 1968 Holly Creek Place | |
| **Dispatched:** 0220 | **En Route:** 0222 | **At Scene:** 0226 | **Transport:** 0240 | **At Hospital:** 0249 | **In Service:** 0301 |

| Patient Information | |
|---|---|
| **Age:** 17<br>**Sex:** F<br>**Weight (in kg [lb]):** 49 kg (108 lb) | **Allergies:** No known drug allergies<br>**Medications:** None<br>**Past Medical History:** None<br>**Chief Complaint:** Patient unconscious; mother reports one episode of vomiting |

| Vital Signs | | | | |
|---|---|---|---|---|
| **Time:** 0232 | **BP:** 96/50 | **Pulse:** 116 | **Respirations:** 0 | **Spo$_2$:** 99% |
| **Time:** 0237 | **BP:** 108/52 | **Pulse:** 84 | **Respirations:** 12 | **Spo$_2$:** 100% |
| **Time:** 0243 | **BP:** 108/60 | **Pulse:** 72 | **Respirations:** 14 | **Spo$_2$:** 100% |

| EMS Treatment (circle all that apply) | | | | |
|---|---|---|---|---|
| **Oxygen @** _15_ **L/min via:**<br>NC (NRM) (Bag mask) | | **Assisted Ventilation** | **Airway Adjunct:**<br>(Oral airway) | **CPR** |
| **Defibrillation** | **Bleeding Control** | **Bandaging** | **Splinting** | **Other:** 2 mg Narcan intranasally, blood glucose level |

## YOU are the Provider SUMMARY continued

| Narrative |
| --- |

Dispatched to a single-family home for "flulike symptoms."

Chief Complaint: Patient unconscious; mother reports one episode of vomiting

History: Patient's mother reported she was "sleepy" and had vomited once. Vomit contained colored pill fragments. A bystander stated he and the patient went to a "Skittles party," where the teenagers brought an assortment of pills from home and took as many as they wanted to get high. Bystander also stated they were drinking beer and liquor.

Assessment: Accessed community through security gate and was escorted to scene with Engine 11 by community security guard. Law enforcement was also on scene.

Found the patient, a 17-year-old girl, sitting slouched on a couch with her mother. Assessment of the patient revealed she was unresponsive; her airway was clear of emesis. She had snoring respirations as we entered the home. Subsequently, all respirations ceased.

Treatment (Rx): Patient was moved to floor, her airway was secured manually, and an oral airway was inserted. Ventilation was provided via bag mask and high-flow oxygen. Patient's pulse was weak.

Secondary assessment revealed pinpoint pupils but was otherwise unremarkable. No medical alert bracelets were found on the patient. Blood glucose level was assessed and was noted to read 112 mg/dL. Administered naloxone 2 mg intranasal.

Reassessment of patient revealed that her level of consciousness, heart rate, blood pressure, and oxygen saturation had improved. She no longer tolerated the oral airway or assisted ventilation with a bag-mask device. The patient was placed on high-flow oxygen via nonrebreathing mask.

Transport: Patient was loaded into the ambulance gurney and moved into the ambulance. Departed the scene and continued treatment en route. Reassessment revealed the patient remained conscious but sleepy. Her airway was patent, and her breathing and pulse were adequate. We continued oxygen therapy and monitored patient's vital signs for the duration of the transport.

Patient was delivered to the ED staff without incident; her condition was improving. Gave verbal report to charge nurse. Cleared the hospital and returned to service at 0301.

**End of report**

## Prep Kit

### Ready for Review

- Poisons act acutely or chronically to destroy or impair body cells.
- If you believe a patient may have taken a poisonous substance, support the XABCs and notify medical control.
- Management of the patient also entails collecting any evidence of the type of poison that was used and taking it to the hospital; diluting and physically removing the poisonous agent; providing respiratory support; and transporting the patient promptly to the hospital.
- Emergency treatment may include administration of an antidote, usually at the hospital, if an antidote exists.
- A poison can be introduced into the body in one of four ways:
  - Inhalation
  - Absorption (surface contact)
  - Ingestion
  - Injection
- It is impossible to remove or dilute injected poisons from the body, a fact that makes these cases especially urgent.

- Always consult medical control before you proceed with the treatment of a patient who has been poisoned.
- Move patients who have inhaled poison to fresh air; be prepared to use supplemental oxygen via a nonrebreathing mask and/or ventilatory support via a bag-mask device if necessary.
- With absorbed or surface contact poisons, be sure to avoid contaminating yourself. Remove all contaminated substances and clothing from the patient, and flood the affected part.
- Approximately 80% of all poisonings are by ingestion, including plants, contaminated food, and most drugs. If permitted by local protocol, give activated charcoal to these patients.
- People who abuse a substance can develop a tolerance to it or can develop an addiction.
- One of the most commonly abused drugs in the United States is alcohol. It can depress the CNS and can cause respiratory depression. You must support the airway in such cases, and be prepared for the patient to vomit.
- Opioids, opiates, sedative-hypnotic drugs, and abused inhalants can also depress the CNS and can cause respiratory depression.
- Naloxone is an antidote that reverses the effects of opiate or opioid overdose. Indications for this drug include agonal respirations or apnea. Ventilate the patient prior to administration to minimize hypoxia.
- Take special care with patients who have used inhalants because the drugs may cause seizures or sudden death.
- Sympathomimetics, including cocaine, stimulate the CNS, causing hypertension, tachycardia, seizures, and dilated pupils.

Patients who have taken these drugs may be paranoid, as may patients who have taken hallucinogens.
- Anticholinergic medications, often taken in suicide attempts, can cause a person to become hot, dry, blind, red-faced, and mentally unbalanced. An overdose of tricyclic antidepressants can lead to cardiac dysrhythmias.
- The symptoms of cholinergic medications, which include organophosphate insecticides, can be remembered by the mnemonic DUMBELS, for excessive Diarrhea, Urination, Miosis/muscle weakness, Bradycardia/bronchospasm/bronchorrhea, Emesis, Lacrimation, and Seizures/salivation/sweating; or SLUDGEM, for Salivation/sweating, Lacrimation, Urination, Defecation/drooling/diarrhea, Gastric upset and cramps, Emesis, and Muscle twitching/miosis.
- Two main types of food poisoning cause gastrointestinal symptoms.
  - In one type, bacteria in the food directly cause disease, such as salmonellosis.
  - In the other type, bacteria such as *Staphylococcus* produce powerful toxins, often in leftover food.
  - The most severe form of toxin ingestion is botulism; the first neurologic symptoms may appear as late as 4 days after ingestion.
- Plant poisoning can affect the circulatory system, the gastrointestinal system, and the CNS. Some plants, such as dieffenbachia, irritate the skin or mucous membranes and may cause obstruction of the airway.
- Always remember the importance of scene safety.

## Vital Vocabulary

**addiction** A state of overwhelming obsession or physical need to continue the use of a substance.

**antidote** A substance that is used to neutralize or counteract a poison.

**delirium tremens (DTs)** A severe withdrawal syndrome seen in alcoholics who are deprived of ethyl alcohol; characterized by restlessness, fever, sweating, disorientation, agitation, and seizures; can be fatal if untreated.

**emesis** Vomiting.

**hallucinogen** An agent that produce false perceptions in any one of the five senses.

**hematemesis** Vomiting blood.

**hypnotic** A sleep-inducing effect or agent.

**ingestion** Swallowing; taking a substance by mouth.

**material safety data sheet (MSDS)** A form, provided by manufacturers and compounders (blenders) of chemicals, containing information about chemical composition, physical and chemical properties, health and safety hazards, emergency response, and waste disposal of a specific material; also known as a safety data sheet (SDS).

**narcotic** A drug that produces sleep or altered mental consciousness.

**opiate** A subset of the opioid family, referring to natural, nonsynthetic opioids.

**opioid** A synthetically produced narcotic medication, drug, or agent similar to the opiate morphine, but not derived from opium; used to relieve pain.

**overdose** An excessive quantity of a drug that, when taken or administered, can have toxic or lethal consequences.

**poison** A substance whose chemical action could damage structures or impair function when introduced into the body.

**sedative** A substance that decreases activity and excitement.

**stimulant** An agent that produces an excited state.

**substance abuse** The misuse of any substance to produce a desired effect.

**tolerance** The need for increasing amounts of a drug to obtain the same effect.

**toxicology** The study of toxic or poisonous substances.

**toxin** A poison or harmful substance.

## References

1. Acetaminophen information. US Food and Drug Administration website. http://www.fda.gov/Drugs/DrugSafety/InformationbyDrugClass/ucm165107.htm. Updated November 14, 2017. Accessed April 15, 2020.

2. Alcohol facts and statistics. National Institute on Alcohol Abuse and Alcoholism website. https://www.niaaa.nih.gov/publications/brochures-and-fact-sheets/alcohol-facts-and-statistics. Updated February 2020. Accessed April 16, 2020.

3. All manufacturers of prescription combination drug products with more than 325 mg of acetaminophen have discontinued marketing. US Food and Drug Administration website. http://www.fda.gov/Drugs/DrugSafety/InformationbyDrugClass/ucm390509.htm. Published December 11, 2014. Accessed April 15, 2020.

4. American Heart Association. *Highlights of the 2015 American Heart Association Guidelines Update for CPR and ECC*. Dallas, TX: American Heart Association; 2015:1–29.

5. Aspirin overdose. Medline Plus website. https://www.nlm.nih.gov/medlineplus/ency/article/002542.htm. Updated April 9, 2020. Accessed April 15, 2020.

6. Chemical suicides: the risk to emergency responders. Chemical Hazards Emergency Medical Management website. http://chemm.nlm.nih.gov/chemicalsuicide.htm. Updated March 10, 2020. Accessed April 15, 2020.

7. Cicero TJ, Ellis MS, Surratt HL, Kurtz SP. The changing face of heroin use in the United States: a retrospective analysis of the past 50 Years. *JAMA Psychiatry* 2014;71(7):821–826.

8. Fletcher H. Carbon monoxide poisoning risk rises as temperatures drop. Tennessean website. http://www.tennessean.com/story/news/2015/02/18/carbon-monoxide-poisoning-risk-rises-temps-drop/23624783/. Published February 18, 2015. Accessed April 15, 2020.

9. Gummin DD, Mowry JB, Spyker DA, et al. 2018 annual report of the American Association of Poison Control Centers' National Poison Data System (NPDS): 36th annual report. *Clin Toxicol (Phila)* 2019;57(12):1220–1413.

10. Hampden County Sheriff's Department. Chemical and detergent suicides. Public Intelligence website. https://info.publicintelligence.net/MAchemicalsuicide.pdf. Accessed April 15, 2020.

11. Heroin. National Institute on Drug Abuse website. http://www.drugabuse.gov/publications/drugfacts/heroin. Updated November 2019. Accessed April 15, 2020.

12. MDPV effects. https://www.erowid.org/chemicals/mdpv/mdpv_effects.shtml. The Vaults of Erowid website. Published March 11, 2010. Accessed April 15, 2020.

13. Overdose death rates. National Institute on Drug Abuse website. https://www.drugabuse.gov/related-topics/trends-statistics/overdose-death-rates. Updated March 2020. Accessed April 16, 2020.

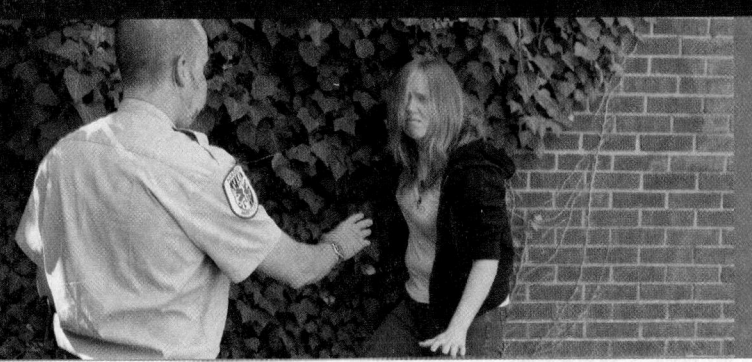

# Chapter 23

# Behavioral Health Emergencies

## NATIONAL EMS EDUCATION STANDARD COMPETENCIES

### Medicine

Applies fundamental knowledge to provide basic emergency care and transportation based on assessment findings for an acutely ill patient.

### Psychiatric

Recognition of
- Behaviors that pose a risk to the EMT, patient, or others (pp 855–856, 862–863, 868–871)

- Basic principles of the mental health system (p 855)
- Assessment and management of
  - Acute psychosis (pp 857–863)
  - Suicidal/risk (pp 857–862, 869–871)
  - Agitated delirium (pp 857–864)

## KNOWLEDGE OBJECTIVES

1. Discuss the myths and realities concerning behavioral health emergencies. (pp 854–855)
2. Discuss general factors that can cause alteration in a patient's behavior. (p 855)
3. Define a behavioral crisis. (p 855)
4. Recognize the magnitude of mental health disorders in society. (p 856)
5. Know the main principles of how the mental health care system functions. (p 855)
6. Know the two basic categories of diagnosis that a mental health professional will use. (p 857)
7. Explain special considerations for assessing and managing a behavioral crisis or behavioral health emergency. (pp 857–862)

8. Define acute psychosis. (p 862)
9. Define schizophrenia. (p 863)
10. Explain the care for a psychotic patient. (pp 862–863)
11. Define excited delirium or agitated delirium. (p 864)
12. Explain the care for a patient with excited delirium. (p 864)
13. Describe methods used to restrain patients. (pp 864–868)
14. Know the main principles of care for the agitated, violent, or uncooperative patient. (pp 868–869)

15. Explain how to recognize the behavior of a patient at risk of suicide, including the management of such a patient. (pp 869–871)

16. Recognize issues specific to posttraumatic stress disorder (PTSD) and the returning combat veteran. (pp 871–873)

17. Discuss the medical and legal aspects of managing a behavioral health emergency. (pp 873–874)

## SKILLS OBJECTIVE

1. Demonstrate the techniques used to mechanically restrain a patient. (pp 866–867, Skill Drill 23-1)

## Introduction

As an EMT, you will care for patients experiencing behavioral health emergencies. A crisis may be the result of an acute medical condition, mental illness, mind-altering substances, stress, or other causes. This chapter discusses various types of behavioral health emergencies, including those involving drug overdoses, violent behavior, and different forms of mental illness. You will learn how to assess a person who exhibits signs and symptoms of a behavioral health emergency and understand what kind of emergency care may be required in these situations. The chapter also covers legal concerns in dealing with behavioral health emergencies, the dangers of suicide, and difficulties related to posttraumatic stress disorder. Finally, you will learn how to identify and manage a potentially violent patient, including the use of patient restraints.

## Myth and Reality

At some point, most people experience an emotional crisis, but only rarely does this crisis result in mental illness. Otherwise healthy people may sustain acute or temporary mental health disorders. Therefore, you should not jump to the conclusion that a patient is mentally ill when exhibiting behaviors discussed in this chapter.

A common misconception about mental illness is that if you are feeling bad or depressed, you must be sick. That is simply not true. There are many perfectly justifiable reasons for feeling depressed, including divorce or the death of a relative or friend. For a teenager who just broke up with his girlfriend of 12 months, it is altogether normal to withdraw from ordinary activities and to feel down for a while. This is a normal reaction to an acute crisis situation. However, when a person finds that the majority of his or her days are characterized by sadness, week after week, he or she may indeed have a behavioral health problem.

Some people believe anyone with a behavioral health disorder is dangerous, violent, or otherwise unmanageable. This is also not true. Only a small percentage of behavioral health patients fall into these categories. However, as an EMT, you may be exposed to a higher proportion of violent patients because you are seeing people who are, by definition, considered to be having a behavioral crisis;

## YOU are the Provider

At 1920 hours, you are dispatched to 517 East Bandera for a man who, according to a neighbor, is sitting in his yard "acting bizarre." Law enforcement is en route to the scene but has not yet arrived. You and your partner acknowledge the call, get into the ambulance, and proceed to the scene. The weather is clear, the temperature is 70°F (21°C), and the traffic is moderate.

1. How should you and your partner proceed to this call?

2. Other than an underlying behavioral health condition, what other conditions can affect a person's behavior?

otherwise, you probably would not be seeing them. You have been called because family members or friends felt unable to manage the person on their own. The situation may be a result of drug or alcohol use or abuse or medication noncompliance, or the individual may have a long history of mental illness and is reacting to a particularly stressful event.

It is easy to assume the patient having a behavioral crisis does not understand the situation or the message you are trying to convey. However, especially during an acute crisis, many patients still have awareness and understanding. Communication is key. Never make disparaging or inappropriate statements. It is not only poor patient care, but inappropriate comments could escalate the situation. You may be able to calm the patient with reassurances and avoid restraints or other physical interactions that can be a danger to you or the patient. In some cases patients will deescalate once a level of trust has been established.

Although you cannot determine what has caused a person's crisis, you may be able to predict whether the person will become violent. The ability to predict violence is one of your more important assessment tools.

## Defining a Behavioral Crisis

Behavior is what you can see of a person's response to the environment: his or her actions. Sometimes, it is obvious what is causing a person's response: A person is punched, and he or she runs away, bursts into tears, or hits back. Sometimes, it is less clear, such as when someone is depressed for complex emotional or biological reasons.

Most of the time, people respond to the environment in reasonable ways. Over the years, people learn to adapt to a variety of situations in daily life, including stress. Stress is managed by the use of coping mechanisms. However, there are times when the stress is so great that the normal means of coping are not enough, or the person uses negative coping mechanisms such as withdrawal or numbing self-medication with drugs and alcohol. In some cases, the reaction is acute, but in other cases it develops over time. Both situations can create a crisis.

The change in behavior may be considered inappropriate or not normal by the person who calls 9-1-1. A behavioral crisis describes the situation involving patients of all ages who exhibit agitated, violent, or uncooperative behavior or who are a danger to themselves or others. EMS is called when behavior has become unacceptable to the patient, family, or community. EMS can be called for an older adult who lives alone and started a kitchen fire when he or she left the burner on or for a person who is in danger from hoarding behavior. In these instances, a patient may have dementia or depression, behavior that may interfere with the activities of daily living. Chronic depression is a persistent feeling of sadness and despair. It may be a symptom of an underlying health disorder. There may not be a medical or traumatic emergency but simply a request for evaluation.

A person who experiences a panic attack after having a heart attack is not necessarily mentally ill. Likewise, you would expect a person who is fired from a job to have some sort of reaction, often sadness and depression. These problems are short-term and isolated events. However, when a person reacts with a fit of rage, attacking people and property, this behavior has gone beyond what society considers within the scope of a normal response to stressful stimulus. That person is likely undergoing a behavioral crisis. Depending on the nature of the response, an abnormal or disturbing pattern of behavior is regarded as a matter of concern from a mental health standpoint.

When a behavioral health emergency arises, patients may show agitation or violence or become a threat to themselves or others. This is more serious than a typical behavioral crisis that causes inappropriate behavior. A behavioral health emergency often leads to severe impairments in the ability to perform activities of daily living and may be accompanied by bizarre behavior.

When there is an immediate threat to the person involved or when a patient's behavior threatens you, family, friends, or bystanders, the situation should be considered a behavioral health emergency. For example, a person might respond to the death of a spouse by attempting suicide. Other patients might respond to an upsetting event by exhibiting bizarre behavior.

## The Magnitude of Mental Health Disorders

According to the National Institute of Mental Health, mental disorders are common throughout the United States, affecting tens of millions of people each year. A **psychiatric disorder** is an illness with psychological or behavioral symptoms that may result in impaired functioning. Anxiety disorders are among the most common mental health disorders and include generalized anxiety disorder, panic disorder, and social and other phobias.

The mental health system in the United States provides many levels of assistance to people with psychological conditions. Common emotional issues such as marital conflict and parenting issues can often be resolved with the assistance of a professional counselor. More serious issues, such as clinical depression, are often handled by a psychologist who has specialized training dealing with

more complex psychological conditions. For the treatment of the most severe conditions, such as schizophrenia or bipolar disorder, a psychiatrist may need to prescribe medication. Most behavioral health disorders can be treated in an outpatient environment; however, some people require hospitalization in specialized behavioral health units.

Behavioral health disorders have many underlying causes. These include social and situational stress, such as divorce or death of a loved one; psychiatric diseases, such as schizophrenia; physical illnesses, such as diabetic emergencies; chemical problems, such as alcohol or drug use; or biologic disturbances, such as electrolyte imbalances. Sometimes these conditions can be compounded by noncompliance with prescribed medication regimens.

## Pathophysiology

As an EMT, you are not responsible for diagnosing the underlying cause of a behavioral crisis or emergency. However, you should understand the two basic categories of diagnosis that a physician will use: organic (physical) and functional (psychological).

## YOU are the Provider

Law enforcement personnel arrive at the scene and inform you that it is safe for you to enter. One of the police officers informs you that the patient allowed them to check him for any weapons and that he does not have any.

You find the patient, a 44-year-old man, sitting on the lawn in front of his house; one of the police officers is trying to talk to him. He appears sad and withdrawn and is rocking back and forth. You introduce yourself to the patient and perform a primary assessment.

| Recording Time:  0 Minutes | |
| --- | --- |
| **Appearance** | Sad, withdrawn appearance |
| **Level of consciousness** | Conscious and alert |
| **Airway** | Open; clear of secretions and foreign bodies |
| **Breathing** | Normal rate; adequate depth |
| **Circulation** | Normal pulse rate; skin pink and moist; no obvious bleeding |

The patient tells you he "has a lot of problems," but nobody will listen to him.

**3.** What should be your most immediate concern with this patient?

**4.** How should you proceed with your assessment of this patient?

## Organic

**Organic brain syndrome** is a temporary or permanent dysfunction of the brain caused by a disturbance in the physical or physiologic functioning of brain tissue. Causes of organic brain syndrome include sudden illness; traumatic brain injury; seizure disorders; drug and alcohol abuse, overdose, or withdrawal; and diseases of the brain, such as Alzheimer dementia or meningitis.

**Altered mental status** can arise from a physiologic issue such as a hypoglycemia, hypoxia, impaired cerebral blood flow, and/or hyperthermia or hypothermia. In the absence of a physiologic cause, altered mental status may be an indicator of a psychiatric disorder such as bipolar disorder.

## Functional

A **functional disorder** is a physiologic disorder that impairs bodily function when the body seems to be structurally normal. Something has gone wrong, but the root cause cannot be identified. Schizophrenia, anxiety conditions, and depression are good examples of functional disorders. The chemical or physical basis of these disorders does not alter the appearance of the patient.

### Words of Wisdom

A patient displaying bizarre behavior may actually have an acute medical illness that is the cause, or a partial cause, of the behavior. Behavioral changes may be the result or a symptom of a treatable medical condition such as diabetes or a stroke. They can also be the result of a head injury or drug or alcohol intoxication. Medical conditions presenting as behavioral disorders must be identified. A patient with hypoglycemia presenting with altered behavior can face a life-threatening situation if the medical condition is not treated. Remember, a psychiatric diagnosis is never made until possible medical causes of altered behavior have been actively excluded as possibilities. This requires evaluation by a physician.

## Safe Approach to a Behavioral Crisis

All routine EMT skills—patient approach, assessment, patient communication, obtaining the history, and providing care—are used in a behavioral crisis. However, other management techniques are also involved. Follow the general guidelines listed in **TABLE 23-1** to ensure your safety at the scene of a behavioral health emergency.

## Patient Assessment

### Scene Size-up

The first things for you to consider at the scene of a behavioral crisis or psychiatric emergency are your safety and the patient's response to the environment. Is the situation potentially dangerous for you and your partner? Do you need immediate law enforcement backup? Should you stage until law enforcement personnel have secured the scene? Does the patient's behavior seem typical or normal for the circumstances? Are there legal issues involved (crime scene, consent, refusal)? Make sure to take appropriate standard precautions. Request any additional resources you may need (law enforcement, additional personnel) early. You can always send them away if they are not needed. Be vigilant and avoid tunnel vision.

Determine the mechanism of injury and/or nature of illness. Remember, certain injuries and medical conditions can cause altered behavior that can be confused with a behavioral health emergency. Note any medications or substances that may contribute to the complaint or that may be for treatment of a relevant medical condition.

### Street Smarts

When attempting to determine the cause of altered behavior in a patient with a behavioral health history, the patient may not know the cause of his or her own behavior. This lack of insight can be frustrating to EMS providers attempting to help. Demonstrate patience when assessing and talking with these patients. The unexplained behavior is confusing and frustrating to the patient as well.

### Words of Wisdom

Never leave a patient alone who may be experiencing a behavioral emergency.

---

**TABLE 23-1** Safety Guidelines for a Behavioral Health Emergency

- **Assess the scene.** Immediately request law enforcement to secure and maintain scene safety. Do not attempt to enter or control a scene where physical violence or weapons are present.
- **Ensure you have a means of communication, such as a radio.** If there is an unexpected problem, you may need to immediately contact help. *Never* let the patient get between you and the door.
- **Know where the exits are.** Park your ambulance in a location that allows you a safe and easy way out if it becomes necessary.
- **Don appropriate personal protective equipment.**
- **Have a definite plan of action.** Decide who will do what. If restraint is needed, how will it be accomplished? Avoid restraint unless your safety is an issue. Ensure you have sufficient help if restraint is required. Consider requesting ALS assistance for chemical restraint if appropriate and possible.
- **Urgently deescalate the patient's level of agitation.** This is imperative in the interest of patient safety as well as for you and others on the scene.
- **Calmly identify yourself.** Try to gain the patient's confidence. Ask questions in a low, calm voice, and be patient. Reassure the patient that you are there to help.
- **Be direct.** State your intentions and what you expect of the patient. Let the patient know what you are doing and maintain good eye contact.
- **Be prepared to spend extra time.** It may take longer than normal to assess, listen to, and prepare the patient for transport.
- **Stay with the patient.** Do not let the patient leave the area. You should not leave the area either unless law enforcement personnel can stay with the patient. Remove any stimulus that is distressing to the patient.
- **Do not get too close to a potentially volatile patient.** Patients may object to you invading their personal space, so avoid unnecessary physical contact. A squatting, 45° angle approach is usually not confrontational, but the position may hinder your movements (**FIGURE 23-1**). Prepare to move quickly if the patient becomes violent; otherwise do not make quick moves. Do not allow anything to hang around your neck like a tie or stethoscope.
- **Express interest in the patient's story.** Let the patient tell you in his or her own words what happened or what is going on now. Listening can be your best skill. Do not tell the patient he or she is not hearing voices; however, do not play along with auditory or visual disturbances, delusions, or hallucinations. Do not tell the patient you understand what he or she is going through. You do not know what he or she is feeling, and this statement can trigger anger and escalate the patient's condition.
- **Avoid fighting with the patient.** Remember, the patient is not responding to you in a normal manner. He or she may be wrestling with internal forces over which neither of you has control. You and others may be stimulating these inner forces without knowing it. If you can respond with empathy to the feeling that the patient is expressing, whether the feeling is anger or fear or desperation, you may be able to gain his or her cooperation. If possible, try to involve a friend or family member whom the patient trusts. Always try to talk the patient into cooperating. Do not threaten the patient. Do not talk down to the patient or directly confront him or her. If the patient verbally attacks you, do not take it personally.
- **Be honest and reassuring.** If the patient asks whether he or she has to go to the hospital, the answer should be, "Yes, that is where you can receive help."
- **Do not judge.** Do not judge a patient by behavior over which she or he may not have control. Set aside personal feelings and concentrate on providing care. Always treat the patient with respect.

© Jones & Bartlett Learning.

## Primary Assessment

Begin your assessment from the doorway or from a distance. How does the patient appear? Calm? Agitated? Awake or sleepy? How is the patient dressed? Is the patient out in the cold wearing only shorts? Is the patient's attire appropriate for the situation? Begin by introducing yourself, and let the patient know you

are there to help. Allow the patient to tell you what happened or how he or she feels. Perform a rapid physical exam if the patient allows you. Look for trauma, especially head trauma. Remember, sometimes a traumatic brain injury (TBI) can take several days to present with symptoms. TBI is discussed further in Chapter 29, *Head and Spine Injuries.*

Closely observe the patient. Does the patient answer slowly with single-word answers or rapidly

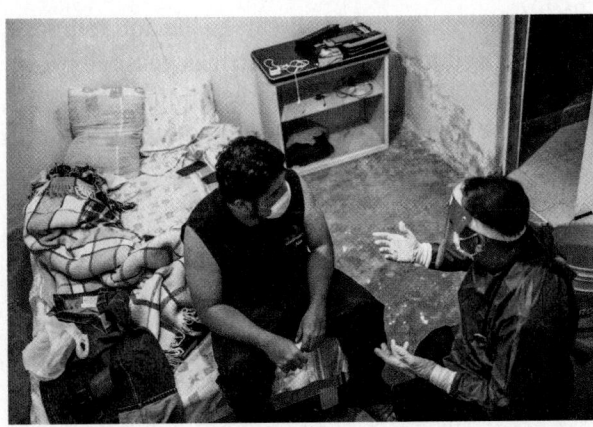

**FIGURE 23-1** When working with a potentially volatile patient, position yourself at a 45° angle, but be aware this position could hinder your movements.

© PEDRO PARDO/AFP/Getty Images.

in long, rambling sentences? Do the patient's words make sense, or do they have no apparent sequence? Is the patient sitting slumped in a chair, hunched and shuffling around the room, or rigid and standing perfectly still? Is the patient alert and oriented? Use the AVPU scale to check for alertness. To determine orientation, ask the patient, "Who are you?," "Where are you?," "What time is it?," "What happened?," and "How can I help?" Asking these questions will allow you to begin to establish a rapport with the patient. This rapport is critical to the success of your interaction. Engage family members or loved ones to encourage the patient's cooperation, if their presence does not worsen the patient's agitation.

### Street Smarts

Family members often experience an emotional response to the patient's actions. They may be frustrated or feel they are the cause of the patient's behavior. Be sensitive to their feelings and concerns.

Most medical or trauma situations will include a behavioral component. Anyone experiencing an emergency will generally have some level of fear or anxiety. A patient with difficulty breathing will be anxious. The parent of a small child who fell out of a second-story window will most likely be hysterical and feeling guilty. An assault victim often experiences fear or anger. It is important to treat the whole patient: the behavioral component as well as the medical or traumatic issue.

If your patient is in physical distress, assess the airway to make sure it is patent and adequate. Next, evaluate the patient's breathing and obtain rate and effort. Use pulse oximetry if available. Provide the appropriate interventions based on your assessment findings. Some behavioral situations will involve a compromised airway or inadequate breathing if a patient has ingested prescription medications, drugs, or alcohol.

Next, you will need to assess the pulse rate, quality, and rhythm. Assessing a patient's circulation includes an evaluation for the presence of shock and bleeding. Assess the patient's perfusion by evaluating skin color, temperature, and capillary refill. Because skin paleness can be difficult to detect in patients with dark skin, instead check for pale mucous membranes inside the inner lower eyelid or slow capillary refill.

Unless your patient is unstable from a medical problem or trauma, prepare to spend time with your patient. It may take time and patience to gain the patient's trust if he or she is fearful or unwilling to cooperate with you.

## History Taking

When a medical patient is conscious, the next step in your assessment is to investigate the chief complaint and then obtain a SAMPLE history. Obtain information about the patient and his or her medical history.

Determine the reason for the patient's behavior; your assessment should consider four major areas as possible contributors:

- Is the patient's central nervous system functioning properly? For example, the patient may be experiencing a diabetic emergency such as hypoglycemia. This situation could cause the patient to behave in an unusual or irrational manner.
- Are hallucinogens or other drugs or alcohol a factor? Does the patient see strange things? Is everything distorted? Do you smell alcohol on the patient's breath? Are there clues at the scene that suggest intoxication?
- Are significant life changes, symptoms, or illness (caused by mental rather than physical factors) involved? These might include the death of a loved one, severe depression,

history of behavioral illness, threats of suicide, or some other major interruption of activities of daily living.

- If a patient has a history of behavioral health illness, has there been a recent change in medications? Often, treatment of functional behavioral health conditions is a trial-and-error process with medications and therapy. Doctors and therapists work with the patient and family to find the most effective course of treatment, with medication changes sometimes causing unexpected or undesirable outcomes. In some cases, the patient may refuse to take a medication.

During the SAMPLE history, you may be able to elicit information that would be helpful to the hospital staff. Ask specifically about previous episodes, treatments, hospitalizations, and medications related to behavioral symptoms (**TABLE 23-2**).

In geriatric patients, consider Alzheimer disease and other causes of dementia as possible causes of abnormal behavior. Determining the patient's baseline mental status will be essential in guiding your treatment and transport decisions and will also be extremely helpful to hospital personnel.

Family, friends, observers, and caregivers may be of great help in answering these questions. Together with your observations and interactions with the patient, they should provide enough data for you to assess the situation. This assessment has two primary

---

**TABLE 23-2 Questions to Ask in Evaluating a Mental Health Disorder**

- Does the patient appropriately answer your questions?
- Does the patient's behavior seem appropriate?
- Does the patient seem to understand you?
- Is the patient withdrawn or detached? Hostile or friendly? Happy or depressed?
- Are the patient's vocabulary and expressions what you would expect under the circumstances?
- Does the patient seem aggressive or dangerous to you or others?
- Is the patient's memory intact? Check orientation to time, place, person, and event: What day, month, and year is it? Who am I?
- Does the patient express disordered thoughts, delusions, or hallucinations?

© Jones & Bartlett Learning.

---

goals: recognizing major threats to life and reducing the stress of the situation as much as possible.

Reflective listening is a technique frequently used by behavioral health professionals to gain insight into a patient's thinking. It involves repeating, in question form, what the patient has said, encouraging the patient to expand on his or her thoughts. Although it often requires more time to be effective than is available in an EMS setting, it may be a helpful tool for you to use when other techniques are unsuccessful at gathering the patient's history.

---

**Words of Wisdom**

When assessing a patient in a behavioral health emergency, it can be very useful to gather information separately from a relative or caregiver. Splitting up the history-taking process in this way often yields valuable information and can help reduce the potential for violence when there is tension between the people involved. However, if the patient is threatening or uncontrollable, do not enter the room with the patient to obtain a more detailed history unless additional help, such as law enforcement personnel, is present.

---

## Secondary Assessment

In an unconscious patient, begin with a physical exam to look for a reason for the unresponsiveness. Rule out trauma, especially to the head. Follow this rapid exam for hidden life threats with a detailed physical exam and obtain a complete set of vital signs. Obtain vital signs only if you are able to do so without worsening your patient's emotional condition. Make every effort to assess blood pressure, pulse, respirations, skin, and pupils. Then gather what history you can from others. Consider whether prior events such as physical agitation, use of stimulants, alcohol withdrawal, or TASER exposure may be contributing to the patient's condition. (Many law enforcement agencies use TASER devices to immobilize people who are behaving in a violent or aggressive manner.) When physically examining a patient with a history of behavioral crises, check for track marks indicating drug abuse and for signs of self-mutilation.

Sometimes even a conscious patient in a behavioral health emergency will not respond to your questions. In those cases, you may be able to tell a

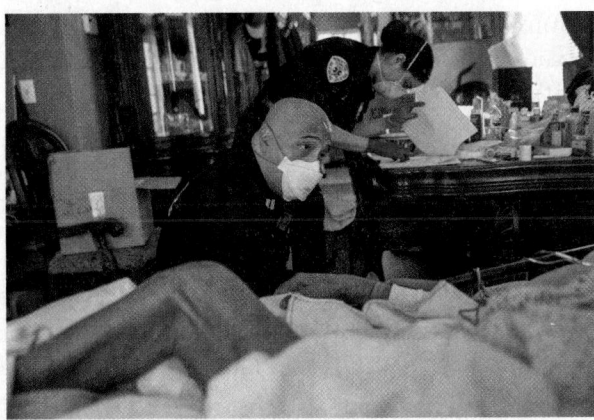

**FIGURE 23-2** Making eye contact with a patient can provide useful clues about a patient's emotional state.

© John Moore/Getty Images News/Getty Images.

lot about the patient's emotional state from facial expressions, pulse rate, and respirations. Tears, sweating, and blushing may be significant indicators of state of mind such as sadness, nervousness, or embarrassment. Also, make sure you look at the patient's eyes; a patient who has a blank gaze or rapidly moving eyes may be experiencing central nervous system dysfunction (**FIGURE 23-2**).

## Words of Wisdom

In many patients with autism or autism spectrum disorder, making eye contact can be very stressful for the patient and may cause the patient to become agitated. Do not force eye contact.

A behavioral health emergency puts tremendous stress on a person's coping mechanisms. The person is actually incapable of responding reasonably to the demands of the environment. This state may be temporary, as in an acute illness such as drug-induced hallucinations, or more chronic, as in a complex, mental illness such as schizophrenia. The patient's perception of reality may be compromised or distorted.

If you feel transport may put you at risk, ask law enforcement personnel to accompany you. This provides you with additional assistance should the patient's behavior change rapidly. If a police officer restrains the patient with handcuffs, the officer must ride in the back of the ambulance to release the cuffs in the case of an emergency. Always follow local protocols regarding the use of physical restraints.

There may be a specific facility to which patients with behavioral health emergencies are transported. Transport by ground rather than by air. Try to make the patient comfortable, but require that he or she ride on the stretcher with all straps secured. Stretchers with foam padding around the head allow the patient to position his or her head for adequate airway patency. Placing the stretcher in Fowler or high Fowler position helps prevent aspiration and reduces physical exertion by relaxing the abdominal muscles.

## Reassessment

Never let your guard down. Most patients you treat and transport with emotional complaints pose no danger to you or others, but it is not always possible to determine this while on scene. Remember, many patients experiencing a behavioral crisis may act spontaneously. Be prepared to intervene quickly. If restraints are necessary, reassess and document the patient's respirations, as well as pulse, motor, and sensory functions in all restrained extremities, every 5 minutes. Restraint is discussed later in this chapter.

In terms of interventions, as much as your heart may go out to an emotionally distressed patient, there often is little you will be able to do during the short time you will be treating the patient. Your job is to defuse and control the situation and safely transport your patient to the hospital. The best treatment may be to be a good listener. Often these patients are happy if someone will listen to their problem. Intervene only as much as it takes to accomplish these tasks. Be caring and careful. Be aware of standard precautions. If the patient is spitting, place a surgical mask loosely over his or her mouth, and make sure you are wearing appropriate PPE including adequate eye protection and a mask. Continually reassess the patient's ability to protect the airway and breathe.

In many areas, local protocol allows ALS providers to administer medications to calm a combative patient. This will often make the situation safer for you and your patient. If you encounter a situation where you think chemical (pharmacologic) restraint might be necessary, request ALS as early as possible.

> ### Words of Wisdom
>
> The medicolegal issues associated with responses to a behavioral crisis increase emphasis on the importance of providing thorough and specific documentation. Record detailed, objective findings that support the conclusion of abnormal behavior (eg, withdrawn, will not talk, crying uncontrollably) and quote the patient's own words when appropriate—for example, "Life isn't worth it anymore" or "The voices are telling me to kill people." Avoid judgmental statements that may create the impression you based your care on personal bias rather than the patient's needs.

Give the receiving hospital advance warning when a patient experiencing a behavioral health emergency is coming in. Many hospitals require extra preparation to ensure the appropriate staff and rooms are available. Report whether restraints will be required when the patient arrives.

Thoroughly and carefully document your actions. Think about what you are going to write before you write it, so that you can describe as clearly as possible what are often confusing scenes.

Communicate to the hospital the things you observed at the scene that may help explain the patient's situation. These are important facts the hospital will not know unless you tell them. Include observed behaviors or items seen such as medications or weapons. Medications may have contributed to the crisis or may give you information about an otherwise undisclosed medical condition. Because behavioral health emergencies have few or no physical signs, you may have the only documentation clarifying the patient's distress. Because these emergencies are also fraught with legal dangers, document everything that occurred on the call, particularly situations that required restraint. When restraints are required to protect you or the patient from harm, include why and what type of restraints were used. This information is essential if the case is reviewed for medicolegal reasons.

## Acute Psychosis

**Psychosis** is a state of delusion in which the person is out of touch with reality. Affected people live in their own reality of ideas and feelings. To the person experiencing a psychotic episode, the line between reality and fantasy is blurred. That reality may make patients belligerent and angry toward others. Patients may become silent and withdrawn as they give all their attention to the voices and feelings within.

## YOU are the Provider

The patient tells you his wife was killed in a car accident 1 year ago today, and even though he has been to numerous counseling sessions over the past year they have not seemed to help. He further tells you his employer does not seem to care about his problems and has threatened to fire him unless he "snaps out of it." He allows your partner to take his vital signs but refuses to allow you to perform any other assessment or treatment.

| Recording Time: 9 Minutes | |
| --- | --- |
| **Respirations** | 16 breaths/min; adequate depth |
| **Pulse** | 88 beats/min; strong and regular |
| **Skin** | Pink, warm, and moist |
| **Blood pressure** | 144/84 mm Hg |
| **Oxygen saturation (Spo$_2$)** | 98% (on room air) |

The patient denies chest pain, shortness of breath, or any other physical symptoms. He tells you it is extremely difficult for him to even get out of bed and face each day and he feels as though his life no longer serves any purpose.

**5.** What is your field impression of this patient?

**6.** What care can you provide to this patient in the field?

Psychotic episodes occur for many reasons; the use of mind-altering substances is a common cause, and that experience may be limited to the duration of the substance within the body. Other causes include intense stress, delusional disorders, and, more commonly, schizophrenia. Some psychotic episodes last for brief periods; others last a lifetime.

## Schizophrenia

Schizophrenia is a complex disorder that is not easily defined or easily treated. It affects how a person thinks, feels, and behaves. The typical onset occurs during early adulthood, between the ages of 16 and 30 years. Symptoms of the illness become more prominent over time. Some people in whom schizophrenia has been diagnosed display signs during early childhood; their disease may be associated with brain damage or may have other causes. Other influences thought to contribute to this disorder include genetics and psychological and social influences. Patients with schizophrenia may experience symptoms including delusions, hallucinations, paranoia, a lack of interest in pleasure, and erratic speech.

Dealing with a psychotic patient is difficult. The usual methods of reasoning with a patient are unlikely to be effective because the psychotic person has his or her own rules of logic that may be quite different from nonpsychotic thinking. Follow these guidelines in dealing with a psychotic patient:

- Determine if the situation is a danger to yourself or others.
- Clearly identify yourself. ("I'm Gloria. I'm an EMT with the ambulance service, and this is my partner, Stan. We've come to see if we can help. Can you tell us what is happening?")
- Be calm, direct, and straightforward. Your composure and confidence can do a great deal toward calming the patient.
- Maintain an emotional distance. Do not touch the patient, and do not patronize the patient or be overly reassuring.
- Do not argue. Do not challenge patients regarding the reality of their beliefs or the validity of their perceptions. Do not go along with their delusions simply to humor them, and do not make an issue of the delusions. Talk about real things.
- Explain what you would like to do. ("Let's walk downstairs to the ambulance.")

- Involve people the patient trusts, such as family or friends, to gain the patient's cooperation.

## Delirium

*Delirium* is a condition of impairment in cognitive function that can present with disorientation, hallucinations, or delusions. *Agitation* is a behavior characterized by restless and irregular physical activity. Although patients experiencing delirium are generally not dangerous, if they exhibit agitated behavior they may strike out irrationally. One of the most important factors to consider in these cases is your personal safety.

If you think you can safely approach the patient, be calm, supportive, and empathetic. Be an active listener by nodding, indicating understanding, and by limiting your interruptions of the patient's comments. It is extremely important to approach the patient slowly and purposefully and to respect the patient's personal space. Limit physical contact with the patient as much as possible. It is also imperative that you do not leave the patient unattended, unless the situation becomes unsafe for you or your partner.

Use careful interviewing to assess the patient's cognitive functioning. Try to indirectly determine the patient's orientation, memory, concentration, and judgment by asking simple questions such as "When did you first begin to notice these feelings?" Through interviewing, try to determine what the patient is thinking. Are the patient's thoughts disorganized? For example, does the patient begin to answer your question and then drift off only to begin discussing a childhood friend? Is the patient experiencing delusions or hallucinations? Does the patient have any unusual worries or fears? For example, does the patient express anxiety if you go too close to a pile of old newspapers?

Pay particular attention to the patient's ability to communicate clearly and make notes on the patient's apparent mood. Is the patient anxious, depressed, elated (extremely happy or joyful), or agitated? Pay attention to the patient's appearance, dress, and personal hygiene.

If the patient appears to be experiencing a drug overdose, take all medication bottles or illegal substances with you to the medical facility. The patient should be transported to a hospital with behavioral health facilities capable of handling the condition. Whenever possible, refrain from using lights and siren because these may aggravate the patient's condition.

## Excited Delirium

A medical emergency sometimes encountered in an EMS response is excited delirium. **Excited delirium** is also known as agitated delirium or exhaustive mania.

The symptoms of excited delirium may include hyperactive irrational behavior with possible vivid hallucinations, which can create the potential for violent behavior. Common physical symptoms include hypertension, hyperthermia, tachycardia, diaphoresis, and dilated pupils. Because hallucinations are erroneous perceptions of reality, the patient may perceive you as a threat. Agitation is recognized as a biologic attempt to release nervous tension and can produce sudden, unpredictable physical actions in your patient.

If the patient's agitation continues, request ALS assistance so chemical restraint can be considered. Uncontrolled or poorly controlled patient agitation and physical violence can place the patient at risk for sudden cardiopulmonary arrest. Physical agitation can lead to sudden death, thought to result from metabolic acidosis, though the cause of death is not clear. Physical control measures (including TASERs) can contribute to sudden death in these patients. Also, this condition can be worsened by stimulant drugs (eg, cocaine) or alcohol withdrawal. Finally, **positional asphyxia** occurs when a patient's physical position restricts chest wall movements or causes airway obstruction. It can also cause sudden death. This condition can occur unintentionally when a patient is being physically restrained.

## Restraint

In situations when a patient engages in combative behavior, your safety and that of your partner must be your top priority. Therefore, it may be necessary for the patient to be physically restrained.

Prehospital patient restraint reduces the possibility of patient injury and the potential for injury to EMS providers, and allows for safe and appropriate treatment of an uncooperative patient. The National Association of Emergency Medical Services Physicians (NAEMSP) recommends that every prehospital care transport provider create and follow a

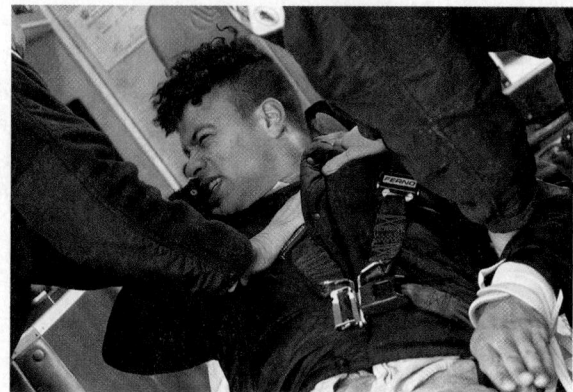

**FIGURE 23-3** Restraints should be used when necessary only to prevent injury and in the least restrictive manner that achieves the needed result.

© Jones & Bartlett Learning.

prehospital patient restraint protocol. Such protocols consider the appropriateness of restraint, the types of restraints, and care provided to the patient following restraint. Legislation regarding restraints ensures the safety of individuals who are an immediate threat to themselves or others. Your protocol must consider the laws of your state as they pertain to an individual's rights and processes for involuntarily restraining patients.

There is wide variation in prehospital patient restraint protocols throughout the country. Protocols should include only the use of restraint devices that have been approved by the state health department or local EMS agency. Restraint types can be soft, leather, or cloth. Soft restraints can include sheets, wide wristlets, and chest harnesses. Hard restraints can include plastic ties, handcuffs, or leather restraints. EMS protocols should avoid the use of hard restraints if possible. If hard restraints are approved, they will most likely be limited to the use of leather wrist restraints. The type of restraints used should not occlude circulation in the extremity and should allow the EMT to quickly remove them if the patient vomits or respiratory distress develops.

The method of restraint chosen should be the least restrictive method that will ensure the safety of the patient and providers (**FIGURE 23-3**).

### Risks Associated With Patient Restraint

Personnel must be properly trained in the use of restraints. Improperly applied restraints can result in severe and potentially life-threatening complications, such as positional asphyxia, aspiration, severe acidosis, and sudden cardiac death.

If you restrain a person without authority in a nonemergency situation, you expose yourself to a possible lawsuit and to personal danger. Legal actions against you can involve charges of assault, battery, false imprisonment, and violation of civil rights. You may use restraints only to protect yourself or others from bodily harm or to prevent the patient from injuring himself or herself. In either case, you may use reasonable force only as necessary to control the patient, something that courts may define differently. For this reason, follow local protocols and your company prehospital restraint policy, and consult medical control if needed.

You should always involve law enforcement personnel if you are called to assist a patient in a severe behavioral health emergency, especially when restraining a competent individual against his or her will. Law enforcement may provide physical backup in managing the patient and serve as the necessary witnesses. A patient who is restrained by law enforcement personnel is in their custody.

Before you consider physical restraint, make a significant effort to use verbal deescalation techniques to ease the situation and avoid the need for physical restraint. Also, consider asking the family to assist you in calming and reasoning with the patient. Verbal deescalation is safest because it does not require any physical contact with the patient. Be honest and straightforward with the patient and talk in a calm and friendly tone.

---

### Street Smarts

Sometimes the way we stand when speaking to patients can be misinterpreted as being aggressive. Do not stand in a rigid position or with your arms crossed over your chest. If used well, nonverbal communication can help calm a tense situation.

---

## The Process of Restraining a Patient

Once the decision has been made to restrain a patient, you should carry it out as quickly as is safely possible. Make sure you have adequate help to safely restrain a patient. Ideally, five people should

be present to carry out the restraint, each being responsible for one extremity and the head. There should also be a team leader who directs the restraining process, as well as a person to assist with applying the restraints. Before you begin, discuss the plan of action. As you prepare to restrain the patient, stay outside the patient's range of motion. Use the minimum force that is necessary to control a patient. Avoid acts of physical force that may cause injury to the patient. The level of force will vary, depending on the following factors:

- The degree of force that is necessary to keep the patient from injuring himself or herself, and others.
- A patient's sex, size, strength, and mental status, including the possibility of drug-induced states. Phencyclidine (PCP) use may make the patient especially difficult to restrain.
- The type of abnormal behavior the patient is exhibiting.

Other important considerations include:

- Somebody, preferably you or your partner, should talk to the patient throughout the process.
- Remember to treat the patient with dignity and respect at all times.
- Wear appropriate barrier protection during patient restraint activities.
- Never leave a restrained patient unattended.

Physically uncooperative patients should be restrained in the supine position with one arm restrained up and one restrained down. The head can be elevated at a 30° angle, if possible, to help prevent airway compromise. Both legs and both arms should be restrained. Restraining the hips, thighs, and chest inhibits movement. Restraining the thighs just above the knees prevents kicking and is more effective than only restraining the ankles. Do not place anything over the patient's face, head, or neck. If the patient is spitting, a surgical mask may be placed loosely over the patient's mouth.

Patients should never be transported while hobbled, hog-tied, or restrained in a prone position with hands and feet behind the back, as positional asphyxia could occur. It is impossible to adequately monitor the patient in this position, and it may inhibit the breathing of an impaired or exhausted patient. Patients should never be transported while

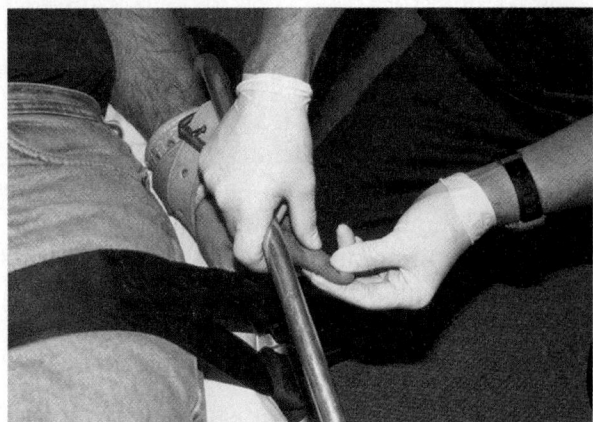

**FIGURE 23-4** Frequently assess circulation while a patient is restrained.

© Jones & Bartlett Learning.

sandwiched between backboards or mattresses. Stretcher straps should be applied during transport as the standard procedure for all patients. Sheets can be used as additional stretcher straps if necessary. Stretcher straps and sheets should never restrict the patient's chest wall motion.

Respiratory and circulatory problems have been known to occur in combative patients who are restrained. A physically restrained patient struggling against restraints can experience severe acidosis or fatal dysrhythmia. Monitor the patient for vomiting, airway obstruction, respiratory status, circulatory status (blood pressure), and changes in level of consciousness. Drug or alcohol intoxication may initially cause violent behavior that may lead to physical deterioration. Reassess airway and breathing continuously. You should make frequent checks of circulation on all restrained extremities, regardless of patient position (**FIGURE 23-4**).

Chemical restraint administered by ALS personnel is an effective way to safely transport and treat the violent, combative, or agitated patient. Physical restraint should be reserved for situations where chemical restraint is unavailable or otherwise ineffective or contraindicated.

Restraints applied in the field should not be removed until the patient is evaluated at the receiving facility. Release the restraints only if necessary to provide emergency patient care and only if you have assistance. Be especially careful if a combative patient suddenly becomes calm and cooperative.

This is not the time to relax but to be vigilant. The patient may suddenly become combative again and injure someone. Keep in mind that you may use reasonable force to defend yourself against an attack by an emotionally disturbed patient. It is extremely helpful to have (and document) witnesses in attendance, even during transport, to protect against false accusations. EMTs have been accused of sexual misconduct and other physical abuse in such circumstances. Also document the reason for the restraint, the type of restraint used, and the technique that was used.

## Performing Patient Restraint

The steps in **SKILL DRILL 23-1** show an example of the four-point restraint technique.

1. Bring down the patient into the supine position.
2. Acting at the same time, secure the patient in the supine or left lateral position.
3. Secure the patient's extremities with wrist and ankle restraints (**Step 1**).
4. Use stretcher straps or sheets to secure the legs (**Step 2**).
5. Fasten the remaining straps, including chest and pelvis straps if available (**Step 3**). Do not use multiple knots.
6. Continue to verbally reassure and calm the patient following chemical/physical restraints.
7. Regularly check circulation to the extremities (**Step 4**).

# Skill Drill 23-1 Restraining a Patient

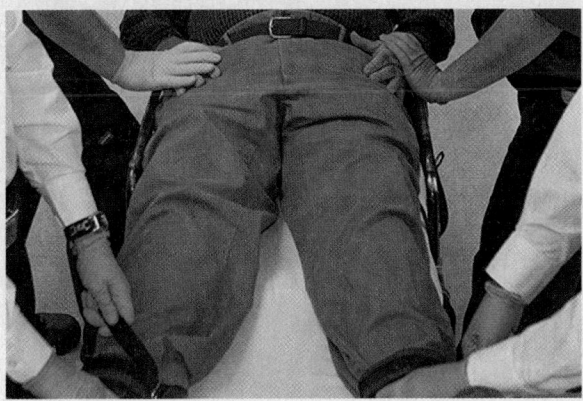

## Step 1

Bring down the patient into the supine position. Acting at the same time, secure the patient in the supine or left lateral position with wrist and ankle restraints.

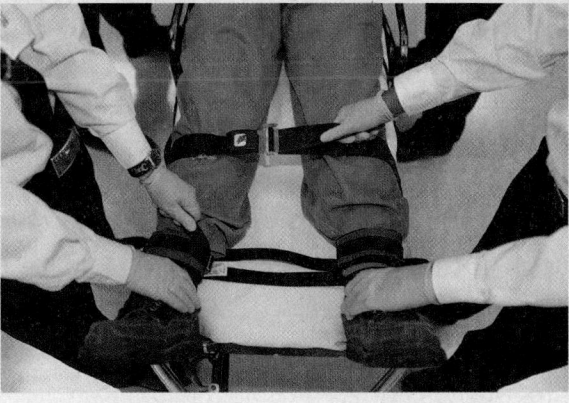

## Step 2

Use stretcher straps or sheets to secure the legs.

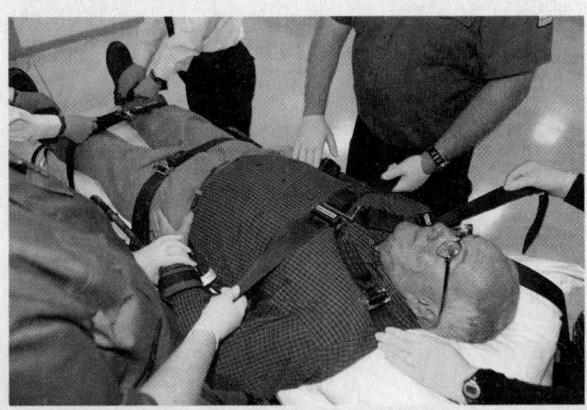

## Step 3

Fasten the remaining stretcher straps.

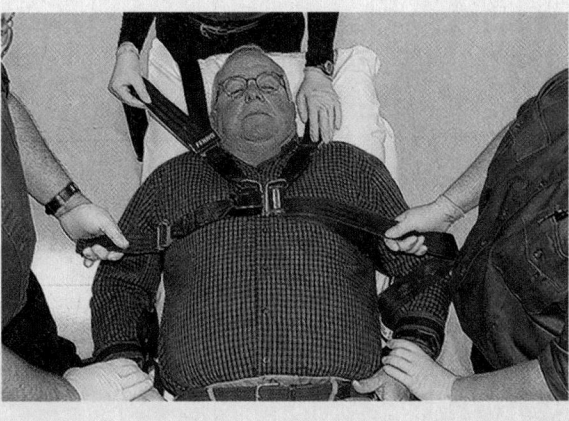

## Step 4

Continue to verbally reassure and calm the patient following chemical/physical restraints. Regularly check circulation to the extremities.

© Jones & Bartlett Learning.

A two-point restraint technique is an option if allowed per local protocols. This technique is performed in the same way as four-point restraint, except instead of restraining all four extremities to the stationary frame of the stretcher, one arm is placed upward toward the head and the other is placed downward toward the waist (**FIGURE 23-5**).

Once a patient has been restrained, reassess the airway and breathing. Document this information in your patient care report.

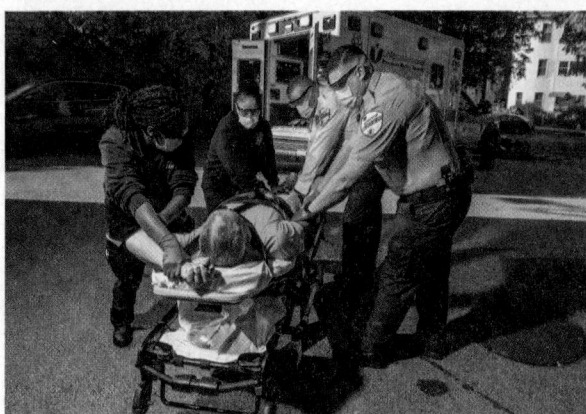

**FIGURE 23-5** In two-point restraint, one arm is placed upward while the other is placed downward.

© Jones & Bartlett Learning.

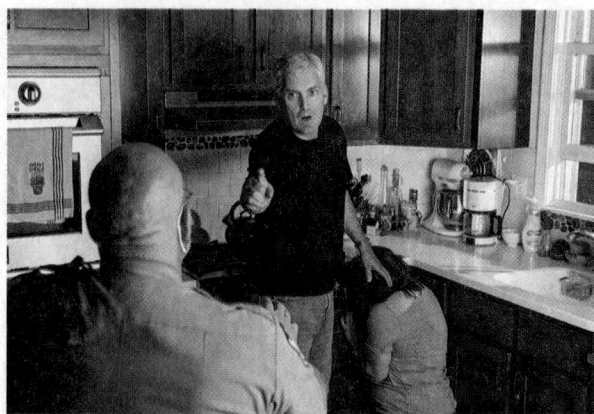

**FIGURE 23-6** Watch for indicators of potential violence when approaching the scene.

© Jones & Bartlett Learning.

# The Potentially Violent Patient

Violent patients account for only a small percentage of the patients experiencing a behavioral crisis. However, the potential for violence should always be a critical consideration for you (**FIGURE 23-6**).

Use the following list of risk factors to assess the level of danger:

- **History.** Has the patient previously exhibited hostile, overly aggressive, or violent behavior? Ask people at the scene, or request this information from law enforcement personnel or family.

- **Posture.** How is the patient sitting or standing? Is the patient tense, rigid, or sitting on the edge of his or her seat? Such physical tension is often a warning signal of impending hostility.
- **The scene.** Is the patient holding or near potentially lethal objects such as a knife, gun, glass, poker, or bat (or near a window or glass door)?
- **Vocal activity.** What type of speech is the patient using? Loud, obscene, erratic, and bizarre speech patterns usually indicate emotional distress. Someone using quiet, ordered speech is not as likely to strike out as someone who is yelling and screaming.

## YOU are the Provider

The patient is initially reluctant to allow you to transport him to the hospital. However, after you express your concern about his safety and well-being, he consents to transport. Other than allowing you to reassess his vital signs, he tells you he would prefer to just be taken to the hospital; he does not want to be physically assessed.

| Recording Time: 20 Minutes | |
| --- | --- |
| **Level of consciousness** | Conscious and alert |
| **Respirations** | 16 breaths/min; adequate depth |
| **Pulse** | 76 beats/min; strong and regular |
| **Skin** | Pink, warm, and moist |
| **Blood pressure** | 138/86 mm Hg |
| **Spo$_2$** | 98% (on room air) |

**7.** Should you perform a physical assessment of this patient despite the fact that he requested you not to? Why or why not?

- **Physical activity.** The motor activity of a person undergoing a psychiatric emergency may be the most telling factor of all. A patient who has tense muscles, clenched fists, or glaring eyes; is pacing or cannot sit still; or is fiercely protecting personal space requires careful watching. Agitation may predict a quick escalation to violence.

## Words of Wisdom

When working with a potentially hostile or violent patient, remove everyone from the scene who is not needed, such as family, friends, or bystanders. This will prevent injury or the likelihood of someone agitating the patient. Conversely, if a family member has a positive influence on the patient, you may consider allowing him or her to help.

Other factors to consider in assessing a patient's potential for violence include the following:

- Poor impulse control
- A history of truancy, fighting, and uncontrollable temper

- History of substance abuse
- Depression, which accounts for 20% of violent attacks
- Functional disorder (If the patient tells you voices are telling him or her to kill, believe it.)

## Suicide

The single most significant factor that contributes to suicide is depression. Anytime you encounter an emotionally depressed patient, you must consider the possibility of suicide. The risk factors for suicide are listed in **TABLE 23-3**.

It is a common misconception that people who threaten suicide never act on the threat. Suicide is a cry for help. Threatening suicide is an indication that someone is in a crisis that he or she cannot handle alone. Immediate intervention is necessary. Whether the patient has any of these risk factors, you must be alert to the following warning signs:

- Does the patient have an air of tearfulness, sadness, deep despair, or hopelessness that suggests depression?

## Special Populations

In general, children experience behavioral crises as commonly as adults; but often, the children's situations are managed by their parents or caregivers. If you are called to help with a child experiencing a behavioral crisis, it is imperative to listen to the caregiver and follow his or her lead on how to best approach the child. Aggressive behavior in children, especially when it seems to be a pattern, may be a symptom of an underlying medical or psychological condition. As a precaution against them hurting themselves or others, children need a thorough evaluation from a mental health professional. Although some children with a behavioral crisis may be physically large, do not make the mistake of assuming you can treat them like adults.

One specific behavioral crisis that is common among teenagers is suicide. According to the Centers for Disease Control and Prevention, suicide is the second leading cause of death for people 15 to 24 years of age. Although we sometimes tend to view a teenager's problems as minor, problems often appear insurmountable to them. Never discount a teenager's comments about suicide as being "just an attempt to get attention."

Common factors that lead to suicide attempts in adults are often also found in teenagers. One of them

is dealing with the end of a relationship. Teenagers are just beginning to relate to others in an intimate way, so when a relationship ends, they often do not know how to handle the apparent rejection. Adults who attempt suicide may have a drug or alcohol addiction, and this is common among teenagers as well. Teenage suicide victims may have a history of disciplinary problems or may have a very unstable home life. Another factor that is sometimes involved with teenage suicide victims is social pressures. Peer approval is one of the most important aspects of a teenager's life, and teenagers who seem to have poor relationships with their peers may be at a higher risk for suicide. In other cases, teenagers can be influenced by peers to commit suicide either individually or as part of a pact. Another risk factor to consider is that children of parents who committed suicide are more likely to attempt it themselves.

Expression of thoughts of suicide and attempts at suicide by teenagers should always be taken seriously. Never disregard suicidal comments, even if a parent insists the child "is faking." Take action to ensure that teenagers are evaluated by a professional after attempting or considering suicide because it is very important for their long-term emotional well-being.

| **TABLE 23-3** Risk Factors for Suicide |
|---|
| • Depression at any age, feeling trapped or purposeless |
| • Feelings of helplessness and hopelessness |
| • Previous suicide attempt (Approximately 80% of successful suicides were preceded by at least one prior attempt.) |
| • Current expression of wanting to commit suicide or sense of hopelessness |
| • Specific plan for suicide |
| • Family history of suicide |
| • People older than 40 years, particularly if single, widowed, divorced, alcoholic, or depressed (Men who are older than 55 years have an especially high risk and are often successful if they make an attempt.) |
| • Recent loss of spouse, significant other, family member, or support system |
| • Chronic debilitating illness or recent diagnosis of serious illness |
| • Feeling anxious, agitated, angry, reckless, or aggressive; also, dramatic mood changes such as from depression to agitation |
| • Financial setback, loss of job, police arrest, imprisonment, or some sort of social embarrassment |
| • Alcohol and substance abuse, particularly with increasing use |
| • Children of an alcoholic or abusive parent |
| • Withdrawal from family and friends or a lack of social support, resulting in isolation |
| • Significant anniversaries of sentinel events |
| • Unusual collection or acquisition of things that can cause death, such as a gun or a large volume of pills |

© Jones & Bartlett Learning.

## Special Populations

Geriatric patients may be struggling with the loss of loved ones, health issues including the diagnosis of a serious illness such as cancer or dementia, living on a fixed income, and fear of losing their independence. Depression is understandable and not uncommon. When you visit the home of a geriatric patient, especially one who lives alone, ensure that the patient is living in a safe and healthy environment. If you have concerns, contact adult protective services or an equivalent community resource that can conduct an investigation and provide appropriate assistance.

## Street Smarts

People who are depressed may not realize that there are resources available to help them through a difficult time. Keep a list of helpful numbers, such as the local crisis center, psychiatric units, and suicide hotline, to provide to patients. Your simple act of caring may save a life.

- Does the patient avoid eye contact, speak slowly or haltingly, and project a sense of vacancy, as if he or she really is not there?
- Does the patient seem unable to talk about the future? Ask the patient whether he or she has any vacation plans. Suicidal people consider the future so uninteresting that they do not think about it; people who are seriously depressed consider the future so distant that they may not be able to think about it at all.
- Is there any suggestion of suicide? Even vague suggestions should not be taken lightly, even if presented as a joke. If you think that suicide is a possibility, do not hesitate to bring up the subject. You will not give the patient ideas if you ask directly, "Are you considering suicide?"
- Does the patient have any specific plans related to death? Has the patient recently prepared a will? Has the patient given away significant possessions or told close friends what he or she would like done with them? Arranged for a funeral service? These are critical warning signs.

You should also consider the following additional risk factors for suicide:

- Are there any unsafe objects in the patient's hands or nearby (a sharp knife, glass, poisons, or a gun)?
- Is the environment unsafe (an open window in a high-rise building, a patient standing on a bridge or precipice)?
- Is there evidence of self-destructive behavior (partially cut wrists, excessive alcohol or drug use)?

- Is there an imminent threat to the patient or others?
- Is there an underlying medical problem?
- Are there cultural, religious, or social beliefs promoting suicide?
- Has there been trauma?

On the basis of your observations and conversations with the patient, you may need to determine if interventions such as restraints are needed. Remember, a suicidal patient may be homicidal as well. Do not jeopardize your life or the lives of your partners. If you have reason to believe that you are in danger, you must obtain police intervention. In the meantime, try not to frighten the patient or make him or her suspicious. Remember, the most important service you can provide for a suicidal patient is compassionate transportation to a medical facility where the patient can receive proper treatment.

### Safety Tips

Patients with suicidal thoughts, especially patients who have made a threat or unsuccessful attempt, may not be thinking clearly and may behave in unpredictable ways. Some recognize that if they get into the ambulance or enter the hospital, they will not have the opportunity to complete their threat or intent. Therefore, they may make a last effort to kill themselves. Suicidal/homicidal patients will not hesitate to hurt you or your partner. Be careful how you assess the situation; make certain you, your team, and the patient are safe.

## Posttraumatic Stress Disorder and Returning Combat Veterans

**Posttraumatic stress disorder (PTSD)** can occur after exposure to, or injury from, a traumatic event. Such events may include sexual or physical assault, child abuse, a serious accident, a natural disaster, war, loss of a loved one, or stressful life changes. People may have experienced fear of danger, helplessness, or a severe reaction during the event. The reaction could be to trauma that occurred long ago or may be the result of multiple traumatic events over time. It is not necessarily the result of one isolated or recent event.

It is estimated that 7% to 8% of the general population will experience signs of PTSD at some point in their lives. For health care workers returning from a warfare environment, which could include disaster workers, threat of personal harm is considered a predictive factor in determining in whom PTSD will develop.

Military personnel who experienced combat have a high incidence of PTSD. PTSD occurred in up to 20% of veterans of the Iraq and Afghanistan Wars, 10% of Gulf War veterans, and 30% of Vietnam War veterans. Reminders of their experiences in the military such as news coverage or gatherings of veterans can also be triggers.

### Street Smarts

Posttraumatic stress disorder affects those working in EMS, fire service, and police agencies. In a 2016 report published by the National Association of EMTs, *National Survey on EMS Mental Health Services*, the majority of EMS providers surveyed felt affected personally by mental health issues. Take care of yourself, and watch those you work with for signs of depression and other mental illness. Take care of each other. Helpful resources on this subject include EMS Strong (www.emsstrong.org) and the Code Green Campaign (codegreencampaign.org).

### Signs and Symptoms of PTSD

Symptoms of PTSD include feelings of helplessness, anxiety, anger, and fear. People with PTSD may avoid things that remind them of the trauma, including loud noises or smells, and sometimes avoid interactions with other people. This emotional and physical distancing from others can have a negative effect on one's quality of life. Memories of the trauma linger and continue to be disruptive. Symptoms of PTSD may be made worse in the context of other mental health challenges.

The sympathetic nervous system provides the fight-or-flight mechanism to help protect us in a perceived dangerous situation. It is not intended to last any longer than required to mitigate the threat. People with PTSD suffer nervous system arousal that continues and is not easily suppressed. Heart rate increases to channel blood into the heart, lungs, and brain; pupils dilate; and systolic blood pressure is increased. Senses are sharpened and mental acuity is heightened. The victim may be hypervigilant or display an exaggerated startle response to perceived danger.

People with PTSD can relive the traumatic event through intrusive thoughts, nightmares, or even flashbacks. *Flashbacks* are uncontrollable events triggered by a sound, sight, or smell. The patient may experience the same visceral response as when he or she initially encountered the stress. These episodes can last seconds or hours and can occur at any time, even years after the exposure. The person fears this inability to control a flashback and worries that it will present as irrational behavior. Recent traumatic events may also trigger old memories and create a reflex reaction of preparing for the worst. A person who has experienced flashbacks may become preoccupied with the perception of danger. Hypervigilance and trouble sleeping are not unusual.

Dissociative PTSD occurs when the person attempts to escape from constant internal distress or a particularly disturbing event. His or her altered consciousness allows him or her to continue functioning under negative conditions. Some people may undergo an out-of-body experience. Others experience delusions. Other psychological conditions such as personality disorders and increased functional impairment can develop in those with a dissociative subtype of PTSD.

Guilt, shame, paranoia, hostility, and depression are not uncommon for combat veterans. Alcohol and/or drug use is a common way to suppress the sympathetic nervous system activity and slow down the body. This attempt at anesthesia can easily become addictive. Suicide is sometimes sought to end the pain. Veterans are much more likely to harm themselves or try to harm themselves. They also sustain a host of physical conditions, some from injuries sustained in combat, and sometimes vague, unfocused pain not associated with any specific part of the body. This perception of physical pain may be a sign of their anguish. In particular, combat veterans may have heart disease at a younger age than expected, a higher incidence of type 2 diabetes, and a loss of brain gray matter. High cholesterol and hypertension are not uncommon and are often undiagnosed or misdiagnosed.

Another consideration for the combat veteran is the higher incidence of TBI sustained from trauma secondary to explosion of an improvised explosive device (IED). In some cases, the TBI may go undiagnosed due to similarities with the symptoms of PTSD or because the patient downplays the symptoms. People with TBI can sustain sensory dysfunction, confusion headaches, memory loss, and general disorientation. Memory loss can include retrograde and anterograde amnesia (before and after the event). Try to eliminate excess noise. Do not touch or do anything to the veteran without an explanation.

## YOU are the Provider

You depart the scene and begin transport to a hospital located 8 miles away. The patient remains conscious and alert but is still withdrawn and sad. You ask him additional questions about his present situation, but he does not answer you; he briefly looks up at you and then looks back down. You reassess his vital signs and then call in your report to the receiving facility.

| Recording Time:    30 Minutes | |
| --- | --- |
| **Level of consciousness** | Conscious and alert |
| **Respirations** | 16 breaths/min; adequate depth |
| **Pulse** | 72 beats/min; strong and regular |
| **Skin** | Pink, warm, and dry |
| **Blood pressure** | 130/80 mm Hg |
| **Spo$_2$** | 99% (on room air) |

You arrive at the destination hospital and give your verbal report to the charge nurse. After transferring patient care to the hospital staff, you return to service.

**8.** What factors should you consider before transporting a patient with a behavioral health emergency?

**9.** If the patient does not answer your questions, should you continue to encourage him to talk? Why or why not?

Interestingly, diesel fumes often can be a trigger for combat veterans. Keep your diesel equipment far enough away.

## Caring for the Combat Veteran

How do you recognize returning veterans? They often continue to adhere to their military identity with short haircuts and wearing military clothing with combat patches, and often have tattoos. Their homes may have flags, memorials, commendations, and military photos. They may have a military appearance and use military vocabulary. They tend to show respect for authority but may be reluctant to talk to you about PTSD. They may not be aware that they have it, or do not want to be considered "mental." They might have trouble asking for help. Asking, "How do you want me to help you?" or "What is it you need right now?" is a good way to open the conversation.

The returning combat veteran is a patient who will require a unique level of understanding, compassion, and specialized attention. These patients experience pain that is emotional as well as physical. You will need to take time to establish the history of this patient and listen to his or her concerns. Approach this patient with sensitivity and respect. Be careful how you phrase your questions. "Were you in combat?" is an appropriate question, but, in some cases, veterans may be in denial or do not believe they were in combat. A better question might be, "Were you shot at or under fire?" If you served in combat, you can create trust by letting the patient know. Ask questions about the patient's service (branch, rank, etc). You may get enough information out of that conversation to eliminate the need to probe further with specific questions.

Use a calm, firm voice, but be in charge. Respect a veteran's personal space. Limit the number of people involved or move to a private and quiet space. In some cases, supportive family or friends can be helpful. Ask about suicidal intentions. This might create an opportunity for the patient to reach out. Military veterans are trained to use weapons and are also resourceful in improvising weapons. If you are concerned about suicide, ensure there is nothing the patient can access and use as a weapon.

Physical restraint will not be effective with this population and may only escalate the problem. Even seat belts on the stretcher can aggravate a patient. If it is necessary to calm the patient, especially in the face of safety considerations, chemical restraints administered by ALS should be considered.

# Medicolegal Considerations

The medical and legal aspects of emergency medical care become more complicated when the patient is experiencing a behavioral health emergency. Nevertheless, legal challenges are greatly reduced when an emotionally disturbed patient consents to care. Gaining the patient's confidence is, therefore, a critical task for you.

Mental incapacity can take many forms: unconsciousness (as a result of hypoxia, alcohol, or drugs), temporary but severe stress, and depression. Once you have determined that a patient has impaired mental capacity, you must decide whether he or she requires immediate emergency medical care. A patient in a mentally unstable condition may resist your attempts to provide care. Nevertheless, you must not leave the patient alone. Doing so may result in harm to the patient and expose you to civil action for abandonment or negligence. In such a case, consult medical control. If medical control believes that an involuntary emergency petition is in order, then taking the patient into protective custody is appropriate, and you should request law enforcement personnel to help restrain the patient and transport under involuntary circumstances.

Each state has different processes for involuntary emergency petitioning for a person in a behavioral health emergency situation. Be familiar with your state's protocols. For example, in some states two physician signatures are necessary on the petition to make it valid. It is therefore imperative to get the first physician to agree to the appropriateness of petitioning a patient prior to initiating protective custody in the field.

## Consent

When a patient is not mentally competent to grant consent for emergency medical care, the law assumes that there is implied consent. For example, the consent of an unconscious patient is implied if life or health is at risk. The law refers to this as the emergency doctrine: Consent is implied because of the necessity for immediate emergency treatment. In a situation that is not immediately life threatening, emergency medical care or transportation may be delayed until the proper consent is obtained.

In cases involving behavioral health emergencies, however, the matter is not always clear. Does a life-threatening emergency exist or not? If you are not sure, contact your supervisor if available or appropriate based on local protocols, or contact medical control. Only with the concurrence of medical control can the patient be taken into custody with an emergency petition. Once the emergency petition is in place, law enforcement personnel can be used to help achieve restraint and transport.

## Limited Legal Authority

As an EMT, you do not have legal authority to require a patient to undergo emergency medical care if the patient is competent and understands the risks and benefits of transport versus refusal. Patients have the right to refuse care. However, most states have legal statutes regarding the emergency care of mentally ill and drug-impaired people. These statutory provisions may permit law enforcement personnel to place the person in protective custody so that emergency care can be given. You should be familiar with your local and state laws regarding these situations.

A typical provision may state the following:

*Any police officer who has reasonable cause to believe that a person is mentally ill and dangerous to himself, herself, or others or gravely disabled... may take such person into custody and take or cause such person to be taken to a general hospital for emergency examination...*

The general rule of law is that a competent adult has the right to refuse treatment, even if lifesaving care is involved. However, in psychiatric cases, a court of law would probably consider your actions in providing lifesaving care to be appropriate, particularly if you have a reasonable belief that the patient would harm himself or herself, or others, without your intervention. If you decide a patient must be transported against his or her will, make sure you have the appropriate resources on scene to avoid unnecessary injury to the patient, you, or your partner. In addition, a patient who is impaired in any way, whether by mental illness, medical condition, or intoxication, may not be considered competent to refuse treatment or transportation. These situations are among the most perilous you will encounter from a legal standpoint. When in doubt, consult with your supervisor or medical control. Always maintain a high index of suspicion regarding your patient's condition—assume the worst and hope for the best. Err on the side of treatment and transport. Carefully document the patient's statements and behavior to support your actions.

## Special Populations

As the population ages, you will begin to see more patients older than 65 years. In responding to an increasing number of geriatric patients, you will probably notice some behavioral or psychiatric symptoms, including depression, dementia, and delirium. These changes in mental status can affect your ability to thoroughly assess and treat an ill or injured geriatric patient. Understanding the causes of altered behavior in geriatric patients will help you with patient care.

For example, consider a woman in her 80s who has suffered the loss of her spouse of 40 years and the loss of her parents, siblings, and friends. Her children may live far away. Her only income may be a small pension and social security. More than anything, she wants to stay in the home she shared with her husband. When she has medical concerns, she does not call 9-1-1 because she is afraid that she will be taken to the hospital and then forced into a care home.

When you visit the home of an older adult, especially one who lives alone, ensure the person is living in a safe and healthy environment. Does he or she have food and medications? Is the home sanitary or overrun with bugs or rodents? Is there hoarding behavior? Is the person's mental status in question? If you have concerns, call adult protective services.

Depression is one of the mental health symptoms that you will see in older adults. Depression has many causes. A diagnosis of major illness such as cancer or dementia can lead to depression. Medications can induce a feeling of depression, possibly because of an interaction with other drugs. In addition, changes in the endocrine system such as menopause can cause depression. Depression might also be caused by an imbalance in brain chemicals.

With all the possible causes of depression, an older adult can feel helpless and hopeless. A depressed person may be argumentative or passive. He or she might trivialize complaints, not wanting to be a bother to anyone. Someone who sees no way out of his or her situation may turn to suicide. Be alert for a suicidal gesture or ideation, even though it may not be obvious. As an EMT, your interaction with a depressed older person might prevent a suicide.

Although depression can create a behavioral crisis in geriatric patients, dementia is another more common cause of abnormal behavior. According to the Alzheimer's Association, more than 5 million people are afflicted with this condition; it is the sixth leading cause of death in the United States. Each year, 500,000 people die from complications of it, and 1 in 3 older adults die of Alzheimer disease or some other form of dementia.

Currently, there is no cure for Alzheimer dementia, but there are medications that can slow the progression of the disease. Openly hostile behavior can develop in patients with Alzheimer dementia, including kicking, yelling, pinching, and hitting you, your partner, or the patient's caregiver. You might need to restrain a violent patient, but do so gently and only to the point at which the violent behavior stops.

As with any patient, you want to rule out medical causes for altered behavior, especially those you can treat. Causes of altered behavior include diabetic emergencies, heat- and cold-related illnesses, poisoning and overdose, strokes and transient ischemic attacks, infection, hypoxia, and head injury. Urinary tract infection and constipation can alter an older person's behavior.

As the EMT responding to a call for help, you should accept the possibility of depression in a geriatric patient. Do not discount the patient's feelings or devalue the patient's emotions. Be alert for a suicidal gesture and pay attention to any statements about death. To get the patient's cooperation, you can elicit the patient's help in providing care for the acute illness or injury. A smile and a touch can go a long way toward alleviating fear in all of your patients, especially older patients.

## YOU are the Provider SUMMARY

**1. How should you and your partner proceed to this call?**

The patient's reported behavior, "acting bizarre," is a broad description that could indicate any number of conditions. In the interest of your safety, you should assume that the patient is a danger to himself/herself, or others. This is not a scene that you should enter without the protection of law enforcement. Never approach a scene of actual or potential violence until law enforcement personnel have arrived and deemed the scene safe for you to enter. In this case, you and your partner should stage a few blocks away from the scene and wait for law enforcement personnel to arrive. Proceed to the scene *only* after they have notified you and given you the all clear.

**2. Other than an underlying psychiatric condition, what other conditions can affect a person's behavior?**

A multitude of factors can affect a person's behavior; the presence of an underlying psychiatric condition is only one. Conditions such as hypoxemia, hypoglycemia, metabolic disorders, drug- or alcohol-related problems, stress-related issues, head trauma, and brain tumors (among others) can profoundly affect a person's behavior; these conditions may even cause the patient to become violent.

**3. What should be your most immediate concern with this patient?**

Personal safety should be your primary concern when caring for *any* patient. This is especially true when caring for patients who are displaying abnormal or bizarre behavior. When caring for a patient who is experiencing a behavioral crisis, you must always consider his or her potential for violence. There are certain behaviors and risk factors that you should look for when assessing a patient's potential for violence: patient history, posture, and verbal and physical activity.

Does the patient have a history of hostile, overly aggressive, or violent behavior? Observe the patient's speech. Loud, obscene, erratic, or bizarre speech patterns are clear indicators of emotional distress.

Your patient is sitting on the ground, rocking back and forth; this could indicate a general state of nervousness or increasing agitation.

**4. How should you proceed with your assessment of this patient?**

The patient has something to say; he states he "has a lot of problems," but also notes that nobody will listen to him. Therefore, use the most important assessment tool you have: listening. Actively listen to what the patient is saying. It may give you clues as to the underlying cause of his behavior; it also reassures him that you *are* listening.

Express sincere interest in what the patient is saying. Let him tell you in his own words what happened or what is going on. Do not interrupt him. Allow him to finish what he is saying before you ask him any questions—just as you would with any other patient.

When you are caring for a patient with a behavioral crisis, you must be prepared to spend extra time with him or her. It often takes longer to assess, listen to, and prepare the patient for transport.

**5. What is your field impression of this patient?**

The field impression of the patient is based on many factors, including physical assessment, medical history, and chief complaint. On the basis of your field impression, you can begin the treatment most appropriate for the situation.

Your patient is displaying clear signs of depression. Despite attending counseling sessions, he is unable to cope with the loss of his wife; this has brought him to the point of lacking the desire to even get out of bed in the morning. He no longer feels as though he has a purpose in life. He has experienced emotional distress for a year, and today—the anniversary of his wife's death—has precipitated an acute emotional crisis.

**6. What care can you provide to this patient in the field?**

Although the patient does not appear to be experiencing any physical problems, clearly he is emotionally overwhelmed. The fact that your patient is severely depressed places him in a high-risk category for suicide. He should *not* be left alone! Patients who are experiencing a behavioral crisis require a great deal of emotional support and active listening.

**7. Should you perform a physical assessment of this patient despite the fact that he requested you do not? Why or why not?**

The patient—although severely depressed—still has decision-making capacity. He is conscious and alert, able to answer your questions appropriately, and is not displaying any psychotic behavior (eg, hallucinations, delusions). Therefore, he maintains the legal right to refuse a physical examination; touching him without his consent could lead to allegations of assault against you.

Unless there is an accompanying physical complaint, a detailed physical exam is rarely indicated in a patient with an emotional crisis; in fact, it may be detrimental to your gaining the patient's trust.

**8. What factors should you consider before transporting a patient with a behavioral health emergency?**

On arriving at the scene of a patient with a behavioral health emergency, you must assess him or her for signs of potential violence. These observations should continue throughout the *entire* patient encounter. Even though this patient is calm right now, this could easily change and he could become acutely violent. The worst time for this to happen is in the back of the ambulance, where you will be the only EMT. Do not let your guard down when caring for a patient with an emotional crisis; continuously monitor his or her behavior. Stay attentive at all times.

If you have reason to believe that the patient is at an increased risk for becoming violent, you should have other authorized personnel, such as a police officer or firefighter, ride in the back of the ambulance. If it is necessary to restrain the patient, use just enough force to effectively accomplish the task. Unless it is absolutely necessary to provide patient care, do not release the restraints—regardless of any promises to calm down the patient makes. Never hesitate to call for ALS assistance if available for consideration of use of medications to provide chemical restraint.

**9. If the patient does not answer your questions, should you continue to encourage him to talk? Why or why not?**

Some patients who are experiencing a behavioral health emergency talk excessively, while others talk little or not at all (as in depression). If the patient wants to talk, you should encourage him or her to do so. Many patients find relief—even if it is only temporary—by simply having someone to talk to. If the patient prefers not to talk, *do not force the issue*.

Depressed patients are typically withdrawn and are not very talkative. Instead of persistently encouraging a patient to talk, you should continue to monitor the patient's behavior.

## YOU are the Provider SUMMARY *continued*

### EMS Patient Care Report (PCR)

| Date: 11-23-20 | Incident No.: 012009 | Nature of Call: Behavioral crisis | | Location: 517 E. Bandera | |
|---|---|---|---|---|---|
| Dispatched: 1920 | En Route: 1921 | At Scene: 1937 | Transport: 2000 | At Hospital: 2011 | In Service: 2021 |

#### Patient Information

**Age:** 44
**Sex:** M
**Weight (in kg [lb]):** 79 kg (175 lb)

**Allergies:** No known drug allergies
**Medications:** Paxil, Ambien
**Past Medical History:** None
**Chief Complaint:** Apparent emotional distress

#### Vital Signs

| Time: 1946 | BP: 144/84 | Pulse: 88 | Respirations: 16 | Spo$_2$: 98% |
|---|---|---|---|---|
| Time: 1957 | BP: 138/86 | Pulse: 76 | Respirations: 16 | Spo$_2$: 98% |
| Time: 2007 | BP: 130/80 | Pulse: 72 | Respirations: 16 | Spo$_2$: 99% |

#### EMS Treatment (circle all that apply)

| Oxygen @ ___ L/min via:  NC   NRM   Bag mask | | Assisted Ventilation | Airway Adjunct | CPR |
|---|---|---|---|---|
| Defibrillation | Bleeding Control | Bandaging | Splinting | Other: Emotional support |

#### Narrative

Medic 1780 dispatched to a residence for a man who is "acting bizarre."

Chief Complaint: Possible depression

History: The patient advised that today is the anniversary of his wife's death and that he finds it extremely difficult to even get out of bed in the morning. He further advised he feels as though his life has no purpose anymore. According to the patient, he has been to several counseling sessions over the past year, but they have not seemed to help him. He further said his employer does not seem to care about his problems and has threatened to fire him unless his depressed behavior improves. Staged at 5th Street and Elm until law enforcement arrived on scene and advised that it was safe to enter. A law enforcement official advised EMS that the patient had been checked for any weapons on his person and that none were found.

Assessment: On arriving at the scene, found the patient, a 44-year-old man, sitting on the lawn in front of his house, rocking back and forth. He was conscious and alert; however, he appeared sad and was clearly withdrawn. Introduced EMS crew to patient and performed primary assessment. His airway was patent, and his breathing was adequate. No gross abnormalities noted during this examination.

Treatment (Rx): Patient would only consent to assessment of his vital signs; he would not consent to further assessment or treatment. Visual examination did not reveal any gross injuries or life-threatening conditions, and the patient continued to remain conscious, alert, calm, and oriented and was able to answer questions appropriately.

Transport: Initially, patient refused EMS transport; however, after explaining to him that there could be an underlying medical problem contributing to his depression, he consented to transport and vital signs monitoring only; he maintained his refusal of a physical examination. Careful assessment of the patient did not reveal any gross indicators of potential violence. Patient walked to the ambulance on his own accord and was safely secured to the stretcher. Began transport to the hospital and continued to monitor the patient's behavior and vital signs en route. No changes in the patient's status were noted en route, and he remained calm but did not want to talk. Remainder of transport was uneventful. Delivered patient to ED staff and gave verbal report to charge nurse Caron RN. After transferring patient care to the hospital staff, Medic 1780 returned to service.

**End of report**

# Prep Kit

## Ready for Review

- A behavioral crisis is any reaction to events that interferes with the activities of daily living or has become unacceptable to the patient, family, or community.
- During a psychiatric emergency, a patient may show agitation or violence or become a threat to himself, herself, or others. This is more serious than the more typical behavioral crisis that causes inappropriate behavior such as interference with activities of daily living or bizarre behavior.
- According to the National Institute of Mental Health, mental health disorders are common throughout the United States, affecting tens of millions of people each year. Psychiatric disorders are illnesses with psychologic or behavioral symptoms that may result in impaired functioning.
- Behavioral disorders have many possible underlying causes including social or situational stress such as divorce or death of a loved one; mental illnesses such as schizophrenia; physical illnesses such as diabetic emergencies; chemical problems such as alcohol or drug use; or biologic disturbances such as electrolyte imbalances. Sometimes these conditions can be compounded by noncompliance with prescribed medication regimens.
- As an EMT, you are not responsible for diagnosing the underlying cause of a behavioral health emergency. Your job is to diffuse and control the situation and safely transport your patient to the hospital. Intervene only as much as it takes to accomplish these tasks. Be caring and careful.
- To the person experiencing a behavioral health emergency, the line between his or her reality and fantasy may be blurred.
- The threat of suicide requires immediate intervention. Depression is the most significant risk factor for suicide.
- A patient with PTSD has experienced fear of danger, helplessness during the event, or a severe reaction during the event. In PTSD, memories of the trauma linger and continue to be disruptive. It can be made worse with the existence of concurrent mental illness.
- Patients experiencing delirium are generally not dangerous, but if they exhibit agitated behavior they may strike out irrationally. One of the most important factors to consider in these cases is your personal safety. Excited delirium is a medical emergency.
- A patient in a mentally unstable condition may resist your attempts to provide care. In such situations, consult medical control and request that law enforcement personnel help you handle the patient. Another reason for seeking law enforcement support is for a patient who resists treatment; such a patient often threatens you and others. Violent or dangerous people must be taken into custody by the police before emergency care can be rendered.
- Always consult medical control and contact law enforcement personnel for help before restraining a patient. If restraints are required, use the minimum force necessary. Assess the airway and circulation frequently while the patient is restrained.

## Vital Vocabulary

**activities of daily living** The basic activities a person usually accomplishes during a normal day, such as eating, dressing, and bathing.

**altered mental status** A change in the way a person thinks and behaves that may signal disease in the central nervous system or elsewhere in the body.

**behavior** How a person functions or acts in response to his or her environment.

**behavioral crisis** The point at which a person's reactions to events interfere with activities of daily living; this becomes a psychiatric emergency when it causes a major life interruption, such as attempted suicide.

**behavioral health emergency** An emergency in which abnormal behavior threatens a person's own health and safety or the health and safety of another person—for example, when a person becomes suicidal or homicidal, or has a psychotic episode.

**depression** A persistent mood of sadness, despair, and discouragement; may be a symptom of many different mental and physical disorders, or may be a disorder on its own.

**excited delirium** A serious behavioral condition in which a person exhibits agitated behavior combined with disorientation, hallucinations, or delusions; also called agitated delirium or exhaustive mania.

**functional disorder** A disorder in which there is no known physiologic reason for the abnormal functioning of an organ or organ system.

**organic brain syndrome** Temporary or permanent dysfunction of the brain, caused by a disturbance in the physical or physiologic functioning of brain tissue.

**positional asphyxia** Restriction of chest wall movements and/or airway obstruction; can rapidly lead to sudden death.

**posttraumatic stress disorder (PTSD)** A delayed reaction to a prior incident. Often the result of one or more conditions concerning the incident, and may relate to an incident that involved physical harm or the threat of physical harm.

**psychiatric disorder** An illness with psychological or behavioral symptoms and/or impairment in functioning caused by a social, psychological, genetic, physical, chemical, or biologic disturbance.

**psychosis** A mental disorder characterized by the loss of contact with reality.

**schizophrenia** A complex, difficult-to-identify mental disorder whose onset typically occurs during early adulthood. Symptoms typically become more prominent over time and include delusions, hallucinations, a lack of interest in pleasure, and erratic speech.

# References

1. Alzheimer's Association. Facts and figures. https://www.alz.org/alzheimers-dementia/facts-figures. Accessed February 28, 2020.

2. Belviso M, De Donno A, Vitale L, Introna F Jr. Positional asphyxia: reflection on 2 cases. *Am J Forensic Med Pathol* 2003;24(3):292–297.

3. Gibbons SW, Hickling EJ, Watts DD. Combat stressors and post-traumatic stress in deployed military healthcare professionals: an integrative review. *J Adv Nurs* 2012;68(1):3–21.

4. Hsieh A. Seven tips to remember when restraining patients. EMS1.com. https://www.ems1.com/patient-handling/articles/7-tips-to-remember-when-restraining-patients-HXtosXLkeKvR1pDm/. Published December 23, 2010. Accessed February 28, 2020.

5. Kupas DF, Wydro GC. Patient restraint in emergency medical services systems. *Prehosp Emerg Care* 2002;6(3):340–345.

6. McGuire JM. The incidence of and risk factors for emergence delirium in US military combat veterans. *J Perianesth Nurs* 2012;27(4):236–245.

7. National Association of Emergency Medical Technicians. 2016 National Survey on EMS Mental Health Services. http://www.naemt.org/docs/default-source/ems-health-and-safety-documents/mental-health-grid/2016-naemt-mental-health-report-8-14-16.pdf. Published 2016. Accessed February 28, 2020.

8. National Association of State EMS Officials. *National Model EMS Clinical Guidelines: Version 2.0.* https://nasemso.org/wp-content/uploads/National-Model-EMS-Clinical-Guidelines-2017-Distribution-Version-05Oct2017.pdf. Updated September 2017. Accessed February 28, 2020.

9. National Highway Traffic Safety Administration. *National Emergency Medical Services Education Standards.* DOT HS 811 077A. www.ems.gov/pdf/811077a.pdf. Published January 2009. Accessed February 28, 2020.

10. National Institute of Mental Health. Schizophrenia. https://www.nimh.nih.gov/health/topics/schizophrenia/index.shtml. Updated February 2016. Accessed February 28, 2020

11. Schoenly L. Excited delirium: medical emergency—not willful resistance. EMS1.com. https://www.ems1.com/ems-products/patient-handling/articles/excited-delirium-medical-emergency-not-willful-resistance-3B8xLHBK7myikoFx/. Published July 10, 2015. Accessed February 28, 2020.

12. Suicide Awareness Voices of Education. Suicide facts. https://save.org/about-suicide/suicide-facts/. Accessed February 28, 2020.

13. Takeuchi A, Ahern TL, Henderson SO. Excited delirium. *West J Emerg Med*. 2011;12(1):77-83.

14. US Department of Veterans Affairs. PTSD: National Center for PTSD. https://www.ptsd.va.gov/. Updated July 1, 2019. Accessed February 28, 2020.

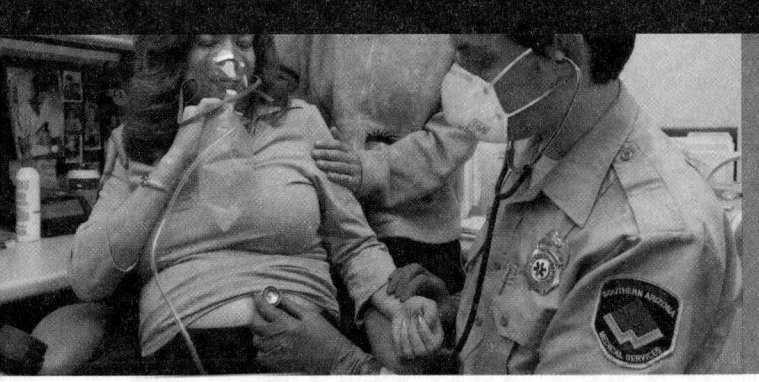

# Chapter 24

# Gynecologic Emergencies

## NATIONAL EMS EDUCATION STANDARD COMPETENCIES

### Medicine
Applies fundamental knowledge to provide basic emergency care and transportation based on assessment findings for an acutely ill patient.

### Gynecology
- Recognition and management of shock associated with
  - Vaginal bleeding (pp 885–889)

- Anatomy, physiology, assessment findings, and management of
  - Vaginal bleeding (pp 882–883, 885–889)
  - Sexual assault (to include appropriate emotional support) (pp 890–893)
  - Infections (pp 882–890)

## KNOWLEDGE OBJECTIVES

1. Describe the anatomy and physiology of the female reproductive system; include the developmental changes that occur during puberty and menopause. (pp 882–883)
2. Discuss the special, age-related patient management considerations EMTs should provide for both younger and older female patients who are experiencing gynecologic emergencies. (pp 883–884)
3. List common examples of gynecologic emergencies; include the causes, risk factors, assessment findings, and patient management considerations. (pp 884–886)
4. Explain how an EMT would recognize conditions associated with hemorrhage during pregnancy. (pp 885–886)
5. Discuss the assessment and management of a patient who is experiencing a gynecologic

   emergency; include a discussion of specific assessment findings. (pp 886–889)
6. Explain the general management of a patient who is experiencing a gynecologic emergency in relation to privacy and communication. (pp 886–889)
7. Give examples of the personal protective equipment EMTs should use when treating patients with gynecologic emergencies. (p 889)
8. Discuss the special considerations and precautions EMTs must observe when arriving at the scene of a suspected case of sexual assault or rape. (pp 890–892)
9. Discuss the assessment and management of a patient who has been sexually assaulted or raped; include the additional steps EMTs must take on behalf of the patient. (pp 890–893)

## SKILLS OBJECTIVES

There are no skills objectives for this chapter.

## Introduction

The most obvious difference between men and women is that women are uniquely formed to conceive and give birth. This difference makes women susceptible to many conditions that do not occur in men. This chapter examines a few of those conditions. Female anatomy is discussed first, followed by conditions that may be encountered in the prehospital setting. Vaginal bleeding causes are reviewed. Health concerns specific to the very young and the very old are discussed. The principles of treating a woman who has been the victim of sexual assault or rape, as well as recognizing the potential use of date rape drugs, are also discussed.

## Anatomy and Physiology

The female reproductive system includes internal and external structures. The external female genitalia consist of the vaginal opening just posterior to the urethral opening (**FIGURE 24-1**). The **labia majora** and **labia minora** are folds of tissue that surround the urethral and vaginal openings. At the anterior end of the labia is the clitoris, and at the posterior end is the anus. The **perineum** is the area of tissue between the vagina and the anus. The labia are extremely vascular and can be injured, but because of their location, they seldom are damaged except in cases of sexual abuse.

In terms of internal structures, the **ovaries** are the primary female reproductive organ (**FIGURE 24-2**).

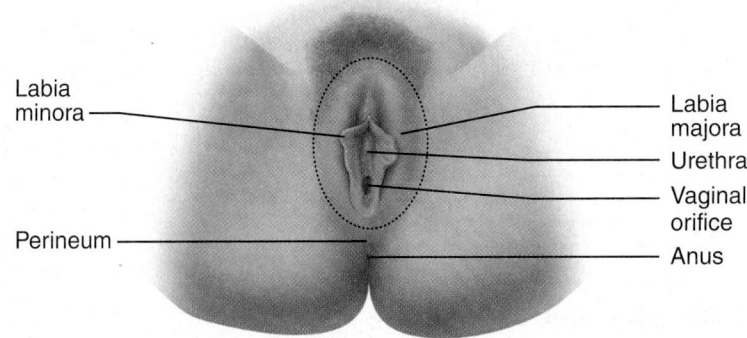

**FIGURE 24-1** The external genitalia of the female reproductive system.

© Jones & Bartlett Learning.

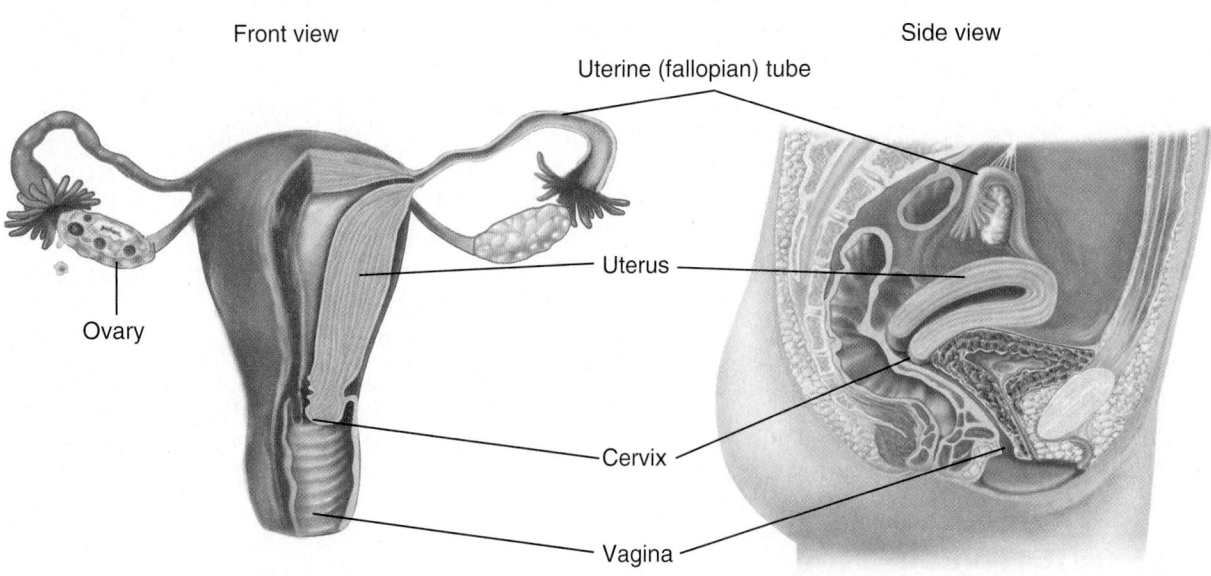

**FIGURE 24-2** Anterior and lateral views of the female reproductive system.

© Jones & Bartlett Learning.

The ovaries are located on each side of the lower abdomen and produce an ovum, or egg, that, if fertilized, will develop into a fetus. The **fallopian tubes** connect each ovary to the uterus. The **uterus** is the muscular organ where the fetus grows during pregnancy. The narrowest portion of the uterus, the **cervix**, opens into the vagina. The **vagina** is the outermost cavity of a woman's reproductive system and forms the lower part of the birth canal.

When a female reaches puberty, she begins to ovulate and experience menstruation. **Ovulation** is the cycle in which the ovum is released. The onset of menstruation is called *menarche* and usually occurs between the ages of 11 and 16 years, although it can occur earlier or later. Any female who has reached menarche is capable of becoming pregnant. Women continue to experience the cycle of ovulation and menstruation until they reach *menopause*, which marks the end of menstrual activity. Women reach menopause at widely varying ages, but it commonly occurs around the age of 50 years.

Each ovary produces an ovum during each menstrual cycle, although not necessarily in an orderly pattern that alternates back and forth between each ovary, and releases it into the fallopian tube. Some women experience minor cramping pain during ovulation when an ovum is released. The pain is sometimes described as a dull pain on one side of the lower abdomen. The quality and severity of the pain vary for each woman.

The process of fertilization begins in the vagina, where sperm from the male penis are deposited in the female reproductive tract. The sperm pass through the cervix into the uterus and eventually up the fallopian tubes. As the ovum moves slowly down the fallopian tube, sperm moving up the tube can surround it, and one sperm fertilizes it. When an ovum is fertilized in the fallopian tube, the developing embryo travels into the uterus, where the lining of the walls of the uterus has become engorged with blood in anticipation of receiving a fertilized ovum. Here, the embryo attaches to the uterine wall and continues to grow.

If the ovum is not fertilized in the fallopian tube, it continues to travel into the uterus. When fertilization has not occurred within about 14 days of ovulation, the lining of the uterus begins to separate and menstruation occurs. The menstrual flow consists of blood from the separated lining of the uterus and lasts about 1 week. Female hormones produced primarily in the ovaries control the process of ovulation and menstruation.

## Street Smarts

The onset of menarche in girls can be an emotionally and physically disturbing event. It is not uncommon for this event to be preceded by cramping pain that can be misinterpreted by the girl who has not yet experienced menstruation. Most girls have learned about the menstrual process from their parents or from health classes at school, but some are still unprepared when it occurs. Girls who have led a sheltered life or who do not have a female parent in the home are more likely to be surprised by the onset of their menstruation. Parents may also be in denial, insisting that their little girl is too young to be experiencing menstruation.

Approach the patient (and her parents) in the most professional manner possible. Empathize with their concerns. If transport is necessary for some reason, consider having a female EMT or a female family member accompany the patient.

## YOU are the Provider

At 0555 hours, law enforcement personnel request your assistance at 4300 West Avenue for a young woman who was assaulted. You and your partner respond to the scene, which is located about 4 miles away. While you are en route, an on-scene law enforcement officer radios you over a private channel and informs you the patient has been sexually assaulted and that the scene is safe. The weather is overcast, the temperature is 78°F (26°C), and the traffic is light.

**1.** What factors should you consider based on the nature of this call?

**2.** What are some unique aspects about assessing and treating a woman who has been sexually assaulted?

# Pathophysiology

The causes of gynecologic emergencies are varied and range from sexually transmitted diseases to trauma. You should recognize and properly manage female patients with any kind of abdominal or pelvic pain and consider problems that could be potentially life threatening.

## Pelvic Inflammatory Disease

**Pelvic inflammatory disease (PID)** is an infection of the upper female reproductive organs—specifically, the uterus, ovaries, and fallopian tubes—that occurs almost exclusively in sexually active women. Disease-causing organisms enter the vagina during sexual activity and migrate through the opening of the cervix and into the uterine cavity. The infection may then expand to the fallopian tubes and can cause scarring that can increase the risk of life-threatening conditions such as ectopic pregnancy or sterility. If the ovaries are affected, it can lead to the development of a life-threatening abscess. Although PID itself is seldom a threat to life, it can lead to an ectopic pregnancy or an abscess, which can cause death. *Ectopic pregnancy* is a pregnancy that develops outside the uterus, most often in the fallopian tube. The most common presenting sign of PID is generalized lower abdominal pain. Other signs and symptoms include an abnormal and often foul-smelling vaginal discharge, increased pain during sexual intercourse, fever, general malaise, and nausea and vomiting. Risk factors associated with PID include having multiple sex partners and/or a partner who

## Special Populations

Menopause is the permanent cessation of a woman's menstrual cycle. The process of menopause is complicated. As menopause approaches, menstrual periods may become irregular and vary in severity. It is not uncommon for women at this stage to continue to have irregular menstrual periods for several months to a year as the process progresses. It is important to recognize that during this time it is still possible for women to become pregnant. If a woman and her partner no longer use birth control methods because they believe pregnancy cannot occur, they may be in denial when they do see signs of pregnancy. Treat patients with compassion and reassure them, but also transport them for examination by a physician to determine if this or something else (such as a tumor or cyst) is causing the problem

## YOU are the Provider

You arrive at the scene and find the patient, a 25-year-old woman, sitting on the ground near her car. She is conscious and alert but is crying. Her shirt is torn, and she is nude from the waist down. A police officer has covered her with a blanket. After introducing yourself and your partner, you perform a primary assessment.

**Recording Time:   0 Minutes**

| | |
|---|---|
| **Appearance** | Obvious emotional distress |
| **Level of consciousness** | Conscious and alert |
| **Airway** | Open; clear of secretions and foreign bodies |
| **Breathing** | Normal rate; adequate depth |
| **Circulation** | Radial pulses normal rate and strong; skin is pink, warm, and moist; no obvious bleeding |

A police officer informs you the patient was apparently assaulted in her vehicle and the last thing she remembered was talking to a young man she met while listening to music and drinking a margarita with her friends at a local nightclub at about 2100 hours last night.

**3.** What immediate medical treatment, if any, does this patient require?

**4.** On the basis of the police officer's report, what should you suspect regarding the events that preceded the patient's assault?

has had sex with multiple people, having an untreated sexually transmitted disease, having a past history of PID, being sexually active, being younger than 26 years, douching, and using an intrauterine device for birth control.

## Sexually Transmitted Diseases

Sexually transmitted diseases can lead to more serious conditions. For example, untreated gonorrhea and chlamydia often progress to PID.

**Chlamydia** is caused by the bacterium *Chlamydia trachomatis*. According to the Centers for Disease Control and Prevention (CDC), chlamydia is currently the most commonly reported sexually transmitted disease in the United States. Although the symptoms of chlamydia are usually mild or absent, some women may report lower abdominal pain, low back pain, nausea, fever, pain during sexual intercourse, and/or bleeding between menstrual periods. Chlamydial infection of the cervix can spread to the rectum, leading to rectal pain, discharge, or bleeding. If it is left untreated, the disease can progress to PID. In rare cases, chlamydia causes arthritis that may be accompanied by skin lesions and inflammation of the eye and urethra.

**Bacterial vaginosis** is the most common vaginal infection in women age 15 to 44 years, according to the CDC. In this infection, normal bacteria in the vagina are replaced by an overgrowth of other bacterial forms. Symptoms may include itching, burning, or pain and may be accompanied by a "fishy," foul-smelling discharge. Pregnant women with bacterial vaginosis may have premature babies or babies born with low birth weight. If it is left untreated, bacterial vaginosis can lead to more serious infections or result in PID.

**Gonorrhea** is caused by *Neisseria gonorrhoeae*, a bacterium that can grow and multiply rapidly in the warm, moist areas of the reproductive tract, including the cervix, uterus, and fallopian tubes in women and in the urethra in women and men. The bacterium can also grow in the mouth, throat, eyes, and anus. Symptoms, which are generally more severe in men than in women, appear approximately 2 to 10 days after exposure. Women may be infected with gonorrhea for months but not have any symptoms, or only mild ones, until the infection has spread to other parts of the reproductive system. When symptoms do appear in women, they generally present as painful urination, with associated burning or itching; a yellowish or bloody vaginal discharge, usually with a foul odor; and blood associated with vaginal sexual intercourse. More severe infections may present with cramping and abdominal pain, nausea and vomiting, and bleeding between menstrual periods; these symptoms indicate that the infection has progressed to PID. Rectal infections generally present with anal discharge and itching and occasional painful bowel movements with fecal blood spotting. Infection of the throat (for which oral sex is the introducing factor) usually results in mild symptoms consisting of painful or difficult swallowing, sore throat, swollen lymph glands, and fever. Headache and nasal congestion may also be present. If the infection is not treated, the bacterium may enter the bloodstream and spread to other parts of the body, including the brain.

## Vaginal Bleeding

Because menstrual bleeding occurs monthly in most women, vaginal bleeding that is the result of other causes may initially be overlooked. Some possible causes of vaginal bleeding include abnormal menstruation, vaginal trauma, ectopic pregnancy, spontaneous abortion (miscarriage), cervical polyps, and cancer. Trauma to the internal female genitalia from any cause other than vaginal penetration is rare because these organs are located deep within the pelvis. Injuries to the vagina and external genitalia are painful and serious because of the large number of nerves and blood vessels in this area. In contrast, internal bleeding from polyps or cancer, while also serious, may be relatively painless.

Ectopic pregnancy and spontaneous abortion are two conditions that can cause vaginal bleeding in women early in pregnancy who may not realize they are pregnant. These potentially life-threatening conditions are covered in Chapter 34, *Obstetrics and Neonatal Care*. All cases of vaginal bleeding should be taken seriously, and the patient should be evaluated by a physician for a thorough gynecologic examination.

## Patient Assessment

Obtaining an accurate and detailed patient assessment is critically important when dealing with gynecologic issues. You will be able to gain only a primary impression of the problem in the field, yet a thorough patient assessment will help determine just how sick the patient is and whether you should initiate life-saving measures. This is especially true when dealing with abdominal pain.

Women experience many of the same conditions that cause abdominal pain in men—for example, ulcers and appendicitis. In addition, there are numerous gynecologic causes of abdominal pain. An old medical axiom states, "Anyone who neglects to consider a gynecologic cause in a woman of childbearing age who reports abdominal pain will miss the diagnosis at least 50% of the time." Missing the diagnosis may be fatal for the patient.

## Scene Size-up

Every emergency call—including calls involving gynecologic emergencies—begins with a thorough scene size-up. Is the scene safe? Will you need assistance? How many patients do you have? What is the nature of illness (NOI) or mechanism of injury (MOI)? Have you taken standard precautions? Gynecologic emergencies can be messy, sometimes involving significant amounts of blood and body fluids contaminated with organisms that can potentially cause communicable diseases.

Where and in what position is the patient found (**FIGURE 24-3**)? If she is at home, what is the condition of the residence? Is it clean or dirty? Do you see evidence of a fight? Is there evidence of alcohol, tobacco products, or drug use present? Does the patient live alone or with other people? All of the information you obtain contributes to your assessment of the patient's overall health and the safety of the scene. In the case of a crime scene, you may also be required to testify in court regarding the conditions on your arrival. Your documentation needs to

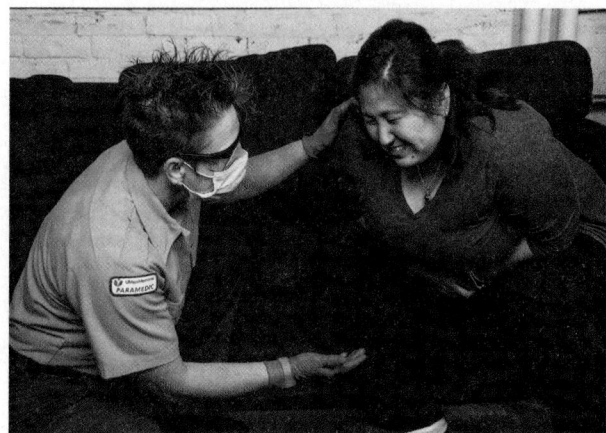

**FIGURE 24-3** Note the position of the patient during your assessment.

© Jones & Bartlett Learning.

be accurate and thorough. Involve law enforcement if any type of assault is suspected. In cases of sexual assault, it is important to have a female EMT provide patient care, if possible, so consider calling for a female provider early if you and your partner are both men.

Often, the NOI or MOI in patients with gynecologic emergencies will be understood from the dispatch information, such as in cases of sexual assault. In other patients, the exact nature of the condition will not emerge until you gather patient history information. For example, your patient may present with vague symptoms such as abdominal pain, and you will not be able to determine the exact nature of the problem until you gather more information during the patient history.

## Primary Assessment

The general impression is an important aspect of all patient assessments. As you approach the patient, you should quickly determine if her condition is stable or unstable. Use this information to help you as you proceed further with the assessment. Use the AVPU scale to determine the patient's level of consciousness.

Always evaluate the airway and breathing immediately to ensure they are adequate and treat any airway or breathing problem that is identified according to established guidelines and local protocol. Identifying and treating life threats takes precedence over all other assessment and treatment.

It is important to carefully assess circulation in all patients. Palpate a pulse and evaluate skin color, temperature, and moisture to help identify the patient who might have blood loss. Because skin paleness can be difficult to detect in patients with dark skin, check for pale mucous membranes inside the inner lower eyelid or slow capillary refill. On general observation, the patient may appear ashen or gray. If the patient has experienced significant blood loss because of vaginal bleeding, she may not demonstrate obvious signs of shock but may still be hypovolemic. If the patient has a weak or rapid pulse or has pale, cool, or diaphoretic skin, place the patient in a supine position. Cover the patient to keep her warm, and then transport to the nearest appropriate hospital for treatment.

Most cases of gynecologic emergencies are not life threatening; however, if signs of shock exist because of bleeding, then rapid transport is necessary. The remainder of the assessment can be performed en route to the hospital.

## History Taking

Begin by asking about the patient's chief complaint, but realize some of the questions you must ask may be considered extremely personal. Be sensitive to the patient's feelings and ensure that her privacy and dignity are protected. Gynecologic emergencies can be highly embarrassing for the patient, and many women may be extremely uncomfortable with discussing their sexual history in front of strangers or even close family members. An adolescent girl may want to keep her sexual history from her parents.

For a report of abdominal pain, ask specific questions about onset, duration, quality, and radiation. Provoking or relieving factors and associated symptoms such as syncope, lightheadedness, nausea, vomiting, and fever are also relevant. For a report of vaginal bleeding, ask about onset, duration, quantity (number of sanitary pads or tampons soaked), and associated symptoms such as syncope and lightheadedness.

Obtain a SAMPLE history beginning with her current symptoms. Make note of any allergies she has or any over-the-counter or prescription medications she is taking, such as birth control pills and any birth control devices she uses. Ask the patient about medical conditions, and ask specifically about her last menstrual period. This will help determine if the patient is possibly pregnant. Not every woman has a menstrual cycle every month, which may make determining the possibility of

pregnancy challenging. Do not let your guard down by ruling out pregnancy as a possibility. Ask about the possibility of sexually transmitted diseases and the possibility of pregnancy. Find out when she last ate or drank and what events led up to her calling for EMS. Use her history of events, her chief complaint, and her answers to your other questions to lead further questioning. For example, if she answers that she is sexually active, ask her about birth control and about symptoms of pregnancy. If she has vaginal bleeding, ask how many sanitary pads or tampons she is using per hour. This information can help create an estimate of blood loss.

## Secondary Assessment

The secondary assessment may be performed on scene, en route to the emergency department (ED), or, in some instances, not at all. If the patient is critically ill or injured or the transport time is short, you may not have time to conduct this part of the patient assessment process.

Pertinent secondary assessment findings should include:

- **Vital signs.** Blood pressure, pulse, skin color, orthostatic vital signs
- **Abdomen.** Distention and tenderness
- **Genitourinary.** Visible bleeding
- **Neurologic.** Mental status

Your physical examination of a gynecologic patient should be limited and professional. Only examine the genitalia if it is necessary to do so to treat the patient. Protect the woman's privacy during the physical examination. Few women are comfortable with having their body exposed to a crowd of family, neighbors, EMTs, police officers, or firefighters. Limit the personnel present to only those required to perform the necessary tasks; show the patient you respect her by being an advocate for her modesty. You also serve as a role model for other EMS providers when you act this way.

The population of women older than 65 years is increasing, and although they are past their childbearing years, many will have other gynecologic problems. They may have concerns specific to hormone replacement therapy, have an increased risk of cancer, or could be suffering from internal physical changes in the female organs associated with aging—for example, pelvic floor prolapse and urinary incontinence. Although these problems cannot be treated in the prehospital environment, perform and record a thorough assessment and treat any of the patient's immediate needs.

Focus your physical examination on the history of events and the patient's chief complaint. If vaginal bleeding is present, you should ask about its quality and quantity. You need to look at vaginal bleeding when it is sufficient to cause shock. If questioning suggests less aggressive bleeding and no evidence of shock, privacy takes precedence, and examination is deferred to the emergency department. Use external sanitary pads to absorb the bleeding and keep the possibility of hypoperfusion or shock in mind. Always ask if there is pain associated with the vaginal bleeding or discharge. Never insert anything into the vagina to control bleeding, including a tampon.

Vaginal discharge is a condition that does not need to be visualized if no bleeding is noted by the patient. Make observations about the discharge and ask the patient about any qualities she noticed and the history of the discharge. A transport decision is based on the patient's vital signs, which, if they are normal, confirm that visualizing is not necessary.

Fever, nausea, and vomiting are common with many medical conditions but should be considered especially significant with gynecologic emergencies. Fever should always be considered a sign of an infectious process. Any report of syncope on the part of the patient, especially if she reports vaginal bleeding, is considered significant. Treat the patient reporting this symptom as being in shock until proven otherwise.

Assess the patient's vital signs, including heart rate, rhythm, and quality; respiratory rate, rhythm, and quality; skin color, temperature, and condition; capillary refill time; and blood pressure. Consider obtaining orthostatic vital signs if bleeding is known or suspected. Pay special attention to the presence

## YOU are the Provider

The patient remains conscious and alert but is still in obvious emotional distress. She gives you consent to take her vital signs. A female police officer is present when you ask the patient if she is injured. She tells you she is experiencing vaginal pain and has a small amount of vaginal bleeding. The only obvious injuries you can see are minor abrasions to her forearms and legs.

| Recording Time:    8 Minutes | |
| --- | --- |
| **Respirations** | 14 breaths/min; adequate depth |
| **Pulse** | 72 beats/min; strong and regular |
| **Skin** | Pink, warm, and moist |
| **Blood pressure** | 110/70 mm Hg |
| **Oxygen saturation (Spo$_2$)** | 98% (on room air) |

The patient tells you she wants to take a shower and change her clothes. She also tells you she needs to urinate. She asks a police officer to call a friend of hers and ask the friend to come to the scene.

**5.** What additional assessment should you perform on this patient?

**6.** How should you respond to the patient's request to take a shower, change her clothes, and use the bathroom?

of tachycardia and hypotension, which could indicate hemorrhagic shock.

Monitor the patient's condition frequently to watch for changes in vital signs and mental status. Consider using noninvasive blood pressure monitoring to continuously track the patient's blood pressure. Remember, pulse oximetry readings may not be accurate in the setting of hypovolemia.

## Reassessment

Repeat the primary assessment. Reassess the patient's vital signs and the chief complaint. Reassess the patient's vital signs every 5 minutes to identify hypoperfusion from excessive blood loss. If the patient shows signs of shock, begin treatment and rapid transport.

How is the patient's condition improving with the interventions? Identify and treat any changes in the patient's condition. For example, if the patient appears to be losing consciousness, position her in the supine position and reassess. Finally, pay specific attention to the needs of your patient, and respect her desire for conversation or silence. Provide her with calm reassurance. Explain to her that the hospital staff will be sympathetic to her condition and will be well qualified to treat her.

There are few interventions that can or should be done for a patient with a gynecologic emergency. If the patient has vaginal bleeding, treat her for hypoperfusion or shock. Keep her warm, place her in a supine position, and provide her with supplemental oxygen even if she is not experiencing difficulty breathing. Consider advanced life support intercept for fluid replacement depending on transport times and local protocols, then transport to the nearest appropriate receiving facility.

Notify staff at the receiving hospital of all relevant information, including the possibility of pregnancy, so a proper response can be prepared. Carefully document the patient's condition, her chief complaint, the scene, and all interventions, especially in cases of sexual assault.

### Words of Wisdom

Gynecologic emergencies can occur at any age during a woman's lifetime. Focus on assessing and correcting the patient's ABCs and consider rapid transport as an important part of the call.

## Emergency Medical Care

Whenever you care for patients with gynecologic emergencies, you must maintain the patient's privacy as much as possible. If the patient is in a public place, move her to the ambulance. Gain the patient's confidence by communicating appropriately. If possible, have a female EMT participate in the patient's care.

Excessive internal vaginal bleeding can have many causes and can possibly lead to hypoperfusion or shock. Determining the cause of the bleeding should be considered less important than treating for shock and transporting the patient to an appropriate facility. Use sanitary pads on the external genitalia to absorb the blood. Most women will use sanitary pads before you arrive, so you may continue that approach. Document the number of sanitary pads that were saturated with blood. If the woman has a tampon in place, it is not necessary to have her remove it. Vaginal bleeding is rarely significant enough to cause hemorrhagic shock, but the patient should be treated for shock nevertheless. Apply oxygen, keep the patient supine and warm, and promptly transport to the hospital.

The genitals have a rich nerve supply, making injuries very painful. Treat any external lacerations, abrasions, and tears with sterile compresses, using local pressure to control bleeding and a diaper-type bandage to hold the dressings in place. Leave any foreign bodies in place after stabilizing them with bandages. Under no circumstances should you pack or place dressings inside the vagina. Continue to assess the patient while transporting her to the ED. Contusions and other blunt trauma will require careful in-hospital evaluation.

### Words of Wisdom

Gynecologic emergencies may involve significant blood and body fluids. PPE, including gloves, eye protection, and a mask, must be considered.

## Assessment and Management of Specific Conditions
### Pelvic Inflammatory Disease

A patient with PID will report abdominal pain. The pain generally starts during or after normal menstruation, so inquiring about the date of the patient's last menstrual period is an important detail of the patient's history. The pain may be described as achey and may be made worse by walking. Other symptoms may include vaginal discharge, fever and chills, and pain or burning on urination. Patients often present with a distinctive gait that appears as a shuffle when they walk.

### Safety Tips

Remember that many sexually transmitted diseases can also be transmitted by contact with blood. Some examples of these diseases include syphilis, many types of hepatitis, and human immunodeficiency virus.

Prehospital treatment is limited, and nonemergency transport is usually recommended. As stated earlier, PID itself is seldom life threatening, but it is serious enough to require transport and evaluation in the hospital.

## Sexual Assault and Rape

Unfortunately, sexual assault and rape are all too common occurrences. According to a government survey, approximately 18% of women (or 1 in 5) in

the United States reported being raped during their lifetime, and 1 in every 3 have been sexually abused in some form, often before the age of 12 years. EMTs called to treat a victim of sexual assault, sexual abuse, or actual or alleged rape face many complex issues, ranging from obvious medical ones to serious psychological and legal issues. You may be the first person the victim has contact with after the encounter, and how you manage the situation from first contact throughout treatment and transport may have a lasting effect for the patient and you. Being professional, respectful, and sensitive is important.

When performing your assessment, be aware of information suggesting the potential use of date rape or club drugs. The patient may or may not be aware of the use of drugs in the assault but an inability to remember the event should create suspicion. While alcohol is the most frequently used date rape drug, drugs such as Rohypnol (flunitrazepam), known as roofies; GHB (gamma-hydroxybutyric acid), known as Liquid Ecstasy; Ketalar (ketamine), known as Special K; Klonopin (clonazepam); MDMA, known as Ecstasy; and Xanax (alprazolam) are drugs typically used during sexual assault and rape for the intended purpose of incapacitating a person.

Drugs that are added into a person's drink may go undetected because they often do not have a

### YOU are the Provider

The patient refuses to go to the hospital and tells you all she wants to do is take a shower and change her clothes. Her friend arrives at the scene and asks if she can talk to the patient alone. After a brief conversation, the patient tells you she will go to the hospital, but only if her friend can come with her. You tell her that will be fine. You secure her to the stretcher, reassess her vital signs, and begin transport. You also bring along her torn underpants and skirt, which were found at the scene nearby, in a paper bag.

| Recording Time: 28 Minutes | |
| --- | --- |
| Level of consciousness | Conscious and alert |
| Respirations | 14 breaths/min; adequate depth |
| Pulse | 80 beats/min; strong and regular |
| Skin | Pink, warm, and dry |
| Blood pressure | 118/68 mm Hg |
| Spo₂ | 99% (on room air) |

**7.** How should you respond to the patient's refusal to go to the hospital?

**8.** What information can you as an EMT share with the patient's friend?

color, smell, or taste. The effects may be immediate and are made more active with alcohol. The person may become weak and confused and may even have a loss of consciousness. These drugs cause muscle relaxation and loss of muscle compliance, which may make the victim more compliant during a sexual assault. If these drugs are still in the patient's system, during your assessment you may see hypotension, bradycardia, abdominal complaints, difficulty breathing, seizures, coma, and even death.

Because sexual assault and rape are crimes, you can generally expect law enforcement to be involved early in the situation. In many cases, EMS may be called by law enforcement. Police officers generally have basic medical training; many states require at least basic training at the first responder (emergency medical responder) level. Nevertheless, primary training for police officers focuses on crime investigation, not patient care.

A rape victim has just experienced a major trauma of the body and mind. The last thing a victim wants to do is give a concise, detailed report of what has just occurred. If you attempt to gather patient information in this manner, it will most likely cause the victim to shut down. Whenever possible, a female rape victim should be given the option of being treated by a female EMT, because the patient may be experiencing mixed feelings toward men; these feelings will hinder the patient assessment and the patient's well-being.

The job of law enforcement is to solve the crime, arrest the perpetrator, and see justice served. Your job, as the EMT, is to handle the medical and psychological aspects of the case and to act as the patient advocate. In this capacity, it is important for you to focus on several key components.

The first component is the medical treatment of the patient. Is the victim physically injured? Are any life-threatening injuries present? Does the patient report any pain?

The second component is your psychological care of the patient. Do not cross-examine the patient or attempt to obtain information for the benefit of the police. These issues will be handled later by the hospital staff and police. Do not pass judgment on the patient, and protect the patient from the judgment of others on the scene. A crime may have been committed, and you need to remain aware of that fact. Many women report feeling violated when subjected to interrogation, criticism, or disbelief.

Last, remember that you are at a crime scene and the victim's body is part of that crime scene. Although your job is to treat the medical aspects of the incident and not to collect evidence, you still have a responsibility to preserve evidence. Do not cut through any clothing or throw away anything from the scene. Place bloodstained clothing and anything else that could be evidence in separate paper (not plastic) bags. Obtain evidence bags from the police if necessary. Paper bags allow wet items to dry naturally, whereas plastic allows mold to grow and may destroy biologic evidence.

It may be necessary to gently discourage the patient from cleaning herself. Victims tend to want to wash away the humiliation and embarrassment of the assault. Valuable evidence can be destroyed in this process. Also discourage the patient from urinating, changing clothes, moving her bowels, or rinsing out her mouth. She will be photographed and examined by nurses trained in sexual assault examination and management (sometimes called Sexual Assault Nurse Examiners [SANE nurses]) or law enforcement personnel as well, and the evidence needs to be as accurate as possible. If you cannot discourage the patient from taking these actions, respect her feelings. Some patients may refuse transport altogether, and they have the right to do so. In such cases, follow your system's refusal of treatment policy or procedure for sexual assault victims without judging or talking down to the patient. Your compassion is the best tool you have to gain the patient's confidence and encourage her to get help.

If the patient refuses transport, offer to call the local rape crisis center for her. Many communities have rape crisis centers with victim advocacy hotlines. Having a professional advocate at the scene may help the patient deal with the trauma, and the advocate can better explain in more compassionate detail the necessity of preserving evidence.

## Street Smarts

Keep a list of local resources that you can provide to someone who has experienced a sexual assault. Although your patient may not feel comfortable speaking at the moment, knowing there are people who can help when he or she is ready can provide reassurance and courage at a later time.

Many victim advocates are rape-trauma survivors themselves. They can provide support to the patient in the hospital during any additional physical examinations.

Take the patient's history, and limit any physical examination to a brief survey for life-threatening injuries. Treat all other injuries such as contusions or lacerations according to the appropriate procedures and protocols for your EMS system. Follow standard precautions. Expose and examine the vaginal area only if there is evidence of bleeding that needs to be treated. Cover and protect the patient from curious onlookers. Examine and interview the patient with a minimum of people present; move her to the ambulance if necessary.

The patient report is a legal document and, should the case result in an arrest and subsequent trial, may be subpoenaed. Keep the report concise, and record only what the patient stated in her own words. Use quotation marks to indicate you are reporting the patient's version of events. Do not insert your own opinion as to whether the patient was sexually assaulted or raped or offer any conclusions that would prove or disprove the patient's account of the event. Focus on the facts. Record all of your observations during the physical examination—the patient's emotional state, the condition of her clothing, obvious injuries, and so forth. Remember

that rape is a legal diagnosis, not a medical diagnosis. The medical team can establish only whether sexual intercourse occurred; a court must decide whether sexual intercourse was forcibly inflicted against her will. **TABLE 24-1** lists the treatment principles you should use when dealing with a victim of sexual assault.

Often the most important intervention for sexual assault patients is comforting reassurance and transport to a facility that has employees who are certified to perform the proper physical examination in this type of case. Reminding the patient that she is safe with you and that the hospital staff and the police will take good care of her may help reassure her. Sometimes just the presence of a female EMT can be emotionally helpful. Do not insist that the patient talk to you, but listen carefully and do not be judgmental if she does want to talk. Remember that victims of sexual assault may also need medical assistance; therefore, treat the medical injuries, but also remember to ensure the patient's privacy and provide her with emotional support.

Although most cases of sexual assault are on women by men, it is important to remember that it is possible for a man to be sexually assaulted or for the assailant to be either a woman or a man. The principles of care above still apply and the likelihood of psychological trauma is just as strong.

## YOU are the Provider

You reassess the patient en route to the hospital; her mental status and vital signs indicate that she is stable. Her friend provides emotional support to her and assures her that what happened was not her fault. You call your radio report to the receiving facility and give them your estimated time of arrival.

| Recording Time: 38 Minutes | |
| --- | --- |
| Level of consciousness | Conscious and alert |
| Respirations | 16 breaths/min; adequate depth |
| Pulse | 76 beats/min; strong and regular |
| Skin | Pink, warm, and dry |
| Blood pressure | 122/72 mm Hg |
| Spo$_2$ | 98% (on room air) |

**9.** Why is it important to transport a sexual assault victim to the hospital, even if she does not have any obvious injuries?

**TABLE 24-1** Treatment Principles for Sexual Assault

In addition to the usual treatment principles that apply to all victims, follow these special steps when treating patients who have been sexually assaulted:

1. Document the patient's history, assessment, treatment, and response to treatment in detail because you may have to appear in court many years later. Do not speculate. Record only the facts.
2. Complete the SAMPLE history objectively.
3. Follow any crime scene policy established by your system to protect the scene and any potential evidence for police, particularly policies regarding evidence collection. If the patient will tolerate being wrapped in a sterile burn sheet, this may help investigators find any hair, fluid, or fiber from the alleged offender.
4. Do not examine the genitalia unless there is major bleeding. If an object has been inserted into the vagina or rectum, do not attempt to remove it.
5. Whenever possible, reduce the patient's anxiety by using an EMT who is the same gender as the patient.
6. Discourage the patient from bathing, voiding, or cleaning any wounds until after the hospital staff has completed an assessment. Handle the patient's clothes as little as possible, placing clothing and any other evidence in paper bags. If the patient insists on urinating, ask the patient to do so in a sterile urine container (if available). Also, deposit the toilet paper in a paper bag. Seal and label the bag for law enforcement. This can be critically important evidence.
7. If possible, transport the patient to a hospital with specialized staff such as Sexual Assault Nurse Examiners (SANE) who can fully evaluate these patients, perform medical and forensic examinations, and provide all aspects of medical and supportive care for these patients.

© Jones & Bartlett Learning.

# YOU are the Provider SUMMARY

**1. What factors should you consider based on the nature of this call?**

As with any call, your first priority should be to ensure the scene is safe for you to enter; this is especially true when you respond to an assault or any other call that has a higher than usual risk for violence. Although an on-scene law enforcement officer has informed you that the scene is safe, you must still remain aware of your surroundings when you arrive. While the scene may initially be safe, it can quickly turn violent.

Your next consideration should be for the patient. Although you should avoid asking specific questions over the radio regarding a sexual assault, you should determine if the patient is conscious and if she appears to have any life-threatening injuries or major bleeding. As with any patient, the more information you obtain while en route to the scene, the better prepared you will be to provide immediate care when you arrive.

Finally, you should consider the fact that you are responding to a crime scene. Although your job is to treat the *medical* aspects of the incident and not to collect evidence, you still have a responsibility to preserve evidence, to the extent possible, without sacrificing patient care.

**2. What are some unique aspects about assessing and treating a woman who has been sexually assaulted?**

The initial medical treatment you provide to a sexual assault victim follows the same principles as with any other patient—identify and treat life-threatening injuries. However, it is important to remember that the emotional effects on the patient are devastating.

When you are called to treat a victim of sexual assault, you face many challenges, which range from obvious medical concerns to serious psychological and legal matters. Be professional and sensitive at all times.

You should expect that the victim will not want to talk about the details of what happened. Do not force the victim to talk about the experience if the victim does not want to talk. Whenever possible, a female sexual assault victim should be assessed and treated by a female EMT.

**3. What immediate medical treatment, if any, does this patient require?**

Your primary assessment has not revealed any obvious immediately life-threatening injuries or conditions; therefore, immediate emergency medical treatment is not indicated *at this point.*

The patient is conscious and alert, although she is emotionally distressed. Her airway is patent, and her breathing is adequate. Her radial pulses are strong and a normal rate. There is no significant obvious bleeding that requires your attention, and her skin is pink, warm, and moist.

**4. On the basis of the police officer's report, what should you suspect regarding the events that preceded the patient's assault?**

Sexual assault is an acutely overwhelming emotional and traumatic event, and some patients experience amnesia as an involuntary emotional protective reflex. However, this type of amnesia is typically limited to the sexual assault itself, not several hours before the assault occurred. It is now 0555 hours, and the patient has absolutely no recollection of the events that occurred after 2100 hours the night before. You should be suspicious that the patient was unknowingly given a drug by the person who perpetrated this crime; this may have been the young man she met at the nightclub or a random person—man or woman.

**5. What additional assessment should you perform on this patient?**

As with any patient, the extent of your secondary assessment is based on your suspicion of injuries or conditions that may not have been grossly apparent during the primary assessment. In sexual assault victims, it is unlikely that patients will consent to a physical examination of their entire body at the scene and doing so could disturb evidence. More importantly, such an examination would not impact the care you would provide. Therefore, you should limit any physical examination of the patient to a brief survey for life-threatening injuries.

The patient in this scenario reports vaginal pain but denies vaginal bleeding. The external genitalia should not be exposed and examined—whether the EMT is a man or woman—unless there is evidence of severe bleeding that requires immediate treatment. Asking the patient questions rather than performing a hands-on examination will be enough for your assessment. Because she has reported minor bleeding, you offered her a menstrual pad to wear.

**6. How should you respond to the patient's request to take a shower, change her clothes, and use the bathroom?**

It is common for victims of sexual assault to want to take a shower, change their clothes, rinse their mouth out, or douche. These actions stem from the desire to wash away the humiliation and embarrassment of the assault.

However, remember that valuable evidence may be lost if the patient takes any measures to clean up; therefore, you should discourage—*not disallow*—her from doing so. The patient should also be discouraged from urinating or moving her bowels; doing so may destroy any DNA evidence that may remain from vaginal or anal penetration. Make every attempt to explain to the patient that she has potential evidence on or inside of her body that may be used to identify the perpetrator. If, despite your best efforts, you cannot convince the patient not to clean herself, you must respect her feelings and avoid forcing the issue.

**7. How should you respond to the patient's refusal to go to the hospital?**

In many cases, sexual assault victims will refuse EMS transport, and some will refuse *any and all* assessment and treatment. Provided the patient has decision-making capacity, the patient has the legal right to refuse transport.

If the patient refuses EMS transport, do not simply accept the refusal and leave. You must still ensure she is aware of the potential consequences of refusing treatment. She reports vaginal pain and minor external bleeding; this could indicate a significant internal injury that could be potentially fatal. She *must* be made aware of this fact.

Although the patient in this case does not recall being sexually assaulted, her signs and symptoms (eg, vaginal pain and bleeding) and the way she presents—torn shirt and nude from the waist down—are clear indicators that suggest she was sexually assaulted. Patients who recall being sexually assaulted often benefit from being removed from the scene where the assault occurred so they have decreased exposure to visual or auditory reminders present in the environment where the traumatic

# YOU are the Provider SUMMARY *continued*

event occurred. The best way to do this is to convince her to go to the hospital; doing so will remove her from the scene *and* allow her to be examined by a physician. Sometimes a victim of sexual assault may be more comfortable with a relative or friend along during transport, especially if the crew is of the opposite gender.

**8. What information can you as an EMT share with the patient's friend?**

In all patient encounters, you are an advocate for the patient and patient confidentiality is a priority. Allow the friend to talk to the patient if the patient agrees. Do not share any information about your assessment findings or information about the assault as HIPAA confidentiality guidelines apply.

**9. Why is it important to transport a sexual assault victim to the hospital, even if she does not have any obvious injuries?**

Sexual assault victims should be transported to the hospital for several reasons. First, the patient should have a medical examination by a physician to rule out injuries or conditions that were not detected or not present in the field. Injuries such as internal abdominal bleeding can have a delayed onset of symptoms for up to several hours. Additionally, evidence will need to be collected during the examination. Many hospitals have professionally trained sexual assault nurse investigators trained in evidence collection and psychological support of these patients. Furthermore, the patient will need initial and follow-up screening for any sexually transmitted diseases.

## EMS Patient Care Report (PCR)

| Date: 11-11-20 | Incident No.: 211109 | Nature of Call: Assault | | Location: 4300 West Avenue | |
|---|---|---|---|---|---|
| Dispatched: 0555 | En Route: 0557 | At Scene: 0602 | Transport: 0647 | At Hospital: 0657 | In Service: 0665 |

### Patient Information

| | |
|---|---|
| **Age:** 25<br>**Sex:** F<br>**Weight (in kg [lb]):** 50 kg (110 lb) | **Allergies:** None<br>**Medications:** No known drug allergies<br>**Past Medical History:** None<br>**Chief Complaint:** Vaginal pain; amnesia |

### Vital Signs

| Time: 0610 | BP: 110/70 | Pulse: 72 | Respirations: 14 | Spo$_2$: 98% |
|---|---|---|---|---|
| Time: 0630 | BP: 118/68 | Pulse: 80 | Respirations: 14 | Spo$_2$: 99% |
| Time: 0640 | BP: 122/72 | Pulse: 76 | Respirations: 16 | Spo$_2$: 98% |

### EMS Treatment (circle all that apply)

| Oxygen @ ___ L/min via:<br><br>NC   NRM   Bag mask | | Assisted Ventilation | Airway Adjunct | CPR |
|---|---|---|---|---|
| Defibrillation | Bleeding Control:<br>(Menstrual pad) | Bandaging | Splinting | Other: Limited assessment, emotional support |

## YOU are the Provider SUMMARY *continued*

### Narrative

Medic 86 was requested by law enforcement to respond to a residence for a woman who was assaulted.

Chief Complaint: Vaginal pain; amnesia

History: While en route to the scene, law enforcement informed that the patient appeared to have been sexually assaulted. Prior to EMS arrival, the patient informed law enforcement personnel she did not recall the events that occurred after 2100 the night before, when she was at a nightclub with her friends. Law enforcement found her with her shirt torn and she was nude from the waist down, so they wrapped her with a blanket before EMS arrival. On EMS arrival, patient reported vaginal pain and some minor vaginal bleeding. She denied significant medical history and medication allergies.

Assessment: Arrived on scene and found the patient, a 25-year-old woman, sitting on the ground next to her car with a blanket wrapped around her. She was conscious and alert, although clearly emotionally upset. Her airway was patent, her breathing was adequate, and no obvious bleeding was noted. The only obvious injuries noted were several small abrasions to her forearms and legs.

Treatment (Rx): The patient would not consent to a secondary assessment or treatment; she would allow only assessment of her vital signs. She was given a menstrual pad for minor vaginal bleeding.

Transport: The patient stated she did not want to go to the hospital, via EMS or any other method of transportation. She further stated she wanted to take a shower and change her clothes. Advised patient this was not recommended because of the possibility of destroying potential evidence; however, she stated she did not care and only wanted to clean herself. Further advised the patient of the need for a physical examination at the hospital because hidden injuries, some of which could be life threatening, could not be ruled out in the prehospital setting. The patient requested law enforcement to summon a friend of hers to the scene. After talking to her friend, she consented only to EMS transport and agreed not to shower or otherwise clean herself; she further requested her friend accompany her in the back of the ambulance. Patient walked several steps to the ambulance. Transported to the hospital on the stretcher with her friend in the back. She remained conscious and alert, and her vital signs remained stable. Provided emotional support, with the assistance of her friend, until delivery at the emergency department. Delivered patient to hospital and gave verbal report to staff nurse, Yuan. Police remain in custody of a bag with the patient's clothes found at the scene. Medic 86 cleared the hospital and returned to service at 0650.

**End of report**

## Prep Kit

### Ready for Review

- A woman's body is uniquely formed to conceive and give birth. This difference makes women susceptible to a number of conditions that do not occur in men.
- If fertilization of the ovum does not occur within about 14 days of ovulation, the lining of the uterus begins to separate and menstruation occurs and lasts for about 1 week.
- When a girl reaches puberty, she begins to ovulate and experience menstruation.
- Women continue to experience the cycle of ovulation and menstruation until they reach menopause.
- The causes of gynecologic emergencies are varied and range from sexually transmitted diseases to trauma.
- Pelvic inflammatory disease (PID) is an infection of the upper female reproductive organs: the uterus, ovaries, and fallopian tubes. PID can lead to an ectopic pregnancy or an abscess, which can cause death.
- Sexually transmitted diseases can lead to more serious conditions, such as pelvic inflammatory disease.
- Because menstrual bleeding occurs every month in most women, vaginal bleeding that is the result of other causes may initially be overlooked. Some possible causes of vaginal bleeding include abnormal menstruation, vaginal trauma, ectopic pregnancy, spontaneous abortion, cervical polyps, ectopic pregnancy, miscarriage, and even cancer.

- There are few interventions that can or should be done in the prehospital setting to treat a gynecologic emergency.
- Whenever you deal with patients who have a gynecologic emergency, you must maintain the patients' privacy as much as possible.
- EMTs called to treat a victim of sexual assault, sexual abuse, or actual or alleged rape face

many challenges, ranging from obvious medical ones to serious psychological and legal issues. You may be the victim's first contact after the encounter, and how the situation is managed from first contact throughout treatment and transport may have lasting effects for the patient and you. It is very important to always be professional, sensitive, and kind.

## Vital Vocabulary

**bacterial vaginosis** An overgrowth of bacteria in the vagina; characterized by itching, burning, or pain, and possibly a "fishy"-smelling discharge.

**cervix** The lower third, or neck, of the uterus.

**chlamydia** A sexually transmitted disease caused by the bacterium *Chlamydia trachomatis*.

**fallopian tubes** The tubes that connect each ovary with the uterus and are the primary location for fertilization of the ovum.

**gonorrhea** A sexually transmitted disease caused by *Neisseria gonorrhoeae*.

**labia majora** Outer fleshy "lips" covered with pubic hair that protect the vagina.

**labia minora** Inner fleshy "lips" devoid of pubic hair that protect the vagina.

**ovaries** The primary female reproductive organs that produce an ovum, or egg, that, if fertilized, will develop into a fetus.

**ovulation** The process in which an ovum is released from a follicle.

**pelvic inflammatory disease (PID)** An infection of the fallopian tubes and the surrounding tissues of the pelvis.

**perineum** The area of skin between the vagina and the anus.

**rape** Sexual intercourse forcibly inflicted on another person, against that person's will.

**sexual assault** An attack against a person that is sexual in nature, the most common of which is rape.

**uterus** The muscular organ where the fetus grows, also called the womb; responsible for contractions during labor.

**vagina** The outermost cavity of a woman's reproductive tract; the lower part of the birth canal.

## References

1. American Forensic Nurses. FAQ. http://amrn.com/faq.html. Accessed November 17, 2019.

2. Centers for Disease Control and Prevention. Bacterial vaginosis—statistics. https://www.cdc.gov/std/bv/stats.htm. Updated December 15, 2015. Accessed November 17, 2019.

3. Centers for Disease Control and Prevention. Pelvic inflammatory disease—CDC fact sheet. https://www.cdc.gov/std/pid/stdfact-pid.htm. Updated December 11, 2015. Accessed November 17, 2019.

4. Centers for Disease Control and Prevention. Preventing sexual violence. https://www.cdc.gov/violenceprevention/sexualviolence/fastfact.html. Reviewed January 17, 2020. Accessed January 24, 2020.

5. Centers for Disease Control and Prevention. Sexual violence. https://www.cdc.gov/violenceprevention/sexualviolence. Reviewed January 17, 2018. Accessed January 24, 2020.

6. Centers for Disease Control and Prevention. Sexual violence is preventable. https://www.cdc.gov/injury/features/sexual-violence/index.html. Updated August 28, 2019. Accessed November 17, 2019.

7. Centers for Disease Control and Prevention. Sexually transmitted diseases: disease and related conditions. https://www.cdc.gov/std/general/default.htm. Updated November 4, 2016.

8. Ecochard R, Gougeon A. Side of ovulation and cycle characteristics in normally fertile women. In: *Human Reproduction*. April 2000; vol 15(4):752–755. https://doi.org/10.1093/humrep/15.4.752. Accessed March 24, 2020.

9. Harvard Health Publishing. Sexually transmitted disease? At my age? health.harvard.edu. https://www.health.harvard.edu/diseases-and-conditions/sexually-transmitted-disease-at-my-age. Published February 2018. Accessed February 6, 2020.

10. National Association of State EMS Officials. National Model EMS Clinical Guidelines. https://nasemso .org/wp-content/uploads/National-Model-EMS -Clinical-Guidelines-2017-PDF-Version-2.2.pdf. Published January 2019. Accessed November 17, 2019.

11. National Highway Traffic Safety Administration. *National Emergency Medical Services Education Standards*. DOT HS 811 077A. ems.gov. http://www.ems.gov /pdf/811077a.pdf. Published January 2009. Accessed November 17, 2019.

12. National Highway Traffic Safety Administration. *National Emergency Medical Services Education Standards: Emergency Medical Technician Instructional Guidelines*. DOT HS 811 077C. ems.gov. www.ems.gov/pdf /811077a.pdf. Published January 2009. Accessed November 17, 2019.

13. National Sexual Violence Resource Center. Get statistics: sexual assault in the United States. https://www.nsvrc.org/node/4737. Accessed February 6, 2020.

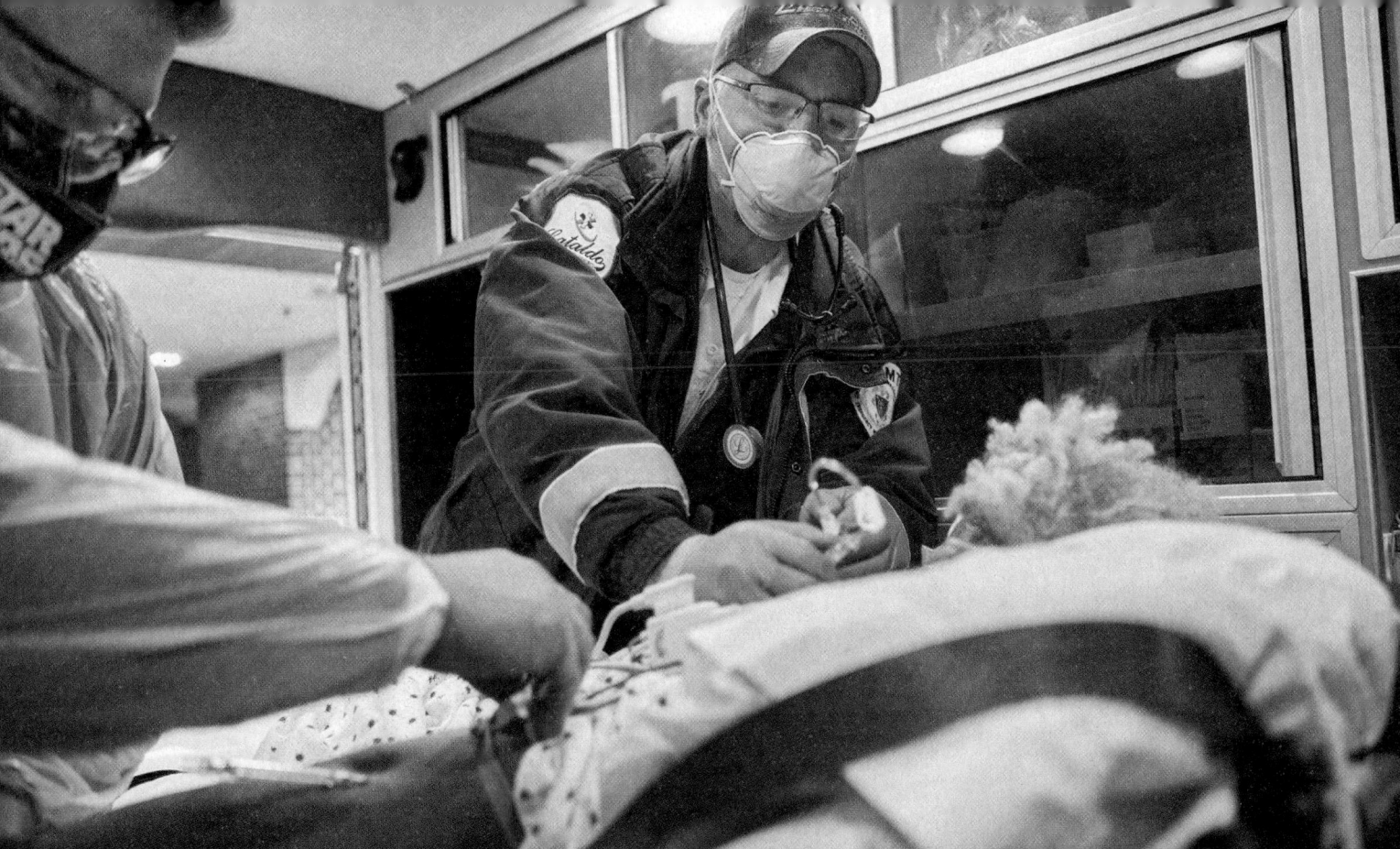

# Trauma

**25** Trauma Overview

**26** Bleeding

**27** Soft-Tissue Injuries

**28** Face and Neck Injuries

**29** Head and Spine Injuries

**30** Chest Injuries

**31** Abdominal and Genitourinary Injuries

**32** Orthopaedic Injuries

**33** Environmental Emergencies

# Chapter 25

# Trauma Overview

## NATIONAL EMS EDUCATION STANDARD COMPETENCIES

### Trauma

Applies fundamental knowledge to provide basic emergency care and transportation based on assessment findings for an acutely injured patient.

### Trauma Overview

Pathophysiology, assessment, and management of the trauma patient

- Trauma scoring (p 924)
- Rapid transport and destination issues (pp 922–926)
- Transport mode (pp 924–926)

### Multisystem Trauma

Recognition and management of
- Multisystem trauma (pp 918–919)

Pathophysiology, assessment, and management of
- Multisystem trauma (pp 918–919)
- Blast injuries (pp 915–918)

## KNOWLEDGE OBJECTIVES

1. Define the terms *mechanism of injury* (MOI), *blunt trauma*, and *penetrating trauma*. (pp 901, 904)
2. Explain the relationship of the MOI to potential energy, kinetic energy, and work. (pp 901–902)
3. Provide examples of the MOI that would cause blunt and penetrating trauma to occur. (pp 904–915)
4. Describe the five types of motor vehicle crashes, the injury patterns associated with each one, and how each relates to the index of suspicion of life-threatening injuries. (pp 904–911)
5. Discuss the three specific factors to consider during assessment of a patient who has been injured in a fall, plus additional considerations for pediatric and geriatric patients. (pp 912–913)
6. Discuss the effects of high-, medium-, and low-velocity penetrating trauma on the body and how an understanding of each type helps EMTs form an index of suspicion about unseen life-threatening injuries. (pp 913–915)
7. Discuss primary, secondary, tertiary, and miscellaneous blast injuries and the anticipated damage each one will cause to the body. (pp 915–918)
8. Describe multisystem trauma and the special considerations that are required for patients who fit this category. (pp 918–919)
9. Explain the major components of trauma patient assessment; include considerations related to whether the MOI was significant or nonsignificant. (p 920)
10. Discuss the special assessment considerations related to a trauma patient who has injuries in each of the following areas: head, neck and throat, chest, and abdomen. (pp 920–922)
11. Provide a general overview of multisystem trauma patient management. (pp 922–924)
12. Explain trauma patient management in relation to scene time and transport selection. (pp 922–926)
13. List the criteria for the appropriate use of helicopter emergency medical services. (p 924)

14. Discuss the American College of Surgeons Committee on Trauma classification of trauma centers. (pp 922–924)

15. Explain the American College of Surgeons Committee on Trauma and the Centers for Disease Control and Prevention field triage decision scheme as it relates to making an appropriate destination selection for a trauma patient. (pp 922–925)

## SKILLS OBJECTIVE

There are no skills objectives for this chapter.

## Introduction

According to the National Center for Health Statistics, traumatic injuries and unintentional injuries are the leading causes of death in the United States among people from 1 to 44 years of age. Proper prehospital evaluation and care has the capability to reduce a patient's suffering, long-term disability, and risk of death from trauma. Patients who need EMS assistance are generally categorized as either a medical or trauma emergency, although one may result from the other or both may exist. This is discussed further in Chapter 15, *Medical Overview*.

**Trauma emergencies** occur as a result of physical forces applied to the body. **Medical emergencies** include illnesses or conditions; these are not caused by an outside force. Traumatic injuries may be caused by underlying medical conditions (a patient has a stroke and veers off the road, striking a tree). Similarly, medical illnesses may result from recent or remote traumatic injuries (pneumonia develops in a patient a few days after a fall that fractured the patient's ribs). This chapter introduces the basic physical concepts that dictate how traumatic injuries occur and how they affect the human body. When you understand these concepts, you will be better prepared to size up a vehicular crash scene and assess a patient.

This chapter begins with a basic discussion of energy and trauma. Next, different types of vehicle crashes and their effect on the body are explained. By assessing a vehicle that has crashed, you can often determine what happened to the passengers at the time of impact. This may allow you to predict what injuries the passengers sustained at the time of impact. Evaluation of the mechanism of injury for the trauma patient will provide you with an index of suspicion for different types of serious and/or life-threatening underlying injuries. Certain injury patterns occur with certain types of injury events. The **index of suspicion** is your awareness and concern for potentially serious underlying and unseen injuries.

## Energy and Trauma

Traumatic injury occurs when the body's tissues are exposed to energy levels beyond their tolerance (**FIGURE 25-1**). The **mechanism of injury (MOI)** is the way in which traumatic injuries occur; it describes the forces (or energy transmission) acting on the body that cause injury. Three concepts of energy are typically associated with injury (not including thermal energy, which causes burns): potential energy, kinetic energy, and the energy of work. When considering the effects of energy on the human body, it is important to remember that energy can be neither created nor destroyed: it can only be converted or transformed. It is not the objective of this section to help you reconstruct the scene of a motor vehicle crash. Rather, you should have a sense of the effects of the event on the human body and understand, in

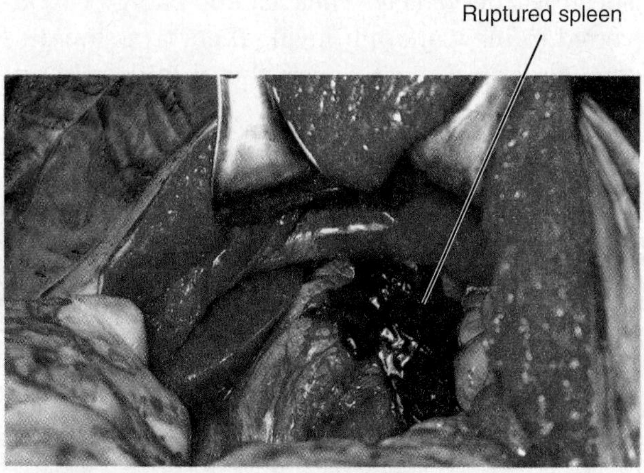

Ruptured spleen

**FIGURE 25-1** Traumatic injury occurs when the body's tissues are exposed to energy levels beyond their tolerance. This photo shows a ruptured spleen.

© Pthawatc/Shutterstock.

a broad sense, how that event is related to potential and kinetic energy.

For example, when assessing a patient who fell, you need not calculate the speed at which the person hit the ground. Instead, focus on the factors of the impact and how those relate to the potential for injury. For example, it is important to estimate the height from which the patient fell, as well as the surface he or she landed on, to fully appreciate the injury potential of the fall.

**Work** is defined as force acting over a distance. For example, the force needed to bend metal multiplied by the distance over which the metal is bent is the work that crushes the front end of a vehicle that is involved in a frontal impact. Similarly, forces that bend, pull, or compress tissues beyond their inherent limits result in the work that causes injury.

The energy of a moving object is called **kinetic energy**. Kinetic energy reflects the relationship between the mass (weight) of the object and the velocity (speed) at which it is traveling. Kinetic energy is expressed as:

$$\text{Kinetic energy} = \tfrac{1}{2}\ \text{mass} \times \text{velocity}^2 \text{ or}$$
$$\text{KE} = \tfrac{1}{2}\ \text{m} \times \text{v}^2$$

Remember, energy cannot be created or destroyed, only converted. In the case of a motor vehicle crash, the kinetic energy of the speeding vehicle is converted into the work of stopping the vehicle, usually by crushing the vehicle's exterior (**FIGURE 25-2**). Similarly, the passengers of the vehicle have kinetic energy because they were traveling at the same speed as the vehicle. Their kinetic energy is converted to the work of bringing them to a stop. It is this work on the passengers that results in injury. Notice that, according to the equation for kinetic

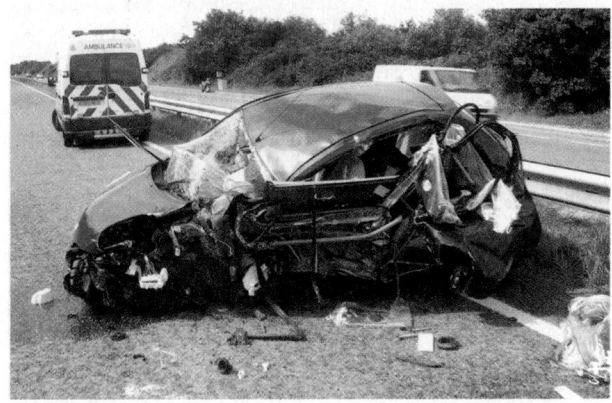

**FIGURE 25-2** The kinetic energy of a speeding car is converted into the work of stopping the car, usually by crushing the car's exterior and damaging the point of impact.

Courtesy of Mark Woolcock.

energy, the energy that is available to cause injury *doubles* when an object's weight doubles but *quadruples* when its speed doubles. When a car's speed increases from 50 to 70 mph, the energy that is available to cause injury nearly doubles. This point is even clearer when considering gunshot wounds. The speed of the bullet (high-velocity compared with low-velocity) has a greater impact on producing injury than the mass (size) of the bullet. Therefore, it is important to report to the hospital the type of firearm that was used in a shooting. The amount of kinetic energy that is converted to do work on the body dictates the severity of the injury. High-energy injuries often produce such severe damage that patients require immediate transport to an appropriate facility to have any hope of survival.

**Potential energy** is the product of mass (weight), force of gravity, and height and is mostly associated with the energy of falling objects. A worker on a

## YOU are the Provider

At 1520 hours, you and your partner are dispatched to a motor vehicle crash in which a passenger vehicle reportedly struck a tree head-on at an unknown rate of speed. The emergency medical dispatcher (EMD) reports that the patient is still in the vehicle, but it is unknown if the person is trapped. Law enforcement personnel and two engine companies have also been dispatched to the scene. Your response time is 8 minutes, the weather is clear, and the traffic is heavy.

**1.** On the basis of the information provided by the EMD, can you predict the potential types of injuries the patient may have? If so, how?

**2.** Why is it important to determine the speed at which a vehicle was traveling at the time of impact?

## Words of Wisdom

### Newton's Laws of Motion

#### Newton's First Law

Newton's first law of motion states that objects at rest tend to stay at rest and objects in motion tend to stay in motion unless acted on by some force. The first part of the law is fairly clear. An object such as an empty soda can will not move spontaneously unless some force, such as a gust of wind, acts on it. An example will help to illustrate the second part. In a car traveling at 30 mph, the passengers and the car are moving at 30 mph. The passengers do not feel as though they are moving because they are not moving relative to the car. However, when the car strikes a concrete barrier and comes to a sudden stop, the passengers continue to travel at 30 mph. They stay in motion until they are acted on by an external force—most likely the windshield, steering wheel, or dashboard. To appreciate the severity of the impact, think of the driver as sitting motionless while a steering wheel rams into his or her chest at 30 mph. Now consider that the same thing happens to the driver's internal organs. They also are in motion, traveling at 30 mph relative to the ground, until they are acted on by an external force, in this case the sternum, rib cage, or other body structure. This scenario illustrates the three collisions that are associated with blunt trauma.

#### Newton's Second Law

Newton's second law of motion states that force (F) equals mass (m) times acceleration (a), that is, $F = m \times a$, in which acceleration is the change in velocity (speed) that occurs over time. Therefore, it is not so much that speed kills, but that the change in velocity with respect to time generates the forces that cause injury. Simply put, it is not the fall, but the sudden stop at the bottom, that causes the injury.

In the example of the car traveling at 30 mph, it takes about 3 seconds for the car to decrease its speed from 30 to 0 mph when the driver applies the brakes smoothly. If he or she is properly restrained by well-adjusted seat belts, the driver slows, or decelerates, at the same rate as the car. But if the car is stopped not by braking but by hitting a large tree and the driver is not restrained, his or her body will continue to stay in motion at 30 mph until it is stopped by an external force, in this case, the steering wheel. Although the change in the body's velocity is the same as when the car was braking smoothly in 3 seconds (30 to 0 mph), that change now takes place in about 0.01 second. Because the period of deceleration is 300 times less, the average force of impact is 300 times greater. This means that the force

is approximately 150 times the force of gravity. Imagine a force 150 times your body weight slamming into your chest.

Now consider the same car striking the same tree, but this time, the driver is restrained with a shoulder and lap belt. The driver is essentially tied to the car and stops during the same period the car stops. It takes some time, although brief, to crush the front of the car and bring it to a halt. The car comes to a stop in approximately 0.05 second. The change in the driver's velocity is the same (30 to 0 mph), but the longer period of deceleration results in a g force of 30 times that of gravity (one g force is the normal acceleration due to gravity). This is still a substantial force, but it is much less than the force experienced by the unrestrained driver.

In a final example, the car and driver, as before, are traveling at 30 mph, and the driver is properly restrained with a three-point seat belt. In this case, however, the car is also equipped with an airbag. When the car hits the tree and suddenly stops, the driver's upper body initially continues forward at 30 mph. The body is partially slowed by the lap and shoulder belts but is finally brought to rest by the airbag. The upper body compresses the airbag, which stops the body's forward motion in about 0.1 second. Thanks to the airbag, the force of impact is applied over a much larger area. The dual action of the airbag (distributing the force of impact over a greater area and increasing the duration of impact) results in less severe injuries.

#### Newton's Third Law

Newton's third law of motion states that for every action, there is an equal and opposite reaction. Therefore, if you push on a door, the door pushes back (reacts) with an equal force but in the opposite direction. In the case of a dented A-pillar, the force of the driver's head was sufficient to dent the strong metal. But in terms of patient assessment, the more important point is the reaction force of the pillar on the head. Newton's third law states that the two forces are equal but occur in opposite directions. In other words, the head was essentially hit by an A-pillar traveling at 30 mph. Similarly, it takes a substantial force to collapse a steering wheel. When you notice a collapsed steering wheel during scene size-up, suspect serious chest injuries even if the driver initially has no visible signs of chest injury. Often, reading the scene and understanding the basic principles of energy transfer will give you as clear a picture of the patient's potential injuries and injury severity as the actual physical patient assessment.

scaffold has potential energy because he or she is some height above the ground. If the worker falls, potential energy is converted into kinetic energy. As the worker hits the ground, the kinetic energy is converted into work—that is, the work of bringing the body to a stop and thereby fracturing bones and damaging tissues.

## MOI Profiles

Different types of MOIs will produce many types of injuries. Examples of nonsignificant injuries include injury to an isolated body part or a fall without the loss of consciousness. Examples of significant MOIs include injury to more than one body system (**multisystem trauma**), falls from heights, motor vehicle and motorcycle crashes, car versus pedestrian (or bicycle or motorcycle), gunshot wounds, and stabbings. Whether one or more body systems are involved, maintain a high index of suspicion for serious unseen injuries.

## Blunt and Penetrating Trauma

Traumatic injuries can be considered in two categories: blunt trauma and penetrating trauma. **Blunt trauma** is the result of force (or energy transmission) to the body that causes injury without anything penetrating the soft tissues or internal organs and cavities. **Penetrating trauma** results in injury by objects that pierce and penetrate the surface of the body and injure the underlying soft tissues, internal

organs, and body cavities. Either type of trauma may occur from a variety of MOIs. It is important to consider unseen as well as visible, obvious injuries with either type of trauma. Damage to the underlying deeper tissues is often more significant.

## Blunt Trauma

Blunt trauma results from an object making contact with the body. Any object, such as a baseball bat, can cause blunt trauma if it is moving fast enough. Motor vehicle crashes and falls are two of the most common MOIs for blunt trauma. When providing care for your patient, be alert to signs of skin discoloration or reports of pain because these may be the only signs of blunt trauma. During assessment, maintain a high index of suspicion for hidden (internal) injuries in patients with blunt trauma.

### Vehicular Crashes

Motor vehicle crashes are traditionally classified as frontal (head-on), rear-end, lateral (T-bone), rollover, and rotational (spins). The principal difference among these crash types is the direction of the force of impact; also, with spins and rollovers, there is the possibility of multiple impacts. Motor vehicle crashes typically consist of a series of three collisions. Understanding the events that occur during each one of these three collisions will help you be alert for certain types of injury patterns.

The three collisions in a typical impact are as follows:

1.  The collision of the car against another car, a tree, or some other object. Damage to the car is perhaps the most dramatic part of the collision, but it does not directly affect patient care, except possibly to make extrication difficult (**FIGURE 25-3**). However, it does provide information about the severity of the collision, and therefore has an indirect effect on patient care. The greater the damage to the car, the greater the energy that was involved and, therefore, the greater the potential to cause injury to the patient. By assessing the vehicle that has crashed, you can often determine the MOI, which may allow you to predict what injuries may have happened to the passengers at the time of impact according to forces that acted on their bodies. When you arrive at the crash scene and

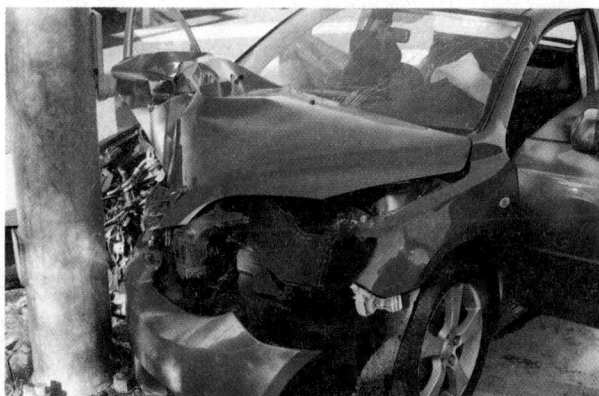

**FIGURE 25-3** The first collision in a typical impact is that of the vehicle against another object (in this case, a utility pole). The appearance of the vehicle can provide you with critical information about the severity of the crash. The greater the damage to the vehicle, the greater the energy that was involved.

© Rocketegg/iStock /Getty Images Plus/Getty Images.

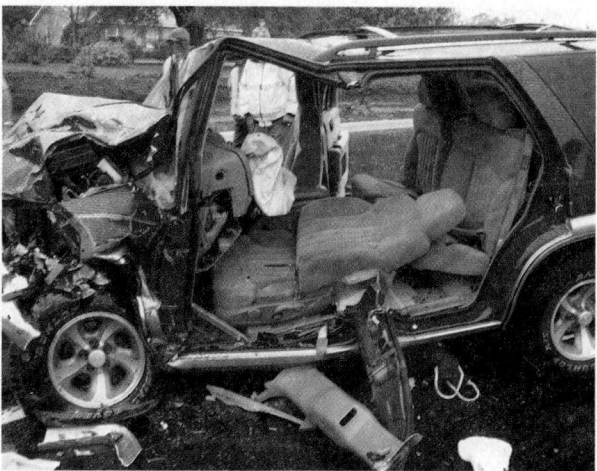

**FIGURE 25-4** The second collision in a typical impact is that of the passenger against the interior of the car. The appearance of the interior of the car can provide you with information about the severity of the patient's injuries.

Courtesy of Rhonda Hunt.

perform your scene size-up, quickly inspect the severity of damage to the vehicle or vehicles. If there is significant damage to a vehicle, your index of suspicion for the presence of life-threatening injuries should automatically increase. A great amount of force is required to crush and deform a vehicle, cause intrusion into the passenger compartment, tear seats from their mountings, and collapse steering wheels. Such damage suggests the presence of high-energy trauma.

2. The collision of the passenger against the interior of the car. Just as the kinetic energy produced by the vehicle's mass and velocity is converted into the work of bringing the vehicle to a stop, the kinetic energy produced by the passenger's mass and velocity is converted into the work of stopping his or her body (**FIGURE 25-4**). Just like the obvious damage to the exterior of the car, the injuries that result are often dramatic and usually immediately apparent during your scene size-up or primary assessment. Common passenger injuries include lower extremity fractures (knees into the dashboard), rib fractures (rib cage into the steering wheel), and head trauma (head into the windshield). Such injuries occur more frequently if the passenger is not restrained. But even when the passenger is restrained with a properly adjusted seat belt, injuries can occur, especially in lateral and rollover impacts.

3. The collision of the passenger's internal organs against the solid structures of the body. The injuries that occur during the third collision may not be as obvious as external injuries, but they are often the most life threatening. For example, as the passenger's head hits the windshield, the brain continues to move forward until it comes to rest by striking the inside of the skull. This results in a compression injury (or bruising) to the anterior portion of the brain and a tension injury (stretching) of the posterior portion of the brain (**FIGURE 25-5**). This is an example of a **coup-contrecoup brain injury** (**FIGURE 25-6**). Similarly, traumatic aortic transection or rupture is associated with a sudden and rapid deceleration of the heart and the aorta within the thoracic cavity, which may rupture the aorta and cause fatal bleeding.

## Special Populations

Children and pregnant women are also at risk when seatbelts are applied inappropriately or they are too close to airbags.

Understanding the relationships among the three collisions will help you make the connections between the amount of damage to the exterior of

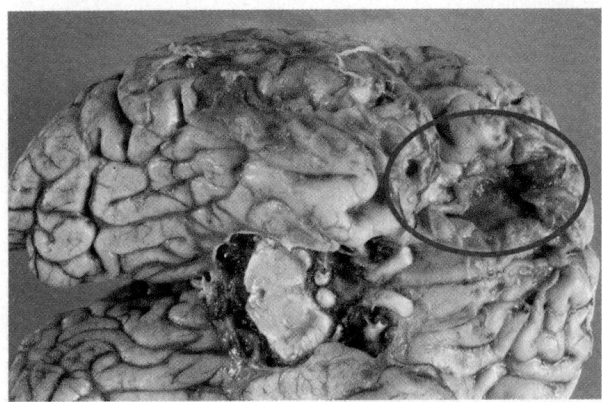

**FIGURE 25-5** The discolored spots show injuries (contusions) in this brain.

© Dr. E. Walker/Science Source.

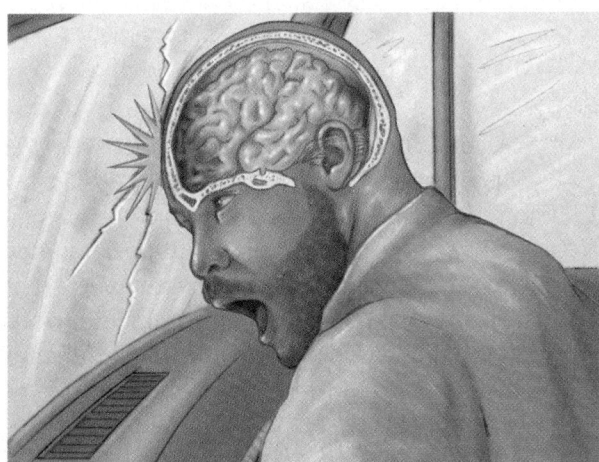

**FIGURE 25-6** The third collision in a typical impact is that of the passenger's internal organs against the solid structures of the body. A coup-contrecoup injury occurs when the brain continues its forward motion and strikes the inside of the skull (the coup), resulting in a compression injury to the anterior portion of the brain and a tension injury (stretching) of the posterior portion (the contrecoup).

© Jones & Bartlett Learning.

the vehicle and potential injury to the passenger. For example, in a high-speed crash that results in massive damage to the vehicle, you should suspect serious injuries to the passengers, even if the injuries are not readily apparent. Several potential physical problems may develop as a result of traumatic injuries. Your initial general impression of the patient and evaluation of the MOI can help direct life-saving care and provide critical information to the hospital staff. Therefore, if you see a contusion on the patient's forehead and the windshield

is starred and pushed out, you should strongly suspect an injury to the brain. After you inform medical control about the damage to the windshield, hospital staff can prepare for the patient by being ready to perform a computed tomography (CT) scan of the brain. Without your input, the physician might have found the brain injury anyway, but it might not have been detected until the brain had swollen sufficiently to cause clinical signs of the injury. Whenever there is a significant impact to the head, also suspect a spinal injury and take cervical spine precautions if indicated.

### Words of Wisdom

Others in the patient's chain of care are relying on you to pass on important information about the mechanism of injury. Use your observations to paint an accurate picture of the scene in written and verbal communication. Some agencies take digital images of the vehicles to show emergency department workers the mechanisms involved.

The amount of damage considered significant varies, depending on the type of crash, but any substantial deformity of the vehicle should be enough cause for you to consider transporting the patient to a trauma center. Significant MOIs are suggested by the following findings:

- Death of an occupant in the vehicle
- Severe deformity of the vehicle or intrusion into the vehicle
  - Severe deformities of the frontal part of the vehicle, with or without intrusion into the passenger compartment
  - Moderate intrusions from a lateral (T-bone) type of accident
  - Severe damage from the rear
  - Crashes in which rotation is involved (rollovers and spins)
- Ejection from the vehicle

Damage to the vehicle that was involved and information obtained during the scene size-up are not the only clues you can use to determine crash severity. Clearly, if one or more of the passengers are dead, you should suspect that the other passengers have sustained serious injuries, even if the injuries are not obvious. Therefore, focus on treating life-threatening injuries and providing rapid transport to a trauma center, because these passengers have likely experienced the same amount of force that caused the death of the others. Digital photos of the crash scene may provide valuable information to the staff and treating physicians at the trauma center; however, photos should be shown or transmitted only to appropriate personnel and should never be shared over social media. Photos containing patient images or other identifiable patient information may become part of the medical record or may need to be deleted after review by the receiving health care providers, depending on protected health information policies developed by the department privacy officer.

## Safety Tips

Anything in the back of the ambulance that is not secured, including you and the patient, can become projectiles during a crash. Secure everyone and everything!

## Frontal Crashes

Understanding the MOI after a frontal crash first involves evaluation of the supplemental restraint system, including seat belts and airbags. Determine whether the passenger was restrained by a full and properly applied three-point restraint. Also determine whether the airbag was deployed. Identifying the types of restraints used and whether airbags were deployed will help you identify injury patterns related to the supplemental restraint systems.

When properly applied, seat belts are successful in restraining the passengers in a vehicle and preventing a second collision inside the motor vehicle. According to the Centers for Disease Control and Prevention (CDC), seat belt use saved an estimated 15,000 lives in 2016. Seat belts may also decrease the severity of the third collision, that of the passenger's organs with the chest or abdominal wall. The protective abilities of seat belts are further enhanced by deployment of the airbags. Airbags provide the final capture point of the passengers and decrease the severity of **deceleration** injuries by allowing seat belts to be more compliant and by gently cushioning the occupant as the body slows, or decelerates.

Remember that airbags decrease injury to the chest, face, and head very effectively. However, you should still suspect that other serious injuries to the extremities (resulting from the second collision) and to internal organs (resulting from the third collision) have occurred. Airbags have been standard equipment in most motor vehicles

## YOU are the Provider

When you arrive at the scene, fire and law enforcement personnel are already present. An air transport helicopter is available with a 10-minute ETA upon dispatch. The front of the vehicle has been crushed all the way up to the windshield. The driver, a young man, was unrestrained and is still in the driver's seat; he appears to be unconscious and his face is covered with blood. As your partner accesses the patient from the backseat and manually stabilizes his head, you perform a primary assessment.

| Recording Time: 0 Minutes | |
| --- | --- |
| Appearance | Bleeding from the head, face, and mouth; pale skin; labored breathing |
| Level of consciousness | Responsive only to pain |
| Airway | Blood in the nasopharynx and oropharynx |
| Breathing | Rapid and labored |
| Circulation | Radial pulses weak and rapid; skin cool, pale, and clammy |

Despite the severity of exterior damage to the vehicle, the patient is not entrapped and there is no interior intrusion into the passenger compartment. You suction the patient's mouth, apply a cervical collar, and prepare to rapidly extricate him from the vehicle. Responders from one of the engine companies have prepared a backboard to move him to the stretcher.

**3.** What damage in the vehicle's interior may have caused the patient's signs and symptoms?

since 1999. These safety devices enhance the safety and survival of forward-facing occupants inside the vehicle during a crash. In an emergency braking event, or crash, the airbag inflates very quickly. Because a rear-facing car seat is in proximity to the dashboard, rapid inflation of the airbag could cause serious injury or death to an infant. All children who are shorter than 4 feet 9 inches (145 cm) should ride in the rear seat or, in the case of a pickup truck or other single-seated vehicle, the airbag should be turned off.

When providing care to an occupant inside a motor vehicle, it is important to remember that if the airbag did not inflate during the accident, it may deploy during extrication. If this occurs, you may be seriously injured. Extreme caution must be used when extricating a patient in a vehicle with an airbag that has not deployed.

Supplemental restraint systems can also cause harm depending on whether they are used properly or improperly. For example, some older vehicle models have seat belts that buckle automatically at the shoulder but require the passengers to buckle the lap portion; not buckling the lap portion can cause the occupant to travel down and under the shoulder strap as the body continues forward, resulting in the lower body striking the dashboard. This movement of the body can cause the lower extremities and the pelvis to crash into the dashboard because that part of the body is unrestrained. Seat belts may also cause unseen abdominal injuries, particularly in pediatric patients. Seat belts are designed to be worn over the iliac crests of the pelvis to distribute the force over the bony surface. Hip dislocations may result if seat belts are worn too low. Internal injuries can occur when the belt is worn too high, resulting in damage to abdominal organs (**FIGURE 25-7**). Lumbar spine fractures are also possible, particularly in children and older patients.

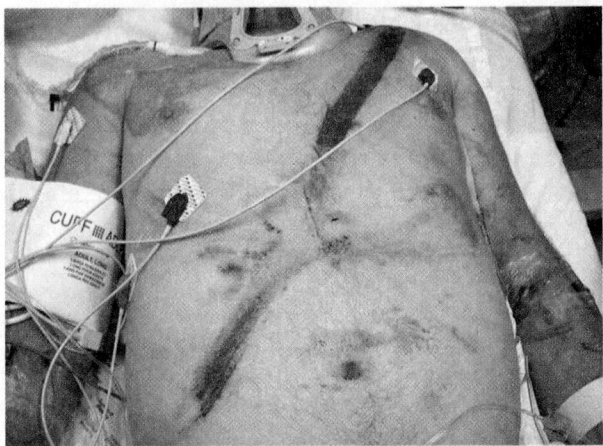

**FIGURE 25-7** Injuries can result if the seat belt is worn too high or too low across the waist. Although less common, injuries can also result from seat belts worn in the correct position across the torso.

Courtesy of ED, Royal North Shore Hospital/NSW Institute of Trauma & Injury.

---

## Words of Wisdom

Know your local protocols for spinal motion restriction. They have likely been updated to reflect current research and national guidelines.

---

When passengers are riding in vehicles equipped with airbags but are not restrained by seat belts, they are often thrown forward in the act of emergency braking. As a result, they come into contact with the airbag and/or the doors at the time of deployment. This MOI is also responsible for some severe injuries to children who are riding unrestrained in the front seats of vehicles, unrestrained passengers, and those sitting too close to the airbag. Today's motor vehicles often have multiple airbags and side curtains. These are designed to protect the occupants of the vehicle, but can also alter injury patterns. Certain areas of a vehicle's body may have airbags that will deploy when impacted. Pushing on or using extrication tools in those areas may cause airbags to unexpectedly deploy. This can happen even after the car battery has been disengaged.

In addition, some passengers may pass out before impact, and you may find them lying against the deployed airbag. When you encounter these types of situations, look for abrasions and/or traction-type injuries on the face, lower part of the neck, and chest (**FIGURE 25-8**).

Contact points are often obvious as you perform a simple, quick evaluation of the interior of the vehicle. If there is no intrusion into the passenger compartment, you might see that an unrestrained front-seat passenger in a frontal crash has come into contact with the dashboard or the instrument panel at the knees, thus transferring loads from the knees through the femur to the pelvis and hip joint (**FIGURE 25-9A**). The chest and/or abdomen may

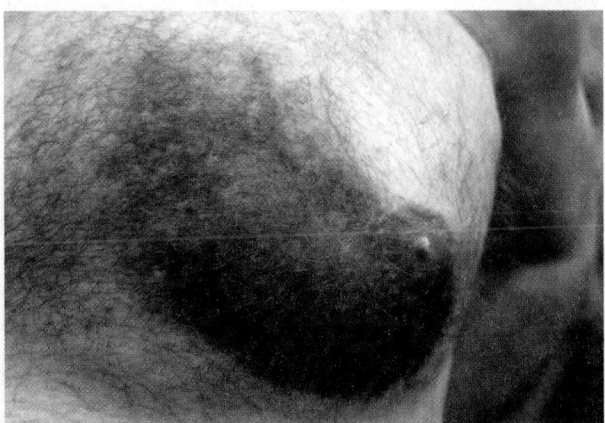

**FIGURE 25-8** Airbags can cause injury in frontal crashes, specifically, abrasions, contusions, and traction-type injuries to the face, neck, chest, and inner arms.

© crozstudios/Alamy Stock Photo.

also hit the steering wheel (**FIGURE 25-9B**). In addition, the passenger's face often hits the steering wheel, or the passenger may launch forward and up, hitting the windshield and/or the roof header in the area of the visors (**FIGURE 25-9C**). Signs of most of these injuries can be found by inspecting the interior of the vehicle during extrication of the patient.

## Rear-End Crashes

Rear-end impacts are known to cause whiplash injuries, particularly when the passenger's head and/or neck is not restrained by an appropriately placed headrest (**FIGURE 25-10**). On impact, the passenger's body and torso move forward. As the body is propelled forward, the head and neck are left behind because the head is relatively heavy, and they appear to be whipped back relative to the torso. As the vehicle comes to rest, the unrestrained passenger moves forward, striking the dashboard. In this type of crash, the cervical spine and surrounding area may be injured. The cervical spine is less tolerant of damage when it is bent back. Headrests decrease extension of the head and neck during a crash and, therefore, help reduce injury. Other parts of the spine and the pelvis may also be at risk for injury. In addition, the patient may sustain an acceleration injury to the brain—that is, the third collision of the brain within the skull. Passengers in the backseat wearing only a lap belt might have a higher incidence of injuries to the thoracic and lumbar spine.

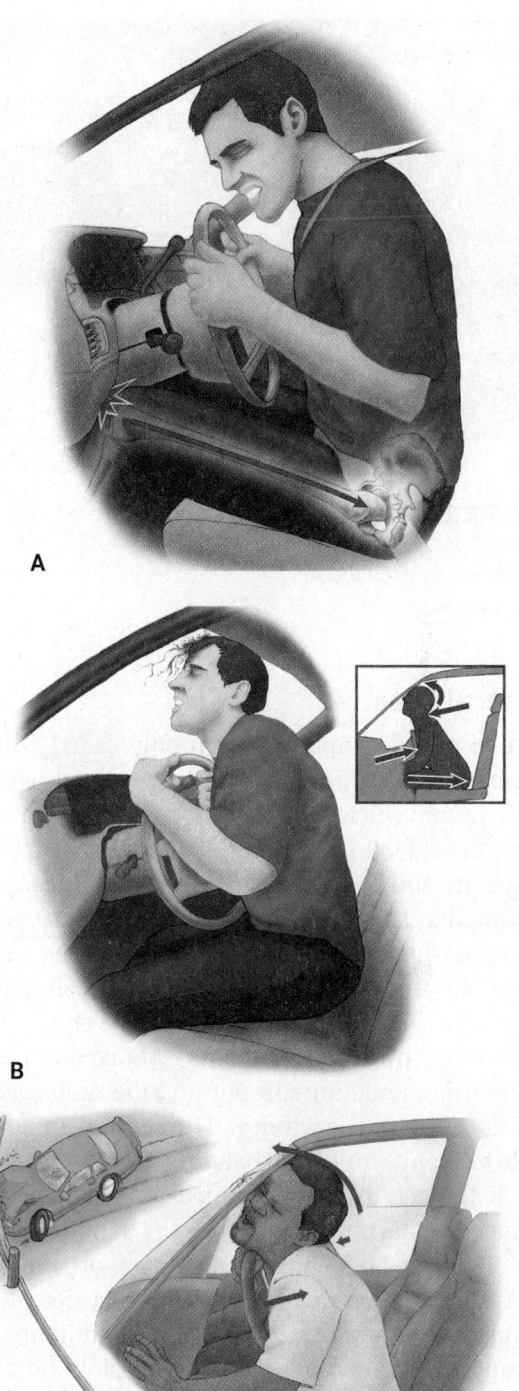

A

B

C

**FIGURE 25-9** Mechanism of injury and condition of the vehicle interior suggest likely areas of injury. **A.** The knees can strike the dashboard, resulting in a hip fracture or dislocation. **B.** Serious chest and abdominal injuries can result from striking the steering wheel. **C.** Head and spinal injuries can result when the face and head strike the windshield.

**A, B, C:** © Jones & Bartlett Learning.

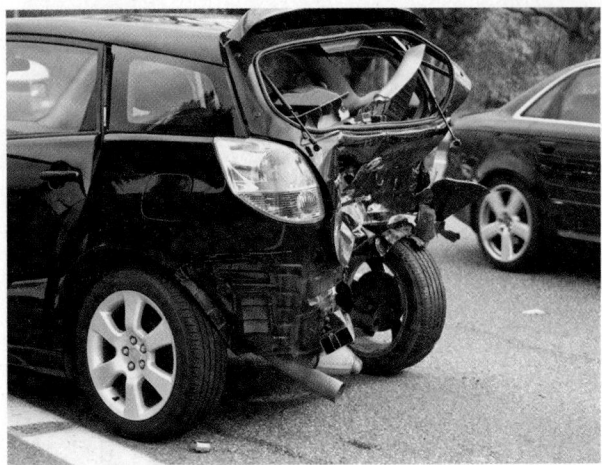

**FIGURE 25-10** Rear-end impacts often cause whiplash injuries, particularly when the head and/or neck is not restrained by a headrest.

© Crystalcraig/Dreamstime.com.

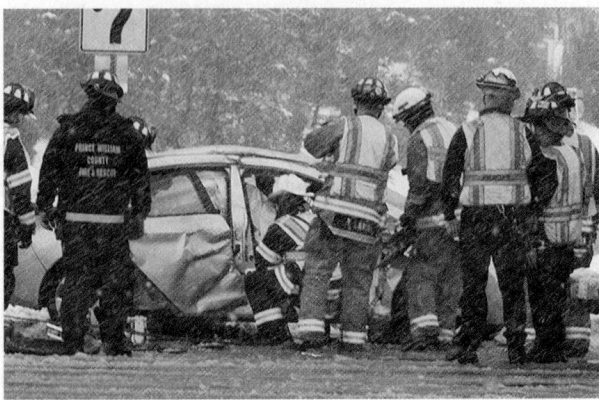

**FIGURE 25-11** In a lateral crash, the car is typically struck above its center of gravity and begins to rock away from the side of impact. This causes a type of lateral whiplash in which the passenger's shoulders and head whip toward the intruding vehicle.

© KAREN BLEIER/Staff/AFP/Getty Images.

## Lateral Crashes

Lateral or side impacts (commonly called T-bone crashes) are a common cause of death associated with motor vehicle crashes. When a vehicle is struck from the side, it is typically struck above its center of gravity and begins to rock away from the side of the impact. This results in the passenger sustaining a lateral whiplash injury (**FIGURE 25-11**). The movement is to the side, and the passenger's shoulders and head whip toward the intruding vehicle. This action may thrust the shoulder, thorax, and upper extremities, and, more important, the skull against the doorpost or the window. The cervical spine has little tolerance for lateral bending.

If there is substantial intrusion into the passenger compartment, suspect your patient to have lateral chest and abdomen injuries on the side of the impact, as well as possible fractures of the lower extremities, pelvis, and ribs. In addition, the organs within the abdomen are at risk because of a possible third collision. According to the *Journal of Safety Research*, lateral crashes cause approximately 25% of all severe injuries to the aorta and approximately 30% of all fatalities that occur in motor vehicle crashes.

## Rollover Crashes

Certain vehicles, such as large trucks and some sport utility vehicles, are more susceptible to rollover crashes because of their high center of gravity.

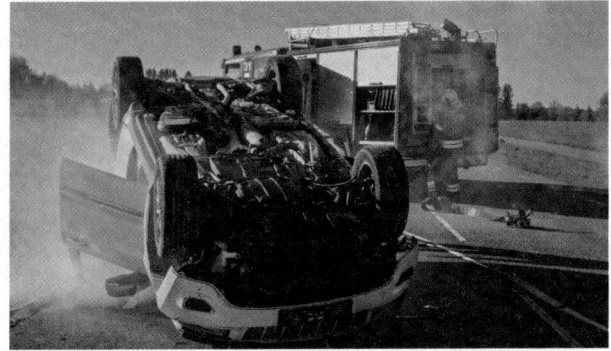

**FIGURE 25-12** Passengers who have been ejected or partially ejected may have struck the interior of the car many times before ejection.

© Gorodenkoff/Shutterstock.

Injury patterns that are commonly associated with rollover crashes differ, depending on whether the passenger was restrained or unrestrained. The most unpredictable types of injuries are caused by rollover crashes in which an unrestrained passenger may have sustained multiple strikes within the interior of the vehicle as it rolled one or more times. The most common life-threatening event in a rollover is ejection or partial ejection of the passenger from the vehicle (**FIGURE 25-12**). Passengers who have been ejected may have struck the interior of the vehicle many times before ejection. The passenger may also have struck several objects, such as trees, a guardrail, or the vehicle's exterior, before landing. Passengers who have been partially ejected may have struck both the interior and exterior of the vehicle and may have been sandwiched between the exterior of the vehicle and the environment as the vehicle rolled. Ejection and partial ejection are significant MOIs; in these cases, prepare to care for life-threatening injuries.

Even when restrained, passengers can sustain severe injuries during a rollover crash, although the patterns of injury tend to be more predictable, and when the restraint system is properly used, ejection from the vehicle is less likely. A passenger on the outboard side of a vehicle that rolls over is at high risk for injury because of the centrifugal force (the patient is pinned against the door of the vehicle). Rollover crashes can also cause injury when the roof of the vehicle hits the ground during the rollover; a passenger who is restrained can still move far enough toward the roof to make contact and sustain a spinal cord injury. Therefore, rollover crashes are dangerous for both restrained and, to a greater degree, unrestrained passengers because these crashes provide multiple opportunities for second and third collisions.

## Rotational Crashes

Rotational crashes (spins) are conceptually similar to rollovers. The rotation of the vehicle as it spins provides opportunities for the vehicle to strike objects such as utility poles. For example, as a vehicle spins and strikes a pole, the passengers experience not only the rotational motion, but also a lateral impact.

## Car Versus Pedestrian

Car-versus-pedestrian crashes often result in patients who have graphic and apparent injuries, such as broken bones; however, this type of crash can cause serious unseen injuries to underlying body systems. Therefore, you must maintain a high index of suspicion for unseen injuries. A thorough evaluation of the MOI is critical. First, estimate the speed of the vehicle that struck the patient; next, determine whether the patient was thrown, what surface the patient landed on, and at what distance or whether the patient was struck and pulled under the vehicle. Evaluate the vehicle that struck the patient for structural damage that might indicate contact points with the patient and alert you to potential injuries. Multisystem injuries are common after this type of event. If available, consider summoning advanced life support (ALS) backup for any patients who have or are thought to have sustained a significant MOI.

## Car Versus Bicycle

In a car-versus-bicycle crash, evaluate the MOI in much the same manner as car-versus-pedestrian crashes. However, additional evaluation of damage to and the position of the bicycle is warranted. If the patient was wearing a helmet, inspect the helmet for damage and suspect potential injury to the head (**FIGURE 25-13**). Presume that the patient has sustained an injury to the spinal column, or spinal cord, until proven otherwise at the hospital. Initiate and maintain appropriate spinal motion restriction during the encounter. When practical, roll the patient on to his or her side to allow for an appropriate assessment of the posterior side of the body.

## Car Versus Motorcycle

In a motorcycle crash, any structural protection afforded to the victim is not derived from a steel cage, as is the case in an automobile, but from protective

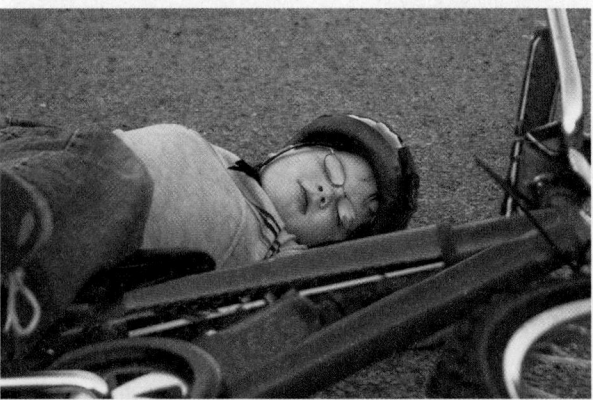

**FIGURE 25-13** If the patient's bike helmet is damaged, suspect head and spine injuries.

devices worn by the rider—that is, helmet, leather or abrasion-resistant clothing, and boots. Although helmets are designed to protect against impact forces to the head, they do not protect from cervical spinal injury. Patients who have experienced a motorcycle crash should undergo cervical spine assessment and have a cervical collar placed if indicated. Leather and synthetic gear worn over the body was initially designed to protect professional riders in competition, where falls tend to be controlled and result in long sliding mechanisms on hard surfaces rather than multiple collisions against road objects and other vehicles. Leather clothing will mostly protect against road abrasion but offers no protection against blunt trauma from secondary impacts. In a street crash, collisions usually occur against other larger vehicles or stationary objects.

When assessing the scene of a motorcycle crash, look for deformity of the motorcycle, the side of most damage, the distance of skid in the road, the deformity of stationary objects or other vehicles, and the extent and location of deformity in the helmet. These findings can be helpful in estimating the extent of trauma sustained by a patient.

> ### Words of Wisdom
>
> If possible, bring the helmet to the hospital for the trauma staff to see. The helmet will provide them with critical information about the type and extent of potential head injury.

There are four types of motorcycle impacts.

- **Head-on crash.** The motorcycle strikes another object and stops its forward motion while the rider and parts of the motorcycle that are broken off continue their forward motion until stopped by an outside force, such as drag from the road or another opposing force from a secondary collision.
- **Angular crash.** The motorcycle strikes an object or another vehicle at an angle so that the rider sustains direct crushing injuries to the lower extremity between the object and the motorcycle. This usually results in severe open and comminuted lower extremity injuries with severe neurovascular compromise, often resulting in traumatic amputation or otherwise requiring surgical amputation.

- **Ejection.** The rider will travel at high speed until stopped by a stationary object, another vehicle, or road drag. Severe abrasion injuries (road rash) down to bone can occur with drag. An unpredictable combination of blunt injuries can occur from secondary collisions.
- **Controlled crash.** A technique used to separate the rider from the body of the motorcycle and the object to be hit is referred to as laying the bike down. It was developed by motorcycle racers and adapted by street bikers as a means of achieving a controlled crash. As a crash approaches, the motorcycle is turned flat and tipped sideways at 90° to the direction of travel so that one leg is dropped to the grass or asphalt. This slows the occupant faster than the motorcycle, allowing the rider to become separated from the motorcycle. If properly protected with leather or synthetic abrasion-resistant gear, injuries should be limited to those sustained by rolling over the pavement and any secondary collision that may occur. When executed properly, this maneuver prevents the rider from being trapped between the bike and the object. However, a rider unable to clear the bike will continue into the vehicle, often with devastating results.

## Falls

The injury potential of a fall is related to the height from which the patient fell. Falls are common MOIs for blunt trauma. The greater the height of the fall, the greater the potential for injury. A fall from more than 20 feet (6 m) is considered significant. The patient lands on the surface just as an unrestrained passenger smashes into the interior of a vehicle. The internal organs travel at the speed of the patient's body before it hits the ground and stop by smashing into the interior of the body. Again, as in a motor vehicle crash, it is these internal injuries that are the least obvious during assessment but pose the gravest threat to life. Therefore, suspect internal injuries in a patient who has fallen from a significant height, just as you would in a patient who has been in a high-speed motor vehicle crash. Always consider syncope or other underlying medical causes of the fall.

Patients who fall and land on their feet may have less severe internal injuries because their

## Special Populations

When your patient is a child, the following constitute a significant MOI:

1. Falls of greater than 10 feet (3 m; or two to three times the height of the child)
2. Medium- to high-speed vehicle crash (>25 mph)

Also note that young children are top-heavy, so they tend to land on their heads even from short falls. Triage children to a pediatric trauma center if possible.

legs may have absorbed much of the energy of the fall (**FIGURE 25-14**). However, as a result, they may have serious injuries to the lower extremities and pelvic and spinal injuries from energy that was transmitted through the legs. Patients who impact head first, as in diving accidents, will likely have serious head and/or spinal injuries. In either case, a fall from a significant height is a serious event with great injury potential, and the patient should be evaluated thoroughly. Take the following factors into account:

- The height of the fall
- The type of surface struck
- The part of the body that hit first, followed by the path of energy displacement

Many falls, especially those sustained by older patients, are not the result of high-energy trauma, even though broken bones may result. Older patients often have osteoporosis, a condition in which the bones can fail under relatively low stress because they are structurally weakened. Because of this condition, an older patient can sustain a fracture as a result of a fall from a standing position. These cases do not constitute true high-energy trauma unless the patient fell from a significant height.

## Special Populations

Many older patients are seriously injured from standing, ground-level falls. Completely assess older patients for all possible injuries, even from low-impact falls.

## Penetrating Trauma

Penetrating trauma is the second leading cause of trauma death in the United States after blunt trauma. In 2017, the CDC reported over 38,000 deaths from firearms, which is just under the number of deaths related to motor vehicles. Low-energy penetrating trauma may be caused accidentally by impalement or intentionally by a knife, ice pick, or other weapon (**FIGURE 25-15**). Often, it is difficult to determine the entrance and exit wounds from a **projectile** in a prehospital setting. First, determine the number of penetrating injuries and then combine that information with the important things you already know about the potential pathway of penetrating projectiles to form an index of suspicion about unseen life-threatening injuries. With low-energy penetrations, injuries are caused by the sharp edges of the object moving through the body and are, therefore, close to the object's path. However, weapons such as knives may have been deliberately moved around internally, causing more damage than the external wound might suggest. Try to determine the length of the penetrating object.

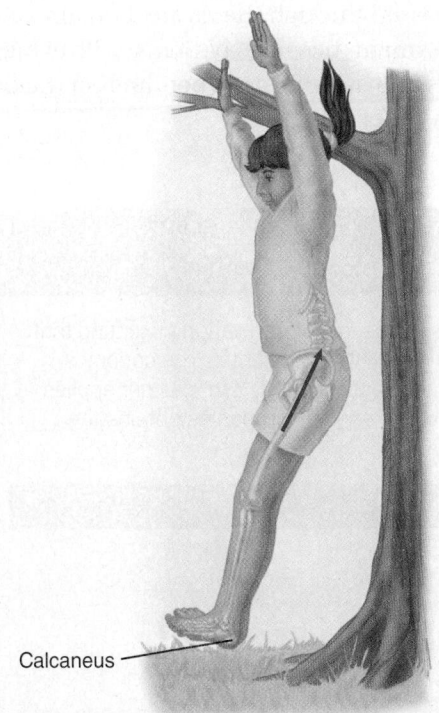

Calcaneus

**FIGURE 25-14** When a patient falls and lands on his or her feet, the energy is transmitted to the spine, sometimes producing a spinal injury in addition to injuries to the legs and pelvis.

© Jones & Bartlett Learning.

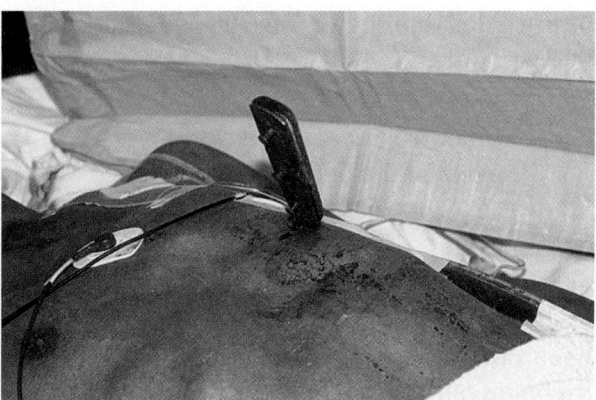

**FIGURE 25-15** Injuries from low-energy penetrations, such as a stab wound, are caused by the sharp edges of the object moving through the body.

© Andrew Pollak, MD. Used with permission.

## Words of Wisdom

Do not waste time trying to determine whether a penetrating wound is an entrance or exit wound; this can be difficult. Instead, focus on identifying all wounds and providing appropriate care.

In medium- and high-velocity (speed) penetrating trauma, the path of the projectile (usually a bullet) may not be as easy to predict. This is because the bullet may flatten out, tumble, or even ricochet within the body before exiting. The path the projectile takes is referred to as a **trajectory**. Fragmentation, especially frangible bullets that are designed to disintegrate into tiny particles on impact, will increase damage as multiple fragments increase the likelihood of multiple organs/vessels sustaining injury. Full metal jacket bullets cause less damage than fragmented rounds because of their tendency to pass through the body's tissues. The bullet's speed is another factor in the resulting injury pattern; there is often additional damage caused by the object moving inside the body, but not along the suspected pathway. This phenomenon, called **cavitation**, results from the rapid changes in tissue and fluid pressure that occur with the passage of the projectile, and it can result in serious injury to internal organs distant to the actual path of the bullet (**FIGURE 25-16**). Consequences of cavitation can be temporary or permanent. Temporary cavitation injury results from a stretching of the tissues that occurs with the pressure changes. Permanent cavitation injury results along the path where the projectile, such as a bullet, has passed through the tissue. Remain alert during assessment because patients will exhibit various signs and symptoms depending on the organ or organs affected.

## YOU are the Provider

The decision is made to transport the patient by helicopter based on injuries and based on information indicating that heavy traffic would result in a significant delay in ground transportation to the Level 1 trauma center. The patient is removed from the vehicle onto the backboard, and you perform a quick secondary assessment. Your partner applies high-flow oxygen via a nonrebreathing mask while one of the EMTs from one of the engine companies obtains the patient's vital signs.

| Recording Time: 5 Minutes | |
| --- | --- |
| **Respirations** | 22 breaths/min; labored |
| **Pulse** | 120 beats/min; weak radial pulses |
| **Skin** | Cool, clammy, and pale |
| **Blood pressure** | 84/64 mm Hg |
| **Oxygen saturation (Spo$_2$)** | 97% (with supplemental oxygen) |

The patient's level of consciousness is still markedly decreased; he responds only to pain. He has a large hematoma and laceration to his forehead, which is covered with a sterile dressing. He also has crepitus and bruising to his chest. A Level I trauma center is 30 miles away, but there is a Level III trauma center only 15 miles away.

**4.** Should the patient be transported to the Level I trauma center or the Level III trauma center? Why?

**5.** What other transport factors should you consider with this patient?

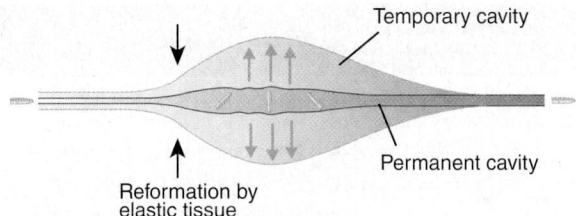

**FIGURE 25-16** Two types of injury are caused by cavitation—temporary and permanent.

© Jones & Bartlett Learning.

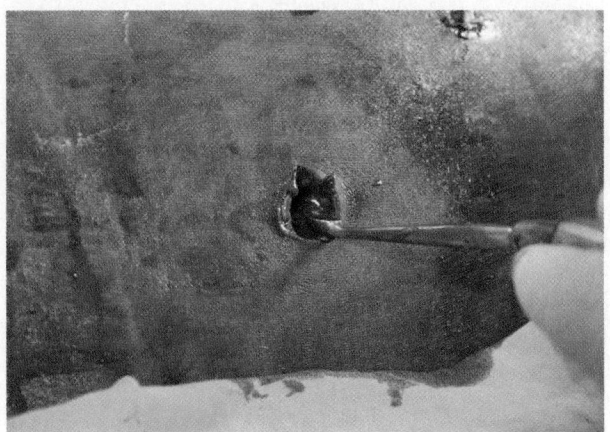

**FIGURE 25-17** An entry wound from a gunshot injury.

© Medicimage/Universal Images Group North America LLC/Alamy Stock Photo.

The relationship between distance and the severity of injury varies depending on the type of weapon involved, such as a rifle, pistol, or shotgun. Air resistance, often referred to as **drag**, slows the projectile, decreasing the depth of penetration and energy of the projectile and thus reducing damage to the tissues. Much like a boat moving through water, the bullet disrupts not only the tissues that are directly in its path but also those in its wake. Therefore, the area that is damaged by medium- and high-velocity projectiles is typically many times larger than the diameter of the projectile itself (**FIGURE 25-17**). This is one reason that exit wounds are often many times larger than entrance wounds.

As with motor vehicle crashes, the energy available for a bullet to cause damage is more a function of its speed than its mass (weight). If the mass of the bullet is doubled, the energy that is available to cause injury is doubled. If the velocity of the bullet is doubled, the energy that is available

to cause injury is quadrupled. For this reason, it is important for you to try to determine the type of weapon that was used. Although it is not necessary (or always possible) for you to distinguish between medium- and high-velocity injuries, any information regarding the type of weapon that was used should be relayed to medical control. Medium-velocity injuries may be caused by handguns and some rifles, whereas high-velocity injuries may be caused by a military weapon. Police at the scene may be a useful source of information regarding the caliber of weapon. Most civilian gunshot wound injuries in the United States are the result of low-velocity weapons.

An important factor for the seriousness of a gunshot wound is the type of tissue through which the projectile passes. Tissue of high elasticity, such as muscle, is better able to tolerate stretch than tissue of low elasticity, such as the liver. In a gunshot wound, shotgun wadding, bits of clothing, skin, and hair driven into the wound can cause massive contamination, leading to increased potential for infection should the patient survive the initial trauma.

**TABLE 25-1** summarizes how to recognize developing problems in trauma patients.

## Blast Injuries

Although most commonly associated with military conflict, blast injuries are also seen in civilian practice in mines, shipyards, and chemical plants and, increasingly, in association with terrorist activities. As with any explosion, there is a risk of contamination of patients from environmental contaminants, toxic chemicals, or dirty bombs. People who are injured in explosions may be injured by any of four different mechanisms (**FIGURE 25-18**).

- **Primary blast injuries.** These injuries are due entirely to the blast itself; that is, damage to the body is caused by the pressure wave generated by the explosion. When the victim is close to the blast, the blast wave may cause disruption of major blood vessels and rupture of eardrums and major organs, including the lungs. Hollow organs are the most susceptible to the pressure wave. In some cases, pressure wave injuries can amputate limbs.

**TABLE 25-1** Recognizing Developing Problems in Trauma Patients

| Mechanism of Injury | Signs and Symptoms | Index of Suspicion |
|---|---|---|
| Blunt or penetrating trauma to the neck | • Noisy or labored breathing<br>• Increased respiratory rate<br>• Swelling of the face or neck<br>• Altered gag reflex<br>• Decreasing/low GCS score (<9 is severe)<br>• Decreasing/low Spo$_2$<br>• Rapid, weak pulse<br>• Decreasing/low blood pressure | • Significant bleeding or foreign bodies in the upper or lower airway, causing obstruction<br>• Be alert for airway compromise |
| Significant chest wall blunt trauma from motor vehicle crashes, car-versus-pedestrian, and other crashes; penetrating trauma to the chest wall | • Significant chest pain<br>• Shortness of breath<br>• Increased respiratory rate<br>• Asymmetric chest wall movement<br>• Subcutaneous emphysema<br>• Decreasing GCS score (<9 is severe)<br>• Decreasing/low Spo$_2$<br>• Presence of jugular vein distention<br>• Rapid, weak pulse<br>• Decreasing/low blood pressure<br>• Loss of peripheral pulses during inspiration<br>• Narrowing pulse pressures | • Cardiac or pulmonary contusion<br>• Pneumothorax (accumulation of air or gas in the pleural cavity) or hemothorax (accumulation of blood in the pleural cavity)<br>• Broken ribs, causing respiratory compromise |
| Any significant blunt force trauma from motor vehicle crashes or penetrating injury | • Blunt or penetrating trauma to the neck, chest, abdomen, or groin<br>• Blows to the head sustained during motor vehicle crashes, falls, or other incidents, producing loss of consciousness, altered mental status, inability to recall events, combativeness, or changes in speech patterns<br>• Inability to maintain airway<br>• Difficulty moving extremities; headache, especially with nausea and vomiting<br>• Decreasing GCS score (<9 is severe)<br>• Decreasing/low Spo$_2$<br>• Rapid, weak pulse<br>• Decreasing/low blood pressure or increasing blood pressure with slow pulse | • Injuries in these regions may tear and cause damage to the large blood vessels located in these body areas, resulting in significant internal and external bleeding<br>• Be alert to the possibility of bruising to the brain and bleeding in and around the brain tissue, which may cause the development of excess pressure inside the skull around the brain |
| Any significant blunt trauma, falls from a significant height, or penetrating trauma | • Severe back and/or neck pain, history of difficulty moving extremities, loss of sensation or tingling in the extremities<br>• Decreasing GCS score (<9 is severe)<br>• Rapid, weak pulse or slow pulse | • Injury to the bones of the spinal column or to the spinal cord |

Abbreviation: GCS, Glasgow Coma Scale

- **Secondary blast injuries.** Damage to the body results from being struck by flying debris, such as shrapnel from the device or from glass or splinters, which have been set in motion by the explosion. Objects are propelled by the force of the blast wave and strike the victim, causing injury. These objects can travel great distances and be propelled at tremendous speeds, up to almost 3,000 mph for conventional military explosives.

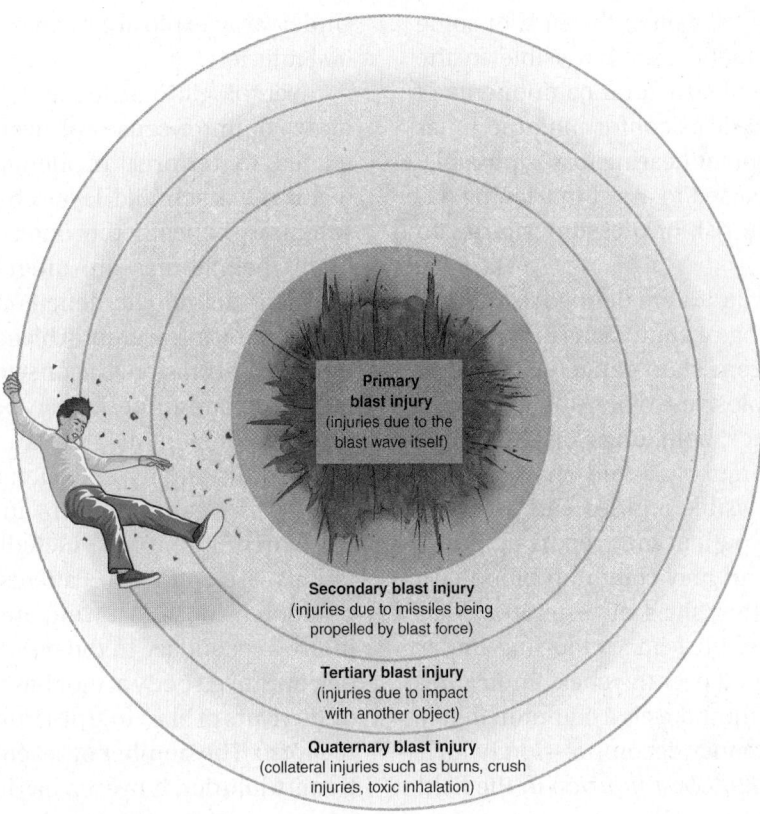

Primary
blast injury
(injuries due to the
blast wave itself)

Secondary blast injury
(injuries due to missiles being
propelled by blast force)

Tertiary blast injury
(injuries due to impact
with another object)

Quaternary blast injury
(collateral injuries such as burns, crush
injuries, toxic inhalation)

**FIGURE 25-18** Mechanisms of blast injuries.

© Jones & Bartlett Learning.

- **Tertiary blast injuries.** These injuries occur when the patient is hurled by the force of the explosion against a stationary object. A blast wind (sudden change in the surrounding atmosphere) creates a pressure wave. This can cause the patient's body to be hurled or thrown, resulting in further injury. This physical displacement of the body is also referred to as ground shock when the body impacts the ground.
- **Quaternary blast injuries.** This category of miscellaneous injuries includes burns from hot gases or fires started by the blast; respiratory injury from inhaling toxic gases; suffocation; poisoning; medical emergencies incurred as a result of the explosion; crush injuries from the collapse of buildings; contamination of wounds from environmental, chemical, or toxic substances; radiation injury from dirty bombs; and mental health emergencies. Essentially, all injuries due to the blast event that are not attributable directly to a primary, secondary, or tertiary mechanism are categorized as quaternary blast injuries.

Most patients who survive an explosion will have some combination of the four types of injuries mentioned. The remainder of the discussion will be confined to primary blast injuries because while secondary blast injuries account for most of the trauma, primary injuries are the ones that are most easily overlooked.

## Tissues at Risk

Hollow organs (those that contain air), such as the middle ear, lung, and gastrointestinal tract, are most susceptible to pressure changes. The junction between tissues of different densities and exposed areas such as head and neck tissues are also susceptible to injury. The ear is the organ system that is most sensitive to blast injuries. The **tympanic membrane** evolved to detect minor changes in pressure and will rupture at pressures of 5 to 7 pounds per square inch above atmospheric pressure. Thus, the tympanic membranes are a sensitive indicator that you can use to help determine the possible presence of other blast injuries. The patient may report ringing in the ears, pain in the ears, or some loss of hearing, and blood may be visible in the ear canal. Dislocation of structural components of the ear, such as the ossicles conforming the inner ear, may occur. Permanent hearing loss is possible. These findings can be used to assist in triaging patients as they indicate risk of pressure injuries to the lungs.

**Pulmonary blast injuries** are defined as pulmonary trauma (consisting of contusions and hemorrhages) that results from short-range exposure to the detonation of explosives. When the explosion occurs in an open space, both lungs are usually injured. Primary blast injury is often characterized by a lack of external visible injuries and thus can go unrecognized. The patient may report tightness or pain in the chest and may cough up blood and have tachypnea or other signs of respiratory distress. Subcutaneous emphysema (crackling under the skin) can be palpated over the chest, indicating air in the thorax. Pneumothorax is a common injury and may require emergency decompression (which is covered in Chapter 30, *Chest Injuries*) in the field for your patient to survive. Pulmonary edema may ensue rapidly. If there is any reason to suspect lung injury in a blast victim (even just the presence of a ruptured eardrum), administer oxygen to maintain $Sao_2$ of 94% to 99%. Avoid giving oxygen under positive pressure, however, because that may simply increase the damage to the lung or increase the size of a pneumothorax.

One of the most concerning pulmonary blast injuries is **arterial air embolism**, which occurs on alveolar disruption with subsequent air embolization into the pulmonary vasculature. Even small air bubbles can enter a coronary artery and cause myocardial injury. Air embolisms to the cerebrovascular system can produce disturbances in vision, changes in behavior, changes in state of consciousness, and a variety of other neurologic signs.

Solid organs are relatively protected from shock wave injury but may be injured by secondary missiles or a hurled body. Hollow organs, however, may be injured by the same mechanisms that damage lung tissue. Skin injuries, ranging from petechiae, or pinpoint red-purple hemorrhages that show up on the skin, to large hematomas may be found. Perforation or rupture of the bowel and colon is a risk.

Underwater explosions can result in severe abdominal injuries.

Neurologic injuries and head trauma are the most common causes of death from blast injuries related to terrorist incidents. Subarachnoid (beneath the arachnoid layer covering the brain) and subdural (beneath the outermost covering of the brain) hematomas are often seen. Permanent or transient neurologic deficits may be secondary to concussion, intracerebral bleeding, or air embolism. Instant but transient unconsciousness, with or without retrograde amnesia, may be initiated not only by head trauma, but also by cardiovascular problems. Bradycardia and hypotension are common after an intense pressure wave from an explosion.

Extremity injuries, including traumatic amputations, are common. Patients with traumatic amputation by postblast wind are likely to sustain fatal injuries secondary to the blast. In present-day combat, improved body armor has increased the number of survivors of blast injuries from shrapnel wounds to the torso. The number of severe orthopaedic and extremity injuries, however, has increased. In addition, whereas body armor may limit or prevent shrapnel from entering the body, it also catches more energy from the blast wave, possibly resulting in the victim being thrown backward, thus increasing the potential for spine and spinal cord injury.

Although blast injuries have usually occurred in war zones, they often occur in industrial settings and are, unfortunately, currently more common because of the increased use of explosives as a tool for urban terrorism and, in the United States, from methamphetamine laboratory explosions. Although civilian blast injuries in an industrial or mining setting used to be mostly characterized by blast injuries and burns, terrorist bombs often contain shrapnel. As an EMT, you and other EMS and trauma services personnel should be fully educated and aware of what to expect in these scenarios.

## Multisystem Trauma

*Multisystem trauma* is a term that describes a person who has been subjected to multiple traumatic injuries involving more than one body system, such as head and spinal trauma, chest and abdominal trauma, or chest and multiple extremity trauma. You must recognize patients who fit into this classification and provide rapid treatment and transportation, and alert medical control as to the nature of the patient's injuries so that the trauma center is prepared prior to your arrival. Multisystem trauma patients have a high level of morbidity and mortality; therefore, they require teams of physicians to treat their injuries.

## Golden Principles of Prehospital Trauma Care

As with any EMS call, your main priority in managing multisystem trauma is to ensure your safety and the safety of your crew and patient. Next, you must determine the need for additional personnel or equipment, evaluate the MOI, and identify and appropriately manage life threats. Once these steps have been completed, you can focus on patient care. Hemorrhage control has the highest priority. Severe bleeding from partial or complete amputations or other large wounds must be stopped. A tourniquet should be applied when bleeding from an extremity cannot be controlled using direct pressure (as discussed in Chapter 26, *Bleeding*). Assessing and managing the airway and breathing, including ventilatory support and high-flow oxygen, while maintaining appropriate spinal motion restriction is the second priority. Ensure that other shock therapy, such as keeping the patient warm, is completed. Initiate spinal motion restriction precautions as indicated.

If the patient is entrapped, consider the use of rapid extrication techniques. In most patients with multisystem trauma, definitive care requires surgical intervention; therefore, on-scene time should be limited to 10 minutes or less, referred to as the platinum 10. During transport, obtain a SAMPLE history and complete a secondary assessment. Most care can be provided during transport. However, keep in

### Words of Wisdom

Rapid transport decisions are needed for patients who have sustained significant trauma. If definitive care is not provided after the first 60 minutes from the time of injury, referred to as the Golden Hour, the body has increasing difficulty in compensating for shock and traumatic injuries. Because many injured patients require definitive care in less than 1 hour, this concept is also referred to as the Golden Period.

## YOU are the Provider

Based on information indicating that heavy traffic would result in a significant delay in ground transportation to the Level 1 trauma center, the patient is loaded into the ambulance with appropriate spinal precautions and immediately reassessed.

| Recording Time: 10 Minutes | |
|---|---|
| **Level of consciousness** | Responds only to pain |
| **Respirations** | 30 breaths/min; extremely labored |
| **Pulse** | 130 beats/min; absent radial pulses |
| **Skin** | Cool, clammy, and pale |
| **Blood pressure** | 80/50 mm Hg |
| **Spo₂** | 89% (supplemental oxygen) |

Your partner begins assisting the patient's ventilations with a bag-mask device and high-flow oxygen, and oral suctioning is performed as needed to keep the patient's airway clear of blood. The patient flexes his arms in response to pain, but does not open his eyes or respond verbally when you talk to him. An EMT from one of the engine companies drives the ambulance to the landing zone, which is about a mile away.

**6.** What trauma scoring systems are commonly used to assess the severity of a trauma patient's condition? How would you apply them to this patient?

mind that your patient has sustained multisystem trauma, and the order in which you usually provide treatment and care may need to be adjusted depending on the needs of the patient. For critically injured patients, consider ALS intercept and/or air medical transportation. Regardless of the mode of transport, ensure that the patient is transported to an appropriate facility and that the facility is notified as soon as possible. Specific standards of care regarding multisystem trauma are addressed in detail in the respective chapters.

## Patient Assessment

Identifying life-threatening illnesses and injuries as soon as possible has proven to improve patient outcomes. As an EMT, you must apply this knowledge as well as the appropriate assessment skills to assess, triage, manage, and transport patients with traumatic injuries to the most appropriate facility. The major components of patient assessment include the following:

- Scene size-up
- Primary assessment
- History taking
- Secondary assessment
- Reassessment

When you are caring for a patient who has experienced a significant MOI and the patient is considered to be in serious or critical condition, you should rapidly perform a physical examination. With a patient who has experienced a nonsignificant MOI, focus on the chief complaint while assessing the patient as a whole. The human body is divided into areas (or systems) based on body function, and its internal organs are subject to unseen injuries when force is applied to the body. For example, the brain may have bruising, the heart and lungs may have bruising or unseen bleeding, and

### Street Smarts

Work on building and maintaining strong communication skills within your team. With good communication, your entire team (and the patient) benefits from the observations of each member. Poor communication can lead to mistakes that at least one team member could have prevented.

the organs of the abdomen may have life-threatening bleeding. The following sections discuss the assessment of various body systems.

## Injuries to the Head

The brain lies well protected within the skull. However, when the head is injured from trauma, disability and unseen injury to the brain may occur. The brain itself may tear or become bruised, causing bleeding. The blood vessels around the brain may also tear and produce bleeding. Bleeding or swelling inside the skull from brain injury is often life threatening; therefore, your assessment must include conducting frequent neurologic examinations. Neurologic assessments, coupled with the patient's level of consciousness, will often provide details on subtle changes in the patient's condition. Some patients will not have obvious signs or symptoms, such as changes in pupillary size and reactivity, of unseen brain injury until minutes or hours after the injury has occurred.

## Injuries to the Neck and Throat

The neck and throat contain many structures that are susceptible to injuries from trauma that could be serious or deadly to your patients. In this region of the human body, the trachea (or windpipe) may become torn or swell after an injury to the neck or deviate after an injury to the lungs. These types of injuries may result in an airway problem that could quickly become a serious life threat because they interfere with the patient's ability to breathe; therefore, your assessment must include frequent physical examination looking for DCAP-BTLS in the neck region. In addition, you should assess for jugular venous (vein) distention and tracheal deviation (late sign of injury).

The neck also contains large blood vessels that supply the brain with oxygen-rich blood. When a neck injury occurs, swelling may prevent blood flow to the brain and cause injury to the central nervous system, even though the brain may not have been directly affected by the initial force that caused the injury to the neck. If a penetrating injury to the neck results in an open wound, the patient may have significant bleeding or air may be drawn into the circulatory system. If air enters the veins, this may result in air embolism, which may lead to cardiac arrest if the air enters the heart. Occlusive dressings must be used to keep this from happening. A crushing injury to the upper part of the neck may cause the cartilages of the upper airway and larynx to fracture. This can lead to air leaking into the soft tissue of the neck. When air is trapped in subcutaneous tissue (subcutaneous emphysema), it produces a crackling sound or feeling when palpated, called subcutaneous crepitation. Either air in the circulation or an airway cartilage fracture may cause rapid death.

## Injuries to the Chest

The chest contains the heart, the lungs, and the large blood vessels of the body. When injury occurs to this area of the body, many life-threatening injuries may occur. For example, blunt trauma to the chest can fracture ribs or the sternum. When ribs are broken and the chest wall does not expand normally during breathing, this interferes with the body's ability to obtain sufficient amounts of oxygen for the cells. Bruising may occur to the heart and cause an irregular heartbeat. Depending on the severity of the trauma, the large vessels of the heart may be torn inside the chest, causing massive unseen bleeding that can quickly kill the trauma patient. In some chest injuries the lungs become bruised, thus interfering with normal oxygen exchange in the body.

Some chest injuries result in air collecting between the lung tissue and the chest wall. As air accumulates in this space, the lung tissue becomes compressed, again interfering with the body's ability to effectively exchange oxygen. This injury is called a pneumothorax. If left untreated or unrecognized, the lung tissue becomes squeezed under pressure until the heart is also squeezed and can no longer pump blood. This condition is called a tension pneumothorax and is a life-threatening emergency. In some patients, bleeding develops in this portion of the chest. Instead of air collecting in this space, blood collects and causes interference with breathing. This condition is called a hemothorax, and it also poses a threat to the patient's life.

A penetration or perforation of the integrity of the chest is called an open chest wound. As air enters the chest cavity, the natural pressure balance within the chest cavity is no longer equal. If left untreated, shock and/or death will result. Regardless of the particular injury, it is imperative

that you reassess a trauma patient's chest region every 5 minutes. The assessment should include DCAP-BTLS, lung sounds, and chest rise and fall. Some patients will not have obvious signs or symptoms such as absent breath sounds or respiratory difficulty immediately.

## Injuries to the Abdomen

The abdomen is an area of the human body that contains many organs vital to body function. These organs also require a high blood flow so they can perform the functions necessary for life. The organs of the abdomen and retroperitoneum (the space immediately behind the true abdomen) can be classified into two simple categories: solid and hollow. The solid organs include the liver, spleen, pancreas, and kidneys. The hollow organs include the stomach, large and small intestines, and urinary bladder.

When injuries from trauma occur in this region of the body, serious and life-threatening problems may occur. The solid organs may tear, lacerate, or fracture. This causes serious bleeding into the abdomen that can quickly cause death. Be alert for a trauma patient who reports abdominal pain—it may be a symptom of abdominal bleeding. Also be alert to vital signs that begin to worsen; this can be a sign of serious, unseen bleeding inside the abdominal region of the body.

When the hollow organs of the body have been injured, they may rupture and leak toxic chemicals used for digestion into the abdomen. This not only causes pain, but a life-threatening infection also may eventually develop.

The abdomen also contains large blood vessels that supply the organs of this region and the lower extremities with oxygen-rich blood. Occasionally these vessels rupture or tear and cause serious

### Street Smarts

Combine your assessment skills with critical thinking in order to provide the patient with excellent care. For example, remember that a multisystem trauma patient with associated traumatic brain injury (TBI) has twice the risk of death when compared with a trauma patient without associated TBI. Maintain a high index of suspicion for all multisystem trauma patients, especially those with associated TBI.

unseen bleeding that may cause death. Some patients, particularly healthy young adults, are able to compensate longer than others from blood loss; therefore, you should always maintain a high index of suspicion when the MOI suggests injury to the abdominal region. This is best accomplished by reassessing the abdominal region.

# Management: Transport and Destination

Caring for victims of traumatic injuries requires a solid understanding of the trauma system in the United States. You need a good working knowledge of the resources available to you, including the most optimal methods of rapid transport and trauma centers that can best provide definitive care. Call for ALS and helicopter assistance early, possibly even before you arrive on scene, to avoid delays in treatment and transport.

## Scene Time

Because survival of critically injured trauma patients is time dependent, limit on-scene time to the minimum amount necessary to correct life-threatening injuries and package the patient. Optimally, on-scene time for critically injured patients should be less than 10 minutes—the platinum 10. The following criteria will help you identify a critically injured patient:

- Dangerous MOI
- Decreased level of consciousness
- Any threats to airway, breathing, or circulation

Patients who present with these criteria or who are very young or old or have chronic illnesses should also be considered to be high risk, thus requiring rapid treatment and transport.

## Destination Selection

You will often be summoned to injury scenes to transport critically ill trauma patients to definitive care. For this reason, it is important for you to be familiar with how the American College of Surgeons Committee on Trauma (ACS-COT) classifies trauma care. Trauma centers are classified into Levels I through IV, with Level I having the most resources, followed by Levels II, III, and IV (**TABLE 25-2**).

A Level I facility is a regional resource center and generally serves large cities or heavily populated areas. Level I facilities must be capable of providing every aspect of trauma care from prevention through rehabilitation; therefore, the facility must have adequate personnel and resources. Because of the extensive requirements, most Level I facilities are university-based teaching hospitals.

## YOU are the Provider

The air transport helicopter arrives at the landing zone approximately 5 minutes after your unit. After reassessing the patient, you give your verbal report to the flight paramedic and transfer patient care.

| Recording Time:   15 Minutes | |
| --- | --- |
| Level of consciousness | Responds only to pain |
| Respirations | 30 breaths/min; extremely labored |
| Pulse | 140 beats/min; absent radial pulses |
| Skin | Cool, clammy, and pale |
| Blood pressure | 74/50 mm Hg |
| Spo$_2$ | 95% (supplemental oxygen) |

After further assessment and treatment, the helicopter crew loads the patient into the aircraft and departs the scene. You later learn that the patient had bleeding in the brain and chest and multiple rib fractures. He was taken to surgery, and was in critical condition in the surgical intensive care unit.

**7.** How does the level of trauma care provided by the paramedic differ from that of the EMT?

| TABLE 25-2 Key Elements for Trauma Centers | | |
|---|---|---|
| **Level** | **Definition** | **Key Elements** |
| Level I | A comprehensive regional resource that is a tertiary care facility; capable of providing total care for every aspect of injury—from prevention through rehabilitation | 1. 24-hour in-house coverage by general surgeons<br>2. Availability of care in specialties such as orthopaedic surgery, neurosurgery, anesthesiology, emergency medicine, radiology, internal medicine, and critical care<br>3. Should also include cardiac, hand, pediatric, and microvascular surgery and hemodialysis<br>4. Provides leadership in prevention, public education, and continuing education of trauma team members<br>5. Committed to continued improvement through a comprehensive quality assessment program and organized research to help direct new innovations in trauma care |
| Level II | Able to initiate definitive care for all injured patients | 1. 24-hour immediate coverage by general surgeons<br>2. Availability of orthopaedic surgery, neurosurgery, anesthesiology, emergency medicine, radiology, and critical care<br>3. Tertiary care needs such as cardiac surgery, hemodialysis, and microvascular surgery may be referred to a Level I trauma center<br>4. Committed to trauma prevention and continuing education of trauma team members<br>5. Provides continued improvement in trauma care through a comprehensive quality assessment program |
| Level III | Able to provide prompt assessment, resuscitation, and stabilization of injured patients and emergency operations | 1. 24-hour immediate coverage by emergency medicine physicians and prompt availability of general surgeons and anesthesiologists<br>2. Program dedicated to continued improvement in trauma care through a comprehensive quality assessment program<br>3. Has developed transfer agreements for patients requiring more comprehensive care at a Level I or Level II trauma center<br>4. Committed to continuing education of nursing and allied health personnel or the trauma team<br>5. Must be involved with prevention and have an active outreach program for its referring communities |
| Level IV | Able to provide advanced trauma life support before transfer of patients to a higher level trauma center | 1. Includes basic emergency department facilities to implement ATLS protocols and 24-hour laboratory coverage<br>2. Transfer to higher level trauma centers follows the guidelines outlined in formal transfer agreements<br>3. Committed to continued improvement of these trauma care activities through a formal quality assessment program<br>4. Involved in prevention, outreach, and education within its community |

© Jones & Bartlett Learning.

A Level II facility is typically located in less populated areas. Level II centers are expected to provide initial definitive care, regardless of injury severity. These facilities can be academic institutions or a public/private community facility. Because of its location and resources, a Level II trauma center may not be able to provide the same comprehensive care as a Level I trauma center.

Level III facilities serve communities that do not have access to Level I or II facilities. Level III facilities provide assessment, resuscitation, emergency care, and stabilization. A Level III facility must have transfer agreements with a Level I or II trauma center and must have protocols in place to transfer patients whose needs exceed the resources of the facility.

Level IV facilities are typically found in remote outlying areas where no higher level of care is available. These facilities provide ATLS prior to transfer to a higher level trauma center. Such a facility may be a clinic urgent care facility, with or without a physician.

Although an inclusive trauma system should leave no facility without a direct link to a Level I or II facility, all facilities are expected to provide the same high quality of initial care regardless of the classification level.

Trauma centers are categorized as either adult trauma centers or pediatric trauma centers, but not necessarily both. Pediatric trauma centers are not nearly as common as adult trauma centers. When transporting a pediatric trauma patient, you must be certain to transport your patient to a pediatric trauma center if there is one in your area; do not make the mistake of transporting a pediatric patient to an adult trauma center when a pediatric trauma center is available.

In 2011, the ACS-COT and the CDC published an updated field triage decision scheme (**FIGURE 25-19**). These criteria are intended to help prehospital care providers recognize injured patients who are likely to benefit from transport to a trauma center compared with transport to an emergency department. The decision scheme is not intended to serve as a mass-casualty or disaster triage tool; it is intended only for individual patients.

## Type of Transport

Modes of transport ultimately come in one of two categories: ground or air. Transport modes are discussed further in Chapter 15, *Medical Overview*. Ground transportation EMS units are generally staffed by EMTs and paramedics. Air transportation EMS units or critical care transport units are often staffed by critical care transport professionals such as critical care nurses and paramedics.

You should be familiar with your local protocols defining indications for use of helicopter emergency medical services (HEMS) transport. In 2014, an expert panel developed evidence-based guidelines for the appropriate use of emergency air medical services for trauma patients.

- Field triage criteria for trauma patients should include anatomic, physiologic, and situational components based on the CDC's 2011 Guidelines for the Field Triage of Injured Patients. These guidelines help predict injury severity to determine the need for helicopter or ground ambulance transport.
- When it is not clear that the patient meets the guidelines for severity, medical direction should be consulted to determine the appropriate means of transport for the patient.

## Words of Wisdom

### Trauma Scoring Systems

The numeric scoring of trauma patients for determining the severity of their injury is common practice in the health care profession. When the various scoring systems were created, it was thought that the implementation of the scoring system would assist in rapidly identifying the severity of the patient's injuries. There are several different trauma scoring systems.

### Trauma Score

The **trauma score** calculates a number from 1 to 16, with 16 being the best possible score. It accounts for the **Glasgow Coma Scale (GCS) score**, respiratory rate, respiratory expansion, systolic blood pressure, and capillary refill. The GCS is an evaluation tool used to determine level of consciousness (**TABLE 25-3**). It evaluates and assigns point values (scores) for eye opening, verbal response, and motor response; these scores are then totaled and help to effectively predict patient outcomes. Note that the lower the score, the more severe the extent of brain injury.

The trauma score relates to the likelihood of patient survival. However, this scoring system does not accurately predict survivability in patients with severe head injuries because motor and verbal deficits make those criteria difficult to assess; in its place, the Revised Trauma Score, discussed next, is used.

### Revised Trauma Score

The **Revised Trauma Score (RTS)** is most commonly used for patients with head trauma because it is weighted to compensate for major head injury without multisystem injury or major physiologic changes.

The RTS is a physiologic scoring system that is also used to assess the severity of a trauma patient's injuries. Objective data used to calculate the RTS include the GCS score, systolic blood pressure (SBP), and respiratory rate (RR). In addition to assessing injury severity, the RTS has demonstrated reliability in predicting survival in patients with severe injuries. The highest RTS a patient can receive is 12; the lowest is 0. The RTS is calculated as shown in **TABLE 25-4**.

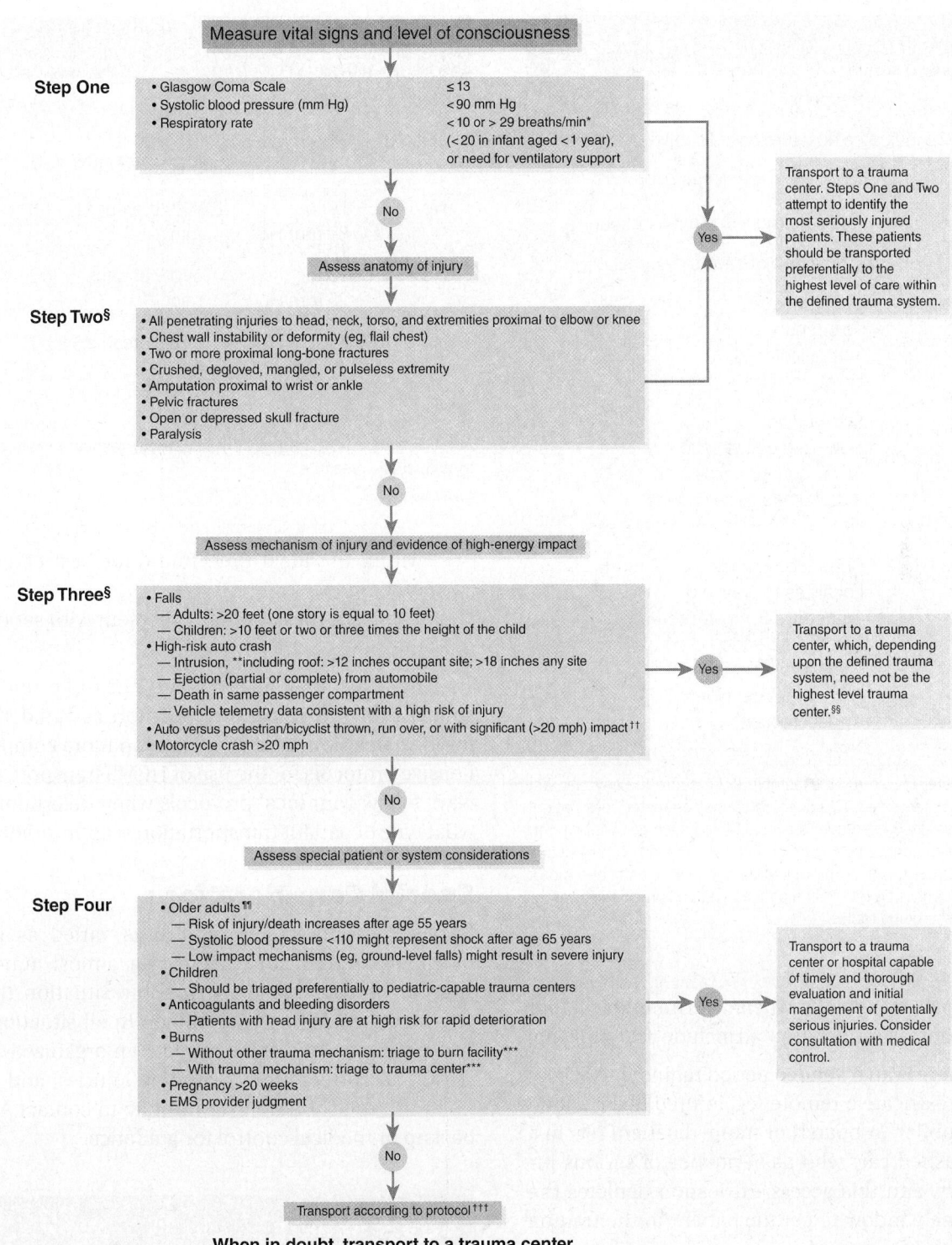

**Measure vital signs and level of consciousness**

**Step One**
- Glasgow Coma Scale — ≤13
- Systolic blood pressure (mm Hg) — <90 mm Hg
- Respiratory rate — <10 or > 29 breaths/min*
  (<20 in infant aged <1 year),
  or need for ventilatory support

No

**Assess anatomy of injury**

**Step Two§**
- All penetrating injuries to head, neck, torso, and extremities proximal to elbow or knee
- Chest wall instability or deformity (eg, flail chest)
- Two or more proximal long-bone fractures
- Crushed, degloved, mangled, or pulseless extremity
- Amputation proximal to wrist or ankle
- Pelvic fractures
- Open or depressed skull fracture
- Paralysis

No

**Assess mechanism of injury and evidence of high-energy impact**

**Step Three§**
- Falls
  — Adults: >20 feet (one story is equal to 10 feet)
  — Children: >10 feet or two or three times the height of the child
- High-risk auto crash
  — Intrusion, **including roof: >12 inches occupant site; >18 inches any site
  — Ejection (partial or complete) from automobile
  — Death in same passenger compartment
  — Vehicle telemetry data consistent with a high risk of injury
- Auto versus pedestrian/bicyclist thrown, run over, or with significant (>20 mph) impact††
- Motorcycle crash >20 mph

No

**Assess special patient or system considerations**

**Step Four**
- Older adults¶¶
  — Risk of injury/death increases after age 55 years
  — Systolic blood pressure <110 might represent shock after age 65 years
  — Low impact mechanisms (eg, ground-level falls) might result in severe injury
- Children
  — Should be triaged preferentially to pediatric-capable trauma centers
- Anticoagulants and bleeding disorders
  — Patients with head injury are at high risk for rapid deterioration
- Burns
  — Without other trauma mechanism: triage to burn facility***
  — With trauma mechanism: triage to trauma center***
- Pregnancy >20 weeks
- EMS provider judgment

No

**Transport according to protocol†††**

Yes → Transport to a trauma center. Steps One and Two attempt to identify the most seriously injured patients. These patients should be transported preferentially to the highest level of care within the defined trauma system.

Yes → Transport to a trauma center, which, depending upon the defined trauma system, need not be the highest level trauma center.§§

Yes → Transport to a trauma center or hospital capable of timely and thorough evaluation and initial management of potentially serious injuries. Consider consultation with medical control.

**When in doubt, transport to a trauma center**

**Abbreviation:** EMS = emergency medical services.
  * The upper limit of respiratory rate in infants is >29 breaths per minute to maintain a higher level of overtriage for infants.
  § Any injury noted in Step Two or mechanism identified in Step Three triggers a "yes" response.
  ¶ Age <15 years.
  ** Intrusion refers to interior compartment intrusion, as opposed to deformation, which refers to exterior damage.
  †† Includes pedestrians or bicyclists thrown or run over by a motor vehicle or those with estimated impact >20 mph with a motor vehicle.
  §§ Local or regional protocols should be used to determine the most appropriate level of trauma center within the defined trauma system; need not be the highest-level trauma center.
  ¶¶ Age >55 years.
  *** Patients with both burns and concomitant trauma for whom the burn injury poses the greatest risk for morbidity and mortality should be transferred to a burn center. If the nonburn trauma presents a greater immediate risk, the patient may be stabilized in a trauma center and then transferred to a burn center.
  ††† Patients who do not meet any of the triage criteria in Steps One through Four should be transported to the most appropriate medical facility as outlined in local EMS protocols.

**FIGURE 25-19** 2011 decision scheme for field triage of injured patients.

Adapted from Centers for Disease Control and Prevention, *Morbidity and Mortality Weekly Report*, January 13, 2012.

**TABLE 25-3** Glasgow Coma Scale[a]

| Test | Response | Score |
|------|----------|-------|
| Score: 15 indicates no neurologic disabilities. | | |
| Score: 13–14 may indicate mild dysfunction. | | |
| Score: 9–12 may indicate moderate dysfunction. | | |
| Score: 8 or less is indicative of severe dysfunction. | | |
| Eye opening | Spontaneous | 4 |
| | To sound | 3 |
| | To pressure | 2 |
| | None | 1 |
| Verbal | Oriented conversation | 5 |
| | Confused conversation | 4 |
| | Inappropriate words | 3 |
| | Incomprehensible sounds | 2 |
| | None | 1 |
| Motor | Obeys commands | 6 |
| | Localizes to pressure | 5 |
| | Withdraws from pressure | 4 |
| | Abnormal flexion (decorticate) | 3 |
| | Abnormal extension (decerebrate) | 2 |
| | None | 1 |

[a]Some systems use a "Not testable (NT)" score for any element that cannot be tested. Eye opening cannot be tested in a patient whose eyes are closed due to a local factor, such as swelling; verbal response cannot be tested in a patient who has a preexisting factor interfering with communication, such as mutism; and motor response cannot be tested in a patient who has preexisting paralysis or other limiting factor.

© Jones & Bartlett Learning.

**TABLE 25-4** Revised Trauma Score

| GCS | SBP | RR | Value |
|-----|-----|-----|-------|
| 13 to 15 | >89 mm Hg | 10 to 29 breaths/min | 4 |
| 9 to 12 | 76 to 89 mm Hg | >29 breaths/min | 3 |
| 6 to 8 | 50 to 75 mm Hg | 6 to 9 breaths/min | 2 |
| 4 to 5 | 1 to 49 mm Hg | 1 to 5 breaths/min | 1 |
| 3 | 0 | 0 | 0 |

Abbreviations: GCS, Glasgow Coma Scale; RR, respiratory rate; SBP, systolic blood pressure

© Jones & Bartlett Learning.

Factors to consider when determining whether the patient is seriously injured include the following:

- There is an extended period required to access or extricate a remote (eg, injured hiker, snowmobiler, or boater) or trapped patient (eg, in a crashed car) who has evidence of serious injury, and this access/extrication depletes the time window to get the patient to the trauma center by ground.
- The patient needs medical care and stabilization at the ALS level, and there is no ALS-level ground ambulance service available within a reasonable time frame.
- Traffic conditions or hospital availability make it unlikely that the seriously injured patient will get to a trauma center via ground ambulance

within the ideal time frame for best clinical outcome.
- There is a mass-casualty incident with serious injuries.

These recommendations are not to be understood as fully encompassing, but more as a guideline for local decision makers to develop more comprehensive protocols for the use of HEMS transport. Always follow your local protocols when determining what type of patient transportation is appropriate.

## Special Considerations

Because traumatic injuries are as varied as the mechanisms that cause them, it is almost impossible to prepare for every possible situation that you may face during your career. In all situations, you must remain calm, complete an organized assessment, correct life-threatening injuries, and do no harm. You should never hesitate to contact ALS backup or medical control for guidance.

## Street Smarts

Most EMS professionals will experience some type of traumatic incident while on duty. About one-third of EMS professionals will be diagnosed with depression or posttraumatic stress disorder. The risk of suicide among EMS professionals is double that of non–public safety personnel. Take care of yourself. Know the resources that are available to you. Seek help when needed.

# YOU are the Provider SUMMARY

**1. On the basis of the information provided by the EMD, can you predict the potential types of injuries the patient may have? If so, how?**

Although you will not ultimately know the type and severity of injuries the patient has until you arrive at the scene, information provided by the dispatch operator can influence your index of suspicion.

En route to this scene, you know that the incident involves a head-on (frontal) crash with a tree, and the patient is still in the vehicle. What you do not know is the speed of the vehicle at the time of impact, whether the patient was restrained, or whether any airbags deployed. *Just because the patient is still in the vehicle does not indicate that he was restrained.* Until you arrive at the scene and gather more information, you should assume the worst.

The patient has experienced three collisions: collision of the vehicle against another object, collision of himself against the interior of the vehicle, and collision of his internal organs against the solid structures of the body.

Damage to the vehicle (the first collision) provides information about the severity of the collision. The greater the damage is to the vehicle, the greater the energy that was involved and, therefore, the greater the potential to cause injury. If there is significant damage to the vehicle, your index of suspicion for serious injury to the patient should increase, even if injuries are not immediately apparent.

Just like the obvious damage that occurs to the exterior of the vehicle during the first collision, the injuries that result from the second collision are often obvious during the primary assessment. Common injuries that occur during the second collision include lower extremity and pelvic fractures (when the knees impact the dashboard), rib fractures, pneumothoraces (when the chest impacts the steering wheel), and head and neck trauma (when the head impacts the windshield).

The type of injury experienced by the unrestrained occupant depends on the path he or she took at the time of impact. There may be injuries to the abdomen, pelvis, and lower extremities if the patient's body took the down-and-under path causing the abdomen to impact the lower part of the steering wheel and the knees to impact the dashboard. Head, neck, or chest trauma may be present if the patient was propelled over the steering wheel. Blunt chest and/or abdominal trauma may result from direct impact with the steering wheel.

The injuries that occur during the third collision may not be as obvious as external injuries, but these injuries may be the most life threatening. For example, if the chest impacts the steering wheel, the thoracic organs continue their forward motion until they collide with the inside of the chest cavity. As a result of these forces, shearing injuries of the great vessels (eg, aorta, vena cava) or injury to the heart as it impacts with the sternum may occur. If the occupant's head strikes the windshield, the brain continues its forward motion until it strikes the inside of the skull; this results in compression injuries to the anterior part of the brain and stretching or tearing of the posterior part of the brain.

**2. Why is it important to determine the speed at which a vehicle was traveling at the time of impact?**

A vehicle's speed affects the potential for injury to its occupant or occupants. According to the equation for kinetic energy ($KE = \frac{1}{2}mv^2$), the energy available to cause injury doubles when the object's weight doubles, but *quadruples when the object's speed doubles*.

The relationship between a vehicle's speed and its deceleration is best described in these terms: The faster the vehicle is traveling and the quicker it stops, the greater the potential for serious injury to the occupant(s).

**3. What damage in the vehicle's interior may have caused the patient's signs and symptoms?**

The patient's signs and symptoms indicate, at a minimum, injury to his head and chest. He is bleeding from the head, face, and mouth; his level of consciousness is markedly decreased; and his respirations are rapid and labored.

Inspection of the interior of the vehicle in this incident will most likely reveal a deformed steering wheel (top, bottom, or both) that occurred when the patient's chest—and maybe abdomen—impacted it. You will also likely find an outward bulge of the windshield with a typical starburst fracture where the patient's head and face made impact with it. You may also find some of the patient's hair caught in the windshield, and this is a clear indicator of patient impact. Keep in mind that these may not be the only contact points; they are simply the most likely areas based on the patient's injuries.

**4. Should the patient be transported to the Level I trauma center or the Level III trauma center? Why?**

You are caring for a multisystem trauma patient; that is, he has experienced trauma that affects more than one body system. The obvious trauma to his head and his level of consciousness indicate a TBI. The bruising and crepitus to his chest and his labored breathing indicate intrathoracic trauma, and his vital signs indicate a general state of shock. He requires the highest level of trauma care available—a Level I trauma center if possible. There are several reasons you may consider the Level III center, however. If you are unable to achieve an adequate airway to be able to maintain ventilation throughout the time of transport to the Level I center, you should consider going to the Level III center first for stabilization prior to transfer to the Level I center. Similarly, if the patient's condition is otherwise sufficiently grave from the standpoint of his head injury or blood pressure, going to the Level III center first might be warranted. Be familiar with transport times and options to minimize those times (ie, HEMS transport) in your area.

**5. What other transport factors should you consider with this patient?**

The patient should be transported to a Level I trauma center; however, the closest one is 30 miles away. Ground transport in heavy traffic will cause a delay in patient care. This situation requires you to make a decision regarding how to best transport the patient to a Level I facility in the most expedient manner.

In this scenario, you are faced with two transport options: Try to coordinate a paramedic intercept and transport by ground to the Level I facility or request HEMS transport. Coordinating a paramedic intercept and transporting the patient by ground will get ALS care to the patient quicker, but it will not get him to the Level I facility and therefore to definitive care any quicker. Conversely, air medical transport via a helicopter will get ALS personnel (ie, paramedic, critical care nurse) to the patient *and* get him to the Level I facility in less time. You should also be prepared for the situation where you are faced with the same patient but no access to HEMS for some reason, such as bad weather. Your priorities remain the same, but the best option for achieving the fastest access to resuscitative care may be less obvious.

**6. What trauma scoring systems are commonly used to assess the severity of a trauma patient's condition? How would you apply them to this patient?**

The two most commonly used numeric trauma scoring systems are the GCS and the RTS.

To assess the patient in this scenario, you must first calculate his GCS. The patient does not open his eyes, even when a painful stimulus is applied; therefore, he receives a 1 for eye opening. For verbal response, he also receives a 1 because he does not respond when you talk to him. For motor response, he receives a 3; he responds to pain by flexing his arms (decorticate posturing). Currently, the patient's GCS score is 5, which indicates a severe brain injury.

To calculate the patient's RTS, you will use his GCS, along with his systolic blood pressure and respiratory rate. He has already been assigned a GCS score of 5; therefore, he is assigned a numeric value of 1. His systolic blood pressure is 80 mm Hg; therefore, he is assigned a numeric value of 3. His respiratory value is 34 breaths/min; therefore, he is assigned a numeric value of 3. Given these parameters, the patient's RTS is 7.

Note that *a single assessment of a trauma patient's GCS and RTS scores cannot reliably capture his or her clinical progression.* Obtain baseline scores and then frequently (at least every 5 minutes) reassess them. Document all scores you obtained in the field, including the times they were obtained.

**7. How does the level of trauma care provided by the paramedic differ from that of the EMT?**

The level of trauma care you provide as an EMT versus personnel with a higher level of training, such as AEMTs and paramedics, differs mainly in the emergency treatment interventions that can be performed. For example, paramedics are trained to provide advanced airway management and intravenous therapy, and to administer certain emergency medications, among others. Although these additional skills can be of great benefit to the patient, they are not definitive care interventions. Paramedics cannot repair a lacerated liver or stop bleeding in the brain; therefore, their focus on trauma care should not be significantly different from yours. Trauma care is based on identifying injuries, stabilizing the patient, and rapid transport to the appropriate medical facility, in this case, a trauma center. In many cases, you will be called on to assist the paramedic in performing advanced level skills. Depending on local protocols, you may even be able to perform additional skills as deemed necessary by the EMS system medical director.

## YOU are the Provider SUMMARY continued

### EMS Patient Care Report (PCR)

| Date: 9-1-20 | Incident No.: 012109 N | Nature of Call: Motor vehicle crash | | Location: 2100 Block Hwy 46 | |
|---|---|---|---|---|---|
| Dispatched: 1520 | En Route: 1520 | At Scene: 1528 | Transport: 1538 | At Hospital: 1552 | In Service: 1630 |

#### Patient Information

**Age:** 20
**Sex:** M
**Weight (in kg [lb]):** estimated at 68 kg (150 lb)

**Allergies:** Unknown
**Medications:** Unknown
**Past Medical History:** Unknown
**Chief Complaint:** Multiple traumatic injuries

#### Vital Signs

| Time: 1533 | BP: 84/64 | Pulse: 120 | Respirations: 22 | Spo$_2$: 97% |
|---|---|---|---|---|
| Time: 1538 | BP: 80/50 | Pulse: 130 | Respirations: 30 | Spo$_2$: 89% |
| Time: 1543 | BP: 74/50 | Pulse: 140 | Respirations: 30 | Spo$_2$: 95% |

#### EMS Treatment (circle all that apply)

| Oxygen @ _15_ L/min via: NC (NRM) (Bag mask) | | Assisted Ventilation | Airway Adjunct | CPR |
|---|---|---|---|---|
| Defibrillation | (Bleeding Control) | Bandaging | Splinting | Other: (Thermal management, suction, spinal motion restriction) |

#### Narrative

Dispatched for a motor vehicle versus tree head-on crash. Rescue assignment and law enforcement were dispatched as well.

Chief Complaint: Multiple traumatic injuries

History: Arrived at the scene and noted that a small passenger vehicle made frontal impact with a large tree. Damage to the front of the vehicle was significant. The driver, a 20-year-old man, was still in the vehicle; however, he was unrestrained. Driver- and passenger-side airbags both deployed, and patient was not entrapped. Medevac requested after initial assessment give ground transport time and patient condition. Partner accessed patient through backseat and manually stabilized his head. Engine 3 fire fighter reported interior damage to the steering wheel and a starburst fracture to the windshield with evidence of human hair.

Assessment: Primary assessment revealed that the patient was responsive only to pain. He had blood in his oropharynx, a large hematoma and laceration with active bleeding to his forehead, and facial bleeding. His respirations were rapid and labored.

Treatment (Rx): Suctioned the patient's oropharynx, controlled the bleeding on his forehead, applied cervical collar, and rapidly extricated him from the vehicle. Applied oxygen @ 15 L/min via nonrebreathing mask and performed secondary assessment, which revealed diffuse bruising and crepitus to the chest. Breath sounds were diminished over the left side of the chest. Pelvis and upper and lower extremities were unremarkable for gross injury. Pupils were dilated to approximately 6 mm, and sluggish to react.

Transport: Applied spinal motion restriction precautionsand a blanket for warmth, and loaded patient into the ambulance. Engine 3 EMT drove ambulance to landing zone (LZ) to meet with air transport helicopter.

Reassessment: Reassessment revealed that his respiratory rate had increased, his breathing effort was more labored, and his oxygen saturation had decreased. Began assisting his ventilations with a bag-mask device and high-flow oxygen. Continued to reassess patient every 3 to 5 minutes and noted no change in his clinical status. Contacted air medical helicopter via radio and provided patient status update. Continued to assist patient's ventilations and suctioned his oropharynx as needed to maintain airway patency. Vital signs were also reassessed, as noted above. After a 3-minute wait at the LZ, air transport helicopter arrived. Gave verbal report to flight paramedic, and transferred patient care to the flight crew.

**End of report**

# Prep Kit

## Ready for Review

- Determine the mechanism of injury (MOI) as quickly as possible; this will assist you in developing an index of suspicion for the seriousness of your patient's unseen injuries.
- Three concepts of energy are typically associated with injury: potential energy, kinetic energy, and work.
- Traumatic injuries can be described as blunt trauma or penetrating trauma.
- Motor vehicle crashes are classified traditionally as frontal (head-on), lateral (T-bone), rear-end, rotational (spins), and rollover.
- In every crash, there are three collisions that occur:
  - The collision of the vehicle against some type of object
  - The collision of the passenger against the interior of the vehicle
  - The collision of the passenger's internal organs against the solid structures of the body
- Maintain a high index of suspicion for serious injury in the patient who has been involved in a motor vehicle crash with significant damage to the vehicle, has fallen from a significant height, or has sustained penetrating trauma to the body.
- Communicate MOI findings in the written patient care report and verbally to hospital staff; this will ensure that appropriate treatment of potential serious injuries continues for the patient at the hospital.
- People who are injured in explosions may have injuries that are classified as primary blast injuries, secondary blast injuries, tertiary blast injuries, and/or quaternary blast injuries.
- A patient who has sustained a significant MOI and is considered to be in serious or critical condition should receive a secondary assessment including a rapid examination of the entire body. Any patient who has sustained a nonsignificant MOI should receive an assessment more focused on the chief complaint while still assessing the patient as a whole.
- Caring for victims of traumatic injuries requires a solid understanding of the trauma system in the United States. This includes transport time, transport destination, and selection of type of transport.
- The criteria for transport to a trauma center vary from system to system. Key variables define the level rating of a trauma center. There are four categories of trauma centers. Your system may include a Level I trauma center, the highest-level trauma center.
- The field triage decision scheme from the American College of Surgeons Committee on Trauma and the Centers for Disease Control and Prevention outlines criteria to help prehospital care providers recognize injured patients who are likely to benefit from transport to a trauma center.

## Vital Vocabulary

**arterial air embolism**  Air bubbles in the arterial blood vessels.

**blunt trauma**  An impact on the body by objects that cause injury without penetrating soft tissues or internal organs and cavities.

**cavitation**  A phenomenon in which speed causes a bullet to generate pressure waves, which cause damage distant from the bullet's path.

**coup-contrecoup brain injury**  A brain injury that occurs when force is applied to the head and energy transmission through brain tissue causes injury on the opposite side of original impact.

**deceleration**  The slowing of an object.

**drag**  Resistance that slows a projectile, such as air.

**Glasgow Coma Scale (GCS) score**  An evaluation tool used to determine level of consciousness, which evaluates and assigns point values (scores) for eye opening, verbal response, and motor response, which are then totaled; effective in helping predict patient outcomes.

**index of suspicion** Awareness that unseen life-threatening injuries may exist when determining the mechanism of injury.

**kinetic energy** The energy of a moving object.

**mechanism of injury (MOI)** The forces, or energy transmission, applied to the body that cause injury.

**medical emergencies** Emergencies that require EMS attention because of illnesses or conditions not caused by an outside force.

**multisystem trauma** Trauma that affects more than one body system.

**penetrating trauma** Injury caused by objects, such as knives and bullets, that pierce the surface of the body and damage internal tissues and organs.

**potential energy** The product of mass, gravity, and height, which is converted into kinetic energy and results in injury, such as from a fall.

**projectile** Any object propelled by force, such as a bullet by a weapon.

**pulmonary blast injuries** Pulmonary trauma resulting from short-range exposure to the detonation of explosives.

**Revised Trauma Score (RTS)** A scoring system used for patients with head trauma.

**trajectory** The path a projectile takes once it is propelled.

**trauma emergencies** Emergencies that are the result of physical forces applied to a patient's body.

**trauma score** A score calculated from 1 to 16, with 16 being the best possible score. It relates to the likelihood of patient survival with the exception of a severe head injury. It takes into account the Glasgow Coma Scale (GCS) score, respiratory rate, respiratory expansion, systolic blood pressure, and capillary refill.

**tympanic membrane** The eardrum; a thin, semitransparent membrane in the middle ear that transmits sound vibrations to the internal ear by means of auditory ossicles.

**work** The measure of force over distance.

# References

1. Achildi O, Betz RR, Grewal H. Lapbelt injuries and the seat belt syndrome in pediatric spinal cord injury. *J Spinal Cord Med.* 2007;30(Suppl 1):S21-S24.

2. Centers for Disease Control and Prevention. Explosions and blast injuries: a primer for clinicians. http://www.cdc.gov/masstrauma/preparedness/primer.pdf. Accessed February 5, 2020.

3. Centers for Disease Control and Prevention. Key injury and violence data. http://www.cdc.gov/injury/wisqars/overview/key_data.html. Updated June 10, 2016. Accessed November 12, 2019.

4. Centers for Disease Control and Prevention. Policy impact: seat belts. https://www.cdc.gov/motorvehiclesafety/seatbeltbrief/index.html. Updated January 21, 2014. Accessed November 17, 2019.

5. Centers for Disease Control and Prevention, National Center for Health Statistics. Firearm mortality by state. https://www.cdc.gov/nchs/pressroom/sosmap/firearm_mortality/firearm.htm. Reviewed January 10, 2019. Accessed February 5, 2020.

6. Centers for Disease Control and Prevention, National Center for Injury Prevention and Control. Seat belts: get the facts. https://www.cdc.gov/motorvehiclesafety/seatbelts/facts.html. Reviewed June 5, 2018. Accessed February 5, 2020.

7. Centers for Disease Control and Prevention. Ten leading causes of death by age group, United States—2017. https://www.cdc.gov/injury/wisqars/pdf/leading_causes_of_death_by_age_group_2017-508.pdf. Accessed February 9, 2020.

8. Floccare DJ, Stuhlmiller DF, Brathwaite SA, et al. Appropriate and safe utilization of helicopter emergency medical services: a joint position statement with resource document. *Prehospital Emergency Care.* 2013. https://www.ncbi.nlm.nih.gov/pubmed/23834231. Accessed November 17, 2019.

9. Laberge-Nadeau C, Bellavance F, Messier S, Vézina L, Pichette F. Occupant injury severity from lateral collisions: a literature review. *J Safety Res.* 2009;40(6):427-435.

10. Masudi T, McMahon HC, Scott JL, Lockey AS. Seat belt–related injuries: a surgical perspective *J Emerg Trauma Shock.* 2017;10(2):70-73. Accessed March 25, 2020. https://www.ncbi.nlm.nih.gov/pubmed/28367011.

11. McMahon C, Yates D, Campbell F, Hollis S, Woodford M. Unexpected contribution of moderate traumatic brain injury to death after major trauma. *J Trauma.* 1999;47(5):891-895.

12. National Association of Emergency Medical Technicians. Guide to building an effective EMS wellness and

resilience program. http://www.naemt.org/docs
/default-source/ems-preparedness/naemt-resilience
-guide-01-15-2019-final.pdf?Status=Temp&sfvrsn
=d1edc892_2. Accessed November 17, 2019.

13. National Association of State EMS Officials. National
model EMS clinical guidelines: version 2.2. https://
nasemso.org/wp-content/uploads/National-Mode
l-EMS-Clinical-Guidelines-2017-PDF-Version-2.2.pdf.
Updated January 5, 2019. Accessed February 5, 2020.

14. National Center for Health Statistics. All injuries. Centers
for Disease Control and Prevention website. http://www
.cdc.gov/nchs/fastats/injury.htm. Updated April 27,
2016. November 17, 2019.

15. National Highway Traffic Safety Administration. Air bags.
https://www.nhtsa.gov/equipment/air-bags. Accessed
February 5, 2020.

16. National Highway Traffic Safety Administration. *National
Emergency Medical Services Education Standards. Emer-
gency Medical Technician Instructional Guidelines*. DOT
HS 811 077C. ems.gov.www.ems.gov/pdf/811077c.pdf.
Published January 2009. Accessed November 17, 2019.

17. National Registry of Emergency Medical Technicians.
*2015 Paramedic Psychomotor Competency Portfolio
(PPCP)*. Columbus, OH: National Registry of Emergency
Medical Technicians Inc; 2015.

18. National Registry of Emergency Medical Technicians.
Emergency Medical Technician Psychomotor Examination. https://www.nremt.org/nremt/about/psychomo-
tor_exam_emt.asp. Accessed November 12, 2019.

19. Palanca S, Taylor DM, Bailey M, Cameron PA. Mechanisms of motor vehicle accidents that predict major injury. *Emerg Med (Fremantle)*. 2003;15(5-6):423-428.

20. Sasser SM, Hunt RC, Faul M, et al. Guidelines for field tri-
age of injured patients: recommendations of the National
Expert Panel on Field Triage, 2011. Centers for Disease
Control and Prevention website. http://www.cdc.gov
/mmwr/preview/mmwrhtml/rr6101a1.htm. Published
January 13, 2012. Accessed January 19, 2015.

21. Thomas SH, Brown KM, Oliver ZJ, et al. An evidence-
based guideline for the air medical transportation
of prehospital trauma patients. *Prehosp Emerg
Care*. 2014;18(Suppl 1):35-44.

22. Volunteer Firemen's Insurance Service. Manage your risk.
Vehicle rollovers: lessons learned from past incidents.
https://www.vfis.com/Portals/vfis/fire-truck-safety
/Vehicle-Rollover-Prevention-VFIS.pdf. Published 2019.
Accessed February 5, 2020.

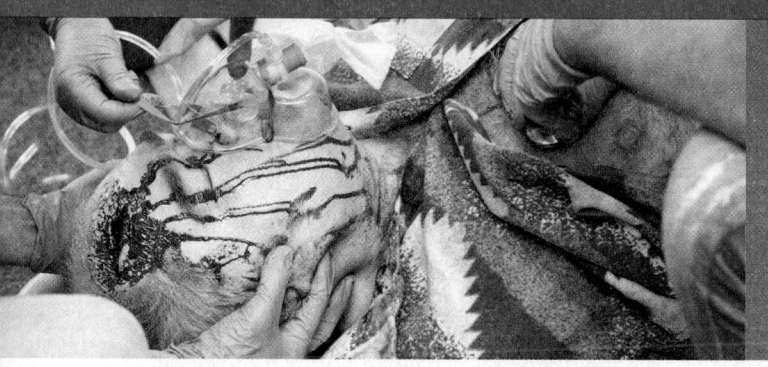

# Chapter 26

# Bleeding

## NATIONAL EMS EDUCATION STANDARD COMPETENCIES

### Trauma
Applies fundamental knowledge to provide basic emergency care and transportation based on assessment findings for an acutely injured patient.

### Bleeding
Recognition and management of
• Bleeding (pp 938–956)

Pathophysiology, assessment, and management of
• Bleeding (pp 937–956)

### Pathophysiology
Applies fundamental knowledge of the pathophysiology of respiration and perfusion to patient assessment and management.

## KNOWLEDGE OBJECTIVES

1. Describe the general structure of the circulatory system and the function of its parts, including the heart, arteries, veins, and capillaries. (pp 934–937)

2. Explain the significance of bleeding caused by blunt force trauma, including the importance of perfusion. (pp 937–941)

3. Discuss hypovolemic shock as a result of bleeding, including the signs of shock. (pp 940–941)

4. Explain the importance of following standard precautions when treating a patient with external bleeding. (p 938)

5. Describe the characteristics of external bleeding, including the identification of the following types of bleeding: arterial, venous, and capillary. (pp 938–940)

6. Explain how to determine the nature of the illness (NOI) for internal bleeding,

including identifying possible traumatic and nontraumatic sources. (p 940)

7. Identify the signs and symptoms of internal bleeding. (pp 940–941)

8. Discuss internal bleeding in terms of the different mechanisms of injury (MOIs) and their associated internal bleeding sources. (p 940)

9. Explain how to conduct a primary assessment, including identification of life threats beyond bleeding, ensuring a patent airway, and making a transport decision. (pp 942–944)

10. Explain how to assess a patient with external or internal bleeding, including the physical examination, vital signs, and the use of monitoring devices. (pp 943–944)

11. Explain the emergency medical care of the patient with external bleeding. (pp 944–954)

12. Explain the emergency medical care of the patient with internal bleeding. (pp 955–956, Skill Drill 26-5)

1. Demonstrate the emergency medical care of the patient with external bleeding. (p 947, Skill Drill 26-1)
2. Demonstrate the emergency medical care of the patient with external bleeding using wound packing. (p 948, Skill Drill 26-2)
3. Demonstrate the emergency medical care of the patient with external bleeding using

a commercial tourniquet. (p 950, Skill Drill 26-3)
4. Demonstrate emergency medical care of the patient with epistaxis, or nosebleed. (p 953, Skill Drill 26-4)
5. Demonstrate the emergency medical care of the patient who shows signs and symptoms of internal bleeding. (pp 955–956, Skill Drill 26-5)

## Introduction

In addition to airway management, two of the most important skills you will learn as an EMT are to recognize and manage life-threatening bleeding. Bleeding can be external and obvious or internal and hidden. Either type of bleeding is potentially dangerous, first causing weakness and eventually, if left uncontrolled, shock and death. Uncontrolled bleeding (hemorrhage) is the most common cause of hypoperfusion (shock) following a traumatic injury.

### Words of Wisdom

Hypoperfusion (shock) due to severe bleeding (hemorrhage) is a common cause of hypovolemia; however, not all forms of hypovolemic shock are due to hemorrhage (eg, vomiting, diarrhea, burns).

This chapter will help you understand how the cardiovascular system reacts to blood loss. The chapter begins with a brief review of the anatomy and function of the cardiovascular system. It then describes the signs, symptoms, and emergency medical care of both external and internal bleeding. The chapter concludes with a discussion about the relationship between bleeding and hypovolemic shock.

## Anatomy and Physiology of the Cardiovascular System

The cardiovascular system circulates blood to the body's cells and tissues, delivering oxygen and nutrients and carrying away metabolic waste products (**FIGURE 26-1**). Refer to Chapter 6, *The Human Body*, for further details.

The cardiovascular system is the main system responsible for supplying and maintaining adequate blood flow. It consists of three parts:

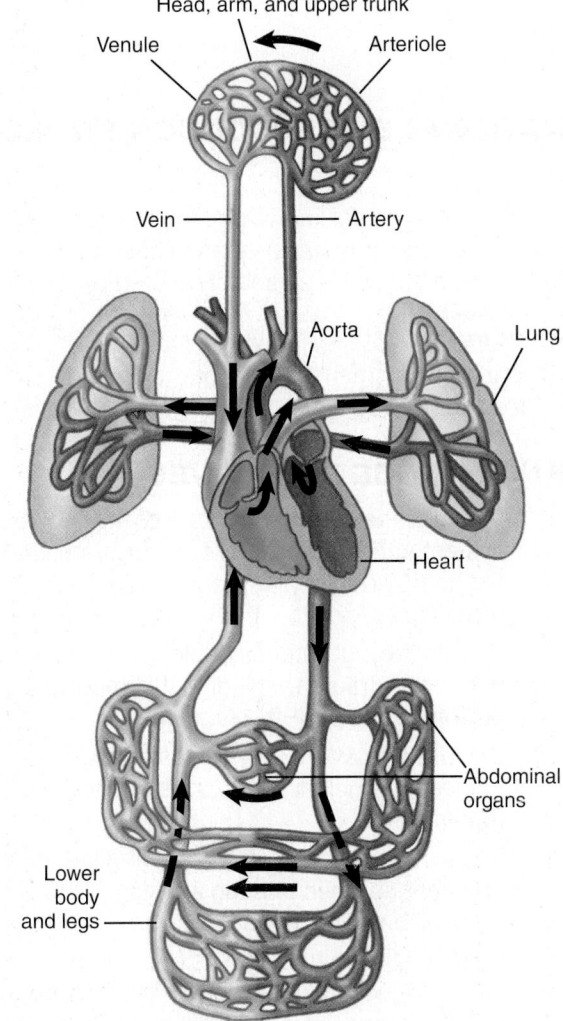

**FIGURE 26-1** The cardiovascular system includes the heart, arteries, veins, and interconnecting capillaries.

© Jones & Bartlett Learning.

- The pump (the heart)
- A container (the blood vessels that reach the cells of the body)
- The fluid (blood and body fluids)

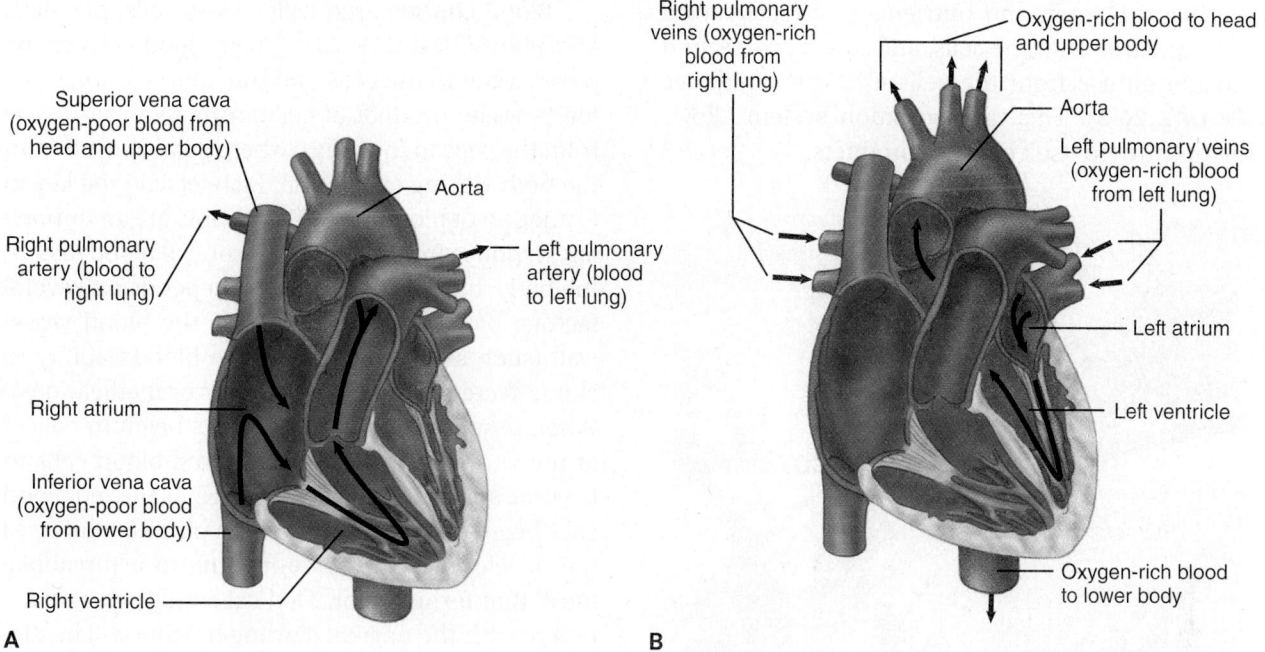

**FIGURE 26-2 A.** The right side of the heart circulates blood from the body to the lungs. **B.** The left side of the heart circulates oxygen-rich blood from the lungs to the rest of the body. It is the more muscular of the two pumps because it must pump blood into the aorta and arteries in order to reach all cells of the body.

A, B: © Jones & Bartlett Learning.

## The Heart

All organs depend on the heart to provide a rich blood supply. For this reason, the heart muscle has several unique features. First, because the heart cannot tolerate a disruption of its blood flow for more than a few minutes, the heart muscle needs a rich and well-distributed blood supply. Second, the heart works as two paired pumps (**FIGURE 26-2**). Each side of the heart has an upper chamber (atrium) and a lower chamber (ventricle), both of which pump blood. Blood leaves each chamber of a normal heart through a one-way valve, which keeps the blood moving in the proper direction by preventing backflow.

## Blood Vessels and Blood

As blood flows out of the heart, it passes into the aorta, the largest artery in the body. The arteries become smaller the farther they are from the heart. The smaller blood vessels that connect the arteries and capillaries are arterioles. Capillaries are small tubes, with the diameter of a single red blood cell, that pass among all the cells in the body, linking the arterioles and the venules. Blood leaving the distal side of the capillaries flows into the venules. These small, thin-walled vessels empty into the veins, and the veins then empty into the inferior and superior venae cavae. This is the process that returns blood in the venous portion of the circulatory system to

## YOU are the Provider

At 1620 hours, you are dispatched to a woodworking shop at 517 East Graham Street for a 32-year-old man with severe bleeding from the arm. The exact mechanism of injury (MOI) is unknown. You and your partner proceed to the scene with a response time of approximately 6 minutes.

**1.** What are the functions of arteries? What major arteries are located in the upper extremity?

**2.** Why is arterial bleeding more severe than venous bleeding?

the heart. Oxygen and nutrients easily pass from the capillaries into the cells, and waste and carbon dioxide diffuse from the cells into the capillaries (**FIGURE 26-3**). This transportation system allows the body to rid itself of waste products.

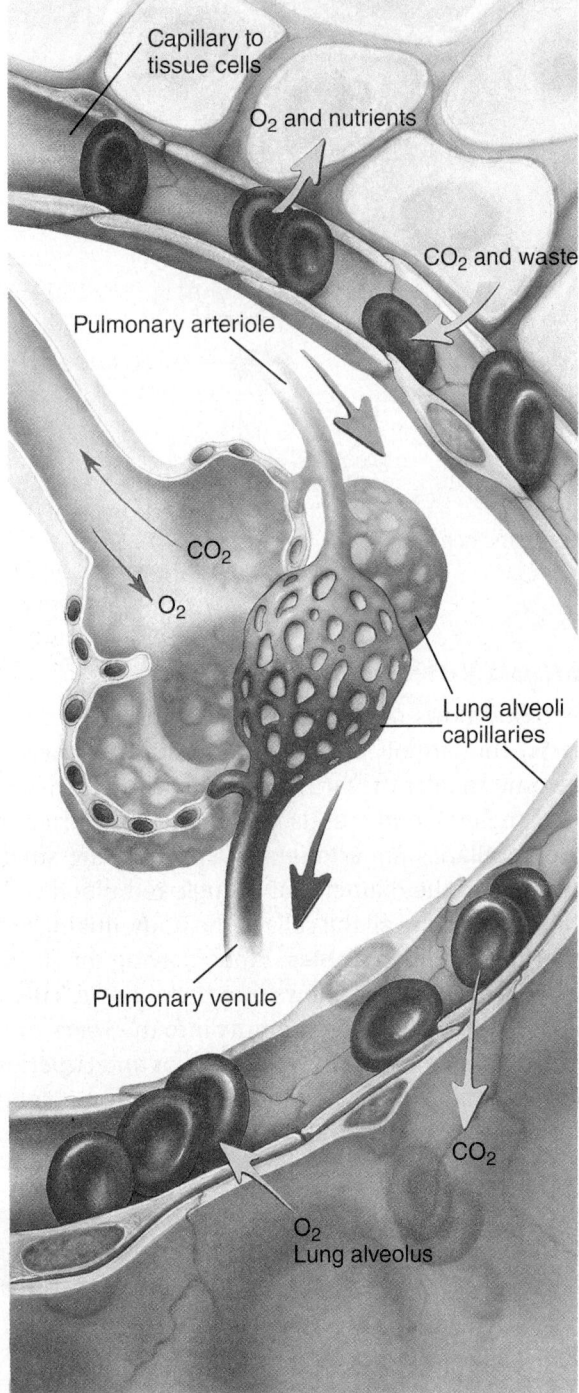

**FIGURE 26-3** Oxygen and nutrients pass easily from the capillaries into the cells, and waste and carbon dioxide diffuse from the cells into the capillaries (top). Oxygen and carbon dioxide pass freely between the lungs and capillaries (bottom).

Blood contains red cells, white cells, platelets, and plasma (**FIGURE 26-4**). Red blood cells transport oxygen to the cells and transport carbon dioxide (a waste product of cellular metabolism) away from the cells to the lungs, where it is removed from the body during exhalation. Platelets are the key to formation of blood clots. Blood clots are an important response from the body to control blood loss. In the body, blood clot formation depends on several factors: blood stasis, changes in the blood vessel wall (such as a wound), and the blood's ability to clot (affected by disease processes or medications). When tissues are injured, platelets begin to collect at the site of injury; this causes red blood cells to become sticky and clump together. As the red blood cells begin to clump, a protein in plasma reinforces the developing clot by converting to a threadlike mesh that forms a clot. Medical conditions that interfere with the normal clotting process will be discussed later in this chapter.

The autonomic nervous system monitors the body's needs and adjusts the blood flow by constricting or dilating blood vessels as required. During an emergency, the autonomic nervous system automatically redirects blood away from other organs to the heart, brain, lungs, and kidneys. Thus, the cardiovascular system adapts to changing conditions in the body to maintain homeostasis and perfusion. If blood volume is significantly diminished and the system fails to provide sufficient circulation for every body part to perform its function, then **hypoperfusion**, or **shock**, results. See

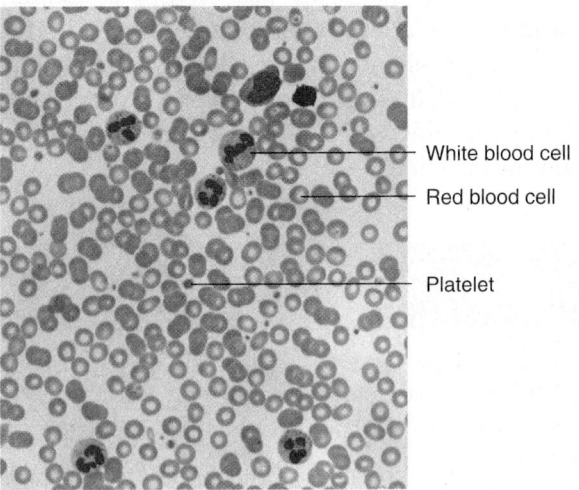

**FIGURE 26-4** The microscopic appearance of the three major elements in blood: red blood cells, white blood cells, and platelets.

Chapter 13, *Shock*, for a more detailed discussion of this process.

## Pathophysiology and Perfusion

**Perfusion** is the circulation of blood within an organ or tissue to allow it to meet the cells' current needs for oxygen, nutrients, and waste removal. Blood enters an organ or tissue first through the arteries, then the arterioles, and finally, the capillary beds (**FIGURE 26-5**). As it passes through the capillaries, the blood delivers nutrients and oxygen to the surrounding cells and picks up the wastes they have generated.

Blood must pass through the cardiovascular system fast enough to maintain adequate circulation throughout the body and to avoid clotting, yet slow enough to allow each cell time to exchange oxygen and nutrients for carbon dioxide and other waste products. Although some tissues never rest and require a constant blood supply, most require a large volume of circulating blood only intermittently, with less required when at rest. For example, skeletal muscles require a minimal blood supply during sleep, as opposed to a large blood supply during exercise. Another example is the gastrointestinal tract, which requires a high flow of blood after a meal. After digestion is completed, however, the gastrointestinal tract functions well with a small fraction of that blood flow.

All organs and organ systems of the human body depend on adequate perfusion to function properly. Some organs require a rich supply of blood and do not tolerate interruption of blood supply for even a few minutes without sustaining damage. If perfusion to these organs is interrupted, then dysfunction and failure of that organ system will occur. The death of an organ system can quickly lead to the death of the patient. Emergency medical care is designed to support adequate perfusion of these critical organs and organ systems, listed in **TABLE 26-1**, until the patient arrives at the hospital.

The heart requires constant perfusion to function optimally; without it, cells in the brain and spinal cord start to die after 4 to 6 minutes. (Remember that cells of the central nervous system do not have the capacity to regenerate.) Without adequate perfusion, the lungs can survive only 15 to 20 minutes and kidneys can be damaged after 45 minutes. Skeletal muscle demonstrates evidence of injury after 2 to 3 hours of inadequate perfusion, while the gastrointestinal tract can tolerate slightly longer periods. These times are based on a normal core body temperature (98.6°F [37.0°C]). An organ or tissue that is kept at a considerably lower temperature may be better able to resist damage from hypoperfusion.

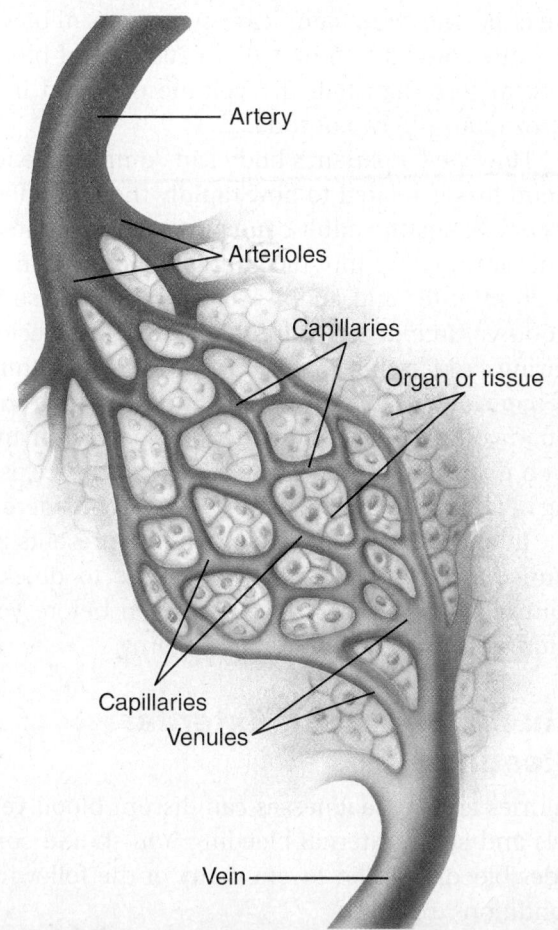

**FIGURE 26-5** Perfusion occurs when blood circulates through tissues or an organ to provide the necessary oxygen and nutrients and remove waste products.

© Jones & Bartlett Learning.

| TABLE 26-1 Critical Organs and Corresponding Organ Systems | |
| --- | --- |
| **Organ** | **Organ System** |
| Heart | Cardiovascular system |
| Brain | Central nervous system |
| Lungs | Respiratory system |
| Kidneys | Renal system |

© Jones & Bartlett Learning.

# External Bleeding

**Hemorrhage** means bleeding. External bleeding is visible hemorrhage. Examples include nosebleeds and bleeding from open wounds. As an EMT, you must understand how to control external bleeding.

## The Significance of External Bleeding

With serious external bleeding, it is often difficult to determine the amount of blood loss because blood will look different on different surfaces, such as when it is absorbed in clothing, when it has been diluted in water, or when the environment is dark. It is important to estimate the amount of external blood loss; however, treatment should be based on the patient's presentation and mechanism of injury (MOI).

The typical adult male body contains approximately 70 mL of blood per kilogram of body weight, whereas the adult female body contains approximately 65 mL of blood per kilogram of body weight. Therefore, a typical adult man weighing 175 pounds (79 kg) has a total blood volume of about 10 to 12 pints (6 L). The body cannot tolerate an acute blood loss of greater than 20% of this total blood volume, or more than 2 pints (approximately 1 L) in the average adult. With significant blood loss, adverse changes in vital signs will occur, including increased heart and respiratory rates and decreased blood pressure. Because infants and

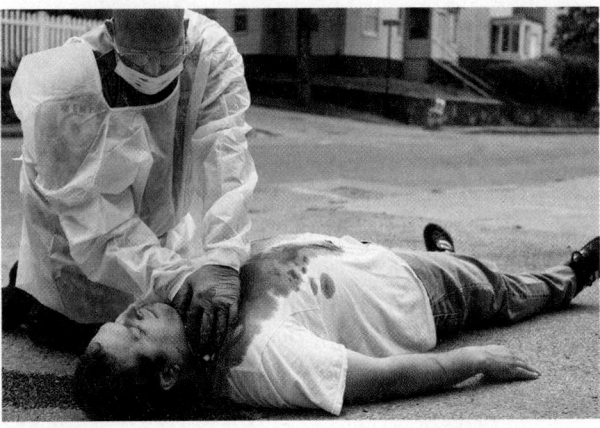

**FIGURE 26-6** Your safety is paramount. Always wear proper protective equipment when caring for a patient who is bleeding.

© Jones & Bartlett Learning.

children have less blood volume compared with adults, these effects are seen with smaller amounts of blood loss. For example, a 1-year-old has a typical total blood volume of about 27 oz (800 mL); the child will show significant symptoms of blood loss after only 3 to 6 oz (100 to 200 mL) of blood loss, or less than half the volume of liquid in a 12-oz (350-mL) can of soda.

How well a patient's body can compensate for blood loss is related to how rapidly the blood loss occurs. A healthy adult can comfortably donate 1 unit, or roughly 1 pint (500 mL) of blood within 15 to 20 minutes and adapt well to this decrease in blood volume. If this volume of blood loss occurs during a much shorter period, however, symptoms of **hypovolemic shock**, a condition in which low blood volume results in inadequate perfusion and even death, might develop. The age and preexisting health of the patient should also be considered.

In any situation, severe blood loss presents an immediate life threat. Your priority is to quickly control major external bleeding, even before you address airway and breathing concerns.

## Characteristics of External Bleeding

Injuries and some illnesses can disrupt blood vessels and cause external bleeding. You should consider bleeding to be severe if any of the following conditions exist:

- The patient has a poor general appearance and has no response to external stimuli.

## Safety Tips

Remember that a bleeding patient may expose you to potentially infectious body fluids; therefore, always follow standard precautions when treating patients with external bleeding. Wear gloves and eye protection in all situations, and wear a gown and mask if there is a risk of blood splatter (**FIGURE 26-6**). Always keep spare gloves with you. Avoid direct contact with body fluids if possible. Take special care if you have an open sore, cut, scratch, or ulcer. Also remember that frequent, thorough handwashing between patients and after every call is a simple yet important protective measure. When you care for multiple patients, remember to wash your hands frequently and don clean gloves between patients to avoid cross-contamination of body fluids and blood. If soap and water are unavailable, use a waterless hand sanitizer, and wash with soap and water as soon as possible.

- Assessment reveals signs and symptoms of shock (hypoperfusion).
- You note a significant amount of blood loss.
- The blood loss is rapid and ongoing.
- You cannot control the bleeding.
- The bleeding is associated with a significant MOI.

Typically, arterial bleeding from an open artery is bright red (because it is oxygen rich) and spurts in time with the pulse. The pressure that causes the blood to spurt also makes this type of bleeding difficult to control. As the amount of blood circulating in the body drops, so does the patient's blood pressure and, eventually, the arterial spurting.

Venous bleeding from an open vein is darker than arterial blood (because it is oxygen poor) and can flow slowly or rapidly, depending on the size of the vein. Because it is under less pressure, most venous blood does not spurt and is easier to manage; however, it can be profuse and life threatening. Capillary bleeding from damaged capillary vessels is dark red and oozes from a wound steadily but slowly. Venous and capillary blood is more likely to clot spontaneously than arterial blood (**FIGURE 26-7**).

On its own, bleeding tends to stop rather quickly, within about 10 minutes, in response to internal mechanisms and exposure to air. When a person's skin is broken, blood flows rapidly from the open blood vessel. Soon afterward, the cut ends of the blood vessel begin to narrow (**vasoconstriction**), reducing the amount of bleeding. Then a clot forms, plugging the hole and sealing the injured portions of the blood vessel. This process is called **coagulation**. With a severe injury, the damage to the blood vessel may be so great that a clot cannot completely block the hole. Bleeding will never stop if an effective clot does not form, unless the injured blood vessel is completely cut off from the main blood supply by direct pressure or a tourniquet.

Despite the efficiency of the circulatory system, it may fail in certain situations. Movement, disease process, certain medications (such as blood thinners), removal of bandages, the external environment, or body temperature commonly affect the blood's clotting factors. Occasionally, blood loss is very rapid. In these cases, the patient might die before clotting occurs.

A small portion of the population lacks one or more of the blood's clotting factors, a condition

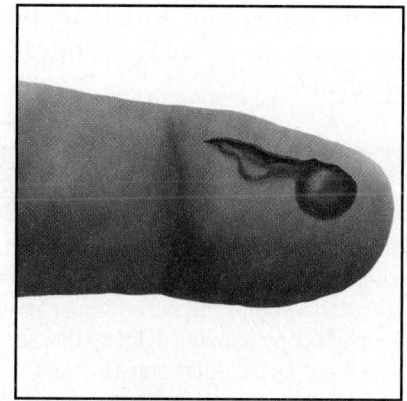

A

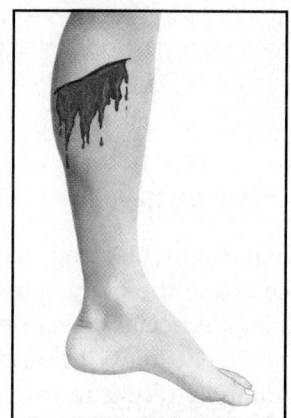

B

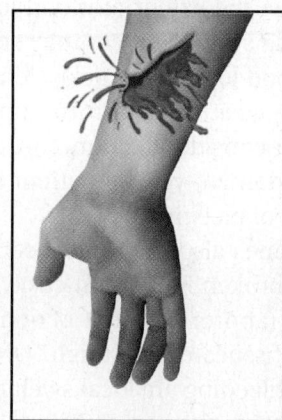

C

**FIGURE 26-7 A.** Bleeding from capillary vessels is dark red and oozes from the wound slowly but steadily. **B.** Venous bleeding is darker than arterial bleeding and flows steadily. **C.** Arterial bleeding is characteristically bright red and spurts in time with the pulse.

A, B, C: © Jones & Bartlett Learning.

called **hemophilia**. There are several forms of hemophilia, most of which are hereditary and some of which are severe. Sometimes bleeding occurs spontaneously in patients with hemophilia. Because the patient's blood does not clot effectively, all injuries, no matter how trivial, are potentially serious. Transport any injured patient with hemophilia immediately.

## Internal Bleeding

Internal bleeding is any bleeding that occurs in a cavity or space inside the body. Internal bleeding can be very serious, especially because it is not easy to detect immediately. Injury or damage to internal organs commonly results in extensive internal bleeding, which can cause hypovolemic shock before you realize the extent of blood loss. A person with a bleeding stomach ulcer may sustain a large amount of blood loss very quickly. Similarly, a person who has a lacerated liver or a ruptured spleen may sustain a considerable amount of blood loss within the abdomen, yet the patient may have no outward signs of bleeding.

Broken bones also may cause serious internal blood loss. A broken femur can easily result in the loss of 2 pints (approximately 1 L) or more of blood into the soft tissues of the thigh. Often, the only signs of such bleeding are local swelling and bruising (called a **contusion**, or **ecchymosis**) caused by the accumulation of blood around the ends of the broken bone. Severe pelvic fractures may result in life-threatening hemorrhage.

Always be alert to the possibility of internal bleeding. Assess the patient for related signs and

symptoms, particularly if the MOI is significant. If you suspect that a patient is bleeding internally, treat for shock and promptly transport him or her to the hospital.

## Mechanism of Injury for Internal Bleeding

A high-energy MOI should increase your index of suspicion for the possibility of serious, unseen injuries such as internal bleeding in the abdominal cavity. Internal bleeding is possible whenever the MOI suggests that severe forces affected the body. These forces include blunt and penetrating trauma. Internal bleeding commonly occurs as a result of falls, blast injuries, motor vehicle crashes, and other blunt trauma. Remember that internal bleeding can also result from penetrating trauma.

As you assess a patient, look for signs of injury using the DCAP-BTLS as well as any other signs of injury. Always suspect internal bleeding in a patient who has sustained a penetrating injury or blunt trauma.

## Nature of Illness for Internal Bleeding

Internal bleeding is not always caused by trauma. Many illnesses can cause internal bleeding. Some of the more common causes of nontraumatic internal bleeding include bleeding ulcers, bleeding from the colon, ruptured ectopic pregnancy, and aneurysms.

Abdominal tenderness, guarding, rigidity, pain, and distention are frequent in these situations but are not always present. In older patients, dizziness, faintness, or weakness may be the first sign of nontraumatic internal bleeding. Ulcers or other gastrointestinal problems may cause vomiting of blood or bloody diarrhea.

It is not as important for you to know the specific organ involved as it is to recognize that the patient is in shock. When combined with prompt transport decisions and limited time spent at the scene, the rapid recognition of a patient in shock should result in the rapid administration of potentially life-saving treatments.

## Signs and Symptoms of Internal Bleeding

The most common symptom of internal bleeding is pain. Significant internal bleeding will generally cause swelling in the area of bleeding, but swelling is often undetected until massive blood loss has occurred. Internal bleeding is most common in head, extremity, and pelvic injuries and is often associated with significant abdominal trauma. Intra-abdominal bleeding will often cause pain and abdominal distention. Bleeding into the chest cavity or lung may cause dyspnea, tachycardia, **hemoptysis** (the coughing up of bright red blood), and hypotension. A **hematoma**, a mass of blood that has collected in the soft tissues beneath the skin, indicates bleeding into soft tissues and may be the result of a minor or a severe injury. Bruising or ecchymosis may not be present initially, and the only sign of severe pelvic or abdominal trauma may be redness, skin abrasions, or pain.

Bleeding from any body opening, however slight, is serious. It usually indicates internal bleeding that is not easy to see or control. Bright red bleeding from the mouth or rectum or blood in the urine (**hematuria**) may suggest serious internal injury or disease. Nonmenstrual vaginal bleeding is always significant.

## Street Smarts

EMTs must be able to provide emotional support to patients in an emergency, especially patients who are in life-threatening situations or extreme mental distress or pain.

Other signs and symptoms of internal bleeding in trauma and medical patients include the following:

- **Hematemesis.** The vomiting of blood. The vomitus may be bright red or dark red. If the blood has been partially digested, the vomitus may look like coffee grounds.
- **Melena.** Black, foul-smelling, tarry stool that contains digested blood.
- **Pain, tenderness, bruising, guarding, or swelling.** These signs and symptoms, particularly in an extremity, may mean that a closed fracture is bleeding.
- **Broken ribs, bruises over the lower part of the chest, or a rigid, distended abdomen.** These signs and symptoms may indicate a lacerated spleen or liver. Patients with an injury to one of these organs may have referred pain in the right shoulder (indicating the liver is injured) or left shoulder (indicating the spleen is

injured). Suspect internal abdominal bleeding in a patient with referred pain.

The first sign of hypovolemic shock is a change in mental status, such as anxiety, restlessness, or combativeness. In nontrauma patients, weakness, faintness, or dizziness on standing can all be early signs. Changes in skin color or pallor (pale skin) are often seen in both trauma and medical patients with severe bleeding. Later signs of hypovolemic shock suggesting internal bleeding include the following:

- Tachycardia
- Weakness, fainting, or dizziness at rest
- Thirst
- Nausea and vomiting
- Cold, moist (clammy) skin
- Shallow, rapid breathing
- Dull eyes
- Slightly dilated pupils that are slow to respond to light
- Capillary refill time longer than 2 seconds in infants and children
- Weak, rapid (thready) pulse
- Decreasing blood pressure
- Altered level of consciousness

Patients with these signs and symptoms, particularly in the setting of significant MOI, require prompt transport, preferably to a trauma center. See Chapter 13, *Shock*, for a review of hypovolemic shock.

## Patient Assessment for External and Internal Bleeding

### Scene Size-Up

As you approach the patient, be alert to potential hazards to yourself and the crew, bystanders, and the patient. At vehicle crashes, ensure there are no fluids leaking from the vehicle or energized power lines in the area where you will be working. In incidents involving violence, such as assaults or patients with gunshot wounds, make sure that police have advised the scene is safe. You may need to stage several blocks away until law enforcement personnel have secured the area.

Follow standard precautions. Place several spare pairs of gloves in your pocket for easy access in case your gloves tear or there are multiple patients with bleeding. If you enter a residence, be alert for anxious bystanders, family members, and even pets, as they may become hostile. Determine the number of patients needing care. Consider early on what additional resources you may need, and verify as you begin your assessment.

Determine the nature of the illness (NOI) by observing signs (such as bloody emesis) or the MOI (such as an upturned step stool). Consider the need for spinal motion restriction and/or additional resources, such as an advanced life support unit. Be sure to also consider environmental factors in your decision making. For example, caring for a sick or injured victim of a motor vehicle crash on a clear, sunny day is different from treating the same victim during a snowstorm. Extremely hot or cold weather can worsen a patient's overall condition.

## Special Populations

In older patients, dizziness, syncope, or weakness may be the first sign of nontraumatic internal hemorrhage.

## Primary Assessment

When you treat a patient who has experienced significant blood loss from a visible wound or with suspected internal bleeding, do not be distracted from identifying and managing life threats, which is the focus of your primary assessment. As you approach a trauma patient, note important indicators that may signal the seriousness of the patient's condition. For example, a patient with external bleeding may have bloodstains on his or her clothing. Be aware of obvious signs of injury and distress, such as facial grimace. Determine the patient's sex and age.

Perform a rapid exam of the patient, look for life threats, and treat them as you find them. If the patient has obvious, life-threatening external bleeding, remember to address it *first* (even before airway and breathing) by controlling it quickly; then assess the XABCs and provide treatment. If direct pressure is ineffective in controlling massive hemorrhage from an arm or leg, the patient may require a tourniquet before the airway is opened. Next, assess skin color: cool, moist skin that is pale or gray suggests a perfusion problem. Because skin paleness can be difficult to detect in patients with dark skin, instead check for pale mucous membranes inside the inner lower eyelid or slow capillary refill. Determine the patient's level of consciousness using the AVPU scale. Does the patient have a patent (open) airway? If the patient is able to speak, this indicates that the airway is patent. What is the mental status of the patient? These indicators will help you assess how sick the patient is, which will help you develop an index of suspicion for serious illness or injuries related to internal bleeding.

Consider the need for spinal motion restriction. At the same time, ensure a patent airway, look for adequate breathing, and check for breath sounds. If necessary, provide the patient with high-flow oxygen or assist ventilation with a bag-mask device or nonrebreathing mask, depending on the patient's level of consciousness and rate and quality of breathing. If the patient is unconscious, the airway may be obstructed. Insert an oropharyngeal (oral) airway to secure the airway.

## Words of Wisdom

Non–life-threatening bleeding, such as from an abrasion, can be bandaged later in the assessment as necessary. However, significant and ongoing bleeding, whether internal or external, is an immediate life threat.

Quickly assess pulse rate and quality; determine the condition, color, and temperature of the skin; and check the capillary refill time to help establish the potential for internal bleeding and shock. Treat the patient for shock, if needed, by applying oxygen, improving circulation, and maintaining a normal body temperature.

The results of your initial general impression and your assessment of the XABCs will help you decide whether to manage the patient on scene or transport immediately and manage the patient en route to the hospital. If the patient has signs and symptoms of internal bleeding or airway or breathing problems, provide rapid transport to the most appropriate facility. The condition of patients with significant bleeding may quickly become unstable. Signs such as tachycardia, tachypnea, low blood pressure, weak pulse, and clammy skin are signs of impending circulatory collapse and indicate the need for rapid transport.

## History Taking

After the primary assessment is complete, investigate the chief complaint and be alert for signs or symptoms of other injuries based on the MOI and/or NOI. Remember, internal bleeding can be found in both medical and trauma patients. For example, ectopic pregnancy, gastrointestinal bleeding, bleeding from a dialysis shunt, and severe nosebleed are medical causes of potential internal bleeding. If signs and symptoms of internal bleeding are not obvious, look more carefully during the patient assessment process. In a responsive trauma patient with an isolated injury and a limited MOI, consider a detailed physical examination of the specific area after you assess vital signs and obtain a history.

### Street Smarts

Practice good communication skills. If you're thinking something, say so. If you know something, share it. If your patient is telling you something, listen. Good communication can reduce duplication of effort, decrease scene time, and improve patient care.

When you encounter a patient with minor or superficial bleeding, avoid focusing solely on the bleeding. With significant trauma, assess the entire patient, looking for the source of the problem, any preexisting illnesses, and other issues.

If the patient is responsive, obtain a SAMPLE history. It is important to ask the patient if he or she takes blood-thinning medications because bleeding is generally more profuse and difficult to control in patients who take blood thinners. Blood thinners are often prescribed for patients with a history of stroke, pulmonary embolism, or heart attack. Common blood thinners include antiplatelets such as aspirin, clopidogrel (Plavix), and ticagrelor (Brilinta), and anticoagulants such as warfarin (Coumadin), rivaroxaban (Xarelto), dabigatran (Pradaxa), apixaban (Eliquis), and edoxaban (Savaysa).

If the patient is unresponsive, obtain medical history information from medical alert tags or ask family members or bystanders if they have any information. Look for signs and symptoms of hypoperfusion and determine how much blood loss has occurred.

### Secondary Assessment

Unless you discover a life-threatening condition during the primary assessment, next conduct a secondary assessment, which is a detailed, comprehensive examination of the patient to uncover injuries or illness that may have been missed during the primary assessment. Record vital signs, complete an assessment of pain, and attach appropriate monitoring devices to quantify oxygenation and circulatory status. In some instances, such as a critically injured patient or a short transport time, there may not be time to conduct a secondary assessment, as this is generally conducted en route to the hospital.

Assess all areas of the body for DCAP-BTLS to identify underlying or secondary injuries. For

### YOU are the Provider

You arrive at the scene and find the patient standing outside in front of the shop. He has a towel wrapped around his left wrist; it is soaked in blood and you can see a large amount of blood on the ground. He is conscious and alert but anxious. He tells you he cut his wrist on a table saw when his arm slipped and ran into the blade.

| Recording Time: 0 Minutes | |
| --- | --- |
| **Appearance** | Anxious |
| **Level of consciousness** | Conscious and alert |
| **Airway** | Open; clear of secretions or foreign bodies |
| **Breathing** | Increased rate; adequate depth |
| **Circulation** | Bleeding from the left wrist; skin is cool, pale, and dry; pulse is rapid and strong |

**3.** Is the patient effectively controlling the bleeding from his injury?

**4.** What should be your initial treatment priority?

isolated injuries such as pain in the ankle, assess that area only (detailed physical examination). When examining the head, be alert for uncontrolled bleeding from large scalp lacerations. In the abdomen, feel all four quadrants for tenderness or rigidity. In the extremities, record pulse, motor, and sensory function.

Obtain baseline vital signs; this allows you to more easily identify any changes that may occur during treatment. In an adult patient, a systolic blood pressure of less than 100 mm Hg with a weak, rapid pulse and cool, moist skin that is pale or gray are signs of hypoperfusion that require immediate attention. In patients with dark skin, because skin paleness may be difficult to detect, you may instead need to assess for paleness of the mucous membranes or slow capillary refill.

## Special Populations

In geriatric patients and patients who take certain blood pressure medications, the pulse rate may not increase with early shock; therefore, try to determine the patient's baseline blood pressure and quickly obtain a medical history and list of medications to help you better assess the patient's condition.

## Reassessment

Because the signs and symptoms of internal bleeding are often slow to develop, it is important to reassess the patient frequently. Children especially will compensate well for blood loss and then crash quickly. The reassessment is your best opportunity to determine whether your patient's condition is improving or getting worse and to determine the effectiveness of any interventions and treatments. Reassess an unstable patient every 5 minutes and a stable patient every 15 minutes.

Whenever you suspect significant bleeding, either external or internal, and signs of shock are present provide high-flow oxygen. If significant bleeding is visible, control external bleeding (shown later in Skill Drill 26-1). Using multiple methods to control external bleeding usually works best. If the patient has signs of hypoperfusion, provide aggressive treatment for shock and rapid transport to the appropriate hospital. If internal bleeding is suspected, apply high-flow oxygen via a nonrebreathing mask and provide rapid transport to the hospital. (See Skill Drill 26-5 for additional steps.)

Do not delay transport of a patient to complete an assessment, particularly when significant bleeding is present, even if the bleeding is controlled. The assessment can be started during transport.

In patients with severe external bleeding, it is important to recognize, estimate, and report the amount of blood loss that has occurred and how rapidly or over what period of time it occurred. For example, you may report that approximately 2 pints (approximately 1 L) of blood loss occurred or that the bleeding soaked through three trauma dressings. Report this information to hospital personnel during transport to allow the hospital to evaluate needed resources, such as the availability of surgical suites, surgeons, and other specialty providers. Your transfer report at the hospital should update hospital personnel on how your patient has responded to your care. Be sure your paperwork reflects all of the patient's injuries and the care you have provided.

## Emergency Medical Care for External Bleeding

Before you care for a patient with obvious external bleeding, remember to follow standard precautions. This includes gloves and eye protection at a minimum and may include a mask and gown. As with all patient care, make sure the patient has an open airway and is breathing adequately. Provide high-flow oxygen, if indicated, and control bleeding. If obvious, life-threatening bleeding is present, control it as quickly as possible. These assessments and interventions should, ideally, take place simultaneously in situations where adequate resources are available.

## Words of Wisdom

It is best to don gloves and eye protection before you enter the scene. By the time you realize that you need them, it is often too late.

Several methods are available to control external bleeding:

- Direct pressure
- Pressure dressings and/or splints
- Tourniquets
- Junctional tourniquet
- Hemostatic dressing
- Wound packing

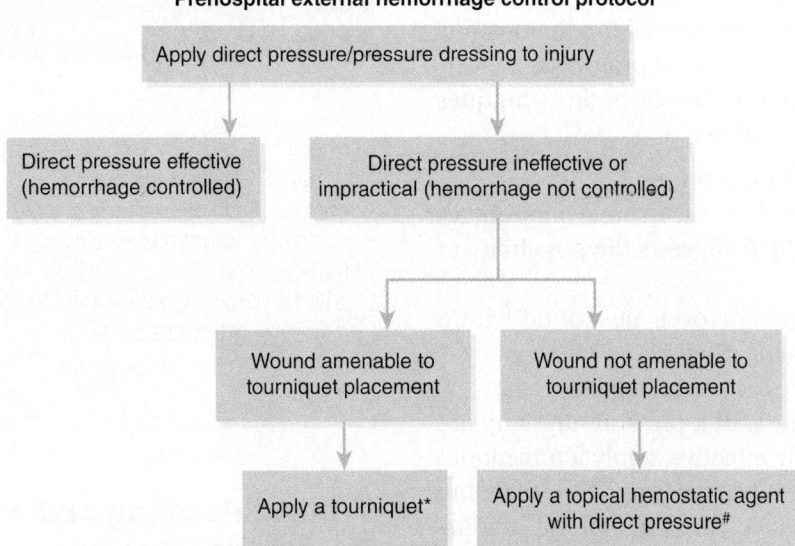

*Use of tourniquet for extremity hemorrhage is strongly recommended if sustained direct pressure is ineffective or impractical; Use a commercially-produced, windlass, pneumatic, or ratcheting device, which has been demonstrated to occlude arterial flow and avoid narrow, elastic, or bungee-type devices; Utilize improvised tourniquets only if no commercial device is available; Do not release a properly-applied tourniquet until the patient reaches definitive care.

#Apply a topical hemostatic agent, in combination with direct pressure, for wounds in anatomic areas where tourniquets can not be applied and sustained direct pressure alone is ineffective or impractical; Only apply topical hemostatic agents in a gauze format that supports wound packing; Only utilize topical hemostatic agents which have been determined to be effective and safe in a standardized laboratory injury model.

**FIGURE 26-8** Steps of bleeding control.

To control bleeding, follow the steps shown in **FIGURE 26-8**. Begin with direct pressure, and move to the next steps if direct pressure does not control the bleeding.

Most cases of external bleeding can be controlled simply by applying direct, local pressure to the bleeding site. This method is by far the most common way to control external bleeding and is usually effective. (Previously, elevation of the extremity was also recommended, but there is no evidence it helps control bleeding and it may aggravate other injuries.) Pressure stops the flow of blood and permits normal coagulation to occur. You may apply pressure with your gloved fingertip or hand over the top of a sterile dressing if one is immediately available. If there is an object protruding from the wound, never remove it unless it is in the cheek and blocking the patient's airway. Apply bulky dressings to stabilize the impaled object in place, and apply pressure as best you can for at least 5 minutes without interruption.

In most cases, direct pressure will stop the bleeding. Once you have applied a dressing to control bleeding, create a pressure dressing to maintain the pressure by firmly wrapping a sterile, self-adhering roller bandage around the entire wound. Use 4 × 4–inch (101 × 101–mm) sterile gauze pads for small wounds and sterile universal dressings for larger wounds.

Cover the entire dressing with the bandage above and below the wound and stretch the bandage tight enough to control bleeding. If you were able to palpate a distal pulse before applying the dressing, then you should still be able to palpate a distal pulse on the injured extremity after applying the pressure dressing. If bleeding continues, then the dressing is insufficient. If the bleeding oozes slowly through the dressing, then reinforce it by applying more dressings on top of it. Do not remove a dressing until a physician has evaluated the patient.

Bleeding will almost always stop when the pressure of the dressing exceeds arterial pressure. This will assist in controlling bleeding and helping blood to clot.

If direct pressure fails to immediately stop hemorrhage, then apply a tourniquet above the level of the bleeding. If this is not possible because the bleeding is too proximal, then consider a junctional tourniquet or wound packing with a hemostatic dressing if available (follow local protocols).

**SKILL DRILL 26-1** illustrates the basic techniques to control external bleeding:

1. Follow standard precautions.
2. Maintain the airway with spinal motion restriction if the MOI suggests the possibility of spinal injury.
3. Apply direct pressure over the wound with a dry, sterile dressing (**Step 1**).
4. Apply a pressure dressing (**Step 2**).
5. If direct pressure and a pressure dressing are not immediately effective, apply a tourniquet to an extremity above the level of the bleeding (**Step 3**). NOTE: For life-threatening hemorrhage in an area where standard tourniquet application is not possible (such as axial or inguinal sites), consider wound packing or a junctional tourniquet per local protocols.
6. Tighten the tourniquet until bleeding stops (**Step 4**). Position the patient supine unless there is a reason not to—for example, underlying respiratory distress.
7. Apply high-flow oxygen, as necessary, once hemorrhage is controlled. Keep the patient warm. Transport promptly.

## Words of Wisdom

Much of the bleeding associated with broken bones occurs because the sharp ends of the bones cut muscles and other tissues. As long as a fracture remains unstable, the bone ends will move and continue to injure partially clotted blood vessels. Therefore, immobilizing a fracture and decreasing movement will help control bleeding. Often, a simple splint will quickly reduce the bleeding associated with a fracture (**FIGURE 26-9**). If the patient is unstable, however, do not spend excess time splinting a fracture.

## Wound Packing and Hemostatic Dressings

Gauze can be packed into larger wounds to control hemorrhage when direct pressure is not adequate or application of a tourniquet is not possible. A **hemostatic dressing** is a dressing impregnated with a chemical compound that slows or stops bleeding by promoting clot formation.

Hemostatic dressings can be used together with wound packing and direct pressure when direct pressure alone is ineffective, such as with massive abdominal injuries, or when tourniquet placement

## YOU are the Provider

You immediately apply direct pressure to the patient's wrist with a dry, sterile dressing, and apply a pressure dressing. This effectively controls the patient's bleeding. While you further assess the patient and apply a splint, your partner applies high-flow oxygen, obtains the patient's vital signs, and inquires about his medical history. The patient denies having any medical problems and states he does not take any medications.

| Recording Time: 5 Minutes | |
| --- | --- |
| **Respirations** | 24 breaths/min; regular and adequate |
| **Pulse** | 120 beats/min; strong and regular |
| **Skin** | Cool, pale, and dry |
| **Blood pressure** | 104/60 mm Hg |
| **Oxygen saturation (SpO$_2$)** | 94% (on oxygen) |

5. What are the components of the cardiovascular system and how are they affected by the patient's injury?
6. What factors determine the severity of external bleeding?

## Skill Drill 26-1 Controlling External Bleeding

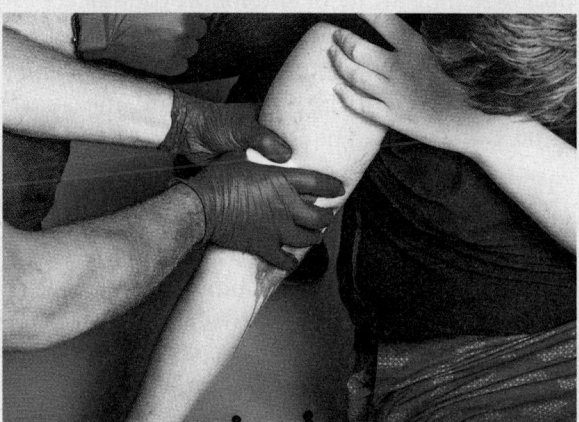

### Step 1

Take standard precautions. Apply direct pressure over the wound with a dry, sterile dressing.

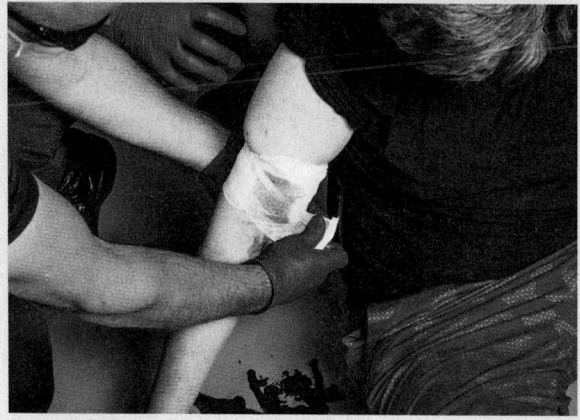

### Step 2

Apply a pressure dressing.

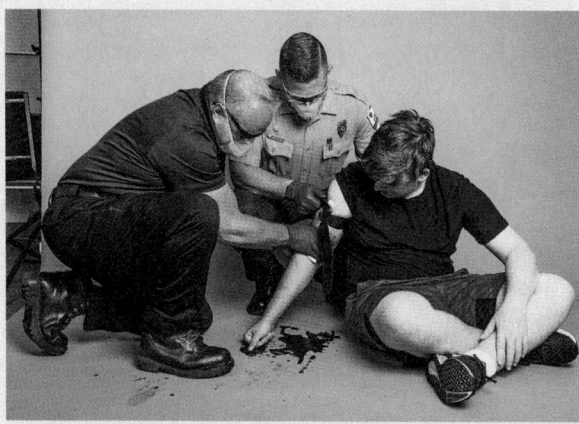

### Step 3

If direct pressure with a pressure dressing does not control bleeding, apply a tourniquet above the level of the bleeding.

© Jones & Bartlett Learning.

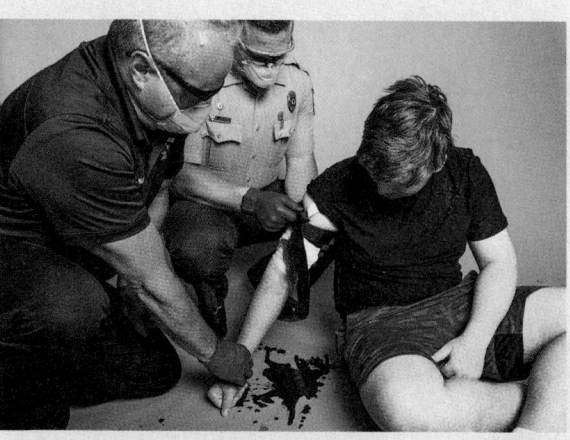

### Step 4

Tighten the tourniquet until bleeding is controlled and pulses are no longer palpable distal to the tourniquet. Properly position the patient. Apply high-flow oxygen as necessary. Keep the patient warm. Transport promptly.

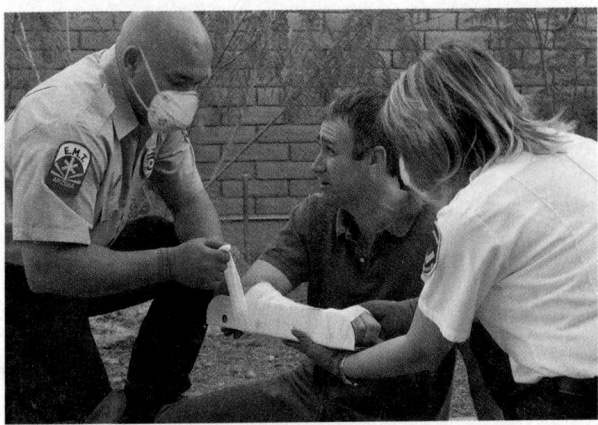

**FIGURE 26-9** Use of a simple splint will often quickly control bleeding associated with a fracture. If a fracture is not immobilized, then the bone ends are free to move and may continue to injure partially clotted blood vessels.

© Jones & Bartlett Learning. Courtesy of MIEMSS.

is otherwise impossible. These dressings have the potential to improve prehospital bleeding control, especially when transport time to definitive care is prolonged. Be aware of and follow your local protocols regarding use of wound packing and hemostatic dressings.

Follow your local protocols and the steps in **SKILL DRILL 26-2** to pack a wound.

1. Follow standard precautions.
2. Remove or open the patient's clothing as needed to expose the wound (**Step 1**).
3. Wipe away any pooled blood.
4. Pack the wound tightly with hemostatic gauze (preferred) or plain gauze (**Step 2**).
5. Apply steady pressure by pressing with both hands directly on top of the bleeding wound. Push down as hard as you can (**Step 3**).

# Skill Drill 26-2 Packing a Wound

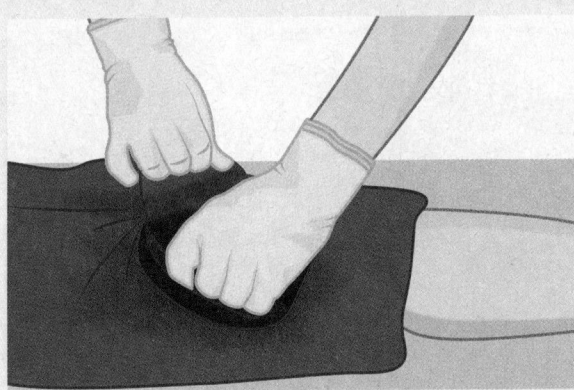

**Step 1**

Expose the wound and wipe away any pooled blood.

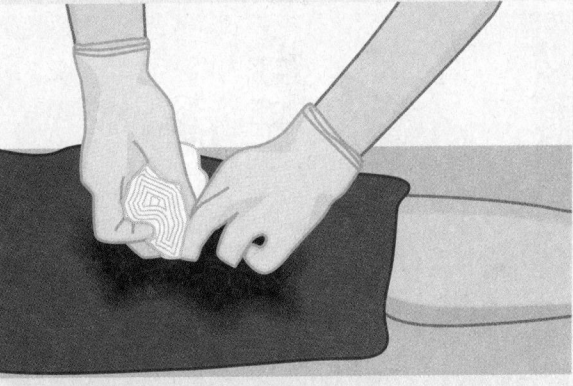

**Step 2**

Pack the wound tightly with hemostatic gauze (preferred), plain gauze, or a clean cloth.

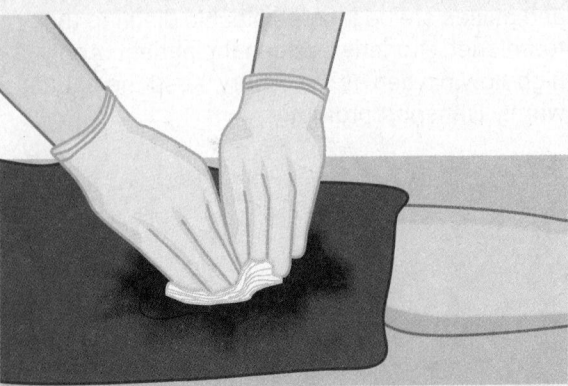

**Step 3**

Apply steady pressure by pressing with both hands directly on top of the bleeding wound. Push down as hard as you can.

© Jones & Bartlett Learning.

6. Continue holding pressure until relieved by another prehospital provider or the patient is delivered to definitive care.

## Tourniquets

If direct pressure does not control extremity bleeding, then use a tourniquet. The tourniquet is only useful if a patient has substantial bleeding from an extremity injury. Several different types of commercial tourniquets are available (**FIGURE 26-10**). Make sure you are familiar with the type of tourniquet used by your service.

Follow the manufacturer's instructions for the specific type of tourniquet used by your service.

Follow the steps in **SKILL DRILL 26-3** to apply a commercial tourniquet.

1. Follow standard precautions.
2. Apply direct pressure over the bleeding site.
3. Place the tourniquet around the extremity high and tight, proximal to the bleeding site (in the axillary region for upper extremity injuries and at the groin for lower extremity injuries) (**Step 1**).

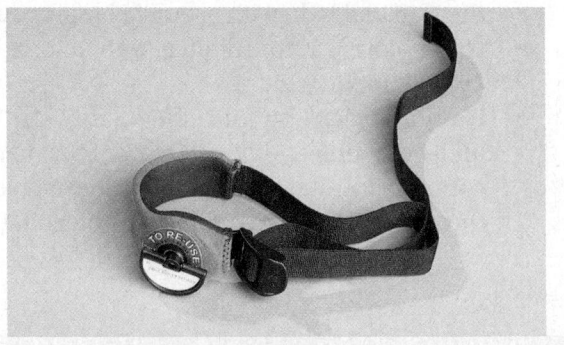

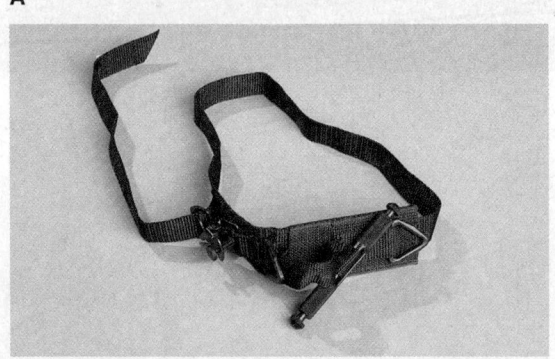

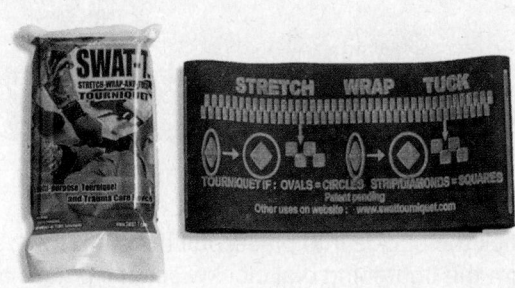

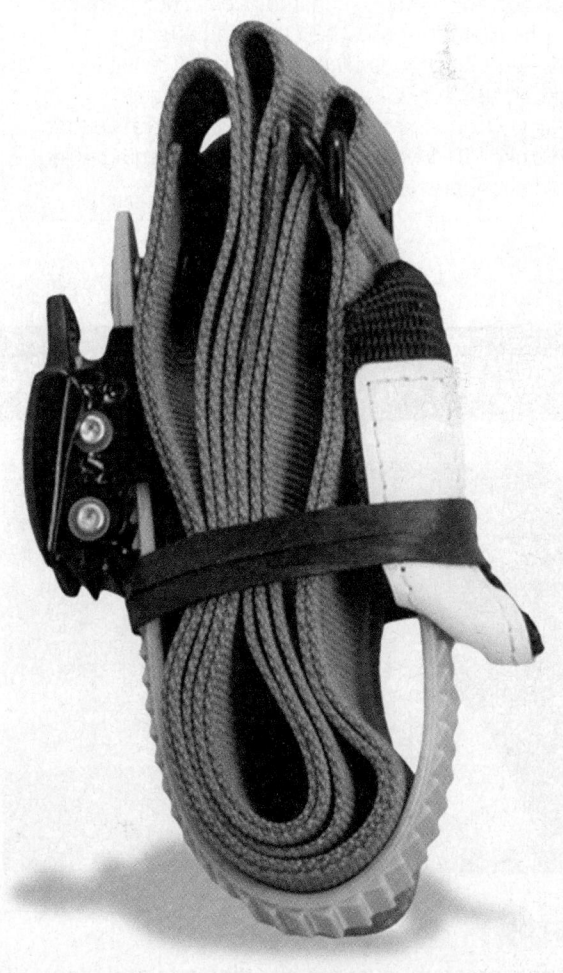

**FIGURE 26-10** Different examples of commercial tourniquets. **A.** Mechanical advantage tourniquet (MAT). **B.** Combat application tourniquet (CAT). **C.** Ratcheting medical tourniquet (RMT). **D.** Special weapons and tactics tourniquet (SWAT-T).

A, B: © Jones & Bartlett Learning; C, D: Photo by Diane Zahorodny. Courtesy of Chinook Medical Gear.

4. Click the buckle into place and pull the strap tight.
5. Turn the tightening dial or windlass clockwise until pulses are no longer palpable distal to the tourniquet or until bleeding has been controlled (**Step 2**).
6. Do not release a tourniquet once applied, unless instructed to do so by medical control.

### Words of Wisdom

If the patient has an open fracture of an extremity, bleeding can be substantial. Consider a tourniquet early if bleeding is not easily controlled with direct pressure or if pressure results in excessive pain. The method used to control severe external bleeding may be governed by local protocols, but regardless of the method, it must be quick and effective. Remember, uncontrolled bleeding may result in shock and death. Patients can bleed to death quickly from extremity injuries. It is imperative that you use effective techniques to stop bleeding when you encounter it.

Whenever you apply a tourniquet, make sure you observe the following precautions:

- Do not apply a tourniquet directly over any joint. Always place the tourniquet proximal to the injury (in the axillary region for upper extremity injuries and at the groin for lower extremity injuries).
- If the tourniquet does not immediately control bleeding, apply a second one adjacent to the first.
- Make sure the tourniquet is tightened securely.
- Never use wire, rope, a belt, or any other narrow material that could cut into the skin.
- If it is possible to do so without causing a delay, consider placing padding under the tourniquet as you apply it. This step may protect the skin and help with arterial compression.
- Never cover a tourniquet with a bandage. Leave it in full view.
- Do not loosen the tourniquet after you have applied it, unless directed to do so by medical control. Hospital personnel will loosen it once they are prepared to manage the bleeding.

## Skill Drill 26-3 Applying a Commercial Tourniquet

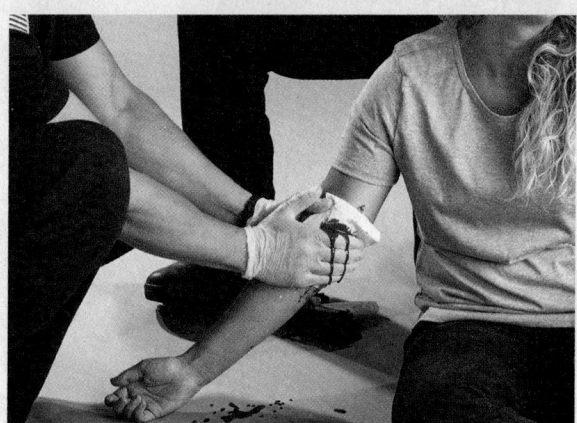

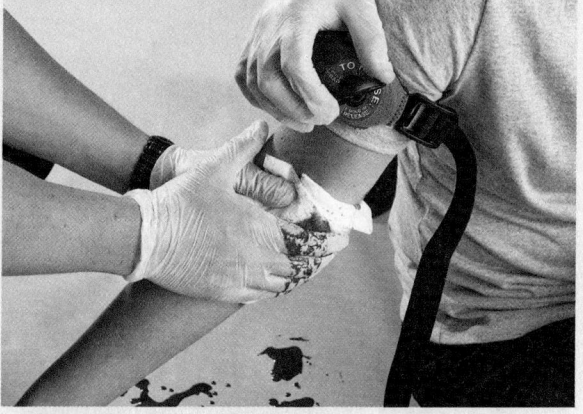

**Step 1**

Apply pressure over the bleeding site and place the tourniquet proximal to the injury (in the axillary region for upper extremity injuries and at the groin for lower extremity injuries).

© Jones & Bartlett Learning.

**Step 2**

Click the buckle into place, pull the strap tight, and turn the tightening dial clockwise until pulses are no longer palpable distal to the tourniquet and until bleeding has been controlled.

Mark the exact time the tourniquet was applied and be sure to communicate the time of application, the site of application, and the rationale for application clearly and specifically to hospital personnel on arrival.

## Junctional Tourniquets

A **junctional tourniquet** allows for proximal compression of life-threatening bleeding in areas where standard tourniquet application is not possible, such as the groin or the axilla. A junctional tourniquet may be indicated for severe hemorrhage at the junction of the torso with the arms (axillary area) or legs (inguinal area). Use of junctional tourniquets have been approved by the Food and Drug Administration for use in prehospital medicine and have been shown to be at least 75% effective in controlling hemorrhage when used properly. Some junctional tourniquets may also be used as a pelvic binder for suspected unstable pelvic fractures. Junctional tourniquets are presently used primarily in military and tactical settings.

## Splints

Air splints (commonly known as soft splints or pressure splints) can help control internal or external bleeding associated with severe extremity injuries, such as fractures (**FIGURE 26-11**). They also immobilize the fracture itself. An air splint acts in a manner similar to a pressure dressing applied to an entire extremity rather than to a small, local area. Use only approved, clean, or disposable valve stems when orally inflating air splints.

## Pelvic Binder

Use of a pelvic binder (pelvic compression device) is now common in prehospital care (**FIGURE 26-12**). A **pelvic binder** is a type of splint that may be indicated for a suspected closed unstable pelvic fracture. Research indicates that a pelvic binder is an effective method to reduce the width of and to stabilize pelvic ring injuries. This helps to control internal bleeding, specifically bleeding associated with a life-threatening **open-book pelvic fracture**. It is applied when pelvic fracture is suspected and the patient has signs of shock.

To apply a pelvic binder, slide the binder under the supine patient with the device centered over the trochanters (hips). Secure and tighten the device according to manufacturer's instructions. It is important to provide the correct amount of force when applying a compression device.

Pediatric patients who weigh less than 50 pounds (23 kg) may be too small for an adult pelvic binder; however, there are commercial pediatric pelvic binders available. Follow local protocols regarding use of a pelvic binder.

Rigid splints will help immobilize fractures as well as reduce pain and further damage to soft tissues. After you have applied a splint, be sure to monitor pulse and motor and sensory function in the distal extremity.

## Bleeding From the Nose, Ears, and Mouth

Bleeding around the face always presents a risk for airway obstruction or aspiration. Maintain a clear

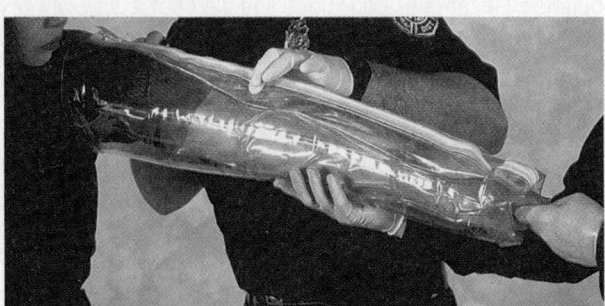

**FIGURE 26-11** Air splints can also be used to control bleeding because they act as a pressure bandage for the entire extremity. They are not as effective as tourniquets, however, and should never be used when a tourniquet is otherwise indicated.

© Jones & Bartlett Learning. Courtesy of MIEMSS.

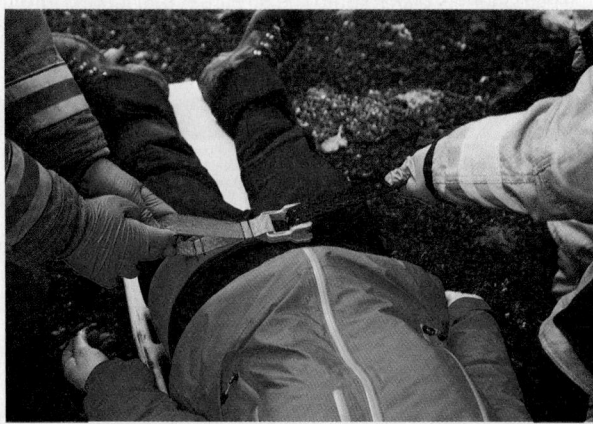

**FIGURE 26-12** A pelvic compression device or binder.

SAM Medical Products®.

airway by positioning the patient appropriately and using suction when indicated. Several conditions can result in bleeding from the nose, ears, and/or mouth, including the following:

- Fracture of the base of the skull
- Facial injuries, including those caused by a direct blow to the nose
- Sinusitis, infections, nose drop use and abuse, dried or cracked nasal mucosa, intranasal use of street drugs (snorting), or other abnormalities
- High blood pressure
- Coagulation disorders
- Digital trauma (nose picking)
- Cancer

**Epistaxis**, or nosebleed, is a common emergency. Occasionally, it can cause blood loss great enough to send a patient into shock. Keep in mind that the blood that is visible may be only a small part of the total blood loss. Much of the blood may pass down the throat into the stomach as the patient swallows. A person who swallows a large amount of blood may become nauseated and start vomiting the blood, which is sometimes confused with internal bleeding. Most nontraumatic nosebleeds occur from sites in the septum (the tissue dividing the nostrils). You can usually handle this type of bleeding effectively by pinching the nostrils together. **SKILL DRILL 26-4** illustrates the basic techniques to control epistaxis.

1. Follow standard precautions.
2. Help the patient to sit, leaning forward, with the head tilted forward. This position stops the blood from trickling down the throat or being aspirated into the lungs.
3. Apply direct pressure for at least 15 minutes by pinching the fleshy part of the nostrils together. This is the preferred method. This technique may also be performed by the patient (**Step 1**).
4. Another option is to place a rolled 4 × 4–inch (101 × 101–mm) gauze bandage between the upper lip and the gum. Have the patient apply pressure by stretching the upper lip tightly against the rolled bandage and pushing it up into and against the nose. If the patient is unable to do this effectively, use your gloved fingers to press the gauze against the gum (**Step 2**).
5. Keep the patient calm and quiet, especially if he or she has high blood pressure or is anxious. Anxiety tends to increase blood pressure, which could worsen the nosebleed.
6. Apply ice over the nose.
7. Maintain the pressure until the bleeding is completely controlled, usually no more than 15 minutes if this is the patient's only problem. Most often, failure to stop a nosebleed is the result of releasing the pressure too soon (**Step 3**).

## YOU are the Provider

The patient is placed onto the stretcher and loaded into the ambulance. He remains conscious and alert but is still anxious. You place him in a supine position and cover him with a blanket. Shortly before departing the scene, you reassess him and obtain another set of vital signs.

| Recording Time: 10 Minutes | |
| --- | --- |
| **Level of consciousness** | Conscious and alert; anxious |
| **Respirations** | 24 breaths/min; regular and adequate |
| **Pulse** | 116 beats/min; strong and regular |
| **Skin** | Cool, pale, and dry |
| **Blood pressure** | 112/70 mm Hg |
| **Spo$_2$** | 98% (on oxygen) |

**7.** How might a patient's outcome be affected if bleeding is internal rather than external?

**8.** What are the signs and symptoms of internal bleeding?

## Skill Drill 26-4 Controlling Epistaxis

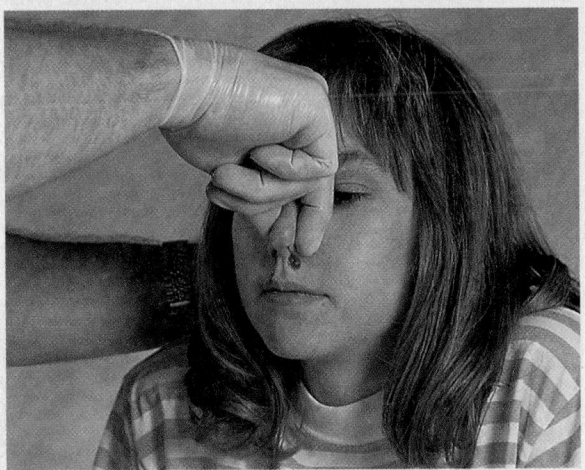

### Step 1

Position the patient sitting, leaning forward. Apply direct pressure, pinching the fleshy part of the nostrils together.

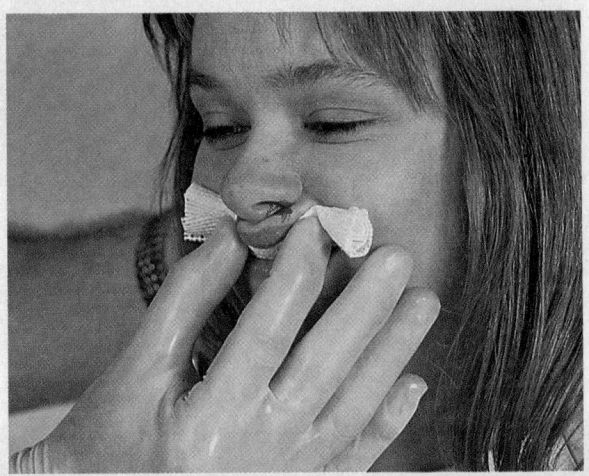

### Step 2

Alternative method: Apply pressure with a rolled gauze bandage between the upper lip and gum. Calm the patient.

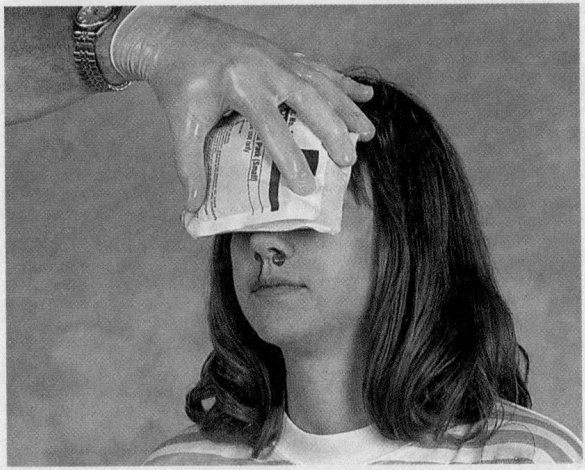

### Step 3

Apply ice over the nose. Maintain pressure until bleeding is controlled. Initiate prompt transport while you or the patient applies pressure. Assess and treat for shock, including oxygen, as needed.

8. Provide prompt transport. You can initiate transport while having the patient maintain direct pressure or while maintaining pressure yourself.

9. Assess the patient for signs and symptoms of shock and treat appropriately.

Bleeding from the nose or ears following a head injury may indicate a skull fracture. In these cases, do not attempt to stop the blood flow. This bleeding may be difficult to control. Applying excessive pressure to the injury may force the blood leaking through the ear or nose to collect within the head. This could increase the pressure on the brain and possibly cause permanent damage. If you suspect a skull fracture, loosely cover the bleeding site with a sterile gauze pad to collect the blood and help keep contaminants away from the site. Apply light compression by wrapping the dressing loosely around the head (**FIGURE 26-13**). If blood or drainage contains cerebrospinal fluid, you will see a characteristic staining of the dressing much like a target or halo shape (**FIGURE 26-14**).

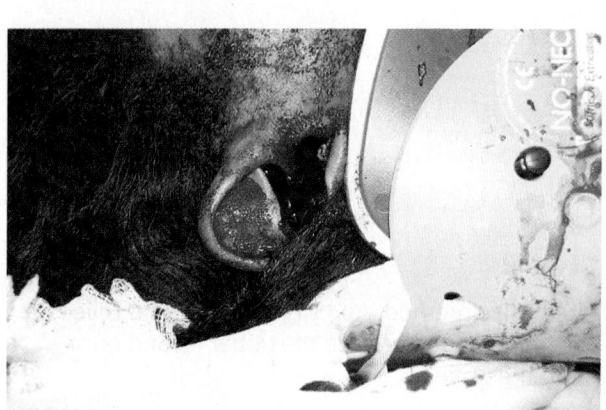

**FIGURE 26-13** Bleeding from the ear after a head injury may indicate a skull fracture. Loosely cover the bleeding site with a sterile gauze pad and apply light compression by wrapping the dressing loosely around the head.

© E.M. Singletary, MD. Used with permission.

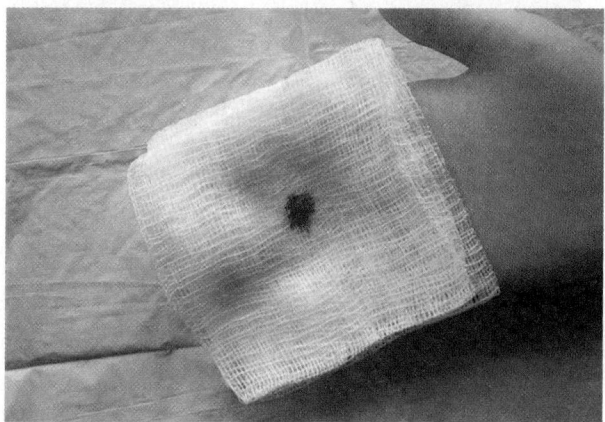

**FIGURE 26-14** When cerebrospinal fluid is present in blood or drainage, a stain in the shape of a target or halo will appear.

Courtesy of Rhonda Hunt.

## YOU are the Provider

You continue to monitor the patient en route to the hospital and reassess his condition as appropriate. After reassessing the patient and his vital signs, you call your radio report into the receiving facility.

| Recording Time: 17 Minutes | |
| --- | --- |
| **Level of consciousness** | Conscious and alert; restless |
| **Respirations** | 20 breaths/min; regular and adequate |
| **Pulse** | 110 beats/min; strong and regular |
| **Skin** | Cool, pale, and dry |
| **Blood pressure** | 114/68 mm Hg |
| **Spo$_2$** | 97% (on oxygen) |

The patient is delivered to the hospital and you give your report to the attending physician. An intravenous line is started, and the patient is given a small amount of medication to address his pain and anxiety. He is taken to the operating room for repair of severed tendons, nerves, and an artery as a result of the injury.

**9.** How does the body typically respond to blood loss?

## Emergency Medical Care for Internal Bleeding

Controlling internal bleeding or bleeding from major organs usually requires surgery or other procedures that must be done in the hospital. It is important for you to remain calm and reassure the patient. Keeping the patient as still and quiet as possible assists the body's clotting process. Provide high-flow oxygen, if indicated, and cover the patient with a blanket to maintain body temperature. You can usually control internal bleeding into the extremities in the field simply by splinting the extremity, usually most effectively with an air splint. Never use a tourniquet to control the bleeding from closed, internal, soft-tissue injuries. Follow the steps in **SKILL DRILL 26-5** to care for patients with possible internal bleeding.

1. Follow standard precautions.
2. Control all obvious external bleeding. Treat suspected internal bleeding in a extremity by applying a splint (**Step 1**).
3. Maintain the airway with spinal motion restriction if the MOI suggests the possibility of spinal injury.
4. Administer high-flow oxygen and provide artificial ventilation as necessary (**Step 2**).
5. Depending on local protocols, use a pelvic compression device or splint to control suspected internal bleeding from the pelvic area (**Step 3**).
6. Monitor and record the vital signs at least every 5 minutes.
7. Keep the patient warm (**Step 4**).
8. Give the patient nothing by mouth, not even small sips of water.
9. Provide prompt transport for all patients with signs and symptoms of hypoperfusion. Report any changes in the patient's condition to emergency department personnel.

## Skill Drill 26-5 Controlling Internal Bleeding

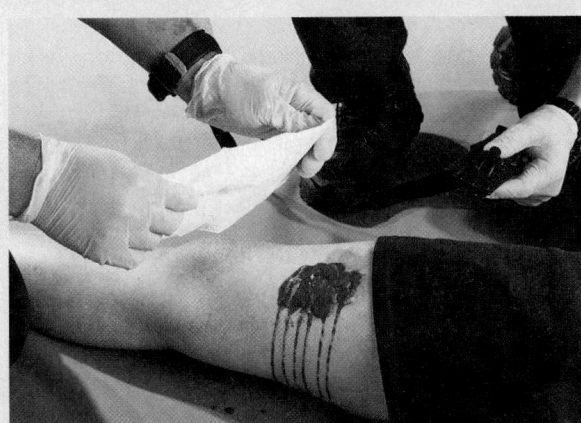

### Step 1

Control obvious external bleeding and treat suspected internal bleeding using a splint. Apply a tourniquet for severe external bleeding that cannot be controlled with direct pressure.

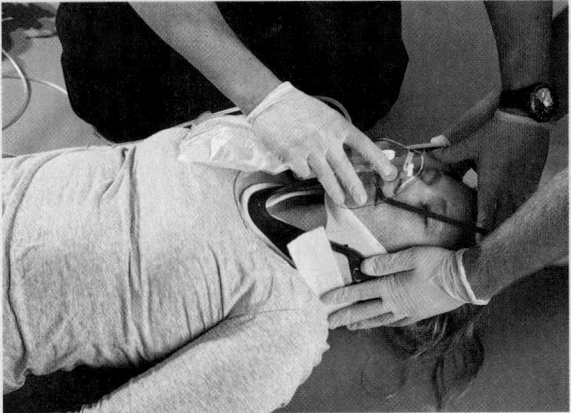

### Step 2

Follow standard precautions. Maintain the airway and be alert for cervical spine injury. Administer oxygen if indicated and provide ventilation as necessary.

*(continues)*

## Skill Drill 26-5 Controlling Internal Bleeding *(continued)*

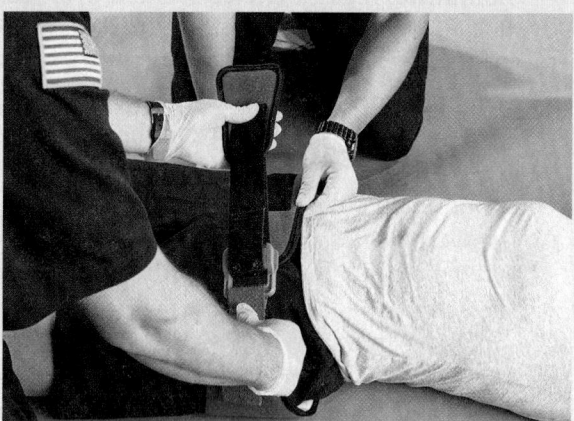

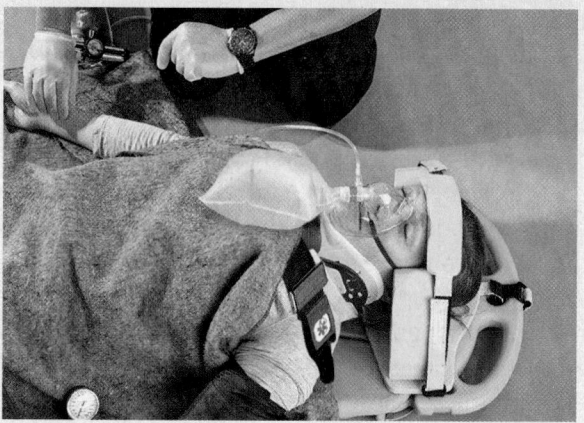

**Step 3**

Depending on local protocols, use a pelvic compression device or splint to control suspected internal bleeding in the pelvic region.

© Jones & Bartlett Learning.

**Step 4**

Monitor vital signs and keep the patient warm.

## YOU are the Provider SUMMARY

**1. What are the functions of arteries? What major arteries are located in the upper extremity?**

Arteries are high-pressure blood vessels that distribute oxygenated blood throughout the body. The major arteries located in the upper extremity include the brachial artery, located on the inner (medial) aspect of the arm; the radial artery, located on the thumb-side (lateral) aspect of the wrist and forearm, proximal to the hand; and the ulnar artery, located on the opposite side of the forearm from the radial artery. The radial and ulnar arteries are the two terminal branches of the brachial artery.

**2. Why is arterial bleeding more severe than venous bleeding?**

Blood flow through the arteries is driven by contraction of the left ventricle. Pressure in the arteries is much higher than pressure in the veins, so blood loss from an artery is generally more rapid and severe. Arterial bleeding is also more difficult to control than venous bleeding.

**3. Is the patient effectively controlling the bleeding from his injury?**

As evidenced by the blood-soaked towel and large amount of blood on the ground, the patient clearly

is *not* effectively controlling the bleeding from his injury. Further, you do not know how much blood loss he has sustained because he is standing outside—not in the area where the injury occurred. The fact that he is anxious and has cool, pale skin suggests significant external blood loss.

**4. What should be your initial treatment priority?**

You must take immediate action to control the patient's bleeding. His airway is patent, as evidenced by the fact that he is conscious, alert, and talking.

In most cases, direct pressure will control both venous and arterial bleeding. If direct pressure and a pressure dressing are ineffective in immediately controlling severe external bleeding, apply a tourniquet and transport. Your partner can apply oxygen while you are attempting to manage the bleeding but if you are alone, administration of oxygen should be delayed until after the bleeding is controlled. Other treatment such as splinting the arm, would also be delayed.

**5. What are the components of the cardiovascular system and how are they affected by the patient's injury?**

The cardiovascular system—the system responsible for supplying and maintaining adequate blood

## YOU are the Provider **SUMMARY** *continued*

flow to the body's tissues and cells—consists of three components: the pump (the heart), the container (the blood vessels), and the fluid (blood and body fluids). These components of the cardiovascular system are interdependent—that is, they rely on each other to perform a common function. Because the patient is bleeding significantly, the intravascular volume is markedly decreased in all of the blood vessels, potentially leading to hypovolemic shock. The heart increased its rate to compensate for the decreased blood volume to keep perfusion adequate. If it was not able to compensate adequately or the bleeding could not be controlled and the blood pressure decreased further (below 90 mm Hg systolic), decompensated shock would have developed.

**6. What factors determine the severity of external bleeding?**

The single most influential factor is the type and size of the blood vessel that is injured. A lacerated brachial artery, for example, will bleed more severely than a small vein in the leg. The patient's blood pressure and heart rate can also affect the severity of external bleeding. The greater the pressure on the arterial wall and the faster the heart rate, the more rapid the bleeding tends to be. The patient's medical history also should be considered. Bleeding in patients who take blood-thinning medications or in those with a bleeding disorder tends to be more difficult to control and may result in more blood loss because it takes longer for the blood to clot.

**7. How might a patient's outcome be affected if bleeding is internal rather than external?**

Internal bleeding is hidden and cannot be controlled in the prehospital setting. Many patients with internal bleeding do not have signs or symptoms of shock until a significant amount of blood loss has occurred. Overall, patients with internal bleeding have a higher mortality rate than those with external bleeding. Most of these deaths are the result of intrathoracic or intra-abdominal bleeding, in which

surgical intervention is delayed. Internal bleeding can also be caused by multiple long bone fractures and pelvic fractures.

**8. What are the signs and symptoms of internal bleeding?**

Because internal bleeding is not visible, you must rely on your assessment skills and careful evaluation of the MOI. Signs and symptoms of internal bleeding are essentially those of shock: restlessness or anxiety; cool, pale, clammy skin; tachycardia; rapid, shallow breathing; and thirst. A late sign is hypotension. External indicators of internal bleeding in both medical and trauma patients include hematemesis (vomiting blood), melena (dark, tarry stools), and hemoptysis (coughing up blood). Other indicators of internal bleeding, which are more common in trauma patients, include redness or bruising, swelling, or tenderness over the injured area. Always be alert to the possibility of internal bleeding, particularly if the MOI is significant. Remember that if a trauma patient is in shock but does not have any obvious external signs of injury, suspect internal bleeding!

**9. How does the body typically respond to blood loss?**

If the typical adult sustains more than approximately 2 pints (approximately 1 liter) of blood loss, significant changes in vital signs will occur, including increased heart and respiratory rates (compensatory phase) and, as a later sign, decreased blood pressure (indicating decompensation).

A loss of circulating blood volume is sensed by receptors in the body that send messages to the nervous system. In response, the sympathetic nervous system releases epinephrine and norepinephrine. Norepinephrine constricts the peripheral blood vessels (vasoconstriction), thus shunting blood from areas of lesser need (eg, skin and muscles) to areas of greater need (eg, heart, brain, kidneys, liver). If blood loss continues, however, the body's compensatory mechanisms will eventually fail, the patient's blood pressure will fall, and he or she will die.

### EMS Patient Care Report (PCR)

| **Date:** 6-30-20 | **Incident No.:** 220109 | **Nature of Call:** Laceration | | **Location:** 517 E. Graham St. | |
|---|---|---|---|---|---|
| **Dispatched:** 1620 | **En Route:** 1621 | **At Scene:** 1627 | **Transport:** 1635 | **At Hospital:** 1655 | **In Service:** 1704 |

#### Patient Information

**Age:** 32
**Sex:** M
**Weight (in kg [lb]):** 82 kg (180 lb)

**Allergies:** No known drug allergies
**Medications:** None
**Past Medical History:** None
**Chief Complaint:** Laceration to left wrist

## YOU are the Provider SUMMARY *continued*

### Vital Signs

| Time: 1637 | BP: 104/60 | Pulse: 120 | Respirations: 24 | Spo$_2$: 94% |
| Time: 1642 | BP: 112/70 | Pulse: 116 | Respirations: 24 | Spo$_2$: 89% |
| Time: 1649 | BP: 114/68 | Pulse: 110 | Respirations: 20 | Spo$_2$: 97% |

### EMS Treatment (circle all that apply)

| Oxygen @ _15_ L/min via:<br><br>NC (NRM) Bag mask | Assisted Ventilation | Airway Adjunct | CPR |
| Defibrillation | (Bleeding Control) | (Bandaging) | Splinting | Other: (Shock treatment) |

### Narrative

Dispatched to a business with lights and siren for a patient with severe bleeding from the arm.

Chief Complaint: Laceration to left wrist

History: Patient stated that his hand slipped while he was working with a table saw and his left wrist ran across the blade. Patient denied significant past medical history and further denied taking any medications.

Assessment: Arrived on scene to find the patient, a 32-year-old male, standing in front of his place of employment, a woodworking shop. He was conscious and alert, but notably anxious. His airway was patent and his breathing, although increased, was producing adequate tidal volume. Patient had blood-soaked towel wrapped around his left wrist and a significant amount of blood was on the ground where he was standing. Approximately 4 cm gaping wound on left arm with brisk bleeding noted.

Treatment (Rx): Immediately applied direct pressure to patient's wrist with sterile dressing to control the bleeding and then applied a pressure dressing followed by a splint. Applied oxygen at 15 L/min via nonrebreathing mask and obtained vital signs, as noted above.

Reassessment: Further assessment revealed that patient's skin was cool, pale, and dry.

Transport: Bleeding remains controlled throughout transport.

Placed patient onto stretcher, covered him with a blanket, and placed him into the ambulance. Reassessed patient's vital signs and began transport to the hospital. Continued to monitor patient's condition en route; he remained conscious and alert, although anxious, and his vital signs remained stable. Reassessed bandaged wound and noted that the bleeding remained controlled. Called report to receiving facility and informed them of our arrival. Delivered patient to hospital without incident. Assisted patient's move onto hospital bed. Verbal report given to charge nurse.

**End of report**

# Prep Kit

## Ready for Review

- Perfusion is the circulation of blood in adequate amounts to meet the cells' current needs for oxygen, nutrients, and waste removal.
- The cardiovascular systems contains three main parts: a working pump (heart), a container (blood vessels), and fluid (oxygen-carrying blood).
- Hypoperfusion, or shock, occurs when one or more of these three components is not working properly and the cardiovascular system fails to provide adequate perfusion.
- Always ask the patient if he or she takes blood-thinning medications (aspirin, warfarin) because bleeding is generally more profuse and difficult to control in these patients.

- Both internal and external bleeding can cause shock. You must know how to recognize and control both.
- The methods to control bleeding, in order, are:
  - Direct pressure
  - Pressure dressing
  - Tourniquet
  - Splinting device
- Bleeding from the nose, ears, and/or mouth may result from a skull fracture. Other causes include high blood pressure and sinus infection. Evaluate the MOI and consider the more serious problem of skull fracture.
- Bleeding around the face always presents a risk for airway obstruction or aspiration. Maintain a clear airway by positioning the patient appropriately and using suction when indicated.
- If bleeding is present at the nose and a skull fracture is suspected, place a gauze pad loosely under the nose.
- If bleeding from the nose is present and a skull fracture is not suspected, pinch both nostrils together for 15 minutes. If the patient is awake and has a patent airway, place a gauze pad inside the upper lip against the gum.
- Promptly transport any patient you suspect of having internal bleeding or significant external bleeding.
- If the MOI is significant, be alert to signs and symptoms of internal bleeding in the chest or abdomen, such as serious bruising or complaints of difficulty breathing or abdominal pain.
- Signs of serious internal bleeding include the following:
  - Vomiting blood (hematemesis)
  - Black, tarry stools (melena)
  - Coughing up blood (hemoptysis)
  - Distended abdomen
  - Broken ribs
- The signs and symptoms of internal bleeding are often slow to develop; therefore, reassess an unstable patient every 5 minutes and a stable patient every 15 minutes.

## Vital Vocabulary

**aorta** The main artery that receives blood from the left ventricle and delivers it to all the other arteries that carry blood to the tissues of the body.

**arterioles** The smallest branches of arteries leading to the vast network of capillaries.

**artery** A blood vessel, consisting of three layers of tissue and smooth muscle, that carries blood away from the heart.

**capillaries** The small blood vessels that connect arterioles and venules; various substances pass through capillary walls, into and out of the interstitial fluid, and then on to the cells.

**coagulation** The formation of clots to plug openings in injured blood vessels and stop blood flow.

**contusion** A bruise from an injury that causes bleeding beneath the skin without breaking the skin; also see *ecchymosis*.

**ecchymosis** A buildup of blood beneath the skin that produces a characteristic blue or black discoloration as the result of an injury; also see *contusion*.

**epistaxis** A nosebleed.

**hematemesis** Vomited blood.

**hematoma** A mass of blood that has collected within damaged tissue beneath the skin or in a body cavity.

**hematuria** Blood in the urine.

**hemophilia** A hereditary condition in which the patient lacks one or more of the blood's normal clotting factors.

**hemoptysis** The coughing up of blood.

**hemorrhage** Bleeding.

**hemostatic dressing** A dressing impregnated with a chemical compound that slows or stops bleeding by assisting with clot formation.

**hypoperfusion** A condition in which the circulatory system fails to provide sufficient circulation to maintain normal cellular functions; also called shock.

**hypovolemic shock** A condition in which low blood volume, due to massive internal or external bleeding or extensive loss of body water, results in inadequate perfusion.

**junctional tourniquet** A device that provides proximal compression of severe bleeding near the axial or inguinal junction with the torso.

**melena** Black, foul-smelling, tarry stool containing digested blood.

**open-book pelvic fracture** A life-threatening fracture of the pelvis caused by a force that displaces one or both sides of the pelvis laterally and posteriorly.

**pelvic binder** A device to splint the bony pelvis to reduce hemorrhage from bone ends, venous disruption, and pain.

**perfusion** The circulation of blood within an organ or tissue in adequate amounts to meet the current needs of the cells.

**shock** A condition in which the circulatory system fails to provide sufficient circulation to maintain normal cellular functions; also called hypoperfusion.

**tourniquet** The bleeding control method used when a wound continues to bleed despite the use of direct pressure; useful if a patient is bleeding severely from a partial or complete amputation.

**vasoconstriction** The narrowing of a blood vessel, such as with hypoperfusion or cold extremities.

**veins** The blood vessels that carry blood from the tissues to the heart.

**venules** Very small, thin-walled blood vessels.

# References

1. Bulger EA, Snyder D, Schoelles K, et al. An evidence-based prehospital guideline for external hemorrhage control: American College of Surgeons Committee on Trauma. Prehosp Emerg Care. 2014;18(2). https://www.facs.org/~/media/files/quality%20programs/trauma/education/acscot%20evidencebased%20prehospital%20guidelines%20for%20external%20hemmorrhage%20control.ashx. Accessed February 6, 2020.

2. Hsu SD, Chen CJ, Chou YC, Wang SH, Chan DC. Effect of early pelvic binder use in the emergency management of suspected pelvic trauma: a retrospective cohort study. Int J Environ Res Public Health. 2017;14(10): 1217. Published October 12, 2017. doi:10.3390/ijerph14101217.

3. National Association of Emergency Medical Technicians. PHTLS: Prehospital Trauma Life Support. 8th ed. Burlington, MA: Jones & Bartlett Learning; 2016.

4. National Association of State EMS Officials. National Model EMS Clinical Guidelines. https://nasemso.org/projects/model-ems-clinical-guidelines/. Accessed February 6, 2020.

5. National Highway Traffic Safety Administration. National Emergency Medical Services Education Standards. DOT HS 811 077A. ems.gov. www.ems.gov/pdf/811077a.pdf. Published January 2009. Accessed February 6, 2020.

6. National Highway Traffic Safety Administration. National Emergency Medical Services Education Standards. Emergency Medical Technician Instructional Guidelines. DOT HS 811 077C. ems.gov. www.ems.gov/pdf/811077c.pdf. Published January 2009. Accessed February 6, 2020.

7. National Registry of Emergency Medical Technicians. 2015 Paramedic Psychomotor Competency Portfolio (PPCP). Columbus, OH: National Registry of Emergency Medical Technicians Inc; 2015.

8. National Registry of Emergency Medical Technicians. Psychomotor Exams. https://www.nremt.org/nremt/about/psychomotor_exam_emt.asp. Accessed February 6, 2020.

9. New York State Department of Health. Prehospital Bleeding/External Hemorrhage Control. https://www.health.ny.gov/professionals/ems/pdf/t-2_bleeding_external.pdf. Updated March 10, 2016. Accessed February 6, 2020.

10. SAM Medical Products. SAM Junctional Tourniquet for battlefield and trauma injuries. https://www.sammedical.com/assets/uploads/SJT-203-05-f.pdf. Accessed February 6, 2020.

11. SAM Medical Products. SAM Junctional Tourniquet (SJT). https://www.fda.gov/media/89465/download. Accessed February 6, 2020.

12. San Francisco General Hospital. Pelvic Binder Guideline. https://anesthesia.ucsf.edu/sites/anesthesia.ucsf.edu/files/wysiwyg/pdfs/PelvicBinderProtocol.pdf. Accessed February 6, 2020.

13. Scott I, Porter K, Laird C, Greaves I, Bloch M. The prehospital management of pelvic fractures: initial consensus statement. Emerg Med J. 2013;30(12). https://emcrit.org/wp-content/uploads/2013/12/pelvic-binders.pdf. Accessed February 6, 2020.

14. Stop the Bleed, American College of Surgeons. Stop the Bleed homepage. https://www.stopthebleed.org/. Accessed February 6, 2020.

15. Stop the Bleed, American Heart Association. Stop the Bleed Save A Life. https://www.stopthebleed.org/-/media/stop-the-bleed/files/basics_of_bleeding_control_booklet.ashx. Published 2017. Accessed February 6, 2020.

16. Vaidya R, Roth M, Zarling B, et al. Application of circumferential compression device (binder) in pelvic injuries: room for improvement. West J Emerg Med. 2016;17(6):766-774. doi:10.5811/westjem.2016.7.30057.

17. WikiEM. Tourniquet (junctional). https://wikem.org/wiki/Tourniquet_(junctional). Updated February 20, 2018. Accessed February 6, 2020.

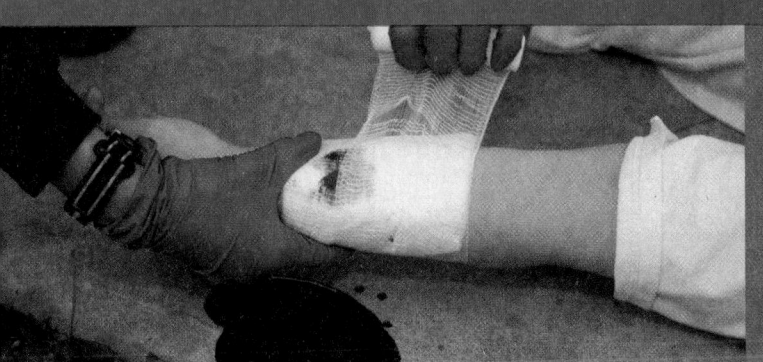

# Chapter 27

# Soft-Tissue Injuries

## NATIONAL EMS EDUCATION STANDARD COMPETENCIES

### Trauma

Applies fundamental knowledge to provide basic emergency care and transportation based on assessment findings for an acutely injured patient.

### Soft-Tissue Trauma

Recognition and management of
- Wounds (pp 964–980)
- Burns
  - Electrical (pp 964, 986–989, 994–996)
  - Chemical (pp 964, 986–989, 993–994)
  - Thermal (pp 991–992)
- Chemicals in the eye and on the skin (pp 981–989, 994)

Pathophysiology, assessment, and management
- Wounds
  - Avulsions (pp 966, 967–968, 986–989)
  - Bite wounds (pp 964, 970–976, 980–981)
  - Lacerations (pp 964, 966–967, 970–976)
  - Puncture wounds (pp 964, 966–977, 996)
  - Incisions (pp 964, 967, 970–976)
- Burns
  - Electrical (pp 964, 981–989, 994–996)
  - Chemical (pp 964, 981–989, 993–994)
  - Thermal (pp 964, 981–989, 991–992)
  - Radiation (pp 964, 981–989, 996–997)
- Crush syndrome (pp 964–966, 970–976)

## KNOWLEDGE OBJECTIVES

1. Describe the anatomy of the skin; include the layers of the skin. (pp 962–964)
2. Know the major functions of the skin. (p 964)
3. Name the three types of soft-tissue injuries. (p 964)
4. Describe the types of closed soft-tissue injuries. (pp 965–966)
5. Describe the types of open soft-tissue injuries. (pp 966–970)
6. Explain patient assessment of closed and open injuries. (pp 970–976)
7. Explain patient assessment of closed and open injuries in relation to airway management. (pp 971–973)
8. Explain the emergency medical care for closed and open injuries. (pp 976–977)
9. Explain the emergency medical care for an open wound to the abdomen. (pp 977–978)
10. Explain the emergency medical care for an impaled object. (p 978)
11. Explain the emergency medical care for neck injuries. (pp 978–980)
12. Describe the steps of the emergency treatment of small animal bites, human bites, and rabies. (pp 980–981)
13. Explain how the seriousness of a burn is related to its depth and extent. (pp 984–986)
14. Define superficial, partial-thickness, and full-thickness burns; include the characteristics of each burn. (pp 983–985)
15. Explain the primary assessment of a patient with a burn. (pp 986–989)

16. Explain the emergency medical care for burn injuries. (pp 989–991)
17. Describe the emergency management of chemical, electrical, thermal, inhalation, and radiation burns. (pp 991–997)
18. Know the functions of sterile dressings and bandages. (pp 997–998)

## SKILLS OBJECTIVES

1. Demonstrate the emergency medical care of an open chest wound. (pp 976–977)
2. Demonstrate the emergency medical care of closed soft-tissue injuries. (p 976)
3. Demonstrate how to control bleeding from an open soft-tissue injury. (pp 976–977)
4. Demonstrate the emergency medical care of an open abdominal wound. (pp 977–978)
5. Demonstrate how to stabilize an impaled object. (pp 978, 979, Skill Drill 27-1)
6. Demonstrate how to care for a burn. (pp 989–991, Skill Drill 27-2)
7. Demonstrate the emergency medical care of a chemical, electrical, thermal, inhalation, or radiation burn. (pp 991–997)

## Introduction

As an EMT, you will be regularly called to care for victims with soft-tissue injuries. These injuries can be as simple as a cut or scrape or as serious as a life-threatening internal injury. It is important to not allow yourself to become distracted by dramatic wounds and make the critical mistake of neglecting more life-threatening conditions such as airway obstructions. It is your responsibility as an EMT to assess and treat each of these injuries within the current standard of care guidelines.

The soft tissues of the body can be injured through a variety of mechanisms. A blunt injury occurs when the energy exchange between the patient and an object is more than the tissues can tolerate. This is discussed in greater detail in Chapter 25, *Trauma Overview*. Whereas a blunt injury does not penetrate the skin, a penetrating injury occurs when an object, such as a bullet or knife, breaks through the skin and enters the body. Barotrauma, commonly seen in blast injury victims, refers to injuries that result from sudden or extreme changes in air pressure. Burns may also result in soft-tissue injuries.

Soft-tissue trauma is a common form of injury. In fact, wound care is one of the most frequently performed procedures in emergency departments (EDs) across the United States. Most of these injuries require basic interventions such as wound irrigation, dressing, bandaging, and limited suturing.

Death resulting from soft-tissue injury is often related to hemorrhage or infection. Uncontrolled hemorrhage can quickly lead to shock and death. When the skin barrier is breached, invading pathogens—bacteria, fungi, and viruses—can cause local or systemic infection. Infection can be life or limb threatening, especially in children, older adults, and people with diabetes or other conditions that may compromise the immune system.

Soft-tissue injuries and their associated complications can often be prevented by using simple protective actions. For example, wearing gloves when working with abrasive materials helps prevent skin injuries. To reduce injuries in the workplace, safety measures have been implemented that include the use of safety devices to prevent interaction between machine parts and body parts. Using plastic scissors, plastic knives, and plastic drinking cups at home will reduce the risk of cuts and other skin injuries among children. Effective strategies that have reduced injury and death from burns include using smoke alarms, controlling the temperature of hot water heaters, and enforcing building codes that regulate electrical and construction practices.

This chapter discusses the various types of soft-tissue injuries and the appropriate assessment and treatment of this classification of injuries.

## Anatomy and Physiology of the Skin

The skin is our first line of defense against external forces and infection. It is also the largest organ in the body. Although it is relatively tough, skin is still

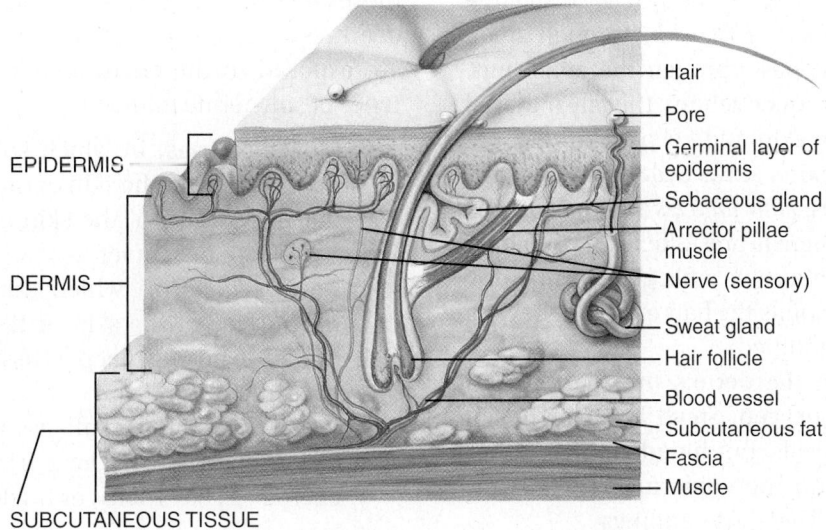

EPIDERMIS

DERMIS

SUBCUTANEOUS TISSUE

Hair
Pore
Germinal layer of epidermis
Sebaceous gland
Arrector pillae muscle
Nerve (sensory)
Sweat gland
Hair follicle
Blood vessel
Subcutaneous fat
Fascia
Muscle

**FIGURE 27-1** The skin comprises a tough external layer called the epidermis and a vascular inner layer called the dermis.

© Jones & Bartlett Learning.

quite susceptible to injury. Injuries to soft tissues range from simple bruises and abrasions to serious lacerations and amputations. Soft-tissue injury may result in exposure of deep structures such as blood vessels, nerves, and bones. In all instances, you must control bleeding, prevent further contamination to decrease the risk of infection, and protect the wound from further damage. Therefore, you must know how to apply dressings and bandages to various parts of the body.

Skin varies in thickness, depending on a person's age and the area the skin covers. The skin of the very young and the very old is thinner than the skin of a young adult. The skin covering the scalp, the back, and the soles of the feet is quite thick, whereas the skin of the eyelids, lips, and ears is very thin. Thin skin is more easily damaged than thick skin.

## Anatomy

The skin has two principal layers: the epidermis and the dermis (**FIGURE 27-1**). The **epidermis** is the tough, external layer that forms a watertight covering for the body. The epidermis contains several layers. The cells on the surface layer of the epidermis are constantly worn away. They are replaced by cells that are pushed to the surface when new cells form in the germinal layer at the base of the epidermis. Deeper cells in the germinal layer contain pigment granules. Along with blood vessels in the dermis, these granules produce skin color.

The **dermis** is the inner layer of the skin. It lies below the germinal cells of the epidermis. The dermis contains the structures that give the skin its characteristic appearance: hair follicles, sweat glands, and sebaceous glands. The sweat glands' primary function is to cool the body. They discharge sweat onto the surface of the skin through small pores, or ducts, that pass through the epidermis. Sebaceous glands produce sebum, the oily material that waterproofs the skin and keeps it supple. Sebum travels to the skin's surface along the shaft of adjacent hair follicles. *Hair follicles* are small organs that produce hair. There is one follicle for each hair, each connected with a sebaceous gland and a tiny muscle. This muscle pulls the hair erect whenever a person is cold or frightened.

Blood vessels in the dermis provide the skin with nutrients and oxygen. Small branches reach up to the germinal cells, but blood vessels do not penetrate farther into the epidermis. The dermis also contains specialized nerve endings.

The skin covers all external surfaces of the body. The various openings in the body, including the mouth, nose, anus, and vagina, are not covered by skin. Instead, these openings are lined with mucous membranes. Similar to skin, these membranes provide a protective barrier against bacterial invasion, but mucous membranes differ from skin in that they secrete a watery substance that lubricates the openings. Therefore, mucous membranes are moist, whereas skin is generally dry.

## Physiology

The skin serves many functions. It protects the body by keeping pathogens out and fluids in, and it helps regulate body temperature. The nerves in the skin report to the brain on the environment and on many sensations. It is this nerve pathway connection that allows the body to adapt to environments through responses in the skin and surrounding tissues.

The skin is the body's major organ for regulating temperature. In a cold environment, the blood vessels in the skin constrict, diverting blood away from the skin and decreasing the amount of heat that radiates from the body's surface. In hot environments, the vessels in the skin dilate. The skin becomes flushed or red, and heat radiates from the body's surface. In addition, sweat glands secrete sweat to help cool the body. As the sweat evaporates from the skin's surface, the body temperature drops, and the person begins to cool down.

Any break in the skin allows bacteria to enter and increases the possibilities of infection, fluid

loss, and loss of temperature control. Any one of these conditions can cause serious illness and even death. Soft tissues are often injured because they are exposed to the environment. There are three types of soft-tissue injuries:

- Closed injuries, in which soft-tissue damage occurs beneath the skin or mucous membrane but the surface of the skin or mucous membrane remains intact.
- Open injuries, in which there is a break in the surface of the skin or the mucous membrane, exposing deeper tissues to potential contamination.
- Burns, in which the soft-tissue damage occurs as a result of thermal heat, frictional heat, toxic chemicals, electricity, or nuclear radiation.

## Pathophysiology of Closed and Open Injuries

Wounds heal in a natural process that involves several overlapping stages, all directed toward the larger goal of maintaining homeostasis or balance. Ultimately, the goal is for the body to return to a functional state, although the injured area may not always be restored to its preinjury state.

Among the primary concerns in wound healing is the cessation of bleeding. Loss of blood, internal or external, hinders the provision of vital nutrients and oxygen to the affected area. It also impairs the tissue's ability to eliminate wastes. The result is abnormal or absent function, which interferes with homeostasis. To stop the flow of blood, the vessels, platelets, and clotting cascade must work in unison.

During inflammation (the next stage of wound healing), additional cells move into the damaged area to begin repair. White blood cells migrate to the area to combat pathogens that have invaded exposed tissue. Foreign products and bacteria are also removed from the body. Similarly, lymphocytes (a type of white blood cell) destroy bacteria and other pathogens. Mast cells release histamine as part of the body's response in the early stages of inflammation. Histamine dilates blood vessels, increasing blood flow to the injured area and resulting in a reddened, warm area immediately around the site. Histamine makes capillaries more permeable, and swelling may occur as fluid seeps out of these "leaky" capillaries. Inflammation ultimately leads to the removal of foreign material, damaged cellular parts, and invading microorganisms from the wound site.

In the outer layer of skin, cells are stacked in layers. To replace the area damaged in a soft-tissue injury, a new layer of cells must be moved into this region. This is the next stage of wound healing. Cells quickly multiply and redevelop across the edges of the wound. Except in cases of clean incisions, the appearance of the restructured area seldom returns to the preinjury state. For example, large wounds or injuries that result in significant disruption of the skin will often not complete this process. People with lightly pigmented skin may see a pink line of scar tissue signaling the presence of collagen, a structural protein that has reinforced the damaged tissue. Despite the changed appearance, the function of the area may be restored to near normal. Tissue injuries may be difficult to detect in dark skin.

During the next stage of wound healing, new blood vessels form as the body attempts to bring oxygen and nutrients to the injured tissue. New capillaries bud from intact capillaries that lie adjacent to the damaged skin. These vessels provide a channel for oxygen and nutrients and serve as a pathway for waste removal. Because they are new and delicate, bleeding might result from a very minor injury. It may take weeks to months for the new capillaries to be as stable as preexisting vessels.

Collagen is a tough, fibrous protein found in scar tissue, hair, bones, and other connective tissues. In the last stage of wound healing, collagen provides stability to the damaged tissue and joins wound borders, thereby closing the open tissue. Unfortunately, collagen cannot restore damaged tissue to its original strength.

## Closed Injuries

Closed soft-tissue injuries are characterized by a history of blunt trauma, pain at the site of injury, swelling beneath the skin, and discoloration. Such injuries can vary from mild to quite severe.

A **contusion**, or bruise, is an injury that causes bleeding beneath the skin but does not break the skin. Contusions result from blunt forces striking the body. The epidermis remains intact, but cells within the dermis are damaged, and small blood vessels are usually torn. The depth of the injury varies, depending on the amount of energy absorbed. As fluid and blood leak into the damaged area, the patient may have swelling and pain. The buildup of blood produces a characteristic blue or black discoloration called **ecchymosis** (**FIGURE 27-2**).

A **hematoma** is blood that has collected within damaged tissue or in a body cavity (**FIGURE 27-3**). A

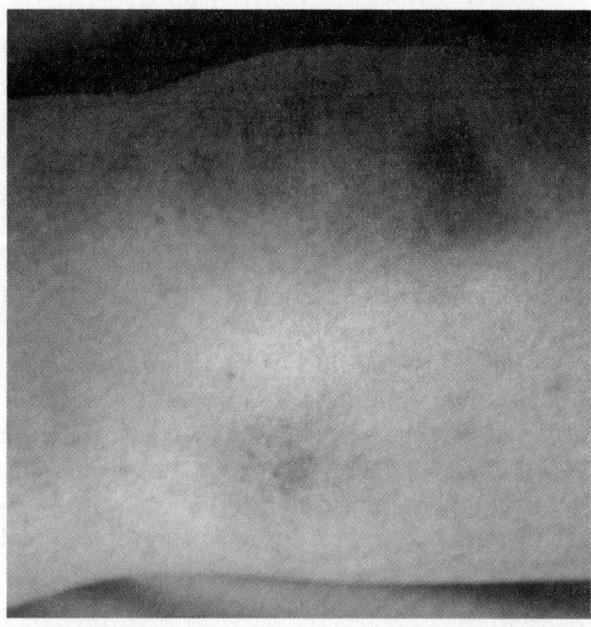

**FIGURE 27-2** Contusions, more commonly known as bruises, occur as a result of a blunt force striking the body. The characteristic blue or black discoloration (ecchymosis) signifies bleeding underneath the skin.

© Jones & Bartlett Learning. Courtesy of MIEMSS.

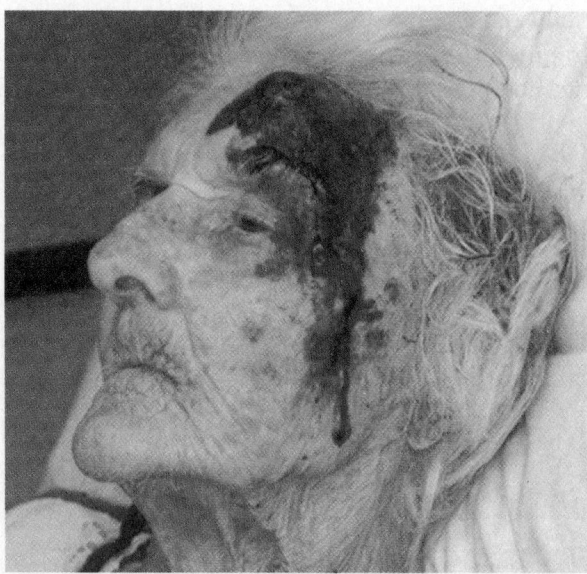

**FIGURE 27-3** A hematoma develops whenever a blood vessel is damaged and bleeds into surrounding tissues.

Courtesy of Rhonda Hunt.

hematoma occurs whenever a blood vessel is damaged and bleeds into the surrounding tissues. It is often associated with extensive tissue damage. A hematoma can result from a soft-tissue injury, a fracture, or any injury to a blood vessel. In severe cases, the hematoma may contain more than 1 liter of blood.

A **crushing injury** occurs when significant force is applied to the body (**FIGURE 27-4**). The extent of the damage depends on how much force is applied and how long it is applied. In addition to causing direct soft-tissue damage, continued compression of the soft tissues cuts off circulation, producing further tissue destruction. For example, if a patient's legs are trapped under a collapsed pile of rocks, damage to the leg tissues will continue until the rocks are removed.

When an area of the body is trapped for longer than 4 hours and arterial blood flow is compromised, **crush syndrome** can develop. When a patient's tissues are crushed beyond repair, muscle cells die and release harmful substances into the surrounding tissues. The oppressing force prevents blood from returning to the injured body part, so these harmful substances are released into the body's circulation only *after* the limb is freed and blood flow is returned. For this reason, when possible, if a patient has been trapped with a crushing object for a prolonged period of time, advanced life support (ALS) providers should administer intravenous (IV) fluid *before* the crushing object is lifted off the body. Freeing the limb or other body part from entrapment results in the release of the by-products of metabolism and harmful products of tissue

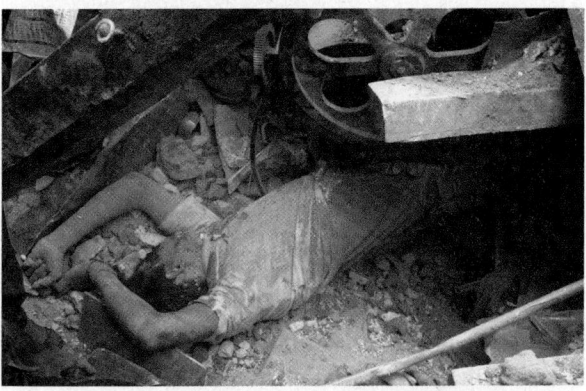

**FIGURE 27-4** The damage associated with a crushing or compression injury varies depending on the direct damage to the soft tissues and how long the tissue was cut off from circulation.

© SAM PANTHAKY/Stringer/AFP/Getty Images.

destruction, and as a result it can create the potential for cardiac arrest and renal failure. Consider requesting ALS assistance for situations of prolonged entrapment prior to extrication.

**Compartment syndrome** develops when edema and swelling result in increased pressure within a closed soft-tissue compartment. Because tissues are limited in the amount they can stretch or expand, pressure increases within the compartment, which interferes with circulation. Compartment syndrome commonly develops in the extremities and may occur in conjunction with open or closed injuries or when swelling occurs under restrictive immobilization devices such as a cast. As pressure develops, delivery of nutrients and oxygen is impaired and by-products of normal metabolism accumulate. This causes pain that worsens with passive movement of the tissues within the compartment. Signs of impaired circulation may also be present. The longer this situation persists, the greater the chance for tissue death. Continually reassess skin color, temperature, and pulses distal to the injury site during transport if compartment syndrome is suspected.

Severe closed injuries can also damage internal organs. The greater the amount of energy absorbed from the blunt force, the greater the risk of injury to deeper structures. Therefore, you must assess all patients with closed injuries for more serious hidden injuries. Remain alert for signs of shock or internal bleeding, and begin treatment of these conditions if necessary.

## Open Injuries

Open injuries differ from closed injuries in that the protective layer of skin is damaged. This can produce extensive bleeding. A break in the protective skin layer or mucous membrane also means that the wound is contaminated and may become infected. **Contamination** is the presence of infectious organisms (pathogens) or foreign bodies, such as dirt, gravel, or metal, in the wound. You must address excessive bleeding and contamination in your treatment of open soft-tissue wounds. There are four types of open soft-tissue wounds that you must be prepared to manage:

- Abrasions
- Lacerations
- Avulsions
- Penetrating wounds

An **abrasion** is a wound of the superficial layer of the skin, caused by friction when a body part rubs or scrapes across a rough or hard surface. An abrasion usually does not penetrate completely through the dermis, but blood may ooze from the injured capillaries in the dermis. Also known as road rash, road burn, strawberry, and rug burn, abrasions can be extremely painful because the nerve endings are located in this area (**FIGURE 27-5**).

A **laceration** is a jagged cut in the skin caused by a sharp object or a blunt force that tears the tissue, whereas an **incision** is a sharp, smooth cut. The depth of the injury can vary, extending through the skin and subcutaneous tissue, even into the underlying muscles and adjacent nerves and blood vessels (**FIGURE 27-6**). Lacerations and incisions may appear linear (regular) or stellate (irregular) and may occur along with other types of soft-tissue injury. Lacerations or incisions that involve arteries or large veins may result in severe bleeding.

An **avulsion** is an injury that separates various layers of soft tissue (usually between the subcutaneous layer and **fascia**) so they become either completely detached or hang as a flap (**FIGURE 27-7**). Often there is significant bleeding. If the avulsed tissue is hanging from a small piece of skin, the circulation through the flap may be at risk. If you can, replace the flat avulsed flap in its original position as long as it is not visibly contaminated with dirt and/or other foreign materials. If an avulsion is

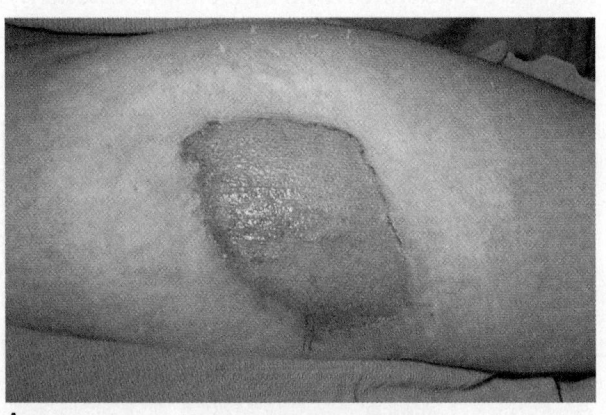

**A**

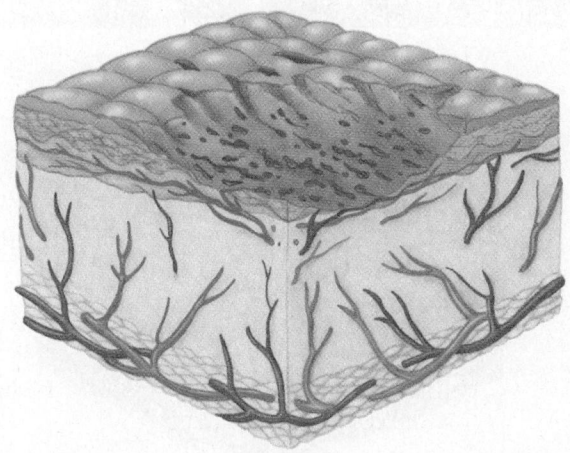

**B**

**FIGURE 27-5** Abrasions usually do not penetrate completely (**A**) through the dermis, but blood may ooze from the capillaries (**B**). These wounds are typically superficial and result from rubbing or scraping across a hard, rough surface.

A: © American Academy of Orthopaedic Surgeons. B: © Jones & Bartlett Learning.

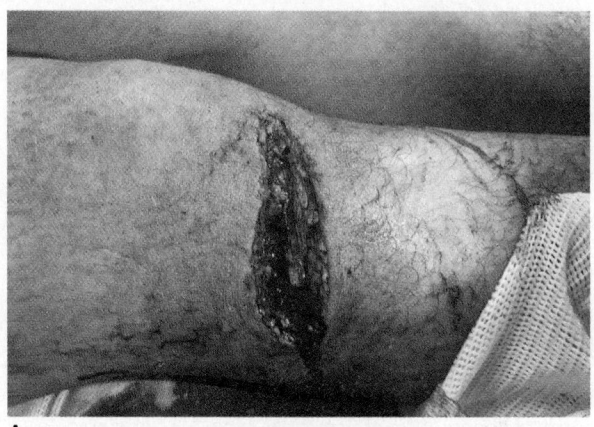

**A**

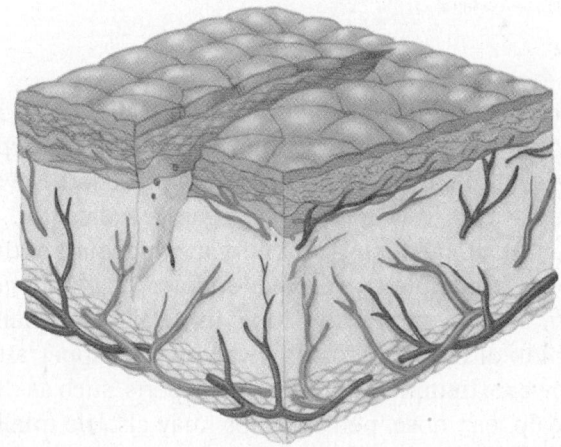

**B**

**FIGURE 27-6** Lacerations vary in depth (**A**) and can extend through the skin and subcutaneous tissue to the underlying muscles, nerves, and blood vessels (**B**). These wounds can be smooth or jagged, depending on the object that caused the injury.

A: © AUYNantapon/Shutterstock; B: © Jones & Bartlett Learning.

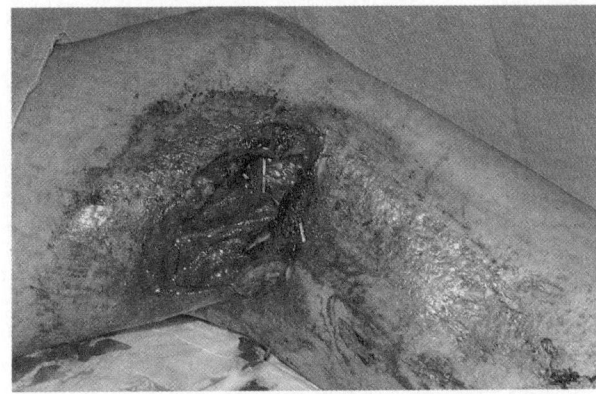

**A**

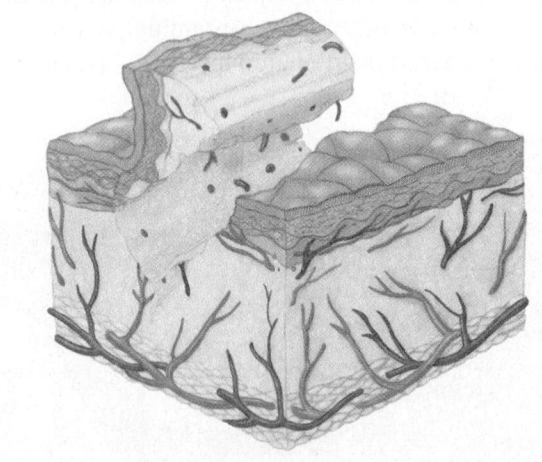

**B**

**FIGURE 27-7** Avulsions are injuries characterized by complete separation of tissue (**A**) or tissue hanging as a flap (**B**). Significant bleeding is common.

**A, B:** © Jones & Bartlett Learning.

complete, you should wrap the separated tissue in sterile gauze and take it with you to the ED. This type of avulsion often has serious risk for infection. Never remove an avulsion skin flap, regardless of its size.

An **amputation** is an injury in which part of the body is completely severed. Chapter 32, *Orthopaedic Injuries*, covers this topic in detail. We usually think of amputations as involving the upper and lower extremities. But other body parts, such as the scalp, ear, nose, penis, or lips, may also be totally avulsed or amputated. You can easily control the bleeding from some amputations, such as a finger, with direct pressure and pressure dressings. If an amputation involves a large area of muscle mass, such as a thigh, there may be massive bleeding. In this situation, you should stop the bleeding, which often requires a tourniquet, and treat the patient

for hypovolemic shock. For more information see Chapter 26, *Bleeding*.

A **penetrating wound** (or puncture wound) is an injury resulting from a piercing object, such as a knife, ice pick, splinter, or bullet. Such objects leave relatively small entrance wounds, so there may be little external bleeding (**FIGURE 27-8**). However, these objects can damage structures deep within the body and cause unseen bleeding. If the wound is to the chest or abdomen, the injury can cause rapid, fatal bleeding. Assessing the amount of damage caused by a puncture wound is difficult and is reserved for the physician at the hospital.

Objects that penetrate the skin but remain in place are referred to as **impaled objects**. The concerns with this type of injury include the amount of damage to structures deep inside the body and the presence of foreign materials deep inside the tissue.

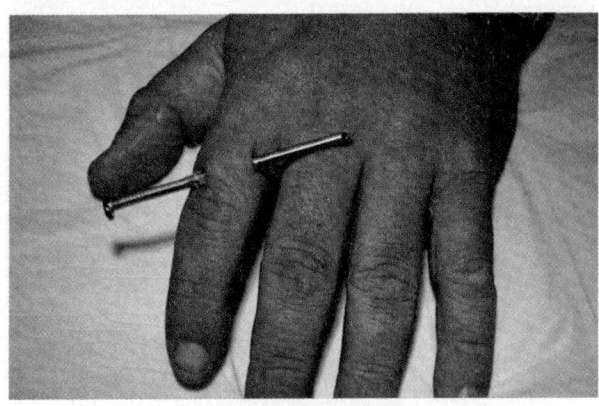

**A**

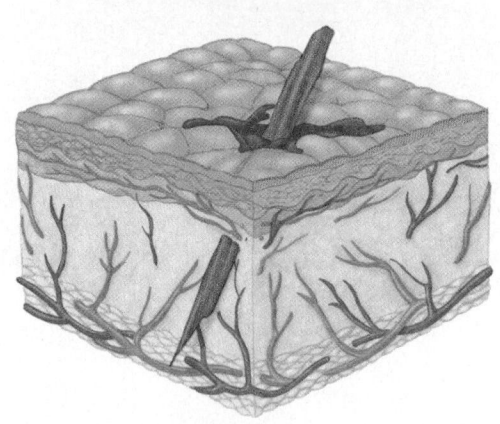

**B**

**FIGURE 27-8** Penetrating wounds and impaled objects (**A**) may cause very little external bleeding but can damage structures deep within the body (**B**).

**A, B:** © Jones & Bartlett Learning.

The damage to underlying structures is difficult to determine and manage, and the presence of foreign materials inside the tissue results in a significantly higher risk of infection. An impaled object also requires specific treatments and care, described later in this chapter.

> ### Words of Wisdom
>
> Treat all penetrating wounds of the neck, chest, back, and upper abdomen with an occlusive dressing to prevent the possible movement of air into the vascular space, thoracic cavity, and/or abdominal cavity.

Stabbings and shootings often result in multiple penetrating injuries. You must assess these patients carefully to identify all wounds. Because a penetrating object can pass completely through the body, always count the number of penetrating injuries (or holes), especially with gunshot wounds. Knowing the difference between entrance wounds and exit wounds may be difficult in a prehospital setting, especially when considering different types of ammunition. Although entrance wounds are often smaller than exit wounds (**FIGURE 27-9**), it is better to simply count the number of penetrating injuries, and leave the distinction between entrance and exit to the physician who is working in a more controlled environment. Gunshot wounds have unique characteristics that require special care. The amount of energy transmitted by a gunshot injury is directly related to the speed of the bullet. When possible, determine the type of gun used in the shooting, but do not let this delay patient transport. Sometimes, the patient or bystanders can tell you how many rounds were fired, but given the stress of the environment, their information may be unreliable; however, it may help hospital personnel to better care for the patient. Shotgun wounds create multiple paths of missiles (shot) and create a larger surface area and volume of tissue damage.

Many cases involving shootings go to court at some point, and you may be called to testify. Therefore, you must carefully document the circumstances surrounding any gunshot injury, the patient's condition, and the treatment you give.

As with closed wounds caused by crushing forces, open crush wounds may involve damaged internal organs or broken bones, as well as extensive soft-tissue damage (**FIGURE 27-10**). Whereas external bleeding may be minimal, internal bleeding may be severe, or even life threatening. The crushing force damages soft tissues as well as vessels and nerves. This frequently results in a painful, swollen, deformed area.

Blast injuries (discussed in Chapter 25, *Trauma Overview*) may also result in multiple penetrating injuries. The mechanism of injury (MOI) from a blast is generally caused by three factors:

- **Primary blast injury:** Injuries to the body caused by the blast wave itself; damage to the body is caused by the sudden pressure changes generated by the explosion.

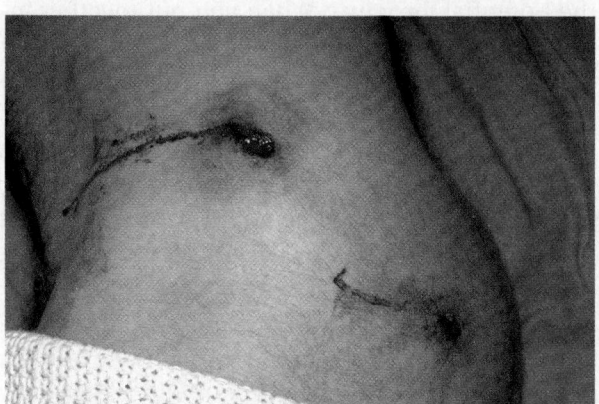

**FIGURE 27-9** An entrance and exit wound from a gunshot. An entrance wound may have burns around the edges. An exit wound can be larger than an entrance wound and is associated with greater damage to soft tissues locally.

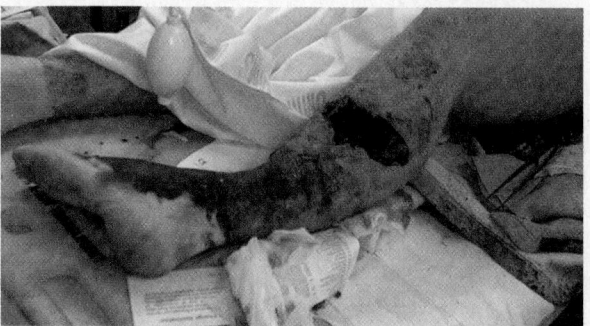

**FIGURE 27-10** An open crush wound is characterized by extensive tissue damage and deformity that is often accompanied by swelling and extreme pain.

- **Secondary blast injury:** Injuries caused to the body from being struck by flying debris propelled by the force of the blast. These small objects may cause multiple penetrating wounds.
- **Tertiary blast injury:** Injuries to the body from being thrown or hurled by the force of the explosion into an object or onto the ground.

It is important to conduct a complete primary and secondary assessment to determine what types of injuries are sustained from a blast injury and treat them appropriately.

## Patient Assessment of Closed and Open Injuries

Assessing closed injuries is often more difficult than assessing open injuries. Therefore, anytime you observe bruising, swelling, or deformity, or the patient reports pain, the possibility of a closed injury should be considered.

Assessing an open injury in some ways is easier than assessing a closed injury because you can see the injury. Open wounds are defined as injuries in which there is a break in the surface of the skin or the mucous membrane, exposing deeper tissues to potential contamination. You must use caution to avoid letting a patient's non–life-threatening gruesome injury distract you from recognizing another injury that is more of a threat to his or her life.

### Words of Wisdom

Extremities that are painful, swollen, or deformed should be splinted whenever time allows. When you splint these types of injuries, remember to assess the patient's pulses and motor and sensory functions before and after applying the splint. You should also evaluate the MOI. Because diffuse or generalized soft-tissue injuries can be life threatening, all patients with a significant MOI should be considered to have internal bleeding and shock until proven otherwise by the ED staff.

### Scene Size-Up

As you arrive on scene, observe the scene for hazards and threats to the safety of the crew, bystanders, and the patient. Assess the effect of hazards on patient care and address the hazards. As always,

ensure the scene is safe, and consider the need for additional resources.

Ensure that you and your crew have taken the necessary standard precautions before you approach the scene—a minimum of gloves and eye protection. Eye exposures may occur from splashes and droplets at a busy scene. Eye and mask protection are required when managing open injuries to avoid potential splashing. Place several pairs of gloves in your pocket for easy access in case your gloves tear or there are multiple patients with bleeding.

Open soft-tissue injuries can be very messy but should not take priority over more serious life-threatening injuries. Controlling bleeding and bloody contaminants can be difficult because of the nature of the wounds. Be careful where you put your hands or place your equipment and how you package the patient for transport. Because of the color of blood and how well it soaks through clothing, you can often identify patients with an open injury as you approach the scene. However, blood can be hidden under thick, dark clothing, such as denim and leather, or in the environment, such as sand, grass, or carpeting. Do not spend time trying to estimate blood loss; focus on controlling the bleeding.

As you observe the scene, look for indicators of the MOI. This helps you develop an early index of suspicion for underlying injuries in a patient who has sustained a significant MOI. Remember, the MOI alone does not necessarily describe the true extent of injuries but it helps you understand the potential for injury. When you put together information from dispatch and your observations of the scene, consider how the MOI produced the injuries expected. Remember, medical emergencies may result in trauma, so there may be conditions to consider beyond the traumatic injuries. Your interactions with the patient and your assessment will ultimately provide you with additional information about the extent of the actual injuries. For example, in a vehicle crash, a patient who has sustained abrasions and lacerations to the face from an impact with the steering wheel or windshield may have experienced enough force to injure the cervical spine as well. In this case, spinal motion restriction should be maintained throughout your care of the patient. The MOI may also provide information about potential safety threats. For example, gunshot wounds may indicate the presence of an angry and violent offender in the area or a dangerous scene. Make sure you use all available information to evaluate scene safety and consider whether additional resources may be necessary.

## Primary Assessment

The primary assessment of a patient with a closed or open injury should focus on identifying and managing life-threatening concerns and identifying transport priority.

Your general impression will help you develop an index of suspicion for serious injuries and determine how urgently your patient needs care. As you approach the patient, important indicators will alert you to the seriousness of the patient's condition, including the following:

- Is the patient awake and interacting with his or her surroundings, or lying still and not making sounds?
- Is the patient appropriately or inappropriately responding to you?
- Is the patient's breathing pattern rapid or slow, deep or shallow?
- What is the color and condition of the patient's skin? Although paleness, or a decrease in blood flow, can be difficult to detect in dark-skinned people, it may be observed by examining mucous membranes inside the inner lower eyelid

and capillary refill. On general observation, the patient may appear ashen or gray.
- Does the patient have any apparent life threats?

The answers to these questions contribute to your general impression and help to determine your treatment priorities and the urgency of care needed. A good question to ask yourself is, "How sick is my patient based on what I know right now?"

Closed soft-tissue injuries may appear to be minor; however, they may indicate serious internal injuries. For example, a patient with a hematoma on the head and a decreased level of consciousness may have a serious brain injury. Open injuries may be obvious and significant, likely indicating a serious condition. However, other injuries may not be as obvious but may still indicate a serious condition.

Check for responsiveness. If the patient is alert, ask about the chief complaint to help direct you

### Words of Wisdom

It is easy to become distracted when a patient has significant soft-tissue injuries, there is a large amount of blood, or the patient is frightened or screaming. However, this is when you need to focus on the problems at hand and manage life-threatening injuries.

## YOU are the Provider

The patient is ambulatory, so you immediately move him to the ambulance that is parked a short distance away and complete your primary assessment. Your partner obtains additional information from the firefighters who rescued him.

| Recording Time: 2 Minutes | |
| --- | --- |
| **Appearance** | Shivering; in obvious pain |
| **Level of consciousness** | Conscious and alert |
| **Airway** | Open; clear of secretions or foreign bodies; no signs of swelling or redness |
| **Breathing** | 14 breaths/min; adequate depth; unlabored |
| **Circulation** | Increased pulse rate; strong at the radial site; no obvious bleeding |

You apply high-flow oxygen via a nonrebreathing mask and then carefully remove clothing that is not adhered to his skin so you can assess the severity of his burns.

**3.** What additional information should you obtain from the firefighters who rescued the patient?

**4.** How are thermal burns classified? What are the characteristics of each type of burn?

to any apparent life threats. If the patient is not alert, determine if he or she responds to verbal or painful stimuli or if he or she is unresponsive. An unresponsive patient may indicate a life-threatening condition. Administer high-flow oxygen via a nonrebreathing mask to patients whose level of consciousness is less than alert and oriented, treat for potential shock, and provide immediate transport to the ED.

If significant trauma has likely affected multiple body systems, start with a rapid exam of the patient to be sure you have found all of the problems and injuries. A rapid 60- to 90-second exam may identify factors that assist you in determining whether a patient requires rapid transport. Begin with the head and neck while manually holding the head in place. When you are done, apply a cervical collar if it is indicated.

When performing the rapid exam, look for life threats and treat them as you find them. Significant bleeding is an immediate life threat and must be controlled quickly using appropriate methods. A patient with massive hemorrhage may require a tourniquet *before* the airway is opened. If the patient has obvious life-threatening external bleeding, control the bleeding first, *before* airway and breathing, then assess and treat the XABCs, and treat for shock.

> ### Words of Wisdom
>
> As you consider the MOI and form suspicions about where bleeding is occurring, expose that part of the body. Blood flowing freely from veins in a large gash can be as much of a threat as blood spurting from an artery.

Providing high-flow oxygen may help reduce the effects of shock and assist in oxygenation of damaged tissues, particularly in crush injuries. If the patient has signs of hypoperfusion, treat him or her aggressively for shock: Place the patient supine, prevent heat loss with a blanket, and provide rapid transport to the hospital. Request ALS as necessary to assist with more aggressive shock management.

Ensure the patient has a clear and patent airway. If the airway is not patent, take the necessary steps to make it clear and patent. Protect the patient from further spinal injury as you manage the airway by preventing the head and torso from moving. If the patient is unresponsive or has a significantly altered level of consciousness, consider inserting an oropharyngeal airway or nasopharyngeal airway, and suction the airway as needed.

You must quickly assess the patient for adequate breathing. Inspect and palpate the chest wall for DCAP-BTLS. If a soft-tissue injury is discovered on the chest or abdomen, auscultate for clear and symmetric breath sounds, and look at the structure of the chest wall to ensure equal expansion and rise and fall of the chest. Provide high-flow oxygen, or provide assisted ventilations using a bag-mask device as needed, depending on the level of consciousness and if your patient is breathing inadequately.

Open soft-tissue injuries of the face and neck have the potential to interfere with the effectiveness of the airway and breathing. Evaluate the patient's voice and ability to speak to identify throat injuries. If an open injury is found on the chest, evaluate for air movement through the wound in the form of bubbling or sucking sounds, which indicate a deep, penetrating injury. Assess the patient's back for injuries that might need treatment. Quickly place an occlusive dressing over the wound. Provide high-flow oxygen or assisted ventilations with a bag-mask device as needed, depending on the patient's level of consciousness and on the adequacy of the patient's breathing. Monitor the patient for signs of increasing respiratory distress that may require you to relieve pressure built up under the dressing (caused by a pneumothorax).

Quickly assess the patient's pulse rate, rhythm, and quality; determine the skin condition, color, and temperature; and check the capillary refill time. These assessments will help you determine the presence of circulatory problems or shock. Closed soft-tissue injuries may not always have visible signs of bleeding because most of the bleeding is occurring inside the body. Your assessment of the pulse and skin will indicate how aggressively you need to treat your patient for shock.

Determine whether your patient needs immediate transport or stabilization on scene. If the patient you are treating has an airway or breathing problem or signs and symptoms of shock or internal bleeding, you must consider rapid transport to the hospital for treatment or request ALS support. Also, if you identify conditions that have the potential to become unstable, such as a distended abdomen or femur fractures, the patient requires rapid and immediate transport.

You should also consider whether transport to the closest hospital is appropriate or whether the patient would be better served by transport to a trauma center that might be farther away. In some situations it may be appropriate to request aeromedical transport to expedite transfer to a trauma or specialty center. Each consideration requires that you clearly and completely understand your local resources and protocols.

Most patients do not require immediate, rapid transportation, but there are certain conditions for which treatment is limited in the field, and, therefore, immediate transport is the better choice. The following list will help guide you in determining the types of patients that need immediate transportation:

- Poor initial general impression
- Altered level of consciousness
- Dyspnea
- Abnormal vital signs
- Shock
- Severe pain

Do not delay transport of a seriously injured trauma patient to complete non–life-saving treatments in the field, such as splinting extremity fractures or treating minor bleeding such as abrasions; instead, complete these types of treatments en route to the hospital during the secondary assessment.

Patients who have visible significant bleeding or signs of significant internal bleeding may quickly become unstable. Stay alert for signs of hypoperfusion (tachycardia; tachypnea; weak pulse; cool, moist skin), and reassess your priority and transport decision if these signs develop.

## History Taking

After you manage life threats during the primary assessment, investigate the chief complaint or history of present illness. Obtain a medical history and be alert for injury-specific signs and symptoms as well as any pertinent negatives such as no pain or loss of sensation.

Make every attempt to obtain a SAMPLE history from your patient. Using OPQRST may provide some background on isolated extremity injuries. When you use SAMPLE, OPQRST, and DCAP-BTLS together, your assessment will be well rounded and provide significant insight into the patient's

## YOU are the Provider

The patient tells you he sustained the burns when he was trying to escape from the burning house. Both of the exits were blocked by fire and debris, so he ran into the bedroom. However, he was unable to exit through the window because of burglar bars he had installed; this was when the firefighters found him. He denies losing consciousness. Your partner assesses his vital signs as you perform a secondary assessment.

| Recording Time: 6 Minutes | |
| --- | --- |
| **Respirations** | 14 breaths/min; adequate depth; unlabored |
| **Pulse** | 108 beats/min; strong and regular |
| **Skin** | Red, warm, and dry; burns to the torso and arms |
| **Blood pressure** | 166/86 mm Hg |
| **Oxygen saturation (Spo$_2$)** | 98% (on oxygen) |

Your secondary assessment reveals partial-thickness burns to his anterior chest and abdomen, and partial- and full-thickness burns to both of his arms, including his hands. His face is covered with soot, and his facial hair and the hair just above his hairline are singed. You do not see any obvious skin burns to his facial area, and the remainder of your assessment does not reveal any other injuries. The patient denies having difficulty breathing or any other symptoms other than pain.

**5.** What percentage of the patient's body surface area has been burned?

**6.** What factors should you consider to determine the severity of a burn?

condition. You have the opportunity to interview the patient well before the ED physician's examination. Any information you receive will be valuable if the patient loses consciousness.

If the patient is not responsive, attempt to obtain the history from other sources, such as friends, family members, or even bystanders who might have witnessed the event. Medical identification jewelry and wallet cards may also provide information about the patient's medical history or alert you to the presence of implanted medical devices. Although these items may not seem significant, they can provide information about the patient's underlying medical conditions. This information, in conjunction with the physical assessment, may help provide an overview of the patient's overall status.

Typical signs of an open injury include bleeding, a break in the skin, shock, hemorrhage, and disfigurement or loss of a body part. Typically, symptoms include pain and/or burning at the injury site. Chronic medical conditions such as anemia (low quantity of hemoglobin in the blood) and hemophilia (a disorder in which blood has a diminished ability to clot) as well as a host of other medical conditions can complicate open soft-tissue injuries. Medications such as aspirin or others that impair the blood's ability to clot and are frequently taken by older patients may make it more difficult to control bleeding.

## Secondary Assessment

After you evaluate the XABCs and identify and treat immediate life threats, a more detailed assessment should follow. The secondary assessment is a more systematic full-body scan or focused examination of the patient that is used to reveal injuries or medical conditions that may have been missed during the primary assessment. In some instances, such as with a critically injured patient or a short transport time, you may not have time to conduct a full secondary assessment. Typically, the secondary assessment, which includes assessing interventions and repeating vital signs, occurs en route to the ED.

Listen to breath sounds with a stethoscope. Breath sounds should be clear and equal bilaterally, anteriorly, and posteriorly. Determine the patient's respiratory rate and note the pattern and quality of the respiratory effort. Assess for asymmetric chest wall movement.

Assess the neurologic system to gather baseline data on your patient. This examination should include the level of consciousness, pupil size and reactivity, and motor and sensory response.

Assess the musculoskeletal system by performing a detailed exam of the entire body. Look for DCAP-BTLS. Assess the chest, abdomen, and extremities for hidden bleeding and injuries. Log roll the patient and assess the posterior torso for injuries. Once the back has been assessed, the patient can be log rolled back down onto a backboard, followed by spinal motion restriction if indicated. Log rolling and maintaining spinal motion restriction should take into consideration injuries found during the primary assessment as well as local protocols.

Assess all anatomic regions, looking for the following signs/symptoms:

- Check the neck for jugular vein distention and tracheal deviation. Be alert for patients with a stoma or tracheostomy.
- Check the pelvis for stability.
- Check the abdomen; feel all four quadrants for tenderness or rigidity and inspect for bruising. If the abdomen is tender, expect internal bleeding.
- Check the extremities and record the pulse and motor and sensory function.

Patients who have hidden internal injuries under a closed soft-tissue injury may have internal bleeding and may rapidly become unstable. It is important to reassess the vital signs to identify how quickly the patient's condition is changing; a single vital sign will not always provide the necessary information to evaluate the patient's condition. Make sure you obtain a series of vital signs to ensure subtle changes are evident as soon as possible. Signs such as tachycardia, tachypnea, low blood pressure, weak pulse, and cool, moist, and pale skin indicate hypoperfusion and imply the need for rapid transport and treatment at the hospital. Remember that soft-tissue injuries can cause shock, even without a significant MOI. The reassessment of your patient's vital signs will give you a good understanding of how well or how poorly your patient is tolerating the injury and whether your interventions have been effective.

## Reassessment

Reassessment of a patient is just as important as your original assessment and should be regularly conducted during transport to ensure your patient's condition is not declining. Repeat the primary assessment completely, but pay extra attention to areas of concern that you identified during your initial assessment and assess the effectiveness of prior treatments. Reassess vital signs and the chief complaint. Are the airway, breathing, and circulation still adequate? Recheck patient interventions. Are the treatments you provided for problems with the XABCs still effective? Reassessing a patient with an open soft-tissue injury is extremely important, especially if you did not put the bandage on the patient's injury. Frequently, other emergency care personnel may have dressed and bandaged the wound before your arrival. You may need to place additional dressings over the original dressing or bandages. If so, frequently reassess the effectiveness of the bandaging. If blood continues to soak through bandages, use additional methods to control bleeding as discussed later in the chapter. How is the patient's condition improving with the interventions? Identify and treat changes in the patient's condition.

Closed soft-tissue injuries can be life threatening if not appropriately treated. Assess and manage all threats to the patient's airway, breathing, and circulation. Supplemental oxygen via a nonrebreathing mask is commonly given to all patients with traumatic injuries affecting airway or ventilation or those with a potential for shock.

Although most open soft-tissue injuries are not serious, they tend to be graphic and can be distracting to the patient. If not appropriately treated, they can lead to substantial blood loss and even shock. By appropriately treating open soft-tissue injuries, you can decrease the risk of common complications such as bleeding, shock, pain, and infection. Expose all wounds, control bleeding, and be prepared to treat the patient for shock. Consider flushing small wound surfaces *without* significant bleeding with sterile saline prior to applying a dressing. If any material is stuck in the wound, do not remove it because this may worsen bleeding and shock.

Extremities that are painful, swollen, or deformed should be splinted. Take great care when splinting these types of injuries. If done correctly, splinting can assist with pain management and bleeding control; if done poorly, it may cause greater harm. When splinting these types of injuries, remember to assess the patient's pulse and motor and sensory functions distal to the injury zone both before and after applying the splint.

### Words of Wisdom

Estimating blood loss is very difficult, and even the most skilled providers are often not able to accurately estimate blood loss, especially when blood has been absorbed into fabrics or porous surfaces. Note that blood has soaked through a towel, an article of clothing, or the number of bandages used to control the patient's bleeding as these are valuable descriptors for the ED staff.

## YOU are the Provider

After caring for the patient's burns, you cover him with a blanket and begin transport to the hospital. You contact medical control as soon as you leave the scene, and you are advised to provide transport to the ED because the closest burn center is 75 miles away. You reassess the patient, including his vital signs.

| Recording Time: 12 Minutes | |
| --- | --- |
| Level of consciousness | Conscious and alert, but anxious |
| Respirations | 22 breaths/min; becoming labored; voice is becoming hoarse |
| Pulse | 120 beats/min; strong and regular |
| Skin | Red, warm, and dry |
| Blood pressure | 158/84 mm Hg |
| Spo₂ | 99% (on oxygen) |

**7.** What is the proper treatment for the patient's burns?

**8.** How has the patient's condition changed? What should you do now?

Your communication and documentation must include a description of the MOI and the position in which you found the patient when you arrived on scene. This will provide key information to the hospital staff that may affect the patient care plan provided at the hospital. You should attempt to report blood loss using terms that you are comfortable with and that will be easily understood by other personnel. For example, you may say "the bleeding soaked through the patient's jeans prior to our arrival" or "the bleeding soaked through three trauma dressings during our time with the patient." Include the location and description of any soft-tissue injuries or other wounds you have located and treated. Describe the size and depth of the injury. Provide an accurate account of how you treated these injuries. Your ability to clearly and accurately communicate and document enables the physicians and nurses at the hospital to continue to deliver quality care.

## Emergency Medical Care for Closed Injuries

Small contusions generally do not require special emergency medical care, but you should note their presence when trying to determine the true extent of the patient's injuries. More extensive closed injuries may involve significant swelling and bleeding beneath the skin, which could lead to hypovolemic shock. Depending on the time the injury occurred and the response time, the injuries might not have had time to cause swelling or bruising. Closely watch any area of injury throughout the time you are caring for the patient, no matter how minor it may look on initial assessment.

Treat a closed soft-tissue injury by applying the mnemonic RICES:

- **Rest.** Keep the patient as quiet and comfortable as possible.
- **Ice.** Use ice or cold packs to slow bleeding by causing blood vessels to constrict and to reduce pain.
- **Compression.** Apply pressure over the injury site to slow bleeding by compressing the blood vessels.
- **Elevation.** Raise the injured part just above the level of the patient's heart to decrease swelling.
- **Splinting.** Immobilize a soft-tissue injury or an injured extremity to decrease bleeding and reduce pain.

In addition to using these measures to control bleeding and swelling, you should be alert for signs of developing shock. Look for anxiety or agitation and changes in mental status, as these can be early signs of developing shock. An increased heart rate, increased respiratory rate, diaphoresis, cool or clammy skin, and eventual decreases in blood pressure may not develop until late in your care of the patient. Any or all of these signs may indicate internal bleeding resulting from injuries to internal organs. If the patient exhibits signs and symptoms of shock, treat accordingly and aggressively.

## Emergency Medical Care for Open Injuries

Before you begin caring for a patient with an open wound, be sure to protect yourself by following standard precautions. If life-threatening bleeding is observed, assign a team member to apply direct pressure over the wound to control the bleeding. Then assess the severity of the wound. If the wound is in the chest, upper abdomen, or upper back, cover it with an occlusive dressing.

### Words of Wisdom

Although most wounds can be managed with direct pressure, do not waste time with a wound in an arm or leg that is hemorrhaging profusely. Apply a tourniquet early when there is life-threatening hemorrhage.

Your treatment priorities are performing the primary assessment and beginning life-saving interventions. This includes controlling the bleeding, which can be extensive and severe. Several methods are available to control open injuries or external bleeding. Start with the most commonly used; these include the following:

- Direct, even pressure and elevation
- Pressure dressings and/or splints
- Tourniquets

It will often be useful to combine these methods. Different types of tourniquets are shown in **FIGURE 27-11**.

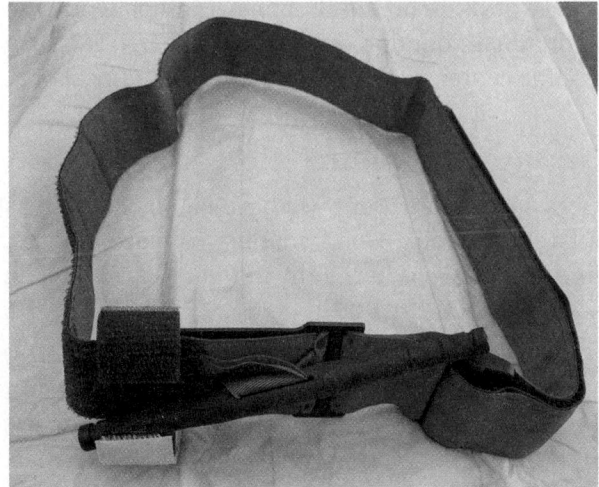

**A**

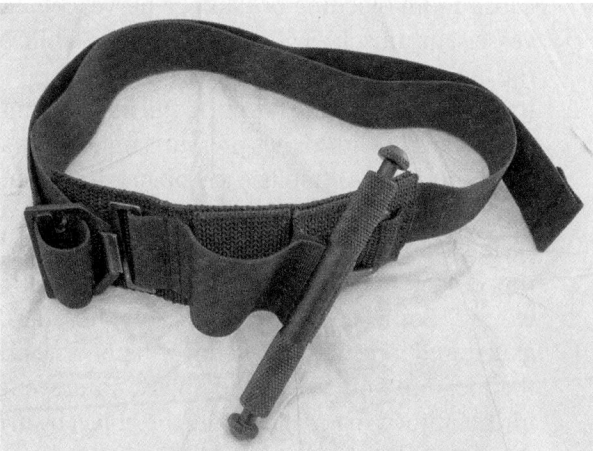

**B**

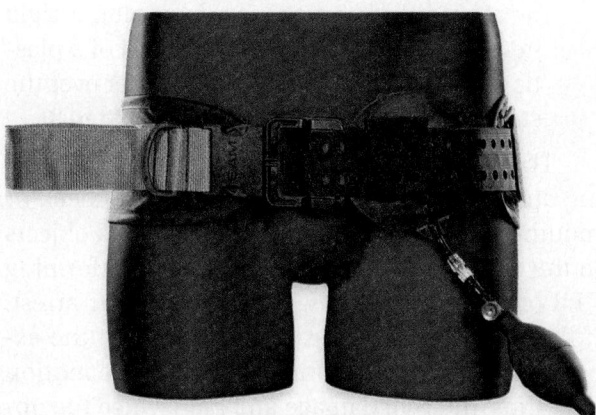

**C**

**FIGURE 27-11** If bleeding continues or reoccurs, apply a tourniquet above the site of bleeding in an extremity—preferably the groin for leg wounds and the axilla for arm wounds. **A.** CAT tourniquet. **B.** SOF-T tourniquet. **C.** Junctional tourniquet.

A, B: Courtesy of Peter T. Pons, MD, FACEP; C: Used with permission from SAM medical.

All open wounds are assumed to be contaminated and present a risk of infection. By applying a sterile dressing, you are reducing the risk of further contamination. This keeps foreign material, such as hair, clothing, and dirt, out of the wound and decreases the risk of infection. In general, you should not remove material from an open wound, no matter how dirty the wound is. Rubbing, brushing, or washing an open wound can cause additional bleeding, but small wound surfaces without significant bleeding can be flushed with sterile saline prior to applying a dressing. Chemical burns and contamination should be flushed to remove remaining chemicals. In most circumstances, hospital personnel, rather than EMTs, will clean open wounds. To prevent a wound from drying, you may apply sterile dressings moistened with sterile saline solution and then cover the moist dressing with a dry, sterile dressing.

In some cases, you can better control bleeding from open soft-tissue wounds by splinting the extremity, even if there is no fracture. Splinting can help you keep the patient calm and quiet, as it typically reduces pain. Splinting also keeps sterile dressings in place, minimizes damage to an already injured extremity, and makes it easier to move the patient.

### Words of Wisdom

Hypovolemic shock is a risk for any patient who has had significant bleeding or bleeding that cannot be controlled. Be alert for this potential and treat aggressively to reduce the risk.

## Abdominal Wounds

An open wound in the abdominal cavity may expose internal organs. In some cases, the organs may even protrude through the wound, an injury called an **evisceration** (**FIGURE 27-12**). Do not touch or move the exposed organs. Instead, cover the wound with sterile gauze moistened with sterile saline solution and secure it with an occlusive dressing (**FIGURE 27-13**). Because the open abdomen radiates body heat very effectively and quickly, and because exposed organs lose fluid rapidly, you must keep the organs moist and warm. If you do not have gauze compresses, you may use moist sterile dressings, covered and secured in place with a bandage

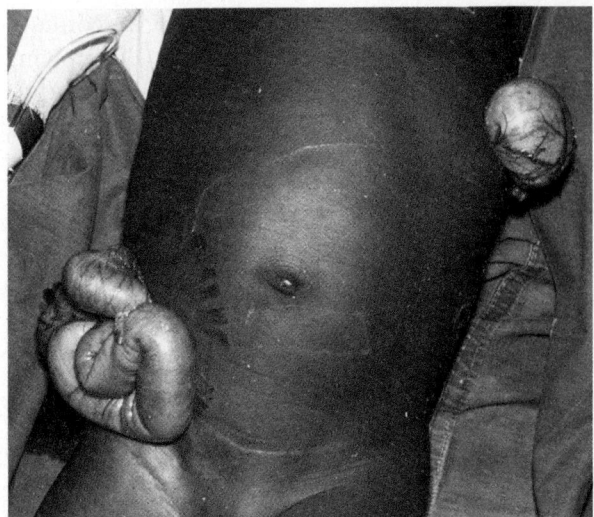

**FIGURE 27-12** An abdominal evisceration is an open wound to the abdomen in which organs protrude through the wound.

© Dr. M. A. Ansary/Science Source.

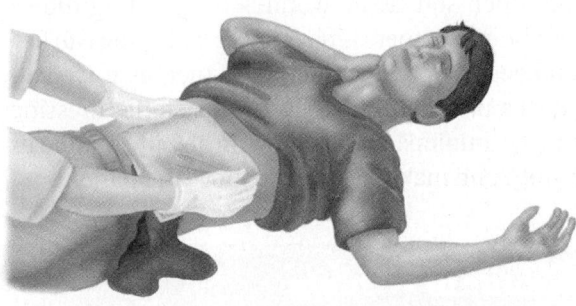

**A**

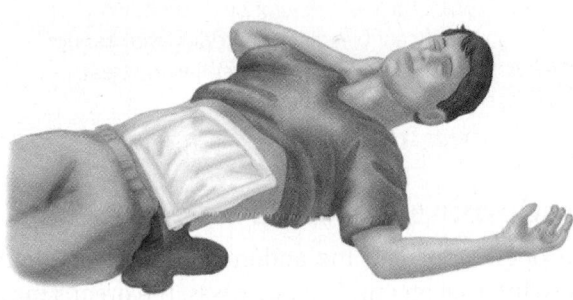

**B**

**FIGURE 27-13 A.** Cover exposed organs with sterile gauze compresses moistened with sterile saline solution. **B.** Place an occlusive dressing over the compresses and secure it in place by taping all four sides.

© Jones & Bartlett Learning.

and tape. Do not use any material that is adherent or loses its substance when wet, such as toilet paper, facial tissue, paper towels, or absorbent cotton. If the patient's legs and knees are uninjured, flex them to

relieve pressure on the abdomen. Most patients with abdominal wounds require immediate transport to a trauma center, depending on the local protocol.

## Impaled Objects

Occasionally, a patient will have an object, such as a knife, fishhook, wood splinter, or piece of glass, impaled in his or her body. To treat this, follow the steps in **SKILL DRILL 27-1**:

1. Do not attempt to move or remove the object unless it is impaled through the cheek or mouth and is causing airway obstruction, or if the patient is pulseless and you must remove it to perform CPR. In most cases, a surgeon will have to remove the object; removing it in the field may cause more bleeding or damage nerves, blood vessels, or muscles within the wound. Stabilize the impaled body part (**Step 1**).
2. Remove any clothing covering the injury. Control bleeding with direct pressure, and apply a bulky dressing to stabilize the object. If the object is in the chest, neck, or back, consider applying a base layer of occlusive dressing around the object to prevent air from entering the wound. Some combination of soft dressings, gauze, and tape may be effective, depending on the location and size of the object. To prevent further injury, manually secure the object by incorporating it into the dressing (**Step 2**).
3. Protect the impaled object from being bumped or moved during transport by taping a rigid item such as a plastic cup, a section of a plastic water bottle, or a supply container over the stabilized object and its bandaging (**Step 3**).

The only exceptions to the rule of not removing an impaled object are objects in the cheek or mouth that actively obstruct breathing and objects in the chest that directly interfere with performing CPR on a patient who is already in cardiac arrest. If the object is very long, cut off (shorten) the exposed portion, first securing it to minimize motion and, thus, internal damage and pain. Once the object has been properly secured and the bleeding is under control, provide prompt transport.

## Neck Injuries

An open neck injury can be life threatening. If the veins of the neck are open to the environment,

## Skill Drill 27-1 Stabilizing an Impaled Object

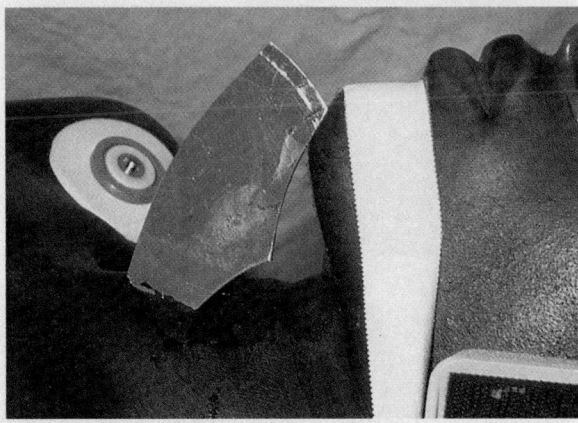

### Step 1

Do not attempt to move or remove the object. Stabilize the impaled body part.

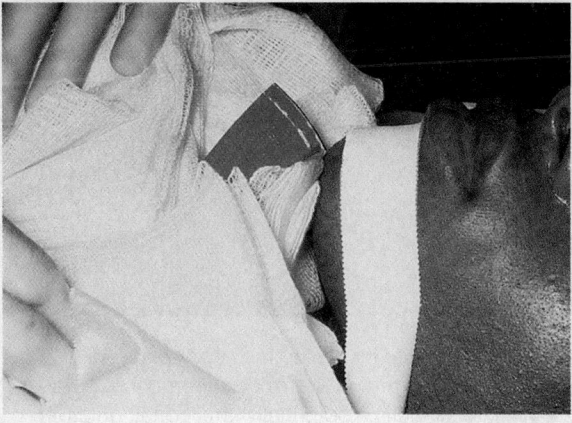

### Step 2

Control bleeding, and stabilize the object in place using soft dressings, gauze, and/or tape.

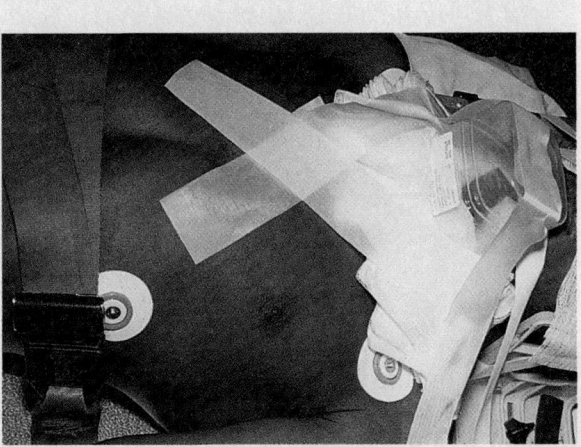

© Jones & Bartlett Learning. Courtesy of MIEMSS.

### Step 3

Tape a rigid item over the stabilized object to prevent it from moving during transport.

they may suck in air (**FIGURE 27-14**). If enough air is sucked into a blood vessel, it can block the flow of blood into the lungs and cause cardiac arrest. This condition is called air embolism. To control bleeding and prevent the possibility of air embolism, cover the wound with an occlusive dressing. Apply manual pressure, but do not compress both carotid vessels at the same time; if you do, this may impair circulation to the brain and cause a stroke.

Secure a pressure dressing over the wound by wrapping roller gauze loosely around the neck and then firmly through the opposite axilla (**FIGURE 27-15**).

Use caution with patients who have sustained a neck injury, depending on the MOI involved. Immobilize the cervical spine if indicated, including placing a cervical collar. The cervical collar may assist with holding a dressing in place over a neck wound.

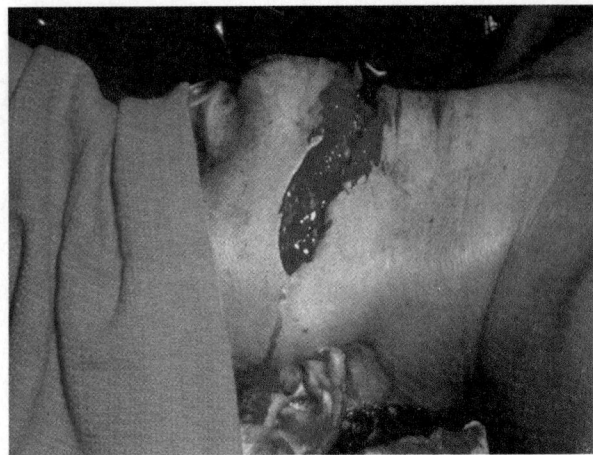

**FIGURE 27-14** Open injuries to the neck can be very dangerous. If veins are open to the environment, they can suck in air, resulting in a potentially fatal condition called air embolism.

© American Academy of Orthopaedic Surgeons.

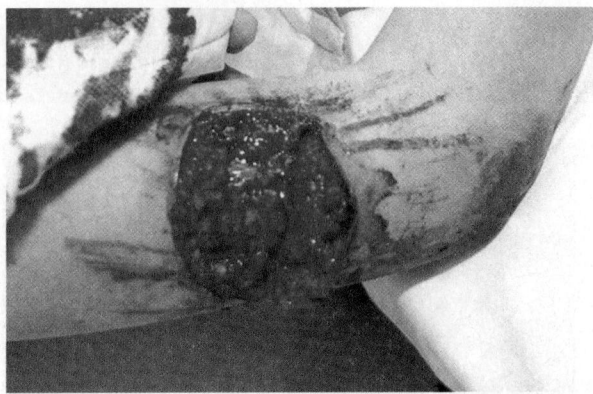

A

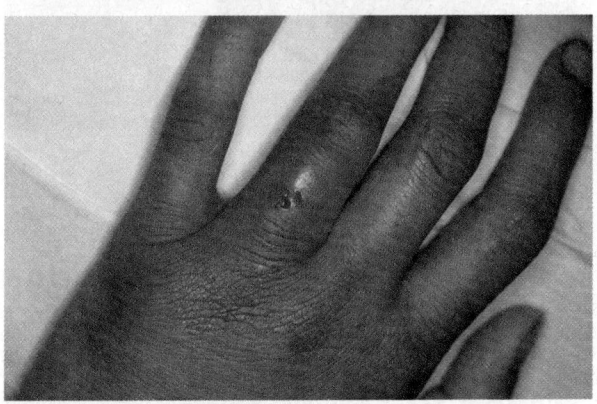

B

**FIGURE 27-16** Small animal bite wounds should be examined at the hospital, as these wounds are heavily contaminated with bacteria. **A.** Dog bite. **B.** Cat bite.

A: Courtesy of Moose Jaw Police Service; B: © Chuck Stewart, MD.

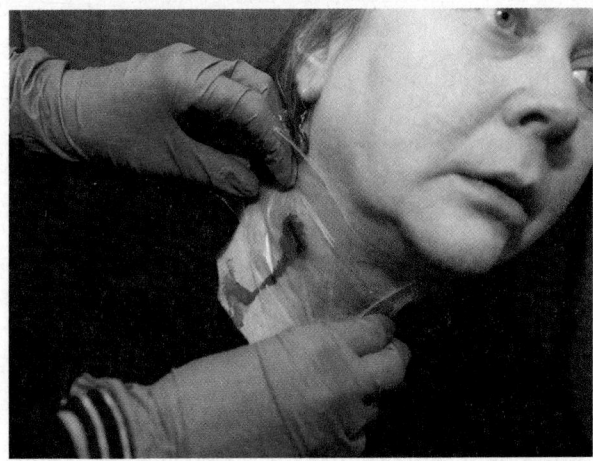

**FIGURE 27-15** Cover neck wounds with an airtight dressing and apply manual pressure. Do not compress both carotid arteries at the same time, as this may impair circulation to the brain.

© Jones & Bartlett Learning.

# Bites
## Small Animal Bites and Rabies

At times you may be called to care for a person who has been bitten by a small animal such as a dog, cat, raccoon, squirrel, or other small nonlivestock animal. Be sure to consider scene and crew safety prior to entering the environment.

Most people who are bitten by small animals do not report the incident to a physician, believing that these bites are not serious; however, they can be very serious. A small animal's mouth is heavily contaminated with bacteria. You should consider all small animal bites as contaminated and potentially infected wounds that may require débridement (the removal of damaged tissue), antibiotics, and tetanus prophylaxis (**FIGURE 27-16**). Occasionally, small animal bites result in mangled, complex wounds that require surgical repair. For these reasons, all small animal bites should be evaluated by a physician. Place a dry, sterile dressing over the wound, and promptly transport the patient to the ED. If an arm or leg was injured, splint that extremity. Often, the patient will be extremely upset and frightened, a situation that calls for reassurance on your part.

A major concern with small animal bites is the spread of rabies, an acute, potentially fatal viral infection of the central nervous system that can affect all warm-blooded animals. Although rabies is currently extremely rare, particularly with widespread vaccination of pets, it still exists. Stray dogs that have not been vaccinated can be carriers of the disease, as can squirrels, bats, foxes, skunks, and raccoons. The virus is in the saliva of a rabid, or infected, animal and is transmitted through biting or licking an open wound. Infection can be prevented in a person who has been bitten by such an animal only by a series of special vaccine injections, a painful procedure that must be started soon after the bite. Because animals that have rabies do not always demonstrate symptoms immediately, a person's only chance to avoid the vaccine is to find the animal and turn it over to the health department for observation and/or testing. Refer to your local animal control procedures.

Children, particularly young ones, may be seriously injured or even killed by dogs. These dogs are not always vicious or **rabid**; sometimes a child unknowingly provokes the animal. However, you must assume the animal may turn and attack you as well. Therefore, you generally should not enter the scene until the animal has been secured. Then you may carry out the necessary emergency care and transport the child to the ED.

### Words of Wisdom

In many locations, reporting animal bites to public health officials is mandatory. Based on your protocols you may need to have law enforcement respond to the scene or to the hospital.

## Human Bites

The human mouth, more so than even the small animal's mouth, contains an exceptionally wide range of bacteria and viruses. For this reason, you should regard any human bite that has penetrated the skin as a serious injury. Similarly, any laceration caused by a human tooth can result in a serious, spreading infection (**FIGURE 27-17**). Remember this if you treat someone who has been punched in the mouth; the person who delivered the punch may also need treatment.

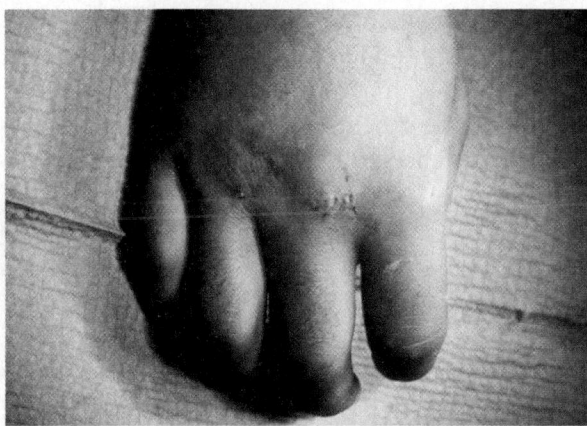

**FIGURE 27-17** Human bites can result in a serious, spreading infection. Thus, patients must be evaluated at the hospital.
© American Academy of Orthopaedic Surgeons.

The emergency treatment of bites consists of the following steps:

1. Apply a dry, sterile dressing.
2. Promptly immobilize the area with a splint or bandage.
3. Provide transport to the ED for surgical cleansing of the wound and antibiotic therapy.

## Burns

As an EMT, you will provide care to patients who have been burned. Often, these calls involve pediatric patients. Burns are among the most serious and painful of all injuries. A severe burn injury presents several simultaneous life threats, including hypovolemic shock, sepsis, hypothermia, and respiratory failure. Management of severe burn injuries has improved over the years, including an emphasis on the psychological challenges that survivors face. Burn units typically employ social workers, vocational counselors, and psychologists as part of a multidisciplinary approach to patient care.

A burn occurs when the body, or a body part, receives more radiant energy than it can absorb, resulting in an injury. Potential sources of this energy include heat, toxic chemicals, and electricity. The proper emergency care of a burn may increase a patient's chances of survival and decrease the risk or duration of a long-term disability. Although a burn may be the patient's most obvious injury, you should always perform a complete assessment to determine whether there are other serious injuries. Finally, keep in mind that children, older patients, and patients with chronic illnesses are more likely to experience shock from burn injuries. Be prepared to treat accordingly.

## Pathophysiology of Burns

Burns are soft-tissue injuries spread out over a large area created by the transfer of radiation, thermal, or electrical energy. Thermal burns can occur when skin is exposed to temperatures higher than 111°F (44°C). In general, the severity of a thermal injury directly correlates with temperature, concentration, or amount of heat energy possessed by the object or substance and the duration of exposure. For example, solids generally have higher heat content than gases, so exposure to a hot solid (such as the rack inside an oven) typically causes a more significant burn than exposure to hot gases (such as those coming out of an oven). Burn injuries are progressive—the greater the heat energy, the deeper the wound.

Exposure time is another important factor. Thermal injury can occur to unresponsive or paralyzed patients from seemingly innocent heat sources such as heating pads or heat lamps if the patient is left unattended and exposed for long periods of time. It may be difficult to evaluate the amount of heat energy or the amount of exposure time in many cases. There can be a vast difference in the temperature of a fire from the floor to the ceiling. Although most people naturally limit the amount of time they are exposed to such heat, if clothing is on fire or the person is trapped or unconscious, exposure time can be extended.

## Complications of Burns

Several complications can result from a burn injury, all of which can be life threatening. The skin serves as a barrier between the environment and the body. When a person is burned, this barrier is destroyed; the victim is now at a high risk for infection, hypothermia, hypovolemia, and shock. Burns to the airway are of great importance because the loose mucosa in the hypopharynx can swell and result in complete airway obstruction. Circumferential burns of the chest can compromise breathing. Circumferential burns of an extremity can lead to compartment syndrome, resulting in neurovascular compromise and irreversible damage if not appropriately treated. If you suspect any complications, call for ALS backup if available or provide rapid transport to the emergency department.

### Words of Wisdom

Burns can cause hypothermia and acidosis and can prevent the blood from clotting effectively. These conditions increase the likelihood of death. Therefore, in the field and during transport, keep the patient warm and provide supplemental oxygen.

### Words of Wisdom

Burn centers have different protocols and criteria for burn classification. The information provided is based on national criteria. Follow local protocols regarding how burns should be treated in the field and where these patients should be transported.

### Words of Wisdom

An isolated burn injury should not cause an altered level of consciousness in your patient. If your patient with a burn has an altered level of consciousness, you should suspect other potential complications, such as hypoperfusion, hypoxia, hypoglycemia, or head injury.

### Words of Wisdom

Burns of 20% total body surface area (TBSA) or more will likely require IV fluid resuscitation. Burns of 30% TBSA or more (less than 15% in older adults) may be fatal without appropriate treatment. Inhalation injury can double the risk of death from a burn injury.

## Burn Severity

The seriousness of a burn may influence the choice of a treatment facility. Five factors will help you to determine the severity of a burn.

1. What is the depth of the burn?
2. What is the extent of the burn?

These first two factors are the most important. After gauging these, ask yourself the following questions.

3. Are any critical areas (face, upper airway, hands, feet, genitalia) involved? Also included in critical areas are any circumferential burns, which are burns that go completely around a body part such as an arm, foot, or chest.
4. Does the patient have any preexisting medical conditions or other injuries?
5. Is the patient younger than 5 years or older than 55 years?

If the answer to any of these three questions is yes, you should upgrade the classification (**TABLE 27-1**).

The American Burn Association and the American College of Surgeons recommend transfer to a designated burn center for any patient with an acute burn with any of the following:

1. Partial-thickness burns of 20% TBSA or greater in patients 10 to 50 years of age.
2. Partial-thickness burns of 10% TBSA or greater in children younger than 10 years or adults older than 50 years.
3. Full-thickness burns of 5% TBSA or greater in patients of any age.
4. Partial- or full-thickness burns to the hands, face, feet, genitalia, or major joints.
5. High-voltage electrical injuries.
6. Significant chemical burns.
7. Concomitant traumatic injury. Note: If the trauma causes a greater immediate risk than the burn injury, consider stabilizing the patient at a trauma center and then transferring to a burn unit (per local protocol).
8. Inhalation injury.

| **TABLE 27-1** Classification of Burns in Adults |
| --- |
| **Severe Burns** |
| • Full-thickness burns involving the hands, feet, face, genitalia, airway, or circumferential burns |
| • Full-thickness burns covering more than 5% TBSA in any patient |
| • Partial-thickness burns covering more than 20% TBSA (age 10 to 50 years) and 10% TBSA (younger than 10 years and older than 50 years) |
| • Burns with concomitant traumatic injuries |
| • Burns to patients younger than 5 years or older than 50 years that would otherwise be classified as "moderate" |
| **Moderate Burns** |
| • Full-thickness burns involving 2% to 10% TBSA (excluding hands, feet, face, genitalia, and upper airway) |
| • Partial-thickness burns covering 15% to 30% TBSA |
| • Superficial burns covering more than 50% TBSA |
| **Minor Burns** |
| • Full-thickness burns covering less than 2% TBSA |
| • Partial-thickness burns covering less than 15% TBSA |
| • Superficial burns covering less than 50% TBSA |

Abbreviation: TBSA, total body surface area

## Special Populations

### Abuse

When you are treating older adults, pediatric patients, or special needs patients with burns, it is important to be alert for the possibility of abuse. Older adult patients who are institutionalized, disoriented, or incapable of clear communication are particularly susceptible to abuse. Pediatric and special needs patients are similarly susceptible to abuse.

Signs of abuse include evidence of multiple injuries in various stages of healing (eg, multiple bruises of different colors, new and old fractures involving more than one extremity), injuries that do not seem to correspond to the history provided by caregivers, and burns associated with a suspicious history.

Burns that appear in a pattern are suspicious for intentional injuries. Multiple small, circular burns may be indicative of cigarette or cigar injuries. Other patterns may indicate irons, stovetops, or other hot surfaces not easily encountered accidentally. Scalding injuries to the buttocks, hands, or feet may also be indicative of abuse. Remember, these injuries are often inflicted in areas not readily seen. If you are suspicious that an older adult has been abused, fully examine the patient under his or her clothing for signs of abuse. As always, your priority is to provide appropriate support and transport the patient in a timely manner.

9.  Significant ongoing medical problems.
10. Special social/emotional or long-term reha-bilitative support (eg, victims of abuse or substance abuse).

Remember, burns to the face are high risk due to the risk of airway involvement. Burns to the hands, feet, or genitalia, or over joints, are also serious due to potential loss of function from scarring.

## Depth

Burns are first classified according to their depth (**FIGURE 27-18**). You must be able to identify the following three types of burns:

- **Superficial (first-degree) burns** involve only the top layer of skin, the epidermis. The skin turns red but does not blister or burn through this top layer. The burn site is often painful. Sunburn is a good example of a superficial burn.
- **Partial-thickness (second-degree) burns** involve the epidermis and some portion of the dermis. These burns do not destroy the entire thickness of the skin, nor is the subcutaneous tissue injured. Typically, the skin is moist, mottled, and white to red. Blisters are present. Partial-thickness burns cause intense pain.
- **Full-thickness (third-degree) burns** extend through all skin layers and may involve

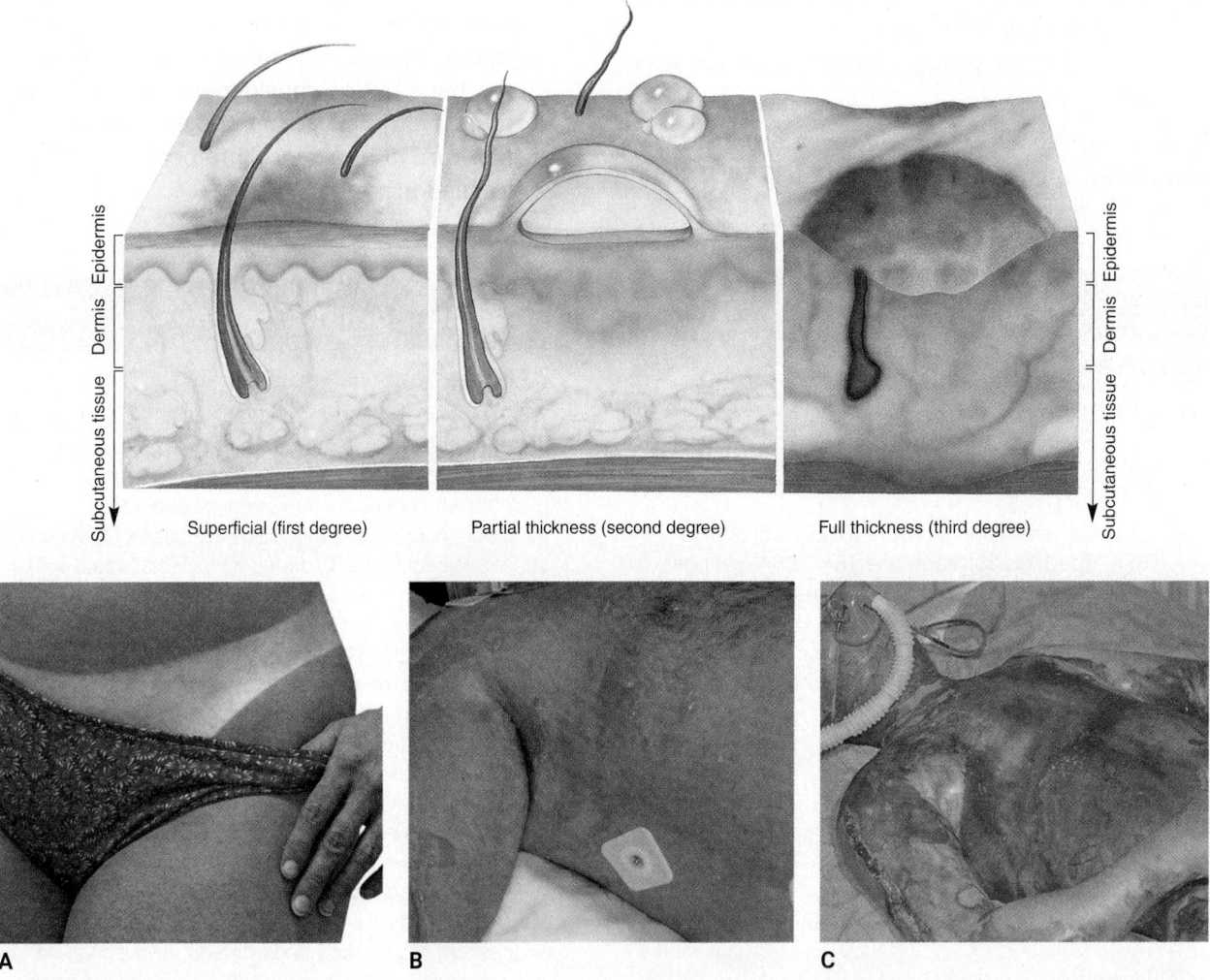

**FIGURE 27-18** Classification of burns. **A.** Superficial (first-degree) burns involve only the epidermis. The skin turns red but does not blister or actually burn through. **B.** Partial-thickness (second-degree) burns involve some of the dermis, but they do not destroy the entire thickness of the skin. The skin is mottled, white to red, and is often blistered. **C.** Full-thickness (third-degree) burns extend through all layers of the skin and may involve subcutaneous tissue and muscle. The skin is dry, leathery, and often either white or charred.

subcutaneous layers, muscle, bone, or internal organs. The burned area is dry and leathery and may appear white, dark brown, or even charred. Some full-thickness burns feel hard to the touch. Clotted blood vessels or subcutaneous tissue may be visible under the burned skin. If the nerve endings have been destroyed, a severely burned area may not have feeling and the surrounding less severely burned areas may be extremely painful.

## Words of Wisdom

The depth of burns can vary. A full-thickness burn may be surrounded by areas of partial-thickness and superficial burns. So, although the area of the full-thickness burn is painless, the patient can still experience pain due to the extent of damage to the surrounding tissues. Request ALS for assistance with pain management if appropriate.

A pure full-thickness burn is unusual. Severe burns are typically a combination of superficial, partial-thickness, and full-thickness burns. Superficial burns heal well without scarring. Small partial-thickness burns also heal without scarring. However, deep partial-thickness burns and all full-thickness burns are prone to scarring and may be best managed surgically.

Significant airway burns are also serious. They may be associated with singed hair within the nostrils, soot around the nose and mouth, hoarseness, and hypoxia. These patients should be rapidly transported to an ED or facility capable of advanced airway management. It becomes increasingly difficult to achieve airway control once swelling begins.

It may be impossible to accurately estimate the depth of a burn shortly after injury. Even experienced burn surgeons sometimes underestimate or overestimate the extent of a burn.

## Extent

One quick way to estimate the surface area that has been burned is to compare it to the size of the patient's palm, including their fingers, which is roughly equal to 1% of the patient's TBSA. This technique is called the rule of palm. Another useful measurement system is the **rule of nines**, which divides the body into sections, each of which is approximately

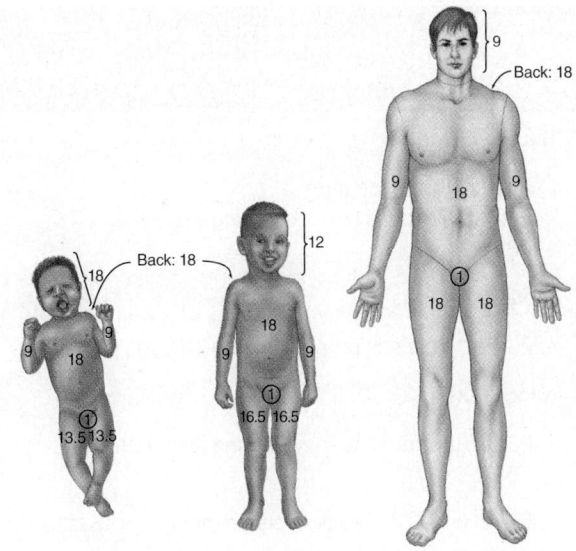

**FIGURE 27-19** The rule of nines is a quick way to estimate the amount of surface area that has been burned; it divides the body into sections, each representing approximately 9% of the total body surface area. The proportions differ for infants, children, and adults.

© Jones & Bartlett Learning.

9% of TBSA (**FIGURE 27-19**). Remember that the head of an infant or child is relatively larger than the head of an adult, and the legs are relatively smaller. When you calculate the extent of burn injury, include only partial-thickness (second-degree) and full-thickness (third-degree) burns. Document

## Special Populations

Burns to children are generally considered more serious than burns of similar size and severity to adults (**TABLE 27-2**). This is because infants and children have more surface area relative to total body mass, which means greater fluid and heat loss. In addition, children do not tolerate burns as well as adults do. Children are also more likely to go into shock, experience the development of hypothermia, and experience airway difficulties because of the unique differences associated with their ages and anatomy.

Many burns in infants and children result from child abuse. The classic burn resulting from deliberate immersion involves the hands and wrists, as well as the feet, lower legs, and buttocks. Similarly, burns around the genitals and multiple cigarette burns should be viewed as possible abuse. Report all suspected cases of abuse to the proper authorities. (See Chapter 35, *Pediatric Emergencies*.)

**TABLE 27-2 Classification of Burns in Infants and Children**

**Severe Burns**

- Any full-thickness burn
- Partial-thickness burns covering more than 20% TBSA

**Moderate Burns**

- Partial-thickness burns covering 10% to 20% TBSA

**Minor Burns**

- Partial-thickness burns covering less than 10% TBSA

Abbreviation: TBSA, total body surface area

© Jones & Bartlett Learning.

superficial (first-degree) burns, but do not include them in the body surface area estimation of extent of burn injury.

## Patient Assessment of Burns

When you assess a burn, it is important to classify the patient's burns. Classifying burns involves determining the source of the burn, the depth of the burn, and its severity. Assessing a patient with a burn is essentially the same as assessing any other trauma patient. Again, be careful to focus not on the dramatic appearance of the injury, but rather on potential life threats that require treatment.

## Scene Size-up

As you arrive on scene, observe the scene for hazards and threats to the safety of you and your crew, bystanders, and the patient. Ensure that the factors that led to the patient's burn injury do not pose a hazard to you and your crew. Is the electricity turned off? Is the chemical leak secure? Has the fire been extinguished? Is there any potential for violence? Has the patient been decontaminated, if needed?

When possible, determine the type of burn that has been sustained and the MOI. What the patient reports will often provide some important information about the extent of the injury. Patients with burn injuries can be a challenge to treat both physically and emotionally. It is easy to become overwhelmed by the sights, sounds, and smells of burn victims.

Assess the scene for any environmental hazards. If the patient is the victim of a lightning strike, is the weather still a threat to your safety? Wear gloves and eye protection when treating any patient with a burn and gowns when serious injuries are expected. Determine the number of patients; the possibility for multiple patients grows if you are responding to a lightning strike or a vehicle crash. At vehicle crashes, ensure the scene is safe from energized electrical lines or leaking fuel in the area where you will be working. If you determine the power company, the fire department, or ALS units are needed, call for additional resources early. Remember, the patient with a burn is a trauma patient. Consider the potential for spinal injuries, broken bones, inhalation injuries, and other injuries.

## Primary Assessment

The primary assessment includes a rapid exam of the patient to identify and manage life-threatening concerns and to assist with transport decisions. The primary assessment begins when you approach the patient and form a general impression.

As you approach the burn trauma patient, simple clues can help identify how serious the injuries are and how quickly you need to assess and treat them. If your patient greets you with a hoarse voice or reports being in an enclosed space with a fire or intense heat source, these should be indications of a significant MOI. The presence of stridor means your patient's airway is significantly swollen and can signal impending complete airway obstruction. Similarly, if the patient has singed facial hair, eyebrows, or nasal hair, your initial general impression might be the patient has a potential airway and/or breathing problem.

Child abuse and elder abuse are unpleasant situations to handle. Unfortunately, they are often situations that involve burns. As you enter a scene where burns are involved, be suspicious of clues that may indicate abuse.

The burned patient you encounter may have graphic injuries; however, stay focused on the primary assessment. As you begin, always consider the need for manual spinal stabilization.

Check for responsiveness using the AVPU scale. Assess a patient's mental status by asking the patient about his or her chief complaint. If the patient is alert, this should help direct you to any apparent life threats. If the patient is not alert, determine if he or she responds to verbal or painful stimuli or if he or she is unresponsive. An unresponsive patient may very well have a life-threatening condition. In all patients whose level of consciousness is less than alert and oriented, you should administer high-flow oxygen via a nonrebreathing mask and provide immediate transport to the ED.

Ensure the patient has a clear and patent airway. If the patient is unresponsive or has a significantly altered level of consciousness, consider inserting a properly sized oropharyngeal or nasopharyngeal airway. Be alert to signs that the patient has inhaled hot gases or vapors, such as singed facial hair or soot present in or around the airway. Heavy amounts of secretions and frequent coughing may also indicate a respiratory burn.

Quickly assess for adequate breathing. Inspect and palpate the chest wall for DCAP-BTLS. Check for clear and symmetric breath sounds, and provide high-flow oxygen or provide assisted ventilations using a bag-mask device as needed, depending on the level of consciousness and breathing rate/quality of your patient. Patients with burns are trauma patients. Evaluate and treat them for spinal injuries and airway problems concurrently. How you open the airway depends on whether a neck injury is suspected. Could the patient have fallen? Do the circumstances surrounding the MOI suggest a possible spinal injury?

Quickly assess the pulse rate and quality and determine perfusion based on the patient's skin condition, color, temperature, and capillary refill time. If you see significant bleeding, take the necessary steps to control it. Significant bleeding is an immediate life threat. If the patient has obvious life-threatening external hemorrhage, control the bleeding first (before airway and breathing); then treat the patient for shock as quickly as possible. Shock frequently develops in patients with burns. Treat the shock by preventing heat loss. This is important because the damaged skin has only a limited ability to regulate body temperature. After the burning process has stopped, cover the patient with a blanket to prevent heat loss.

If the patient you are treating has an airway or breathing problem, significant burn injuries, significant external bleeding, or signs and symptoms of internal bleeding, consider rapid transport to the nearest hospital, trauma center, or burn center for treatment. Consulting with ALS providers may be appropriate for patients with moderate or severe burns and burns of the airway or inhalation injury. ALS providers can treat these patients with endotracheal intubation and intravenous fluids to support airway, breathing, and circulation (shock) difficulties. These can progress so rapidly that immediate ALS assistance can make the difference between life and death.

## History Taking

Investigate the chief complaint or history of present illness. Next, be alert for signs or symptoms of other injuries due to the MOI. If the patient was burned

## YOU are the Provider

You reassess the patient and then call your radio report to the receiving facility. The patient is still experiencing respiratory distress, but he is moving air adequately. Your estimated time of arrival at the hospital is 6 minutes.

| Recording Time: 17 Minutes | |
| --- | --- |
| **Level of consciousness** | Conscious and alert, but anxious |
| **Respirations** | 22 breaths/min; labored; hoarse voice |
| **Pulse** | 116 beats/min; strong and regular |
| **Skin** | Red, warm, and dry |
| **Blood pressure** | 160/80 mm Hg |
| **Spo₂** | 99% (on oxygen) |

**9.** What, if any, additional treatment is indicated for this patient?

in a confined space, suspect an inhalation injury. When burns result from explosive forces, be alert for other internal injuries and fractures.

Obtain a medical history and be alert for injury-specific signs and symptoms as well as any pertinent negatives such as no pain. Typical signs of a burn are pain, redness, swelling, blisters, or charring. Typically, symptoms include pain and/or burning at the injury site. Regardless of the type of burn injury, it is important to stop the burning process, apply dressings to prevent contamination, and treat the patient for shock.

Obtain a SAMPLE history from your patient. In addition, ask the following questions of a patient with a burn:

- Are you having any difficulty breathing?
- Are you having any difficulty swallowing?
- Are you having any pain?

When you assess a patient with a burn, check to see whether the patient has an emergency medical identification device—a wallet card, necklace, or bracelet—or ask the patient or a family member about preexisting conditions, which may increase the chances of a poor outcome. Remember that the environment, bystanders, and medical identification devices may provide important clues about your patient's condition.

## Secondary Assessment

The secondary assessment is a more detailed, comprehensive, or focused examination of the patient that is conducted to reveal injuries that may have been missed during the primary assessment. In some instances where the patient is critically injured or the transport time is short, you may not have time to conduct a secondary assessment. In other instances, the secondary assessment may occur en route to the ED.

After you complete the primary assessment, perform an exam of the entire body. Quickly assess the patient from head to toe looking for DCAP-BTLS to ensure you have found all of the problems and injuries. Make a rough estimate, using the rule of nines, of the extent of the burned area to report to medical control. Determine what classification of burns the victim has sustained. The patient may report pain depending on the amount of nerve damage. Before you package your patient, determine the severity of the burns the victim has sustained.

Severity is calculated by considering what caused the burn, the body region that is burned, the depth and extent of the burn, the patient's age, and preexisting illness or injuries. Follow your local protocols for criteria for transport to a burn center. Package the patient for transport based on your findings. Remember to immobilize your patient for spinal injuries as appropriate.

Assessing the respiratory system involves looking, listening, and feeling. A patient who is conscious, alert, and talking does not have immediate airway or breathing difficulties. When you assess the respiratory system of a patient with a burn, look specifically for the following findings:

1. Soot around the mouth
2. Soot around the nose
3. Singed nasal hairs

If any of these findings are present, open the patient's mouth and examine for burns or swelling of the tongue. Ask the patient to cough, and assess for black sputum, which indicates smoke inhalation.

Next, listen to breath sounds with a stethoscope. Breath sounds should be clear and equal bilaterally, anteriorly, and posteriorly. Determine the patient's rate and quality of respiration. Finally, assess the chest for DCAP-BTLS and asymmetric chest wall movement. Patients with burns who present with any type of airway problem should be considered critical.

Quickly assess pulse rate and quality; determine the skin condition, color, and temperature; and check the capillary refill time. If you see visible significant bleeding, you must begin the steps necessary to control bleeding. Significant bleeding, internal or external, is an immediate life threat. If the patient has obvious life-threatening bleeding, quickly control it and treat for shock as quickly as possible. Non–life-threatening bleeding, such as in abrasions, can be bandaged later in your assessment as necessary.

Assess the patient's neurologic system to formulate baseline data for further decisions on patient management. This examination should include assessing for the following:

- Level of consciousness—use AVPU
- Pupil size and reactivity
- Motor response
- Sensory response

Assess the musculoskeletal system by performing a detailed full-body scan. Assess all anatomic regions looking for DCAP-BTLS. Specifically look for the following features:

- In the head, check for singed nasal or facial hair, burns or swelling of the face or ears, or burns or swelling in the mouth. If the patient sustained an electrical injury, examine the scalp for signs of an entrance or exit wounds.
- In the neck, check for burns, especially if they encircle the entire neck, which can impair circulation.
- In the chest, check for burns that encircle the entire chest, which can impair normal chest rise.
- In the abdomen and pelvis, feel all four quadrants for tenderness or rigidity. If the abdomen is tender, expect internal bleeding. Look for burns of the genitalia, as burns to this area are considered high risk.
- Look for burns that encircle an extremity, as they can impair circulation. If the patient sustained an electrical injury, assess thoroughly for entry or exit burn wounds. This should include the axilla and the area between digits. Record the pulse and motor and sensory function.
- Examine the posterior surface of the body, as large burns or electrical exit burns may be located in this body area.

A systematic examination helps you understand what has happened to the outside of your patient. Vital signs are a good indication of how your patient is doing on the inside. If you obtain an early set of vital signs, you will know how your patient is tolerating his or her injuries while en route to the hospital. Because shock is often pronounced in a patient with a burn, blood pressure, pulse, and skin assessment for perfusion are important vital signs to obtain.

In addition to hands-on assessment, use monitoring devices, including oxygen saturation monitors and carbon monoxide monitors, to quantify oxygenation and circulatory status.

## Reassessment

Repeat the primary assessment and reassess the patient's vital signs. Reassess the patient's chief complaint. Reevaluate interventions and treatment you have provided to the patient, particularly those used to treat shock. Identify and treat any changes in the patient's condition.

The goals in treating patients with burns are to stop the burning process, assess and treat breathing, support circulation, and provide rapid transport. Because patients with burns are also trauma patients, provide spinal motion restriction consistent with your local protocol if you suspect spinal injuries. Oxygen is mandatory for inhalation burns and large body surface area burns. If the patient has signs of hypoperfusion, treat aggressively for shock and provide rapid transport to the appropriate hospital. Cover all burns according to your local protocols. The risk of infection is very high and can be reduced if you cover large burn areas with sterile burn sheets or clean linen. Do not delay transport of a seriously injured patient to complete non–life-saving treatments in the field such as splinting extremity fractures. Instead, complete these types of treatment en route to the hospital.

Provide hospital personnel with a description of how the burn occurred. Often, the ED staff can determine the appropriate dilutant for chemical burns or calculate appropriate treatments for other types of burns with enough advanced notice. Report and document the extent of the burns. This should include the amount of body surface area involved, the depth of the burn, and the location. For example, you may say 10% full-thickness burns, 15% partial-thickness burns, and 25% superficial burns to the chest, abdomen, and left lower extremity. If special areas are involved (genitalia, feet, hands, face, or circumferential), they should be specifically mentioned and documented.

## Emergency Medical Care for Burns

Your first responsibility in caring for a patient with a burn is to stop the burning process and prevent additional injury. When caring for a patient with a burn, follow the steps in **SKILL DRILL 27-2**:

1. Follow standard precautions. Because a burn destroys the patient's protective skin layer, always wear gloves and eye protection when treating a patient with a burn.
2. Move the patient away from the burning area. If any clothing is on fire, wrap the patient in a blanket or follow the specific guidelines outlined by your local fire department protocol to put out the flames, and then remove any smoldering clothing and/or jewelry.

## Skill Drill 27-2 Caring for Burns

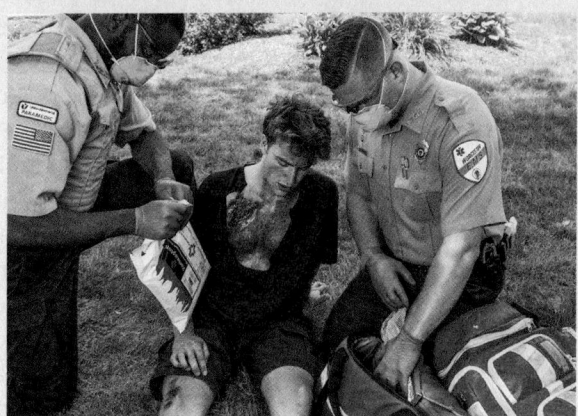

### Step 1

Follow standard precautions to help prevent infection. Remove the patient from the burning area; extinguish or remove hot clothing and jewelry as necessary. If the wound is still burning or hot, immerse the hot area in cool, sterile water, or cover with a wet, cool dressing.

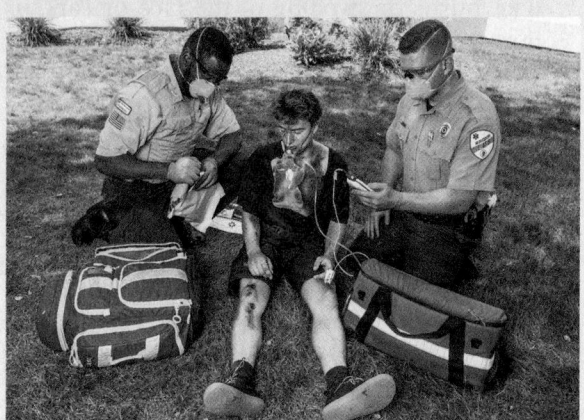

### Step 2

Provide high-flow oxygen, and continue to assess the airway.

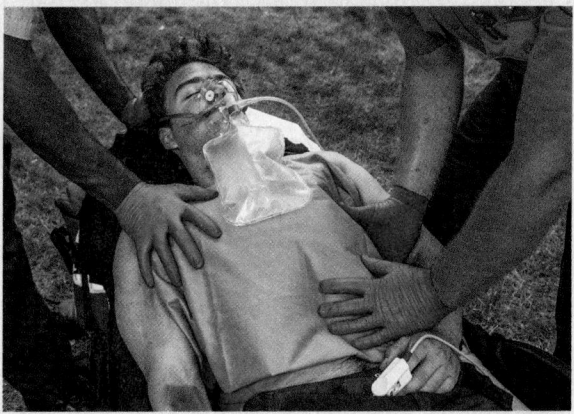

### Step 3

Estimate the severity of the burn, and then cover the area with a dry, sterile dressing or clean sheet. Assess and treat the patient for any other injuries.

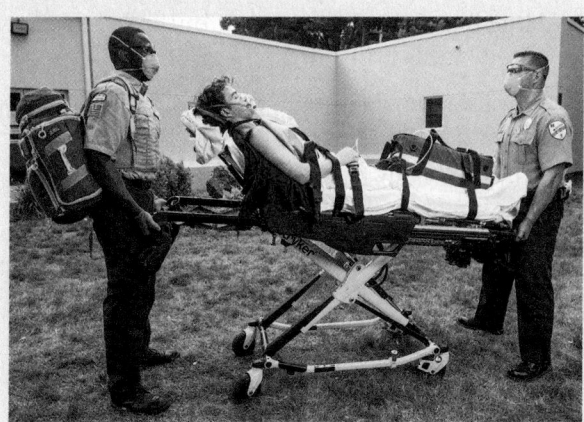

### Step 4

Prepare for transport. Treat for shock. Cover the patient with blankets to prevent loss of body heat. Transport promptly.

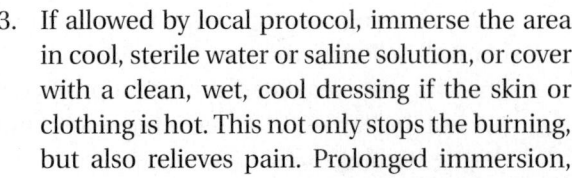

© Jones & Bartlett Learning.

3. If allowed by local protocol, immerse the area in cool, sterile water or saline solution, or cover with a clean, wet, cool dressing if the skin or clothing is hot. This not only stops the burning, but also relieves pain. Prolonged immersion, however, may increase the risk of infection and hypothermia. For this reason, you should not keep the affected part submersed in water for more than 10 minutes. If the burning has stopped before you arrive, do not immerse the

affected part at all. As an alternative to immersion, irrigate the burned area until the burning stops; next apply a sterile dressing (**Step 1**).

Cover large (greater than 10% BSA) burns with a dry, sterile, nonadherent dressing (eg, a sterile burn sheet). Other than for the purpose of stopping the burning process, do not apply water or saline to large surface burn areas.

4. Provide high-flow oxygen. Remember that more fire victims die of smoke inhalation than of skin burns. A patient who has facial burns or has inhaled smoke or fumes may experience respiratory distress. Therefore, provide high-flow oxygen to the patient. Keep in mind that a patient who appears to be breathing well at first may suddenly experience severe respiratory distress. Therefore, continually assess the airway for possible problems (**Step 2**).

5. Rapidly estimate the burn's severity. Cover the burned area with a dry, sterile dressing to prevent further contamination. Sterile gauze is best if the area is not too large. You may cover larger areas with a clean, white sheet. Do not put anything else on the burned area. Never use ointments, lotions, or antiseptics of any kind and do not intentionally break any blisters.

6. Check for traumatic injuries or other medical conditions that may be immediately life threatening. Most patients who have been burned have normal vital signs and can communicate at first, which will make your assessment easier (**Step 3**).

7. Treat the patient for shock.

8. An extensive burn can produce hypothermia (loss of body heat). Prevent further heat loss by covering the patient with warm blankets.

9. Provide prompt transport by local protocol. Do not delay transport to perform a prolonged assessment or to apply coverings to burns in a critical patient (**Step 4**).

## Words of Wisdom

The key to initial burn treatment is to stop the burning process. Using cool water and not cold water is crucial. Using cold water or ice water can cause further injury to the tissue. Once you have stopped the burning process, you must remember to prevent heat loss to reduce the risk of hypothermia.

## Street Smarts

Being burned is a scary experience for most patients. They experience pain, odors associated with burning flesh and hair, and the fear of disfigurement. In your interaction with these patients, be supportive and empathetic. Do your best to make them comfortable while managing life-threatening injuries and transporting to the closest appropriate facility.

## Management of Specific Burns
### Thermal Burns

A **thermal burn** is caused by heat (as opposed to electricity, chemicals, or radiation). Many different situations can cause thermal burns, and all pose a safety hazard to responding emergency care providers. Most commonly, thermal burns are caused by scalds or an open flame. A **flame burn** is very often a deep burn, especially if a person's clothing catches fire. Hot liquids produce scald injuries. A **scald burn** is most commonly seen in children and handicapped adults but can happen to anyone, particularly while cooking. Scald burns often cover large surface areas of the body because liquids can spread quickly. Coming in contact with hot objects produces a **contact burn**. Ordinarily, reflexes protect a person from prolonged exposure to a very hot object, so contact burns are rarely deep unless the patient was prevented from drawing away from the hot object (eg, unconscious, intoxicated, restrained, or impaired).

A **steam burn** can produce a topical (scald) burn. Minor steam burns are common when uncovering the plastic wrap from microwaved food. When the plastic is peeled away, hot steam escapes directly onto the person's hand. Steam (ie, gaseous water) may also cause airway burns.

Another important source of thermal burns is the **flash burn** produced by an explosion, which may briefly expose a person to very intense heat. Lightning strikes can also cause a flash burn. These injuries are usually minor compared with the potential for trauma from whatever caused the flash.

Manage thermal burns mostly the same as you would manage any other burn. Stop the burning source, cool the burned area if appropriate, and remove all jewelry. Maintain a high index of suspicion for inhalation injuries. Increased exposure time will increase damage to the patient. The larger the burn, the more likely the patient will be susceptible to hypothermia and/or hypovolemia. All patients with large surface burns should have a dry sterile dressing applied to help maintain body temperature, prevent infection, and provide comfort.

## Inhalation Burns

Inhalation injuries can occur when burning takes place in enclosed spaces without ventilation. When the upper airway is exposed to excessive heat, the patient can experience rapid and serious airway compromise. The heat can be an irritant to the lungs and the airway, causing coughing, wheezing, and rapid swelling or edema of the mucosa of the upper airway tissues, often evidenced by stridor. Upper airway damage is often associated with the inhalation of superheated gases. Lower airway damage is more often associated with the inhalation of chemicals (eg, acids, aldehydes) and particulate matter. When treating a patient for inhalation injuries, you may encounter severe upper airway swelling that requires immediate intervention. Sometimes airway swelling and compromise will develop more slowly and not manifest until transport. You should consider requesting ALS backup if the patient has signs or symptoms of edema, such as stridor, a hoarse voice, singed nasal hairs, singed facial hairs, burns of the face, or carbon particles in the sputum. Alternatively, expediting transport to the nearest emergency department capable of advanced airway management should be considered if faster than waiting for ALS arrival at the scene. Remember that these patients can deteriorate quickly. Apply cool mist, aerosol therapy, or humidified oxygen to help reduce some minor edema.

## Inhalation of Toxic Gases

The combustion process produces a variety of toxic gases. The less efficient the combustion process, the more toxic the gases—such as carbon monoxide and carbon dioxide—that may be created. When furnaces, kerosene heaters, and other heating devices are in poor repair, they may emit unsafe levels of these toxic gases. Internal combustion engines may emit many of the same gases and, consequently, should always have their exhaust vented to the outdoors. A common cause of carbon monoxide exposure is running a small engine in an enclosed space such as a garage or basement. For this reason, many ambulance services and fire departments have added carbon monoxide detectors to their garages or ambulance bays. Firefighters who are performing an overhaul after a fire may be exposed to high levels of carbon monoxide, as may people who are exposed to large amounts of car exhaust (such as toll takers and auto mechanics).

Carbon monoxide intoxication should be considered whenever a group of people in the same place all report a headache or nausea (a malfunctioning furnace or car exhaust being sucked into the air-handling system can cause carbon monoxide intoxication in groups of people). Similarly, you should be suspicious when people complain of feeling sick at home but not when they go to work or school.

Carbon monoxide can displace oxygen from the alveolar air and from its attachment sites on hemoglobin molecules contained in circulating red blood cells. Because carbon monoxide binds to receptor sites on hemoglobin at least 250 times more easily than oxygen does, the patient's hemoglobin may become saturated with the wrong chemical. Being exposed to relatively small concentrations of carbon monoxide (such as in cigarette smoke) will result in progressively higher blood levels of carbon monoxide. Most people have approximately 2% carbon monoxide attached to their hemoglobin, but these levels may be as high as 4% to 8% in heavy smokers. Levels of 50% or higher may be fatal.

Patients with severe carbon monoxide intoxication usually have an oxygen saturation ($Spo_2$) level that is normal. For this reason, patients who have potentially inhaled toxic gases should receive a high concentration of supplemental oxygen regardless of pulse oximetry readings. New devices that can measure a patient's carbon monoxide level are becoming more widespread in EMS systems, allowing providers to recognize and treat low-level carbon monoxide intoxication rapidly.

The gaseous form of cyanide is hydrogen cyanide. It is generated by the combustion of commonly encountered substances such as paper, cotton, and wool. Hydrogen cyanide is colorless and has the smell of bitter almonds; however, it can be difficult to detect at the scene of a fire. Prehospital diagnosis of hydrogen cyanide poisoning is difficult because laboratory studies are necessary. Signs and symptoms involve the central nervous, respiratory, and cardiovascular systems of the body and include faintness, anxiety, abnormal vital signs, headache, seizures, paralysis, and coma.

In situations in which you have patients who have sustained inhalation injuries, you must first ensure your own safety and the safety of your co-workers. Once you have taken precautions, prehospital treatment of a patient with suspected hydrogen cyanide poisoning may include decontamination and supportive care according to signs and symptoms displayed by the patient until an antidote can be administered by ALS providers.

Exposure to other toxic gases can also cause damage to organs and systems and may cause death. Care for any toxic gas exposure includes recognition, identification, and supportive treatment as necessary according to the patient's signs and symptoms.

## Chemical Burns

A chemical burn can occur whenever a toxic substance contacts the body. Most chemical burns are caused by strong acids or strong alkalis. The eyes are particularly vulnerable to chemical burns (**FIGURE 27-20**). Sometimes the fumes alone from strong chemicals can cause burns, especially to the respiratory tract. The severity of the burn is directly related to the type of chemical, the concentration of the chemical, and the duration of the exposure.

In cases of severe chemical burns or exposure, consider mobilizing a hazardous materials (hazmat) team, if appropriate. To prevent exposure to hazardous materials, determine if you can safely approach the patient. In some cases, you will need to wait to provide care until hazardous materials technicians have decontaminated the patient. You must wear the appropriate chemical-resistant gloves and eye protection whenever you are caring for a patient with a chemical burn. Be particularly careful not to get any chemical, dry or liquid, on yourself or on your uniform; consider wearing a protective gown when this is a possibility. Remember that exposure risk is also present when you are cleaning up after a call.

Treatment of chemical burns can be specific to the chemical agent. If available, read all of the labels of the chemical agent. Do not risk exposure while attempting to gather information on the chemical. If the exposure occurs at an industrial site, such as a chemical manufacturing plant, an expert should be on site and should be able to provide you with valuable information on the chemical.

The emergency care of a chemical burn is basically the same as that for a thermal burn, discussed earlier in the chapter. The severity of the burn will depend on the type of chemical, its strength, the duration of exposure, and the area of the body exposed. To stop the burning process, remove any chemical from the patient. A dry chemical that is activated by contact with water may damage the skin more when it is wet than when it is dry. Therefore, always brush off dry chemicals from the skin and clothing before flushing the patient with water (**FIGURE 27-21**). Remove the patient's clothing,

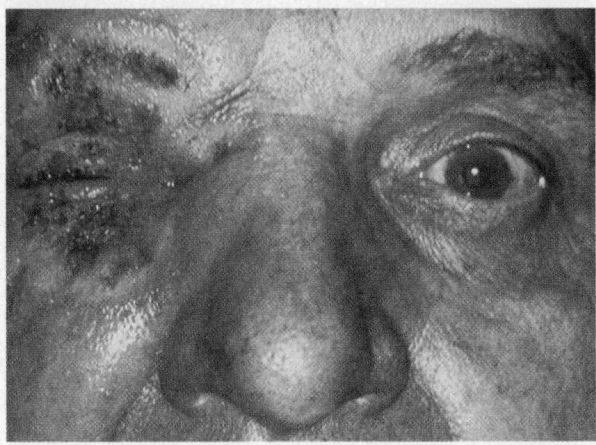

**FIGURE 27-20** The eyes are particularly vulnerable to chemical burns.

© Western Ophthalmic Hospital/Science Source.

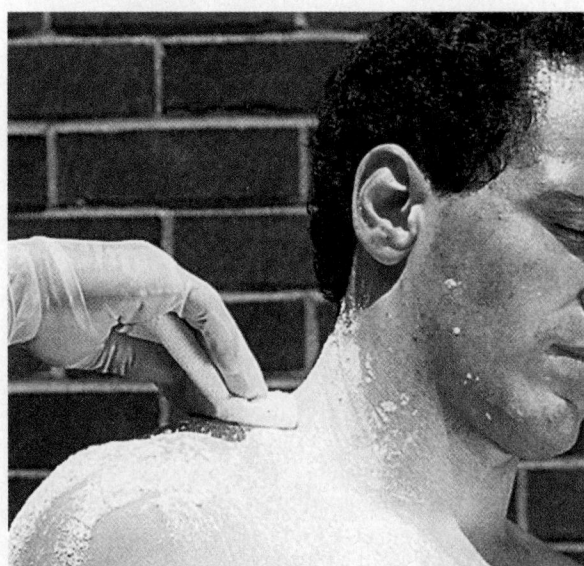

**FIGURE 27-21** Brush off dry chemicals before you flush the burned area with water.

© Jones & Bartlett Learning.

including shoes, stockings, gloves, and any jewelry or eyeglasses, because there may be small amounts of chemicals in the creases. Take great care to ensure you do not come in contact with the chemical. The patient should be properly decontaminated by properly trained personnel.

For liquid chemicals, immediately flush the burned area with large amounts of water (**FIGURE 27-22**). Take care not to contaminate uninjured areas or make the patient hypothermic. Never direct a forceful stream of water from a hose at the patient; the extreme water pressure may mechanically injure the burned skin. Continue flooding the area with gallons of water for 15 to 20 minutes after the patient says the burning pain has stopped. If the patient's eye has been burned, hold the eyelid open (without applying pressure over the globe of the eye) while flooding the eye with a gentle stream of water (**FIGURE 27-23**). Flush the eyes from the inside corners to the outside to prevent cross contamination. If only one eye has been affected, turn the patient's head to that side and flush. If both eyes are affected, consider hooking up a nasal cannula to a bag of saline to flush both eyes simultaneously. The prongs can be placed on the bridge of the nose to flush from the inside corners of the eyes to the outside corners. Be careful not to touch the prongs to the eye or surrounding tissue. Continue flushing the contaminated area en route to the hospital.

As with any substance, once the fluid has been contaminated with the chemical, collect it and properly dispose of it. Conduct a proper decontamination prior to loading any patient into the ambulance and again prior to entering a hospital.

## Electrical Burns

Electrical burns may be the result of contact with high- or low-voltage electricity. High-voltage burns may occur when utility workers make direct contact with power lines. Ordinary household current is still powerful enough to cause severe burns as well as cardiac dysrhythmias.

There must be a complete circuit between the electrical source and the ground for electricity to flow. Any substance that prevents this circuit from being completed, such as rubber, is called an insulator. Any substance that allows a current to flow

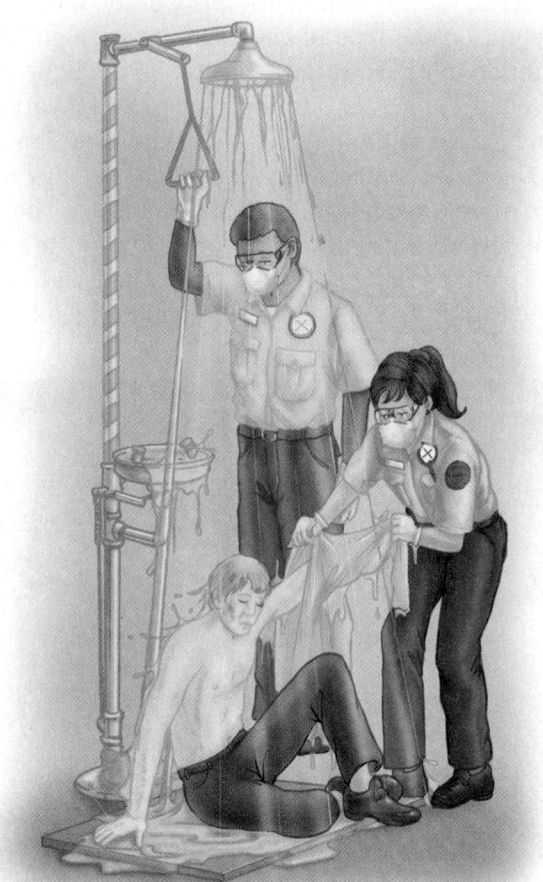

**FIGURE 27-22** Flush the burned area with large amounts of water for 15 to 20 minutes after the patient says that the burning pain has stopped. Avoid contaminating uninjured areas.

© Jones & Bartlett Learning.

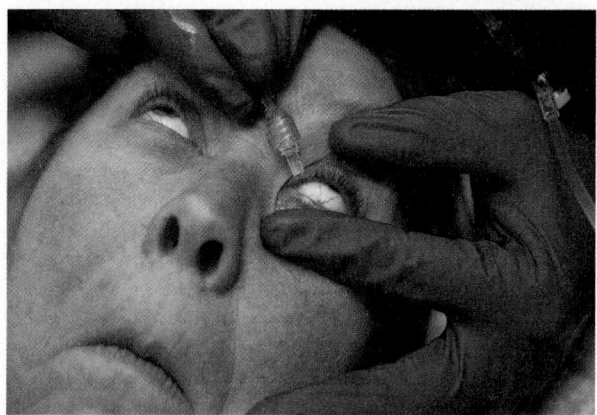

**FIGURE 27-23** Flood the affected eye with a gentle stream of water. Hold the eyelids open, a challenging task because the patient's reflex is to keep the eye shut. Take care to prevent any of the chemical from getting into the other eye during flushing.

© Jones & Bartlett Learning.

through it is called a conductor. The human body, which is primarily water, is a good conductor. Thus, electrical burns occur when the body, or a part of it, completes a circuit connecting a power source to the ground (**FIGURE 27-24**).

The type of electric current, magnitude of current (amperage), and voltage have effects on the seriousness of burns. When an electric current enters the body, the skin is burned at the entrance wound as well as everywhere along the path until the current grounds and exits the body. In addition to tissues damaged by the heat, significant chemical changes take place in the nervous, cardiovascular, and muscular systems of the body, causing disruption of the body's normal functions and/or even system failure.

Your safety is particularly important when you are called to the scene of an emergency involving electricity. Obviously, you can be fatally injured by coming into contact with power lines. But you can also be fatally injured by touching a patient who is still in contact with a live power line or any other electrical source. For this reason, never attempt to remove someone from an electrical source unless you are specially trained to do so. Likewise, never move a downed power line unless you have the special training and equipment necessary for the job. Before even approaching someone who may still be in contact with a power line or an electrical appliance, make certain the power is turned off. Always assume that any downed power line is live.

A burn injury appears where the electricity enters (an entrance wound) and exits (an exit wound)

the body. The entrance wound may be quite small (**FIGURE 27-25A**), but the exit wound can be extensive and deep (**FIGURE 27-25B**). Always look for both entrance and exit wounds. There are two dangers specifically associated with electrical burns. First, there may be a large amount of deep tissue injury. Electrical burns are often more severe than the external signs indicate. The patient may have only a small burn to the skin but may have massive damage to the deeper tissues, organs, and the nervous system (**FIGURE 27-26**). The force of the electrical energy can also cause fractures or joint dislocations. Second, the patient may go into cardiac or respiratory arrest from the electric shock.

Electrical current can cross the chest and cause cardiac arrest or dysrhythmias. Cardiac arrest can also occur after a lightning strike, which is a form of an electrical burn. If indicated, begin CPR on the patient and apply the AED. Although CPR may need to

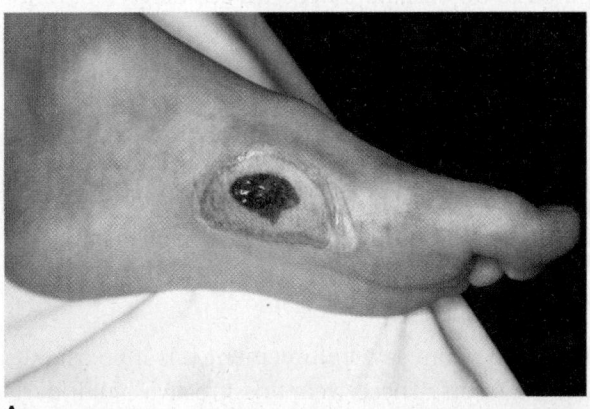

**A**

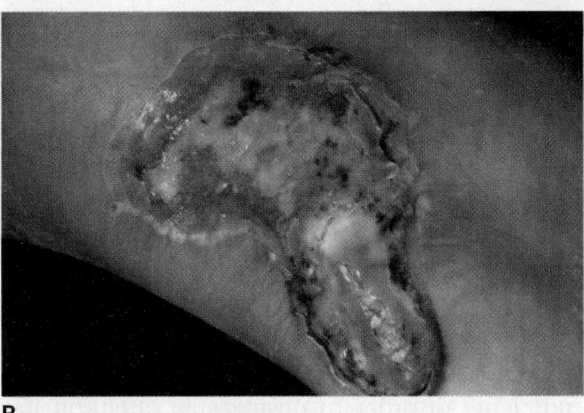

**B**

**FIGURE 27-25** Electrical burns, like gunshot wounds, have entrance and exit wounds. **A.** An entrance wound is often quite small. **B.** The exit wound can be extensive and deep.

A, B: © Chuck Stewart, MD.

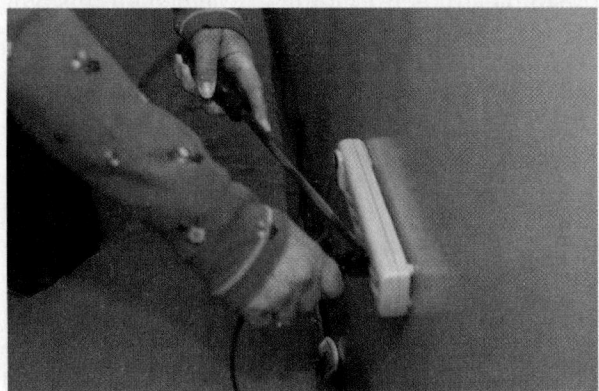

**FIGURE 27-24** The human body is a good conductor of electricity. An electrical burn usually occurs when the body, acting as a conductor, completes a circuit.

© Jones & Bartlett Learning.

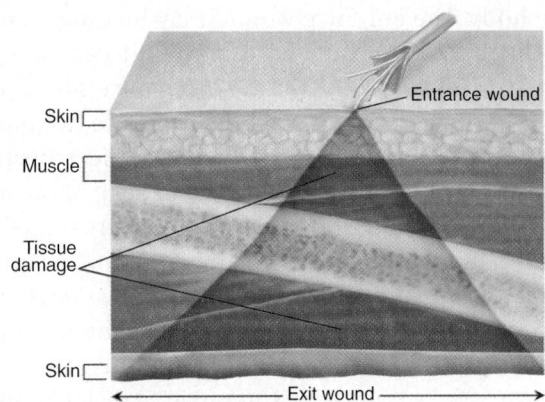

**FIGURE 27-26** External signs of an electrical burn may be deceiving. The entrance wound may be a small burn, whereas the damage to deeper tissue may be massive.

© Jones & Bartlett Learning.

be quite prolonged in patients with electrical burns, it has a high success rate if started promptly. Be prepared to defibrillate if necessary. If neither CPR nor defibrillation is indicated, give supplemental oxygen, and monitor the patient closely for respiratory and cardiac arrest. Treat the soft-tissue injuries by placing dry, sterile dressings on all burn wounds and splinting suspected fractures. Provide prompt transport; all electrical burns are potentially severe injuries that require further treatment in the hospital.

## Taser Injuries

In recent years, law enforcement has increased its use of Tasers. These weapons fire two small darts (electrodes) that puncture the patient's skin. Taser injuries are generally treated as impaled objects and the electrodes are removed by a physician; however, in some jurisdictions, EMTs are permitted to remove these barbs from patients, depending on local protocol. The barbs are approximately 0.5 inch (13 mm) in length, and although they produce wounds, they are small and easily managed unless they penetrate the eye.

When a Taser has been used, the patient can experience potential complications, particularly when he or she is already experiencing certain underlying disorders. Considerable attention has focused on a condition known as **excited delirium**, which is often characterized by extreme agitation, reduced pain sensitivity, hallucinations, persistent struggling, and elevated temperature. This condition is commonly associated with illegal drug ingestion. Excited delirium is a true emergency and warrants assisted ALS response.

Previously, using a Taser in patients with true excited delirium has been associated with dysrhythmias and sudden cardiac arrest. Other studies have found that the risk of sudden death is related to the excited delirium condition, rather than being associated with Taser use. Regardless, be aware of this possibility, and be certain you have access to an AED when you respond to calls for patients who have been exposed to Taser shots.

## Radiation Burns

Acute radiation exposure has become more than a theoretical issue because the use of radioactive materials has increased in industry and medicine; therefore, you must understand it to effectively manage patients exposed to radiation. Potential threats include incidents related to the use and transportation of radioactive isotopes and intentionally released radioactivity in terrorist attacks. To be effective, first determine if there has been a radiation exposure, and then determine whether ongoing exposure continues to exist. Increasingly, special response units are equipped with pager-size radiation detectors, or such detection devices may be provided by other public safety services.

There are three types of ionizing radiation: alpha, beta, and gamma. Alpha particles have little penetrating energy and are easily stopped by the skin. Beta particles have greater penetrating power and can travel much farther in air than alpha particles. They can penetrate the skin but can be blocked by simple protective clothing designed for this purpose. The threat from gamma radiation is directly proportional to its wavelength. This type of radiation is very penetrating and easily passes through the body and solid materials.

Radiation is measured in units of radiation absorbed dose (rad) or radiation equivalent in man (rem): 100 rad = 1 gray (Gy). Small amounts of everyday background radiation are measured in rad; the amount of radiation released in a major incident may be measured in gray. The average human exposure from background radiation is 0.31 rem per year. Mild radiation sickness can be expected with exposures of 1 to 2 Gy (100 to 200 rad), moderate sickness at 2 to 5 Gy, and severe sickness at 4 to 6 Gy. Exposure to more than 10 Gy may result in death within 2 to 4 weeks.

Most ionizing radiation accidents involve gamma radiation, or x-rays. People who have sustained a radiation exposure generally do not pose a risk to the people around them. However, in some types of incidents—particularly those involving explosions—patients may be contaminated with radioactive particulate matter. It is speculated that after a nuclear explosion, most patients will have sustained some type of trauma in addition to the radiation exposure.

Being exposed to a radiation source does not make a patient contaminated or radioactive. However, when patients have a radioactive source on their body (such as debris from a bomb that dispersed radioactive material), they are contaminated and must be initially cared for by a hazmat responder. Maintain a safe distance and wait for the hazmat team to decontaminate the patient before initiating care. Once decontaminated by the hazmat team, care is often transferred to the EMT. Most contaminants can be removed by simply removing the patient's clothes. Call for additional resources to manage this situation. Once the patient is decontaminated and there is no threat to you, begin treating the XABCs and treat the patient for any burns or trauma.

Irrigate open wounds. Washing should be gentle to avoid further damage to the skin, which could result in additional internal radiation absorption. Irrigate the head and scalp the same way. The ED should be notified as soon as practical if you are transporting a potentially contaminated patient. In contrast with other types of contamination, radioactive particulate matter probably poses a relatively small risk to the provider. Consider providing basic care to the patient before decontamination if you are wearing protective clothing.

Increasing your and the patient's distance from the source by even a few feet may dramatically decrease your exposure. Therefore, it is important to identify the radioactive source and the length of the patient's exposure to it, if this information is available without putting you or your patient at risk for exposure. If not readily available, rely on the hazmat team to obtain this information. Limit your duration of exposure, increase your distance from the source, and attempt to place shielding between yourself and sources of gamma radiation.

With contact radiation burns, decontaminate the wound as if it were a chemical burn to remove any radioactive particulate matter, then treat it as a burn.

Many radioactive isotopes are used in medicine and industry, some of which can be absorbed or have their toxic effects blunted by another substance. Like their radioactive effects, the toxic effects of these isotopes vary. Antidotes may help bind an isotope, enhance its elimination from the body, or reduce the toxic effects on other organs. Such antidotal therapy should be considered only under the guidance of a knowledgeable physician or public health agency.

# Dressing and Bandaging

All wounds require bandaging. In most instances, splints help to control bleeding and provide firm support for the dressing. There are many different types of dressings and bandages (**FIGURE 27-27**). You should be familiar with the function and proper application of each.

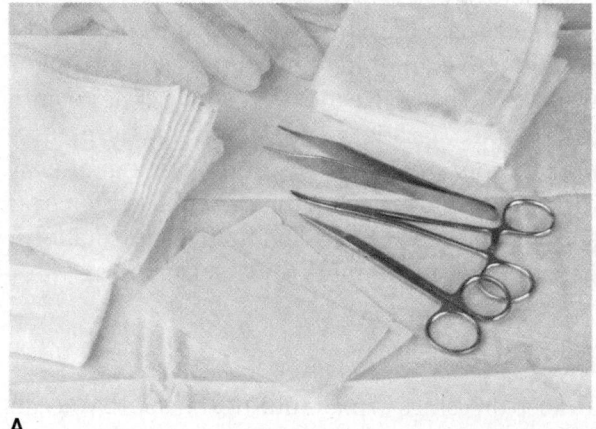

A

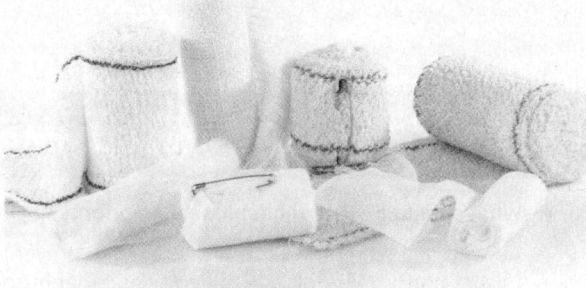

B

**FIGURE 27-27 A.** Many types of sterile dressings are used for covering open wounds, including universal dressings, gauze pads, adhesive dressings, and occlusive dressings. **B.** Bandages keep dressings in place and include soft roller bandages, triangular bandages, and adhesive tape. Splints may also be used to hold dressings in place.

In general, dressings and bandages have three primary functions:

- To control bleeding
- To protect the wound from further damage
- To prevent further contamination and infection

## Sterile Dressings

Universal dressings, conventional 4 × 4–inch (10 × 10–cm) and 4 × 8–inch (10 × 20–cm) gauze pads, and assorted small adhesive-type dressings and soft self-adherent roller dressings will cover most wounds. The universal dressing measures 9 × 36 inches (23 × 91 cm), is made of thick, absorbent material, and is ideal for covering large open wounds. It also makes an efficient pad for rigid splints. These dressings are available in compact, commercially sterilized packages.

Gauze pads are appropriate for smaller wounds, and adhesive-type dressings are useful for minor wounds. An **occlusive dressing**, made of petroleum jelly-based (Vaseline) gauze, aluminum foil, or plastic, prevents air and liquids from entering (or exiting) the wound. These dressings are used to cover sucking chest wounds, abdominal eviscerations, penetrating back wounds, and neck injuries.

## Bandages

To keep dressings in place during transport, you can use soft roller bandages, rolls of gauze, triangular bandages, or adhesive tape. The self-adherent, soft roller bandages are probably easiest to use. They are slightly elastic, which makes them easy to apply, and you can tuck the end of the roll into a deeper layer to secure it in place. The layers adhere somewhat but should not be applied too tightly to one another.

Adhesive tape holds small dressings in place and helps secure larger dressings. Some people, however, are allergic to adhesive tape. If you know your patient is allergic, use paper or plastic tape instead.

Do not use elastic bandages to secure dressings. If the injury swells, the bandage may become a tourniquet and cause further damage. Any improperly applied bandage that impairs circulation can result in additional tissue damage or even the loss of a limb. Always check a limb distal to a bandage for signs of impaired circulation and loss of sensation. Air splints and vacuum splints are useful in stabilizing broken extremities, and they can be used with dressings to help control bleeding from soft-tissue injuries.

If a wound continues to bleed despite the use of direct pressure, quickly use a tourniquet. This is discussed further in Chapter 26, *Bleeding*. Research from the Iraq war has taught us that use of a tourniquet is rarely harmful. If you cannot control bleeding from a major vessel in an extremity, a properly applied tourniquet may save a patient's life. Specifically, the tourniquet is useful if a patient is bleeding severely from any limb injury. Furthermore, the tourniquet is most effective as a life-saving measure if applied prior to the onset of shock from blood loss.

## YOU are the Provider SUMMARY

**1. What should be your most immediate priority?**

As with any patient, your first priority is to prevent further harm. Although the patient was brought to you wrapped in a blanket, this does not mean that his skin or clothing have stopped burning. First, remove the blanket to ensure that his clothes are not smoldering and that the burning process has stopped.

If the patient's clothes are still smoldering or if there is any other evidence to indicate the burning process is ongoing, pour sterile water or saline over the affected areas. Alternatively, apply moist, sterile dressings to extinguish the burning areas. These actions not only stop the burning process, but also help relieve pain. If the burning process has stopped, do not apply any water, saline, or moist dressings until you further assess the patient.

Once you have stopped the burning process, airway and breathing assessment is essential, as the soot on the patient's face indicates a strong risk of smoke or toxic gas inhalation or potential airway injury from inhaling heated air.

## YOU are the Provider **SUMMARY** *continued*

**2. What is a thermal burn? What are the causes of thermal burns?**

A thermal burn is a burn caused by heat, as opposed to radiation, chemicals, or electricity; however, many different situations can cause thermal burns.

Most commonly, thermal burns are caused by an open flame (flame burn), but thermal burns can result whenever the skin is exposed to temperatures higher than 111°F (44°C)—even prolonged exposure to sunlight. In general, the severity of a thermal burn correlates directly with the temperature of the heat source, the amount of heat energy possessed by the object or substance, and the duration of exposure.

Other sources of heat energy, other than fire, include scald burns, which occur from exposure to boiling liquids; contact burns, which occur when a person comes in contact with a heated surface; steam burns, which occur when the body is exposed to superheated gaseous water; and flash burns, which occur when a person is briefly exposed to very intense heat (eg, explosion).

**3. What additional information should you obtain from the firefighters who rescued the patient?**

It has already been established that the patient was trapped in an enclosed space because the firefighters rescued him from the structure. However, you should determine an approximate length of exposure; this is usually a gross estimate at best.

Determine if the patient was conscious or unconscious when he was found. Conscious patients are often able to extinguish themselves unless they are completely engulfed in flames. If the patient is unconscious, however, he or she does not have control over the duration of exposure to the fire itself or the quantity of superheated air that he or she inhales.

Determine how the patient was found. Was the patient in an open area of a room or was he or she trapped beneath a collapsed ceiling beam or other heavy structure? Although you should always assess the patient for traumatic injuries, information provided by the firefighters regarding any MOI can help you focus on a particular area (or areas) of the body. Do not assume the patient's injuries are limited to skin burns and toxic gas exposure; the patient may have experienced other injuries (eg, blunt trauma with internal bleeding, head injury) that could also be life threatening.

**4. How are thermal burns classified? What are the characteristics of each type of burn?**

Burns are classified according to their depth—that is, how far the burn injury extends through the layers of the skin (ie, epidermis, dermis). The types of burns you must be able to identify are superficial (first degree), partial-thickness (second degree), and full-thickness (third degree).

Superficial (first-degree) burns involve only the outer layer of the skin (the epidermis). The skin turns red and is often painful, but it does not blister or the burn does not extend below the epidermis.

Partial-thickness (second-degree) burns involve the epidermis and some portion of the dermis. These burns do not destroy the entire thickness of the skin, nor is the subcutaneous (fatty) tissue injured. Usually these burns are very painful and have blisters that may or may not be intact.

Full-thickness (third-degree) burns extend through all layers of the dermis and epidermis and may involve the subcutaneous skin layers, muscle, bone, or internal organs. The burned area may appear dry and leathery and may appear white, dark brown, or even charred. However, because the nerve endings in the dermis have been destroyed, the areas of full-thickness burn are painless.

**5. What percentage of the patient's body surface area has been burned?**

After you identify the depth of a burn, you must rapidly estimate the extent of the burns—that is, the percentage of the patient's TBSA that is burned.

Your patient has experienced burns to his anterior torso (chest and abdomen); this represents 18% of his TBSA. Additionally, both upper extremities are burned, which represents 18% (9% per extremity) of his TBSA. Therefore, *your patient has burns that cover approximately 36% of his TBSA.*

**6. What factors should you consider to determine the severity of a burn?**

When determining the severity of a burn, the two most important factors to consider initially are the depth and extent of the burn.

The American Burn Association classifies burns as being minor, moderate, or severe. However, your local protocols or regional burn center may have slightly different criteria.

Minor burns in an adult include full-thickness burns that cover less than 2% of BSA, partial-thickness burns that cover less than 15% of BSA, and superficial burns that cover less than 50% of BSA. Moderate burns include full-thickness burns that cover between 2% to 10% of BSA (excluding burns to critical areas of the body), partial-thickness burns that cover 15% to 30% of BSA, and superficial burns that cover more than 50% of BSA. Severe burns include *any* full-thickness burn to a critical area of the body, full-thickness burns that cover more than 10% of BSA to noncritical areas of the body, and partial-thickness burns that cover more than 30% of BSA.

In addition to the depth and extent of the burn, you must determine if the burns are located in any critical areas of the body. Critical areas of the body include the face, upper airway, hands, feet, and genitalia. Also, airway burns or circumferential burns (ie, burns that completely go around an extremity (causing compartment syndrome with the edema compressing and decreasing blood flow distal to the burn), or that go around the chest (causing decreased chest expansion and diminished ventilation) are considered critical burns. The same burn that this patient has would be considered critical in infants, young children, or older adults. Additional nonburn injuries may also move a burn level from moderate (as determined by depth and extent) to severe.

**7. What is the proper treatment of the patient's burns?**

Large (greater than 10% BSA) burns should be covered with a dry, sterile, nonadherent dressing (eg, a sterile burn sheet); *your patient has burns that cover approximately 36% of his BSA.* Other than for the purpose of stopping the burning process, do not apply water or saline to large surface area burns. The larger the burn area, the greater the risks of hypothermia, hypovolemia, and infection.

Dry, sterile dressings applied to large surface area burns help maintain body temperature (reduce the risk of hypothermia), prevent further contamination of the burn (reduce the risk of infection), and provide comfort.

Use further treatment to prevent hypothermia (cover the patient with a blanket); closely monitor the patient's airway and ventilation status and monitor for signs of shock. An ALS provider, if available, can provide pain management and treat complications such as airway swelling.

**8. How has the patient's condition changed? What should you do now?**

The patient's breathing is becoming labored. Respiratory distress in a patient with a burn, especially in a patient without other injuries that would cause breathing difficulties (eg, blunt chest trauma), indicates upper airway swelling secondary to inhaling excessive heat (inhalation injury).

Patients who are trapped in an enclosed space with poor ventilation, especially if they have a loss of consciousness, are at highest risk for an inhalation injury. Although your patient denies a loss of consciousness, you should still suspect some degree of upper airway swelling because he was in an enclosed space.

If the patient is breathing adequately, continue to administer high-flow oxygen and closely observe the patient. Cool mist or aerosol therapy may help reduce mild airway swelling. If the patient is not breathing adequately (eg, shallow breathing [reduced tidal volume], labored respirations, falling oxygen saturation, decreasing level of consciousness), assist his or her ventilations with a bag-mask device.

Depending on your transport time to the closest appropriate hospital and the availability of ALS resources in your area, you should consider an intercept with an ALS unit. Some patients with inhalation injuries require advanced airway management, such as endotracheal intubation, to protect the airway before it closes completely.

**9. What, if any, additional treatment is indicated for this patient?**

Continuous, careful monitoring of this patient is essential. Although his condition does not seem to have worsened, it also has not improved. Continue to administer high-flow oxygen, closely monitor the adequacy of his breathing, and be prepared to assist his ventilations. Monitor him for altered mental status and signs of shock and treat accordingly.

Any patient who is experiencing respiratory distress will be anxious. Provide emotional support and let the patient assume a position of comfort; this is usually a full Fowler (90° angle) position.

## YOU are the Provider SUMMARY *continued*

### EMS Patient Care Report (PCR)

| Date: 10-14-20 | Incident No.: 012309 | Nature of Call: Burns | | Location: 511 Bandera Rd. | |
|---|---|---|---|---|---|
| Dispatched: 1500 | En Route: 1500 | At Scene: 1500 | Transport: 1514 | At Hospital: 1530 | In Service: 1556 |

#### Patient Information

| | |
|---|---|
| **Age:** 45 <br> **Sex:** M <br> **Weight (in kg [lb]):** 77 kg (170 lb) | **Allergies:** No known drug allergies <br> **Medications:** None <br> **Past Medical History:** None <br> **Chief Complaint:** Burns to the torso and arms |

#### Vital Signs

| Time: 1506 | BP: 166/86 | Pulse: 108 | Respirations: 14 | SpO$_2$: 98% |
|---|---|---|---|---|
| Time: 1512 | BP: 158/84 | Pulse: 120 | Respirations: 22 | SpO$_2$: 99% |
| Time: 1517 | BP: 160/80 | Pulse: 116 | Respirations: 22 | SpO$_2$: 99% |

#### EMS Treatment (circle all that apply)

| Oxygen @ _15_ L/min via: <br><br> NC (NRM) Bag mask | Assisted Ventilation | Airway Adjunct | CPR |
|---|---|---|---|
| Defibrillation | Bleeding Control | (Bandaging) | Splinting | **Other:** Thermal management, sterile burn sheet application |

#### Narrative

EMS crew was standing by at the scene of a residential fire when firefighters rescued a 45-year-old man from the burning structure. They presented the patient wrapped in a blanket; he was ambulatory and the burning process was stopped before EMS contact was made. The approximate time of exposure to the burning environment was 8 to 10 minutes.

Chief Complaint: Burns to the torso and arms

History: Patient denies significant past medical history and states he does not take any medications. He states he did not have a loss of consciousness during entrapment.

Assessment: The patient was conscious and alert, his airway was patent, his breathing was adequate, and his face was covered with soot. He reported severe pain to his chest, abdomen, and arms. Immediately moved patient into ambulance, applied high-flow oxygen via nonrebreathing mask, and assessed his burns. Assessment revealed burns that covered approximately 36% of his BSA. Partial-thickness burns were noted to the entire anterior torso, and partial- and full-thickness burns were noted to both of his upper extremities. Additional assessment revealed that his facial hair and the hair just above his hairline were singed; no facial skin burns were noted. The patient denied shortness of breath or any other symptoms other than severe pain from his burns. Secondary assessment did not reveal any other obvious injuries.

Treatment (Rx): Applied dry, sterile burn sheets to patient's burns, covered him with a blanket for warmth, and began transport to the hospital.

Transport: En route, notified medical control, who advised us to transport to the ED because the closest burn center was located 75 miles away. Reassessment revealed that the patient's respirations were becoming labored and his voice was becoming hoarse. Continued high-flow oxygen and continued to monitor his airway and breathing status. Notified the receiving facility of the patient's status and our impending arrival. The patient's vital signs remained stable throughout the duration of the transport. Delivered patient to the ED without incident and gave verbal report to the attending physician, Dr Koteras. Medic 4 returned to service at 1541.

**End of report**

# Prep Kit

## Ready for Review

- The skin protects the body by keeping pathogens out and water in and assisting in body temperature regulation.
- There are three types of soft-tissue injuries:
  - Closed injuries (Soft-tissue damage occurs beneath the skin or mucous membrane but the surface remains intact.)
  - Open injuries (There is a break in the surface of the skin or the mucous membrane, exposing deeper tissue to potential contamination.)
  - Burns (The soft tissue receives more energy than it can absorb without injury; the source of this energy can be thermal, toxic chemicals, electricity, or radiation.)
- Closed soft-tissue injuries are characterized by a history of blunt trauma, pain at the site of injury, swelling beneath the skin, and discoloration. Contusions, hematomas, and crushing injuries are classified as closed injuries. Treat a closed soft-tissue injury by applying the mnemonic RICES: *Rest, Ice, Compression, Elevation,* and *Splinting*.
- Open injuries differ from closed injuries in that the protective layer of skin is damaged. Abrasions, lacerations, avulsions, and penetrating wounds are classified as open injuries. Treat an open soft-tissue injury by applying direct pressure with a sterile bandage using a roller bandage, and splint the extremity. Use a tourniquet when necessary to control bleeding.
- It is generally easier to assess an open injury than it is to assess a closed injury because you can see the injury.
- Small animal and human bites can lead to serious infection and must be evaluated by a physician. Small animals can carry rabies.
- Burns are serious and painful soft-tissue injuries caused by heat (thermal), chemicals, electricity, and radiation.
- Burns are classified primarily by the depth and extent of the burn injury and the body area involved.
- Burns are considered to be superficial, partial-thickness, or full-thickness based on the depth of tissue involved.
- When providing emergency care for burns, do the following:
  - Use standard precautions to protect yourself from potentially contaminated body fluid and to protect the patient from potential infection.
  - Ensure you have cooled the burned area to prevent further cellular damage.
  - Remove jewelry and constrictive clothing; never attempt to remove any synthetic material that may have melted into the burned skin.
  - Ensure an open and clear airway, provide high-flow oxygen, and be alert to signs and symptoms of inhalation injury such as difficulty breathing, stridor, or wheezing.
  - Place sterile dressings over the burn areas; to prevent hypothermia, cover the patient with a clean blanket. Provide prompt transport.
- Dressings and bandages are designed to control bleeding, protect the wound from further damage, prevent further contamination, and prevent infection.

## Vital Vocabulary

**abrasion** Loss or damage of the superficial layer of skin as a result of a body part rubbing or scraping across a rough or hard surface.

**amputation** An injury in which part of the body is completely severed.

**avulsion** An injury in which soft tissue is torn completely loose or is hanging as a flap.

**burns** Injuries in which soft-tissue damage occurs as a result of thermal heat, frictional heat, toxic chemicals, electricity, or nuclear radiation.

**closed injuries** Injuries in which damage occurs beneath the skin or mucous membrane but the surface of the skin remains intact.

**compartment syndrome** Swelling in a confined space that produces dangerous pressure; may cut off blood flow or damage sensitive tissue.

**contact burn** A burn caused by direct contact with a hot object.

**contamination** The presence of infective organisms or foreign bodies such as dirt, gravel, or metal.

**contusion** A bruise from an injury that causes bleeding beneath the skin without breaking the skin.

**crushing injury** An injury that occurs when a great amount of force is applied to the body.

**crush syndrome** Significant metabolic derangement that develops when crushed extremities or body parts remain trapped for prolonged periods. This can lead to renal failure and death.

**dermis** The inner layer of the skin, containing hair follicles, sweat glands, nerve endings, and blood vessels.

**ecchymosis** A buildup of blood beneath the skin that produces a characteristic blue or black discoloration as the result of an injury.

**epidermis** The outer layer of skin, which is made up of cells that are sealed together to form a watertight protective covering for the body.

**evisceration** The displacement of organs outside the body.

**excited delirium** A serious behavioral condition in which a person exhibits agitated behavior combined with disorientation, hallucinations, or delusions; also called agitated delirium or exhaustive mania.

**fascia** The fiber-like connective tissue that covers arteries, veins, tendons, and ligaments.

**flame burn** A burn caused by an open flame.

**flash burn** A burn caused by exposure to very intense heat, such as in an explosion.

**full-thickness (third-degree) burns** Burns that affect all skin layers and may affect the subcutaneous layers, muscle, bone, and internal organs, leaving the area dry, leathery, and white, dark brown, or charred.

**hematoma** A mass of blood that has collected within damaged tissue beneath the skin or in a body cavity.

**impaled objects** Objects that penetrate the skin but remain in place.

**incision** A sharp, smooth cut in the skin.

**laceration** A deep, jagged cut in the skin.

**mucous membranes** The linings of body cavities and passages that communicate directly or indirectly with the environment outside the body.

**occlusive dressing** An airtight dressing that protects a wound from air and bacteria; a commercial vented version allows air to passively escape from the chest, while an unvented dressing may be made of petroleum jelly–based (Vaseline) gauze, aluminum foil, or plastic.

**open injuries** Injuries in which there is a break in the surface of the skin or the mucous membrane, exposing deeper tissue to potential contamination.

**partial-thickness (second-degree) burns** Burns that affect the epidermis and some portion of the dermis but not the subcutaneous tissue, characterized by blisters and skin that is white to red, moist, and mottled.

**penetrating wound** An injury resulting from a sharp, piercing object.

**rabid** Infected with rabies.

**rule of nines** A system that assigns percentages to sections of the body, allowing calculation of the amount of skin surface involved in the burn area.

**scald burn** A burn caused by hot liquids.

**steam burn** A burn caused by exposure to hot steam.

**superficial (first-degree) burns** Burns that affect only the epidermis, characterized by skin that is red but not blistered or actually burned through.

**thermal burn** A burn caused by heat.

# References

1. Burn injuries in child abuse. National Criminal Justice Reference Service website. https://www.ncjrs.gov /pdffiles/91190-6.pdf. Published June 2001. Accessed April 3, 2020.

2. Burn triage and treatment—thermal injuries. Chemical Hazards Emergency Medical Management website. https://chemm.nlm.nih.gov/burns.htm. Accessed April 3, 2020.

3. Criteria for referral: guideline for transfer of patients to burn centers. UC San Diego School of Medicine website. https://medschool.ucsd.edu/som/surgery/divisions /trauma-burn/about/burn-center/Pages/referral.aspx. Accessed April 3, 2020.

4. *National Emergency Medical Services Education Standards*. US Department of Transportation. National Highway Traffic Safety Administration. DOT HS 811 077A. January 2009. www.ems.gov/pdf/811077a.pdf.Accessed April 3, 2020.

5. *National Emergency Medical Services Education Standards. Emergency Medical Technician Instructional Guidelines*. US Department of Transportation. National Highway Traffic Safety Administration. DOT HS 811 077C. January 2009. www.ems.gov/pdf/811077c.pdf. Accessed April 3, 2020.

6. Pitts SR, Niska RW, Xu J, Burt CW. National Hospital Ambulatory Medical Care Survey: 2006 emergency department summary. *Natl Health Stat Report* 2008;(7):1–38.

7. US fire statistics. US Fire Administration website. http:// www.usfa.fema.gov/data/statistics/. Accessed April 3, 2020.

8. Weichman SA. Psychological aspects of burn injuries. *BMJ* 2004;329(7462):391–393.

9. World Health Organization. *Burn Prevention: Success Stories and Lessons Learned*. Geneva, Switzerland: World Health Organization; 2011. http://whqlibdoc.who.int /publications/2011/9789241501187_eng.pdf. Accessed April 3, 2020.

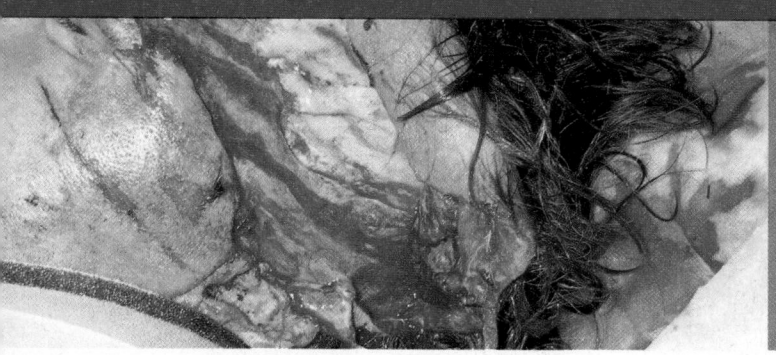

# Chapter 28

# Face and Neck Injuries

## NATIONAL EMS EDUCATION STANDARD COMPETENCIES

### Medicine

Applies fundamental knowledge to provide basic emergency care and transportation based on assessment findings for an acutely ill patient.

### Diseases of the Eyes, Ears, Nose, and Throat

Recognition and management of
- Nosebleed (pp 1027–1028)

### Trauma

Applies fundamental knowledge to provide basic emergency care and transportation based on assessment findings for an acutely injured patient.

### Head, Facial, Neck, and Spine Trauma

- Recognition and management of
  - Life threats (pp 1009–1016)

- Spine trauma (Chapter 29, *Head and Spine Injuries*)
- Pathophysiology, assessment, and management of
  - Penetrating neck trauma (pp 1009–1016, 1032–1033)
  - Laryngotracheal injuries (pp 1009–1016, 1033)
  - Spine trauma (Chapter 29, *Head and Spine Injuries*)
  - Facial fractures (pp 1009–1016, 1030–1031)
  - Skull fractures (Chapter 29, *Head and Spine Injuries*)
  - Foreign bodies in the eyes (pp 1016–1021)
  - Dental trauma (pp 1010–1011, 1031)

## KNOWLEDGE OBJECTIVES

1. Describe the anatomy and physiology of the head, face, and neck; include major structures and specific important landmarks of which EMTs must be aware. (pp 1006–1009)
2. Describe the factors that may cause obstruction of the upper airway following a facial injury. (pp 1009–1011)
3. Discuss the different types of facial injuries and the patient care considerations related to each one. (pp 1009–1011)
4. Explain the emergency care of a patient who has sustained face and neck injuries; include assessment of the patient, review of signs and symptoms, and management of care. (pp 1009–1016)
5. Explain emergency medical care of a patient with soft-tissue wounds of the face and neck. (pp 1015–1016)
6. Explain the emergency medical care of a patient with an eye injury based on the following scenarios: foreign object, impaled object, burns, lacerations, blunt trauma, closed head injuries, and blast injuries. (pp 1016–1027)
7. Describe the three different causes of a burn injury to the eye and the patient management

considerations related to each one.
(pp 1021–1023)

8. Explain emergency medical care of a patient with injuries of the nose. (pp 1027–1028)

9. Explain the emergency medical care of a patient with injuries of the ear, including lacerations and foreign body insertions. (pp 1028–1030)

10. Explain the physical findings and emergency care of a patient with a facial fracture. (pp 1030–1031)

11. Explain the emergency medical care of the patient with dental and cheek injuries; include how to deal with an avulsed tooth. (p 1031)

12. Explain the emergency medical care of a patient with an upper airway injury caused by blunt trauma. (pp 1030–1032)

13. Explain the emergency medical care of the patient with a penetrating injury to the neck; include how to control regular and life-threatening bleeding. (pp 1032–1033)

## SKILLS OBJECTIVES

1. Demonstrate the removal of a foreign object from under a patient's upper eyelid. (pp 1016–1019, Skill Drill 28-1)

2. Demonstrate the stabilization of a foreign object that has been impaled in a patient's eye. (pp 1016–1020, Skill Drill 28-2)

3. Demonstrate irrigation of a patient's eye using a nasal cannula, bottle, or basin. (pp 1021–1023)

4. Demonstrate the care of a patient who has a penetrating eye injury. (pp 1020, 1023)

5. Demonstrate how to control bleeding from a neck injury. (pp 1032–1033, Skill Drill 28-3)

# Introduction

The face and neck are particularly vulnerable to injury because of their relatively unprotected positions on the body. Soft-tissue injuries and fractures to the bones of the face are common and vary greatly in severity. Some are potentially life threatening, and many leave disfiguring scars if not treated properly. Penetrating trauma to the neck may cause severe bleeding. An open injury may allow an air embolism to enter the circulatory system. If a hematoma forms in this area, it may stop or slow blood flow to the brain, causing a stroke. Appropriate prehospital and hospital care can sometimes allow a seemingly devastating injury to result in a surprisingly good outcome.

As an EMT, your objectives when treating a patient with face and neck injuries include preventing further injury, particularly to the cervical spine; managing any acute airway problems; and controlling bleeding. This chapter first reviews the anatomy of the head and neck and then examines the factors that can produce upper airway obstruction. A discussion follows that includes emergency medical care of soft-tissue wounds of the face, nose, and ear; facial fractures; penetrating injuries of the neck; and dental injuries.

# Anatomy and Physiology

The head is divided into two parts: the cranium and the face. The cranium, or skull, contains the brain, which connects to the spinal cord through the foramen magnum, a large opening at the base of the skull. The most posterior portion of the cranium is called the occiput. On each side of the cranium, the lateral portions are called the temples or temporal regions. Between the temporal regions and the occiput lie the parietal regions. The forehead is called the frontal region. Just anterior to the ear, in the temporal region, you can feel the pulse of the superficial temporal artery.

The face is composed of the eyes, ears, nose, mouth, and cheeks. Six bones—the nasal bone, the two maxillae (upper jaw bones), the two zygomas (cheek bones), and the mandible (jaw bone)—are the major bones of the face (**FIGURE 28-1**).

The orbit of the eye is composed of the lower edge of the frontal bone of the skull, the zygoma, the maxilla, and the nasal bone. The bony orbit protects the eye from injury. By viewing the face from the side, you can see the eyeball recessed in the orbit. Only the proximal third of the nose—the bridge—is formed by bone. The remaining two-thirds are composed of cartilage.

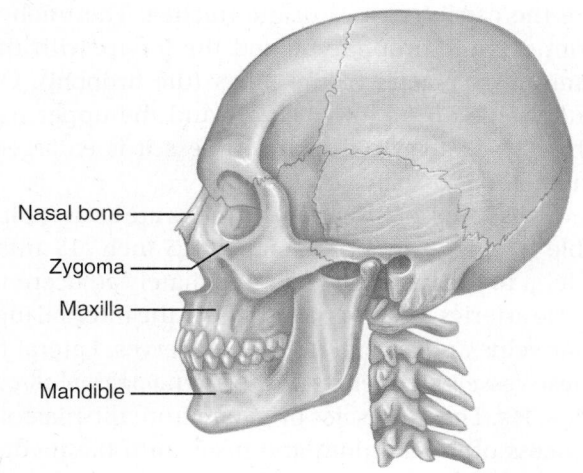

**FIGURE 28-1** The face is composed of six bones: the nasal bone, two maxillae, two zygomas, and the mandible.

© Jones & Bartlett Learning.

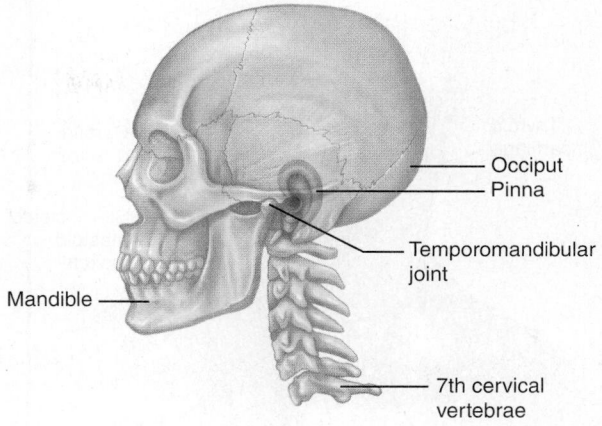

**FIGURE 28-2** Specific landmarks of the head and neck include the pinna, the mandible, the occiput, the seventh cervical vertebra, and the temporomandibular joint.

© Jones & Bartlett Learning.

The exposed portion of the ear is composed entirely of cartilage that is covered by skin. The external, visible part of the ear is called the pinna (**FIGURE 28-2**). The ear lobes are the fleshy portions at the bottom of each ear. The tragus is a small, rounded, fleshy bulge immediately anterior to the ear canal. The superficial temporal artery can be palpated just anterior to the tragus. About 1 inch (2.5 cm) posterior to the external opening of the ear is a prominent bony mass at the base of the skull called the mastoid process.

The mandible forms the jaw and chin. The jaw is the lower border of the mouth, where the tongue and 32 teeth are located. Motion of the mandible occurs at the temporomandibular joint, which lies just in front of the ear on either side of the face. Below the ear and anterior to the mastoid process, the angle of the mandible is easily palpated.

The neck also contains many important structures. It is supported by the cervical spine, or the first seven vertebrae in the spinal column (C1 through C7). The spinal cord exits from the foramen magnum and lies within the spinal canal formed by the vertebrae. The upper part of the esophagus and the trachea lie in the midline of the neck. The carotid arteries are found on either side of the trachea, along with the jugular veins and several nerves.

Several useful landmarks can be palpated and seen in the neck (**FIGURE 28-3**). The most obvious is the firm prominence in the center of the anterior surface, commonly known as the Adam's apple. Specifically, this prominence is the upper part of the larynx, formed by the thyroid cartilage. It is more prominent in men than in women. The other portion of the larynx is the cricoid cartilage, a firm ridge of cartilage (the only complete circular cartilage

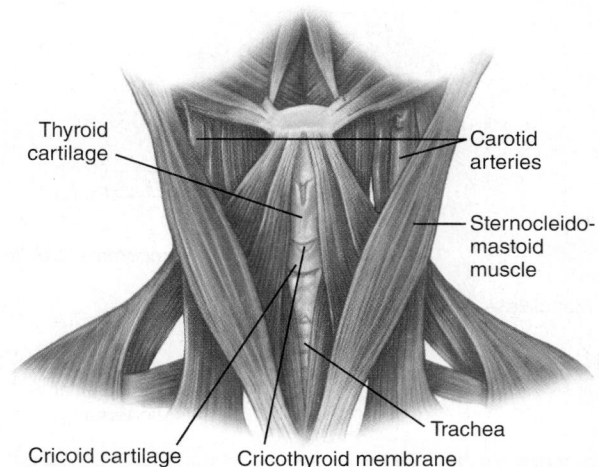

**FIGURE 28-3** Important landmarks in the neck include the cricoid cartilage, the thyroid cartilage, the carotid arteries, the cricothyroid membrane, and the sternocleidomastoid muscles.

© Jones & Bartlett Learning.

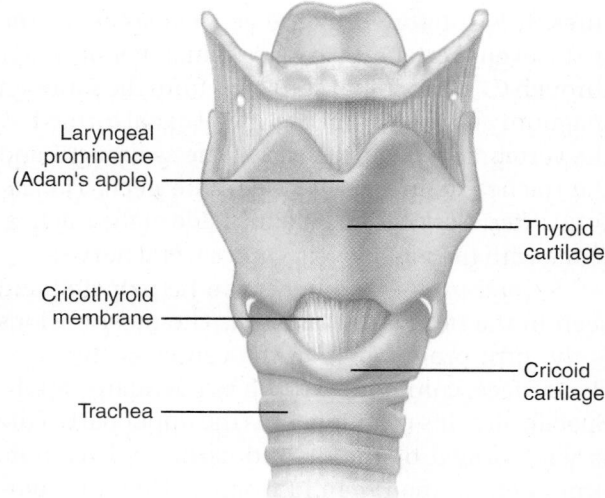

**FIGURE 28-4** The larynx.

© Jones & Bartlett Learning.

structure of the trachea) below the thyroid cartilage, which is somewhat more difficult to palpate. Between the thyroid cartilage and the cricoid cartilage in the midline of the neck is a soft depression, the cricothyroid membrane. This is a thin sheet of connective tissue (fascia) that joins the two cartilages (**FIGURE 28-4**). The cricothyroid membrane is covered at this point only by skin.

Below the larynx, several additional firm ridges are palpable in the anterior midline. These ridges

are the cartilage rings of the trachea. The trachea connects the oropharynx and the larynx with the main air passages of the lungs (the bronchi). On either side of the lower larynx and the upper trachea lies the thyroid gland. Unless it is enlarged, this gland is usually not palpable.

Pulsations of the carotid arteries are easily palpable in a groove approximately 0.5 inch (13 mm) lateral to the larynx. Lying immediately adjacent to these arteries, but not palpable, are the internal jugular veins and several important nerves. Lateral to these vessels and nerves lie the **sternocleidomastoid muscles**. These muscles originate from the mastoid process of the cranium and insert into the medial border of each collarbone and the sternum at the base of the neck. They allow movement of the head.

A series of bony prominences lie posteriorly, in the midline of the neck. They are the spines of the cervical vertebrae. The lower cervical spines are more prominent than the upper ones. They are more easily palpable when the neck is in flexion. At the base of the neck posteriorly, the most prominent spine is the seventh cervical vertebra.

## The Eye

The eye is globe-shaped, approximately 1 inch (2.5 cm) in diameter, and located within a bony socket in the skull called the orbit **FIGURE 28-5**. The orbit is composed of the adjacent bones of the face and skull; the orbit forms the base of the floor of the cranial cavity, and directly above it are the frontal lobes of the brain. In the adult, more than 80% of the eyeball is protected within this bony orbit. Between and below the orbits are the nasal bone and

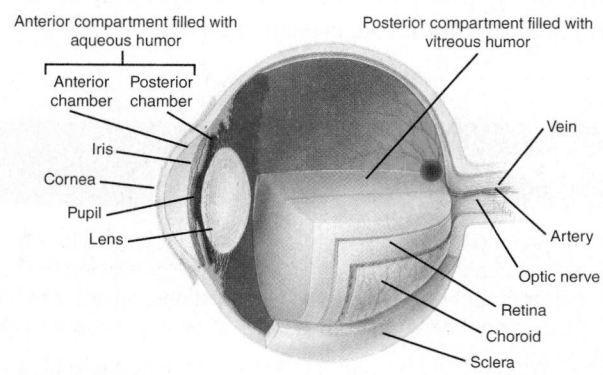

**FIGURE 28-5** The major structures of the eye.

© Jones & Bartlett Learning.

the sinuses, respectively. Therefore, any severe injury to the face or head can potentially damage the eyeball or the muscles attached to the eyeball that cause the eye to move.

The eyeball, or globe, keeps its global shape as a result of the pressure of the fluid contained within its two chambers. The clear, jellylike fluid near the back of the eye is called the vitreous humor. In front of the lens is a clear fluid called the aqueous humor, named for its watery appearance; in Latin, aqua means water. In penetrating injuries of the eye, aqueous humor can leak out, but with time and appropriate medical treatment, the body can make more.

The inner surface of the eyelids and the exposed surface of the eye itself, which are covered by a delicate membrane, the conjunctiva, are kept moist by fluid produced by the lacrimal glands, often called tear glands (**FIGURE 28-6**). Humans blink unconsciously many times per minute. This action sweeps fluid from the lacrimal glands over the surface of the eye, cleaning it. The tears drain on the inner side of the eye through two lacrimal (tear) ducts into the nasal cavity. This is why people sometimes need to blow their nose when they cry.

The white of the eye, called the sclera, extends over the surface of the globe. This extremely tough, fibrous tissue helps maintain the eye's globular shape and protects the more delicate inner structures. On the front of the eye, the sclera is replaced by a clear, transparent membrane called the cornea, which allows light to enter the eye. A circular muscle lies behind the cornea with an opening in its center. Like the shutter in a camera, this muscle adjusts the size of the opening to regulate the amount of light that enters the eye. This circular muscle and surrounding tissue are called the iris. The iris is pigmented, giving the eye its characteristic brown, green, or blue color.

The opening in the center of the iris, which allows light to move to the back of the eye, is called the pupil. Normally, the pupil appears black. Like the opening in a camera, the pupil becomes smaller in bright light and larger in dim light. The pupil also becomes smaller and larger when the person is looking at objects near at hand and farther away; these adjustments occur almost instantaneously. Normally, the pupils in both eyes are equal in size. Some people are born with pupils that are not equal (anisocoria); however, particularly in unconscious patients, unequal pupil size may indicate serious injury or illness of the brain or eye.

Behind the iris is the lens. Like the lens of a camera, this lens focuses images on the light-sensitive area at the back of the globe, called the retina. Within the retina are numerous nerve endings that respond to light by transmitting nerve impulses through the optic nerve to the brain. In the brain, the impulses are interpreted as vision.

The retina is nourished by a layer of blood vessels between it and the sclera at the back of the globe. This layer is called the choroid. If, as sometimes happens, the retina detaches from the underlying choroid and sclera, the nerve endings are not nourished, and the patient experiences blindness. This may be partial blindness, depending on how much of the retina is separated. This condition is called retinal detachment.

## Injuries of the Face and Neck

Injuries about the face and neck can often lead to partial or complete obstruction of the upper airway. Several factors may contribute to the obstruction. Bleeding from facial injuries can be heavy, producing large blood clots in the upper airway. These clots can lead to complete obstruction, particularly in a patient who is not fully conscious. In particular, direct injuries to the nose and mouth, the larynx, or the trachea are often the source of significant bleeding

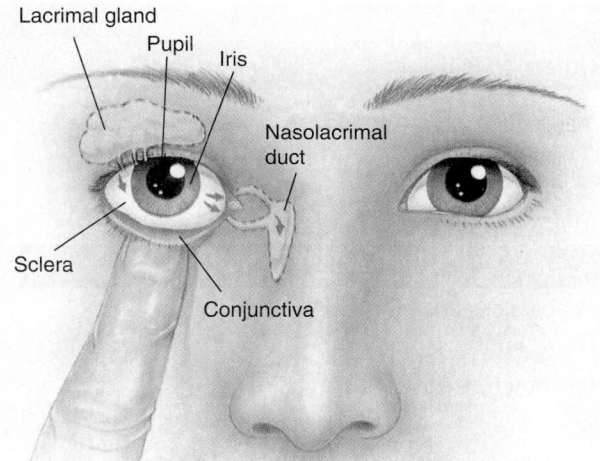

**FIGURE 28-6** The lacrimal system consists of tear glands and ducts. Tears act as a lubricant and keep the front of the eye from drying out.

and/or respiratory compromise. You may need to suction the airway if you are unable to control the bleeding. In addition, the injuries may cause loosened teeth or dentures to become dislodged into the throat, where they may be swallowed or aspirated. The swelling that often accompanies direct and indirect injury to the soft tissues in these areas can also contribute to airway obstruction.

The airway may also be affected when the patient's head is turned to the side, as often is done when the patient has an altered level of consciousness or is unconscious. Other factors that interfere with normal respirations include possible injuries to the brain and/or cervical spine that may be associated with facial injuries. If the great vessels in the neck are injured, significant bleeding and pressure on the upper airway are common; these can result in airway obstruction as well.

Depending on the mechanism of injury (MOI), there may be a cervical spine injury. If there is significant impact to the face, suspect accompanying cervical spine injury and follow your agency's protocol for spinal motion restriction.

## Soft-Tissue Injuries

Soft-tissue injuries of the face and neck are common. Because the face and neck are extremely vascular, swelling from soft-tissue injuries in this area may be more severe than in other injured parts of the body. The skin and underlying tissues in these

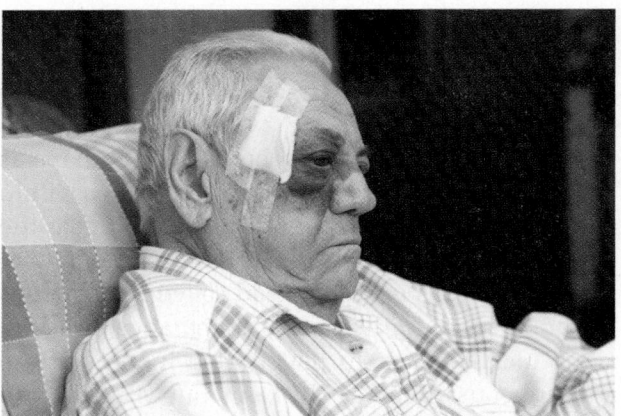

**FIGURE 28-7** Facial hematoma.
© Willowpix/E+/Getty Images.

areas have a rich blood supply, so bleeding from penetrating injuries may be heavy. Even minor soft-tissue wounds of the face and neck may bleed profusely. A blunt injury that does not break the skin may cause a break in a blood vessel wall, causing blood to collect under the skin; this is called a hematoma (**FIGURE 28-7**). In some situations, a flap of skin is peeled back, or avulsed, from the underlying muscle and fascia (**FIGURE 28-8**).

## Dental Injuries

Mandible (lower jaw) fractures are relatively common because of the prominence of the mandible itself. These fractures are second only to nasal

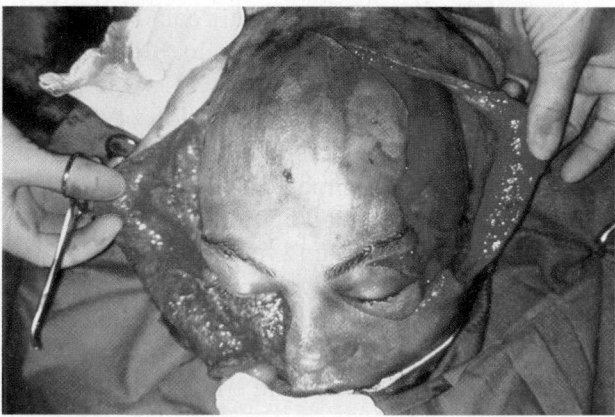

**FIGURE 28-8** A major avulsion injury is characterized by a large flap of skin that is peeled back from the underlying muscle and tissue.

© American Academy of Orthopaedic Surgeons.

fractures in frequency. Most of these fractures are the result of vehicle collisions and assaults. If your patient has a mandibular fracture, then consider the major force necessary to cause that fracture—there is a strong probability your patient will have additional facial trauma and/or cervical injuries. Signs of a mandibular fracture include a misalignment of the teeth, numbness of the chin, and an inability to open the mouth. The patient will most likely have swelling, bruising, and loosened or missing teeth.

Maxillary fractures are predominantly found after blunt-force, high-energy impacts such as an unrestrained driver striking the steering wheel, a fall, or a direct blow from an object such as a pipe. The signs include massive facial swelling, instability of the facial bones, and misalignment of the teeth.

Fractured and avulsed teeth are common following facial trauma. Dental injuries may be associated with motor vehicle crashes or an assault. Always assess the patient's mouth following a facial injury, especially if your examination reveals fractured or avulsed teeth. Teeth fragments (or even whole teeth) can become an airway obstruction and should be removed from the patient's mouth immediately.

## Patient Assessment

### Scene Size-Up

As you arrive on the scene, observe for hazards and threats to the safety of the crew, bystanders, and the patient. Assess the effect of hazards on patient care,

and address those hazards. Assess for the potential for violence and for environmental hazards.

Patients who are conscious and supine and have oral or facial bleeding may protect their airway by coughing, projecting the blood at you. Therefore, standard precautions require eye protection and a face mask. Also, put several pairs of gloves in your pocket for easy access in the event your gloves tear or there are multiple patients with bleeding.

If your response is to a motor vehicle crash, you may be confronted with more than one patient in a vehicle. Determine the number of patients and consider whether you will need additional or specialized resources on the scene.

As you observe the scene, look for indicators of the MOI. This assessment helps you develop an early index of suspicion for underlying injuries in the patient who has sustained a significant MOI. As you put together information from dispatch and your observations of the scene, consider how the MOI produced the injuries expected. Common MOIs for face and neck injuries include motor vehicle collisions, sports participation, falls, penetrating trauma, and blunt trauma. In motor vehicle collisions, the probability of injury increases if the vehicle rolled over or came to an abrupt stop when striking an immovable object, such as a tree. During sports participation, injuries can occur in a player without a helmet who was struck by a baseball or two players who sustained a helmet-to-helmet collision in football.

### Primary Assessment

The primary assessment focuses on identifying and managing life-threatening concerns. Threats to airway, breathing, or circulation must be treated immediately. When there is obvious, active, life-threatening external hemorrhage, it should be addressed before airway and breathing.

As you approach the patient, look for important indicators to alert you to the seriousness of the patient's condition. Is the patient interacting with the environment or lying still, making no sounds? Does the patient have any apparent life threats such as significant bleeding? How is the patient's skin color? The general impression will help you develop an index of suspicion for serious injuries and determine your sense of urgency for medical intervention.

Injuries to the face and throat, such as bleeding and significant swelling, may be obvious but may also be hidden under collars and hats. Because of the likelihood of respiratory distress with these injuries, they should be recognized as early as possible.

As with any injury with life-threatening bleeding, control the blood loss with direct pressure. Always consider the need for manual spinal stabilization and check for responsiveness using the AVPU scale.

Ensure that the patient has a clear and patent airway. If the patient is unresponsive or has a significantly altered level of consciousness, consider inserting a proper-size oropharyngeal airway. The use of a nasopharyngeal airway is controversial, as many believe that inserting a nasopharyngeal airway into the nares of a patient with facial or head trauma carries the risk of introducing the device into the cranial vault and brain tissue. However, recent research suggests this risk is extremely small. As always, be aware of and follow your local protocols.

### Words of Wisdom

Face and throat injuries increase the need for airway and breathing maintenance, so do not hesitate to place a nonrebreathing mask over facial injuries. The seal may not be as easy to maintain, but airway and breathing take priority over soft-tissue injuries.

Quickly assess the pulse rate and quality; determine the skin condition, color, and temperature; and check the capillary refill time. Significant bleeding is an immediate life threat. If the patient has obvious life-threatening bleeding, you must control it quickly.

If the patient you are treating has an airway or a breathing problem or significant bleeding, you must consider quickly transporting the patient to the hospital for treatment or requesting ALS support if that will result in faster access to someone who will be able to intubate the patient. Stabilization and maintenance of airway and breathing and controlling bleeding can be difficult in patients with facial or neck injuries. Avoid delays in transport and consider ALS backup if the transport time is long. A patient with signs and symptoms of internal bleeding must be transported quickly to the appropriate hospital for treatment by a physician.

Internal bleeding in face and throat injuries may compromise blood flow to the brain. Bleeding from major vessels of the throat can have a serious effect on the patient's airway. The condition of a patient with visible significant bleeding or signs of significant internal bleeding may quickly become unstable. Treatment is directed at quickly addressing life threats and providing rapid transport to the closest appropriate hospital. Signs such as tachycardia, tachypnea, low blood pressure, weak pulse, and cool, moist, pale skin are signs of hypoperfusion and imply the need for rapid transport. Note that because skin paleness can be difficult to detect in patients with dark skin, you may need to check for pale mucous membranes inside the inner lower eyelid or slow capillary refill. The patient who has a significant MOI but whose condition appears stable should also be transported promptly to the closest appropriate hospital. Remember that any significant blow to the face or throat should increase your suspicion of spinal or brain injury. Be alert to these signs and reconsider your priority and transport decision if they develop.

Even if the patient has no signs of hypoperfusion or other life-threatening injuries, if the patient has an injury involving the eye it should be considered potentially serious. Consider transporting the patient with serious, isolated eye injuries to an eye care specialty center depending on local protocol. Do not delay transport of a seriously injured patient, particularly one with significant bleeding, even if it is controlled, to take a patient's history or perform a secondary assessment. Further assessment can continue during transport.

### History Taking

After the life threats have been managed during the primary assessment, investigate the chief complaint or history of present illness. Obtain a medical history and be alert for injury-specific signs and symptoms, as well as any pertinent negatives such as no pain or no loss of sensation.

Next, obtain a SAMPLE history from your patient. If the patient is not responsive, attempt to obtain the SAMPLE history from friends or family members who may be present.

In an unresponsive patient you will only be able to notice the signs of the patient's injuries. Any other information will need to be obtained by someone who is knowledgeable about the patient. Keep in mind that the information you obtain may or may not be accurate and may be incomplete. The person providing the information may not be able to give you the actual names of the patient's medications but might be able to provide some pertinent medical history and possibly known allergies.

## Secondary Assessment

The secondary assessment is a comprehensive examination of the patient that is used to uncover injuries that may have been missed during the primary assessment. In some instances, such as when a patient is critically injured or a short transport time, you may not have time to conduct a secondary assessment.

If there is significant trauma that likely affects multiple systems, start with an assessment of the entire body looking for DCAP-BTLS to be sure that you have found all life threats and injuries. When this is completed, perform a detailed examination of specific areas. However, do not delay transport to complete a thorough physical examination.

In the responsive patient who has an isolated injury with a limited MOI, consider focusing your physical examination on the isolated injury, the patient's chief complaint, and the body region affected, which, in this case, is the face and throat. Ensure that control of bleeding is maintained and note the location of the injury. Inspect open wounds for any foreign matter and stabilize impaled objects if they do not obstruct the airway.

During the physical examination, use your eyes and your hands. Your eyes will be looking for swelling, deformities of the bones, contusions, and discoloration, whereas your hands will be gently palpating the face, looking and feeling for any abnormalities such as deformity or tenderness. Ask yourself the following questions:

1. Do the facial bones seem to be in alignment?
2. Does the nasal bone seem to deviate from the midline?
3. Note any variations from the normal facial examination; is there any facial drooping?
4. Does one eye appear to be lower than the other? If so, this is an indication of an orbital fracture.
5. Does the mandible appear to deviate toward one side or the other?

If your patient is responsive, explain exactly what you are doing and what you are looking for. Your discovery of what you consider to be an abnormality may actually be an old injury that the patient can tell you more about.

Assess all underlying systems. This should include the neurologic system, including the brain and major nerves; sensory organs, including the eyes and nose; the respiratory system, including the mouth, nose, sinuses, and airway; and the circulatory system, particularly focusing on the carotid arteries and jugular veins.

When you are evaluating the eyes, start at the outer aspect of the eye and work your way in toward the pupils. Examine the eye for any obvious foreign matter. Your patient may relay this information to you ("I have something in my eye"). Visual acuity, or the clarity of the patient's vision in each eye, is considered the vital sign of the eye. Quickly assess the patient's visual acuity by gently covering one eye and holding fingers up at arm's length in front of the open eye. Test for the ability to see fingers in both the injured and uninjured eyes and document your findings. Note any discoloration of the eye, bleeding in the iris area, or redness. Look for eye symmetry because asymmetry is a possible indication of a brain injury.

Look at each pupil for equal size and reaction to light. If the pupils are not symmetric, ask the patient if he or she has undergone any previous eye surgeries or sustained any injuries. Previous surgery or injury, rather than brain injury, may be the root cause of the pupils not appearing the same. Cataract surgery can cause unequal pupils, but when you have a patient with a suspected head injury or ocular injury, anisocoria (unequal pupils in dim light) may be present. Determine whether the unequal pupils are caused by physiologic or pathologic issues. Use of over-the-counter eye drops can change pupil size, and certain asthma inhalers can have the same effect if inadvertently sprayed into the eye. Brain injury, nerve disease, glaucoma, and meningitis are all possible causes of unequal pupils.

Does the patient have the ability to follow your finger from side to side as well as up and down? Can the patient read normal print? Does the patient report blurry vision in either eye? Is there a new sensitivity to light?

Assess vital signs to obtain a baseline so that you can observe any changes a patient may display during treatment. A systolic blood pressure reading of less than 100 mm Hg with a weak, rapid pulse and cool, moist skin that is pale or gray should alert you to the presence of hypoperfusion in a patient who may have significant bleeding. Remember, you must be concerned with visible bleeding and unseen bleeding inside a body cavity. With facial and throat injuries, baseline information about the rate and quality of respirations and pulse is very important, as is monitoring throughout patient care.

In addition to hands-on assessment, use monitoring devices to quantify your patient's oxygenation and circulatory status.

## Reassessment

Repeat the primary assessment. Reassess vital signs and the chief complaint. Continually reassess the adequacy of the patient's airway, breathing, and circulation. Recheck patient interventions. Are the treatments you provided for problems with ABCs still effective? This is particularly important in patients with facial or neck injuries because of the ease with which injuries can affect associated systems, such as the respiratory (airway and breathing), circulatory, and nervous systems. The patient's condition should be reassessed at least every 5 minutes.

If you suspect possible spinal injury, follow local protocols regarding spinal motion restriction precautions. Spinal injuries should be suspected any-time there is significant trauma to the face or neck. Maintain an open airway, be prepared to suction the patient, and consider an oropharyngeal airway if the patient becomes unresponsive. Whenever you suspect significant bleeding, provide high-flow oxygen. Adequate oxygenation and airway maintenance are important for all patients with face and neck injuries. If needed, provide assisted ventilation using a bag-mask device with high-flow oxygen.

Control any significant visible bleeding. If the patient has signs of hypoperfusion, treat the patient aggressively for shock and provide rapid transport to the appropriate hospital. Do not delay transport of a seriously injured trauma patient to complete non–life-saving treatments in the field, such as splinting extremity fractures. Instead, complete these treatments en route to the hospital. If there is no cervical spine injury suspected, the patient may be more comfortable in the sitting position during transport.

## Street Smarts

Conscious patients who have oral trauma may prefer to use the hard tip suction themselves. Allowing these patients to do so can lessen their anxiety and give them a sense of control over their airway.

## YOU are the Provider

As your partner continues to manually stabilize the patient's head, you perform a secondary assessment of the entire body, which reveals bruising and mild swelling to the anterior part of the neck, directly over the trachea. The remainder of your assessment does not reveal any obvious injuries. You apply a cervical collar and assess his vital signs.

The patient tells you that he was struck in the face with a steel pipe. After he fell to the ground, he was kicked in the face and throat several times. His face is severely swollen, three of his front teeth are missing, and he tells you that it "doesn't feel right" when he closes his mouth.

| Recording Time: | 5 Minutes |
| --- | --- |
| **Respirations** | 22 breaths/min; adequate depth |
| **Pulse** | 118 breaths/min; strong and regular |
| **Skin** | Pink, warm, and dry |
| **Blood pressure** | 132/68 mm Hg |
| **Oxygen saturation (Spo$_2$)** | 97% (on room air) |

**5.** On the basis of the MOI, what type of injuries should you suspect and assess for?

In your documentation, describe the MOI and the position in which you found the patient when you arrived at the scene. Document difficulties that occurred when removing the patient from the vehicle—for example, "prolonged extrication." In patients with severe external bleeding, it is important to recognize, estimate, and report the amount of blood loss that has occurred and how rapidly or how much time has passed since the bleeding started. This can be a challenge for you, especially if the patient is on a surface that is wet or absorbs fluids or if the environment is dark. Inform the hospital personnel about all injuries involving the patient's head and neck.

## Emergency Medical Care

The emergency care of soft-tissue injuries to the face and neck is the same as treatment of soft-tissue injuries elsewhere on the body. You should assess the XABCs and care for any life threats first. Remember also to follow standard precautions in all cases.

In the absence of life-threatening bleeding, your first step is to open and clear the airway. Securing and maintaining a patent airway is paramount. Remember that blood draining into the throat can produce vomiting and airway obstruction; therefore, the patient may need frequent suctioning. Avoid moving the neck if you suspect that the patient may have sustained a cervical spine injury. Use the jaw-thrust maneuver to open the patient's airway, and then suction the mouth. Once spinal motion restriction is achieved, you can tilt the patient or backboard to one side to allow any blood or vomitus to drain out of the mouth rather than pool in the pharynx and obstruct the airway.

Control bleeding by applying direct manual pressure with a dry, sterile dressing. Use roller gauze, wrapped around the circumference of the head, to hold a pressure dressing in place (**FIGURE 28-9**). Do not apply excessive pressure if there is a possibility of an underlying skull fracture. When an injury exposes the brain, eye, or other structures, cover the exposed parts with a moist, sterile dressing to protect them from further damage. For injuries in which the skin is not broken, apply ice or a cold pack locally to help control the swelling of bruised tissues.

For soft-tissue injuries around the mouth, always check for bleeding inside the mouth. Broken

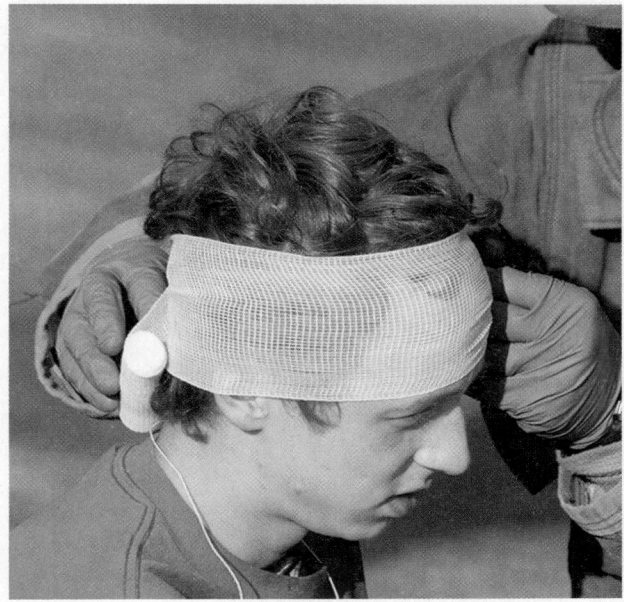

**FIGURE 28-9** Use roller gauze, wrapped around the circumference of the head, to hold a pressure dressing in place.

© Nancy G Fire Photography, Nancy Greifenhagen/Alamy Stock Photo.

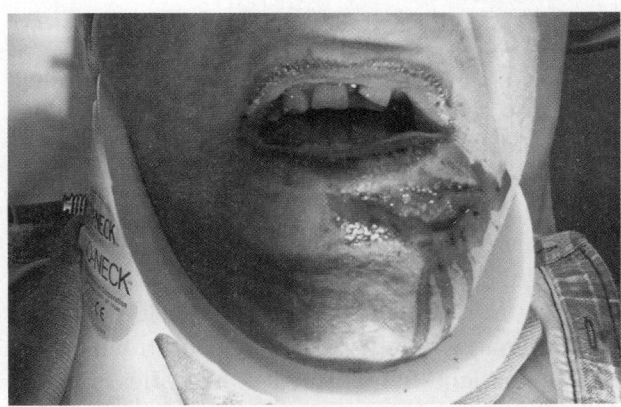

**FIGURE 28-10** Soft-tissue injuries around the mouth can be associated with profuse bleeding inside the mouth and obstruction of the airway.

© E. M. Singletary, MD. Used with permission.

teeth and lacerations to the tongue may cause profuse bleeding and obstruction of the upper airway (**FIGURE 28-10**). Often, the patient will swallow the blood from lacerations inside the mouth, so the hemorrhage may not be apparent. You should also inspect the inside of the mouth for bleeding and hidden injuries in patients who have sustained facial trauma. Remember that patients who swallow significant amounts of blood are prone to vomiting.

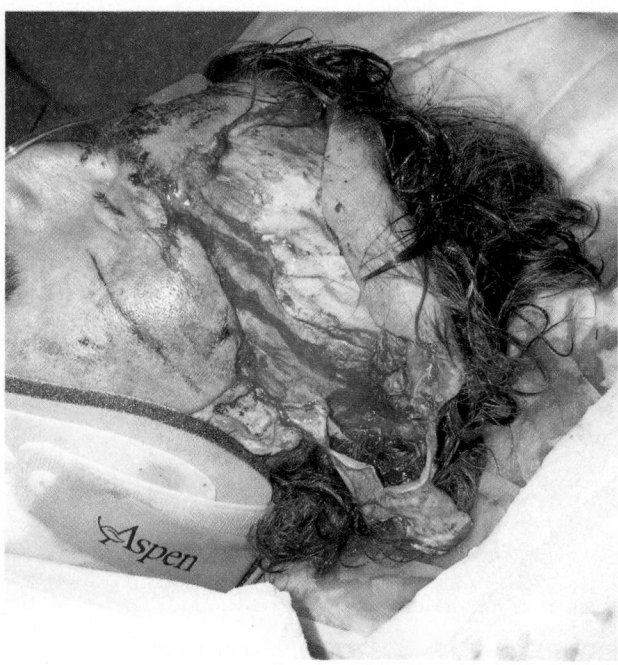

**FIGURE 28-11** If avulsed skin is still attached, place the flap in a position that is as close to normal as possible, and hold it in place with a dry, sterile dressing.

© E. M. Singletary, MD. Used with permission.

Often, physicians will be able to graft a piece of avulsed skin back into the appropriate position. For this reason, if you find portions of avulsed skin that have become separated, wrap them in a sterile dressing, place them in a plastic bag, and keep them cool. Never place tissue directly on ice because freezing will cause further injury to the tissue and make it unusable. Deliver the bag labeled with the patient's name to the emergency department along with the patient. In many avulsion injuries, the skin will still be attached in a loose flap (**FIGURE 28-11**). Place the flap in a position that is as close to normal as possible, and hold it in place with a dry, sterile dressing. These steps will help to increase the patient's chances of having his or her normal appearance restored.

# Emergency Medical Care for Specific Injuries
## Injuries of the Eyes

Eye injuries are common, particularly in sports. An eye injury can produce severe, lifelong

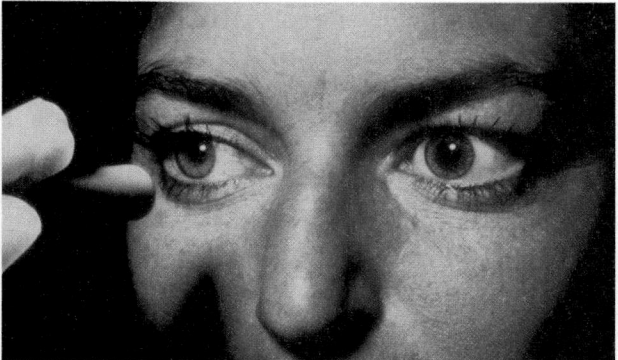

**FIGURE 28-12** Normally, the pupils are round, equal in size, and equally reactive when exposed to light. The pupils shown here appear unequal.

© American Academy of Orthopaedic Surgeons.

complications, including blindness. Proper emergency treatment will minimize pain and may very well help to prevent a permanent loss of vision.

In a normal, uninjured eye, the entire circle of the iris is visible. The pupils are round, usually equal in size, and react equally when exposed to light (**FIGURE 28-12**). Both eyes move together in the same direction when following your moving finger. After an injury, pupil reaction or shape and eye movement are often disturbed. Any of these conditions should cause you to suspect an injury of the globe or its associated tissues. Remember, though, in patients who are unconscious or who have a significantly altered mental status, abnormal pupil reactions sometimes are a sign of brain injury rather than eye injury.

Treatment starts with a thorough examination to determine the extent and nature of any damage. Perform your examination using standard precautions, taking care to avoid aggravating any problems. You are looking for specific abnormalities or conditions that may suggest the nature of the injury (**FIGURE 28-13**). For example, blunt or penetrating injuries can produce swollen or lacerated eyelids. Bleeding soon after irritation or injury can result in a bright red conjunctiva. A damaged cornea quickly loses its smooth, wet appearance.

## Foreign Objects

Large objects are prevented from penetrating the eye by the protective orbit that surrounds it. However, moderately sized and smaller foreign

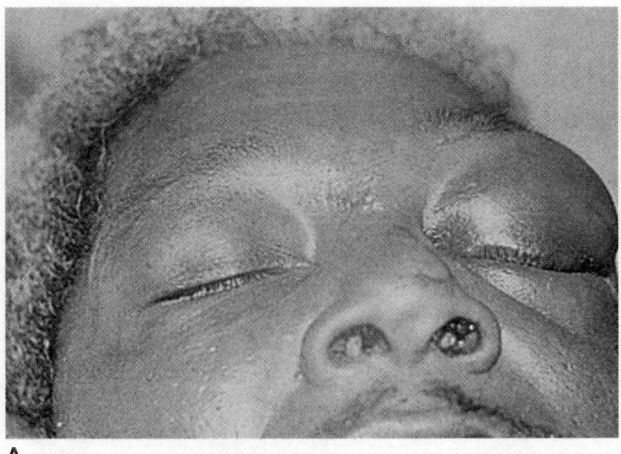

**A**

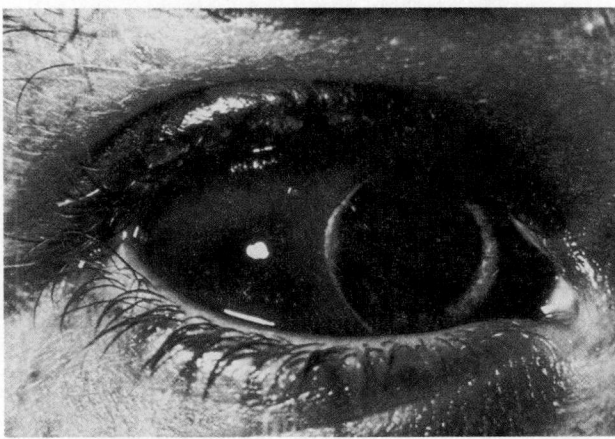

**B**

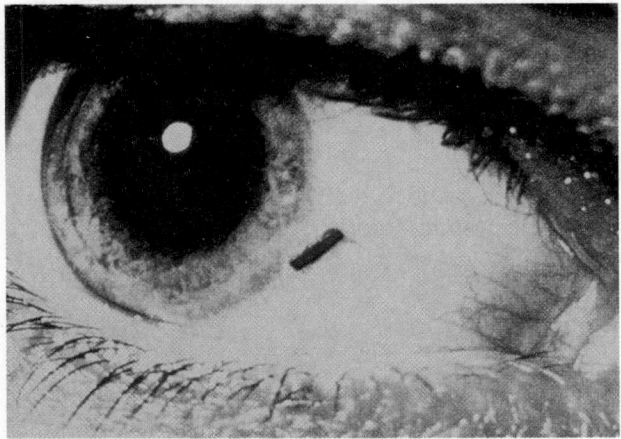

**C**

**FIGURE 28-13** Injuries to the eyes are easily detected by swelling (**A**), bleeding (**B**), and the presence of foreign objects in the eye (**C**).

A: © Jones & Bartlett Learning; B, C: © American Academy of Orthopaedic Surgeons.

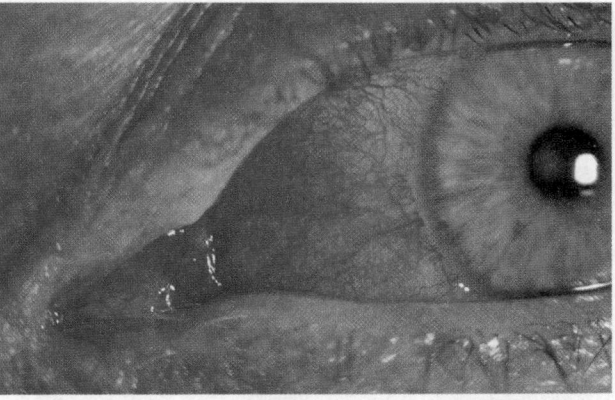

**FIGURE 28-14** Conjunctivitis can result from the presence of a foreign object in the eye.

Courtesy of John T. Halgren, MD, University of Nebraska Medical Center.

objects of many different types can enter the eye and cause significant damage. Even a tiny foreign object, such as a grain of sand lying on the surface of the conjunctiva, may produce severe irritation (**FIGURE 28-14**). The conjunctiva becomes inflamed and red—a condition known as conjunctivitis—almost immediately, and the eye begins to produce tears to flush out the object. Irritation of the cornea or conjunctiva causes intense pain. The patient may have difficulty keeping the eyelids open, because the irritation is further aggravated by bright light.

If a small foreign object is lying on the surface of the patient's eye, you should use a normal saline solution to gently irrigate the eye. Irrigation with a sterile saline solution will frequently flush away loose, small particles. If a small bulb syringe is available, you can use this, or a nasal airway or cannula, to direct the saline into the affected eye. Always flush from the nose side of the eye toward the outside to avoid flushing material into the other eye. After it has been flushed away, a foreign body will often leave a small abrasion on the surface of the conjunctiva. For this reason, the patient will report irritation even when the particle itself is gone. It is always a good idea to transport the patient to the hospital for further assessment to ensure appropriate medical care to the affected eye.

Gentle irrigation usually will not wash out foreign bodies that are stuck to the cornea or lying

## Skill Drill 28-1 Removing a Foreign Object From Under the Upper Eyelid

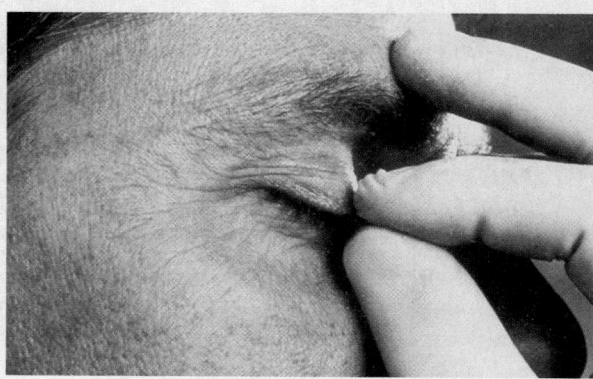

### Step 1

Have the patient look down, grasp the upper lashes, and gently pull the lid away from the eye.

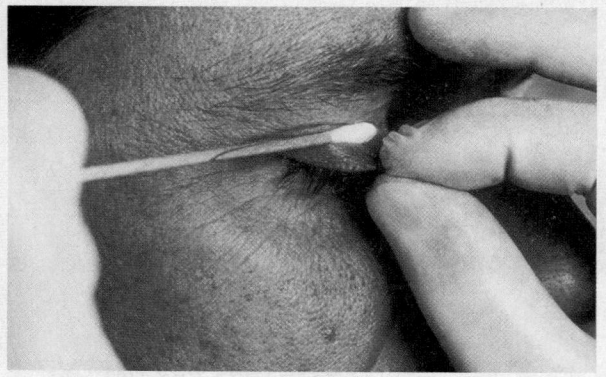

### Step 2

Place a cotton-tipped applicator on the outer surface of the upper lid.

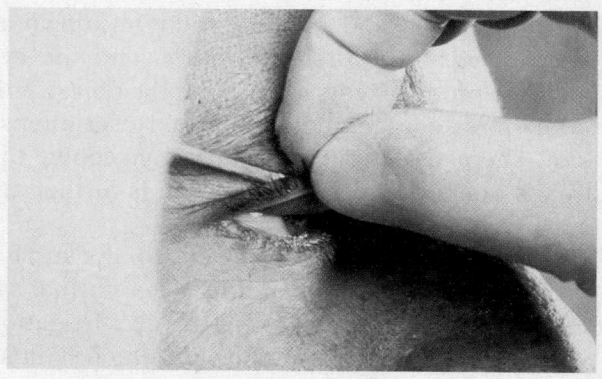

### Step 3

Pull the lid forward and up, folding it back over the applicator.

© Jones & Bartlett Learning. Courtesy of MIEMSS.

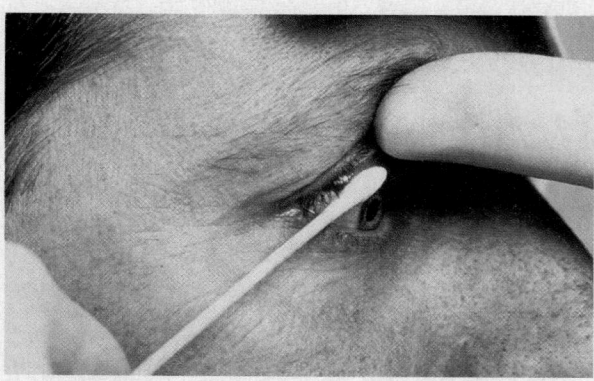

### Step 4

Gently remove the foreign object from the eyelid with a moistened, sterile cotton-tipped applicator.

under the upper eyelid. To examine the undersurface of the upper eyelid, pull the lid upward and forward. If you spot a foreign object on the surface of the eyelid, you may be able to remove it with a moist, sterile cotton-tipped applicator (**SKILL DRILL 28-1**). Never attempt to remove a foreign body that is stuck to the cornea.

1. Tell the patient to look down while you grasp the lashes of the upper eyelid with your thumb and index finger. Gently pull the eyelid away from the eyeball (**Step 1**).
2. Gently place a cotton-tipped applicator horizontally along the center of the outer surface of the upper eyelid (**Step 2**).

3. Pull the eyelid forward and up, which causes it to roll or fold back over the applicator, exposing the undersurface of the eyelid (**Step 3**).
4. If you see a foreign object on the surface of the eyelid, gently remove it with a moistened, sterile cotton-tipped applicator (**Step 4**).

Foreign bodies ranging in size from a pencil to a sliver of metal may be impaled in the eye (**FIGURE 28-15**). These objects must be removed by a physician. Your care involves stabilizing the object and preparing the patient for transport to definitive care. The greater the length of the foreign object you can see sticking out of the eye, the more important stabilization becomes in avoiding further damage. Bandage the object in place to support it. Cover the eye with a moist, sterile

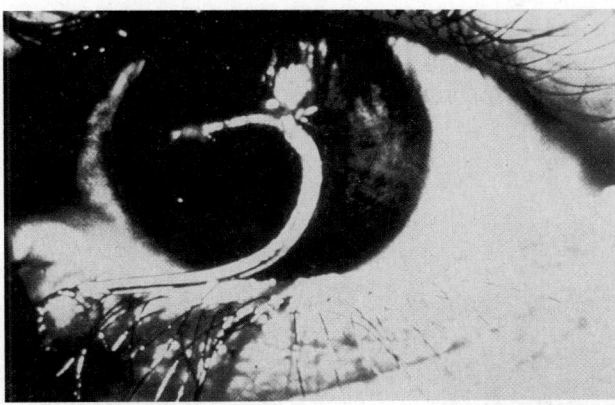

**A**

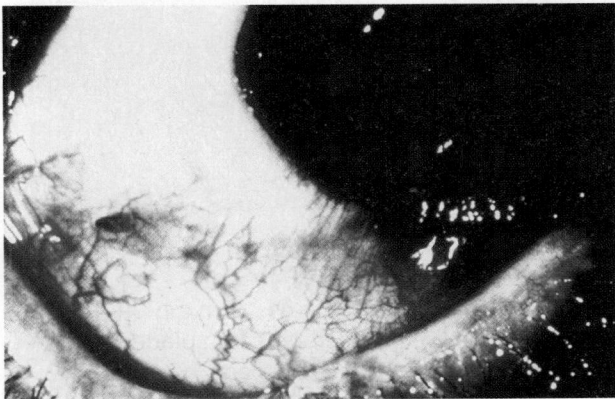

**B**

**FIGURE 28-15** Any number of objects can become impaled in the eye. **A.** Fishhook. **B.** Sharp metal sliver.

A, B: © American Academy of Orthopaedic Surgeons.

dressing, and then surround the object with an eye shield or doughnut-shaped collar made from roller gauze or a small gauze pack. Follow the steps in **SKILL DRILL 28-2**:

1. Begin to prepare the doughnut ring by wrapping a 2-inch (5-cm) gauze roll circumferentially around your fingers and thumb enough times to make a thick dressing layer. You can adjust the inner diameter of what will become the ring by spreading your fingers or squeezing them together (**Step 1**).
2. Remove the gauze from your hand and wrap the remainder of the gauze roll radially around the ring that you have created (**Step 2**).
3. Work your way around the ring until you have wrapped all the way around it and finished the doughnut (**Step 3**).
4. Carefully place the ring over the eye and impaled object, without bumping the object. You can then stabilize the object with a cup or other protective barrier over the object, and secure the object with a roller bandage surrounding the head. Bandage both the injured and uninjured eyes to minimize eye movement and prevent further damage to the globe because when one eye moves, so does the other. Transport to an appropriate medical facility for treatment (**Step 4**).

Sometimes, a variety of types of large and small foreign bodies, particularly small metal fragments, become completely embedded within the eye itself. The patient may not even be aware of the cause of the problem. Suspect such an injury when the history includes metal work (such as hammering, exposure to splinters, grinding, vigorous filing) and when there are other signs of ocular injury. When you see or suspect an impaled object in the eye, place an eye shield over the affected eye and then bandage both eyes with soft, bulky dressings to prevent further injury to the affected eye. Your bandage should be loose enough to hold the eyelid closed but not cause pressure on the eye itself. Using this technique prevents sympathetic motion (the movement of one eye causing both eyes to move), which may cause additional damage to the injured eye. This type of injury must be handled by an ophthalmologist on an urgent basis. Radiographs and special equipment may be required to find the foreign body.

## Skill Drill 28-2 Stabilizing a Foreign Object Impaled in the Eye

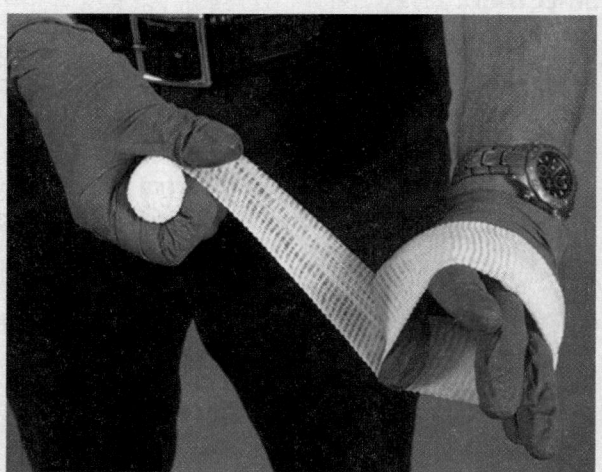

### Step 1

To prepare a doughnut ring, wrap a 2-inch (5-cm) gauze roll around your fingers and thumb seven or eight times. Adjust the diameter by spreading your fingers or squeezing them together.

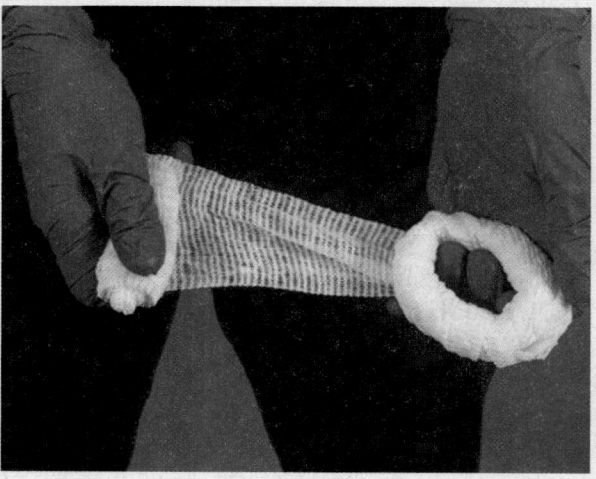

### Step 2

Remove the gauze from your hand and wrap the remainder of the gauze roll radially around the ring that you have created.

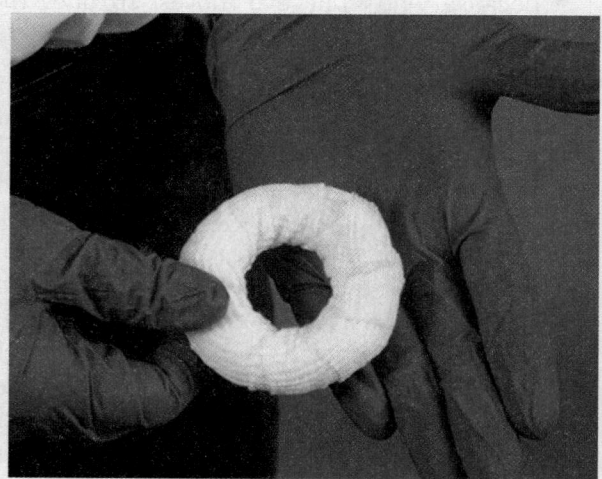

### Step 3

Work around the entire ring to form a doughnut.

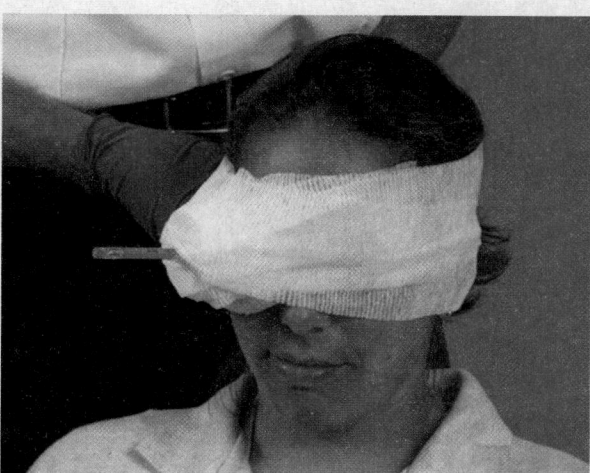

### Step 4

Place the dressing over the eye with a protective barrier to hold the impaled object in place, and then secure it with a roller bandage.

## Burns of the Eye

Chemicals, heat, and light rays all can burn the delicate tissues, such as the cornea, often causing permanent damage. Your role is to stop the burn and prevent further damage.

### Chemical Burns

Chemical burns, usually caused by acid or alkaline solutions, require immediate emergency care (**FIGURE 28-16**). This consists of flushing the eye with water or a sterile saline irrigation solution. If sterile saline is not available, you can use any clean water.

The idea is to direct the greatest amount of irrigating solution or water into the eye as gently as possible (**FIGURE 28-17**). Because opening the eye spontaneously may cause the patient pain, you may have to force the lids open to irrigate the eye adequately. Ideally, you will use a bulb or irrigation syringe, a nasal cannula, or some other device that will allow you to control the flow. In some circumstances, you may have to resort to pouring water into the eye by holding the patient's head under a gently running faucet. You can even have the patient immerse his or her face in a large pan or basin of water and rapidly blink the affected eyelid. If only one eye is affected, care must be taken to avoid contaminated water from getting into the unaffected eye.

Be sure to flush from the inner corner of the affected eye toward the outside corner. Never flush from the outside corner as this may cause the substance to contaminate the unaffected eye. If the burn was caused by an alkali or a strong acid, irrigate the eye continuously for 20 minutes. Follow local protocols or consult with medical control as to whether to try to irrigate while transporting or to stay on scene until flushing is complete. Strong acids and all alkaline solutions can penetrate deeply, requiring a prolonged flush. Again, always take care to protect the uninjured eye and prevent irrigation fluid from running into it.

After you have completed irrigation, apply a clean, dry dressing to cover the eye, and transport the patient promptly to the hospital for further care (**FIGURE 28-18**). If the irrigation can be carried out

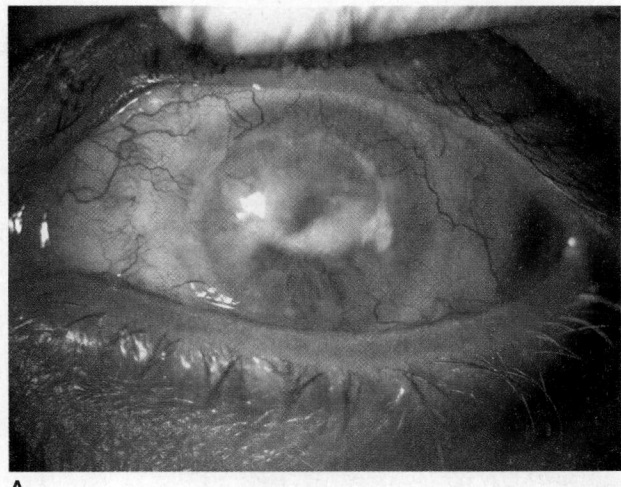

A

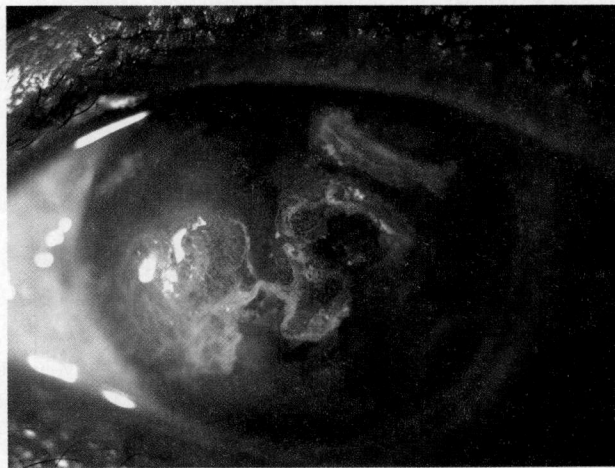

B

**FIGURE 28-16 A.** Chemical burns typically occur when an acid or alkali is splashed into the eye. **B.** This figure shows a chemical burn from lye, an alkaline solution. Because lye can continue to damage the eye even when diluted, fast action is needed.

A, B: © Paul Whitten/Science Source.

satisfactorily in the ambulance, it should be done during transport to save time.

### Thermal Burns

When a patient is burned on the face during a fire, the eyes usually close rapidly because of the heat. This reaction is a natural reflex to protect the eye from

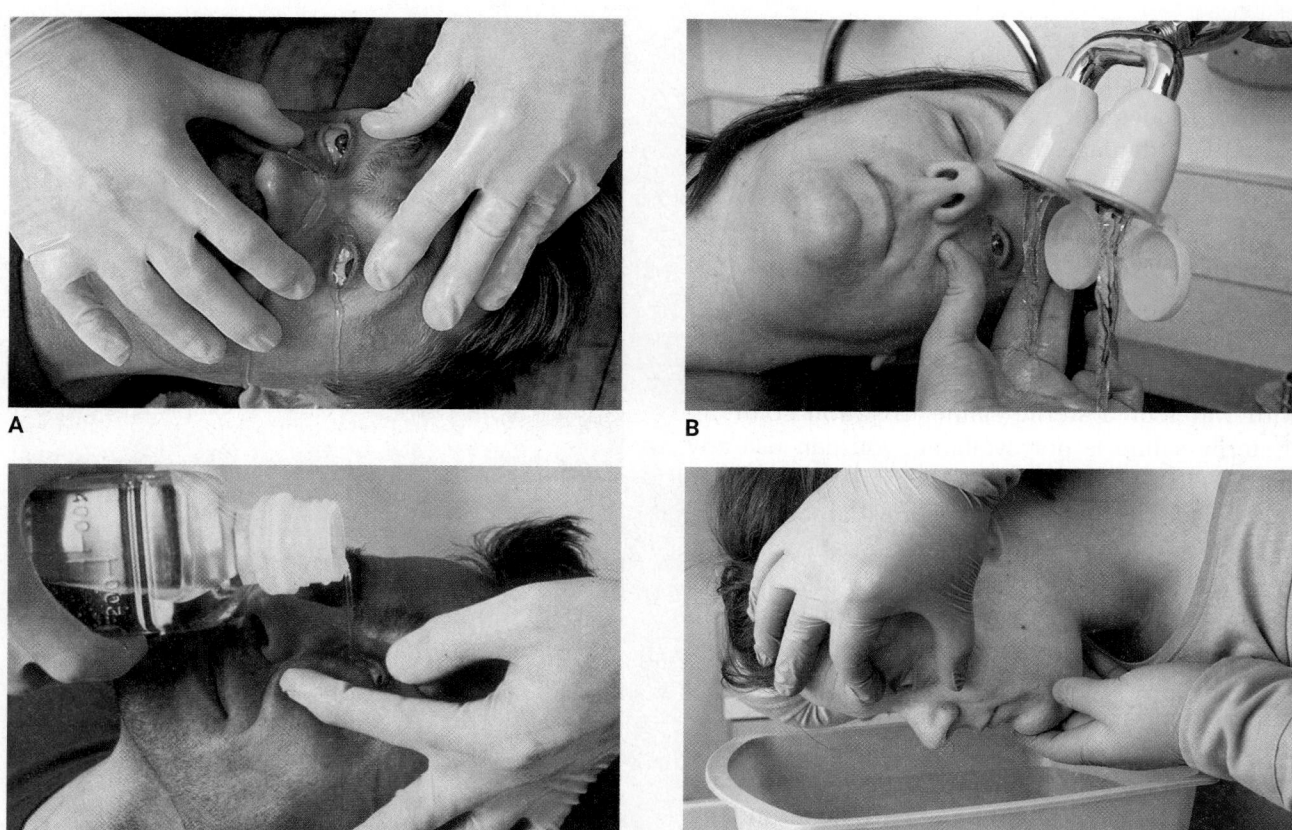

**FIGURE 28-17** The following are four ways to effectively irrigate the eye. **A.** Nasal cannula. **B.** Shower. **C.** Bottle. **D.** Basin. Remember, you must protect the uninjured eye from the irrigating solution to prevent exposure of the unaffected eye to the substance.

**A, C:** © American Academy of Orthopaedic Surgeons; **B, D:** © Jones & Bartlett Learning.

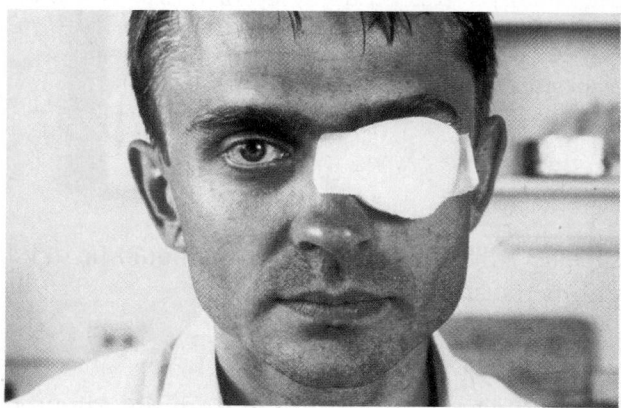

**FIGURE 28-18** Apply a clean, dry dressing to cover the eye after you have finished irrigation.

© American Academy of Orthopaedic Surgeons.

further injury. However, the eyelids remain exposed and are frequently burned (**FIGURE 28-19**). Burns of the eyelids require highly specialized care. It is best to provide prompt transport for these patients without further examination. First, however, you should cover both eyes with a sterile dressing moistened with sterile saline. You may apply eye shields over the dressing. Consider transporting these patients

## Words of Wisdom

With thermal burns to the face, inhalation burns may also occur.

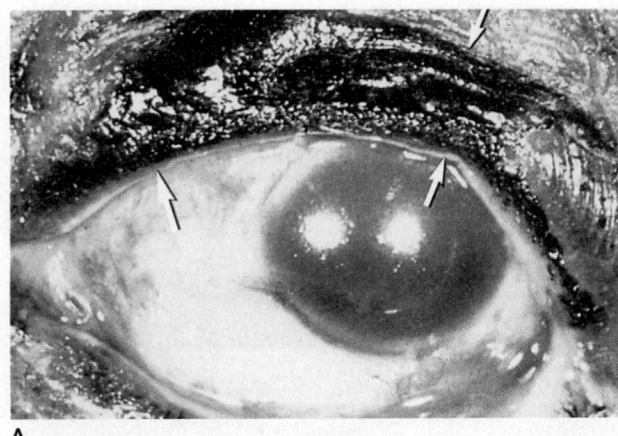

A

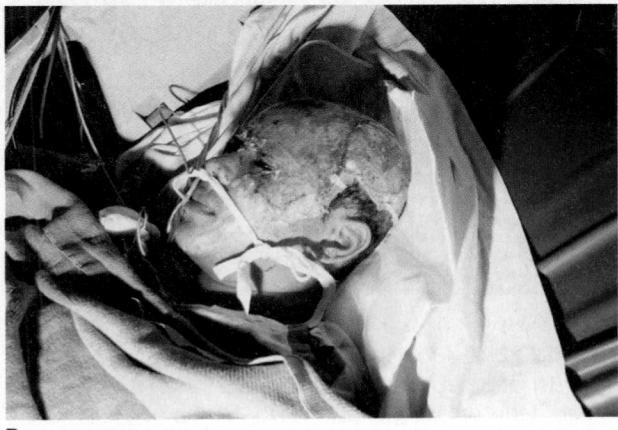

B

**FIGURE 28-19** Thermal burns occasionally cause significant damage to the eyelids. **A.** Arrows show some full-thickness burns. **B.** Burns of the eyelids require immediate hospital care.

to a designated burn center depending on local protocol or medical control recommendations.

### Light Burns

Infrared rays, the light from a solar eclipse (if the patient has looked directly at the sun), and laser burns all can cause significant damage to the sensory cells of the eye when rays of light become focused on the retina. Retinal injuries that are caused by exposure to extremely bright light are generally not painful but may result in permanent damage to vision.

Superficial burns of the eye can result from ultraviolet rays from an arc welding unit, light from prolonged exposure to a sun lamp, or reflected light from a bright, snow-covered area (snow blindness). This kind of burn often is not painful at first but may become so 3 to 5 hours later, when the damaged cornea responds to the injury. Severe conjunctivitis usually develops, with redness, swelling, and excessive tear production. You can ease the pain from these corneal burns by covering each eye with a sterile, moist pad and an eye shield. Have the patient lie down during transport to the hospital and protect him or her from further exposure to bright light.

The patient should be examined by a physician as soon as possible.

### Lacerations

Lacerations of the eyelids require careful repair to restore appearance and function (**FIGURE 28-20**). Bleeding may be heavy, but it usually can be controlled by gentle, manual pressure. If there is a laceration of the globe itself, apply no pressure to the eye. Compression can interfere with the blood supply to the back of the eye and result in loss of vision from damage to the retina. Furthermore, pressure may squeeze the vitreous humor, iris, lens, or even the retina out of the eye and cause irreparable damage or blindness.

Follow these three important guidelines in treating penetrating injuries of the eye:

1. Never exert pressure on or manipulate the injured eye (globe) in any way.
2. If part of the eyeball is exposed, gently apply a moist, sterile dressing to prevent drying.
3. Cover the injured eye with a protective metal eye shield, cup, or sterile dressing. Apply soft dressings to both eyes, and provide prompt transport to the hospital.

On rare occasions following a serious injury, the eyeball may be displaced out of its socket. Do not attempt to reposition it. Simply cover the eye and stabilize it with a moist, sterile dressing (**FIGURE 28-21**). Remember to cover both eyes to prevent further injury because of sympathetic movement. Have the patient lie in a supine position en route to the hospital to prevent further loss of fluid from the eye.

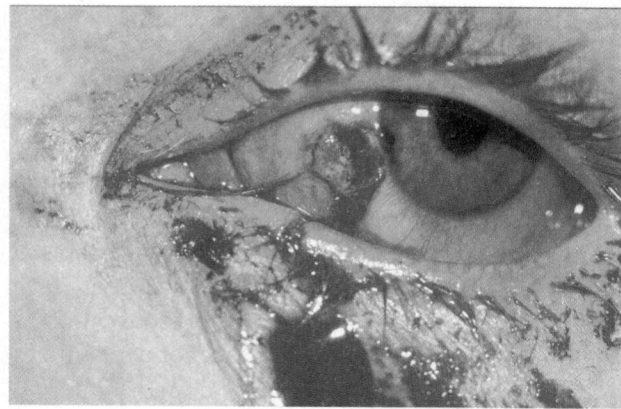

A

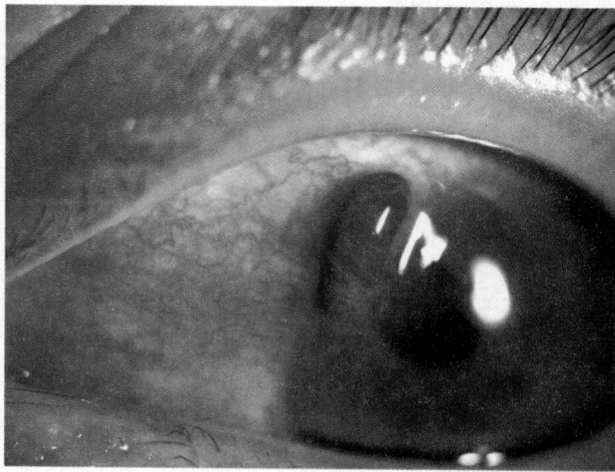

B

**FIGURE 28-20** Lacerations are serious injuries that require prompt transport. **A.** Although bleeding can be heavy, never exert pressure on the eye. **B.** Pressure may squeeze the vitreous humor, iris, lens, or even the retina out of the eye.

A: © Chris Barry/Phototake; B: Paul Whitten/Science Source.

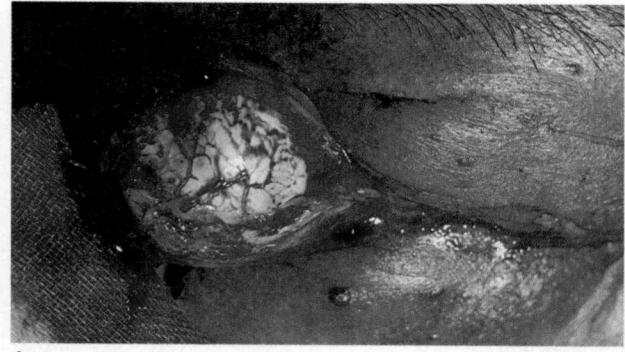

A

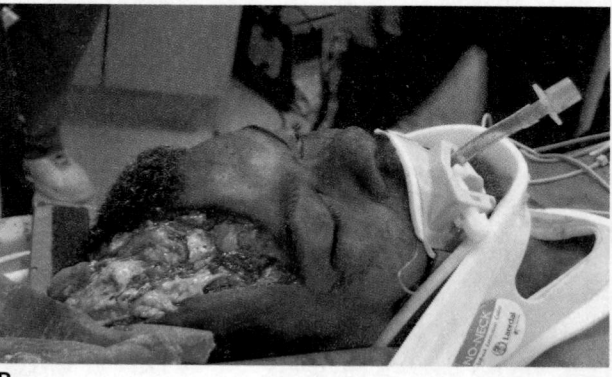

B

**FIGURE 28-21** An injury that exposes the eye (**A**), brain (**B**), or other structures should be covered with a moist, sterile dressing to prevent further damage.

A: © Bob Masini/Phototake; B: © E.M. Singletary, M.D. Used with permission.

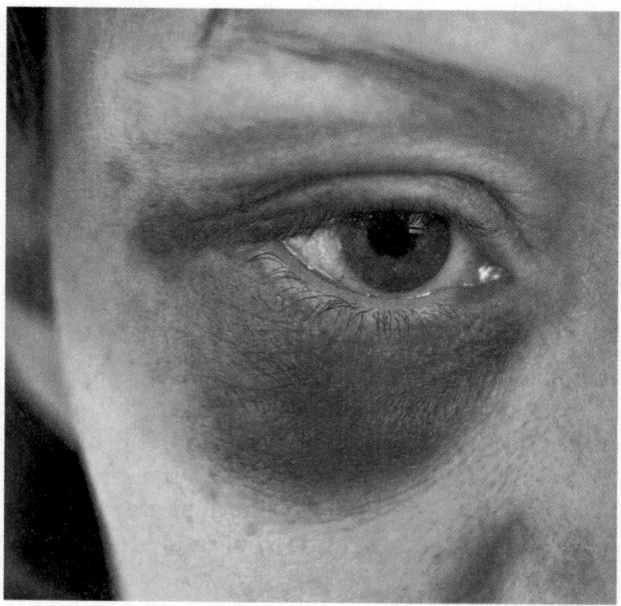

**FIGURE 28-22** The typical "black eye" is caused by bleeding into the tissue around the orbit.

© Berit Skogmo/iStock/Thinkstock.

## Blunt Trauma

Blunt trauma can cause many serious eye injuries. These range from the ordinary black eye, a result of bleeding into the tissue around the orbit, to a severely damaged globe (**FIGURE 28-22**). You may see an injury called hyphema, or bleeding into the anterior chamber of the eye, that obscures part or all of the iris (**FIGURE 28-23**). This injury is common in blunt trauma and may seriously impair vision. Twenty-five percent of hyphemas are associated with underlying globe injuries, a serious injury to the eye. Cover the eye to protect it from further injury and provide transportation to the hospital for further medical evaluation.

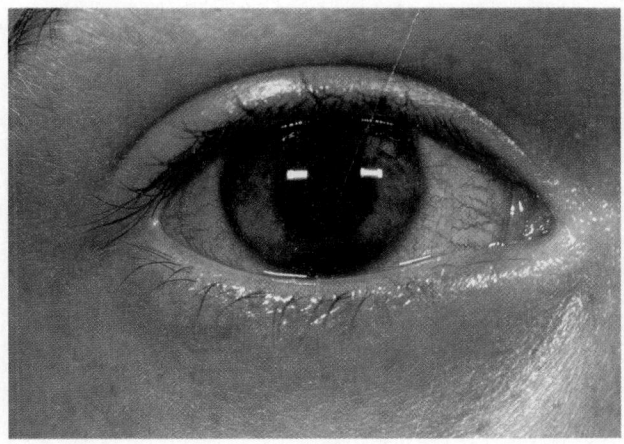

A

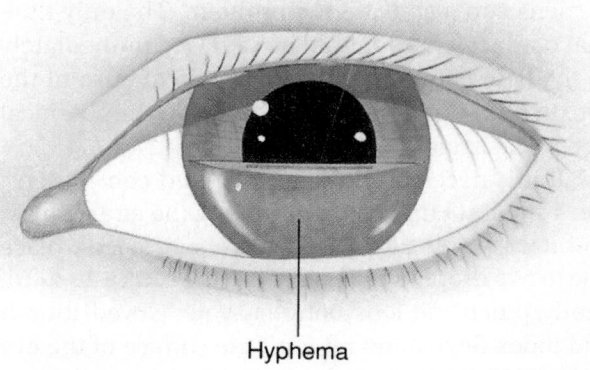

Hyphema

B

**FIGURE 28-23 A.** A hyphema, characterized by bleeding into the anterior chamber of the eye, is common following blunt trauma to the eye. This condition may seriously impair vision and should be considered a sight-threatening emergency. **B.** Illustration of hyphema.

A: © Dr. Chris Hale/Science Source; B: © Jones & Bartlett Learning.

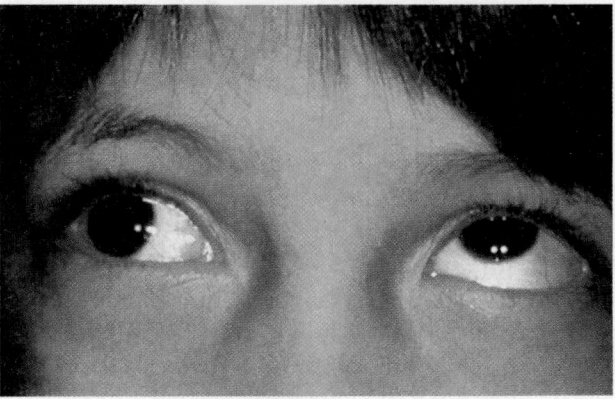

**FIGURE 28-24** A patient with a blow-out fracture may not move his or her eyes together because of muscle entrapment. Therefore, the patient sees double images of any object.

© American Academy of Orthopaedic Surgeons.

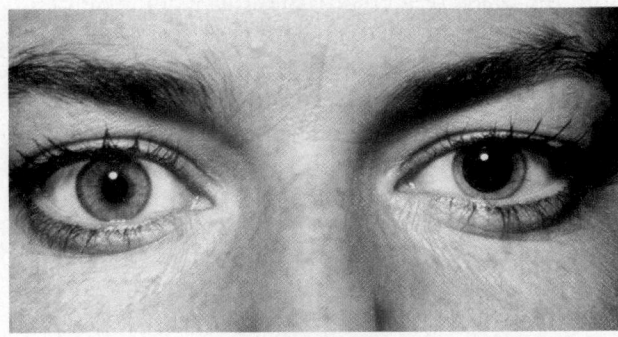

**FIGURE 28-25** Variation of pupil size may indicate a brain injury.

© American Academy of Orthopaedic Surgeons.

Blunt trauma can also cause a fracture of the orbit, specifically of the bones that form its floor and support the globe. When associated with displacement, this injury is sometimes referred to as a **blow-out fracture**. The fragments of fractured bone can entrap some of the muscles that control eye movement, causing double vision (**FIGURE 28-24**). Any patient who reports pain, double vision, or decreased vision following a blunt injury about the eye should be placed on a stretcher and promptly transported to the emergency department. Protect the eye from further injury with a metal shield; cover the other eye to minimize movement on the injured side.

Another possible result of blunt eye injury is retinal detachment. This injury is often seen in sports, especially boxing. It is painless but produces flashing lights, specks, or floaters in the field of vision and a cloud or shade over the patient's vision. Because the retina is separated from the nourishing choroid, this injury requires prompt medical attention to preserve vision in the eye.

## Eye Injuries Following Head Injury

Abnormalities in the appearance or function of the eyes often occur following a brain injury. Any of the following eye findings should alert you to the possibility of a head injury:

- One pupil larger than the other in an unconscious patient (**FIGURE 28-25**)
- The eyes not moving together or pointing in different directions

- Failure of the eyes to follow the movement of your finger as instructed
- Bleeding under the conjunctiva, which obscures the sclera (white portion) of the eye
- Protrusion or bulging of one eye

Record any of these observations, along with the time that you make them. For an unconscious patient, remember to keep the eyelids closed; drying of the ocular tissue can cause permanent injury and may result in blindness. Cover the lids with moist gauze, or hold them closed with clear tape. Normal tears will then keep the tissues moist.

## Blast Injuries

The signs and symptoms of blast injuries range from severe pain and loss of vision to foreign bodies within the globe. Before responding to patients after the blast, first ensure that the scene is safe.

Management of blast injuries to the eye depends on the severity of the injury. If there is a foreign body within the globe, do not attempt to remove it. Use a clean cup or similar item to protect the area. If only one eye is injured, follow local protocols, which may include covering the other eye to eliminate sympathetic motion. Patients with a sudden loss or decrease of vision will need to be verbally instructed on what actions are taking place around them. If the patient has severe swelling or a hematoma to the eyelid, do not attempt to force the eyelid open to examine the eye because this increases the pressure already present within the globe.

## Contact Lenses and Artificial Eyes

Small, hard contact lenses usually are tinted, making them relatively easy to see. Large, soft contact lenses are clear and can be very difficult to see. In general, you should not attempt to remove either type of lens from a patient's eye. You should never attempt to remove a lens from an eye that has been—or may have been—injured because manipulating the lens can aggravate the problem. The only time that contact lenses should be removed immediately in the field is in the case of a chemical burn of the eye. In this situation, the lens can trap the chemical and make irrigation difficult.

If it is necessary to remove a hard contact lens, use a small suction cup, moistening the end with saline (**FIGURE 28-26A**). To remove soft lenses, place one to two drops of saline in the eye (**FIGURE 28-26B**), gently pinch the lens between your gloved thumb and index finger, and lift it off the surface of the eye (**FIGURE 28-26C**). Place the contact lens in a container

---

**YOU** are the Provider

After taking appropriate spinal precautions, you place the patient onto the stretcher and load him into the ambulance. You recovered his teeth and placed them in a commercial tooth-saver container. While you reassess the interventions you have performed thus far, your partner reassesses the patient's vital signs.

| Recording Time:  11 Minutes | |
| --- | --- |
| **Level of consciousness** | Conscious and alert |
| **Respirations** | 20 breaths/min; adequate depth |
| **Pulse** | 108 beats/min; strong and regular |
| **Skin** | Pink, warm, and dry |
| **Blood pressure** | 128/62 mm Hg |
| **Spo$_2$** | 98% (on room air) |

Reassessment of the patient's mouth reveals that it is clear of blood. You begin transport to a trauma center, which is located 15 miles away. En route, the patient tells you that he is becoming nauseated. You call in your radio report and give an estimated time of arrival of 18 to 20 minutes.

**6.** What should you do if this patient begins to vomit?

**7.** How should you treat a patient with active oral bleeding and inadequate ventilation?

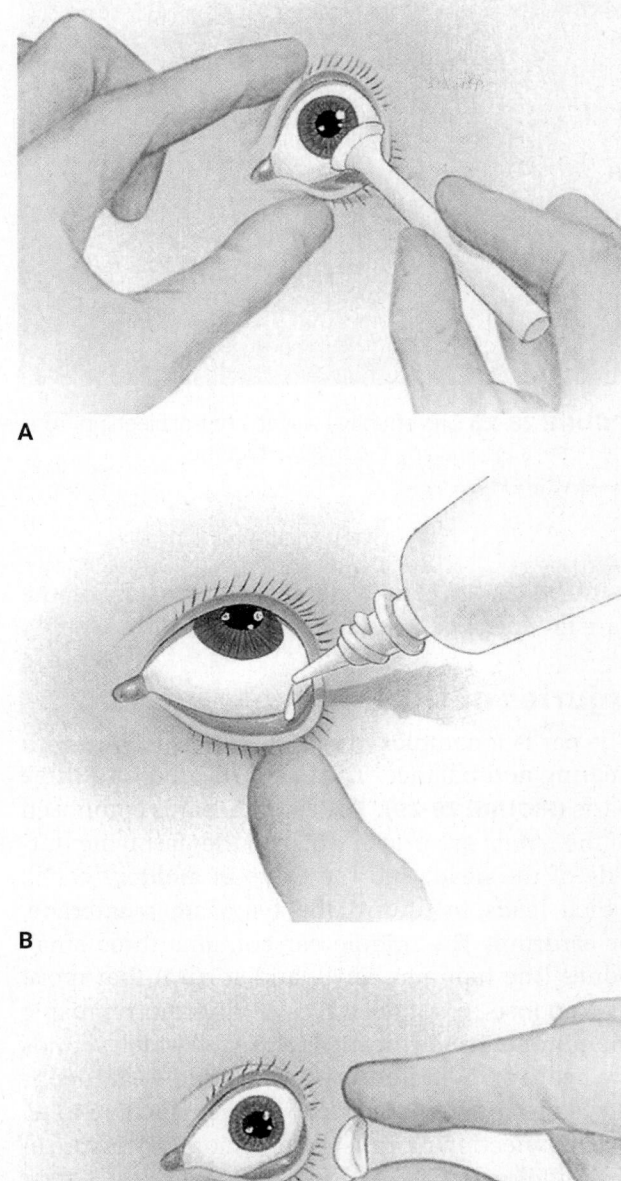

**A**

**B**

**C**

**FIGURE 28-26** Removing contact lenses should be limited to patients with chemical burn injuries to the eye. **A.** To remove hard contact lenses, use a specialized suction cup moistened with sterile saline solution. **B.** To remove soft contact lenses, instill one or two drops of saline or irrigating solution. **C.** Next, pinch off the lens with your gloved thumb and index finger.

A, B, C: © Jones & Bartlett Learning.

filled with sterile saline solution to prevent damage to the contact lens. Always advise the emergency department staff if a patient is wearing contact lenses.

Occasionally, you may find yourself caring for a patient who is wearing an eye prosthesis (an artificial eye). Many people are surprised to find that it can be difficult to distinguish a prosthesis from a natural eye. You should suspect that an eye is artificial when it does not respond to light, move in concert with the opposite eye, or appear quite the same as the opposite eye. If you think that a patient may have an artificial eye but you are not sure, go ahead and ask about it. Although no harm will be done if you care for an artificial eye as you would a normal one, you need to clearly understand the patient's eye function.

## Injuries of the Nose

Nosebleeds (epistaxis) are a common problem that can occur spontaneously or from trauma. One of the most common causes of nosebleeds is digital trauma (picking the nose with a finger). Nosebleeds are further classified into anterior and posterior epistaxis. Anterior nosebleeds usually originate from the area of the septum and bleed slowly. They are usually self-limited and resolve quickly. Posterior nosebleeds are usually more severe and often cause the patient to swallow blood, which can lead to nausea and vomiting. Trauma to the face and skull that results in a basilar skull fracture can cause the posterior wall of the nasal cavity to become unstable. Due to this risk, attempting to place a nasopharyngeal airway in a patient with significant facial trauma, or a suspected basilar skull fracture, is controversial. Follow local protocols regarding insertion of a nasopharyngeal airway in a patient with head or facial trauma.

When you are assessing injuries involving the nose, it helps to picture the inside of the nose itself (**FIGURE 28-27**). The nasal cavity is divided into two sections or chambers by the nasal septum, which is made of cartilage. Within each nasal chamber, there are layers of bone called the **turbinates**, which are covered with a moist lining. Both chambers have a superior turbinate, a middle turbinate, and an inferior turbinate. As a person breathes, air moves through the nasal chambers and is humidified as it passes over the turbinates. Directly above the nose are the frontal sinuses and, on either side, the orbit of the eye.

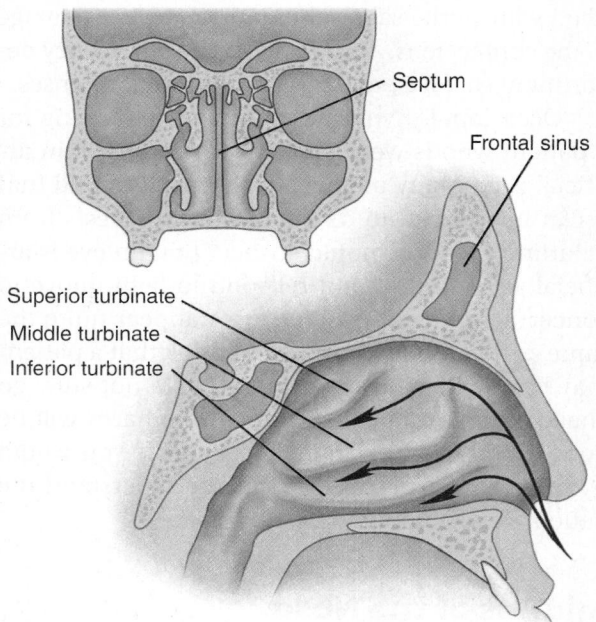

**FIGURE 28-27** The nose has two chambers, divided by the septum. Each chamber is composed of layers of bone called turbinates. Above the nose are the frontal sinuses and, on either side, the orbits of the eyes.

© Jones & Bartlett Learning.

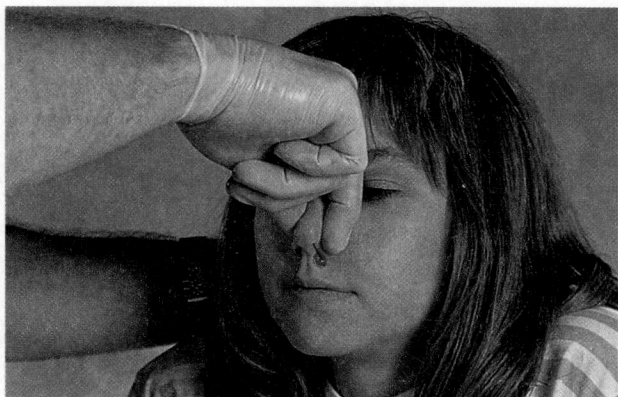

**FIGURE 28-28** One effective way to control bleeding from the nose is by pinching the nostrils together.

© American Academy of Orthopaedic Surgeons.

In patients with severe nasal injury, there may also be injury to the cervical spine. Keep in mind that cerebrospinal fluid (CSF) may escape down through the nose (or ears) following a fracture at the base of the skull. If blood or drainage contains CSF, a characteristic staining of the dressing will occur. This can be seen by using a piece of gauze to absorb blood that is flowing from the nose or ears. If CSF is present, the blood will be surrounded by a lighter ring of fluid. This is often called the halo test. Do not delay care or transportation of a priority patient to perform the halo test.

You can control bleeding from abrasions and lacerations to the nose by applying a sterile dressing. If the patient is bleeding heavily from the nose, this is most likely caused by significant trauma, and you must consider cervical spine injury. The patient should not be moved if the airway can be managed in the patient's current position. For a nontrauma patient who is bleeding from the nose, one effective way to control bleeding is to place the patient in a sitting position, leaning forward, and pinch his or her nostrils together for 10 to 15 minutes

(**FIGURE 28-28**). For a detailed discussion of the care for epistaxis, see Chapter 26, *Bleeding*.

## Injuries of the Ear

The ear is a complex organ that is associated with hearing and balance. The ear is divided into three parts (**FIGURE 28-29**). The external ear is composed of the **pinna**, or auricle, which is the part lying outside of the head, and the **external auditory canal**, which leads in toward the **tympanic membrane**, or eardrum. The middle ear contains three small bones (the hammer, anvil, and stirrup) that move in response to sound waves hitting the tympanic membrane. This is the mechanism by which sounds are heard and differentiated. The middle ear is connected to the nasopharynx by the **eustachian tube**. This connection permits equalization of pressure in the middle ear when external atmospheric pressure changes. The inner ear is composed of bony chambers filled with fluid. As the head moves, so does the fluid. In response, fine nerve endings within the fluid send impulses to the brain indicating the position of the head and the rate of change of position.

Ears are often injured, but they usually do not bleed very much. If local pressure does not control the bleeding, you can apply a roller dressing (**FIGURE 28-30**). First, however, you should place a soft, padded dressing between the back of the ear and the scalp because bandaging the ear against the tender underlying scalp can be extremely painful for the patient. In the case of an ear avulsion, you

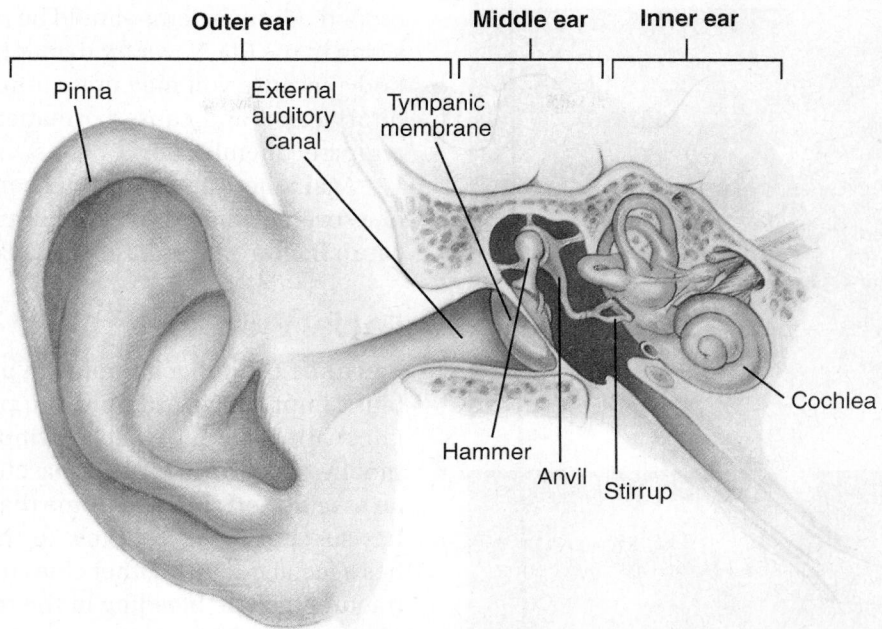

**Outer ear**    **Middle ear**    **Inner ear**

Pinna

External
auditory
canal

Tympanic
membrane

Hammer

Anvil

Stirrup

Cochlea

**FIGURE 28-29** The ear has three principal parts: the external, or outer, ear,
composed of the pinna, external auditory canal, and tympanic membrane; the middle
ear, including the hammer, anvil, and stirrup; and the inner ear, composed of bony
chambers filled with fluid.

© Jones & Bartlett Learning.

# YOU are the Provider

You reassess the patient en route, including his vital signs, and note that his breathing is becoming increasingly labored.
His airway remains clear of secretions and blood, but his neck appears to be more swollen than it was during previous
assessments.

| Recording Time:  16 Minutes | |
| --- | --- |
| **Level of consciousness** | Conscious and alert; anxious |
| **Respirations** | 26 breaths/min; labored |
| **Pulse** | 124 beats/min; strong and regular |
| **Skin** | Cool and moist; perioral cyanosis is developing |
| **Blood pressure** | 122/58 mm Hg |
| **Spo$_2$** | 88% (on room air) |

The hospital staff are notified of the change in the patient's condition. The nurse tells you to bring him straight to the
trauma room on your arrival.

**8.** What is the most likely cause of your patient's labored breathing?

**9.** What adjustments, if any, should you make to your current treatment?

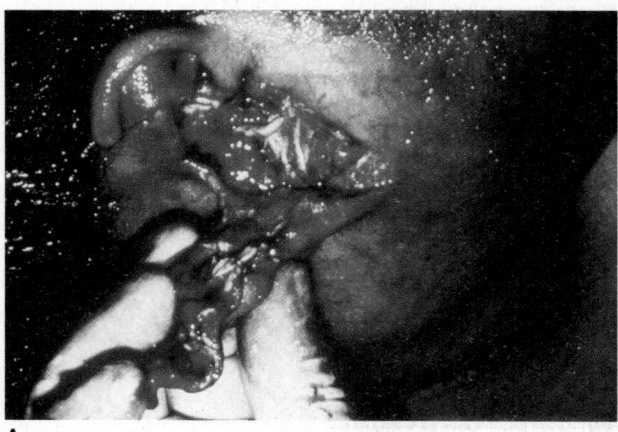

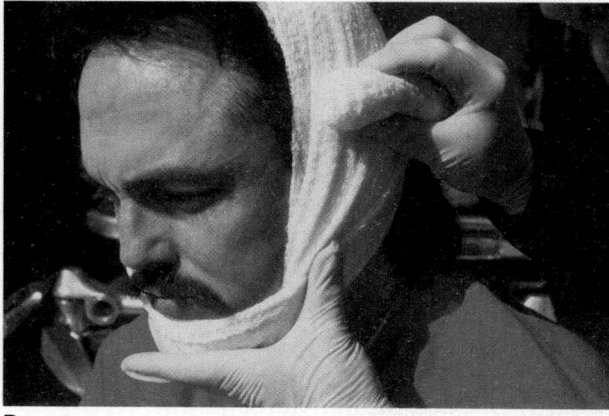

**FIGURE 28-30 A.** A major laceration of the ear. **B.** Proper treatment includes use of a soft, sterile pad behind the ear, between it and the scalp. Then wrap a roller gauze dressing around the head to include the entire ear.

A: © American Academy of Orthopaedic Surgeons; B: © Jones & Bartlett Learning.

should wrap the avulsed part in a dry sterile dressing and put it in a plastic bag labeled with the patient's name. Keep the avulsed part cool and transport it to the hospital with the patient. Often, avulsed tissue from the ear can be reattached.

Sudden changes in pressure created by a blast wave may rupture one or both tympanic membranes. Patients with a ruptured tympanic membrane will often report severe ear pain, difficulty hearing, or ringing in the affected ear. The tympanic membrane may also be perforated by insertion of objects (such as a cotton swab) too far into the ear. Any patient with a suspected tympanic membrane injury should be transported to the hospital for a more detailed evaluation.

The external auditory canal is a favorite place for children to place foreign bodies such as crayons or food. All such items should be removed by a physician in the ED. Never try to manipulate the foreign body because you may press it further into the auditory canal and cause permanent damage to the tympanic membrane.

Again, note any clear fluid coming from the ear of a severely injured patient because this may indicate a fracture at the base of the skull.

## Facial Fractures

Fractures of the facial bones typically result from blunt impact. For example, the patient's head collides with a steering wheel or windshield in an automobile crash or is hit by a baseball bat or pipe in an assault. You should assume that any patient who has sustained a direct blow to the mouth or nose has a facial fracture. Other clues to the possibility of fracture include bleeding in the mouth, inability to swallow or talk, absent or loose teeth, and/or loose or movable bone fragments. Patients may also report that "it doesn't feel right" when they close their jaw, signaling an irregularity of bite.

Facial fractures alone are not acute emergencies unless there is serious bleeding; however, they are an indication of significant blunt force trauma applied to that region of the body. Serious bleeding from a facial fracture can be life threatening. In addition to external hemorrhage, there is the danger of blood clots lodging in the upper airway and causing an obstruction (**FIGURE 28-31**).

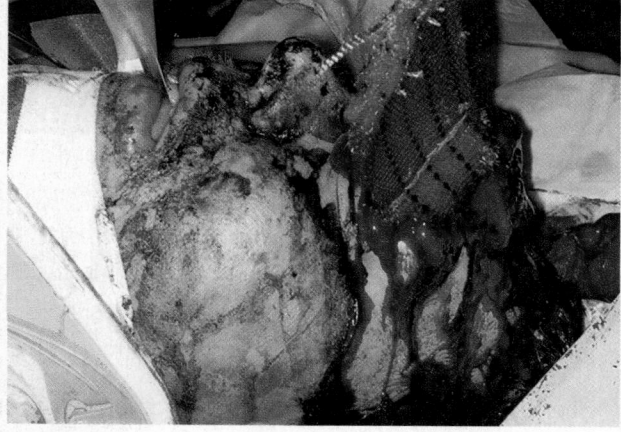

**FIGURE 28-31** Bleeding following a crushing injury to the face can be life threatening because, in addition to the external hemorrhage, blood clots in the airway can cause a complete obstruction.

© Chuck Stewart, MD.

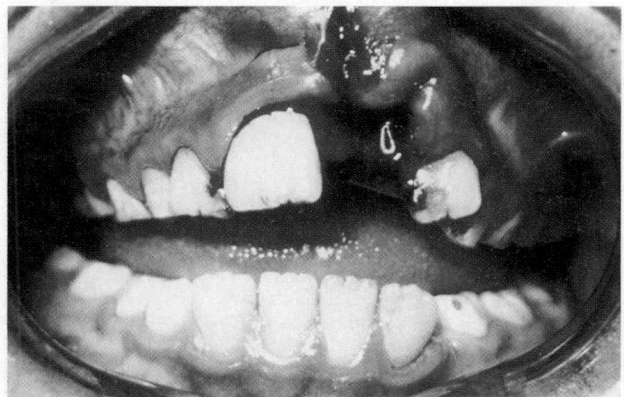

**A**

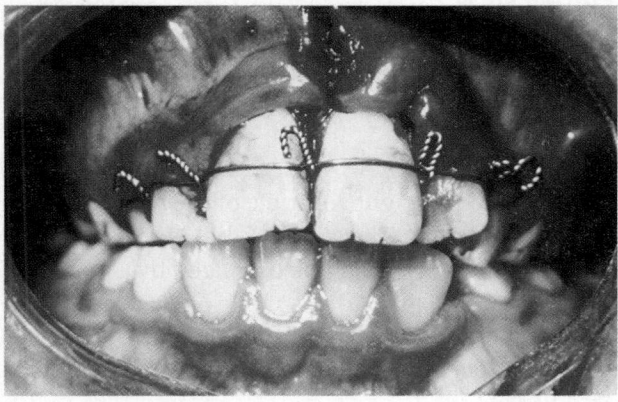

**B**

**FIGURE 28-32 A.** Save any lost teeth or bone fragments following an injury to the mouth. **B.** Even with traumatic loss of a tooth, the possibility of successful reimplantation is very good, especially if the tooth is stored in an appropriate tooth-storage solution, cold milk, or sterile saline.

**A, B:** © American Academy of Orthopaedic Surgeons.

Fractures around the face and mouth can also produce deformity and loose bone fragments. However, plastic surgeons can repair the damage if the injuries are treated within 7 to 10 days of the injury. Be sure to remove and save loose teeth or bone fragments from the mouth; it is often possible to reimplant them (**FIGURE 28-32**). It is also important to remove them as well as any loose dentures or dental bridges to protect against airway obstruction. The removal of dentures will affect the apparent shape of the patient's jaw.

Another source of potential airway obstruction is swelling, which can be extreme within the first 24 hours after injury. If you notice swelling during assessment or at any time while the patient is in your care, check for airway obstruction.

## Dental Injuries

Dental injuries can be traumatic to a patient. Not only is the injury itself traumatic, but the patient's permanent teeth may also be lost—affecting everything from eating to smiling. Keep this in mind when providing care.

Bleeding will occur whenever a tooth is violently displaced out of its socket; therefore, apply direct pressure to stop the bleeding. To keep the airway patent, perform suctioning if needed. Also keep in mind that cracked or loose teeth can potentially obstruct the airway; therefore, suctioning may be necessary.

When dealing with an avulsed tooth, handle it by its crown and not by the root. When transporting the patient, bring along the tooth, placing it in a special tooth storage solution if available in your supplies, or in cold milk or sterile saline. There are also commercially available kits that may be used. Notify the receiving facility about the avulsed tooth because reimplantation is recommended within 1 hour after the trauma.

## Injuries of the Cheek

You may encounter an object that is impaled in the patient's cheek. If you are unable to control the bleeding and it is compromising the patient's airway, remove the impaled object if possible and provide direct pressure on the inside and outside of the cheek. The amount of bandaging should not be so overwhelming that it occludes the mouth and makes it difficult for the patient to breathe.

## Injuries of the Neck

The neck contains many structures that are vulnerable to injury by blunt trauma, such as from a steering wheel in a car crash, or by penetrating injury, such as a stab or gunshot wound. These structures include the upper airway, the esophagus, the carotid arteries and jugular veins, the thyroid cartilage or Adam's apple, the cricoid cartilage, and the upper part of the trachea. Any injury to the neck is serious and should be considered life threatening until proven otherwise in the ED.

### Blunt Injuries

Any crushing injury of the upper part of the neck has the potential to involve the larynx or trachea.

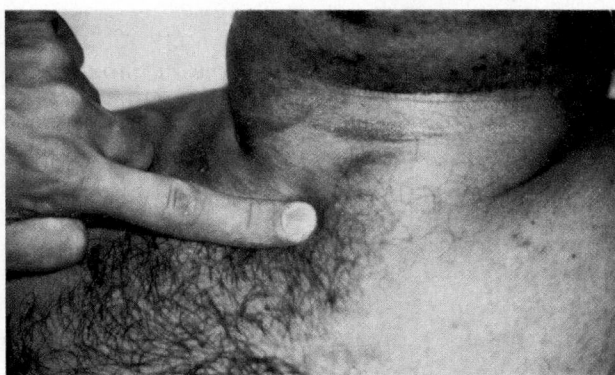

**FIGURE 28-33** Fractures of the larynx or trachea can cause air to leak from the airway into the subcutaneous tissues. The presence of air in the soft tissues produces a crackling sensation called subcutaneous emphysema.

© American Academy of Orthopaedic Surgeons.

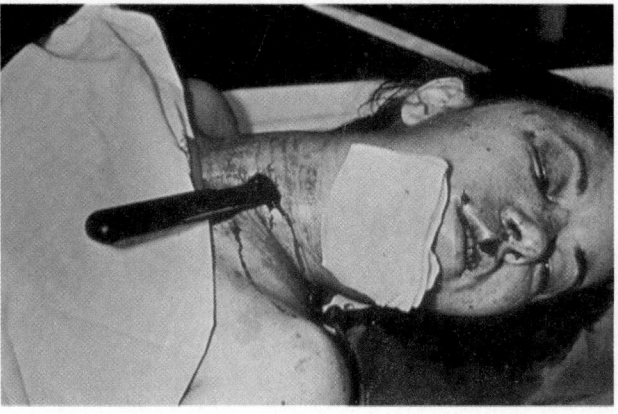

**FIGURE 28-34** Penetrating injuries to the neck can result in profuse bleeding if a carotid artery or jugular vein is damaged.

© American Academy of Orthopaedic Surgeons.

Examples include a collision with a steering wheel, an attempted suicide by hanging, and a clothesline injury sustained while riding a bicycle. Once the cartilages of the upper airway and larynx are fractured, they do not spring back to their normal position. This type of fracture can lead to loss of voice, difficulty swallowing, severe and sometimes fatal airway obstruction, and leakage of air into the soft tissues of the neck (**FIGURE 28-33**). The presence of air in the soft tissues produces a characteristic crackling sensation called subcutaneous emphysema. If you feel this sensation when you palpate the neck, you should maintain the airway as best you can and provide immediate transport. Be aware that complete airway obstruction can develop rapidly in these patients as a result of swelling or bleeding into the underlying tissues. It may be difficult to manage the airway in patients with these injuries; therefore, ALS support should be considered early if available. An incident involving an injury to the throat may also have caused a cervical spinal injury; therefore, spinal motion restriction may be indicated.

## Penetrating Injuries

Penetrating injuries to the neck can cause profuse bleeding from laceration of the great vessels in the neck—the carotid arteries or the jugular veins (**FIGURE 28-34**). Injuries to the carotid and jugular vessels in the neck can cause the body to bleed out, also known as exsanguination. Injuries to these large vessels may also allow air to enter the circulatory system. If a vein has been punctured, air may be sucked through it to the heart, a clinical situation

called an air embolism. A large amount of air in the right atrium and right ventricle of the heart can lead to cardiac arrest. The airway, the esophagus, and even the spinal cord can be damaged by a penetrating injury.

Direct pressure over the bleeding site will control most neck bleeding. Follow the steps in **SKILL DRILL 28-3**:

1. Apply direct pressure to the bleeding site using a gloved fingertip. if necessary, to control bleeding (**Step 1**).
2. Apply a sterile occlusive dressing to ensure that air does not enter a vein (**Step 2**).
3. Secure the dressing in place with roller gauze, adding more dressings if needed.
4. Wrap the gauze around and under the patient's shoulder. To avoid possible airway and circulation problems, do not wrap the gauze around the neck.

Despite the use of these measures, the tissues within the neck may continue to bleed and compress the upper airway, so you should look for signs of airway obstruction.

You might find it necessary to apply pressure both above and below the penetrating wound to control life-threatening bleeding from the carotid artery (above) and the jugular vein (below). You may also need to treat the patient for shock.

If indicated, initiate spinal motion restriction precautions and provide prompt transport. Ensure that the airway remains open en route and apply high-flow oxygen.

## Skill Drill 28-3 Controlling Bleeding From a Neck Injury

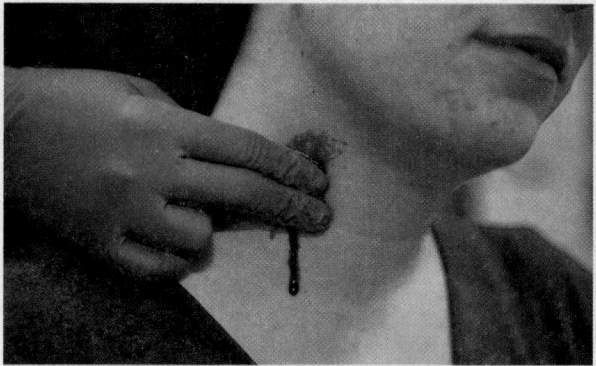

**Step 1**

Apply direct pressure to the bleeding site using a gloved fingertip, if necessary, to control bleeding.

© Jones & Bartlett Learning.

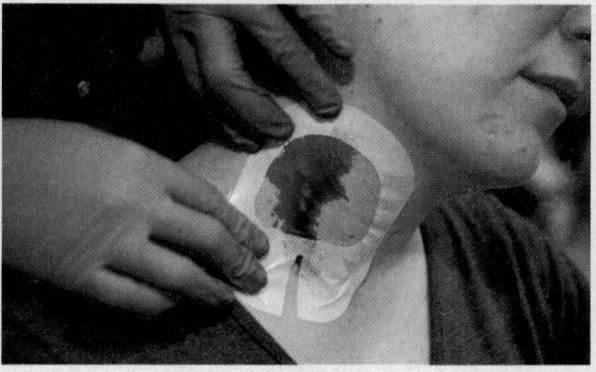

**Step 2**

Apply a sterile occlusive dressing to ensure that air does not enter a vein.

## Laryngeal Injuries

Blunt force trauma to the larynx can occur when an unrestrained driver strikes the steering wheel or when a snowmobile rider or off-road biker strikes a clothesline or a fixed wire strung across a property line. The larynx becomes crushed against the cervical spine, resulting in soft-tissue injury, fractures, and/or separation of the fascia that connects the thyroid and cricoid cartilages. These strangulation injuries can also be found in either intentional or unintentional hangings. Anytime there is suspected injury to the larynx, you should suspect possible cervical spine injury.

Open injuries to the larynx can occur as a result of a stabbing or penetration by a similar object. Penetrating and impaled objects should not be removed unless they interfere with CPR. Stabilize all impaled objects if they are not obstructing the airway (see Chapter 27, *Soft-Tissue Injuries*).

Significant injuries to the larynx pose an immediate risk of airway compromise because of disruption of the normal passage of air, soft-tissue swelling, or aspiration (entry of solids or fluids from the oropharynx or nasopharynx into the airway) of blood. The signs and symptoms of larynx injuries include respiratory distress, hoarseness, pain, difficulty swallowing (dysphagia), cyanosis, pale skin, sputum in the wound, subcutaneous emphysema, bruising on the neck, hematoma, or bleeding.

To manage a laryngeal injury, secure the patient's airway and provide oxygenation and ventilation as needed. Follow local protocols regarding use of spinal precautions.

## YOU are the Provider SUMMARY

**1. What should be your most immediate concern after receiving this initial patient information?**

The presence of severe facial trauma should immediately increase your index of suspicion for potential airway and ventilation compromise, including partial or complete upper airway obstruction. Direct trauma to the nose and mouth can be a source of significant

bleeding. Severe swelling and bleeding can occur in the oropharynx. Crushing injuries to the larynx and trachea are associated with a high incidence of airway and ventilation compromise. The risk of upper airway obstruction is significantly higher if the patient has a decreased level of consciousness and is unable to expel blood from the mouth on his or her own. Also, if the patient swallows large amounts of blood, the risk of vomiting and subsequent aspiration is high.

Dislodged teeth can fall to the back of the throat and be aspirated into the lungs or cause complete obstruction of the upper airway.

Crushing injuries to the throat should increase your index of suspicion for a spinal injury. In addition, when trauma is severe enough to fracture facial bones, the possibility of an underlying brain injury should be considered as well.

**2.  What should your initial actions consist of when you arrive at the scene?**

First, conduct a scene size-up. Although law enforcement personnel have advised you that the scene is secure, you must remain aware of your surroundings at all times. Your patient has been assaulted, which means that the perpetrator, if he or she is not in custody, could return to the scene. Ascertain the total number of patients and call for additional resources if you think you will need them.

As you are approaching the patient, form a general impression.

As you make physical contact with the patient, introduce yourself and manually stabilize his head. Next, assess the status of the patient's airway. If he can talk to you, he has no *immediate* airway problems, although this can quickly change. If there is any blood in his oropharynx, remove it with suction. If he is conscious and alert, consider allowing him to suction his own mouth. Follow standard precautions, including facial protection.

After ensuring a patent airway, assess the quality of the patient's breathing and intervene at once. If he is breathing adequately, monitor his oxygen saturation and administer high-flow oxygen via a nonrebreathing mask if he becomes hypoxic. If he has signs of inadequate breathing (eg, fast or slow rate, shallow breathing [reduced tidal volume]), assist his ventilations.

Complete your primary assessment by assessing the rate and quality of his radial and carotid pulses and looking for and immediately controlling any severe external bleeding. If signs of shock are present, begin immediate shock treatment.

**3.  Does this patient have a patent airway? How can you tell?**

Because the patient is conscious, alert, and talking, he has a patent airway—at least, for the time being. Although he has blood in his mouth, he is able to keep his airway clear by spitting it out. The patient's voice is hoarse; this should concern you because it could indicate upper airway swelling or a crushing injury to the structures of the anterior neck (ie, trachea, larynx).

At this point in the primary assessment, you have not yet determined if he has any injuries that could

affect his level of consciousness, such as a closed head injury. Therefore, you must pay meticulous attention to his mental status and be prepared to suction the blood from his mouth. If he has a loss of consciousness, he will not be able to maintain his airway and you need to be prepared to intervene immediately. *Regardless of the situation, a patient's airway must remain patent at all times!*

**4.  What should be your initial treatment priorities for this patient?**

The goal of the primary assessment is to *find and quickly treat* problems associated with the XABCs. Further assessment and treatment must focus on injuries or conditions that will kill your patient *first*.

Your patient has severe facial trauma and his voice is hoarse. Although he is able to maintain his own airway right now, do not assume that he will be able to continue to do this until you get him to a hospital. Closely monitor his airway and ventilation status!

Your partner is providing manual stabilization of the patient's head based on the assumption that trauma significant enough to cause massive facial trauma can just as easily fracture or dislocate a spinal vertebra.

Closely monitor his airway for continued oral bleeding. If he remains conscious and can easily follow commands, you can allow him to hold the rigid suction catheter and suction the blood from his mouth himself.

Carefully monitor the patient's level of consciousness and breathing adequacy, keep his airway clear of blood, and be prepared to assist his ventilations if his condition deteriorates.

**5.  On the basis of the MOI, what type of injuries should you suspect and assess for?**

On the basis of your assessment, the patient's injuries appear to be isolated to his face and anterior part of the neck. However, a more in-depth assessment by a physician is needed to rule out occult injuries. Facial swelling, which is common following blunt force facial trauma, can make assessment difficult.

On the basis of the MOI, you should be suspicious for facial bone fractures and injury to his trachea and/or larynx. Indicators of facial fractures include oropharyngeal bleeding, loose or absent teeth, difficulty talking or swallowing, and loose or obviously movable bone fragments. Your patient's report that it "doesn't feel right" when he tries to close his mouth signals an irregular bite (dental malocclusion) and is a sign of a mandibular fracture. This is a significant finding because it takes *a lot* of force to fracture the mandible!

Any crushing injury to the anterior part of the neck is likely to involve the larynx or trachea. During your assessment, you detected bruising and swelling of the throat, and the patient's voice is hoarse. These are red-flag indicators of significant anterior neck trauma.

Suspect fracture of the trachea if you detect subcutaneous emphysema, a crackling sensation that is felt when palpating the soft tissues of the neck.

Fractures of the zygomas (cheek bones) often present with a flattened appearance of the cheek bones; however, if the face is severely swollen, this may not be grossly apparent.

When caring for a patient with blunt facial trauma, assess the ability of the patient to move his or her eyes in all directions. Inability of the patient to look up (paralysis of upward gaze) suggests an orbital (blow-out) fracture, in which case a bone fragment has entrapped one of the oculomotor nerves.

A brain injury cannot be ruled out. During your assessment, you should look in and behind the ears. Bruising over the mastoid bone (Battle sign) indicates a basilar skull fracture. Blood that is draining from the ears may contain CSF. This is also an indicator of a basilar skull fracture. Blood or clear fluid drainage from the nose is also a sign of an underlying skull fracture.

Sudden hyperextension of the head during trauma can cause fractures or dislocations of the vertebrae of the cervical spine. Initiate spinal motion restriction precautions when caring for a patient with significant blunt facial trauma.

### 6. What should you do if this patient begins to vomit?

If aspiration occurs, the risk of mortality increases significantly so you *must* have a plan of action to prevent aspiration while transporting a patient who is supine and immobilized on a backboard or other device.

If the patient begins to vomit, *immediately* place him on his side to allow vomitus to drain from his mouth. It is imperative that you protect the patient's airway, but as you turn the entire backboard onto its side, you must also avoid aggravating any possible spinal injury by ensuring that spinal alignment and motion restriction are properly maintained.

While the patient is on his side, suction his mouth to remove any remaining vomitus that did not drain with gravity. Before returning the patient to a supine position, make sure that *all* vomitus and other secretions are removed from his mouth!

### 7. How should you treat a patient with active oral bleeding and inadequate ventilation?

Not only is the patient's airway in immediate jeopardy from obstruction from blood clots and aspiration, but inadequate ventilation will result in hypoxia and may lead to respiratory or cardiopulmonary arrest. Therefore, you must treat both problems simultaneously.

If blood has pooled in the patient's mouth, immediately place the patient onto his or her side to allow the blood to drain from the mouth. Suction

the airway for up to 15 seconds. Then assist the patient's ventilations if they are not adequate.

Continue this alternating pattern of suctioning and assisting ventilations as needed, until the bleeding in the oropharynx is minimal or stops altogether. The patient's airway must remain patent at all times and adequate ventilation must be ensured.

Patients with this type of airway and ventilation predicament would benefit from advanced airway management, especially if they are unconscious. Paramedics can intubate the patient, thus isolating the trachea and preventing aspiration, while manually ventilating the patient with a bag-mask attached to the endotracheal tube. Request ALS, if possible, when caring for patients with this type of complex airway and breathing problem.

### 8. What is the most likely cause of your patient's labored breathing?

Reassessment reveals that his airway remains clear of blood. However, the anterior part of his neck is more swollen so you should suspect that the swelling in his upper airway is increasing—most likely because of injury to his trachea or larynx, thus making it increasingly difficult for him to breathe. His oxygen saturation of 88% reflects significant hypoxemia, and perioral cyanosis (cyanosis around the mouth) is developing.

It is important to note that not all patients with significant injuries deteriorate at the scene. Many of them deteriorate en route to the hospital or shortly after you arrive at the hospital. Therefore, it is critical to *frequently reassess* any patient with injuries that could jeopardize airway patency and impair ventilation.

### 9. What adjustments, if any, should you make to your current treatment?

Your patient's ventilation status has clearly deteriorated. You should consider assisting his ventilations with a bag-mask device and high-flow oxygen. Try to assist the patient's breathing, but do not be too aggressive. If he becomes combative and pushes the bag-mask device away from his face, apply a nonrebreathing mask and carefully monitor his breathing.

If he tolerates assisted ventilation, use extreme caution. Although you must maintain adequate minute volume, a tracheal or laryngeal injury can be exacerbated by aggressive positive-pressure ventilation. Squeeze the bag-mask device just enough to improve the amount of tidal volume with each breath; observe for visible chest rise.

You should *not* use any type of mechanical ventilation device, such as a flow-restricted, oxygen-powered ventilation device, when ventilating a patient with tracheal or laryngeal trauma. These devices deliver oxygen under high pressure and can cause further injury to patients with fractures of the trachea or larynx.

## YOU are the Provider SUMMARY continued

### EMS Patient Care Report (PCR)

| Date: 12-3-20 | Incident No.: 012509 | Nature of Call: Assault | | Location: 1505 Eagle Rock Dr. | |
|---|---|---|---|---|---|
| Dispatched: 1926 | En Route: 1927 | At Scene: 1930 | Transport: 1941 | At Hospital: 2001 | In Service: 2021 |

### Patient Information

| | |
|---|---|
| Age: 30<br>Sex: M<br>Weight (in kg [lb]): 80 kg (175 lb) | Allergies: Penicillin<br>Medications: None<br>Past Medical History: None<br>Chief Complaint: Face and neck injury secondary to assault |

### Vital Signs

| Time: 1935 | BP: 132/68 | Pulse: 118 | Respirations: 22 | Spo$_2$: 97% |
|---|---|---|---|---|
| Time: 1941 | BP: 128/62 | Pulse: 108 | Respirations: 20 | Spo$_2$: 98% |
| Time: 1946 | BP: 122/58 | Pulse: 124 | Respirations: 26 | Spo$_2$: 88% |

### EMS Treatment (circle all that apply)

| Oxygen @ _15_ L/min via:<br>NC   NRM   (Bag mask) | | Assisted Ventilation | Airway Adjunct | CPR |
|---|---|---|---|---|
| Defibrillation | Bleeding Control | Bandaging | Splitting | Other: (Suctioning, spinal precautions) |

### Narrative

Ambulance 12 dispatched to a commercial parking lot for an assault.

Chief Complaint: Face and neck injury

History: The scene was secured by law enforcement prior to EMS arrival. Patient stated that he was struck across the face with a steel pipe, fell to the ground, and was kicked in the face and throat. He denies loss of consciousness. Patient states that it "doesn't feel right" when he tries to close his mouth.

Assessment: On arrival at the scene, found the patient, a 30-year-old male, sitting on the ground; his face was covered with blood and his face was swollen. He was conscious but appeared anxious. He was spitting out small amounts of blood from his mouth, but was maintaining his own airway; his breathing was adequate. Several teeth were missing. Manual c-spine stabilization was applied as patient was assessed further.

Treatment (Rx): Suctioned the patient's mouth as needed to remove blood. Secondary assessment revealed severe swelling of the entire face, and bruising and mild swelling of the anterior part of the neck. No gross evidence of head or C-spine injury was noted during secondary assessment. Initiated spinal motion restriction precautions, and applied a cervical collar. Recovered pt's teeth and placed them in a commercial tooth-saver container.

Transport: Lifted patient onto stretcher, loaded him into the ambulance, and began transport to the hospital. Reassessment en route revealed that his airway was free of blood or other secretions and his vital signs were stable. After radio report was called to receiving facility, patient became more anxious and nauseated and began experiencing respiratory distress. Immediate reassessment revealed that his airway remained free of blood or other secretions, but the anterior part of his neck appeared more swollen than in previous assessments. Further reassessment revealed that perioral cyanosis was developing, and his oxygen saturation had decreased significantly. Began assisting the patient's ventilations with a bag-mask device and high-flow oxygen; he was initially resistant but became more compliant with coaching. Notified hospital of patient status change. Continued to assist patient's ventilations and monitor his airway status for the duration of the transport. Noted improvement in patient's oxygen saturation and skin condition with assisted ventilation. Delivered patient to the ED staff and gave verbal report to Dr. Wheeler. Ambulance 12 cleared the hospital and returned to service at 2021 hrs.

**End of report**

# Prep Kit

## Ready for Review

- Soft-tissue injuries and fractures of the bones of the face and neck are common and vary in severity.
- For face and neck injuries, your priorities are to prevent further injury to the cervical spine, manage the airway and ventilation of the patient, and control bleeding.
- Airway compromise may be caused by heavy bleeding into the airway, swelling in and around the structures of the airway located in the face and neck, and injuries to the central nervous system that interfere with normal respiration.
- To control heavy bleeding from soft-tissue injuries to the face, use direct pressure with a dry, sterile dressing. If brain tissue is exposed, use a moist, sterile dressing.
- Check for bleeding inside the mouth because this may produce airway obstruction.
- Open the airway using the jaw-thrust maneuver (when indicated), and clear the airway in all patients with facial injuries.
- Save avulsed pieces of skin and tissue, and transport them with the patient for possible reattachment at the hospital.
- Maintain a high index of suspicion for unconscious patients with unequal pupils— this sign may indicate an illness or an injury to the brain. Remember, some people are born with one pupil larger than the other.
- Foreign bodies on the surface of the eye should be irrigated gently with normal saline solution. Always flush from the region of the eye closest to the nose toward the outside, away from the midline.
- If a foreign body is on the underside of the eyelid, remove it gently with a cotton-tipped applicator. Never remove foreign bodies stuck to the cornea.
- Chemicals, heat, and light rays all can cause burn injury to the eyes, resulting in permanent damage.
- Be alert to clear fluid draining from the ears or nose. This may indicate a basilar skull fracture.
- Blunt and penetrating trauma to the neck can produce life-threatening injuries. Palpate the neck for signs of subcutaneous emphysema. In patients with this sign, complete airway obstruction may develop in minutes.
- If bleeding is present from a penetrating injury, direct pressure over the site will usually control most forms of bleeding.
- Be alert to the possibility of an air embolism from an open neck injury. Place an occlusive dressing over the site, and provide direct pressure.

## Vital Vocabulary

**air embolism** The presence of air in the veins, which can lead to cardiac arrest if it enters the heart.

**anisocoria** Naturally occurring uneven pupil size.

**blow-out fracture** A fracture of the orbit or of the bones that support the floor of the orbit.

**conjunctiva** The delicate membrane that lines the eyelids and covers the exposed surface of the eye.

**conjunctivitis** Inflammation of the conjunctiva.

**cornea** The transparent tissue layer in front of the pupil and iris of the eye.

**eustachian tube** A tube that connects the middle ear to the oropharynx.

**external auditory canal** The ear canal; leads to the tympanic membrane.

**globe** The eyeball.

**iris** The muscle and surrounding tissue behind the cornea that dilate and constrict the pupil, regulating the amount of light that enters the eye; pigment in this tissue gives the eye its color.

**lacrimal glands** The glands that produce fluids to keep the eye moist; also called tear glands.

**lens** The transparent part of the eye through which images are focused on the retina.

**mastoid process** The prominent bony mass at the base of the skull about 1 inch (2.5 cm) posterior to the external opening of the ear.

**optic nerve** A cranial nerve that transmits visual information to the brain.

**pinna** The external, visible part of the ear.

**pupil** The circular opening in the middle of the iris that admits light to the back of the eye.

**retina** The light-sensitive area of the eye where images are projected; a layer of cells at the back of the eye that changes the light image into electric impulses, which are carried by the optic nerve to the brain.

**retinal detachment** Separation of the retina from its attachments at the back of the eye.

**sclera** The tough, fibrous, white portion of the eye that protects the more delicate inner structures.

**sternocleidomastoid muscles** The muscles on either side of the neck that allow movement of the head.

**subcutaneous emphysema** A characteristic crackling sensation felt on palpation of the skin, caused by the presence of air in soft tissues.

**temporomandibular joint** The joint formed where the mandible and cranium meet, just in front of the ear.

**tragus** The small, rounded, fleshy bulge that lies immediately anterior to the ear canal.

**turbinates** Layers of bone within the nasal cavity.

**tympanic membrane** The eardrum; a thin, semi-transparent membrane in the middle ear that transmits sound vibrations to the internal ear by means of auditory ossicles.

## References

1. National Association of Emergency Medical Technicians. *PHTLS: Prehospital Trauma Life Support*. 9th ed. Burlington, MA: Jones & Bartlett Learning; 2019.

2. National Association of State EMS Officials. *National Model EMS Clinical Guidelines: Version 2.2*. https://nasemso.org/wp-content/uploads/National-Model-EMS-Clinical-Guidelines-2017-PDF-Version-2.2.pdf. Updated January 5, 2019. Accessed February 6, 2020.

3. National Highway Traffic Safety Administration. *National Emergency Medical Services Education Standards*. DOT HS 811 077A. www.ems.gov/pdf/811077a.pdf. Published January 2009. Accessed February 6, 2020.

4. National Highway Traffic Safety Administration. *National Emergency Medical Services Education Standards. Emergency Medical Technician Instructional Guidelines*. DOT HS 811 077C. www.ems.gov/pdf/811077c.pdf. Published January 2009. Accessed February 6, 2020.

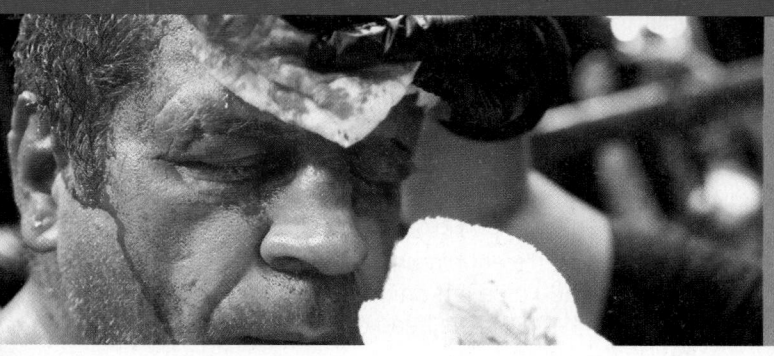

# Chapter 29

# Head and Spine Injuries

## NATIONAL EMS EDUCATION COMPETENCIES

### Trauma

Applies fundamental knowledge to provide basic emergency care and transportation based on assessment findings for an acutely injured patient.

### Head, Facial, Neck, and Spine Trauma

Recognition and management of
- Life threats (pp 1054–1055)
- Spine trauma (pp 1052–1061, 1064–1079)

Pathophysiology, assessment, and management of
- Penetrating neck trauma (Chapter 28, *Face and Neck Injuries*)
- Laryngotracheal injuries (Chapter 28, *Face and Neck Injuries*)

- Spine trauma (pp 1052–1061, 1064–1079)
- Facial fractures (Chapter 28, *Face and Neck Injuries*)
- Skull fractures (pp 1046–1048, 1053–1063)
- Foreign bodies in the eyes (Chapter 28, *Face and Neck Injuries*)
- Dental trauma (Chapter 28, *Face and Neck Injuries*)

### Nervous System Trauma

Pathophysiology, assessment, and management of
- Traumatic brain injury (pp 1048–1052, 1053–1063)
- Spinal cord injury (pp 1052–1061, 1064–1079)

## KNOWLEDGE OBJECTIVES

1. Describe the anatomy and physiology of the nervous system, including its divisions into the central nervous system (CNS) and peripheral nervous system (PNS) and the structures and functions of each. (pp 1040–1045)
2. Explain the functions of the somatic and autonomic nervous systems. (p 1044)
3. List the major bones of the skull and spinal column and their related structures; include their functions as they relate to the nervous system. (pp 1044–1045)
4. Explain the different types of head injuries, their potential mechanism of injury (MOI), and general signs and symptoms of a head injury that EMTs should consider when performing a patient assessment. (pp 1045–1052)
5. Define traumatic brain injury (TBI). (p 1048)

6. Explain the difference between a primary (direct) injury and a secondary (indirect) injury; include examples of possible MOIs that may cause each one. (pp 1048–1049)
7. Describe the different types of brain injuries and their corresponding signs and symptoms, including increased intracranial pressure (ICP), concussion, contusion, and injuries caused by medical conditions. (pp 1048–1052)
8. Describe the different types of injuries that may damage the cervical, thoracic, or lumbar spine; include examples of possible MOIs that may cause each one. (p 1052)
9. Explain the steps in the patient assessment process for a person who has a suspected head or spine injury; include specific variations that may be required as related to the type of injury. (pp 1053–1061)

10. List the MOIs that cause a high index of suspicion for the possibility of a head or spinal injury. (p 1053)

11. Explain emergency medical care of a patient with a head injury; include the three general principles designed to protect and maintain the critical functions of the CNS and ways to determine if the patient has a TBI. (pp 1061–1063)

12. Explain emergency medical care of a patient with a spinal injury; include the implications of not properly caring for patients with injuries of this nature, the steps for performing manual in-line stabilization, implications for sizing and using a cervical collar, and key symptoms that contraindicate in-line stabilization. (pp 1064–1067)

13. Explain the process of preparing patients who have suspected head or spinal injuries for transport; include the use and functions of a long backboard, vacuum mattress, short backboard, and other short spinal extrication devices to immobilize the patient's cervical and thoracic spine. (pp 1067–1079)

14. Explain the different circumstances in which a helmet should be left on or taken off a patient with a possible head or spinal injury. (pp 1079–1080)

15. List the steps EMTs must follow to remove a helmet, including the removal of a football helmet. (pp 1079–1084)

16. Discuss age-related variations that are required when providing emergency care to a pediatric patient who has a suspected head or spine injury. (pp 1083–1084)

## SKILLS OBJECTIVES

1. Demonstrate how to perform a jaw-thrust maneuver on a patient with a suspected spinal injury. (p 1064)

2. Demonstrate how to perform manual in-line stabilization on a patient with a suspected spinal injury. (pp 1064–1065, Skill Drill 29-1)

3. Demonstrate how to apply a cervical collar to a patient with a suspected spinal injury. (pp 1065–1067, Skill Drill 29-2)

4. Demonstrate how to secure a patient with a suspected spinal injury to a long backboard. (pp 1067–1070, Skill Drill 29-3)

5. Demonstrate how to secure a patient with a suspected spinal injury using a vacuum mattress. (pp 1070–1075, Skill Drill 29-4)

6. Demonstrate how to secure a patient with a suspected spinal injury who was found in a sitting position. (pp 1075–1077, Skill Drill 29-5)

7. Demonstrate how to remove a helmet from a patient with a suspected head or spinal injury. (pp 1079–1082, Skill Drill 29-6)

8. Demonstrate the method for removal of a football helmet from a patient with a suspected head or spinal injury. (p 1083)

# Introduction

The nervous system is a complex network of nerve cells that enables all parts of the body to function. It includes the brain, the spinal cord, and several billion nerve fibers that carry information to and from all parts of the body. Because the nervous system is so vital, it is well protected. The brain lies within the skull, and the spinal cord is inside the bony spinal canal. Despite this protection, serious injuries can damage the nervous system.

This chapter briefly reviews the anatomy and function of the central and peripheral nervous systems and of the skeletal system. Discussion of specific head, brain, and spinal injuries follows, including signs, symptoms, assessment, and treatment. Extrication of patients with possible spinal injuries and removal of helmets are also described.

# Anatomy and Physiology
## Nervous System

The nervous system is divided into two anatomic parts: the central nervous system (CNS) and the peripheral nervous system (PNS) (**FIGURE 29-1**). The CNS is composed of the brain and the spinal cord, including the nuclei and cell bodies of most nerve cells. Long nerve fibers link these cells to the body's various organs through openings in the spinal column. These nerve fibers constitute the PNS.

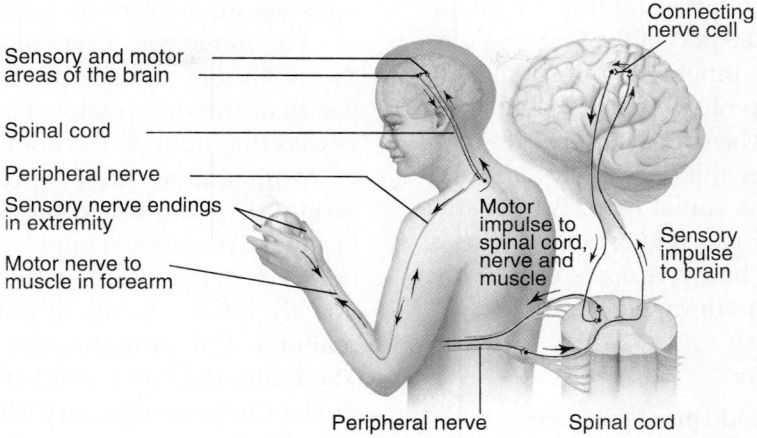

FIGURE 29-1 The nervous system has two anatomic components: the central nervous system and the peripheral nervous system. The central nervous system is composed of the brain and the spinal cord. The peripheral nervous system conducts sensory and motor impulses from the skin and other organs to the spinal cord.

© Jones & Bartlett Learning.

## Central Nervous System

The CNS is composed of the brain and spinal cord. The brain is the organ that controls the body; it is also the center of consciousness. It is divided into three major areas: the cerebrum, the cerebellum, and the brainstem (**FIGURE 29-2**).

The cerebrum, which contains about 75% of the brain's total volume, controls a wide variety of activities, including most voluntary motor function and conscious thought. It is the main part of the brain and is divided into two hemispheres with four lobes. Underneath the cerebrum lies the cerebellum, which coordinates balance and body movements. The most primitive part of the CNS, the brainstem, controls virtually all the functions that are necessary for life, including the cardiac and

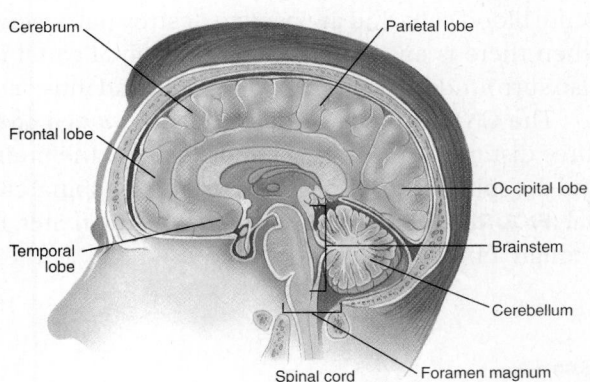

FIGURE 29-2 The brain is part of the central nervous system and is the organ that controls the body. It is divided into three major areas: the cerebrum, the cerebellum, and the brainstem.

© Jones & Bartlett Learning.

## YOU are the Provider

At 0220 hours, you receive a call for a man who was assaulted outside a nightclub. Law enforcement personnel are present and have secured the scene. While you are en route, one of the police officers radios you and informs you the patient was struck on the side of the head with a baseball bat and is unconscious. Your response time to the scene is less than 5 minutes.

**1.** What are the potential concerns surrounding the structure of the cranium and potential brain swelling?

**2.** What is the difference between a primary and a secondary brain injury?

respiratory systems and nerve function transmissions. Located deep within the cranium, the brainstem is the best-protected part of the CNS.

The spinal cord, the other major portion of the CNS, is mostly made up of fibers that extend from the brain's nerve cells. The spinal cord carries messages between the brain and the body via the gray and white matter of the spinal cord. Gray matter is composed of neural cell bodies and synapses, which are connections between nerve cells. White matter consists of fiber pathways.

### Protective Coverings

The cells of the brain and spinal cord are soft and easily injured. Once damaged, they cannot be regenerated or reproduced. Therefore, the entire CNS is contained within a protective framework.

The thick, bony structures of the skull and spinal canal withstand injury very well. The skull is covered by layers of muscle, superficial fascia, and thick skin, which usually bears hair. Superficial fascia connects the muscle to the skin and contains white blood cells that are used to destroy pathogens when there is an open wound. The spinal canal is also surrounded by a thick layer of skin and muscles.

The CNS is further protected by the **meninges**, three distinct layers of tissue that suspend the brain and the spinal cord within the skull and the spinal canal (**FIGURE 29-3**). The outer layer, the dura mater, is a tough, fibrous layer that closely resembles leather.

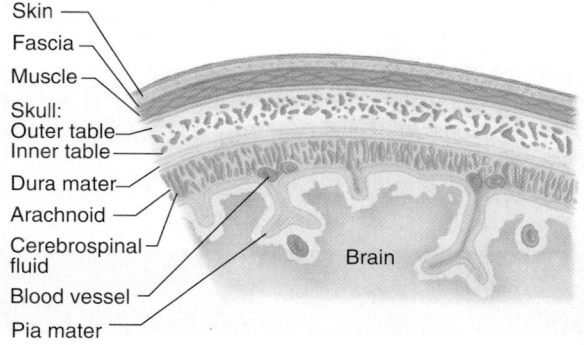

Skin
Fascia
Muscle
Skull:
Outer table
Inner table
Dura mater
Arachnoid
Cerebrospinal fluid
Blood vessel
Pia mater
Brain

**FIGURE 29-3** The central nervous system has several layers of protective coverings: the skin, muscles and their fascia, bone, and the meninges. The three layers of the meninges are the dura mater, the arachnoid, and the pia mater.

This layer forms a sac to contain the CNS, with small openings through which the peripheral nerves exit.

The inner two layers of the meninges, called the arachnoid and the pia mater, are much thinner than the dura mater. They contain the blood vessels that nourish the brain and spinal cord. Cerebrospinal fluid (CSF) is produced in a chamber inside the brain, called the third ventricle. CSF is located in the subarachnoid space below the arachnoid, which is a weblike structure. There is approximately 125 to 150 mL of CSF in the brain at any one time. CSF primarily acts as a shock absorber. The brain and spinal cord essentially float in this fluid, buffered from injury. The brain depends on a rich supply of oxygenated blood to function properly. When this supply is interrupted, even for short periods of time, serious damage to the brain tissue may occur.

When an injury does penetrate all of these protective layers, clear, watery CSF may leak from the nose, the ears, or an open skull fracture. Therefore, if a patient with a head injury has what looks like a runny nose or reports a salty taste at the back of the throat, you should assume that the fluid is CSF.

Ironically, the closed bony structure of the skull (which is similar to a vault) and the meninges, the layers of tissue that isolate and protect the CNS, may lead to serious problems in closed head injuries. Severe injury may cause bleeding within the skull, referred to as intracranial hemorrhage. Such bleeding increases pressure inside the skull and compresses softer brain tissue. In many cases, only prompt surgery can prevent permanent brain damage.

## Peripheral Nervous System

The PNS has two anatomic parts: 31 pairs of spinal nerves and 12 pairs of cranial nerves (**FIGURE 29-4**).

The 31 pairs of spinal nerves conduct sensory impulses from the skin and other organs to the spinal cord. They also conduct motor impulses from the spinal cord to the muscles. Because the arms and legs have so many muscles, the spinal nerves serving the extremities are arranged in complex networks. The brachial plexus controls the arms, and the lumbosacral plexus controls the legs.

Cranial nerves are the 12 pairs of nerves that emerge from the brainstem and transmit information directly to or from the brain. For the most part, they perform special functions in the head and face, including sight, smell, taste, hearing, and facial expressions.

There are two major types of peripheral nerves. The sensory nerves, with endings that perceive only one type of information, carry that information from the body to the brain via the spinal cord. The motor nerves, one for each muscle, carry information from the CNS to the muscles. The connecting nerves, found only in the brain and spinal cord, connect the sensory and motor nerves with short fibers, which allow the cells on either end to exchange simple messages.

## How the Nervous System Works

The nervous system controls virtually all of the body's activities, including reflex, voluntary, and involuntary activities.

In connecting the sensory and motor nerves of the limbs, the connecting nerves in the spinal cord form a reflex arc. If a sensory nerve in this arc detects an irritating stimulus, such as heat, it will bypass the brain and send a message directly to a motor nerve, causing a response such as pulling away from the heat (**FIGURE 29-5**).

**Voluntary activities** are the actions that we consciously perform, in which sensory input determines the specific muscular activity—for example, reaching across the table for a salt shaker or to pass a dish. **Involuntary activities** are the actions that are not under our conscious control, such as breathing; in most instances, we inhale and exhale without consciously thinking about it. Many of our body's functions occur independently of thought, or involuntarily.

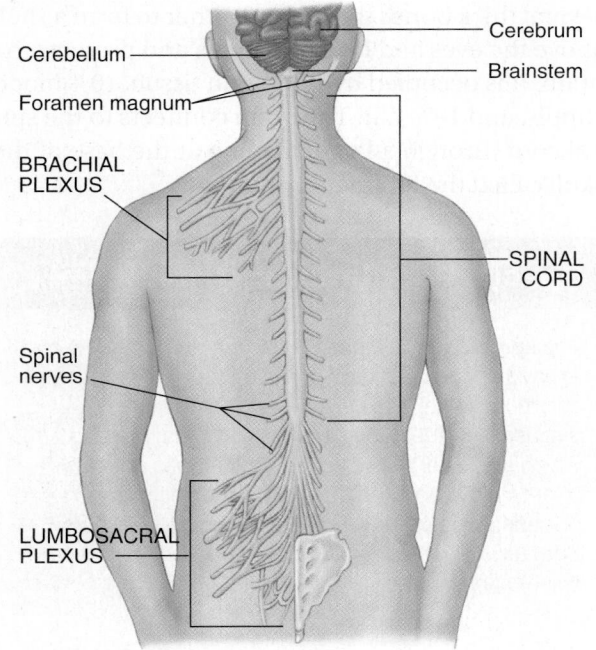

**FIGURE 29-4** The peripheral nervous system is a complex network of motor and sensory nerves. The brachial plexus controls the arms, and the lumbosacral plexus controls the legs.

© Jones & Bartlett Learning.

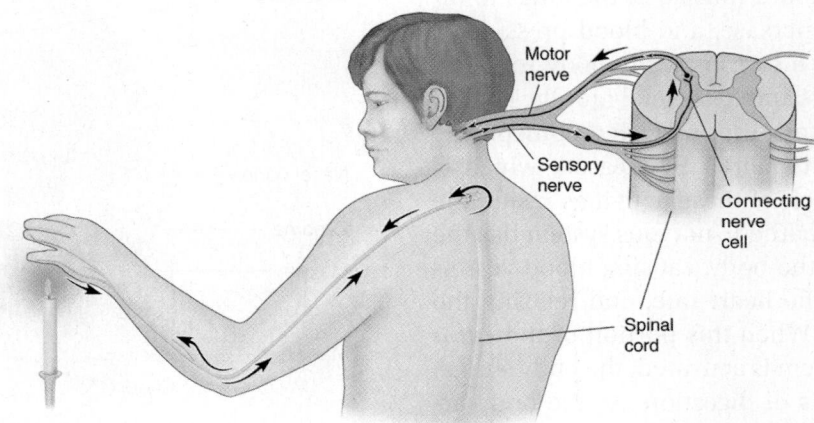

**FIGURE 29-5** The connecting nerves in the spinal cord form a reflex arc. If a sensory nerve in this arc detects an irritating stimulus, it will bypass the brain and send a direct message to a motor nerve.

© Jones & Bartlett Learning.

The part of the nervous system that regulates or controls our voluntary activities, including almost all coordinated muscular activities, is called the somatic (voluntary) nervous system. The mechanism of the somatic nervous system is simple. The brain interprets the sensory information that it receives from the peripheral and cranial nerves and responds by sending signals to the voluntary muscles.

The body functions that occur without conscious effort are regulated by the much more primitive autonomic (involuntary) nervous system. The autonomic nervous system controls the functions of many of the body's vital organs, over which the brain has no voluntary control.

The autonomic nervous system is divided into two sections: the sympathetic nervous system and the parasympathetic nervous system. When confronted with a threatening situation, the sympathetic nervous system reacts to the stress with the fight-or-flight response. This response causes the pupils to dilate, smooth muscle in the lungs to dilate, heart rate to increase, and blood pressure to rise. This response also causes the body to shunt blood to vital organs and to skeletal muscle. During this time of stress, a hormone called epinephrine (also known as adrenaline) is released, which is responsible for much of these activities inside the body. The parasympathetic nervous system has the opposite effect on the body, causing blood vessels to dilate, slowing the heart rate, and relaxing the muscle sphincters. When this portion of the autonomic nervous system is activated, the body shunts blood to the organs of digestion. As the body attempts to maintain homeostasis (balance), these two divisions of the autonomic nervous system tend to balance each other so that basic body functions remain stable and effective.

## Skeletal System

### Skull

The skull is composed of two groups of bones: the cranium, which protects the brain, and the facial bones (**FIGURE 29-6**). The cranium is composed of several thick bones that fuse together to form a shell above the eyes and ears that holds and protects the brain. It is occupied by 80% brain tissue, 10% blood supply, and 10% CSF. The brain connects to the spinal cord through a large opening at the base of the skull called the foramen magnum.

Four major bones make up the cranium. The most posterior portion of the cranium is called the occiput. On each side of the cranium, the lateral portions are called the temples or temporal regions.

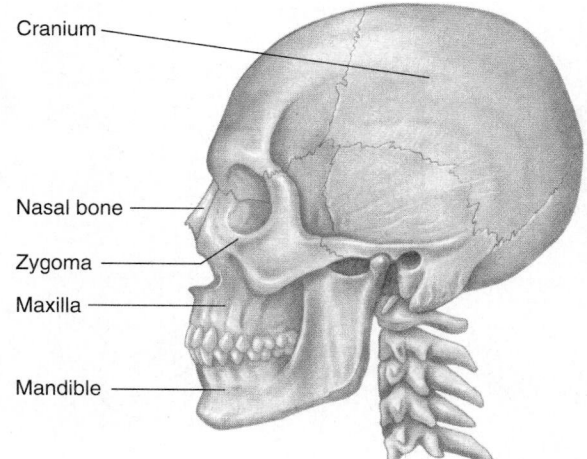

**FIGURE 29-6** The skull includes two large structures: the cranium and the face.

© Jones & Bartlett Learning.

Between the temporal regions and the occiput lie the parietal regions. The forehead is called the frontal region.

The face is composed of 14 bones. The upper immobile jawbones are called the maxillae, the cheek bones are called the zygomas, and the mandible is the lower, moveable portion of the jaw.

The orbit (eye socket) is made up of two facial bones: the maxilla and the zygoma. The orbit also includes the frontal bone of the cranium. Together, these bones form a solid bony rim that protrudes around the eye to protect it. The nose mostly consists of flexible cartilage; in fact, only the proximal third of the nose is formed by bone, with very short bones forming the bridge of the nose.

## Spinal Column

The spinal column is the body's central supporting structure. It has 33 bones, called vertebrae, and is divided into five sections: cervical, thoracic, lumbar, sacral, and coccygeal (**FIGURE 29-7**). Injury to the vertebrae, depending on the level at which the injury occurs, may result in paralysis if the underlying spinal cord or nervous structures are also damaged.

The front part of each vertebra consists of a round, solid block of bone called the vertebral body; the back part forms a bony arch. From one vertebra to the next, the series of arches form a tunnel running the length of the spinal column. This tunnel is the spinal canal, which encases and protects the spinal cord (**FIGURE 29-8**).

The vertebrae are connected by ligaments and separated by cushions, called **intervertebral disks**. These ligaments and disks allow the trunk to bend forward and back, but they also limit motion so that the spinal cord is not injured. When the spine is injured or fractured, the spinal cord and its nerves are left unprotected. Therefore, keep the spine aligned throughout transport, using manual stabilization, as necessary. The spinal column itself is almost entirely surrounded by muscles. However, you can usually palpate the posterior spinous process of some of the vertebrae, which lie just under the skin in the midline of the back. The most prominent and most easily palpable spinous process is at the seventh cervical vertebra at the base of the neck.

## Head Injuries

A head injury is a traumatic insult to the head that may result in injury to soft tissue, bony structures, or the brain. Approximately 4 million people

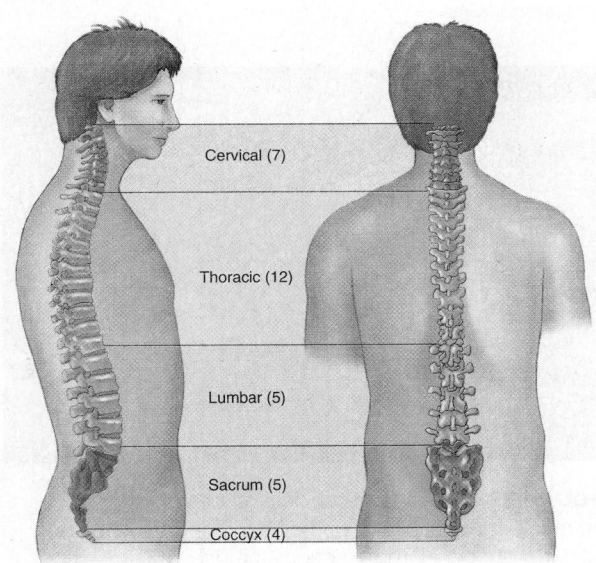

**FIGURE 29-7** The spinal column is the body's central supporting system and consists of 33 bones divided into five sections. Injury to the vertebrae may cause paralysis.

© Jones & Bartlett Learning.

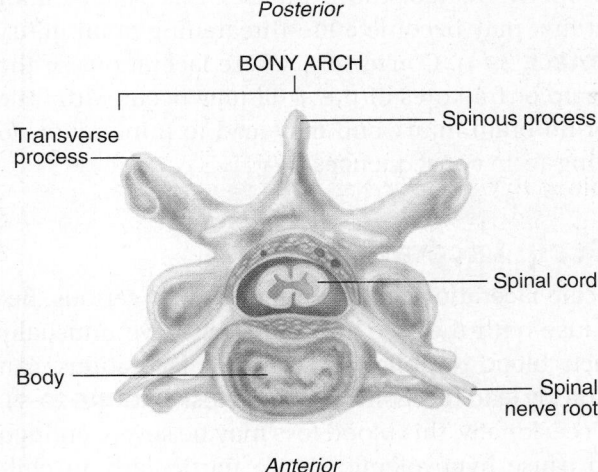

**FIGURE 29-8** The spinal canal is formed by the vertebral body in the front (or anteriorly) and the bony arch in the back (or posteriorly).

© Jones & Bartlett Learning.

experience head injuries of varied severity in the United States each year. According to the Brain Trauma Foundation, 50,000 deaths occur annually as a result of severe head injury and 80,000 people sustain permanent disability. More than 50% of all traumatic deaths result from a head injury. When head injuries are fatal, invariably the cause is associated injury to the brain. In addition to the head injury, and dependent on the mechanism of injury (MOI), you should be alert to the fact that the patient may have sustained additional trauma such as cervical spine injuries, pelvic injuries, and chest injuries.

There are two types of head injuries. In a **closed head injury**, the brain has been injured but there is no opening to the brain. For example, a severe blow that fractures the skull but does not create an open wound would be considered a closed head injury. In an **open head injury**, an opening exists from the outside world to the brain. Obvious skull deformity with a break in the skin is a sign of an open head injury, which is often caused by penetrating trauma. There may be bleeding and exposed brain tissue.

Falls and motor vehicle crashes are among the most common MOIs resulting in head and brain injuries. Head injuries also occur commonly in victims of assault, during sports-related incidents, and in a variety of incidents involving children.

Any head injury is potentially serious. If not properly treated, those injuries that seem minor at first may become a life-threatening brain injury (**TABLE 29-1**). Conversely, severe lacerations of the scalp or fractures of the skull may occur with little or no brain injury and may lead to minimal or no long-term consequences.

## Scalp Lacerations

Scalp lacerations can be minor or very serious. Because both the face and the scalp have unusually rich blood supplies, even small lacerations can quickly lead to significant blood loss (**FIGURE 29-9**). Occasionally, this blood loss may be severe enough to cause hypovolemic shock, particularly in children. In any patient with multiple injuries, bleeding from scalp or facial lacerations may contribute to hypovolemia. In addition, because scalp lacerations are usually the result of direct blows to the head, they are often an indicator of deeper, more serious injuries.

| **TABLE 29-1** General Signs and Symptoms of a Head Injury |
| --- |

Following a head injury, any patient who exhibits one or more of these signs or symptoms has potentially sustained a very serious underlying brain injury:

- Lacerations, contusions, or hematomas to the scalp
- Soft area or skull depression on palpation
- Visible fractures or deformities of the skull
- Decreased mentation, confusion
- Irregular breathing pattern
- Widening pulse pressure
- Slow heart rate
- Ecchymosis about the eyes or behind the ear over the mastoid process
- Clear or pink CSF leakage from a scalp wound, the nose, or the ear
- Failure of the pupils to react to light
- Unequal pupil size
- Loss of sensation and/or motor function
- A period of unconsciousness
- Amnesia
- Seizures
- Numbness or tingling in the extremities
- Dizziness
- Visual complaints
- Combative or other abnormal behavior
- Nausea or vomiting
- Posturing (decorticate or decerebrate)

© Jones & Bartlett Learning.

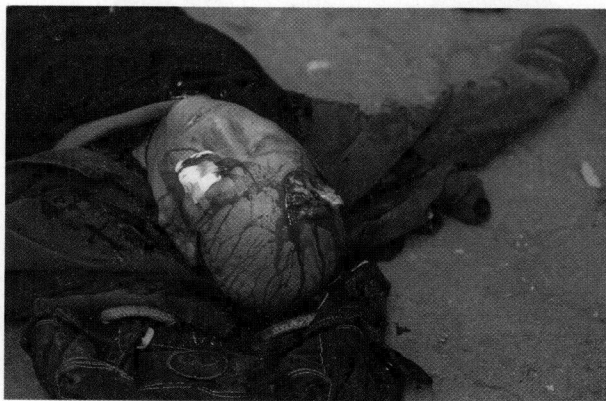

**FIGURE 29-9** Because scalp lacerations are usually the result of direct blows to the head, they are often an indicator of deeper, more serious injuries.

© Marco Ugarte/AP/Shutterstock.

## Skull Fracture

Significant force applied to the head may cause a skull fracture. As with any fracture, a skull fracture may be open or closed, depending on whether there is an overlying laceration of the scalp. Injuries from bullets or other penetrating weapons frequently result in fracture of the skull. The diagnosis of a skull fracture is usually made in the hospital with a computed tomography (CT) scan, but maintain a high index of suspicion that a fracture is present if the patient's head appears deformed or if there is a visible crack in the skull within a scalp laceration. Additional signs of skull fracture that you may see include ecchymosis (bruising) that develops under the eyes (raccoon eyes) (**FIGURE 29-10A**) or behind one ear over the mastoid process (Battle sign) (**FIGURE 29-10B**). These signs may be less obvious in dark-skinned persons.

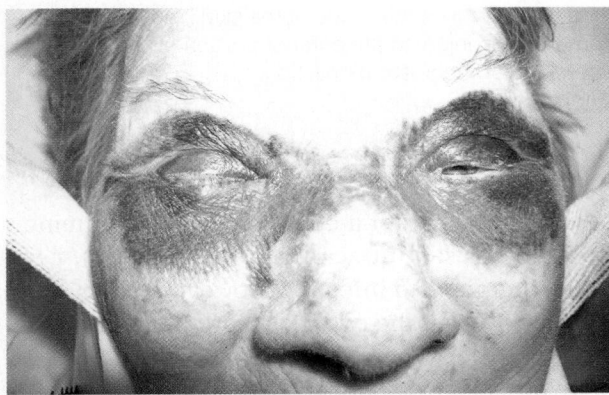

**A**

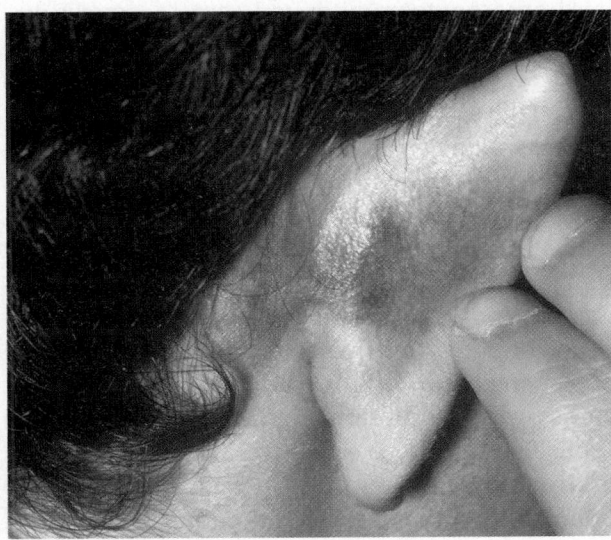

**B**

**FIGURE 29-10** Signs of skull fracture include ecchymosis under the eyes (raccoon eyes) (**A**) or behind one ear over the mastoid process (Battle sign) (**B**).

**A:** © E. M. Singletary, MD. Used with permission; **B:** © Mediscan/Alamy Stock Photo.

## Linear Skull Fractures

Linear skull fractures (nondisplaced skull fractures) account for approximately 80% of all fractures to the skull (**FIGURE 29-11A**). Radiographs are required to diagnose a linear skull fracture because there are often no physical signs such as deformity. If the brain is uninjured and there are no scalp lacerations, then linear fractures are not life threatening. However, if there is a scalp laceration with the linear fracture—making it an open fracture—there is a risk of infection and bleeding inside the brain.

## Depressed Skull Fractures

Depressed skull fractures result from high-energy direct trauma to the head with a blunt object (such as a baseball bat to the head) (**FIGURE 29-11B**). The frontal and parietal bones of the skull are most susceptible to these types of fractures because the bones in these areas are relatively thin. As a consequence, bony fragments may be driven into the brain, resulting in injury. The scalp may or may not be lacerated. Patients with depressed skull fractures often present with signs of neurologic injury (such as loss of consciousness).

## Basilar Skull Fractures

Basilar skull fractures are also associated with high-energy trauma, but they usually occur following diffuse impact to the head (eg, falls, motor vehicle crashes). These injuries generally result from extension of a linear fracture to the base of the skull and are usually diagnosed with a CT scan of the head (**FIGURE 29-11C**).

Signs of a basilar skull fracture include CSF drainage from the nose or the ears, which indicates rupture of the tympanic membrane in the ear, and freely flowing CSF through the ear. Patients with leaking CSF from either the nose or the ear are at risk for bacterial meningitis.

Other signs of a basilar skull fracture include raccoon eyes or Battle sign. Depending on the extent of the damage, raccoon eyes and Battle sign may appear relatively quickly, but in many patients, they may not appear until up to 24 hours following the injury, so their absence in the field does not rule out a basilar skull fracture.

## Open Skull Fractures

Open fractures of the cranial vault result when severe forces are applied to the head and are often

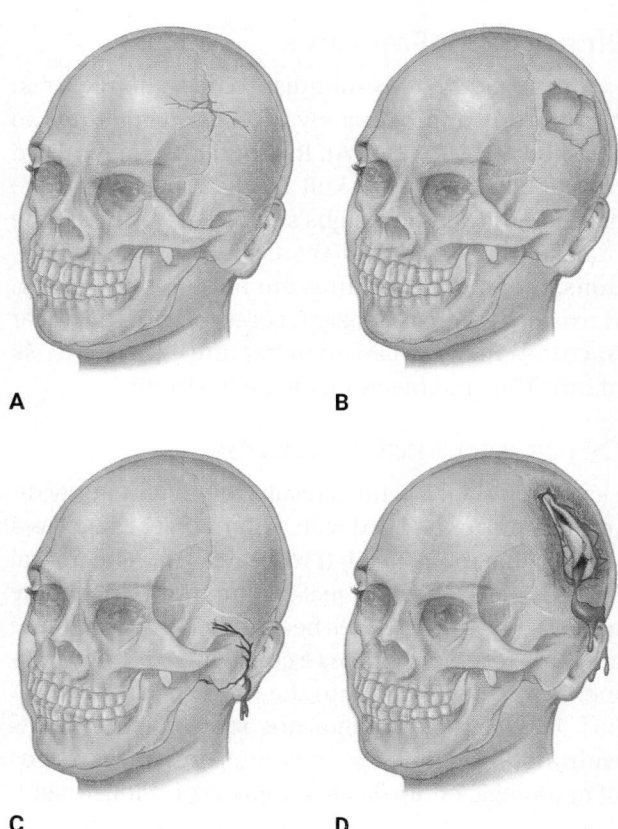

**A** **B**

**C** **D**

**FIGURE 29-11** Types of skull fractures. **A.** Linear.
**B.** Depressed. **C.** Basilar. **D.** Open.

© Jones & Bartlett Learning.

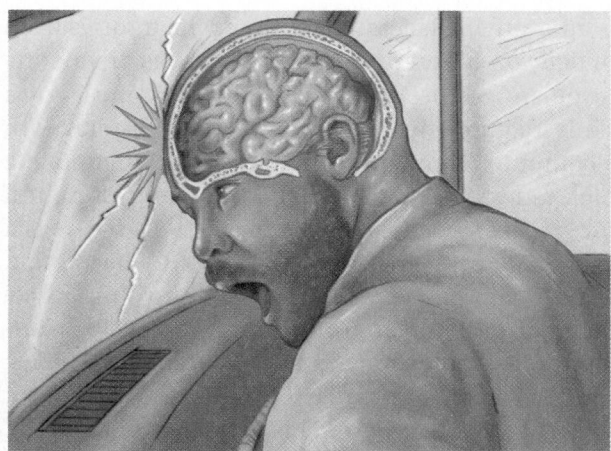

**FIGURE 29-12** For the unrestrained driver or passenger
in a motor vehicle crash, the brain continues its forward
motion and strikes the inside of the skull, resulting in
compression injury to the anterior portion of the brain and
stretching of the posterior portion.

© Jones & Bartlett Learning.

associated with trauma to multiple body systems
(**FIGURE 29-11D**). Brain tissue may be exposed to the
environment, which significantly increases the risk
of a bacterial infection (such as bacterial meningitis). Open cranial vault fractures have a very high
mortality rate.

## Traumatic Brain Injuries

The National Head Injury Foundation defines a
**traumatic brain injury (TBI)** as "a traumatic insult
to the brain capable of producing physical, intellectual, emotional, social, and vocational changes."
TBIs are classified into two broad categories: **primary
(direct) injury** and **secondary (indirect) injury**. Primary brain injury is injury to the brain and its associated structures that results instantaneously from
impact to the head. Secondary brain injury refers
to a multitude of processes that increase the severity of a primary brain injury and, therefore, negatively affect the outcome. Secondary injuries may

be caused by cerebral edema, intracranial hemorrhage, increased intracranial pressure (ICP), cerebral ischemia, and infection; however, hypoxia and
hypotension are the two most common causes. According to the Brain Trauma Foundation, hypoxia
or hypotension significantly increases the risk of
death and disability in a patient with a head injury.
It is important to monitor and address hypoxia and
hypotension when identified. Secondary brain injury may occur anywhere from a few minutes to
several days following the initial head injury.

The brain can be injured directly by a penetrating object, such as a bullet, knife, or other sharp
object. More commonly, brain injuries occur indirectly, as a result of external forces exerted on the
skull. Consider the most common cause of brain injury, the motor vehicle crash. When the passenger's
head hits the windshield on impact with a fixed
object, the brain continues to move forward until it
comes to an abrupt stop by striking the inside of the
skull. This rapid deceleration results in compression
injury (or bruising) to the anterior portion of the
brain along with stretching or tearing of the posterior portion of the brain (**FIGURE 29-12**). As the brain
strikes the front of the skull, the body begins its path
of moving backward. The head falls back against the
headrest and/or seat, and the brain slams into the
rear of the skull. This type of front-and-rear injury is

## Words of Wisdom

Based on the mechanism involved with a coup-contrecoup injury, it is possible for a patient to receive a brain injury without directly hitting his or her head. A rapid change in direction of movement of the head can cause the brain to move forward and then back with such force that it impacts the inside of the skull. Do not exclude the possibility of brain injury simply because the patient has no external head injuries.

known as a **coup-contrecoup injury**. The same type of injury may occur on opposite sides of the brain in a lateral collision.

The injured brain starts to swell, initially because of cerebral vasodilation. An increase in cerebral water (cerebral edema) then contributes to further brain swelling. **Cerebral edema** (swelling of the brain) may not develop until several hours following the initial injury, however.

Low oxygen levels in the blood aggravate cerebral edema. Therefore, patients with cerebral edema may be at particular risk if hypoxemia is not adequately corrected. In fact, the brain consumes more oxygen than any other organ in the body. For this reason, you must make sure that the airway is open and that adequate ventilations and high-flow oxygen are given to any patient with significant head injury. This is especially true if the patient is unconscious. Do not wait for cyanosis or other obvious signs of hypoxia to develop. Similarly, do not wait for pulse oximetry to confirm hypoxia.

It is not uncommon for the patient with a head injury to have a convulsion, or seizure. This is the result of excessive excitability of the brain, caused by direct injury or the accumulation of fluid within the brain (edema). Be prepared to manage seizures in all patients who have had a head injury because the brain may have sustained an injury as well.

## Intracranial Pressure

For adults, the skull is a rigid, unyielding globe that allows little, if any, expansion of the intracranial contents. It also provides a hard and somewhat irregular surface against which brain tissue and its blood vessels can be injured when the head sustains trauma.

Accumulations of blood within the skull or swelling of the brain can rapidly lead to an increase in **intracranial pressure (ICP)**, the pressure within the cranial vault. Increased ICP squeezes the brain against bony prominences within the cranium. Cheyne-Stokes respirations (respirations that are fast and then become slow, with intervening periods of apnea) or ataxic (Biot) respirations (characterized by irregular rate, pattern, and volume of breathing with intermittent periods of apnea) are signs of increased ICP. **Central neurogenic hyperventilation** is another abnormal breathing pattern associated with increased ICP that is characterized by deep, rapid breathing; this pattern is similar to Kussmaul respirations, but without an acetone breath odor. Other signs and symptoms include decreased pulse rate, headache, nausea, vomiting, decreased alertness, bradycardia, sluggish or nonreactive pupils, decerebrate posturing, and increased or widened pulse pressure (the difference between the systolic and diastolic blood pressures). Signs and symptoms will increase and become more severe as the level of pressure increases.

The triad of increased systolic blood pressure, decreased heart rate, and irregular respirations is called Cushing reflex, and signifies increased ICP.

## Intracranial Hemorrhage

The closed compartment of the skull has no extra room for an accumulation of blood, so bleeding inside the skull also increases the ICP. Bleeding can occur between the skull and dura mater, beneath the dura mater but outside the brain, or within the tissue of the brain itself.

## Epidural Hematoma

An **epidural hematoma** is an accumulation of blood between the skull and dura mater (**FIGURE 29-13**). An epidural hematoma is nearly always the result of a blow to the head that produces a linear fracture of the thin temporal bone. The middle meningeal artery runs along a groove in that bone; therefore, it is vulnerable when the temporal bone is fractured. Arterial bleeding into the epidural space will result in rapidly progressing symptoms.

Often, the patient has an immediate loss of consciousness following the injury; this is often followed by a brief period of consciousness (lucid interval), after which the patient lapses back into

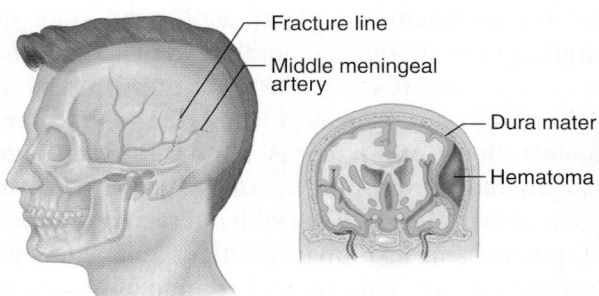

**FIGURE 29-13** An epidural hematoma is usually the result of a blow to the head that produces a linear fracture of the temporal bone and damages the middle meningeal artery. Blood accumulates between the dura mater and the skull.

© Jones & Bartlett Learning.

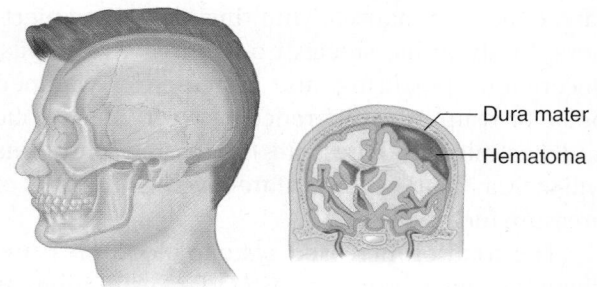

**FIGURE 29-14** In a subdural hematoma, venous bleeding occurs beneath the dura mater but outside the brain.

© Jones & Bartlett Learning.

unconsciousness. Meanwhile, as the ICP increases, the pupil on the side of the hematoma becomes fixed and dilated. Death will follow rapidly without surgery to evacuate the hematoma.

## Subdural Hematoma

A subdural hematoma is an accumulation of blood beneath the dura mater but outside the brain (**FIGURE 29-14**). It usually occurs after falls or injuries involving strong deceleration forces. Subdural hematomas are more common than epidural hematomas and may or may not be associated with a skull fracture. Bleeding within the subdural space typically results from rupture of the veins that bridge the cerebral cortex and dura.

A subdural hematoma is associated with venous bleeding, so this type of hematoma and the signs of increased ICP typically develop more gradually than with an epidural hematoma. The patient with a subdural hematoma often experiences a fluctuating level of consciousness or slurred speech. Any

patient who you suspect has a subdural hematoma needs to be evaluated by a physician.

## Intracerebral Hematoma

An intracerebral hematoma involves bleeding within the brain tissue itself (**FIGURE 29-15**). This type of injury may occur following a penetrating injury to the head or because of rapid deceleration forces.

Many small, deep intracerebral hemorrhages are associated with other brain injuries. The progression of increased ICP depends on several factors, including the presence of other brain injuries, the region of the brain involved (frontal and temporal lobes are the most common locations), and the size of the hemorrhage. Once symptoms appear, the patient's condition often deteriorates quickly. Intracerebral hematomas have a high mortality rate, even if the hematoma is surgically evacuated.

## Subarachnoid Hemorrhage

In a subarachnoid hemorrhage, bleeding occurs into the subarachnoid space, where the CSF circulates. It results in bloody CSF and signs of meningeal irritation (such as neck rigidity or headache).

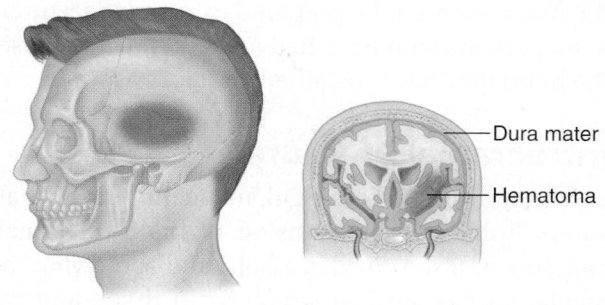

**FIGURE 29-15** An intracerebral hematoma involves bleeding within the brain tissue itself.

© Jones & Bartlett Learning.

Common causes of a subarachnoid hemorrhage include trauma or rupture of an aneurysm.

The patient with a subarachnoid hemorrhage reports a sudden, severe headache. As bleeding into the subarachnoid space increases, the patient experiences the signs and symptoms of increased ICP: decreased level of consciousness, changes in the pupils, vomiting, and seizures. A sudden, severe subarachnoid hemorrhage usually results in death. People who survive often have permanent neurologic impairment.

## Concussion

A blow to the head or face may cause concussion of the brain. Concussions are also known as mild TBIs. There is no universal definition of a concussion, but in general, it is a TBI with a temporary loss or alteration of part or all of the brain's abilities to function without demonstrable physical damage to the brain. For example, a person who "sees stars" after being struck on the head has sustained a concussion that affects the occipital portion of the brain. A concussion may result in unconsciousness and even the inability to breathe for short periods of time; however, approximately 90% of patients who sustain a concussion do not experience a loss of consciousness. A concussion is a functional change, not a structural change, in the brain.

A patient with a concussion may be confused or have amnesia (loss of memory). Occasionally, the patient can remember everything but the events leading up to the injury; this is called retrograde amnesia. Inability to remember events after the injury is called anterograde (posttraumatic) amnesia.

Usually, a concussion lasts only a short time. In fact, it has often resolved by the time you arrive. Nevertheless, you should ask about symptoms of concussion in any patient who has sustained an injury to the head because a concussive injury may exist; these symptoms include dizziness, weakness, visual changes, or changes in mood. Additional signs and symptoms you may encounter with a patient who has sustained a concussion may include nausea or vomiting, and the patient may report ringing in the ears. Slurred speech and the inability to focus may also be present. Depending on the severity of the concussion, you may also notice that the patient has a lack of coordination, has delayed motor functions, displays inappropriate emotional responses, or reports feeling "in a fog" or "just not right." Patients may also report a temporary headache and may appear to be disoriented.

Patients with symptoms consistent with concussion may also have more serious underlying brain injury. A CT scan is necessary to differentiate between these conditions. Always assume that a patient with signs or symptoms of concussion has a more serious injury until proven otherwise. All patients with signs or symptoms of a concussion should be evaluated by a physician or other qualified health care provider.

### Words of Wisdom

Be aware that all athletes who sustain a concussion should be evaluated by a qualified health care provider prior to being allowed to return to play. Some of the tools these health care providers use are specific, commercially available computerized tests to assess concussion and recovery from it. Often the results of the test are compared to baseline evaluations conducted prior to injury. EMTs are not qualified to conduct these types of assessments or to determine when it is safe to return to play after a concussion. A history of severe or repeated concussions, particularly in athletes, has been associated with decrease in brain function and severe dementia in later life and death.

## Contusion

Like any other soft tissue in the body, the brain can sustain a contusion, or bruise, when the skull is struck. A contusion is often far more serious than a concussion because it involves physical injury to the brain tissue, which may sustain long-lasting and even permanent damage. As with contusions that occur elsewhere in the body, there is associated bleeding and swelling from injured blood vessels. Injury of brain tissue or bleeding inside the skull causes an increase of pressure within the skull. A patient who has sustained a brain contusion may exhibit any or all of the signs of brain injury.

## Other Brain Injuries

Brain injuries are not always a result of trauma. Certain medical conditions, such as blood clots or hemorrhages, can also cause brain injuries that produce significant bleeding or swelling. Problems with the blood vessels themselves, high blood pressure, or any number of other problems may cause spontaneous bleeding into the brain, affecting the patient's level of consciousness. This is known as altered mental status. The signs and symptoms of nontraumatic injuries are often the same as those of TBIs, except that there is no obvious history of MOI or any external evidence of trauma. Altered mental status is discussed in Chapter 18, *Neurologic Emergencies*.

## Spine Injuries

The cervical, thoracic, and lumbar portions of the spine can be injured in a variety of ways. Compression injuries can occur as a result of a fall, regardless of whether the patient landed on his or her feet or experienced a direct blow to the crown of the skull, coccyx, or top of the head. The forces that compress the patient's vertebral body can cause the herniation of disks, subsequent compression of the spinal cord and nerve roots, and fragmentation into the spinal canal. Motor vehicle crashes or other types of trauma can overextend or hyperflex the cervical spine and damage the ligaments and joints. Rotation-flexion injuries of the spine result from rapid acceleration forces. This is more likely to happen at C1 and C2. Injuries to this area of the spine are considered unstable because of the location on the spine and the lack of bony and soft-tissue support. Any one of these unnatural motions, as well as excessive lateral bending, can result in fractures or neurologic deficit.

When the spine is pulled along its length (hyperextension), it can cause fractures in the spine as well as ligament and muscle injuries. For example, hangings often result in fracture of the vertebrae in the upper portion of the cervical spine.

When the bones of the spine are altered from traumatic forces, they can fracture or move out of place. When these injuries pinch, pull, or penetrate the spinal cord, permanent damage may occur. Common findings include pain and tenderness on palpation of the region. Less commonly you may feel or observe a deformity of the spine, sometimes referred to as a "step-off" where the spinous process may be palpable on physical examination. If you suspect these types of injuries, take extra precautions when immobilizing the spine, both manually and with adjuncts.

### Words of Wisdom

When assessing the spine, be aware of the possibility of open wounds from the associated trauma. These open wounds can be penetrating injuries or lacerations. If you follow the mnemonic DCAP-BTLS, you will discover any open wounds prior to securing the patient to a backboard. Spinal motion restriction is not indicated in patients with penetrating trauma injuries. Taking the time to do this may delay lifesaving care.

Peter E. Fischer, Debra G. Perina, Theodore R. Delbridge, Mary E. Fallat, Jeffrey P. Salomone, Jimm Dodd, Eileen M. Bulger & Mark L. Gestring (2018) Spinal Motion Restriction in the Trauma Patient – A Joint Position Statement, Prehospital Emergency Care, 22:6, 659-661, DOI: 10.1080/10903127.2018.1481476

## YOU are the Provider

When you arrive at the scene you find a 22-year-old man lying supine on the ground; he is motionless and his head is lying in a large pool of blood. Your partner manually stabilizes his head in a neutral position and opens his airway with the jaw-thrust maneuver as you perform a primary assessment.

| Recording Time: 0 Minutes | |
|---|---|
| Appearance | Motionless; large pool of blood under his head |
| Level of consciousness | Responsive only to deep painful stimuli |
| Airway | Open; clear of secretions or foreign bodies |
| Breathing | Slow and irregular |
| Circulation | Radial pulses slow and bounding; skin warm and dry; bleeding from a large laceration to the right side of his head |

**3.** What are your most immediate treatment priorities for this patient?

**4.** Where should you focus your secondary assessment of this patient?

## Patient Assessment

You should suspect a possible head or spinal injury anytime you encounter one of the following MOIs:

- Motor vehicle crashes (including motorcycles, snowmobiles, and all-terrain vehicles)
- Pedestrian–motor vehicle crashes
- Fall >20 feet (>6 m) (adult)
- Fall >10 feet (>3 m) (pediatric)
- Blunt trauma
- Penetrating trauma to the head, neck, back, or torso
- Rapid deceleration injuries
- Hangings
- **Axial loading injuries** (injuries where load is applied along the vertical or longitudinal axis of the spine; for example, falling from a height and landing on the feet in an upright position)
- Diving accidents

Motor vehicle crashes, direct blows, falls from heights, assault, and sports injuries are common causes of head and spinal injury. A deformed windshield or dented helmet may indicate a major blow to the head, which is likely to have caused TBI (**FIGURE 29-16**). It is especially important to evaluate and monitor the level of consciousness in patients with suspected head injuries, paying particular attention to any changes that may occur.

## Scene Size-Up

Evaluate every scene for hazards to your health and the health of your team or bystanders. Motor

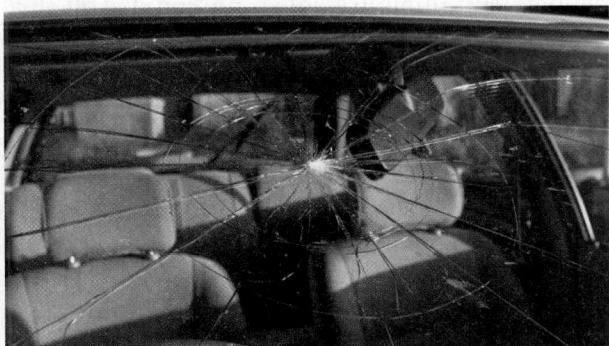

**FIGURE 29-16** The classic "star" on the windshield after an automobile crash is a significant indicator of head injury. Be alert for the signs and symptoms of head injury.

© Joe Gough/Shutterstock.

### Words of Wisdom

Many mechanisms of injury that cause head and spine injuries may also pose a risk to EMTs. Before you approach the patient, get the "big picture" of scene safety and take any actions necessary to ensure your own well-being. Do not rely entirely on assistance from fire or police personnel; maintain your own awareness of the scene.

vehicle crashes are a common cause of head and spinal injuries. These situations have the potential to cause injury to rescuers and bystanders as well. Be prepared with appropriate standard precautions before you approach the patient. You will be spending a great deal of time at the head of the patient. Gloves, a mask, and eye protection should be the minimum standard precautions that you use. Because these patients can have very complicated injuries, call for advanced life support (ALS) as soon as possible when a serious MOI or complicated presentation is evident. Law enforcement may be needed to control traffic or unruly people.

### Words of Wisdom

Proper care of a patient with a possible spinal injury requires assessment of motor and sensory functions both before and after stabilizing the patient. Likewise, careful observation of level of consciousness at different stages of your care for a head-injured patient can provide crucial information. Document your detailed findings of these repeated neurologic examinations to make the information available to hospital personnel and to help establish that your care has been thorough and appropriate.

As you observe the scene, look for indicators of the MOI. This helps you develop an early index of suspicion for underlying injuries in the patient who has sustained a significant MOI. As you put together information from dispatch and your observations of the scene, consider how the MOI produced the injuries suspected. For example, if you respond to a baseball field for a patient who was knocked unconscious by a foul ball, you may begin to suspect that the patient may have a depressed skull fracture and perform a neurologic assessment during the physical examination. Continue to consider the MOI while assessing a patient.

## Primary Assessment

The primary assessment should focus on identifying and managing life-threatening concerns. Threats to circulation, airway, or breathing are considered life threatening and must be treated immediately to prevent mortality. Life-threatening external hemorrhage must be addressed before airway and breathing concerns.

Most head injuries are considered mild and result in no or limited permanent disability. A small percentage of head injuries are considered moderate, and the patient is left with some permanent disabilities. Even fewer head injuries are considered severe, and many patients with a severe head injury die before ever reaching the hospital. There will be patients with head or spine injuries that will not require much intervention other than a thorough assessment and continued observation while being transported to the hospital. In these patients, you may choose to take some time at the scene to provide careful spinal motion restriction before transport. In patients who have airway, breathing, and circulation problems or have other conditions for which you decide a rapid transport to the closest appropriate hospital is needed, rapid spinal motion restriction and quick loading into the ambulance may be indicated. Reduction of on-scene time and recognition of a critical patient increase the patient's chances for survival or a reduction in the amount of irreversible damage.

### Spinal Motion Restriction Considerations

When assessing a patient with suspected head and/or spine injuries, be aware that any unnecessary movement of the patient can cause additional injury. Assess the patient in the position found. After determining and correcting any life-threatening injuries, determine whether a cervical collar needs to be applied. Begin by assessing the scene to determine the risk of injury, then form a general impression of your patient based on his or her level of consciousness and the chief complaint.

MOI alone is not a reason to perform spinal motion restriction. If the patient is absolutely clear in his or her thinking and does not have any neurologic deficits, spinal pain or tenderness, evidence of intoxication, or other illnesses or injuries that may mask a spinal injury or otherwise cause you to believe that the patient's reports may be unreliable, you may consider not performing spinal motion restriction. Follow your local protocols regarding use of spinal motion restriction.

Physicians are typically considered to be the appropriate people to assess and clear patients with potential spinal injuries (cervical-spine clearance refers to assessing and determining whether a spinal injury is actually present). Many jurisdictions allow their EMTs to screen patients and to refrain from initiating spinal motion restriction based on specific criteria.

The backboard is rigid and often places the patient in an anatomically incorrect position for a long period of time. During that time, the back is pressed against the board, compromising circulation to areas of skin. The patient may report pain, and in rare circumstances when a patient remains on a board for a prolonged period of time (typically several hours), decubitus ulcers can develop. Some patients, especially patients who are obese, could experience respiratory compromise while lying flat. Consider moving the patient on a scoop stretcher or vacuum splint board or placing padding under the patient to help minimize the risk of injury and try to minimize the amount of time a patient is on a long backboard. Always follow your local protocols. For more discussion on methods of transferring patients, see Chapter 8, *Lifting and Moving Patients*.

Apply a cervical collar as soon as you have addressed possible airway and breathing problems and provided necessary treatments. A cervical collar may help minimize spinal motion as you treat the airway and breathing. The best time to apply the cervical collar depends on the patient's injuries and the seriousness of his or her condition. For some patients, you may have to apply the collar early, while managing the ABCs. Always look for evidence of exsanguinating hemorrhage and then assess airway, breathing, and circulation (the XABCs). In other patients, manual stabilization may be adequate until you complete your assessment and determine if you need to place the patient on a backboard or other spinal motion restriction device. The key to managing spinal injuries and airway and breathing problems is to move the patient as little as possible and as carefully as possible, maintaining spinal alignment throughout. Place an appropriate-size cervical collar on the patient when indicated. Once the cervical collar is on, do not remove it unless it causes a problem with maintaining the airway or the patient shows signs of increasing ICP. If you must remove the cervical collar, you will have to maintain manual stabilization of the cervical spine until it can be replaced.

## Assessing for Signs and Symptoms of a Head or Spine Injury

Patients with head injuries frequently have spinal injuries, and vice versa. When assessing a patient for possible head or spinal injury, begin by asking the responsive patient the following questions to determine his or her chief complaint:

- What happened?
- Where does it hurt?
- Does your neck or back hurt?
- Can you move your hands and feet?
- Did you hit your head?

Confused or slurred speech, repetitive questioning, or amnesia in responsive patients is an indication of a head injury. Whereas other problems may cause similar symptoms, in the setting of trauma, assume your patient has a head injury until your assessment proves otherwise. A decreased blood glucose level can mimic these same symptoms.

If the patient is found unresponsive, emergency responders, family members, or bystanders may have helpful information, including when the patient lost consciousness or what was his or her previous level of consciousness. Unresponsive patients with any trauma should be assumed to have a spinal injury. Patients with a decreased level of responsiveness on the AVPU scale (responds to verbal stimulus or responds to painful stimulus) should also be considered to have a spinal injury based on their chief complaint.

## Airway, Breathing, and Circulation Considerations

In patients with head and spinal injuries, airway and breathing problems are common and may result in death if not recognized and treated immediately. When a spinal injury is suspected, how you open and assess the airway is important. Begin by manually holding the patient's head still while you assess the airway. Use a jaw-thrust maneuver

to open the airway. When performed correctly, this will prevent movement of the cervical spine. If, however, you are unable to provide a patent and open airway using the jaw-thrust maneuver, it is acceptable to use the head tilt–chin lift maneuver. The patient cannot survive if the airway is not functioning, and even though this maneuver may cause further injury to the spine, it is considered the last resort to provide an airway for your patient. An oropharyngeal or nasopharyngeal airway may assist in maintaining an airway; proper basic life support (BLS) maneuvers have been shown to adequately protect the patient's airway. When it becomes difficult to maintain the airway with BLS techniques, advanced airway techniques, usually employed by AEMTs and paramedics, can be used. The decision to use an oropharyngeal or nasopharyngeal airway is based on the patient's ability to maintain his or her own airway, the presence of a gag reflex, and the extent of facial injuries. Review the indications and contraindications for these airway adjuncts in Chapter 11, *Airway Management.*

Vomiting may occur in the patient with a head injury. With large amounts of emesis, the patient may need to be log rolled to the side and the mouth swept of secretions. When it is necessary to log roll the patient to clear the airway, roll the patient while keeping the body in as straight a line as possible to minimize spinal injuries. Suctioning should be performed immediately to remove smaller amounts of secretions.

Irregular breathing, such as Cheyne-Stokes respirations, may result from increased pressure on the brain because of bleeding or swelling in the cranium. If the ICP increases, there will be more periods of apnea. In either situation, determine whether breathing is present and adequate and continue to monitor the patient's respiratory rate and depth. Prehospital administration of high-flow oxygen is indicated for patients with head and spinal injuries. A single episode of hypoxia in a patient with a head injury significantly increases the risk of death or permanent disability. Pulse oximeter values should not fall below 90% and, ideally, should be 95% or higher. Positive pressure ventilations are not always necessary; however, if the patient's breathing rate is too slow or too fast and shallow, provide positive pressure ventilations using a bag-mask device (see Chapter 11, *Airway Management*). The rate of ventilations should be based on the age of the patient and established BLS guidelines.

Do not hyperventilate the patient. Hyperventilation is controversial because it can increase the severity of head injuries; therefore, it should be avoided except in cases where signs of imminent brainstem herniation have been identified. Even when used, hyperventilation should be used with caution and only when capnography is available to ensure an end-tidal carbon dioxide ($ETCO_2$) level between 30 and 35 mm Hg. Be sure to know your local protocols on this subject.

When approaching a patient who is unconscious, the obvious question is, "Is this person alive?" Whereas checking immediately to determine whether a pulse is present is tempting, it is more important for you to remember the XABCs. Always look for evidence of exsanguinating hemorrhage and then assess airway and breathing prior to moving on to assessment of circulation. Patients who are responsive and moving obviously have a pulse; however, you should still check to see if the pulse is weak or strong and if it is generally too fast or too slow. A pulse that is too slow in the setting of a head injury can indicate a serious condition in your patient. If the pulse is present and adequate, continue your evaluation of the patient.

A single episode of hypoperfusion in a patient with a head injury can lead to significant brain damage and even death. Assess for signs and symptoms of shock and treat appropriately. Neurogenic (spinal) shock is discussed in Chapter 13, *Shock*.

Bleeding may also be present from the same injury that caused the spine and/or head injury. That injury may involve blunt or penetrating forces. Consider again the MOI and the effects it has had on your patient. Control bleeding as previously discussed. When bandaging the head, be careful that you do not move the neck if spinal injuries are suspected and do not apply pressure if a skull fracture is suspected. Remember that head and spine injuries often occur together.

## Manner of Transport

Several transport considerations should be kept in mind for patients with head trauma. Patients with impaired airways, open head wounds, or abnormal vital signs and patients who do not respond to painful stimuli may need to be rapidly extracted from a motor vehicle and transported. During transport, providing the patient with a patent airway and high-flow oxygen is paramount. Because of the potential for increasing ICP, there is an increased risk of vomiting

and seizures, so suction should be readily available. A patient with head trauma may deteriorate rapidly, thus requiring aeromedical transport depending on your local protocols. In supine patients, the head should be elevated 30°, if possible, to help reduce ICP. Remember to maintain spinal motion restriction.

### Words of Wisdom

A blanket or one or two towels placed under the long backboard will elevate the head.

### Street Smarts

Patients who are paralyzed by a spinal cord injury but are conscious and aware of the inability to move their limbs need to be offered emotional support. Remember that it can be very traumatizing for a patient to realize that he or she may now have a debilitating and life-altering injury; therefore, you need to be careful in your choice of words. A patient may ask you difficult questions, such as "Will I be able to walk?" It is best to tell the patient that you are providing immediate care and you cannot predict the outcome.

## History Taking

After the life threats have been managed during the primary assessment, investigate the chief complaint. Obtain a medical history and be alert for injury-specific signs and symptoms as well as any pertinent negatives such as no pain or no loss of sensation.

Using OPQRST may provide some background on isolated extremity injuries. Does the patient have any recall of the incident? Inability to recall events is an important finding in patients with head injuries. You have the opportunity to interview the patient well in advance of the emergency physician. Any information you receive will be valuable if the patient has a loss of consciousness.

If the patient is not responsive, attempt to obtain the history from other sources, such as friends or family members. Medical identification jewelry and cards in wallets may also provide information about the patient's medical history (follow local protocols regarding the removal of items from a patient's wallet). Does the patient have a recent or previous history of unresponsiveness? These key indicators may lead you to suspect a developing TBI.

Make every attempt to obtain a SAMPLE history from your patient. History may be difficult to obtain when a person is confused from a head injury or frightened from a spinal injury. Whereas the prehospital environment is an excellent place to obtain important history, do not delay rapid transport for patients who need hospital intervention. Gather as much SAMPLE history as you can while preparing for transport. In less urgent situations, you should have enough time to gather a complete SAMPLE history without compromising patient care.

## Secondary Assessment

Remember that the ability to walk, move the extremities, or feel sensation does not necessarily rule out a spinal cord or spinal column injury. Similarly, the absence of pain does not always indicate that a spinal injury has not occurred. Do not ask patients with possible spinal injuries to move their necks as a test for pain. Instead, instruct the patient to keep still and not to move the head or neck.

The physical examination may be a systematic full-body scan or a systematic assessment that focuses on a certain area or region of the body, often determined through the chief complaint.

Patients with moderate or severe head injuries associated with a significant MOI should receive life-saving medical or surgical intervention at the closest appropriate trauma hospital without delay. If time allows, perform a secondary assessment to identify and treat injuries that may have been missed during the primary assessment en route to the emergency department (ED). Extremities can be stabilized using the backboard and splinted individually while in the back of the ambulance as time and conditions permit.

Obtaining a complete set of baseline vital signs is essential in patients with head and spine injuries. Significant head injuries may cause the pulse to slow and the blood pressure to rise. With neurogenic shock, the blood pressure may decrease and the heart rate may increase to compensate. Respirations can become erratic with complications from both head and spine injuries. Hypotension may be present with cervical or high thoracic spine injuries. The heart rate may become slow or fail to increase in response to hypotension.

In addition to hands-on assessment, you should use monitoring devices to quantify your patient's oxygenation and circulatory status if available. Pulse oximetry and $ETCO_2$ monitoring should be utilized, if available, on all patients suspected of having a head injury to ensure the patient is not hypoventilating or hyperventilating. Maintain $ETCO_2$ between 35 and 40 mm Hg and a pulse oximetry reading above 94%. Monitor blood pressure. Hypotension can decrease blood supply to the head and cause further injury. It is recommended that you always assess the patient's first blood pressure manually with a sphygmomanometer (blood pressure cuff) and stethoscope.

### Physical Examination Considerations

Examine the entire body using DCAP-BTLS, and examine the head, chest, abdomen, extremities, and back. Check perfusion, motor function, and sensation in all extremities prior to moving the patient. Determine whether the strength in each extremity is equal by asking the patient to squeeze your hands and to gently push each foot against your hands (**FIGURE 29-17**).

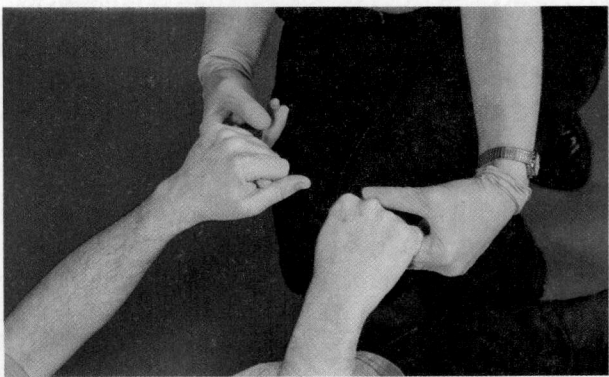

A

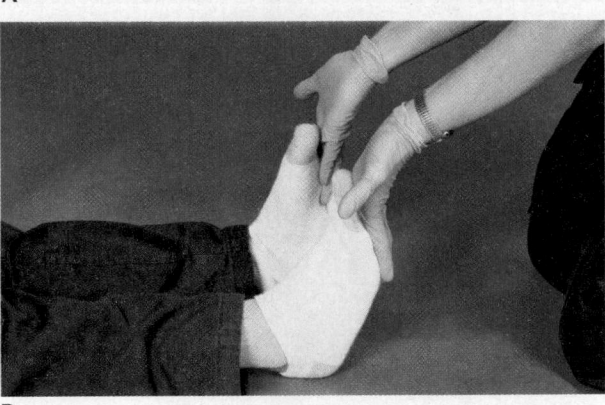

B

**FIGURE 29-17 A.** Assess the equality of strength in each extremity by asking the patient to squeeze your hands. **B.** Next, ask the patient to gently push each foot against your hands.

A decreased or altered level of consciousness is the most reliable sign of a head injury. Monitor the patient for changes in level of consciousness, including signs of confusion, disorientation, or deteriorating mental status. Is the patient unresponsive or repeating questions? Experiencing seizures? Nauseous or vomiting?

Determine whether there is decreased movement and/or numbness and tingling in the extremities. Is there any posturing? Is the patient able to perform motor functions such as squeezing your hands appropriately and equally? Part the patient's hair and inspect the scalp for bruising. Look for blood or CSF leaking from the ears, nose, or mouth and for bruising around the eyes and behind the ears.

Assess pupil size and reaction to light. Unequal pupil size after a head injury in an unconscious patient often signals a serious problem. The brain controls the diameter of pupils and how quickly they react. If an injury has occurred on one side of the brain, just one pupil will dilate. Developing blood clots may be compressing the brain, causing one pupil to dilate and indicating that the brain is at extreme risk of sustaining catastrophic damage (**FIGURE 29-18**). The pupils are windows to the brain and should be assessed as soon as possible to establish a baseline from which to monitor changes.

As soon as you have assessed the patient's level of consciousness, determine the reaction of each pupil to light. Sketch the size of both pupils on the ambulance report to indicate any difference between the two eyes. Continue to monitor the pupils. Any change in their reactions over time may indicate progressive brain injury.

Do not probe open scalp lacerations with your gloved finger because this may push bone fragments into the brain. Do not remove an impaled object from an open head injury.

## Neurologic Examination

For a patient with a head injury, perform a neurologic examination. Perform a baseline assessment using the Glasgow Coma Scale (GCS) and record the time (**TABLE 29-2**). The GCS helps you to identify the

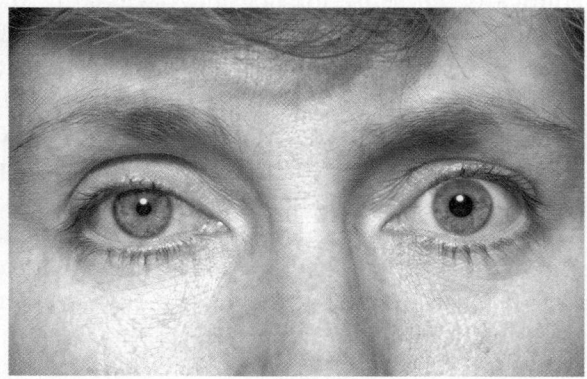

**FIGURE 29-18** Assess pupil size and reaction to light in all patients at least once.

### TABLE 29-2 Glasgow Coma Scale[a]

| Eye Opening | | Best Verbal Response | | Best Motor Response | |
|---|---|---|---|---|---|
| Spontaneous | 4 | Oriented conversation | 5 | Obeys commands | 6 |
| In response to sound | 3 | Confused conversation | 4 | Localizes to pressure | 5 |
| In response to pressure | 2 | Inappropriate words | 3 | Withdraws from pressure | 4 |
| None | 1 | Incomprehensible sounds | 2 | Abnormal flexion | 3 |
| | | None | 1 | Abnormal extension | 2 |
| | | | | None | 1 |

[a]Some systems use a "Not testable (NT)" score for any element that cannot be tested. Eye opening cannot be tested in a patient whose eyes are closed due to a local factor, such as swelling; verbal response cannot be tested in a patient who has a preexisting factor interfering with communication, such as mutism; and motor response cannot be tested in a patient who has preexisting paralysis or other limiting factor.

Score: 13–15 may indicate mild dysfunction, although 15 is the score a person with no neurologic disabilities would receive.

Score: 9–12 may indicate moderate dysfunction.

Score: 8 or less is indicative of severe dysfunction.

patient's speech and ability to follow commands. Always use simple, easily understood terms when reporting the level of consciousness, such as "does not remember events immediately before the injury" or "confused about date and time." Terms such as "obtunded" or "dazed" have different meanings to different people and should not be used in either written or verbal reports.

If your jurisdiction uses the Revised Trauma Score, then the findings from the GCS will be used to determine the Revised Trauma Score value. See Chapter 25, *Trauma Overview*, for a discussion of this scoring system.

Frequently, the level of consciousness will fluctuate—improving, deteriorating, and improving again over time. On other occasions, there may be a gradual, progressive deterioration in the patient's response to stimuli; this usually indicates serious brain injury that may need aggressive medical and/or surgical treatment. The physicians who treat the patient will need to know when a loss of consciousness occurred. They will want to compare their neurologic evaluation with the one you performed in the field.

As you proceed with your assessment, ask yourself these questions: Is the patient's speech clear and appropriate? Does the patient answer in a logical manner, and is the patient able to make decisions? Is the patient aware of his or her current location? Is the patient alert to person, place, time, and why you are at the scene? Can the patient recall the events leading up to the incident, or is there a period of memory lapse? Can the patient recall major current events?

### Special Populations

A modified GCS for pediatric and nonverbal patients assesses eye opening, verbal response, and motor response. The scoring indicators are the same as the GCS but the modified scale takes into consideration responses of coos and babbling, scoring these responses as oriented and appropriate.

### Words of Wisdom

A change in the level of consciousness is the single most important observation that you can make in assessing the severity of brain injury. Level of consciousness usually corresponds to the extent of loss of brain function.

## YOU are the Provider

Your secondary assessment reveals an area of depression to the right side of the patient's head over the temporal bone and dilated and sluggishly reactive pupils. The rest of his body is unremarkable for gross injury. He opens his eyes in response to pain, is making unrecognizable sounds, and his arms are flexed and drawn in toward his body. An engine company arrives at the scene to provide assistance. You ask them to prepare the backboard and straps while you quickly assess the patient's vital signs.

| Recording Time: 5 Minutes | |
|---|---|
| **Respirations** | 6 breaths/min and irregular (baseline); ventilations are being assisted |
| **Pulse** | 60 beats/min; regular and bounding |
| **Skin** | Pink, warm, and dry |
| **Blood pressure** | 190/104 mm Hg |
| **Oxygen saturation (Spo₂)** | 94% (on oxygen) |

There are numerous bystanders present; however, no one knows the patient. During your physical assessment, you did not find any medical alert bracelets or any other evidence of a past medical history.

**5.** What is this patient's GCS score?

**6.** What is the likely explanation for the patient's vital signs?

Any person with a head injury that has resulted in a change in level of consciousness, progressive development of signs or symptoms of a concussion, or other causes of concern should be evaluated. This evaluation should occur soon after injury and must be conducted by a qualified health care provider. EMTs are not qualified to conduct these evaluations in the field.

## Spine Examination

If there is a potential spine injury, examine the spine. To start, inspect for DCAP-BTLS and check the extremities for circulation, motor, or sensory problems. If there is impairment, note the level. You do not need to know the exact nerve impairment because this will not change your treatment.

Pain or tenderness when you palpate the spinal area is certainly a warning sign that a spinal injury may exist. Patients with spinal injuries may report constant or intermittent pain along the spinal column or in the extremities. A spinal cord injury may also produce pain independent of movement or palpation.

Other signs and symptoms of spinal injury include an obvious deformity as you gently palpate the spine; numbness, weakness, or tingling in the extremities; and soft-tissue injuries in the spinal region. Patients with severe spinal injury may lose sensation or experience paralysis below the suspected level of injury or be incontinent (loss of urinary or bowel control) (**FIGURE 29-19**). Obvious injury to the head and neck may indicate injury to the cervical spine.

Injuries to the cervical area may limit the ability of the diaphragm to function fully and minimize the ability of the chest wall to fully expand. Additional signs of spinal cord trauma are an inability to maintain body temperature, priapism (a prolonged erection), and a loss of bowel or bladder control.

## Reassessment

Repeat the primary assessment. Reassess vital signs and the chief complaint. Are the airway, breathing, and circulation still adequate? Recheck patient interventions. Are the treatments you provided for problems with the XABCs still effective? This is particularly important in patients with head or spinal injuries because these injuries can suddenly affect the respiratory, circulatory, and nervous systems.

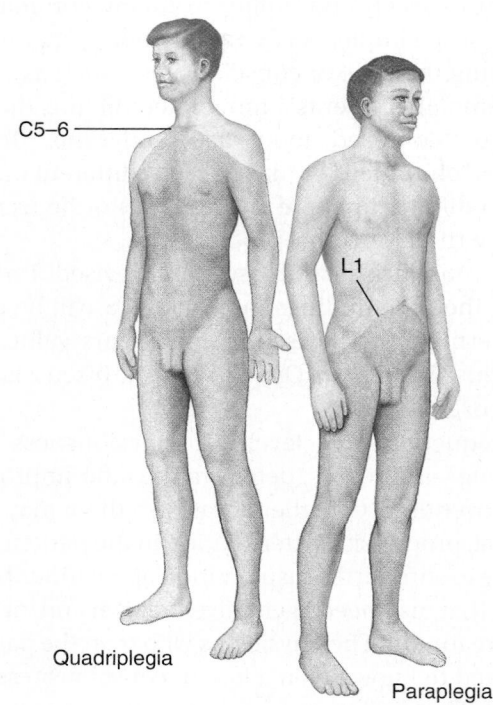

**FIGURE 29-19** With severe spinal injuries, patients may lose sensation or experience paralysis below the suspected level of Injury.

© Jones & Bartlett Learning.

The patient's condition should be reassessed at least every 5 minutes.

Multiple interventions may be necessary in patients with head and spinal injuries. The effectiveness of positive pressure ventilations, spinal motion restriction, and treatments for shock may be determined only with both immediate and continuous observation after providing the intervention. If something is not working, try something else.

You have already established baseline vital signs as part of your assessment. Now is the time to compare those baseline vital signs with repeated vital signs. These changes will often tell you if treatments have been effective. For example, a dilated pupil may constrict with effective positive pressure ventilations in an apneic head injury patient. Watch carefully for changes in the pulse, blood pressure, and respirations. If the ICP increases, the pulse may slow, blood pressure may rise, and respirations may become irregular. Document changes in the level of consciousness and vital signs.

Rapid deterioration of neurologic signs following a head injury is a sign of an expanding intracranial hematoma or rapidly progressing brain swelling. You will notice a deterioration in a conscious patient's awareness of time, place, and person (self), in that order. You must act quickly to evaluate and treat these patients. The trauma patient with signs and symptoms of head injury who also displays signs of shock may have blood loss in another body cavity if hemorrhage is not seen externally. Neurogenic shock due to spinal cord injury without hemorrhage may also cause hypotension.

As discussed earlier, the appearance of clear or pink watery CSF from the nose, the ear, or an open scalp wound indicates that the dura and the skull have both been penetrated. You should make no attempt to pack the wound, ear, or nose in this situation. Cover the scalp wound, if there is one, with sterile gauze to prevent further contamination, but do not bandage it tightly.

Your local protocol for treatment of a suspected head injury should include the administration of high-flow oxygen and the application of a cervical collar, if indicated, as part of spinal motion restriction. Reassessment should take place as the patient is transported to an appropriate trauma facility. Monitor the patient's condition and vital signs and relay this information to the receiving facility, especially if there is a significant or noteworthy change.

### Special Populations

Infants, children, and adults all may have enough blood loss due to scalp lacerations to produce shock; however, this is more common in infants than in older children and adults. Provide oxygen, monitor the airway, treat for shock, and provide immediate transport.

A common response to head injuries, even among children with only very slight head injuries, is vomiting. This is sometimes the result of increased ICP. In managing such vomiting, pay particular attention to protecting the patient's airway.

When providing care for patients with suspected head and spinal injuries, it is essential to maintain good communication with other providers and give complete and detailed information to the destination facility. Key observations that you relay will help in the assessment and eventual treatment of your patient. Hospitals may better prepare for seriously injured patients with more advance warning and a description of the most serious problems found during your assessment, and additional resources can be made available when you arrive. For example, a helicopter may be standing by for transport from a smaller hospital to a Level I trauma center. Larger hospitals may have trauma specialists or neurosurgeons available to meet you on arrival.

Your documentation should include the history you were able to obtain at the scene, your findings during your assessment, treatments you provided, and how the patient responded to them. How frequently you document repeat vital signs depends on the condition of your patient. More seriously injured patients should have documented vital signs every 5 minutes, whereas more stable patients should have documented vital signs every 15 minutes. Always follow local protocols. Take time after your verbal report to hospital staff to sit and make a complete and accurate record of the situation. This will be your only accepted legal memory of the call.

Many events that cause spinal or head injuries may eventually result in some type of litigation. As with all responses, proper documentation of what you observed and the treatment provided will be beneficial as time passes. You may be requested to testify years later in court as a witness at incidents, and proper and complete documentation recorded at the time of the incident will lay the framework for answering any questions that may be asked of you.

## Emergency Medical Care of Head Injuries

Treat the patient with a head injury according to three general principles that are designed to protect and maintain the critical functions of the CNS:

1. Establish an adequate airway. If necessary, begin and maintain ventilation and provide supplemental oxygen. Avoid hyperventilation.
2. Control bleeding and provide adequate circulation to maintain cerebral perfusion. Begin CPR if necessary. Be sure to follow standard precautions.
3. Assess the patient's baseline level of consciousness, and continuously monitor it.

As you continue to treat the patient, do not apply pressure to an open or compressed skull injury. In addition, you must assess and treat other injuries, dress and bandage open wounds as indicated in the treatment of soft-tissue injuries, splint fractures, anticipate and manage vomiting to prevent aspiration, be prepared for convulsions and changes in the patient's condition, and transport the patient promptly and with extreme care.

## Managing the Airway

The most important step in the treatment of patients with head injury, regardless of the severity, is to establish an adequate airway. If the patient has an airway obstruction, perform the jaw-thrust maneuver to open the airway. Once the airway is open, maintain the head and cervical spine in a neutral, in-line position until you have placed a cervical collar and stabilized the patient on a backboard or other spinal motion restriction device (**FIGURE 29-20**). Remove

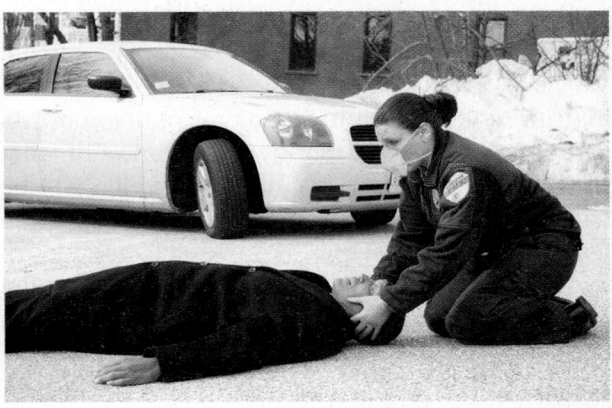

**A**

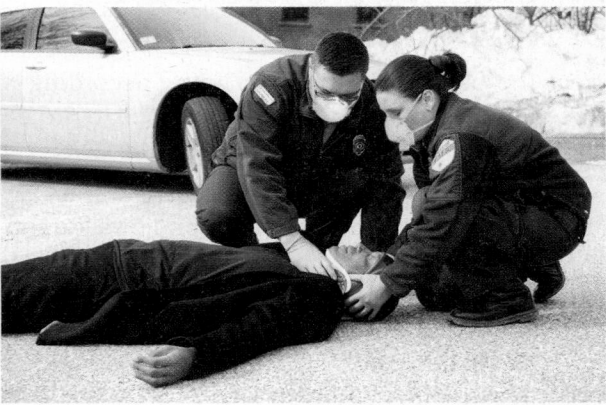

**B**

**FIGURE 29-20 A.** Maintain the head and cervical spine in a neutral in-line position. **B.** Apply a cervical collar as you finish the primary assessment.

any foreign bodies, secretions, or vomitus from the airway. Make sure a suctioning unit is available, because you will often need to clear blood, saliva, or vomitus from the airway.

Once you have cleared the airway, check ventilation. If the respiratory control center of the brain has been injured, the rate and/or depth of breathing may be ineffective. Ventilation may also be limited by chest injuries or, if the spinal cord is injured, by paralysis of some or all of the muscles of respiration. Give supplemental oxygen to any patient with suspected head injury, particularly anyone who is having trouble breathing. This reduces hypoxia and possible cerebral edema. Evaluate the patient's rate and depth of breathing. If the patient is breathing too slowly or too shallowly, use a bag-mask device to assist ventilations. Placement of an oropharyngeal airway, supraglottic airway, or endotracheal tube may be necessary to maintain an open airway. Consider calling for ALS if the patient's airway is compromised. An injured brain is even less tolerant of hypoxia than a healthy brain, and studies have shown that supplemental oxygen can reduce the risk of hypoxic episodes; to be effective, however, it must be started as soon as possible. Do not wait until the patient becomes cyanotic. Continue to assist ventilations and administer supplemental oxygen until the patient reaches the hospital. Avoid hyperventilation.

## Circulation

If the heart is not beating, providing airway maintenance, ventilation, and oxygen accomplishes nothing. You must also begin CPR if the patient is in cardiac arrest.

Active blood loss aggravates hypoxia by reducing the available number of oxygen-carrying red blood cells. Although scalp lacerations rarely cause shock except in infants and children, they often cause the loss of large volumes of blood, which must be controlled. Bleeding inside the skull may cause the ICP to rise to life-threatening levels, even though the actual volume of blood loss inside the skull is relatively small.

You can almost always control bleeding from a scalp laceration by applying direct pressure over the wound. Remember to follow standard precautions. Use a dry, sterile dressing, folding any torn skin flaps back down onto the skin bed before applying pressure (**FIGURE 29-21A**). In some instances, you will have to apply firm compression for several minutes to control bleeding (**FIGURE 29-21B**). If you suspect a skull fracture, do not apply excessive pressure to the open wound. Otherwise, you may increase the ICP or push bone fragments into the brain. If the bandage covers the patient's ears, remember that communication may become difficult because the patient's ability to hear will be decreased. To avoid limiting access to the patient's airway, do not cover the patient's mouth, nose, or jaw.

If the dressing becomes soaked, do not remove it. Instead, place a second dressing over the first.

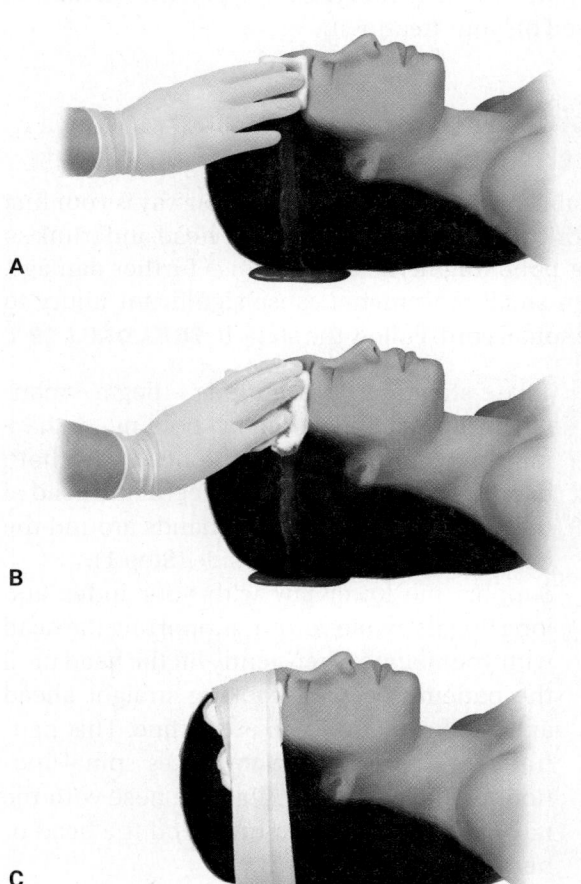

**FIGURE 29-21 A.** Use a dry sterile dressing to fold torn skin flaps back down onto the skin bed before applying pressure. **B.** If you do not suspect an open brain injury or skull fracture, apply firm compression for several minutes to control the bleeding. **C.** Secure the compression dressing in place with a soft, self-adhering roller bandage.

A, B, C: © Jones & Bartlett Learning.

Continue applying manual pressure until the bleeding has been controlled, then secure the dressing in place with a soft, self-adhering roller bandage (**FIGURE 29-21C**).

Shock that develops in a patient with a head injury is usually the result of hypovolemia caused by bleeding from other injuries. As with other trauma patients, shock in these cases indicates that the situation is critical. Such patients must be transported immediately to a trauma center. Maintain the airway while you protect the patient's cervical spine, ensure adequate ventilation, administer 100% oxygen, control obvious sites of bleeding with direct pressure, place the patient supine on a backboard, keep the patient warm, and provide immediate transport.

If the patient becomes nauseated or begins to vomit, elevate one side of the backboard to prevent aspiration. Be sure to maintain the head in the in-line neutral position, with the cervical collar in place. You should also have a suctioning unit available.

## Cushing Triad

If the patient's head injuries are significant enough to cause a TBI, the patient may begin to exhibit the signs of Cushing triad: increased blood pressure (hypertension), decreased heart rate (bradycardia), and irregular respirations such as Cheyne-Stokes respiration or Biot respiration. The Cushing triad identifies the effects seen as the pressure in the skull increases secondary to brain swelling or bleeding. As the pressure in the skull increases, the brainstem and the midbrain may be pushed through the foramen magnum, the hole at the base of the skull. If this process is allowed to continue, the patient will die. Patient outcomes can be worse if the patient is in shock, becomes hypoxic, or is hyperventilated. Manage shock, administer oxygen, and ventilate as necessary, avoiding hyperventilation. If monitoring is available, maintain ETCO$_2$ between 30 and 35 mm Hg (20 breaths/minute for adults, 25 breaths/minute for children, and 30 breaths/minute for infants less than 1 year of age).

### Words of Wisdom

Hypoxemia is one of the key indicators, along with hypotension, of a poor outcome in patients with TBIs.

# Emergency Medical Care of Spinal Injuries

Emergency medical care of a patient with a possible spinal injury begins, as does all patient care, with your protection; therefore, you must remember to follow standard precautions. Next, you must maintain the patient's airway while manually keeping the spine in the proper position, assess respirations, and give supplemental oxygen.

## Managing the Airway

Knowing that improper handling of a spinal injury can leave a patient permanently paralyzed must not prevent you from properly and promptly addressing an airway obstruction. Remember, all patients without an airway will die. If a patient with a spinal injury has an airway obstruction, perform the jaw-thrust maneuver to open the airway (**FIGURE 29-22**).

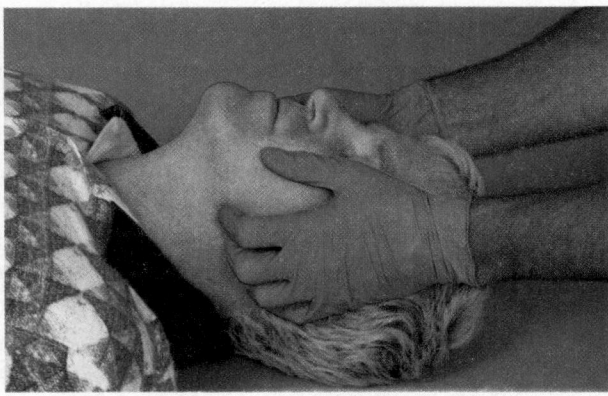

**A**

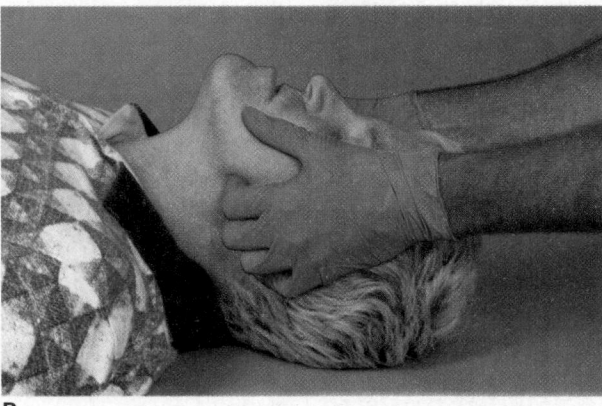

**B**

**FIGURE 29-22** Jaw-thrust maneuver. **A.** Stabilize the neck in a neutral, in-line position. **B.** Push the angle of the lower jaw upward.

**A, B:** © Jones & Bartlett Learning. Courtesy of MIEMSS.

Do not use the head tilt–chin lift maneuver because it extends the neck and may further damage the cervical spine. If the patient is unconscious, you can lift or pull the tongue forward so that you do not have to move the neck. Once the airway is open, hold the head still in a neutral, in-line position until it can be fully immobilized.

After you open the airway, consider inserting an oropharyngeal airway. If your patient accepts an oropharyngeal airway, be sure to monitor the airway closely. Have a suctioning unit available because you will often need to clear away blood, saliva, or vomitus. Provide supplemental oxygen. Continuously monitor the patient's airway and be prepared for any changes in the patient's condition based on your treatment.

## Spinal Motion Restriction of the Cervical Spine

Establishing and maintaining the airway is your first priority. You must immobilize the head and trunk so that bone fragments do not cause further damage. Even small movements cause significant injury to the spinal cord. Follow the steps in **SKILL DRILL 29-1**:

1. Take standard precautions. Begin manual in-line stabilization by holding or having someone firmly hold the head with both hands. Whenever possible, kneel at the head of the patient, and place your hands around the base of the skull on either side (**Step 1**).

2. Support the lower jaw with your index and long fingers, while you are supporting the head with your palms. Then gently lift the head until the patient's eyes are looking straight ahead and the head and torso are in line. This neutral **eyes-forward position** makes spinal motion restriction easier. Align the nose with the navel. Never twist, flex, or extend the head or neck excessively (**Step 2**).

3. Manually maintain this position as you continue to maintain the airway. Have your partner place a rigid cervical collar around the neck to provide more stability. Do not remove your hands from the patient's head until the patient's torso and head have been completely secured to a backboard or other device. The patient must remain immobilized until he or she has been examined at the hospital (**Step 3**).

## Skill Drill 29-1 Performing Manual In-Line Stabilization

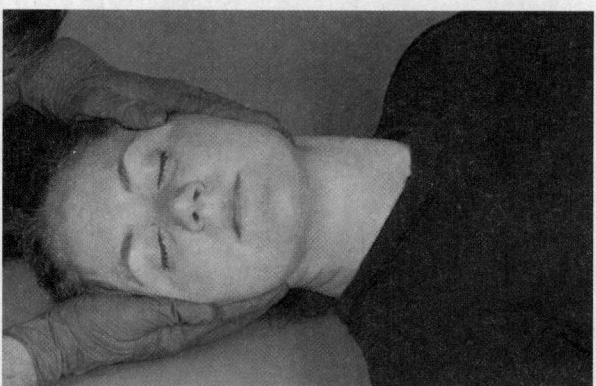

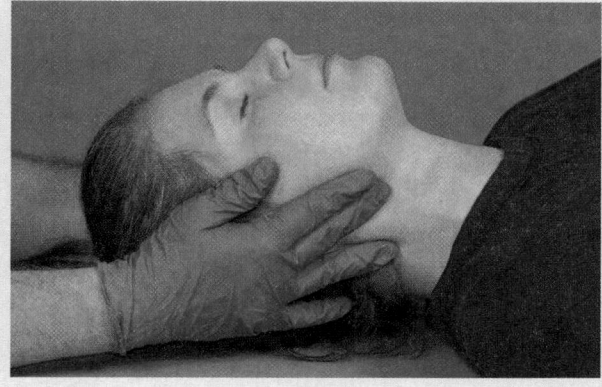

### Step 1

Take standard precautions. Kneel behind the patient and firmly place your hands around the base of the skull on either side.

### Step 2

Support the lower jaw with your index and long fingers, and the head with your palms. Gently lift the head into a neutral, eyes-forward position, aligned with the torso. Do not move the head or neck excessively, forcefully, or rapidly.

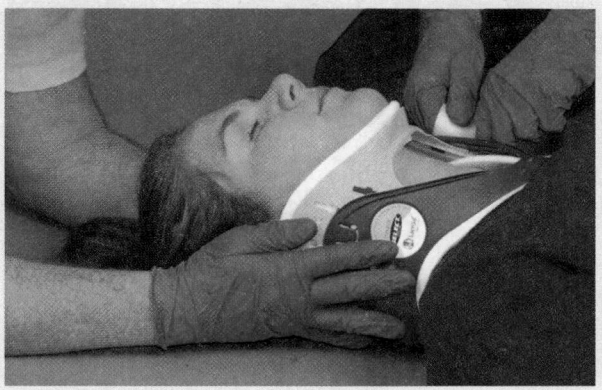

### Step 3

Continue to manually support the head while your partner places a rigid cervical collar around the neck. Maintain manual support until you have completely secured the patient to a backboard.

© Jones & Bartlett Learning. Courtesy of MIEMSS.

You should never force the head into a neutral, in-line position. Do not move the head any farther if the patient reports any of the following symptoms:

- Muscle spasms in the neck
- Substantial increased pain
- Numbness, tingling, or weakness in the arms or legs
- Compromised airway or ventilations

In these situations, immobilize the patient in his or her current position.

### Cervical Collars

Rigid cervical collars provide preliminary, partial support. A cervical collar should be applied to every patient who has a possible spinal injury based on the MOI, history, or signs and symptoms. Keep in mind, however, that cervical collars do not fully immobilize the cervical spine. Therefore, you must maintain manual support until the patient has been completely secured to a board or vacuum mattress.

To be effective, a rigid cervical collar must be the correct size for the patient. The method for determining the correct size is provided by the manufacturer. Make sure you are familiar with the types of collars your service carries. The cervical collar should rest on the shoulder girdle and provide firm support under both sides of the mandible, without obstructing the airway or ventilation efforts in any way (**FIGURE 29-23**). To apply a cervical collar, follow the steps in **SKILL DRILL 29-2**:

1. One EMT provides continuous manual in-line support of the head while the other EMT prepares the collar (**Step 1**).
2. Measure the proper-size collar according to the manufacturer's specifications. It is essential

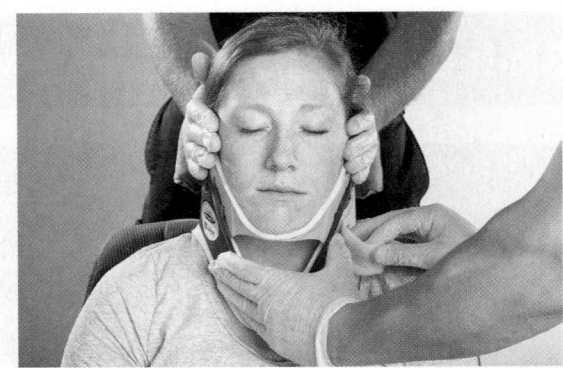

**FIGURE 29-23** Proper fit is essential in applying a cervical collar. The collar should rest on the shoulder girdle and provide firm support under both sides of the mandible without obstructing the airway or any ventilation efforts.
© Jones & Bartlett Learning.

## Skill Drill 29-2 Application of a Cervical Collar

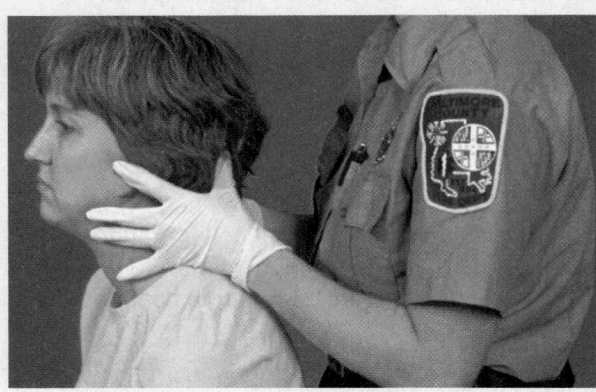

**Step 1**

Apply in-line stabilization.

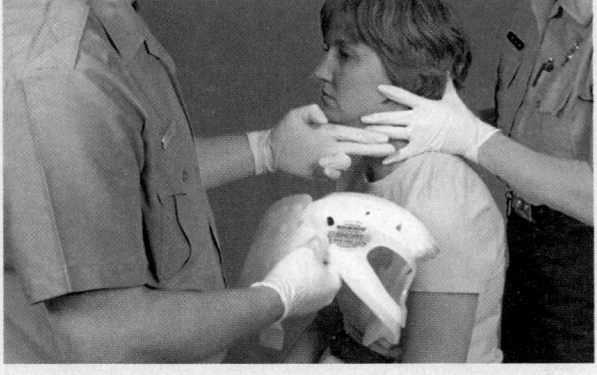

**Step 2**

Measure the proper collar size.

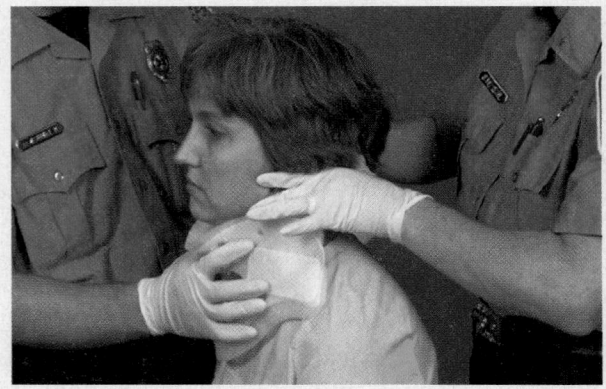

**Step 3**

Place the chin support first.

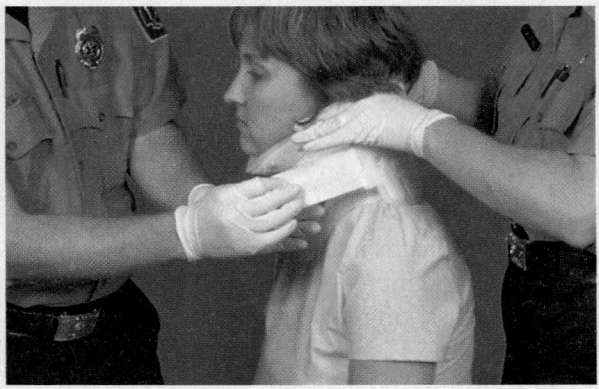

**Step 4**

Wrap the collar around the neck, and secure the collar.

## Skill Drill 29-2 Application of a Cervical Collar (*continued*)

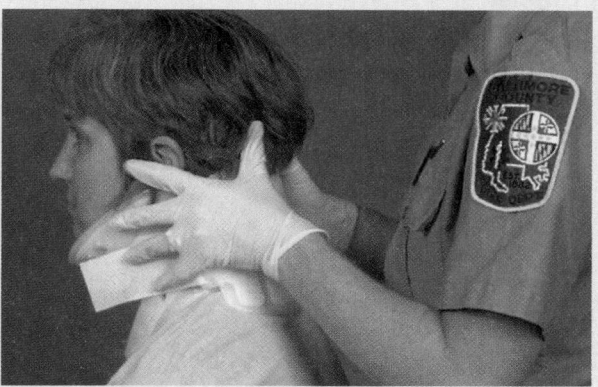

© Jones & Bartlett Learning. Courtesy of MIEMSS.

### Step 5

Ensure proper fit, and maintain neutral, in-line stabilization until the patient is secured to a backboard.

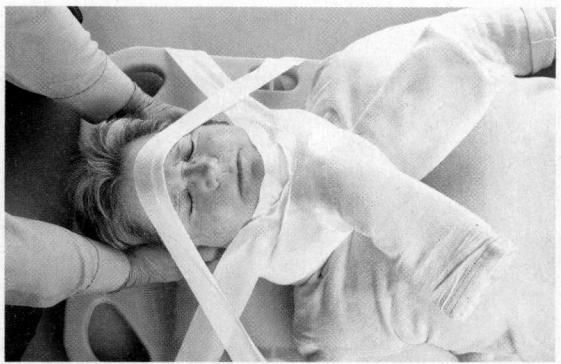

**FIGURE 29-24** If you do not have an appropriate-size cervical collar, you may use a rolled towel around the patient's head. Tape the towel to the backboard or mattress and provide continuous manual support.

© Jones & Bartlett Learning. Photo by Darren Stahlman.

that the cervical collar fits properly. If you do not have the correct-size collar, use a rolled towel around the patient's head; tape it to the backboard and provide supplemental continuous manual support (**FIGURE 29-24**) (**Step 2**).

3. Begin by placing the chin support snugly underneath the chin (**Step 3**).

4. Maintain head stabilization and neutral neck alignment, wrap the collar around the neck, and secure the collar to the far side of the chin support (**Step 4**).

5. Ensure that the collar fits properly, and recheck that the patient is in a neutral, in-line position. Maintain in-line stabilization until the patient has been completely secured to the backboard (**Step 5**).

Once the patient's head and neck have been manually stabilized, assess the pulse, motor, and sensory function in all extremities. Then assess the cervical spine area and neck. Keep in mind that the cervical collar is used to provide increased stability to the neck. It is used in addition to, not instead of, manual cervical stabilization. An improperly fitting collar will do more harm than good. In any case, maintain manual support until the patient has been fully secured to the backboard or vacuum mattress.

## Preparation for Transport
### Supine Patients

A patient who is supine can be effectively immobilized by securing him or her to a long backboard or vacuum mattress. One procedure for moving a patient from the ground to a backboard or vacuum mattress is the four-person log roll. In other cases, you may choose instead to slide the patient onto a backboard or vacuum mattress. The patient's condition, the scene, and the available resources will dictate the method you choose.

You should first take the necessary precautions and then direct the team from a kneeling position at the patient's head so that you can maintain manual in-line cervical stabilization. Your job is to ensure that the head, torso, and pelvis move as a unit, with your teammates controlling the movement of the body. If necessary, you may recruit bystanders to assist the team, but be sure to instruct them fully before moving the patient. To secure a patient to a backboard, follow the steps in **SKILL DRILL 29-3**:

1. Maintain in-line stabilization from a kneeling position at the patient's head. The EMT at the head will direct the log roll.

## Skill Drill 29-3 Securing a Patient to a Long Backboard

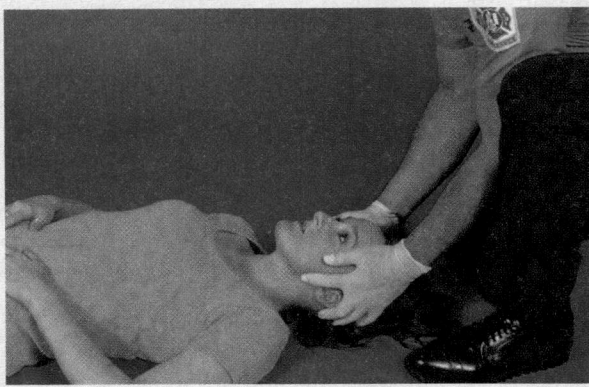

### Step 1

Apply and maintain manual cervical stabilization. Assess distal functions in all extremities.

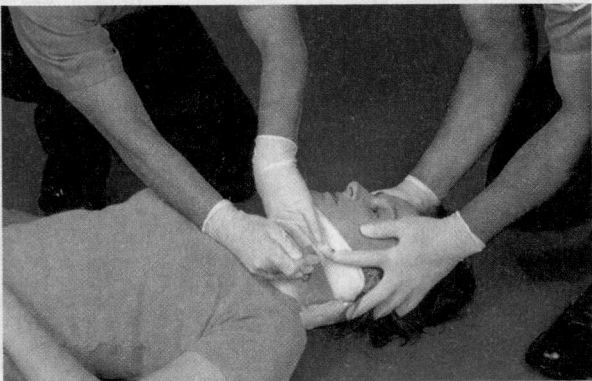

### Step 2

Apply a cervical collar.

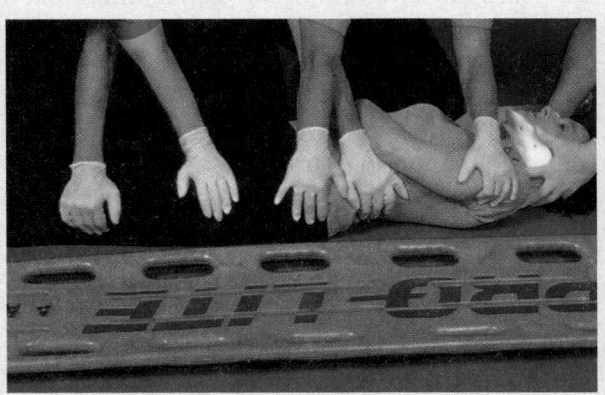

### Step 3

Rescuers kneel on one side of the patient and place hands on the far side of the patient.

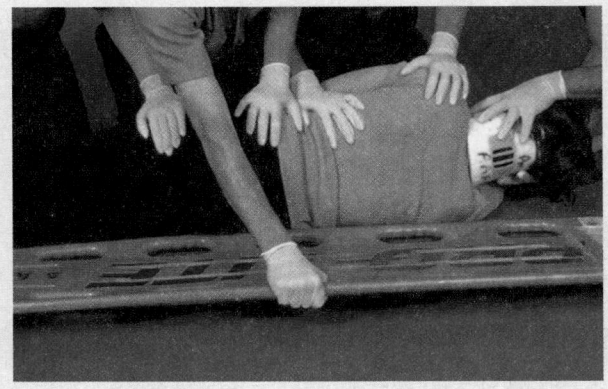

### Step 4

On command, rescuers roll the patient toward themselves, quickly examine the back, slide the backboard under the patient, and roll the patient onto the backboard.

### Step 5

Center the patient on the backboard.

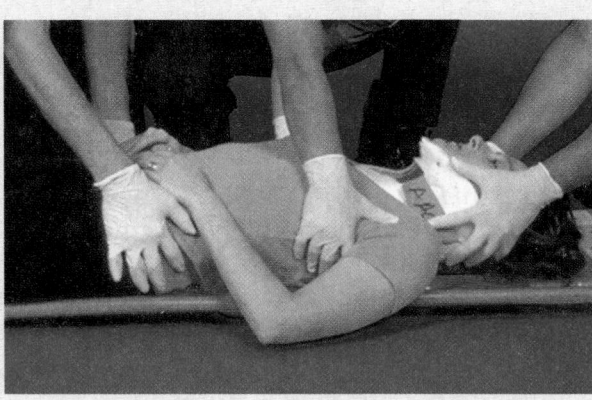

## Skill Drill 29-3 Securing a Patient to a Long Backboard (*continued*)

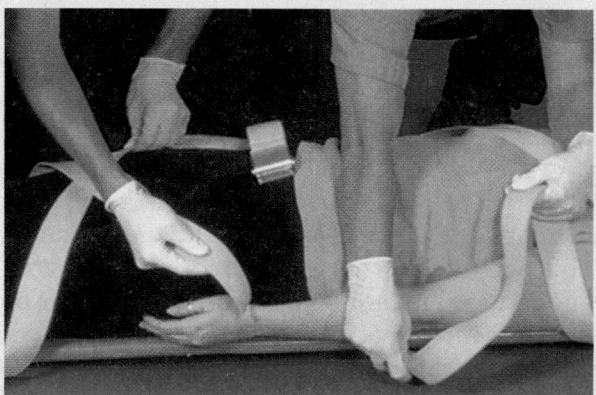

### Step 6

Secure the upper torso first.

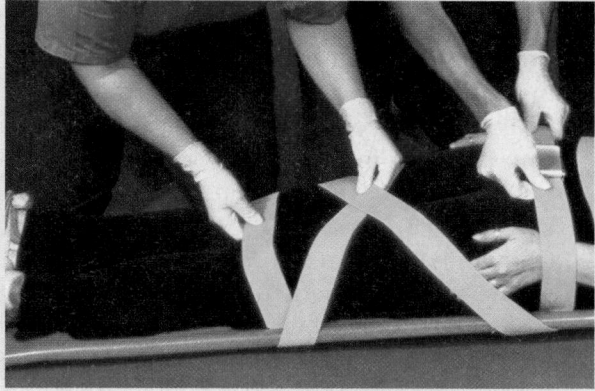

### Step 7

Secure the pelvis and upper legs.

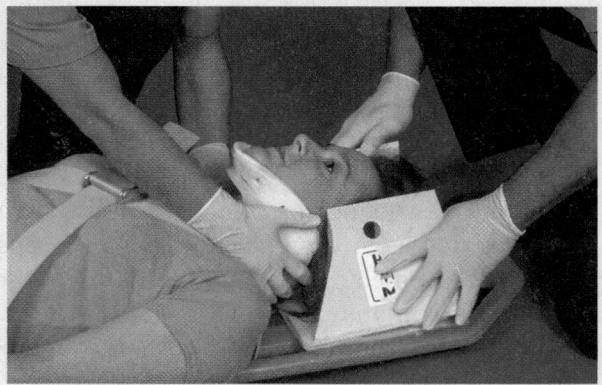

### Step 8

Begin to secure the patient's head using a commercial securing device or rolled towels.

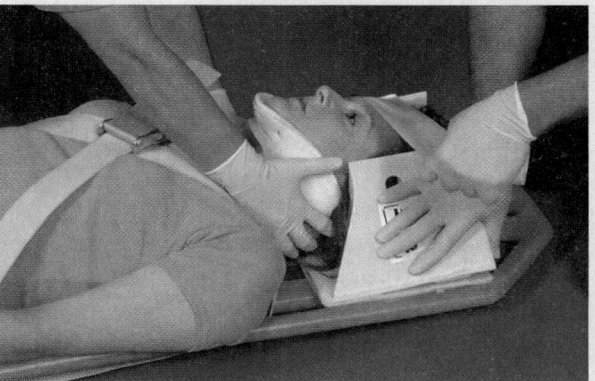

### Step 9

Place tape or a soft strap across the patient's forehead to secure the commercial device or towel rolls (do *not* place the adhesive side of medical duct tape directly onto the patient's skin or eyebrows). Check all straps and readjust as needed. Reassess distal functions in all extremities.

2. Assess pulse, motor, and sensory function in each extremity (**Step 1**).

3. Apply an appropriate-size cervical collar (**Step 2**).

4. The other team members should position the backboard and place their hands on the far side of the patient to increase their leverage. Instruct them to use their body weight and their shoulders and back muscles to ensure a smooth, coordinated pull, concentrating their pull on the heavier portions of the patient's body (**Step 3**).

5. On command from the EMT at the head, the rescuers roll the patient toward themselves. One rescuer quickly examines the back while the patient is rolled on the side, and then slides the backboard behind and under the patient. The team rolls the patient back onto the backboard, avoiding independent rotation of the head, shoulders, or pelvis (**Step 4**).

6. Ensure the patient is centered on the backboard (**Step 5**).

7. Secure the upper torso to the backboard (without restricting the patient's breathing with the straps) once the patient is centered on the backboard (**Step 6**). Consider padding voids between the patient and the backboard to make transport more comfortable and protect the patient.

8. Secure the pelvis and upper legs, using padding as needed. For the pelvis, use straps over the iliac crests and/or groin loops (**Step 7**).

9. Begin to secure the head to the backboard by positioning a commercial securing device or towel rolls (**Step 8**).

10. Secure the head by taping the towels across the forehead. To prevent airway problems and leave access to the airway, do not tape over the throat or chin. Avoid placing the sticky side of the tape on the patient's head (**Step 9**).

11. Check and readjust straps as needed to ensure that the entire body is snugly secured and will not slide during patient movement, but breathing is not restricted.

12. Reassess pulse, motor, and sensory function in each extremity, and continue to do so periodically (**Step 10**).

An alternative to the long backboard or scoop stretcher is to place the patient on a vacuum mattress. The vacuum mattress molds to the specific

## Words of Wisdom

When using a long backboard, ensure that the straps are tight enough to secure the patient but not so tight as to limit the movement of the patient's chest. Pulling the straps too tight may result in hypoventilation.

contours of the patient's body, reducing pressure point tenderness and therefore providing better comfort. The mattress also provides thermal insulation, potentially decreasing the risk of hypothermia, and is the standard equipment used to transport patients with spinal injuries in the United Kingdom. It is an excellent alternative to a backboard for older adults or patients with abnormal curvature of the spine. A drawback to the device is its thickness, requiring careful patient movement to maintain spinal stabilization during the application procedure. The vacuum mattress cannot be used for patients who weigh more than 350 pounds (159 kilograms).

Like a backboard, a vacuum mattress can be used on a supine, sitting, or standing patient.

A patient can be moved onto the vacuum mattress with a scoop stretcher or a log roll. For the scoop stretcher method, the mattress does not need to be partially rigid.

It is important to secure the patient sufficiently but without restricting the patient's breathing. If the patient is not secured sufficiently, this can cause excessive movement, increasing the risk of subsequent spinal cord injury.

Follow the steps in **SKILL DRILL 29-4** to immobilize a patient with a vacuum mattress:

1. Place the mattress on a flat surface near the patient. Make sure the head end of the mattress is at the patient's head (**Step 1**).

2. Allow air to enter the mattress (**Step 2**). The valve stem can remain open until the mattress is soft and pliable.

3. Smooth the mattress so that it is flat and level (**Step 3**).

4. Remove any sharp or bulky items that may damage the vacuum mattress.

5. Connect the pump to the mattress (**Step 4**).

6. Determine which method you will use to move the patient onto the mattress. If you will use the log roll method, evacuate the mattress until it is partially rigid (**Step 5**). (This step

is not needed if using the scoop stretcher method.) The surface should be smooth and the beads inside the mattress should be spread out as evenly as possible.

7. Move the patient onto the vacuum mattress using one of the two methods: scoop stretcher or log roll (**Step 6**). Throughout this procedure, maintain spinal alignment.

8. Scoop stretcher method (for this method, the mattress does not need to be partially rigid):
   a. Apply the scoop stretcher to the patient, then lift and transfer the patient onto the mattress.
   b. Position the patient so his or her head is in the head area of the mattress or very close to the mattress's top edge.

---

## Skill Drill 29-4 Placing a Patient on a Full-Body Vacuum Mattress

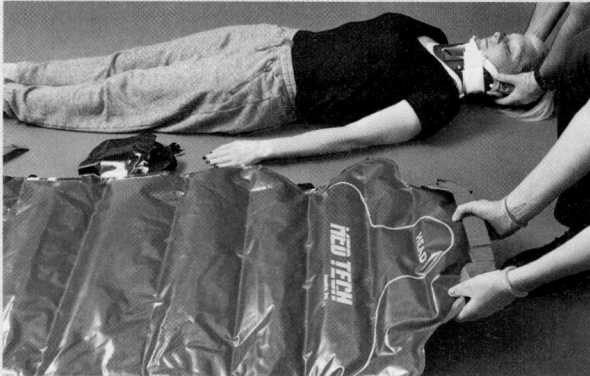

**Step 1**

Place the mattress on a flat surface near the patient, with the head end of the mattress at the patient's head.

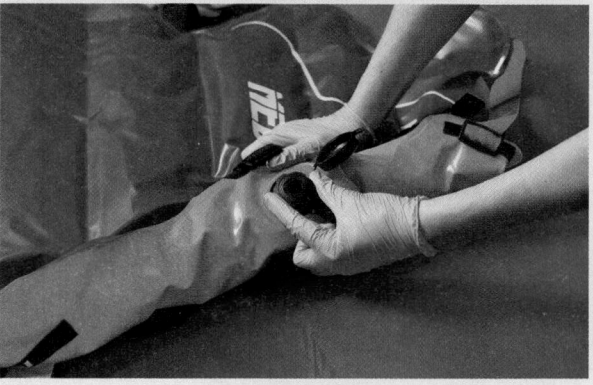

**Step 2**

Allow air to enter the mattress. Keep the valve stem open until the mattress is soft and pliable.

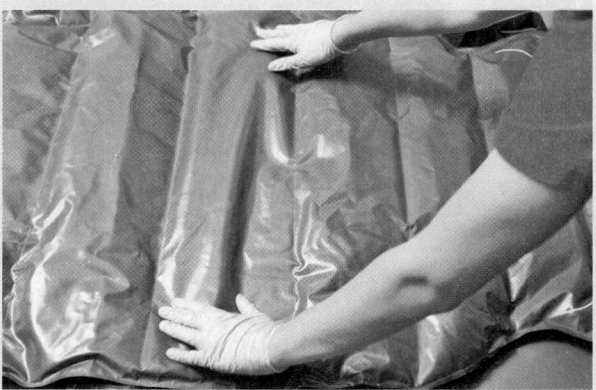

**Step 3**

Smooth the mattress. Remove any sharp or bulky items that may damage the mattress.

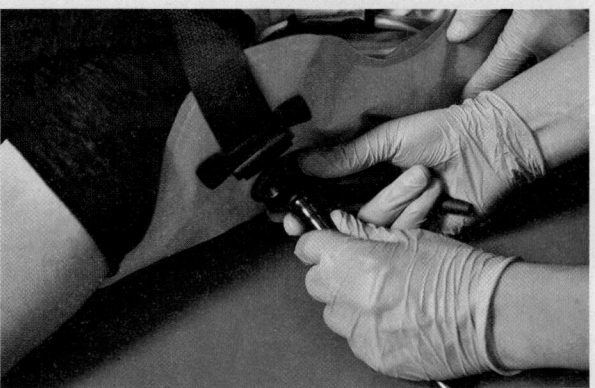

**Step 4**

Connect the pump to the mattress.

*(continues)*

## Skill Drill 29-4 Placing a Patient on a Full-Body Vacuum Mattress (*continued*)

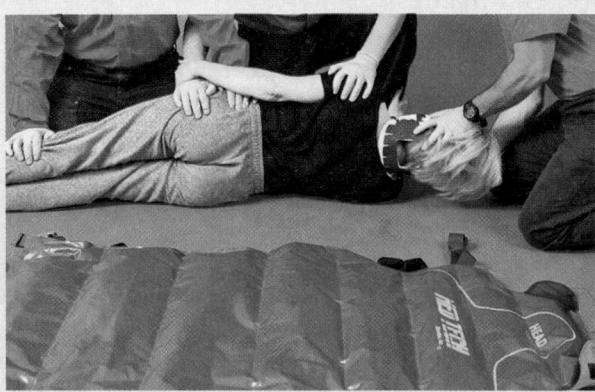

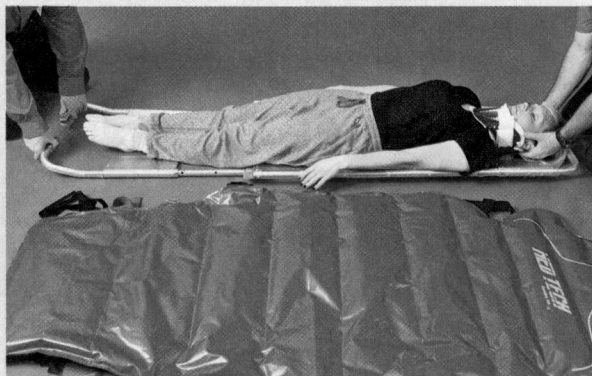

### Step 5

Determine which method you will use to move the patient onto the mattress. If you use the log roll method, evacuate the mattress until it is partially rigid (this step is not needed if using the scoop stretcher method). The surface should be smooth and the beads should be spread out as evenly as possible.

If using a scoop stretcher, you do not need to partially evacuate the mattress at this stage.

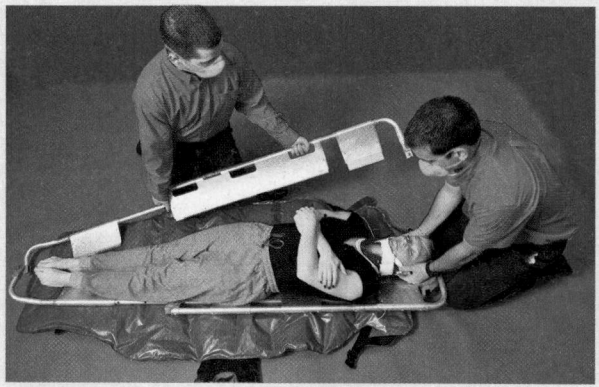

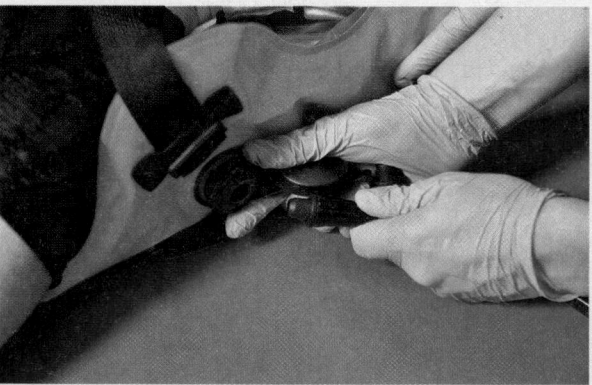

### Step 6

Move the patient onto the vacuum mattress using the method you determined during the previous step. Maintain spinal alignment.

### Step 7

If the vacuum mattress is partially rigid, open the valve to allow air to enter. Keep the valve open until the mattress is pliable.

## Skill Drill 29-4 Placing a Patient on a Full-Body Vacuum Mattress (*continued*)

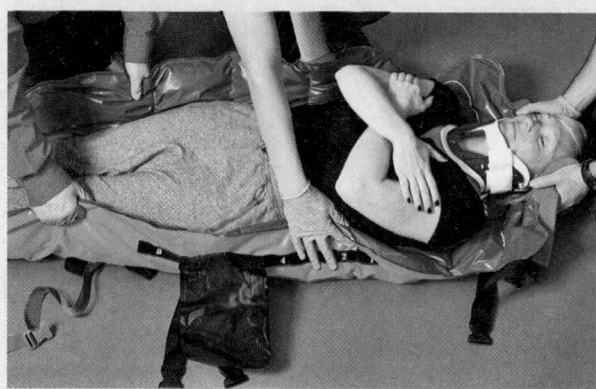

### Step 8

Conform the mattress to each side of the patient's head, close to the shoulders but not the top of the head. Continue to hold these "head blocks" that you have formed and have a second person hold up the sides of the mattress to the patient's hips until the mattress is evacuated of air completely.

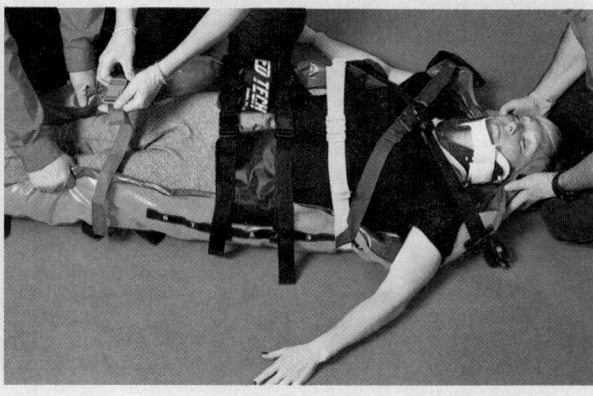

### Step 9

Secure the patient's chest, hips, and legs.

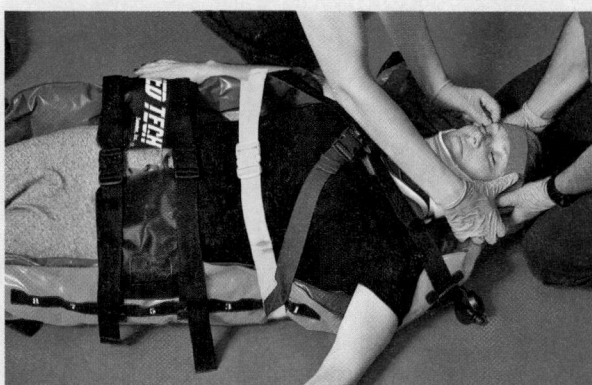

### Step 10

Secure the patient's head. Pad any voids at the top of the shoulders.

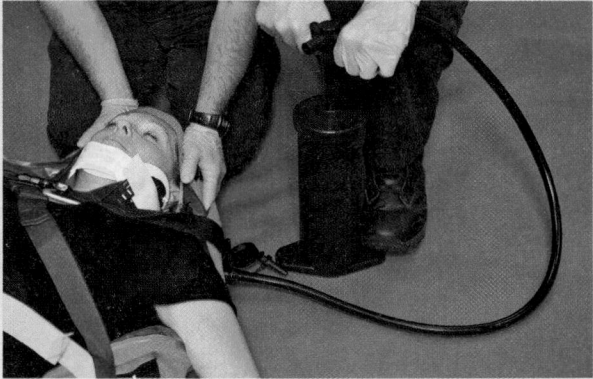

### Step 11

Ensure the patient is as comfortable as possible, then evacuate the remaining air to achieve effective spinal motion restriction.

(*continues*)

## Skill Drill 29-4 Placing a Patient on a Full-Body Vacuum Mattress (*continued*)

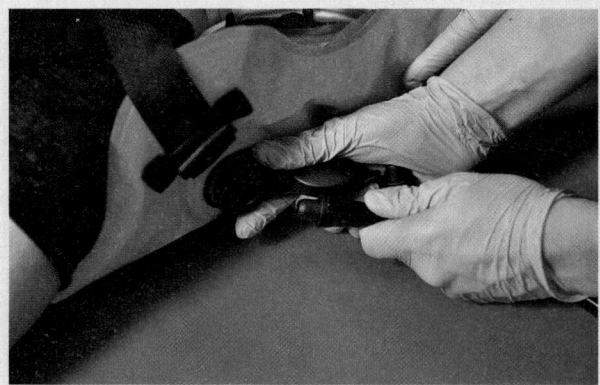

### Step 12

Disconnect the vacuum pump and ensure that the valve is closed or secured.

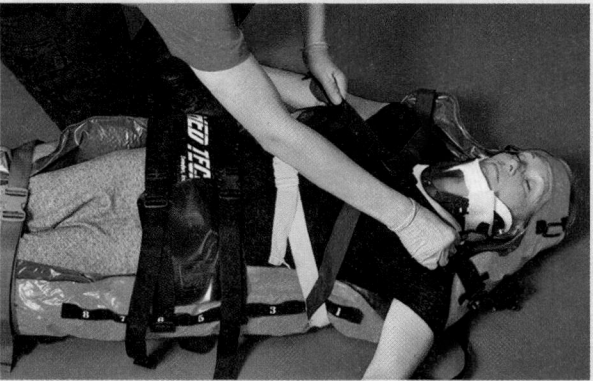

### Step 13

Reassess and adjust the straps around the chest, hips, and legs.

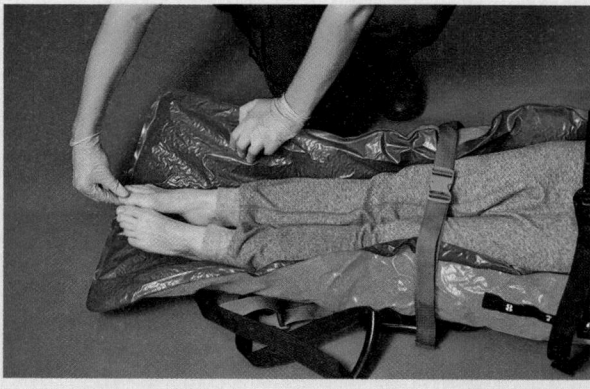

© Jones & Bartlett Learning.

### Step 14

Check the patient's neurovascular status and recheck all straps prior to lifting or moving the patient.

---

    c. Remove the scoop stretcher from around the patient and proceed with application of the vacuum mattress.

9. Log roll method (for this method, the mattress should be partially rigid):

    a. Place the mattress on a backboard or transfer device.

    b. Hold the mattress in place on the backboard, and log roll the patient onto the backboard with the mattress on top of it. (The long backboard is used only for stabilization.)

    c. Position the patient so his or her head is very close to the top edge.

10. If the vacuum mattress is partially rigid, open the valve to allow air to enter (**Step 7**). Keep the valve open until the mattress is pliable.

11. Conform the mattress to each side of the patient's head close to the shoulders, but not the top of the head (**Step 8**). Continue to hold these "head blocks" that you have formed and have a second person hold up the sides of the mattress to the patient's hips until the mattress is evacuated of air completely. Always form the mattress to meet the needs of the patient. Use additional rescuers if needed. Some patients may be more comfortable with their knees slightly bent.

12. Secure the patient's chest, hips, and legs in the mattress (**Step 9**).
13. Secure the patient's head with medical tape (**Step 10**). Pad any voids at the top of the shoulders.
14. If the patient is as comfortable as possible, evacuate the remaining air from the mattress to achieve rigid spinal motion restriction (**Step 11**). (A portable suction unit can be used to evacuate some mattresses; see the manufacturer's recommendations.)
15. Disconnect the vacuum pump and ensure that the valve is closed or secured so the mattress is not accidentally deflated (**Step 12**).
16. Reassess and adjust the straps around the chest, hips, and legs (**Step 13**).
17. Check the patient's neurovascular status and recheck all straps prior to lifting or moving the patient (**Step 14**).

## Sitting Patients

Some patients with a possible spinal injury will be in a sitting position, such as after a vehicle crash. If they are unable to stand and pivot to the stretcher, you should use a short backboard or other short spinal extrication device to restrict movement of the cervical and thoracic spine. The short backboard is then secured to the long backboard.

The exceptions to this rule are situations in which you do not have time to first secure the patient to the short backboard, including the following situations:

- You or the patient is in danger.
- You need to gain immediate access to other patients.
- The patient's injuries justify urgent removal.

In these situations, your team should lower the patient directly onto a long backboard, using the rapid extrication technique. This technique is described in Chapter 8, *Lifting and Moving Patients*. Be sure that you provide manual stabilization of the cervical spine as you move the patient. Rapid extrication is indicated only in cases of life-threatening or limb-threatening injury. In all other cases, proceed with spinal motion restriction with the patient in a seated position. Follow the steps in **SKILL DRILL 29-5** to secure a sitting patient's cervical spine using a commercial device.

1. Take standard precautions. As with the supine patient, you must first stabilize the head and then maintain manual in-line stabilization until

## Skill Drill 29-5 Securing a Patient Found in a Sitting Position

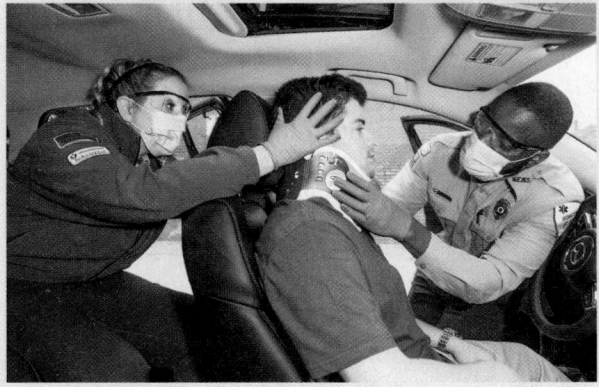 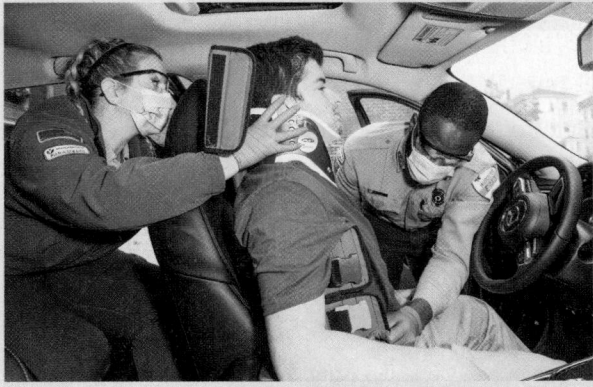

**Step 1**

Take standard precautions. Stabilize the head and neck in a neutral, in-line position. Assess pulse, motor, and sensory function in each extremity. Apply a cervical collar.

**Step 2**

Insert a spinal motion restriction device between the patient's upper back and the seat.

*(continues)*

## Skill Drill 29-5 Securing a Patient Found in a Sitting Position (*continued*)

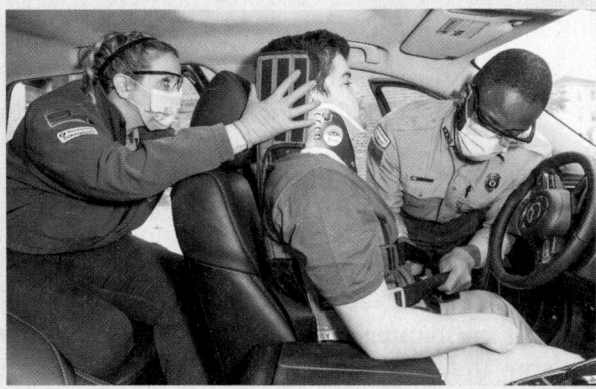

### Step 3

Open the side flaps, and position them around the patient's torso, snug around the armpits.

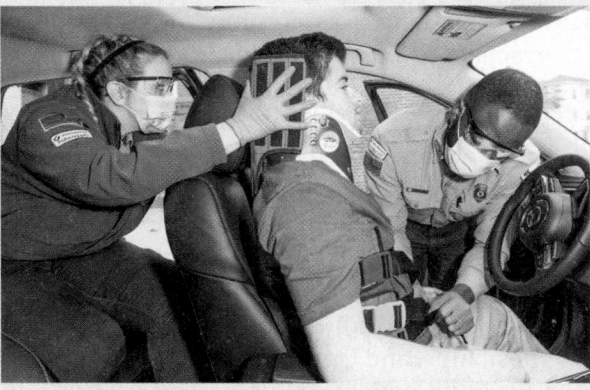

### Step 4

Secure the upper torso flaps, then the mid-torso flaps.

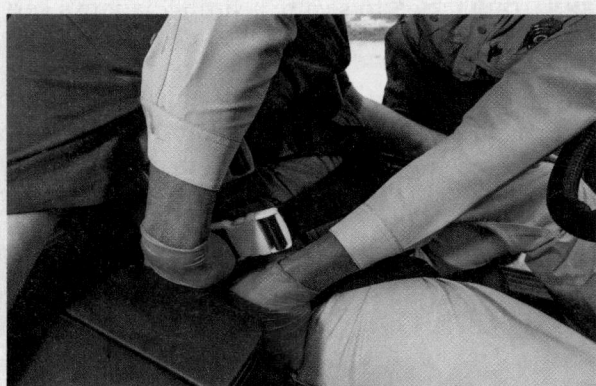

### Step 5

Secure the groin (leg) straps. Check and adjust the torso straps.

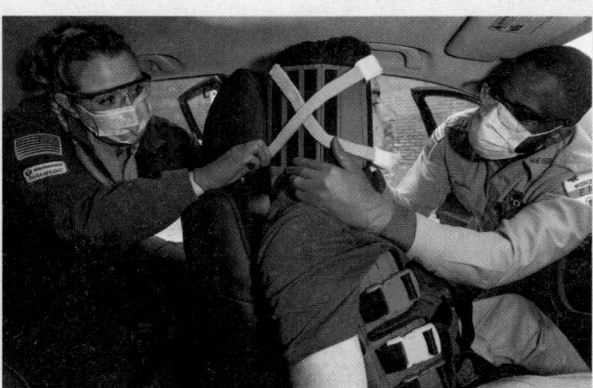

### Step 6

Pad between the head and the device as needed. Secure the forehead strap and fasten the lower head strap around the cervical collar.

### Step 7

Place a long backboard next to the patient's buttocks, perpendicular to the trunk.

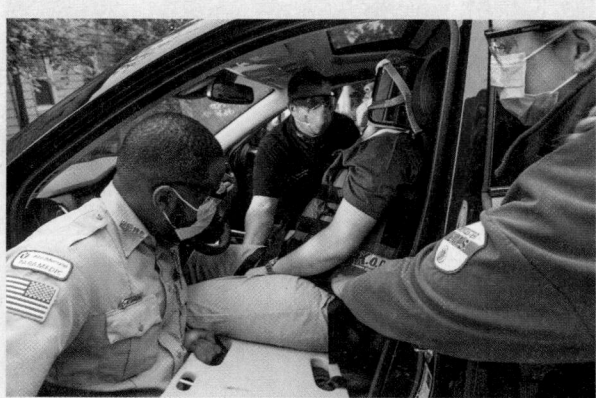

## Skill Drill 29-5 Securing a Patient Found in a Sitting Position (*continued*)

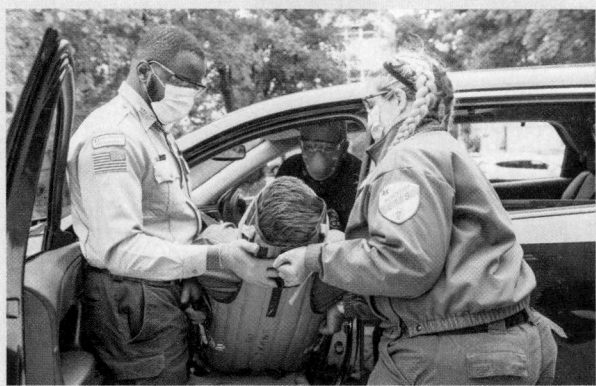

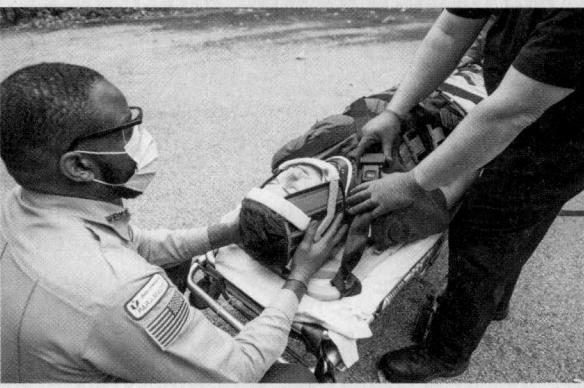

**Step 8**

Turn and lower the patient onto the long backboard. Lift the patient and slip the long backboard under the securing device.

© Jones & Bartlett Learning.

**Step 9**

Secure the spinal precaution device and long backboard to each other. Loosen or release the groin straps. Reassess pulse, motor, and sensory function in each extremity.

the patient has been secured to the long backboard or vacuum mattress.

2. Assess pulse, motor, and sensory function in each extremity.

3. Apply the cervical collar (**Step 1**).

4. Insert an extrication device between the patient's upper back and the seat back (**Step 2**).

5. Open the side flaps (if present), and position them around the patient's torso and snug to the armpits (**Step 3**).

6. Once the extrication device has been properly positioned, secure the upper torso straps and then the midtorso straps (**Step 4**).

7. Position and fasten both groin (leg) straps. Check all torso straps to make sure they are secure. Make any adjustments necessary without excessive movement of the patient (**Step 5**).

8. Pad any space between the patient's head and the extrication device as necessary.

9. Secure the forehead strap, and then fasten the lower head strap around the cervical collar (**Step 6**).

10. Place the long backboard next to the patient's buttocks, perpendicular to the trunk (**Step 7**).

11. Turn the patient parallel to the long backboard, and slowly lower the patient onto it.

12. Lift the patient (without rotating him or her), and slip the long backboard under the short board (**Step 8**).

13. Secure the extrication device and long backboard together. Loosen or release the groin straps.

14. Reassess the pulse, motor, and sensory function in all four extremities. Document your findings, and prepare for immediate transport (**Step 9**).

## Standing Patients

You may arrive at a scene in which you find a patient standing or wandering around after a crash or injury. A patient who is already standing and walking should be able to sit down gently and be transferred to a position in which spinal motion restriction can be maintained.

If the MOI and clinical indications suggest spinal injury or the patient's inability to protect his or her spine, establish spinal motion restriction. Clinical indications may include the following:

- Spinal tenderness or pain
- An altered level of consciousness
- Neurologic deficits

- Obvious anatomic deformity of the spine
- High-energy trauma in a patient intoxicated from drugs, alcohol, or a distracting injury

## Spinal Motion Restriction Devices

An injured spine is often difficult to evaluate in a patient with a head injury. Sometimes, the patient has no neurologic loss. During assessment, pain in the spine may be missed because of shock or because the patient's attention is directed to more painful injuries. Evaluation is even more difficult if the patient is unconscious. Because any manipulation of the unstable spinal column may cause permanent damage to the spinal cord, you must assume the presence of spinal injury in all patients who have sustained significant head injuries. Use manual in-line stabilization or a cervical collar and long backboard.

## Short Backboards

There are several types of short backboards. The most common are the vest-type device (**FIGURE 29-25**) and the rigid short backboard. These devices are designed to immobilize and restrict movement of the head, neck, and torso. They are used to immobilize noncritical patients who are found in a sitting position and have possible spinal injuries.

As described earlier in this chapter, the first step in securing a patient to a short backboard is to provide manual, in-line support of the cervical spine. Assess the pulse, motor function, and sensation in all extremities; next assess the cervical area; and then apply an appropriate-size cervical collar.

Position the device behind the patient and secure it to the torso. Evaluate how well the torso and groin are secured and make adjustments as necessary. Avoid excessive movement of the patient. Next, evaluate the position of the patient's head. Pad behind the head as needed to maintain neutral, in-line stabilization.

Now secure the patient's head to the device. Once the head is secured, you may release manual support of the head. Rotate or lift the patient to the long backboard. At this point, you must reassess the pulse, motor function, and sensation in all four extremities to determine whether the change in position has affected the patient's vital signs or neurologic status. Finally, you should secure the patient to the long backboard.

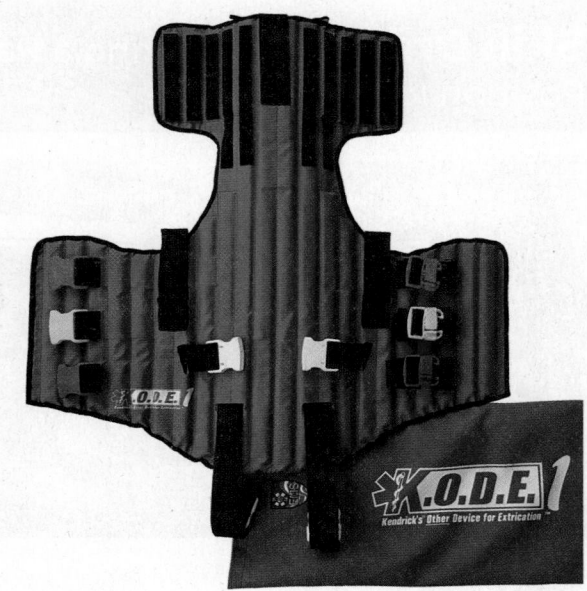

**FIGURE 29-25** A common short-board spinal precaution device is a vest-type device.

© Kendrick EMS.

## Long Backboards

There are several types of long backboards that provide full-body spinal motion restriction (**FIGURE 29-26**), including the head, neck, torso, pelvis, and extremities. Long backboards are used to minimize cervical spine motion in patients who are found in any position (standing, sitting, supine), sometimes in conjunction with short backboards.

Securing a patient to a long backboard was described in detail earlier in this chapter. Briefly, you should begin by providing manual, in-line support of the head. Assess pulse, motor function, and sensation in all extremities, and assess the cervical area. Then apply an appropriate-size cervical collar, and proceed as follows:

1. Position the device.
2. Log roll the patient onto the device. You may also move the patient onto the device using a suitable lift or slide or by using a scoop stretcher. As you maintain in-line support, your partner should kneel by the patient's head and direct the other two EMTs as you roll the patient. Your partner's job is to make sure that the head, torso, and pelvis move as a unit. As the patient's back comes into view,

quickly assess its condition if you did not do so during the initial assessment. One EMT should position the device under the patient. Then, at your partner's command, roll the patient onto the backboard.

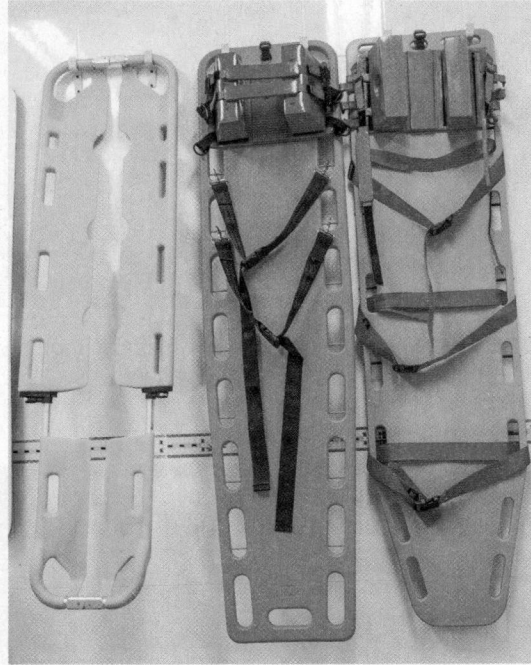

**FIGURE 29-26** Long backboards provide full-body spinal motion restriction, including the head, neck, torso, pelvis, and extremities.

© meenon/iStock/Getty Images Plus/Getty Images.

3. If there are spaces between the patient's head and torso and the backboard, fill them with padding.
4. Secure the torso to the device by applying straps across the chest, pelvis, and legs. Adjust these straps as needed. Then secure the patient's head to the board.
5. Reassess pulse, motor function, and sensation in all extremities.
6. When the patient has been properly secured, you can safely lift the backboard or turn it on its side, if necessary.

## Helmet Removal

As you plan your care of a patient wearing a helmet, ask yourself the following questions:

- Is the patient's airway clear?
- Is the patient breathing adequately?
- Can you maintain the airway and assist ventilations if the helmet remains in place?
- Can the face guard be easily removed to allow access to the airway without removing the helmet?
- How well does the helmet fit?
- Can the patient move within the helmet?
- Can the spine be immobilized in a neutral position with the helmet on?

A helmet that fits well prevents the patient's head from moving and should be left on, provided

### YOU are the Provider

Full spinal motion restriction is established, assisted ventilations are continued, and the patient is loaded into the ambulance. An EMR from the engine company drives the ambulance so your partner can help you with the patient in the back. You begin transport to a local trauma center and reassess the patient's vital signs en route.

| Recording Time: 11 Minutes | |
| --- | --- |
| **Level of consciousness** | Responsive only to deep painful stimuli |
| **Respirations** | 6 breaths/min and irregular (baseline); ventilations are being assisted |
| **Pulse** | 64 beats/min; regular and bounding |
| **Skin** | Pink, warm, and dry |
| **Blood pressure** | 192/100 mm Hg |
| **Spo₂** | 96% (on oxygen) |

**7.** What further treatment is indicated for this patient?

**8.** What should you specifically monitor this patient for during transport?

(1) there are no impending airway or breathing problems, (2) it does not interfere with assessment and treatment of airway or ventilation problems, and (3) you can properly immobilize the spine. You should also leave on the helmet if there is any chance that removing it will further injure the patient.

Remove a helmet if (1) it is a full-face helmet (**FIGURE 29-27**), (2) it makes assessing or managing airway problems difficult and removal of a face guard to improve airway access is not possible, (3) it prevents you from properly immobilizing the spine, or (4) it allows excessive head movement. Finally, always remove a helmet from a patient who is in cardiac arrest.

Sports helmets are typically open in the front and may or may not include an attached face mask. The mask can be removed without affecting helmet position or function by simply removing or cutting the straps that hold it to the helmet, thus allowing

easy access to the airway (**FIGURE 29-28**). A patient who is involved in full-contact sports may be wearing bulky pads to protect various body regions, such

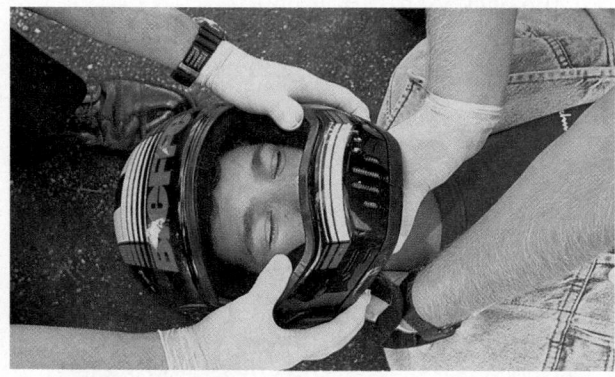

**FIGURE 29-27** A full-face helmet, such as this motorcycle helmet, should be removed from the patient.

© Jones & Bartlett Learning. Courtesy of MIEMSS.

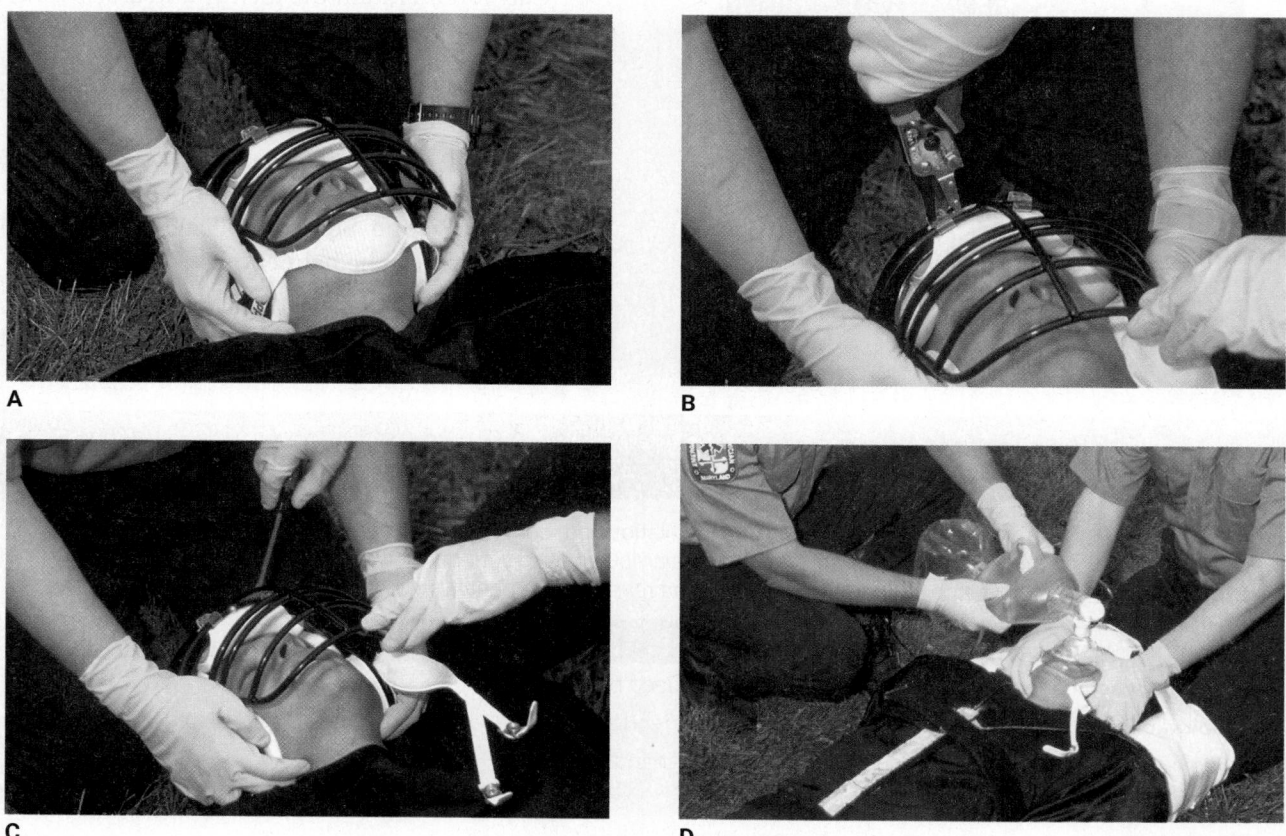

**FIGURE 29-28** The mask on most sports helmets can be removed without affecting helmet position or function.
**A.** Stabilize the patient's head and helmet. Remove the face mask in one of two ways: **B.** Use a trainer's tool designed for cutting retaining clips, or **C.** Unscrew the retaining clips from the face mask. **D.** After the face mask is removed, the helmet can be immobilized against the backboard and a bag-mask device can be used effectively.

**A-D:** © Jones & Bartlett Learning. Courtesy of MIEMSS.

as shoulder pads. Leaving a helmet in place whenever possible is preferred because it helps the body maintain an in-line neutral position. If the helmet is removed, be sure to remove the shoulder pads also or to provide padding to compensate for the shoulder pads and maintain in-line positioning of the body.

## Preferred Method

Removing a helmet should always be at least a two-person job; however, the technique for helmet removal depends on the actual type of helmet worn by the patient. One EMT provides constant in-line support as the other EMT performs the various moves; you and your partner should not move at the same time. You should first consult with medical control, if possible, about your decision to remove a helmet. When you decide to do so, follow the steps in **SKILL DRILL 29-6**:

1. Begin by kneeling at the patient's head. Your partner should kneel on one side of the patient, at the shoulder area.
2. Open the face shield, if there is one, and assess the patient's airway and breathing. Remove eyeglasses if the patient is wearing them (**Step 1**).
3. Stabilize the helmet by placing your hands on either side of it, with your fingers on the patient's lower jaw to prevent movement of the head. Once your hands are in position, your partner can loosen the face strap (**Step 2**).
4. Once the strap has been loosened, your partner should place one hand on the patient's lower jaw at the angle of the jaw and the other behind the head at the occipital region. Once your partner's hands are in position, you may pull the sides of the helmet away from the patient's head (**Step 3**).
5. Gently slip the helmet halfway off the patient's head, stopping when the helmet reaches the halfway point (**Step 4**).
6. Your partner then slides his or her hand from the occiput to the back of the head. This will prevent the head from snapping back once the helmet has been completely removed (**Step 5**).
7. With your partner's hand in place, remove the helmet, and stabilize the cervical spine.
8. Apply the cervical collar, and then secure the patient to the backboard.
9. With large helmets or small patients, you may need to pad under the shoulders to prevent flexion of the neck. If shoulder pads or heavy clothing are in place, you may need to pad behind the patient's head to prevent extension of the neck (**Step 6**).

## YOU are the Provider

Your partner continues to assist the patient's ventilations while you reassess his condition and vital signs. His GCS score remains unchanged from the previous readings. You call the trauma center to give your radio report and advise the center of your estimated time of arrival.

| Recording Time:  16 Minutes | |
| --- | --- |
| **Level of consciousness** | Responsive only to deep painful stimuli |
| **Respirations** | 6 breaths/min and irregular (baseline); ventilations are being assisted |
| **Pulse** | 70 beats/min; regular and bounding |
| **Skin** | Pink, warm, and dry |
| **Blood pressure** | 188/98 mm Hg |
| **Spo$_2$** | 98% (on oxygen) |

You deliver the patient to the ED and give your verbal report to the attending physician. After further assessment and treatment in the ED, the patient is taken to radiology for a CT scan, which reveals an epidural hematoma.

**9.** What is an epidural hematoma?

## Skill Drill 29-6 Removing a Helmet

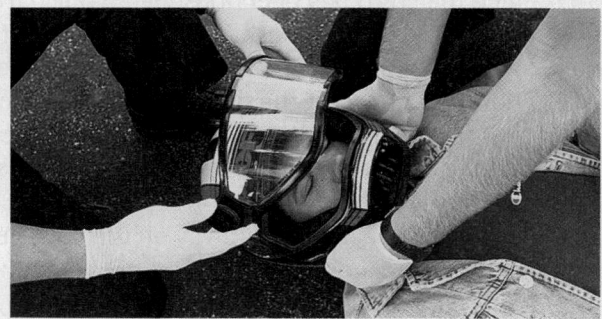

### Step 1

Kneel at the patient's head with your partner at one side. Open the face shield to assess airway and breathing. Remove eyeglasses if present.

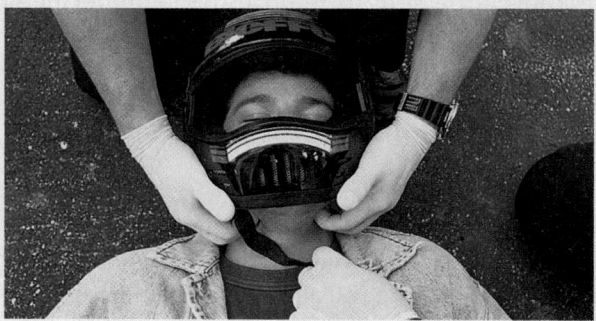

### Step 2

Prevent head movement by placing your hands on either side of the helmet and fingers on the lower jaw. Have your partner loosen the strap.

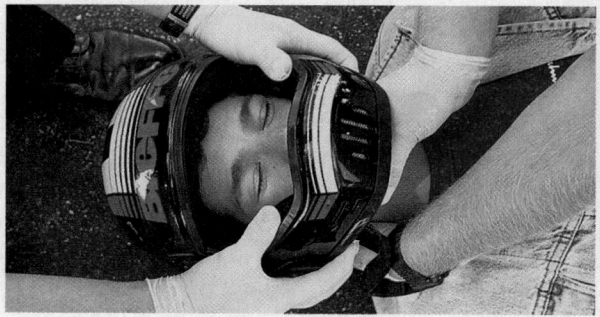

### Step 3

Have your partner place one hand at the angle of the lower jaw and the other at the occiput.

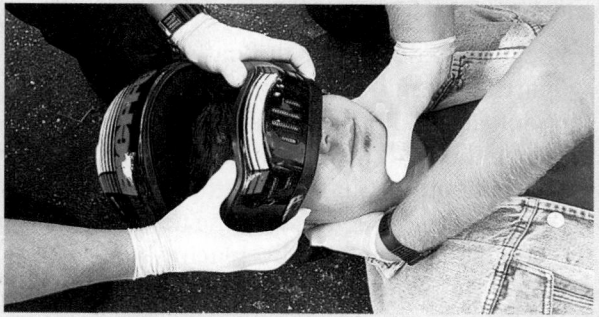

### Step 4

Gently slip the helmet about halfway off, then stop.

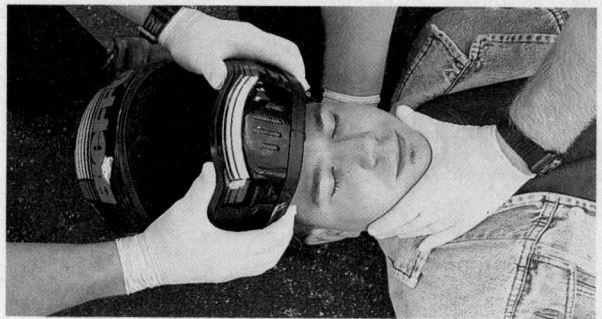

### Step 5

Have your partner slide the hand from the occiput to the back of the head to prevent the head from snapping back.

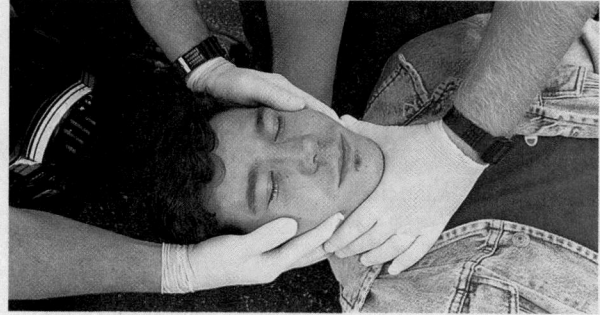

### Step 6

Remove the helmet and stabilize the cervical spine. Apply a cervical collar and secure the patient to a long backboard. Pad as needed to prevent neck flexion or extension.

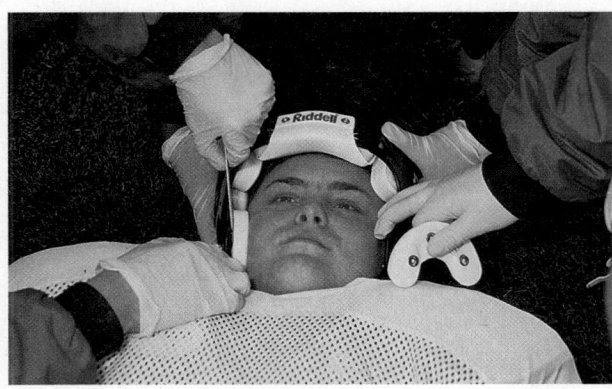

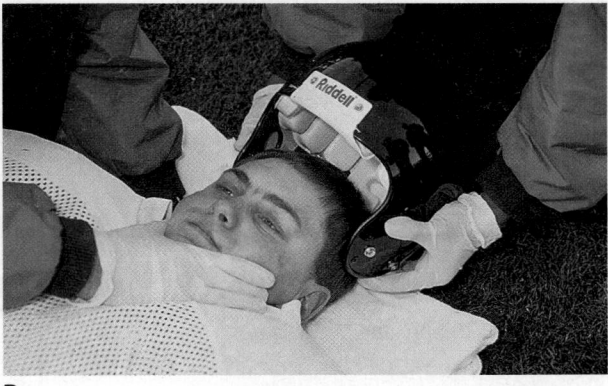

**A**    **B**

**FIGURE 29-29 A.** The jaw pads can be removed from the inside of a football helmet with the aid of a tongue depressor.
**B.** Place the fingers inside the helmet and gently rock it out of place. The person at the side controls the lower jaw with one hand and the occiput with the other. Insert padding behind the occiput to prevent neck extension.

A, B: © Jones & Bartlett Learning. Courtesy of MIEMSS.

## Alternative Method

An alternative method for removal of football helmets has also been used. The advantage of this method is that it allows the helmet to be removed with the application of less force, therefore reducing the likelihood of motion occurring at the neck. The disadvantage of this method is that it is slightly more time consuming. The first step involves removal of the chin strap. This can be cut or carefully unsnapped. Be careful during removal of the chin strap to avoid jarring the neck or head and causing excessive motion. Next, remove the face mask. The face mask is anchored to the helmet by plastic clips (loop straps) secured by screws. These can be removed with a screwdriver or cut with a knife. After the face mask has been removed, the jaw pads can be popped out of place. This can be accomplished with the use of a tongue depressor (**FIGURE 29-29A**). You can then place your fingers inside the helmet, allowing greater control of the helmet during removal as the helmet is gently rocked back off the top of the head. The person at the side of the patient controls the head by holding the jaw with one hand and the occiput with the other (**FIGURE 29-29B**). Padding is inserted behind the occiput to prevent neck extension. If the shoulder pads are in place, appropriate padding must be placed behind the head to prevent hyperextension. As with the previously described method, the person at the side of the patient's chest is responsible for making sure that the head and neck do not move during removal of the helmet.

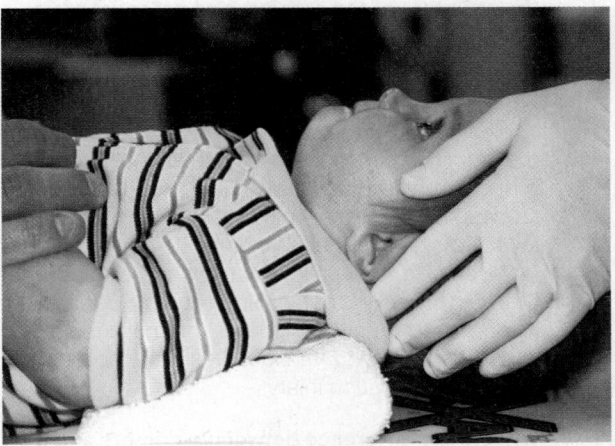

**FIGURE 29-30** Children have proportionately larger heads than adults, so you may need to place padding under the shoulders to avoid excessive flexion of the head.

© American Academy of Orthopaedic Surgeons.

Remember that small children may require additional padding to maintain the in-line neutral position. Children are not small adults. They have smaller airways and proportionately larger heads, so padding is important to maintain the airway. Pad under the shoulders to the toes, as needed, to avoid excessive neck flexion (**FIGURE 29-30**). In addition, place blanket rolls between the child and the sides of an adult-size backboard to prevent the child from slipping to one side or the other (**FIGURE 29-31**). Appropriate-size backboards are available for children.

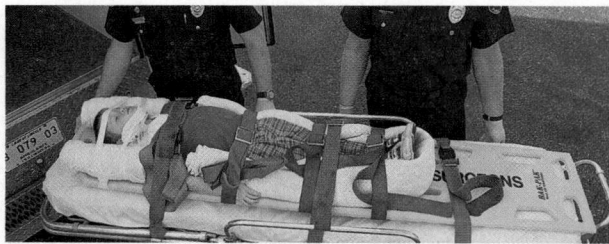

**FIGURE 29-31** Place blanket rolls between the child and the sides of an adult-size backboard to prevent the child from slipping to one side or the other.

© American Academy of Orthopaedic Surgeons.

## Special Populations

You are likely to find infants and children who have been in motor vehicle crashes and are still in their car seats. Follow your local protocols regarding spinal motion restriction techniques. See Chapter 35, *Pediatric Emergencies*, for a complete discussion of removing pediatric patients from car seats and performing spinal stabilization maneuvers.

# YOU are the Provider SUMMARY

**1. What are the potential concerns surrounding the structure of the cranium and potential brain swelling?**

The cranium does an excellent job of protecting the brain from direct trauma following minor injuries. The hard shell of the cranium provides protection for the brain from the bumps and blows that occur as a part of everyday life. However, the very fact that the cranium is a hard shell makes it a mixed blessing following a significant head injury. The cranium's rigid, unyielding structure allows little, if any, expansion of the brain if swelling or bleeding occurs. Furthermore, its hard and somewhat irregular internal surface can injure the brain and its blood vessels following significant deceleration injury.

**2. What is the difference between a primary and a secondary brain injury?**

A TBI can be classified into one of two categories: primary (direct) injury and secondary (indirect) injury.

Primary brain injury is injury to the brain and its associated structures that occurs immediately on impact to the head. It can occur following a penetrating injury, such as a stabbing or a gunshot wound, or if a bone fragment is driven into the brain following a skull fracture; however, it more commonly occurs following blunt-forcce trauma.

Secondary brain injury refers to the aftereffects of the primary head injury. It includes abnormal processes such as cerebral edema, increased ICP, cerebral ischemia and hypoxia, and infection. Secondary brain injury can occur anywhere from a few minutes to several days following the initial head injury.

**3. What are your most immediate treatment priorities for this patient?**

As with any patient, your initial treatment must focus on what will kill him or her *first*. Your patient's breathing rate and quality—slow and irregular—is not adequate and requires immediate treatment. You should instruct your partner to maintain in-line spinal position while he assists the patient's ventilations with a bag-mask device and high-flow oxygen. If a law enforcement officer is available, ask him or her to stabilize the patient's head while your partner assists his ventilations.

Consider inserting a simple airway adjunct. If the patient does not have a gag reflex, insert an oropharyngeal (oral) airway. Use of a nasopharyngeal (nasal) airway should be avoided in patients with a head injury, especially if you observe fluid drainage from the nose. This sign could indicate a mid-face fracture, in which case a nasal airway could inadvertently penetrate the brain. If a simple airway adjunct is not an option, keep the airway open with the jaw-thrust maneuver and maintain the patient's head in a neutral position.

While your partner is managing the patient's airway, you should control the bleeding from the laceration to his head. Use just enough pressure to control the bleeding; if a skull fracture is present, too much pressure could drive fractured bone fragments into his brain. Quickly scan the rest of the patient's body for any other external bleeding and control it as well. Remember the objective of the primary assessment: to find life threats, fix them, and move on.

**4. Where should you focus your secondary assessment of this patient?**

When the patient is unconscious or has experienced a significant MOI, the entire body should be assessed to look for life-threatening injuries that were not grossly apparent in the primary assessment. If immediate threats to the patient's life are found, they should be treated immediately.

Emphasis should be placed on the patient's head and face because this area appears to be where the patient experienced the most injury. Assess the integrity of the skull by *gently* palpating it and noting any areas of deformity, crepitus, or instability. Although you have already bandaged the laceration on the patient's head, you should reassess the bandage to ensure that the bleeding is controlled.

Look in the ears for fluid drainage and look behind the ears for bruising (Battle sign). Fluid or blood drainage from the ears may contain CSF, which would indicate a basilar skull fracture.

Assess the size, equality, and reactivity of the patient's pupils. The nerves that control the dilation and constriction of the pupils are extremely sensitive to increased ICP. Normally, both pupils should briskly constrict when a light is shone into either of the eyes. Pupils that are sluggish (slow) to react could indicate early increased ICP and/or cerebral hypoxia. Unequal or bilaterally fixed and dilated (blown) pupils are later, more ominous signs of increased ICP and indicate pressure on one or both oculomotor nerves. Also observe if there is any sign of blood in the eyes or bruising under the eye orbits (raccoon eyes—another sign of potential basilar skull fracture).

Palpate the facial bones for stability and note any deformities or crepitus.

Patients with a significant head injury should also be assumed to have a cervical spine injury until proven otherwise. Blunt-force trauma that is significant enough to render the patient unconscious could easily fracture a cervical vertebra. Palpate the cervical spine for obvious deformities and then apply a cervical collar. Manually stabilize the patient's head until other spinal motion restriction precautions have been completed (eg, cervical collar, backboard, scoop stretcher, or other spinal motion restricting devices).

Your secondary assessment of *any* critically injured patient should not take long. Address only life-threatening injuries and remain focused on preparing the patient for immediate transport.

**5. What is this patient's GCS score?**

Your patient opens his eyes in response to painful stimuli; therefore, you should assign a score of 2 for eye opening. He is making unrecognizable sounds; therefore, you should assign a score of 2 for verbal response. You noted that his arms were flexed and drawn in toward his body (decorticate posturing); therefore, you should assign a score of 3 for motor response. Based on these findings, the patient's current GCS score is 7, which indicates a severe TBI.

**6. What is the likely explanation for the patient's vital signs?**

Your patient's current vital signs represent a classic trio of findings in patients with a TBI and increased ICP. Hypertension, bradycardia, and irregular respirations—called Cushing triad—indicate significant cerebral edema and increased ICP.

A predictable response of the injured brain is swelling; this causes cerebral edema and a decrease in cerebral perfusion pressure (CPP) because there is little room in the cranium for the brain to swell, causing compression of cerebral blood vessels and decreased blood flow. In an attempt to maintain cerebral blood flow, and thus CPP, arterial blood pressure increases, which presents with hypertension, and the cerebral blood vessels attempt to dilate against the exterior pressure from compression of the vessels. Bradycardia occurs as a reflex response to the increase in the patient's blood pressure.

Pressure on the respiratory centers of the brainstem causes a variety of abnormal respiratory patterns. Irregular respirations—slow or fast—are the third component of Cushing triad. Cheyne-Stokes respirations are characterized by a pattern of rapid breathing (tachypnea), followed by slow breathing (bradypnea) and periods of apnea. Central neurogenic hyperventilation is characterized by deep, rapid breathing; this pattern is similar to Kussmaul respirations, but without an acetone breath odor. Biot respirations, also called ataxic respirations, are characterized by an irregular rate, pattern, and depth of breathing with intermittent periods of apnea.

**7. What further treatment is indicated for this patient?**

Continue to ensure adequate oxygenation and ventilation, and take steps to decrease the ICP and maximize cerebral blood flow.

Continue to assist the patient's ventilations; however, do *not* hyperventilate him. Hyperventilation with high-flow oxygen constricts the blood vessels in the brain, and although this *may* cause a slight decrease in the ICP, it also pushes oxygenated blood away from the brain, potentially causing a decrease in CPP and further brain injury.

Consider elevating the head of the backboard to a 30° angle to reduce the ICP. However, elevating the backboard greater than 30° may cause blood (and oxygen) to leave the brain by gravity, thus causing a decrease in cerebral perfusion, and should be avoided.

Notifying the receiving facility early is critical in the treatment of a patient with a TBI. Report your findings, any treatment that you provided, the patient's response to your treatment, and your estimated time of arrival. This will allow the receiving facility adequate time to prepare to receive the patient.

**8. What should you specifically monitor this patient for during transport?**

The importance of reassessing the brain-injured patient cannot be overemphasized.

Patients with increased ICP commonly vomit and experience seizures. Be prepared to turn the patient to the side and suction the patient's airway if vomiting occurs. If the patient experiences a seizure, continue to assist his ventilations and do not attempt to restrain him.

Carefully and frequently monitor the patient's vital signs, specifically the blood pressure and oxygen saturation. A *single* episode of hypotension (a systolic blood pressure of less than 90 mm Hg) in the adult with a TBI is associated with a significant increase in mortality because it causes a decrease in cerebral perfusion. A *single* drop in the patient's oxygen saturation to below 90% is also associated with a significant increase in mortality; ensure the continual delivery of high-flow oxygen and adequate ventilation!

Frequently reassess the patient's GCS score and pupils and observe for signs of brain herniation. If directed by local protocol or online medical control, ventilate the patient at a rate of 20 breaths/min if signs of brain herniation are observed.

If possible, request an ALS ambulance at the scene to assist with airway management or seizure control as needed, if it does not delay your scene time, or consider an ALS intercept during transport, if it does not cause a delay in transport. The most important intervention for the patient with a TBI, however, is to rapidly transport the patient to a definitive care facility as soon as possible.

**9. What is an epidural hematoma?**

Your patient has an epidural hematoma, which is an accumulation of blood between the skull and dura mater. An epidural hematoma is almost always the result of a blow to the head that produces a fracture of the thin temporal bone (recall that the patient had a compressed area over the temporal region of his skull). The middle meningeal artery courses along the groove in the temporal bone, so it is susceptible to laceration or rupture when the temporal bone is fractured. When this occurs, brisk arterial bleeding will result in rapidly progressing symptoms. The patient with an epidural hematoma typically has an immediate loss of consciousness; this may be followed by a brief return of consciousness (lucid interval), after which the patient's level of consciousness rapidly declines and he or she manifests with signs and symptoms of increasing ICP. *This is consistent with how your patient presented.*

## EMS Patient Care Report (PCR)

| Date: 1-13-20 | Incident No.: 012609 | Nature of Call: Head injury | | Location: 147 Scottie Dr. | |
|---|---|---|---|---|---|
| Dispatched: 0220 | En Route: 0221 | At Scene: 0225 | Transport: 0236 | At Hospital: 0245 | In Service: 0256 |

### Patient Information

**Age:** 22
**Sex:** M
**Weight (in kg [lb]):** 155 lb (70 kg)

**Allergies:** Unknown
**Medications:** Unknown
**Past Medical History:** Unknown
**Chief Complaint:** Head injury; decreased LOC

### Vital Signs

| Time: 0230 | BP: 190/104 | Pulse: 60 | Respirations: 6 | Spo$_2$: 94% |
|---|---|---|---|---|
| Time: 0236 | BP: 192/100 | Pulse: 64 | Respirations: 6 | Spo$_2$: 96% |
| Time: 0241 | BP: 188/98 | Pulse: 70 | Respirations: 6 | Spo$_2$: 98% |

### EMS Treatment (circle all that apply)

Oxygen @ _15_ L/min via:    (Assisted Ventilation)    Airway Adjunct    CPR

NC    NRM    (Bag mask)

Defibrillation    (Bleeding Control)    (Bandaging)    Splinting    Other: (Full spinal motion restriction)

### Narrative

EMS dispatched to a nightclub for a male patient who was assaulted.

Chief Complaint: Head injury; decreased LOC

History: En route, law enforcement personnel, who were present at the scene, advised that the patient was struck on the side of the head with a baseball bat and was unconscious.

Assessment: On arrival at the scene, found the patient, a 22-year-old man, lying supine on the ground; a large pool of blood was under his head. He was motionless and his breathing appeared slow and irregular. Manual cervical-spine stabilization was initiated immediately and the patient's airway was opened with the jaw-thrust maneuver. Primary assessment revealed that he was responsive only to deep painful stimuli. His airway was clear of secretions or foreign bodies, his breathing was slow and irregular, and he was bleeding from a large laceration to the temporal region of his skull.

Treatment (Rx): The patient's gag reflex was intact, so an oral airway was not inserted. A nasal airway was avoided because of the potential for occult skull fracture. Patient's ventilations were assisted with a bag-mask and high-flow oxygen, and bleeding from the scalp laceration was controlled with a light pressure dressing.

Secondary assessment revealed no gross trauma to the rest of the body. Assessment of the head revealed a depression over the area of the laceration. Pupils were bilaterally dilated and sluggish to react to light. There was no evidence of Battle sign or fluid drainage from the ears or nose. Facial bones were stable. Initial GCS score of 7 was assigned (eye opening, 2; verbal response, 2; motor response, 3).

Engine Company 4 arrived to provide assistance.

Transport: Established full spinal motion restriction, loaded patient into ambulance, and began transport. EMR from assisting engine company drove the ambulance because of patient care demands that required two EMTs. En route to the hospital, reassessed vital signs and elevated the head end of the backboard to a 30° angle. Continued to assist ventilations at a rate of 10 breaths/min and noted that ventilations consistently produced adequate chest rise. Oxygen saturation remained greater than 95%. Notified trauma center of the patient's condition and estimated time of arrival. Reassessment revealed no change in patient's condition; he remained responsive only to deep painful stimuli and his GCS score remained at 7. Pupils remained bilaterally dilated and sluggish to react to light. Delivered patient to emergency department and gave verbal report to attending physician. EMS cleared the hospital and returned to service at 0256.

**End of report**

# Prep Kit

## Ready for Review

- The nervous system of the human is divided into two anatomic parts: the CNS and the PNS.
- The CNS is composed of the brain and the spinal cord; the PNS includes a network of nerve fibers, like cables, that transmit information between the body's organs and the brain.
- The CNS is well protected by bony structures; the brain is protected by the skull, and the spinal cord is protected by the bones of the spinal column.
- The CNS is also covered and protected by three layers of tissue called the meninges. The layers are called the dura mater, the arachnoid, and the pia mater.
- A head injury is a traumatic injury to the head that may result in injury to soft tissue, bony structures, or the brain.
- A TBI is a severe head injury that can be a life threat or leave the patient with life-altering injuries.
- The cervical, thoracic, and lumbar portions of the spinal column can be injured through compression such as in a fall, unnatural motions such as overextension from trauma, pulling forces such as from a hanging, or a combination of mechanisms. Each of these may also cause injury to the spinal cord encased in these regions of bone, causing permanent neurologic injury or death.
- Motor vehicle crashes, direct blows, falls from heights, assault, and sports injuries are common causes of spinal injury. A patient who has experienced any of these events may have also sustained a head injury.
- Treat the patient with a head injury according to three general principles that are designed to protect and maintain the critical functions of the CNS: establish an adequate airway, control bleeding, and reassess the patient's baseline level of consciousness.
- Treat the patient with a spinal injury by maintaining the airway while keeping the spine in proper alignment, assess respirations, and give supplemental oxygen.
- In those situations in which your patient has problems with the XABCs or has other conditions for which you decide rapid transport to the hospital is needed, immediate spinal restriction precautions and quick loading into the ambulance may be indicated. Reduction of on-scene time and recognition of a critical patient increases the patient's chances for survival or a reduction in the amount of irreversible damage.
- Infants and young children are more susceptible to shock. Provide oxygen, monitor the airway, treat for shock, and provide immediate transport.
- Older people are at higher risk for a subdural hematoma developing. Signs and symptoms of the condition may not occur for several hours, days, or weeks. Be sure to get a thorough history of any previous trauma.

## Vital Vocabulary

**anterograde (posttraumatic) amnesia**  Inability to remember events after an injury.

**axial loading injuries**  Injuries in which load is applied along the vertical or longitudinal axis of the spine, which results in load being transmitted along the entire length of the vertebral column; for example, falling from a height and landing on the feet in an upright position.

**basilar skull fractures**  Fractures that usually occur following diffuse impact to the head (eg, falls, motor vehicle crashes); generally result from extension of a linear fracture to the base of the skull and can be difficult to diagnose with a radiograph.

**Battle sign**  Bruising behind an ear over the mastoid process that may indicate a skull fracture.

**central neurogenic hyperventilation** An abnormal breathing pattern associated with increased ICP that is characterized by deep, rapid breathing; this pattern is similar to Kussmaul respirations, but without an acetone breath odor.

**cerebral edema** Swelling of the brain.

**closed head injury** Injury in which the brain has been injured but the skin has not been broken and there is no obvious bleeding.

**concussion** A temporary loss or alteration of part or all of the brain's abilities to function without actual physical damage to the brain.

**coup-contrecoup injury** A brain injury that occurs when force is applied to the head and energy transmission through brain tissue causes injury on the opposite side of original impact.

**epidural hematoma** An accumulation of blood between the skull and the dura mater.

**eyes-forward position** A head position in which the patient's eyes are looking straight ahead and the head and torso are in line.

**four-person log roll** The recommended procedure for moving a patient with a suspected spinal injury from the ground to a long backboard or other spinal precaution device.

**intervertebral disks** Tough, elastic structures between adjoining vertebrae that act as shock absorbers.

**intracerebral hematoma** Bleeding within the brain tissue (parenchyma) itself; also referred to as an intraparenchymal hematoma.

**intracranial pressure (ICP)** The pressure within the cranial vault.

**involuntary activities** Actions of the body that are not under a person's conscious control.

**linear skull fractures** Fractures that commonly occur in the temporoparietal region of the skull and that are not associated with deformities to the skull; account for 80% of skull fractures; also referred to as nondisplaced skull fractures.

**meninges** Three distinct layers of tissue that surround and protect the brain and the spinal cord within the skull and the spinal canal.

**open head injury** Injury to the head often caused by a penetrating object in which there may be bleeding and exposed brain tissue.

**primary (direct) injury** An injury to the brain and its associated structures that is a direct result of impact to the head.

**raccoon eyes** Bruising under the eyes that may indicate a skull fracture.

**retrograde amnesia** The inability to remember events leading up to a head injury.

**secondary (indirect) injury** The aftereffects of the primary injury; includes abnormal processes such as cerebral edema, increased intracranial pressure, cerebral ischemia and hypoxia, and infection; onset is often delayed following the primary brain injury.

**subarachnoid hemorrhage** Bleeding into the subarachnoid space, where the cerebrospinal fluid circulates.

**subdural hematoma** An accumulation of blood beneath the dura mater but outside the brain.

**traumatic brain injury (TBI)** A traumatic insult to the brain capable of producing physical, intellectual, emotional, social, and vocational changes.

**voluntary activities** Actions that we consciously perform, in which sensory input or conscious thought determines a specific muscular activity.

## References

1. Alson R, Copeland D. Long backboard use for spinal motion restriction of the trauma patient. International Trauma Life Support website. https://www.itrauma .org/wp-content/uploads/2014/07/SMR-Resource -Document-FINAL-Publication-6-28-14.pdf. Published 2014. Accessed April 1, 2020.

2. Frequently asked questions. Brain Trauma Foundation website. https://www.braintrauma.org/faq. Accessed April 2, 2020.

3. National Association of Emergency Medical Technicians. *PHTLS: Prehospital Trauma Life Support*. 9th ed. Burlington, MA: Jones & Bartlett Learning; 2019.

4. National Association of State EMS Officials. *National EMS Scope of Practice Model 2019*. Washington, DC: National Highway Traffic Safety Administration; February 2019. Report No. DOT HS 812-666. https://www.ems .gov/pdf/National_EMS_Scope_of_Practice_Model_2019. pdf. Accessed April 1, 2020.

5. *National Emergency Medical Services Education Standards*. US Department of Transportation. National Highway Traffic Safety Administration. DOT HS 811 077A. January 2009. www.ems.gov/pdf/811077a.pdf. Accessed April 1, 2020.

6. *National Emergency Medical Services Education Standards. Emergency Medical Technician Instructional Guidelines*. US Department of Transportation. National Highway Traffic Safety Administration. DOT HS 811 077C. January 2009. www.ems.gov/pdf/811077c.pdf. Accessed April 1, 2020.

7. National Registry of Emergency Medical Technicians. *2015 Paramedic Psychomotor Competency Portfolio (PPCP)*. Columbus, OH: National Registry of Emergency Medical Technicians; 2015.

8. Psychomotor exams. National Registry of Emergency Medical Technicians website. https://www.nremt.org /nremt/about/psychomotor_exam_emt.asp. Accessed March 27, 2020.

9. TBI-related deaths. Centers for Disease Control and Prevention website. Reviewed March 29, 2019. Accessed April 2, 2020.

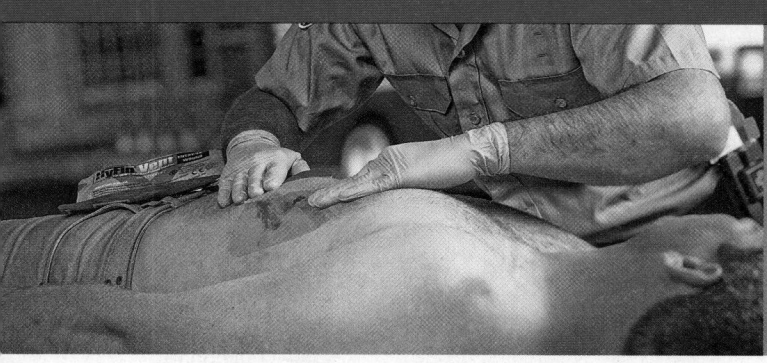

# Chapter 30

# Chest Injuries

## NATIONAL EMS EDUCATION STANDARD COMPETENCIES

### Trauma

Applies fundamental knowledge to provide basic emergency care and transportation based on assessment findings for an acutely injured patient.

### Chest Trauma

Recognition and management of
- Blunt versus penetrating mechanisms (pp 1095–1097, 1102–1110)
- Open chest wound (pp 1095–1096)
- Impaled object (pp 1095–1096)

Pathophysiology, assessment, and management of
- Blunt versus penetrating mechanisms (pp 1095–1102)
- Hemothorax (pp 1097–1102, 1105)
- Pneumothorax (pp 1102–1105)
  - Open (pp 1102–1104)
  - Simple (p 1104)
  - Tension (pp 1104–1105)
- Cardiac tamponade (pp 1105–1107)
- Rib fractures (p 1107)
- Flail chest (pp 1107–1108)
- Commotio cordis (p 1109)

## KNOWLEDGE OBJECTIVES

1. Explain the mechanics of ventilation in relation to chest injuries. (pp 1094–1095)
2. Describe the differences between an open and closed chest injury. (pp 1095–1096)
3. Recognize the signs of chest injury. (pp 1096–1097)
4. Describe the management of a patient with a suspected chest injury, including pneumothorax, hemothorax, cardiac tamponade, rib fractures, flail chest, pulmonary contusion, traumatic asphyxia, blunt myocardial injury, commotio cordis, and laceration of the great vessels. (pp 1102–1110)
5. Recognize the complications that can accompany chest injuries. (pp 1102–1110)

6. Explain the complications of a patient with an open pneumothorax (sucking chest wound). (pp 1102–1104)
7. Differentiate between a pneumothorax (open, simple, and tension) and a hemothorax. (pp 1102–1105)
8. Describe the complications of cardiac tamponade. (pp 1105–1107)
9. Describe the complications of rib fractures. (p 1107)
10. Describe the complications of a patient with a flail chest. (pp 1107–1108)

## SKILLS OBJECTIVES

1. Describe the steps to take in the assessment of a patient with a suspected chest injury. (pp 1097–1102)
2. Demonstrate the management of a patient with a sucking chest wound. (pp 1103–1104)

## Introduction

EMTs commonly encounter chest injuries. According to the Centers for Disease Control and Prevention (CDC), chest trauma causes more than 1.2 million emergency department (ED) visits in the United States annually. Given the location of the heart, lungs, and great blood vessels within the chest cavity, potentially serious injuries may occur. Chest injuries may be the result of blunt trauma, penetrating trauma, or both. Blunt trauma may occur from motor vehicle crashes or falls. Penetrating trauma may be due to shootings, stabbings, or other mechanisms, such as industrial or construction incidents.

Any injury that interferes with breathing must be treated without delay to minimize or prevent permanent damage to tissues that depend on a continuous supply of oxygen. Another major problem with chest injuries may be internal bleeding. Blood from lacerations of the thoracic organs or major blood vessels can collect in the chest cavity, compressing the lungs or heart. This may also occur when air collects in the chest and prevents the lungs from expanding. Your ability to act quickly to care for patients with these injuries can make the difference between a successful outcome and death.

This chapter begins with a review of the anatomy of the chest and the physiology of respiration. It then describes the common signs and symptoms of chest injuries and the proper emergency medical treatment for specific injuries.

## Anatomy and Physiology

To understand and evaluate chest injuries in the prehospital setting, you must first understand the anatomy of the chest and the mechanism by which gases are exchanged during breathing. A quick review will help you understand the logic in the emergency treatment of chest injuries and the potential complications of that treatment.

A key point to remember is the difference between ventilation and oxygenation. Ventilation is the body's ability to move air in and out of the chest and lung tissue. This is described in the section on mechanics of ventilation. Any injury that affects the patient's ability to move air in and out of the chest is serious and may be life threatening. Oxygenation is the process of delivering oxygen to the blood by

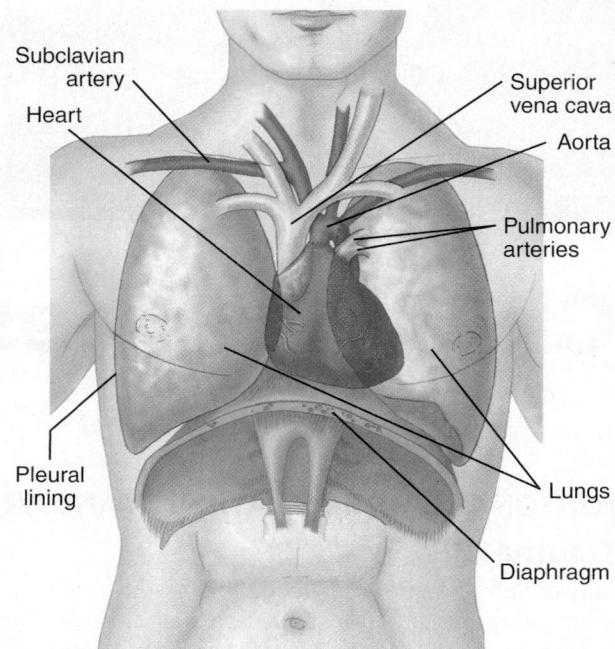

**FIGURE 30-1** A view of the anterior aspect of the chest shows the major organs beneath the surface.

© Jones & Bartlett Learning.

diffusion from the alveoli following inhalation into the lungs. Oxygen must be delivered to the cells, and carbon dioxide (a waste product of cell function) must be removed from the body for proper organ system function.

The chest (thoracic cage) extends from where the neck and chest meet to the diaphragm (**FIGURE 30-1**). In a person who is lying supine or who has just completed exhalation, the diaphragm may rise as high as the nipple line. Thus, a penetrating injury to the chest, such as a gunshot or stab wound, may also penetrate the lung and diaphragm and injure the liver, spleen, or stomach.

The skin, muscle, and bones of the thoracic region have some unique features to allow for the ventilation process. Just under the normal three layers of skin, the epidermis, dermis, and subcutaneous layers, lies striated, or skeletal muscle. This muscle extends between the ribs, forming the intercostal muscles. These muscles, innervated from the spinal nerves originating in the lower cervical or upper thoracic region, contract to expand the rib cage during inhalation. In very young children, the intercostal muscles are not yet developed. Children therefore tend to breathe with their diaphragm,

Anterior

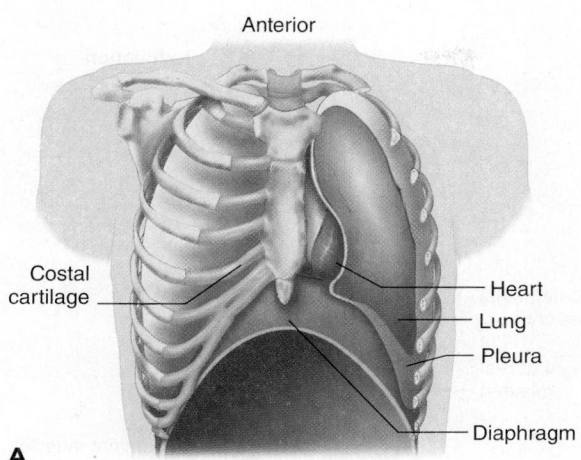

Posterior

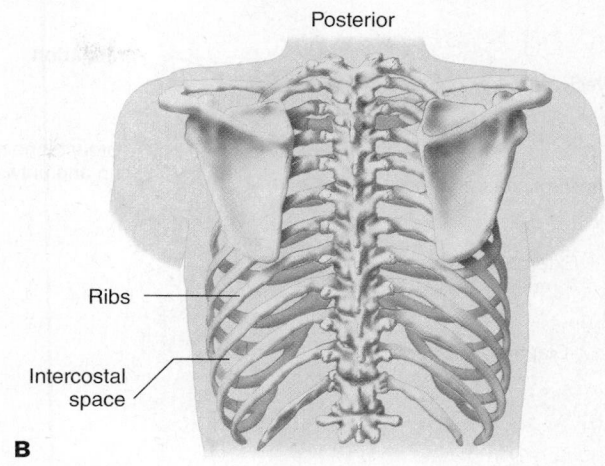

Costal
cartilage

Heart

Lung

Pleura

Diaphragm

**A**

Ribs

Intercostal
space

**B**

**FIGURE 30-2** The organs within the chest are protected by the ribs, which are connected in front (**A**) to the sternum and in back (**B**) to the vertebrae.

**A, B:** © Jones & Bartlett Learning.

referred to as belly breathing, which is normal for their age group.

Lying on the inferior and slightly posterior part of each rib is the neurovascular bundle, composed of a network of nerves, arteries, and veins. When punctured by fractured ribs, bleeding from these vessels can cause a hemothorax. The ribs themselves create a protective and functional cage around the vital organs. Each side of the chest (hemithorax) contains lung tissue that is separated into lobes. The right lung has three lobes, and the left lung has two lobes. The left lobe formation allows space for the heart to reside; this is called the cardiac notch. A thin membrane called the pleura covers each of the lungs and the thoracic cavity. The inner chest wall has a lining called the parietal pleura, and a lining called the visceral pleura covers the lung. Between these two linings is a small amount of pleural fluid that allows the lungs to move freely against the inner chest wall as a person breathes. Pleural fluid also creates surface tension to allow the lungs to adhere to the rib cage, thus allowing the mechanics of ventilation to occur.

The contents of the chest are partially protected by the ribs, which are connected in the back to the vertebrae and in the front, through the costal cartilages, to the sternum (**FIGURE 30-2**). The trachea, in the middle of the neck, divides into the left and right mainstem bronchi, which supply air to the lungs. The thoracic cage also contains the heart and the great vessels: the aorta, the right and left subclavian arteries and their branches, the pulmonary arteries, and the superior and inferior venae cavae. The esophagus runs through the back of the chest, connecting the pharynx above with the stomach and the abdomen below. The esophagus, trachea, and great vessels lie in the mediastinum, a cavity or space centrally located in the thorax. At the bottom of the chest, the diaphragm is a muscle that separates the thoracic cavity from the abdominal cavity.

## YOU are the Provider

At 1020 hours, you are dispatched to 7100 Douglas Avenue for a man with a chest injury. The caller is unsure what has occurred but reports that the address is a construction site. You respond to the scene, which is located about 5 miles away.

**1.** What major organs and structures lie within the chest cavity?

**2.** What injuries commonly result from blunt chest trauma? Penetrating chest trauma?

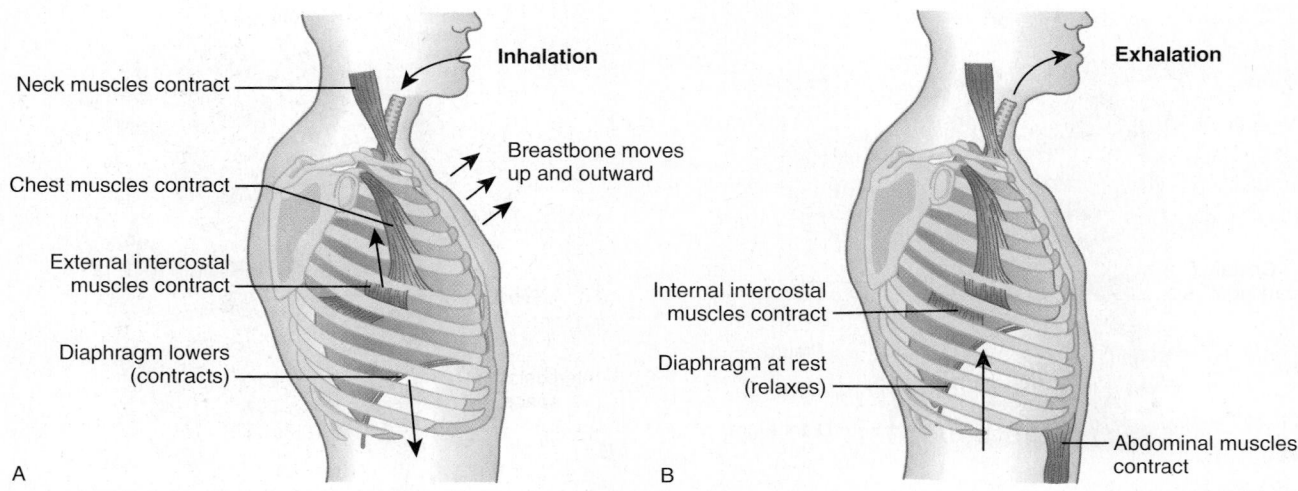

**FIGURE 30-3** The mechanics of inhalation (**A**) and exhalation (**B**).

# Mechanics of Ventilation

When you inhale, the intercostal muscles between the ribs contract, elevating and expanding the rib cage. At the same time, the diaphragm contracts or flattens, increasing the inferior-superior diameter of the chest. The intrathoracic pressure inside the chest decreases, creating a negative pressure differential. Air then enters the lungs through the nose and mouth, which is the path of least resistance from the ambient air space to the upper and lower airway. When you exhale, the intercostal muscles and diaphragm relax, and the tissues move back to their normal positions, forcing the air out, referred to as exhalation (**FIGURE 30-3**). In a normal respiratory system, relaxation of the thoracic muscles and the diaphragm is a relatively passive function. When you are assessing the patient, you should be able to recognize when there is an increase in the work of breathing and equate that with respiratory distress.

Note that the nerves supplying the diaphragm (the phrenic nerves) exit the spinal cord at C3, C4, and C5. Refer to Chapter 6, *The Human Body*, for a review of the spinal column. A patient whose spinal cord is injured below the C5 level may lose the power to move the intercostal muscles, but the diaphragm should still be able to contract. The patient will still be able to breathe because the phrenic nerves remain intact, but the injury may cause belly breathing. Patients with spinal cord injuries at C3 or above can lose their ability to breathe entirely (**FIGURE 30-4**).

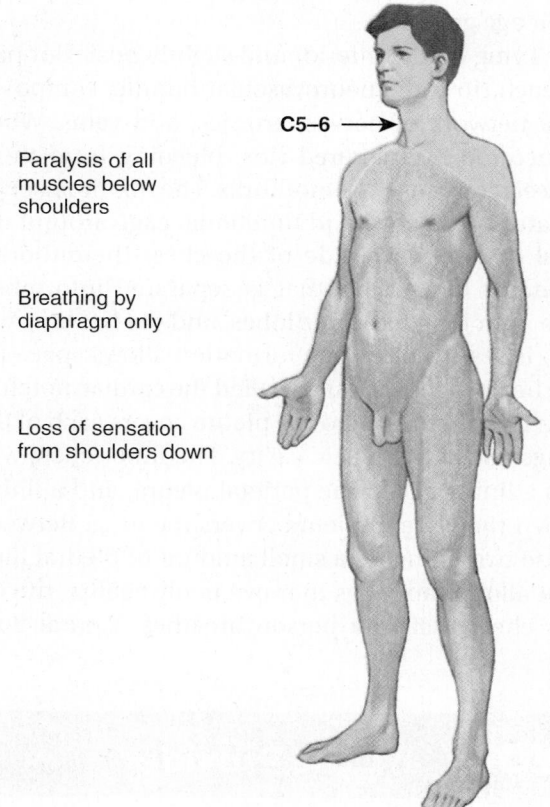

C5–6

Paralysis of all muscles below shoulders

Breathing by diaphragm only

Loss of sensation from shoulders down

**FIGURE 30-4** A patient who sustains a spinal cord injury below the level of C5 and is paralyzed can still breathe spontaneously because the phrenic nerves, which cause the diaphragm to contract, originate at the C3, C4, and C5 levels.

Tidal volume is the amount of air moved into or out of the lungs during a single breath (discussed further in Chapter 11, *Airway Management*). The average tidal volume is approximately 500 mL. If you multiply this amount of air by the number of breaths/min, the result is called the minute ventilation or minute volume. Changing either of these numbers (increasing or decreasing the rate or volume) affects the amount of air moving through the system. For example, if you ventilate a patient with 500 mL at the normal rate of 12 breaths/min, then the minute volume is 6,000 mL (6 L). If you increase the ventilation rate by four extra breaths per minute, then the minute volume increases to 8,000 mL (8 L). Conversely, if the amount of tidal volume decreases, then the minute volume will drop.

This information is important because if the patient is only able to inhale small amounts of air (in the case of a chest injury), the patient will need to exceed the normal respiratory rate of 12 to 20 breaths/min to make up the difference in the minute volume. Remember that the average bag-mask device consists of a self-inflating bag that contains 1,000 to 1,500 mL of air. This device can quickly overinflate the lungs, causing gastric distention, and impair the function of the lungs. Overventilation can also increase intrathoracic pressure (pressure inside the chest), reducing venous return to the chest and secondarily reducing cardiac output. It can also potentially worsen chest injuries such as pneumothorax. In addition, there is the risk of causing acid–base imbalance by blowing off too much carbon dioxide if the rate of artificial ventilation is too high.

## Injuries of the Chest

Recall the discussion of kinematics in Chapter 25, *Trauma Overview*. There are two basic types of chest injuries: open and closed. As the name implies, a closed chest injury is one in which the skin is not broken. This type of injury is generally caused by blunt trauma, such as when a person strikes a steering wheel or an airbag in a motor vehicle crash, is struck by a falling object, or is struck in the chest by some object during a fight (**FIGURE 30-5**). These types of injuries often cause significant contusions in both the cardiac muscle (cardiac contusion) and the lung tissue (pulmonary contusion), thus impairing the function of those organs.

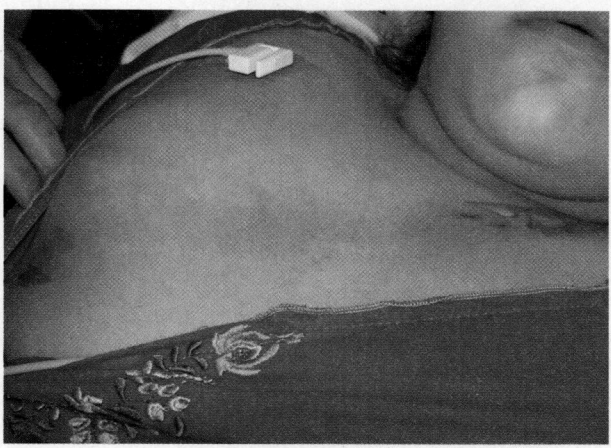

**FIGURE 30-5** Closed chest injuries usually result from blunt trauma, such as when a patient strikes the steering wheel or an airbag in a motor vehicle crash, or is struck by a falling object. A closed chest injury can occur even when a seat belt is worn.

Courtesy of ED, Royal North Shore Hospital/NSW Institute of Trauma & Injury.

If the heart is damaged in this manner, it may not be able to refill with blood or blood may not be pumped with enough force out of the heart, creating a form of inadequate tissue oxygenation called cardiogenic shock. Any bruising of the lung tissue may result in the affected alveoli not functioning. This impairment can cause a decrease in available oxygen (hypoxia) and an increase in carbon dioxide in the blood (hypercarbia). Rib fractures create sharp broken bone ends that can lacerate lung tissue and cause further vessel damage with every movement of the chest wall. This type of bleeding can be hidden from external view and rapidly lead to hypovolemic shock.

An open chest injury is generally caused by penetrating trauma. Some objects, such as a knife, a bullet, a piece of metal, or the broken end of a fractured rib, penetrate the chest wall itself (**FIGURE 30-6**). The damage occurring from this type of trauma typically is instant. However, the symptoms of these injuries may take time to develop as the damaged vessels continue to bleed or the lung collapses from a puncture that results in an expanding pneumothorax. Occasionally, the object that penetrates and creates an open chest injury remains in place. This is referred to as an impaled object. When you have a patient with an impaled object, do not attempt to move or remove the object because it may be occluding the hole in the vessel that has been punctured. Removing the object can lead to severe

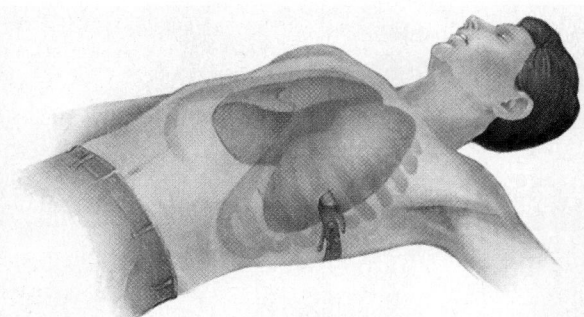

**FIGURE 30-6** Open chest injuries can occur when an external object or the broken end of a fractured rib penetrates the chest wall.

© Jones & Bartlett Learning.

bleeding. Another reason not to remove the impaled object from the chest is that the objects that cause tissue damage on entry will likely cause damage on removal, resulting in further injury. The removal is best left for the surgeon. Any alteration from this standard should come directly from online medical control.

In blunt trauma, a blow to the chest may fracture the ribs, the sternum, or whole areas of the chest wall, bruise the lungs and the heart, and even damage the aorta. Almost one-third of people who are killed immediately in car crashes die as a result of traumatic rupture of the aorta when it is torn from its attachment to the chest cavity. Although the skin and chest wall are not penetrated in a closed injury, broken ribs may lacerate the contents of the chest. Damage to the chest wall structures may impair patients' ability to ventilate on their own.

## Street Smarts

If the patient's oxygen saturation was normal initially and begins to drop rapidly, suspect tension pneumothorax and immediately communicate your suspicions to the team. This life threat must be treated rapidly by a paramedic or physician. Rapid transport or intercept with an advanced life support (ALS) unit is essential.

## Signs and Symptoms of Chest Injury

Important signs and symptoms of chest injury include the following:

- Pain at the site of injury
- Pain localized at the site of injury that is aggravated by or increased with breathing
- Bruising to the chest wall
- Crepitus (the sensation felt when broken bone ends grind together) with palpation of the chest
- Any penetrating injury to the chest

## YOU are the Provider

You arrive at the scene and ensure it is safe. You are directed to the patient by a coworker. The patient, a 19-year-old man, was struck in the left side of the chest by a piece of lumber that was thrown from a piece of equipment operated by a coworker. You find the patient sitting on the ground; he is conscious and alert, but restless and is experiencing respiratory distress. He tells you that it hurts to take a breath.

| Recording Time: 0 Minutes | |
|---|---|
| **Appearance** | Restless; obvious respiratory distress |
| **Level of consciousness** | Conscious and alert, but restless |
| **Airway** | Open; clear of secretions and foreign bodies |
| **Breathing** | Increased rate; labored |
| **Circulation** | Radial pulses strong and rapid; skin is pink and moist; no obvious external bleeding |

Your partner applies high-flow oxygen via nonrebreathing mask as you perform a secondary assessment. The patient denies any other injuries, and coworkers confirm that he did not lose consciousness.

**3.** How should you proceed with your secondary assessment?

- Dyspnea (difficulty breathing, shortness of breath)
- Hemoptysis (coughing up blood)
- Failure of one or both sides of the chest to expand normally with inspiration
- Rapid, weak pulse and low blood pressure
- Cyanosis around the lips or fingernails
- Diminished breath sounds on one side
- Low oxygen saturation

After a chest injury, any change in normal breathing is a particularly important sign. A healthy, uninjured adult usually breathes at a rate from 12 to 20 breaths/min without difficulty and without pain. The chest should rise and fall in a symmetric pattern with each breath. Respirations of fewer than 10 breaths/min or of more than 20 breaths/min may indicate inadequate breathing. Patients with chest injuries often have tachypnea (rapid respirations) and shallow respirations because it hurts to take a deep breath. Shallow breathing or chest wall trauma may interfere with the actual ability to move air. Check the respiratory rate and see if there is actual air movement from the mouth and/or nose. This is best accomplished through visualizing the chest wall for rise and fall.

As with any other injury, pain and tenderness are common at the point of impact as a result of a bruise or fracture. The normal process of breathing usually aggravates pain. Irritation or damage to the pleural surfaces causes a characteristic sharp or sticking pain with each breath when these normally smooth surfaces slide on one another. This sharp pain is called *pleuritic pain* and is typical of chest injuries.

In an injured patient, dyspnea, or difficulty breathing, has many causes, including airway obstruction, damage to the chest wall, poor chest expansion because of the loss of normal control of breathing, or lung compression because of accumulated blood or air in the chest cavity.

Hemoptysis, the spitting or coughing up of blood, usually indicates that the lung itself or the air passages have been damaged. With a laceration of the lung tissue, blood can enter the bronchial passages and is coughed up as the patient tries to clear the airway.

A rapid, weak pulse and low blood pressure are the principal signs of hypovolemic shock, which can result from extensive bleeding from lacerated structures within the chest cavity. Shock following a chest injury may also result from insufficient oxygenation of the blood by the poorly functioning lungs, from an increase in intrathoracic pressure from air or blood in the chest, or from direct injury to the heart itself.

Cyanosis in a patient with a chest injury is a sign of inadequate respiration. The classic blue or ashen gray appearance around the lips and fingernails indicates that blood is not being oxygenated sufficiently. Patients with cyanosis are unable to provide a sufficient supply of oxygen to the blood through the lungs and require immediate ventilation and oxygenation.

Many of these signs and symptoms occur simultaneously. When any one of these develops as a result of a chest injury, the patient requires prompt hospital care.

## Patient Assessment

### Scene Size-Up

As you arrive on the scene, observe for hazards and threats to the safety of the crew, bystanders, and the patient. Ensure that the police are on scene at incidents involving violence, such as assaults or gunshot wounds. Begin the encounter with scene safety as the highest priority. If you determine the power company, fire department, or advanced life support (ALS) units are needed, call for them early.

Ensure that you and your crew take standard precautions; at a minimum, put on gloves and eye protection. Because of the color of blood and the fact that it easily soaks through clothing, you can often identify patients with bleeding as you approach the scene. However, darker clothing may mask signs of bleeding, so you must remain vigilant when the mechanism of injury (MOI) suggests the patient may be bleeding.

As you observe the scene, look for indicators and significance of the MOI. This helps you develop an early index of suspicion for underlying injuries in a patient who has sustained a significant

### Words of Wisdom

Airbags can cause significant chest injuries in patients who are not wearing seat belts. Maintain a high degree of suspicion for severe injuries in unrestrained patients when an airbag has deployed.

MOI. Chest injuries are common in motor vehicle crashes, falls, industrial incidents, and assaults. Determine the number of patients and consider spinal stabilization.

## Primary Assessment

During your primary assessment, you must quickly identify and treat potential life threats and determine priority of patient care and transport. Life-threatening hemorrhage, when present, should be addressed immediately, even before airway concerns.

As you approach, note the patient's level of consciousness. Responsive patients may be able to tell you their chief complaint. Note not only what they say, but also how they say it. Difficulty speaking may indicate several problems, and chest injury is an important one. Perform a rapid physical examination of the patient. Look for obvious injuries, the appearance of blood, and difficulty breathing. Look for cyanosis, irregular breathing, and chest rise and fall on only one side. The initial general impression will help you develop an index of suspicion for serious injuries and determine your sense of urgency for medical intervention. A good question to ask yourself is, "How sick is this patient?" Patients with significant chest injuries will look sick and are often frightened or anxious. Keep in mind that you are rapidly searching for life threats and you will repeat the physical examination in a more detailed manner later in the assessment if time and patient condition allow.

Addressing life threats begins with the assessment of airway and breathing unless life-threatening uncontrolled bleeding is seen. Ensure that the patient has a clear and patent airway. Normal breathing should be effortless, and any deviation from this pattern should be cause for concern. How you assess and manage the airway depends a great deal on whether you suspect a spinal injury. Be suspicious,

## Words of Wisdom

Be sure to assess the neck before applying the cervical collar. Jugular vein distention cannot be observed after the collar is applied. The presence of jugular vein distention may indicate tension pneumothorax (significant ongoing air accumulation in the pleural space) or pericardial tamponade, an injury to the heart that results in blood accumulating in the pericardial sac.

and protect the spine early in your care if indicated. Further measures to ensure spinal motion restriction can be performed after you have secured the XABCs and completed your secondary assessment.

Once you have determined the patient has a patent airway, determine whether breathing is present and adequate. With chest injuries, begin by inspecting for DCAP-BTLS, and look for equal expansion of the chest wall. Listen with a stethoscope to each side of the chest. Absent or decreased breath sounds on one side usually indicate significant damage to a lung, preventing it from expanding properly. Be alert to the pattern of symmetric rise and fall of the patient's chest wall. If the chest wall does not expand on each side when the patient inhales, the chest muscles may have lost their ability to work appropriately. Loss of muscle function may be the result of a direct injury to the chest wall, or it may be related to an injury of the nerves that control those muscles. Check for **paradoxical motion**, an abnormality associated with multiple fractured ribs, in which one segment (often referred to as a flail segment) of the chest wall moves opposite the rest of the chest—that is, out with expiration and in with inspiration.

If you determine the patient has penetrating trauma, address this life threat at once. This condition may interfere with the normal mechanics of breathing and can cause the patient's condition to worsen quickly. For quick initial care, you can use your gloved hand to occlude an open chest wound. When further dressings can be applied, use a **vented chest seal** or an **occlusive dressing** for all penetrating injuries to the chest. An occlusive dressing should be taped on three sides. Leaving one side open allows air to escape but not enter the chest. Apply oxygen with a nonrebreathing mask at 15 L/min. Provide positive-pressure ventilation with 100% oxygen if breathing is inadequate based on the patient's level of consciousness and breathing rate and quality. Positive-pressure ventilation is important for the patient with a flail chest that compromises ventilation. Be diligent with auscultation of breath sounds, and evaluate the effectiveness of your ventilatory support with signs of circulation to the skin. Be aware of decreasing oxygen saturation ($Spo_2$) values because they may indicate the development of hypoxia. Watch for signs of an impending tension pneumothorax, such as increasingly poor compliance during ventilation (difficulty delivering breaths to the patient). If you believe a tension pneumothorax has developed in a patient with an open chest wound, the occlusive dressing should be burped (briefly removed to allow air to escape) and then placed back over the wound.

### Words of Wisdom

Penetrating wounds on the patient's back are easy to miss. Be sure to assess both the anterior surface and the posterior surface of the chest so you do not miss a potentially lethal wound.

Assess the patient's pulse. Determine whether it is present and adequate. If the pulse is too fast or too slow, or if the skin is pale, cool, or clammy, consider your patient to be in shock. Note that because skin paleness can be difficult to detect in patients with dark skin, you may need to check for pale mucous membranes inside the inner lower eyelid or slow capillary refill. You need to treat aggressively to reverse the cause of shock and support the patient's circulatory system. In the early stage of shock, the body compensates for blood loss by increasing the heart rate. Be alert for this change, especially if tachycardia is still present beyond a few minutes after the initial adrenaline rush from the incident or injury. External bleeding may or may not be significant, but if it is considered life threatening, address this threat immediately. Bleeding inside the chest can be significant and, as discussed earlier, can be a quick cause of death. Control external bleeding with direct pressure and a bulky trauma dressing.

Priority patients are considered patients who have a problem with their XABCs. Sometimes the priority is obvious, and the decision to transport quickly is also easy. At other times, what is happening outside the body may not provide obvious clues to the seriousness of what is happening inside the body. Pay attention to subtle clues such as the appearance of the skin, level of consciousness, or a sense of impending doom in the patient. When you find signs of poor perfusion or inadequate breathing, transport quickly and perform the remainder of the assessment en route to the ED. A delay on the scene to perform a lengthy assessment will reduce your patient's chances of survival. With chest injuries, when in doubt, transport rapidly to a trauma center. **TABLE 30-1** lists the "deadly dozen" chest injuries.

**TABLE 30-1** Deadly Dozen Chest Injuries

1. Airway obstruction
2. Bronchial disruption
3. Diaphragmatic tear
4. Esophageal injury
5. Open pneumothorax
6. Tension pneumothorax
7. Massive hemothorax
8. Flail chest
9. Cardiac tamponade
10. Thoracic aortic dissection (leakage from a traumatic aneurysm of the portion of the aorta that lies within the chest)
11. Myocardial contusion
12. Pulmonary contusion

© Jones & Bartlett Learning.

## History Taking

Once you have identified and treated life threats, you can gather the patient's history. If you have not yet done so, determine and investigate the patient's chief complaint and further investigate the MOI. Identify any associated signs and symptoms and pertinent negatives. If the patient was assaulted with a blunt object such as a bat, further evaluate the spinal region for injury because the force may have been transferred through the body from the point of impact. If the patient fell from a great height and is reporting chest discomfort or dyspnea, this may distract the patient from recognizing that he or she has fractures or is bleeding from the extremities. Palpation of the chest will typically cause direct pain at the site of the fracture. When a patient reacts to the pain, be certain to verify where the pain was located relative to the area being touched.

Pertinent negatives when examining the chest include no associated shortness of breath, no rapid breathing, no absent or abnormal breath sounds, and no areas of deformity or abnormal movement. In a patient with a suspected spinal cord injury, equal expansion of the chest and movement of the rib cage and the diaphragm can confirm that there is nerve conduction to that region of the body.

A basic evaluation of signs and symptoms, allergies, medications, pertinent medical history, including respiratory or cardiovascular disease, and last oral intake should be completed when time allows. The events leading to the emergency should also be identified. Questions about the events surrounding the incident should focus on the MOI: the speed of the vehicle or height of the fall, the use of safety equipment such as a helmet, airbag, seat belt, or life jacket, the type of weapon used, the number of penetrating wounds, and so on. A SAMPLE history can be obtained quickly in most situations and can certainly be obtained while accomplishing other tasks. However, if the patient has a loss of consciousness, it will no longer be possible to obtain the information directly. Interviewing witnesses briefly in these circumstances is important.

## Secondary Assessment

In a patient who has an isolated injury to the chest with a limited MOI, such as in a stabbing, you should focus your assessment on the isolated injury, the patient's chief complaint, and the body region affected. Ensure that wounds are identified and that any bleeding is controlled. Note the location and extent of the injury. Assess all underlying systems. Examine the anterior and posterior aspects of the chest wall, and be alert to changes in the patient's ability to maintain adequate respirations.

It is important in patients with a chest injury not to focus only on a chest wound. With significant trauma, you should quickly assess the entire patient from head to toe. If there is significant trauma (such as a blunt trauma or gunshot wound) likely affecting multiple systems, start with a rapid physical examination of the body, looking for DCAP-BTLS to determine the nature and extent of thoracic injury. This examination will help to determine all injuries and the extent of these injuries. Inspection or visualization of the region looking for deformities, such as asymmetry of the left and right sides of the chest or shoulder girdle, may reveal the presence of multiple rib fractures, crush injuries, or significant chest wall injury. Identification of discrete areas of contusion or abrasion may pinpoint a specific point of impact. The presence of puncture wounds or other penetrating injuries indicates a possible open chest injury that should be managed accordingly. Be alert for burns that encircle the chest, which may alter respiratory mechanics. Palpate for tenderness to localize the injury and the presence of fractures. Look for lacerations and local swelling. Application of this systematic approach to patient assessment minimizes the chance of missing a significant injury.

Once you have stabilized the XABCs and have checked the patient from head to toe to identify injuries, obtain a baseline set of vital signs. This activity should include assessment of pulse, respirations, blood pressure, skin condition, oxygen saturation, and pupils. Each of these is considered a sign indicating how your patient is tolerating the injuries. Consider these signs as a window to the functioning of the vital organs. This baseline set of vital signs will be used to evaluate changes in the patient's condition. Because patients with chest injury have so much potential for rapid deterioration,

## YOU are the Provider

Your secondary assessment reveals bruising and crepitus on the left side of the chest and diminished breath sounds over that same side; no paradoxical chest wall movement is noted. The trachea is midline, and the jugular veins are nondistended. Abdominal exam is unremarkable. Your partner takes the patient's vital signs and reports them to you.

| Recording Time: 5 Minutes | |
| --- | --- |
| **Respirations** | 24 breaths/min; labored |
| **Pulses** | 110 beats/min; strong and regular |
| **Skin** | Pink, warm, and moist |
| **Blood pressure** | 138/88 mm Hg |
| **Oxygen saturation (SpO$_2$)** | 95% (on oxygen) |

**4.** On the basis of your assessment findings, what injury or injuries should you suspect?

**5.** How should you proceed with your treatment of this patient?

they should be reevaluated every 5 minutes. This will allow you to quickly recognize changes in the vital sign numbers or trends.

## Special Populations

In older patients with reduced bone density or more fragile bones, even minor trauma to the chest wall can cause significant injury to the underlying tissues and organs. Older patients may have also sustained several fractures to the rib cage. Be alert for these injuries and for signs and symptoms of respiratory compromise, even in lower-energy MOIs. Older patients also have a decreased amount of physiologic reserve and are likely to decompensate more quickly following an injury.

If you find an accelerated pulse rate or respiratory rate, the chest injury may be causing either a decrease in available oxygen (hypoxia) or blood loss that results in a decreased number of red blood cells that can carry oxygen (hypoxemia). The increased respiratory rate is often associated with an obvious increase in work of breathing. This can be identified by noting increased use of the accessory muscles in the face, neck, and chest to assist in the movement of air. In the later stages of injuries, the pulse rate can slow as the myocardium becomes starved for oxygen and the body is no longer able to keep up with the demands. The respiratory rate may drop as the brain becomes starved for oxygen and overloaded with carbon dioxide and other waste products. These are usually signs of impending cardiopulmonary arrest. In the case of increasing pressure on the heart from air in the pleural space or blood in the pericardial space, the blood pressure may exhibit a narrowing pulse pressure as the systolic and diastolic pressures come closer together. This is a result of the inability of the heart to fill with an adequate volume of blood and contract normally.

## Reassessment

The reassessment identifies how your patient's condition is changing. It should focus on repeating the primary assessment, reassessing the chief complaint, and reassessing interventions performed. Reevaluate the patient's airway, breathing, pulse, perfusion, and bleeding. Has breathing improved now that the wound is sealed, or has it become more difficult? If assisting ventilations with a bag-mask device, is it becoming increasingly difficult to deliver breaths to the patient? Other interventions should also be assessed to determine if they are effective. For example, are pulse oximeter values rising now that the patient is receiving oxygen? Reassess vital signs and compare them to vital signs taken earlier. Vital signs are a snapshot in time. Reassessing them frequently allows you to trend the patient's status and determine if the patient is compensating versus decompensating. Many chest injuries will worsen during transport to the hospital because of the seriousness of the injuries. An astute reassessment will help identify worsening conditions in a timely manner so that they can be addressed.

Provide appropriate spinal motion restriction of any patient who has blunt trauma with suspected spinal injuries. If the patient's shortness of breath is worsened in the supine position, place the patient in a position of comfort by elevating the head if necessary while still maintaining spinal motion restriction (**FIGURE 30-7**). Maintain an open airway, be prepared to suction the patient, and consider an oropharyngeal or nasopharyngeal airway. Whenever you suspect significant bleeding, provide high-flow oxygen. If needed, provide assisted ventilation using a bag-mask device with high-flow oxygen. If significant bleeding is visible, you must control the bleeding. If you find penetrating trauma to the chest wall, place a vented chest seal or semiocclusive dressing over the wound. Be prepared to provide positive-pressure ventilation if the patient's efforts are not effective. If the patient

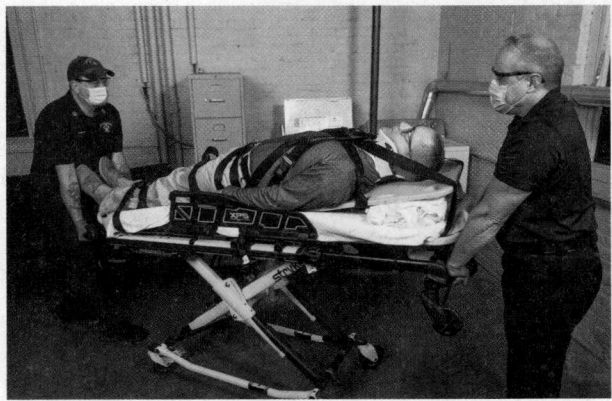

**FIGURE 30-7** Spinal motion restriction with a supine patient.

© Jones & Bartlett Learning.

has signs of hypoperfusion, treat aggressively for shock and provide rapid transport to the appropriate hospital. Do not delay transport of a seriously injured trauma patient to complete non–life-saving treatments such as splinting extremity fractures; instead, complete these types of treatments en route to the hospital.

Communicating with hospital staff early when your patient has a significant MOI to the chest can help them be prepared with appropriate equipment and personnel when you arrive. If a penetrating injury is present, describe it in your report, along with what you have done to care for it. Your documentation should be complete and thorough. Describe all injuries and the treatment given. Remember, your documentation is your legal record of what happened.

## Special Populations

In young children, the rib cage is very flexible and does not provide the same level of protection that the adult rib cage provides. This flexibility can allow any significant injury or compression of the rib cage to be masked because the ribs give way to the pressure and do not fracture. Because the ribs do not fracture, which would help dissipate the force from the blunt object, the force transfers more directly to the organs beneath the ribs. It is important to remember that the organs that underlie the rib cage have been exposed to that force and are likely injured. This flexibility of the ribs may result in fractures that are hidden on examination, and the only indication you may have of compromise is increased work of breathing or alterations in vital signs. This age group is often injured in pedestrian or bicycle collisions that involve vehicles. In car-versus-pedestrian crashes, children often turn toward the vehicle instead of away as adults do, thus resulting in direct impact to the chest by the bumper or hood. Children also may not be cognizant of height or distances and, therefore, may be prone to falls from distances greater than twice their height, resulting in severe trauma.

## Complications and Management of Chest Injuries
### PPE in Chest Injuries

Movement of air out of an open chest wound can aerosolize droplets from the lung. If the patient is at risk for a communicable respiratory virus, extra PPE precautions are needed. When treating these patients, providers should wear an N95 mask, eye protection including goggles or face shield, a gown, and gloves. The unit needs to be thoroughly decontaminated after these calls if there is any ongoing suspicion of COVID-19 or other respiratory virus in the commmunity.

## Pneumothorax

In any chest injury, damage to the heart, lungs, great vessels, and other organs in the chest can be complicated by the accumulation of air in the pleural space. This is a dangerous condition called a **pneumothorax** (commonly called a collapsed lung). In this condition, air enters through a hole in the chest wall or the surface of the lung as the patient attempts to breathe, causing the lung on that side to collapse (**FIGURE 30-8**). As a result, any blood that passes through the collapsed portion of the lung is not oxygenated, and hypoxia can develop. If the lung is collapsed past 30% to 40%, you may hear

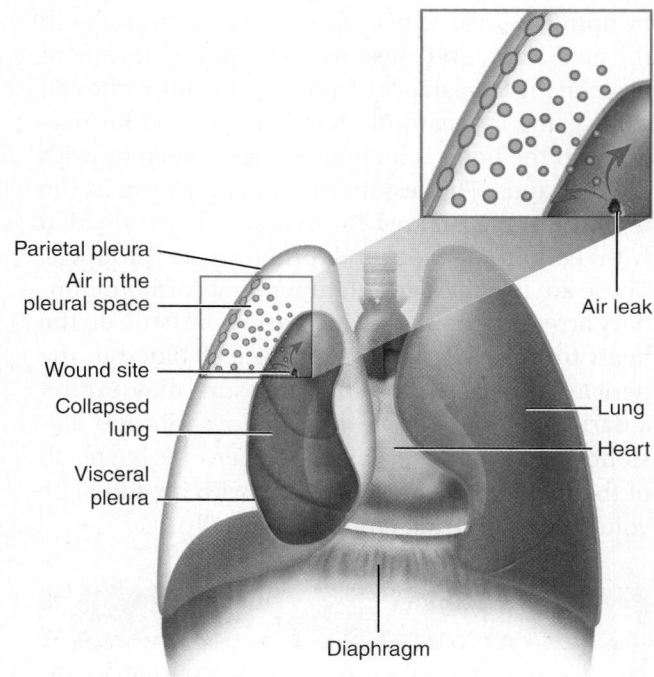

**FIGURE 30-8** Pneumothorax occurs when air leaks into the space between the pleural surfaces from an opening in the chest wall or the surface of the lung. Air in the pleural space causes the lung to collapse.

© Jones & Bartlett Learning.

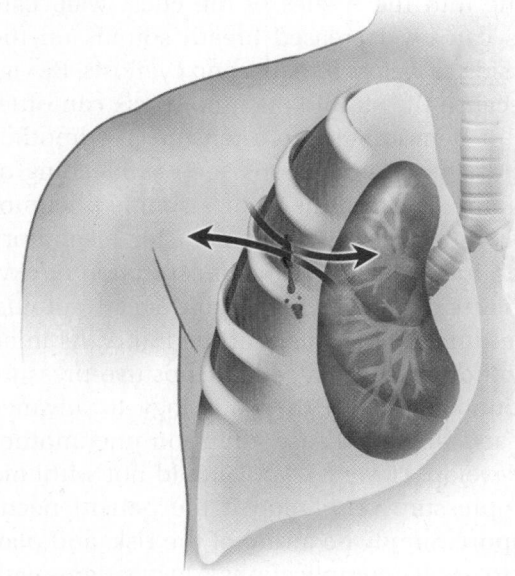

**FIGURE 30-9** With a sucking chest wound, air passes from the outside into the pleural space and back out with each breath, creating a sucking sound.

© Jones & Bartlett Learning.

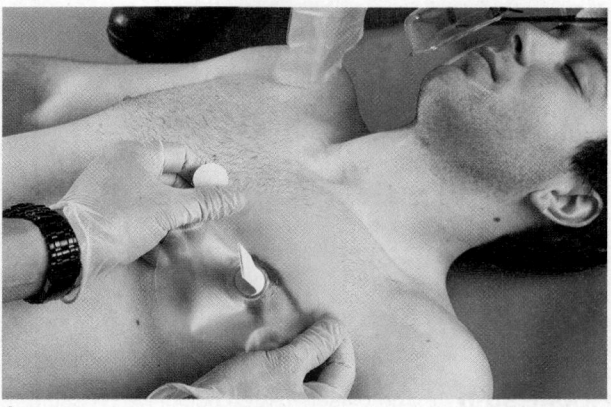

**A**

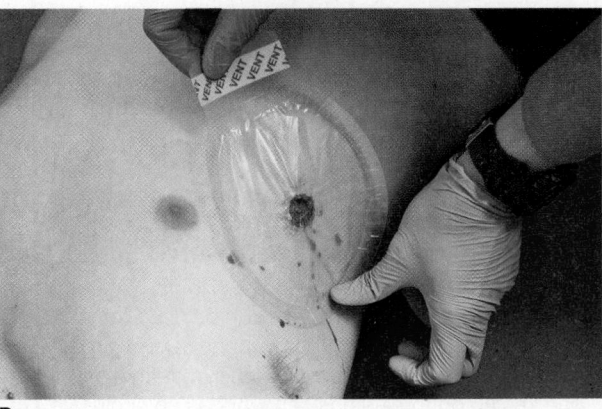

**B**

**FIGURE 30-10** A commercial occlusive dressing may be used to seal all four sides of a sucking chest wound. **A.** An Asherman Chest Seal, which is vented. **B.** A HALO Chest Seal, which is unvented.

A, B: © Jones & Bartlett Learning.

diminished breath sounds on that side of the chest. Absent breath sounds are a significant finding in chest trauma and may indicate the development of a tension pneumothorax, discussed later. Depending on the size of the hole and the rate at which air fills the cavity, the lung may collapse in a few seconds or a few hours. In the uncommon situation when the hole is in the chest wall, you may hear a sucking sound as the patient inhales and the sound of rushing air as he or she exhales. For this reason, an open or penetrating wound to the chest wall is often called an open pneumothorax or a sucking chest wound (**FIGURE 30-9**).

This type of injury is a true emergency requiring immediate emergency medical care and transport. Initial emergency care, after clearing and maintaining the airway and then providing oxygen, is to rapidly seal the open wound with a vented chest seal or semiocclusive dressing. The purpose of the dressing is to seal the wound and prevent air from being sucked into the pleural space through the wound. Vented chest seals are designed to allow air to escape through the dressing but not be sucked back in, thus preventing the development of a pneumothorax. If a vented chest seal is not available, an occlusive dressing can be used. Vented chest seal dressings contain a one-way valve, called a flutter

valve, that allows air to leave the chest cavity but not return (**FIGURE 30-10**). Follow local protocol and the manufacturer's guidelines if you use such a dressing. An occlusive dressing without a flutter valve may be taped to the patient on three sides of the dressing, allowing air to leak from the fourth side (**FIGURE 30-11**). Regardless of which type of dressing you carry, use a dressing that is large enough so that it is not pulled or sucked into the chest cavity.

Careful observation is required after placing an occlusive dressing. The occlusive seal or a clot in the injury may allow a tension pneumothorax to develop. If signs of a tension pneumothorax develop, it is suggested that the occlusive dressing be partially removed to allow air to escape and to then be resecured. You may hear a sudden release of air

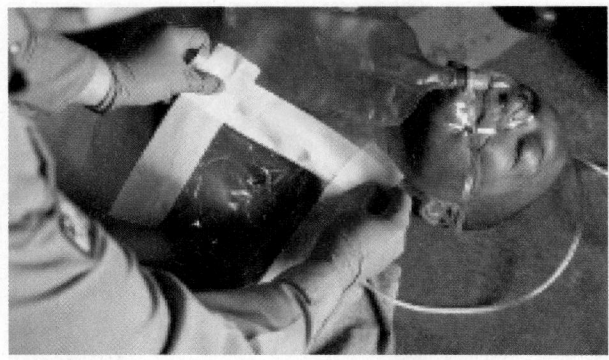

**FIGURE 30-11** An improvised vented occlusive dressing seals three sides of a sucking chest wound, with the fourth left open to allow air to escape.

© Jones & Bartlett Learning.

pressure when you remove one side of the dressing. This situation can develop even after a flutter valve has been applied.

> ### Words of Wisdom
>
> When a vented chest seal is not available, plastic wrap, foil, or petrolatum gauze can be used for the semiocclusive dressing. If the wound is very large and no suitable material is available, a defibrillation pad sealed on three sides can work as an occlusive dressing. When you use an occlusive dressing to seal an open chest wound, record the type of material used and any changes noted afterward: skin color, vital signs, breath sounds, and particularly the patient's level of anxiety.

## Simple Pneumothorax

Any pneumothorax that does not result in major changes in the patient's cardiac physiology is referred to as a simple pneumothorax. These are commonly the result of blunt trauma that results in fractured ribs. As in the spontaneous pneumothorax, the simple pneumothorax is often difficult to diagnose. The lung has to collapse significantly before the effects will be heard as decreased breath sounds. The more common findings are similar to those of other types of pneumothoraces: pleuritic chest pain; dyspnea or increased work of breathing exhibited as increased rate; tachypnea and accessory muscle use; and decreasing oxygen saturation on the pulse oximeter. Another sign of pneumothorax can be a crackling sensation felt on palpation of the skin (called subcutaneous emphysema), which indicates that air escaping from a lacerated lung

is leaking into the tissues of the chest wall. Late findings can be decreased breath sounds on the injured side as well as lethargy and cyanosis. Be vigilant because the simple pneumothorax can often worsen or deteriorate into a tension pneumothorax or develop complications such as bleeding or hemothorax. The treatment for a simple pneumothorax is much like any treatment for respiratory compromise; provide a high concentration of oxygen. Monitor oximeter readings and breath sounds, and treat underlying causes of the injury. As in all pneumothorax treatment, adding positive-pressure ventilation may cause the pathology to advance rapidly and possibly cause a tension pneumothorax to develop. However, you should not withhold positive-pressure ventilation if the patient needs the support. Simply be aware of the risk, and plan on how to resolve complications. Most patients with this problem require ALS intervention, so call for it early or transport rapidly to the nearest hospital or trauma center, depending on which is the fastest way to get your patient to a higher level of care.

## Tension Pneumothorax

A potential complication that may develop following chest injuries with pneumothorax is a tension pneumothorax (**FIGURE 30-12**). This can occur when there is significant ongoing air accumulation in the pleural space. This air gradually increases the pressure in the chest, first causing the complete collapse of the affected lung and then pushing the mediastinum (the central part of the chest containing the heart and great vessels) into the opposite pleural cavity. This prevents blood from returning through the venae cavae to the heart, decreasing cardiac output, causing shock, and ultimately leading to death.

Tension pneumothorax occurs more commonly as a result of closed, blunt injury to the chest in which a fractured rib lacerates a lung or bronchus. Only rarely does a tension pneumothorax arise spontaneously.

> ### Words of Wisdom
>
> The conscious, spontaneously breathing patient in whom tension pneumothorax is developing may exhibit a slower onset of signs and symptoms of tension pneumothorax. In this patient, complaints of chest pain, increasing dyspnea, and dropping oxygen saturation levels, despite administration of oxygen, may be noted before the blood pressure drops.

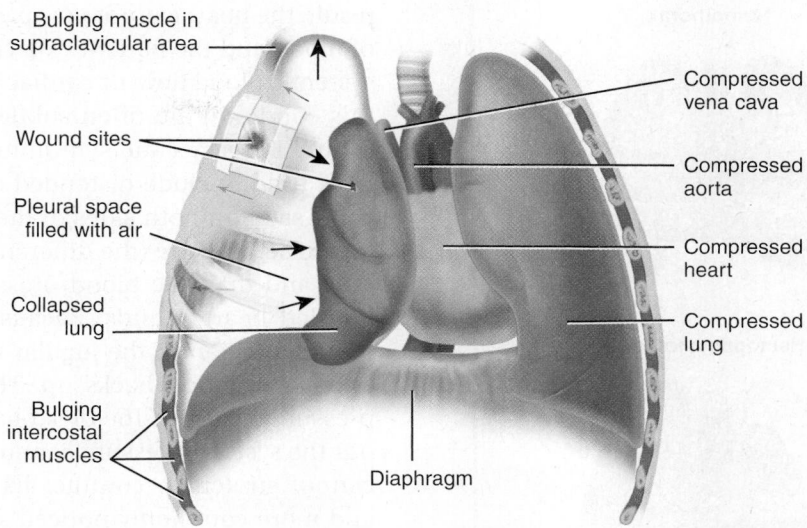

Bulging muscle in supraclavicular area

Wound sites

Pleural space filled with air

Collapsed lung

Bulging intercostal muscles

Compressed vena cava

Compressed aorta

Compressed heart

Compressed lung

Diaphragm

**FIGURE 30-12** A tension pneumothorax can develop if a penetrating chest wound is bandaged tightly and air from a damaged lung cannot escape. The air then accumulates in the pleural space, eventually causing compression of the heart and great vessels. If a dressing sealed on four sides with no vent is used, monitor for signs of tension pneumothorax developing and prepare to vent one side of the dressing.

© Jones & Bartlett Learning.

A patient with a tension pneumothorax will have chest pain, tachycardia, marked respiratory distress, low or rapidly dropping oxygen saturation, and absent or severely decreased lung sounds on the affected side, with signs of shock such as hypotension or altered mental status. The patient may also exhibit jugular vein distention, cyanosis, or tracheal deviation, but these signs are not always present. Jugular vein distention is best assessed for with the patient sitting at a 45° angle. Tracheal deviation, if seen, is a late and grave finding and is a sign that the patient requires immediate intervention.

Relieving a tension pneumothorax that is the result of blunt trauma is often done by inserting a needle through the rib cage into the pleural space, called a needle thoracotomy; however, this procedure typically is performed by ALS personnel or ED staff, depending on local protocols. A tension pneumothorax is a life-threatening condition. Be prepared to support ventilation with high-flow oxygen, and request ALS support or transport immediately to the closest hospital.

## Hemothorax

In blunt and penetrating chest injuries, blood can collect in the pleural space from bleeding around the rib cage or from a lung or great vessel. This condition is called a hemothorax (**FIGURE 30-13**). Suspect a hemothorax if the patient has signs and symptoms of shock without any obvious external bleeding or apparent reason for the shock state, or decreased breath sounds on the affected side, an indication that the lung is being compressed by the blood in the cavity. Because the bleeding is typically caused by severe damage within the chest cavity, there is virtually no way to control the bleeding in the prehospital setting. The only person who can treat this condition is often a surgeon. The presence of air and blood in the pleural space is known as a hemopneumothorax. Again, because the injury has occurred within the walls of the chest, the treatment involves providing rapid transport to the nearest facility capable of inserting a chest tube and potentially performing surgery.

## Cardiac Tamponade

Cardiac tamponade (pericardial tamponade) occurs when the pericardial sac, the space between the protective membrane around the heart (pericardium) and the heart, fills with blood or fluid, perhaps from a ruptured, torn, or lacerated coronary artery or vein (**FIGURE 30-14**). The pericardial sac can also fill with fluid as a result of cancer or an

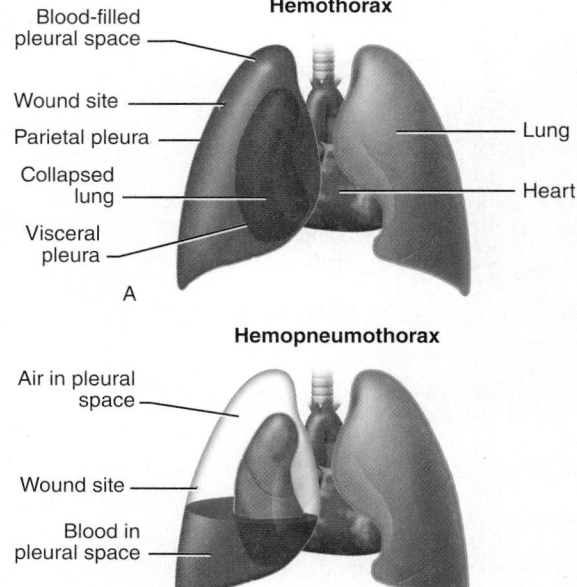

**FIGURE 30-13 A.** A hemothorax is a collection of blood in the pleural space produced by bleeding within the chest. **B.** When both blood and air are present, the condition is a hemopneumothorax.

A, B: © Jones & Bartlett Learning.

autoimmune disease such as lupus. As the amount of blood or fluid increases, the heart is less able to fill with blood during each relaxation phase. As a result, the heart cannot pump an adequate amount of blood and the patient experiences a decrease in systemic blood flow, or cardiac output. The signs of this condition are often subtle until the situation is dire. The signs and symptoms, referred to as the Beck triad, include distended or engorged jugular veins seen on both sides of the trachea, a narrowing pulse pressure (the difference between the systolic and diastolic blood pressure numbers), and muffled heart sounds. Because the heart cannot pump sufficiently, the jugular veins fill with blood and, thus, blood backs up. The narrowing pulse pressure occurs as the diastolic pressure increases but the systolic pressure cannot, because the heart cannot stretch to contract harder. An associated and more commonly noticed sign is a decrease in mental status as blood flow decreases to the brain. The heart muscle is unique in that it needs to be stretched to create a good contraction to pump blood out of the ventricles. This mechanism can fail because of tamponade and can be directly related to a decrease in blood returning to the heart.

Treatment for this condition involves recognition and supportive care. Oxygen should never be withheld from a patient who needs it; provide positive-pressure ventilation to any patient who is hypoventilating or apneic. Rapidly transport the patient to a facility that is capable of intervention.

## YOU are the Provider

The patient is placed onto the stretcher and loaded into the ambulance. While continuing to provide high-flow oxygen via nonrebreathing mask, you reassess his condition and vital signs shortly before departing the scene.

| Recording Time: 10 Minutes | |
| --- | --- |
| Level of consciousness | Conscious, but confused and restless |
| Respirations | 28 breaths/min; labored and shallow |
| Pulse | 124 beats/min; weak at the radial artery |
| Skin | Cool, clammy, and pale; cyanosis around the mouth |
| Blood pressure | 104/58 mm Hg |
| SpO$_2$ | 88% (on oxygen) |

Breath sounds are now inaudible on the entire left side of his chest, and you note that cyanosis is developing around his mouth. His jugular veins appear somewhat distended, and his trachea is midline. The closest appropriate facility is about 10 minutes away, so you instruct your partner to begin transport at once.

**6.** What is most likely happening to your patient?

**7.** Should you adjust your current treatment? If so, how?

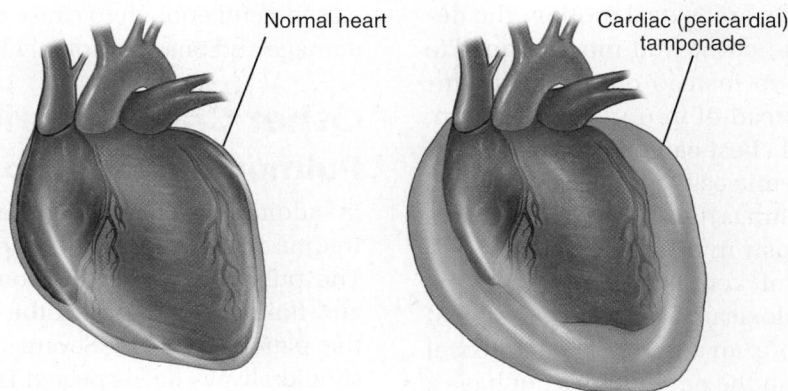

**FIGURE 30-14** Cardiac tamponade, also known as pericardial tamponade, is a potentially fatal condition in which fluid or blood builds up within the pericardial sac, causing compression of the heart's chambers and dramatically impairing its ability to pump blood to the body.

© Jones & Bartlett Learning.

## Words of Wisdom

In a trauma situation, even a small amount of fluid or blood in the pericardial sac is enough to cause fatal pericardial tamponade. Occasionally, fluid in surprisingly large amounts may collect slowly in the pericardial sac as a result of chronic medical conditions, such as cancers and autoimmune diseases or due to infection. Fluid that builds up over time is tolerated much better than fluid from injury that accumulates rapidly within the pericardial sac.

## Rib Fractures

Rib fractures are very common, particularly in older people, whose bones can be more brittle. Because the upper four ribs are well protected by the bony girdle of the clavicle and scapula, a fracture of one of these upper ribs is a sign of a substantial MOI.

Be aware that a fractured rib that penetrates into the pleural space may lacerate the surface of the lung, causing a pneumothorax, a tension pneumothorax, a hemothorax, or a hemopneumothorax.

Patients with one or more cracked ribs will report localized tenderness and pain when breathing. The pain is the result of broken ends of the fracture rubbing against each other with each inspiration and expiration. Patients will tend to avoid taking deep breaths, and their breathing will be rapid and shallow instead. They will often hold the affected portion of the rib cage to minimize the discomfort.

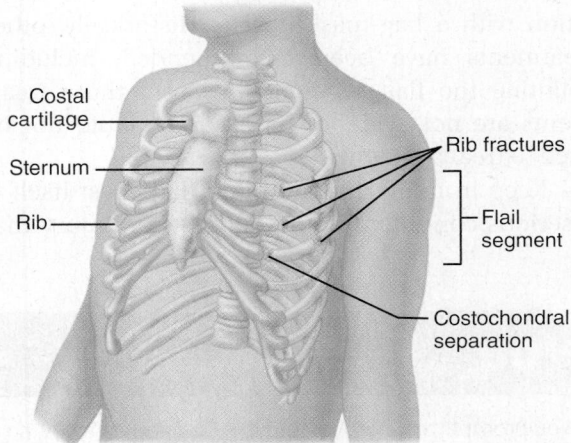

**FIGURE 30-15** When two or more adjacent ribs are fractured in two or more places, a flail chest results. A flail segment will move paradoxically when the patient breathes.

© Jones & Bartlett Learning.

Patients with rib fractures should receive supplemental oxygen during assessment and transport if they are experiencing any respiratory distress.

## Flail Chest

Ribs may be fractured in more than one place. If two or more adjacent ribs are fractured in two or more places, a segment of chest wall may be detached from the rest of the thoracic cage (**FIGURE 30-15**). This condition, known as **flail chest**, can also occur if the sternum is fractured along with several ribs. In what is called paradoxical motion, the detached portion of the chest wall moves opposite of normal: It moves in instead of out during inhalation and out instead of in during exhalation. Breathing with a flail chest can be painful and ineffective, and hypoxemia easily results as air is circulated between the lungs due to the flail segment. A flail segment seriously interferes with the body's normal mechanics of ventilation and must be treated quickly. Paradoxical motion is a late sign of flail segment; therefore, an absence of paradoxical motion does not mean the patient does not have a flail segment.

Treatment of a patient with a flail chest should include maintaining the airway, providing respiratory support if necessary, giving supplemental oxygen, and performing ongoing assessments for possible pneumothorax or other respiratory complications. Treatment may also require positive-pressure ventilation with a bag-mask device. Historically, other treatments have been recommended, including splinting the flail segment; however, these treatments are not evidence-based and should not be used to treat a patient.

Keep in mind that although flail chest itself is a serious condition, it also suggests an injury that was forceful enough to cause other serious internal damage and possible spinal injury.

## Other Chest Injuries
### Pulmonary Contusion

In addition to fracturing ribs, any severe blunt trauma to the chest can injure or bruise the lung. The pulmonary alveoli become filled with blood, and fluid accumulates in the injured area, leaving the patient hypoxic. Severe **pulmonary contusion** should always be suspected in patients with a flail chest and usually develops over a period of hours following the injury. If you believe that a patient may have a pulmonary contusion, provide supplemental oxygen and positive-pressure ventilation as needed to ensure adequate oxygenation and ventilation.

## Other Fractures

In addition to the rib fractures you have already learned about, there are other types of fractures that should be discussed.

### Sternal Fractures

Any suspected fracture of the sternum should increase your index of suspicion for injuries to the

## YOU are the Provider

You promptly call for ALS, but it is 15 minutes away, so you elect to continue treatment and transport. After reassessing the patient's condition, you call a radio report to the receiving facility.

| Recording Time: 15 Minutes | |
| --- | --- |
| Level of consciousness | Conscious, but confused and restless |
| Respirations | 28 breaths/min; labored and shallow |
| Pulse | 128 beats/min; weak at the radial artery |
| Skin | Cool and clammy; cyanosis around the mouth |
| Blood pressure | 90/60 mm Hg |
| Spo₂ | 85% (on oxygen) |

You arrive at the hospital and find a physician and nurse waiting for you in the ambulance bay. The patient is quickly taken into a treatment room, where further assessment is performed. After the physician performs a needle decompression, the patient's condition improves. After returning to service, you follow up with the hospital and learn that the patient had a tension hemopneumothorax which required a chest tube. They report the patient will likely recover after a stay in the intensive care unit.

**8.** What is a tension hemopneumothorax?

**9.** Should you attempt to distinguish a tension pneumothorax from a tension hemopneumothorax? Why or why not?

underlying organs because the amount of force required to break the sternum is significant. There may be involvement of the lungs, great vessels, and the heart.

### Clavicle Fractures

Whereas this fracture is also covered under skeletal injuries, it is important to mention here that the clavicle overlies the first rib and protects a large neurovascular bundle (nerve, artery, and vein) that can be significantly damaged or disrupted should injury to the clavicle occur. The pain, deformity, and swelling that accompany a clavicle fracture can also detract from assessment of the first and second ribs in proximity to the fracture. Suspect upper rib fractures in medial clavicle fractures, and be alert to possible signs of pneumothorax development.

### Traumatic Asphyxia

Sometimes a patient will experience a sudden, severe compression of the chest, which produces a rapid increase in pressure within the chest. This may occur in a pedestrian who is compressed between a vehicle and a wall, or a patient who is pinned under a vehicle. The sudden increase in intrathoracic pressure results in a characteristic appearance, including distended neck veins, cyanosis in the face and neck, and hemorrhage into the sclera of the eye, signaling the bursting of small blood vessels (**FIGURE 30-16**). This is called traumatic asphyxia. These findings suggest an underlying injury to the

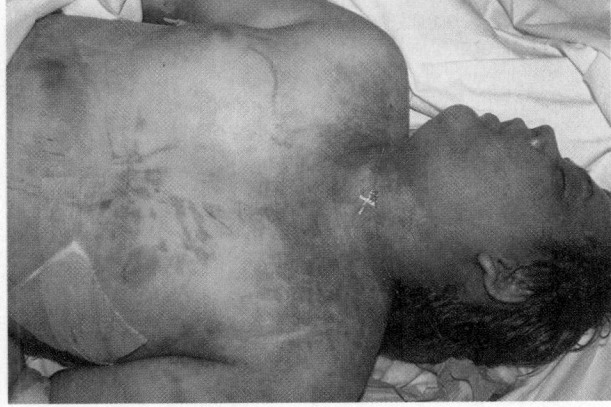

**FIGURE 30-16** Traumatic asphyxia.
© Charles Stewart MD, EMDM MPH.

heart and possibly a pulmonary contusion. Provide ventilatory support with supplemental oxygen and monitor the patient's vital signs as you provide immediate transport.

### Blunt Myocardial Injury

Blunt trauma to the chest may injure the heart itself, making it unable to maintain adequate blood pressure. There is much debate in the medical literature about how to assess myocardial contusion, or bruising of the heart muscle. Often the pulse is irregular, but dangerous rhythms such as ventricular tachycardia and ventricular fibrillation are uncommon. Currently, there is no specific diagnostic test in the prehospital setting, and there is no prehospital treatment for the condition. Still, you should suspect myocardial contusion in all cases of severe blunt injury to the chest. Carefully check the patient's pulse and note any irregularities. Also note any change in blood pressure because this can be a direct result of the injury to the myocardium. Often the patient's signs and symptoms can mimic a heart attack in which the patient may report chest pain or discomfort that is similar in nature to cardiac symptoms. Provide supplemental oxygen, and transport immediately.

### Commotio Cordis

Commotio cordis is a blunt chest injury caused by a sudden, direct blow to the chest (over the heart) that occurs during a critical portion of a person's heartbeat. The result may be immediate cardiac arrest. This phenomenon has occurred after patients were struck with softballs, baseballs, bats, snowballs, fists, and even kicks during kickboxing. The force of the blow to the chest is commonly at speeds of 35 to 40 miles per hour. The blunt force, at a single specific point in the cardiac cycle, causes a lethal abnormal heart rhythm called ventricular fibrillation. The ventricular fibrillation is often responsive to defibrillation and early initiation of CPR. Commotio cordis is more commonly associated with sports-related injuries, although it should be suspected in all cases in which the person is unconscious and unresponsive after a blow to the chest. These patients present in cardiac arrest and should be managed as any other cardiac arrest, understanding that they may be particularly responsive to early defibrillation.

## Laceration of the Great Vessels

The chest contains several large blood vessels: the superior vena cava, the inferior vena cava, the pulmonary arteries, four main pulmonary veins, and the aorta, with its major branches distributing blood throughout the body. Injury to any of these vessels may be accompanied by massive, rapidly fatal hemorrhage. Any patient with a chest wound who shows signs of shock may have an injury to one or more of these vessels. Frequently, significant blood loss is unseen because it remains within the chest cavity. Remain alert to signs and symptoms of shock and to changes in the baseline vital signs, such as tachycardia and hypotension.

Emergency treatment in these cases includes CPR, if appropriate; ventilatory support; and supplemental oxygen. Immediate transport to the trauma center may be critical. Occasionally, some of these patients can be treated. The overwhelming majority of injuries to the great vessels in the chest are rapidly fatal.

### Words of Wisdom

Transection of the aorta may cause up to 15% of deaths that occur on scene from motor vehicle crashes. Given that the body's entire blood volume passes through this vessel, the high mortality associated with such an injury comes as no surprise. Many aortic injuries are rapidly fatal, often causing cardiac arrest prior to hospital arrival, or even prior to arrival of EMS. Local protocols are specific to when CPR should *not* be started in traumatic arrests; however, the survival rate is very low in patients who are pulseless and apneic and have no pupillary response on arrival of EMS.

## YOU are the Provider SUMMARY

**1.** **What major organs and structures lie within the chest cavity?**

Critical organs and structures in the chest cavity include the trachea, large bronchi, lungs, great vessels (eg, aorta, venae cavae), heart, and left and right subclavian arteries and their branches. The heart, trachea, great vessels, and a portion of the esophagus reside within the mediastinum—the space between the lungs.

A thin lining called the visceral pleura covers the lungs, and the parietal pleura covers the inner chest wall. A small amount of pleural fluid is found between the pleurae. The space in between the visceral and parietal pleurae—the pleural space—is only a potential space because the two pleural layers are in direct contact with each other in normal circumstances. However, if trauma occurs to the chest wall, the layers can separate, creating an actual space that becomes filled with air, blood or both.

**2.** **What injuries commonly result from blunt chest trauma? Penetrating chest trauma?**

Blunt (closed) chest trauma occurs when an object strikes the chest (eg, a steel pipe during an assault) or when the chest strikes an object (eg, chest impacts the steering wheel during a car crash). The severity of the injury depends on the amount of energy that the chest wall absorbs. Although the skin and chest wall are not penetrated by blunt force trauma, injury to the intrathoracic organs may be severe.

Rib fractures are common injuries associated with blunt chest trauma. In some cases, a single rib is fractured; in other cases, several adjacent ribs are fractured in more than one place (flail chest). A flail chest can impair ventilation because the section of fractured ribs collapses and puts pressure on the lung during inhalation. A fractured rib can also perforate an internal chest organ, such as the lung, causing air to leak out of the lung and into the pleural space (pneumothorax). If air moves freely between the pleural space and lung, the injury is called a simple pneumothorax. In a tension pneumothorax, the lung is completely collapsed, and the heart and great vessels (eg, aorta, venae cavae) are compressed as pressure shifts across the mediastinum. This causes further ventilatory compromise, decreased cardiac output, shock, and death if untreated. A hemothorax, which may be caused by blunt or penetrating chest trauma, occurs when blood, rather than air, fills the pleural space.

Blunt force chest trauma can also cause bruising of the lung (pulmonary contusion) or the heart muscle (myocardial contusion). Other injuries include shearing injuries of the aorta, traumatic asphyxia, and commotio cordis.

In a penetrating (open) chest injury, the chest wall itself is penetrated by an object such as a knife or bullet, resulting in injury to vital organs in the thoracic cavity. A common injury associated with penetrating chest trauma is a sucking chest wound (open pneumothorax). Sucking chest wounds cause various degrees of ventilatory compromise, depending on the size of the hole in the chest wall.

**3. How should you proceed with your secondary assessment?**

For patients with an isolated injury, your secondary assessment should focus on that area of the body—in this case, the chest and adjacent structures. However, remember that even with an isolated injury, the patient may have other injuries worthy of a head-to-toe trauma assessment.

Expose the patient's chest, and assess for obvious signs of injury, such as bruising, lacerations, or abrasions. Observe the chest wall for symmetry. Asymmetrical chest movement indicates decreased airflow into one lung. Look for any sections of the rib cage that collapse during inhalation and bulge during exhalation (paradoxical chest movement); this is an indication of flail chest injury.

Palpate the chest wall to determine if it is stable, if there are any deformities, or if you feel crepitus—the sensation felt when broken bone ends grind together. Chest wall crepitus is a clear indicator of one or more fractured ribs.

Auscultate the apices (top) and bases (bottom) of both lungs. Decreased or absent breath sounds over the injured side of the chest indicate decreased or absent airflow into that lung and should immediately increase your index of suspicion for a pneumothorax.

Based on the MOI—blunt chest trauma—you should also assess the trachea and jugular veins. Note whether the trachea is in the midline position or if it appears to be deviated to one side or the other. Bear in mind that if the patient has a tension pneumothorax, tracheal deviation is a relatively late sign; a midline trachea does not rule out such an injury. Observe the jugular veins to determine if they appear to be normal, distended, or flat. Jugular vein distention (JVD) is best assessed with the patient sitting at a 45° angle. Do not move the patient to this position solely for the purpose of assessing JVD. Remember that patients who lie flat may naturally have JVD. The presence of JVD in the context of chest trauma suggests a tension pneumothorax or cardiac tamponade, although it is often not present until the injury is well progressed. In addition, collapsed jugular veins suggest shock.

Chest injuries, especially if located below the nipple line, often also involve abdominal injuries. Abdominal assessment therefore may be beneficial, especially as the signs and symptoms of abdominal injury may appear later and the pain from the chest injury may distract from any pain from the abdominal injury. Further assessment beyond that discussed is based on any other symptoms the patient may report and any obvious injuries that you observe.

**4. On the basis of your assessment findings, what injury or injuries should you suspect?**

On the basis of the MOI—blunt trauma to the chest—and the findings of your primary and secondary assessments, you should suspect that your patient has rib fractures and a pneumothorax. He has obvious chest wall bruising, labored breathing, crepitus on palpation, and diminished breath sounds on the same side that the injury occurred.

Depending on the size of the lung perforation and the rate at which air fills the pleural space, the lung may collapse in a few seconds. Breath sounds on the injured side are diminished because the collapsing lung is not fully expanding during inhalation.

Because a pneumothorax impairs oxygenation and ventilation, begin treatment immediately and prepare for rapid transport to the hospital. If the lung on the injured side collapses totally, pressure will shift to the opposite side of the chest—compressing the heart, aorta, and venae cavae in the process—and begin collapsing the unaffected lung; this condition is called a tension pneumothorax and is an immediately life-threatening condition that can result in profound shock and cardiac arrest.

**5. How should you proceed with your treatment of this patient?**

Patients with a pneumothorax need high-flow oxygen, continual close monitoring, and prompt transport to the hospital.

Be especially concerned about the adequacy of the patient's breathing, and continuously monitor it. Your patient is tachypneic, which is common in patients with chest injuries; his respirations are labored, and it hurts when he breathes. Patients with chest injuries often take shallow breaths to minimize the pain. You should consider calling for ALS, particularly if it leads to intervention that is faster than transporting the patient to the hospital, as ALS providers can administer pain medication that can ease the patient's pain and potentially allow the patient to breathe more easily.

If his respirations become too shallow, he will not move adequate amounts of air into his lungs during inhalation; this will only worsen any hypoxemia that already exists from the pneumothorax itself. If this occurs, begin assisting his ventilations with a bag-mask device attached to high-flow oxygen. Other signs of inadequate breathing, which may also necessitate assisted ventilations, include a falling oxygen saturation (despite administration of high-flow oxygen), cyanosis, and a decreasing level of consciousness.

Continue to monitor the patient's level of consciousness and vital signs. If he begins experiencing signs of shock, suspect a developing tension pneumothorax.

**6. What is most likely happening to your patient?**

Compared with previous assessments, your patient's clinical condition has obviously deteriorated. He is now confused; is more tachypneic; his respirations are still labored, but are now shallow; cyanosis is developing around his mouth (perioral cyanosis); his radial pulses are weak; and his oxygen saturation has fallen to 88% despite high-flow oxygen via nonrebreathing mask. Although his systolic blood pressure is still above 100 mm Hg, compared with your previous reading of 138/88 mm Hg, this is a significant decrease. The patient's signs and symptoms indicate he is deteriorating and is in respiratory failure.

The additional signs of inaudible (absent) breath sounds on the injured side of his chest and the appearance of cyanosis indicate that the left lung has collapsed or is filling with blood and air, and pressure is now shifting across the mediastinum toward the unaffected lung. You should suspect your patient has a tension pneumothorax and will continue to deteriorate until he can receive definitive treatment.

**7. Should you adjust your current treatment? If so, how?**

A tension pneumothorax is an immediate life threat and requires aggressive treatment.

The patient now has clear evidence of respiratory failure (decreased level of consciousness [confusion]), which is causing inadequate oxygenation and ventilation. Begin assisting his ventilations with a bag-mask device. Avoid hyperventilating the patient, as doing so may worsen the pneumothorax

and ultimately decrease cardiac output. You must also initiate shock treatment. At a minimum, cover the patient with a blanket to keep him warm. Patients with any injury or condition that impairs their ability to breathe are often resistant to being placed in a supine position; this is especially true if they are conscious. Elevating the head of the stretcher while maintaining spinal motion restriction as indicated may result in an improved ability of the patient to exchange air. If the patient becomes unconscious, however, place him in a supine position and continue to assist his ventilations.

Patients with a tension pneumothorax need an immediate needle thoracentesis (chest decompression). If it will not delay your transport time, intercept an ALS unit, if possible. Otherwise, notify the receiving facility, continue assisting ventilations and shock treatment, and get the patient to the ED as soon as possible.

**8. What is a tension hemopneumothorax?**

In some cases, when a fractured rib perforates a lung, blood from the injured lung also accumulates in the pleural space; this is called a hemopneumothorax because the pleural space contains both blood and air. The amount of blood that accumulates in the pleural space depends on the size and severity of the lung injury.

As blood and air continue to accumulate in the pleural space, the lung on the injured side collapses and pressure shifts across the mediastinum toward the uninjured lung. In a tension hemopneumothorax, the patient experiences respiratory impairment from both blood and air in the pleural space, but also experiences internal blood loss of varying severity.

**9. Should you attempt to distinguish a tension pneumothorax from a tension hemopneumothorax? Why or why not?**

It is impractical to attempt to distinguish a tension pneumothorax from a tension hemopneumothorax in the prehospital setting. Both conditions cause impaired ventilation and perfusion; this is what you should focus on when treating the patient. Provide high-flow oxygen, assist ventilations as needed, initiate shock treatment, and transport without delay. Attempting to distinguish one injury from the other may only delay treatment and transport, thereby increasing the chance of a negative outcome.

## YOU are the Provider SUMMARY *continued*

### EMS Patient Care Report (PCR)

| **Date:** 11-5-20 | **Incident No.:** 012709 | **Nature of Call:** Chest injury | | **Location:** 7100 Douglas Ave. | |
|---|---|---|---|---|---|
| **Dispatched:** 1020 | **En Route:** 1020 | **At Scene:** 1028 | **Transport:** 1035 | **At Hospital:** 1045 | **In Service:** 1115 |

#### Patient Information

**Age:** 19
**Sex:** M
**Weight (in kg [lb]):** 66 kg (145 lb)

**Allergies:** Penicillin
**Medications:** None
**Past Medical History:** None
**Chief Complaint:** Difficulty breathing secondary to chest injury

#### Vital Signs

| Time: 1030 | BP: 138/88 | Pulse: 110 | Respirations: 24 | Spo$_2$: 95% |
|---|---|---|---|---|
| **Time:** 1035 | **BP:** 104/58 | **Pulse:** 124 | **Respirations:** 28 | **Spo$_2$:** 88% |
| **Time:** 1040 | **BP:** 90/60 | **Pulse:** 128 | **Respirations:** 28 | **Spo$_2$:** 85% |

#### EMS Treatment (circle all that apply)

| Oxygen @ _15_ L/min via: NC (NRM) Bag mask | | Assisted Ventilation | Airway Adjunct | CPR |
|---|---|---|---|---|
| **Defibrillation** | **Bleeding Control** | **Bandaging** | **Splinting** | **Other:** Shock treatment, blanket for warmth |

#### Narrative

Medic 414 dispatched to a construction site for a 19-year-old male who sustained a chest injury.

Chief Complaint: Difficulty breathing secondary to chest injury

History: On scene the patient was seated on the ground. Patient reports chest pain and difficulty breathing after being struck in the left anterior part of the chest by a 2 by 4 board, which was thrown from a table saw when a coworker was cutting it. He denies any other injuries, and coworkers confirm that there was no loss of consciousness.

Assessment: The airway is patent; breathing is rapid and labored, with noted shortness of breath and diminished breath sounds on the left; radial pulse is strong and regular; skin is pink, warm, and dry; mental status is alert and oriented to time, place, self. Obvious bruising was noted to left anterior part of the chest, as was crepitus on palpation. No paradoxical chest wall movement was noted, jugular veins were nondistended, and trachea was midline. Abdominal exam was unremarkable.

Treatment (Rx): Oxygen administered via nonrebreathing mask at 15 LPM and vital signs monitored. On reassessment patient became confused, more tachypneic, and his respirations were markedly shallow. Oxygen saturation read 88%, and skin was now cool and clammy, with perioral cyanosis. Breath sounds were absent on the left side of the chest.

Transport: Lifted patient onto stretcher, secured with four straps, and loaded him into the ambulance. Intercept with ALS unit was not possible because it would have caused a significant delay in transport. Covered patient with a blanket for warmth, continued ventilation assistance, and reassessed patient every 5 minutes throughout transport. Delivered patient to hospital, gave verbal report to attending physician, and transferred patient care to hospital staff. Medic 414 returned to service at 1115.

**End of report**

# Prep Kit

## Ready for Review

- A penetrating chest injury has the potential to penetrate the lung and diaphragm and injure the liver or stomach.
- Chest injuries are classified as closed or open. Closed injuries are often the result of blunt force trauma, and open injuries are the result of an object penetrating the skin and/or chest wall.
- Blunt trauma may result in fractures to the ribs and the sternum.
- Life-threatening external hemorrhage must be addressed immediately during the primary assessment, even before airway or breathing concerns.
- During the primary assessment, if an injury is encountered that interferes with the ability of the patient to oxygenate or ventilate, the injury must be addressed quickly.
- Any penetrating injury to the chest may result in air entering the pleural space and may cause pneumothorax. A vented chest seal should be placed on this injury as soon as it is identified.
- When a penetrating injury creates a hole in the chest wall, you may hear a sucking sound as the patient inhales. This is called an open pneumothorax.
- A simple pneumothorax is a result of blunt trauma, such as fractured ribs.
- A spontaneous pneumothorax may be the result of rupture of a weak spot on the lung, allowing air to enter the pleural space and accumulate. This often results from nontraumatic injuries and may occur during times of physical activity such as exercise.
- A pneumothorax may progress to a tension pneumothorax and potentially cause cardiac arrest.
- Hemothorax is the result of blood accumulating in the pleural space after a traumatic injury when the vessels of the lung are lacerated and leak blood.
- A flail chest segment is two or more adjacent ribs broken in two or more places. Positive-pressure ventilation may be particularly important for the patient with a flail chest that compromises ventilation.
- All patients with chest injuries should receive high-flow oxygen or ventilation with a bag-mask device.
- Pulmonary contusion, which is bruising of or injury to lung tissue after traumatic injury, may interfere with oxygen exchange in the lung tissue.
- Myocardial contusion is bruising of the heart muscle after traumatic injury. This condition may have the same signs and symptoms as a heart attack, including an irregular pulse. Remember that this is an injury to the heart muscle from trauma, not from a heart attack.
- Commotio cordis occurs from a direct blow to the chest during a critical portion of the patient's heartbeat. It may result in immediate cardiac arrest.
- Cardiac tamponade is when blood collects in the space between the pericardial sac and the heart. This condition results in pressure building up inside the pericardial sac until the heart cannot pump effectively; cardiac arrest may occur quickly.
- The great vessels of the body are located in the mediastinum. These large vessels may be lacerated or tear after traumatic injury and cause heavy, unseen bleeding inside the patient's chest cavity.
- Any patient who has signs of shock with a chest injury, even with unseen bleeding, should make you suspicious of unseen, life-threatening bleeding inside the chest cavity.

# Vital Vocabulary

**cardiac tamponade (pericardial tamponade)** Compression of the heart as the result of buildup of blood or other fluid in the pericardial sac, leading to decreased cardiac output.

**closed chest injury** An injury to the chest in which the skin is not broken, usually caused by blunt trauma.

**commotio cordis** A blunt chest injury caused by a sudden, direct blow to the chest that occurs only during the critical portion of a person's heartbeat.

**crepitus** A grating or grinding sensation caused by fractured bone ends or joints rubbing together.

**flail chest** A condition in which two or more adjacent ribs are fractured in two or more places or in association with a fracture of the sternum so that a segment of the chest wall is effectively detached from the rest of the thoracic cage.

**flutter valve** A one-way valve that allows air to leave the chest cavity but not return; formed by taping three sides of an occlusive dressing to the chest wall, leaving the fourth side open as a valve; may also be part of a commercial vented occlusive dressing.

**hemopneumothorax** The accumulation of blood and air in the pleural space of the chest.

**hemothorax** A collection of blood in the pleural cavity.

**myocardial contusion** Bruising of the heart muscle.

**occlusive dressing** An airtight dressing that protects a wound from air and bacteria; a commercial vented version allows air to passively escape from the chest, while an unvented dressing may be made of petrolatum gauze, aluminum foil, or plastic.

**open chest injury** An injury to the chest in which the chest wall itself is penetrated by a fractured rib or, more frequently, by an external object such as a bullet or knife.

**open pneumothorax** An open or penetrating chest wall wound through which air passes during inspiration and expiration, creating a sucking sound; also referred to as a sucking chest wound.

**paradoxical motion** The motion of the portion of the chest wall that is detached in a flail chest; the motion—in during inhalation, out during exhalation—is exactly the opposite of normal chest wall motion during breathing.

**pericardium** The fibrous sac that surrounds the heart.

**pneumothorax** An accumulation of air or gas in the pleural cavity.

**pulmonary contusion** Injury or bruising of lung tissue that results in hemorrhage.

**simple pneumothorax** Any pneumothorax that is free from significant physiologic changes and does not cause drastic changes in the vital signs of the patient.

**spontaneous pneumothorax** A pneumothorax that occurs when a weak area on the lung ruptures in the absence of major injury, allowing air to leak into the pleural space.

**sucking chest wound** An open or penetrating chest wall wound through which air passes during inspiration and expiration, creating a sucking sound. See also *open pneumothorax*.

**tachypnea** Rapid respirations.

**tension pneumothorax** An accumulation of air or gas in the pleural cavity that progressively increases pressure in the chest that interferes with cardiac function with potentially fatal results.

**traumatic asphyxia** A pattern of injuries seen after a severe force is applied to the chest, forcing blood from the great vessels back into the head and neck.

**vented chest seal** An occlusive dressing designed to allow air to escape through the dressing but not be drawn back in.

# References

1. Khouzam RN, Al-Mawed S, Farah V, Mizeracki A. Next-generation airbags and the possibility of negative outcomes due to thoracic injury. *Can J Cardiol.* 2014 Apr;30(4):396-404.

2. National Association of Emergency Medical Technicians. *PHTLS: Prehospital Trauma Life Support.* 9th ed. Burlington, MA: Jones & Bartlett Learning; 2019.

3. National Highway Traffic Safety Administration. *National Emergency Medical Services Education Standards.* DOT HS 811 077A. *ems.gov.* www.ems.gov/pdf/811077a.pdf. Published January 2009. Accessed February 6, 2020.

4. National Highway Traffic Safety Administration. *National Emergency Medical Services Education Standards.*

*Emergency Medical Technician Instructional Guidelines.* DOT HS 811 077C. *ems.gov.* www.ems.gov/pdf/811077c.pdf. Published January 2009. Accessed February 6, 2020.

5. Prêtre R, Chilcott M. Blunt trauma to the heart and great vessels. *N Engl J Med.* 1997;336(9):626-632.

6. US Department of Health and Human Services, Centers for Disease Control and Prevention, National Center for Health Statistics. National Hospital Ambulatory Medical Care Survey: 2016 emergency department summary tables. https://www.cdc.gov/nchs/data/nhamcs/web_tables/2016_ed_web_tables.pdf. Accessed February 11, 2020.

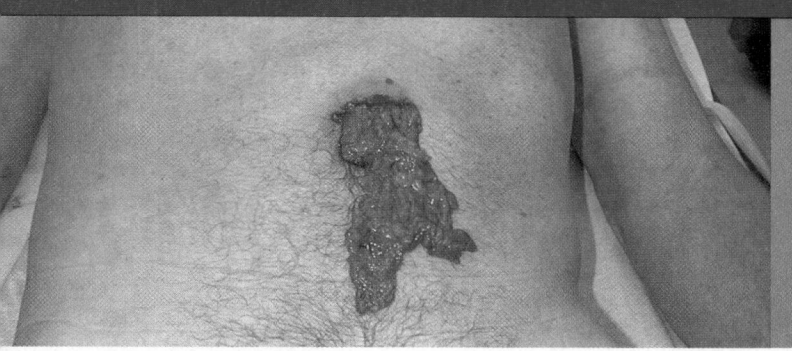

# Chapter 31

# Abdominal and Genitourinary Injuries

## NATIONAL EMS EDUCATION STANDARD COMPETENCIES

### Trauma

Applies fundamental knowledge to provide basic emergency care and transportation based on assessment findings for an acutely injured patient.

### Abdominal and Genitourinary Trauma

- Recognition and management of
  - Blunt versus penetrating mechanisms (pp 1121–1123, 1129–1130, 1133–1134, 1137–1139)
  - Evisceration (pp 1123, 1130–1131)

- Impaled object (pp 1128, 1137)
- Pathophysiology, assessment, and management of
  - Solid and hollow organ injuries (pp 1123–1125)
  - Blunt versus penetrating mechanisms (pp 1121–1123, 1125–1131, 1133–1134, 1137–1139)
  - Evisceration (pp 1123, 1125–1129, 1130–1131)
  - Injuries to the external genitalia (pp 1134–1139)
  - Vaginal bleeding due to trauma (pp 1134–1139)
  - Sexual assault (pp 1138–1139)

## KNOWLEDGE OBJECTIVES

1. Describe the anatomy and physiology of the abdomen; include an explanation of abdominal quadrants and boundaries and the difference between hollow and solid organs. (pp 1118–1121)

2. Describe some special considerations related to the care of pediatric patients and geriatric patients who have experienced abdominal trauma. (pp 1121, 1125)

3. Define closed abdominal injuries; provide examples of the mechanisms of injury (MOIs) likely to cause this type of trauma, and common signs and symptoms exhibited by patients who have experienced this type of injury. (pp 1121–1122)

4. Define open abdominal injuries; include the three common velocity levels that distinguish these injuries, provide examples of the MOIs that would cause each, and describe common signs and symptoms exhibited by patients

   who have experienced this type of injury. (pp 1122–1123)

5. Describe the different ways hollow and solid organs of the abdomen can be injured, and include the common signs and symptoms exhibited by patients depending on the organ or organs involved. (pp 1123–1125)

6. Explain assessment of a patient who has experienced an abdominal injury; include common indicators that help determine the MOI and whether it is a significant MOI. (pp 1125–1129)

7. Explain the emergency medical care of a patient who has sustained a closed abdominal injury, including blunt trauma caused by a seat belt or airbag. (p 1129)

8. Explain the emergency medical care of a patient who has sustained an open abdominal

injury, including penetrating injuries and abdominal evisceration. (pp 1129–1130)

9. Describe the anatomy and physiology of the female and male genitourinary systems; include the differences between the hollow and solid organs. (pp 1131–1133)

10. Discuss the types of traumatic injuries sustained by the male and female genitourinary systems, including the kidneys, urinary bladder, and internal and external genitalia. (pp 1133–1135)

11. Explain assessment of a patient who has experienced a genitourinary injury; include special considerations related to patient privacy and determining the MOI. (pp 1135–1137)

12. Explain the emergency medical care of a patient who has sustained a genitourinary injury to the kidneys, urinary bladder, external male genitalia, female genitalia, or rectum. (pp 1137–1138)

13. Explain special considerations related to a patient who has experienced a genitourinary injury caused by a sexual assault, including patient treatment, criminal implications, and evidence management. (pp 1138–1139)

## SKILLS OBJECTIVES

1. Demonstrate proper emergency medical care of a patient who has experienced a blunt abdominal injury. (p 1129)

2. Demonstrate proper emergency medical care of a patient who has a penetrating abdominal injury with an impaled object. (pp 1129–1130)

3. Demonstrate how to apply a dressing to an abdominal evisceration wound. (pp 1130–1131)

# Introduction

The abdomen is the major body cavity extending from the diaphragm to the pelvis. It contains organs from the digestive, urinary, and genitourinary systems. Although any of these organs can be injured, some are better protected than others. Being well acquainted with the anatomy and positions of abdominal and pelvic organs is important for EMS providers. In the presence of traumatic injury to these areas, providers must understand the functions of these organs if they are to determine the severity.

Significant abdominal trauma can arise from blunt and/or penetrating forces. In the absence of obvious external trauma, internal injuries in this region may be overlooked. Indeed, unrecognized and untreated abdominal injuries are a leading cause of traumatic death. Despite the fact that 10% of all trauma patients have some form of genitourinary injury, such injuries are frequently missed. These oversights may increase the patient's risk for incontinence, infertility, impotence, or other life-altering consequences. Therefore, when assessing patients with a mechanism of injury (MOI) capable of causing abdominal or genitourinary injury, the EMT must maintain a high index of suspicion. Relevant findings should be relayed to the receiving hospital expeditiously to ensure prompt delivery of definitive care.

## YOU are the Provider

You and your partner are working a special event—the annual rodeo. While on standby, you witness a rider being thrown and trampled by a bull. After a rodeo clown distracts and corrals the bull, the rider, a 20-year-old man, slowly gets up and begins to walk. He is clutching his abdomen with one hand and rubbing his lower back with the other hand.

1. How do hollow organ injuries differ from solid organ injuries?

2. How should you focus your assessment of a patient with potential intra-abdominal bleeding?

# Anatomy and Physiology of the Abdomen

## Abdominal Quadrants

By visualizing two imaginary lines (one horizontal and one vertical) that intersect at the umbilicus, the abdomen can be divided into four quadrants: the right upper quadrant (RUQ), left upper quadrant (LUQ), right lower quadrant (RLQ), and left lower quadrant (LLQ) (**FIGURE 31-1**). Remember, "right" and "left" are from the *patient's* point of view.

Bruising or pain in one of these quadrants can help the EMT ascertain which organs are most likely to have been affected. For example, the right upper quadrant contains the gallbladder, the duodenum of the intestines, the majority of the liver, and a small portion of the pancreas. The left upper quadrant contains the spleen, most of the stomach, and the larger portion of the pancreas. The left lower quadrant contains portions of the large and small intestines (most notably, the descending colon and the left half of the transverse colon). The right lower quadrant also contains large portions of the large and small intestines (including the ascending colon and the right half of the transverse colon), as well as the appendix, which is situated at the proximal end of the ascending colon.

## Hollow and Solid Organs

The abdomen contains hollow and solid organs. Hollow organs include the stomach, large and small intestines, gallbladder, ureters, and urinary bladder (**FIGURE 31-2**). It is through these hollow structures that an assortment of materials pass, with most containing food in various stages of digestion. Exceptions include the urinary bladder and ureters, through which urine passes for release, and the gallbladder, which plays a supportive role in the breakdown of fats passing through the intestine.

When ruptured or lacerated, these organs may spill their contents into the abdominal cavity,

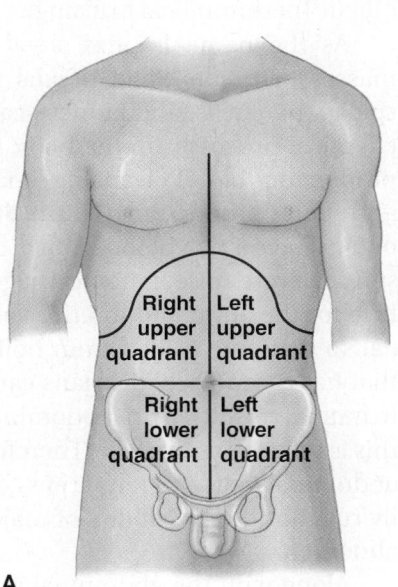

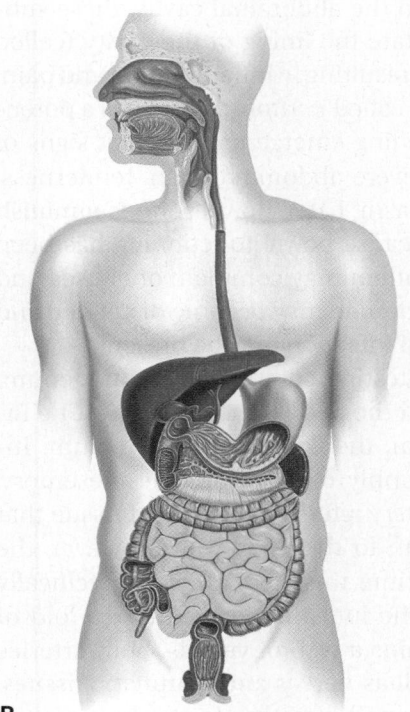

**A**　　　　　　　　**B**

**FIGURE 31-1 A.** Locations on the abdomen are often designated according to four quadrants. **B.** Many organs lie in more than one quadrant.

A: © Jones & Bartlett Learning; B: © leonello calvetti/Shutterstock.

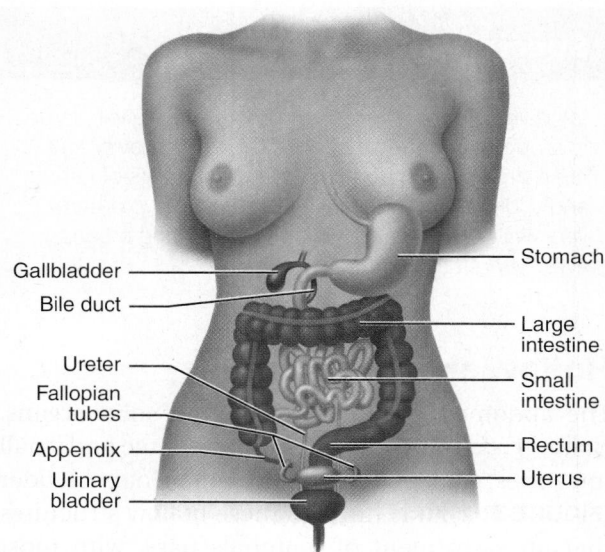

**FIGURE 31-2** The hollow organs in the abdominal cavity are structures through which materials pass.

© Jones & Bartlett Learning.

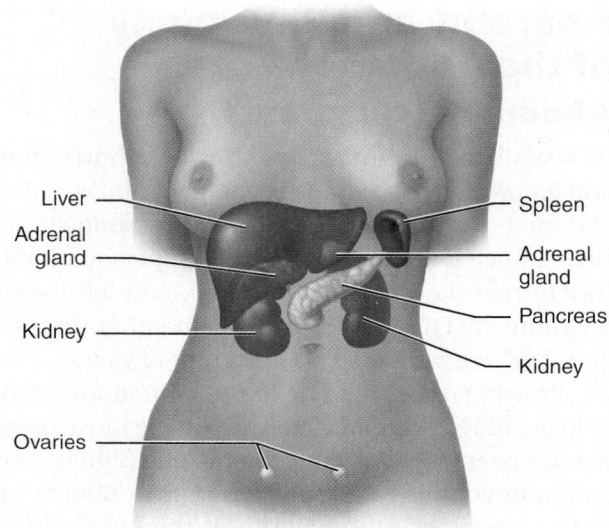

**FIGURE 31-3** The solid organs are solid masses of tissue that do much of the chemical work in the body and receive a large, rich supply of blood.

© Jones & Bartlett Learning.

resulting in intense inflammation and possible infection. For example, the intestines and stomach contain acidic substances that aid in digestion, but when leaked into the abdominal cavity, these substances may irritate the lining of the cavity (called the **peritoneum**), resulting in inflammation and pain. This condition is called *peritonitis*, and it is a potentially life-threatening emergency. The first signs of peritonitis are severe abdominal pain, tenderness, and muscular spasm. Later, bowel sounds diminish or disappear, because bowel functioning has been impaired. The patient may complain of nausea and vomiting, the abdomen may become distended and rigid, and signs of infection may be present.

The small intestine comprises the duodenum, the jejunum, and the ileum. The large intestine includes the cecum, the colon, and the rectum. Intestinal blood supply comes from the mesentery. The term *mesentery* refers to any fold of tissue that attaches an organ to the body wall. However, the majority of the time this term is used specifically in reference to the intestinal mesentery: a fold of tissue that contains a web of vessels, both arteries and veins, as well as nerves and lymphatic tissues. It connects the small intestine to the posterior of the abdominal wall. Both blunt and penetrating abdominal injuries can affect this vasculature, and

patients with injuries to the mesentery can bleed significantly into the **peritoneal cavity**. Although abdominal distention and rigidity may be indicative of inflammation, they can also alert the attentive EMT to the possibility that the patient is bleeding internally into the peritoneal cavity. Occasionally, bruising or ecchymosis may appear around the umbilicus (periumbilical bruising).

As the name implies, **solid organs** are solid masses of tissue. Solid organs such as the liver, spleen, pancreas, and kidneys carry out numerous chemical processes in the body, including enzyme production, blood cleansing, endocrine functions, and energy production (**FIGURE 31-3**). Because these organs have a rich blood supply, their injury can result in severe unseen hemorrhage. The same holds true for the aorta and inferior vena cava. And similar to contents spilled from hollow organs, blood that has escaped solid organs can cause peritoneal irritation, resulting in abdominal pain; however, this is not always the case. Therefore, the absence of abdominal pain and tenderness does not necessarily rule out the possibility of major bleeding in the abdomen.

Along with the abdominal aorta and a portion of the inferior vena cava, many solid organs are considered *retroperitoneal* (*retro-* means "behind"), because they are situated primarily in the posterior aspect of the abdominal cavity and behind the peritoneum. This region is referred to as the **retroperitoneum**. It also houses the kidneys, ureters, and urinary bladder. The majority of the pancreas is located in this region, which is why the pancreas is referred to as a retroperitoneal organ. The last portion of a hollow organ, the colon, occupies the lowest portion of the retroperitoneal space.

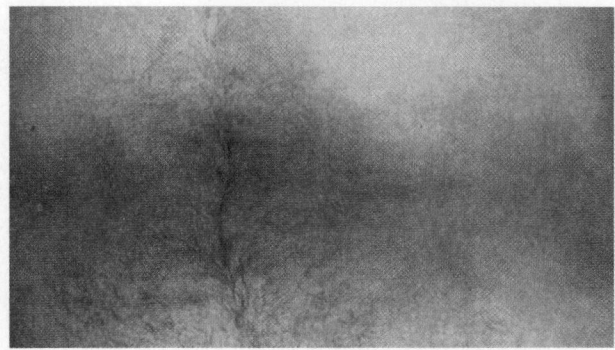

**FIGURE 31-4** Blunt trauma to the abdomen can occur when a patient strikes the steering wheel of a vehicle as a result of a crash.
© American Academy of Orthopaedic Surgeons.

### Special Populations

Falls are the most common mechanism of injury in geriatric patients. The trauma sustained in a fall is not limited to musculoskeletal injuries. For a number of reasons, the EMT should maintain a high index of suspicion for internal injuries, even in patients who have experienced relatively "minor" falls. With advancing age, the abdominal organs lose some of their elasticity, making them more prone to injury when exposed to the forces present in a fall. The aorta, liver, and spleen are particularly vulnerable. Furthermore, if the geriatric patient's bones are brittle, they can fracture even with falls from standing height. The sharp edges of broken bones have the potential to puncture internal organs.

### Words of Wisdom

Rib fractures are common traumatic injuries. When your assessment leads you to suspect lower rib fractures, remember that any trauma forceful enough to break the ribs may also have damaged underlying internal organs.

## Abdominal Injuries

Abdominal injuries can be as obvious as loops of intestines protruding from an open wound, or they can be as covert as a liver laceration, hidden beneath unbroken skin.

## Closed Abdominal Injuries

When a traumatic injury to the abdomen occurs without breaking the skin, it is considered a **closed abdominal injury**. Examples include an assault victim struck in the abdomen by a baseball bat or a rapid deceleration injury from a fall or front-end motor vehicle collision (**FIGURE 31-4**). MOIs capable of causing closed injuries include the following:

- Motor vehicle collisions
- Motorcycle crashes
- Falls
- Blast injuries (barotrauma)
- Pedestrian versus vehicle

- Rapid deceleration
- Compression

Closed abdominal injuries may initially appear as abrasions to the surface of the skin, depending on the MOI, such as a physical assault or a pedestrian struck by a motor vehicle. In some circumstances, depending on how deep in the abdomen the injury occurs, it may take several minutes to hours for the contusion or hematoma to become visible on the surface. Therefore, an EMT cannot rule out the possibility of injury merely on the basis of absence of these findings.

### Injuries From Seat Belts and Airbags

Seat belts have prevented countless injuries and deaths, protecting against ejections from motor vehicles involved in collisions. Despite the undeniable benefits, seat belts occasionally contribute to blunt trauma to abdominal organs. Worn properly, a seat belt lies below the anterior superior iliac spines of the pelvis and against the hip joints. Positioned too high, it can squeeze abdominal organs

Incorrect position

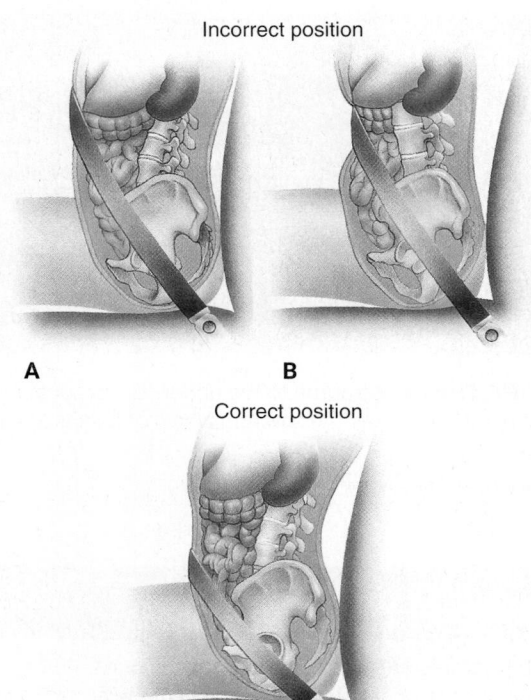

**A**        **B**

Correct position

**C**

**FIGURE 31-5** Diagrams **A** and **B** show improper positioning of lap seat belts. The proper position for a seat belt is below the anterior superior iliac spines of the pelvis and against the hip joints, as shown in diagram **C**.

**A, B, C:** © Jones & Bartlett Learning.

or great vessels against the spine when the vehicle rapidly decelerates or comes to a sudden stop (**FIGURE 31-5**). Fractures of the lumbar spine have also been reported. In later stages of pregnancy, the gravid uterus displaces the urinary bladder to the anterior, making it more susceptible to injury. Pregnant patients who adjust the lap belt for comfort as opposed to functionality can sustain further injuries.

In all current-model vehicles, the lap and diagonal (shoulder) safety belts are combined into one so that they may not be used independently. Of course, people can still place the diagonal portion of the belt behind their back, significantly reducing the effectiveness of this design. Remember to inspect beneath the airbag for signs of damage to the steering column.

## Open Abdominal Injuries

As the name implies, in an **open abdominal injury** the peritoneal cavity has been opened to the outside.

Penetrating traumatic injuries such as stab wounds and gunshot wounds are examples of open injuries. Although some open wounds may not extend any deeper than the muscular wall of the abdomen, this cannot be reliably determined in the prehospital setting. Therefore, the EMT should maintain a high index of suspicion for unseen injuries and potential life threats and expedite transport to the nearest appropriate hospital, usually a designated trauma center.

A major determining factor in the severity of a penetrating MOI is the velocity of the object that penetrated the abdominal wall. The velocity correlates to the amount of energy transmitted to the tissues and therefore to the amount of damage incurred. There are three levels of velocity commonly used in the discussion of traumatic injuries:

- **Low velocity.** Caused by handheld or hand-powered objects such as knives and other edged weapons
- **Medium velocity.** Caused by small-caliber handguns and shotguns
- **High velocity.** Caused by more powerful weapons such as high-powered rifles and handguns of higher caliber

In addition to entrance and exit wounds, medium- and high-velocity projectiles create temporary wound channels or cavities. Cavitation occurs as the pressure wave from the projectile is transferred to the tissues. This causes microscopic tears to blood vessels and nerves, expanding the width and length of the wound beyond what can be seen on physical examination. Depending on the velocity of the projectile, cavitation can produce significant tissue destruction and bleeding. The higher the velocity, the larger the cavity created and, subsequently, the greater the extent of damaged tissue.

Despite the absence of cavitation, low-velocity penetrations can cause substantial damage to underlying organs. A visual inspection of the entry wound does not necessarily convey the severity of the internal damage. This is an especially important consideration when treating patients with penetrating trauma in the region of the diaphragm, the muscle that separates the thoracic cavity from the peritoneal cavity. Because the diaphragm rises and falls as we breathe, its location is somewhat variable from one moment to the next. For that reason, it should be assumed that any penetrating abdominal injury at or below the xiphoid process may have punctured the diaphragm. The resulting opening could create a passageway through which abdominal contents might pass, or *herniate*, into the thoracic cavity, potentially hindering chest expansion and causing respiratory complications.

An open abdominal injury that goes through the skin and muscle layer and through the fascia or the interior covering of the abdomen, such that organs now protrude from the peritoneum, is an **evisceration**. This visually shocking injury can be extremely painful. Do not push down on the patient's abdomen, and perform only a visual assessment when there is any suspicion of this type of injury. If there is clothing close to the wound, carefully cut the clothing around the wound, leaving a border of intact cloth outside the injured area.

Always be certain you can see exactly where the tips of your scissors are when cutting clothing. The risk of injury to the underlying exposed abdominal contents is extremely high. Never pull, even gently, on any clothing stuck to or inside the wound channel because doing so may remove even more of the abdominal contents.

## Hollow Organ Injuries

Injuries that involve the hollow organs often have delayed signs and symptoms. The hollow organs commonly spill their contents into the abdomen and then an infection occurs, which can take a few hours to days to develop. When the stomach and the intestines are injured, they can spill gastrointestinal contents such as food, waste, and digestive liquids that are highly toxic and acidic. These substances cause significant tissue damage to the entire peritoneum.

Both blunt and penetrating trauma can cause injuries to the hollow organs. Blunt trauma causes the organ to "pop," thus releasing fluids or air. Penetrating trauma causes direct injury such as laceration and punctures. In open wounds, patients typically report an intense pain that can be out of character for the size of the injury. Patients may also report intense pain with open wounds of the stomach or small bowel.

## YOU are the Provider

When you reach the patient, he is lying supine on the ground outside of the arena area. The scene is safe, and the bull has been penned up. The patient is conscious, but restless. He reports pain over his entire abdomen, both flank areas, and the back of his head. Your partner manually stabilizes his head while you perform a primary assessment.

| Recording Time: 0 Minutes | |
| --- | --- |
| **Appearance** | In obvious pain; restless |
| **Level of consciousness** | Conscious and alert; restless |
| **Airway** | Open, clear of secretions or foreign bodies |
| **Breathing** | Increased rate; adequate depth |
| **Circulation** | Radial pulses rapid and weak; skin pale, cool, and moist; no obvious bleeding |

**3.** How should you interpret your primary assessment findings?

**4.** What immediate treatment is indicated for this patient?

The gallbladder and the urinary bladder, which are filled with bile and urine, are two additional hollow organs whose contents are potentially irritating and damaging to the tissues of the abdomen if ruptured by injury. These fluids move via gravity into the loose spaces and voids in the peritoneal cavity, eventually leading to infection.

Free air in the peritoneal cavity is abnormal, and it usually indicates that a hollow organ or loop of bowel has perforated. Perforation with free air is usually very painful. If the site of perforation is not rapidly identified and repaired, severe infection and septic shock may develop. Any air in the peritoneal cavity seeks the most superior space or void; thus the location of the air can change with positioning of the patient.

## Solid Organ Injuries

Solid organs (liver, spleen, diaphragm, kidneys, and pancreas) can bleed significantly and cause rapid blood loss that can be hard to identify from a physical examination, because the patient is not experiencing significant pain. Conversely, solid organs can slowly ooze blood into the peritoneal cavity, causing pain to increase slowly over time and increasing the chance for toxicity to develop. Blood in the peritoneal cavity irritates tissue and fills any voids or spaces, which can make it difficult for you to determine the exact source of the bleeding. Because of the structures in the retroperitoneal space (the kidneys, adrenal gland, pancreas, nerve roots, lymph nodes, abdominal aorta, and inferior vena cava) and the spaces in the abdominal cavity, the peritoneal cavity can hold a large volume of blood following traumatic injuries of solid organs and major blood vessels.

The liver is the largest organ in the abdomen. It is very vascular; therefore, it can contribute to hypoperfusion if it is injured. It is often injured by a fractured lower right rib or a penetrating injury, such as a stab wound. A common finding during assessment of patients with an injured liver is referred pain to the right shoulder.

Like the liver, the pancreas and spleen are organs responsible for filtering blood and are therefore very vascular. Both organs are prone to heavy bleeding when fractured by blunt force or lacerated or punctured by penetrating injury. The spleen is often injured during motor vehicle crashes, especially in the cases of improperly placed seat belts or impact from the steering wheel, falls from heights or onto sharp objects, and bicycle and motorcycle crashes where the patient hits the handlebars on impact. Referred left shoulder pain also occurs in some cases of splenic injury.

If the diaphragm is penetrated or ruptured, loops of bowel may herniate into the thoracic cavity. Because the bowel will now be displacing lung tissue and vital capacity, patients will exhibit dyspnea or feel short of breath. Patients with a ruptured diaphragm after a motor vehicle crash may become very anxious and short of breath if placed in the supine position on a backboard. Change in position from upright to supine results in more abdominal contents spilling into the thoracic cavity and compressing the lungs, prohibiting the lungs from fully expanding.

In the retroperitoneal space, the kidneys can be impacted or penetrated by trauma. The kidneys are filtration organs; therefore, they are supplied with large quantities of blood. They can be sheared from their base, crushed, or fractured—causing significant blood loss. If a kidney is injured, a common finding is **hematuria**, or blood in the urine. This may be obvious to the naked eye or impossible to detect in the field. You may find drops of blood or blood-tinged urine on the patient's underwear, leading you to inspect the exterior of the genitals. Blood visible on inspection of the urinary meatus (opening of the urethra situated on the glans penis in men and in the vulva in women) indicates significant trauma to the genitourinary system. If blood is not present, do not take this as a sign that the patient is free from injury; the blood may not be visible yet.

## Patient Assessment of Abdominal Injuries

The assessment findings in patients with potential abdominal injuries can be challenging to interpret. Some abdominal injuries are obvious and graphic; however, many are subtle and easy to overlook. On the surface, injuries may appear minor (eg, abrasions, bruising) when in fact these outward signs may be the only visible clues that a more severe internal injury exists. Sometimes, coexisting injuries, such as a fractured bone, may cause so much pain that the patient is distracted from perceiving the abdominal discomfort. Other times, the pain may begin subtly and worsen gradually over time. In some cases, the traumatic event may have occurred hours or even days prior to your receiving the call to respond, because the pain has only recently grown severe enough to drive the patient to seek help.

### Scene Size-Up

Your scene size-up begins at the time of dispatch. The initial information you receive may be vague or incomplete, but it still provides a place to start your mental preparation en route to the scene. Is the patient injured or ill? What equipment should you bring to the patient's side? Are additional resources, such as law enforcement, hazardous materials personnel, or an advanced life support (ALS) unit, necessary? As always, standard precautions should be in place prior to exiting the ambulance.

As you inspect the scene, consider the MOI and the need for spinal motion restriction. The MOI may supply you with clues as to what underlying injuries are most likely. If the MOI is a motor vehicle collision, inspect the inside and outside of the vehicle. Is the windshield starred? Is the dashboard deformed? Was the patient wearing a seat belt?

In the case of an assault, your first priority is to ensure that law enforcement has rendered the scene safe. Do not approach a questionable scene; your safety must come first. Once the scene has been secured, gather more detailed information about the assault. For blunt trauma, where and how many times was the patient struck? If a weapon was used, was it low-, medium-, or high-velocity? If an edged weapon was used, was it serrated, smooth, or jagged? Was it clean or dirty? How long was it? Such specifics can be especially helpful to hospital staff; however, do not delay transport for the sake of locating a weapon, and be careful not to contaminate evidence in the process.

### Special Populations

In pediatric patients, a common mechanism of injury is a motor vehicle versus pedestrian or motor vehicle versus bicycle. In young children, the chest and abdomen are less protected by bony structures than in the adult. The pediatric patient may experience significant transfer of energy on impact. In the pediatric patient, the rib cage is so flexible that the chest can be flattened almost to the spine before rib fractures occur. This extensive compression can involve not only the organs of the chest, but also the abdomen. The ribs then recoil to their normal position, and the patient is left with very few outward signs that an injury has occurred.

### Primary Assessment

As you approach the patient, quickly form a general impression of his or her condition, and note the patient's level of consciousness. Is the patient awake and alert, interacting with his or her surroundings, or is the patient lying motionless and silent?

The purpose of the primary assessment is to quickly evaluate the patient's airway, breathing, circulation, and mental status, while treating all immediate life threats. Severe external hemorrhage must be controlled immediately upon discovery, even ahead of airway and breathing problems. Next, ensure the patient has a clear and patent airway. A patient experiencing nausea and/or vomiting may be at risk for aspiration, especially if his or her level of consciousness is diminished. Have suction ready, and be prepared to turn the patient onto his or her side should sudden vomiting occur.

Trauma to the kidneys, liver, and spleen can cause profound internal bleeding, posing a substantial risk for shock. One of the earliest signs of shock is tachycardia, as the heart attempts to compensate for the loss of blood. Later signs include hypotension; pale, cool, moist skin; and an altered mental status. In some cases, the abdomen may become distended from an accumulation of blood. If present, shock must be treated aggressively by administering oxygen, positioning the patient supine, and keeping the patient warm.

For critical patients, quickly scan the body from head to toe for additional injuries and initiate rapid transport to the closest appropriate facility without further delay. If the patient's condition is stable, you may opt to gather additional information prior to departure.

## History Taking

Once you have identified and treated immediate life threats, attempt to gather more information from the patient (eg, SAMPLE history). Building upon the chief complaint, apply the OPQRST mnemonic as you seek details about the patient's symptoms. Specifically, have the patient describe the pain in his or her own words. Ask if the pain travels (ie, radiates) to any other part of the body. Has the patient experienced nausea, vomiting, or diarrhea? If the answer is yes, how many times has the patient vomited or had an unusual stool? How long has this problem persisted? And what did it look like? As an example, a patient who describes having black and tarry stools (**melena**) may be experiencing gastrointestinal bleeding. Coffee-ground emesis could be the result of partially digested blood. If the patient is unresponsive or otherwise unable to answer your questions, collect as much information as you can from friends and family.

Unfortunately, a patient's complaint of pain in the abdomen can be deceiving. Injured organs tend to irritate surrounding tissues. As a result, the pain is often diffuse, making it difficult for the patient to pinpoint a specific spot on the abdomen where the pain is felt. Instead, the patient may report having pain "all over" the abdomen. To further complicate matters, it is not uncommon for patients with abdominal trauma to report pain coming from an altogether different part of the body. This *referred* pain is the result of interconnecting sensory neurons that serve multiple tissues. When the nerves from one part of the body converge with those coming from another site, the result is—in a manner of speaking—a distortion in the patient's perception of the pain's location. However, the relationship between a given injury site and the location where pain is perceived often can provide the attentive

provider with valuable insight. For example, bleeding from an injury to the spleen frequently presents with pain referred to the left shoulder. When a patient complains of tearing pain that travels from the abdomen to the back, he or she could be experiencing a dissecting abdominal aneurysm. Pain that radiates from the lateral hip to the midline of the groin might be a sign of damage to the kidneys or ureter. Pain located predominantly in the right lower quadrant might be indicative of an inflamed or ruptured appendix. When the gallbladder is injured or inflamed, the patient may report having pain just under the margin of the ribs on the right side or pain between the shoulder blades.

As blood and fluid from damaged organs flow into the peritoneal cavity, the common response is acute pain that gradually spreads across the entire abdomen. The resulting inflammation of the peritoneum, called *peritonitis*, can result in pain provoked by removal of pressure, a finding commonly referred to as *rebound tenderness*. It is often discovered while rescuers are in the process of moving the patient onto the stretcher or while palpating the abdomen during the physical examination. If the EMT suspects rebound tenderness, he or she should not attempt to reproduce it. Note the finding but then refrain from aggravating the site further.

Making your assessment even more challenging is that the patient may present with voluntary or involuntary **guarding**. Voluntary guarding occurs when the patient tenses up or stiffens his or her abdominal muscles in a conscious effort to splint the area, *guarding* against movements that would provoke additional pain. By contrast, involuntary guarding persists even when the patient is distracted; it is the result of muscle spasms from peritonitis. Additionally, the patient with abdominal pain may prefer to lie still with the knees drawn up toward the chest. If taking a deep breath causes the pain to intensify, the patient's breathing may be rapid and shallow.

If the patient has been subjected to a significant MOI, an exam of the entire body is warranted. Moving from head to toe, quickly but thoroughly survey for additional injuries. If a life-threatening injury is discovered, the EMT must treat it immediately. Assess the patient's need for spinal motion restriction and apply it in accordance with local protocol. Immobilizing a patient with penetrating trauma is not indicated. Spinal column instability after gunshot wounds is uncommon, whereas delaying transport to a trauma center could prove fatal. Do not delay the transport of seriously injured trauma patients for the sake of completing non–life-saving treatments, such as splinting extremity fractures or dressing superficial wounds. Secondary injuries should be managed en route to the hospital.

## Secondary Assessment

In some instances, whether due to a short transport time or the need to manage life-threatening injuries en route to the hospital, the EMT may not have sufficient time to complete a secondary assessment. However, when time and circumstances permit it, perform a systematic physical examination:

- As much as practical, protect the patient's dignity and privacy. If the patient's condition permits, wait until you are in the back of the ambulance before removing clothing.
- Unless spinal injury is suspected, transport the patient in his or her position of comfort. For some, the fetal position may provide the greatest degree of comfort, as it reduces abdominal tension and subsequently provides measure of pain relief.

- For a patient with a suspected spinal injury, place padding such as blankets or pillows under the knees to help alleviate tension on the abdominal wall.
- Remove or loosen clothing to expose the injured regions of the body. Use care in situations where blood may have adhered to the material, and avoid causing further damage to exposed tissues, such as in the case of an evisceration.

### Words of Wisdom

For a number of reasons, bowel sounds are not typically auscultated in the field. The noise often found at an out-of-hospital scene makes it incredibly difficult to hear and interpret these sounds. Even in a relatively quiet environment, those trained in the performance of this skill will rarely have sufficient time to do it properly. Ultimately, bowel sounds are of limited value in the prehospital evaluation of trauma patients.

Inspect and palpate the abdomen, looking for signs of injury (DCAP-BTLS). Palpation should be systematic, assessing each of the four abdominal

## YOU are the Provider

After applying high-flow oxygen to the patient, you perform a secondary assessment. Your partner continues to manually stabilize the patient's head in a neutral position. During your physical examination, you find numerous abrasions to his anterior abdomen and flanks, and he has pain to palpation of his right upper abdominal quadrant. The rest of your secondary assessment is unremarkable for gross injuries. An off-duty EMT from your agency, who was a spectator at the rodeo, provides assistance and obtains a set of vital signs.

| Recording Time: 6 Minutes | |
|---|---|
| **Respirations** | 24 breaths/min; adequate depth |
| **Pulse** | 120 beats/min; weak and regular |
| **Skin** | Pale, cool, and clammy |
| **Blood pressure** | 104/54 mm Hg |
| **Oxygen saturation (Spo$_2$)** | 97% (on oxygen) |

Spinal motion restriction is maintained and the patient is loaded into the ambulance. He is still, conscious, and alert, but is restless and reports being very thirsty. You begin transport to the hospital while continuing to assess and treat the patient en route.

**5.** What are some common bruising patterns and clinical signs associated with intra-abdominal bleeding?

quadrants individually, preferably beginning with an area in which the patient does not report having pain. This approach allows you to investigate the possibility of radiation and extension of the pain into other quadrants without causing the patient to voluntarily guard the rest of the abdomen. Palpation should begin with light touch, slowly progressing deeper into the tissues. The objective is to pinpoint the pain's location, not to increase its intensity. If a light touch produces pain, deep palpation is unnecessary and may actually aggravate the underlying trauma. Likewise, if the abdomen is obviously injured (eg, impaled object, evisceration), palpation is unlikely to yield information of value and may therefore be bypassed.

Closed injuries from blunt trauma may be evidenced by bruises (often reddened areas of skin at this early stage), abrasions, or other visible marks. The location or locations of these indicators should guide you to consider the underlying structures (**FIGURE 31-6**). For example, bruises in the right upper quadrant, left upper quadrant, or flank (the region below the rib cage and above the hip) might suggest an injury to the liver, spleen, or kidney, respectively (**FIGURE 31-7**). Bruises around the umbilicus may signify severe internal bleeding in the abdomen (**FIGURE 31-8**).

Obtain and record the patient's vital signs early, and repeat them every 5 minutes in the patient whom you suspect has a serious injury. This regular monitoring will help you to quickly identify changes in the patient's condition, including signs of decompensation from blood loss. Patients experiencing external or internal hemorrhaging should be monitored closely. Generally, the first blood pressure reading should be obtained manually with a sphygmomanometer (blood pressure cuff) and stethoscope. Subsequent blood pressure values may be assessed using an automated device. Remember that hypotension is a late sign of shock. Therefore, be on the alert for earlier signs, such as tachycardia and pale, cool, clammy skin.

## Assessment of an Isolated Abdominal Injury

If the evidence suggests the injury is isolated to the abdomen, you may limit the focus of your physical examination to the affected area. Visually

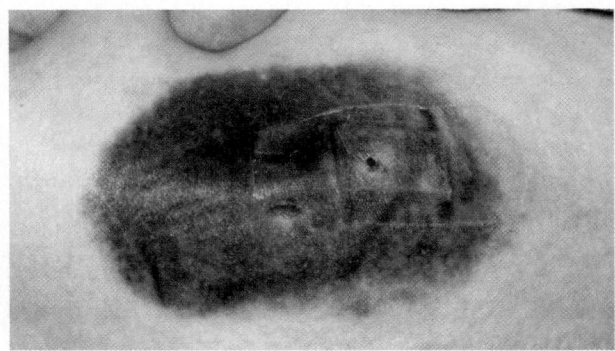

**FIGURE 31-6** Bruising on the abdomen can provide clues to the possible injury of underlying organs.
© Dr. P. Marazzi/Science Source.

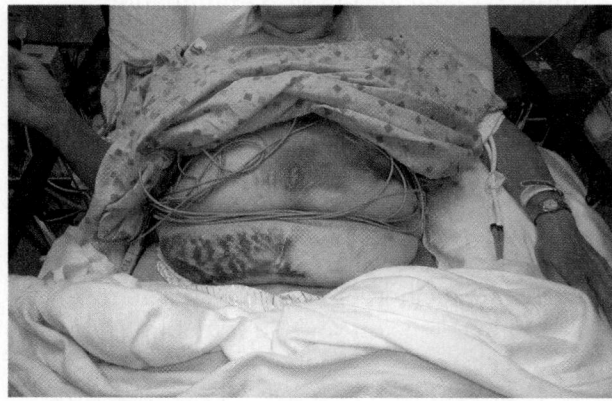

**FIGURE 31-7** Bruises in the right upper quadrant, left upper quadrant, or flank suggest an injury to the liver, spleen, or kidney, respectively.
© E.M. Singletary, M.D. Used with permission.

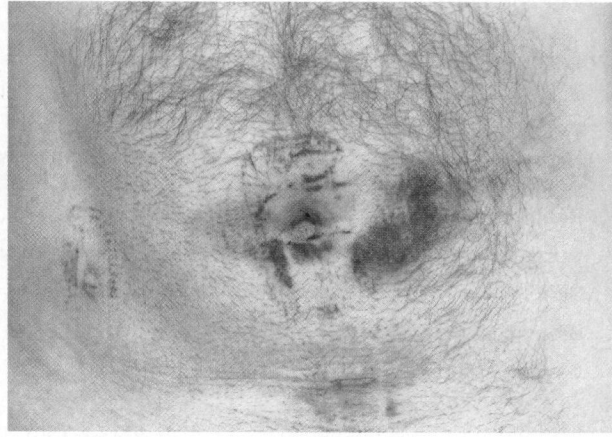

**FIGURE 31-8** Bruising around the umbilicus indicates the possibility of significant bleeding inside the abdomen.
© Peter Dazeley/The Image Bank/Getty Images.

inspect the abdomen for penetrating wounds (eg, gunshots, stabbings). As mentioned previously, you should not be deceived by a seemingly small wound; the outward appearance does not necessarily reflect the extent of the underlying injuries. If an entry wound is discovered, check for a corresponding exit wound. If the injury was caused by a high-velocity missile from a rifle, you may see a small, harmless-looking entrance wound with a large, gaping exit wound. For patients who have a knife or other object embedded in the abdomen, stabilize the object with supportive bandaging. Do not attempt to remove it.

### Words of Wisdom

Occasionally, you will have a patient who is extremely sensitive to palpation or is ticklish. This can make the physical examination process more difficult. Because it is difficult for a patient to tickle himself or herself, use the technique of placing the patient's hand on the surface of his or her abdomen and then palpate and compress the abdomen with the patient's hand between your hand and the patient's skin.

### Words of Wisdom

Roll the patient onto his or her side to examine the back for signs of injury. Avoid log rolling a patient with an evisceration; doing so may cause more abdominal contents to protrude from the wound. Keep such patients supine. When safe to do so, allow them to flex their knees to reduce tension in the abdominal muscles.

### Reassessment

Repeat the primary assessment, and reassess the vital signs. Evaluate the status of interventions performed as well as the patient's response to treatment. Note trends in the patient's mental status, pain level, and vital signs, and determine whether the patient's condition is improving or deteriorating. Make adjustments in care as needed.

Contact the receiving hospital, and outline the patient's MOI, injuries, and relevant vital signs. Use approved medical and anatomic terminology correctly, but when in doubt, avoid jargon and simply describe what you see. Include pertinent negatives and details about the scene.

## Emergency Medical Care of Abdominal Injuries

### Closed Abdominal Injuries
#### Blunt Abdominal Injuries

A patient with blunt abdominal trauma may have one or more of the following:

- Severe bruising of the abdominal wall
- Laceration of the liver and spleen
- Rupture of the intestine
- Tears in the mesentery, the membranous folds that attach the intestines to the walls of the body, and injury to blood vessels within them
- Kidney rupture or avulsion from its arteries and veins
- Rupture of the urinary bladder, especially in a patient who had a full and distended bladder at the time of the injury
- Severe intra-abdominal hemorrhage
- Peritoneal irritation and inflammation in response to the rupture of hollow organs

A patient who has sustained blunt abdominal trauma should be monitored closely and evaluated for progression into shock. The patient with blunt abdominal trauma may experience nausea and vomiting. Be prepared to protect the airway with suctioning as needed. Administer oxygen to patients who are unconscious or who are in shock. Cover patients with a blanket to keep them warm. If the patient's diaphragm has ruptured and abdominal organs are in the chest cavity, ventilatory assistance with a bag-mask device may be necessary. Consider calling ALS for placement of an oral or nasal gastric tube.

### Open Abdominal Injuries
#### Penetrating Abdominal Injuries

Patients with penetrating injuries generally have obvious wounds and external bleeding (**FIGURE 31-9A**). For example, a large wound may have protrusions of bowel, fat, or other structures. However, not all open injuries will present with significant external bleeding. The EMT should maintain a high index of

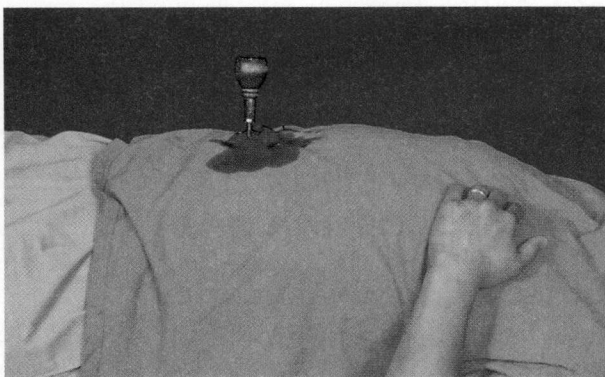

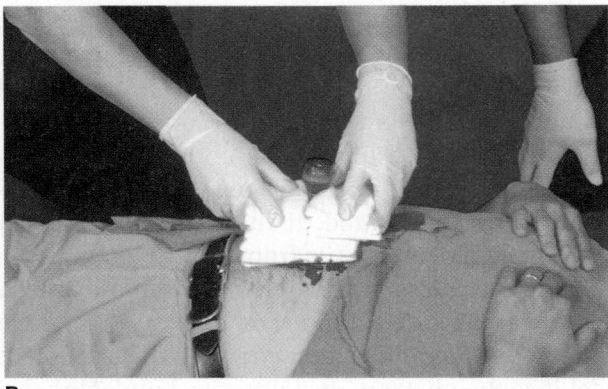

**A**

**B**

**FIGURE 31-9 A.** Penetrating injuries have obvious wounds and may also have external bleeding. **B.** If the penetrating object is still in place, use a roller bandage to stabilize the object and to control bleeding.

A, B: © Jones & Bartlett Learning. Courtesy of MIEMSS.

suspicion that these patients have substantial, albeit unseen, internal hemorrhage.

In caring for a patient with a penetrating wound to the abdomen, follow the general procedures previously described for care of a blunt abdominal injury as well as following the specific steps for the penetrating wound. Inspect the patient's back and sides for exit wounds, and apply a dry, sterile dressing to any open wounds. If the penetrating object is still in place, apply a stabilizing bandage around it to control external bleeding and to minimize movement of the object (**FIGURE 31-9B**).

## Abdominal Evisceration

Severe lacerations of the abdominal wall may produce an evisceration, a wound from which internal organs protrude (**FIGURE 31-10**). If an evisceration is discovered, place a sterile dressing moistened with normal saline over the wound, apply a bandage, and transport. Never attempt to push eviscerated tissue or organs back into the abdominal cavity. Because body heat escapes quickly from open abdominal wounds, and because exposed organs lose fluid rapidly, the affected area should be kept warm and moist (**FIGURE 31-11**). Avoid using adherent materials and those that lose substance when wet,

## YOU are the Provider

You reassess the patient en route and note that his clinical status has deteriorated. You ask your driver to notify the receiving facility as you continue to treat the patient. Given your relatively short transport time to the hospital, you determine that ALS rendezvous would not result in earlier appropriate care for the patient.

| Recording Time: 12 Minutes | |
| --- | --- |
| **Level of consciousness** | Responsive to pain only |
| **Respirations** | 28 breaths/min; shallow |
| **Pulse** | 134 beats/min; absent radial pulses |
| **Skin** | Cool, pale, and clammy |
| **Blood pressure** | 82/54 mm Hg |
| **Spo$_2$** | 88% (on oxygen) |

**6.** Why is your patient's condition deteriorating? How should you modify your treatment?

such as toilet paper, facial tissue, paper towels, or absorbent cotton. Protocols in some EMS systems direct that an occlusive dressing be placed over the top of the other dressings.

The abdomen of a patient with a ruptured diaphragm may have a sunken anterior wall, as

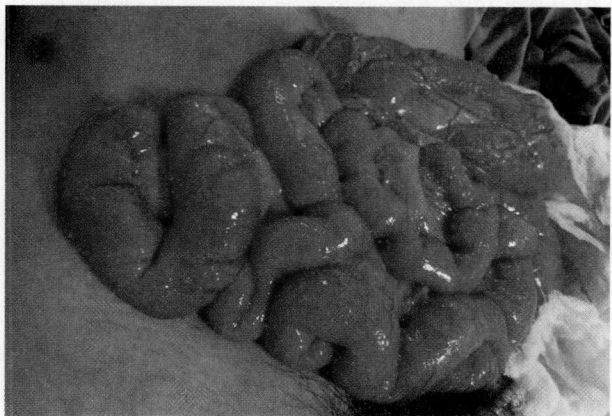

**FIGURE 31-10** An abdominal evisceration is an open abdominal wound from which internal organs protrude.

© Arucha Srimuang/Shutterstock.

abdominal contents have shifted up into the chest cavity. The added pressure on the lungs may lead to impaired lung expansion and difficulty breathing, necessitating positive pressure ventilation by bag-mask device.

## Anatomy of the Genitourinary System

The organs of the genitourinary system play a role in waste removal and sexual reproduction.

The urinary system controls the discharge of certain waste materials filtered from the blood by the kidneys. The kidneys are solid organs, whereas the ureters, urinary bladder, and urethra are hollow organs (**FIGURE 31-12**).

With the exception of the prostate gland and the seminal vesicles, the male genitalia lie outside the pelvic cavity (**FIGURE 31-13**). The structures of the female genitalia, except for the vulva, clitoris, and labia, are contained entirely within the pelvis (**FIGURE 31-14**). The male and female reproductive organs have certain similarities and, of course,

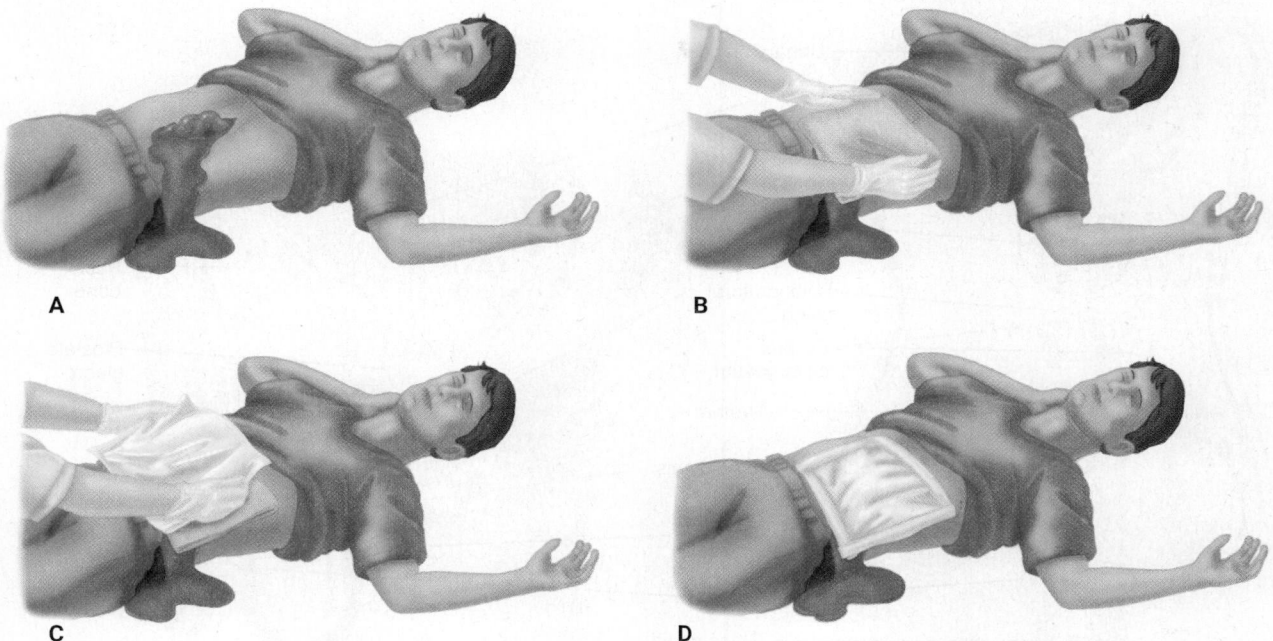

**A**

**B**

**C**

**D**

**FIGURE 31-11 A.** The open abdomen radiates body heat rapidly and must be covered. **B.** Cover the wound with moistened, sterile dressings and with an occlusive dressing, depending on local protocol. **C.** Secure the dressing with a bandage. **D.** Secure the bandage with tape.

**A-D:** © Jones & Bartlett Learning.

basic differences. They allow for the production of sperm and egg cells and their respective hormones, the act of sexual intercourse, and, ultimately, reproduction.

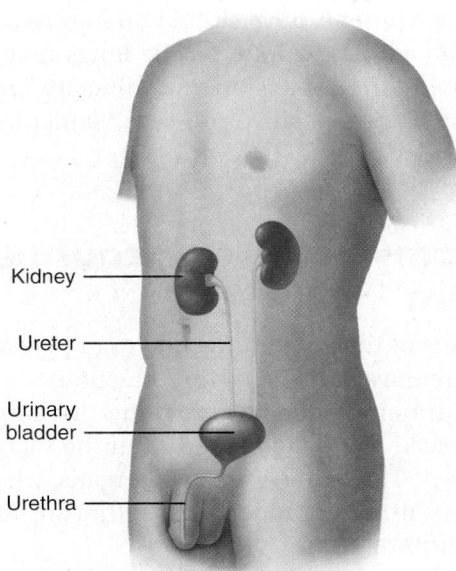

**FIGURE 31-12** The urinary system lies behind the digestive tract. The kidneys are solid organs; the ureter, urinary bladder, and urethra are hollow organs.

© Jones & Bartlett Learning.

## Street Smarts

As health care professionals trained in the management of life-threatening emergencies, EMTs and paramedics have learned how to respond in situations others would find terrifying. Over time, what you consider to be an "emergency" and what that word means to a layperson may differ greatly. What has become a routine sight for you may be unfamiliar and frightening for a patient or his or her family. In fact, your routine day may be the worst day of their lives. For this reason, we in EMS must continually remind ourselves to put ourselves in our patients' shoes. Of all the types of care we provide, one of the most meaningful is often overlooked: empathy.

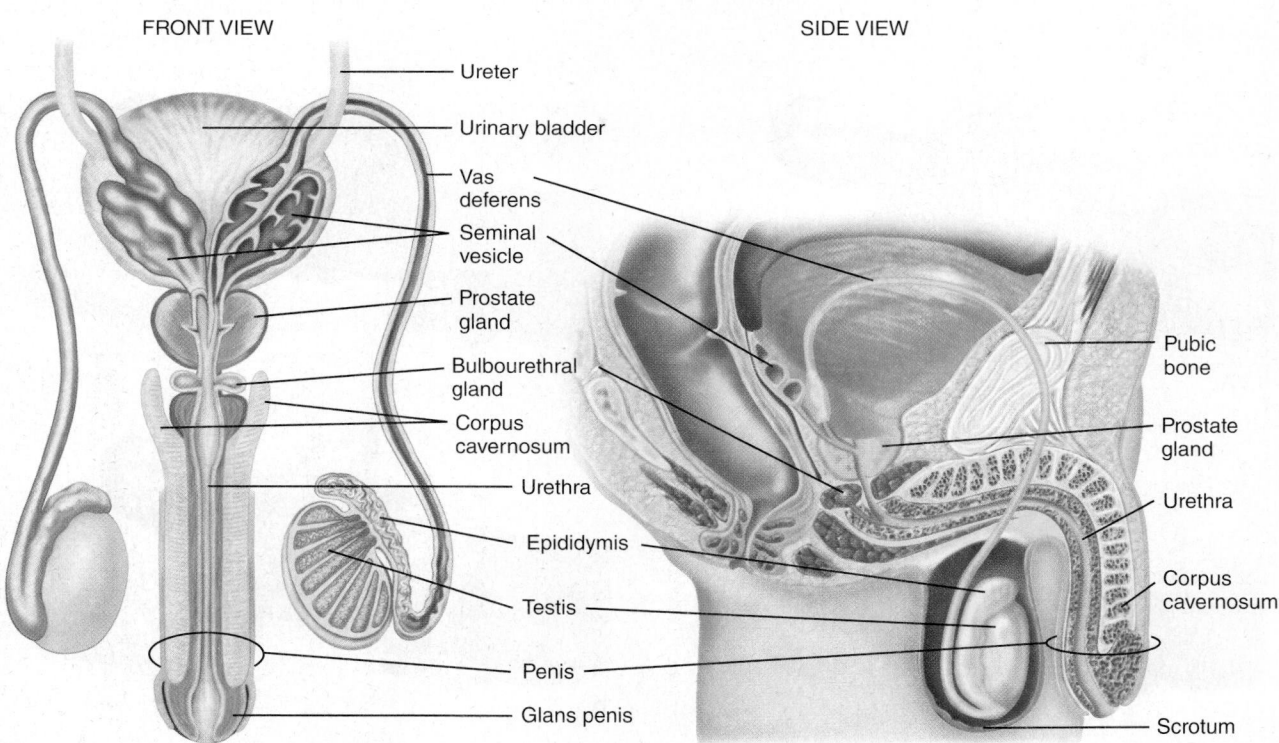

**FIGURE 31-13** The male reproductive system includes the testicles, vas deferens, seminal vesicles, prostate gland, urethra, and penis.

© Jones & Bartlett Learning.

FRONT VIEW         SIDE VIEW

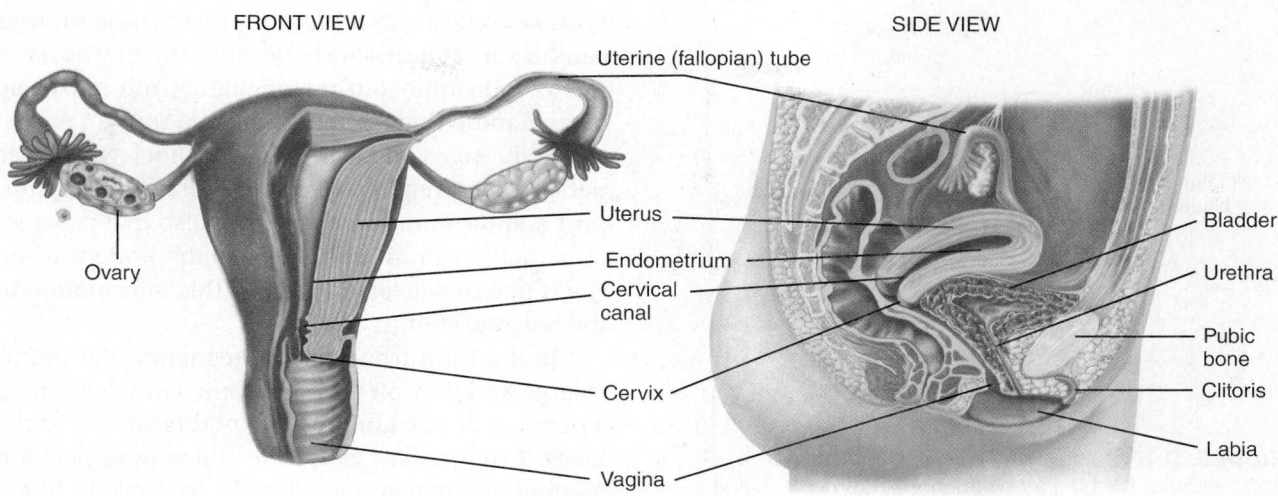

**FIGURE 31-14** The female reproductive system includes the ovaries, fallopian tubes, uterus, cervix, and vagina.

© Jones & Bartlett Learning.

# Injuries of the Genitourinary System

## Injuries of the Kidneys

Injuries of the kidneys are not uncommon, and they rarely occur in isolation. This is because the kidneys lie in such a well-protected area of the body that for them to sustain damage from blunt or penetrating mechanisms, the structures that surround them would almost certainly have to be damaged as well. Less significant injuries to the kidneys may result from a smaller yet concentrated direct blow or from something as innocuous as being tackled while playing football (**FIGURE 31-15**). Suspect kidney damage if the patient has a history or physical evidence of any of the following:

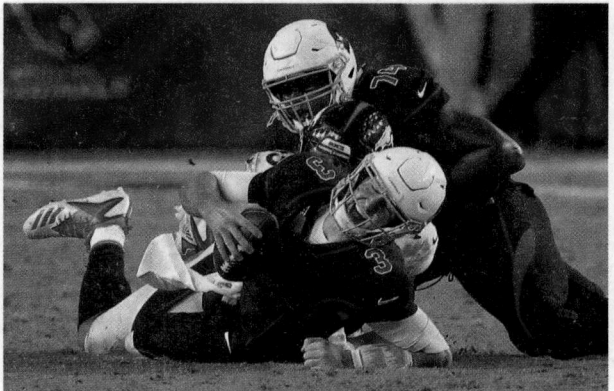

**FIGURE 31-15** A tackle in football that results in blunt trauma to the lower rib cage or the flank can cause kidney injury.

© Rick Scuteri/AP/Shutterstock.

- An abrasion, laceration, or contusion in the flank
- A penetrating wound in the flank (the region below the rib cage and above the hip) or the upper abdomen
- Fractures on either side of the lower rib cage or of the lower thoracic or upper lumbar vertebrae
- A hematoma in the flank region

## Injuries to the Urinary Bladder

Injury to the urinary bladder, either blunt or penetrating, may result in its rupture. When this happens, urine spills into the surrounding tissues, and any urine that passes through the urethra is likely to be bloody. Blunt injuries of the lower abdomen or pelvis often cause rupture of the urinary bladder, particularly when the bladder is full and distended. Sharp, bony fragments from a fracture of the pelvis often perforate the urinary bladder (**FIGURE 31-16**). Penetrating wounds of the lower midabdomen or the perineum (the pelvic floor and associated structures that occupy the pelvic outlet) can directly involve the urinary bladder. In men, sudden deceleration from a motor vehicle or motorcycle crash can literally shear the bladder from the urethra. Remember, in the second and third trimesters

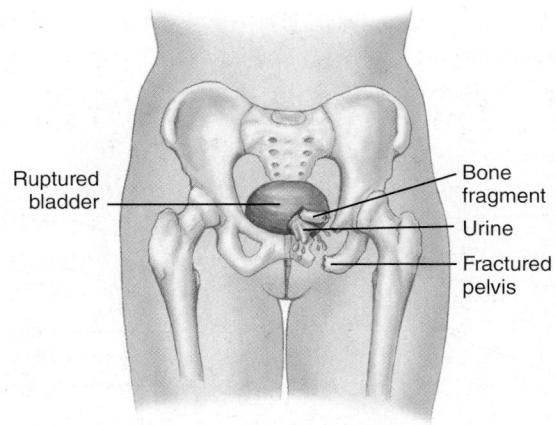

Ruptured
bladder

Bone
fragment

Urine

Fractured
pelvis

**FIGURE 31-16** Fracture of the pelvis can result in perforation of the bladder by the bony fragments. Urine then leaks into the pelvis.

© Jones & Bartlett Learning.

of pregnancy, the incidence of injury to the urinary bladder is increased by displacement of the uterus.

## Injuries of the External Male Genitalia

Injuries of the external male genitalia include all types of soft-tissue wounds. Although these injuries are uniformly painful and generally a source of great concern to the patient, they are rarely considered life threatening. They should not be given priority over other, more severe wounds, unless the rich blood supply causes significant bleeding. It is important to know that pain from an injury to the testicles or another cause, such as infection or cancer, may be referred to the lower abdomen. As a result, when assessing men with lower abdominal pain you should also consider injury or other causes of pain to the testicles.

## Injuries of the Female Genitalia

### Internal Female Genitalia

The uterus, ovaries, and fallopian tubes are subject to the same kinds of injuries as any other internal organ. However, they are rarely damaged because they are small, deep in the pelvis, and well protected by the pelvic bones. Unlike the urinary bladder, which lies adjacent to the bony pelvis, they are usually not injured as a result of a pelvic fracture.

An exception is the pregnant uterus. As pregnancy progresses, the uterus enlarges substantially and rises out of the pelvis, becoming vulnerable to both penetrating and blunt injuries. These injuries can be particularly severe because the uterus has a rich blood supply during pregnancy. You must also keep in mind that the fetus is at risk. You can expect to see the signs and symptoms of shock with these patients; be prepared to provide all necessary support and prompt transport. Note also that contractions may begin. If possible, ask the patient when she is due to deliver, and report this information to the hospital staff.

In the third trimester of pregnancy, the uterus is large and may obstruct the vena cava, leading to a decrease in the amount of blood returning to the heart if the patient is placed in a supine position (supine hypotensive syndrome). As a result, blood pressure may decrease. The patient should be carefully placed on her left side so that the uterus will not lie on the vena cava. If the patient is secured to a backboard, tilt the board to the left. Chapter 24, *Gynecologic Emergencies*, and Chapter 34, *Obstetrics and Neonatal Care*, cover gynecologic emergencies and the special considerations for pregnant trauma patients in detail.

### External Female Genitalia

The external female genitalia include the vulva, the clitoris, and the major and minor labia (lips) at the entrance of the vagina. Injuries of the external female genitalia can include all types of soft-tissue injuries. Because these genital parts have a rich nerve supply, injuries are very painful. Vaginal bleeding may occur because of penetrating or blunt trauma. These injuries can be accidental, as in the case of straddle injuries from bicycles or motorcycles; or they can be intentional, as in the case of assaults. Determining the MOI will assist you in deciding if you need to call for additional resources, as in the case of sexual assault.

In any case of trauma, it is important to determine the possibility of pregnancy. Ask the patient for the date of her last known menstrual period or if she has been sexually active. Assume all women of childbearing age are possibly pregnant. This information is medically relevant because some medications and tests may be harmful for a fetus, and there is the potential for another source of blood loss in the gravid uterus.

In cases of external bleeding and trauma, a sterile absorbent sanitary napkin or pad may be applied to the labia. Do not insert instruments, gloved fingers, or a tampon into the vagina because this can cause further damage.

## Patient Assessment of the Genitourinary System

Being examined after sustaining a genitourinary injury can be embarrassing for the patient. Therefore, the EMT should maintain a professional presence at all times when interacting with these patients. As much as is practical, provide the patient with privacy during the assessment process. If possible, the assessment should be performed by a provider of the same sex.

### Scene Size-up

Assess the scene for anything that could jeopardize the safety of the crew, the patient, or bystanders. Do not approach until all threats have been mitigated by the appropriate personnel (eg, law enforcement, hazmat). Apply standard precautions to minimize your direct exposure to body fluids. Be aware that while visible blood on the patient's clothing or surroundings can be apparent as you approach, blood can also be hidden under thick clothing such as denim and leather. In addition to gloves, eye protection is required whenever treating a patient with open injuries. Determine the number of patients and consider if you need additional or specialized resources on the scene.

By integrating the information supplied by dispatch with your observations of the scene and the MOI, you may be able to anticipate the presence of certain injuries. Be cognizant of the possibility that the patient may be reluctant to discuss his or her injuries or consent to a physical examination. It is also possible that the patient may withhold or understate the details of the MOI for fear of embarrassment. Only by maintaining a professional demeanor, respecting the patient's privacy, and protecting the patient's dignity will you be able to gain the patient's trust. Having that trust increases the likelihood that the patient will disclose important pieces of information that may have an impact on his or her care.

### Primary Assessment

Upon reaching the patient, quickly identify and treat immediate life threats, establish the priority level of the patient's condition, and prepare for transport. The genitourinary system is highly vascular. Consequently, genitourinary injuries can precipitate a substantial loss of blood. Because life-threatening

## YOU are the Provider

The patient is becoming combative and resists your attempts to assist his ventilations, but he will tolerate oxygen via a nonrebreathing mask. During your reassessment, you note blood on the front of the patient's underwear, which was not there during previous assessments. You examine the area more carefully but do not see any open injuries to the genitalia or adjacent areas. You call your radio report in to the receiving facility.

| Recording Time:  17 Minutes | |
| --- | --- |
| Level of consciousness | Responsive to pain only |
| Respirations | 28 breaths/min; shallow |
| Pulse | 128 beats/min; weak and regular |
| Skin | Cool, pale, and clammy |
| Blood pressure | 90/58 mm Hg |
| Spo$_2$ | 93% (on oxygen) |

The patient begins vomiting bright red blood. You quickly turn the backboard to the side to allow the vomitus to drain and then suction his mouth to ensure that his airway remains clear.

**7.** On the basis of your reassessment, what additional injuries should you suspect?

**8.** How will your reassessment findings change your current treatment plan?

hemorrhage must be addressed immediately, even before airway or breathing concerns, do not circumvent examining this area of the body. Look externally at the patient's undergarments for signs of bleeding and injury. Make every effort to protect the patient's privacy and dignity as you inspect the exterior genitalia for visible signs of injury.

Once severe bleeding has been controlled, ensure the patient has a clear and patent airway. Consider the need for spinal motion restriction, and use caution to avoid excessive manipulation of the cervical spine as you manage the patient's airway. If the patient is unresponsive or has a significantly altered level of consciousness, consider inserting an oropharyngeal or nasopharyngeal airway. Ensure the patient is breathing adequately. Provide assisted ventilations using a bag-mask device as needed.

Check the patient's pulse rate and quality; determine the skin condition, color, and temperature; and assess the capillary refill time. If signs of shock are present, treat accordingly. Remember that because internal bleeding may be well hidden in patients with closed injuries, you must have a high index of suspicion for shock in such cases.

Also during the primary assessment, note the patient's level of alertness. Is the patient awake and interacting with his or her surroundings? By contrast, is the patient lying motionless and silent? If so, does the patient respond when you say his or her name? If not, will the patient react to physical stimuli such as a sternal rub?

A patient with a genitourinary system injury should be taken to a trauma center for evaluation and treatment. Even when these injuries do not become life-*ending*, they can nevertheless be life-*altering*—often dramatically so, requiring specialized medical care. When possible and when protocol permits, these patients should be transported to a facility capable of treating this subset of injuries.

## History Taking

When attempting to ascertain the chief complaint, your goal is to understand why the patient felt he or she needed medical assistance. Why did he or she call 9-1-1? Ask about associated complaints, but avoid putting words in the patient's mouth by asking closed-ended questions. For example, when asking the patient to describe his or her discomfort, do not ask, "Is it a stabbing pain?" or "Do you also have pain in your shoulder?" Instead, ask open-ended

questions such as "How would you describe the discomfort?" or "Is anything else bothering you?" Common associated complaints with genitourinary injuries are nausea, vomiting, diarrhea, blood in the urine (hematuria), vomiting of blood (hematemesis), and abnormal bowel and bladder habits such as an increase in frequency or the absence of the need to void.

You can use the SAMPLE history to gain further insight into the specifics of the chief complaint. Use OPQRST to learn more about the patient's pain experience. Inquire about urine output; specifically, did the patient notice the presence of blood in the urine? Note, however, that occult bleeding into the urine may still exist even though it was not severe enough for the patient to see it with the naked eye. Therefore, just because bleeding has not been obvious, that fact alone does not preclude the possibility that your patient has internal genitourinary injuries.

Ask your patient if he or she is allergic to any medications and other triggers. Medications may mask the signs and symptoms of injuries or make them more severe, so it is important to know what your patient takes, whether prescribed, over-the-counter, or "natural" (eg, herbal remedies). The importance of past medical history cannot be overstated. The incidence of previous injuries or illnesses affecting the genitourinary system may be a key element to understanding the patient's present condition. The last oral intake is important to ascertain as well, as this information may aid physicians in determining whether the symptoms are related to the ingestion of specific foods and/or fluids. Finally, addressing the events that led to the injury may supply you with valuable clues.

## Secondary Assessment

The secondary assessment is a more thorough physical examination used to uncover injuries that may have been missed during the primary assessment. As previously mentioned, there are times when the EMT is unable to conduct a secondary assessment. Most often, this is due to one of two conditions: (1) the need to provide ongoing life-saving treatment to a patient with critical injuries or (2) an especially short duration of transport to the emergency department (ED).

Generally, when your patient's injuries are isolated to the genitourinary system and the MOI is relatively minor, you can forego a full head-to-toe exam and instead focus solely on the affected region. By contrast, if trauma is extensive, likely affecting multiple systems, the physical exam should include the entire body. Applying a systematic approach while assessing for DCAP-BTLS reduces the risk that a significant injury will be missed.

Finally, obtain the patient's vital signs and reassess them frequently, observing for trends in the patient's condition. As previously mentioned, signs such as tachycardia, tachypnea, low blood pressure, weak pulse, and cool, moist, and pale skin should lead you to suspect shock. Although paleness, or a decrease in blood flow, can be difficult to detect in dark-skinned people, it may be observed by examining mucous membranes inside the inner lower eyelid and capillary refill. On general observation, the patient may appear ashen or gray. Treat accordingly.

## Reassessment

Repeat the primary assessment, and obtain additional sets of vital signs. Reassess all interventions performed and determine how the patient is responding to care. Adjust interventions as necessary. As early as possible, communicate your suspicions, concerns, and assessment findings to receiving facility staff. Giving timely advance notice ensures ED staff are prepared.

# Emergency Medical Care of Genitourinary Injuries

## Kidneys

Damage to the kidneys may not be obvious on inspection of the patient. You may or may not see bruises or lacerations on the overlying skin. However, if the injury is associated with significant blood loss, you will see signs of shock. Another potential sign of kidney damage is blood in the urine (hematuria). Treat shock and associated injuries in the appropriate manner. Provide rapid transport to the hospital, carefully monitoring the patient's vital signs en route.

## Urinary Bladder

If you discover blood at the urethral opening or physical signs of trauma on the lower abdomen, pelvis, or perineum, the urinary bladder may be damaged. There may be blood at the tip of the penis or a bloodstain on the patient's underwear.

## External Male Genitalia

A few general rules apply to the treatment of injuries involving the external male genitalia:

- Because these injuries can be very painful, do whatever possible to make the patient comfortable.
- Cover abrasions with sterile, moist compresses.
- To control bleeding, apply direct pressure with dry, sterile gauze dressings.
- Never remove or manipulate objects impaled through or embedded in the urethra.
- If possible, retrieve avulsed skin and transport it along with the patient. However, any search for missing tissue should not delay transport, and it should never distract the providers from providing emergency care.

After controlling serious bleeding, the EMT who encounters a patient with an avulsion of the penis should wrap the tissue in a soft, sterile dressing moistened with sterile saline solution; place it in a bag or other container labeled with the patient's name; and rapidly transport it along with the patient.

When caring for a patient who has sustained an amputation of the penile shaft, whether partial or complete, the EMT's first concern must be bleeding control. Using a sterile dressing, he or she should apply direct pressure to the site. Constricting devices (ie, tourniquets) are not appropriate for the control of penile bleeding. As with avulsions, a completely amputated penis should be retrieved, as surgical reconstruction is possible. Wrap it in a moist, sterile dressing; place it in a plastic bag; and transport it along with the patient if possible. It should be kept cool but not placed into direct contact with ice.

When an erect penis is bent sharply, the shaft can be severely damaged, sometimes requiring surgical repair. This injury is associated with intense pain and bleeding into the tissues, and it can be quite frightening for the patient. Provide rapid transport to the ED.

Accidental laceration of the skin about the head of the penis usually occurs when the penis is erect and is associated with heavy bleeding. Local pressure with a sterile dressing is usually sufficient to stop the hemorrhage.

It is not uncommon for the skin of the shaft of the penis or the foreskin to get caught in the zipper of pants. If a small segment of the zipper is involved (one or two teeth), you can try to unzip the pants. However, if a longer segment is involved, or if the patient is agitated, do not attempt to unzip the pants. Instead, use heavy scissors to cut the zipper out of the pants to make the patient more comfortable during transport. Prior to cutting, explain to the patient what you are about to do. Be particularly careful not to cause injury to the scrotum while cutting the zipper away. Always be certain that you are able to see exactly what you are cutting with your scissors.

Urethral injuries in men are not uncommon. Lacerations of the urethra can result from straddle injuries, pelvic fractures, or penetrating wounds of the perineum. These injuries may bleed profusely; however, the bleeding may not be apparent externally. Direct pressure with a dry, sterile dressing usually controls any external hemorrhage. Because the urethra is the channel for urine, it is very important to know whether the patient can urinate and whether hematuria is present. For this reason, you should save any voided urine for later examination at the hospital. Any foreign bodies that may be protruding from the urethra will have to be removed in a surgical setting.

Avulsion of the skin of the scrotum may damage the scrotal contents. If possible, preserve the avulsed skin in a moist, sterile dressing for possible use in reconstruction. Wrap the scrotal contents or the perineal area with a sterile, moist compress, and use a local pressure dressing to control bleeding. Promptly transport the patient to the ED.

Direct blows to the scrotum can result in the rupture of a testicle or significant accumulation of blood around the testes. In either case, you should apply an ice pack to the scrotal area while transporting the patient.

## Female Genitalia

Lacerations, abrasions, and avulsions should be treated with moist, sterile compresses. Use local pressure to control bleeding and a diaper-type bandage to hold dressings in place. Under no circumstances should you pack or place dressings into the vagina. Leave any foreign bodies in place after you stabilize them with bandages.

In general, although these injuries are painful, they are seldom life threatening. Bleeding may be heavy but is usually controllable with local compression. Contusions and other blunt injuries all require careful in-hospital evaluation. However, the urgency for transport will be determined by associated injuries, the amount of hemorrhage, and the presence of shock.

## Rectal Bleeding

Rectal bleeding is a common complaint and something that you may hear as a chief complaint or secondary to abdominal or pelvic complaints. Bleeding from the rectum may present as bloodstains or blood soaking through underwear, or patients may report blood in the toilet after a bowel movement or attempted bowel movement. Rectal bleeding can be caused by a sexual assault, rectal foreign bodies, hemorrhoids, colitis, or ulcers of the digestive tract. Significant rectal bleeding can occur after hemorrhoid surgery and can lead to significant blood loss and shock.

## Sexual Assault and Rape

Sexual assault and rape are all too common. In the United States, an average of 433,648 individuals aged 12 years or older become victims of rape or sexual assault each year. The definition of rape, sexual assault, and similar terms differs by state. Although most victims are women, men and children are also victimized. Often, you can do little beyond providing compassion and transportation to the ED. On some occasions, patients will have sustained multiple-system trauma and will also need treatment of shock.

Do not examine the genitalia of a victim of sexual assault unless obvious bleeding requires you to apply a dressing. Treat all other injuries according to appropriate procedures and protocols for your EMS system. Observe standard precautions. Take care to shield the patient from curious onlookers. Because you may have to appear in court as much as several years later, you must document in detail the patient's history, assessment, treatment, and response to treatment. Do not speculate. Record only the facts.

Follow any crime scene policy established by your system to protect the scene and any potential evidence for police. Advise the patient not to wash, bathe, shower, douche (if female), urinate, or defecate until after a physician has examined him or her; this will help preserve any evidence of a crime. If oral penetration has occurred, advise the patient not to eat, drink, brush teeth, or use mouthwash until he or she has been examined. If the patient will tolerate being wrapped in a sterile burn sheet, this may help investigators find any hair, fluid, or fiber from the alleged offender. Handle the patient's clothes as little as possible, placing articles and any other evidence in paper bags. Do not use plastic bags. If a female patient insists on urinating, have

her do so in a sterile urine container (if available). Also, have her deposit the toilet paper in a paper bag. Seal and label the bag for the police because these items can be critical evidence.

To reduce the patient's anxiety, whenever possible the EMT who is caring for the patient should be the same sex as the patient. Remember, a victim of rape or sexual assault, whether a man or a woman, may need medical assistance. In these cases, you must treat the medical injuries but also provide privacy, support, and reassurance. Chapter 24, *Gynecologic Emergencies*, covers this topic in detail.

## YOU are the Provider SUMMARY

**1. How do hollow organ injuries differ from solid organ injuries?**

Hollow organs—such as the stomach, intestines, and urinary bladder—are structures through which materials pass. When hollow organs are ruptured or lacerated, they release their contents into the pelvis or peritoneal (abdominal) cavity. The release of hollow organ contents into the peritoneal cavity causes an intense inflammatory response (peritonitis), which can result in a life-threatening infection. Hollow organ injury may be associated with some internal bleeding; however, the major cause of death is sepsis, which typically occurs later in the hospital.

Solid organs—such as the liver, spleen, pancreas, and kidneys—are highly vascular and tend to bleed profusely when injured by blunt or penetrating trauma. Unlike hollow organ injury, the major cause of death following injury to the solid organs is internal hemorrhage, which can very quickly lead to death.

**2. How should you focus your assessment of a patient with potential intra-abdominal bleeding?**

When you are caring for a patient with blunt or penetrating abdominal trauma, you should focus on recognizing signs and symptoms of shock, initiating treatment without delay, and providing rapid transport to the hospital.

If your patient sustained blunt abdominal trauma, has external evidence of injury (eg, bruising, distention, rigidity), or signs of shock—all signs that clearly suggest intra-abdominal bleeding—does the origin of the hemorrhage affect the treatment that you provide in the field? The answer, of course, is no. What

*does* matter is that *the patient is bleeding from a source that you cannot control*, and that his or her outcome depends on you recognizing the situation, initiating prompt treatment, and providing rapid transport.

**3. How should you interpret your primary assessment findings?**

Rarely do EMS providers actually witness the injury when it occurs; this is why it is so important for you to pay attention to clues that suggest a particular mechanism of injury (MOI). However, in this situation you did witness the patient being trampled by a bull and were able to see that his injuries appear to be to the abdomen and flanks.

On the basis of the MOI and your primary assessment findings, your initial impression should be that your patient is in shock, which is likely the result of intra-abdominal bleeding. Although you will need to perform a head-to-toe secondary assessment to identify any other injuries, intra-abdominal bleeding is the most plausible field impression given the information that you have. You should quickly identify this patient as a "load and go," begin immediate treatment, and arrange for rapid transport to the hospital.

**4. What immediate treatment is indicated for this patient?**

Apply high-flow oxygen via a nonrebreathing mask. Oxygen is a critical treatment for any patient with signs and symptoms of shock and should be administered as soon as possible. Carefully monitor the patient's breathing, and be ready to assist his ventilations if signs of inadequate breathing (eg, shallow breaths [reduced tidal volume], decreased mental status) are observed.

Cover the patient with a blanket to keep him warm. Some body functions, such as blood clotting, are negatively affected by decreased body temperature; therefore keeping the patient warm is essential. Patients in shock are also less able to maintain body temperature because heat production requires energy, and energy requires oxygen, so diminished heat production is made worse by a lack of oxygen. In this case, oxygen is also needed as the loss of oxygen-carrying red blood cells reduces perfusion to the vital organs.

**5. What are some common bruising patterns and clinical signs associated with intra-abdominal bleeding?**

As blood accumulates in the abdominal cavity, the abdomen typically becomes distended and rigid. Palpation of the patient's abdomen can be challenging in the presence of abdominal guarding. Guarding is a conscious (voluntary) or unintentional (involuntary) response to abdominal trauma, and it is characterized by stiffening of the rectus abdominis muscles in an attempt to minimize the pain. Although guarding may be seen in patients who do not have significant intra-abdominal injury, *any abdominal rigidity following trauma should be assumed to be the result of internal bleeding*.

If bruising is observed following abdominal trauma, there are several patterns that you should look for during your assessment of the abdomen. Periumbilical (around the umbilicus) bruising is an indicator of blood in the peritoneal cavity. Bruising to the flank area is an indicator of blood behind the peritoneal cavity and suggests injury to the kidneys, pelvis, or bladder.

Injury to the liver or spleen may present with referred pain to the shoulders. Unlike radiating pain, which is characterized by pain that "moves" from one area of the body to another, referred pain is characterized by pain in two separate locations.

It is important to note that some patients with intra-abdominal bleeding may not present with external signs of injury. The retroperitoneal space is a common location for hidden bleeding and can accommodate a large volume of blood.

**6. Why is your patient's condition deteriorating? How should you modify your treatment?**

Your patient was exhibiting signs of shock on initial contact with him. His level of consciousness has decreased, he is hypotensive, his breathing is inadequate, and his oxygen saturation is falling despite the use of high-flow oxygen. This indicates that he is now in decompensated shock; the compensatory mechanisms that help maintain adequate perfusion to the tissues and cells of the body are failing.

Any deterioration in a patient's clinical status should prompt you to immediately repeat the primary assessment. His oxygen saturation is falling, which is likely the result of the combined effects of internal bleeding and inadequate breathing. At this point, you should begin assisting his ventilations with a bag-mask device attached to high-flow oxygen. Consider inserting a nasopharyngeal airway; his level of consciousness has decreased to the point that he may not be able to completely maintain his own airway.

Patients who have experienced trauma and who are in shock should be transported in the supine position.

As you continue to treat the patient, you must continuously monitor his XABCs. His condition is critical, and he is at high risk for cardiac arrest. If he becomes apneic and pulseless, begin cardiopulmonary resuscitation and ask your partner to update the receiving facility. An ALS unit would be beneficial for airway management and IV fluid administration if it could be arranged without delaying transport.

**7. On the basis of your reassessment, what additional injuries should you suspect?**

Bloodstains on the front of the patient's underwear without evidence of any open genitalia injuries indicates that he has blood in his urine (hematuria) and suggests injury to his kidneys, urinary bladder, or both. Remember, the patient had diffuse abdominal pain and abrasions to *both* the anterior part of his abdomen and flanks. In addition to injury to his liver or spleen, which is likely the cause of his shock, it is clearly possible that he experienced injury to his genitourinary organs as well.

As you will recall from your evaluation of the patient, he had pain and abrasions of his flanks; this indicates direct trauma to that area, which overlies the kidneys. Injury to the kidneys may not be obvious during your assessment. If anything, you may see only abrasions or redness over the flanks; flank bruising typically does not manifest until later. Because one of the functions of the kidney is the formation of urine, another sign of kidney injury is hematuria.

Hematuria can also indicate rupture of the urinary bladder. Blood at the urethral opening should also make you suspicious for urinary bladder rupture.

## YOU are the Provider SUMMARY *continued*

Hematemesis, the vomiting of blood, indicates bleeding within the gastrointestinal tract. More specifically, vomiting bright red blood indicates injury to some part of the upper gastrointestinal tract. You should suspect injury to the patient's stomach.

**8. How will your reassessment findings change your current treatment plan?**

Despite the presence of indicators that suggest injury to both solid and hollow abdominal and genitourinary organs, you should concentrate on maintaining the patient's airway, ensure adequate oxygenation and ventilation, and treat for shock. There are no other prehospital treatments for the patient's suspected specific injuries. Rapid transport to a trauma center is critical! If the scene location is a distance from the hospital, air transport should be considered. Blunt trauma with internal bleeding is often more likely to be fatal than penetrating abdominal trauma with external bleeding. Blunt trauma with internal bleeding is often more significant than penetrating abdominal trauma with external bleeding. Open injuries are obvious, whereas internal injuries are often hidden and may be missed. In the absence of obvious external injury, a trauma patient with signs of shock should be assumed to be bleeding into his or her abdomen.

### EMS Patient Care Report (PCR)

| **Date:** 12-16-20 | **Incident No.:** 012809 | **Nature of Call:** Traumatic injury | | **Location:** 1333 Rodeo Blvd. |
|---|---|---|---|---|
| **Dispatched:** 1904 | **En Route:** 1904 | **At Scene:** 1904 | **Transport:** 1914 | **At Hospital:** 1925 | **In Service:** 1934 |

#### Patient Information

**Age:** 20
**Sex:** M
**Weight (in kg [lb]):** 61 kg (135 lb)

**Allergies:** No known drug allergies
**Medications:** None
**Past Medical History:** None
**Chief Complaint:** Pain in abdomen, flanks, and back of head

#### Vital Signs

| **Time:** 1910 | **BP:** 104/54 | **Pulse:** 120 | **Respirations:** 24 | **Spo₂:** 97% |
|---|---|---|---|---|
| **Time:** 1916 | **BP:** 82/54 | **Pulse:** 134 | **Respirations:** 28 | **Spo₂:** 88% |
| **Time:** 1921 | **BP:** 90/58 | **Pulse:** 128 | **Respirations:** 28 | **Spo₂:** 93% |

#### EMS Treatment (circle all that apply)

**Oxygen @ 15 L/min via:**
NC (NRM) Bag mask

(Assisted Ventilation) | Airway Adjunct | CPR

| Defibrillation | Bleeding Control | Bandaging | Splinting | **Other:** Thermal management, shock treatment, spinal motion restriction, suctioning |

| Narrative |
| --- |

EMS was standing by at a rodeo event when a bull rider was thrown from a bull and trampled.

Chief Complaint: Pain in abdomen, flanks, and back of head

History: Patient reports pain in the RUQ of his abdomen, his flank areas, and the back of his head.

Assessment: On contact with the patient, a 20-year-old man, he was found to be conscious, but restless, and in severe pain. He had initially walked away from the injury site. His airway was patent and his breathing was adequate; radial pulses were rapid and weak. Manual cervical-spine stabilization was initiated immediately.

Treatment (Rx): Administered high-flow oxygen via nonrebreathing mask and performed secondary assessment. Assessment revealed abrasions of the anterior part of the abdomen and both flanks and palpable tenderness in the RUQ. Breath sounds were clear to auscultation bilaterally, and the remainder of the assessment was unremarkable.

Transport: Maintained spinal motion restriction, covered patient with a blanket, loaded him into the ambulance, obtained vital signs, and began transport to the hospital. En route, patient's mental status and vital signs deteriorated; he was now responsive only to pain; his respirations increased in rate, but decreased in depth; a marked decrease in his blood pressure was observed; and his oxygen saturation decreased. Began assisting the patient's ventilations with a bag-mask device attached to high-flow oxygen. Patient became somewhat combative and would no longer tolerate assisted ventilation. However, he would tolerate oxygen via nonrebreathing mask.

Reassessment of patient revealed little improvement in his vital signs. Noted blood on patient's underwear, which was previously not present. Assessment of genitalia and adjacent areas revealed no signs of open injury. Continued to monitor patient and contacted receiving facility. Patient then began vomiting bright red blood, so the patient was immediately turned to the side and the patient's mouth was suctioned to prevent aspiration and to ensure airway patency. Suctioned remaining vomitus from the patient's mouth and returned the patient to a supine position.

Called radio report to receiving facility to provide update on patient's status, and closely monitored his condition throughout the duration of the transport. Patient was delivered to ED staff without further incident, and verbal report was given to attending physician Givens. EMS cleared the hospital and returned to service at 1934.

**End of report**

# Prep Kit

## Ready for Review

- Abdominal injuries are categorized as either open (penetrating trauma) or closed (blunt force trauma).
- Either classification of injury can result in injury to the hollow or solid organs of the abdomen and cause significant life-threatening bleeding.
- Blunt force trauma that causes closed injuries results from an object striking the body without breaking the skin, such as being hit with a baseball bat or when the patient's body strikes the steering wheel during a motor vehicle crash.
- Penetrating trauma is often a result of a gunshot wound or stab wound. Other mechanisms of injury such as a fall on an object can also cause penetrating trauma to the abdomen.
- Injury to the solid organs often causes significant internal bleeding that can be life threatening.
- Injury to the hollow organs of the abdomen may cause irritation and inflammation to the

peritoneum as caustic digestive juices leak into the peritoneum. A serious infection may also occur over several hours.

- Always maintain a high index of suspicion for serious intra-abdominal injury in the trauma patient, particularly in the patient who exhibits signs of shock.
- Assess the abdomen for signs of bruising, rigidity, penetrating injuries, and reports of pain.
- Never remove an impaled object from the abdominal region. Secure it in place with a large bulky dressing and provide rapid transport. When the MOI is penetrating trauma, spinal immobilization is usually not indicated (follow local protocol).
- Be prepared to treat the patient for shock. Place the patient supine, keep the patient warm, and provide high-flow oxygen.
- Never replace an organ that protrudes from an open injury to the abdomen (evisceration).

Instead, keep the organ moist and warm. Cover the injury site with a large, sterile, moist, bulky dressing and an occlusive dressing, if specified by local protocol.

- Injuries to the kidneys may be difficult to detect because they are located in the well-protected region of the body. Be alert to bruising or a hematoma in the flank region.
- Injury to the external male or female genitalia is very painful for patients but is usually not life threatening.
- In the case of sexual assault or rape, treat for shock if necessary, and record all the facts in detail. Follow any crime scene policy established by your system to protect the scene and any potential evidence. Advise the patient not to wash, bathe, shower, douche (if female), or void until after a physician has examined him or her.

## Vital Vocabulary

**closed abdominal injury** An injury in which there is soft-tissue damage inside the body but the skin remains intact.

**evisceration** The displacement of organs outside of the body.

**flank** The region below the rib cage and above the hip.

**guarding** Involuntary muscle contractions of the abdominal wall to minimize the pain of abdominal movement; a sign of peritonitis.

**hematuria** Blood in the urine.

**hollow organs** Structures through which materials pass, such as the stomach, small intestines, large intestines, ureters, and urinary bladder.

**melena** Black, foul-smelling, tarry stool containing digested blood.

**open abdominal injury** An injury in which there is a break in the surface of the skin or mucous membrane, exposing deeper tissue to potential contamination.

**peritoneal cavity** The abdominal cavity.

**peritoneum** The membrane lining the abdominal cavity (parietal peritoneum) and covering the abdominal organs (visceral peritoneum).

**retroperitoneum** The potential space located posterior to the peritoneal cavity of the abdomen.

**solid organs** Solid masses of tissue where much of the chemical work of the body takes place (eg, the liver, spleen, pancreas, and kidneys).

## References

1. McGready JB, Breyer BN. Current epidemiology of genitourinary trauma. *Urol Clin North Am.* 2013;40(3):323–334.

2. *National Emergency Medical Services Education Standards.* US Department of Transportation. National Highway Traffic Safety Administration. DOT HS 811 077A. January 2009. www.ems.gov/pdf/811077a.pdf. Accessed April 6, 2020.

3. *National Emergency Medical Services Education Standards. Emergency Medical Technician Instructional Guidelines.* US Department of Transportation. National Highway Traffic Safety Administration. DOT HS 811 077C. January 2009. www.ems.gov/pdf/811077c.pdf. Accessed April 6, 2014.

4. Victims of sexual violence: statistics. RAINN website. https://www.rainn.org/statistics/victims-sexual-violence. Accessed April 6, 2020.

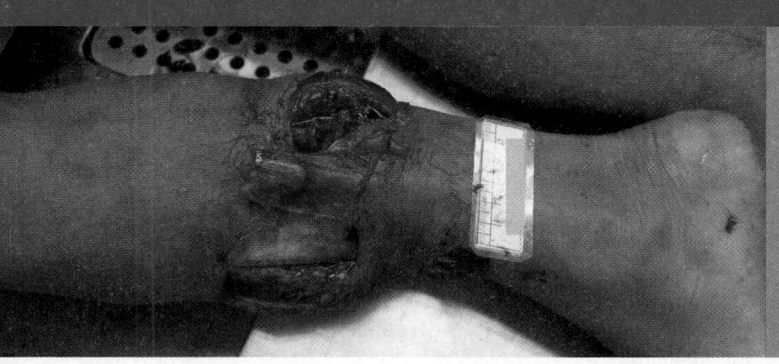

# Chapter 32

# Orthopaedic Injuries

## NATIONAL EMS EDUCATION STANDARD COMPETENCIES

### Trauma

Applies fundamental knowledge to provide basic emergency care and transportation based on assessment findings for an acutely injured patient.

### Orthopaedic Trauma

- Recognition and management of
  - Open fractures (pp 1152–1155, 1163–1191)
  - Closed fractures (pp 1152–1155, 1163–1191)
  - Dislocations (pp 1155–1156, 1155–1191)
  - Amputations (pp 1158, 1176, 1191)
- Pathophysiology, assessment, and management of
  - Upper and lower extremity orthopaedic trauma (pp 1151–1192)
  - Open fractures (pp 1152–1155, 1159–1191)
  - Closed fractures (pp 1152–1153, 1159–1191)

- Dislocations (pp 1155–1156, 1159–1190)
- Sprains/strains (pp 1156–1157, 1159–1193)
- Pelvic fractures (pp 1152–1155, 1158–1163, 1168–1169, 1178–1179)
- Amputations/replantation (pp 1158, 1176, 1191)

### Medicine

Applies fundamental knowledge to provide basic emergency care and transportation based on assessment findings for an acutely ill patient.

### Nontraumatic Musculoskeletal Disorders

Anatomy, physiology, pathophysiology, assessment, and management of
- Nontraumatic fractures (pp 1152–1155, 1159–1191)

## KNOWLEDGE OBJECTIVES

1. Describe the anatomy and physiology of the musculoskeletal system. (pp 1146–1151)
2. Name the four mechanisms of injury. (pp 1151–1152)
3. Describe the different types of musculoskeletal injuries, including fractures, dislocations, amputations, sprains, and strains. (pp 1151–1158)
4. Recognize the characteristics of specific types of musculoskeletal injuries. (pp 1151–1158, 1169–1191)
5. Differentiate between open and closed fractures. (pp 1152–1153)
6. Explain how to assess the severity of an injury. (p 1158)

7. Describe the emergency medical care of the patient with an orthopaedic injury. (pp 1163–1192)
8. Describe the emergency medical care of the patient with a swollen, painful, deformed extremity (fracture). (pp 1163–1191)
9. Discuss the need for, general rules of, and possible complications of splinting. (pp 1164–1165)
10. Explain the reasons for splinting fractures, dislocations, and sprains at the scene versus transporting the patient immediately. (pp 1164–1165)
11. Describe the emergency medical care of the patient with an amputation. (p 1191)

1. Demonstrate the care of musculoskeletal injuries. (pp 1163–1164, Skill Drill 32-1)
2. Demonstrate how to apply a rigid splint. (pp 1165–1167, Skill Drill 32-2)
3. Demonstrate how to apply a vacuum splint. (pp 1167–1168, Skill Drill 32-3)
4. Demonstrate how to splint the hand and wrist. (pp 1176–1177, Skill Drill 32-4)
5. Demonstrate how to apply a Hare traction splint. (pp 1183–1185, Skill Drill 32-5)
6. Demonstrate how to apply a Sager traction splint. (pp 1185–1186, Skill Drill 32-6)
7. Demonstrate how to splint the clavicle, the scapula, the shoulder, the humerus, the elbow, and the forearm. (pp 1169–1176)
8. Demonstrate how to care for a patient with an amputation. (p 1191)

# Introduction

The human body is a well-designed system in which form, upright posture, and movement are provided by the musculoskeletal system. This system also protects the vital internal organs of the body. The term *musculoskeletal* refers to the bones and voluntary muscles of the body. However, the bones and muscles are susceptible to external forces that can cause injury. Also at risk are the tendons, cartilage, and ligaments.

Musculoskeletal injuries are among the most common reasons why patients seek medical attention. Complaints related to the musculoskeletal system result in almost 60 million visits to physicians annually in the United States. Approximately one in seven Americans will experience some type of musculoskeletal impairment, leading to millions of missed days of work or school and costing hundreds of billions of dollars yearly. An estimated 70% to 80% of all patients with multisystem trauma have one or more musculoskeletal injuries.

Musculoskeletal system injuries are often easily identified because of pain, swelling, and deformity. Although these injuries are less frequently fatal, they often result in short- and long-term disability. By providing prompt assessment and treatment such as splinting, EMTs may help reduce disability. Although these injuries can appear dramatic, do not focus solely on a musculoskeletal injury without first determining that no life-threatening injuries exist. Never forget the XABCs!

As an EMT, you must be familiar with the basic anatomy of the musculoskeletal system. Although muscles are technically soft tissue, they are discussed in this chapter because of their close relationship with the skeleton. Therefore, the chapter begins with a review of the musculoskeletal anatomy. Various types and causes of musculoskeletal injuries in general are identified, and the assessment and treatment process for each is explained, followed by a detailed discussion of splinting. The chapter then focuses on specific musculoskeletal injuries, beginning at the clavicle and ending at the feet.

# Anatomy and Physiology of the Musculoskeletal System

## Muscles

The muscular system includes three types of muscles: skeletal, smooth, and cardiac. Skeletal muscle, also called striated muscle because of its characteristic stripes, attaches to the bones and usually crosses at least one joint. This type of muscle is also called voluntary muscle because it is under direct voluntary control of the brain, responding to commands to move specific body parts (**FIGURE 32-1**). Usually, movement is the result of several muscles contracting and relaxing simultaneously. Skeletal muscle makes up the largest portion of the body's muscle mass. Its primary functions are movement and posture. Cardiac muscle contributes to the cardiovascular system, and smooth muscle is a component of other body systems, including the digestive system and the cardiovascular system.

All skeletal muscles are supplied with arteries, veins, and nerves. Blood from the arteries brings oxygen, glucose, and nutrients to the muscles (**FIGURE 32-2**). Waste products, including carbon dioxide and lactic acid, are carried away in the veins. Disease or trauma can result in the loss of a muscle's nervous supply; this, in turn, can lead to weakness

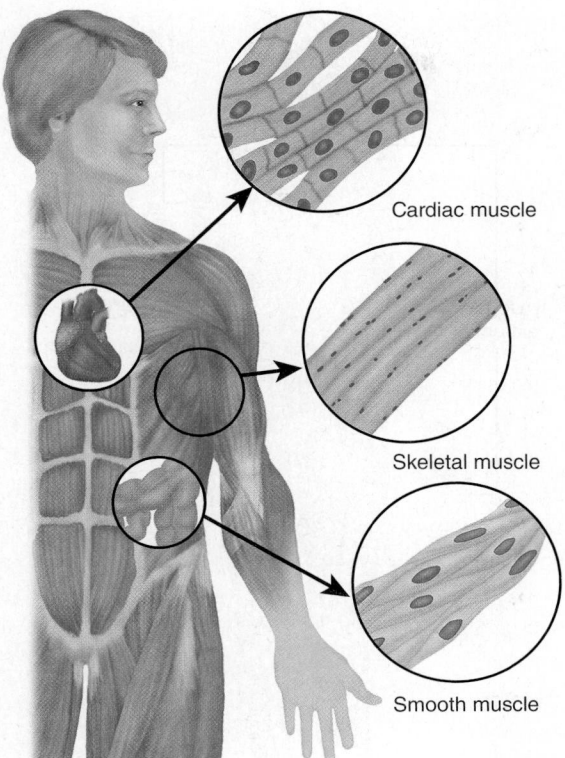

**FIGURE 32-1** For musculoskeletal injuries, the major muscle type involved is skeletal muscle.

© Jones & Bartlett Learning.

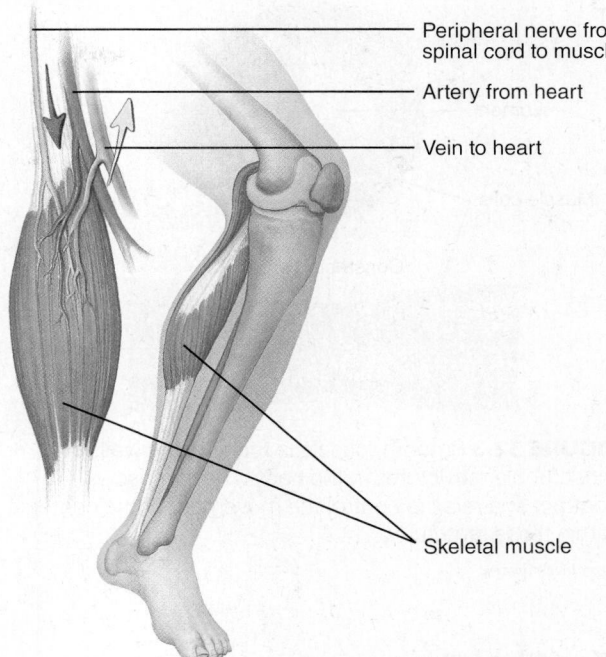

**FIGURE 32-2** Skeletal muscles are supplied by arteries, veins, and nerves that bring oxygen and nutrients, carry away waste products, and conduct nervous stimuli.

© Jones & Bartlett Learning.

and eventually atrophy, or a decrease in the size of the muscle and its inherent ability to function. Skeletal muscle tissue is directly attached to the bone by tough, ropelike structures known as tendons, which are extensions of the fascia (fibrous tissue) that covers all skeletal muscle. Fascia surrounds and supports the muscles and neurovascular structures.

Smooth muscle, also called involuntary muscle because it is not under voluntary control of the brain, performs much of the automatic work of the body. This type of muscle is found in the walls of most tubular structures of the body, such as the gastrointestinal tract and the blood vessels. Smooth muscle contracts and relaxes to control the movement of the contents within these structures (**FIGURE 32-3**).

The heart neither looks nor acts like skeletal or smooth muscle. It is composed largely of cardiac muscle, a specifically adapted involuntary muscle with its own regulatory system. The remainder of this chapter is concerned exclusively with skeletal muscle.

**YOU** **are the Provider**

At 1620 hours, you are dispatched to a soccer field for a player with a possible broken leg. You and your partner proceed to the scene, with a response time of about 5 minutes. En route, dispatch advises you that the patient is conscious, alert, and breathing. The weather is overcast, the temperature is 88°F (31°C), and the traffic is moderate.

**1.** Under which circumstances can orthopaedic injuries pose a threat to a patient's life?

**2.** Given the information you have, can you rule out a critical injury?

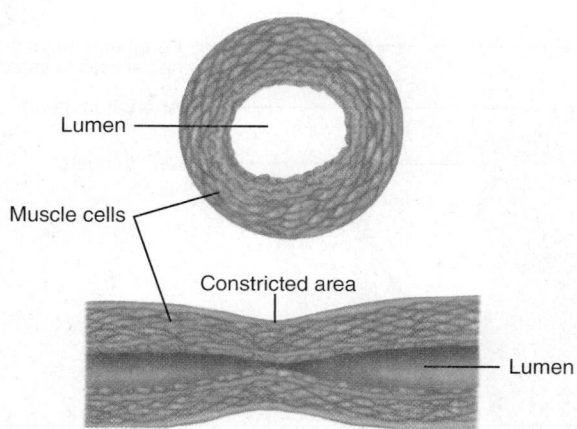

**FIGURE 32-3** Smooth muscle is found in the walls of most tubular structures in the body. These muscles contract and relax to control the movement of the contents within these structures.

© Jones & Bartlett Learning.

## The Skeleton

The skeleton, which gives us our recognizable human form, protects our vital internal organs, and allows us to move, is composed of approximately 206 bones (**FIGURE 32-4**). The bones in the skeleton also produce blood cells (in the bone marrow) and serve as a reservoir for important minerals and electrolytes.

The skull is a solid, vaultlike structure that surrounds and protects the brain. The thoracic cage protects the heart, lungs, and great vessels; the lower ribs protect the liver and spleen. The bony spinal canal encases and protects the spinal cord.

The pectoral girdle, also referred to as the shoulder girdle, consists of two scapulae and two clavicles (**FIGURE 32-5**). The scapula (shoulder blade) is a flat, triangular bone held to the rib cage by powerful muscles that buffer it against injury. The clavicle (collarbone) is a slender, S-shaped bone attached by ligaments to the sternum on one end and to the acromion process on the other. The clavicle acts as a strut to keep the shoulder propped up; however, because it is slender and very exposed, this bone is vulnerable to injury.

The upper extremity extends from the shoulder to the fingertips. The arm is composed of the upper arm (humerus), elbow, and forearm (radius and ulna) (**FIGURE 32-6**). The upper extremity joins the shoulder girdle at the glenohumeral joint. The

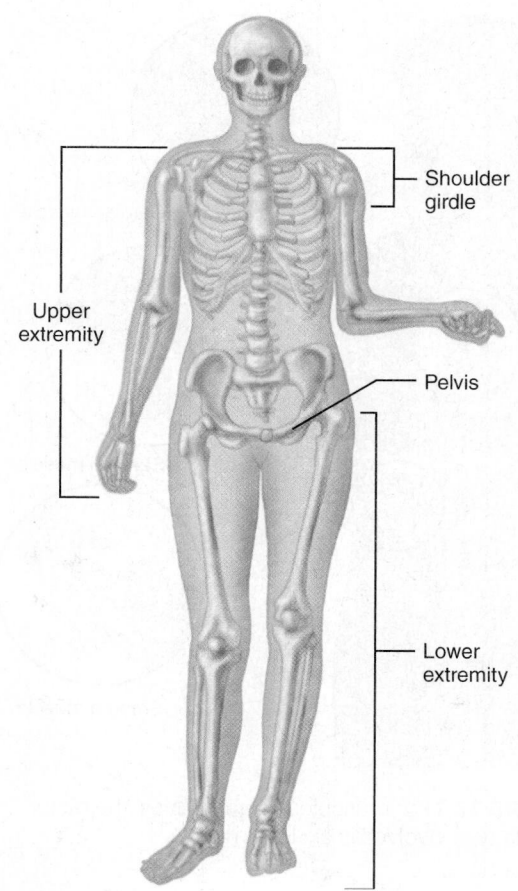

**FIGURE 32-4** The human skeleton, consisting of approximately 206 bones, gives us our form and protects our vital organs.

© Jones & Bartlett Learning.

upper extremity begins with the humerus. The humerus connects with the bones of the forearm at the elbow—the radius and ulna—to form the hinged elbow joint.

The radius and ulna make up the forearm. The radius, the larger of the two forearm bones, lies on the thumb side of the forearm. The ulna is narrow and is on the little finger side of the forearm. Because the radius and the ulna are connected by relatively stiff ligaments at both ends, when one is broken, the other is often broken as well.

The hand contains three sets of bones: carpals (wrist bones), metacarpals (hand bones), and phalanges (finger bones) (**FIGURE 32-7**). The carpals are vulnerable to fracture when a person falls on an outstretched hand. Phalanges are more apt to be

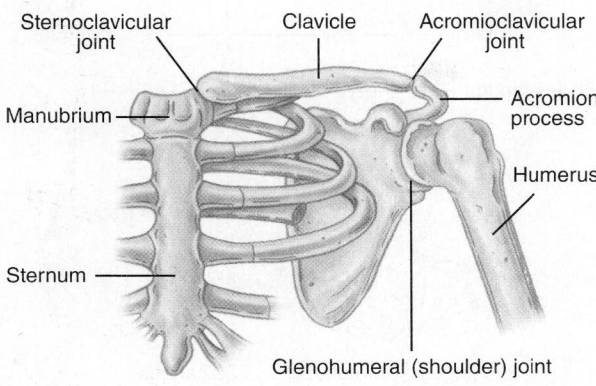

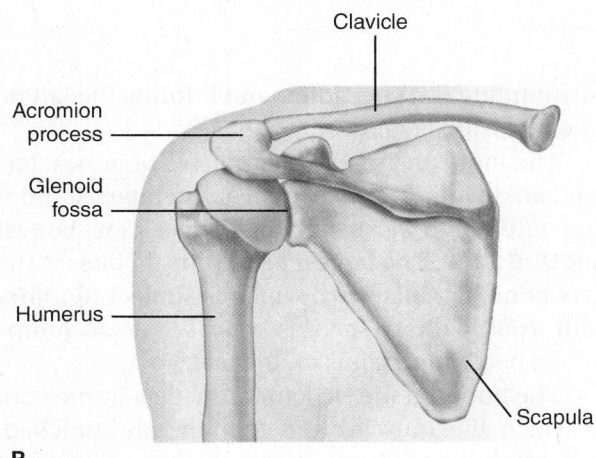

**FIGURE 32-5** The pectoral girdle. **A.** Anterior view, including the clavicle. **B.** Posterior view, including the scapula.

A, B: © Jones & Bartlett Learning.

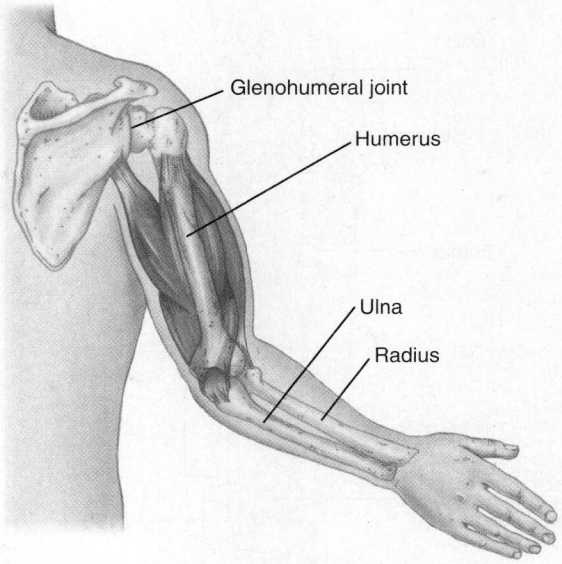

**FIGURE 32-6** The anatomy of the arm.

© Jones & Bartlett Learning.

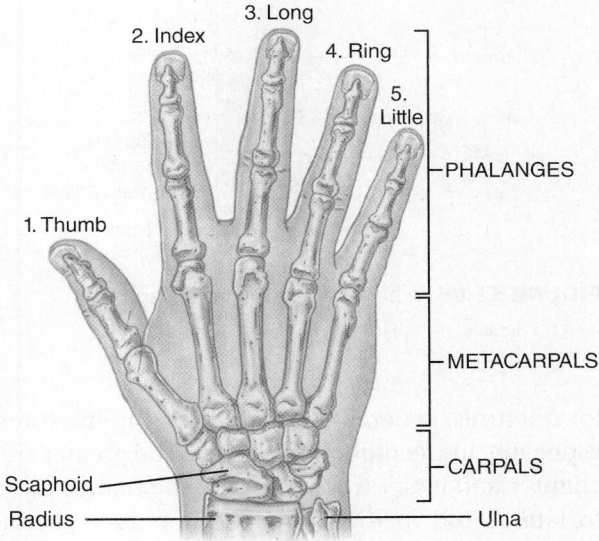

**FIGURE 32-7** The anatomy of the wrist and hand.

© Jones & Bartlett Learning.

injured by a crush injury, such as being slammed in a door.

The pelvis supports the body weight and protects the structures within the pelvis: the bladder, rectum, and female reproductive organs. The pelvic girdle is three separate bones—the ischium, ilium, and pubis—fused together to form the innominate (or hip) bone. The two iliac bones are joined posteriorly by tough ligaments to the sacrum at the sacroiliac joints; the two pubic bones are connected anteriorly by equally tough ligaments to one another at the pubic symphysis. These joints allow very little motion, so the pelvic ring is strong and stable.

The lower extremity consists of the bones of the thigh, leg, and foot (**FIGURE 32-8**). The femur

(thighbone) is a long, powerful bone that connects in the ball-and-socket joint of the hip and in the hinge joint of the knee. The femoral *head* is the ball-shaped part that fits into the acetabulum (hip socket). It is connected to the *shaft* (diaphysis), or long tubular portion of the femur, by the femoral *neck*. The femoral neck is a common site

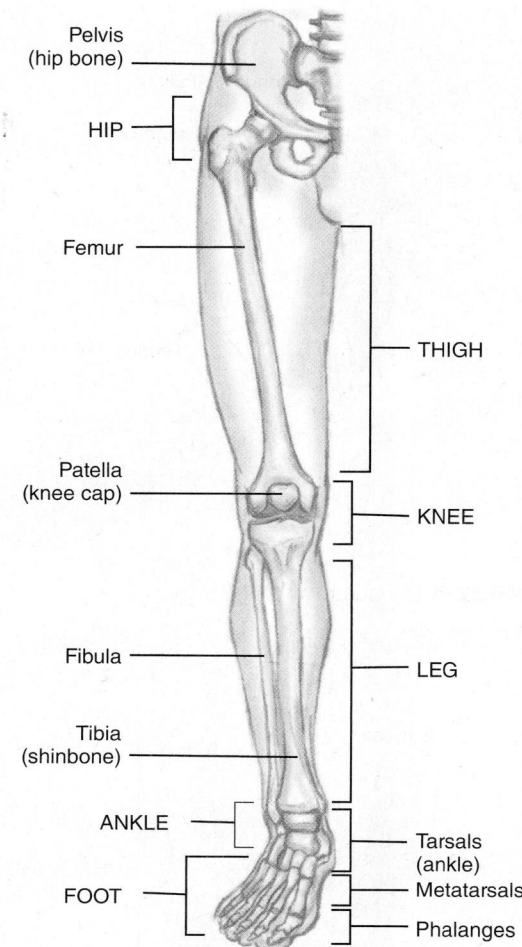

**FIGURE 32-8** The bones of the thigh, leg, and foot.

© Jones & Bartlett Learning.

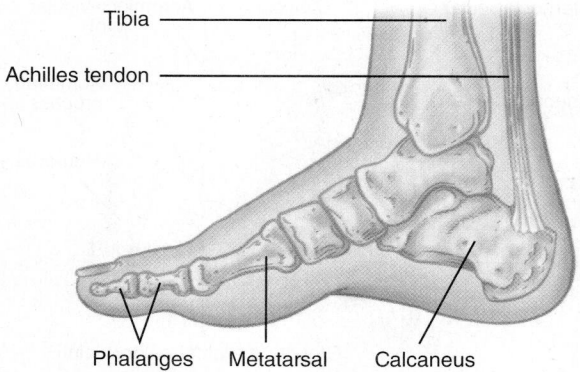

**FIGURE 32-9** The bones of the foot and ankle.

© Jones & Bartlett Learning.

for fractures, generally referred to as hip fractures, especially in the older population. The greater trochanter and lesser trochanter are the names given to lateral and medial bony protuberances below the femoral neck and just above the shaft of the femur.

The lower leg consists of two bones, the tibia and the fibula. The **tibia** (shinbone) is the larger of the two leg bones and is responsible for supporting the major weight-bearing surfaces of the knee and ankle. The tibia connects to the patella (kneecap) via the patellar tendon just below the knee joint and runs down the front of the lower leg. The tibia is vulnerable to direct blows and can be felt just beneath the skin. The much smaller **fibula** runs along the lateral side of the tibia and slightly posterior to it. The fibula is an important anchor for ligaments

surrounding the knee joint, and it forms the lateral side of the ankle joint.

The foot consists of three classes of bones: tarsals (ankle and hindfoot bones), metatarsals (foot and forefoot bones), and phalanges (toe bones) (**FIGURE 32-9**). The largest of the tarsal bones is the heel bone, or **calcaneus**, which is subject to injury with axial loading, such as when a person jumps from a height and lands on the feet.

The bones of the skeleton provide a framework to which the muscles and tendons are attached. Bone is a living tissue that contains nerves and receives oxygen and nutrients from the arterial system. Therefore, when a bone breaks, a patient typically experiences severe pain and bleeding. Bone marrow, located in the center of each bone, produces red and white blood cells and platelets.

A **joint** is formed wherever two bones come into contact. The sternoclavicular joint, for example, is where the sternum and the clavicle come together. Joints are held together in a tough, fibrous structure known as a capsule, which is supported and strengthened in certain key areas by bands of fibrous tissue called **ligaments**. In moving joints, the ends of the bones are covered with a thin layer of cartilage known as **articular cartilage**. This cartilage is a pearly white substance that allows the ends of the bones to glide easily. Joints are bathed and lubricated by synovial (joint) fluid.

Some joints, such as the shoulder, allow motion to occur in a circular manner. Other joints, such as the knee and elbow, act as hinges. Still other joints, including the sacroiliac joint in the lower back and the sternoclavicular joints, allow only a minimum amount of motion. Certain joints, such as the

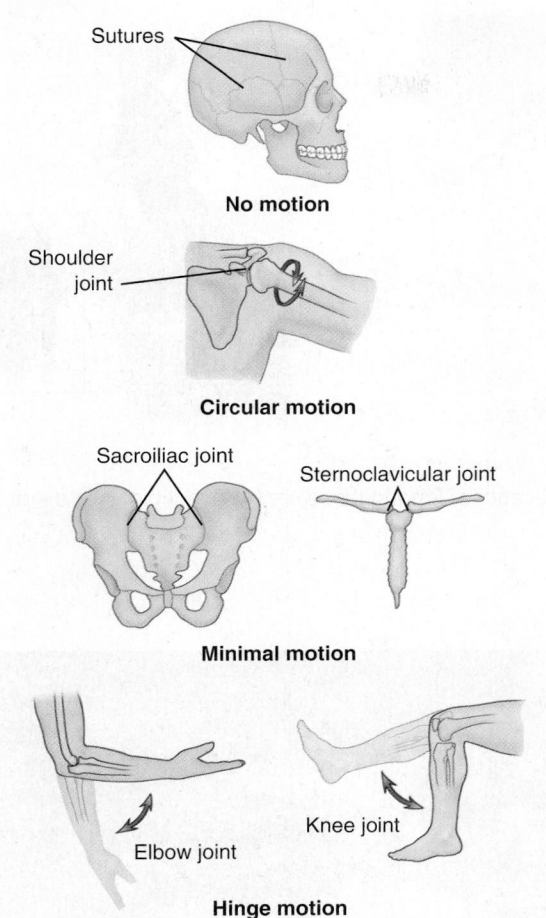

**FIGURE 32-10** Joints have many functions. Some joints allow for motion to occur in a circular manner; others act as hinges. Still others allow only minimal motion or none at all.

© Jones & Bartlett Learning.

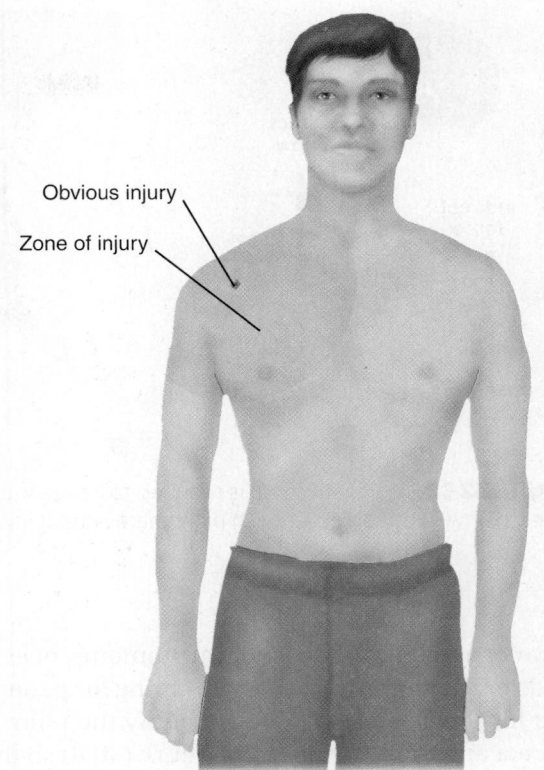

**FIGURE 32-11** The zone of injury is the area of soft tissue, including the adjacent nerves and blood vessels, that surrounds the obvious injury of a bone or joint.

© Jones & Bartlett Learning.

sutures in the skull (present until about 18 months of age), fuse together during growth to create a solid, immobile, bony structure (**FIGURE 32-10**).

## Musculoskeletal Injuries

Injury to bones and joints is often associated with injury to the surrounding soft tissues, especially to the adjacent nerves and blood vessels. The entire area is known as the zone of injury (**FIGURE 32-11**). Depending on the amount of kinetic energy the tissues absorb from forces acting on the body, the zone may extend to a distant point. For this reason, you should not become distracted by a patient's obvious injury; you must first complete a primary assessment to check for life-threatening injuries.

This is especially true in assessing damage from high-energy trauma, which is discussed next.

## Mechanism of Injury

Significant force is generally required to cause fractures and dislocations. This force may be applied to the limb in any of the following ways (**FIGURE 32-12**):

- Direct blows
- Indirect forces
- Twisting forces
- High-energy injuries

A direct blow can result in fracture of the bone at the point of impact. An example is the patella (kneecap) that fractures when it strikes the dashboard in a motor vehicle crash.

Alternatively, the resultant force may cause a fracture or dislocation at a distant point, as when a person falls and lands on an outstretched hand. The direct impact may cause a wrist fracture, but the resultant force can also cause dislocation of the

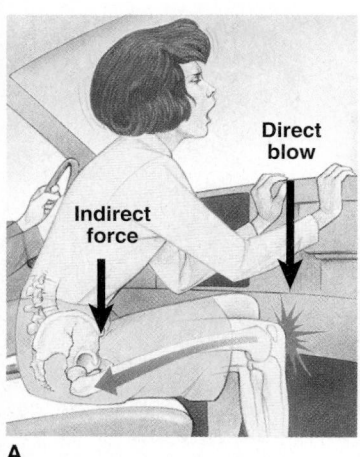

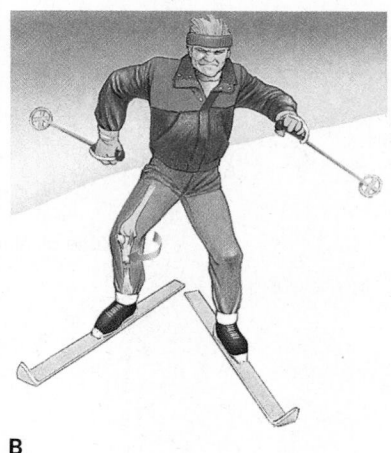

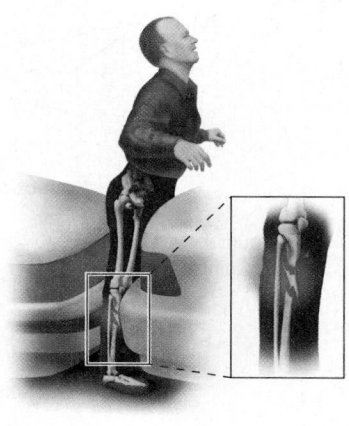

**A**                              **B**                              **C**

**FIGURE 32-12** Significant force is required to cause fractures or dislocations. Among these are (**A**) direct blows and indirect forces, (**B**) twisting forces, and (**C**) high-energy crush injuries.

A, B, C: © Jones & Bartlett Learning.

elbow or a fracture of the forearm, humerus, or even clavicle. Therefore, when you are caring for patients who have fallen, immediately identify the point of contact and the mechanism of injury (MOI) so that you decrease the chance of overlooking any associated injuries.

Twisting forces are a common cause of musculoskeletal injury, especially to the anterior cruciate ligament (ACL) or the medial cruciate ligament (MCL) in the knee. Skiing injuries often happen because of twisting: A ski becomes caught, and the skier falls, applying a twisting force to the lower extremity.

High-energy injuries, such as those that result from motor vehicle crashes, falls from heights, gunshot wounds, and other extreme forces, produce severe damage to the skeleton, surrounding soft tissues, and vital internal organs. A patient may have multiple injuries to many body parts, including more than one fracture or dislocation in a single limb.

A significant MOI is not always necessary to fracture a bone. A slight force can easily fracture a bone that is weakened by a tumor, infection, or osteoporosis, a generalized bone disease that is common among postmenopausal women. In geriatric patients with osteoporosis, minor falls or simple twisting injuries can cause a fracture, most often of the wrist, spine, or hip. You should suspect the presence of a fracture in any older patient who reports pain and has sustained even a mild injury.

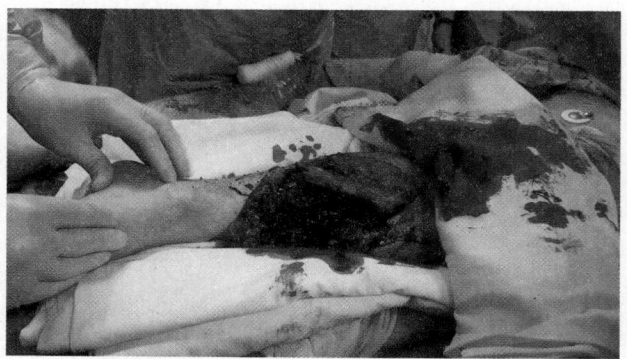

**FIGURE 32-13** A fracture can occur anywhere on the surface of a bone and may or may not break the skin.

© Courtesy of Andrew N. Pollak, MD, FAAOS.

## Fractures

A **fracture** is a broken bone. More precisely, it is a break in the continuity of the bone, often occurring as a result of an external force (**FIGURE 32-13**). The break can occur anywhere on the surface of the bone and in many different types of patterns. Contrary to a common misconception, there is no difference between a broken bone and a fractured bone. A potential complication of fractures is compartment syndrome (discussed later in the chapter), which refers to elevated pressure within a fascial compartment.

Fractures are classified as either closed or open. In assessing and treating patients with possible fractures or dislocations, your first priority is to

### Words of Wisdom

The terms *fracture* and *break* mean the same thing. You may often hear that a limb was both fractured and broken. As an EMT, you should understand that there is no difference. If a bone is fractured, it is by definition broken, and if it is broken, it is by definition fractured. Don't get stuck in the semantics of trying to find a difference between these terms as there is none.

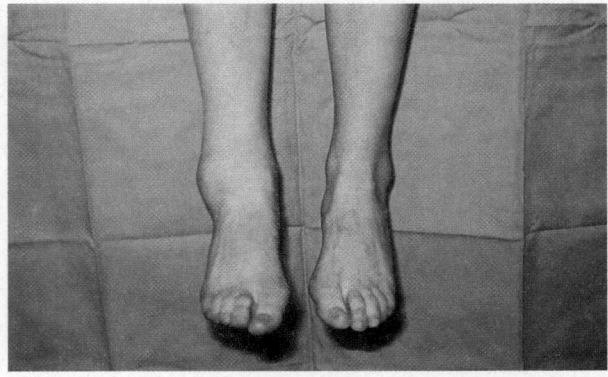

**FIGURE 32-14** Always compare the injured limb with the uninjured limb when checking for deformity.

© Courtesy of Andrew N. Pollak, MD, FAAOS.

determine whether the overlying skin is damaged. If it is not, the patient has a **closed fracture**. However, making this determination is not always as easy as it sounds. With an **open fracture**, there is an external wound, caused either by the same blow that fractured the bone or by the broken bone ends lacerating the skin. The wound may vary in size from a small puncture to a gaping tear that exposes bone and soft tissue. Regardless of the extent and severity of the damage to the skin, you should treat any injury that breaks the skin as a possible open fracture. Complications of open fractures include increased blood loss and a higher likelihood of infection. Be sure to wear gloves if there are any open wounds.

Fractures are also described by whether the bone is moved from its normal position. A **nondisplaced fracture** (sometimes called a hairline fracture) is a simple crack of the bone that may be difficult to distinguish from a sprain or simple contusion. Radiographic examinations are required for physicians to diagnose a nondisplaced fracture. A **displaced fracture** produces actual deformity, or distortion, of the limb by shortening, rotating, or angulating it. Often, the deformity is obvious and can be associated with crepitus. However, in some cases the deformity is minimal. Be sure to look for differences between the injured limb and the opposite uninjured limb in any patient with a suspected fracture of an extremity (**FIGURE 32-14**).

Medical personnel use special terms to describe specific types of fractures (**FIGURE 32-15**):

- **Comminuted.** A fracture in which the bone is broken into more than two fragments.
- **Epiphyseal.** A fracture that occurs in a growth section of a child's bone and may result in growth abnormalities.
- **Greenstick.** An incomplete fracture that passes only partway through the shaft of a bone but

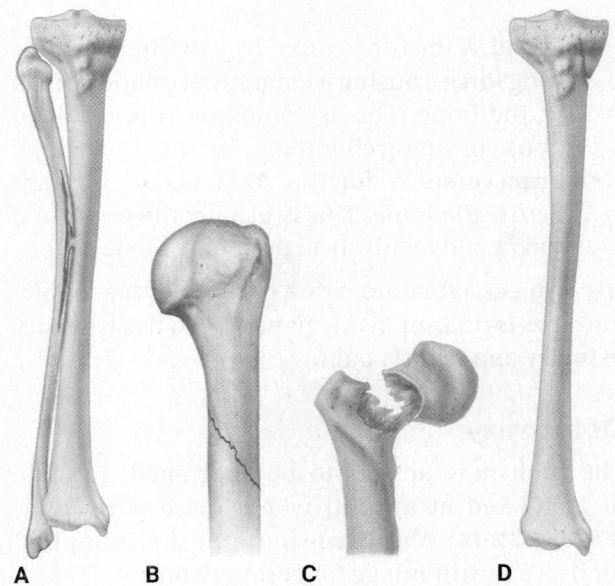

**FIGURE 32-15** Special terms to describe fractures. **A.** Greenstick fracture. **B.** Oblique fracture. **C.** Pathologic fracture. **D.** Incomplete fracture.

A-D: © Jones & Bartlett Learning.

may still cause substantial angulation; occurs in children.

- **Incomplete.** A fracture that does not run completely through the bone; a nondisplaced partial crack.
- **Oblique.** A fracture in which the bone is broken at an angle across the bone. This is usually the result of a sharp, angled blow to the bone.
- **Pathologic.** A fracture of weakened or diseased bone, seen in patients with osteoporosis, infection, or cancer; often produced by minimal force.

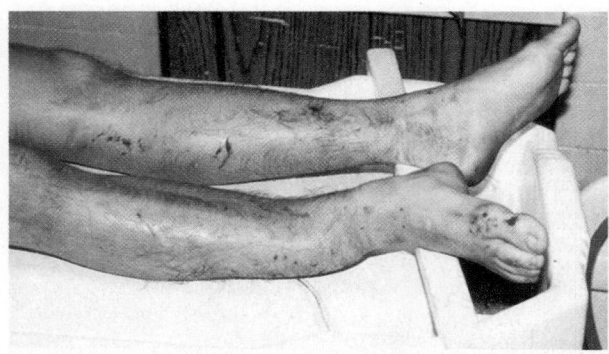

**FIGURE 32-16** Obvious deformity, shortening, rotation, or angulation should increase your index of suspicion for a fracture.

© Charles Stewart MD, EMDM MPH.

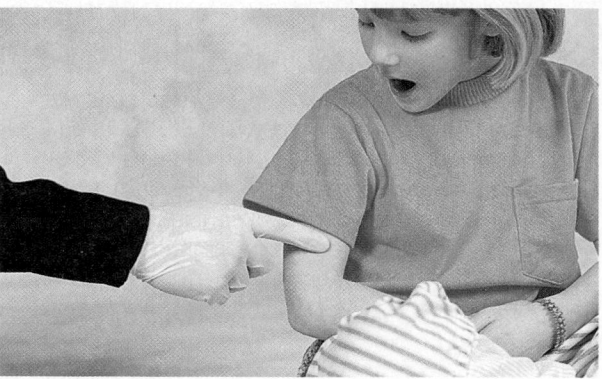

**FIGURE 32-17** Point tenderness is pain elicited by palpation with a finger at the site of an injury.

© Jones & Bartlett Learning. Courtesy of MIEMSS.

- **Spiral.** A fracture caused by a twisting or spinning force, causing a long, spiral-shaped break in the bone. This is sometimes the result of abuse in young children.
- **Transverse.** A fracture that occurs straight across the bone. This is usually the result of a direct and relatively high-energy blow.

Suspect a fracture if one or more of the following signs is present in any patient who has a history of injury and reports pain.

## Deformity

The limb may appear to be shortened, rotated, or angulated at a point where there is no joint (**FIGURE 32-16**). Always use the opposite, uninjured limb as a mirror image for comparison.

## Tenderness

**Point tenderness** on palpation in the zone of injury is the most reliable indicator of an underlying fracture, although it does not tell you the type of fracture (**FIGURE 32-17**).

## Guarding

An inability to use the extremity is the patient's way of immobilizing it to minimize pain. The muscles around the fracture contract to prevent any movement of the broken bone. Guarding does not occur with all fractures; some patients may continue to use the injured part for a time. Occasionally, nondisplaced fractures are less painful, and there is minimal soft-tissue damage.

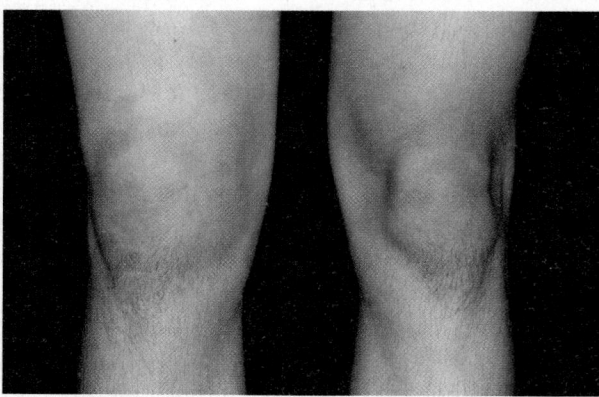

**FIGURE 32-18** Swelling that occurs in association with a fracture can often mask deformity of the limb.

© Dr. P. Marazzi/Science Source.

## Swelling

Rapid swelling usually indicates bleeding from a fracture and is typically followed by substantial pain. Often, if the swelling is severe, it may mask deformity of the limb (**FIGURE 32-18**). Generalized swelling from fluid buildup may occur several hours after an injury.

## Bruising

Fractures are almost always associated with **ecchymosis** (discoloration) of the surrounding soft tissues (**FIGURE 32-19**). Bruising may be present after almost any injury and may take hours to develop; it is not specific to bone or joint injuries. The discoloration associated with acute injuries is usually redness, as you may have seen with someone

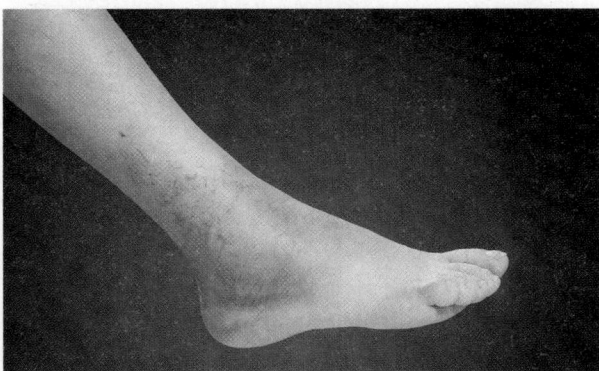

**FIGURE 32-19** Fractures almost always have associated bruising into the surrounding soft tissue.

© fotokostic/iStockphoto.

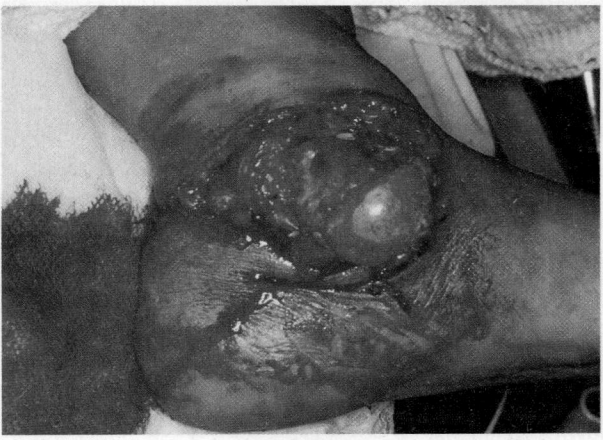

**FIGURE 32-20** Bone ends may protrude through the skin or be visible within the wound of an open fracture.

© Charles Stewart MD, EMDM MPH.

who has been punched. Within hours or days, blue, purple, and black discoloration will appear, followed by yellow and green.

## Crepitus

A grating or grinding sensation known as **crepitus** can be felt and sometimes even heard when fractured bone ends rub together.

## False Motion

Also called free movement, **false motion** is any motion at a point in the limb where there is no joint and therefore motion is not expected to occur. It is an indication of a fracture.

## Exposed Fragments

In open fractures, bone ends may protrude through the skin or be visible within the wound (**FIGURE 32-20**). *Never* attempt to push the end of a protruding bone back into place. This could increase the risk for infection.

## Pain

Pain, along with tenderness, bruising, and bleeding, commonly occurs in association with fractures. Remember to use the OPQRST mnemonic to assess pain: Onset; Provocation/palliation; Quality; Region/Radiation; Severity; and Time (duration).

## Locked Joint

A joint that is locked into position is difficult and painful to move. Keep in mind that crepitus and false motion appear only when a limb is moved or manipulated and are associated with injuries that are extremely painful. Do not manipulate the limb excessively in an effort to elicit these signs. This sign is more commonly the result of a soft-tissue injury within the joint (typically the knee or elbow), but the presence of a locked joint should alert you to the possibility of an underlying fracture or cartilage injury.

## Dislocations

A **dislocation** is a disruption of a joint in which the bone ends are no longer in contact. The supporting ligaments are often torn, usually completely, allowing the bone ends to separate from each other (**FIGURE 32-21**). A fracture-dislocation is a combination injury at the joint, in which the joint is dislocated and there is a fracture of the end of one or more of the bones.

A dislocated joint may sometimes spontaneously **reduce**, or return to its normal position before your assessment. In this situation, you will be able to confirm the dislocation only by taking a patient history. However, the joint surfaces often remain completely separated from one another. A dislocation that does not spontaneously reduce is a serious problem. The ends of the bone can be locked in a displaced position, making any motion of the joint difficult and painful. Commonly dislocated joints include the fingers, shoulder, elbow, hip, and knee.

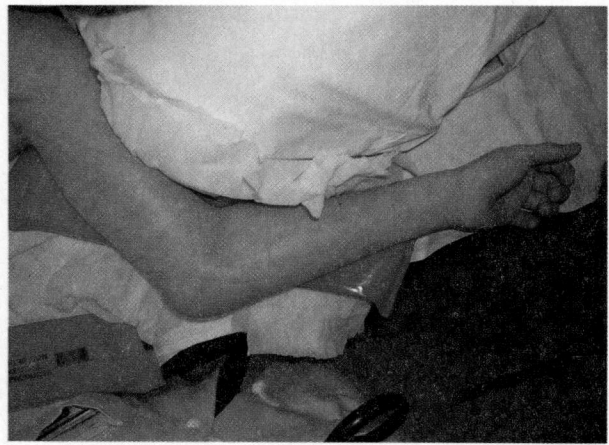

**A**

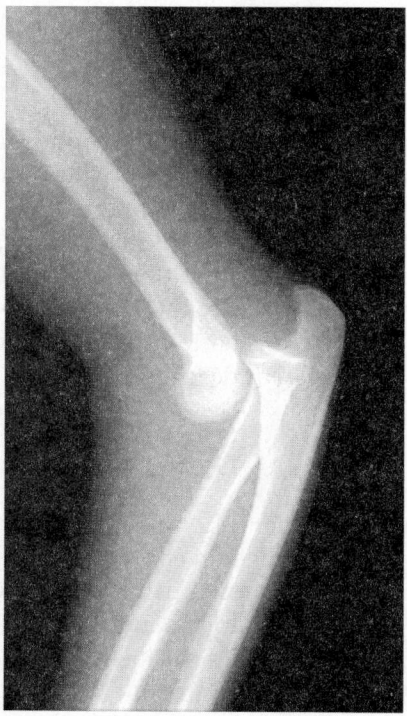

**B**

**FIGURE 32-21** A dislocation is a disruption of a joint in which the bone ends are no longer in contact. **A.** The clinical appearance of an elbow dislocation. **B.** Radiographic appearance of the same elbow.

**A:** © E. M. Singletary, M.D. Used with permission; **B:** © Medical Body Scans/Science Source.

The signs and symptoms of a dislocated joint are similar to those of a fracture (**FIGURE 32-22**):

- Marked deformity
- Swelling
- Pain that is aggravated by any attempt at movement

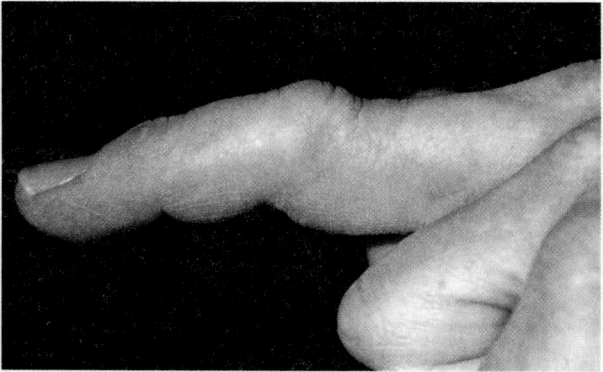

**FIGURE 32-22** Joint dislocations, such as this finger, are characterized by deformity, swelling, pain with any movement, tenderness, locking, and impaired circulation.
© Dr. P. Marazzi/Science Source.

- Tenderness on palpation
- Loss of normal joint motion
- Numbness or impaired circulation to the limb or digit

## Sprains

A **sprain** occurs when a joint is twisted or stretched beyond its normal range of motion. As a result, the supporting capsule and ligaments are stretched or torn, resulting in injury to the ligaments, articular capsule, synovial membrane, and tendons crossing the joint. A sprain can be thought of as a partial dislocation.

Sprains can range from mild to severe, depending on the amount of damage done to the supporting ligaments. The most severe sprains involve actual tearing of the ligament and may allow transient joint dislocation. Mild sprains are caused by ligament stretching rather than tearing. A sprain can occur in any joint, but sprains most often occur in the knee, shoulder, and ankle. Many sprains occur after a person misjudges a step or landing. Evasive moves, such as those done during a sporting event, commonly cause sprains in athletes. Some patients might report hearing a "snap" when the injury occurred.

After the injury, the joint alignment generally returns to a somewhat normal position, so the joint is not significantly displaced. In contrast with fractures and dislocations, sprains usually do not involve deformity, and joint mobility is usually limited by pain, not by joint incongruity. The following

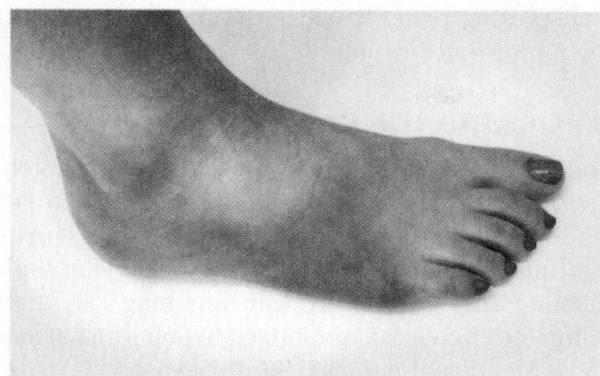

**FIGURE 32-23** Sprains often occur in the knee or ankle and are characterized by swelling, bruising, point tenderness, pain, and joint instability.

© Sean Gladwell/Dreamstime.com.

signs and symptoms often indicate that the patient may have a sprain (**FIGURE 32-23**):

- The patient is unwilling to use the limb (guarding).
- Swelling and ecchymosis are present at the injured joint as a result of torn blood vessels.
- Pain prevents the patient from moving or using the limb normally.
- Instability of the joint is indicated by increased motion, especially at the knee; however, this may be masked by severe swelling and guarding.

A fracture can look like a sprain, and vice versa. You will frequently not be able to distinguish a non-displaced fracture from a sprain. Therefore, it is important to document the MOI, because certain sprains and fractures occur more consistently with certain mechanisms. Your approach should always be to determine the MOI. The basic principles of prehospital management for sprains, dislocations, and fractures are essentially the same and are discussed later in the chapter.

## Strain

A **strain** (pulled muscle) is a stretching or tearing of the muscle and/or tendon, causing pain, swelling, and bruising of the soft tissues in the area. It occurs because of an abnormal contraction or from excessive stretching. Strains may range from minute separation to complete rupture. Unlike with a sprain, no ligament or joint damage typically occurs.

Often, no deformity is present and only minor swelling is noted at the site of the injury. Some patients may report a "snap" when a muscle tears. Some may report increased sharp pain with passive movement of the injured extremity. Patients may report severe weakness of the muscle. Many patients also have some tenderness. The general treatment of strains is similar to the prehospital management for sprains, dislocations, and fractures.

## YOU are the Provider

When you arrive at the scene, you find the patient, a 21-year-old woman, sitting on the ground with an ice pack over her left tibia. She is conscious and alert and tells you that another player fell against her leg.

| Recording Time: 0 Minutes | |
|---|---|
| **Appearance** | Anxious; in obvious pain; no sign of severe bleeding |
| **Level of consciousness** | Conscious and alert |
| **Airway** | Open; clear of secretions and foreign bodies |
| **Breathing** | Increased rate; adequate depth |
| **Circulation** | Radial pulses increased rate, strong and regular |

The patient denies having any other injuries and tells you that she heard a "snap" when the other player fell against her leg. She is in severe pain.

**3.** What initial treatment should you provide to this patient?

**4.** What are some indicators of a fractured bone?

## Amputations

A limb amputation is an injury in which an extremity is completely severed from the body. This injury is associated with every aspect of the musculoskeletal system—from bone to ligament to muscle. Amputations can occur as a result of trauma or a surgical intervention.

## Complications

Orthopaedic injuries can lead to numerous complications—not just those involving the skeletal system, but also systemic changes or illness. It is essential that you do not focus all of your attention on the skeletal injury. Keep in mind that there is a patient attached to the injured extremity! For example, pregnant women who sustain pelvic fractures tend to have higher mortality rates. Therefore, it is imperative to treat not only the fracture, but also the other needs of the woman and fetus.

The likelihood of a complication is often related to the strength of the force that caused the injury, the injury's location, and the patient's overall health. Any injury to a bony structure is likely to be accompanied by bleeding. In general, the greater the force that caused the injury, the greater the hemorrhage will be. Following a fracture, the sharp ends of the bone may damage muscles, blood vessels, arteries, and nerves, or the ends may penetrate the skin and produce an open fracture. A significant loss of tissue may occur at the fracture site if the muscle is severely damaged or if the penetration of the bone through the skin results in a large open wound.

To prevent contamination following an open fracture, brush away any obvious debris on the skin surrounding an open fracture before applying a dressing. Do not enter or probe the open fracture site to retrieve debris because this may lead to further contamination.

Long-term disability is one of the most devastating consequences of an orthopaedic injury. In many cases, a severely injured limb can be repaired and made to look almost normal. Unfortunately, many patients cannot return to work for long periods because of the extensive rehabilitation required and because of pain. As an EMT, you have a critical role in mitigating the risk of long-term disability. You can help reduce the risk or duration of long-term disability by preventing further injury, reducing the risk of wound infection, and

transporting patients with orthopaedic injuries to an appropriate hospital.

## Assessing the Severity of Injury

You must become skilled at quickly and accurately assessing the severity of an injury. The Golden Period (the time from injury to definitive care) is critical not only for life, but also for preserving limb viability. In an extremity with anything less than complete circulation, prolonged hypoperfusion can cause significant damage. For this reason, any suspected open fracture or vascular injury is considered an emergency. In a patient who has multisystem trauma, any additional bleeding can increase problems with underlying injuries or overall perfusion.

Remember that most injuries are not critical; you can identify critical injuries by using the musculoskeletal injury grading system shown in **TABLE 32-1** as a guideline.

---

**TABLE 32-1** Musculoskeletal Injury Grading System

**Minor Injuries**
- Minor sprains
- Fractures or dislocations of digits

**Moderate Injuries**
- Open fractures of digits
- Nondisplaced long bone fractures
- Nondisplaced pelvic fractures
- Major sprains of a major joint

**Serious Injuries**
- Displaced long bone fractures
- Multiple hand and foot fractures
- Open long bone fractures
- Displaced pelvic fractures
- Dislocations of major joints
- Multiple digit amputations
- Laceration of major nerves or blood vessels

**Severe, Life-Threatening Injuries (Survival Is Probable)**
- Multiple closed fractures
- Limb amputations
- Fractures of both long bones of the legs (bilateral femur fractures)

**Critical Injuries (Survival Is Uncertain)**
- Multiple open fractures of the limbs
- Suspected pelvic fractures with hemodynamic instability

## Patient Assessment

As an EMT, your assessments, attempts to splint, and efforts to stabilize the patient's condition are very important. However, always look at the big picture, evaluating the overall complexity of the situation to determine and treat any life threats. For example, overlooking an obstructed airway to splint a lower leg fracture could be deadly for the patient. Always carefully assess the MOI to try to determine the amount of kinetic energy that an injured limb has absorbed, and maintain a high index of suspicion for associated injuries.

It is not important to distinguish among fractures, dislocations, sprains, and contusions. In most cases, your assessment will be reported as an extremity injury. However, you must be able to distinguish mild injuries from severe injuries because some severe injuries may compromise neurovascular function, which could threaten long-term function.

### Scene Size-up

Information from dispatch may indicate the MOI, the number of patients involved, and any first aid procedures used prior to your arrival. This will be useful information for you to think about as you travel to the scene. Remember, the information given by the dispatcher is only as accurate as the patient's or bystander's report. In addition, the situation may change prior to your arrival at the incident. Dispatch information can still be used to help you consider whether spinal immobilization will be needed, the equipment you may need, and whether hazards might be present.

As you arrive at the scene, try to identify the forces associated with the MOI. Could they have produced injuries other than the musculoskeletal injuries reported by dispatch? Consider the possibility of hidden bleeding; internal injuries that you cannot see and closed fractures of the femur are examples. Standard precautions may be as simple as wearing gloves. With a severe MOI or other risk factors, a mask and gown may be necessary. Eye protection may also be indicated. Evaluate the need for law enforcement support, advanced life support (ALS), or additional ambulances, and request them early based on your initial scene assessment.

When you assess a patient who has experienced a significant MOI, look for indicators of the MOI and be alert for both primary and secondary injuries. Primary injuries occur as a result of the MOI, whereas secondary injuries are the result of what happens after the initial injury. For example, being hit by a motor vehicle will often result in a primary pelvic injury and often a secondary head injury when the patient rolls onto the hood of the car. As you put together information from dispatch and your observations of the scene, consider what injuries the MOI would lead you to expect. For example, when you approach a rear-end motor vehicle crash, you should suspect head, neck, and chest injuries.

### Primary Assessment

The primary assessment should focus on identifying and managing life threats. Treating the patient according to his or her level of consciousness and XABCs is always the priority. Exsanguinating hemorrhage as well as threats to airway, breathing, and circulation are considered life threatening and must be treated immediately to prevent mortality. Significant bleeding, internal or external, is an immediate life threat. If the patient has obvious life-threatening external hemorrhage, it should be addressed first (even before airway and breathing), and then begin treating the patient for shock as quickly as possible. For example, if you are unable to control arterial bleeding from extremities by using direct pressure, apply a **tourniquet** (if possible). Arterial bleeding from an open fracture should be treated prior to giving oxygen.

When evaluating the patient's level of consciousness and orientation, check for responsiveness using the AVPU scale, and assess mental status by asking the patient about his or her chief complaint. If the patient is alert, this should help direct you to any apparent life threats. An unresponsive patient may have an underlying life-threatening condition. You should administer high-flow oxygen via a nonrebreathing mask (or a bag-mask device, if indicated) to all patients whose level of consciousness is less than alert and oriented, and provide rapid transport to the emergency department (ED).

Perform a primary assessment of the patient and ask about the MOI. Was it a direct blow, indirect force, twisting force, or high-energy injury? In many situations, the musculoskeletal complaints will be simple and usually not life threatening; however, some situations, such as those with a significant

MOI, will include multiple problems that include musculoskeletal injuries. The initial interaction with your patient will provide you with a starting point and help you to distinguish the simple from the complex injuries. If there was significant trauma and multiple body systems were affected, the musculoskeletal injuries may be a lower priority. Scene time should not be wasted on prolonged musculoskeletal assessment or splinting fractures that are otherwise not life threatening. The expression "splinting to death" is used to describe such a situation; you are so involved in splinting fractures that the patient dies from other injuries.

Fractures and sprains usually do not create airway and breathing problems. Other problems, such as injuries to the head, intoxication, or other related illnesses and injuries, may cause inadequate breathing. Evaluating the chief complaint and MOI will help you to identify whether the patient has an open airway and whether breathing is present and adequate. In a conscious patient, this is as simple as noting whether the patient can speak normally. In an unconscious patient, it is as simple as opening the airway using the appropriate technique to check for breathing. Remember, little else matters if the patient's airway and breathing are inadequate.

Your circulatory assessment should focus on determining whether the patient has a pulse, has adequate perfusion, or is bleeding. If your patient is conscious, he or she will have a pulse. If the patient is unconscious, make sure there is a pulse by palpating the carotid artery. Hypoperfusion (shock) and bleeding problems will most likely be your primary concern. If the skin is pale, cool, or clammy and capillary refill time is slow, immediately treat your patient for shock. Maintain a normal body temperature, because trauma patients can rapidly become hypothermic even in warm environments. If musculoskeletal injuries in the extremities are suspected, they must be at least initially stabilized, if not splinted, prior to moving. This cause of shock may need to be eliminated later in your assessment.

If the patient has an airway or breathing problem, or significant bleeding, provide rapid transport to the hospital after quickly treating these life threats. A patient who has a significant MOI but whose condition appears otherwise stable should also be transported promptly to the closest appropriate hospital. Patients with bilateral fractures of the long bones (humerus, femur, or tibia) have been subjected to a high amount of kinetic energy, which should dramatically increase your index of suspicion for serious unseen injuries. When a decision for rapid transport is made, you can use a long backboard as a splinting device to splint the whole body rather than splinting each extremity individually. If you take time to splint the patient's arms and legs individually, you may delay the prompt surgical intervention that may be needed for other injuries when a significant MOI has occurred. Individual splints should be applied en route if the XABCs are stable and time permits.

Patients with a simple MOI, such as twisting of an ankle or dislocating a shoulder, may be further assessed and their condition stabilized on scene prior to transport if no other problems exist.

## Handling Injured Extremities During Assessment and Transport

Recall that fractures can break through the skin and cause external bleeding. This may occur during the initial injury or during manipulation of the extremity while preparing for splinting or transport. Careful handling of the extremity minimizes this risk. If external bleeding is present, bandage the extremity quickly to control bleeding. The dressings that cover the wound and bone should be kept clean to reduce the potential for bone infection. The bandage should be secure enough to control bleeding without restricting circulation distal to the injury. Monitor bandage tightness by assessing the circulation, sensation, and movement distal to the bandage. Swelling from fractures and internal bleeding may cause bandages to become too tight. If bleeding cannot be controlled, quickly apply a tourniquet.

Also handle fractures carefully while preparing for transport. Careful handling is necessary to limit pain and prevent sharp bone ends from breaking through the skin or damaging nerves and blood vessels in the extremity.

## History Taking

After the life threats have been managed during the primary assessment, investigate the chief complaint. Obtain a medical history and be alert for injury-specific signs and symptoms and for any pertinent negatives, such as no pain or loss of sensation.

Obtain a SAMPLE history for all trauma patients. How much and in what detail you explore this history depends on the patient's condition and how quickly you need to transport the patient to the hospital. For patients with simple fractures, dislocations, or sprains, it is easier to obtain a SAMPLE history. At the scene you may have access to family members and others who have information about the patient's history. Attempt to obtain this history without delaying time to definitive care.

OPQRST can be of limited use in cases of severe injury and is usually too lengthy when matters of exsanguinating hemorrhage, airway, breathing, circulation, and rapid transport require immediate attention. However, OPQRST may be useful when the MOI is unclear, the patient's condition is stable, or details of the injury are uncertain. This more detailed questioning for simple trauma may help you and the hospital staff to better understand the specific injury.

## Secondary Assessment

If significant trauma has likely affected multiple systems, start with a secondary assessment of the entire body to be sure that you have identified all problems and injuries. Begin with the head and work systematically toward the feet, checking the head, chest, abdomen, extremities, and back. The goal is to identify hidden and potentially life-threatening injuries. This secondary assessment will also help you to prepare for packaging and rapid transport. Knowing if an arm or leg is broken will be important when log rolling and securing the patient prior to transport.

Use the DCAP-BTLS approach to assess the musculoskeletal system. Identify any extremity deformities that likely represent significant musculoskeletal injury, and stabilize them appropriately. Contusions and abrasions may overlie more subtle injuries and should prompt you to carefully evaluate the stability and neurovascular status of the limb. The presence of puncture wounds or other signs of penetrating injury should alert you to the possibility of an open fracture. Associated burns must be identified and treated appropriately. Palpate for tenderness, which, like contusions or abrasions, may be the only significant sign of an underlying musculoskeletal injury.

When lacerations are present in an extremity, an open fracture must be considered, bleeding controlled, and dressings applied. Careful inspection for swelling and comparison with the opposite limb may also reveal otherwise occult musculoskeletal injury. You may find a hematoma in the zone of injury during the assessment.

If your assessment reveals no external signs of injury, ask the patient to move each limb carefully, stopping immediately if a movement causes pain. Skip this step in your evaluation if the patient reports neck or back pain; excess motion could cause permanent damage to the spinal cord.

When nonsignificant trauma has occurred and you suspect that your patient has a simple strain, sprain, dislocation, or fracture, take the time to focus your secondary assessment on that specific injury. Look for DCAP-BTLS. Be sure to assess the entire zone of injury by removing clothing from the area and looking and palpating for injuries. In musculoskeletal injuries, this zone generally extends from the joint above (proximal) to the joint below (distal), front and back.

### Words of Wisdom

If the patient has two or more injured extremities, treat the patient as a significant trauma patient and provide rapid transport to the hospital. The likelihood of other more severe injuries is greater when two or more bones have been broken.

Remember to evaluate the circulation, motor function, and sensation distal to the injury. Many important blood vessels and nerves lie close to the bone, especially around the major joints. Therefore, any injury or deformity of the bone may be associated with vessel or nerve injury. For this reason, you must assess neurovascular function every 5 to 10 minutes during the assessment, depending on the patient's condition, until the patient is at the hospital. Always recheck the neurovascular function before and after you splint or otherwise manipulate the limb. Manipulation can cause a bone fragment to press against or compress a nerve or vessel. Failure to restore circulation in this situation can lead to death of the limb. Always give priority to patients with impaired circulation that develops or remains present after a manipulation.

Because many of the steps require patient cooperation, you will not be able to assess sensory and motor functions in an unconscious patient, but you can evaluate the limb for deformity, swelling, ecchymosis, false motion, and crepitus.

Evaluation of the injured limb should include the 6 Ps of musculoskeletal assessment—pain, paralysis, paresthesia (numbness or tingling), pulselessness, pallor, and pressure. Assess neurovascular status as described in Chapter 10, *Patient Assessment*.

## Words of Wisdom

Extremity injuries that impair circulation or nerve function in distal tissues are urgent conditions. Patients with these injuries need careful assessment, prompt transport, and frequent reassessment of distal functions. It is also valuable to report this information in your initial radio contact with the hospital to allow personnel to prepare.

Determine a baseline set of vital signs, including pulse rate, rhythm, and quality; respiratory rate, rhythm, and quality; blood pressure; skin condition; and pupil size and reaction to light. These need to be obtained as soon as possible. Your patient may appear to be tolerating the injury well until you reassess these vital signs and they indicate otherwise. Trending these vital signs helps you to understand whether your patient's condition is improving or worsening over time, particularly during long transports. Shock or hypoperfusion is common in musculoskeletal injuries; therefore, this baseline information is a very important part of your initial assessment.

## Reassessment

Repeat the primary assessment to ensure your interventions are working as they should. Perform a reassessment every 5 minutes for an unstable patient and every 15 minutes for a stable patient.

Because trauma patients often have multiple injuries, you must assess their overall condition, stabilize the XABCs, and control any serious bleeding before further treating the injured area. In a critically injured patient, secure the patient to a backboard to immobilize the spine, pelvis, and extremities, and provide prompt transport to a trauma center. In this situation, a secondary assessment with extensive evaluation and splinting of limb injuries in the field is a waste of valuable time. Perform the primary assessment and transport, reassessing the patient en route to the ED.

If the patient has no life-threatening injuries, you may take extra time at the scene to stabilize the patient's overall condition and more completely evaluate the injury. If time permits, remove or cut away the patient's clothing to look for open fractures or dislocations, severe deformity, swelling, and/or ecchymosis.

When you have finished assessing the extremity, apply a secure splint to stabilize the injury prior to transport. The joints above and below the site of injury should be included in the splint. To minimize the potential for complications, the splint should be well padded. A comfortable and secure splint will reduce pain, reduce shock, and minimize compromised circulation. A good rule is to check the patient's circulation, motor function, and sensation before and after splinting. Splint application will be discussed later in the chapter.

The main goal in providing care for musculoskeletal injuries is stabilization in the most comfortable position that allows for maintenance of good circulation distal to the injury. This should be done whether you are preparing the patient for rapid transport or you have as much time as you need to assess and treat the patient.

Your radio report to the hospital should include a description of the problems found during your assessment. Particularly, you should report problems with the patient's XABCs, open fractures, and compromised circulation that occurred before or after splinting. Often, the hospital staff can arrange for specialists or consider antibiotics early if they are aware of problems. How much information you include in your radio report will depend on your local protocols. Additional details, such as the mandated reporting of situations involving elder or child abuse, can be given during your verbal report at the hospital when you transfer care to the nursing staff or physician.

It is important to document the presence or absence of circulation, motor function, and sensation distal to the injury before you move an extremity, after manipulation or splinting of the injury, and on arrival at the hospital. Hospital staff may refer to your notes to clarify confusing situations or communication problems. Your careful documentation becomes part of the patient's permanent medical record and may protect you from legal action that the patient may pursue later. Do not rely on your memory for details about situations; your memory is unreliable. Always document your findings.

## Emergency Medical Care

Your first steps in providing care for any patient are the primary assessment and stabilizing the patient's XABCs. If needed, perform a secondary assessment

of either the entire body or the specific area of injury. Always follow standard precautions and be alert for signs and symptoms of internal bleeding. Internal bleeding should be suspected whenever the MOI suggests that severe forces have impacted the body.

Follow the steps in **SKILL DRILL 32-1** when caring for patients with musculoskeletal injuries:

1. Remove jewelry. Expose the entire zone of injury by removing or cutting away clothing. Cover open wounds with dry, sterile dressings, and apply direct pressure to control bleeding. If bleeding cannot be controlled, quickly apply

## Skill Drill 32-1 Caring for Musculoskeletal Injuries

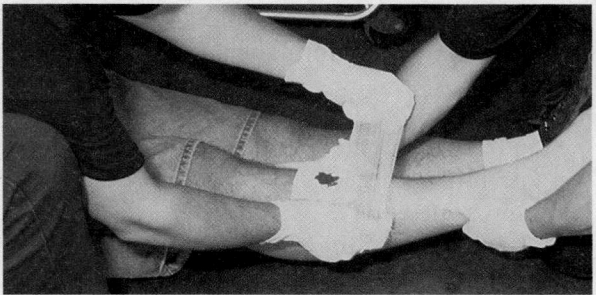

### Step 1

Cover open wounds with dry, sterile dressings, and apply pressure to control bleeding. Assess distal pulse and motor and sensory function. If bleeding cannot be controlled, quickly apply a tourniquet.

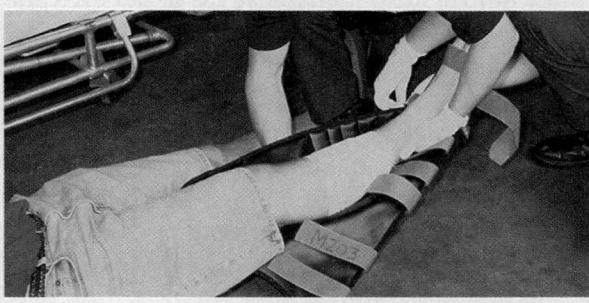

### Step 2

Apply a splint, and elevate the extremity approximately 6 inches (15 cm) (slightly above the level of the heart). Assess distal pulse and motor and sensory function.

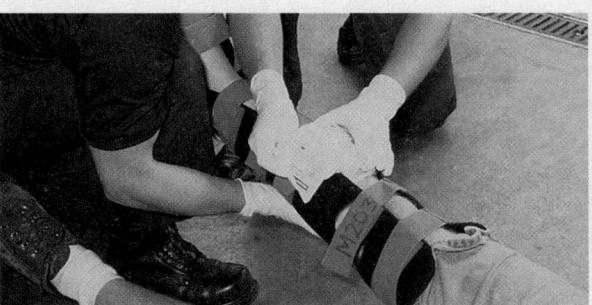

### Step 3

Apply cold packs if there is swelling, but do not place them directly on the skin.

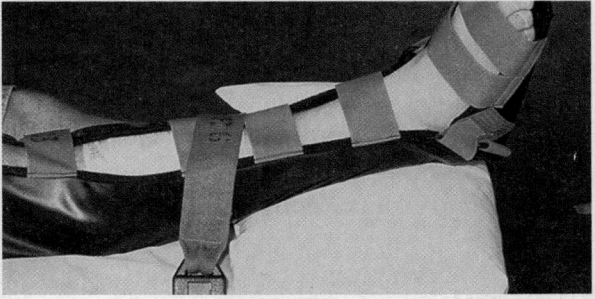

### Step 4

Position the patient for transport, and secure the injured area.

a tourniquet. Assess distal motor, sensory, and circulatory function. Once dressed, open fractures may be managed in the same manner as a closed fracture (**Step 1**).

2. Apply the appropriate splint and elevate the extremity. For fractures, it is essential to splint the joints above and below the injury to ensure adequate stabilization. Position injured limbs slightly above the level of the heart. Patients with lower extremity injuries should lie supine with the affected limb elevated about 6 inches (15 cm) to minimize swelling. Never allow the injured limb to flop about or dangle from the edge of the backboard. Always reassess distal motor, sensory, and circulatory function following the application of splints. Evaluate motor function by asking the patient to move his or her fingers and toes. Assess sensation by having the patient close his or her eyes and state which finger or toe you are touching. Examine circulatory status by palpating the distal pulse and checking capillary refill time. Additionally, note the color and condition of the patient's skin (**Step 2**).

3. If swelling is present, apply cold packs to the affected area. However, cold packs should never be placed directly on exposed skin or other tissues (**Step 3**).

4. Prepare for transport. A patient with an isolated upper extremity injury will likely prefer to sit in the semi-Fowler position rather than lie supine on the stretcher. Assuming there is no risk of spinal injury, either position is acceptable. Continue to keep the extremity elevated above the level of the heart, and secure it so that it does not dangle from the edge of the backboard or stretcher (**Step 4**).

5. Transport your patient to the most appropriate facility and consider the need to request advanced life support for pain management.

6. Advise hospital personnel of the patient's injuries and all interventions performed.

## Splinting

A **splint** is any flexible or rigid device used to prevent motion in an injured bone or joint (**FIGURE 32-24**). Unless the patient's life is in immediate danger, the EMT should splint all fractures, dislocations, and sprains prior to moving the patient. By preventing

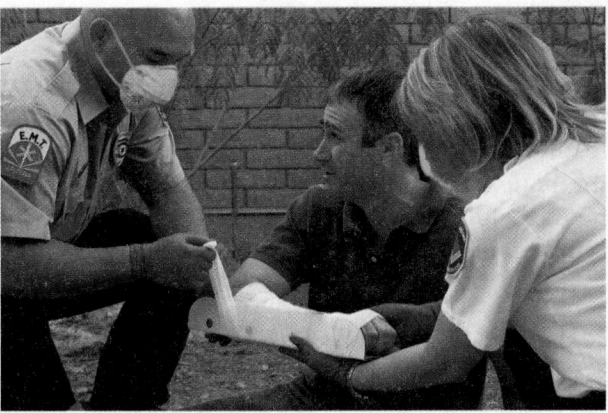

**FIGURE 32-24** Splinting reduces pain and prevents additional damage to the injured extremity.
© Jones & Bartlett Learning. Courtesy of MIEMSS.

movement of bone fragments, joint dislocations, and soft-tissue trauma, splinting reduces pain and makes it easier to transfer and transport the patient. In addition, splinting will help to prevent the following:

- Further damage to muscles, the spinal cord, peripheral nerves, and blood vessels from broken bone ends
- Laceration of the skin by broken bone ends. One of the primary indications for splinting is to prevent a closed fracture from becoming an open fracture (conversion).
- Restriction of distal blood flow resulting from compression of blood vessels
- Excessive bleeding of the tissues at the injury site caused by broken bone ends
- Increased pain from movement of bone ends

## General Principles of Splinting

The following principles of splinting apply to most situations:

1. Remove clothing from the area of any suspected fracture or dislocation so that you can inspect the extremity for DCAP-BTLS.

2. Note and record the patient's neurovascular status distal to the site of the injury, including pulse, sensation, and movement. Continue to monitor the neurovascular status until the patient reaches the hospital.

3. Cover open wounds with a dry, sterile dressing before splinting. Be sure to follow standard

precautions. Do not intentionally replace protruding bones. Notify the receiving hospital of all open wounds.

4. Do not move the patient before splinting an extremity unless there is an immediate danger to the patient or you or unless there are threats defined in the primary assessment of XABCDE that you are unable to correct.

5. In a suspected fracture of the shaft of any bone, be sure to stabilize the joints above and below the fracture.

6. With injuries in and around the joint, be sure to stabilize the bones above and below the injured joint.

7. Pad all rigid splints to prevent local pressure and patient discomfort.

8. While applying the splint, maintain manual stabilization to minimize movement of the limb and to support the injury site.

9. If fracture of a long bone shaft has resulted in severe deformity, use constant, gentle manual traction to align the limb so that it can be splinted. This is especially important if the distal part of the extremity is cyanotic or pulseless.

10. If you encounter resistance to limb alignment, splint the limb in its deformed position.

11. Immobilize all suspected spinal injuries in a neutral in-line position on a backboard or other spinal motion restriction device such as a vacuum mattress.

12. If the patient has signs of shock (hypoperfusion), align the limb in the normal anatomic position, and provide transport (total body immobilization).

13. When in doubt, splint.

## Words of Wisdom

Straightening or splinting an injured limb can compromise distal functions, as can the initial injury. Record the status of distal circulation and nervous function (neurovascular status) before and after straightening or splinting. At a minimum, your written record should describe these functions before splinting and confirm whether they were normal immediately after splinting and on hospital arrival. For all but the shortest transports, also indicate the results of reassessments while en route.

## Types of Splints

Although a splint can be improvised using a variety of materials, the EMT must be competent in utilizing the commercial devices on the ambulance that are frequently used. The basic types of splints are rigid splints, formable splints, traction splints, and pelvic binders.

### Rigid Splints

Rigid (nonformable) splints are made from firm material and are applied to the sides, front, and/or

## YOU are the Provider

A nurse present at the scene assists by stabilizing the leg above the ankle and below the knee while you expose the injury. The patient has an obvious deformity in the midshaft area of her tibia/fibula; however, there are no open wounds. As you further assess the injury, your partner obtains the patient's vital signs.

| Recording Time: 5 Minutes | |
| --- | --- |
| **Respirations** | 22 breaths/min; adequate depth |
| **Pulse** | 112 beats/min; strong and regular |
| **Skin** | Pink, warm, and moist |
| **Blood pressure** | 130/78 mm Hg |
| **Oxygen saturation (Spo$_2$)** | 98% (on ambient air) |

**5.** How should you proceed with your assessment of this patient's injury?

**6.** How should you treat an injured extremity in which distal perfusion is absent?

back of an injured extremity to prevent motion at the injury site. Common examples of rigid splints include padded board splints, molded plastic and metal splints, padded wire ladder splints, and folded cardboard splints. As always, be sure to follow standard precautions. It takes two people to apply a rigid splint. Follow the steps in **SKILL DRILL 32-2**:

1. Gently support the limb at the site of injury as your partner prepares and begins to position the equipment. Apply steady, in-line traction if necessary. Maintain this support until the splint is completely applied (**Step 1**). Assess distal pulse and motor and sensory function.
2. Place the rigid splint under or alongside the limb.
3. Place padding between the limb and the splint to make sure there is even pressure and even contact. Look for bony prominences, and pad them (**Step 2**).
4. Apply bindings to hold the splint securely to the limb (**Step 3**).

## Skill Drill 32-2 Applying a Rigid Splint

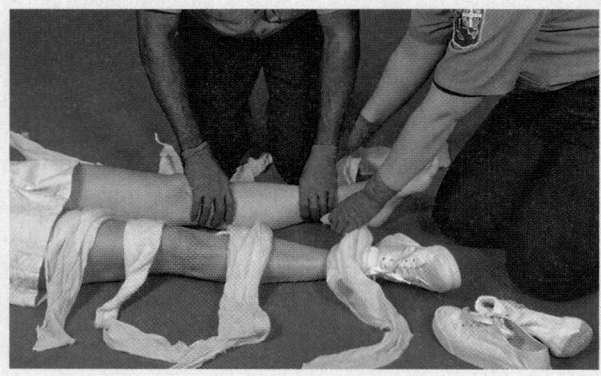

### Step 1

Provide gentle support and in-line traction for the limb. Assess distal pulse and motor and sensory function.

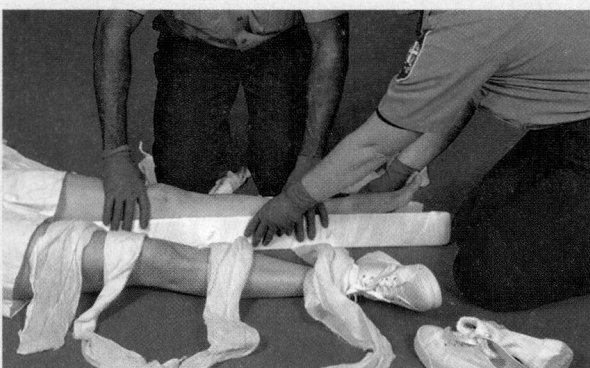

### Step 2

Place the splint alongside or under the limb. Pad between the limb and the splint as needed to ensure even pressure and contact.

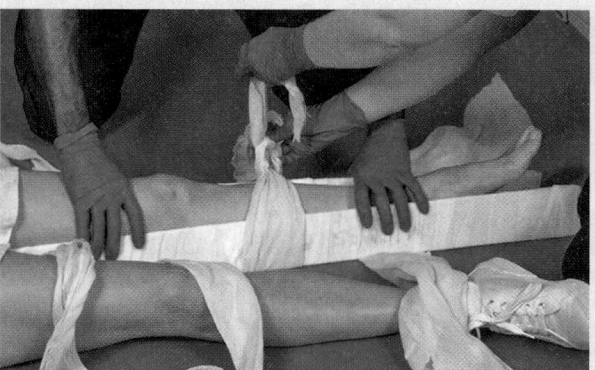

### Step 3

Secure the splint to the limb with bindings.

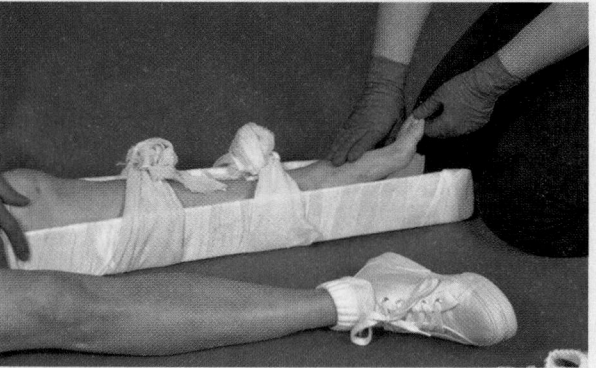

### Step 4

Assess and record distal neurovascular function.

5. Check and record the distal nervous and circulatory (neurovascular) function (**Step 4**).

There are two situations in which you must splint the limb in the position of deformity—when the deformity is severe, as is the case with many dislocations, and when you encounter resistance or extreme pain when applying gentle traction to the fracture of a shaft of a long bone. In either situation, apply padded board splints to each side of the limb and secure them with soft roller bandages (**FIGURE 32-25**). Most dislocations should be splinted as found, but follow local protocols. Attempts to realign or reduce dislocations may lead to more damage.

### Formable Splints

The formable splints you are most likely to use as an EMT are structural aluminum malleable (SAM) splints and vacuum splints. Other formable splints include air splints, pillow splints, and sling and swathe bandages. Technically, pelvic binders are also a type of formable splint, but are discussed later as a distinct type of splint later in this section.

A SAM splint consists of a moldable aluminum core encased in layers of foam padding. It usually comes packaged in a roll and can quickly be shaped, folded, or cut to serve numerous splinting needs. When curved or molded into a "T" shape, the splint becomes rigid (**FIGURE 32-26**). It can be molded and remolded as needed. Because there are several ways to use the splint, depending on

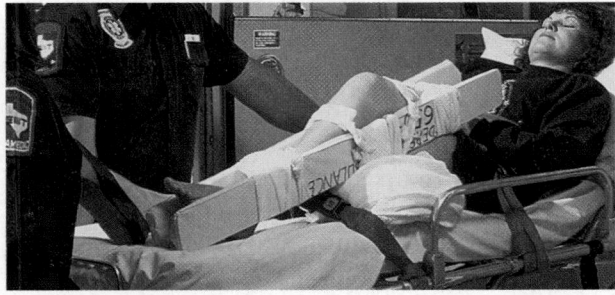

**FIGURE 32-25** If you encounter resistance or extreme pain when applying traction to a long bone, apply padded board splints to each side of the limb, and secure them with soft roller bandages, stabilizing the limb in its deformed position.

© American Academy of Orthopaedic Surgeons.

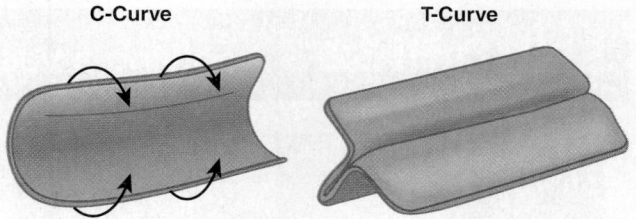

**FIGURE 32-26** A structural aluminum malleable splint becomes rigid when molded into a "T" shape.

© Jones & Bartlett Learning.

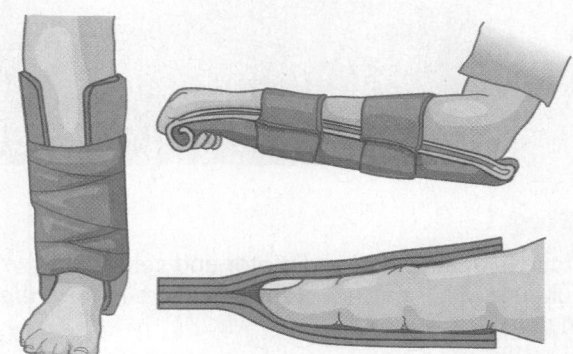

**FIGURE 32-27** Structural aluminum malleable splints can be used in various ways.

© Jones & Bartlett Learning.

the area to be stabilized, the EMT must be familiar with its application in a variety of scenarios (**FIGURE 32-27**).

### Street Smarts

Test your problem-solving skills. Practice using the SAM splint for a variety of injuries. With a partner, try splinting fractures and dislocations of sites such as a thumb, finger, wrist, forearm, elbow, humerus, shoulder, ankle, lower leg, knee, and cervical spine. Remember to follow the basic rules of splinting discussed earlier in this chapter.

A vacuum splint can be easily shaped to fit around a deformed limb. Instead of pumping air in, however, you can use a hand pump to pull the air out through a valve. Follow the steps in **SKILL DRILL 32-3** to apply a vacuum splint:

1. Assess distal pulse and motor and sensory function.
2. Your partner supports and stabilizes the injured limb, applying traction if needed (**Step 1**).

## Skill Drill 32-3 Applying a Vacuum Splint

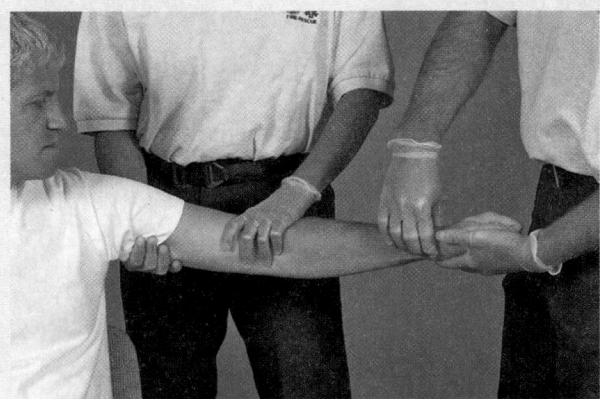

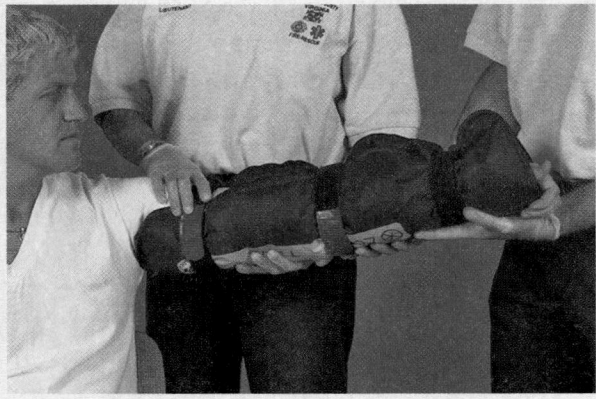

### Step 1

Assess distal pulse and motor and sensory function. Your partner stabilizes and supports the injury.

### Step 2

Place the splint, and wrap it around the limb.

### Step 3

Draw the air out of the splint through the suction valve, and then seal the valve. Assess distal pulse and motor and sensory function.

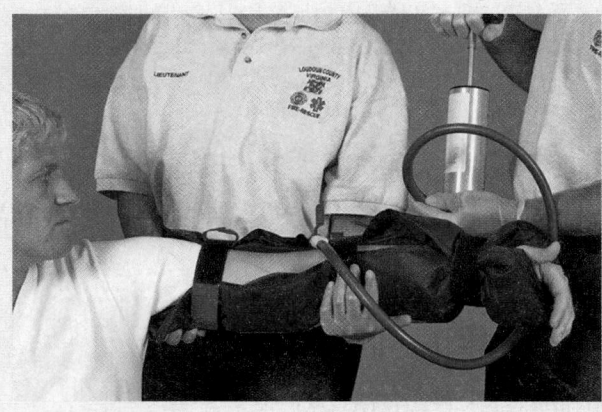

© Jones & Bartlett Learning. Courtesy of MIEMSS.

3. Gently place the injured limb onto the vacuum splint and wrap the splint around the limb (**Step 2**).
4. Draw the air out of the splint through the suction valve, and then seal the valve. Once the air has been drawn out, the vacuum splint becomes rigid, conforming to the shape of the deformed limb and stabilizing it. The splint will remain rigid as long as the valve remains closed (**Step 3**).
5. Check distal circulation and nervous functions and monitor them en route.

### *Pelvic Binders*

A **pelvic binder** is used to splint the bony pelvis to reduce hemorrhage from bone ends, venous disruption, and pain (**FIGURE 32-28**). Generally, pelvic binders are lightweight, made of soft material, easily applied by one EMT, and should allow access to the abdomen, perineum, anus, and groin for examination and diagnostic testing. Because multiple manufacturers produce pelvic binder devices, you should be familiar with the manufacturer's instructions for your specific device.

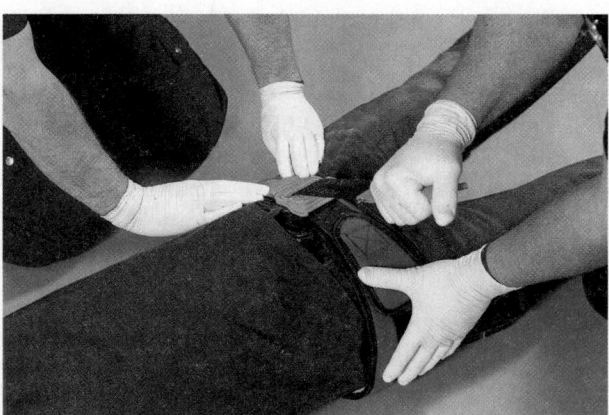

**FIGURE 32-28** Pelvic binders are meant to provide temporary stabilization until definitive immobilization can be achieved. Note: On a real patient, the clothing would be cut away prior to application of the splint.

© Jones & Bartlett Learning.

## Hazards of Improper Splinting

You must be aware of the hazards associated with the improper application of splints, including the following:

- Compression of nerves, tissues, and blood vessels
- Delay in transport of a patient with a life-threatening injury
- Reduction of distal circulation
- Aggravation of the injury
- Injury to tissue, nerves, blood vessels, or muscles as a result of excessive movement of the bone or joint

## Transportation

Once an injured limb is adequately splinted, the patient is ready to be transferred to a backboard or stretcher and transported.

Very few, if any, musculoskeletal injuries justify the use of excessive speed during transport. The limb will be stable once a dressing and splint have been applied. However, a patient with a pulseless limb must be given a higher priority. Still, if the hospital is only a few minutes away, speeding to the ED will not make an important difference to the patient's time to definitive treatment. If the treatment facility is a more substantial distance away, a patient with a pulseless limb should be transported by helicopter or urgent ground transportation. If circulation in the distal limb is impaired, always notify medical control so that proper steps can be taken quickly once the patient arrives in the ED.

# Specific Musculoskeletal Injuries

## Injuries of the Clavicle and Scapula

The clavicle, or collarbone, is one of the most commonly fractured bones in the body. Fractures of the clavicle occur commonly in children when they fall on an outstretched hand. They can also occur with crush injuries of the chest. A patient with a fracture of the clavicle will report pain in the shoulder and will usually hold the arm across the front of his or her body (**FIGURE 32-29**). A young child often reports pain throughout the entire arm and is unwilling to use any part of that limb. These complaints may make it difficult to localize the point of injury, but, generally, swelling and point tenderness occur over the clavicle. Because the clavicle is subcutaneous (just beneath the skin), the skin will occasionally tent over the fracture fragment. The clavicle lies directly over major arteries, veins, and nerves; therefore, fracture of the clavicle may lead to neurovascular compromise.

### Words of Wisdom

Point tenderness and severe pain with or without gross instability are the most reliable indicators of an underlying fracture.

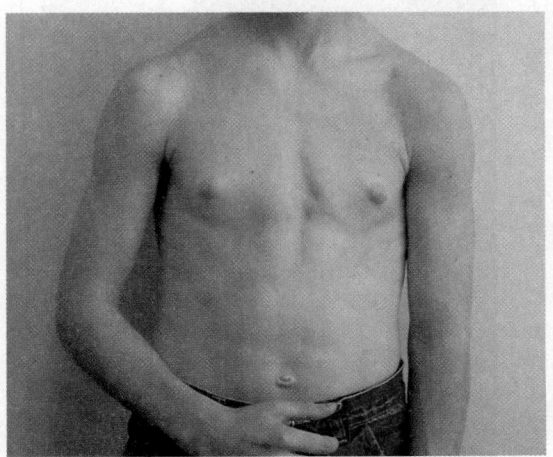

**FIGURE 32-29** A patient with a fracture of the clavicle will usually hold the arm across the front of his or her body.

© American Academy of Orthopaedic Surgeons.

Fractures of the scapula, or shoulder blade, occur much less frequently because this bone is well protected by many large muscles. Fractures of the scapula are almost always the result of a forceful, direct blow to the back, directly over the scapula, which may also injure the thoracic cage, lungs, and heart. For this reason, you must carefully assess the patient for signs of breathing problems. Provide supplemental oxygen and prompt transport for patients who are having difficulty breathing. Remember, it is the associated chest injuries, not the fractured scapula itself, that pose the greatest threat of long-term disability.

Abrasions, contusions, and significant swelling may also occur, and the patient will often limit use of the arm because of pain at the fracture site. The scapula also has bony projections that may be fractured with less force than required to fracture the body of the scapula.

The joint between the outer end of the clavicle and the acromion process of the scapula is called the **acromioclavicular (AC) joint**. This joint is frequently separated during sports, such as football or hockey, when a player falls and lands on the point of the shoulder, driving the scapula away from the outer end of the clavicle. This dislocation is often called an AC separation. The distal end of the clavicle will often stick out, and the patient will report pain, including point tenderness over the AC joint (**FIGURE 32-30**).

Fractures of the clavicle and scapula and AC separations can all be splinted effectively with a sling and swathe. A **sling** is any bandage or material that helps support the weight of an injured upper extremity, relieving the downward pull of gravity on the injured site. To be effective, a sling must apply gentle upward support to the olecranon process of the ulna. The knot of the sling should be tied to one side of the neck so that it does not press uncomfortably on the cervical spine (**FIGURE 32-31A**).

To fully stabilize the shoulder region, a **swathe**, a bandage that passes completely around the chest, must be used to bind the arm to the chest wall. The swathe should be tight enough to prevent the arm from swinging freely, but not so tight as to compress the chest and compromise breathing. Leave the patient's fingers exposed so that you can

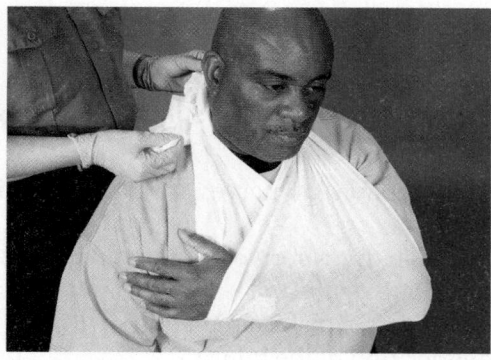

**A**

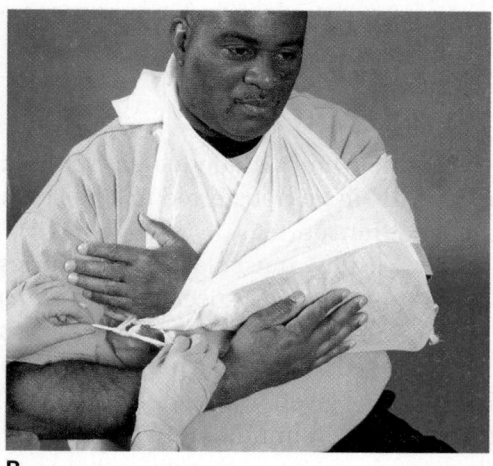

**B**

**FIGURE 32-31 A.** Apply a sling so that the knot is tied to one side of the neck. **B.** Bind the arm to the chest wall with a swathe so that the arm cannot swing freely. Leave the patient's fingers exposed so that you can assess distal circulation.

**A, B:** © Jones & Bartlett Learning. Courtesy of MIEMSS.

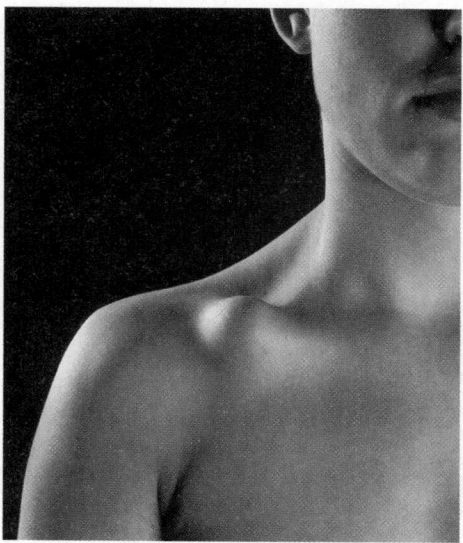

**FIGURE 32-30** With acromioclavicular separations, the distal end of the clavicle usually sticks out.

© Mike Devlin/Science Source.

assess neurovascular function at regular intervals (**FIGURE 32-31B**).

Commercially available shoulder stabilizers or slings will provide adequate splinting for injuries of the shoulder region, as will triangular bandage slings.

## Dislocation of the Shoulder

The glenohumeral joint (shoulder joint) is where the head of the humerus, the supporting bone of the upper arm, meets the glenoid fossa of the scapula. The glenoid fossa joins with the humeral head to form the glenohumeral joint. In shoulder dislocations, the humeral head most commonly dislocates anteriorly, coming to lie in front of the scapula as a result of forced abduction (away from the midline) and external rotation of the arm (**FIGURE 32-32**).

Shoulder dislocations are extremely painful. The patient will guard the shoulder and try to protect it by holding the dislocated arm in a fixed position away from the chest wall (**FIGURE 32-33**). The shoulder joint will usually be locked, and the shoulder will appear squared off or flattened. The humeral head will protrude anteriorly underneath the pectoralis major on the anterior chest wall. As a result, the axillary nerve may be compressed, causing a numb patch on the outer aspect of the shoulder. Be sure to document this finding. Some patients may also report some numbness in the hand because of either nervous or circulatory compromise.

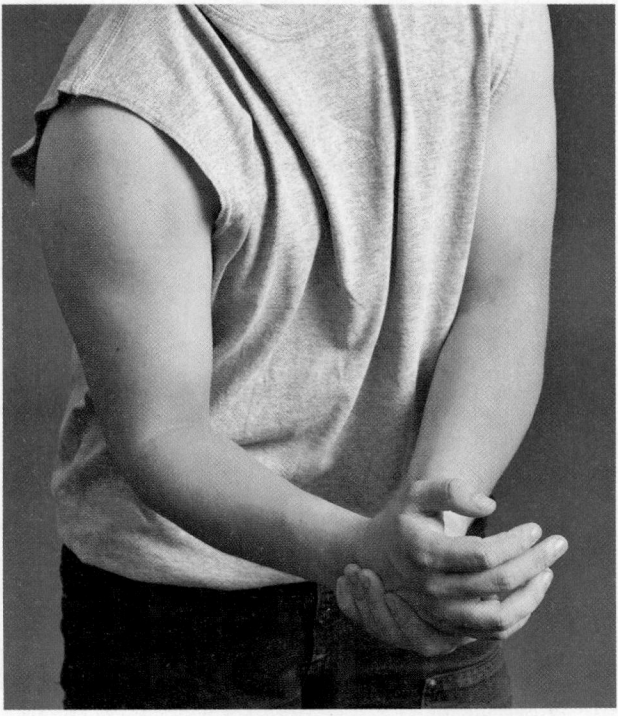

**FIGURE 32-33** A patient with a dislocated shoulder will guard the shoulder, trying to protect it by holding the arm in a fixed position away from the chest wall.

© Jones & Bartlett Learning.

Stabilizing an anterior shoulder dislocation is difficult because any attempt to bring the arm in toward the chest will produce pain. You must splint the joint in whatever position is most comfortable for the patient. If necessary, place a pillow or rolled blankets or towels between the arm and chest to fill up the space between them (**FIGURE 32-34**). Once the arm has been stabilized in this way, the elbow can usually be flexed to 90° without causing further pain. At this point, you can apply a sling to the forearm and wrist to support the weight of the arm. Finally, secure the arm in the sling to the pillow and chest with a swathe. Transport the patient in a seated or semiseated position.

Dislocation of the shoulder disrupts the supporting ligaments. Often, these ligaments fail to heal properly, so dislocation recurs, causing further joint injury with each dislocation. In certain cases, surgical repair may be required. Some patients are able to reduce (set) their own dislocated shoulders. However, this maneuver must be done in a hospital setting and only after radiograph films have been obtained confirming the nature and direction of the dislocation.

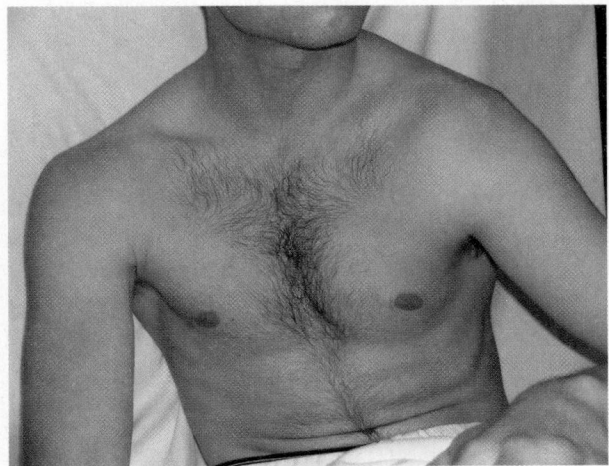

**FIGURE 32-32** Most shoulder dislocations are anterior. Note the absence of the normal rounded appearance of the shoulder.

© E. M. Singletary. Used with permission.

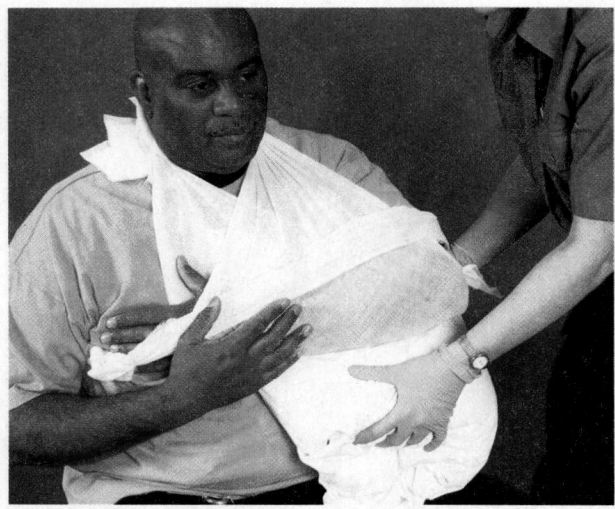

**FIGURE 32-34** Splint the shoulder joint in a position of comfort, and place a pillow or towel between the arm and the chest wall to stabilize the arm, after which the elbow can be flexed to 90°. Apply a sling and secure the arm to the chest with a swathe.

© Jones & Bartlett Learning. Courtesy of MIEMSS.

### Words of Wisdom

When you assess a patient with a possible shoulder dislocation, position yourself behind the patient and compare the shoulders. The dislocated side is often lower than the uninjured side.

Posterior dislocation is less common than anterior shoulder dislocation. Football players, especially linemen, are susceptible to this injury. The arm will often be locked in adduction (toward the midline), so it cannot be rotated. Reducing dislocated shoulders usually requires medical supervision.

## Fracture of the Humerus

Fractures of the humerus occur either proximally, in the midshaft, or distally at the elbow (**TABLE 32-2**). Fractures of the proximal humerus resulting from falls are common among older people. Fractures of

**TABLE 32-2** Characteristics and Treatment of Fractures of the Humerus

| Type | Characteristics | Treatment |
| --- | --- | --- |
| Proximal humeral fractures | • Significant swelling, but no significant deformity of the upper arm<br>• Neurovascular compromise uncommon<br>• If neurologic compromise present, any or all of the brachial plexus may be affected, depending on the degree of displacement<br>• Concurrent soft-tissue injuries possible<br>• Possible rotator cuff injury (If radiograph films show no fracture, a tear of the rotator cuff is possible, especially if the patient cannot rotate the arm.) | • Stabilize in a sling and swathe or a shoulder stabilizer.<br>• Use the chest wall as a splint, and secure the injured arm to the chest wall.<br>• Place a short, padded board splint on the lateral side of the arm under the sling and swathe for additional support. |
| Midshaft fractures | • Gross angulation of the arm<br>• Marked instability and crepitus of fracture fragments<br>• Possible neurovascular compromise<br>• Possible entrapment of the radial nerve (The patient cannot extend or dorsiflex the wrist or fingers and may report numbness on the dorsum of the hand; classic wrist drop.) | • Stabilize with a sling and swathe or a shoulder stabilizer.<br>• Use the chest wall as a splint, and secure the injured arm to the chest wall.<br>• Place a short, padded board splint on the lateral side of the arm under the sling and swathe for additional support. |
| Distal humeral fractures | • Significant swelling at the elbow<br>• Possible neurovascular compromise<br>• Possible injury to the ulnar or median nerve (Document nerve status before and after any attempt to reduce or stabilize the fracture.) | • Stabilize in a splint, in addition to a sling and swathe or a shoulder stabilizer. |

© Jones & Bartlett Learning.

the midshaft occur more often in young patients, usually as the result of a violent injury.

With any severely angulated fracture, consider applying traction to realign the fracture fragments before splinting them. Check your local protocols for indications and techniques for applying traction to a severely angulated fracture. Support the site of the fracture with one hand, and with the other hand, grasp the two humeral condyles (its lateral and medial protrusions) just above the elbow. Pull gently in line with the normal axis of the limb (**FIGURE 32-35**). Once you achieve gross realignment of the limb, splint the arm with a sling and swathe, supplemented by a padded board splint on the lateral aspect of the arm (**FIGURE 32-36**). If

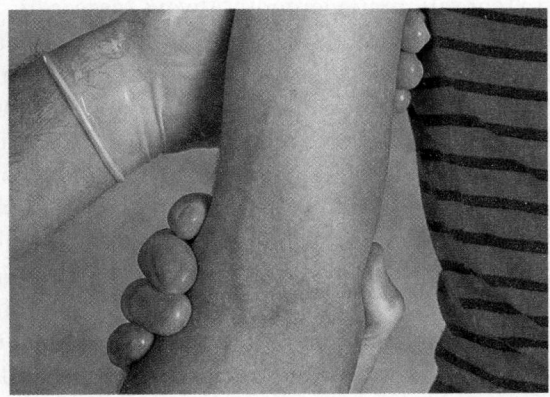

**FIGURE 32-35** To align a severe deformity associated with a humeral shaft fracture, apply gentle pressure to the humeral condyles, as shown in this uninjured arm.

© Jones & Bartlett Learning. Courtesy of MIEMSS.

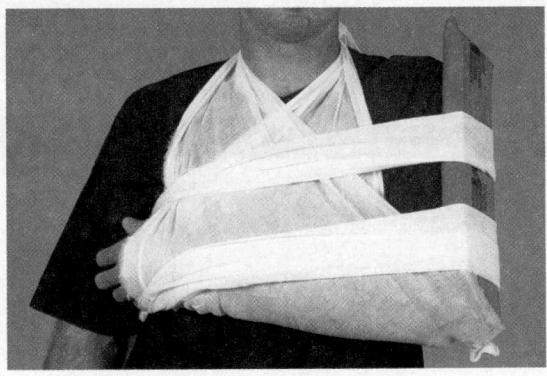

**FIGURE 32-36** Splint a humeral shaft fracture with a sling and swathe supplemented by a padded board splint on the lateral aspect of the arm.

© Jones & Bartlett Learning. Courtesy of MIEMSS.

the patient reports significant pain or resists gentle traction, splint the fracture in the deformed position with a padded wire ladder or a padded board splint, using pillows to support the injured limb. Note that compartment syndrome, discussed later in this chapter, can develop in the forearm in children with these fractures. When compartment syndrome occurs, it typically begins to develop several hours after injury and can evolve over the course of days. Once present, it represents a surgical emergency requiring emergent operative treatment to avoid catastrophic and permanent muscle and nerve damage in the arm.

## Elbow Injuries

Fractures and dislocations often occur around the elbow, and the different types of injuries are difficult to distinguish without radiographic examinations. However, they all produce similar limb deformities and require the same emergency care. Injuries to nerves and blood vessels are quite common in this region. Such injuries can be worsened or even caused by inappropriate emergency care, particularly by excessive manipulation of the injured joint.

### Fracture of the Distal Humerus

This type of fracture, also known as a supracondylar or intercondylar fracture, depending on its location, is common in children. Frequently, the fracture fragments rotate significantly, producing deformity and causing injuries to nearby vessels and nerves. Swelling occurs rapidly and is often severe.

### Dislocation of the Elbow

This type of injury typically occurs in athletes and rarely in young children. The ulna and radius are most often displaced posteriorly relative to the humerus. The ulna, the bone on the little finger side of the forearm, and the radius, the bone on the thumb side of the forearm, both join the distal humerus at the elbow joint. The posterior displacement makes the olecranon process of the ulna much more prominent (**FIGURE 32-37**). The joint is usually locked, with the forearm moderately flexed on the arm; this position makes any attempt at motion extremely painful. As with a fracture of the distal humerus, there is swelling and significant potential for vessel or nerve injury.

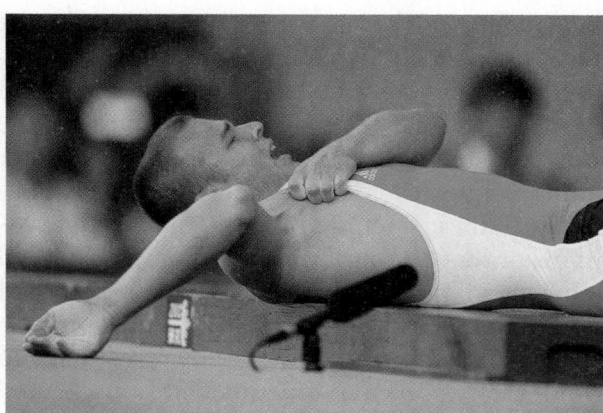

**FIGURE 32-37** Posterior dislocation of the elbow makes the olecranon process of the ulna much more prominent.

© JUNG YEON-JE/AFP/Getty Images.

### Words of Wisdom

Toddlers can sustain an injury similar to an elbow dislocation when they are lifted or pulled by the arm. This injury, which is sometimes called nursemaid's elbow, is actually a soft-tissue impingement condition, not a joint dislocation.

## Elbow Joint Sprain

This diagnosis is often mistakenly applied to an occult, nondisplaced fracture, because it can be difficult to distinguish between sprains and fractures.

## Fracture of the Olecranon Process of the Ulna

This fracture can result from direct or indirect forces and is often associated with lacerations and abrasions. The patient will be unable to actively extend the elbow.

## Fractures of the Radial Head

Often missed during diagnosis, this fracture generally occurs as a result of a fall on an outstretched arm or a direct blow to the lateral aspect of the elbow. Attempts to rotate the forearm will cause discomfort.

## Care of Elbow Injuries

All elbow injuries are potentially serious and require careful management. Always assess distal neurovascular functions periodically in patients with elbow injuries. If you find strong pulses and good capillary refill, splint the elbow injury in the position in which you found it, adding a wrist sling if this seems helpful. Two padded board splints, one applied to each side of the limb and secured with soft roller bandages, usually are enough to stabilize the arm (**FIGURE 32-38A**). Make sure the board extends from the shoulder joint to the wrist joint, stabilizing the entire bone above and below the injured joint. Alternatively, you can mold a padded wire ladder splint or a SAM splint to the shape of

## YOU are the Provider

As the nurse continues to manually stabilize the patient's leg, you retrieve the splinting supplies from the ambulance, and your partner reassesses her vital signs.

| Recording Time: 13 Minutes | |
| --- | --- |
| Level of consciousness | Conscious and alert |
| Respirations | 22 breaths/min; adequate depth |
| Pulse | 110 beats/min; strong and regular |
| Skin | Mucous membranes in inner lower eyelid and capillary refill normal; warm and moist |
| Blood pressure | 134/80 mm Hg |
| Spo$_2$ | 99% (on ambient air) |

**7.** How should you splint this patient's injury?

**8.** What are some methods for providing pain relief from orthopaedic trauma?

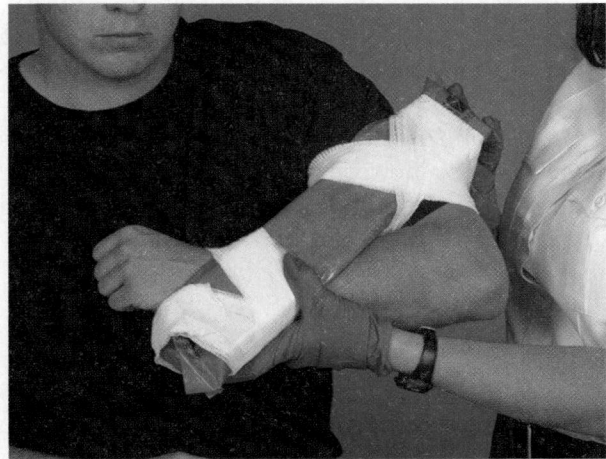

**A**

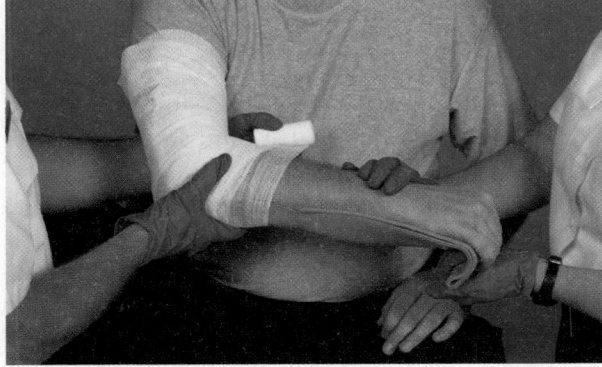

**B**

**FIGURE 32-38 A.** Two padded board splints provide adequate stabilization for an injured elbow. **B.** A structural aluminum malleable splint can be molded to the shape of the limb so that you can splint it in the position in which it was found.

A, B: © Jones & Bartlett Learning. Courtesy of MIEMSS.

the limb (**FIGURE 32-38B**). If necessary, you may add further support to the limb with a pillow.

A cold, pale hand or a weak or absent pulse and poor capillary refill indicate that the blood vessels have likely been injured. Further care of this patient must be dictated by a physician. Notify medical control immediately. If you are within 10 to 15 minutes of the hospital, splint the limb in the position in which you found it, and provide prompt transport. Otherwise, medical control may direct you to try to realign the limb to improve circulation in the hand.

If the limb is pulseless and significantly deformed at the elbow, apply gentle manual traction in line with the long axis of the limb to decrease the

deformity. This maneuver may restore the pulse. Be careful, because excessive manipulation may only worsen the vascular problem. If no pulse returns after one attempt, splint the limb in the most comfortable position for the patient. If the pulse is restored by gentle longitudinal traction, splint the limb in whatever position allows the strongest pulse. Provide prompt transport for all patients with impaired distal circulation.

### Special Populations

Growth plate injuries in children are common, especially around the wrist, elbow, knee, and ankle. Injuries tend to occur through these cartilaginous growth centers because they are inherently weaker than the surrounding bone. Because longitudinal growth of the limb depends on the function of the growth plate, it is extremely important to recognize the possibility of growth plate injuries, stabilize the injured limb, and transport the patient in a timely manner to an appropriate center. Proper functioning of the injured growth plate throughout the remainder of skeletal growth may depend on timely anatomic reduction of the fracture and close follow-up by a pediatric orthopaedic surgeon.

Any deformity close to a joint in children younger than 16 years should be assumed to be a growth plate injury. Treat and transport the patient appropriately.

## Fractures of the Forearm

Fractures of the shaft of the radius and ulna are common in people of all age groups but are seen most often in children and older people. Usually, both bones break at the same time when the injury is the result of a fall on an outstretched hand (**FIGURE 32-39**). An isolated fracture of the shaft of the ulna may occur as the result of a direct blow to it; this is known as a nightstick fracture.

Fractures of the distal radius, which are especially common in older patients with osteoporosis, are known as Colles fractures. The term "silver fork deformity" is used to describe the distinctive

### Special Populations

In the United States, more than 80,000 distal radial fractures occur each year in people older than 65 years.

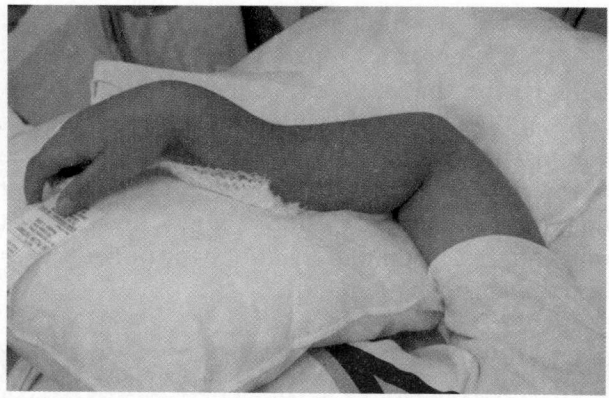

**FIGURE 32-39** Fractures of the forearm often occur in children as a result of a fall on an outstretched hand.

© E. M. Singletary. Used with permission.

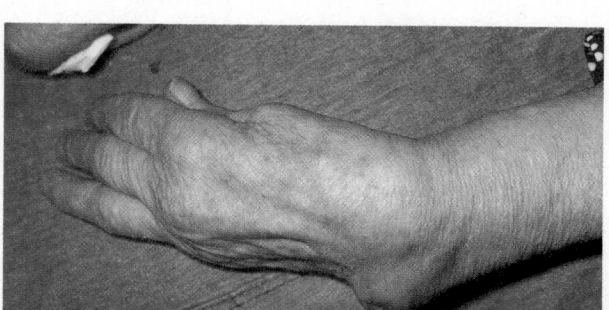

**A**

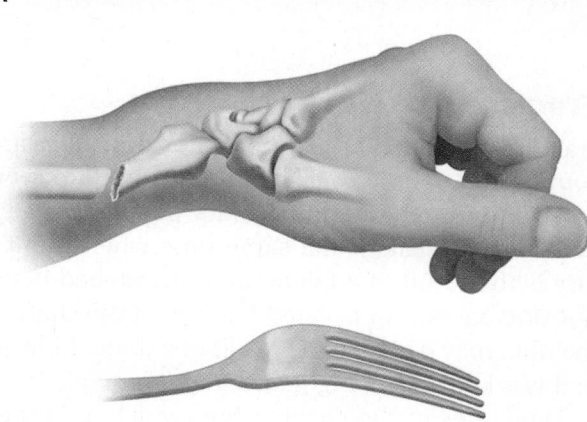

**B**

**FIGURE 32-40 A.** Fractures of the distal radius produce a characteristic silver fork deformity. **B.** An artist's illustration.

**A:** © Dr. M.A. Ansary/Science Source; **B:** © Jones & Bartlett Learning.

appearance of the patient's arm (**FIGURE 32-40**). In children, this fracture may occur through the growth plate and can have long-term consequences.

To stabilize fractures of the forearm or wrist, you can use a padded board, air, vacuum, or pillow splint. If the shaft of the bone has been fractured, be sure to include the elbow joint in the splint. Splinting of the elbow joint is not essential with fractures near the wrist; however, the patient will be more comfortable if you add a sling or pillow for more support. If possible, elevate the injured extremity above the heart to help alleviate swelling.

## Injuries of the Wrist and Hand

Injuries of the wrist, ranging from dislocations to sprains, are common after falls. Dislocations are usually associated with a fracture, resulting in a fracture dislocation. Another common wrist injury is the isolated, nondisplaced fracture of a carpal bone, especially the scaphoid. Any questionable wrist sprain or fracture should be splinted and evaluated in the ED or an orthopaedic surgeon's office.

Hand injuries vary widely, and some may have potentially serious consequences. Industrial, recreational, and home accidents often result in dislocations, fractures, lacerations, burns, and amputations. Because the fingers and hands are required to function in intricate ways, any injury that is not treated properly may result in permanent disability, as well as deformity. For this reason, all injuries to the hand, including simple lacerations, should be evaluated by a physician. For example, do not attempt to "pop" a dislocated finger joint back in place (**FIGURE 32-41**). Always take any amputated parts to the hospital with the patient. Be sure to wrap the amputated part in

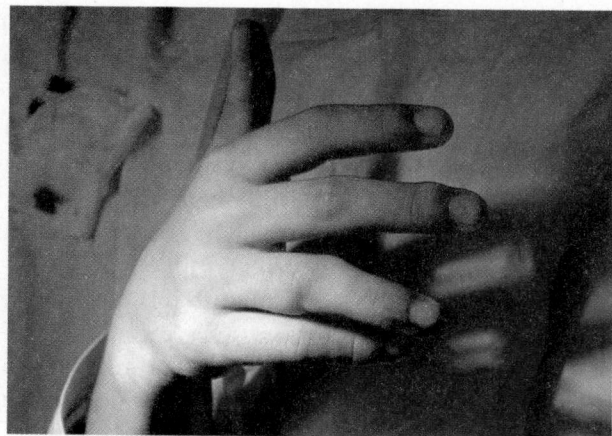

**FIGURE 32-41** Dislocation of the finger joint. Do not try to "pop" the joint back into place.

© E. M. Singletary, MD. Used with permission.

a dry or moist sterile dressing, depending on your local protocol, and place it in a dry plastic bag. Put the bag in a cooled container; do not soak the part in water or allow it to freeze.

A bulky forearm dressing makes an effective splint for any hand or wrist injury. Follow the steps in **SKILL DRILL 32-4**:

1. Follow standard precautions.
2. Cover open wounds with a dry, sterile dressing.
3. Assess distal pulse and motor and sensory function.
4. Supporting the injured limb, form the injured hand into the position of function, with the

wrist slightly bent down and all finger joints moderately flexed. This is the position that is used to hold a can most comfortably.

5. Place a soft roller bandage into the palm of the hand (**Step 1**).
6. Apply a padded board splint to the palmar side of the wrist, leaving the fingers exposed (**Step 2**).
7. Secure the entire length of the splint with a soft roller bandage (**Step 3**). Assess distal pulse and motor and sensory function.
8. Apply a sling and swathe, or prop the splinted hand and wrist on a pillow or on the patient's chest during transport to the hospital.

---

## Skill Drill 32-4 Splinting the Hand and Wrist

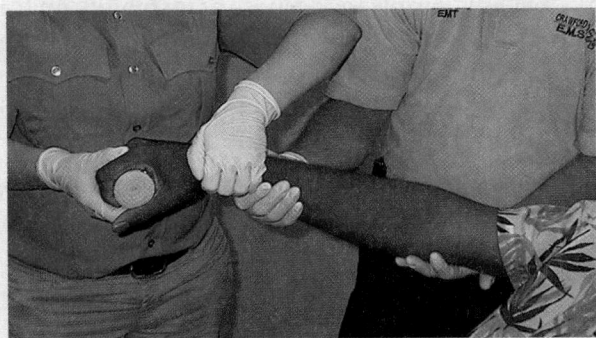

### Step 1

Support the injured limb and move the hand into the position of function. Place a soft roller bandage in the palm.

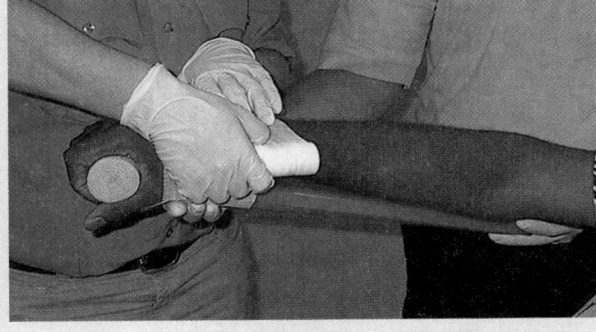

### Step 2

Apply a padded board splint on the palmar side with fingers exposed.

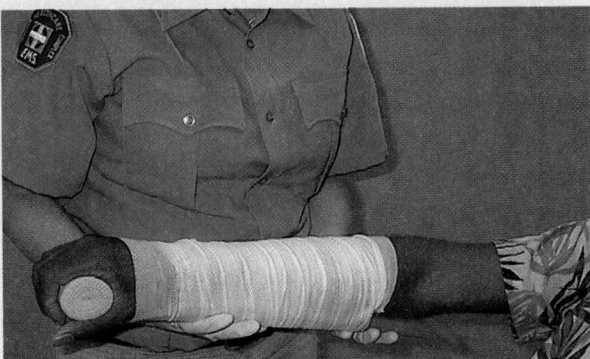

### Step 3

Secure the splint with a roller bandage.

## Fractures of the Pelvis

Fractures of the pelvis often result from direct compression in the form of a heavy blow that literally crushes the pelvis. The blow may be from a motor vehicle crash, a weapon, a falling object, or a fall from a height. Injuries to the pelvis can also be caused by indirect forces. For example, when the knee strikes the dashboard in a motor vehicle crash, the impact of the force is transmitted along the line of the femur (thighbone), which is the longest and largest bone in the body. The head of the femur is driven into the pelvis, causing a fracture of the acetabulum, the portion of the pelvis that forms the socket of the hip joint. However, not all pelvic fractures result from violent trauma. Even a simple fall can produce a fracture of the pelvis, especially in older people with osteoporosis.

Certain types of pelvic fractures may be accompanied by life-threatening loss of blood from the laceration of blood vessels affixed to the pelvis at certain key points. Up to several liters of blood may drain into the pelvic space and the retroperitoneal space, which lies between the abdominal cavity and the posterior abdominal wall. The result is significant hypotension, shock, and sometimes death. For this reason, you must take immediate steps to treat shock, even if there is no visible swelling.

Often, there is no evidence of bleeding until severe blood loss has occurred. Be prepared to resuscitate the patient rapidly if this becomes necessary.

Because the pelvis is surrounded by heavy muscle, open fractures of the pelvis are uncommon. However, pelvis fracture fragments can lacerate the rectum and vagina, creating an open fracture that is often overlooked. Once the protective pelvic ring is broken, the structures it is designed to protect, including the urinary bladder, are more susceptible to injury. The bladder may be lacerated by pelvic bone fragments, or it may tear as a result of direct pressure on the bladder itself or tension on the urethra.

You should suspect a fracture of the pelvis in any patient who has sustained a high-velocity injury and reports discomfort in the lower back or abdomen. Because the area is covered by heavy muscle and other soft tissue, deformity or swelling may be difficult to see. The most reliable sign of fracture of the pelvis is simple tenderness or instability on firm compression and palpation. Firm compression on the two iliac crests will produce pain at a fracture site in the pelvic ring. Assess for tenderness by taking the following steps (**FIGURE 32-42**):

1. Place the palms of your hands over the lateral aspect of each iliac crest, and apply firm but gentle inward pressure on the pelvic ring.

## YOU are the Provider

After properly splinting the patient's leg, you place her onto the stretcher, load her into the ambulance, and begin transport to the hospital. You reassess her condition and vital signs en route and note that her condition remains stable. You call your radio report in to the receiving facility; your estimated time of arrival is 8 minutes.

| Recording Time: 23 Minutes | |
| --- | --- |
| **Level of consciousness** | Conscious and alert |
| **Respirations** | 20 breaths/min; adequate depth |
| **Pulse** | 115 beats/min; strong and regular |
| **Skin** | Mucous membranes in inner lower eyelid and capillary refill normal; warm and dry |
| **Blood pressure** | 128/76 mm Hg |
| **SpO$_2$** | 98% (on ambient air) |

During transport, the patient reports numbness and tingling in her left foot. Your reassessment reveals that her pedal pulse is weaker than it was before and that her foot looks pale and feels cool.

9. What is the most likely cause of the patient's complaint? What can you do to remedy the situation?

10. What factors increase the risk of complications following orthopaedic trauma?

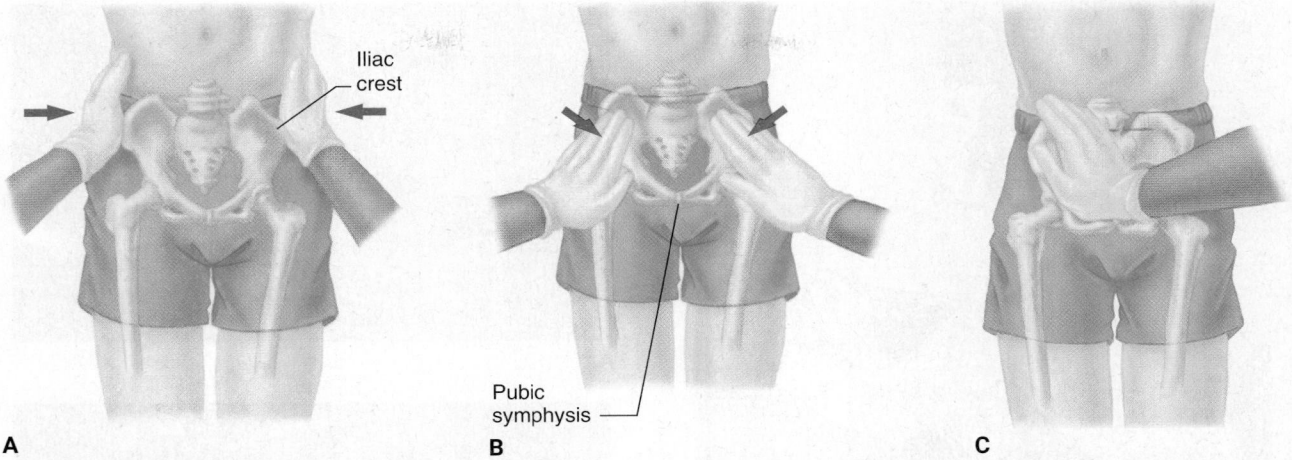

**FIGURE 32-42 A.** To assess for tenderness or instability in the pelvic region, place your hands over the lateral aspect of each iliac crest, and gently compress the pelvis. **B.** With the patient in a supine position, place your palms over the anterior aspect of each iliac crest, and apply firm but gentle downward pressure. **C.** Palpate the pubic symphysis with the palm of your hand.

A, B, C: © Jones & Bartlett Learning.

2. With the patient lying supine, place a palm over the anterior aspect of each iliac crest, and apply firm downward pressure.
3. Use the palm of your hand to firmly but gently palpate the pubic symphysis, the firm cartilaginous joint between the two pubic bones. This area will be tender if there is injury to the anterior portion of the pelvic ring.

If there has been injury to the bladder or the urethra, the patient will have lower abdominal tenderness and may have evidence of hematuria (blood in the urine) or blood at the urethral opening.

Perform the primary assessment, and carefully monitor the general condition of any patient whom you suspect has a pelvic fracture, because the patient is at high risk for hypovolemic shock. Patients in stable condition can be secured to a backboard or a scoop stretcher to stabilize isolated fractures of the pelvis.

## Dislocation of the Hip

The hip joint is a stable ball-and-socket joint that dislocates only after significant injury. Most dislocations of the hip are posterior. The femoral head is displaced posteriorly to lie in the muscles of the buttock. Posterior dislocation of the hip commonly occurs as a result of a motor vehicle crash in which the knee meets with a direct force, such as the dashboard, and the entire femur is driven posteriorly,

dislocating the hip joint (**FIGURE 32-43**). Thus, you should suspect a hip dislocation in any patient who has been in a motor vehicle crash and has a contusion, laceration, or obvious fracture in the knee region. Very rarely does the femoral head dislocate anteriorly; in this circumstance, the legs are suddenly and forcibly spread wide apart and locked in this position.

Posterior dislocation of the hip is frequently complicated by injury to the sciatic nerve, which is located directly behind the hip joint. The sciatic nerve is the largest peripheral nerve in the body; it controls the activity of muscles in the posterior thigh and below the knee and the sensation in most of the leg and foot. When the head of the femur is forced out of the hip socket, it may compress or stretch the sciatic nerve, leading to partial or complete paralysis of the nerve. The result is decreased sensation in the leg and foot and frequently weakness in the foot muscles. Generally, only the dorsiflexors, the muscles that raise the toes or foot, are involved, causing the foot drop that is characteristic of damage to the peroneal portion of the sciatic nerve.

Patients with a posterior dislocation of the hip typically lie with the hip joint flexed (the knee joint drawn up toward the chest) and the thigh rotated inward toward the midline of the body over the top of the opposite thigh (**FIGURE 32-44A**). With the less common anterior dislocation, the limb is in the opposite position, extended straight out, externally

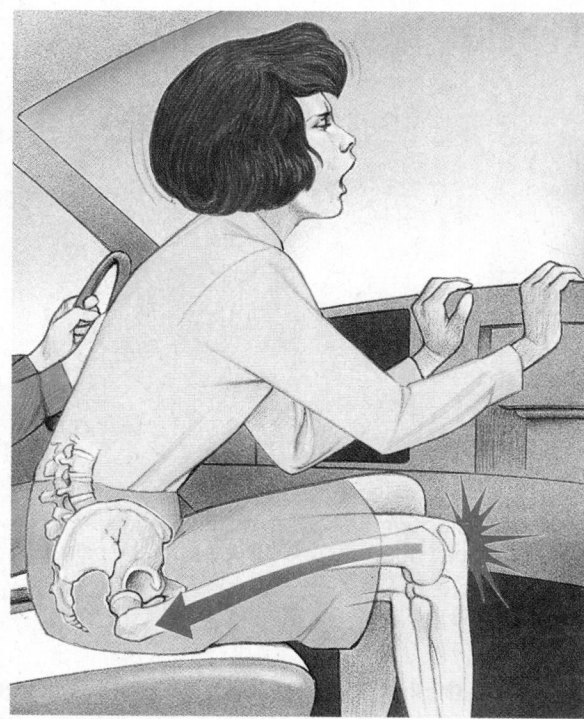

**FIGURE 32-43** Posterior dislocation of the hip can occur as a result of the knee hitting the dashboard in a motor vehicle crash. The impact drives the femur posteriorly (see arrow), dislocating the joint.

© Jones & Bartlett Learning.

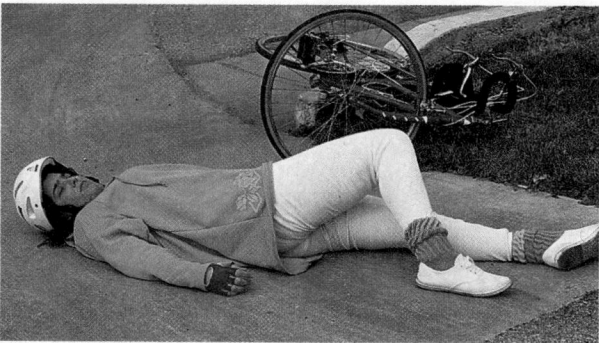

**A**

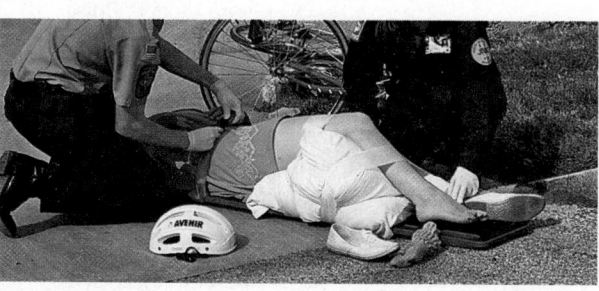

**B**

**FIGURE 32-44 A.** The usual position of a patient with a posterior dislocation of the hip. The hip joint is flexed, and the thigh is rotated inward and adducted across the midline of the body. **B.** Support the affected limb with pillows and blankets, particularly under the flexed knee. Secure the entire limb to a backboard with long straps to prevent movement during transport.

**A, B:** © Jones & Bartlett Learning. Courtesy of MIEMSS.

rotated, and pointing away from the midline of the body.

Dislocation of the hip is associated with distinctive signs. The patient will have severe pain in the hip and will strongly resist any attempt to move the joint. The lateral and posterior aspects of the hip region will be tender on palpation. With some thin patients, you can palpate the femoral head deep within the muscles of the buttock. Check for a sciatic nerve injury by carefully assessing sensation and motor function in the lower extremity. Occasionally, sciatic nerve function will be normal at first and then slowly diminish.

As with any other extremity injury, do not attempt to reduce the dislocated hip in the field. Splint the dislocation in the position of the deformity, and place the patient supine on a backboard. Support the affected limb with pillows and rolled blankets, particularly under the flexed knee (**FIGURE 32-44B**). Then secure the entire limb to the backboard with long straps so that the hip region will not move, and provide prompt transport.

## Fractures of the Proximal Femur

Fractures of the proximal (upper) end of the femur are common, especially in older people and patients with osteoporosis. Although these fractures are usually called hip fractures, they rarely involve the hip joint. Instead, the break goes through the neck of the femur, the intertrochanteric (middle) region, or across the proximal shaft of the femur (subtrochanteric fractures). These three fracture types may also be a result of high-energy injuries in younger patients.

Patients with displaced fractures of the proximal femur display a very characteristic deformity. They lie with the leg externally rotated, and the injured leg is usually shorter than the opposite, uninjured limb. When the fracture is not displaced, this deformity is not present. With any kind of hip fracture, patients typically are unable to walk or move the leg because of pain in the hip region or in the groin or inner aspect of the thigh. The hip region may be tender on palpation, and gentle rolling of the leg will cause pain but will not do further damage. On occasion, the pain is referred to the knee, and it is not uncommon for a geriatric patient with a hip fracture to report knee pain after a fall. Assess the pelvis for any soft-tissue injury and bandage appropriately. In addition, assess pulses and motor and sensory functions, looking for signs of vascular and nerve damage. Once your assessment is complete, splint the lower extremity of an older patient who has fallen and reports pain in either the hip or the knee, even if there is no deformity, and then transport the patient to the ED.

The age of the patient and the severity of the injury will dictate how you splint the fracture. A geriatric patient with an isolated hip fracture does not require a traction splint. You can effectively stabilize such a fracture by placing the patient on a backboard, vacuum mattress, or scoop stretcher, using pillows or rolled blankets to support the injured limb in the deformed position. Then secure the injured limb carefully to the device with long straps.

Patients with hip fractures may have a significant amount of blood loss. Therefore, you should treat with high-flow oxygen, monitor vital signs frequently, and be alert for signs of shock.

> ## Special Populations
>
> As the population of older adults in the United States continues to increase, emergency calls for older adults will constitute an ever-growing proportion of the EMT's workload.

## Femoral Shaft Fractures

Fractures of the femur can occur in any part of the shaft, from the hip region to the femoral condyles just above the knee joint. Following a fracture, the large muscles of the thigh spasm to "splint" the unstable limb. The muscle spasm often produces significant deformity of the limb, with severe angulation or external rotation at the fracture site. Usually, the limb also shortens significantly. Fractures of the femoral shaft may be open, and fragments of bone may protrude through the skin. As with any other open fracture, never attempt to push the bone or bones back into the skin.

There is often a significant amount of blood loss, as much as 500 to 1,000 mL, after a fracture of the shaft of the femur. With open fractures, the amount of blood loss may be even greater. Thus, it is not unusual for hypovolemic shock to develop. Handle patients with these fractures with extreme care because any extra movement or fracture manipulation may increase the amount of blood loss.

Because of the severe deformity that occurs with these fractures, bone fragments may impinge on important nerves and vessels and produce significant damage. For this reason, you must carefully and periodically assess the distal neurovascular function in patients who have sustained a fracture of the femoral shaft. Remove the clothing from the affected limb so that you can adequately inspect the injury site for any open wounds. Remember to follow standard precautions when any blood or body fluids are present. Monitor the patient's vital signs closely, and continue to watch for the onset of hypovolemic shock. You must provide rapid transport in this situation.

Cover any open wound with a dry, sterile dressing. If the foot or leg below the level of the fracture shows signs of impaired circulation (is pale, cold, or pulseless), apply gentle longitudinal traction to the deformed limb in line with the long axis of the limb. Gradually turn the leg from the deformed position to restore the limb's overall alignment. Often, this restores or improves circulation to the foot. If it does not, the patient may have sustained a serious vascular injury and may be in need of prompt medical attention.

A fracture of the femoral shaft is best stabilized with a traction splint, such as a Sager splint.

## Traction Splints

Application of in-line traction is the act of pulling on a body structure in the direction of its normal alignment. It is the most effective way to realign a fracture of the shaft of a long bone so that the limb can be splinted more effectively. Traction splints are used primarily to secure fractures of the shaft of the femur, which are characterized by pain, swelling, and deformity of the midthigh.

Excessive traction can be harmful to an injured limb. When applied correctly, however, traction stabilizes the bone fragments and improves the overall alignment of the limb. Do not attempt to force the bone fragments back into alignment. In the field, the goals of in-line traction are as follows:

1. Stabilize the fracture fragments to prevent excessive movement.
2. Align the limb sufficiently to allow it to be placed in a splint.
3. Avoid potential neurovascular compromise.

Several different types of lower extremity traction splints are commercially available, such as the Hare traction splint, the Sager splint, the Reel splint, and the Kendrick splint (**FIGURE 32-45**). Each has its own unique method of application; therefore, it is important to practice using the device or devices your agency carries.

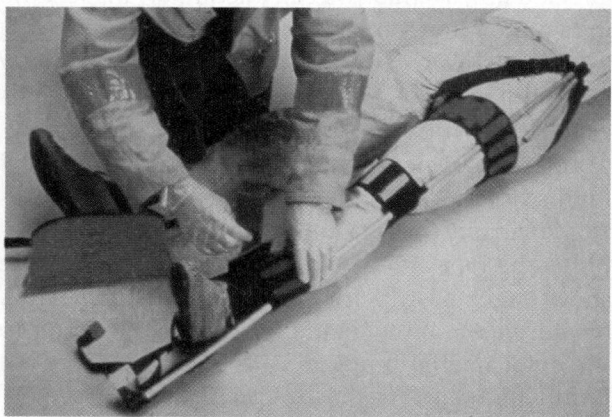

**FIGURE 32-45** The Kendrick traction splint.

Courtesy of Kendrick EMS. Used with permission.

Traction splints are not suitable for use on the upper extremity because the major nerves and blood vessels in the patient's axilla cannot tolerate countertraction forces.

Do not use traction splints for, or in the presence of, any of the following conditions:

- Injuries of the upper extremity
- Injuries close to or involving the knee
- Injuries of the pelvis
- Partial amputations or avulsions with bone separation
- Lower leg, foot, or ankle injuries

Proper application of a traction splint requires a minimum of two EMTs. Before you apply a traction splint, be sure to control any external bleeding. The amount of traction that is required varies but often does not exceed 15 pounds (7 kg). Use the least amount of force necessary. Grasp the foot or hand at the end of the injured limb firmly; once you start pulling, do not stop until the limb is fully splinted. Releasing manual traction before the limb is secured will allow the muscles to contract, allowing the bone fragments to cause more damage to surrounding tissue. Always apply traction along the long axis of the limb. Imagine where the uninjured limb would lie, and pull gently along the line of that imaginary limb until the injured limb is in approximately that position (**FIGURE 32-46**). Grasping the foot or hand and the initial pull of traction usually causes the patient some discomfort as the bone

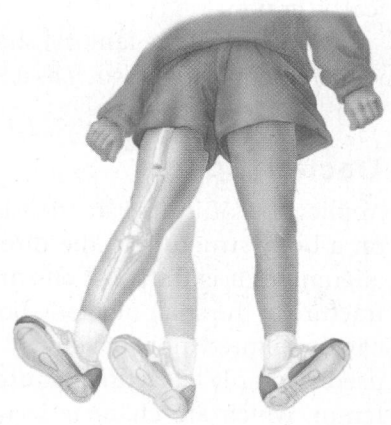
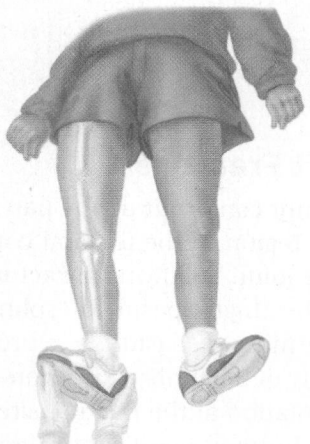

**FIGURE 32-46** To apply traction, imagine the position where the uninjured limb would lie, and then gently pull along that line until the injured limb is in that position. Do not release traction once you have applied it.

© Jones & Bartlett Learning.

fragments move. A second EMT should support the injured limb directly under the site of the fracture. This initial discomfort quickly subsides, and you can then apply further gentle traction. However, if the patient strongly resists the traction or if it causes more pain that persists, stop and splint the limb in the deformed position.

To apply a Hare traction splint, follow the steps in **SKILL DRILL 32-5**:

1. Cut open the patient's pant leg, or otherwise expose the injured lower extremity. Remove the patient's shoe. Follow standard precautions as needed. Be sure to assess and record

---

## Skill Drill 32-5 Applying a Hare Traction Splint

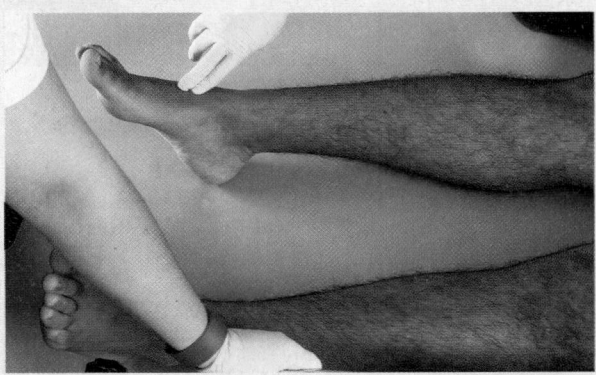

### Step 1

Expose the injured limb and check pulse and motor and sensory function. Place the splint beside the uninjured limb, adjust the splint to the proper length, and prepare the straps.

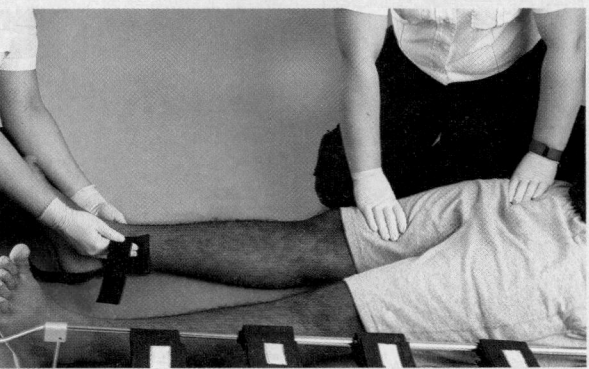

### Step 2

Support the injured limb as your partner fastens the ankle hitch about the foot and ankle.

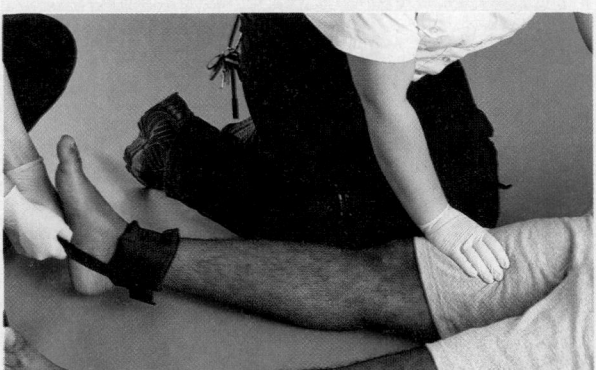

### Step 3

Continue to support the limb as your partner applies gentle in-line traction to the ankle hitch and foot.

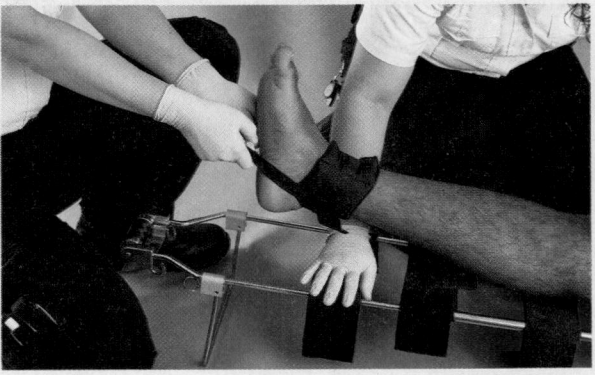

### Step 4

Slide the splint into position under the injured limb.

*(continues)*

## Skill Drill 32-5 Applying a Hare Traction Splint (*continued*)

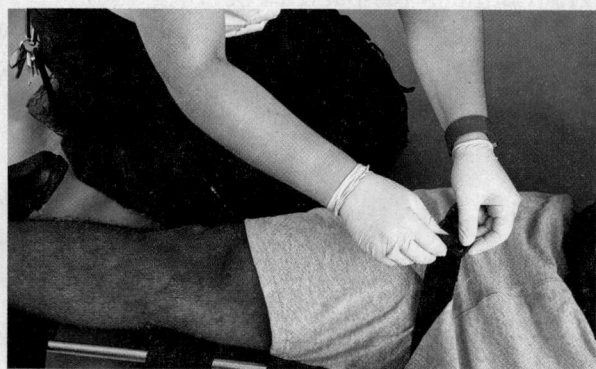

### Step 5

Pad the groin and fasten the ischial strap.

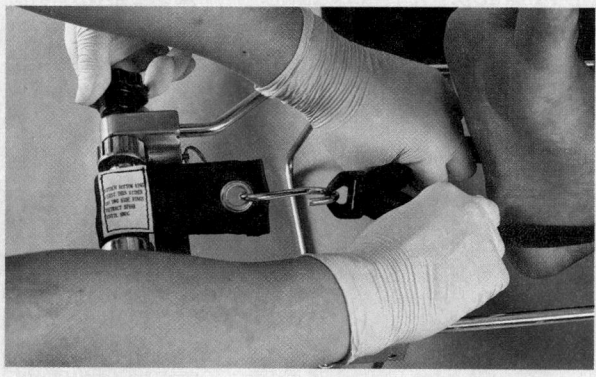

### Step 6

Connect the loops of the ankle hitch to the end of the splint as your partner continues to maintain traction. Carefully tighten the ratchet to the point that the splint holds adequate traction.

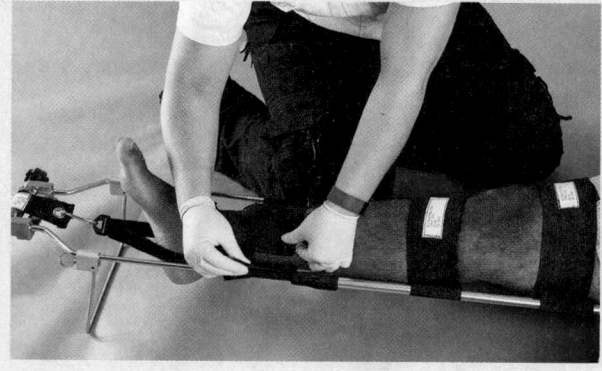

### Step 7

Secure and check support straps. Assess pulse and motor and sensory functions.

© Jones & Bartlett Learning.

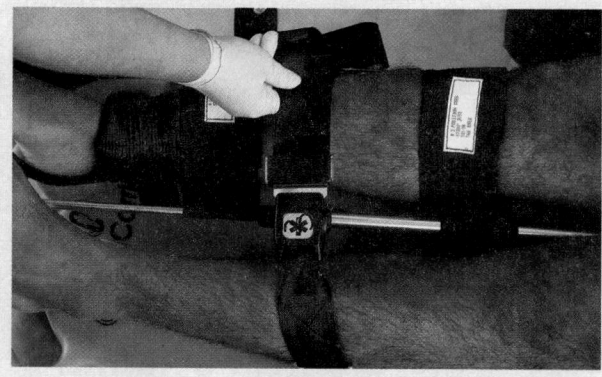

### Step 8

Secure the patient and splint to the backboard in a way that will prevent movement of the splint during patient movement and transport.

the pulse and motor function and sensation distal to the injury.

2. Place the splint beside the patient's uninjured leg, and adjust it to the proper length, with the ring at the ischial tuberosity and the splint extending 12 inches (30 cm) beyond

the foot. Open and adjust the four Velcro support straps, which should be positioned at the midthigh, above the knee, below the knee, and above the ankle (**Step 1**).

3. Manually support and stabilize the injured limb so that no motion will occur at the

fracture site while your partner fastens the appropriate-size ankle hitch about the patient's ankle and foot (**Step 2**).

4. Support the leg at the site of the suspected injury while your partner manually applies gentle longitudinal traction to the ankle hitch and foot. Use only enough force to align (reposition) the limb so that it will fit into the splint; do not attempt to align the fracture fragments anatomically (**Step 3**).

5. Slide the splint into position under the patient's injured limb, making certain that the ring is seated well on the ischial tuberosity (**Step 4**).

6. Pad the groin area, and gently apply the ischial strap (**Step 5**).

7. While your partner continues to maintain traction, connect the loops of the ankle hitch to the end of the splint. Then apply gentle traction to the connecting strap between the ankle hitch and the splint, just strongly enough to maintain limb alignment. Use caution. This splint comes with a ratchet mechanism to tighten the strap. Overtightening can theoretically overstretch the limb and further injure the patient. Adequate traction has been applied when the leg is the same length as the other leg and the patient feels relief (**Step 6**).

8. Once proper traction has been applied, fasten the support straps so that the limb is securely held in the splint. Check all proximal and distal support straps to make sure they are secure (**Step 7**).

9. At this point, reassess distal pulses and motor function and sensation.

10. Place the patient securely on a backboard or other stabilization device for transport to the ED. You may need to load the patient feetfirst into the ambulance so that you do not shut the door against the splint (**Step 8**).

Because the traction splint stabilizes the limb by producing countertraction on the ischium and in the groin, pad these areas well. Avoid excessive pressure on the external genitalia. Always use commercially available padded ankle hitches rather than pieces of rope, cord, or tape. Such improvised hitches can sometimes be painful and can potentially impair circulation in the foot.

The Sager splint is lightweight, is easy to store, and applies a measurable amount of traction. Unlike the Hare device, the Sager splint can be applied by a single rescuer when necessary. As with any splint, in addition to knowing the precise sequence of steps to apply the splint properly, you must practice the splinting technique frequently to remain competent. Follow the steps below to apply a Sager splint (**SKILL DRILL 32-6**):

1. Having taken standard precautions, expose the injured extremity. Assess distal motor, sensory, and circulatory function in the injured leg.

2. Position the splint against the medial aspect of the injured leg, with the perineal cushion resting against the ischial tuberosity. Note that the shorter, articulating end of the cushion should be oriented toward the ground (**Step 1**).

3. Slip the thigh strap behind the knee, then slide it up the thigh. Once in position, secure the thigh strap (**Step 2**).

4. As needed, raise the spring clip and extend the inner metal shaft so that the crossbar is positioned adjacent to the heel. *Note that in contrast to the Hare device, the Sager splint does not require a preapplication measurement that extends the distal end of the device a certain distance beyond the foot.*

5. Apply the padded ankle harness just above the malleoli (ankle).

6. Pull the cable ring snugly up against the bottom of the foot, and attach the harness to the crossbar (**Step 3**).

7. Grasp the padded outer shaft with one hand while using the other to pull the handle of the inner shaft until the appropriate amount of traction is achieved: approximately 10% of the patient's body weight, up to a maximum of 15 pounds (7 kg) (**Step 4**).

8. Slip the elastic cravats under the leg (behind the knee), slide them to their proper positions, and secure the device to the leg (**Step 5**).

9. Make sure to use the pedal pinion strap to secure the feet together to prevent rotation of the injured leg. This component is often neglected.

10. Move the patient to the stretcher.

11. Assess distal motor, sensory, and circulatory function in the injured leg (**Step 6**).

## Skill Drill 32-6 Applying a Sager Traction Splint

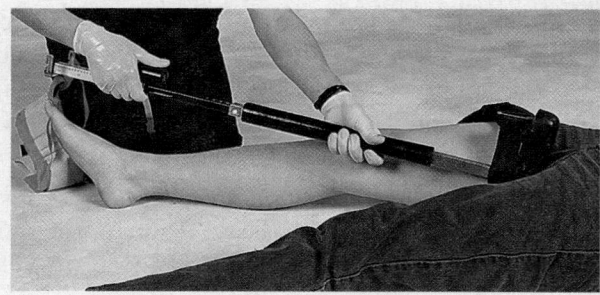

### Step 1

After exposing the injured area, assess distal motor, sensory, and circulatory function. Position the splint against the medial aspect of the injured leg, with the perineal cushion resting against the ischial tuberosity. Adjust the thigh strap so that it lies anteriorly when secured.

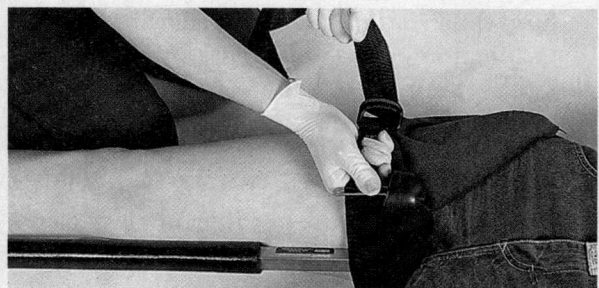

### Step 2

Secure the thigh strap.

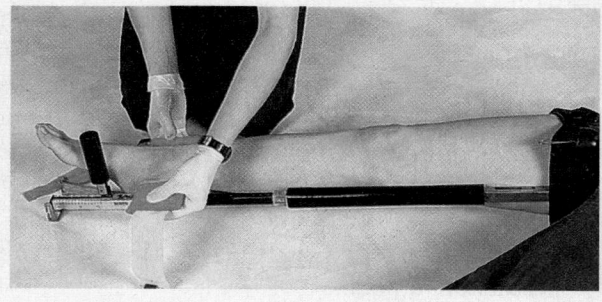

### Step 3

Apply the padded ankle harness just above the ankle. Attach the harness to the crossbar.

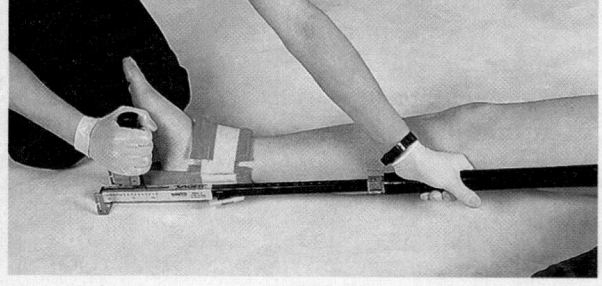

### Step 4

Extend the splint's inner shaft to apply traction of about 10% of body weight, up to a maximum of 15 pounds (7 kg).

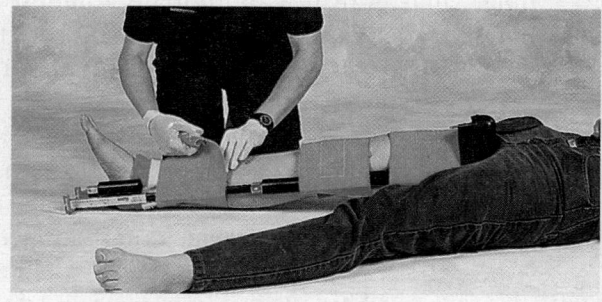

### Step 5

Secure the splint with elasticized cravat bandages.

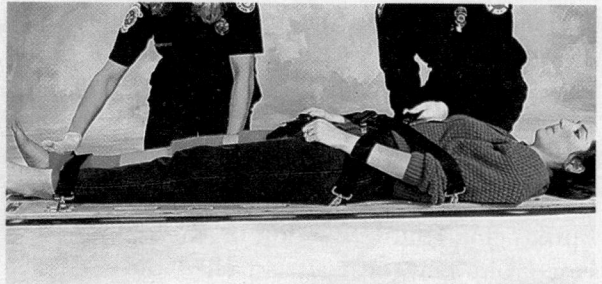

### Step 6

Secure the patient to a backboard. With a figure of eight configuration, use the pedal pinion strap to secure the feet together. Reassess distal motor, sensory, and circulatory function.

## Injuries of Knee Ligaments

The knee is very vulnerable to injury; therefore, many different types of injuries occur in this region. Ligament injuries, for example, range from mild sprains to complete dislocation of the joint. The patella can also dislocate. In addition, all the bony elements of the knee (distal femur, upper tibia, and patella) can fracture.

The knee is especially susceptible to ligament injuries, which occur when abnormal bending or twisting forces are applied to the joint. Such injuries are often seen in both recreational and competitive athletes. The ligaments on the medial side of the knee are most frequently injured, typically when the foot is fixed to the ground and the lateral aspect of the knee is struck by a heavy object, such as when a football player is tackled from the side.

Usually, a patient with a knee ligament injury will report pain in the joint and be unable to use the extremity normally. When you examine the patient, you will generally find swelling, occasional ecchymosis, point tenderness at the injury site, and a joint effusion (excess fluid in the joint).

Splint all suspected knee ligament injuries. The splint should extend from the hip joint to the foot, stabilizing the bone above the injured joint (the femur) and the bone below it (the tibia). A variety of splints can be used, including a padded rigid long leg splint or two padded board splints securely applied to the medial and lateral aspects of the limb. A backboard, a pillow splint, or simply binding the injured limb to its uninjured mate is an acceptable—but less effective—splinting technique. The patient will usually be able to straighten the knee to allow you to apply the splint. However, if you encounter resistance or pain when trying to straighten the knee, splint it in the flexed position. Then continue to monitor the distal neurovascular function until the patient reaches the hospital.

## Dislocation of the Knee

Dislocations of the knee are true emergencies that may be associated with vascular occlusion or injury that may threaten the limb. When the knee is dislocated, the ligaments that provide support to it may be damaged or torn. When this happens, the proximal end of the tibia completely displaces from its juncture with the lower end of the femur, usually producing a significant deformity. Although substantial ligament damage always occurs with a knee dislocation, the more urgent injury is often to the popliteal artery, which is frequently lacerated or compressed by the tibia, which typically displaces posteriorly. When gross deformity, severe pain, and an inability to move the joint cause you to suspect a dislocation of the knee, always check the distal circulation carefully before taking any other step. If the distal pulses are absent, contact medical control immediately for further stabilization and transport instructions.

The direction of dislocation refers to the position of the tibia with respect to the femur. Posterior knee dislocations, which result from extreme hyperextension of the knee, are the most common, occurring in almost one-half of all cases. Commonly, the anterior and posterior cruciate ligaments are damaged, but there is also a high risk of injury to the popliteal artery.

Medial dislocations result from a direct blow to the lateral part of the leg. Because the deforming force causes the medial aspect of the knee to stretch apart, there is a high likelihood of injury to the medial ligaments. When the force is applied from the medial direction, a lateral dislocation occurs and the lateral part of the knee is stretched apart, injuring the lateral ligament. Lateral and medial dislocations happen far less commonly and are less likely to injure the popliteal artery.

Patients with a knee dislocation will typically report pain in the knee and report that the knee "gave out." If the knee did not spontaneously reduce, there may be evidence of significant deformity and decreased range of motion. Complications may include limb-threatening popliteal artery disruption, injuries to the nerves, and joint instability. Do not confuse this injury with a relatively minor patella dislocation, discussed later.

If adequate distal pulses are present, splint the knee in the position in which you found it, and transport the patient promptly. Do not attempt to manipulate or straighten any severe knee injury if there are good distal pulses. If the limb is straight, apply standard rigid long leg splints to at least two sides of the limb to stabilize it (**FIGURE 32-47A**). If the knee is bent and the foot has a good pulse, splint the joint in the bent position, using parallel padded board splints secured at the hip and ankle joint to provide a stable A-frame (**FIGURE 32-47B**). Secure the limb to a backboard or stretcher with pillows and straps to eliminate any motion during transport.

On rare occasions, and depending on local protocol in the context of a very prolonged

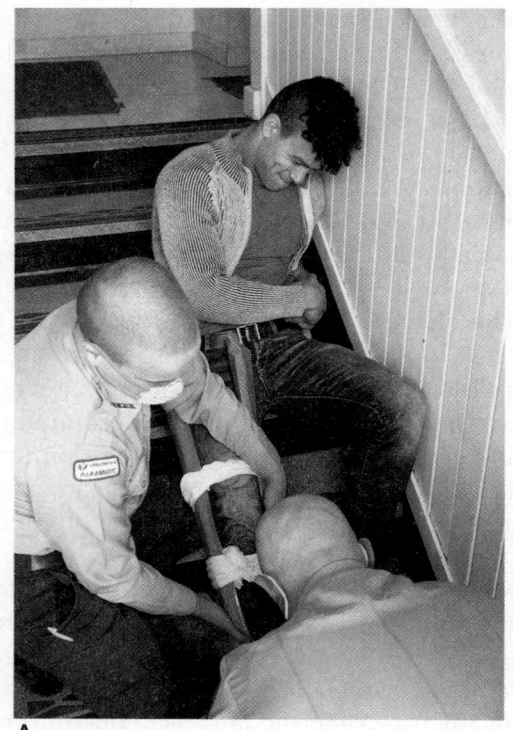

**A**

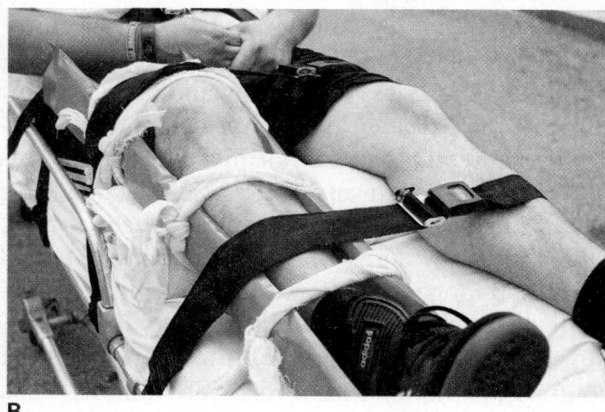

**B**

**FIGURE 32-47 A.** When the injured knee is straight, apply padded board splints extending from the hip to the ankle. **B.** If the knee is flexed and the foot has good pulses, apply padded board splints with the knee in the flexed position.

A, B: © Jones & Bartlett Learning.

anticipated transport time to the hospital, medical control may instruct you to attempt to realign a deformed, pulseless limb to reduce compression of the popliteal artery and, thus, restore distal circulation. Only make one attempt to do this. First, straighten the limb by applying gentle longitudinal traction in the axis of the limb. Once you apply manual traction, maintain it until the limb is fully

splinted; otherwise, the limb might return to its deformed position. If traction significantly increases the patient's pain, do not continue. As you apply traction, monitor the posterior tibial pulse to see whether it returns. Splint the limb in the position in which you feel the strongest pulse. If you are unable to restore the distal pulse, splint the limb in the position that is most comfortable for the patient, and then provide prompt transport to the hospital. Notify medical control of the status of the distal pulse so that treatment can be arranged in advance.

## Fractures About the Knee

Fractures about the knee may occur at the distal end of the femur, at the proximal end of the tibia, or in the patella. Because of local tenderness and swelling, it is easy to confuse a nondisplaced or minimally displaced fracture about the knee with a ligament injury. Likewise, a displaced fracture about the knee may produce significant deformity that makes it look like a dislocation. Manage these two types of injuries as follows:

- If there is an adequate distal pulse and no significant deformity, splint the limb with the knee straight.
- If there is an adequate pulse and significant deformity, splint the joint in the position of deformity.
- If the pulse is absent below the level of the injury, suspect possible vascular damage, and contact medical control immediately for further instructions.
- Never use a traction splint if you suspect a fractured knee.

## Dislocation of the Patella

A dislocated patella most commonly occurs in teenagers and young adults who are engaged in athletic activities. Some patients have recurrent dislocations of the patella. As with recurrent dislocation of the shoulder, a minor twisting may be enough to produce the problem. Usually, the dislocated patella displaces to the lateral side. The displacement of the patella produces a significant deformity in which the knee is held in a moderately flexed position, and the patella is displaced to the lateral side of the knee (**FIGURE 32-48**).

Splint the knee in the position in which you found it; most often, this is with the knee flexed to

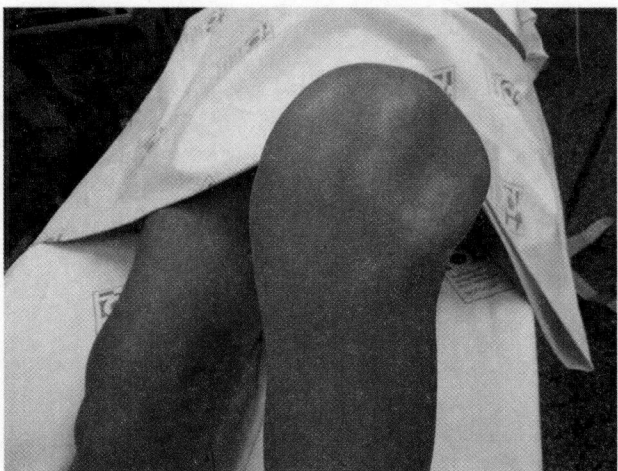

**FIGURE 32-48** Usually, the dislocated patella displaces to the lateral side, and the knee is held in a partially flexed position.

a moderate degree. To stabilize the knee, apply padded board splints to the medial and lateral aspects of the joint, extending from the hip to the ankle. Use pillows to support the limb on the stretcher.

Occasionally, as you apply the splint, the patella will return to its normal position spontaneously. If this occurs, stabilize the limb as for a knee ligament injury in a padded long leg splint, and transport the patient to the ED. Report the spontaneous reduction as soon as you arrive at the hospital so that the medical staff is aware of the severity of the injury.

## Injuries of the Tibia and Fibula

Fracture of the shaft of the tibia or the fibula may occur at any place between the knee joint and the ankle joint. Often both bones fracture at the same time. Even a single fracture may result in severe deformity, with significant angulation or rotation. Because the tibia is located just beneath the skin, open fractures of this bone are relatively common (**FIGURE 32-49**).

Fractures of the tibia and fibula should be stabilized with a padded rigid long leg splint or an air splint that extends from the foot to the upper thigh. Once splinted, the affected leg should be secured to the opposite leg. Traction splints are not indicated for isolated tibial fractures. As with most other fractures of the shaft of long bones, you should correct severe deformity before splinting by applying

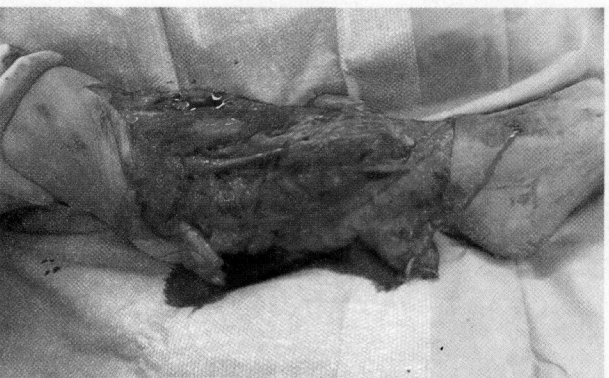

**FIGURE 32-49** Because the tibia is so close to the skin, open fractures are relatively common.

gentle longitudinal traction. The goal is to restore a position that will take a standard splint; it is not necessary to replace the fracture fragments in their anatomic position.

Fractures of the tibia and fibula are sometimes associated with vascular injury as a result of the distorted position of the limb following injury. Realigning the limb frequently restores an adequate blood supply to the foot. If it does not, transport the patient promptly and notify medical control while you are en route.

## Ankle Injuries

The ankle is a commonly injured joint. Ankle injuries occur in people of all ages and range in severity from a simple sprain, which heals after a few days of rest, to severe fracture-dislocations that lead to permanent disability. As with other joints, it is sometimes difficult to tell a nondisplaced ankle fracture from a simple sprain without radiograph examination (**FIGURE 32-50**). Therefore, any ankle injury that produces pain, swelling, localized tenderness, or the inability to bear weight must be evaluated by a physician. The most frequent mechanism of ankle injury is twisting, which stretches or tears the supporting ligaments. A more extensive twisting force may result in fracture of one or both malleoli. Dislocation of the ankle is usually associated with fractures of one or both malleoli.

You can manage the wide spectrum of injuries to the ankle in the same way, as follows:

1. Dress all open wounds.
2. Assess distal neurovascular function.

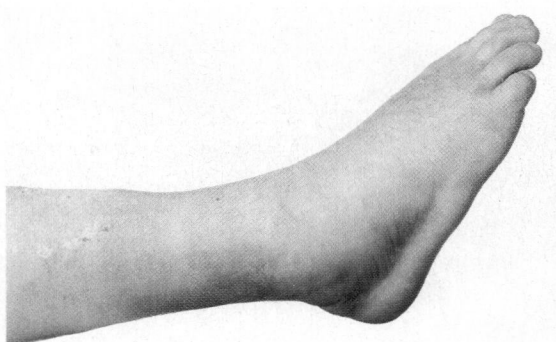

**FIGURE 32-50** Swelling about the ankle is characteristic of sprains and fractures.

© rob_lan/iStockphoto.

3. Correct any gross deformity by applying gentle longitudinal traction to the heel.
4. Before releasing traction, apply a splint.

You can use a padded rigid splint, an air splint, or a pillow splint. Make sure it includes the entire foot and extends up the leg to the level of the knee joint.

## Foot Injuries

Injuries to the foot can result in the dislocation or fracture of one or more of the tarsals, metatarsals, or phalanges of the toes. Toe fractures are especially common.

Of the tarsal bones, the calcaneus, or heel bone, is the most frequently fractured. Injury often occurs when the patient falls or jumps from a height and lands directly on the heel. The force of injury compresses the calcaneus, producing immediate swelling and ecchymosis. If the force of impact is great enough, as from a fall from a roof or tree, there may also be other fractures.

Occasionally, the force of injury is transmitted up the legs to the spine, producing a fracture of the lumbar spine (**FIGURE 32-51**). When a patient who has jumped or fallen from a height reports heel pain, ask him or her about back pain and carefully check the spine for tenderness and deformity.

If you suspect that the foot is dislocated, carefully remove the shoe and immediately assess for pulses and motor and sensory functions. Stabilize the extremity using a commercially available splint or a pillow splint, leaving the toes exposed so that you can periodically assess neurovascular function.

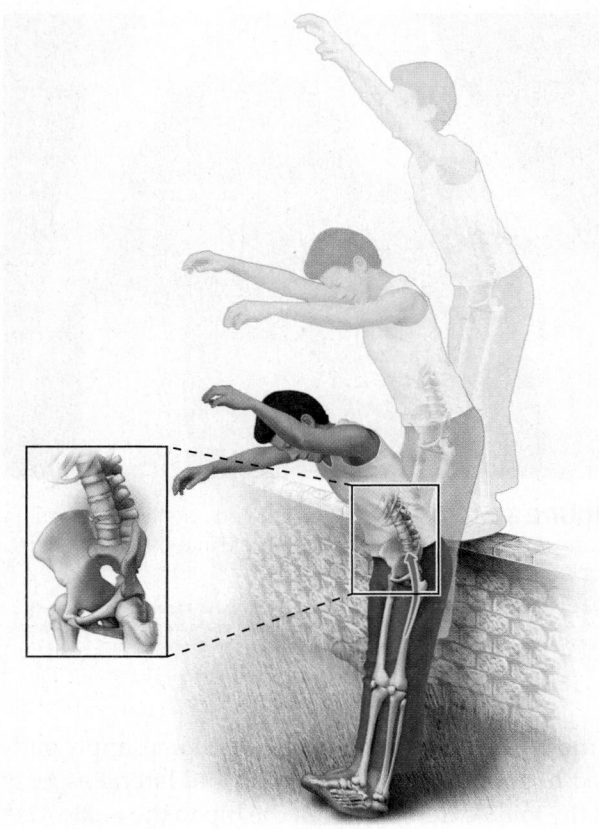

**FIGURE 32-51** After a fall, the force of injury is transmitted up the legs to the spine, sometimes resulting in a fracture of the lumbar spine.

© Jones & Bartlett Learning.

Contact medical control and inform them if pulses are absent.

Injuries of the foot are associated with significant swelling but rarely with gross deformity. Vascular injuries are uncommon. As in the hand, lacerations about the ankle and foot may damage important underlying nerves and tendons. Puncture wounds of the foot are common and may cause serious infection if not treated early. All of these injuries must be evaluated and treated by a physician.

To splint the foot, apply a rigid padded board splint, an air splint, or a pillow splint, stabilizing the ankle joint and the foot (**FIGURE 32-52**). Leave the toes exposed so that you can periodically assess neurovascular function.

When the patient is lying on the stretcher, elevate the foot approximately 6 inches (15 cm) to minimize swelling. All patients with lower extremity injuries should be transported in the supine position to allow for elevation of the limb. Never allow

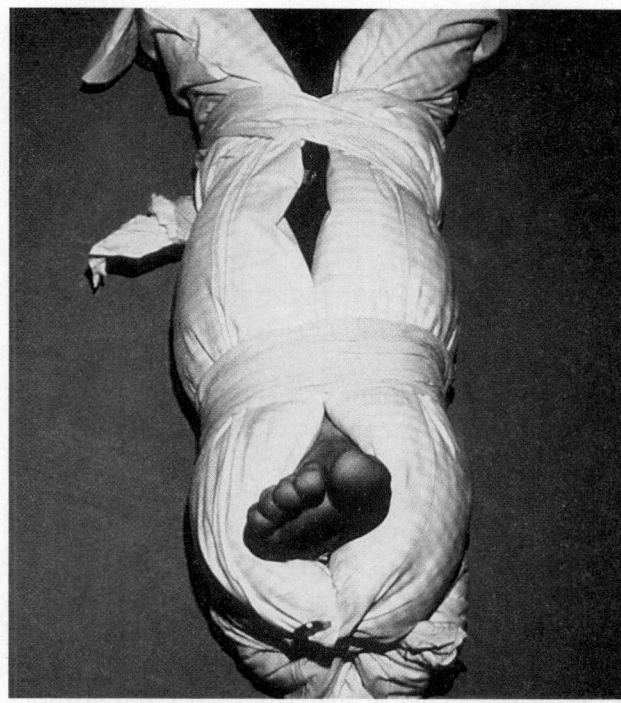

**FIGURE 32-52** A pillow splint provides excellent stabilization of the foot.

© American Academy of Orthopaedic Surgeons.

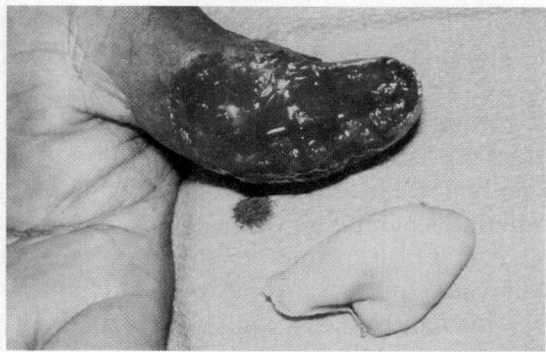

**FIGURE 32-53** Amputated parts can occasionally be reattached, so make every attempt to find the part and transport it to the emergency department along with the patient.

© American Academy of Orthopaedic Surgeons.

the foot and leg to dangle off the stretcher onto the floor or ground.

If a patient has fallen from a height and reports heel pain, use a backboard to immobilize any suspected spinal injury in addition to splinting the foot.

## Sprains and Strains

Because it may be difficult to differentiate among the various types of injuries in the field, it is best to err on the side of caution and treat every severe sprain as if it is a fracture. Therefore, general treatment of sprains and strains is similar to that of fractures and includes RICES (Rest, Ice, Compression, Elevation, and Splinting; this treatment is described in Chapter 27, *Soft-Tissue Injuries*). In addition, reduce or protect the limb from weight-bearing activity. Manage pain as soon as is practical.

## Amputations

You must control bleeding and treat for shock when dealing with traumatic amputations. Complete traumatic amputations may occasionally not bleed much if the cut vessels go into spasm, reducing blood loss.

Currently, surgeons can occasionally reattach amputated parts (**FIGURE 32-53**). However, correct prehospital care of the amputated part is vital to successful reattachment. With partial amputations, make sure to stabilize the part with bulky compression dressings and a splint to prevent further injury. Do not sever any partial amputations; this may complicate later reattachment. Hemorrhage from complete or incomplete amputations can be severe and life threatening. Control any bleeding from the stump. If bleeding is severe, quickly apply a tourniquet.

With a complete amputation, make sure to wrap the clean part in a sterile dressing and place it in a plastic bag. Follow your local protocols regarding how to preserve amputated parts. In some areas, dry sterile dressings are recommended for wrapping amputated parts; in other areas, dressings moistened with sterile saline are recommended. Put the bag in a cool container filled with ice. Lay the wrapped part on a bed of ice; do not pack it in ice. The goal is to keep the part cool without allowing it to freeze or for frostbite to develop. The amputated part should be transported with the patient to the appropriate resource hospital. To prevent injury from direct contact with the ice, never lay the part directly on ice without wrapping it first.

## Compartment Syndrome

Muscles in the extremities are contained within the fascia, which divides the muscles into numerous compartments. Because fascia's ability to stretch or expand is limited, anything that increases pressure within the compartment, such as bleeding and swelling, has the potential to impede blood flow through the muscle inside. **Compartment syndrome** is a limb-threatening condition characterized by localized tissue swelling within a compartment. As blood flow decreases inside a muscle compartment, ischemia results and anaerobic metabolism compensates for the reduction in oxygen. This reduced oxygenation, in turn, damages and eventually kills the muscle cells. Definitive treatment occurs in the hospital, through a surgical procedure called a fasciotomy, which involves an incision through the skin and fascia that allows the swollen muscle to expand, thereby reducing pressure inside the compartment. However, because compartment syndrome can be overlooked, some patients do not receive surgical intervention soon enough. In these unfortunate cases, it may become necessary for the surgeon to amputate the extremity.

Compartment syndrome often develops within 6 to 12 hours after injury, usually as a result of excessive bleeding, a severely crushed extremity, or the rapid return of blood to an ischemic limb. Early signs and symptoms of compartment syndrome include pain that is out of proportion to the injury, pain on passive stretch of muscles within the compartment, and altered sensation (abnormal, reduced, or absent). Additional signs may include pallor (pale skin) and decreased power (ranging from decreased strength and movement of the limb to complete paralysis).

Compartment syndrome can occur with or without an accompanying bone fracture. However, when a fracture is involved, the most commonly occurring fracture site is the tibia for adults, and the forearm in children. If you have a patient with a fracture below the elbow or the knee, be on the lookout for extreme pain; decreased sensation, tingling, or numbness; pain on stretching of affected muscles; and decreased power/paralysis. If you suspect that a patient has compartment syndrome, splint the affected limb, keeping it at the level of the heart (but not above), and provide immediate transport, reassessing neurovascular status frequently during transport.

Be aware that another potential cause of compartment syndrome is a splint that has been applied too tightly. Therefore, after splinting an injured extremity, if signs or symptoms of compartment syndrome appear during transport, try loosening knots or other potentially constricting elements of the splint. Then reassess frequently to determine whether the condition has improved or worsened. It may be easy to dismiss a patient telling you how badly his or her injured extremity hurts as being consistent with a diagnosis of an underlying fracture. Consider the potential for compartment syndrome with all extremity injuries.

## YOU are the Provider SUMMARY

**1. Under which circumstances can orthopaedic injuries pose a threat to a patient's life?**

Sprains, strains, and dislocations are rarely life threatening. Dislocations and isolated closed fractures can cause neurovascular damage and permanent disability if not treated promptly, but typically do not pose a threat to life. However, multiple closed long bone fractures, which can cause severe internal bleeding if bone fragments lacerate major blood vessels, can result in hypovolemic shock and death. Open fractures and extremity amputations (excluding fingers and toes) can also result in hypovolemic shock due to severe external bleeding. Amputation of a leg or arm can quickly lead to exsanguination (bleeding to death) if bleeding is not controlled. Contamination of the wound could also lead to an infection of the underlying tissue, even affecting bone. This infection can lead to gangrene or sepsis.

Pelvic fractures are potentially life threatening because the pelvic cavity can accommodate a large volume of blood. Patients can die of pelvic fractures because hypovolemic shock occurs secondary to severe internal bleeding when a fractured bone fragment or dislocated bone lacerates or severs a major artery or vein or there is significant bleeding from fractured bone ends.

**2. Given the information you have, can you rule out a critical injury?**

No. As concise as the dispatch information can sometimes be, you will not know the extent of a patient's injury (or injuries) until you arrive at the scene and perform a patient assessment. In this case, all you know is that the patient is conscious and alert and breathing and has a possible leg fracture. Although the dispatch information infers that this is an isolated injury secondary to a soccer-related incident, keep an open mind and avoid the preconceived notion that the leg injury is the only injury.

When you approach any patient, regardless of the nature of the call, you must perform a primary assessment to detect and correct immediate threats to airway, breathing, and circulation. Avoid tunnel vision when assessing and treating patients with orthopaedic trauma. A fractured leg may be the most obvious injury; however, it may not be the only injury. Also, it may not be the most life-threatening injury.

**3. What initial treatment should you provide to this patient?**

Because the patient denies having any other injuries— for example, a neck injury, which may require spinal immobilization—your initial action, after taking standard precautions, should be to expose the injury site and perform manual stabilization. With an injury in the tibia-fibula area, you or your partner should manually stabilize above the ankle and below the knee. Manual stabilization will help minimize the potential for further injury by preventing movement of the leg.

After you expose and manually stabilize the injury site, assess the patient for obvious signs of injury, such as swelling, deformity, bruising, and open wounds. The absence of deformity does not rule out an underlying fracture, as the bone may be cracked without any displacement of the bone ends. Also, swelling often masks underlying deformity. Treat any extremity injury as though an underlying fracture is present and stabilize it appropriately.

**4. What are some indicators of a fractured bone?**

A fracture is defined as *any* break in the continuity of a bone and is classified as being open (overlying skin is not intact) or closed (overlying skin is intact). In many cases, the deformity is grossly obvious; in other cases, it is subtle. Signs of a fracture include deformity, point tenderness (pain on palpation directly over the injury), swelling, bruising, and crepitus.

**5. How should you proceed with your assessment of this patient's injury?**

This patient did not experience multisystem trauma or a significant MOI; therefore, a secondary assessment of the entire body is not indicated. Instead, focus on evaluating perfusion and sensory and motor functions distal to the injury. When you assess an extremity injury, remember the 6 Ps of musculoskeletal assessment: pain, paralysis, paresthesia, pulselessness, pallor, and pressure.

First, assess the patient's level of pain using a scale of 0 to 10. Next, assess perfusion. In some cases, a fractured bone end may compress or, in rare cases, sever a blood vessel, resulting in inadequate or absent perfusion distal to the fracture. Compare the color of the skin with that of the uninjured limb. If perfusion is adequate, the skin should be pink and warm. Although paleness, or a decrease in blood flow, can be difficult to detect in dark-skinned people, it may be observed by examining mucous membranes inside the inner lower eyelid and capillary refill. On general observation, the patient may appear ashen or gray. Palpate the dorsalis pedis pulse (on the top of the foot) and the posterior tibial pulse (on the posterior medial aspect of the ankle where the distal tibia ends). Pulses that are weak or absent in comparison with pulses in the uninjured limb also suggest compromised perfusion.

Next, use a blunt object, and stroke it up the bottom and sides of her foot. If she is unable to feel you touching her foot, you should suspect that a nerve has been compressed or otherwise injured by a fractured bone end. To test motor function, simply ask her to wiggle her toes; however, if this increases her pain, discontinue this part of the examination. Paresthesias (numbness or tingling) could indicate compromised perfusion and/or nerve injury. A feeling of pressure distal to the injury site could indicate elevated pressure within a fascial compartment due to internal bleeding; if this continues, it could result in compartment syndrome.

In addition to assessing perfusion and sensory and motor functions, assess the areas above and below the injury (the injury zone); in this case, the injury zone extends above her knee and below her ankle. Remember, her leg may be the most obvious injury, but it may not be the only injury.

**6. How should you treat an injured extremity in which distal perfusion is absent?**

In general, you should splint an orthopaedic injury in the position it was found, provided that distal perfusion is intact. In some cases, an injured extremity may be so severely angulated that gentle longitudinal traction may be required to splint the injury effectively, even if distal perfusion is adequate.

If your assessment reveals that perfusion distal to the injury is compromised or absent (ie, pallor, absent distal pulses, cold skin), apply gentle longitudinal traction to realign the limb until perfusion is restored. The goal is *not* to return the extremity to its normal anatomic position, but rather to restore distal circulation. In many cases, gentle realignment of the limb restores adequate perfusion; however, if one attempt (local protocol may dictate more than one attempt) at realignment is unsuccessful, splint the injury, transport the patient as soon as possible, and notify the receiving facility early.

**7. How should you splint this patient's injury?**

Prior to splinting any extremity injury, assess the patient's distal perfusion and sensory and motor functions. Fractures of the tibia and fibula can be stabilized with a padded rigid leg splint; an air splint; or a vacuum splint that stabilizes the joints above and below the fracture site. In this case, stabilize the knee and ankle. As with most other fractures of the shaft of long bones, correct any severe deformity before applying the splint by applying gentle longitudinal traction. Restore the deformed limb to a position that will accommodate a splint—not necessarily to its normal anatomic position. The affected leg, once splinted, should be secured to the opposite leg.

Immediately after the splint is secured in place, reassess distal perfusion and sensory and motor functions. If perfusion is found to be inadequate, the splint should be loosened or reapplied as necessary to restore this vital function.

**8. What are some methods for providing pain relief from orthopaedic trauma?**

Pain relief is an important aspect in the overall care of a patient with orthopaedic trauma. Pain increases anxiety, which only adds to the patient's problems.

After you apply the splint, which should be padded for comfort, elevate the injured extremity above the level of the heart. This will help reduce pain and swelling by encouraging blood to drain from the extremity.

Chemical cold packs wrapped with gauze or some other type of insulating material can be applied directly over the injury site. A cold stimulus applied to the skin constricts the blood vessels; this can help reduce swelling and pain.

Certain medications can be administered to the patient by a paramedic. In some cases, especially during a prolonged transport, it may be helpful to request ALS intervention.

**9. What is the most likely cause of the patient's complaint? What can you do to remedy the situation?**

On the basis of the patient's complaint of numbness and tingling and your findings of pallor and weak pedal pulses, you should suspect that you applied the splint too tightly and that it is now impairing distal circulation.

Simply loosen the splint if it was applied too tightly. If you used padded board splints and triangular bandages (cravats), loosen the cravats. If you applied an air splint, release some of the air from the

splint. If you applied a vacuum splint, gently attempt to spread the edges of the splint apart to the point at which the patient feels relief. If this is not possible and a prolonged transport time is anticipated, it would not be unreasonable to stop the ambulance and apply a different type of splint, provided that the patient's condition is stable. Regardless of the splint that you used, immediately reassess distal circulation after making any adjustments, and ask the patient whether the numbness and/or tingling has subsided. In most cases, these adjustments will lead to improvement.

**10. What factors increase the risk of complications following orthopaedic trauma?**

Orthopaedic injuries can lead to systemic complications. Do not focus all of your attention on the skeletal injury; after all, there is a patient attached to the injured extremity! The risk of complications following orthopaedic trauma is increased by a variety of factors, such as the amount of force that caused the injury, the injury location, and the patient's overall health. Injuries in patients who smoke cigarettes or who have diabetes, for example, tend to heal poorly and complications are more common.

Any fracture—open or closed—is accompanied by a risk of bleeding. In general, the severity of bleeding is directly related to the force that caused the injury. A significant loss of tissue may occur at the fracture site if the muscle is severely damaged or if the bone's penetration of the skin causes a large wound.

Infection is another potential complication, especially in patients with open fractures or patients with other medical problems such as cigarette smoking or diabetes. To prevent contaminating an open fracture, and to minimize the risk of infection, brush away any obvious debris on the skin surrounding the fracture before covering it with a sterile dressing. Do not probe into an open fracture to retrieve debris.

Long-term disability is one of the most devastating complications of orthopaedic trauma. In many cases, a severely injured limb can be successfully repaired; however, many patients may not be able to work for long periods because of severe, chronic pain and the extensive rehabilitation that is often required.

As an EMT, you can help reduce the risk of complications, thus reducing the risk or duration of long-term disability following orthopaedic trauma, by preventing further injury, properly splinting orthopaedic injuries, reducing the risk of wound infection, and transporting patients to an appropriate medical facility.

# YOU are the Provider SUMMARY *continued*

## EMS Patient Care Report (PCR)

| Date: 12-23-20 | Incident No.: 012909 | Nature of Call: Leg injury | | Location: 404 Field Drive | |
|---|---|---|---|---|---|
| Dispatched: 1620 | En Route: 1620 | At Scene: 1625 | Transport: 1644 | At Hospital: 1656 | In Service: 1707 |

### Patient Information

| | |
|---|---|
| **Age:** 21 <br> **Sex:** F <br> **Weight (in kg [lb]):** 50 kg (110 lb) | **Allergies:** Codeine <br> **Medications:** Birth control pills <br> **Past Medical History:** None <br> **Chief Complaint:** Left leg pain |

### Vital Signs

| Time: 1630 | BP: 130/78 | Pulse: 112 | Respirations: 22 | Spo$_2$: 98% |
|---|---|---|---|---|
| Time: 1638 | BP: 134/80 | Pulse: 110 | Respirations: 22 | Spo$_2$: 99% |
| Time: 1648 | BP: 128/76 | Pulse: 115 | Respirations: 20 | Spo$_2$: 98% |

### EMS Treatment (circle all that apply)

| Oxygen @ ___ L/min via: <br><br> NC   NRM   Bag mask | | Assisted Ventilation | Airway Adjunct | CPR |
|---|---|---|---|---|
| Defibrillation | Bleeding Control | Bandaging | (Splinting) | **Other:** (Cold pack; elevated injured leg) |

### Narrative

Medic 8 dispatched to a soccer field for a patient with a "possible broken leg."

Chief Complaint: Left leg pain

History: The patient denies any other injuries; she further denies any past medical history.

Assessment: Arrived on scene and found the patient, a 21-year-old woman, sitting on the ground with her left leg extended and covered with an ice pack. She was conscious and alert; her airway was patent, and her breathing was adequate. Patient states that she injured her left leg when another player fell against it during the game. Assessment of her leg revealed obvious deformity to the midshaft tibial area. Patient describes pain severity as a "9" on a 0 to 10 scale. No open injuries were noted. Pulse and sensory and motor functions were grossly intact distal to the injury. A nurse was present at the scene and assisted EMS by manually stabilizing the injury site. Secondary assessment was performed and revealed no gross evidence of injury to the areas above her knee and below her ankle on the injured extremity. Her right lower extremity was also normal. Vital signs were obtained and noted above.

Treatment (Rx): Splinted injured extremity with padded board splints; pulse and sensory and motor functions were assessed after splinting and were found to be grossly intact.

Transport: Secured patient onto stretcher, elevated her left leg with pillows, loaded her into the ambulance, and began transport. Applied cold pack to injury site for pain relief. Patient stated that elevation of her leg and the cold pack reduced her pain to a 5/10. Monitored patient's vital signs en route and noted that they remained stable. Patient began reporting paresthesia to her left foot during transport. Reassessment of area distal to the injury revealed that her foot was cool and pale and her pedal pulse was weaker than before. Loosened bandages that were securing splints in place, after which patient stated that the paresthesia resolved; her foot regained a pink color and became warm, and her pedal pulse was stronger following this intervention. Remainder of transport was uneventful. Delivered patient to emergency department and gave verbal report to staff nurse. Medic 8 cleared the hospital and returned to service at 1707.

**End of report**

# Prep Kit

## Ready for Review

- Skeletal or voluntary muscle attaches to bone and forms the major muscle mass of the body. This muscle contains veins, arteries, and nerves.
- There are approximately 206 bones in the human body. When this living tissue is fractured, it can produce bleeding and significant pain.
- A joint is a junction where two bones come into contact. Joints are stabilized in key areas by ligaments.
- A fracture is a broken bone, a dislocation is a disruption of a joint, a sprain is a stretching injury to the ligaments around a joint, and a strain is a stretching of the muscle.
- Depending on the amount of kinetic energy absorbed by tissues, the zone of injury may extend beyond the point of contact. Always maintain a high index of suspicion for associated injuries.
- Fractures of the bones are classified as open or closed. Both are splinted in a similar manner, but remember to control bleeding and apply a sterile dressing to the open extremity injury before splinting.
- Fractures and dislocations are often difficult to diagnose without a radiograph examination.

You will treat these injuries similarly. Stabilize the injury with a splint and transport the patient.
- Signs of fractures and dislocations include pain, deformity, point tenderness, false motion, crepitus, swelling, and bruising.
- Signs of sprains include bruising, swelling, and an unstable joint.
- Compare the unaffected extremity with the injured extremity whenever possible.
- The main types of splints used by EMTs are rigid splints, traction splints, formable splints, and pelvic binders.
- Remember to splint the injured extremity from the joint above to the joint below the injury site for complete stabilization.
- A sling and swathe are commonly used to treat shoulder dislocations and to secure injured upper extremities to the body. Lower extremities can be secured to the unaffected limb or to a backboard.
- The most common life-threatening musculoskeletal injuries are multiple fractures, open fractures with arterial bleeding, pelvic fractures, bilateral femur fractures, and limb amputations.

## Vital Vocabulary

**acromioclavicular (AC) joint** A simple joint where the bony projections of the scapula and the clavicle meet at the top of the shoulder.

**amputation** An injury in which part of the body is completely severed.

**articular cartilage** A pearly white layer of specialized cartilage covering the articular surfaces (contact surfaces on the ends) of bones in synovial joints.

**calcaneus** The heel bone.

**closed fracture** Any break in a bone in which the overlying skin is not broken.

**compartment syndrome** Swelling in a confined space that produces dangerous pressure; may cut off blood flow or damage sensitive tissue.

**crepitus** A grating or grinding sensation or sound caused by fractured bone ends or joints rubbing together.

**dislocation** Disruption of a joint in which ligaments are damaged and the bone ends are no longer in contact.

**displaced fracture** A fracture in which bone fragments are separated from one another, producing deformity in the limb.

**ecchymosis** Bruising or discoloration associated with bleeding within or under the skin.

**false motion** Movement that occurs in a bone at a point where there is no joint, indicating a fracture; also called free movement.

**fascia** The fiberlike connective tissue that covers arteries, veins, tendons, and ligaments.

**fibula** The outer and smaller bone of the two bones of the lower leg.

**fracture** A break in the continuity of a bone.

**glenoid fossa** The part of the scapula that joins with the humeral head to form the glenohumeral joint.

**hematuria** Blood in the urine.

**joint** The place where two bones come into contact.

**ligaments** Bands of fibrous tissue that connect bones to bones. Ligaments support and strengthen a joint.

**nondisplaced fracture** A simple crack in the bone that has not caused the bone to move from its normal anatomic position; also called a hairline fracture.

**open fracture** Any break in a bone in which the overlying skin has been broken.

**pelvic binder** A device to splint the bony pelvis to reduce hemorrhage from bone ends, venous disruption, and pain.

**point tenderness** Tenderness that is sharply localized at the site of the injury, found by gently palpating along the bone with the tip of one finger.

**position of function** A hand position in which the wrist is slightly dorsiflexed and all finger joints are moderately flexed.

**reduce** To return a dislocated joint or fractured bone to its normal position; to set.

**retroperitoneal space** The space between the abdominal cavity and the posterior abdominal wall, containing the kidneys, certain large vessels, and parts of the gastrointestinal tract.

**sciatic nerve** The major nerve to the lower extremities; controls much of muscle function in the leg and sensation in most of the leg and foot.

**sling** A bandage or material that helps to support the weight of an injured upper extremity.

**splint** A flexible or rigid device used to protect and maintain the position of an injured extremity.

**sprain** A joint injury involving damage to supporting ligaments, and sometimes partial or temporary dislocation of bone ends.

**strain** Stretching or tearing of a muscle; also called a muscle pull.

**swathe** A bandage that passes around the chest to secure an injured arm to the chest.

**tibia** The shinbone; the larger of the two bones of the lower leg.

**tourniquet** The bleeding control method used when a wound continues to bleed despite the use of direct pressure; useful if a patient is bleeding severely from a partial or complete amputation.

**traction** Longitudinal force applied to a structure.

**zone of injury** The area of potentially damaged soft tissue, adjacent nerves, and blood vessels surrounding an injury to a bone or a joint.

# References

1. Emergency Medical Technician Psychomotor Examination. National Registry of Emergency Medical Technicians, Inc. website. https://www.nremt.org/nremt/about/psychomotor_exam_emt.asp. Accessed June 18, 2014.

2. *National Emergency Medical Services Education Standards*. US Department of Transportation. National Highway Traffic Safety Administration. DOT HS 811 077A. January 2009. www.ems.gov/pdf/811077a.pdf. Accessed June 14, 2014.

3. *National Emergency Medical Services Education Standards. Emergency Medical Technician Instructional Guidelines*. US Department of Transportation. National Highway Traffic Safety Administration. DOT HS 811

077C. January 2009. www.ems.gov/pdf/811077a.pdf. Accessed June 14, 2014.

4. *National Model EMS Clinical Guidelines*. National Association of State EMS Officials website. https://www.nasemso.org/Projects/ModelEMSClinicalGuidelines/index.asp. Published 2016. Accessed October 23, 2014.

5. National Registry of Emergency Medical Technicians. *2015 Paramedic Psychomotor Competency Portfolio (PPCP)*. Columbus, OH: National Registry of Emergency Medical Technicians, Inc.; 2015.

6. Soles GL, Tornetta P 3rd. Multiple trauma in the elderly: new management perspective. *J Orthop Trauma* 2011;25(Suppl 2):S61–S65.

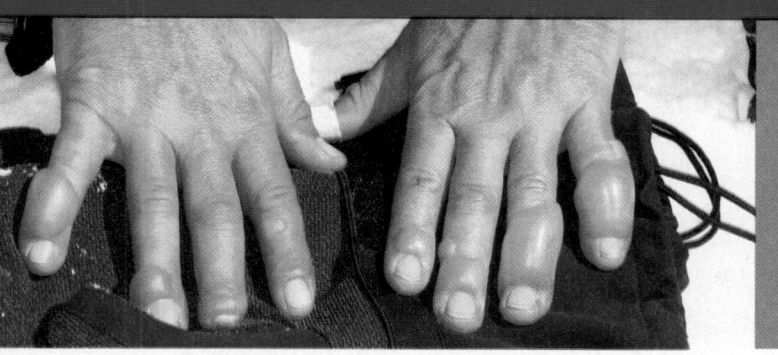

# Chapter 33

# Environmental Emergencies

## NATIONAL EMS EDUCATION STANDARD COMPETENCIES

### Trauma
Applies fundamental knowledge to provide basic emergency care and transportation based on assessment findings for an acutely injured patient.

### Environmental Emergencies
Recognition and management of
- Submersion incidents (pp 1218–1220, 1225–1226)
- Temperature-related illness (pp 1202–1206, 1209–1213, 1215–1217)

Pathophysiology, assessment, and management of
- Near drowning (pp 1218–1220, 1223–1225)
- Temperature-related illness (pp 1202–1217)
- Bites and envenomation (pp 1228–1235)
- Dysbarism (p 1226)
  - High altitude (pp 1226–1227)
  - Diving injuries (pp 1220–1223)
- Electrical injury (p 1227)
- Radiation exposure (Chapter 41, *Terrorism Response and Disaster Management*)

## KNOWLEDGE OBJECTIVES

1. Identify the four factors that affect how a person deals with exposure to a cold or hot environment. (pp 1201–1202)
2. Describe the five ways heat loss occurs in the body, and how the rate and amount of heat loss or gain can be modified in an emergency situation. (pp 1202–1203)
3. Describe the four general stages of hypothermia. (pp 1203–1205)
4. Describe local cold injuries and their underlying causes. (pp 1205–1206)
5. Describe the process of providing emergency care to a patient who has sustained a cold injury, including assessment of the patient, review of signs and symptoms, and management of care. (pp 1209–1210)
6. Explain the importance of following local protocols when rewarming a patient who is experiencing moderate or severe hypothermia. (p 1209)
7. Describe the three emergencies that are caused by heat exposure, including their risk factors, signs, and symptoms. (pp 1211–1213)
8. Describe the process of providing emergency care to a patient who is experiencing a heat emergency, including assessment of the patient, review of signs and symptoms, and management of care. (pp 1213–1217)
9. Describe drowning, including its incidence, risk factors, and prevention. (pp 1218–1220)
10. List the basic rules of performing a water and ice rescue. (p 1219)
11. Explain why EMTs should have a prearranged rescue plan based on the environment in which they work. (p 1219)

12. List five conditions that may result in a spinal injury following a submersion incident and the steps for stabilizing a patient with a suspected spinal injury in the water. (pp 1218–1220)

13. Discuss recovery techniques and resuscitation efforts EMTs may need to follow when managing a patient who has been involved in a submersion incident. (p 1220)

14. Describe the three types of diving emergencies, how they may occur, and their signs and symptoms. (pp 1220–1222)

15. Describe the process of providing emergency care to a patient who has been involved in a drowning or diving emergency, including assessment of the patient, review of signs and symptoms, and management of care. (pp 1223–1226)

16. Discuss the types of dysbarism injuries, including their incidence, risk factors, signs and symptoms, and emergency medical treatment. (pp 1226–1227)

17. Discuss lightning injuries, including their incidence, risk factors, signs and symptoms, and emergency medical treatment. (pp 1227–1228)

18. Describe the process of providing emergency care to patients who have been bitten by each of the following venomous spiders: (pp 1228–1229)
    - Black widow spider
    - Brown recluse spider

19. Describe the process of providing emergency care to a patient who has sustained a bite or sting from each of the following insects and arachnids, including steps the EMT should follow if a patient develops a severe reaction to the sting or bite: (pp 1229–1230, 1233–1234)
    - Hymenoptera (bees, wasps, yellowjackets, and ants)
    - Scorpions
    - Ticks

20. Describe the process of providing emergency care to a patient who has been bitten by each of the following types of snake and is showing signs of envenomation: (pp 1231–1233)
    - Pit viper
    - Coral snake

21. Describe the process of providing emergency care to a patient who has been stung by a coelenterate or other marine animal. (p 1235)

## SKILLS OBJECTIVES

1. Demonstrate the emergency medical treatment of local cold injuries in the field. (p 1210)

2. Demonstrate how to use a warm-water bath to rewarm the limb of a patient who has sustained a local cold injury. (p 1210)

3. Demonstrate how to treat a patient with heat cramps. (p 1215)

4. Demonstrate how to treat a patient with heat exhaustion. (pp 1215–1217, Skill Drill 33-1)

5. Demonstrate how to treat a patient with heatstroke. (p 1217)

6. Demonstrate how to stabilize a patient with a suspected spinal injury in the water. (pp 1218–1221, Skill Drill 33-2)

7. Demonstrate how to care for a patient who is suspected of having an air embolism or decompression sickness following a drowning or diving emergency. (pp 1222–1223)

8. Demonstrate how to care for a patient who has been bitten by a pit viper and is showing signs of envenomation. (pp 1231–1232)

9. Demonstrate how to care for a patient who has been bitten by a coral snake and is showing signs of envenomation. (pp 1232–1233)

10. Demonstrate how to care for a patient who has sustained a coelenterate envenomation. (p 1235)

# Introduction

The human body functions best when all body systems operate in balance, a concept known as homeostasis. Environmental factors such as temperature and atmospheric pressure can overwhelm the body's ability to cope with its surroundings. A variety of medical emergencies can result, particularly in children, older people, people with chronic illnesses, and young adults who overexert themselves. These can lead to mental status changes, functional changes, and possible death. Environmental emergencies can occur in any setting and often accompany other illnesses and injuries that require treatment at the same time. For example, a trauma patient with hypothermia is at a higher risk of death than a patient with a normal body temperature. As an EMT, you can save lives by recognizing and responding properly to these emergencies, most of which require prompt treatment at the scene and in the hospital.

In this chapter you will learn how the body regulates core temperature, and the ways in which heat loss can occur. The various forms of heat-, cold-, and water-related emergencies are described, including how to diagnose and treat hypothermia, frostbite, and hyperthermia. You will also learn about pressure-related emergencies, or dysbarism injuries, caused by diving and high-altitude climbing; injuries caused by lightning; and envenomation, caused by bites and stings.

## Factors Affecting Exposure

The following four factors will affect how a person deals with a cold or hot environment. These can be used as prevention strategies for those who work or play in extreme environmental temperatures. Consider these factors during the assessment of your patient to determine whether he or she was prepared for a cold or hot environment. A hiker prepared for a warm summer hike in the foothills will present and respond to treatment differently than a traveler stranded in a hot vehicle because the radiator boiled over.

1. **Physical condition.** Patients who are ill or in poor physical condition will not be able to tolerate extreme temperatures as well as those whose cardiovascular, metabolic, and nervous systems are all functioning well. For example, an athlete in peak physical condition performs better and is less likely to experience injury or illness than someone with a less active lifestyle. Exertion also plays a role. For instance, a brisk walk will generate body heat when you are out in the cold but will also produce heat when it is not needed, such as walking on a hot asphalt road because your vehicle ran out of gasoline.

2. **Age.** Children and older adults are more likely to experience temperature-related illness. Infants have poor thermoregulation (the body's ability to maintain normal temperature) at birth and do not have the ability to shiver and generate heat when needed until about 12 to 18 months. An infant's surface area-to-mass ratio is larger than an adult's, so infants heat up and cool down faster. When you get cold, you put on a sweater; a small child may not think to do this or may have difficulty finding and putting one on. On the other end of the spectrum, older adults have a loss of subcutaneous tissues as they age, reducing the amount of insulation they have. Poor circulation also contributes to increased heat loss. This is why older people often wear extra layers of clothing. Medications can also affect an older person's body thermostat, putting him or her at increased risk for temperature-related emergencies. Finally, older patients are also at high risk for falls, and lying immobile on a hot or cold surface can rapidly lead to overexposure.

3. **Nutrition and hydration.** Your body needs calories for your metabolism to function. Staying well hydrated provides water as a catalyst for much of this metabolism. A lack of food or water will aggravate both hot and cold stress. Calories provide fuel to burn, creating heat during the cold, and water provides sweat for evaporation and removing heat. Alcohol use may increase fluid loss and place the patient at greater risk for temperature-related emergencies.

4. **Environmental conditions.** Factors such as air temperature, humidity level, and wind can complicate or improve environmental situations. A light breeze helps you stay cool when it is hot outside, but a cold wind when it is cold outside can be uncomfortable. Extremes in temperature and humidity are not needed to produce hot or cold injuries. Many hypothermia cases occur at temperatures between 30°F (–1°C) and 50°F (10°C). Most heatstroke cases occur when the temperature is above 80°F (26.7°C) and the humidity is 80% or higher. When evaluating your patient's condition, consider the environment and whether your patient is prepared for that situation. Older patients may turn the heat down in the winter or neglect to use air conditioning in the summer because of cost concerns. Some people may not open windows in a heat wave for fear of burglars. An understanding of the environmental conditions may help in your treatment decisions and give you an idea about how the patient will respond to your care.

## Cold Exposure

Normal body temperature is 98°F (36.7°C). Complicated regulatory mechanisms keep this internal temperature constant, regardless of the ambient temperature, the temperature of the surrounding environment. If the body, or any part of it, is exposed to cold environments, these mechanisms may be overwhelmed. Cold exposure may cause injury to individual parts of the body, such as the feet, hands, ears, or nose, or to the body as a whole.

Because heat always travels from a warmer place to a cooler place, body heat tends to move into the environment. Heat loss can occur in the following five ways:

- Conduction is the transfer of heat from a part of the body to a colder object or substance by direct contact, such as when a warm hand touches cold metal or ice, or is immersed in water with a temperature of less than 98°F (36.7°C). Heat can also be gained if the object or substance being touched is warm.
- Convection occurs when heat is transferred to circulating air, such as when cool air moves across the body surface. A person who stands

outside in windy, wintry weather and wears only lightweight clothing is mainly experiencing heat loss by convection. A person can gain heat if the air moving across the person's body is hotter than the temperature of the environment, such as in deserts or industrial settings like foundries, but it is more common to see rapid heat gain in spas and hot tubs where the water temperature may be well above body temperature.

- Evaporation is the conversion of any liquid to a gas, a process that requires energy, or heat. Evaporation is the natural mechanism by which sweating cools the body. This is why swimmers coming out of the water feel a sensation of cold as the water evaporates from their skin. People who exercise vigorously in a cool environment may sweat and feel warm at first, but later, as their sweat evaporates, they can become cold.
- Radiation is the transfer of heat by radiant energy. Radiant energy is a type of invisible light that transfers heat. Radiation causes heat loss, such as when a person stands in a cold room. Heat can also be gained by radiation—for example, when a person stands by a fire.
- Respiration causes body heat loss as warm air in the lungs is exhaled into the atmosphere and cooler air is inhaled. In warm climates, the air temperature can be well above body temperature, causing an individual to gain heat with each breath.

The rate and amount of heat loss or gain by the body can be modified in three ways:

1. **Increase or decrease heat production.** One way for the body to increase its heat production is to increase the rate of metabolism of its cells; the body can accomplish this through shivering (active movement of many muscles to generate heat). Also, people often have a natural urge to move around when they are cold. When a person is hot, he or she tends to reduce the level of activity, thus reducing heat production.

2. **Move to an area where heat loss is decreased or increased.** The most obvious way to decrease heat loss from radiation and convection is to move out of a cold environment and seek shelter from the wind. The same holds true for

a patient who is too hot. Simply moving the patient into the shade can reduce the ambient temperature by 10° or more. If you cannot move the patient, create shade and increase air movement by fanning the patient.

3. **Wear the appropriate clothing for the environment.** To avoid heat loss in cold environments, wear layers of clothing that provide good insulation, such as wool, down, and synthetic fabrics. Protective clothing traps perspiration and prevents evaporation, which prevents cooling. Keep the head, hands, and feet covered, and remove wet clothing if possible. To encourage heat loss in hot environments, wear lightweight, loose-fitting clothing, particularly around the head and neck.

## Hypothermia

When the entire body temperature falls, the condition is called hypothermia. Hypothermia means "low temperature." It is diagnosed when the core temperature of the body—the temperature of the heart, lungs, and vital organs—falls below 95°F (35°C). The body can usually tolerate a drop in core temperature of a few degrees. However, below this critical point, the body cannot regulate its temperature and generate body heat. Progressive loss of body heat then begins.

To protect itself against heat loss, the body normally constricts blood vessels in the skin; this results in the characteristic appearance of blue lips and/or fingertips. As a secondary precaution against heat loss, the body tends to create additional heat by shivering. As cold exposure worsens and these mechanisms are overwhelmed, many body functions begin to slow down and mental status deteriorates. Eventually, the functioning of key organs such as the heart begins to slow. Untreated, this can lead to death.

Hypothermia can develop either quickly, as when someone is immersed in cold water, or gradually, as when a person is exposed to the cold environment for several hours or more. Recall that the temperature does not have to be below freezing for hypothermia to occur. In winter, hypothermia at temperatures well above freezing may develop in people experiencing homelessness and those whose homes lack heat. Even in summer, swimmers who remain in the water for a long time are at risk of

hypothermia. Like all heat- and cold-related conditions, hypothermia is more common among young and old people and those with illness, who are less able to adjust to temperature extremes.

Patients with injuries or illness, such as burns, shock, head injury, stroke, generalized infection, injuries to the spinal cord, diabetes, and hypoglycemia, are more susceptible to hypothermia, as are patients who have taken certain drugs or consumed alcohol.

## Signs and Symptoms

Signs and symptoms of hypothermia generally become more severe as the core temperature falls. Hypothermia generally progresses through four stages, as shown in **TABLE 33-1**. Although there is no clear distinction among the stages, the different signs and symptoms of each will help you estimate the severity of the condition. When you assess a patient in the field, you should be able to distinguish between mild and severe hypothermia.

To assess the patient's core body temperature (CBT), pull back on your glove and place the back of your hand on the patient's skin at the abdomen (**FIGURE 33-1**). This area of the body is usually well protected and will give you a quick, general idea of the patient's core temperature. If the skin feels cool, the patient is likely experiencing a generalized cold emergency.

If you work in a cold environment, and/or depending on local protocols, you may carry a hypothermia thermometer, which registers lower core temperatures. It must be inserted in the rectum for an accurate reading. Regular thermometers will not register the temperature of a patient who has significant hypothermia.

Mild hypothermia occurs when the core temperature is greater than 93.2°F (34°C) but less than the normal 98°F (36.7°C). The patient is usually alert and shivering in an attempt to generate more heat through muscular activity. The patient may jump up and down and stamp his or her feet. Pulse rate and respirations are usually rapid. The skin in light-skinned people can be red, but may eventually appear pale, then cyanotic. People in a cold environment may have bluish lips or fingertips because of the body's constriction of blood vessels at the skin to retain heat.

Moderate hypothermia exists when the core temperature is 86°F to 93.2°F (30°C to 34°C). When

**TABLE 33-1** Characteristics of Systemic Hypothermia

| Extent of Hypothermia | Mild 93.2°F (34°C) | Moderate 93.2° to 86°F (34° to 30°C) | | Severe <86°F (30°C) |
|---|---|---|---|---|
| Core Temperature | 95° to 93°F (35° to 33.9°C) | 92° to 89°F (33.3° to 31.7°C) | 88° to 80°F (31.1° to 26.7°C) | <80°F (<26.7°C) |
| Signs and symptoms | Shivering, foot stamping | Loss of coordination, muscle stiffness | Coma | Apparent death |
| Cardiorespiratory response | Constricted blood vessels, rapid breathing | Slowing respirations, slow pulse | Weak pulse, dysrhythmias, very slow respirations | Cardiac arrest |
| Level of consciousness | Withdrawn | Confused, lethargic, sleepy | Unresponsive | Unresponsive |

© Jones & Bartlett Learning.

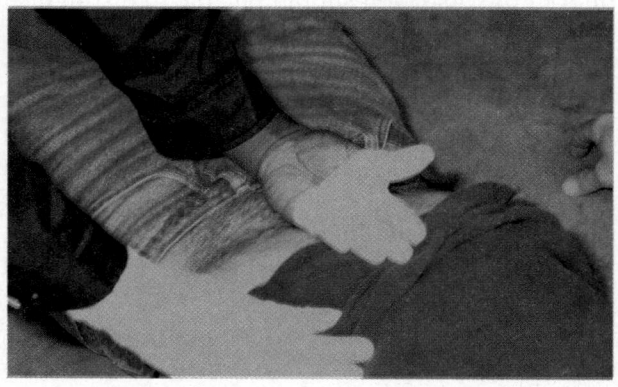

**FIGURE 33-1** To assess a patient's core body temperature, pull back your glove and place the back of your hand on the patient's skin at the abdomen.

© Jones & Bartlett Learning.

the core temperature is less than 90°F (32.2°C), shivering stops and muscular activity decreases. At first, small, fine muscle activity such as coordinated finger motion ceases. Eventually, as the temperature falls further, all muscle activity stops and mental status deteriorates.

Severe hypothermia is considered to be a core temperature of less than 86°F (30°C). As the core temperature drops toward 85°F (29.4°C), the patient becomes lethargic, and usually stops fighting the cold. The level of consciousness decreases, and the patient may try to remove his or her own clothes. Poor coordination and memory loss follow, along with reduced or complete loss of sensation to

touch, mood changes, and impaired judgment. The patient becomes less communicative, experiences joint or muscle stiffness, and has trouble speaking. The patient begins to appear stiff or rigid.

If the core temperature continues to fall to 80°F (26.7°C), vital signs slow; the pulse becomes slower and weaker, and respirations become shallow or absent. Cardiac dysrhythmias may occur as the blood pressure decreases.

At a core temperature of less than 80°F (26.7°C), all cardiorespiratory activity may cease, pupillary reaction is slow, and the patient may appear dead. However, *never assume that a cold, pulseless patient is dead.* Patients may survive severe hypothermia if proper emergency care is provided. It is critical that you perform an extended pulse check (up to a full minute). Assess at the carotid or femoral pulse. A patient in apparent cardiac arrest from

### Words of Wisdom

It is not uncommon for some people to become hypothermic and be unaware they are cold. This situation may occur when patients have consumed alcohol or drugs. For example, a fan at a college football game may consume alcohol, feel warm and remove his shirt, and become hypothermic. These patients may present with altered mental status. Don't assume this presentation is just the alcohol; consider hypothermia even if the patient reports not feeling cold.

hypothermia should not be considered dead until aggressive rewarming has been attempted, along with resuscitation. Remember the saying: "No one is dead unless they are *warm* and dead." It is important to note that patients who have died from a cause other than hypothermia will be cold to the touch; however, there will be additional, obvious signs of death such as rigor mortis. The "warm and dead" rule does not apply to such patients.

## Local Cold Injuries

Most injuries from cold are confined to exposed parts of the body. The extremities, particularly the feet and hands, and the ears, nose, and face are especially vulnerable to cold injury (**FIGURE 33-2**). When exposed parts of the body become very cold but not frozen, injuries such as frostnip and immersion foot (also called trench foot) can result. When the parts become frozen, the injury is called frostbite.

If possible, determine the duration of the exposure, the temperature to which the body part was exposed, and the wind velocity during exposure. These important factors will help you determine the severity of a local cold injury. You should also investigate these potential underlying factors:

- Exposure to wet conditions
- Inadequate insulation from cold or wind
- Restricted circulation from tight clothing or shoes or circulatory disease
- Fatigue
- Poor nutrition
- Alcohol or drug abuse
- Hypothermia
- Diabetes
- Cardiovascular disease
- Age

In hypothermia, blood is shunted away from the extremities to maintain the core temperature. This shunting of blood increases the risk of local cold injury to the extremities, ears, nose, and face. Thus, the patient with hypothermia should also be assessed for frostbite or other local cold injury. The reverse is also true. Remember, both local and systemic cold exposure injuries can occur in the same patient.

## Frostnip and Immersion Foot

After prolonged exposure to the cold, the skin may freeze whereas the deeper tissues are unaffected.

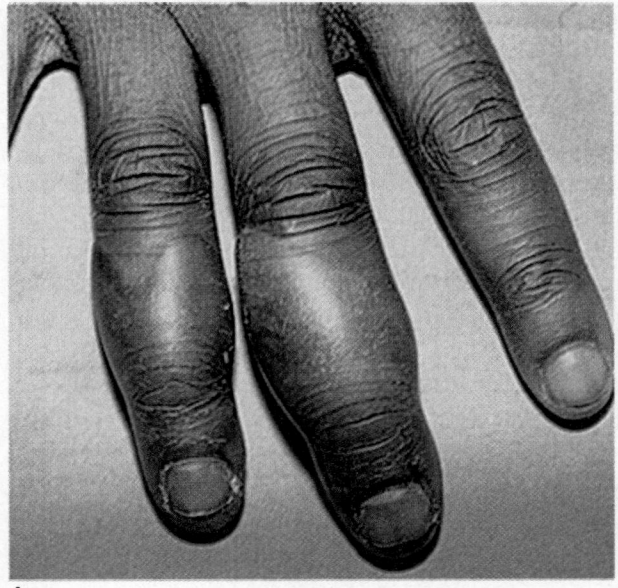

**A**

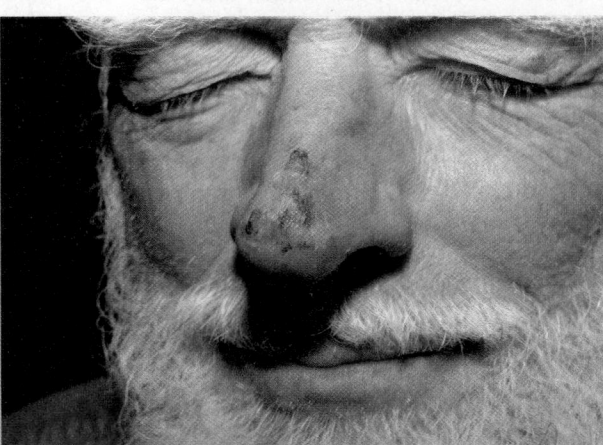

**B**

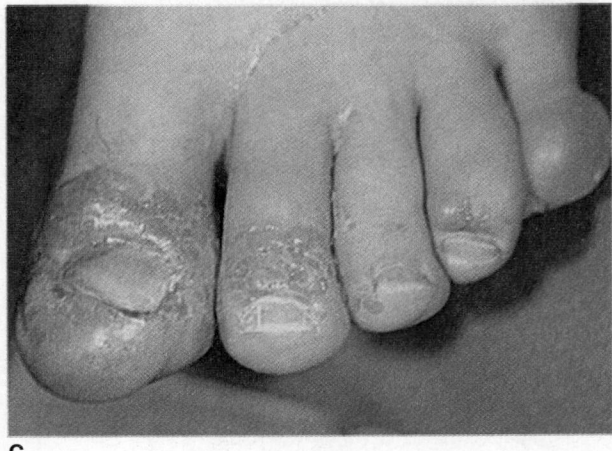

**C**

**FIGURE 33-2** The (**A**) hands, (**B**) nose, and (**C**) feet are particularly susceptible to frostbite.

A: Courtesy of Neil Malcom Winkelmann; B: © Dr. P. Marazzi/Science Source; C: © Charles Stewart MD, EMDM MPH.

This condition, which often affects the ears, nose, and fingers, is called frostnip. Because frostnip is usually painless, the patient often is unaware that a cold injury has occurred. Immersion foot occurs after prolonged exposure to cold water. It is particularly common in hikers or hunters who stand for a long time in a river or lake. With both frostnip and immersion foot, the skin is pale (blanched) and cold to the touch; normal color does not return after palpation of the skin. In some cases, the skin of the foot will be wrinkled, but it can also remain soft. The patient reports loss of feeling and sensation in the injured area.

## Frostbite

Frostbite is the most serious local cold injury because the tissues are actually frozen. Freezing permanently damages cells, although the exact mechanism by which damage occurs is unknown. The presence of ice crystals within the cells may cause physical damage. The change in the water content in the cells may also cause changes in the concentration of critical electrolytes, producing permanent changes in the chemistry of the cell. When the ice thaws, further chemical changes occur in the cell, causing permanent damage or cell death, called necrosis or gangrene (**FIGURE 33-3**). If gangrene occurs, the dead tissue may need to be surgically removed, sometimes by amputation. Following less severe damage, the exposed part will

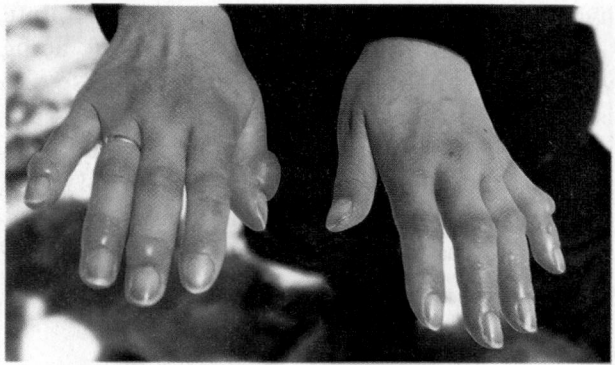

**FIGURE 33-4** Frostbitten parts are usually hard and waxy to the touch.
Courtesy of Neil Malcom Winkelmann.

become inflamed, tender to touch, and unable to tolerate exposure to cold.

Frostbite can be identified by the hard, waxy feel of the affected tissues (**FIGURE 33-4**). The injured part feels firm to frozen as you gently touch it. If the frostbite is only skin deep, it will feel leathery or thick instead of hard. Blisters and swelling may be present. In dark-skinned people, changes may be more subtle and harder to appreciate. Maintain a high index of suspicion for potential frostbite in these patients if the exposure to cold has been substantial and the tissues feel abnormal. In light-skinned people with a deep injury that has thawed or partially thawed, the skin may appear red or white, or it may be mottled and cyanotic (purple and blue).

As with a burn, the depth of skin damage will vary. With superficial frostbite, only the skin is frozen; with deep frostbite, the deeper tissues are frozen as well. You may not be able to tell superficial from deep frostbite in the field. Even an experienced surgeon in a hospital setting may not be able to tell for several days after exposure and injury.

## Assessment of Cold Injuries

Management of hypothermia in the field, regardless of the severity of the exposure, consists of stabilizing the ABCs and preventing further heat loss.

## Scene Size-up

Typically, your scene assessment begins with information provided by dispatch. Note environmental conditions. Air temperature, wind chill, and

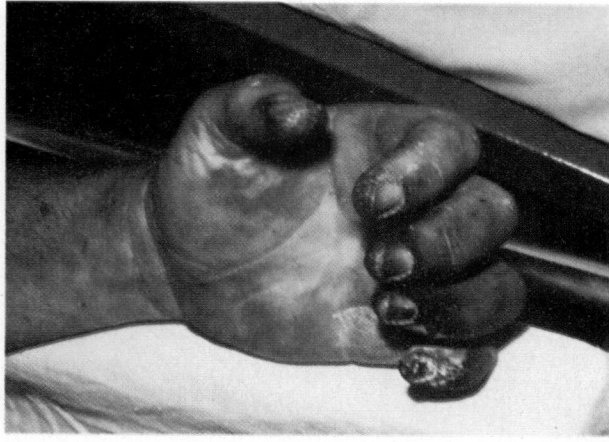

**FIGURE 33-3** Gangrene (necrosis), or permanent cell death, occurs when tissue is frozen and destructive chemical changes occur in the cells.
Courtesy of Dr. Jack Poland/CDC.

whether it is wet or dry are important aspects of scene size-up and will likely affect the patient.

Ensure that the scene is safe for you and other emergency responders. Identify potential safety hazards, such as wet grass, mud, or icy streets. Cold environments may present special challenges both for you and your patient; consider special hazards such as avalanches. Use appropriate standard precautions and consider the number of patients you may have. Summon additional help, such as a search-and-rescue team, as quickly as possible.

As you observe the scene, look for indicators of the mechanism of injury (MOI). For example, if you find a vehicle in a secluded ditch off the highway and the vehicle's roof and hood are covered with fresh snow, then you may assume that the patient was in a motor vehicle crash and has been exposed to the cold for a long period of time.

## Primary Assessment

In a cold emergency, your patient's chief complaint may be only that he or she is cold, or the cold may be an additional complication of an existing medical injury or trauma. Perform a rapid examination to determine whether a life threat exists, and if so, treat it. If the chief complaint is simply feeling cold, quickly assess the patient's core temperature by placing the back of your hand on the abdomen. Evaluate the patient's mental status quickly using the AVPU scale. An altered mental status indicates the intensity of the cold injury. Consider spinal immobilization based on your scene size-up and the chief complaint.

Your assessment should account for the physiologic changes that occur as a result of hypothermia. If you believe the patient is in cardiac arrest, proceed directly to ("C" in ABC) providing high-quality chest compressions, then address airway and breathing ("A" and "B") afterward. Ensure that the patient has an adequate airway and is breathing. If your patient's breathing is slow or shallow, ventilation with a bag-mask device may be necessary. Use warmed and humidified oxygen if it is available, because it helps to warm the patient from the inside out.

If you cannot feel a radial pulse, gently palpate for a carotid pulse and wait for up to 60 seconds before you decide whether the patient is pulseless. Even a pulse rate of 1 or 2 beats/min indicates

cardiac activity, and cardiac activity may spontaneously recover once the body core is warmed. However, there is evidence that CPR, when correctly done, will increase blood flow to the critical parts of the body. For this reason, some authorities recommend starting CPR on a patient with hypothermia and no pulse. The American Heart Association recommends that CPR be started if the patient has no detectable pulse or breathing. Remember, for a patient with hypothermia, this may require a prolonged pulse check of up to 60 seconds.

Perfusion will be compromised based on the severity of the cold exposure. Your assessment of the patient's skin will not be helpful in determining shock. Assume that shock is present and treat it appropriately. Bleeding may be difficult to find because of the slow-moving circulation and thick clothing. If the scene size-up, MOI, or chief complaint suggests the potential for bleeding, look for it carefully, remembering internal bleeding will not be visualized.

Even mild hypothermia can have serious consequences and complications, including cardiac dysrhythmias and blood clotting abnormalities. Therefore, all patients with hypothermia require rapid transport for evaluation and treatment. Assess the scene for the safest way to quickly move your patient from the cold environment. As you package your patient for transport, work quickly, safely, and gently. Rough handling of a patient with hypothermia may cause a cold, slow, weak heart to twitch or fibrillate. If transportation is delayed, protect the patient from further heat loss.

## History Taking

After the life threats have been managed during the primary assessment, investigate the chief complaint. Obtain a medical history and be alert for injury-specific signs and symptoms as well as any pertinent negatives.

Obtaining a patient's history in these situations may be difficult. If possible, find out how long your patient has been exposed to the cold environment, either from the patient or bystanders. Exposures may be short or prolonged in duration. For example, a patient may have acute hypothermia from sudden immersion in cold water or hypothermia that developed over the course of hours during an expedition. Your SAMPLE history can provide important information affecting both your treatment in the field and the treatment your patient will receive in the hospital. Recall that medications and underlying medical conditions may have an impact on the way cold affects the patient's metabolism. The patient's last oral intake and activity prior to the exposure will help to determine the severity of the cold injury.

## Secondary Assessment

The secondary assessment is used to uncover injuries that may have been missed during the primary assessment. In some instances, such as a critically injured patient or a short transport time, you may not have time to conduct a secondary assessment.

Focus your physical examination on the severity of hypothermia, assessing the areas of the body directly affected by cold exposure, and the degree of damage. Is the whole body cold (hypothermia) or just parts (frostbite)? These determinations will affect your treatment decisions. For example, a patient who stops shivering, but remains in a cold environment, will experience a rapid decrease in body temperature—a sign of severe hypothermia and a life-threatening emergency.

Determine the degree and extent of cold injury, as well as any other injuries or conditions that may not have been initially detected. The numbing effect of cold, both on the brain and on the body, may impair your patient's ability to tell you about other injuries or illnesses. Therefore, a careful examination of your patient's entire body will help you avoid missing important clues to your patient's condition.

Keep in mind that vital signs may be altered by the effects of hypothermia and can be an indicator of its severity. Respirations may be slow and shallow, resulting in low oxygen levels in the body. Low blood pressure and a slow pulse also indicate moderate to severe hypothermia. Carefully evaluate your patient for changes in mental status using the AVPU scale.

Determine CBT using a hypothermia thermometer, if local protocols allow. Pulse oximetry will often be inaccurate due to the lack of perfusion in the extremities.

## Reassessment

Repeat the primary assessment. Reassess vital signs and the chief complaint. Has the patient's condition improved with the interventions? Identify and treat changes in the patient's condition. Keep a close eye on your patient's level of consciousness and vital signs. As the body rewarms, the sudden redistribution of fluids and the release of built-up chemicals

## YOU are the Provider

You arrive at the scene and find the patient sitting under a tree in his garden; he is conscious but confused. His wife tells you that he has been working outside all day. She further states that despite her efforts, he refused to take a break and drink some water. As your partner opens the jump kit, you perform a primary assessment.

| Recording Time: 0 Minutes | |
|---|---|
| **Appearance** | Flushed |
| **Level of consciousness** | Conscious, but confused |
| **Airway** | Open, clear of secretions or foreign bodies |
| **Breathing** | Increased rate and depth |
| **Circulation** | Radial pulses weak and rapid; skin hot and moist; no gross bleeding |

Your partner applies high-flow oxygen via a nonrebreathing mask, and the patient's wife tells you that when she went to check on him, she found him sitting under a tree; initially, he did not respond to her. She further tells you that he has hypertension and angina, for which he takes furosemide (Lasix), potassium chloride (K-Dur), lisinopril (Prinivil), and nitroglycerin as needed. He also has insulin-dependent diabetes.

**3.** What risk factors does this patient have that predispose him to a heat emergency?

**4.** What type of heat emergency do you suspect he is experiencing? Why?

can have harmful effects, including cardiac dysrhythmias. Be vigilant even if the patient's condition appears to be improving.

Review all treatments that have been performed. In a cold-related emergency, depending on your local protocols, your treatment may only include oxygen delivery. Reassess oxygen delivery and continue to provide for a warm environment by removing any wet or frozen clothing. Do not remove any clothing frozen to the patient's skin.

Communicate all of the information you have gathered to the receiving facility, which may be essential in evaluating and treating your patient in the hospital. Your documentation should always include the patient's physical status, the conditions at the scene, information gathered from bystanders, and any changes in the patient's mental status during treatment and transport.

## General Management of Cold Emergencies

In most cases, move the patient from the cold environment to prevent further heat loss. To prevent further damage to the feet, do not allow the patient to walk. Remove any wet clothing, and place dry blankets over and under the patient (**FIGURE 33-5**). If available, give the patient warm, humidified oxygen if you have not already done so as part of the primary assessment.

Always handle the patient gently so that you do not cause any pain or further injury to the skin.

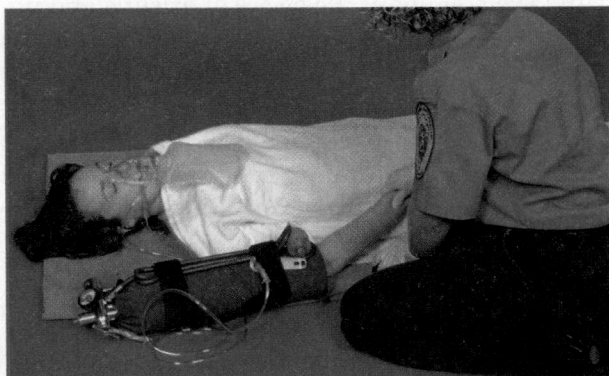

**FIGURE 33-5** Place dry blankets over and under the patient with hypothermia; give warm, humidified oxygen, if available.

© Jones & Bartlett Learning. Courtesy of MIEMSS.

Rough handling of a patient with moderate to severe hypothermia may cause the heart to go into ventricular fibrillation, which may not respond to defibrillation; this condition is characterized by uncontrollable twitching without effective pumping action by the heart. Do not massage the extremities. Do not allow the patient to eat or to use any stimulants, such as coffee, tea, soda, or tobacco products. Stimulants are vasoconstrictors, which may further impair circulation to affected areas.

If the patient is alert, shivering, responds appropriately, and the CBT is between 90°F to 95°F (32.2°C to 35°C), then the hypothermia is mild. Begin passive rewarming slowly, which includes placing the patient in a warm environment, removing wet clothing, and applying heat packs or hot water bottles to the groin, axillary, and cervical regions. Turn the heat up high in the patient compartment of the ambulance. To avoid burns, do not place heat packs directly on the skin. If possible, you may give warm fluids by mouth, as allowed by local protocols, assuming that the patient is alert and can swallow without difficulty.

However, when the patient has moderate or severe hypothermia, active rewarming is best accomplished in the emergency department (ED) utilizing aggressive strategies to introduce heat into the body's core. Such therapies might include warm intravenous fluids, lavage with warm fluids, and rewarming blood outside the body before reintroducing it (extracorporeal rewarming). Rewarming the patient too quickly, or from the extremities rather than the core may cause a fatal cardiac dysrhythmia or other significant complications. For this reason, local protocols may dictate the appropriate type of rewarming strategies based on the patient's CBT.

With a patient with moderate or severe hypothermia, your goal is to prevent further heat loss. Remove the patient immediately from the cold environment, place the patient in the ambulance, remove wet clothing, cover the patient with blankets, and transport. Remember to handle the patient gently to decrease the risk of ventricular fibrillation.

If you cannot get the patient out of the cold immediately, move the patient out of the wind and away from contact with any object that will conduct heat away from the body. Place blankets and a waterproof protective cover on the patient. Remember that body heat loss easily occurs around the head and neck, both of which can be covered with a towel. Regardless of the nature or severity of the cold injury, remember that even an unresponsive patient may be able to hear you. Some patients have reported hearing a provider pronounce them dead—a provider who forgot the saying: "No one is dead unless they are warm and dead."

## Emergency Care of Local Cold Injuries

The emergency treatment of local cold injuries in the field should include the following steps:

1. Remove the patient from further exposure to the cold.
2. Handle the injured part gently, and protect it from further injury.
3. Remove any wet or restricting clothing from the patient, especially over the injured part.

If there is no chance of reinjury or if transport to the ED will be significantly delayed, consider active rewarming if local protocols allow. Consult medical control, if available. With frostnip, contact with a warm object may be all that the patient needs; you can use your hands or the patient's own body (for example, have the patient tuck his or her hands into the armpits). During rewarming, the affected part will often tingle and become red in light-skinned people. With immersion foot, remove wet shoes, boots, and socks, and rewarm the foot gradually, protecting it from further cold exposure. Next, cover it loosely with a dry, sterile dressing. Never rub or massage injured tissues, which could cause further damage. Do not re-expose the injury to cold.

With a late or deep cold injury, such as frostbite, remove any jewelry from the injured part and cover the injury loosely with a dry, sterile dressing. Do not break blisters or rub or massage the area. Do not apply heat or rewarm the part. Unlike with frostnip and trench foot, rewarming of the frostbitten extremity is best accomplished in the ED. You can cause further injury to fragile tissues by attempting to rewarm a frostbitten part. Never apply something warm or hot, such as the exhaust from the ambulance engine or, even worse, an open flame. Do not allow the patient to stand or walk on a frostbitten foot. Evaluate the patient's general condition for the signs or symptoms of systemic hypothermia. Support the vital functions as necessary, and provide rapid transport to the hospital.

If prompt hospital care is unavailable and medical control instructs you to begin rewarming in the field, use a warm-water bath. Immerse the frostbitten part in water with a temperature between 104°F and 105°F (40°C and 41°C). Check the water temperature with a thermometer before immersing the limb, and recheck it frequently during the rewarming process. The water temperature should never exceed 105°F (41°C). Stir the water continuously. Keep the frostbitten part in the water until it feels warm and sensation has returned to the skin. Dress the area with dry, sterile dressings, placing them also between injured fingers or toes. Expect the patient to report severe pain.

Never attempt rewarming if there is any chance that the part may freeze again before the patient reaches the hospital. Some of the most severe consequences of frostbite, including gangrene and amputation, have occurred when parts thawed and then were allowed to refreeze.

Cover the frostbitten part with soft, padded, sterile cotton dressings. If blisters have formed, do not break them. Remember, you cannot accurately predict the outcome of a case of frostbite early in its course. Even body parts that appear gangrenous may recover following proper treatment.

## Cold Exposure and You

As an EMT, you are also at risk for hypothermia if you work in a cold environment. If cold weather search-and-rescue operations are a possibility in your assigned areas, you should receive survival training and precautionary tips. Become familiar with local conditions. Be aware of existing and potential weather conditions, and monitor changes that are forecast for the area. Make sure to wear proper clothing whenever appropriate. Your vehicle, too, must be properly equipped and maintained for a cold environment. You cannot help others if you do not protect yourself. Never allow yourself to become a victim!

## Heat Exposure

Recall that normal body temperature is 98°F (36.7°C). In a hot environment or during vigorous physical activity, the body will try to rid itself of the excess heat. The two most efficient methods to decrease heat are sweating (and evaporation of the sweat) and dilation of skin blood vessels, which brings blood to the skin surface to increase the rate of heat radiation. In addition, a person who becomes overheated can remove clothing and seek a cooler environment.

Ordinarily, the heat-regulating mechanisms of the body work well, and people are able to tolerate significant temperature changes. When heat gain exceeds heat loss, hyperthermia can result. Hyperthermia is a high core temperature, usually 101°F (38.3°C) or higher.

### Words of Wisdom

It is important to keep yourself hydrated while on duty, especially during periods of heavy exertion or when working in the heat. The color of urine (usually darker with dehydration) and frequency of urination correlate directly with the body's hydration status.

When the body's mechanisms to decrease body heat are overwhelmed and the body is unable to tolerate the excessive heat, a heat emergency develops in the patient. High air temperature can reduce heat loss by radiation; high humidity reduces heat loss through evaporation. The inability to acclimate (adjust) to the heat is a risk factor. Another risk factor is vigorous exercise, during which sweat loss can exceed 1 liter per hour, causing loss of fluid and electrolytes.

A heat emergency can take the following three forms:

- Heat cramps
- Heat exhaustion
- Heatstroke

All three forms may be present in the same patient because untreated heat exhaustion may progress to heatstroke. Heatstroke is life threatening.

People at greatest risk for a heat emergency are children; geriatric patients; patients with heart disease, chronic obstructive pulmonary disease (COPD), diabetes, dehydration, and obesity; and those with limited mobility. Older people, newborns, and infants exhibit poor thermoregulation. Newborns and infants often wear too much clothing. Alcohol and certain drugs, including medications that dehydrate the body or decrease the ability of the body to sweat, also make a person more susceptible to heat emergencies. When you are treating

someone for a heat emergency, always obtain a medication history.

## Heat Cramps

Heat cramps are painful muscle spasms that occur after vigorous exercise. They do not occur only when it is hot outdoors. They may be seen in factory workers and even well-conditioned athletes. The exact cause of heat cramps is not well understood. It is known that sweat produced during strenuous exercise, particularly in a warm environment, causes a change in the body's electrolyte balance. The result may be a loss of essential electrolytes from the cells. Dehydration may also play a role in the development of muscle cramps. Large amounts of water loss can result from excessive sweating. This loss of water may affect muscles that are being stressed and cause them to spasm.

Heat cramps usually occur in the leg or abdominal muscles. When the abdominal muscles are involved, the pain and muscle spasm may be so severe that the patient appears to have an acute abdominal condition. If a patient with a sudden onset of abdominal cramps has been exercising vigorously in a hot environment, suspect heat cramps.

## Heat Exhaustion

Heat exhaustion, also called heat prostration or heat collapse, is the most common heat emergency. Heat exposure, stress, and fatigue are causes of heat exhaustion, which is caused by hypovolemia as the result of the loss of water and electrolytes from heavy sweating. Recall that for sweating to be an effective cooling mechanism, the sweat must be able to evaporate from the body. Otherwise, the body will continue to produce sweat, with further loss of body water. People standing in the hot sun and particularly those wearing several layers of clothing, such as sports fans or parade watchers, may sweat profusely but experience little body cooling. The sweat-soaked clothing will actually begin to trap heat, increasing body temperature. High humidity will also decrease the amount of evaporation that can occur. The heat index provided in **FIGURE 33-6** shows how high humidity increases the effects of ambient temperature. For example, if the temperature is 90°F (32.2°C) with 86% humidity, the effect of the atmosphere on a person is the same as being in an environment of 105°F (40.6°C).

Temperature (°F)

| Relative Humidity (%) | 80 | 81 | 84 | 86 | 88 | 90 | 92 | 94 | 96 | 98 | 100 | 102 | 104 | 106 | 108 | 110 |
|---|---|---|---|---|---|---|---|---|---|---|---|---|---|---|---|---|
| 40 | 80 | 81 | 83 | 85 | 88 | 91 | 94 | 97 | 101 | 105 | 109 | 114 | 119 | 124 | 130 | 136 |
| 45 | 80 | 82 | 84 | 87 | 89 | 93 | 96 | 100 | 104 | 109 | 114 | 119 | 124 | 130 | 137 | |
| 50 | 81 | 83 | 85 | 88 | 91 | 95 | 99 | 103 | 108 | 113 | 118 | 124 | 131 | 137 | | |
| 55 | 81 | 84 | 86 | 89 | 93 | 97 | 101 | 106 | 112 | 117 | 124 | 130 | 137 | | | |
| 60 | 82 | 84 | 88 | 91 | 95 | 100 | 105 | 110 | 116 | 123 | 129 | 137 | | | | |
| 65 | 82 | 85 | 89 | 93 | 98 | 103 | 108 | 114 | 121 | 126 | 130 | | | | | |
| 70 | 83 | 86 | 90 | 95 | 100 | 105 | 112 | 119 | 126 | 134 | | | | | | |
| 75 | 84 | 88 | 92 | 97 | 103 | 109 | 116 | 124 | 132 | | | | | | | |
| 80 | 84 | 89 | 94 | 100 | 106 | 113 | 121 | 129 | | | | | | | | |
| 85 | 85 | 90 | 96 | 102 | 110 | 117 | 126 | 135 | | | | | | | | |
| 90 | 86 | 91 | 98 | 105 | 113 | 122 | 131 | | | | | | | | | |
| 95 | 86 | 93 | 100 | 108 | 117 | 127 | | | | | | | | | | |
| 100 | 87 | 95 | 103 | 112 | 121 | 132 | | | | | | | | | | |

Likelihood of Heat Disorders With Prolonged Exposure or Strenuous Activity

☐ Caution ☐ Extreme Caution ☐ Danger ■ Extreme Danger

**FIGURE 33-6** High humidity increases the effects of ambient temperature.

Courtesy of the National Weather Service/NOAA.

People working or exerting themselves in poorly ventilated areas are unable to release heat through convection. Thus, people who work or exercise vigorously and those who wear heavy clothing in a warm, humid, or poorly ventilated environment are particularly susceptible to heat exhaustion.

The signs and symptoms of heat exhaustion and those of associated hypovolemia are as follows:

- Dizziness, weakness, or syncope signifying a change in level of consciousness with accompanying nausea, vomiting, or headache. Muscle cramping may also be present, including abdominal cramping.
- Onset while working vigorously or exercising in a hot, humid, or poorly ventilated environment and sweating heavily.
- Onset, even at rest, in the older and infant age groups in hot, humid, and poorly ventilated environments or extended time in hot, humid environments. People who are not acclimatized to the environment may also experience onset at rest.
- Cold, clammy skin with ashen pallor.
- Dry tongue and thirst.
- Normal vital signs, although the pulse is often rapid and weak (an indication for use of pulse

oximetry) and the diastolic blood pressure may be low.
- Normal or slightly elevated body temperature—on rare occasions, as high as 104°F (40°C).

## Heatstroke

**Heatstroke**, the least common but most serious heat emergency, occurs when the body is subjected to more heat than it can handle and normal mechanisms for getting rid of the excess heat are overwhelmed. The body temperature then rises rapidly to the level at which tissues are destroyed. Untreated heatstroke always results in death.

Heatstroke can develop in patients during vigorous physical activity or when they are outdoors or in a closed, poorly ventilated, humid space. It also occurs during heat waves among people (particularly geriatric patients) who live in buildings with no air conditioning or with poor ventilation. It may also develop in children who are left unattended in a locked vehicle on a hot day.

Many patients with heatstroke have hot, dry, flushed skin because their sweating mechanism has been overwhelmed. However, in the course of heatstroke, the skin may be moist or wet due to exertion by the patient. Keep in mind that a patient can have heatstroke even if he or she is still sweating. This presentation is often seen in endurance athletes, military personnel, or emergency providers who wear personal protective equipment, such as firefighters, SWAT team members, or hazmat workers. The body temperature rises rapidly in patients with heatstroke. It may rise to 106°F (41.1°C) or more. As the body core temperature rises, the patient's level of consciousness decreases, resulting in unconsciousness.

Often, the first sign of heatstroke is confusion or a change in behavior. However, the patient often becomes unresponsive quickly and seizures may occur. The pulse is usually rapid and strong at first, but as the patient becomes increasingly unresponsive, the pulse becomes weaker and the blood pressure falls. The respiratory rate increases as the body attempts to compensate. An important and classically described sign of heatstroke is when the patient no longer perspires, which means the body has lost its thermoregulatory mechanism. If you are perspiring in the environment, your patient should also be perspiring. If any one of these signs is present, suspect heatstroke and act accordingly.

## Assessment of Heat Emergencies

### Scene Size-up

As part of your scene size-up, perform an environmental assessment. How hot is it outside? How hot is it in the room where your patient is located? How well is the patient tolerating the heat? Dispatch may report the call initially as a medical or trauma emergency. The heat emergency may be secondary. Always look for hazards as well as clues as to what may have caused your patient's emergency. If the patient is unconscious, has an altered mental status, or requires intravenous fluids to treat shock, consider calling for advanced life support (ALS) assistance as long as doing so does not delay access to aggressive cooling techniques.

As you observe the scene, look for indicators of the MOI. For example, you arrive on the scene at a shopping mall to find an older man with a decreased level of consciousness inside a parked vehicle on a warm, humid, sunny day. The MOI for this patient is sitting in a warm environment under direct sunlight with no ventilation.

Heat emergencies commonly occur in the context of athletic events and practices, often with athletic trainers present. In those instances, you may find the patient submerged in a cold-water immersion bath inside the athletic training room. It is harmful to allow heat to persist for any amount of time; therefore, cooling prior to transport is indicated if facilities such as an ice bath are available. If the patient is placed in a cold-water immersion bath on your arrival, monitor the patient in the water and assist as necessary. Do not remove the patient until the temperature has normalized to the appropriate level, between 101°F and 102°F (38.3°C and 38.9°C). Do not overcool the patient. Overcooling can lead to shivering, which generates more heat. Monitor the patient closely.

Finally, if you anticipate a prolonged scene time, protect yourself from the heat and remember to stay hydrated. Use appropriate standard precautions, including gloves and eye protection. Long-sleeved shirts and long pants may be uncomfortable in warm weather; however, they can help protect you from being splashed by blood or other body fluids.

### Primary Assessment

As you approach your patient, observe how the patient interacts with you and the environment. This will help identify the patient's degree of distress. Introduce yourself and ask about the chief complaint. A heat emergency may be the primary problem or it may simply be aggravating a medical or trauma condition. Remember, prolonged heat exposure may stress the heart, causing a heart attack. Use this initial interaction to guide you in assessing for immediate life threats and related problems. Perform a rapid scan and avoid tunnel vision.

Assess the patient's mental status using the AVPU scale. Heatstroke is a life-threatening emergency. Gather clues about his or her mental status to identify the severity of your patient's condition. The more altered the patient's mental status is, the more serious the heat emergency.

Assess the patient's airway and breathing and treat any life threats. Unless the patient is unresponsive, the airway should be patent. Nausea and vomiting, however, may occur. Position the patient to protect the airway as necessary. If the patient is unresponsive, be cautious of how you open the airway; consider spinal motion restriction if trauma is a possibility. If your patient is unresponsive, insert an airway and provide bag-mask ventilations.

| TABLE 33-2 Skin Condition | |
|---|---|
| **Skin Condition** | **Indicates** |
| Moist, pale, cool skin | Excessive fluid and salt loss |
| Hot, dry skin | Body is unable to regulate core temperature |
| Hot, moist skin | Body is unable to regulate core temperature |

© Jones & Bartlett Learning.

If circulation is adequate, assess the patient for perfusion and bleeding. Assess the patient's skin condition carefully (**TABLE 33-2**). Treat the patient aggressively for shock by removing the patient from the heat and positioning the patient to improve circulation.

If your patient has any signs of heatstroke, provide rapid transport.

## History Taking

After the life threats have been managed during the primary assessment, investigate the chief complaint. Obtain a medical history and be alert for specific signs and symptoms such as the absence of perspiration, decreased level of consciousness, confusion, muscle cramping, nausea, and vomiting.

Obtain a SAMPLE history. Patients with inadequate oral intake or who are taking diuretics may have difficulty tolerating exposure to heat. Remember, many medications used by geriatric patients affect how well they tolerate heat. Be thorough in your questioning. Determine your patient's exposure to heat and humidity and activities prior to the onset of symptoms.

## Secondary Assessment

The secondary assessment is used to uncover injuries that may have been missed during the primary assessment. In some instances, such as a critically injured patient or a short transport time, you may not have time to conduct a secondary assessment.

If your patient is unresponsive, perform a secondary assessment of the entire body looking for problems or explanations as to what is wrong. Obtain the patient's vital signs to help understand the severity of the emergency.

If the patient is conscious, perform an assessment of specific areas of the body. Heat exposure has significant effects on the metabolism, muscles, and cardiovascular system. Assess the patient for muscle cramps or confusion. Examine the patient's mental status and take the patient's vital signs.

Perform a detailed examination if circumstances and time permit. Pay special attention to the patient's skin temperature, turgor, and level of moisture. Skin turgor is the ability of the skin to resist deformation. It is tested by gently pinching skin on the abdomen or back of the hand. Normally the skin will quickly flatten out. If the patient is dehydrated, the skin will remain tented (poor skin turgor). Perform a careful neurologic examination.

Patients with hyperthermia will often have tachycardia and tachypnea. As long as they maintain a normal blood pressure, their bodies will compensate for the fluid loss. Once their blood pressure begins to fall, it indicates they are no longer able to compensate for fluid loss and are going into shock. Your assessment of the patient's skin will help determine the severity of the emergency. For example, in heat exhaustion, the skin temperature may be normal or may even be cool and clammy; however, in heatstroke, the skin is hot.

Check the patient's body temperature with a thermometer, depending on protocol. Your unit equipment may include disposable or oral thermometers with disposable covers, infrared digital skin thermometers, or tympanic (ear) thermometers. You may not use these devices routinely, so become familiar with how they work. In patients with a heat-related emergency, monitoring of pulse oximetry is also useful.

## Reassessment

Watch your patient's condition carefully for deterioration. Remove your patient as quickly as possible from the hot environment. Patients with heat cramps or exhaustion usually respond well to passive cooling and fluids by mouth. Patients with symptoms of heatstroke should be transported immediately in a cool ambulance, passively cooled with clothing removal, and actively cooled by spraying the patient with water and fanning to enhance evaporation. Any decline in level of consciousness is an ominous sign. Monitor the patient's vital signs at least every 5 minutes. Evaluate the effectiveness

| TABLE 33-3 Symptoms of Heat Exhaustion and Heatstroke | |
|---|---|
| **Heat Exhaustion Symptoms** | **Heatstroke Symptoms (Medical Emergency)** |
| Dizziness or fainting | Headache |
| Heavy sweating | Confusion or delirium |
| Cold, pale, and clammy skin | Possible loss of consciousness |
| Nausea or vomiting | Absence of sweating, or dry skin, except in exertional heat stroke |
| Fast, weak pulse | Hot, red skin |
| Weakness or muscle cramps | Nausea or vomiting |
| Excessive thirst | Rapid heart rate |
| | Body temperature above 104°F (40°C) |

© Jones & Bartlett Learning.

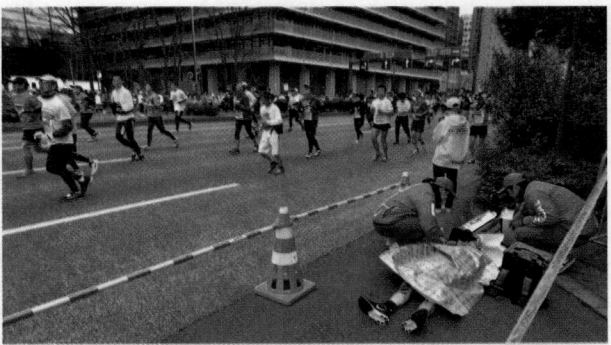

**FIGURE 33-7** A patient with any heat emergency should be moved to a cool environment as you begin your assessment and treatment. A person, suffering muscle cramps, receives treatment during the 12th Tokyo Marathon in Tokyo, Japan on February 25, 2018.

© David Mareuil/Anadolu Agency/Getty Images.

of your interventions. Be careful not to overcool a patient who is experiencing a heat emergency, but the risk of failing to reverse heat stroke by active cooling far exceeds the risk of overcooling. Remember, heat stroke is uniformly fatal if not reversed rapidly and effectively.

Inform the ED staff as soon as possible that your patient is experiencing heatstroke, because additional resources may be required. Document the environmental conditions and the activities the patient was performing prior to the emergency in your patient care report. Consider other possibilities of the altered mental status, such as traumatic brain injury, alcohol consumption, or a low blood glucose level (**TABLE 33-3**).

# Management of Heat Emergencies

## Heat Cramps

Take the following steps to treat heat cramps in the field (**FIGURE 33-7**):

1. Promptly remove the patient from the hot environment, including direct sunlight. Loosen any tight clothing.

2. Administer high-flow oxygen if the patient shows signs of hypoxia or respiratory distress.
3. Rest the cramping muscles. Have the patient sit or lie down until the cramps subside.
4. Replace fluids by mouth. Give water or a diluted (half-strength) balanced electrolyte solution, such as a sports drink. In most cases, plain water is the most useful. Do not give salt tablets or solutions that have a high salt concentration.
5. Cool the patient with cool water spray or mist, and add convection to the cooling method by manually or mechanically fanning the patient.

When the heat cramps are gone, the patient may resume activity. For example, an athlete can return to play once the heat cramps have disappeared. However, heavy sweating may cause the cramps to reoccur. The best strategy for treatment and prevention is hydration by drinking enough water.

If the cramps do not go away after these measures, transport the patient to the hospital. If you are uncertain that the patient's cramps were caused by the heat or you note anything out of the ordinary, contact medical control or transport the patient to the hospital.

## Heat Exhaustion

To treat the patient with heat exhaustion, follow the steps in **SKILL DRILL 33-1**:

1. Promptly remove the patient from the hot environment, preferably into the back of the air-conditioned ambulance. If outdoors, move

## Skill Drill 33-1 Treating for Heat Exhaustion

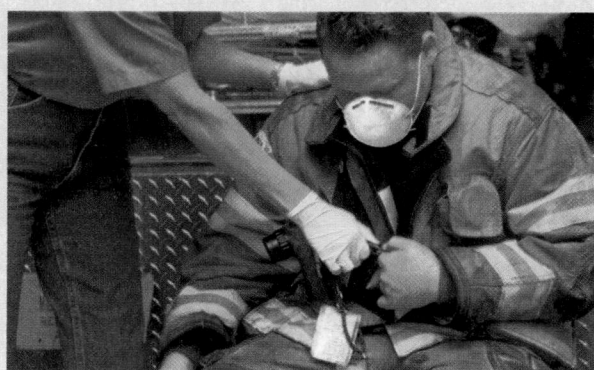

### Step 1

Move the patient to a cooler environment. Remove extra clothing.

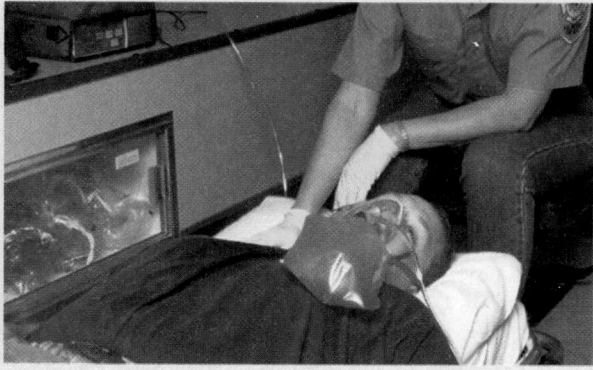

### Step 2

Give oxygen if indicated. Check the patient's blood glucose level if indicated. Perform cold-water immersion or other cooling measures as available. Place the patient in a supine position and fan the patient.

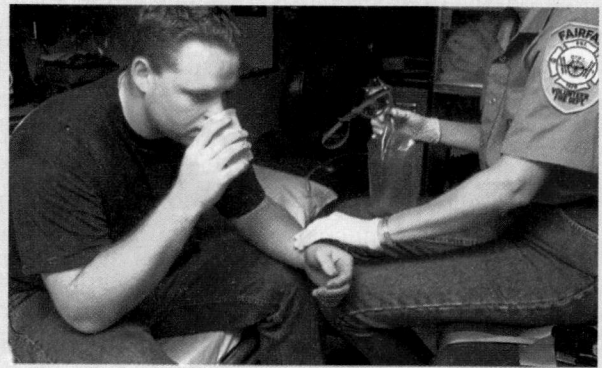

### Step 3

If the patient is fully alert, give water by mouth.

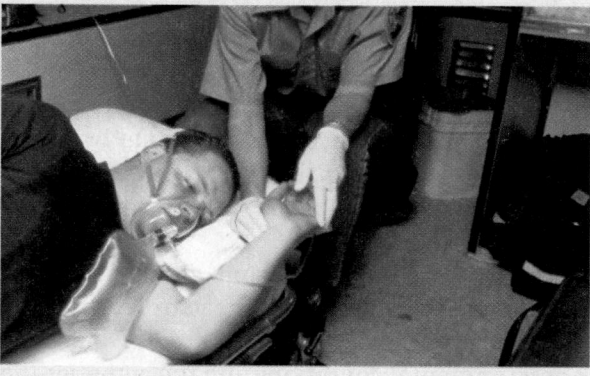

### Step 4

If nausea develops, secure and transport the patient on his or her left side.

© Jones & Bartlett Learning. Courtesy of MIEMSS.

out of direct sunlight. Remove any excessive layers of clothing, particularly around the head and neck (**Step 1**).

2. Administer high-flow oxygen if indicated, if this was not already done as part of the primary assessment.

3. If the patient has an altered mental status, check the blood glucose level.

4. Cool the patient with misting and administration of ice packs to the trunk of the patient's body. If an ice bath or similar facility is available, provide cold-water immersion to the patient if allowed per local protocol. Cold-water (ice bath) immersion is recommended for patients with a core temperature of 104°F (40°C) or an altered mental status.

5. Encourage the patient to lie down. Loosen any tight clothing and cool the patient by manually or mechanically fanning him or her (**Step 2**).

6. If the patient is fully alert, encourage him or her to sit up and slowly drink up to a liter of water, as long as nausea does not develop. Never force fluids by mouth on a patient who is not fully alert, or allow drinking while supine, because the patient could aspirate the fluid into the lungs. If the patient does not become nauseated, transport the patient on the left side to prevent aspiration (**Step 3**).

   In most cases, these measures will reverse the symptoms, causing the patient to feel better within 30 minutes. Prepare to transport the patient to the hospital, and also consider a rendezvous with ALS for more aggressive treatment, such as intravenous fluid therapy and close monitoring, especially in the following circumstances:

   - The symptoms do not clear up promptly.
   - The level of consciousness decreases.
   - The body temperature remains elevated.
   - The person is very young, is older, or has any underlying medical condition, such as diabetes or cardiovascular disease.

7. Transport the patient on his or her left side if you think the patient may be nauseated, but make certain that the patient is secured (**Step 4**).

## Heatstroke

Recovery from heatstroke is only possible if treatment is administered rapidly, so you must identify this patient quickly. Emergency treatment has one objective: lower the body temperature by any means available. Take the following steps when treating a patient with heatstroke:

1. Move the patient out of the hot environment and into the ambulance.
2. Set the air conditioning to maximum cooling.
3. Remove the patient's clothing.
4. Administer high-flow oxygen if indicated, if this was not already done as part of the primary assessment. If needed, assist the patient's ventilations with a bag-mask device and appropriate airway adjuncts as per your protocol. If the patient is unresponsive and unable to protect his or her airway, consider rapid transport and cooling en route. Consult medical control if available.

5. Provide cold-water immersion in an ice bath, if possible. Cooling should begin immediately and continue en route to the hospital (**FIGURE 33-8**). If it is not possible to cool en route and cold-water immersion is available at the scene, continue cold-water immersion at the scene until the CBT is between 101°F and 102°F (38.3°C and 38.9°C).

6. Spray the patient with cool water and fan him or her to quickly evaporate the moisture on the skin.

7. Aggressively and repeatedly fan the patient with or without dampening the skin.

8. Exclude other causes of altered mental status, and check blood glucose level, if possible.

9. Provide rapid transport to the hospital.

10. Notify the hospital as soon as possible so that the staff can prepare to treat the patient immediately on arrival.

11. Do not overcool the patient. Call for ALS assistance if the patient begins to shiver.

### Special Populations

Remember that the aging process alters the body's ability to compensate for its surroundings. Temperature-related emergencies can develop in older people over time, even in indoor environments that may not seem uncomfortable to you. Be vigilant for temperature-related illnesses.

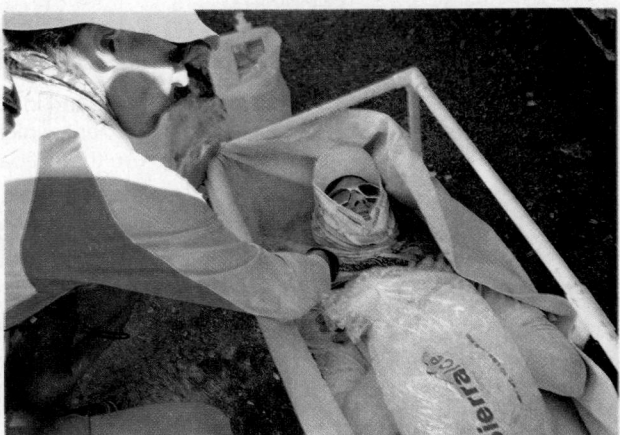

**FIGURE 33-8** As part of treatment of heatstroke, if available, immerse the patient in an ice-water bath if this treatment is consistent with your local protocol.

© Toni L. Sandys/Washington Post/Getty Images.

# Drowning

Drowning is the process of experiencing respiratory impairment from submersion or immersion in liquid. Some agencies previously used the term near-drowning to refer to a patient who survives at least temporarily (24 hours) after suffocation in water. Terms such as near-drowning, and wet, dry, and secondary drowning, are confusing. Although previously popular, they have no effect on care and therefore are no longer used.

According to the Centers for Disease Control and Prevention, an average of 10 people die from unintentional drownings each day. More than 25% are children younger than 14 years. Alcohol consumption, preexisting seizure disorders, geriatric patients with cardiovascular disease, and unsupervised access to water are among the major risk factors.

Drowning is often the last in a cycle of events caused by panic in the water. It can happen to anyone who is submerged in water for even a short period of time. Struggling toward the surface or the shore, the person becomes fatigued or exhausted, which leads him or her to sink even deeper. Most people can only hold their breath for about a minute when submerged under water. After that, water is inhaled and then the person coughs. Without rescue, the person continues to aspirate, becomes hypoxic, loses consciousness, and within a few minutes stops breathing and then suffers a cardiac arrest. In cold water this process is extended. However, drowning also occurs in buckets, puddles, bathtubs, and other places where the person is not completely submerged. Young children can drown in as little as 1 inch (3 cm) of water if left unattended.

## Spinal Injuries in Submersion Incidents

Submersion incidents may be complicated by spinal fractures and spinal cord injuries, which occur in less than 0.5% of persons who are drowning. Assume that spinal injury exists with the following conditions:

- The submersion has resulted from a diving mishap or fall from a significant height.
- The patient is conscious but reports weakness, paralysis, or numbness in the arms or legs.
- You suspect the possibility of spinal injury despite what witnesses say.

Most spinal injuries in diving incidents affect the cervical spine. When spinal injury is suspected, the neck must be protected from further injury. This means that you will have to stabilize the suspected injury while the patient is still in the water. If the situation does not indicate a possible spinal injury, stabilization is not recommended. To stabilize a

## YOU are the Provider

You quickly place the patient onto the stretcher and load him into the ambulance. The air conditioner is on and set to high. You perform a secondary assessment, which does not reveal any gross signs of injury, while your partner assesses the patient's vital signs. You then depart the scene and begin further treatment en route to the hospital.

| Recording Time: 6 Minutes | |
| --- | --- |
| **Respirations** | 24 breaths/min; adequate depth |
| **Pulse** | 130 beats/mm; weak and regular |
| **Skin** | Hot, flushed, and moist |
| **Blood pressure** | 88/66 mm Hg |
| **Oxygen saturation (Spo$_2$)** | 95% (on oxygen) |

**5.** What specific treatment is required for this patient?

**6.** What is the most likely explanation for this patient's vital signs?

## Safety Tips

You must ensure the safety of rescue personnel and request additional rescue resources, as appropriate, before a water rescue can begin. Water rescue is typically handled by specialized rescue personnel, but you may be involved if you arrive first or if water rescue is included in your scope of practice per local protocols. If the patient is conscious and still in the water, perform a water rescue. The saying "Reach, throw, and row, and only then go" (**FIGURE 33-9**) sums up the basic rule of water rescue. First, try to reach for the patient. If that does not work, throw the patient a rope, a life preserver, or any floatable object that is available. For example, an inflated spare tire, rim and all, will float well enough to support two people in the water. Next, use a boat if one is available. Do not attempt a swimming rescue unless you are trained and experienced in the proper

techniques. Even then, you should always wear a helmet and a personal flotation device (**FIGURE 33-10**). Too many well-meaning rescuers have themselves become victims while attempting a swimming rescue. In cold climates or cold-water locations, rapid hypothermia is also a concern for rescuers. Be prepared for this potential event.

The steps for ice rescue are similar and may involve reaching with a pole or ladder or throwing a rope or flotation device. A victim who has fallen through the ice may also be coached into placing his or her arms out of the water and onto the ice, kicking and rolling out of the water, and crawling to safety.

If you work in a recreation area near lakes, rivers, or the ocean, you should have a prearranged plan for water rescue. For colder areas, a plan for ice rescue is also necessary. This plan should include access to and cooperation with local providers who are trained and skilled in water rescue; these providers should help to develop the protocol for water rescue. Because the success of any water rescue depends on how rapidly the patient is removed from the water and ventilated, make sure you always have immediate access to personal flotation devices and other rescue equipment. Survival rates drastically decline the longer a victim is immersed. Cold-water drowning survival rates are somewhat higher.

Skidplate texture: © Photodisc.

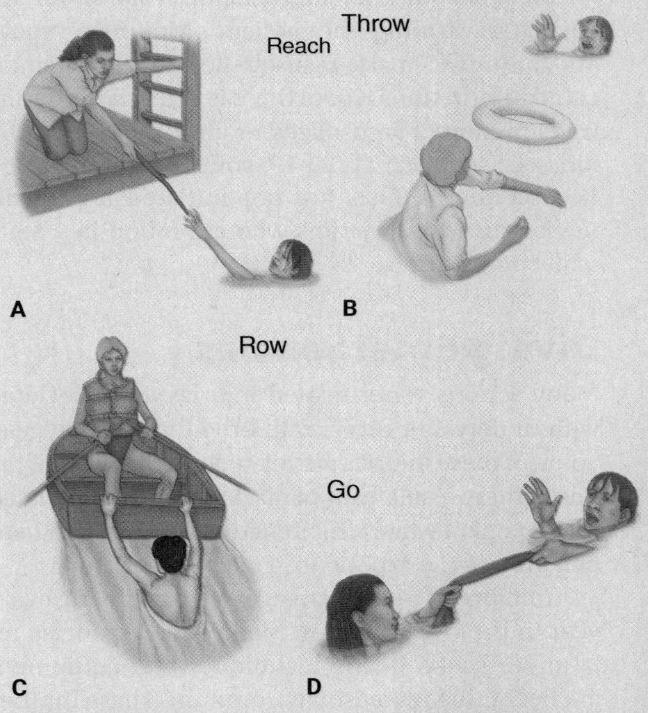

Throw
Reach

**A**

**B**

Row

Go

**C**

**D**

**FIGURE 33-9** Basic rules of water rescue. **A.** Reach for the person from shore. If you cannot reach the person from shore, wade closer. **B.** If an object that floats is available, throw it to the person. **C.** Use a boat if one is available. **D.** If you must swim to the person, use a towel or board for him or her to hold onto. Do not let the person grab you.

© Jones & Bartlett Learning.

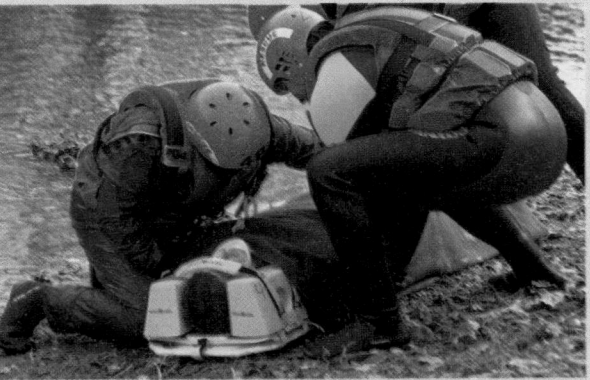

**FIGURE 33-10** When performing a water rescue, you must be properly trained and must wear proper personal protective equipment, including a personal flotation device.

© Ellis & Associates.

suspected spinal injury in water, follow the steps in **SKILL DRILL 33-2**:

1. Turn the patient supine. Two rescuers are usually required to turn the patient safely, although in some cases one rescuer will suffice. Always rotate the entire upper half of the patient's body as a single unit. Twisting only the head, for example, may aggravate any injury to the cervical spine (**Step 1**).
2. Restore the airway and begin ventilation. Immediate ventilation is the primary treatment of all drowning patients as soon as the patient is faceup in the water. Use a pocket mask if it is available. Have the other rescuer support the head and trunk as a unit while you open the airway and begin artificial ventilation (**Step 2**). Prepare for vomiting; 65% of victims requiring rescue breathing vomit and 88% of those receiving chest compressions will vomit.
3. Float a buoyant backboard or spinal restriction device under the patient as you continue ventilation (**Step 3**).
4. Secure the trunk and head to the board or device to restrict spinal motion. Do not remove the patient from the water (**Step 4**).
5. Remove the patient from the water on the backboard (**Step 5**).
6. Cover the patient with a blanket. Give oxygen if the patient is breathing spontaneously. Begin CPR if there is no pulse. Effective cardiac compression or CPR is extremely difficult to perform when the patient is still in the water (**Step 6**).

## Recovery Techniques

On occasion, you may be called to the scene of a drowning and find that the patient is not floating or visible in the water. An organized rescue effort in these circumstances calls for providers who are experienced with recovery techniques and equipment, including snorkel, mask, and scuba gear. Scuba gear (self-contained underwater breathing apparatus) is a system that delivers air to the mouth and lungs at atmospheric pressures that increase with the depth of the dive.

## Resuscitation Efforts

When a person is submerged in water that is colder than body temperature, heat will be conducted from the body to the water. The resulting hypothermia can protect vital organs from the lack of oxygen.

In addition, exposure to cold water will occasionally activate certain primitive reflexes, which may preserve basic body functions for prolonged periods.

If a person is found unconscious in the water, resuscitation may be beneficial to the patient's outcome, but it must be administered by a highly trained rescuer.

Also, whenever a person dives or jumps into very cold water, the diving reflex, slowing of the heart rate caused by submersion in cold water, may cause immediate bradycardia, a slow heart rhythm. Loss of consciousness and drowning may follow. However, the person may be able to survive for an extended period of time under water, thanks to a lowering of the metabolic rate associated with hypothermia. For this reason, local protocols often dictate that resuscitation efforts continue for up to 1 hour after submersion, while simultaneously rewarming the patient. Mouth-to-mouth and mouth-to-mask resuscitation are contraindicated in situations where there is active community transmission of aerosolized or airborne respiratory illnesses such as COVID-19, small pox, or measles. Resuscitation efforts are not initiated for unwitnessed drowning victims who are found in a state of decomposition.

## Diving Emergencies

Many serious water-related injuries are associated with underwater dives, with or without scuba gear. Some of these injuries are related to the nature of the dive; others result from panic. Panic is not restricted to the person who is frightened by water. It can happen even to the experienced diver or swimmer.

Millions of people engage in scuba diving every year in the United States. Medical emergencies relating to scuba diving techniques and equipment are becoming increasingly common. These injuries are separated into three phases of the dive: descent, bottom, and ascent.

### Descent Emergencies

Descent problems are usually caused by the sudden increase in pressure on the body as the person dives deeper into the water. Some body cavities cannot adjust to the increased external pressure of the water; the result is severe pain. The usual areas affected are the lungs, the sinus cavities, the middle ear, the teeth, and the area of the face surrounded by the diving mask. Usually, the pain caused by these "squeeze problems" forces the diver to return

## Skill Drill 33-2 Stabilizing a Suspected Spinal Injury in the Water

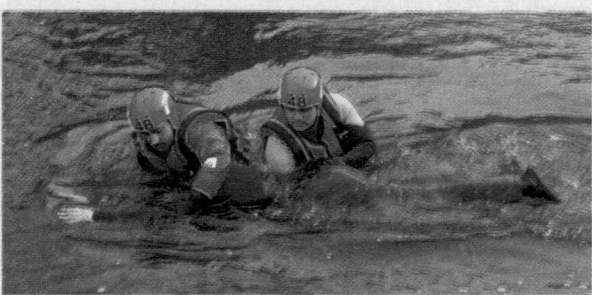

### Step 1

Turn the patient to a supine position by rotating the entire upper half of the body as a single unit.

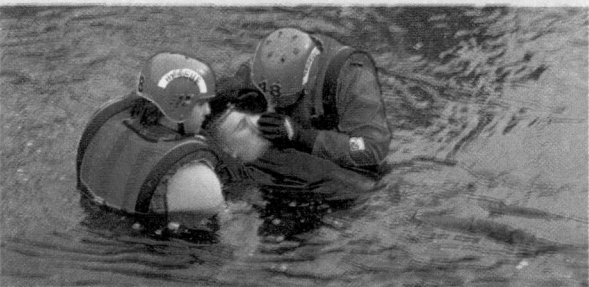

### Step 2

As soon as the patient is turned, begin artificial ventilation using the mouth-to-mouth method or a pocket mask unless you are in a situation where there is active community transmission of aerosolized or airborne respiratory illness.

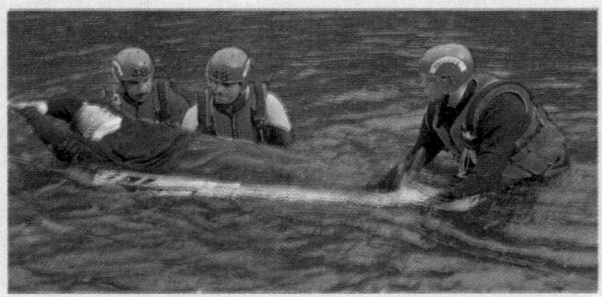

### Step 3

Float a buoyant backboard or appropriate device under the patient.

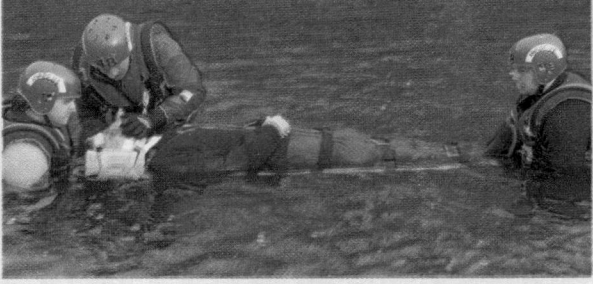

### Step 4

Secure the patient to the backboard or device.

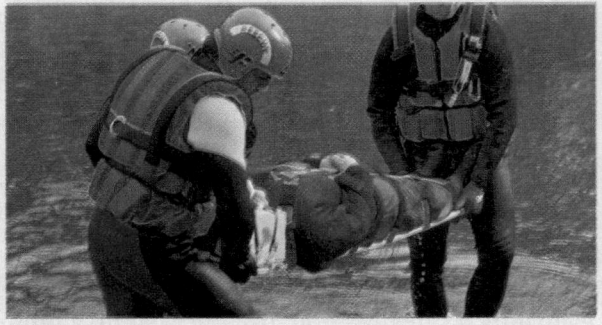

### Step 5

Remove the patient from the water.

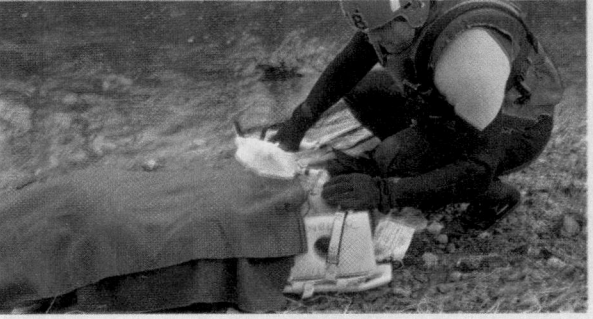

### Step 6

Maintain the body's normal temperature and apply oxygen if the patient is breathing. Begin CPR if breathing and pulse are absent.

to the surface to equalize the pressures, and the problem clears up by itself. A diver who continues to report pain, particularly in the ear, after returning to the surface should be transported to the hospital.

A special problem may develop in a person with a perforated tympanic membrane (ruptured eardrum) while diving. If cold water enters the middle ear through a ruptured eardrum, the diver may sustain a loss of balance and orientation. The diver may then shoot to the surface and experience ascent problems.

## Emergencies at the Bottom

Problems related to the bottom of the dive are rarely seen. They include inadequate mixing of oxygen and carbon dioxide in the air the diver breathes and accidental feeding of poisonous carbon monoxide into the breathing apparatus. Both are the result of faulty connections in the diving gear. These situations can cause drowning or rapid ascent; they require emergency resuscitation and transport of the patient.

## Ascent Emergencies

Most of the serious injuries associated with diving are related to ascending from the bottom and are referred to as ascent problems. These emergencies usually require aggressive resuscitation. Two particularly dangerous medical emergencies are air embolism and decompression sickness.

## Air Embolism

The most dangerous, and most common, emergency in scuba diving is an air embolism, a condition involving bubbles of air in the blood vessels. An air embolism may occur on a dive as shallow as 6 feet (2 m). The problem starts when the diver holds his or her breath during a rapid ascent. The air pressure in the lungs remains at a high level while the external pressure on the chest decreases. As a result, the air inside the lungs expands rapidly, causing the alveoli in the lungs to rupture. The air released from this rupture can cause the following injuries:

- Air may enter the pleural space and compress the lungs (a pneumothorax).
- Air may enter the mediastinum (the space within the thorax that contains the heart and great vessels), causing a condition called pneumomediastinum.

- Air may enter the bloodstream and create bubbles of air in the vessels called air emboli.

Pneumothorax and pneumomediastinum both result in pain and severe dyspnea. An air embolus will act as a plug and prevent the normal flow of blood and oxygen to a specific part of the body. The brain and spinal cord are the organs most severely affected by air embolism because they require a constant supply of oxygen.

The following are potential signs and symptoms of an air embolism:

- Blotching (mottling of the skin)
- Froth (often pink or bloody) at the nose and mouth
- Severe pain in muscles, joints, or abdomen
- Dyspnea and/or chest pain
- Dizziness, nausea, and vomiting
- Dysphasia (difficulty speaking)
- Cough
- Cyanosis
- Difficulty with vision
- Paralysis and/or coma
- Irregular pulse and cardiac arrest

## Decompression Sickness

Decompression sickness, commonly called the bends, occurs when bubbles of gas, especially nitrogen, obstruct the blood vessels. This condition results from too rapid an ascent from a dive, too long of a dive at too deep a depth, or repeated dives within a short period of time. During the dive, nitrogen that is being breathed dissolves in the blood and tissues because it is under pressure. When the diver ascends, the external pressure is decreased, and the dissolved nitrogen forms small bubbles within those tissues. These bubbles can lead to problems similar to those that occur in air embolism (blockage of tiny blood vessels, depriving parts of the body of their normal blood supply), but severe pain in certain tissues or spaces in the body is the most common problem.

Similarly, decompression sickness can occur even after a safe dive from driving a car up a mountain or flying in an unpressurized airplane that climbs too rapidly to a great height. However, the risk of this diminishes after 24 to 48 hours.

The most striking symptom is abdominal and/or joint pain so severe that the patient literally doubles over or bends. Dive tables and diving computers are

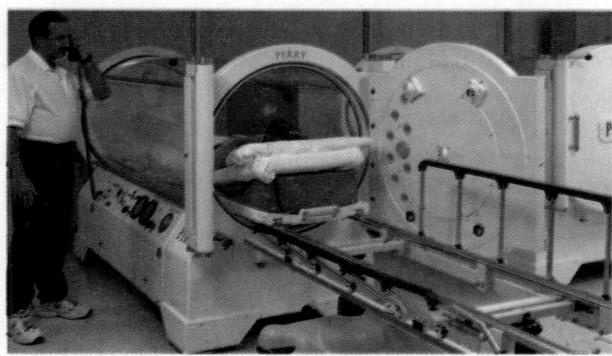

**FIGURE 33-11** A hyperbaric chamber, usually a small room, is pressurized to a level higher than atmospheric pressure and used in the treatment of decompression sickness and air embolism.

Courtesy of Perry Baromedical Corporation.

available to calculate and record the proper rate of ascent from a dive, including the number and length of pauses that a diver should make on the way up. However, even divers who stay within these limits can occasionally experience symptoms of the bends.

You may find it difficult to distinguish between air embolism and decompression sickness. In general, air embolism occurs immediately on return to the surface, whereas the symptoms of decompression sickness may not occur for several hours. The emergency treatment is the same for both. It consists of basic life support (BLS) including supplemental oxygen, followed by recompression in a hyperbaric chamber: a chamber or a small room that is pressurized to a level higher than atmospheric pressure (**FIGURE 33-11**). Recompression treatment allows the bubbles of gas to dissolve into the blood and equalizes the pressures inside and outside the lungs. Once these pressures are equalized, gradual decompression can be accomplished under controlled conditions to prevent the bubbles from re-forming.

## Assessment of Drowning and Diving Emergencies

### Scene Size-up

In managing water emergencies, your standard precautions should include gloves, mask, and eye protection at a minimum. Check for hazards to your crew. Never drive through moving water—even

a small amount can cause the vehicle to be swept away. Use extreme caution when driving through standing water. Never attempt a water rescue without proper training and equipment. Call for additional resources early.

If your patient is still in the water, look for the best, safest means of removal. This may require additional help from search-and-rescue teams or special extrication equipment. Trauma and an associated need to provide spinal motion restriction must be considered when the scene is a recreational setting. Check for additional patients based on where and how the emergency occurred.

As you observe the scene, look for indicators of the MOI. As you put together information from dispatch and your observations of the scene, consider how the MOI produced the injuries suspected.

### Primary Assessment

Use your evaluation of the patient's chief complaint to guide you in your assessment of life threats and determine whether spinal motion restriction is necessary. Pay particular attention to chest pain, dyspnea, and complaints related to sensory changes when a diving emergency is suspected. Determine the patient's level of consciousness using the AVPU scale. Be suspicious of drug and alcohol use and the effects on the patient's level of consciousness.

Standard measures should be taken for any patient found or injured while in the water. Begin with opening the airway and assessing breathing in unresponsive patients. Consider the possibility of spinal trauma and take appropriate actions. The airway may be obstructed with water. Suction according to protocol if the patient has vomited and expect that the patient is likely to vomit during your care and resuscitation. Provide ventilations with a bag-mask device for inadequate breathing. Use an airway adjunct to facilitate bag-mask ventilations as necessary.

If the patient is responsive, provide high-flow oxygen with a nonrebreathing mask. If there is no risk of spinal injury, position the patient to protect the airway from aspiration in the event of vomiting.

Auscultation and frequent reassessment of breath sounds in drowning patients is a key part of your assessment. You may hear diminished sounds or even gurgling sounds from water that has been inhaled. Provide this information, and any changes in the patient's lung sounds, to the ALS providers who may rendezvous with your unit as well as to the receiving facility. Breath sounds are also particularly significant for patients with scuba diving injuries; while the patients ascended to the surface, a pneumothorax or tension pneumothorax may have developed.

Check for a pulse. It may be difficult to find a pulse because of constriction of the peripheral blood vessels and low cardiac output, resulting in cyanosis. Nevertheless, if the pulse is unmeasurable, the patient may be in cardiac arrest. After administering five breaths, begin CPR and apply your automated external defibrillator (AED) according to BLS and the International Liaison Committee on Resuscitation guidelines.

Evaluate the patient for adequate perfusion and treat for shock by maintaining normal body temperature and improving circulation through positioning. The patient's skin may be cold to the touch. If the MOI suggests trauma, assess for bleeding and treat appropriately.

Even if resuscitation in the field appears successful, always transport patients to the hospital. Inhalation of any amount of fluid can lead to delayed complications lasting for days or weeks. Patients with decompression sickness and air embolism must be treated in a recompression chamber. If you live in an area with a significant amount of scuba diving activity, you will have transport protocols for such cases. Usually, the patient will be stabilized in the nearest ED. Perform all interventions en route.

## History Taking

After the life threats have been managed during the primary assessment, investigate the chief complaint. Obtain a medical history and be alert for injury-specific signs and symptoms as well as any pertinent negatives.

Obtain a SAMPLE history with special attention to the dive parameters, including depth, the length of time the patient was underwater, the time of onset of symptoms, and previous diving activity. Note any physical activity, alcohol or drug consumption, and other medical conditions. All of these factors may have an effect on the diving or drowning emergency.

## Secondary Assessment

The secondary assessment is used to uncover injuries that may have been missed during the primary assessment. In some instances, such as a critically injured patient or a short transport time, you may not have time to conduct a secondary assessment.

If the patient is responsive, focus your physical examination on the basis of the chief complaint and the history obtained. This should include a thorough examination of the patient's lungs, including breath sounds.

Prolonged submersion typically results in an unresponsive patient. It is important to begin with a full-body scan in these situations to look for hidden life threats and potential trauma, even if trauma is not suspected. A scuba diver with a possible medical condition should be assessed for indications of decompression sickness or an air embolism. Focus on pain in the joints and the abdomen. Pay attention to whether your patient is getting adequate ventilation and oxygenation, and check for signs of hypothermia.

Time and personnel permitting, complete a detailed assessment en route to the hospital. A careful examination may reveal additional injuries not initially observable. Examine the patient for respiratory, circulatory, and neurologic compromise. A careful distal circulatory, sensory, and motor function examination will be helpful in assessing the extent of the injury. Assess for peripheral pulses, skin color and discoloration, itching, pain, and paresthesia (numbness and tingling).

Check the patient's pulse rate, quality, and rhythm. Pulse and blood pressure may be difficult to palpate in a patient with hypothermia. Check carefully for both peripheral and central pulses, and listen over the chest for a heartbeat if pulses are weak. Check the respiratory rate, quality, and rhythm and listen for breath sounds. Assess and document pupil size and reactivity.

Although it is a valuable tool, oxygen saturation readings may produce a false low reading because of hypoperfusion of the patient's monitoring finger. Shivering also can interfere with obtaining an accurate reading because of excessive movement.

## Reassessment

Repeat the primary assessment. Reassess vital signs and the chief complaint. Are the airway, breathing, and circulation still adequate? Recheck patient interventions. Are your treatments for problems with the ABCs still effective?

The condition of patients who have experienced submersion in water may deteriorate rapidly because of pulmonary injury, fluid shifts in the body, cerebral hypoxia, and hypothermia. Patients with pneumothorax, air embolism, or decompression sickness may decompensate quickly. Assess your patient's mental status constantly, and assess vital signs at least every 5 minutes. Pay particular attention to respirations and breath sounds.

Document the circumstances of the drowning and extrication. The receiving facility personnel will need to know how long the patient was submerged, the temperature of the water, the clarity of the water, and whether there was any possibility of cervical spine injury.

If you respond to a diving incident, the receiving facility personnel will also need a complete dive profile to properly treat your patient. This information may be available in a dive log, on a dive computer, or from the patient's diving partners. If possible, bring all of the diver's equipment to the hospital. It will be helpful in determining the cause of the incident. Be sure to document the disposition of this equipment.

## Emergency Care for Drowning or Diving Emergencies

Treatment for drowning begins with rescue and removal from the water. Provide spinal motion restriction when a fall from a significant height or suspected diving injury has occurred (or if this is a possibility when no information is provided). Artificial ventilation should be provided as soon as possible. Artificial ventilation should only be performed in the water if rapid removal from the water is not possible. Spinal motion restriction must continue while artificial ventilation is being performed. If the patient is not breathing, clear any vomit from the airway manually or with suction and assist ventilations with a bag-mask device or pocket mask. Rolling patients onto their side or performing abdominal thrusts will not remove water from the lungs and should not be done unless the airway is obstructed. Frothy sputum in the patient's airway does *not* require removal with suctioning. When resuscitating a patient who has drowned, the usual CAB order (compressions, airway, breathing) is not used. Rather, address airway and breathing concerns first, beginning with five rescue breaths, then use compressions and use the AED.

If the patient is breathing spontaneously, but has been submerged, administer oxygen (if this was not done as part of the primary assessment). Treat all drowning patients for hypothermia by removing wet clothing and wrapping them in warm blankets.

When treating conscious patients who are suspected of having an air embolism or decompression sickness from scuba diving, follow these accepted treatment steps:

1. Remove the patient from the water. Try to keep the patient calm.

---

## YOU are the Provider

Your partner notifies the hospital and gives the hospital a patient report. You continue active cooling measures and initiate the appropriate shock treatment. When you reassess the patient, you note that his level of consciousness has decreased; he is responsive only to pain. His respirations are still rapid, but are now markedly shallow.

| Recording Time: 11 Minutes | |
| --- | --- |
| Level of consciousness | Responsive only to pain |
| Respirations | 26 breaths/min; shallow |
| Pulse | 126 beats/min; weak and regular |
| Skin | Flushed, hot, and moist |
| Blood pressure | 90/70 mm Hg |
| Spo$_2$ | 89% (on oxygen) |

**7.** How should you adjust your treatment of this patient?

**8.** How will you know when you have adequately cooled the patient?

2. Administer oxygen.
3. Consider the possibility of pneumothorax and monitor the patient's breath sounds for development of a tension pneumothorax.
4. Provide prompt transport to the ED or to the nearest recompression facility for treatment based on local protocols.

Injury from decompression sickness is often reversible with proper treatment. However, if the bubbles block critical blood vessels that supply the brain or spinal cord, permanent central nervous system injury may result. Therefore, the key in emergency management of serious ascent problems is to recognize that an emergency exists and treat as soon as possible. Depending on local protocols, consider transport to a facility with a hyperbaric chamber if there is one near your service area. Remember that aeromedical evacuation for someone who has sustained an injury in ascending from a dive is relatively contraindicated as the decrease in air pressure may worsen the underlying decompression injury.

## Other Water Hazards

Pay close attention to the body temperature of a person who is rescued from cold water. Treat hypothermia caused by immersion in cold water the same way you treat hypothermia caused by cold exposure. Prevent further heat loss from contact with the ground, stretcher, or air, and transport the patient promptly.

A person swimming in shallow water may experience breath-holding syncope, a loss of consciousness caused by a decreased stimulus for breathing. This happens to swimmers who breathe in and out rapidly and deeply before entering the water in an effort to expand their capacity to stay underwater. Whereas this technique increases the swimmer's oxygen level, the hyperventilation involved lowers the carbon dioxide level. Because an elevated level of carbon dioxide in the blood is the strongest stimulus for breathing, the swimmer may not feel the need to breathe even after using up all the oxygen in his or her lungs. This results in drowning. The emergency treatment for a patient with breath-holding syncope is the same as that for a drowning patient.

## Prevention

Each year, many young children drown in residential pools. Appropriate precautions can prevent most submersion incidents. All swimming pools should be surrounded by a fence that is at least 6 feet (2 m) high, with slats no farther apart than 3 inches (8 cm), and self-closing, self-locking gates. The most common problem is a lack of adult supervision. An incident can occur when a child is unattended for only a few seconds. Half of all teenage and adult drownings are associated with alcohol use. As a health care professional, you should be involved in public education efforts to make people aware of the hazards of swimming pools and water recreation.

## High Altitude

High altitudes can cause dysbarism injuries. Dysbarism injuries are any signs and symptoms caused by the difference between the surrounding atmospheric pressure and the total gas pressure in various tissues, fluids, and cavities of the body. Altitude illnesses occur when an unacclimated person is exposed to diminished oxygen pressure in the air at high altitudes. These illnesses affect the central nervous system and pulmonary system, and range from common acute mountain sickness to high-altitude cerebral edema (HACE) and high-altitude pulmonary edema (HAPE).

Acute mountain sickness is caused by diminished oxygen pressure in the air at altitudes above 5,000 feet, resulting in diminished oxygen in the blood (hypoxia). It strikes those who ascend too high too fast and those who have not acclimatized to high altitudes. The signs and symptoms include a headache, lightheadedness, fatigue, loss of appetite, nausea, difficulty sleeping, shortness of breath during physical exertion, and a swollen face. Treatment primarily consists of stopping the ascent and descending to a lower altitude, and administering oxygen if the patient is dyspneic. However, consider other possible causes for the same symptoms, such as hypoglycemia or carbon monoxide poisoning from a camping stove.

With HAPE, fluid collects in the lungs, hindering the passage of oxygen into the bloodstream. It can occur at altitudes of 8,000 feet or greater. The signs and symptoms include shortness of breath, cough with pink sputum, cyanosis, and a rapid pulse.

HACE usually occurs in climbers and may accompany HAPE; it can quickly become life threatening. The signs and symptoms include a severe, constant, throbbing headache; ataxia (lack of muscle coordination and balance); extreme fatigue; vomiting; and loss of consciousness. The symptoms of HACE and HAPE may overlap.

In the field, treatment for HAPE and/or HACE consists of descending to a lower altitude. During the descent, begin providing oxygen, and promptly transport to an appropriate facility. For inadequate respirations, provide positive pressure ventilation with a bag-mask device. If local protocols allow, continuous positive airway pressure may be helpful for a patient with respiratory distress from HAPE.

# Lightning

According to the National Weather Service, there are an estimated 25 million cloud-to-ground lightning flashes in the United States each year. On average, lightning kills between 20 and 30 people per year in the United States based on documented cases. This number has decreased over the past several years. Although documented lightning injuries in the United States average about 300 per year, undocumented lightning injuries are likely much higher. Lightning is the fifth most common cause of death from isolated environmental phenomena.

The energy associated with lightning comprises direct current of up to 200,000 amps and a potential of 100 million volts or more. Temperatures generated from lightning vary between 20,000°F and 60,000°F (11,000°C and 33,000°C).

Most deaths and injuries caused by lightning occur during the summer months when people are enjoying outdoor activities, despite an approaching thunderstorm. Those most commonly struck by lightning include boaters, swimmers, and golfers. Any type of activity that exposes the person to a large, open area increases the risk of being struck by lightning.

Whether or not lightning injures or kills depends on whether a person is in the path of the lightning discharge. The current associated with the lightning discharge travels along the ground. Although some people are injured or killed by a direct lightning strike, many people are indirectly struck when standing near an object that has been struck by lightning, such as a tree (splash effect).

The cardiovascular and nervous systems are most commonly injured during a lightning strike; therefore, respiratory or cardiac arrest is the most common cause of lightning-related deaths. The tissue damage caused by lightning is different from that caused by other electric-related injuries (ie, high-voltage power line injuries) because the tissue damage pathway usually occurs over the skin, rather than through it. During your assessment, look for not only the entrance wound but also the exit wound. The exit wound does not necessarily occur on the same side of the body. Additionally, because the duration of a lightning strike is short, skin burns are usually superficial; full-thickness (third-degree) burns are rare. Lightning injuries are categorized as being mild, moderate, or severe:

- **Mild.** Loss of consciousness, amnesia, confusion, tingling, and other nonspecific signs and symptoms. Burns, if present, are typically superficial.
- **Moderate.** Seizures, respiratory arrest, dysrhythmias that spontaneously resolve, and superficial burns.
- **Severe.** Cardiopulmonary arrest. Because of the delay in resuscitation, often the result of occurrence in a remote location, many of these patients do not survive.

## Emergency Medical Care

As with any scene response, your priority is safety. Take measures to protect yourself and your partner from being struck by lightning, especially if the thunderstorm is still in progress. Contrary to popular belief, lightning can, and does, strike in the same place twice. Move the patient to a place of safety, preferably in a sheltered area.

If you are in an open area and adequate shelter is unavailable, it is important to recognize the signs of an impending lightning strike and take immediate action to protect yourself. If you suddenly feel a tingling sensation or your hair stands on end, the area around you has become charged—a sure sign of an imminent lightning strike. Make yourself as small a target as possible by squatting down into a ball, with as little of your body as possible touching the ground. If you are standing near a tree or other tall object, move away as fast as possible, preferably to a low-lying area. Lightning tends to strike objects that project from the ground (ie, trees, fences, buildings).

The process of triaging multiple victims of a lightning strike is different than the conventional triage methods used during a mass-casualty incident (see Chapter 40, *Incident Management*). When a person is struck by lightning, respiratory or cardiac arrest, if it occurs, usually occurs immediately. Delayed respiratory or cardiac arrest is much less likely to develop in those who are conscious following a lightning strike; most of these people will survive. Therefore, you should focus your efforts on those who are in respiratory or cardiac arrest. This process, called **reverse triage**, differs from conventional triage, where such patients would ordinarily be classified as deceased.

When a person is struck by lightning, it causes massive direct current shock, with the patient experiencing massive muscle spasms (tetany) that can result in fractures of long bones and spinal vertebrae. Therefore, manually stabilize the patient's head in a neutral in-line position and open the airway with the jaw-thrust maneuver. If the patient is in respiratory arrest with a pulse, begin immediate bag-mask ventilations with 100% oxygen. If the patient is in cardiac arrest, begin CPR, attach an AED as soon as possible and provide defibrillation if indicated. If severe bleeding is present, control it immediately.

Transport the patient to the closest appropriate facility. If CPR or ventilations are not required, address other injuries (ie, splint fractures, dress and bandage burns) and provide continuous monitoring while en route to the hospital. A patient with signs and symptoms of a lightning strike, but no obvious life threats, should still be transported to the ED for evaluation.

# Bites and Envenomation

This section discusses bites and stings from spiders, hymenoptera, snakes, scorpions, and ticks, and injuries from marine animals.

## Spider Bites

Spiders are numerous and widespread in the United States. Many species of spiders bite. However, only two, the female black widow spider and the brown recluse spider, are able to deliver serious, even life-threatening bites. When you care for a patient who has had some type of bite, be alert to the possibility that the spider may still be in the area, although it is unlikely. Remember that your safety is of paramount importance.

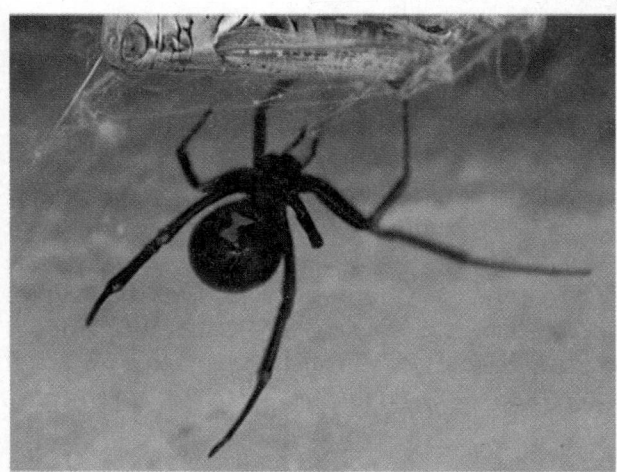

**FIGURE 33-12** Black widow spiders are distinguished by their glossy black color and bright red-orange hourglass marking on the abdomen.

© Crystal Kirk/ShutterStock.

## Black Widow Spider

The female black widow spider (*Latrodectus*) is fairly large, measuring approximately 2 inches (5 cm) long with its legs extended. It is usually black and has a distinctive, bright red-orange marking in the shape of an hourglass on its abdomen (**FIGURE 33-12**). The female black widow spider is larger and more toxic than the male. Black widow spiders are found in every state except Alaska. They prefer dry, dim places around buildings, in woodpiles, and among debris.

The bite of the black widow spider is sometimes overlooked. If the site becomes numb right away, the patient may not even recall being bit. However, most black widow spider bites cause localized pain and symptoms, including agonizing muscle spasms. In some cases, a bite on the abdomen causes muscle spasms so severe that the patient may be thought to have an acute abdominal condition, possibly peritonitis. The main danger with this type of bite, however, is that the black widow's venom can damage nerve tissues (it is a neurotoxin). Other systemic symptoms include dizziness, sweating, nausea, vomiting, and rashes. Tightness in the chest and difficulty breathing develop within 24 hours, as well as severe cramps, with boardlike rigidity of the abdominal muscles. Generally, these signs and symptoms subside over 48 hours.

If necessary, a physician can administer a specific **antivenin**, a serum containing antibodies that counteract the venom, but because of a high incidence of side effects, its use is reserved for severe bites, for older or feeble patients, and for children younger than 5 years. In children, these bites can be fatal. In general, emergency treatment of a black widow spider bite consists of BLS for the patient in respiratory distress. More often, the patient will only require pain relief. Transport the patient to the ED as soon as possible for treatment. If possible, safely bring the spider to the hospital or take a photo of the spider with a cell phone and send it to the hospital ahead of time so that it can be definitively identified.

## Brown Recluse Spider

The brown recluse spider (*Loxosceles*) is dull brown and, at 1 inch (3 cm), smaller than the black widow (**FIGURE 33-13**). The short-haired body has a violin-shaped mark, brown to yellow in color, on its back. Although the brown recluse spider lives mostly in the southern and central parts of the country, it may be found throughout the continental United States. The spider takes its name from the fact that it tends to live in dark areas—in corners of old, unused buildings, under rocks, and in woodpiles. In cooler areas, it moves indoors to closets, drawers, cellars, and clothing.

In contrast to the venom of the black widow spider, the venom of the brown recluse spider is not

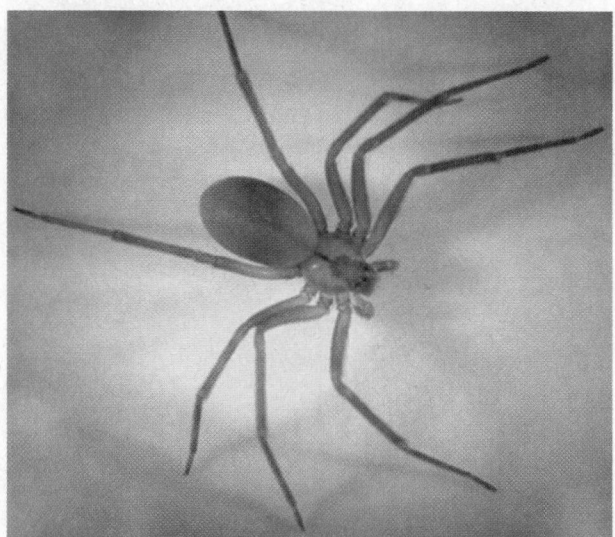

**FIGURE 33-13** Brown recluse spiders are dull brown and have a dark, violin-shaped mark on the back.

Courtesy of Kenneth Cramer, Monmouth College.

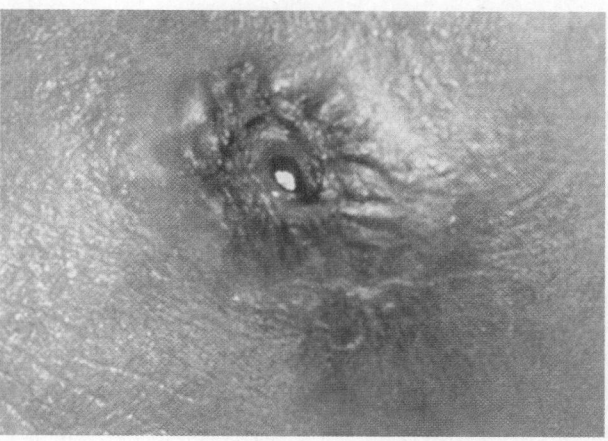

**FIGURE 33-14** The bite of a brown recluse spider is characterized by swelling, tenderness, and a pale, mottled, cyanotic center. There may also be a small blister on the bite.

Courtesy of Department of Entomology, University of Nebraska.

neurotoxic but cytotoxic; that is, it causes severe local tissue damage. Typically, the bite is not painful at first but becomes so within hours. The area becomes swollen and tender, developing a pale, mottled, cyanotic center and possibly a small blister (**FIGURE 33-14**). Over the next several days, a scab of dead skin, fat, and debris forms and digs down into the skin, producing a large ulcer that may not heal unless treated promptly. Transport patients with such symptoms as soon as possible.

Brown recluse spider bites rarely cause systemic symptoms and signs. When they do, provide BLS and prompt transport to the ED. Again, it is helpful if you can identify the spider and either safely bring it to the hospital with the patient, or take a picture of the spider and send it to the hospital ahead of time. Because symptoms do not typically develop for hours after the bite occurs, this is usually not possible.

## Hymenoptera Stings

Typically hymenoptera (bees, wasps, yellowjackets, and ants) stings are painful but are not a medical emergency. Remove the stinger and, if still present, the venom sac. This is best done by using a firm-edged item such as a credit card to scrape the stinger and sac off the skin. Use ice packs to assist in controlling pain from a hymenoptera sting.

If the patient is allergic to the venom, then anaphylaxis may occur. The signs and symptoms of anaphylaxis are flushed skin, low blood pressure, and difficulty breathing that is usually associated with reactive airway sounds such as wheezes, or in severe cases, diminished or absent breath sounds. Hives (urticaria) may develop near the site of envenomation or centrally on the body. The patient can also have swelling to the throat and tongue. Anaphylaxis is a true emergency and can be fatal if not recognized and treated quickly. If anaphylaxis develops, be prepared to assist the patient in administering an epinephrine auto-injector (EpiPen). Also be prepared to support the airway and breathing should the patient experience significant respiratory compromise. Chapter 21, *Allergy and Anaphylaxis,* has a detailed discussion of the treatment of anaphylaxis.

## Snake Bites

Snake bites are a worldwide problem. According to the World Health Organization, more than 400,000 injuries from venomous snake bites occur annually, including at least 20,000 deaths. However, snake bite fatalities in the United States are extremely rare: approximately 15 per year for the entire country.

Of the approximately 115 different species of snakes in the United States, only 19 are venomous. These include the rattlesnake (*Crotalus*); the copperhead (*Agkistrodon contortrix*); the cottonmouth, or water moccasin (*Agkistrodon piscivorus*); and the coral snakes (*Micrurus fulvius* and *Micruroides euryxanthus*) (**FIGURE 33-15**). At least one of these venomous species is found in every state except Alaska, Hawaii, and Maine. As a general rule, these snakes are timid. They usually do not bite unless provoked or accidentally injured, as when they are stepped on. There are a few exceptions to these rules. Cottonmouths are often aggressive, and rattlesnakes are easily provoked. Coral snakes, in contrast, usually bite only when they are being handled.

Most snake bites occur between April and October, when the animals are active, and tend to involve young men who have been drinking alcohol. Texas reports the largest number of bites. Other states with a major concentration of snake bites are Louisiana,

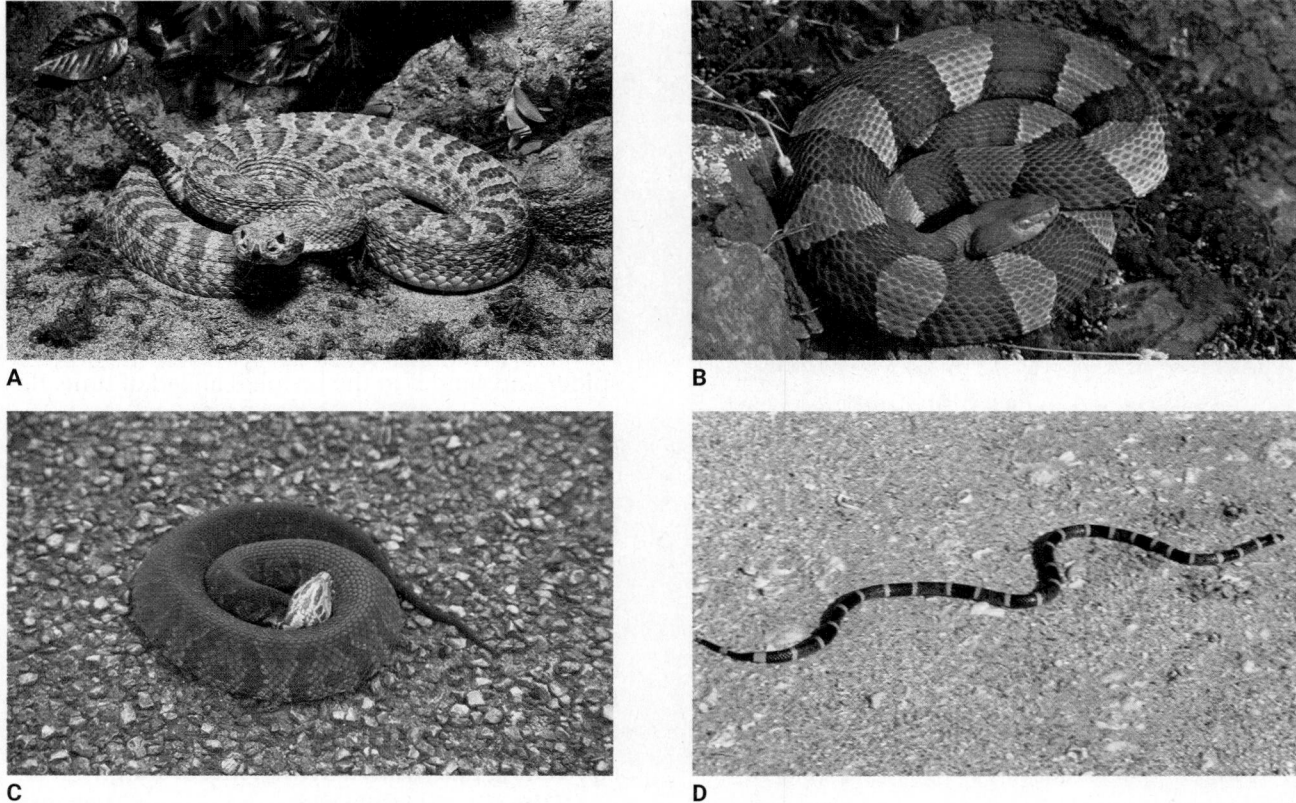

**FIGURE 33-15 A.** Rattlesnake. **B.** Copperhead. **C.** Cottonmouth (water moccasin). **D.** Coral snake.

Georgia, Oklahoma, North Carolina, Arkansas, West Virginia, and Mississippi. If you work in one of these areas, you should be thoroughly familiar with the emergency handling of snake bites. Remember, almost any time you are caring for a patient with a snake bite, another snake may be in the area and create a second victim—you. Therefore, use extreme caution on these calls and be sure to wear the proper protective equipment for the area.

In general, only one-third of snake bites result in significant local or systemic injuries. Often, envenomation does not occur because the snake has recently struck another animal and exhausted its supply of venom for the time being.

Venomous snakes native to the United States all have hollow fangs in the roof of the mouth that inject the venom from two sacs at the back of the head. The classic appearance of the venomous snake bite, therefore, is two small puncture wounds, usually about 0.5 inch (1 cm) apart, with discoloration and swelling, and the patient usually reports pain surrounding the bite (**FIGURE 33-16**). Fang marks are a clear indication of a venomous snake bite. A snake bite with other tooth marks may be from a nonvenomous snake. If you are unsure whether the snake was venomous, proceed as if it was, especially if the patient exhibits other signs and symptoms.

A person who has been bitten by any venomous snake needs prompt transport. Also, notify the hospital as soon as possible if a patient has been bitten by a pit viper or coral snake. Some venoms can cause paralysis of the nervous system, and hospitals may not have appropriate antivenin on hand.

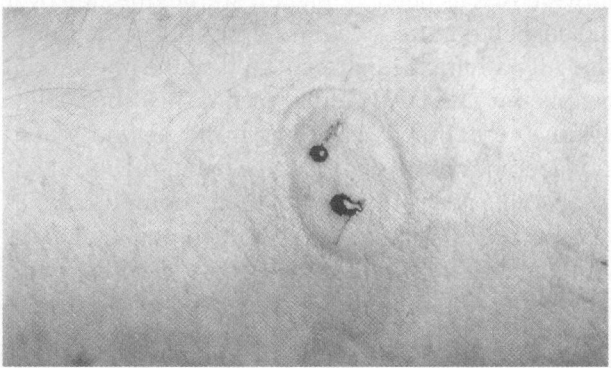

**FIGURE 33-16** A snake bite wound from a poisonous snake has characteristic markings: two small puncture wounds about 0.5 inch (1 cm) apart, discoloration, and swelling.

© Dorling Kindersley ltd/Alamy Stock Photo.

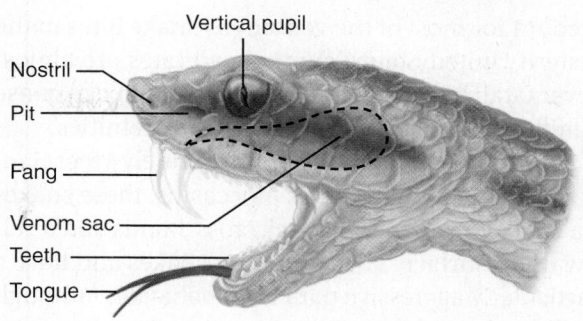

**FIGURE 33-17** Pit vipers have small, heat-sensing organs (pits) located in front of their eyes that allow them to strike at warm targets, even in the dark.

© Jones & Bartlett Learning.

## Pit Vipers

Rattlesnakes, copperheads, and cottonmouths are all pit vipers, with triangular-shaped, flat heads (**FIGURE 33-17**). They take their name from the small pits located just behind each nostril and in front of each eye. The pit is a heat-sensing organ that allows the snake to strike accurately at any warm target, especially in the dark, when it cannot see through its vertical, slit-like pupils.

The fangs of the pit viper normally lie flat against the roof of the mouth and are hinged to swing back and forth as the mouth opens. When the snake strikes, the mouth opens wide and the fangs extend; in this way, the fangs penetrate whatever the mouth strikes. The fangs are hollow teeth that act like hypodermic needles. They are connected to a sac containing a reservoir of venom, which in turn is attached to a poison gland. The gland itself is a specifically adapted salivary gland, which produces enzymes that digest and destroy tissue. The primary purpose of the venom is to kill small animals and facilitate the digestive process.

In the United States, the most common form of pit viper is the rattlesnake. Several different species of rattlesnake can be identified by the rattle on the tail. The rattle is numerous layers of dried skin that were shed but failed to fall off, coming to rest against a small knob on the end of the tail. Rattlesnakes have many patterns of color, often with a diamond pattern. They can grow to 6 feet (2 m) or longer.

Copperheads are smaller than rattlesnakes, usually 2 to 3 feet long (60 to 90 cm) with a red-copper color crossed with brown or red bands. These snakes typically inhabit woodpiles and abandoned dwellings, often close to areas of habitation. Although they account for most of the venomous snake bites in the eastern United States, copperhead bites are almost never fatal; however, note that the venom can cause significant damage to tissues in the extremities.

Cottonmouths grow to approximately 4 feet (1 m) in length. Also called water moccasins, these snakes are olive or brown, with black cross-bands and a yellow undersurface. They are water snakes and have a particularly aggressive pattern of behavior. Although fatalities from these snake bites are rare, tissue destruction from the venom may be severe.

The signs of envenomation by a pit viper are severe burning pain at the site of the injury, followed by swelling and a blue discoloration (ecchymosis) in light-skinned people that signals bleeding under the skin. Bluish discoloration may be more difficult to see in dark-skinned people. These signs are evident within 5 to 10 minutes after the bite has occurred and last over the next 36 hours. In addition to destroying tissues locally, the venom of the pit viper can interfere with the body's clotting mechanism and cause bleeding at various distant sites. This toxin affects the entire nervous system. Other systemic signs, which may or may not occur, include weakness, nausea, vomiting, sweating, seizures, fainting, vision problems, changes in level of consciousness, and shock. If swelling has occurred, use a pen to mark its edges on the skin. This will allow physicians to assess the timing and extent of the swelling with greater accuracy. If the patient has no local signs an hour after being bitten, it is likely that envenomation did not take place.

The toxicity is related to the amount of toxin injected. A bite will affect children more than adults because there is less body mass to absorb the toxin. The same principle holds true for a small-statured adult.

In treating a snake bite from a pit viper, follow these steps:

1. Calm the patient; assure him or her that venomous snake bites are rarely fatal. Place the patient in a supine position and explain that staying still will slow the spread of any venom through the system. Determine the approximate time of the bite and document your time en route to a receiving facility. This time from onset to evaluation at the facility is one of the criteria used in grading the severity of the incident and in determining the amount of antivenin to be used.

2. Locate the bite area; clean it gently with soap and water or a mild antiseptic. Do not apply ice to the area.

3. If the bite occurred on an arm or leg and the transport time to the hospital is anticipated to exceed 2 hours, consider the use of a pressure immobilization bandage of the extremity (eg, 40 to 70 mm Hg in the arms and 55 to 70 mm Hg in the legs) and then place the affected extremity below the level of the heart.

4. Be alert for an anaphylactic reaction to the venom and treat with an epinephrine auto-injector, as appropriate.

5. Do not give anything by mouth, and be alert for vomiting.

6. If, as rarely happens, the patient was bitten on the trunk, keep him or her supine and quiet and transport as quickly as possible.

7. Monitor the patient's vital signs and mark the skin with a pen over the area that is swollen, proximal to the swelling, to note whether swelling is spreading.

8. If there are any signs of shock, place the patient supine and administer oxygen.

9. If the snake has been killed, as is often the case, be sure to bring it with you in a secure, hard-sided container so that physicians can identify it and administer the proper antivenin. Alternatively, take a picture of the snake with a cell phone and send it to the hospital ahead of time.

10. Notify the hospital that you are bringing in a patient who has a snake bite; if possible, describe the snake.

11. Transport the patient promptly to the hospital.

If the patient shows no sign of envenomation, provide BLS as needed, place a sterile dressing over the suspected bite area, and immobilize the injury site. All patients with a suspected snake bite should be taken to the ED, whether or not they show signs of envenomation. Treat the wound as you would any deep puncture wound to prevent infection.

Familiarize yourself with the venomous snakes in your region, as well as local protocols for handling snake bites. There may be specific hospitals where antivenin is more readily available, either in the facility or through zoos, health departments, or other services.

## Coral Snakes

The coral snake is a small reptile with a series of bright red, yellow, and black bands completely encircling the body. Many harmless snakes have similar coloring, but only the coral snake has red and yellow bands next to one another, as this helpful rhyme suggests: "Red on yellow will kill a fellow; red on black, venom will lack."

A rare creature that lives in most southern states and in the Southwest, the coral snake is a relative of the cobra. It has tiny fangs and injects the venom with its teeth by a chewing motion, leaving behind one or more puncture or scratch-like wounds. Because of its small mouth and teeth and limited jaw expansion, the coral snake usually bites its victims on a small part of the body, such as a finger or toe.

Coral snake venom is a powerful toxin that causes paralysis of the nervous system. Within a few hours of being bitten, a patient may exhibit bizarre behavior, followed by progressive paralysis of eye movements and respiration. Often, there are limited or no local symptoms.

Successful treatment, either emergency or long term, depends on positive identification of the snake and support of respiration. Antivenin is also available for coral snake bites, but most hospitals do not stock it. Therefore, you should notify the receiving hospital of the need for it as soon as possible. The steps for emergency care of a coral snake bite are the same as a pit viper bite.

## Scorpion Stings

Scorpions are eight-legged arthropods from the class Arachnida. They have a venom gland and a stinger at the end of their tail (**FIGURE 33-18**).

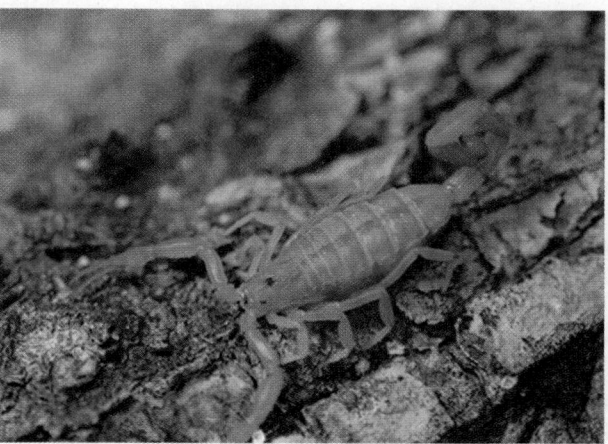

**FIGURE 33-18** The sting of a scorpion is usually more painful than it is dangerous, causing localized swelling and discoloration.
© Visual & Written SL/Alamy Stock Photo.

Scorpions are rare; they live primarily in the southwestern United States and in deserts. With one exception, a scorpion's sting is usually very painful but not dangerous, causing localized swelling and discoloration. The exception is the *Centruroides sculpturatus*. Although it is found naturally in Arizona and New Mexico, as well as parts of Texas, California, and Nevada, it may be kept as a pet by anyone. The venom of this particular species may produce a severe systemic reaction that leads to circulatory collapse, severe muscle contractions, excessive salivation, hypertension, convulsions, and cardiac failure. Antivenin is available but

## YOU are the Provider

The patient's level of consciousness appears to have improved and he is now resisting your attempts to assist his ventilations. After reapplying the nonrebreathing mask, you reassess his vital signs and clinical condition. His skin, although still very warm, does not feel as hot as it did initially; it also appears less flushed. You will arrive at the hospital in approximately 5 minutes.

| Recording Time: 16 Minutes | |
| --- | --- |
| **Level of consciousness** | Confused; somewhat combative |
| **Respirations** | 22 breaths/min; depth has improved |
| **Pulse** | 120 beats/min and regular; appears to be stronger |
| **Skin** | Less flushed, very warm to the touch, moist |
| **Blood pressure** | 98/58 mm Hg |
| **Spo$_2$** | 94% (on oxygen) |

**9.** What other conditions should you consider as potential causes of the patient's altered mental status?

must be administered by a physician. If you are called to care for a patient with a suspected sting from *C sculpturatus*, notify the receiving hospital as early as possible to facilitate the availability of this antivenin. Administer BLS and provide rapid transport to the ED.

## Tick Bites

Found most often on brush, shrubs, trees, sand dunes, or other animals, ticks usually attach themselves directly to the skin (**FIGURE 33-19**). Only a fraction of an inch (about 3 mm) long, they can easily be mistaken for a freckle, especially because their bite is not painful. Indeed, the danger with a tick bite is not from the bite itself, but from the infecting organisms that the tick carries. Two infectious diseases, Rocky Mountain spotted fever and Lyme disease, are transmitted to humans by ticks. Both are spread through the tick's saliva, which is injected into the skin when the tick attaches itself. The longer a tick stays embedded, the greater the chance that a disease will be transmitted.

Rocky Mountain spotted fever, which is not limited to the Rocky Mountains area, occurs within 7 to 10 days after a bite by an infected tick. Its symptoms include nausea, vomiting, headache, weakness, paralysis, and possible cardiorespiratory collapse.

Lyme disease has received extensive publicity. Lyme disease was originally seen only in the town of Lyme, Connecticut. According to the Centers for Disease Control and Prevention, it has now been reported in all states except for Hawaii. It occurs most

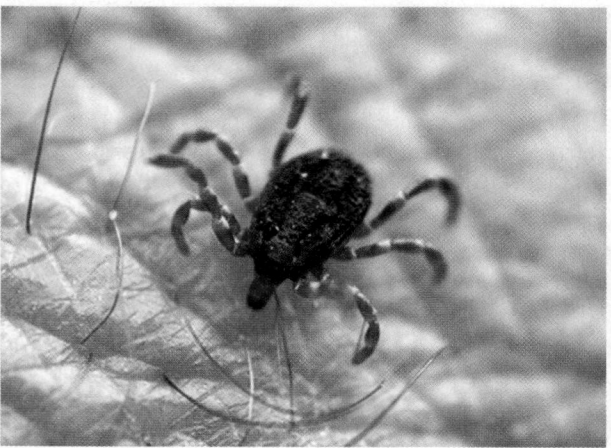

**FIGURE 33-19** Ticks typically attach themselves directly to the skin.

© Joao Estevao A. Freitas (jefras)/ShutterStock.

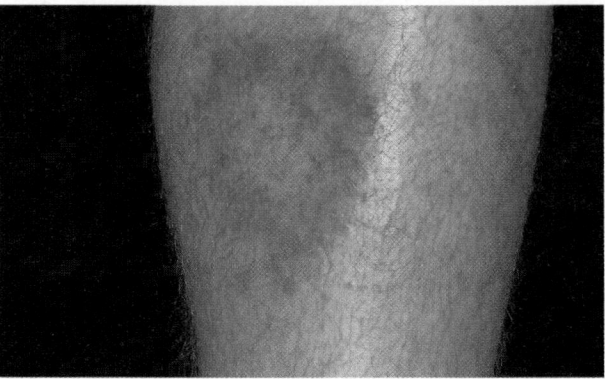

**FIGURE 33-20** The rash associated with Lyme disease has a characteristic bull's-eye pattern.

© E. M. Singletary, MD. Used with permission.

commonly in the Northeast and the Great Lakes states; Pennsylvania reported the largest number of cases from 2011 to 2013. The first symptoms are generally fever and flulike symptoms, sometimes associated with a bull's-eye rash that may spread to several parts of the body (**FIGURE 33-20**). After a few days or weeks, painful swelling of the joints, particularly the knees, occurs. Lyme disease may be confused with rheumatoid arthritis and, like that disease, may result in permanent disability. However, if it is recognized and treated promptly with antibiotics, the patient may recover completely.

Tick bites occur most commonly during the summer months, when people are out in the woods wearing little protective clothing. Do not attempt to suffocate the tick with gasoline or petroleum jelly, or burn it with a lighted match; you will only increase the risk of infection or burn the patient. For patients in conventional EMS settings with tick bites or signs and symptoms of Lyme disease, provide any necessary supportive emergency care and transport the patient for further evaluation. In a situation (such as wilderness EMS) where access to care is delayed, remove the tick from the patient. Using fine tweezers, grasp the tick by the head and pull gently but firmly straight up so that the skin is tented. Hold this position until the tick releases. Special tweezers are available for this, but are unnecessary. This method will usually remove the whole tick. (Partial removal can lead to infection.) Cleanse the area with antiseptic and save the tick in a glass jar or other container so that it can be identified. Do not handle the tick with your fingers. The patient should follow up with his or her health care provider as soon as possible.

# Injuries From Marine Animals

Coelenterates, including fire coral, Portuguese man-of-war, sea wasp, sea nettles, true jellyfish, sea anemones, true coral, and soft coral, are responsible for more envenomations than any other marine animals (**FIGURE 33-21**). The stinging cells of the coelenterate are called nematocysts, and large animals may discharge hundreds of thousands of them. Envenomation causes very painful, red lesions in light-skinned people extending in a line from the site of the sting. These lesions may be more difficult to see in dark-skinned people. Systemic symptoms include headache, dizziness, muscle cramps, and fainting.

To treat a sting from the tentacles of a jellyfish, a Portuguese man-of-war, various anemones, corals, or hydras, remove the patient from the water and

| TABLE 33-4 Common Marine Envenomations | | |
|---|---|---|
| Dogfish | Marine snail | Starfish |
| Dragonfish | Portuguese man-of-war | Stingray |
| Fire coral | Ratfish | Stonefish |
| Hydroid | Scorpion fish | Tiger fish |
| Jellyfish | Sea anemone | Toadfish |
| Lionfish | Sea urchin | Weever fish |

© Jones & Bartlett Learning.

remove the tentacles by scraping them off with the edge of a stiff object, such as a credit card. Do not try to manipulate the remaining tentacles; this will only cause further discharge of the nematocysts. On very rare occasions, a patient may have a systemic allergic reaction to the sting of one of these animals. Treat such a patient for anaphylactic shock and provide rapid transport to the hospital.

Toxins from the spines of urchins, stingrays, and certain spiny fish such as the lionfish, scorpion fish, or stonefish are also heat sensitive (**TABLE 33-4**). Therefore, the best treatment for such injuries is also to soak the affected extremity in hot water for 30 minutes. This will often provide dramatic relief from local pain. However, the patient still needs to be transported to the ED because an allergic reaction or infection, including tetanus, could develop.

If you work near the ocean, you should be familiar with the marine life in your area. The emergency treatment of common coelenterate envenomations consists of the following steps:

1. Limit further discharge of nematocysts by avoiding fresh water, wet sand, showers, or careless manipulation of the tentacles. Keep the patient calm, and reduce motion of the affected extremity.
2. Remove the remaining tentacles by scraping them off with the edge of a stiff object such as a credit card. Do not use your ungloved hand to remove the tentacles, because self-envenomation will occur. Persistent pain may respond to immersion in hot water (110°F to 115°F [43.3°C to 46.1°C]) for 30 minutes. If available, immersion in vinegar may also help alleviate the symptoms.
3. Provide transport to the ED.

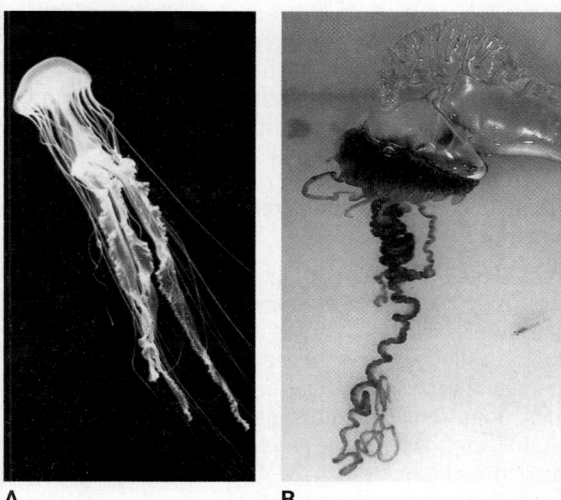

A    B

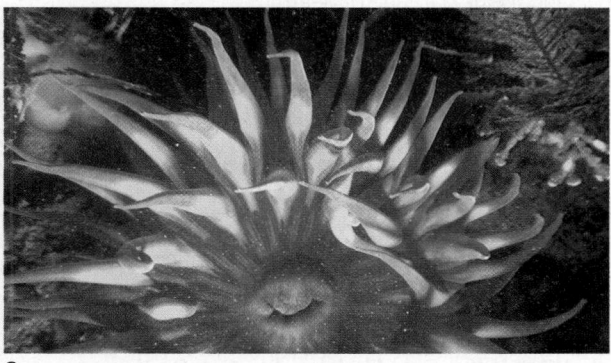

C

**FIGURE 33-21** Coelenterates are responsible for many marine envenomations. **A.** Jellyfish. **B.** Portuguese man-of-war. **C.** Sea anemone.

A: © Creatas/Alamy Stock Photo; B: Courtesy of NOAA; C: Photos.com.

**1. How does the body normally balance heat production and elimination?**

Normal core temperature—the temperature of the heart, lungs, and other vital organs—is usually around 98°F (36.7°C). A series of regulatory mechanisms keep this internal temperature constant, regardless of the ambient temperature (the temperature of the surrounding environment). However, heat elimination must balance heat production; if it does not, a temperature-related emergency occurs.

There are several ways the body removes excess heat, the most efficient of which are sweating (especially through evaporation of the sweat) and dilation of the blood vessels. Ordinarily, the heat-regulating mechanisms of the body work very well and people are able to tolerate significant temperature changes. People can also assist their bodies with heat elimination by removing heat-retaining clothing or by moving to a cooler environment.

**2. What factors can decrease the body's ability to eliminate excess heat?**

Several factors can decrease a person's ability to eliminate excess heat. If air temperature is high, heat loss by radiation is reduced. Heat travels from a warmer place to a cooler place; if the ambient temperature is higher than body temperature, heat will move from the environment and into the body. If the relative humidity, the amount of moisture in the air, is high, heat loss by evaporation is reduced. Heat elimination is most impaired when both the air temperature and relative humidity are high.

Vigorous exercise causes a loss of fluids and electrolytes, resulting in dehydration. People who have an inadequate intake of water can also become dehydrated. Dehydration decreases heat loss through sweating and evaporation.

Small children and older patients exhibit poor thermoregulation; therefore, they are less able to eliminate excess body heat. Additionally, the body's water content decreases with age, which reduces the ability to sweat.

Certain medical conditions, such as heart disease, chronic obstructive pulmonary disease, diabetes, dehydration, and obesity, interfere with the process of body heat elimination. In addition, alcohol and certain drugs, including medications that dehydrate the body (ie, diuretics) or decrease the ability of the body to sweat, reduce heat elimination from the body.

**3. What risk factors does this patient have that predispose him to a heat emergency?**

Your patient has several risk factors for a heat emergency, the single most significant of which is prolonged exertion in a hot, humid environment. Also, the patient has not been drinking any water. Combining his inadequate intake of fluid with the profuse sweating that occurs during exposure to a hot environment, you should suspect that he is dehydrated.

The patient's past medical history also predisposes him to a heat emergency. Diabetes is a systemic condition that impairs many body functions, including thermoregulation, as well as fluid regulation if blood sugar levels are high. The patient also has hypertension, for which diuretics, such as the furosemide in this case, are often prescribed. Diuretics promote urination, further contributing to his dehydration.

**4. What type of heat emergency do you suspect he is experiencing? Why?**

There are several clinical findings that indicate your patient is experiencing the most serious heat illness, heatstroke. Unlike other less severe forms of heat illness (eg, heat cramps, heat exhaustion), patients with heatstroke have an altered level of consciousness, ranging from confusion to coma, and flushed, hot skin. Your patient has both of these. Untreated heatstroke causes permanent brain and tissue damage; in most cases, it causes death.

**5. What specific treatment is required for this patient?**

Immediate treatment of heatstroke includes moving the patient to a cool environment and administering oxygen. Further treatment is aimed at actively cooling the patient. Unless there are extenuating circumstances that will delay your transport, active cooling measures should be performed en route to the hospital. Heatstroke is a true emergency; it requires rapid cooling and rapid transport. Any delays in providing treatment increase the potential for permanent brain and tissue damage or death.

Remove the patient's clothes because they can trap heat or interfere with evaporation of sweat from the skin or with contact of cooler air with the patient's body. Place cold packs at the patient's groin and axillae and behind the neck. Spray or pour saline on the patient and aggressively fan him; this measure, in conjunction with the air conditioner, will facilitate heat loss through convection and evaporation.

Continue to actively cool the patient and notify the receiving facility early so the facility can continue treatment immediately on your arrival.

**6. What is the most likely explanation for this patient's vital signs?**

Your patient's vital signs—tachypnea, tachycardia, and hypotension—indicate shock. This is because heatstroke is associated with a severe loss of fluids and electrolytes, which results in hypovolemia. You should expect that patients with heatstroke will be

## YOU are the Provider SUMMARY *continued*

tachypneic and tachycardic because of all the heat energy they have in their body. This response alone may enable patients to start to compensate for the severe fluid loss that occurs with heatstroke. The presence of hypotension, however, indicates that the body's compensatory mechanisms have failed (decompensated shock).

Patients with hypovolemic shock associated with heatstroke will need intravenous fluids and other treatment aimed at correcting electrolyte abnormalities at the hospital. Consider an ALS intercept, but do not delay transport to do this. AEMTs and paramedics are able to establish intravenous lines and administer fluids, but this is less emergent than cooling. Otherwise, continue high-flow oxygen and closely monitor the patient.

**7. How should you adjust your treatment of this patient?**

Your patient's level of consciousness has deteriorated, and his respirations are now shallow. Furthermore, his oxygen saturation level has decreased to 89%. These clinical signs indicate that your patient is no longer breathing adequately. This can result in hypoxia and a decreased ability to remove heat from the body. Some heat is removed from the body during the exhalation phase of respiration.

Patients with inadequate breathing need assisted breathing with a bag-mask device and high-flow oxygen. In addition to actively cooling the patient, ensure that oxygenation and ventilation remain adequate. Consider inserting an airway adjunct to assist in maintaining airway patency. In this case, a nasal airway is the best choice because the patient is not completely unconscious and likely has an intact gag reflex.

**8. How will you know when you have adequately cooled the patient?**

Ideally, you should monitor the patient's CBT; this is most reliably obtained by assessing the patient's

rectal temperature, if local protocols allow. It is important to note that the CBT increases rapidly in patients with heatstroke, but does not decrease as quickly, even with aggressive cooling measures. Therefore, you will likely have to actively cool the patient throughout the entire transport, unless the destination hospital is a great distance away.

Follow your local protocols or contact online medical control regarding the target temperature that you should attempt to achieve. If your protocols do not allow you to monitor a patient's CBT rectally, an axillary temperature should be assessed, although it is less accurate.

If you are unable to monitor the patient's CBT, frequently reassess his skin temperature during the cooling process. Does it feel as hot as it was initially, or does it seem to be cooler than it was before? It is important to frequently assess the effectiveness of your interventions.

When actively cooling a patient with heatstroke, do not cool him or her to the point of shivering. Shivering generates more heat and can occur when cooling is not monitored closely.

**9. What other conditions should you consider as potential causes of the patient's altered mental status?**

Altered mental status may be associated with heatstroke alone or could be the result of a completely different problem. An increase in heat energy causes the body to expend a lot of glucose; therefore, consider the possibility of hypoglycemia, especially because this patient has diabetes, which increases that risk. You should also consider the possibility of a head injury. Recall that the patient apparently fainted. When this occurred, he may have fallen and struck his head, resulting in a concussion or intracranial hemorrhage. Do not rule out an occult head injury in the absence of obvious signs of trauma.

### EMS Patient Care Report (PCR)

| Date: 8-11-20 | Incident No.: 013010 | Nature of Call: Fainting | | Location: 1102 Rosewood Avenue | |
| --- | --- | --- | --- | --- | --- |
| Dispatched: 1415 | En Route: 1415 | At Scene: 1422 | Transport: 1430 | At Hospital: 1443 | In Service: 1450 |

#### Patient Information

| | |
| --- | --- |
| **Age:** 55 | **Allergies:** Penicillin, erythromycin |
| **Sex:** M | **Medications:** Lasix, K-Dur, Prinivil, nitroglycerin, insulin |
| **Weight (in kg [lb]):** 75 kg (165 lb) | **Past Medical History:** Hypertension, angina, diabetes |
| | **Chief Complaint:** Heat exposure; confused |

## YOU are the Provider SUMMARY *continued*

### Vital Signs

| Time: 1428 | BP: 88/66 | Pulse: 130 | Respirations: 24 | Spo$_2$: 95% |
| Time: 1433 | BP: 90/70 | Pulse: 126 | Respirations: 26 | Spo$_2$: 89% |
| Time: 1438 | BP: 98/58 | Pulse: 120 | Respirations: 22 | Spo$_2$: 94% |

### EMS Treatment (circle all that apply)

| Oxygen @ _15_ L/min via:<br>NC (NRM) (Bag mask) | (Assisted Ventilation) | (Airway Adjunct) | CPR |
| Defibrillation | Bleeding Control | Bandaging | Splinting | Other: (Rapid cooling measures) |

### Narrative

EMS was dispatched to a residence for a man who fainted after working outside in the heat for a prolonged period of time.

Chief Complaint: Heat exposure; confused

History: According to the patient's wife, he would not come out of the heat to take a break and drink some water. When she found him, he did not respond to her initially. Patient's past medical history includes hypertension, diabetes, and angina; medications listed above.

Assessment: Arrived on scene and found the patient, a 55-year-old man, sitting under a tree in his garden. He was conscious but confused. His airway was patent and his breathing, although increased in rate, was producing adequate depth.

Treatment (Rx): Applied high-flow oxygen via nonrebreathing mask and quickly moved the patient via ambulance stretcher to the air-conditioned ambulance. Secondary assessment was performed, but did not reveal any gross signs of injury. Patient's skin was flushed, hot, and moist. Initial axillary temperature read 104.5°F (40.3°C). Removed patient's clothing and began rapid cooling measures by placing cold packs to his groin, axillae, and behind his neck. ALS was unavailable.

Transport: Began transport and continued cooling by spraying the patient with saline and fanning him. Vital signs indicated shock, so high-flow oxygen therapy was continued. Reassessment revealed that patient's mental status had markedly diminished; he was responsive only to pain. His respirations remained rapid, but were markedly decreased in depth. Inserted nasal airway and began assisting patient's ventilations with a bag-mask device and high-flow oxygen. After cooling measures, reassessment revealed that the patient's skin, although very warm, did not feel as hot as it was initially; he also appeared less flushed. Patient became somewhat combative and would no longer tolerate assisted ventilation. Reapplied nonrebreathing mask and reassessed his axillary temperature; it read 102.5°F (39.2°C). Continued to reassess patient's vital signs as indicated and monitored him for signs of overcooling. Remainder of transport was uneventful; patient was delivered to the emergency department and verbal report was given to attending physician Emerson. EMS cleared the hospital and returned to service at 1450.

**End of report**

# Prep Kit

## Ready for Review

- Cold-related emergencies can be either a local or a systemic problem.
- Local cold injuries include frostbite, frostnip, and immersion foot. Frostbite is the most serious because the tissues freeze. All patients with a local cold injury should be removed

from the cold and protected from further exposure.
- If instructed to do so by medical control, rewarm frostbitten parts by immersing them in water at a temperature between 100°F and 112°F (37.8°C and 44.4°C).

- The key to treating patients with hypothermia is to stabilize vital functions and prevent further heat loss. Do not attempt to rewarm patients who have moderate to severe hypothermia because they are susceptible to the development of dysrhythmias.
- Do not consider a patient dead until he or she is "warm and dead." Local protocols will dictate whether such patients receive CPR or defibrillation in the field.
- The body's regulatory mechanisms normally maintain body temperature within a very narrow range around 98°F (36.7°C). Body temperature is regulated by heat loss to the atmosphere via conduction, convection, evaporation, radiation, and respiration.
- Heat emergencies can take three forms: heat cramps, heat exhaustion, and heatstroke.
  - Heat cramps are painful muscle spasms that occur with vigorous exercise. Treatment includes removing the patient from the heat, resting the affected muscles, and replacing fluid loss.
  - Heat exhaustion is essentially a form of hypovolemic shock caused by dehydration. Symptoms include cold and clammy skin, weakness, confusion, headache, and rapid pulse. Body temperature can be high, and the patient may or may not still be sweating. Treatment includes removing the patient from the heat and treating for mild hypovolemic shock.
  - Heatstroke is a life-threatening emergency, usually fatal if untreated. Patients with heatstroke are often dry and will have high body temperatures, typically greater than 104°F (40°C). Patients who have heatstroke due to exertion may have wet skin. Changes in mental status can include coma. Rapid lowering of the body temperature in the field is critical.
- The first rule in caring for drowning victims is to be sure not to become a victim yourself. Protect the spine when removing patients from the water because spinal cord injuries often occur in drownings. Be alert for hypothermia.
- Injuries associated with scuba diving may be immediately apparent or may show up hours later. Patients with an air embolism or decompression sickness may have pain, paralysis, or an altered mental status. Be prepared to transport such patients to a recompression facility with a hyperbaric chamber.
- Venomous spiders include the black widow spider and the brown recluse spider.
- Venomous snakes include pit vipers and coral snakes.
- A person who has been bitten by a venomous snake needs prompt transport; clean the bite area and keep the patient calm to slow the spread of venom.
- Notify the hospital as soon as possible if a patient has been bitten by a pit viper or coral snake. Some venoms can cause paralysis of the nervous system, and hospitals may not have appropriate antivenin on hand.
- Patients who have been bitten by ticks may be infected with Rocky Mountain spotted fever or Lyme disease and should see a doctor within a day or two. Remove the tick using tweezers, and save it for identification.
- Always provide prompt transport to the hospital for any patient who has been bitten by a venomous insect or animal. Remember that vital signs can deteriorate rapidly. Carefully monitor the patient's vital signs en route, especially for airway compromise.

## Vital Vocabulary

**air embolism** The presence of air in the veins, which can lead to cardiac arrest if it enters the heart.

**ambient temperature** The temperature of the surrounding environment.

**antivenin** A serum that counteracts the effect of venom from an animal or insect.

**bends** A common name for decompression sickness.

**breath-holding syncope** Loss of consciousness caused by a decreased breathing stimulus.

**conduction** The loss of heat by direct contact (eg, when a body part comes into contact with a colder object).

**convection**  The loss of body heat caused by air movement (eg, a breeze blowing across the body).

**core temperature**  The temperature of the central part of the body (eg, the heart, lungs, and vital organs).

**decompression sickness**  A painful condition seen in divers who ascend too quickly, in which gas, especially nitrogen, forms bubbles in blood vessels and other tissues; see *bends*.

**diving reflex**  The slowing of the heart rate caused by submersion in cold water.

**drowning**  The process of experiencing respiratory impairment from submersion or immersion in liquid.

**dysbarism injuries**  Any signs and symptoms caused by the difference between the surrounding atmospheric pressure and the total gas pressure in various tissues, fluids, and cavities of the body.

**evaporation**  The conversion of water or another fluid from a liquid to a gas.

**frostbite**  Damage to tissues as the result of exposure to cold; frozen body parts; frozen or partially frozen body parts are frostbitten.

**heat cramps**  Painful muscle spasms usually associated with vigorous activity in a hot environment.

**heat exhaustion**  A heat emergency in which a significant amount of fluid and electrolyte loss occurs because of heavy sweating; also called heat prostration or heat collapse.

**heatstroke**  A life-threatening condition of severe hyperthermia caused by exposure to excessive natural or artificial heat, marked by warm, dry skin; severely altered mental status; and often irreversible coma.

**homeostasis**  A balance of all systems of the body.

**hymenoptera**  A family of insects that includes bees, wasps, ants, and yellowjackets.

**hyperthermia**  A condition in which the body core temperature rises to 101°F (38.3°C) or more.

**hypothermia**  A condition in which the body core temperature falls below 95°F (35°C).

**radiation**  The transfer of heat to colder objects in the environment by radiant energy; for example, heat gain from a fire.

**respiration**  The inhaling and exhaling of air; the physiologic process that exchanges carbon dioxide from fresh air.

**reverse triage**  A triage process used in treating multiple victims of a lightning strike, in which efforts are focused on those who are in respiratory and cardiac arrest. Reverse triage is different from conventional triage, where such patients would be classified as deceased.

**scuba gear**  A system that delivers air to the mouth and lungs at various atmospheric pressures, increasing with the depth of the dive; stands for self-contained underwater breathing apparatus.

**turgor**  The ability of the skin to resist deformation; tested by gently pinching skin on the forehead or back of the hand.

## References

1. Lyme disease: data and statistics. Centers for Disease Control and Prevention website. http://www.cdc.gov/lyme/stats/. Updated September 24, 2015. Accessed November 18, 2014.

2. *National Emergency Medical Services Education Standards.* US Department of Transportation. National Highway Traffic Safety Administration. DOT HS 811 077A. January 2009. www.ems.gov/pdf/811077a.pdf. Accessed June 14, 2014.

3. *National Emergency Medical Services Education Standards. Emergency Medical Technician Instructional Guidelines.* US Department of Transportation. National Highway Traffic Safety Administration. DOT HS 811 077C. January 2009. www.ems.gov/pdf/811077a.pdf. Accessed June 14, 2014.

4. National Model EMS Clinical Guidelines. National Association of State EMS Officials website. https://nasemso.org/projects/model-ems-clinical-guidelines/. Published 2019. Accessed July 28, 2020.

5. The global burden of snakebite: a literature analysis and modelling based on regional estimates of envenoming and deaths. World Health Organization website. http://www.who.int/neglected_diseases/integrated_media_snakebite/en/. Published November 3, 2008. Accessed November 18, 2014.

6. Weather fatalities 2018. National Weather Service website. https://www.weather.gov/hazstat/. Published 2018. Accessed April 7, 2020.

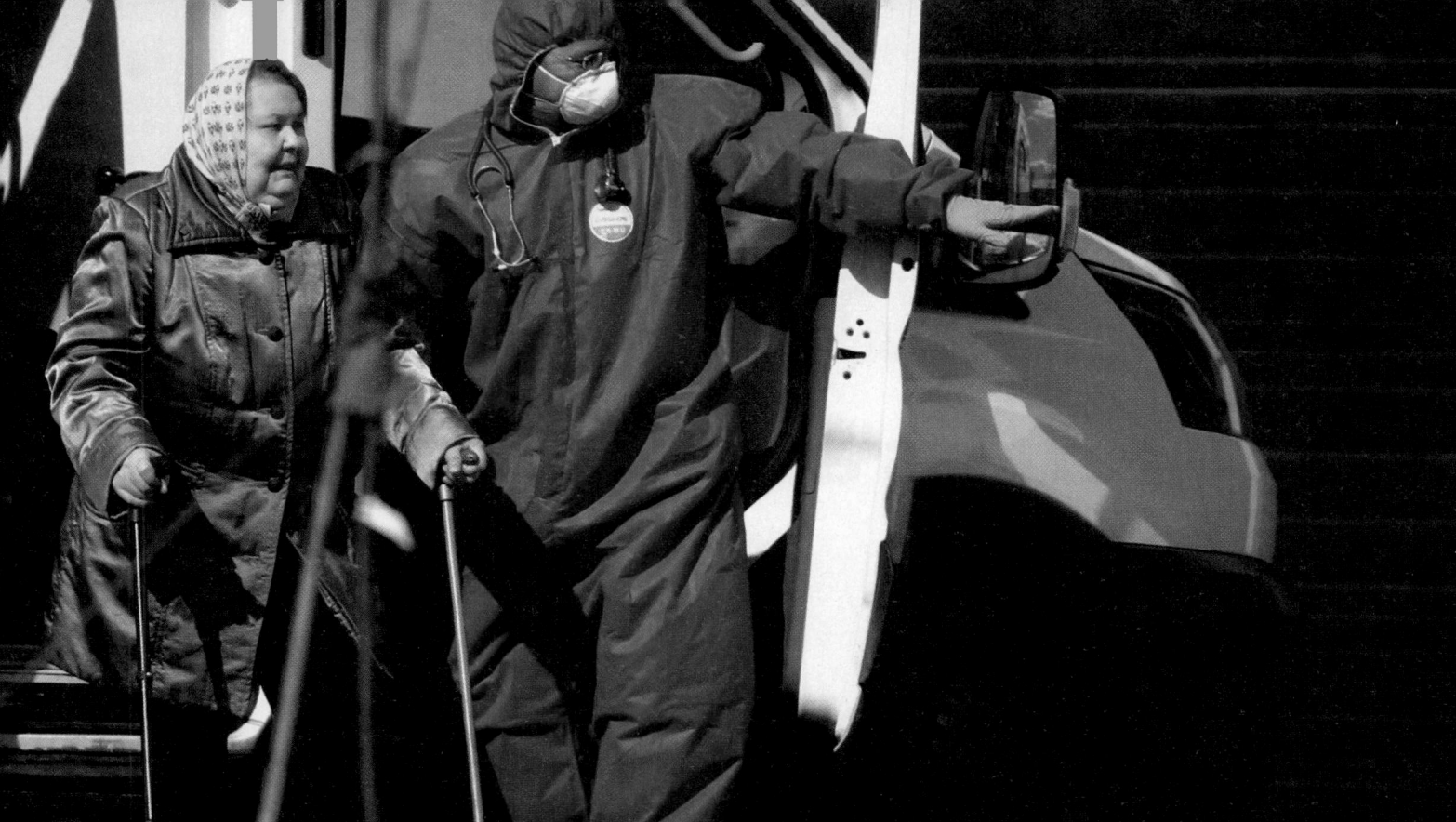

# Special Patient Populations

SECTION

# 8

**34** Obstetrics and Neonatal Care

**35** Pediatric Emergencies

**36** Geriatric Emergencies

**37** Patients With Special Challenges

# Chapter 34

# Obstetrics and Neonatal Care

## NATIONAL EMS EDUCATION STANDARD COMPETENCIES

### Special Patient Populations

Applies a fundamental knowledge of growth, development, and aging and assessment findings to provide basic emergency care and transportation for a patient with special needs.

### Obstetrics

- Recognition and management of:
  - Normal delivery (pp 1256–1265)
  - Vaginal bleeding in the pregnant patient (pp 1248–1251, 1253–1254, 1255)
- Anatomy and physiology of normal pregnancy (pp 1243–1247)
- Pathophysiology of complications of pregnancy (pp 1247–1251)
- Assessment of the pregnant patient (pp 1253–1255)
- Management of
  - Normal delivery (pp 1256–1265)
  - Abnormal delivery (pp 1270–1274)
    - Nuchal cord (p 1263)
    - Prolapsed cord (pp 1271–1272)
    - Breech delivery (pp 1270–1271)
  - Third-trimester bleeding (pp 1248–1250)
    - Placenta previa (pp 1249–1250)
    - Abruptio placentae (pp 1249–1250)
- Spontaneous abortion/miscarriage (p 1250)
- Ectopic pregnancy (p 1249)
- Preeclampsia/eclampsia (p 1248)

### Neonatal Care

Assessment and management
- Newborn care (pp 1264–1270)
- Neonatal resuscitation (pp 1265–1270)

### Trauma

Applies fundamental knowledge to provide basic emergency care and transportation based on assessment findings for an acutely injured patient.

### Special Considerations in Trauma

- Recognition and management of trauma in the:
  - Pregnant patient (pp 1251–1252)
  - Pediatric patient (Chapter 35, *Pediatric Emergencies*)
  - Geriatric patient (Chapter 36, *Geriatric Emergencies*)
- Pathophysiology, assessment, and management of trauma in the:
  - Pregnant patient (pp 1251–1255)
  - Pediatric patient (Chapter 35, *Pediatric Emergencies*)
  - Geriatric patient (Chapter 36, *Geriatric Emergencies*)
  - Cognitively impaired patient (Chapter 37, *Patients With Special Challenges*)

1. Identify the anatomy and physiology of the female reproductive system. (pp 1243–1245)
2. Explain the normal changes that occur in the body during pregnancy. (pp 1246–1247)
3. Recognize complications of pregnancy including abuse, substance abuse, hypertensive disorders, bleeding, spontaneous abortion (miscarriage), and gestational diabetes. (pp 1247–1251)
4. Discuss the need to consider two patients—the woman and the unborn fetus—when treating a pregnant trauma patient. (pp 1251–1252)
5. Discuss special considerations involving pregnancy in different cultures and with teenage patients. (pp 1252–1253)
6. Explain assessment of the pregnant patient. (pp 1253–1255)
7. Explain the significance of meconium in the amniotic fluid. (p 1254)
8. Differentiate among the three stages of labor. (pp 1255–1256)
9. Describe the indications of an imminent delivery. (p 1256)
10. Explain the steps involved in normal delivery management. (pp 1256–1265)
11. List the contents of an obstetrics kit. (p 1257)
12. Explain the necessary care of the fetus as the head appears. (p 1263)
13. Describe the procedure followed to clamp and cut the umbilical cord. (p 1264)
14. Describe delivery of the placenta. (pp 1264–1265)
15. Explain the steps to take in neonatal assessment and resuscitation. (pp 1265–1270)
16. Recognize complicated delivery emergencies, including breech presentations, limb presentations, umbilical cord prolapse, spina bifida, multiple gestation, premature newborns, postterm pregnancy, and fetal demise. (pp 1270–1274)
17. Describe postpartum complications and how to treat them. (p 1274)

1. Demonstrate the procedure to assist in a normal cephalic delivery. (pp 1256–1265, Skill Drill 34-1)
2. Demonstrate care procedures of the fetus as the head appears. (p 1263)
3. Demonstrate how to clamp and cut the umbilical cord. (pp 1262–1264)
4. Demonstrate the steps to follow in postdelivery care of the newborn. (p 1264)
5. Demonstrate how to assist in delivery of the placenta. (pp 1264–1265)
6. Demonstrate the postdelivery care of the woman. (p 1264)
7. Demonstrate procedures to follow for complicated delivery emergencies including vaginal bleeding, breech presentation, limb presentation, and prolapsed umbilical cord. (pp 1270–1273)

# Introduction

While most childbirths in the United States occur in a health care setting with trained medical personnel in attendance, the rate of births occurring in out-of-hospital settings has increased by approximately 77% since 2004. The most recent data available suggest that approximately 2 of every 100 births will occur outside of the hospital environment. In 2017, there were over 60,000 out of hospital births, with just over 38,000 of them taking place in the home. When responding to an obstetric emergency, the EMT is faced with a critical decision: delay transport and assist with the delivery on scene or initiate transport with minimal delay and plan for delivery at the hospital. Multiple factors affect this decision, such as trauma, weather, and distance to the hospital. This chapter explains how to make this decision and how to proceed if on-scene delivery is necessary. It describes the anatomy and physiology of a normal pregnancy and the normal process of childbirth. Also discussed are common complications, including trauma in a pregnant patient, so that you will be prepared to handle normal and abnormal deliveries. Finally, the chapter discusses the evaluation and care of the newborn and neonatal resuscitation.

# Anatomy and Physiology of the Female Reproductive System

The female reproductive system includes the ovaries, fallopian tubes, uterus, cervix, vagina, and breasts. The ovaries are two glands located on either side of the uterus that are similar in function to the male testes. Each ovary contains thousands of follicles, and each follicle contains an egg (the female contribution to conception). Females are born with all the eggs they will release in their lifetime.

During puberty, the maturing female body undergoes multiple physical and hormonal changes, ultimately leading to menarche. After the first menstrual bleeding occurs, periods begin occurring with more regularity. Ultimately, a routine cycle is established, with an average duration of 28 days between menstrual periods. During the typical menstrual cycle, only one follicle (of 10 to 20 that attempt the process each month) will mature and release an egg. The remaining follicles die and are reabsorbed by the body. The processes that the follicle goes through and the actual release of the egg (ovulation) are stimulated by the release of specific hormones in the female body. Ovulation occurs approximately 2 weeks prior to menstruation. Immediately following ovulation, the endometrium (the lining of the inside of the uterus) begins to thicken in preparation for the potential implantation of a fertilized egg. If the egg is not fertilized within 36 to 48 hours after it has been released from the follicle, it will simply die, and the thickened endometrium will be shed because it is not needed. This shedding is the menstrual flow that occurs on the first day of a woman's cycle.

The fallopian tubes extend out laterally from the uterus, with one tube associated with each ovary. When an egg is released from the ovary, it travels through the fallopian tube to the uterus.

Fertilization, which occurs when a sperm meets an egg, usually takes place when the egg is inside the fallopian tube. The fertilized egg then continues to the uterus where, if implantation occurs, the fertilized egg develops into an embryo (the stage from 0 to 10 weeks after fertilization) and then a fetus (the stage from 10 weeks until delivery) and grows until the time of delivery at approximately 9 months (40 weeks) of gestation (**FIGURE 34-1**). The uterus is a muscular organ that encloses and protects the developing fetus. During labor, it produces contractions and ultimately helps to push the fetus through the birth canal. The birth canal is made up of the vagina and the lower third, or neck, of the uterus, called the cervix. During pregnancy, the cervix contains a mucus plug that seals the uterine opening, preventing contamination from the outside. When the cervix begins to dilate, this plug is discharged into the vagina as pink-tinged mucus, sometimes called bloody show. This small amount of bloody discharge often signals the beginning of labor.

The vagina is the outermost cavity of the female reproductive system and forms the lower part of the birth canal. It is about 3 to 5 inches (8 to 12 cm) in length, beginning at the cervix and ending as an external opening of the body. The vagina completes the passageway from the uterus to the outside world for the newborn. The area between the vagina and the anus is called the perineum.

## Words of Wisdom

Documentation of the last menstrual period (often noted as LMP) should be included in the history section of the patient's chart. The last menstrual period is documented as the first day of the patient's last menstrual bleeding. Documentation should also include the average number of days that the patient experiences bleeding and the average number of days between the start of each cycle. For women who have experienced menopause, the month and year of the last known menstrual period should be charted, if possible, particularly when relevant to the chief complaint (eg, vaginal bleeding, abdominal pain).

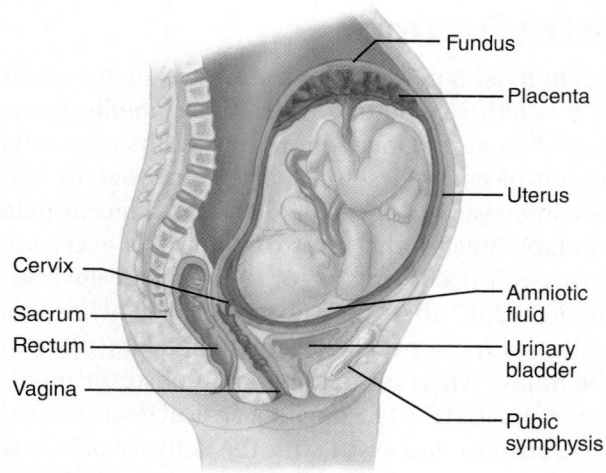

**FIGURE 34-1** Anatomic structures of the pregnant woman.

© Jones & Bartlett Learning.

The breasts are also a part of the female reproductive system. Early signs of pregnancy include increased size and tenderness in the breasts. Shortly after the baby is born, mammary glands within the breasts begin to produce milk, which is carried through small ducts in the nipples.

As the fetus continues to develop, it requires increasingly more nourishment and support. The **placenta** is a disk-shaped structure attached to the uterine wall that provides nourishment to the fetus through the umbilical cord. Blood normally does not mix between the fetus and the pregnant woman because of the placental barrier (**FIGURE 34-2**). This barrier consists of two layers of cells, keeping the circulations of the woman and the fetus separated but allowing nutrients, oxygen, waste, and carbon dioxide to pass between the fetus and woman. Many drugs and toxins are also able to pass through this barrier. Anything ingested by a pregnant woman therefore has the potential to affect the fetus. After delivery of the newborn, the placenta separates from the uterus and is delivered. The **umbilical cord** connects the woman and fetus through the placenta. Oxygenation, nutrition, and waste removal all rely on this connection remaining intact. The umbilical cord contains two arteries and one vein. The flow of oxygen through the fetal circulation is altered while in the womb and transitions to normal physiology within minutes after birth. The umbilical vein carries oxygenated blood from the placenta to the heart of the fetus, and the umbilical arteries carry deoxygenated blood from the heart of the fetus to the placenta. Oxygen and other nutrients cross from the woman's circulation through the placenta and then through the umbilical cord to support the fetus as it grows.

The fetus develops inside a fluid-filled, bag-like membrane called the **amniotic sac**, or bag of waters. The sac contains approximately 500 to 1,000 mL of amniotic fluid, which helps insulate and protect the fetus. When the sac ruptures, usually at the beginning of labor, the amniotic fluid is released in a gush. It is typical for the patient to tell you that her "water broke." Some women may experience a small leak rather than a gush of fluid. This fluid helps to lubricate the birth canal and remove any bacteria.

A pregnancy is considered full term when it reaches 39 weeks but has not gone beyond 40 weeks, 6 days. A pregnancy that has reached full term is referred to as **term gestation**.

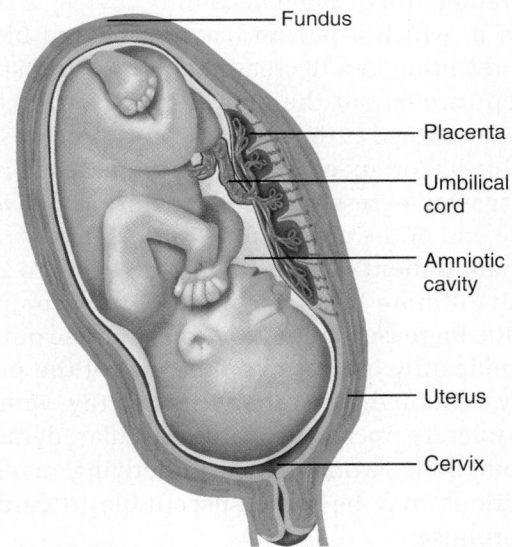

- Fundus
- Placenta
- Umbilical cord
- Amniotic cavity
- Uterus
- Cervix

**FIGURE 34-2** The placental barrier keeps the maternal and fetal blood separate but allows nutrients, oxygen, waste, carbon dioxide, toxins, and most medications to pass between the fetus and pregnant woman.

© Jones & Bartlett Learning.

## YOU are the Provider

At 0625 hours, you are dispatched to a residence at 2505 Landa Park Boulevard for a woman in labor. You and your partner proceed to the scene, which is located a short distance away. While en route, dispatch advises you that the patient is 38 weeks' pregnant and her contractions are 3 minutes apart.

**1.** What anatomic and physiologic changes occur during pregnancy? How will they affect your assessment of the patient?

**2.** How will you determine whether delivery is imminent or if there is enough time to transport the pregnant patient?

## Normal Changes in Pregnancy

Four body systems—the reproductive, respiratory, cardiovascular, and musculoskeletal systems— undergo major physiologic and anatomic changes during pregnancy. Understanding these changes is important when assessing and treating a pregnant patient.

In the reproductive system, hormone levels increase to support fetal development and prepare the body for childbirth. These increased hormone levels also put the pregnant woman at an increased risk for complications from trauma, bleeding, and some medical conditions. As the fetus develops, the uterus grows, stretching to accommodate a full-term fetus. As the size of the uterus increases, so does the amount of fluid it contains. These factors eventually result in displacement of the uterus out of its well-protected position within the pelvic area and may expose it to injury. By the 20th week of pregnancy, the top of the uterus is at or above the belly button. This increases the chance of direct fetal injury in trauma.

In the second trimester of pregnancy, the rapid growth of the uterus leads to changes in the respiratory system. As the uterus grows, it pushes up on the diaphragm, displacing it from its normal position and leading to reduced tidal volume with each breath. To make up for this, the pregnant female's respiratory rate must increase. Pregnancy also increases the patient's overall demand for oxygen as her metabolic demands and workload increase to support the developing fetus. These changes lead to an overall reduction in respiratory reserve and decreased ability to compensate during times of respiratory distress.

Changes also occur in the cardiovascular system. Overall blood volume gradually increases throughout the pregnancy to allow for adequate perfusion of the uterus as the fetus grows and to prepare for the blood loss that will occur during childbirth. Blood volume may increase by as much as 50% by the end of the pregnancy. The number of red blood cells also increases, which increases the woman's need for iron. Pregnant women often take prenatal vitamin supplements containing iron to avoid becoming **anemic**, a condition in which a person has too few red blood cells, resulting in a decreased ability to transport oxygen throughout the body. Blood clotting factors also change as the woman's body prepares for childbirth. The speed of clotting increases to protect against excessive bleeding during delivery. By the end of the pregnancy (third trimester), the pregnant patient's heart rate increases up to 20% (about 20 more beats per minute) to accommodate the increase in blood volume. Cardiac output is significantly increased by the end of the pregnancy. Although an otherwise healthy woman may tolerate increased cardiovascular demand without issue, women with underlying medical conditions may be more susceptible to cardiac compromise.

Pregnant women are at increased risk for gastroesophageal reflux, nausea, vomiting, and potential aspiration. The filling and emptying of the stomach into the small intestine is under the control of key hormones and the nervous system. Changes in these systems and the displacement of the stomach upward because of the increased size of the uterus significantly increase the chance that a pregnant patient will vomit and aspirate. You should be prepared to quickly manage the patient's airway if needed.

Weight gain during pregnancy is normal; however, the increase in body weight eventually challenges the heart and affects the musculoskeletal system. Certain hormones affect the musculoskeletal system by relaxing ligaments that stabilize bones and joints. Women in the third trimester of pregnancy also experience a change in the body's center of gravity, making them prone to slipping and falling.

## Complications of Pregnancy

Although most pregnant women are healthy, some may have preexisting medical conditions when they conceive or become ill during pregnancy. Administering oxygen to a pregnant patient with respiratory distress and/or cardiovascular compromise is safe and can reduce fetal distress.

### Diabetes

Diabetes will develop in approximately 6% of pregnant women during the second half of their pregnancy. This condition, called **gestational diabetes**, resolves in most women after delivery. Treatment of a pregnant woman with diabetes is the same as treatment for any patient who has diabetes. A pregnant woman can control her blood glucose level with diet and exercise or take medication. In some cases, the woman will have to manage her condition with insulin injections. A pregnant woman experiencing hyperglycemia or hypoglycemia should be cared for in the same manner as any patient with diabetes. If a pregnant woman has an altered level of consciousness, your assessment should include determining whether she has a history of diabetes, and you should check the blood glucose level if local protocols permit.

Many women experience nausea before labor and may not have eaten recently. These factors can lead to hypoglycemia and weakness. Consult with medical control if delivery is imminent.

### Hypertension in Pregnancy

Hypertension in pregnancy generally manifests as one of three conditions: gestational hypertension, preeclampsia, or eclampsia. Elevated blood pressure is a feature of all three conditions; however, the degree of hypertension and the presence of systemic effects, such as protein in the urine, altered mental status, or seizures, will aid in determining the patient's specific condition.

**Gestational hypertension** is the presence of high blood pressure in the absence of other systemic effects. High blood pressure in this context is defined as systolic blood pressure higher than 140 mm Hg and diastolic blood pressure higher than 90 mm Hg. The condition is considered severe when the systolic blood pressure is higher than 160 mm Hg

---

## YOU are the Provider

When you arrive at the scene, you are greeted at the door by the patient's husband. He is obviously anxious and tells you, "She's having the baby! I thought I could get her to the hospital in time, but I was wrong." You find the patient, a 28-year-old woman, lying supine in her bed. You introduce yourself and your partner and perform a primary assessment.

| Recording Time: 0 Minutes | |
| --- | --- |
| **Appearance** | Diaphoretic; in obvious pain |
| **Level of consciousness** | Conscious and alert |
| **Airway** | Open; clear of secretions and foreign bodies |
| **Breathing** | Increased rate; adequate depth |
| **Circulation** | Increased pulse rate; strong and regular; no gross bleeding |

The patient tells you that she feels as if she needs to move her bowels and that her contractions are now about 2 minutes apart and last about 45 seconds. A brief visual examination of her perineum does not reveal crowning. According to the patient's husband, this is her third delivery, and she has had gestational diabetes and preeclampsia with this pregnancy. Her amniotic sac ruptured about 5 hours ago.

**3.** What are gestational diabetes and preeclampsia? How can they affect this delivery?

**4.** Is there time to transport this patient, or should you prepare for imminent delivery?

and/or the diastolic blood pressure is higher than 110 mm Hg.

Preeclampsia, a condition that occurs in the second half of pregnancy (after 20 weeks' gestation), involves new-onset hypertension along with other systemic effects, such as protein in the urine. This condition occurs in approximately 3.4% of pregnancies in the United States. The risk of preeclampsia occurring is 1.5 to 2 times higher in a woman's first pregnancy; however, if she experiences preeclampsia with her first pregnancy, the risk is increased in subsequent pregnancies. Preeclampsia is characterized by the following signs and symptoms:

- Hypertension (systolic blood pressure >140 mm Hg, diastolic blood pressure >90 mm Hg)
- Severe or persistent headache
- Visual abnormalities such as seeing spots, blurred vision, or sensitivity to light
- Swelling in the hands and feet (edema)
- Upper abdominal or epigastric pain
- Dyspnea and/or retrosternal chest pain
- Anxiety
- Altered mental status

A related condition, eclampsia, is characterized by the presence of seizures. To treat a patient having seizures caused by eclampsia, lay the patient on her left side, maintain her airway, and administer supplemental oxygen. If vomiting occurs, suction the airway. Provide rapid transport for a pregnant patient having seizures, and call for an advanced life support (ALS) intercept, if available.

Transporting the patient on her left side can also prevent supine hypotensive syndrome. This condition is caused by compression of the inferior vena cava by the pregnant uterus when the patient lies supine, reducing the amount of blood that is returned to the heart. Hypotension (low blood pressure) may result from this compression. Any patient in the third trimester of pregnancy should always be positioned at least leaning slightly to her left side during transport except during delivery.

## Street Smarts

Differentiating between gestational hypertension, preeclampsia, and eclampsia can be difficult, but good clinical decision-making (or critical thinking) skills can help. It may be helpful to think of the conditions as existing along a continuous spectrum of the same disease process. For example, if you are transporting a pregnant patient who has a blood pressure of 148/96 mm Hg, but no other signs or symptoms are present at your initial examination, the patient's condition suggests gestational hypertension. During reassessment, the patient tells you she has blurred vision, a severe headache, and abdominal pain. Her condition has worsened and progressed from gestational hypertension into preeclampsia. As you pull into the ambulance bay of the hospital, the patient begins to experience active seizures. Her condition is eclampsia, because seizure activity is present. This example underscores the importance of continually reassessing your patient, listening to your patient, and communicating changes in the patient's condition to hospital personnel.

## Bleeding

Vaginal bleeding during pregnancy can be the result of a number of conditions (**TABLE 34-1**). The timing

| TABLE 34-1 Conditions That Can Cause Vaginal Bleeding | | | |
|---|---|---|---|
| **Condition** | **Timing** | **Pain** | **Bleeding** |
| Ectopic pregnancy | Early pregnancy—generally 6 to 8 weeks after last missed period. | Severe lower abdominal pain, typically unilateral. May radiate to one shoulder. | Ranges from scant brown spotting to profuse bright red. |
| Abruptio placentae | Later pregnancy—usually after 20 weeks. | Lower abdominal and/or back pain. May be associated with contractions. | Moderate vaginal bleeding. Most bleeding is internal. |
| Placenta previa | Later pregnancy—usually after 20 weeks. | Relatively painless. | May present as moderate bleeding to life-threatening hemorrhage. |

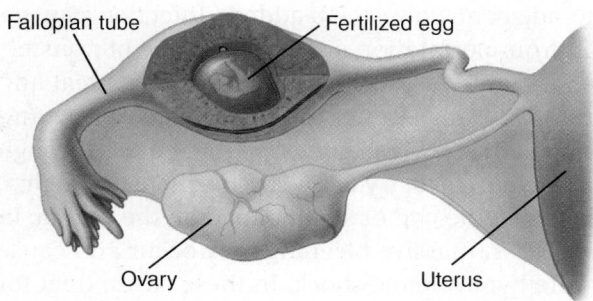

**FIGURE 34-3** In an ectopic pregnancy, a fertilized egg implants somewhere other than in the uterus. Here, it is implanted in one of the fallopian tubes, the most common location for an ectopic pregnancy.

© Jones & Bartlett Learning.

of the bleeding along with the presence and location of pain can help identify the patient's condition.

An **ectopic pregnancy** is when an embryo develops outside of the uterus, most often in a fallopian tube. A patient with an ectopic pregnancy may present with signs of internal bleeding when the fallopian tube ruptures (**FIGURE 34-3**). It is estimated that ectopic pregnancies account for approximately 1.5% of reported pregnancies in the United States. Sudden onset of severe abdominal pain and vaginal bleeding in the first trimester of pregnancy should be considered ectopic pregnancy until proven otherwise. It is also important to consider the possibility of an ectopic pregnancy in a woman who has missed a menstrual cycle and reports sudden, severe, usually unilateral pain in the lower abdomen. A history of pelvic inflammatory disease, tubal ligation, or previous ectopic pregnancies should heighten your suspicion of a possible ectopic pregnancy. Vaginal bleeding in early pregnancy may also be a sign of a spontaneous abortion, which is discussed in more detail in the following section.

In the later stages of pregnancy, vaginal bleeding may indicate a serious condition involving the placenta. In **abruptio placentae**, the placenta separates prematurely from the wall of the uterus (**FIGURE 34-4**). The most common causes are hypertension and trauma. A patient with abruptio placentae often reports severe pain; however, vaginal bleeding may not be heavy. She may also present with signs of shock such as weak, rapid pulse and pale, cool, diaphoretic skin. In **placenta previa**, the placenta develops over and covers the cervix

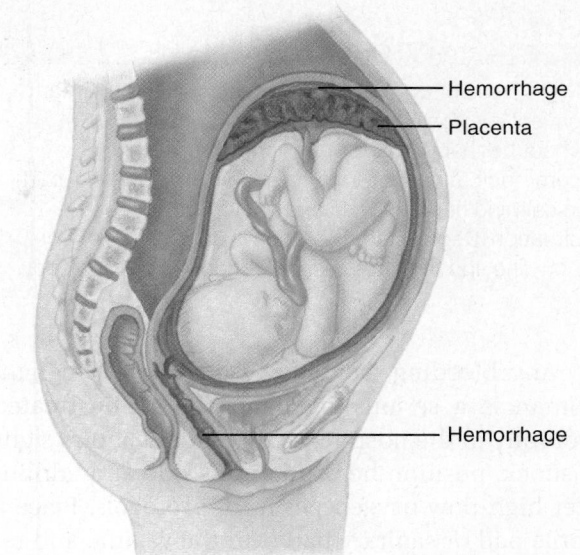

**FIGURE 34-4** In abruptio placentae, the placenta separates prematurely from the wall of the uterus.

© Jones & Bartlett Learning.

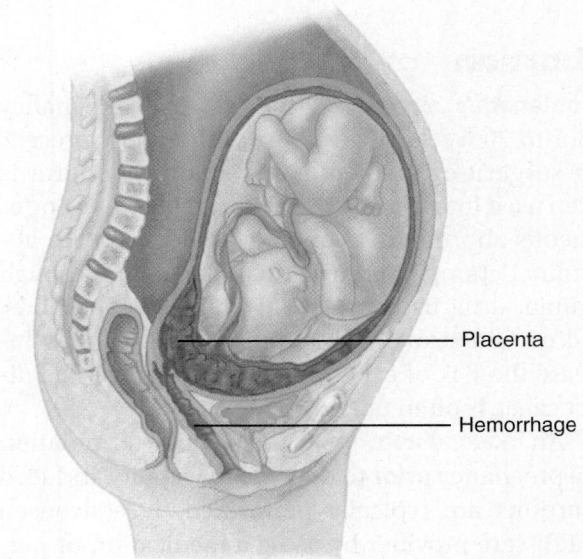

**FIGURE 34-5** In placenta previa, the placenta develops over and covers the cervix.

© Jones & Bartlett Learning.

(**FIGURE 34-5**). When early labor begins and the cervix begins to dilate, the pregnant woman may experience heavy vaginal bleeding, often without significant pain. Both abruptio placentae and placenta previa are life-threatening conditions and require immediate rapid transport.

Any bleeding from the vagina in a pregnant woman is a serious sign and should be treated promptly in the hospital. If the patient shows signs of shock, position her on her left side and administer high-flow oxygen per local protocols. Place a sterile pad or sanitary pad over the vagina, and replace it as often as necessary. Save the pads so that hospital personnel can estimate how much blood loss the patient experienced. Also save any tissue that may be passed from the vagina. Do not put anything into the vagina to control bleeding.

## Abortion

**Spontaneous abortion** is the loss of a pregnancy prior to 20 weeks of gestation without any preceding surgical or medical intervention. The term is often used interchangeably with **miscarriage**. Spontaneous abortion is frequently associated with abdominal cramping and vaginal bleeding. Although trauma, drug use, underlying medical conditions, and certain sexually transmitted diseases may increase the risk of experiencing miscarriage, the direct cause is often unknown.

An **induced abortion** is the elective termination of a pregnancy prior to the time of viability. Induced abortions are typically performed by a licensed health care provider by using a medication or performing a surgical procedure. The abortion may also be induced illegally by an untrained person or by the patient herself, at risk of great harm to the patient. Regardless of the reason or the cause of the abortion, complications are possible.

The most serious complications of abortion, whether it be spontaneous or induced, are bleeding and infection. Bleeding can result when portions of the fetus or placenta remain inside the uterus (incomplete abortion) or when the wall of the uterus is injured (perforation of the uterus and possibly the adjacent bowel or bladder). Infection can result from perforation and from the use of nonsterile instruments. If the patient is in shock, treat and promptly transport her to the hospital. Collect and bring to the hospital any tissue that passes through the vagina. Never try to pull tissue out of the vagina. Place a sterile pad or sanitary pad on the vagina. In rare cases, massive bleeding may occur and cause severe hypovolemic shock. In these cases, treat for shock and provide immediate transport.

## Abuse

Intimate partner violence often begins or worsens during pregnancy. Abuse during pregnancy increases the chance of spontaneous abortion, premature delivery, and low birth weight. The woman is at risk of bleeding, infection, and uterine rupture. A calm, professional approach is especially important if you suspect your patient has been abused. Pay attention to the environment for any signs of abuse. Your attention to detail will be helpful in your documentation and in informing the physicians and staff who will be caring for the patient at the hospital.

Pregnant patients who are abused may be reluctant to explain how their injuries occurred. If possible, talk to the patient in a private area, away from the potential abuser. Suspect abuse when the story of how an injury happened does not make sense. An abused patient who is pregnant will be concerned about her baby. The best way for you to care for the fetus is to treat the pregnant woman. Reassure the patient as you provide treatment. Support the patient's airway, breathing, and circulation (ABCs), control any bleeding, stabilize extremity injuries, treat for shock, and keep her warm.

## Substance Abuse

Overall, drug abuse by pregnant women and the hospitalization of newborns who need care due to intrauterine drug exposure are on the rise in the United States. The use of illicit substances has been reported in up to 6.3% of pregnant women. The incidence of illicit substance use was highest in pregnant females 17 years of age and younger. These women often have had little or no prenatal care. The effects of the addiction on the fetus can include prematurity, low birth weight, and severe respiratory depression. Some of these infants will die. Fetal alcohol syndrome is a condition seen in infants born to women who have abused alcohol.

Opioid use disorder in pregnant women should be considered while obtaining the patient history. If the patient has disclosed her opioid use to her physician, she may be taking an opioid antagonist to treat her disorder and prevent ongoing use during her pregnancy. It is essential to report this history to the receiving facility.

If you are called to handle a delivery of an addicted woman, pay special attention to your own safety. Follow standard precautions. As with all imminent deliveries, personal protective equipment (PPE) should include eye protection, a face mask, and gloves. Clues that you may be dealing with an addicted patient include the presence of drug paraphernalia, empty wine or liquor bottles, and statements made by family or bystanders or by the patient herself. The newborn of an addicted woman will probably need immediate resuscitation. Assist with the delivery, and be prepared to support the newborn's respirations and administer oxygen during transport. Do not judge or lecture the patient. Your job is to help with the delivery, provide treatment to the mother and the newborn, and transport both to the hospital.

## Special Considerations for Trauma and Pregnancy

When you are dispatched to a trauma call that involves a pregnant woman, you have two patients to consider—the woman and the unborn fetus. Trauma to a pregnant woman may have a direct effect on the condition of the fetus. Pregnant women may be victims of many types of trauma, including assaults, motor vehicle crashes, and shootings.

Falls are the third leading cause of trauma in pregnant women, following intimate partner violence and motor vehicle collisions. Contributing factors include hormonal changes that loosen the joints and the increased weight of the uterus and displacement of abdominal organs, which shift the woman's center of gravity. Increased blood volume and elevated resting heart rate, both normal changes during pregnancy, may mask the signs and symptoms of shock until a significant amount of blood has been lost. Fetal distress may also be present well before signs of shock are evident in the pregnant woman. In women who have sustained serious trauma, the blood supply to the fetus is often actively reduced as a physiologic reflex so that the woman receives an adequate amount of blood.

When called to a trauma patient who is pregnant, be alert to additional concerns and be ready to assess and manage unique types of injuries. For example, as a pregnancy progresses, the uterus enlarges substantially, making it especially vulnerable to penetrating trauma and blunt injuries. The fetus may be injured directly from penetrating types of trauma such as gunshot wounds and stabbings. A traumatic injury to the abdomen can be life threatening to the woman and fetus because the pregnant uterus has a rich blood supply. If the woman is hypoxic, is in shock, or has hypovolemia, the fetus will be in distress. In most cases, the only chance to save the fetus is to adequately resuscitate the woman.

When a pregnant woman is involved in a motor vehicle crash or other trauma with a significant mechanism of injury (MOI), severe hemorrhage may result from injuries to the pregnant uterus. Women with severe injuries have been shown to have a six-fold increase in the incidence of abruptio placentae. This condition results in significant intrauterine hemorrhage that can cause life-threatening hypovolemic shock in the woman and also increases the chance of fetal death. In a pregnant trauma patient, suspect abruptio placentae when the MOI is blunt trauma to the abdomen and the patient's signs and symptoms suggest shock. Common symptoms include vaginal bleeding and severe abdominal pain. In this situation, quickly assess and transport the patient, support the airway, administer high-flow oxygen, place sanitary pads on the vagina, position the patient on her left side, and call for ALS backup.

Improper positioning of the seat belt can result in injury to a pregnant woman and the fetus if they are involved in a motor vehicle crash. The lap belt should be placed under the abdomen and over the pelvis (iliac crests), and the shoulder belt should be positioned between the breasts. Carefully assess a pregnant woman's abdomen and chest for seat belt marks, bruising, and obvious trauma. Maintain a high index of suspicion for internal abdominal bleeding in the woman and possible direct injury to the fetus, regardless of seat belt placement.

## Maternal Cardiac Arrest

The most common causes of maternal cardiac arrest in the United States include hemorrhage and severe infection leading to septic shock. It is estimated that 1 in 12,000 pregnant patients who are hospitalized will experience cardiac arrest. One of the key tenets in resuscitation of the pregnant patient is that saving the mother provides the best chance for saving the fetus. Resuscitation efforts should focus on aggressively treating the pregnant patient with high-quality CPR and rapid transport to the closest appropriate facility.

Treatment of cardiac arrest in a pregnant patient may require modifications, depending on how far along the patient is in her pregnancy. If a woman is in the third trimester of pregnancy, manual displacement of the uterus toward the patient's left side may be necessary to facilitate blood return to the right side of the heart. See Chapter 14, *BLS Resuscitation*, for how to perform this procedure. High-quality, minimally interrupted CPR is essential for the pregnant patient, as is early use of an AED. The baby has the best chance to survive if the mother is resuscitated. Use of mechanical CPR devices has not been tested and is not advised in pregnant women.

Notify personnel at the receiving facility as soon as possible that you are en route with a pregnant trauma patient in cardiac arrest so they will have time to prepare. It is possible that a cesarean section may be performed on arrival to the hospital in order to save the fetus. Performing a cesarean section is not within the scope of practice for nonphysician EMS providers.

## Assessment and Management

Although you have two patients to care for when your patient is pregnant, your focus should be on the assessment and management of the woman. It is difficult to assess the extent of internal blood loss in a pregnant patient. The MOI should be the basis for suspicion of shock because the physiologic changes that occur with pregnancy can hide the typical signs and symptoms of shock. As you assess and treat the patient, be prepared for vomiting, and anticipate the

need to manage the airway to protect the patient from aspirating. Attempt to determine the gestational age (in number of weeks). This will help you determine the size of the fetus and the position of the uterus in the patient's abdominal cavity. It is nearly impossible for you to accurately assess or determine the status of the fetus, so you should aggressively provide emergency medical care to the woman to provide the best possible outcome for the fetus.

Follow these guidelines when treating a pregnant trauma patient:

1. **Maintain an open airway.** A pregnant patient has an increased risk of vomiting and aspiration. Be prepared for and anticipate vomiting; keep your suction unit readily available.
2. **Administer high-flow oxygen.** Remember that the patient's body is also supplying oxygen to the fetus. Keep the oxygen saturation level high and administer high-flow, 100% oxygen by nonrebreathing mask.
3. **Ensure adequate ventilation.** Listen to breath sounds, and confirm that bilateral breath sounds are present. If the patient's ventilations are inadequate, provide or assist ventilation with a bag-mask device and 100% oxygen.
4. **Assess circulation.** Control any external bleeding with direct pressure. Maintain a high index of suspicion for internal bleeding and shock based on the MOI. Keep the patient warm.
5. **Transport considerations.** Transport the patient on her left side. Call early for ALS assistance or a medical helicopter for significant MOIs or major traumatic injuries. Transport the patient to a specialty obstetric center or trauma center if one is available in your area; give early notification that you have a pregnant trauma patient in transport.

## Cultural Value Considerations

Cultural sensitivity is important when you are assessing and treating a pregnant patient. Women of some cultures may have a value system that will affect the choice of how they care for themselves during pregnancy and how they have planned the childbirth process. Some cultures may not permit a male health care provider, especially in the prehospital setting, to assess or examine a female patient. Some cultures may view pregnancy differently than you do in terms of social, psychological, and emotional issues. Some may see pregnancy as a means of achieving status and recognition within the family unit, whereas others may experience a drop in self-esteem. Respect these differences and honor requests from the patient. Always remember that your responsibility is to the patient and is limited to providing care and transport. In addition, keep in mind that a competent, rational adult has the right to refuse all or any part of your assessment or care.

## Teenage Pregnancy

The United States has one of the highest teenage pregnancy rates among developed countries. A pregnant teenager may not know that she is pregnant, or she may be in denial about her pregnancy or afraid to seek prenatal care. As you begin to assess any female teenager, you should remember that pregnancy is a possibility, even if she denies being sexually active. Respect the teenager's privacy and need for independence. If possible, perform your assessment and obtain the history away from the teenager's parents. Consider the possibility that the pregnancy resulted from rape or incest. Be aware that in most states, once a teenager becomes pregnant she is considered emancipated, or having the rights of an adult, at least as it relates to giving or refusing consent for medical treatment. Become familiar with the laws in your state so that you will know when pregnant teenagers can give or refuse consent for themselves.

## Patient Assessment

Childbirth is seldom an unexpected event, but there are occasions when it becomes an emergency. Dispatch protocols usually include the dispatcher asking simple questions to determine whether birth is imminent. Some of this information may be passed on to you to help you prepare for the situation. Trauma or medical conditions may cause premature contractions, or your patient may be at full term and experiencing contractions because it is time to deliver.

## Scene Size-up

Take standard precautions; gloves and eye and face protection are a minimum if delivery has already begun or is complete. If the call is going to result in a field delivery and if time allows, a gown should also be used. Do not be lax in your safety observations and precautions because a delivery is in progress or the family is anxious. Rushing may endanger not only you but also the fetus and pregnant woman. Remain calm and professional. Consider calling for additional or specialized resources.

Not every call to a pregnant patient will be because she is in labor, of course, so it is important to determine the MOI or nature of illness in a pregnant patient. Do not develop tunnel vision during a call, assuming that because the patient is pregnant, that is the reason for the call! Because a pregnant woman's balance may be altered, trauma from falls and the need for spinal motion restriction must be considered.

### Words of Wisdom

If the woman in labor is confirmed positive or highly suspicious for an airborne communicable disease, PPE requirements are enhanced. The EMT should wear an N95 mask plus the standard PPE needed in this situation: protective eyewear, a gown, and gloves.

### Primary Assessment

Form a general impression as to whether the patient is in active labor and, if so, whether you have time to assess for imminent delivery and address other possible life threats. Perform a rapid examination of the patient to assess for airway, breathing, or circulation problems. The chief complaint may be, "The baby is coming!" Take a moment to confirm whether the fetus will be delivered in the next few minutes or whether you have time to continue to evaluate the situation. When trauma or medical problems such as vaginal bleeding or seizures are the presenting complaint, evaluate these first and then assess the effect of these problems on the fetus.

During an uncomplicated birth, life-threatening conditions involving the woman's airway and breathing usually are not an issue. However, a motor vehicle crash, an assault, or any number of medical conditions in a pregnant woman may cause a life threat to exist and may result in a complicated delivery. In these situations, assess the airway and breathing to ensure they are adequate. If needed, provide airway management and administer high-flow oxygen.

External and internal bleeding are potential life threats to the patient and should be assessed early. Blood loss after delivery is expected, but significant bleeding is not. Recall that normal changes in pregnancy result in increased overall blood volume, increased heart rate, and changes in blood clotting. These changes can have a significant effect on a pregnant patient who is bleeding, regardless of the cause. Quickly assess for any potential life-threatening bleeding, and begin treatment immediately. Assess the skin for color, temperature, and moisture, and check the pulse to determine whether it is too fast or too slow. Because skin paleness can be difficult to detect in patients with dark skin, you may need to check for pale mucous membranes inside the inner lower eyelid or slow capillary refill. If there are signs of shock, control the bleeding, administer oxygen, and keep the patient warm.

If delivery is imminent, you must prepare to deliver the baby at the scene. The ideal place to deliver the baby is in your ambulance or the privacy of the woman's home. The area should be warm and private, with plenty of room to move around.

If the delivery is not imminent, prepare the patient for transport and perform the remainder of the assessment en route to the hospital. Administer oxygen if necessary. Women in the second and third trimesters of pregnancy should be transported leaning toward their left side when possible to prevent supine hypotensive syndrome. Provide rapid transport for pregnant patients who have significant bleeding and pain, are hypertensive, are having a seizure, or have an altered mental status.

## History Taking

Regardless of whether the patient is in active labor, is having an obstetric emergency, or is a pregnant patient with another complaint (eg, trauma), obtain a thorough history that includes her expected due date, any complications she is aware of, if she has been receiving prenatal care, and a complete medical history. Obtain a SAMPLE history. Some pregnant women will have a history of medical problems for which they take prescription medications. Some women with no history of medical problems will require medications during pregnancy. Pertinent history should include questions related specifically to prenatal care. Identify any complications the patient may have had during the pregnancy or potential complications during delivery that her physician has identified. These complications may include the size or position of the fetus or the position and health of the placenta. Determine the due date, fetal movement, frequency of contractions, and history of previous pregnancies and deliveries and their complications, if any. Determine whether there is a possibility of more than one fetus. Ask whether the woman has taken any drugs or medications during the pregnancy. If her water has broken, ask whether the fluid was green. Green fluid is due to staining from **meconium** (fetal stool). The presence of meconium can indicate newborn distress.

## Secondary Assessment

Perform a complete assessment of the major body systems as needed, with emphasis on the patient's chief complaint. Ask the patient whether she can feel the fetus moving. If the patient is in labor, the physical examination should focus on contractions

## YOU are the Provider

Shortly after your partner assesses the patient's vital signs, you observe the fetus's head crowning at the vaginal opening. As the head delivers, you can feel the umbilical cord wrapped around the fetus's neck.

| Recording Time: 7 Minutes (Mother) | |
| --- | --- |
| **Respirations** | 24 breaths/min; adequate depth |
| **Pulse** | 110 beats/min; strong and regular |
| **Skin** | Pink, warm, and moist |
| **Blood pressure** | 122/82 mm Hg |
| **Oxygen saturation (Spo$_2$)** | 98% (on room air) |

**5.** How should you manage the umbilical cord?

**6.** What would you do if the amniotic sac were still intact?

and possible delivery. Assess the length and frequency of contractions by asking the patient and by placing your hand on the abdomen. Compare what you feel with the patient's experience during each contraction. If at any point you suspect that delivery is imminent, check for crowning. This assessment should be performed only when appropriate and according to local protocol. If you do not suspect that delivery is imminent and the patient reports other problems unrelated to delivery, you should not visually inspect the vaginal area. Be sure to protect the woman's privacy during the physical examination.

The secondary assessment of a pregnant patient should include a complete set of vital signs and pulse oximetry. Vital signs should include pulse; respirations; skin color, temperature, and condition; and blood pressure. Be especially alert for tachycardia and hypotension (which could mean hemorrhage or compression of the vena cava) or hypertension (possibly indicating preeclampsia). A woman's blood pressure typically drops slightly during the first two trimesters of pregnancy but returns to normal during the third trimester. Compare your findings with previous blood pressure readings the patient may know of from prenatal visits. Hypertension, even when mild, may indicate more serious problems.

## Reassessment

As time allows, repeat the primary assessment with a focus on the patient's ABCs and vaginal bleeding, particularly after delivery. Obtain another set of vital signs and compare the results with those obtained earlier. Frequent reassessment of vital signs may identify hypoperfusion from excessive blood loss as a result of delivery. Recheck interventions and treatments to determine whether they were effective. For example, is the vaginal bleeding slowing with uterine massage? Uterine massage, discussed later in this chapter, can slow vaginal bleeding after delivery by stimulating the uterus to contract back towards its prepregnancy size.

In most cases, childbirth is a natural process that does not require your assistance. When childbirth is complicated by trauma or other conditions, however, any interventions you provide for the mother will benefit the fetus. For example, if a pregnant woman has a pulse oximetry level of 94%

or lower, her fetus will be hypoxic, too. Administering oxygen to the mother will improve the oxygen level of the fetus. Administer oxygen if the assessment findings indicate a need, even in the absence of pulse oximetry readings.

If your assessment determines that delivery is imminent, notify staff at the receiving hospital. Provide an update on the status of the woman and newborn after delivery. On the rare occasion that the delivery of the placenta does not occur within 30 minutes or you determine that a complication is occurring that cannot be treated in the field, notify the hospital staff of your findings as you transport. Be sure to notify staff at the receiving hospital of all relevant information so they have time to prepare. The information you provide may help the hospital staff determine whether the patient will be seen in the emergency department or the labor and delivery unit. When a pregnant woman has problems unrelated to childbirth (such as trauma or difficulty breathing), be sure to include the pregnancy status of your patient in your radio report. The hospital staff will want to know the patient's number of weeks of gestation, her due date, and any known complications of the pregnancy.

Thorough documentation is essential, especially in the case of a newborn where delivery occurred in the field. In this situation, you will have two patient care reports to complete. Obstetrics is among the most litigated specialties in medicine; therefore, scrupulous documentation is essential.

## Stages of Labor

The three stages of labor are (1) dilation of the cervix, (2) delivery of the fetus, and (3) delivery of the placenta. The first stage begins with the onset of contractions and ends when the cervix is fully dilated. Because the cervix has to be stretched thin by uterine contractions until the opening is large enough for the fetus to pass through into the vagina, the first stage of labor is usually the longest. In primigravida women, the first stage of labor lasts an average of 12 to 18 hours, compared to an average duration of 6.5 to 13 hours for multigravida women. You will usually have time to transport the woman if she is in the first stage of labor.

The onset of labor starts with contractions of the uterus. Other signs of the beginning of labor are the bloody show (blood-streaked mucus) and

| TABLE 34-2 False Labor Versus True Labor | |
|---|---|
| **False Labor (Braxton-Hicks Contractions)** | **True Labor** |
| Contractions are not regular and do not increase in intensity or frequency. Contractions come and go. | Contractions, once started, consistently get stronger and closer together. |
| Pain and contractions start and stay in the lower abdomen. | Pain and contractions may start in the lower back and "wrap around" to the lower abdomen. |
| Physical activity or a change in position may alleviate the pain and contractions. | Physical activity may intensify the contractions. A change in position does not relieve contractions. |
| Bloody show, if present, is brownish. | The bloody show is pink or red and generally accompanied by mucus. |
| If leakage of fluid occurs, it is usually urine. It will be in small amounts and smell of ammonia. | The amniotic sac may have broken just before the contractions started or it may break during contractions. A moderate amount of fluid that may smell sweet will be present, and fluid will continue to leak. |

© Jones & Bartlett Learning.

the rupture of the amniotic sac (water breaking). These events usually occur near the first contraction or early in the first stage of labor. Initially, the uterine contractions may not occur at regular intervals. The woman may think that she simply has a nagging backache. In true labor, the frequency and intensity of contractions increase with time. The uterine contractions become more regular and last about 30 to 60 seconds each. The length of labor varies greatly.

**TABLE 34-2** lists characteristics of true labor versus false labor, or Braxton-Hicks contractions. With false labor, you should provide transport for the patient. With true labor, you may need to prepare for a delivery, depending on the stage of labor, the patient's condition, and transport time.

Some women experience a premature rupture of the amniotic sac, before the fetus is ready to be born. When this occurs, the patient may or may not go into labor. Some patients may experience this premature rupture of the membranes as long as several months before they are due to deliver. In this situation, you will need to provide supportive care and transport to the hospital. These patients are usually placed on bed rest and followed up closely by an obstetrician.

Toward the end of the third trimester of pregnancy, the head of the fetus normally descends into the woman's pelvis as the fetus positions for delivery. This movement down into the pelvis is called **lightening**. Your patient may tell you that she has felt this. Some women describe this as a relief because once the fetus has moved from under their rib cage, breathing becomes easier. Lightening may also occur gradually and not be noticed by some patients.

The second stage of labor begins when the fetus enters the birth canal, and it ends with delivery of the newborn (spontaneous birth). During this stage, you will have to make a decision about whether to help the woman deliver at the scene or provide transport to the hospital. Because the fetus goes through positional changes as it moves through the birth canal during this stage, the uterine contractions are usually closer together and last longer. Pressure on the rectum may make the woman feel as if she needs to have a bowel movement. Under no circumstances should you let the woman sit on the toilet. She may also have the uncontrollable urge to push down. The perineum will begin to bulge significantly. When the top of the fetus's head begins to appear at the vaginal opening, this is called **crowning**.

The third stage of labor begins with the birth of the newborn and ends with the delivery of the placenta. During this stage, the placenta must separate completely from the uterine wall. Contractions continue, assisting the separation process and clamping down and closing the blood vessels that connected the placenta to the uterine lining. This may take up to 30 minutes.

# Normal Delivery Management
## Preparing for Delivery

Consider delivery at the scene when delivery is imminent (will occur within a few minutes) or when a natural disaster, inclement weather, or other environmental factor makes it impossible to reach the hospital. If the patient has delivered before, she may be able to tell you whether she is about to deliver. Otherwise, her answers to the following questions will help you determine whether delivery is imminent:

- How long have you been pregnant?
- When are you due?
- Is this your first pregnancy?
- Are you having contractions? How far apart are the contractions? How long do the contractions last?
- Have you had any spotting or bleeding?
- Has your water broken?
- Do you feel as though you need to have a bowel movement?
- Do you feel the need to push?

Ask the following questions to help determine any potential complications:

- Were any of your previous deliveries by cesarean section?
- Have you had any problems in this or any previous pregnancy?
- Do you use drugs, drink alcohol, or take any medications?
- Is there a chance you are having more than one baby?
- Does your physician expect any other complications?

If the patient says that she is about to deliver, says she has to move her bowels, or feels the need to push, immediately prepare for a delivery and consider calling for additional resources. The fetus's head is probably pressing on the rectum, and delivery is about to occur. Otherwise, does the patient have an extremely firm abdomen? Visually inspect the vagina to check for crowning. Crowning is an indication that the delivery is occurring. Do not touch the vaginal area until you have determined that delivery is imminent. In general, you should touch the vaginal area only during the delivery and when your partner is present. Gently spread the pregnant woman's legs apart, explaining that you are doing so to decide whether the baby should be delivered immediately or whether she should be transported to the hospital for the delivery.

Once labor has begun, it cannot be slowed or stopped. Never attempt to hold the patient's legs together, because this will only complicate the delivery. Do not let her go to the bathroom. Instead, reassure her that the sensation of needing to move her bowels is normal and that it means she is about to deliver.

### Street Smarts

When a woman pushes during labor, it is not uncommon for her to have a bowel movement. If this happens, discreetly and rapidly remove the feces and place clean towels under her perineum.

If your decision is to deliver the baby at the scene, remember that you are only assisting the woman with the delivery. Your part is to help, guide, and support the baby as it is born. Use standard precautions at all times. Administer oxygen to the patient if indicated. Limit distractions for yourself and the patient. You want to appear calm and reassuring while protecting the woman's privacy. Most important, recognize when the situation is beyond your level of training. If there is any doubt, contact medical control for further guidance. Always recognize your own limitations. If you are unsure about what to do, transport the patient even if delivery might occur during transport.

Your emergency vehicle should always be equipped with a sterile emergency obstetric (OB) kit containing the following items (**FIGURE 34-6**):

- Surgical scissors or a scalpel
- Umbilical cord clamps
- Towels, drapes, or sheets
- 4 × 4–inch (10 × 10–cm) gauze sponges and/or 2 × 10–inch (5 × 25–cm) gauze sponges
- Sterile gloves
- Infant blanket
- Sanitary pads
- A plastic bag

In addition, you should have appropriate PPE and equipment such as an infant bag-mask device to resuscitate the newborn if needed.

Once you have determined that delivery is imminent and you have positioned the patient in an acceptable location, open the OB kit and continue to prepare for the delivery.

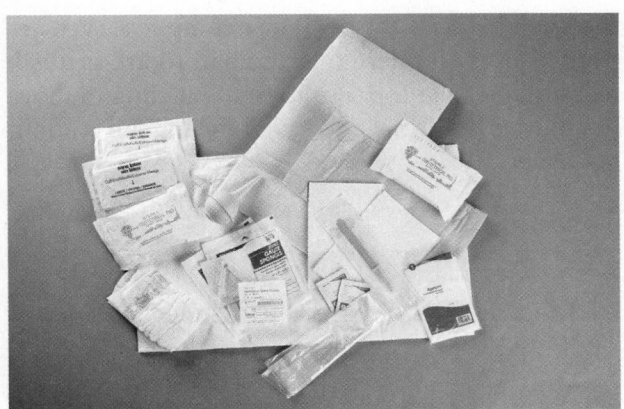

**FIGURE 34-6** Your unit should contain a sterile obstetric kit.

© Jones & Bartlett Learning.

## Patient Position

The patient's clothing and undergarments should be removed or pushed up to her waist. Preserve the patient's privacy as much as you can while helping her to move into position. If the emergency delivery is occurring at home, move the patient to a sturdy, flat surface or the floor if she will allow it. You will find it easier to work with the patient on a firm surface that is padded with blankets, folded sheets, or towels rather than on a bed. Put a pillow or blankets beneath her hips to elevate them about 2 to 4 inches (5 to 10 cm). It is sometimes more comfortable for

### Street Smarts

If you are the team leader during a situation where birth is imminent, communication with your crew members is essential. Do not assume that other members on the crew know what you expect them to do. Communicate effectively and give clear instructions, such as, "I will assist with the delivery of the baby, I want you to stay by the mother's head." Directly point to crew members when addressing them so there is no ambiguity about whom you are speaking to. Communicate with your crew, and have a plan for where you will place the newborn after delivery, who will be responsible for drying the newborn and keeping the newborn warm, and who will be responsible for caring for the mother and the newborn after delivery. Effective communication and strong leadership will go a long way toward calming the nerves of your patient and the crew.

the woman to put a pillow under one hip to allow her to turn to one side. Allow the patient to get comfortable. Support the patient's head, neck, and upper back with pillows and blankets. Have her keep her legs and hips flexed, with her feet flat on the surface beneath her and her knees spread apart. Women who have delivered before may prefer another delivery position, such as on the side. Another position is acceptable if both you and the patient are comfortable with it. You should also begin preparing for the newborn's arrival.

Track the progression of the delivery closely at all times. You want to avoid an explosive delivery, in which the crowning head pops out too quickly and uncontrollably.

## Preparing the Delivery Field

Take the following steps to prepare the area where the delivery will occur:

1. Put on a protective face shield and gown. As time allows, place towels or sheets on the floor around the delivery area to help soak up body fluids and to protect the woman and the newborn.
2. Carefully open the OB kit so its contents remain sterile.
3. Put on the sterile gloves. After this, handle only sterile materials.
4. Use the sterile sheets and drapes from the OB kit to make a sterile delivery field. Place one drape under the patient's buttocks, and unfold it toward her feet. Wrap another behind the patient's back and drape it over each thigh (**FIGURE 34-7A**). Finally, drape a third sheet across her abdomen (**FIGURE 34-7B**).

## The Delivery

Your partner should be at the patient's head to comfort, soothe, and reassure the woman during the delivery. The patient may want to grip someone's hand. She may yell, cry, or say nothing at all. It is common for patients to become nauseated during delivery, and some may vomit. If this occurs, have your partner assist her and ensure that her airway remains clear.

You must continually check for crowning. Some patients, especially those who have previously had children, may experience precipitous (fast) labor and birth. When labor is too fast, the tissues do not have time to stretch, and the patient is at risk for tears in the perineal area (see the section, *Delivering the Head*, in this chapter). Position yourself so that you can see the perineal area at all times. Time the patient's contractions, starting at the beginning of one and ending with the beginning of the next, to determine the frequency of the contractions. In addition, time the duration of each contraction by feeling the patient's abdomen from the moment the contraction begins (uterus and abdomen tightening) to the moment it ends (uterus and abdomen relaxing). Remind the patient to take quick, short breaths during each contraction but not to strain. Encourage the patient to rest and breathe deeply through her mouth between contractions.

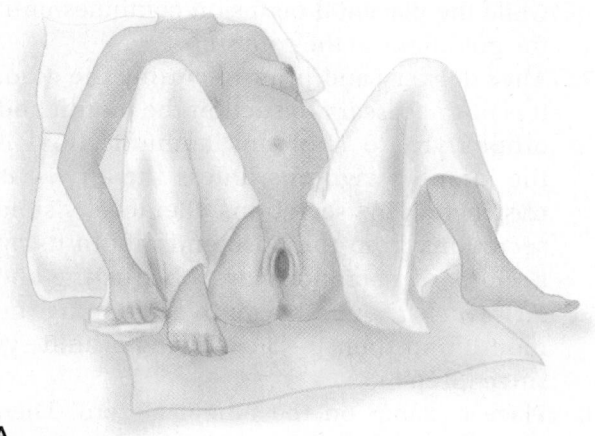

**A**

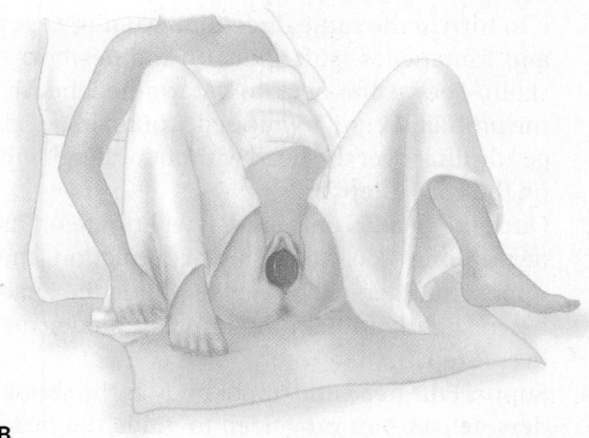

**B**

**FIGURE 34-7** Preparing the delivery field. **A.** Use sterile sheets and drapes from the OB kit to make a clean delivery field. Place one sheet under the woman's buttocks. Wrap another sheet behind her back with either end draped over the thighs. **B.** Drape another sheet over the woman's abdomen.

**A, B:** © Jones & Bartlett Learning.

## YOU are the Provider

You have successfully slipped the umbilical cord from around the neck and have completed delivery of the rest of the body. It is a girl! As you assess the newborn, your partner reassesses the patient's vital signs.

| Recording Time: 12 Minutes (Mother) | |
| --- | --- |
| Level of consciousness | Conscious and alert |
| Respirations | 22 breaths/min; adequate depth |
| Pulse | 114 beats/min; strong and regular |
| Skin | Pink, warm, and moist |
| Blood pressure | 130/60 mm Hg |
| Spo$_2$ | 98% (on room air) |

After providing immediate postdelivery care to the newborn, including clamping and cutting the cord and drying and stimulating the infant, you assess her and note that she is breathing; has a heart rate of 80 beats/min; and has cyanosis of her face, trunk, and extremities.

**7.** What is involved in the routine postdelivery care of a newborn?

**8.** What immediate treatment is indicated for this newborn?

Follow the steps in **SKILL DRILL 34-1** to deliver the newborn:

1.  Crowning is the definitive sign that delivery is imminent and transport should be delayed until after the child has been born (**Step 1**).

2.  Allow the woman to push the head out. Use your hands to support the bony parts of the head as it emerges. The child's body will naturally rotate to the right or left at this point in the delivery. Continue to support the head to allow it to turn in the same direction. Avoid the eyes and fontanelles (soft spots on the newborn's skull). Feel at the neck to determine whether the umbilical cord is wrapped around it. If it is, gently lift it over the head without pulling hard on the cord (**Step 2**).

3.  Once the head is delivered, it will rotate on its own to one side. At the next contraction, the upper shoulder will be visible. Guide the head down slightly to help the upper shoulder deliver (**Step 3**).

4.  Support the head and upper body as the shoulders deliver. You may need to guide the head up slightly to help deliver the lower shoulder (**Step 4**).

5.  Once the body is delivered, support the newborn firmly but gently. The newborn will be very slippery. Support the newborn's head with the neck in a neutral position to keep the airway open (**Step 5**).

6.  If the mother is willing and able, place the newborn directly on the mother's abdomen, with the cord still intact. This skin-to-skin technique keeps the newborn warm and perfused; the mother's skin provides warmth while the placental perfusion continues until the pulsations in the cord stop.

7.  After delivery and prior to cutting the cord, it is not necessary to suction the mouth and oropharynx to clear any amniotic fluid if the infant is vigorous unless the airway is obstructed by secretions. Remove visible secretions from the nose and mouth using a cloth. If secretions are obstructing the airway, clear them by gently suctioning the mouth and then the nose using a bulb syringe (**Step 6**).

8.  Place a clamp on the umbilical cord. Then place a second clamp 2 to 3 inches (5 to 8 cm) away from the first (**Step 7**).

## Skill Drill 34-1 Delivering the Newborn

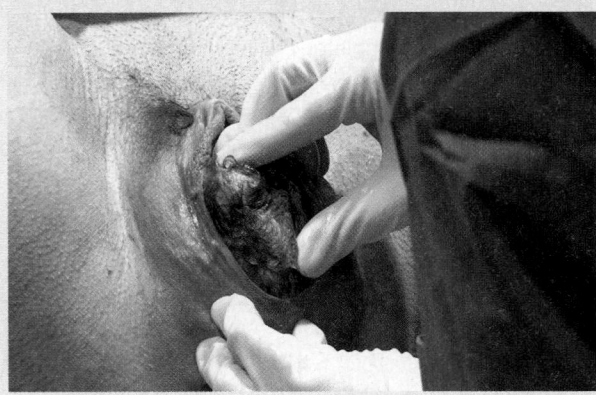

**Step 1**

Crowning is the definitive sign that delivery is imminent and transport should be delayed until after the child has been born.

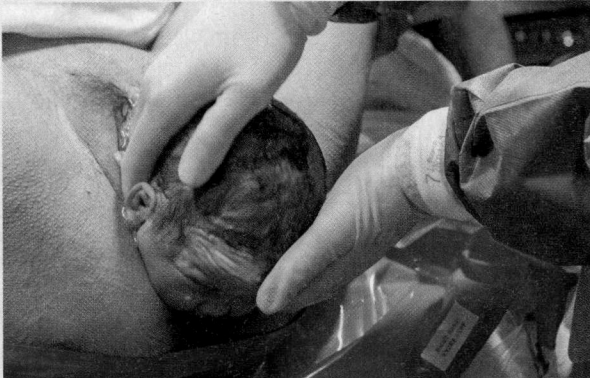

**Step 2**

Use your hands to support the bony parts of the head as it emerges. The child's body will naturally rotate to the right or left at this point in the delivery. Continue to support the head to allow it to turn in the same direction.

## Skill Drill 34-1 Delivering the Newborn (*continued*)

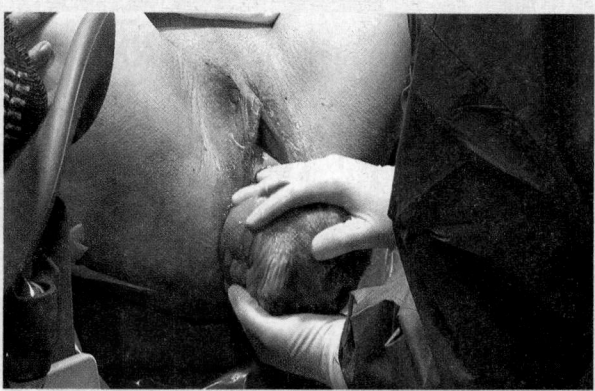

**Step 3**

As the upper shoulder appears, guide the head down slightly to deliver the shoulder.

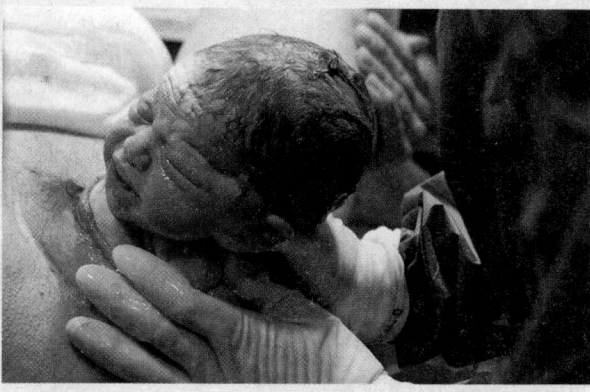

**Step 4**

Support the head and upper body as the lower shoulder delivers, guide the head up if needed.

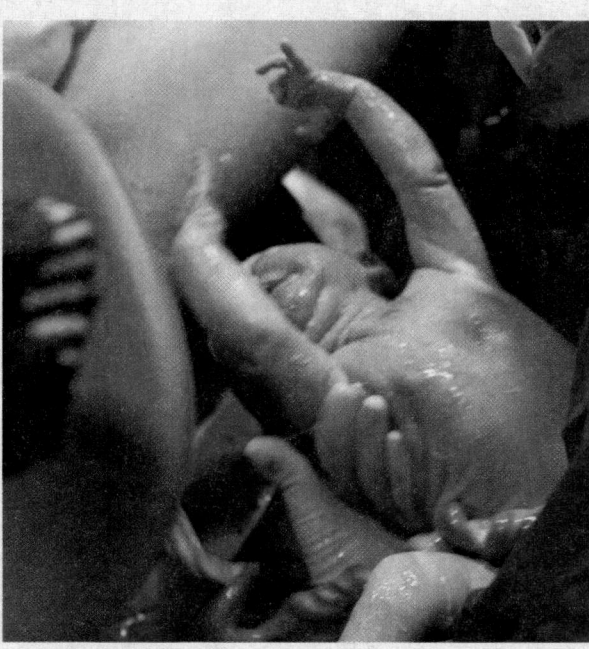

**Step 5**

Handle the newborn firmly but gently, support the head, and keep the neck in a neutral position to maintain the airway. Consider placing the newborn on the mother's abdomen with the umbilical cord still intact, allowing skin-to-skin contact to warm the newborn. Otherwise, keep the newborn approximately at the level of the vagina until the cord has been cut.

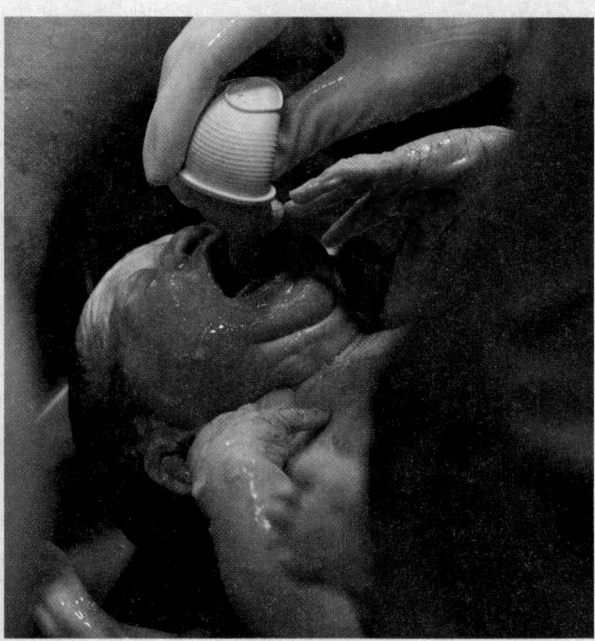

**Step 6**

After delivery and prior to cutting the cord, if the child is gurgling or shows other signs of respiratory distress, suction the mouth and oropharynx gently with a bulb syringe to clear any amniotic fluid and ease the infant's initiation of air exchange.

(*continues*)

## Skill Drill 34-1 Delivering the Newborn (*continued*)

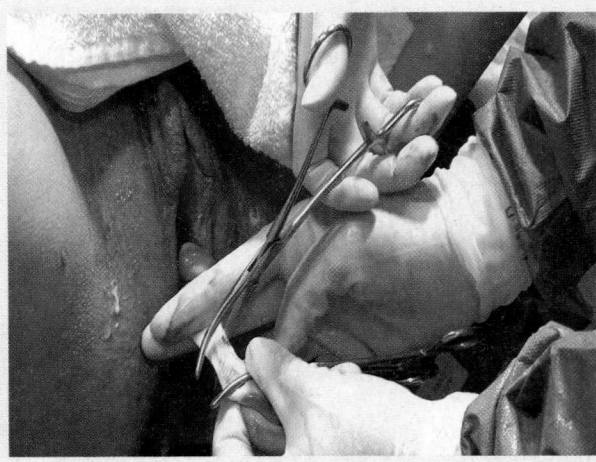

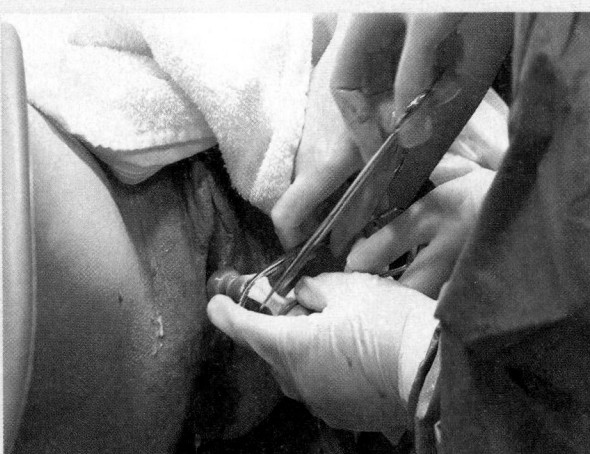

### Step 7

Wait 30 to 60 seconds for the umbilical cord to stop pulsing. Place a clamp on the cord. Place a second clamp 2 to 3 inches (5 to 8 cm) away from the first.

### Step 8

Cut between the clamps.

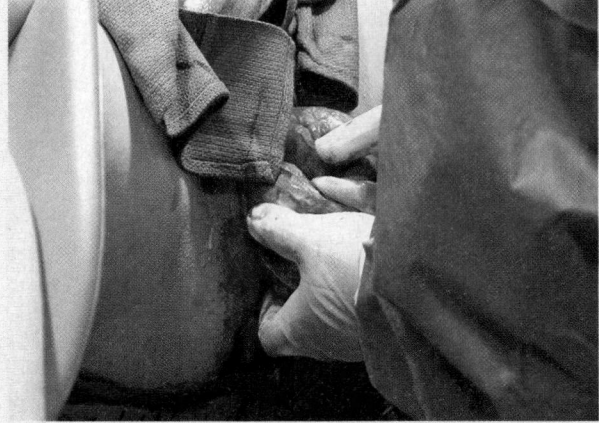

© University of Maryland Shock Trauma Center/MIEMSS.

### Step 9

Allow the placenta to deliver itself. Do not pull on the cord to speed delivery.

9. Cut between the two clamps (**Step 8**).
10. The placenta will deliver itself, usually within 30 minutes of birth. Never pull on the end of the umbilical cord in an attempt to speed delivery of the placenta (**Step 9**).

### Words of Wisdom

When a fetus is positioned headfirst in the birth canal, this is called the cephalic presentation. Most births are cephalic presentation.

## Delivering the Head

Observe the head as it begins to exit the vagina so you can provide support as it emerges. It may take many contractions from the time the head begins to crown until the head delivers. Once it is obvious that the head is coming out farther with each contraction, place your sterile gloved hand over the emerging bony parts of the head, avoid the eyes and fontanelles, and, by exerting minimal pressure, control the delivery of the head. This will allow the head to come out smoothly and prevent it and the rest of the newborn from suddenly popping out during a strong contraction, possibly causing injury to the patient's perineal area and/or to the newborn. Continue to support the head as it rotates.

The risk of perineal tearing during labor can be reduced by applying gentle pressure across the perineum with a sterile gauze pad. Also be prepared for the possibility of the patient having a bowel movement because of the increased pressure on the rectum.

As you assist with the delivery of the head, be careful that you do not poke your fingers into the newborn's eyes or the fontanelles. The fontanelles are soft spots on the newborn's skull that will eventually become covered with bone. At birth, the brain is covered only with skin and membranes at these areas. There are two primary fontanelles, one on the top of the head and one near the back of the head.

### Unruptured Amniotic Sac

The amniotic sac will usually rupture at the beginning of labor; if not, it may rupture during contractions. If the amniotic sac has not ruptured by the time the fetal head is crowning, it will appear as a fluid-filled sac (comparable to a water balloon) emerging from the vagina. This situation is potentially life threatening for the fetus because the sac will suffocate the fetus if it is not removed. If the sac has not ruptured spontaneously, you may puncture it with a clamp or tear it by twisting it between your fingers. Make sure that the puncture site is away from the fetus's face, and perform this procedure only as the head is crowning. Do not puncture the sac if the fetus's head is not crowning. As the sac is punctured, amniotic fluid will gush

out. Push the ruptured sac away from the fetus's face as the head is delivered. Wipe the mouth and nose with gauze. If the airway is obstructed with fluid, clear the newborn's mouth and nose using the bulb syringe. If the amniotic fluid is greenish (indicating meconium staining) instead of clear or has a foul odor, make sure you notify the receiving hospital. Meconium in the amniotic fluid may result in respiratory distress or an airway obstruction in the newborn.

### Umbilical Cord Around the Neck

As soon as the head is delivered, use one finger to feel whether the umbilical cord is wrapped around the neck. This condition is called a **nuchal cord**, and it is present in 15% to 34% of term births. A nuchal cord that is wound tightly around the neck could strangle the fetus so it must be released immediately from the neck. Usually, you can slip the cord gently over the delivered head (or over the shoulder, if necessary). If this is not possible, you must cut the cord by placing two clamps about 2 inches (5 cm) apart on the cord and cutting between the clamps. Once the cord is cut, you must attempt to speed the delivery by encouraging the woman to push harder and possibly more often because the fetus will now have no oxygen supply until it is delivered and breathing spontaneously. Handle the cord very carefully; it is fragile and easily torn.

## Delivering the Body

Once the head has been delivered, it usually rotates to one side or the other. This rotation places the body in a better position for delivery. By this time, the woman will most likely be ready to push again, and the upper shoulder will be visible in the vagina. The head is the largest part of the fetus. Once it is delivered, the body usually delivers easily. Support the head and upper body as the shoulders deliver. Make sure to always support the head with one hand. Lower the head a little to deliver the upper shoulder, and then very gently raise it to deliver the lower shoulder. Do not pull the fetus from the birth canal. Once the shoulders deliver, the abdomen and hips will appear and will slide out easily. The newborn will be extremely slippery, so make sure to support the body with your other hand as it delivers. The newborn may be covered with a white, cheesy substance called **vernix caseosa**. Support and hold the newborn with both of your hands. Handle the newborn firmly but carefully.

## Postdelivery Care

As soon as the newborn is delivered, if the mother is able and willing, hand the newborn to the mother or place the newborn on her chest or abdomen with skin-to-skin contact and cover with a blanket. As described earlier, this helps keep the newborn warm and may improve perfusion. Dry the newborn, then wrap him or her in a clean, dry blanket or towel to maintain warmth. Newborns are very sensitive to temperature, so warm the blanket or towel, if possible, before you use it. Wrap the newborn so that only the face is exposed, making sure that the top of the head is covered. Keep the neck in a neutral position so the airway remains open. Consider placing the newborn on one side. If circumstances prevent placing the newborn on the mother, cradle the newborn in your arms. Use a sterile gauze pad to wipe secretions from the newborn's mouth and nose as needed. If your local protocols specify, keep the

newborn at the same level as the woman's vagina until the umbilical cord has been cut.

Postdelivery care of the umbilical cord is important because infection is easily transmitted through the cord to the newborn. In a full-term newborn who is vigorous and not showing signs of respiratory distress, it has become generally accepted practice to place the newborn on the mother's chest and delay cord clamping for approximately 60 seconds. In any newborn who requires immediate care for respiratory distress or other complication, prompt care takes priority over delayed cord clamping. Using the two clamps in the OB kit, clamp the cord between the woman and the newborn, preferably 6 inches (15 cm) from the newborn's body. Place the clamps about 2 to 4 inches (5 to 10 cm) apart. When they are firmly in place, carefully cut the cord between them with sterile scissors or a scalpel. Remember, the cord is fragile; if handled roughly, it could be torn from the newborn's abdomen, resulting in a fatal hemorrhage. Once the clamps are in place, there is no need to rush.

By now, the newborn should be pink and breathing on his or her own (**FIGURE 34-8**). At this time, evaluate the newborn for term gestation, good muscle tone, and breathing/crying; also obtain the 1-minute Apgar score (see the section, *The Apgar Score*, in this chapter). If the mother is alert and in stable condition and you have not done so already, hand the newborn to her so that skin-to-skin contact can begin while you dry and wrap the newborn. If this is not possible, give the newborn, wrapped in a warm blanket, to your partner, who can monitor the newborn and complete the initial care. You need to return your attention to the woman and the delivery of the placenta.

## Delivery of the Placenta

The placenta is attached to the end of the umbilical cord, which is coming out of the woman's vagina. The placenta usually delivers within a few minutes of the birth, although it may take as long as 30 minutes, so do not delay transport waiting for the placenta to deliver. Again, your job is only to assist. Never pull on the end of the umbilical cord in an attempt to speed delivery of the placenta. You may tear the cord, the placenta, or both and cause serious or perhaps life-threatening hemorrhage in the patient. A gush of bloody fluid, usually less than

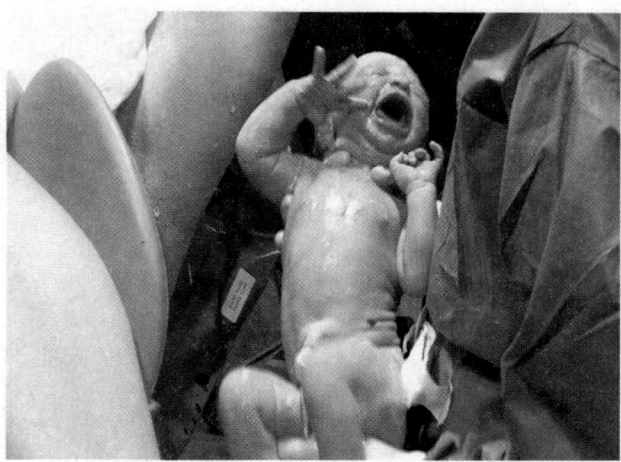

**FIGURE 34-8** When you are holding the infant, use two hands to support the infant's entire body, including the head. One hand should support the back, chest, and head without squeezing or otherwise placing excess pressure on the neck. The second hand should support the buttocks.

© University of Maryland Shock Trauma Center/MIEMSS.

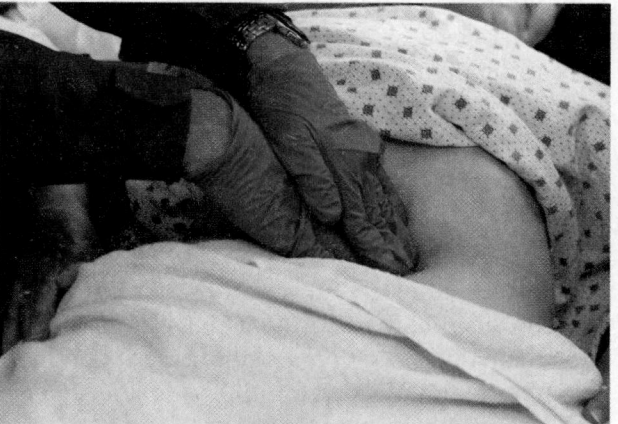

**FIGURE 34-9** After delivery, massage the woman's abdomen in a firm, circular motion.

© Jones & Bartlett Learning.

500 mL, occurs before the placenta delivers and is normal and expected.

The normal placenta is round, about 7 inches (18 cm) in diameter, and about 1 inch (2.5 cm) thick. One surface is smooth and covered with a shiny gray membrane. The other surface is rough, divided into lobes, and is a dark reddish-brown color similar to raw liver. Wrap the entire placenta and cord in a towel, place them into a plastic bag, and take them to the hospital. Hospital personnel will examine the placenta and the cord to make certain that the entire placenta has been delivered. If a piece of the placenta has been retained inside the woman, it could cause persistent bleeding or infection.

After delivery of the placenta and before transport, place a sterile pad or sanitary pad over the vagina and straighten the woman's legs. You can help to slow bleeding by massaging the woman's abdomen using a firm, circular, kneading motion with one hand cupped over the top of the fundus and the other above the pubic bone (**FIGURE 34-9**). The abdominal skin will be wrinkled and very soft. You should be able to feel a firm, grapefruit-sized mass in the lower abdomen; this is called the fundus. The fundus is the upper end of the uterus. As you massage the fundus, the uterus will contract and become firmer. This may be uncomfortable for the

woman. Reassure her and explain that it is necessary to help control the bleeding. Breastfeeding also stimulates the uterus to contract because, like massaging the uterus, it causes the production of oxytocin, a hormone that helps to contract the uterus and slow bleeding. Take a moment to congratulate the new mother and thank anyone who assisted. Be sure to record the time of birth in your patient care report.

The following are emergency situations:

- The placenta has not delivered after 30 minutes.
- More than 500 mL of bleeding occurs before delivery of the placenta.
- Significant bleeding occurs after delivery of the placenta.

If any of these events occur, promptly transport the woman and newborn to the hospital. Never put anything into the vagina. Place a sterile pad or sanitary pad over the woman's vagina, administer oxygen, keep her and the newborn warm by preventing any heat loss, and monitor her vital signs closely.

## Neonatal Assessment and Resuscitation

The American Heart Association and American Academy of Pediatrics have published guidelines on the routine care and resuscitation of newborns. The first minute after birth is often referred to as the "golden minute," and during this time all newborns should be assessed to determine the need for resuscitation. Follow standard precautions, and always wear gloves when handling a newborn.

During the first minute of life, perform the following four initial steps of newborn care:

- Airway positioning and suctioning, if needed
- Drying
- Warming
- Tactile stimulation

These initial steps of newborn care should be carried out in all newborns. If signs of good tone and adequate ventilation are not present after performing the initial steps for approximately 30 seconds, then positive-pressure ventilation with a bag-mask device may be necessary. If the newborn is vigorous with good tone and has adequate respirations (good color, strong cry, and spontaneous respirations) in the first minute of life, then note the Apgar score and place the baby onto the mother's chest for skin-to-skin bonding and routine care. The normal respiratory and cardiovascular physiologic responses expected are that the newborn will begin breathing spontaneously within 30 seconds after birth, and the heart rate will be 100 beats/min or higher.

Many newborns require some form of stimulation that will encourage them to breathe air and begin circulating blood through the lungs (**TABLE 34-3**). The following list provides additional details regarding the initial steps of newborn care.

- Position the newborn on his or her back with a towel or blanket under the shoulders so that the neck is slightly extended in a neutral or sniffing position.
- If necessary, suction the mouth and then the nose using a bulb syringe or suction device with an 8 French or 10 French catheter. Suction both sides of the back of the mouth, where secretions tend to collect, but avoid deep suctioning of the mouth and throat, which can cause the heart rate to slow.
- In addition to vigorously drying the newborn's head, back, and body with dry towels, you may rub the newborn's back and gently flick or slap the soles of his or her feet.

If the newborn does not breathe after 30 seconds of stimulation, then begin positive-pressure ventilation with an appropriately sized bag-mask device.

| **TABLE 34-3** Initial Steps for Newborn Care and Resuscitation | |
|---|---|
| Assess and support | • Airway (position and suction if needed) <br> • Breathing (tactile stimulation) <br> • Circulation (heart rate and skin color) <br> • Temperature (warm and dry) |
| Basic life support interventions | • Dry and warm the newborn. <br> • Provide tactile stimulation while actively drying and warming. <br> • Open the airway and suction with a bulb syringe if needed. <br> • Use a bag-mask device to ventilate the newborn if needed. This is seldom required. <br> • Perform chest compressions if there is no pulse or if the heart rate is <60 beats/min after 30 seconds of ventilation and the heart rate is not increasing. |

© Jones & Bartlett Learning.

You should be properly equipped for resuscitation measures in case the newborn is in distress. Most of the equipment and supplies needed to resuscitate a newborn can be found in your OB kit. Other items you may need are clean, dry towels; an infant blanket; a bag-mask device with a 450-mL reservoir; and masks in both newborn and premature sizes.

## Additional Resuscitation Efforts

Observe the newborn for spontaneous respirations, skin color, and movement of the extremities. If the respiratory effort appears appropriate, evaluate the heart rate by palpating the pulse at the brachial artery or listening to the newborn's chest with a stethoscope. The heart rate is the most important measure in determining the need for further resuscitation (**FIGURE 34-10**).

If chest compressions are required, use the hand-encircling technique for two-person resuscitation (**FIGURE 34-11**). Perform bag-mask ventilation during a pause after every third compression. Avoid giving a compression and a ventilation simultaneously, because one will decrease the effectiveness of the other. Cardiac arrest in neonates is nearly always the result of ventilation compromise. Use a

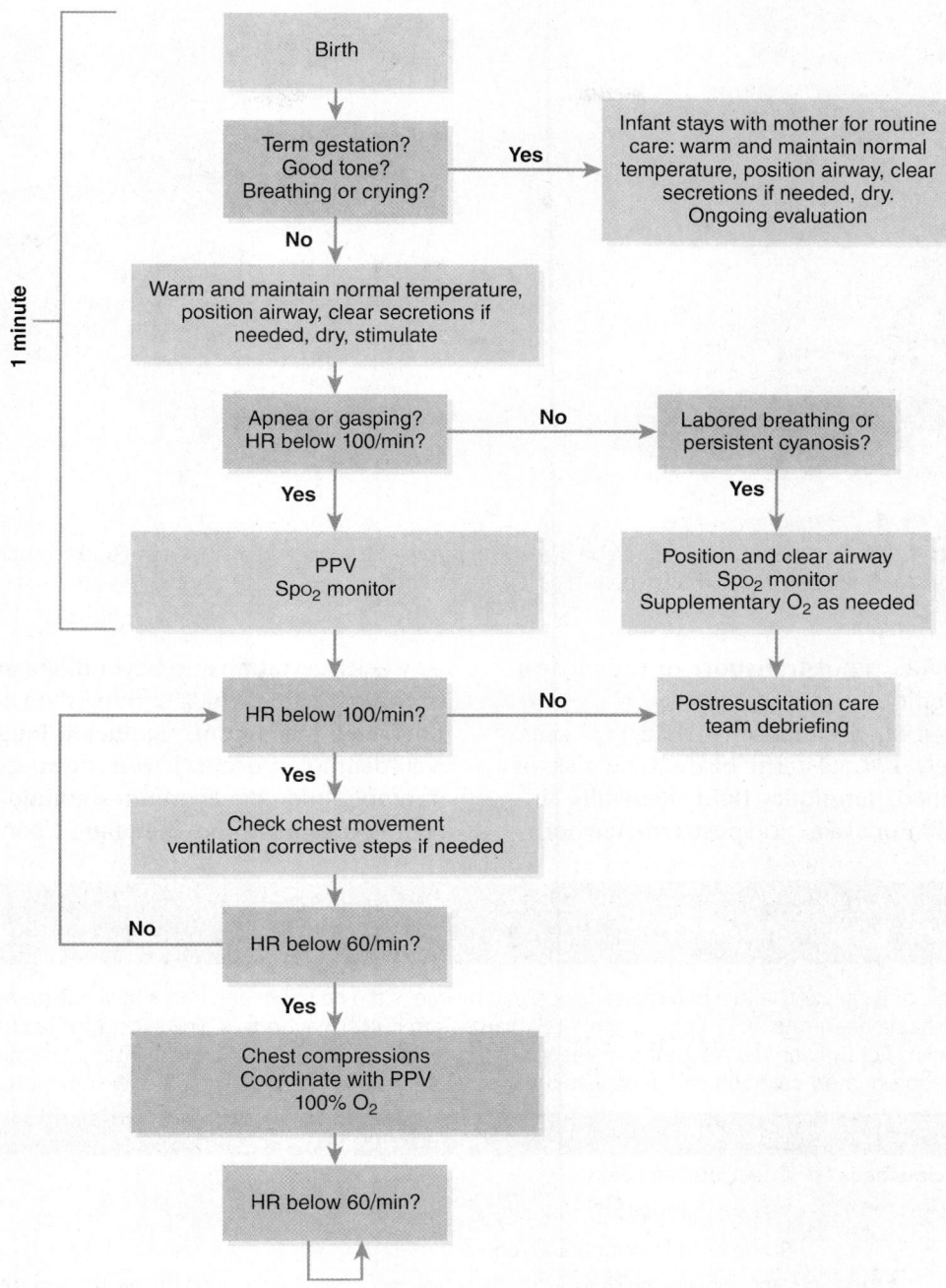

**FIGURE 34-10** Basic Neonatal Resuscitation Program algorithm.

Abbreviations: HR, heart rate; PPV, positive-pressure ventilation; Spo₂, oxygen saturation as measured by pulse oximetry; O₂, oxygen.

© Jones & Bartlett Learning.

compression-to-ventilation ratio of 3:1, which will yield a total of 120 "actions" per minute (90 compressions and 30 ventilations). Hands-only CPR is not as effective as ventilation with CPR. Remember that adequate ventilation is absolutely critical to the successful resuscitation of the neonate.

Transport any newborn who requires more than routine resuscitation to a hospital with a level III neonatal intensive care unit, if available in your area. This type of unit is designed for newborns who require specialized care. If a level III neonatal intensive care unit is not available in

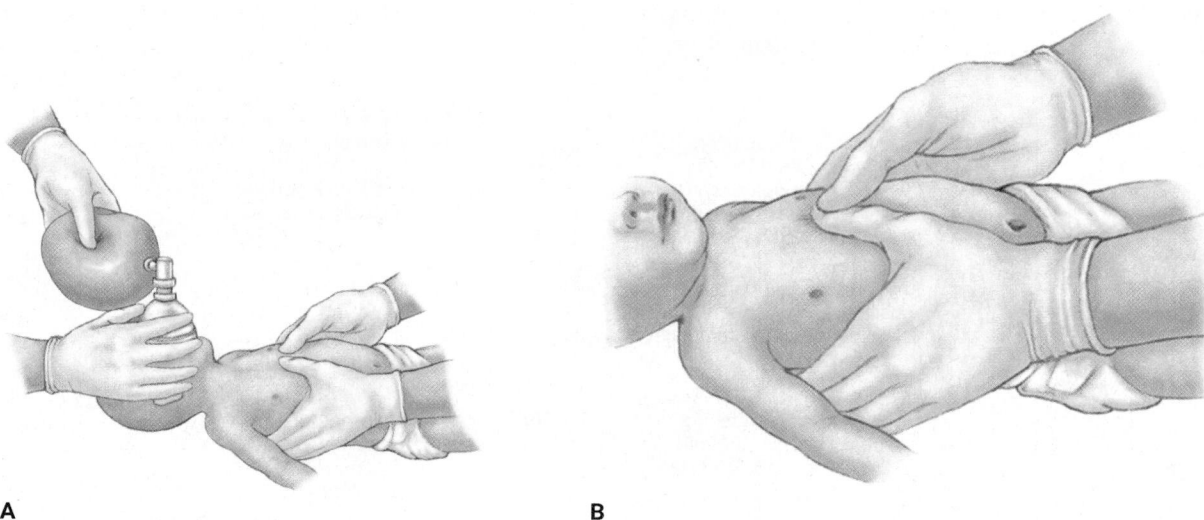

**A**                                        **B**

**FIGURE 34-11 A.** Chest compressions should be given with the hands encircling the newborn and thumbs side by side. **B.** In very small newborns, you may need to overlap the thumbs.

A, B: © Jones & Bartlett Learning.

your area, provide rapid transport to the closest appropriate facility.

Meconium-stained amniotic fluid is seen in approximately 17% of term births. The risk of meconium-stained amniotic fluid generally increases with gestational age, and postterm newborns

(42 weeks' gestation and beyond) are at highest risk. Meconium can be thick or thin. If the newborn aspirates thick meconium, significant lung disease and even death can occur. If you see meconium in the amniotic fluid or meconium staining and the newborn is not breathing adequately, consider quickly

## YOU are the Provider

After 30 seconds of ventilation with a bag-mask device, you reassess the newborn and find that she is breathing adequately and has a heart rate of 120 beats/min. At 5 minutes after birth, her body is pink except for her hands and feet, which remain slightly cyanotic. You hand the newborn to the mother after swaddling the infant. The placenta delivers and is appropriately cared for. You reassess the mother's vital signs and then prepare for transport.

| Recording Time: 20 Minutes (Mother) | |
|---|---|
| **Level of consciousness** | Conscious and alert |
| **Respirations** | 20 breaths/min; adequate depth |
| **Pulse** | 98 beats/min; strong and regular |
| **Skin** | Pink, warm, and moist |
| **Blood pressure** | 126/60 mm Hg |
| **Spo$_2$** | 97% (on room air) |

En route to the hospital, you reassess the newborn and mother. The mother remains conscious and alert and has mild vaginal bleeding. The newborn's body is pink, but her hands and feet remain blue; her heart rate is 130 beats/min, and her respirations are rapid; she pulls her foot away when you flick the sole; and she resists your attempts to straighten her knees. You call the receiving hospital and give your radio report; your estimated time of arrival is 6 minutes.

**9.** What further treatment is indicated for the mother?

**10.** What Apgar score should you assign to this newborn at 5 minutes after birth?

suctioning the newborn's mouth and then nose after delivery before providing rescue ventilations.

## The Apgar Score

The Apgar score is the standard scoring system used to assess the status of a newborn. This system assigns a numeric value (0, 1, or 2) to five areas of activity of the newborn:

- **Appearance.** Shortly after birth, the skin of a light-skinned newborn and the mucous membranes of a dark-skinned newborn should turn pink. Newborns often have cyanosis of the extremities for a few minutes after birth, but hands and feet should "pink up" quickly. Blue skin all over or blue mucous membranes signal a central cyanosis.

- **Pulse.** Measure the pulse by chest auscultation. If a stethoscope is not available, you can measure pulsations with your fingers at the brachial pulse. A newborn with no pulse requires immediate CPR.

- **Grimace or irritability.** Grimacing, crying, or withdrawing in response to stimuli is normal and indicates that the newborn is doing well. Test this by snapping a finger against the sole of the newborn's foot.

- **Activity or muscle tone.** The degree of muscle tone indicates the oxygenation of the tissues. Normally, the hips and knees are flexed at birth, and, to some degree, the newborn will resist attempts to straighten them. A newborn should not be floppy or limp.

- **Respirations.** Normally, a newborn's respirations are regular and rapid, with a good strong cry. If the respirations are slow, shallow, or labored, or if the cry is weak, the newborn may have respiratory insufficiency and need assistance with ventilation. Complete absence of respirations or crying is obviously a very serious sign; in addition to assisted ventilation, CPR may be necessary.

The total of the five numbers is the Apgar score. The highest possible score is 10. The Apgar score should be calculated at 1 minute and again at 5 minutes after birth. Calculation of the Apgar score should not delay resuscitation efforts and is generally deferred when resuscitation is required. A score of 7 or higher is generally considered reassuring. **TABLE 34-4** shows the Apgar scoring system. **FIGURE 34-12** shows a photo of a newborn with an Apgar score of less than 9.

Follow these steps when assessing a newborn:

1. Quickly calculate the Apgar score to establish a baseline on the newborn's status.
2. Stimulation should result in an immediate increase in respiration rate. If not, you must begin ventilations with a bag-mask device. Unlike adults, in whom sudden cardiac arrest may precede respiratory arrest, newborns who are in cardiac arrest usually have had a

**TABLE 34-4** Apgar Scoring System

| Area of Activity | Score | | |
|---|---|---|---|
| | 2 | 1 | 0 |
| Appearance | Entire newborn is pink. | Body is pink, but hands and feet remain blue. | Entire newborn is blue or pale. |
| Pulse | More than 100 beats/min | Fewer than 100 beats/min | Absent pulse |
| Grimace or irritability | Newborn cries and tries to move foot away from finger snapped against sole of foot. | Newborn gives a weak cry in response to stimulus. | Newborn does not cry or react to stimulus. |
| Activity or muscle tone | Newborn resists attempts to straighten hips and knees. | Newborn makes weak attempts to resist straightening. | Newborn is completely limp, with no muscle tone. |
| Respiration | Rapid respirations | Slow respirations | Absent respirations |

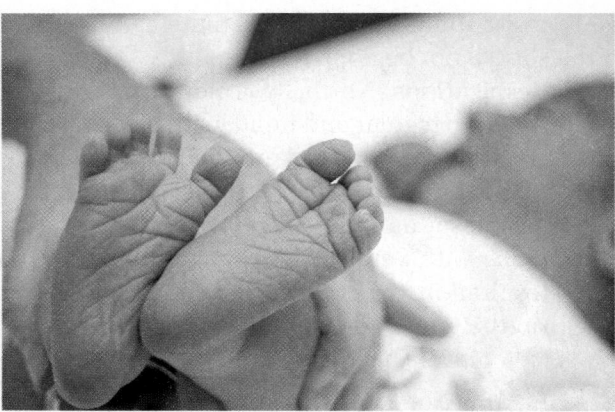

**FIGURE 34-12** Newborns who have blue extremities immediately after delivery would receive only 1 point for "Appearance" on the Apgar scale.

© John Thys/Reporters/Science Source.

respiratory arrest first. Therefore, it is essential to keep the newborn ventilating and oxygenating well.

3. If the newborn is breathing well, check the pulse rate by feeling the brachial pulse or auscultating the chest with a stethoscope. The pulse rate should be at least 100 beats/min. If it is not, begin ventilations with a bag-mask device. Begin ventilations without oxygen attached as the 21% oxygen in the atmosphere is often enough, and a change that is too rapid in oxygen levels from the saturation levels before birth may be detrimental. Ventilation alone may increase the newborn's heart rate. Reassess respirations and heart rate at least every 30 seconds to make sure that the pulse rate is increasing and respirations are becoming spontaneous.

4. Assess the newborn's oxygenation via pulse oximetry, which is best taken at the right wrist, and observe for central cyanosis. Remember that the oxygen saturation does not usually reach the 85% to 95% range until about 10 minutes after birth. If central cyanosis is present or the oxygen saturation does not improve but breathing is adequate, administer blow-by oxygen by holding oxygen tubing or an oxygen mask close to the newborn's face. Set the oxygen flow rate at 5 L/min.

5. Remember that you now have two patients. Request a second unit as soon as possible if you determine that the newborn is in any distress and will require resuscitation.

## Special Populations

Current information on neonatal resuscitation may vary from what you learned in your class on CPR, which usually does not differentiate between CPR for an infant and CPR for a neonate (newborn). Be sure to know your specific local protocols on neonatal resuscitation.

In situations where assisted ventilation is required, you should use a newborn bag-mask device. Cover the newborn's mouth and nose with the mask, and begin ventilation with high-flow oxygen at a rate of 40 to 60 breaths/min. Make sure you have a good mask-to-face seal. Use gentle pressure to make the chest rise with each ventilation. You may need to bypass the pop-off valve to accomplish this, especially during the first few breaths.

If the newborn does not begin breathing on his or her own or does not have an adequate heart rate, continue CPR and rapidly transport. Once CPR has been started, do not stop until the newborn responds with adequate respirations and heart rate or is pronounced dead by a physician. Do not give up! If the newborn presents in distress, do not take time to assess the Apgar score—begin resuscitation immediately.

# Complicated Delivery Emergencies
## Breech Delivery

The position in which an infant is born or the body part that is delivered first is called the **presentation**. Most infants are born head first, in what is called a **vertex presentation**. Occasionally, the buttocks are delivered first. This is called a **breech presentation** (**FIGURE 34-13**). With a breech presentation, the fetus is at great risk for trauma from the delivery. In addition, a prolapsed cord is more common in a breech delivery. Breech deliveries are usually longer than a normal delivery, so there may be time to get the pregnant woman to the hospital. If the buttocks have already passed through the vagina, however, the delivery has begun. You should provide emergency care and call for ALS backup. In general, if the

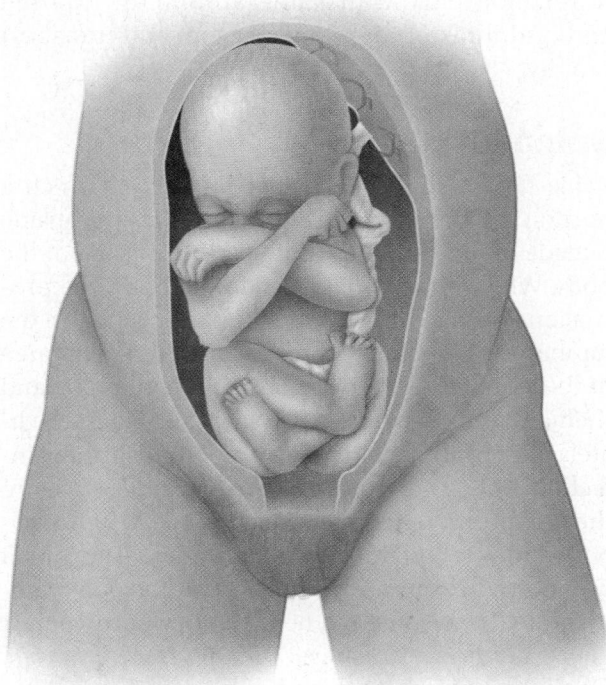

**FIGURE 34-13** In a breech presentation, the buttocks are delivered first. Breech deliveries are usually slow, so you will often have time to transport the woman to the hospital.

© Jones & Bartlett Learning.

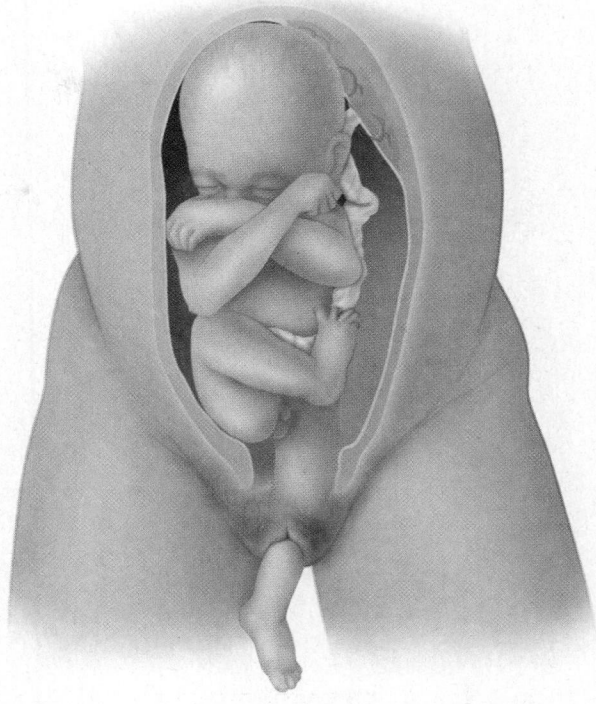

**FIGURE 34-14** In rare cases, a limb, usually a single arm or leg, presents first. This is a life-threatening situation, and you must provide prompt transport for hospital delivery.

© Jones & Bartlett Learning.

woman does not deliver within 10 minutes of the buttocks presentation, provide prompt transport. Consult medical control to guide you in this difficult situation.

Preparing for a breech delivery is the same as for a normal childbirth. Position the pregnant woman, prepare the OB kit, and place yourself and your partner as you would for a normal delivery. Allow the buttocks and legs to deliver spontaneously, supporting them with your hand to prevent rapid expulsion. The buttocks will usually come out easily. Let the legs dangle on either side of your arm while you support the trunk and chest as they are delivered. The head is almost always facedown and should be allowed to deliver spontaneously. As the head is delivering, you will need to perform a potentially life-saving procedure to manage the newborn's airway. Make a "V" with your gloved fingers and position them in the vagina to keep the walls of the vagina from compressing the fetus's airway. This situation and a prolapsed cord are the only two circumstances in which you should insert your fingers into the vagina.

## Presentation Complications

On rare occasions, the presenting part of the fetus is neither the head nor the buttocks but a single arm or leg. This is called a **limb presentation** (**FIGURE 34-14**). You cannot successfully deliver a fetus with a limb presentation in the field. These fetuses usually must be delivered surgically. If you are faced with a limb presentation, you must transport the patient to the hospital immediately. If a limb is protruding, cover it with a sterile towel. Never try to push it back in, and never pull on it. Place the patient on her back, with her head down and pelvis elevated. Because the woman and fetus are likely to be physically stressed, remember to administer high-flow oxygen to the woman.

**Prolapse of the umbilical cord**, a situation in which the umbilical cord comes out of the vagina before the fetus (**FIGURE 34-15**), is another rare presentation that must be treated in the hospital. This situation is dangerous because the fetus's head will compress the cord during birth and cut off circulation, depriving the fetus of oxygenated blood. Do not attempt to push the cord back into the vagina.

towel, moistened with saline, around the exposed cord. Administer high-flow oxygen, and transport rapidly.

## Spina Bifida

Spina bifida is a developmental defect in which a portion of the spinal cord or meninges may protrude outside of the vertebrae and possibly outside of the body. When it protrudes outside the body, the protrusion is seen on the newborn's back, usually in the lumbar area. It is important to cover the open area of the spinal cord with a moist, sterile dressing and then an occlusive dressing to seal the area immediately after birth to help prevent a potentially fatal infection. This treatment will have a positive effect on the newborn's outcome. Maintenance of the newborn's body temperature is important, so if you must use moist dressings, which can lower the body temperature, have someone hold the newborn against his or her body. Chapter 37, *Patients With Special Challenges*, discusses spina bifida in greater detail.

## Multiple Gestation

According to the CDC, twins occur about once in every 30 births; triplets or higher multiples occur much less frequently. The woman will usually know if she is carrying multiple fetuses. Sometimes, there is a family history of twins or the woman suspects that she is having twins because she has an unusually large abdomen. Usually, however, the identification of multiple fetuses is made early in pregnancy with modern ultrasonographic techniques. With multiple fetuses, always be prepared for more than one resuscitation, and call for assistance.

Twins are usually smaller than single fetuses, and delivery is typically not difficult. Consider the possibility that you are dealing with twins any time the first newborn is small or the woman's abdomen remains fairly large and firm after the birth. You should also ask the patient about the possibility of multiples. If twins are present, the second one will usually be born within 45 minutes of the first. About 10 minutes after the first birth, contractions will begin again, and the birth process will repeat itself.

The procedure for delivering twins is the same as that for a single fetus; however, you will need some supplies from an additional OB kit. Clamp and cut the cord of the first newborn as soon as it has been delivered and before the second newborn

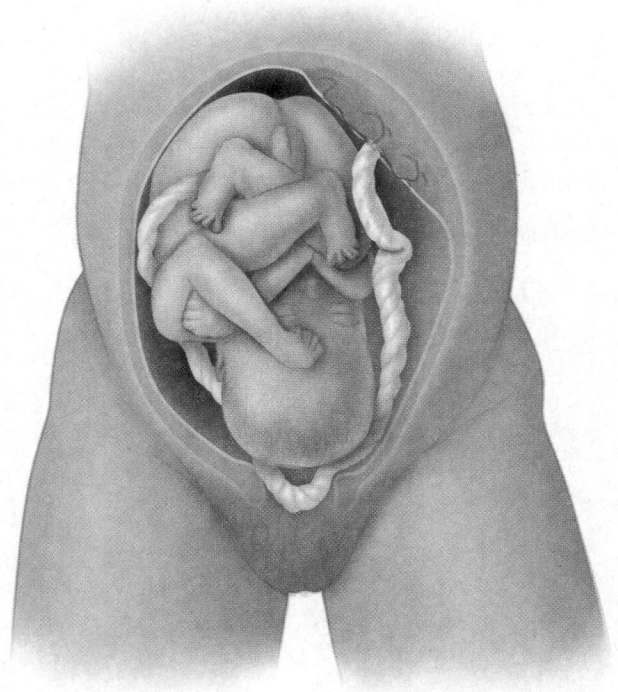

**FIGURE 34-15** A prolapsed umbilical cord is a life-threatening situation for the fetus and must be treated at the hospital.

© Jones & Bartlett Learning.

Prolapse of the umbilical cord usually occurs early in labor when the amniotic sac ruptures. There is usually time to get the patient to the hospital. Your job is to try to keep the fetus's head from compressing the cord.

Place the pregnant woman supine with the foot end of the stretcher raised 6 to 12 inches (15 to 30 cm) higher than the head, with her hips elevated on a pillow or folded sheet. Alternatively, the woman may be placed in the knee-chest position: kneeling and bent forward, facedown. Either of these positions will help keep the weight of the fetus off the prolapsed cord. Carefully insert your sterile gloved hand into the vagina, and gently push the fetus's head away from the umbilical cord. Note that this is one of only two situations (the other being a breech presentation) in which you should place a hand or finger into the vagina. Maintain this position and continue to keep the pressure off of the cord continuously throughout the transport to the hospital and possibly until the patient is in the operating room. Wrap a sterile is delivered. The second fetus may deliver before or after the first placenta. There may be only one placenta, or one for each fetus. When the placenta has been delivered, check whether there is one umbilical cord or two. If you see only one umbilical cord coming out of the first placenta, another placenta is still to be delivered. If both cords are attached to one placenta, the delivery is complete. Identical twins are always the same sex; fraternal twins may be the same or different sexes.

Record the time of birth of each twin separately. Twins may be so small that they look premature; handle them carefully and keep them warm. Identify the first newborn delivered as "Baby A." With the delivery of two or more newborns, you can indicate the order of delivery by writing on a piece of tape and placing it on the blanket or towel that is wrapped around each newborn.

## Premature Birth

Full-term gestation is considered to be between 39 weeks and 40 weeks, 6 days, which is approximately 9 calendar months. A normal, full-term, single newborn will weigh approximately 7 lb (3 kg) at birth. Any newborn who delivers before 8 months (36 weeks of gestation) or weighs less than 5 lb (2 kg) at birth is considered premature. This determination is not always easy to make. Often, the exact gestation time cannot be determined. A premature newborn is smaller and thinner than a full-term newborn, and the head is proportionately larger in comparison with the rest of the body (**FIGURE 34-16**). The

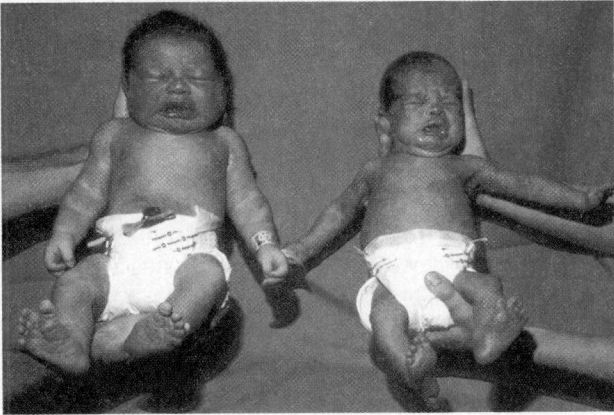

**FIGURE 34-16** Premature newborns (right) are smaller and thinner than full-term newborns.
© American Academy of Orthopaedic Surgeons.

vernix caseosa will be absent or minimal on a premature newborn. There will also be less body hair.

Premature newborns need special care to survive. They often require resuscitation, which should be performed unless physically impossible. With such care, premature newborns as small as 1 lb (0.5 kg) have survived.

## Postterm Pregnancy

In 2018, approximately 6.2% of pregnancies were postterm. Postterm means the gestation period is longer than 41 completed weeks of gestation. The rate of postterm pregnancies has been steadily declining for the past decade.

A true postterm pregnancy can lead to complications in both the woman and fetus. Postterm fetuses can be larger than a typical 40-week fetus, sometimes weighing more than 10 lb (5 kg), which can lead to a more difficult labor and delivery and an increased chance of injury to the fetus as it travels through the birth canal. The likelihood of a cesarean section being required is increased. The woman is also at increased risk for perineal tears and infection. Postterm newborns have an increased risk of meconium aspiration, infection, and being stillborn and may not have developed normally because of the restricted size of the uterus. Be prepared to resuscitate the newborn, as respiratory and neurologic functions may have been affected. The larger size of the fetus causes it to take up more space inside the uterus, resulting in compression of the structures, including the blood vessels of the placenta and the umbilical cord.

## Fetal Death

Unfortunately, you may find yourself delivering a fetus that died in the woman's uterus before labor began. This situation will test your medical, emotional, and social abilities. Grieving parents will be emotionally distraught and may be hostile, requiring all of your professionalism and support skills. Chapter 35, *Pediatric Emergencies*, discusses how to handle the death of a child in detail.

The onset of labor may be premature, but labor will otherwise progress normally in most cases. If an intrauterine infection has caused the death of the fetus, you may note an extremely foul odor. Depending on the stage of decomposition, the delivered fetus may have skin blisters, skin sloughing, and a dark discoloration. The head will be soft and perhaps grossly deformed.

Do not attempt to resuscitate an obviously dead neonate. However, do not confuse this situation with that in which a newborn is in cardiopulmonary arrest as a complication of the birthing process. You must attempt to resuscitate newborns if there is any question about viability.

## Postpartum Complications

Some bleeding always occurs with delivery, but bleeding that exceeds approximately 1,000 mL is considered high risk for maternal mortality and morbidity. If bleeding continues after delivery of the placenta, continue to massage the uterus, but check your technique and hand placement. If the woman appears to be in shock, treat her accordingly and transport, massaging the uterus en route. Excessive bleeding after birth is usually caused by the muscles of the uterus not fully contracting. This can be from delivering more than one infant, a long labor process so the uterus is too "tired" to contract, or parts of the placenta still being inside the uterus. This condition is potentially life threatening for the woman. Cover the vagina with a sterile pad, changing the pad as often as necessary. Do not discard any blood-soaked pads; hospital personnel will use them to estimate the amount of blood loss. Also save any tissue that may have passed from the vagina.

Administer oxygen if necessary, monitor vital signs frequently, and transport the patient immediately to the hospital. Never hold the woman's legs together or pack the vagina with gauze pads in an attempt to control bleeding.

Postpartum patients are also at increased risk of a venous embolism. One reason is the increased clotting ability that is a normal change of pregnancy. Also, a pregnant woman who has been on bed rest for any length of time is more prone to clots. The most common embolism seen in postpartum women is a pulmonary embolism, which is a clot that travels through the bloodstream and becomes lodged in the pulmonary circulation. This obstruction will block blood flow to the lungs and is potentially life threatening. If you deliver a newborn in the field and the woman begins to report sudden difficulty breathing or shortness of breath, consider the possibility that she has a pulmonary embolism.

You should also suspect a pulmonary embolism in patients of childbearing age with respiratory complaints who have recently delivered, especially with the sudden onset of difficulty breathing or altered mental status. Women have died of a postpartum pulmonary embolism from days to several weeks or months after childbirth. Provide supportive care of the ABCs with high-flow oxygen and rapid transport to the hospital.

## YOU    are the Provider **SUMMARY**

**1. What anatomic and physiologic changes occur during pregnancy? How will they affect your assessment of the patient?**

Most pregnancy-related changes are observed in the respiratory and cardiovascular systems. As the uterus enlarges during pregnancy, it is displaced upward from the pelvic cavity, where it is normally protected, and is therefore exposed to potential injury. The enlarged uterus pushes upward on the diaphragm. This decreases the woman's ability to breathe deeply, so the respiratory rate increases slightly to maintain adequate minute volume. Pregnancy also increases maternal oxygen demand and consumption, and the body compensates with the increased rate as well. Blood volume increases throughout pregnancy. To accommodate the increase in total blood volume, the woman's heart rate increases up to 20%, or about 20 beats/min, by the third trimester of pregnancy.

Vital signs changes during pregnancy, such as an increase in heart rate and respiratory rate, should not be assumed to be pregnancy related if the woman experiences an acute illness or injury. Instead, assume them to be signs of shock until proven otherwise.

**2. How will you determine whether delivery is imminent or if there is enough time to transport the pregnant patient?**

Ask the patient how long she has been pregnant, when she is due to deliver, and if this is her first pregnancy. *As a general rule*, labor is longer in women who are pregnant for the first time (primigravida). If the patient is experiencing contractions, ask her how far apart they are and how long they last. Ask if her bag of waters (amniotic sac) has ruptured. This typically occurs toward the end of the first stage of labor, but may not occur until the delivery itself. Ask her if she is experiencing any vaginal spotting or bleeding; during the first stage of labor a plug of mucus—sometimes mixed with blood (bloody show)—is expelled from the dilating cervix and discharged from the vagina. Ask the patient if she feels the urge to push or move her bowels as the pressure of the baby's head on the perineum may be misinterpreted as the need to have a bowel movement. The presence of crowning is an obvious indicator that delivery is in progress. Perhaps one of the most reliable indicators of imminent delivery is when the patient states, "I'm having this baby now!" This is especially true in women who have given birth before.

**3. What are gestational diabetes and preeclampsia? How can they affect this delivery?**

Gestational diabetes, or diabetes of pregnancy, is a condition that develops during pregnancy and typically resolves on its own after delivery. Infants born to women with gestational diabetes are often large for their gestational age, which could lead to shoulder dystocia—a condition in which the fetus's shoulders are too broad to fit through the woman's pelvic opening—or other delivery complications caused by the fetus's size. In addition, many women experience nausea before labor and have not eaten recently—factors that could lead to hypoglycemia and weakness in the woman and fetus.

Preeclampsia, or pregnancy-induced hypertension, is characterized by hypertension; edema of the hands, feet, and face; and protein in the urine. Other symptoms may include visual disturbances (eg, seeing spots, blurred vision), headache, and anxiety.

Untreated preeclampsia may lead to eclampsia, which is characterized by life-threatening seizures. The presence of preeclampsia, as with gestational diabetes, increases the risk of fetal distress, which may necessitate resuscitation of the newborn after delivery.

**4. Is there time to transport this patient, or should you prepare for imminent delivery?**

The patient is experiencing frequent (every 2 minutes) contractions that are lasting 45 seconds, and she has the urge to move her bowels, which indicates that the fetus is in the birth canal. On the basis of these factors, delivery will likely occur within the next few minutes; therefore, you and your partner should prepare for imminent delivery.

**5. How should you manage the umbilical cord situation?**

As soon as the head has delivered, you should assess for the location of the umbilical cord. If wrapped around the newborn's neck, an umbilical cord must be managed immediately because if the cord is wrapped tightly around the newborn's neck, the airway could be constricted. Usually, you can slip the cord gently over the head (or shoulders, if necessary). If not, place two clamps on the cord about 2 inches (5 cm) apart and cut between them. Delivery must proceed quickly if this is necessary, as the infant is no longer receiving oxygen from the mother once the cord is clamped. Handle the cord very carefully; it is fragile and easily torn.

**6. What would you do if the amniotic sac were still intact?**

If you notice that the amniotic sac seems to be intact after the head delivers or as the head is crowning, immediately puncture the membrane and allow the fluid to drain. Avoid using sharp objects to puncture the membrane; first attempt to use your gloved fingers to tear the membrane. Once the membrane ruptures and the fluid drains, wipe the traces of the membrane away from the newborn's mouth and nose and continue with the delivery.

**7. What is involved in the routine postdelivery care of a newborn?**

Immediate postdelivery care of a newborn—regardless of his or her appearance—involves keeping the newborn dry and warm and facilitating effective breathing. The need for further treatment is based on assessment of the newborn's respiratory effort, heart rate, and skin color.

**8. What immediate treatment is indicated for this newborn?**

The newborn is breathing; however, her heart rate is low (80 beats/min) and her trunk and extremities are cyanotic. These clinical signs indicate that she is hypoxemic and will require additional resuscitative measures. Begin positive-pressure ventilations with a bag-mask device. Newborn bradycardia is almost always the result of hypoxemia.

Ventilate the newborn at a rate of 40 to 60 breaths/min for 30 seconds with room air, and

## YOU are the Provider SUMMARY *continued*

then reassess the heart rate. In most cases, a brief period of positive-pressure ventilation is all that is needed to increase the newborn's heart rate. If the heart rate is still less than 100 beats/min after 30 seconds of positive-pressure ventilation, continue ventilations, slowly add oxygen, keep the newborn warm, and transport at once.

**9. What further treatment is indicated for the mother?**

After delivery and before transport, place a sterile pad or sanitary pad over the vaginal opening and straighten the mother's legs. *Never place any pads or dressings into the vagina.* Gently massage the mother's abdomen with a firm, circular kneading motion to cause the uterus to contract and help control bleeding.

If severe bleeding occurs after placental delivery, transport immediately and treat the mother for shock. Place additional sterile pads or sanitary pads over the mother's vaginal opening, administer high-flow oxygen if necessary, and keep her warm with blankets. Closely monitor her vital signs en route.

**10. What Apgar score should you assign to this newborn at 5 minutes after birth?**

This newborn has a pink body but cyanotic hands and feet; therefore, you should assign a score of *1* for appearance. Her heart rate is 120 beats/min; therefore, assign a score of *2* for the pulse. She moves her foot away when you flick the soles; therefore, assign a score of *2* for grimace. She resists your attempts to straighten her knees, which indicates good muscle tone; therefore, assign a score of *2* for activity. Finally, her respirations are rapid (40 to 60 breaths/min is a normal newborn respiratory rate); therefore, assign a score of *2* for respirations. On the basis of your assessment findings, you should assign the newborn an Apgar score of 9 at 5 minutes. Since you were busy with resuscitative measures at 1 minute, no APGAR would likely have been obtained at that time, but because of the low heart rate and generalized cyanosis, it would have been lower than the 5-minute score.

### EMS Patient Care Report (PCR)[a]

| Date: 12-9-20 | Incident No.: 013115 | Nature of Call: Woman in labor | | Location: 2505 Landa Park Blvd | |
|---|---|---|---|---|---|
| Dispatched: 0625 | En Route: 0627 | At Scene: 0631 | Transport: 0655 | At Hospital: 0708 | In Service: 0753 |

#### Patient Information (Mother)

| | |
|---|---|
| Age: 28 <br> Sex: F <br> Weight (in kg [lb]): 70 kg (155 lb) | Allergies: No known drug allergies <br> Medications: Prenatal vitamins <br> Past Medical History: Gestational diabetes, preeclampsia <br> Chief Complaint: Active labor |

#### Vital Signs

| Time: 0638 | BP: 122/82 | Pulse: 110 | Respirations: 24 | Spo$_2$: 98% |
|---|---|---|---|---|
| Time: 0643 | BP: 130/60 | Pulse: 114 | Respirations: 22 | Spo$_2$: 98% |
| Time: 0651 | BP: 126/60 | Pulse: 98 | Respirations: 20 | Spo$_2$: 97% |

#### EMS Treatment (circle all that apply)

| Oxygen @ ___ L/min via: <br><br> NC   NRM   Bag mask | | Assisted Ventilation | Airway Adjunct | CPR |
|---|---|---|---|---|
| Defibrillation | Bleeding Control | Bandaging | Splinting | Other: Assisted with delivery of baby; fundal massage |

## YOU are the Provider SUMMARY *continued*

| Narrative |
|---|

Medic 44 is dispatched to a residence for a female in labor.

Chief Complaint: Active labor

History: On arrival, patient stated, "I am having my baby now!" She stated that this is her third baby. Her husband, who was present at the scene, advised that she has had gestational diabetes and preeclampsia with this pregnancy and has had regular prenatal care. The patient stated that her contractions were 2 minutes apart and lasting about 45 seconds each; she further stated that she had the urge to move her bowels and that her amniotic sac ruptured 5 hours ago.

Assessment: Arrived on scene and found the patient, a 28-year-old female, lying supine in her bed. She was conscious and alert; her airway was patent, and her breathing, although increased in rate, was of adequate depth. Initial visual inspection of the vaginal area did not reveal crowning. After initial set of vital signs was obtained, reassessment of vaginal area revealed crowning.

Treatment (Rx): Properly positioned patient, and prepared for delivery. Husband remained present and provided emotional support and respiratory coaching to his wife. Delivery of head revealed nuchal cord, which was easily corrected by sliding the cord over the shoulders. Delivered the rest of the female infant without difficulty at 0645. Allowed mother to hold the newborn. Clamped and cut the umbilical cord. Placental delivery occurred approximately 5 minutes after the birth of the baby. Reassessed mother's vital signs, and provided fundal massage for mild postpartum bleeding.

Transport: Assisted mother onto ambulance gurney and secured newborn in a car seat for movement to the same ambulance for transport to the hospital. En route, patient remained stable. Reassessment of vaginal bleeding revealed that it had stopped. Transported mother and her baby to the hospital without incident. Assisted mother onto a hospital bed and the infant was placed on a warming bed to be evaluated by nursery staff. Provided verbal report to attending physician. Medic 44 returned to service at 0753.

**End of report**

[a]Note: Even though the mother and newborn are transported together in the same ambulance, two patient care reports are needed—one for the mother and one for the newborn. The specific assessment findings for the infant are noted in the other report.

# Prep Kit

## Ready for Review

- Inside the uterus, the developing fetus is within the amniotic sac. The umbilical cord connects the woman and fetus through the placenta. Eventually, contractions of the uterus will propel the fetus through the birth canal.
- Throughout pregnancy, the body changes to accommodate the fetus. The primary systems involved with these changes are the respiratory, cardiovascular, and musculoskeletal systems.
- As a result of enlargement of the uterus, a pregnant patient's respiratory capacity changes with increased respiratory rates and decreasing minute volumes.
- A pregnant woman's blood volume increases by as much as 50%, and the heart rate increases by 20%.
- Increased hormone levels affect the musculoskeletal system by making the joints looser, or less stable.
- Complications of pregnancy include hypertensive disorders, bleeding, and diabetes.
- During a trauma call that involves a pregnant woman, you have two patients to consider—the woman and the unborn fetus. Trauma to the woman may have a direct effect on the condition of the fetus.
- The first stage of labor, dilation, begins with the onset of contractions and ends when the cervix is fully dilated. The second stage of labor, expulsion of the fetus, begins when the cervix is fully dilated and the fetus enters the birth canal; it ends with delivery of the

newborn. The third stage of labor, delivery of the placenta, begins with the delivery of the newborn and ends with the delivery of the placenta.

- Once labor has begun, it cannot be slowed or stopped; however, there is usually time to transport the patient to the hospital during the first stage of labor. During the second stage of labor, you must decide whether to deliver at the scene or transport the patient. During the third stage of labor, after delivery of the newborn, anticipate delivery of the placenta. This may occur after transport has been initiated and usually is within 30 minutes of delivery of the newborn. Warm, dry, and stimulate the infant after birth.
- Abnormal or complicated deliveries include breech deliveries (buttocks first), limb presentations (arm or leg first), and prolapse of the umbilical cord (umbilical cord first).

Quickly transport the patient with a limb presentation or prolapsed umbilical cord to the hospital.

- You should place a finger or hand into the vagina for only two reasons: to keep the walls of the vagina from compressing the fetus's airway during a breech presentation or to push the fetus's head away from the cord when the cord is prolapsed.
- Assess a newborn for term gestation, good muscle tone, and breathing/crying to determine whether he or she requires resuscitation. Also obtain an Apgar score 1 minute and 5 minutes after birth.
- Excessive bleeding after delivery is a serious emergency. Begin fundal massage. Cover the vagina with a sterile pad. Change the pad as often as necessary and take all used pads to the hospital for examination.

## Vital Vocabulary

**abruptio placentae** Premature separation of the placenta from the wall of the uterus.

**amniotic sac** The fluid-filled, baglike membrane in which the fetus develops.

**anemic** Describes a condition in which the patient has too few red blood cells, resulting in a decreased ability to transport oxygen throughout the body via the bloodstream.

**Apgar score** A scoring system for assessing the status of a newborn that assigns a number value to each of five areas.

**birth canal** The vagina and cervix.

**bloody show** A small amount of blood in the vagina that appears at the beginning of labor and may include a plug of pink-tinged mucus that is discharged when the cervix begins to dilate.

**breech presentation** A delivery in which the buttocks come out first.

**cervix** The lower third, or neck, of the uterus.

**crowning** The appearance of the fetus's head at the vaginal opening during labor.

**eclampsia** A pregnancy complication that is characterized by new-onset hypertension (systolic blood pressure >140 mm Hg or diastolic blood pressure >90 mm Hg) with seizure activity and preceding systemic effects, such as blurred vision, headache, or protein in the urine. It is differentiated from preeclampsia by the presence of seizure activity.

**ectopic pregnancy** A pregnancy that develops outside the uterus, typically in a fallopian tube.

**embryo** The early stage of development after the fertilization of the egg (first 10 weeks).

**endometrium** The lining of the inside of the uterus.

**fetal alcohol syndrome** A condition caused by the consumption of alcohol by a pregnant woman; characterized by growth and physical problems, mental retardation, and a variety of congenital abnormalities in her child.

**fetus** The developing, unborn infant inside the uterus, from 10 weeks after fertilization until birth.

**fundus** The dome-shaped top of the uterus.

**gestational diabetes** Diabetes that develops during pregnancy in women who did not have diabetes before pregnancy.

**gestational hypertension** A blood pressure greater than or equal to 140 mm Hg systolic or 90 mm Hg diastolic in a pregnant female in whom hypertension has not previously been diagnosed.

**induced abortion** The elective termination of a pregnancy prior to the time of viability.

**lightening** The movement of the fetus down into the pelvis late in pregnancy.

**limb presentation** A delivery in which the presenting part is a single arm or leg.

**meconium** Fetal stool. When appearing as a dark green material in the amniotic fluid, it can indicate distress or disease in the newborn; it can be aspirated into the fetus's lungs during delivery.

**menarche** The first menstrual cycle or onset of the first menstrual bleeding in females.

**menopause** The cessation of menstruation, typically in the fourth or fifth decade of life.

**miscarriage** The spontaneous passage of the fetus and placenta before 20 weeks; also called spontaneous abortion.

**multigravida** A woman who has had previous pregnancies.

**nuchal cord** An umbilical cord that is wrapped around the fetus's neck.

**perineum** The area of the skin between the vagina and the anus.

**placenta** The tissue attached to the uterine wall that nourishes the fetus through the umbilical cord.

**placenta previa** A condition in which the placenta develops over and covers the cervix.

**preeclampsia** A pregnancy complication that is characterized by new-onset hypertension (systolic blood pressure >140 mm Hg or diastolic blood pressure >90 mm Hg) along with systemic effects, such as blurred vision, headache, or protein in the urine. Differentiated from eclampsia by the lack of seizure activity.

**presentation** The position in which an infant is born; defined by the part of the body that appears first.

**primigravida** A woman who is experiencing her first pregnancy.

**prolapse of the umbilical cord** A situation in which the umbilical cord comes out of the vagina before the fetus.

**spina bifida** A developmental defect in which a portion of the spinal cord or meninges may protrude outside of the vertebrae and possibly even outside of the body, usually at the lower third of the spine in the lumbar area.

**spontaneous abortion** The loss of a pregnancy prior to 20 weeks of gestation without any preceding surgical or medical intervention. Often called a miscarriage.

**supine hypotensive syndrome** Low blood pressure resulting from compression of the inferior vena cava by the weight of the pregnant uterus when the woman is supine.

**term gestation** A pregnancy that has reached full term, between 39 weeks and 40 weeks, 6 days.

**umbilical cord** The structure that connects the pregnant woman to the fetus via the placenta; contains two arteries and one vein.

**vernix caseosa** A white, cheesy substance that covers the body of the fetus.

**vertex presentation** A delivery in which the head of the newborn comes out first.

## References

1. Abalos E, Cuesta C, Grosso AL, Chou D, Say L. Global and regional estimates of preeclampsia and eclampsia: a systematic review. *Eur J Obstet Gynecol Reprod Biol* 2013;170(1):1-7.

2. American Academy of Pediatrics. Delayed umbilical cord clamping after birth. *Pediatrics* 2017;139(6):e20170957.

3. American Academy of Pediatrics. To suction or not to suction: the meconium debate continues. *NRP.* 2019;28(1). https://downloads.aap.org/DOICH/NRP%20

Instructor%20Update%20Spring_Summer%202019.pdf. Accessed February 15, 2020.

4. American Academy of Pediatrics Committee on Fetus and Newborn, American College of Obstetricians and Gynecologists Committee on Obstetric Practice. The Apgar score. *Pediatrics* 2015;136(4):819-822.

5. Ananth CV, Keyes KM, Wapner RJ. Pre-eclampsia rates in the United States, 1980−2010: age-period-cohort analysis. *BMJ* 2013;347:f6564.

6. Balchin I, Whittaker JC, Lamont JF, Steer PJ. Maternal and fetal characteristics associated with meconium-stained amniotic fluid. *Obstet Gynecol* 2011;117(4):828-835.

7. Beckman CRB, Ling FW, Herbert WNP, et al. *Obstetrics and Gynecology*. 7th ed. Baltimore, MD: Lippincott Williams & Wilkins; 2014.

8. Branson RD, Johannigman JA. Pre-hospital oxygen therapy. *Respir Care* 2013;58(1):86-97.

9. Centers for Disease Control and Prevention, National Center for Health Statistics. Multiple births. https://www.cdc.gov/nchs/fastats/multiple.htm. Reviewed January 18, 2014. Accessed February 15, 2020.

10. Cheng HT, Wang YC, Lo HC, et al. Trauma during pregnancy: a population-based analysis of maternal outcome. *World J Surg* 2012;36(12):2767-2775.

11. Combs CA, Laros RK Jr. Prolonged third stage of labor: morbidity and risk factors. *Obstet Gynecol* 1991;77(6):863-867.

12. Committee on Obstetric Practice. Committee opinion no. 684: delayed umbilical cord clamping after birth. *Obstet Gynecol* 2017;129(1):e5-e10. doi:10.1097/AOG.0000000000001860.

13. Committee on Practice Bulletins—Obstetrics. Practice bulletin no. 183: postpartum hemorrhage. *Obstet Gynecol* 2017;130(4):e168-e186. doi:10.1097/AOG.0000000000002351.

14. Deputy NP, Kim SY, Conrey EJ, Bullard KM. Prevalence and changes in preexisting diabetes and gestational diabetes among women who had a live birth—United States, 2012–2016. *MMWR* 2018;67(43):1201-1207.

15. Division of Reproductive Health, National Center for Chronic Disease Prevention and Health Promotion. Reproductive health: teen pregnancy. Centers for Disease Control and Prevention website. https://www.cdc.gov/teenpregnancy/about/index.htm. Reviewed March 1, 2019. Accessed February 15, 2020.

16. Dombrowski MP, Bottoms SF, Saleh AA, Hurd WW, Romero R. Third stage of labor: analysis of duration and clinical practice. *Am J Obstet Gynecol* 1995;172(4 Pt 1):1279-1284.

17. Gazmararian JA, Lazorick S, Spitz AM, et al. Prevalence of violence against pregnant women. *JAMA* 1996;275(24):1915-1920.

18. Haydon ML, Gorenberg DM, Nageotte MP, et al. The effect of maternal oxygen administration on fetal pulse oximetry during labor in fetuses with nonreassuring fetal heart rate patterns. *Am J Obstet Gynecol* 2006;195(3):735-738.

19. Hillard PJ. Physical abuse in pregnancy. *Obstet Gynecol* 1985;66(2):185-190.

20. Hwang SS, Diop H, Liu CL, et al. Maternal substance use disorders and infant outcomes in the first year of life among Massachusetts singletons, 2003–2010. *J Pediatr* 2017;191:69-75.

21. Jeejeebhoy FM, Zelop CM, Lipman S, et al. Cardiac arrest in pregnancy. *Circulation* 2015;132(18):1747-1773.

22. Larson JD, Rayburn WF, Crosby S, Thurnau GR. Multiple nuchal cord entanglements and intrapartum complications. *Am J Obstet Gynecol* 1995;173(4):1228-1231.

23. Larson JD, Rayburn WF, Harlan VL. Nuchal cord entanglements and gestational age. *Am J Perinatol* 1997;14(9):555-557.

24. MacDorman MF, Declercq E. Trends and state variations in out-of-hospital births in the United States, 2004–2017. *Birth* 2019;46(2):279-288.

25. Martin JA, Hamilton BE, Osterman MJK. Births in the United States, 2018. NCHS Data Brief. No. 346. July 2019. https://www.cdc.gov/nchs/data/databriefs/db346-h.pdf. Accessed February 15, 2020.

26. Mendez-Figueroa H, Dahlke JD, Vrees RA, Rouse DJ. Trauma in pregnancy: an updated systematic review. *Am J Obstet Gynecol* 2013;209(1):1-10.

27. Mhyre JM, Tsen LC, Einav S, et al. Cardiac arrest during hospitalization for delivery in the United States, 1998–2011. *Anesthesiology* 2014;120(4):810.

28. National Association of State EMS Officials. *National EMS Scope of Practice Model 2019*. DOT HS 812-666. Washington, DC: National Highway Traffic Safety Administration. https://www.ems.gov/pdf/National_EMS_Scope_of_Practice_Model_2019.pdf. Accessed February 15, 2020.

29. O'Reilly KB. One in three physicians has been sued; by age 55, 1 in 2 hit with suit. American Medical Association website. https://www.ama-assn.org/practice-management/sustainability/1-3-physicians-has-been-sued-age-55-1-2-hit-suit. Published January 26, 2018. Accessed February 15, 2020.

30. Perlman JM, Wyllie J, Kattwinkel J, et al. Part 7: neonatal resuscitation: 2015 international consensus on cardiopulmonary resuscitation and emergency cardiovascular care science with treatment recommendations. *Circulation* 2015;132(16 Suppl 1):S204-S241.

31. Schäffer L, Burkhardt T, Zimmermann R, Kurmanavicius J. Nuchal cords in term and postterm deliveries—do we need to know? *Obstet Gynecol* 2005;106(1):23-28.

32. Sheiner E, Abramowicz JS, Levy A, et al. Nuchal cord is not associated with adverse perinatal outcome. *Arch Gynecol Obstet* 2006;274(2):81-83.

33. Stewart DE. Incidence of postpartum abuse in women with a history of abuse during pregnancy. *CMAJ* 1994;151(11):1601-1604.

34. Substance Abuse and Mental Health Services Administration. Key substance use and mental health indicators in the United States: results from the 2016 National Survey on Drug Use and Health. https://www.samhsa.gov/data/sites/default/files/NSDUH-FFR1-2016/NSDUH-FFR1-2016.pdf. Published September 2017. Accessed February 15, 2020.

35. Wyckoff MH, Aziz K, Escobedo MB, et al. Part 13: neonatal resuscitation: 2015 American Heart Association guidelines update for cardiopulmonary resuscitation and emergency cardiovascular care. *Circulation* 2015;132(Suppl 2):S543-S560.

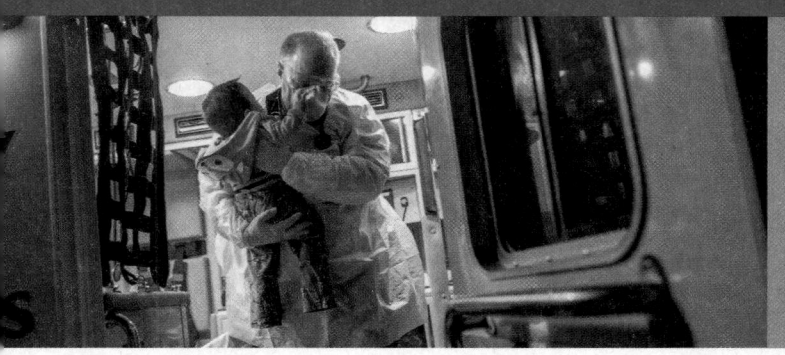

# Chapter 35

# Pediatric Emergencies

## NATIONAL EMS EDUCATION STANDARD COMPETENCIES

### Special Patient Populations

Applies a fundamental knowledge of growth, development, and aging and assessment findings to provide basic emergency care and transportation for a patient with special needs.

### Patients With Special Challenges

- Recognizing and reporting abuse and neglect (pp 1336–1339 and Chapter 36, *Geriatric Emergencies*)

Health care implications of

- Abuse (pp 1336–1339 and Chapter 36, *Geriatric Emergencies*)
- Neglect (pp 1336–1339 and Chapter 36, *Geriatric Emergencies*)
- Homelessness (Chapter 37, *Patients With Special Challenges*)
- Poverty (Chapter 37, *Patients With Special Challenges*)
- Bariatrics (Chapter 37, *Patients With Special Challenges*)
- Technology dependent (Chapter 37, *Patients With Special Challenges*)
- Hospice/terminally ill (Chapter 37, *Patients With Special Challenges*)
- Tracheostomy care/dysfunction (Chapter 37, *Patients With Special Challenges*)
- Home care (Chapter 37, *Patients With Special Challenges*)
- Sensory deficit/loss (Chapter 37, *Patients With Special Challenges*)
- Developmental disability (Chapter 37, *Patients With Special Challenges*)

### Pediatrics

Age-related assessment findings, and age-related assessment and treatment modifications for pediatric-specific major diseases and/or emergencies

- Upper airway obstruction (pp 1294–1300, 1308–1310)
- Lower airway reactive disease (pp 1294–1300, 1310–1312)
- Respiratory distress/failure/arrest (pp 1294–1297, 1308–1320)
- Shock (pp 1296–1300, 1320–1322)
- Seizures (pp 1322–1323, 1328)
- Sudden unexpected infant death and sudden infant death syndrome (p 1339)

Age-related assessment findings, and developmental stage–related assessment and treatment modifications for pediatric-specific major diseases and/or emergencies

- Upper airway obstruction (pp 1308–1310)
- Lower airway reactive disease (pp 1310–1311, 1312)
- Respiratory distress/failure/arrest (pp 1294–1297)
- Shock (pp 1297–1300, 1320–1321)
- Seizures (pp 1322–1323, 1328)
- Sudden infant death syndrome (pp 1339–1342)
- Gastrointestinal disease (pp 1324–1325)

### Trauma

Applies fundamental knowledge to provide basic emergency care and transportation based on assessment findings for an acutely injured patient.

## Special Considerations in Trauma

Recognition and management of trauma in the

- Pregnant patient (Chapter 34, *Obstetrics and Neonatal Care*)
- Pediatric patient (pp 1284–1290, 1293–1307, 1329–1335)
- Geriatric patient (Chapter 36, *Geriatric Emergencies*)

Pathophysiology, assessment, and management of trauma in the

- Pregnant patient (Chapter 34, *Obstetrics and Neonatal Care*)
- Pediatric patient (pp 1286–1290, 1293–1307, 1328–1335)
- Geriatric patient (Chapter 36, *Geriatric Emergencies*)
- Cognitively impaired patient (Chapter 37, *Patients With Special Challenges*)

## KNOWLEDGE OBJECTIVES

1. Explain some of the challenges inherent in providing emergency care to pediatric patients and why effective communication with both the patient and his or her family members is critical to a successful outcome. (p 1284)

2. Discuss the physical and cognitive developmental stages of an infant, including health risks, signs that may indicate illness, and patient assessment. (pp 1285–1286)

3. Discuss the physical and cognitive developmental stages of a toddler, including health risks, signs that may indicate illness, and patient assessment. (pp 1286–1287)

4. Discuss the physical and cognitive developmental stages of a preschool-age child, including health risks, signs that may indicate illness, and patient assessment. (pp 1287–1288)

5. Discuss the physical and cognitive developmental stages of a school-age child, including health risks, signs that may indicate illness, and patient assessment. (pp 1288–1289)

6. Discuss the physical and cognitive developmental stages of an adolescent, including health risks, patient assessment, and privacy issues. (pp 1289–1290)

7. Describe differences in the anatomy and physiology of the pediatric patient compared to the adult patient and their implications for EMTs, with a focus on the following body systems: respiratory, circulatory, nervous, gastrointestinal, musculoskeletal, and integumentary. (pp 1290–1293)

8. Describe differences in the pathophysiology of the pediatric patient compared to the adult patient and their implications for EMTs, with a focus on the following body systems: respiratory, circulatory, nervous, gastrointestinal, musculoskeletal, and integumentary. (pp 1290–1293)

9. Explain the steps in the primary assessment of a pediatric patient, including the elements of the pediatric assessment triangle (PAT), hands-on XABCs, transport decision considerations, and privacy issues. (pp 1294–1303)

10. Explain the steps in the secondary assessment of a pediatric patient, including what EMTs should look for related to different body areas and the method of injury. (pp 1304–1306)

11. Describe the emergency care of a pediatric patient in respiratory distress, including the different causes of pediatric respiratory emergencies, the signs and symptoms of increased work of breathing, and the difference between respiratory distress and respiratory failure. (pp 1294–1297, 1308–1320)

12. List the possible causes of an upper and a lower airway obstruction in a pediatric patient and the steps in the management of foreign body airway obstruction. (pp 1308–1310)

13. Describe asthma, its possible causes, signs, and symptoms, and the steps in the management of a pediatric patient who is experiencing an asthma attack. (pp 1310–1311)

14. Explain how to determine the correct size of an airway adjunct intended for a pediatric patient during an emergency. (p 1313)

15. List the different oxygen delivery devices that are available for providing oxygen to a pediatric patient, including the indications for the use of each and precautions EMTs must take to ensure the patient's safety. (pp 1316–1320)

16. Describe the emergency care of a pediatric patient who is in shock (hypoperfusion), including common causes, signs, and symptoms. (pp 1320–1322)

17. Describe the emergency care of a pediatric patient with an altered mental status, including common causes, signs, and symptoms. (p 1322)

18. Describe the emergency care of a pediatric patient who has experienced a seizure, including

the different types of seizures and the common causes, signs, and symptoms. (pp 1322–1323, 1328)

19. Describe the emergency care of a pediatric patient with meningitis, including common causes, signs, symptoms, and special precautions. (pp 1323–1324)

20. Describe the emergency care of a pediatric patient who is experiencing a gastrointestinal emergency, including common causes, signs, and symptoms. (pp 1324–1325)

21. Describe the emergency care of a pediatric patient who has been poisoned, including common sources of poisoning, signs, and symptoms. (pp 1325–1326)

22. Describe the emergency care of a pediatric patient who is dehydrated, including how to gauge the severity of dehydration based on key signs and symptoms. (pp 1326–1327)

23. Describe the emergency care of a pediatric patient who is experiencing a fever emergency, including common causes. (pp 1327–1329)

24. Describe the emergency care of a pediatric patient who has experienced a drowning emergency, including common causes, signs, and symptoms. (pp 1328–1329)

25. Discuss the common causes of pediatric trauma emergencies; include how to

differentiate between injury patterns in adults, infants, and children. (pp 1329–1335)

26. Discuss the significance of burns in pediatric patients, their most common causes, and general guidelines EMTs should follow when assessing patients who have sustained burns. (pp 1333–1335)

27. Explain the four triage categories used in the JumpSTART system for pediatric patients during disaster management. (pp 1335–1336)

28. Describe child abuse and neglect and its possible indicators, including the medical and legal responsibilities of EMTs when caring for a pediatric patient who is a possible victim of child abuse. (pp 1336–1339)

29. Discuss brief resolved unexplained event (BRUE), sudden unexpected infant death, and sudden infant death syndrome (SIDS), including its risk factors, patient assessment, and special management considerations related to the death of an infant patient. (pp 1339–1342)

30. Discuss the responsibilities of EMTs when communicating with a family or loved ones following the death of a child. (pp 1340–1341)

31. Discuss some positive ways EMTs may cope with the death of a pediatric patient and why managing posttraumatic stress is important for all health care professionals. (pp 1341–1342)

## SKILLS OBJECTIVES

1. Demonstrate how to position the airway in a pediatric patient. (pp 1297–1298, Skill Drill 35-1)

2. Demonstrate how to palpate the pulse and estimate the capillary refill time in a pediatric patient. (pp 1299–1300)

3. Demonstrate how to use a length-based resuscitation tape to size equipment appropriately for a pediatric patient. (p 1313)

4. Demonstrate how to insert an oropharyngeal airway in a pediatric patient. (pp 1313–1314, Skill Drill 35-2)

5. Demonstrate how to insert a nasopharyngeal airway in a pediatric patient. (pp 1314–1316, Skill Drill 35-3)

6. Demonstrate how to administer blow-by oxygen to a pediatric patient. (pp 1316–1317)

7. Demonstrate how to assist ventilation of an infant or child using a bag-mask device. (pp 1317–1318)

8. Demonstrate how to perform one-person bag-mask ventilation on a pediatric patient. (pp 1318, 1319, Skill Drill 35-4)

9. Demonstrate how to perform two-person bag-mask ventilation on a pediatric patient. (pp 1318–1319)

10. Demonstrate how to immobilize a pediatric patient who has been involved in a trauma emergency. (pp 1330, 1331, Skill Drill 35-5)

11. Demonstrate how to immobilize a pediatric patient in a car seat who has been involved in a trauma emergency. (pp 1330–1333, Skill Drill 35-6)

## Introduction

Children differ anatomically, physically, and emotionally from adults. The illnesses and injuries that children sustain, and their responses to them, vary based on age or developmental level. Children are not small adults; therefore, you must tailor your approach to accommodate the unique needs of pediatric patients. Depending on his or her age, the child may not be able to tell you what is wrong. Fear of EMS providers and pain can make the child difficult to assess. In addition, the child's parents or primary caregivers may be stressed, frightened, or behaving irrationally. For these reasons, pediatrics, the specialized medical practice devoted to the care of young patients, can be extremely challenging.

With the proper training and an understanding of this patient population, you will learn the tools necessary to form a baseline assessment and plan of care. Once you learn how to approach children of different ages and what to expect while caring for them, you will find that treating children also offers some special rewards. Not only are their innocence and openness appealing, but they often respond to treatment much more rapidly than adults do.

## Communication With the Patient and the Family

In most situations, caring for an infant or child means that you must care for the parents or caregivers as well (**FIGURE 35-1**). Family members often need emotional support when medical emergencies or problems develop. A calm parent or caregiver usually results in a calm child; he or she can often assist you with the child's care. An agitated parent or caregiver usually means that the child will act the same way, which often will make the child's care more difficult. Make sure that you are calm,

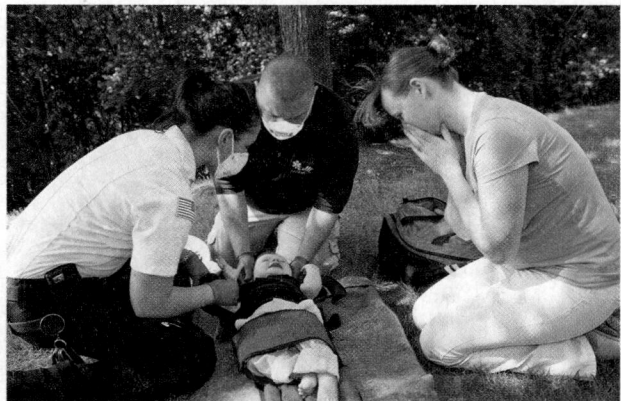

**FIGURE 35-1** Treating a sick or injured child can be extremely challenging. It is important to maintain a calm, professional demeanor as you care for both the child and the parents or caregivers.

© Jones & Bartlett Learning. Photographed by Glen E. Ellman.

efficient, professional, and sensitive as you deal with pediatric patients and their families.

## Growth and Development

Many physical and emotional changes occur during childhood, which extends from birth until age 18 years. Chapter 7, *Life Span Development*, discusses these changes in greater detail. These changes will affect the care you provide to pediatric patients and can create difficulties during your assessment and treatment of the child if you do not expect them. For example, a child's head is proportionally larger than an adult's head, which predisposes the child to heat loss and head injuries from falls and other forms of trauma.

Whereas each child is unique, the thoughts and behaviors of children are often grouped into five stages: infancy, the toddler years, preschool years, school-age years, and adolescence. Children in each stage grapple with different developmental issues. Even though there are specific issues that are important to different age groups, there are also some general rules that apply when you care for children of any age.

## The Infant

Infancy is usually defined as the first year of life; the first month after birth is called the neonatal or newborn period.

### 0 to 2 Months

Infants younger than 2 months spend most of their time sleeping or eating. They experience the world through their bodies and respond mainly to physical stimuli such as light, warmth, hunger, and sound. Infants sleep for up to 16 hours per day between feeding times and parent or caregiver interactions. An infant should be aroused easily from a sleeping state, and it should be considered an emergency if this is not the case.

Infants are unable to tell the difference between parents or caregivers and strangers. Other than crying, infants have a limited ability to communicate pain or discomfort. Infants may cry if certain basic physical needs must be met, such as food, warmth, and comfort. Soothing an infant should be relatively easy for the parent or caregiver, such as by holding, cuddling, or rocking the infant. Hearing is generally well developed at birth, so calm and reassuring talk is often helpful as well. Every reasonable attempt should be made to identify why the infant is crying. If all obvious needs have been addressed and the infant is still inconsolable, then this could be a sign of significant illness.

Infants at this stage have a sucking reflex for feeding. Head control is limited, but infants can turn their heads and focus on faces. Infants have poor thermoregulation (the body's ability to maintain normal temperature). Their heads also have a relatively large surface area. These factors predispose them to hypothermia, so parents or caregivers will often bundle infants to keep them warm. Therefore, it is often necessary to unbundle the infant during your assessment.

### 2 to 6 Months

Infants between ages 2 and 6 months are more active, which makes them easier to evaluate. They spend more time awake, they begin to smile and make eye contact, and they recognize parents or caregivers. Healthy infants in this age group will have a strong sucking reflex, active extremity movement, and a vigorous cry. They may follow a bright light or toy with their eyes or turn their heads toward a loud sound or a familiar voice.

During this stage, the infant has an increased awareness of what is going on around him or her and will use both hands to examine objects and explore the world. About 70% of infants will sleep through the night by 6 months. At this point in development, infants will begin to roll over.

As with younger infants, persistent crying and irritability can be an indicator of serious illness. A lack of eye contact in a sick infant can also be a sign of significant illness, depressed mental status, or a delay in development.

### 6 to 12 months

During this stage, infants begin to babble and by their first year, infants can say their first word. These infants also sit without support, progress to crawling, and finally, begin to walk. This form of locomotion predisposes this age group to increased exposure to physical dangers. At this age, infants are teething and tend to explore their world by picking things up and placing them in their mouths. This behavior increases the risk for choking and poisonings from toxic substances.

At 6 to 12 months, infants may begin to cry if separated from their parents or caregivers. This behavior, called separation anxiety, is common among this age group (**FIGURE 35-2**). One way you can limit the infant's agitation is to let the parent or caregiver hold the infant as you start your physical assessment. As with the younger infants, persistent crying or irritability can be a symptom of serious illness.

### Assessment

Begin your assessment by observing the infant from a distance, preferably in a parent's or caregiver's arms—this will avoid separation anxiety and often make the assessment of the infant easier. Provide as much sensory comfort as you can: Warm your hands and the end of the stethoscope and offer a pacifier if the parent or caregiver allows it. If possible, have a parent or caregiver hold the infant

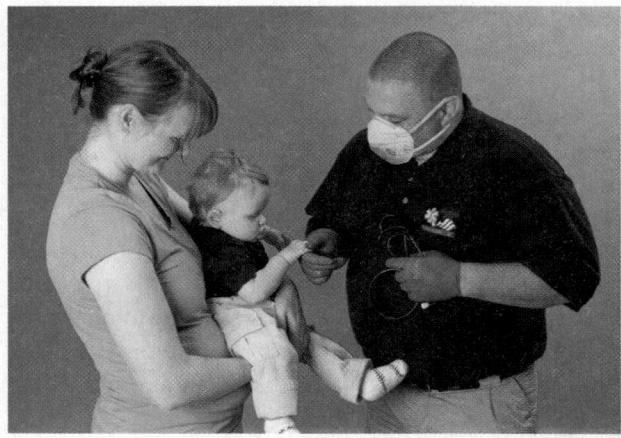

**FIGURE 35-2** Infants are usually not afraid of strangers, but as they reach 6 months to 1 year, they may become irritable or cry if separated from their parents or caregivers.

© Jones & Bartlett Learning. Photographed by Glen E. Ellman.

during all procedures or allow them to stay close to the infant. If possible, plan to do any painful or uncomfortable procedures at the end of the assessment process, so that the infant does not become agitated while you are trying to perform a physical examination. Complete each procedure efficiently and avoid interruptions. Explain each procedure to the parent or caregiver before you perform it, because the procedure and the infant's reaction to it may be upsetting.

## The Toddler

After infancy, until about age 3 years, a child is called a toddler. Toddlers experience rapid changes in growth and development.

### 12 to 18 Months

During this period, toddlers begin to walk and to explore their environment. They are able to open doors, drawers, boxes, and bottles. Because they are explorers by nature and are not afraid, injuries in this age group increase. At 12 to 18 months, toddlers begin to imitate the behaviors of older children and parents and may express a desire to dress like their mommies or daddies. The toddler knows major body parts when you point to them and may speak four to six words. Because of a lack of molars, toddlers may not be able to fully chew their food before swallowing, leading to an increased risk of choking.

### 18 to 24 Months

The mind of the toddler develops rapidly. At the beginning of this stage, the toddler may have a vocabulary of 10 to 15 words. By age 2 years, a toddler should be able to pronounce approximately 100 words. When you point to a common object, toddlers should be able to name it. At this stage, toddlers begin to understand cause and effect with such activities as playing with pop-up toys (jack-in-the-box) and turning on and off a light switch. The toddler's balance and gait also improve rapidly during this period. Running and climbing are two skills that develop. At this stage, toddlers tend to cling to their parents or caregivers and often have a special object such as a blanket or teddy bear that comforts them when they are separated. Be sure to use any comforting objects when available to help calm the toddler.

### Assessment

Stranger anxiety may still develop early in this period. Toddlers may resist separation from parents or caregivers and be afraid to let others come near them. Allow the toddler to hold any special object that brings the toddler comfort ("Would you like to hold your blankie while I listen to your tummy?"). When possible, demonstrate the assessment on a doll or stuffed animal first, which may limit the toddler's anxiety and make it easier to perform the assessment. Because of their newfound independence, they may also be unhappy about being restrained or held for procedures (**FIGURE 35-3**).

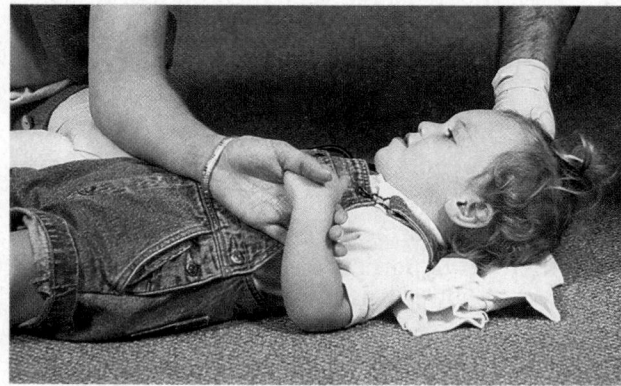

**FIGURE 35-3** Because of their newfound independence, toddlers may be unhappy about being restrained or held for procedures.

© Jones & Bartlett Learning.

Two-year-olds have a well-deserved reputation for having their own ideas about almost everything, which is why these years are often called the "terrible twos."

Toddlers have trouble describing or localizing pain because they do not have the verbal ability to be precise. Pain in the abdomen may be expressed as "My tummy hurts," and the physical examination may reveal tenderness throughout the body. Therefore, the use of visual clues and the Wong-Baker FACES pain rating scale, discussed later in this chapter, can be helpful with this age group.

Toddlers can be curious and adventuresome, so you may be able to distract them (**FIGURE 35-4**). For example, you might allow the toddler to play with a tongue depressor while you assess his or her vital signs. Restrain the toddler for as short a time as possible, and allow him or her to be comforted by the parent or caregiver immediately after a painful procedure. Whenever possible, begin your assessment at the feet or far from the location of any pain to keep from upsetting the toddler.

As with infants, persistent crying or irritability in a toddler can be a symptom of serious illness or injury. Painful procedures make a lasting impression at this stage. Older toddlers may remember negative experiences with physicians or nurses, such as vaccinations or stitches, and fear treatment. Remember to involve the parent or caregiver in any procedures. This not only provides you with an extra set of hands, but the presence of the parent or caregiver will comfort the toddler. If a parent or caregiver is unavailable, reassure the toddler using simple words and a calm, soothing voice.

## The Preschool-Age Child

Preschool-age children (ages 3 to 6 years) are able to use simple language effectively. The most rapid increase in language occurs during this stage of development. These children can walk and run well and begin throwing, catching, and kicking during play. Toilet training is mastered at this stage.

Preschool-age children have a rich imagination, which can make them particularly fearful about pain and change involving their bodies (**FIGURE 35-5**). At this age, they often believe that their thoughts or wishes can cause injury or harm to themselves or to others. They may also believe that an injury is the result of a bad deed they did earlier in the day.

They are also learning which behaviors are appropriate and which behaviors will lead to a "time out." Tantrums may occur when preschool-age children feel they cannot control a situation or its outcomes.

The risk of foreign body airway obstruction continues to be high at this age.

### Assessment

Preschool-age children can understand directions, be more specific in describing their sensations, and identify painful areas when questioned. Despite the increased ability to communicate, much of the

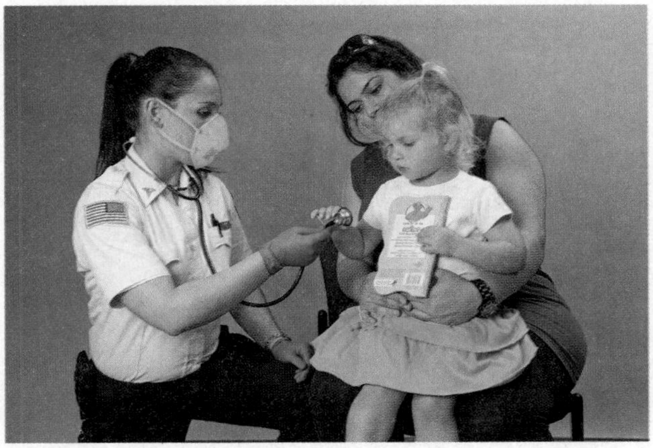

**FIGURE 35-4** Allow a toddler to sit on the parent's or caregiver's lap during your assessment, and use a toy to distract him or her.

© Jones & Bartlett Learning. Photographed by Glen E. Ellman.

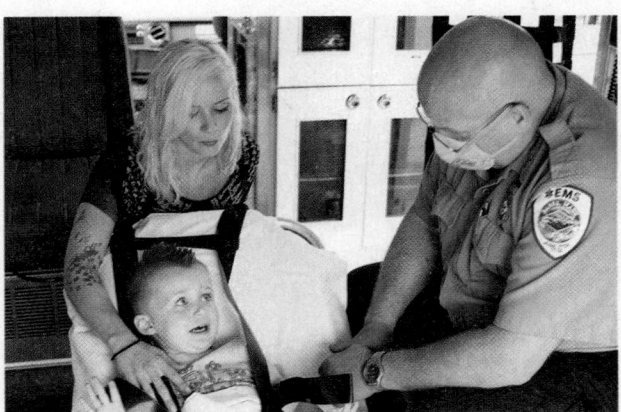

**FIGURE 35-5** Preschool-age children have a vivid imagination, so much of the history must still be obtained from the parent or caregiver.

© Jones & Bartlett Learning.

child's history will still be obtained from parents or caregivers. Remember to communicate simply and directly. Tell the child what you are going to do immediately before you do it; this way, the child has no time to develop frightening fantasies. Also keep in mind that the preschool-age child can be very literal. Asking if you may "take" his or her blood pressure may lead the child to believe that you will not give it back. Use plain language and provide plenty of reassurance.

At this age, preschool-age children are easily distracted with counting games, small toys, or conversation (**FIGURE 35-6**). Appealing to the preschool-age child's imaginative thinking may allow treatment to go a bit smoother. For example, have the child pretend to be a superhero inhaling special powers while breathing in oxygen. Be sure to adjust the level of the game to the developmental level of the child; do not assume that preschool-age children understand more than they actually do.

While caring for this age group and others within the pediatric population, never lie to the patient. Once you have lost your pediatric patient's trust, it will be a challenge to regain it.

Begin your assessment with the feet and move toward the head, similar to assessing a toddler. Use adhesive bandages to cover the site of an injection or other small wound, because the preschool-age child might be worried about keeping his or her body together in one piece. Keep in mind that modesty is developing at this age, so keep the child covered when possible.

## School-Age Years

**School-age** children (ages 6 to 12 years) begin to act more like adults. They can think in concrete terms, respond sensibly to direct questions, and help take care of themselves. School is important at this stage and concerns about popularity and peer pressure occupy a great deal of time and energy. Children with chronic illness or disabilities can become self-conscious because of concerns about fitting in with their peers. At this stage, children begin to understand that death is final, but their understanding of what death is and why it occurs is still unrealistic. This may increase their anxieties about illness or injury.

### Assessment

Your assessment begins to be more like an adult assessment; talk to the child, not just the parent or caregiver, while taking the medical history (**FIGURE 35-7**). This will help you gain the patient's

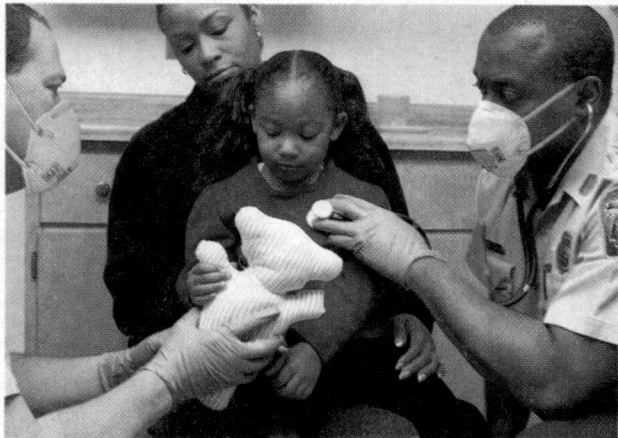

**FIGURE 35-6** A preschool-age child can be easily distracted by games or conversation.

© Jones & Bartlett Learning. Courtesy of MIEMSS.

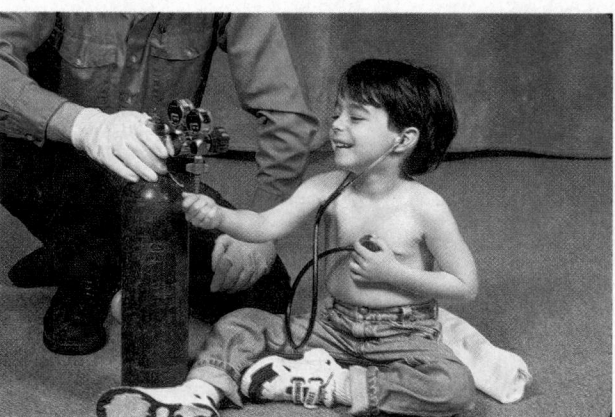

**FIGURE 35-7** School-age children are more like adults in that they can answer your questions and can help to take care of themselves.

© Jones & Bartlett Learning.

trust. At this stage, the child is usually familiar with the process of physical examination through check-ups and immunizations. This may make your job easier or more difficult, depending on whether the child's prior health care experiences have been positive or negative. Begin your assessment at the head and move toward the feet, similar to assessing an adult.

Whenever possible, give the school-age child simple, appropriate choices, such as "Would you like to sit up or lie down?" or "Would you like to take off your clothes yourself?" Only ask the type of questions that let you control the answer and do not bargain or debate with the patient. For example, ask the child if you may find out the blood pressure on the child's right or left arm. Presenting a choice allows you to obtain assessment information and gives the child some control in a frightening situation. Encourage cooperation by allowing the child to listen to his or her own heartbeat through the stethoscope. Ensure the patient's modesty during the examination.

Preschool-age children can understand the difference between emotional and physical pain and have concerns about what pain means. Give them simple explanations about what is causing their pain and what will be done about it. Games and conversation may distract them. Ask them to describe their favorite place, pets, school activities, or toys. Ask the parent's or caregiver's advice in choosing the right distraction. Rewarding the child after a procedure can be helpful in his or her future cooperation and recovery. Often, kind words and a smile make a good reward when toys or books are unavailable.

## Adolescents

Most adolescents (ages 12 to 18 years) are able to think abstractly and can participate in decision making. This is also the stage when personal morals begin to develop. Adolescents are able to discriminate between what is right and wrong. They are now able to incorporate their own values and beliefs into their daily decision-making process. Even though this age group is physically similar to adults, adolescents are still children on an emotional level. They gradually shift from relying on family to relying on friends for emotional psychological support, social development, and acceptance from their peers (especially the opposite sex). Interest in romantic relationships begins.

Adolescence is when puberty begins. Primary and secondary sex characteristics develop (sex organs, facial/axillary hair). This period of change makes the adolescent concerned about his or her appearance. Simple injuries or illnesses can be exaggerated or understated due to anxiety about body image or fear of disfigurement. The adolescent may dislike being observed during procedures and may have strong feelings about privacy.

Adolescence is a time of experimentation and risk-taking behaviors. Adolescents often feel that they are free from danger, and that they are "indestructible." Adolescents struggle with independence, loss of control, body image, sexuality, and peer pressure. They may have mood swings or depression and when ill or injured, may act younger than their age.

### Assessment

Adolescents can often understand complex concepts and treatment options; provide them with information when they request it (**FIGURE 35-8**). When the adolescent's condition is stable, discuss the situation and allow the adolescent to be involved in his or her care. Provide the adolescent with choices regarding his or her health, while also lending guidance if needed. You will find adolescents to be more helpful and understanding of necessary procedures than younger patients.

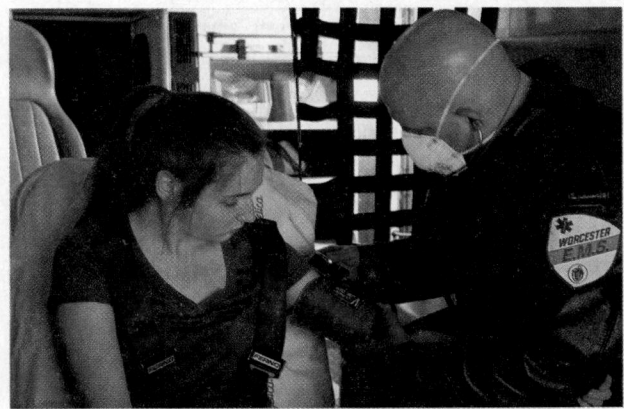

**FIGURE 35-8** Respect the adolescent's privacy at all times; give the patient whatever information he or she requests.
© Jones & Bartlett Learning.

If the adolescent's condition requires him or her to be exposed or partially exposed to be assessed, take every measure to respect the patient's modesty and privacy. If an EMT of the same gender is available to perform the physical examination, it may lessen the stress of the event. Adolescents undergo numerous body changes during puberty, and some adolescents may have a negative or altered body image (an unrealistic sense of what their bodies look like, how it should look, or how society expects them to look). An injury that could result in a scar from a laceration or burn will be challenging for you to address. The best practice is to be honest yet tactful, and to reassure the adolescent that you are doing everything within your training to help in this situation. Allow the adolescent to speak openly about any thoughts and concerns.

Because the adolescent is under the influence of hormonal changes, peer pressure, and emotional highs and lows, risk-taking behaviors are common. Some of the risks that the adolescent takes can ultimately facilitate development and judgment and help to shape his or her identity as an adult. However, some risks can result in unintentional trauma, drug and/or alcohol abuse, unprotected sex, and pregnancy.

Be aware that female adolescents may be pregnant, so ask, "Is there a chance you could be pregnant?" Communicate her answer to the receiving facility and note it on your patient care report. The adolescent might not want this information known to her parents or caregivers and may fear the consequences of her actions. If you suspect that the patient might want to tell you something, but is silent in front of a parent or caregiver, try to interview the adolescent without the parent or caregiver present.

Adolescents have a clear understanding of the purpose and meaning of pain. Whenever possible, explain any necessary procedures well in advance. Assess their level of pain by observing facial and body expression as well as by asking questions; adolescents can be reserved and may not request pain relief even when they need it. To distract them, find out some of their interests, such as sports or movies, and get them talking.

## Anatomy and Physiology

There is no other time in a person's life that his or her body is growing and changing as fast as during childhood. Newborns quickly adapt to the world outside the mother's body (uterus). Toddlers learn to walk and talk. Adolescents transition into sexual maturity. To effectively assess and treat a pediatric patient, you must understand the physical differences between children and adults and alter your patient care accordingly.

## The Respiratory System

To manage the pediatric airway effectively, you must understand the anatomic differences between the adult and pediatric airway. To start with, the pediatric airway is smaller in diameter and shorter in length, the lungs are smaller, and the heart is higher in a child's chest. The glottic opening (vocal cords) is higher and positioned more anteriorly (toward the front), and the neck appears to be nonexistent. As the child develops, the neck gets proportionally longer as the vocal cords and epiglottis achieve their anatomically correct adult position.

The anatomy of a pediatric airway and other important structures differs from that of an adult in the following ways (**FIGURE 35-9**):

- A larger, rounder occiput, or back of the head, which requires more careful positioning of the airway.
- A proportionately larger tongue relative to the size of the mouth and a more anterior location in the mouth. The child's tongue is also larger relative to the small mandible and can easily block the airway.
- A long, floppy, U-shaped epiglottis in infants and toddlers is larger than an adult's, relative to the size of the airway, which extends at a 45° angle into the airway.
- Less-developed rings of cartilage in the trachea that may easily collapse if the neck is flexed or hyperextended.
- A narrowing funnel-shaped (wide to narrow) upper airway compared to that of a cylinder-shaped (same width) lower airway.

These differences will influence the treatment decisions that you make about pediatric patients, including whether intervention is needed and, if so, what procedure to use.

Because of the smaller diameter of the trachea in infants, which is about the same diameter as a drinking straw, their airway is easily obstructed by secretions, blood, or swelling. Infants are obligate

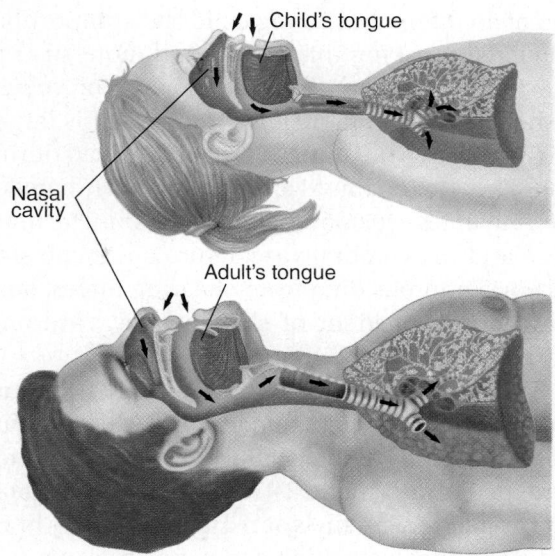

**FIGURE 35-9** The anatomy of a child's airway differs from that of an adult in several ways. The back of the head is larger in a child. The tongue is proportionately larger and is located more anterior in the mouth. The trachea is smaller in diameter and more flexible. The airway itself is lower and narrower (funnel-shaped).

© Jones & Bartlett Learning.

| TABLE 35-1 Pediatric Respiratory Rates | |
|---|---|
| Age | Respirations (breaths/min) |
| Infant: 1 month to 1 year | 30 to 60 |
| Toddler: 1 to 3 years | 24 to 40 |
| Preschool age: 4 to 5 years | 22 to 34 |
| School age: 6 to 12 years | 18 to 30 |
| Adolescent: 13 to 18 years | 12 to 16 |

Data From: *Pediatric Advanced Life Support*, 2015, American Heart Association.

nose breathers, which may require diligent suctioning or reassessment and management to maintain a clear airway.

An infant needs to breathe faster than an older child (**TABLE 35-1**). Children's lungs grow and develop increased abilities to handle the exchange of oxygen as they age. A respiratory rate of 30 to 60 breaths/min is normal for the newborn, whereas the adolescent is expected to have rates closer to the adult range (12 to 20 breaths/min). Children

have not only a higher metabolic rate, but also a higher oxygen demand, which is twice that of an adult. This is partly related to the actual size of the lung tissues and the volume that can be exchanged. Smaller lungs mean that the oxygen reserves are smaller. This higher oxygen demand, combined with a smaller oxygen reserve, increases the risk of hypoxia because of apnea or ineffective ventilation efforts.

Breathing also requires the use of the chest muscles and diaphragm. Because intercostal muscles are not well developed in children, movement of the diaphragm, their major muscle of respiration, dictates the amount of air that they inspire. Young children also experience muscle fatigue much more quickly than older children. This can lead to respiratory failure if a child has to physically fight

### Words of Wisdom

Reference materials such as field guides or mobile device apps can help you with the assessment of a child. Many EMS agencies also maintain copies of specialized pediatric protocols in their system. Refer to these resources during your care, and remember to make notes about your specific observations and treatment decisions. This information-intensive approach to pediatric care helps ensure good care and thorough documentation, and can reduce any anxiety you may feel about assessing children.

### Safety Tips

In a pediatric patient, the lung tissues are susceptible to a simple or tension pneumothorax if excessive ventilatory pressures occur during assisted ventilations with a bag-mask device. To prevent hypoxia and to avoid damaging the lung tissues, use the appropriate-size mask and reservoir bag to avoid administering an excessively large tidal volume. Only use enough force to make the chest rise slightly. Focus your attention on the rise and fall of the chest wall, versus just simply squeezing the reservoir bag. Ventilate with the patient's underlying respiratory rate and be careful not to ventilate against the patient's efforts.

to breathe for long periods of time. Anything that places pressure on the abdomen of a young child can block the movement of the diaphragm and cause respiratory compromise. Gastric distention can also interfere with movement of the diaphragm and lead to hypoventilation. Use caution when applying straps to a spinal motion restriction device because this may hinder full symmetrical chest wall expansion and thus limit tidal volume.

Breath sounds in children are easier to hear because of their thinner chest walls, but because less air is exchanged with each breath, detection of poor air movement or complete absence of breath sounds may be more difficult.

## The Circulatory System

It is important to know the normal pulse ranges when evaluating children (**TABLE 35-2**). An infant's heart can beat as many as 160 times per minute or more if the body needs to compensate for injury or illness. This is the primary method the body uses to compensate for decreased perfusion.

Children are able to compensate for decreased perfusion by constricting the vessels in the skin. Constriction of the blood vessels can be so profound that blood flow to the extremities can be diminished. Signs of vasoconstriction include pallor (early sign), weak distal (eg, radial or pedal) pulses in the extremities, delayed capillary refill time, and cool hands or feet.

## The Nervous System

Compared with the adult nervous system, the pediatric nervous system is immature, underdeveloped, and not well protected. Recall that the head-to-body ratio of an infant and young child is disproportionately larger, making this population more susceptible to head injuries from falls or motor vehicle crashes. The occipital region of the head is larger, which increases the momentum of the head during a fall. The subarachnoid space is relatively smaller, resulting in less cushioning for the brain. The brain tissue and the cerebral vasculature are fragile and susceptible to bleeding from shearing forces, such as during an incident of shaken baby syndrome (discussed later in the chapter).

The pediatric brain requires a higher amount of cerebral blood flow, oxygen, and glucose than does adult brain tissue. Glucose stores are limited in the pediatric patient. These special needs mean that the pediatric brain is at risk for secondary brain damage from hypotension and hypoxic events.

Spinal cord injuries are less common in pediatric patients when compared to adults, with approximately 20% of these injuries occurring in children. If a child's cervical spine is injured, it is most likely to be an injury to the ligaments as the result of a fall. If you suspect a neck injury, perform manual in-line stabilization or follow local protocols.

## The Gastrointestinal System

The abdominal muscle structures are less developed in children, which results in less protection from blunt or penetrating trauma. The internal organs, such as the liver and the spleen, are proportionally larger and situated more anteriorly, so they are susceptible to bleeding and injury. Because the internal organs are positioned in closer proximity to each other, there is a higher risk for multiple organ injury caused by minimal direct impact to this region, such as from a lap belt in a motor vehicle. The liver, spleen, and kidneys are more frequently injured in children than in adults.

## The Musculoskeletal System

A child's bones are softer than those of an adult. The skeletal system contains open growth plates at the ends of long bones, which enable these bones to grow during childhood. As a result of the active growth plates, children's bones are weaker and more flexible, making them susceptible to fracture with stress. The open growth plates are also weaker than ligaments and tendons, leading to a risk of length discrepancies if there is an injury to the

| **TABLE 35-2** Responsive Pediatric Pulse Rates | |
|---|---|
| **Age** | **Pulse Rate (beats/min)** |
| Newborn to 3 months | 85 to 205 |
| 3 months to 2 years | 100 to 190 |
| 2 to 10 years | 60 to 140 |
| >10 years | 60 to 100 |

Data From: *Pediatric Advanced Life Support*, 2015, American Heart Association.

growth plate. Because of these factors, you should immobilize extremities with suspected sprains or strains because they may be fractures through growth plates.

The bones of the infant's head are flexible and soft, which allows the head to be delivered through the birth canal and accommodates the growth of the brain during development. Located on the front (anterior) and back (posterior) portions of the head are soft spots known as **fontanelles**. Each will close at specific stages of development—18 months for the anterior suture and 6 months for the posterior suture. It is important to note that some bulging is a normal assessment finding when the infant is either crying, coughing, or lying on the back or stomach. The fontanelles of an infant can be a useful assessment tool for such issues as increased intracranial pressure (bulging with a noncrying infant) or dehydration (a sunken appearance).

The thoracic cage in young children is highly elastic and flexible because it is primarily composed of cartilaginous connective tissue. The ribs and vital organs are less protected by muscle and fat. The highly flexible ribs mean that fractures in pediatric patients are rare, unless a high-energy impact to the chest wall is encountered, such as during a motor vehicle crash. However, underlying damage may still exist within the thoracic cavity without any exterior markings.

## The Integumentary System

The integumentary system of the child differs from that of the adult in several ways. The child's skin is thinner with less subcutaneous fat; it tends to burn more deeply and easily than that of an adult, as in the case of a sunburn. Infants and children also have a larger body surface area–to–body mass ratio, which can lead to significant fluid and heat losses.

## Patient Assessment

Because a young child might not be able to speak, your assessment of his or her condition must be based largely on what you can see and hear. Family members may be able to provide vital information about an incident or illness. Remember to include parents or caregivers as part of your team. Whenever possible, involve them in decisions and have them help comfort the infant or child during the assessment and any interventions.

## Scene Size-up

The assessment begins at the time of initial dispatch. On the way to the scene, prepare mentally for approaching and treating an infant or child and interacting with the family. This means planning for a pediatric scene size-up, pediatric equipment, and the age-appropriate physical assessment. If possible, collect information from the dispatcher about the age and gender of the child, the location of the scene, the nature of illness (NOI) or mechanism of injury (MOI), and the chief complaint.

As with any EMS call, the scene size-up begins by ensuring that you and your partner have taken the appropriate safety measures and standard precautions. As you enter the scene, note the position in which the child is found. Look for any possible safety threats to the child, parents or caregivers, bystanders, or EMS providers. Keep in mind that the child may be a safety threat if he or she has a communicable disease.

Next, complete an environmental assessment. The environmental assessment will provide important information regarding the chief complaint, number of patients, MOI or NOI, and ongoing health risks. Inspect the physical environment and observe the family–child and/or caregiver–child interactions. Information from the parents or caregivers will be extremely important and may provide clues as to the patient's problem. As with the adult population, document dangerous scene conditions and obtain statements from parents, caregivers, or bystanders; this information will assist child protective services if the child is later determined to be a victim of an intentional injury. On the scene, be like a sponge: soak up as much useful information as possible to ensure scene safety and the delivery of timely care.

At a traumatic scene, when the child is unresponsive or unable to communicate because of his or her developmental age, assume that the MOI was significant enough to cause head or neck injuries. Restrict spinal motion if you suspect the MOI to be severe. Remember to pad under the child's head and/or shoulders and back to facilitate a neutral position for airway management. Always follow local protocols.

## Primary Assessment

As with the adult population, the objective of the primary assessment is to identify and treat immediate or potential threats to life.

### Pediatric Assessment Triangle

When you assess an infant or child, use the pediatric assessment triangle (PAT) to determine if the patient is sick or not sick. The pediatric assessment triangle (PAT) is a structured assessment tool that allows you to rapidly form a general impression of the child's condition without touching the child. This first-glance assessment, which can be performed in less than 30 seconds, will help you to identify the general category of the patient's physical problem and establish urgency for treatment and/or transport.

The PAT consists of three elements: appearance (muscle tone and mental status), work of breathing, and circulation to the skin (**FIGURE 35-10**). The only equipment required for the PAT is your own eyes and ears.

As you evaluate the child's appearance, note the level of consciousness or interactiveness and muscle tone—signs that will provide you with information about the adequacy of the patient's cerebral perfusion (mentation) and overall function of the central nervous system.

Much of the information regarding the child's level of consciousness can be obtained by using the PAT. In addition, you can evaluate the child's level of

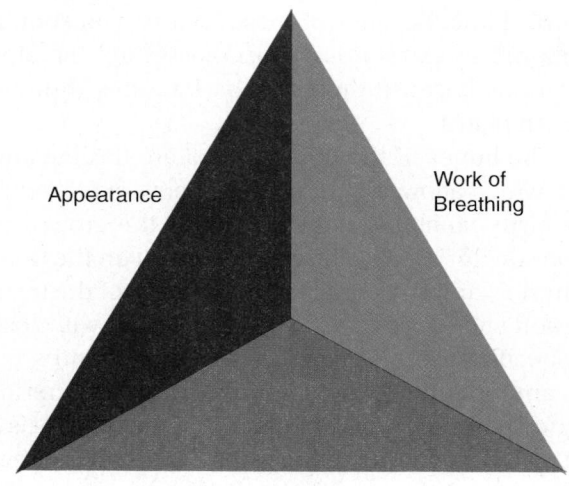

**FIGURE 35-10** The three components of the pediatric assessment triangle (PAT) include appearance, work of breathing, and circulation to the skin.

Used with permission of American Academy of Pediatrics, *Pediatric Education for Prehospital Professionals*, © American Academy of Pediatrics, 2000.

consciousness by using the AVPU scale, modified as necessary for his or her age (**TABLE 35-3**).

An infant or child with a normal level of consciousness will act appropriately for his or her age, exhibiting good muscle tone and maintaining good eye contact (**FIGURE 35-11**). An abnormal level of consciousness is characterized by age-inappropriate behavior or level of interactiveness, poor muscle tone, or poor eye contact with the parent or caregiver or with you (**FIGURE 35-12**).

## YOU are the Provider

You arrive at the scene, enter the residence, and find the child sitting on the couch next to her mother. She immediately makes eye contact with you, appears fearful of your presence, and starts clinging to her mother. You note that she is in obvious respiratory distress. As you approach the child, you make a visual assessment of her.

| Recording Time: 0 Minutes | |
| --- | --- |
| **Appearance** | Obvious increased respiratory effort |
| **Level of consciousness** | Conscious; appears fearful |
| **Airway** | Open, no obvious obstructions |
| **Breathing** | Increased rate; moderate difficulty; nasal flaring; prominent supraclavicular retractions |
| **Circulation** | Skin pink and dry; no gross bleeding |

**3.** Why did you *not* immediately perform a hands-on assessment of this child?

**4.** On the basis of your initial observations, is this child experiencing respiratory distress or respiratory failure?

| **TABLE 35-3** The AVPU Scale | |
|---|---|
| Awake and Alert | Patient is awake; the eyes visually track people and objects |
| Responsive to Verbal Stimuli | Patient opens the eyes or moans, speaks, or moves in response to your voice |
| Responsive to Pain | Patient does not respond to verbal stimuli but moves or cries out in response to pain (eg, pinched trapezius muscle or sternal rub) |
| Unresponsive | No response to any stimulus |

© Jones & Bartlett Learning.

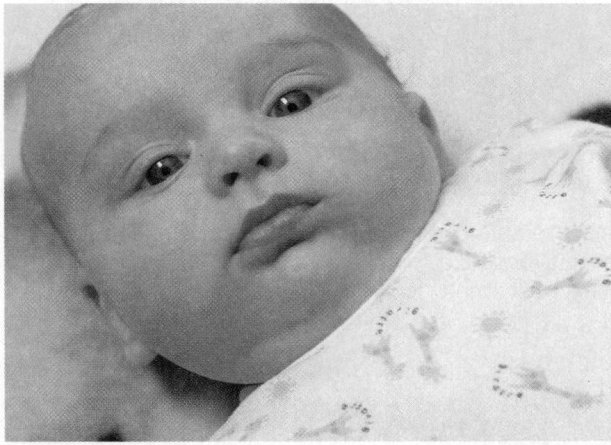

**FIGURE 35-11** An infant or child making good eye contact is most likely not critically ill.

© Photos.com.

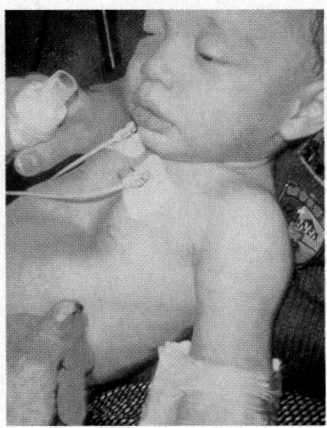

**FIGURE 35-12** A limp child who is unable to maintain eye contact may be critically ill or injured.

Courtesy Health Resources and Services Administration, Maternal and Child Health Bureau, Emergency Medical Services for Children Program.

| **TABLE 35-4** Characteristics of Appearance: The TICLS Mnemonic | |
|---|---|
| **Characteristic** | **Features to Look For** |
| Tone | Is the child moving or resisting examination vigorously? Does the child have good muscle tone? Or is the child limp, listless, or flaccid? |
| Interactiveness | How alert is the child? How readily does a person, object, or sound distract the child or draw the child's attention? Will the child reach for, grasp, and play with a toy or examination instrument, like a penlight or tongue blade? Or, is the child uninterested in playing or interacting with the parent or caregiver or with the EMT? |
| Consolability | Can the child be consoled or comforted by the parent or caregiver or by the EMT? Or is the child's crying or agitation unrelieved by gentle reassurance? |
| Look or gaze | Does the child fix his or her gaze on a face, or is there a vacant, glassy-eyed stare? |
| Speech or cry | Is the child's cry strong and spontaneous or weak or high-pitched? Is the content of speech age-appropriate or confused or garbled? |

© Jones & Bartlett Learning.

The mnemonic TICLS (or tickles) can also help to determine if the pediatric patient is sick or not sick. TICLS includes Tone, Interactiveness, Consolability, Look or gaze, and Speech or cry (**TABLE 35-4**).

A child's work of breathing increases as the body attempts to compensate for abnormalities in oxygenation and ventilation. Increased work of breathing often manifests as follows:

- **Abnormal airway noise.** Grunting or wheezing
- **Accessory muscle use.** Contractions of the muscles above the clavicles (supraclavicular)
- **Retractions.** Drawing in of the muscles between the ribs (intercostal retractions) or of the sternum (substernal retractions) during inspiration (**FIGURE 35-13**)

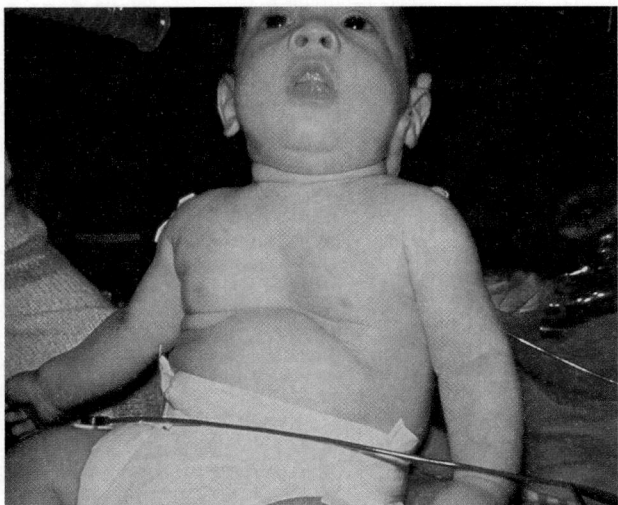

**FIGURE 35-13** Retractions of the intercostal muscles or sternum indicate increased work of breathing.

Courtesy of Health Resources and Services Administration, Maternal and Child Health Bureau, Emergency Medical Service for Children Program.

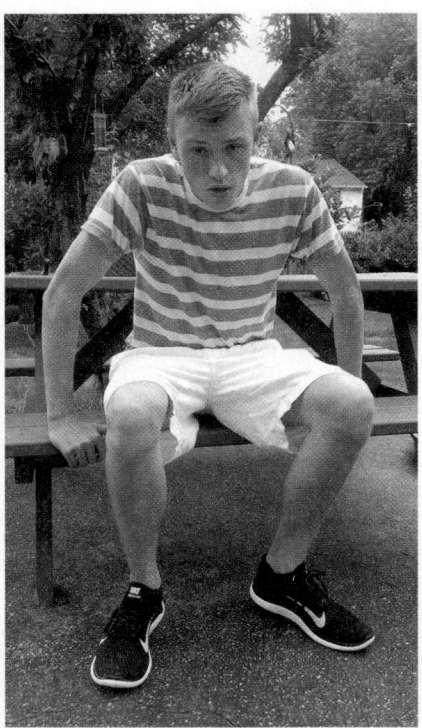

**FIGURE 35-14** A patient in the tripod position will sit leaning forward on outstretched arms with the head and chin thrust slightly forward.

© Jones & Bartlett Learning.

- **Head bobbing.** The head lifting and tilting back during inspiration, then moving forward during expiration
- **Nasal flaring.** The nares (the external openings of the nose) widening; usually seen during inspiration
- **Tachypnea.** Increased respiratory rate
- **Tripod position.** Used by older children to maximize the effectiveness of the airway (**FIGURE 35-14**)

As discussed previously, an important sign of perfusion is circulation to the skin. When cardiac output falls, the body, through vasoconstriction, shunts blood from areas of lesser need (such as the skin) to areas of greater need (such as the brain, heart, and kidneys). Although paleness, or a decrease in blood flow, can be difficult to detect in dark skin, it may be observed by examining mucous membranes inside the inner lower eyelid and capillary refill time. On general observation, the patient may appear ashen or gray.

The PAT is a valuable tool in the field when you are confronted with various etiologies, such as respiratory distress or failure, cardiovascular shock leading to cardiopulmonary failure or arrest, isolated head injury, ingestion of a toxic substance, or neurologic injuries—or even as an approach to a stable pediatric patient.

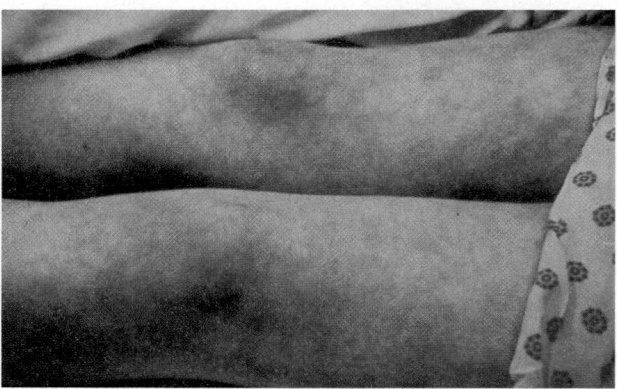

**FIGURE 35-15** Mottling of the skin indicates poor perfusion and is the result of constriction of peripheral blood vessels.

Courtesy of Health Resources and Services Administration, Maternal and Child Health Bureau, Emergency Medical Service for Children Program.

Pallor of the skin and mucous membranes may be seen in compensated shock; it may also be a sign of anemia or hypoxia. Mottling is caused by constriction of peripheral blood vessels and is another sign of poor perfusion (**FIGURE 35-15**).

Cyanosis, a blue discoloration of the skin and mucous membranes, reflects a decreased level of oxygen in the blood. Cyanosis is a late sign of respiratory failure or shock; absence of discoloration, however, does not rule out these conditions. Never wait for the development of cyanosis before administering oxygen!

On the basis of the findings of the PAT triangle, you will decide if the child is in stable condition or requires urgent care. If the patient's condition is unstable, assess for exsanguination and airway, breathing, and circulation (XABCs), treat any life threats, and transport immediately to an appropriate facility. In children with obvious life-threatening external hemorrhage, assess and address the CABs first, including applying tourniquets for arterial hemorrhage from extremities. See Chapter 26, *Bleeding*, for more information.

If the child is in stable condition, then you have time to continue with the remainder of the patient assessment process, perform necessary interventions, and discuss transport options with the parents or caregivers.

## Hands-on XABCs

For pediatric patients, you will now perform a hands-on XABCs assessment. Assess and treat any life threats as you identify them by following the XABCDE format:

    **X** Exsanguination
    **A** Airway
    **B** Breathing
    **C** Circulation
    **D** Disability
    **E** Exposure

If the child's airway is open and the patient can adequately keep it open (as is often the case in conscious pediatric patients), assess respiratory adequacy. However, if the child is unresponsive or has difficulty keeping the airway clear, you must ensure that the airway is properly positioned and that it is clear of mucus, vomitus, blood, and foreign bodies.

If trauma has been ruled out, open the patient's airway with the head tilt–chin lift maneuver (**FIGURE 35-16**). If spinal trauma is suspected, use the jaw-thrust maneuver to open the airway (**FIGURE 35-17**).

Positioning the airway correctly is critical in pediatric emergency care. Always position the airway

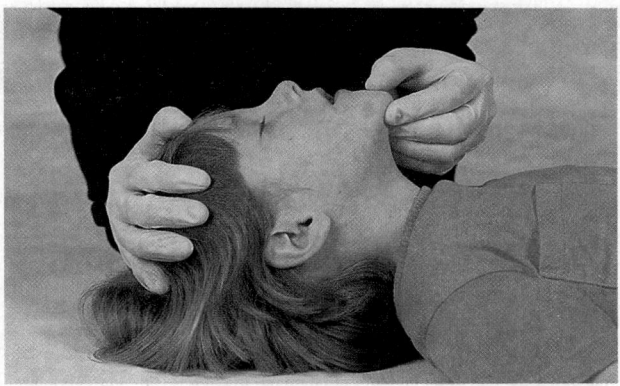

**FIGURE 35-16** Use the head tilt–chin lift maneuver to open the airway of a pediatric patient without trauma.
© Jones & Bartlett Learning. Courtesy of MIEMSS.

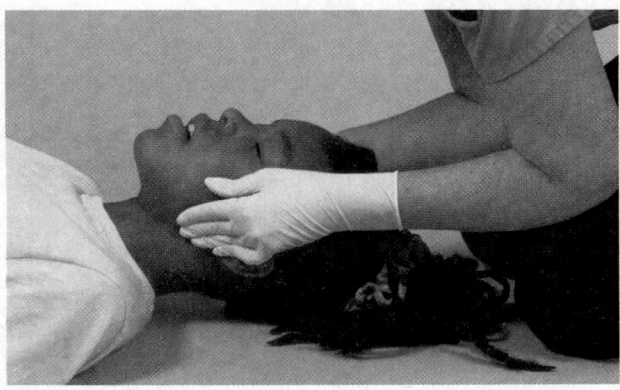

**FIGURE 35-17** Use the jaw-thrust maneuver to open the airway of a child with possible spinal injury.
© Jones & Bartlett Learning. Courtesy of MIEMSS.

in a neutral **sniffing position**. This accomplishes two goals at once, keeping the trachea from kinking and maintaining the proper alignment should you have to restrict spinal motion.

Follow these steps to position the airway in a child without trauma (**SKILL DRILL 35-1**):

1. Place the pediatric patient on a firm surface such as a short backboard or pediatric immobilization device (**Step 1**).
2. Fold a small towel and place it under the patient's shoulders and back (**Step 2**).
3. Stabilize the child's forehead to limit rolling of the head during transport. Use the head tilt–chin lift maneuver to open the airway (**Step 3**).

After the child's airway has been opened, make sure that it is clear of potential obstructions such

## Skill Drill 35-1 Positioning the Airway in a Pediatric Patient

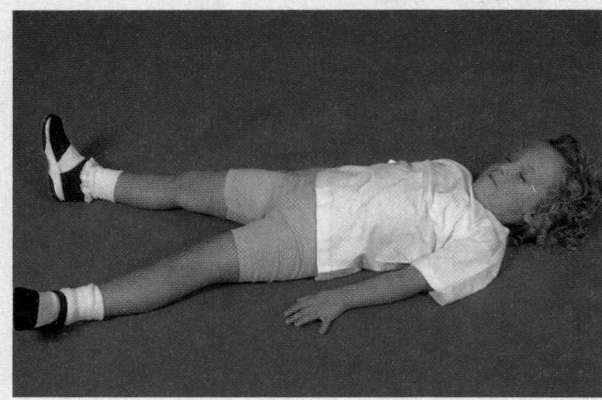

### Step 1

Position the child on a firm surface.

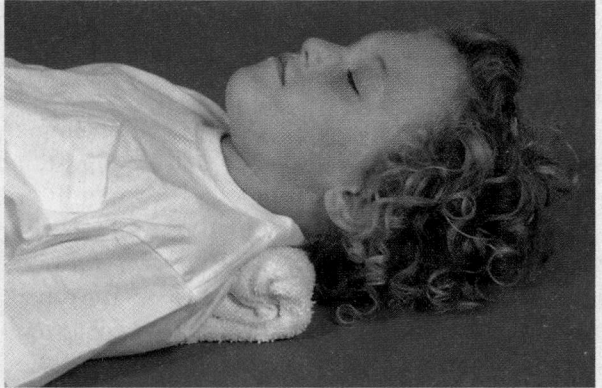

### Step 2

Place a folded towel about 1 inch (2.5 cm) thick under the shoulders and back.

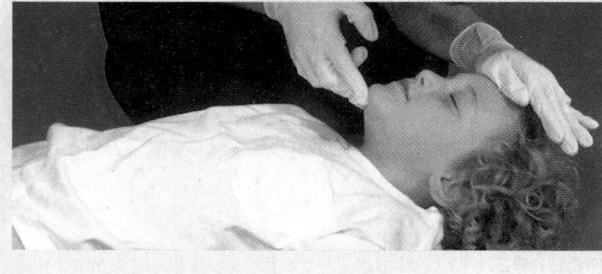

### Step 3

Stabilize the forehead to limit movement, and use the head tilt–chin lift maneuver to open the airway.

© Jones & Bartlett Learning. Courtesy of MIEMSS.

as mucus, blood, or foreign bodies. Next, establish whether the patient can maintain his or her own airway spontaneously (without the use of airway adjuncts) or whether adjuncts will be necessary to maintain airway patency. Techniques for airway management, and how to identify appropriate-size equipment for the patient, are discussed later in this chapter.

Carefully assess the patient's breathing while at the same time feeling for a pulse. Note the degree of air movement at the nose and mouth and determine whether the chest is rising adequately and symmetrically. Assess the respiratory rate and effort with which the child is breathing as well.

When you assess a child, place both hands on the patient's chest to feel for the rise and fall of the chest wall. You will be able to count the actual respiratory rate and assess for symmetry. This assessment maneuver is especially helpful when your patient requires assisted ventilations with a bag-mask device. In infants, belly breathing is considered adequate because of the soft pliable bones of the chest and the strong muscular diaphragm.

If the child is conscious and not in need of immediate intervention (such as suctioning or assisted ventilation), it is usually easier to assess respirations with the patient sitting on the parent's or caregiver's lap. Listen for abnormal breath sounds (**TABLE 35-5**) and note any signs of increased respiratory effort (work of breathing).

As the child begins to tire, retractions often become weak and ineffective and the accessory muscles become less prominent during breathing. Bradypnea, a decrease in the respiratory rate, is an ominous sign and indicates impending respiratory arrest. Do not mistake bradypnea for a sign of improvement; it usually indicates that the child's condition has deteriorated. Therefore, be prepared to begin ventilatory assistance.

When you assess circulation, you must determine if the patient has a pulse, is bleeding, or is in shock. Remember, infants and children can tolerate only small amounts of blood loss before circulatory compromise occurs. Assess and control any active bleeding early in your assessment.

A pulse may be difficult to palpate if it is weak, very fast, or very slow. In infants, palpate the brachial pulse or femoral pulse. In children older than 1 year, palpate the carotid pulse (**FIGURE 35-18**). Note the rate and quality of the pulse: Is it weak or strong? Is it normal, slow, or fast? Strong central pulses usually indicate that the child is not hypotensive; however, this does not rule out the possibility of compensated shock. Weak or absent peripheral

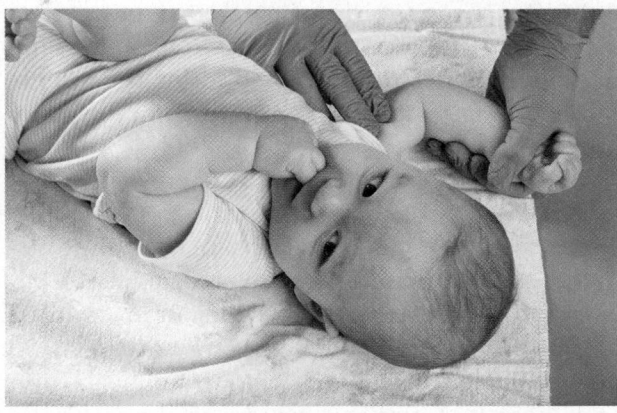

**A**

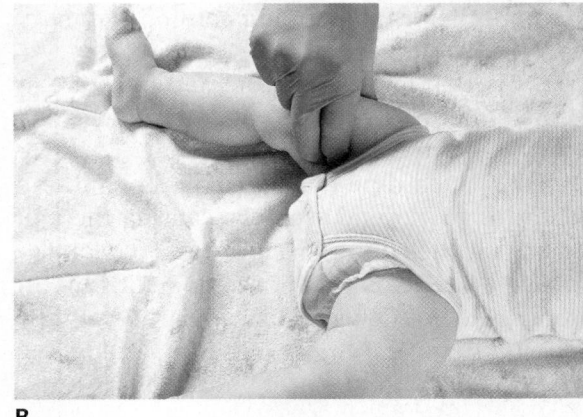

**B**

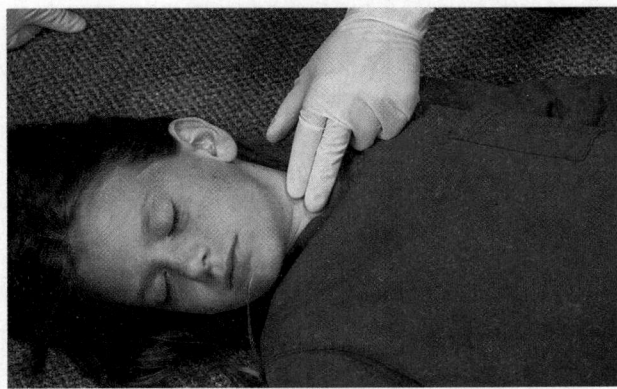

**C**

**FIGURE 35-18 A.** Palpate the brachial pulse in infants. **B.** Palpate the femoral pulse as a second choice. **C.** In children older than 1 year, palpate the carotid pulse.

| TABLE 35-5 Abnormal Breath Sounds | |
| --- | --- |
| Crackles | A crackling or bubbling sound typically heard on inspiration; indicates inflammation or infection (such as in pneumonia) |
| Stridor | High-pitched inspiratory sound; indicates a partial upper airway obstruction (such as in croup or from a foreign body) |
| Wheezing | High- or low-pitched sound heard usually during expiration; indicates a partial lower airway obstruction (such as in asthma, bronchiolitis, or foreign body aspiration) |
| Grunting | An "uh" sound heard during exhalation; reflects the pediatric patient's attempt to keep the alveoli open by increasing pressure in the chest cavity; indicates inadequate oxygenation (such as in pneumonia) |
| Absent breath sounds (silent chest) | Combined with increased work of breathing, absent breath sounds indicate a complete upper or lower airway obstruction (such as from a foreign body, severe asthma, or pneumothorax); an ominous sign of impending respiratory failure that must be quickly addressed |

pulses indicate decreased perfusion. The absence of a central pulse (that is, brachial or femoral in infants, carotid in older children) indicates the need for CPR.

Tachycardia may be an early sign of hypoxia or shock, but it may also reflect less serious conditions such as fever, anxiety, pain, and excitement. Like the respiratory rate and effort, the pulse rate should be interpreted within the context of the overall history, PAT, and the entire primary assessment.

A trend of an increasing or decreasing pulse rate may provide useful information and may suggest worsening hypoxia or shock, or improvement after treatment. When hypoxia or shock becomes critical, bradycardia occurs. Bradycardia is a condition in which the heart rate is less than 80 beats/min in children or less than 100 beats/min in newborns. As with slowing respirations, bradycardia in a pediatric patient is an ominous sign and often indicates impending cardiopulmonary arrest.

Feel the skin for temperature and moisture at the same time you assess the patient's pulse. Is the skin warm and dry, or cold and clammy? Estimate the capillary refill time by squeezing the end of a finger or toe for several seconds, causing the nail bed to blanch, then observing the return of blood to the area (**FIGURE 35-19**). Color should return within 2 seconds after you let go. The capillary refill time is used to assess end-organ perfusion. It is most

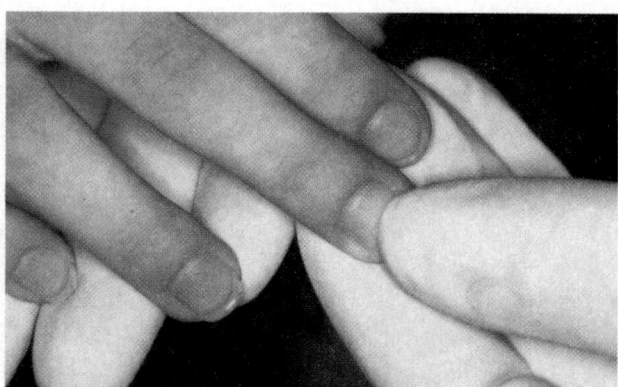

**FIGURE 35-19** Estimate the capillary refill time by squeezing the end of a finger or toe for several seconds until the nail bed blanches. Normal color should return within 2 seconds after you let go.

© Jones and Bartlett Learning.

reliable in children younger than 6 years; however, factors such as cold temperatures may affect the capillary refill time.

Assess the pediatric patient's level of consciousness using the AVPU scale or the Pediatric Glasgow Coma Scale (**TABLE 35-6**).

Check the responses of each pupil to a direct beam of light. A normal pupil constricts after a light stimulus. Pupillary response may be abnormal in the presence of drugs, ongoing seizures, hypoxia, or brain injury. Note if the pupils are dilated, constricted, reactive, or fixed.

Next, look for symmetric movement of the extremities and note any neurologic motor deficit such as the inability to move the upper or lower extremities, an inability to communicate, weakness, or difficulty walking (gait).

---

### Words of Wisdom

Helpful mnemonics to remember:

  B   Blood pressure
  L   Level of consciousness
  S   Skin: color, temperature, moisture
  C   Capillary refill time
  P   Pulse: rate, rhythm, strength
  R   Respiratory rate, effort, pattern

---

Pain is present with most types of injury and many illnesses. When you assess the severity of pain, consider the developmental age of the patient. The ability to recognize pain will improve as patients become older. For example, crying and agitation in an infant may be the result of hunger or a wet diaper. Meanwhile, a 3-year-old child can say, "My tummy really hurts." In children ages 3 and older, pain scales using pictures of facial expressions (Wong-Baker FACES scale) may help assess the level of pain (**FIGURE 35-20**).

Proper exposure of the pediatric patient is necessary to complete the hands-on XABCs. The PAT requires that the parent or caregiver remove part of the pediatric patient's clothing to allow careful observation of the face, chest wall, and skin. Further exposure may be needed to fully evaluate physiologic functions, anatomic abnormalities, and unsuspected injuries or rashes. Be careful to avoid

**TABLE 35-6** Pediatric Glasgow Coma Scale (GCS)

| Activity | Score | Infant | Score | Child |
|---|---|---|---|---|
| Eye opening | 4 | Open spontaneously | 4 | Open spontaneously |
| | 3 | Open to speech or sound | 3 | Open to speech |
| | 2 | Open to pressure | 2 | Open to pressure |
| | 1 | No response | 1 | No response |
| Verbal | 5 | Coos, babbles | 5 | Oriented conversation |
| | 4 | Irritable cry | 4 | Confused conversation |
| | 3 | Cries to pain | 3 | Cries |
| | 2 | Moans to pain | 2 | Moans |
| | 1 | No response | 1 | No response |
| Motor | 6 | Normal spontaneous movement | 6 | Obeys verbal commands |
| | 5 | Localizes to pressure | 5 | Localizes to pressure |
| | 4 | Withdraws from pressure | 4 | Withdraws from pressure |
| | 3 | Abnormal flexion (decorticate) | 3 | Abnormal flexion (decorticate) |
| | 2 | Abnormal extension (decerebrate) | 2 | Abnormal extension (decerebrate) |
| | 1 | No response (flaccid) | 1 | No response (flaccid) |

Data From: *Pediatric Advanced Life Support*, 2015, American Heart Association.

## Wong-Baker FACES® Pain Rating Scale

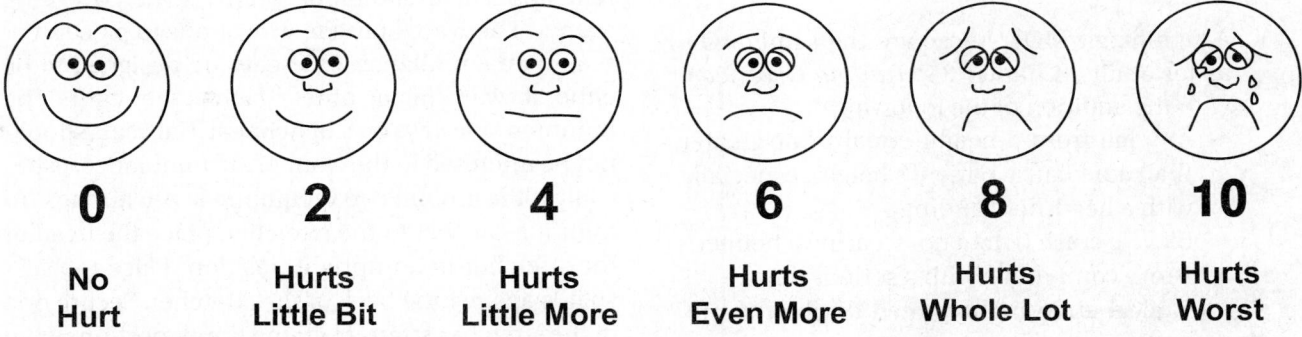

| 0 | 2 | 4 | 6 | 8 | 10 |
|---|---|---|---|---|---|
| No Hurt | Hurts Little Bit | Hurts Little More | Hurts Even More | Hurts Whole Lot | Hurts Worst |

**FIGURE 35-20** The Wong-Baker FACES pain rating scale.

heat loss, especially in infants, by covering the patient as soon as possible.

The thermoregulatory system in the pediatric body is immature. Paired with thinner skin and a lack of subcutaneous fat, this makes children more susceptible to hypothermia. Infants younger than 6 months lack the ability to shiver in response to a cold stimulus and therefore cannot generate body

### Words of Wisdom

Remember that infants and children are susceptible to hypothermia because of poor thermoregulation and a larger surface area–to–mass ratio than adults. You must ensure that a pediatric patient stays warm, especially when he or she is compromised due to illness or trauma.

heat from this protective mechanism. Newborns and infants less than 1 month are the most susceptible to hypothermia.

Keep infants and young children warm (but not overly hot) during transport or when the patient is exposed to assess or reassess an injury. In particular, cover the head because up to 50% of heat loss can occur with a head that is larger in proportion to the rest of the body. Without recognition and treatment of hypothermia, the pediatric patient may become unconscious.

## Transport Decision

After you have completed the primary assessment using hands-on XABCs and initiated any treatment, you must decide when, how, and where to transport the patient. First, determine whether rapid transport to the hospital is indicated. If the child is in stable condition, obtain a patient history, perform a secondary assessment at the scene, transport, and provide additional treatment as needed.

Rapid transport is indicated if the scene is unsafe for the patient or if any of the following conditions exist:

- A significant MOI—these are the same MOIs as for adults (Chapter 25, *Trauma Overview*), with the addition of the following:
  - Any fall from a height equal to or greater than a pediatric patient's height, especially with a head-first landing
  - Bicycle crash (when not wearing a helmet)
- A history compatible with a serious illness
- A physical abnormality noted during the primary assessment
- A potentially serious anatomic abnormality
- Significant pain
- Abnormal level of consciousness, altered mental status, and/or any signs or symptoms of shock

In addition to the preceding factors, consider the following when making a transport decision:

- The type of clinical problem (injury versus illness)
- The expected benefits of advanced life support (ALS) treatment in the field
- Local EMS system treatment and transport protocols

- Your comfort level
- Transport time to the hospital

If the child's condition is urgent, then initiate rapid transport to the closest appropriate facility. Specialty facilities such as trauma centers or children's hospitals have the training, staff, and equipment to provide complete care for all levels of pediatric patients. However, the most appropriate facility is not always the closest facility. To help you determine where to transport a pediatric patient, ask yourself this crucial question: *Can I deliver the pediatric patient to the most appropriate facility without risk or delay to the child?* If you cannot, or if the illness or injury is so extensive that you cannot provide the care that the pediatric patient needs, then transport the child to the closest facility. Additional assessment and treatment should occur en route to the hospital.

Children weighing less than 40 pounds (18 kg) who do not require spinal motion restriction should be transported in a car seat if the situation allows. Many types of car seats are available. A car seat should be chosen to fit the appropriate weight of the pediatric patient and should meet the current applicable standards set by your governing agency. There are only a few locations to place a car seat in an ambulance. Car seats are designed to be either forward-facing or rear-facing; they cannot be mounted sideways on a bench seat. Car seats should not be mounted in the front of an ambulance, especially if the ambulance is equipped with airbags. To mount a car seat to the stretcher, place the head of the stretcher in an upright position. Place the seat so it is against the back of the stretcher. Secure one of the stretcher straps from the upper portion of the stretcher through the seat belt positions on the seat and strap it tightly to the stretcher. Repeat on the lower portion of the stretcher. Push the car seat into the stretcher tightly and retighten the straps.

To secure a car seat to the captain's chair, follow the seat manufacturer's instructions. Remember that children younger than 2 years must be transported in a rear-facing position because of the lack of mature neck muscles.

For pediatric patients who require spinal motion restriction, it is no longer considered appropriate to secure a pediatric patient in a car seat. Immobilize the child on a long backboard or other suitable spinal immobilization device. If the patient's condition is unstable and requires airway or ventilatory support, he or she should be positioned to maximize the ability to manage the airway and ventilatory requirements. Pediatric patients in cardiopulmonary arrest should likewise not be placed in a car seat but instead on a device that can be secured to the stretcher. Follow local protocols.

In a situation involving a high-speed crash with potential for damage to the child's car seat, do not use the patient's own car seat when the child is in stable condition. Instead, transfer the patient to the ambulance's car seat or suitable restraining device. The goal is to secure and protect the patient for transport in the ambulance. The patient should be protected just as if he or she were in any other vehicle on the road.

## Words of Wisdom

Depending on the age or developmental level of the child, he or she may be unable to provide the necessary information for a thorough and complete patient history. Always include parents and primary caregivers in the history-taking process. This is especially true when a child has a chronic, critical, or unique illness; the parents and caregivers will often have more experience and knowledge about the illness and the necessary care than you. Take advantage of their knowledge and their ability to assist you on scene, which will benefit the child's care.

## History Taking

Your approach to the history will depend on the age of the child. Historical information for an infant, toddler, or preschool-age child will need to be obtained from the parent or caregiver. When dealing with an adolescent, you will usually be able to obtain most of the immediate information from the patient; however, consult the parent or caregiver for a complete history.

Information about sexual activity, the possibility of pregnancy, or the use of illicit drugs or alcohol should be obtained from an adolescent patient in private. Adolescents will be reluctant to provide this information in the presence of their parents or caregivers. When asking sensitive questions, assure the adolescent that this information is important and is needed to provide the most appropriate care.

Question the parent or child about the immediate illness or injury based on the child's chief complaint. Together with an evaluation of the child's medical history, this may provide clues to the underlying illness or injury and other conditions that may exist.

When you interview the parent or caregiver or older child about the chief complaint, obtain the following pertinent information:

- The NOI or MOI
- How long the child has been sick or injured
- The key events leading to the injury or illness: Were there any witnesses to the injury? From what height did the patient fall? What surface did the child land on (soft or hard)?
- Presence of fever
- Effects of the illness or injury on the child's behavior
- Pediatric patient's activity level
- Recent eating, drinking, and urine output
- Change in bowel or bladder habits
- Presence of vomiting, diarrhea, abdominal pain
- Presence of rashes

If the parent or caregiver is unable to accompany you to the hospital, obtain a name and phone number so a staff person can call if there are questions. This might be the case when you respond to a day care facility or babysitter's location or when a parent must remain at the scene to care for other children. Most day care facilities require emergency contact information, past medical history, and/or a list of current prescribed medications taken by the child in case of an emergency. Care may be delayed if this information is not discovered early; however, you must never delay care of a critical patient.

Obtaining a SAMPLE history for a child is the same as obtaining an adult's history. However, the questions should be based on the patient's age and developmental stage of life (**TABLE 35-7**).

The OPQRST format can help you gather additional information about a patient's history of present illness and current symptoms. Chapter 10, *Patient Assessment*, describes this process in detail. The process for obtaining the OPQRST information is the same for children and adults. As with the SAMPLE history, the questions should be based on the child's age and developmental stage (**TABLE 35-8**).

**TABLE 35-7** Pediatric SAMPLE Components

| Component | Explanation |
|---|---|
| Signs and symptoms | Onset and nature of symptoms of pain or fever<br>Age-appropriate signs of distress (see OPQRST questions in Table 35-8) |
| Allergies | Known drug reactions or other allergies |
| Medications | Exact names and doses of ongoing drugs (including over-the-counter, prescribed, herbal, and recreational drugs)<br>Timing and amount of last dose<br>Time and dose of analgesics or antipyretics |
| Pertinent past medical history | Previous illness or injuries<br>Immunizations<br>Complications surrounding pregnancy, labor, or delivery, including the route of delivery (infants and toddlers) |
| Last oral intake | Timing of the child's last food or drink, including bottle or breastfeeding |
| Events leading up to the illness or injury | Key events leading up to the current incident<br>Fever history |

© Jones & Bartlett Learning.

**TABLE 35-8** Pediatric OPQRST Components

| Component | Explanation |
|---|---|
| Onset | How long has the patient been experiencing this event? What was the patient doing when the symptoms began? |
| Provocation/palliation | Does anything make the pain or discomfort better or worse? In what position is the patient most comfortable? |
| Quality | What does the pain feel like? "Dull," "sharp," and "cramping" are common descriptions. Does it come in waves? |
| Region/radiation | Where does the patient feel the symptoms? |
| Severity | Observe nonverbal cues (such as wincing or posture). Ask the patient to rate his or her symptoms using the Wong-Baker FACES scale (see Figure 35-20). |
| Timing | When did symptoms begin? Have the symptoms been constant or do they come and go? |

© Jones & Bartlett Learning.

## Special Populations

A lower extremity injury should be suspected in any child who refuses to bear weight. Do not allow a patient with a suspected lower extremity injury to walk—question parents, bystanders, or the child to determine the MOI and symptoms.

## Secondary Assessment

In some instances, such as a critically ill or injured child or a short transport time, you may not have time to conduct a secondary assessment. Perform a secondary assessment of the entire body when pediatric patients have the potential for hidden illnesses or injuries—for example, unresponsive medical patients or trauma patients with a significant MOI. This type of examination may help to identify problems such as a distended abdomen or possible fractures that were not as obvious during the primary assessment, but whose presenting signs and symptoms became more apparent over time.

Use the DCAP-BTLS mnemonic (Deformities, Contusions, Abrasions, Punctures/Penetrations, Burns, Tenderness, Lacerations, and Swelling) to remind you what to assess for on a pediatric patient involved in a traumatic event.

After a physical examination of the whole body has been completed, perform a focused assessment on pediatric patients without life-threatening illnesses or injuries. Focus your physical examination on the area or areas of the body affected by the illness or injury as well as on the chief complaint, MOI or NOI, and the findings of the primary assessment.

Infants, toddlers, and preschool-age children who do not have apparent life-threatening illness or injuries should be assessed starting at the feet and ending at the head; school-age children and adolescents can be assessed using the head-to-toe approach, as with adults. The extent of the physical examination will depend on the situation and may include the following:

- **Head.** The younger the infant or child, the larger the head is in proportion to the rest of the body, increasing the risk for head injury with deceleration (such as in falls or motor vehicle crashes). Look for bruising, swelling, and hematomas. Significant blood loss can occur between the skull and scalp of a small infant. A tense or bulging fontanelle in an upright, non-crying infant suggests elevated intracranial pressure caused by meningitis, encephalitis, or intracranial bleeding. A sunken fontanelle suggests dehydration.
- **Nose.** Young infants are obligate nose breathers, so nasal congestion with mucus can cause respiratory distress. Gentle bulb or catheter suction of the nostrils may bring relief.

- **Ears.** Look for any drainage from the ear canals. Leaking blood suggests a skull fracture. Check for bruises behind the ear or Battle sign, a late sign of skull fracture. The presence of pus may indicate an ear infection or perforation of the eardrum. Bruising or hematomas of the ear may result from abuse, especially if found on both sides.
- **Mouth.** In the trauma patient, look for active bleeding and loose teeth. Note the smell of the breath. Some ingestions are associated with identifiable odors, such as hydrocarbons (eg, gasoline). Acidosis, as in diabetic ketoacidosis, may impart a fruity odor to the breath.
- **Neck.** Examine the area near the trachea for swelling or bruising. Note if the pediatric patient cannot move his or her neck and has a high fever. This may indicate that the child has meningitis.
- **Chest.** Examine the chest for penetrating injuries, lacerations, bruises, or rashes. If the patient is injured, feel the clavicles and every rib for tenderness and/or deformity.
- **Back.** Inspect the back for lacerations, penetrating injuries, bruises, or rashes.
- **Abdomen.** Inspect the abdomen for distention. Gently palpate the abdomen and watch closely for guarding or tensing of the abdominal muscles, which may suggest infection, obstruction, or intra-abdominal injury. Note any tenderness or masses. Look for any seat belt abrasions or bruising.
- **Extremities.** Assess for symmetry. Compare both sides for color, warmth, size of joints, swelling, and tenderness. Put each joint through its full range of motion while watching the child's eyes for signs of pain, unless there is obvious deformity of the extremity suggesting a fracture.

Some of the guidelines used to assess adult circulatory status—heart rate and blood pressure—have important limitations in children. First, normal heart rates vary with age in children. Second, blood pressure is usually not assessed in patients younger than 3 years; it offers little information about the child's circulatory status and is often difficult to obtain. In these patients, assessment of the skin is a better indication of their circulatory status.

It is important to use appropriate-size equipment when you assess a pediatric patient's vital signs. To obtain an accurate reading of a child's blood pressure, use a cuff that covers two-thirds of the patient's upper arm. A blood pressure cuff that is too small may give you a falsely high reading, whereas a cuff that is too large may give you a falsely low reading. A useful tool to determine blood pressure in children ages 1 to 10 years (lower limits) is:

$$70 + (2 \times \text{Child's age in years}) = \text{Lowest expected systolic blood pressure}$$

Respiratory rates may be difficult to interpret. Rapid respiratory rates may simply reflect high fever, anxiety, pain, or excitement. Slow rates (ie, lower than normal for age) often signal rapid deterioration requiring intervention. When time and the patient's condition permit, count the respirations for 30 seconds and then double that number. If the patient yawns, sighs, coughs, or talks during the 30-second period, wait a few seconds and begin again. In infants and children younger than 3 years, evaluate respirations by assessing the rise and fall of the abdomen. Assess the pulse rate by counting at least 1 minute, noting its quality and regularity. When you are more rushed due to the critical nature of the child's condition, count the pulse rate for 15 seconds and multiply by 4 to obtain an approximation of the rate.

Note that normal vital signs in pediatric patients vary with age (**TABLE 35-9**). Remember that your approach to taking vital signs also varies with the age of the pediatric patient. Be gentle, talk to the child, assess respirations and then pulse, and assess blood pressure last. Warm your stethoscope on your hands or a cloth before placing it on the skin. You may also want to let the pediatric patient hold the equipment first; this may help to reduce his or her anxiety.

Evaluate pupils in the child using a small penlight. The response of pupils is a good indication of

**TABLE 35-9** Pediatric Blood Pressure Ranges

| Age | Systolic Blood Pressure (mm Hg) |
|---|---|
| Neonate: 1 to 4 days | 60 to 76 |
| Neonate: 4 days to 1 month | 67 to 84 |
| Infant: 1 to 3 months | 73 to 94 |
| Infant: 3 to 6 months | 78 to 103 |
| Infant: 6 months to 1 year | 82 to 105 |
| Child: 1 to 2 years | 85 to 104 |
| Child: 2 to 7 years | 88 to 106 |
| Child: 7 to 15 years | 96 to 115 |
| Adolescent: 15 to 18 years | 110 to 131 |

Data From: *Pediatric Advanced Life Support*, 2015, American Heart Association.

how well the brain is functioning, particularly when trauma has occurred. Be sure to compare the size of the pupils to one another.

A pulse oximeter is a valuable tool to measure the oxygen saturation in a child with respiratory issues (**FIGURE 35-21**). Adhesive sensors also can be useful on a child's foot or even forehead if needed.

**Reassessment**

Reassess the pediatric patient's condition as necessary—a general rule is to obtain vital signs every 15 minutes for a child in stable condition and at least every 5 minutes for a child in unstable condition. Temperature is a vital sign that should be assessed on all seriously ill pediatric patients. Infants and children can decompensate with alarming unpredictability; therefore, continually monitor respiratory effort, skin color and condition, and

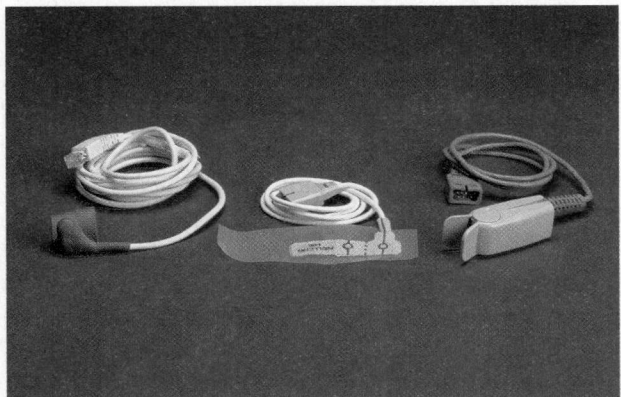

**A**

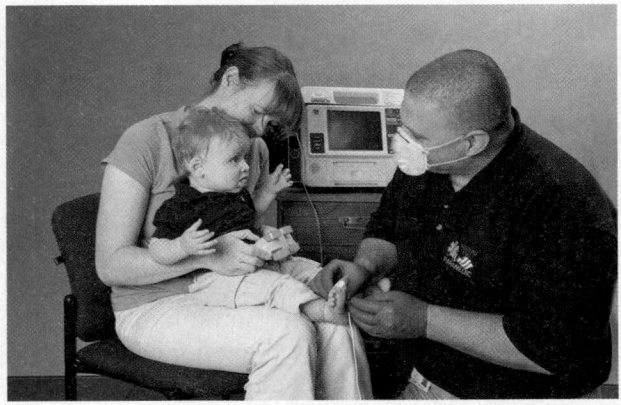

**B**

**FIGURE 35-21** Pulse oximetry, which measures the child's oxygen saturation, can be used to monitor the patient's status. **A.** Pulse oximeter probes can wrap around or clip onto fingers, toes, or ear lobes. **B.** A pulse oximeter being applied to an infant's foot.

**A, B:** © Jones & Bartlett Learning.

level of consciousness or interactiveness. Repeat the primary assessment and adjust your treatment accordingly.

When you provide interventions for a pediatric patient, remember that parents and caregivers may be able to assist you by calming and reassuring the child and are often well educated about their child's medical conditions. They are also able to assist with administering oxygen or medications via a nebulizer. Together you can build a trusting environment for the pediatric patient, who is already in a state of stress.

Communicate with the hospital regarding your findings and the interventions you used to improve the child's condition. Be sure that all of this information is documented and given to emergency department (ED) personnel.

## YOU are the Provider

Your partner hands the child's mother a pediatric nonrebreathing mask with the oxygen flow rate set at 12 L/min, and he asks her to hold the mask near the child's face. Although the child becomes somewhat agitated by the oxygen, she does not push the mask away. After your partner talks to the child and explains what he is going to do, he assesses her vital signs. You gather additional information from the child's parents.

| Recording Time: 5 Minutes | |
|---|---|
| **Respirations** | 34 breaths/min; labored |
| **Pulse** | 124 beats/min; strong and regular |
| **Skin** | Pink, warm, and dry; capillary refill time 1 second |
| **Blood pressure** | 86/56 mm Hg |
| **Oxygen saturation (Spo$_2$)** | 95% (on oxygen) |

The child's mother tells you that her daughter has had a cold for the past 2 days and has slowly developed a low-grade fever and high-pitched cough, which she describes as a "barking seal" sound. She was going to take her to the doctor tomorrow, but called 9-1-1 when the child began experiencing trouble breathing. Further assessment of the child reveals that her breath sounds are clear and equal bilaterally and she has prominent intercostal retractions.

**5.** What is the most likely cause of this child's respiratory distress?

**6.** Should you separate this child from her parents to provide further treatment? Why or why not?

# Respiratory Emergencies and Management

Respiratory problems are the leading cause of cardiopulmonary arrest in the pediatric population. Failure to recognize and treat declining respiratory status will result in death. A pediatric patient in respiratory distress still has the compensatory mechanisms and the ability to exchange oxygen and carbon dioxide. During respiratory distress, the child is working harder to breathe and will eventually go into respiratory failure if left untreated. Respiratory failure occurs when the patient has exhausted all compensatory mechanisms and waste products begin to collect. If this is not treated, a total shutdown of the respiratory system will occur—respiratory arrest.

In the early stages of respiratory distress, you may note changes in the child's behavior, such as anxiety, restlessness, or combativeness. As the body attempts to maximize the amount of air going into the lungs, the work of breathing increases. As discussed previously, the signs and symptoms of increased work of breathing include nasal flaring, abnormal breath sounds, accessory muscle use, and the tripod position.

As the pediatric patient progresses to possible respiratory failure, efforts to breathe decrease; the chest rises less with inspiration and the respiratory rate may slow. The body has used up its available energy stores and cannot continue to support the extra work of breathing under these conditions. At this point, without care, cyanosis may develop (a late sign). Be aware that not all pediatric patients develop cyanosis. You should be just as concerned about a child with pale skin as one with blue skin.

Changes in behavior will also occur until the patient demonstrates an altered level of consciousness. The child may experience periods of apnea (absence of breathing). As the lack of oxygen becomes more serious, the heart muscle itself becomes hypoxic and slows down. This leads to bradycardia—almost always an ominous sign in children. If the heart rate is fast, you need to investigate the cause. However, if the heart rate is slow (less than 60 beats/min) or absent, despite bag-mask ventilation with high-flow oxygen, especially in an unconscious infant or child, you must begin CPR immediately. Without aggressive airway management, bradycardia may quickly progress to cardiopulmonary arrest.

Of course, respiratory failure does not always indicate airway obstruction. It may indicate trauma, nervous system problems, dehydration (often caused by vomiting and diarrhea), or metabolic disturbances. For example, a pediatric patient who ingested a narcotic may have inadequate, slow breathing, or a child might have a pH imbalance, as can happen with some rare pediatric diseases. Regardless of the cause, your first step is always to ensure adequate oxygenation and ventilation.

Never forget that a pediatric patient's condition can progress from respiratory distress to respiratory failure at any time. For this reason, you must reassess the child frequently.

A child or infant in respiratory distress needs supplemental oxygen. Anxiety, agitation, or crying may increase the effort or work of breathing, so use whichever method seems least upsetting—mask, blow-by, or nasal cannula. You may need to get creative by distracting the child with games, a toy, or conversation. Assist ventilation with a bag-mask device and 100% oxygen for infants and children who are in possible respiratory failure.

Allow the pediatric patient to remain in a comfortable position. For a small child, this may mean sitting on the parent's or caregiver's lap. Give nothing by mouth if the patient has severe respiratory distress, in case the patient's condition deteriorates suddenly. If the patient's condition progresses to respiratory failure, begin assisted ventilation immediately, and continue to provide supplemental oxygen.

## Airway Obstruction

Children, especially those younger than 5 years, can (and do) obstruct their airway with any object that they can fit into their mouth, such as hot dogs, balloons, grapes, or coins (**FIGURE 35-22**). In cases of trauma, a child's teeth may have been dislodged into the airway. Blood, vomitus, or other secretions can also cause mild or severe airway obstruction.

Airway obstruction can also be caused by infections, including pneumonia, croup, epiglottitis, and bacterial tracheitis (**FIGURE 35-23**). These conditions are discussed further in Chapter 16, *Respiratory Emergencies*. Consider infection as a possible cause of airway obstruction if a child has congestion, fever, drooling, and cold symptoms. Suspect

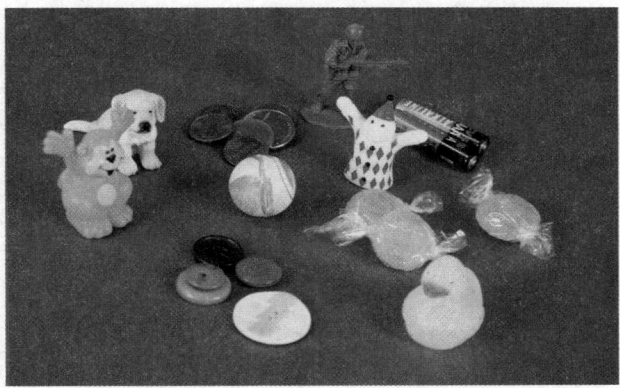

**FIGURE 35-22** Any number of objects can obstruct a child's airway, including batteries, coins, toys, buttons, and candy.

© Jones & Bartlett Learning. Photographed by Kimberly Potvin.

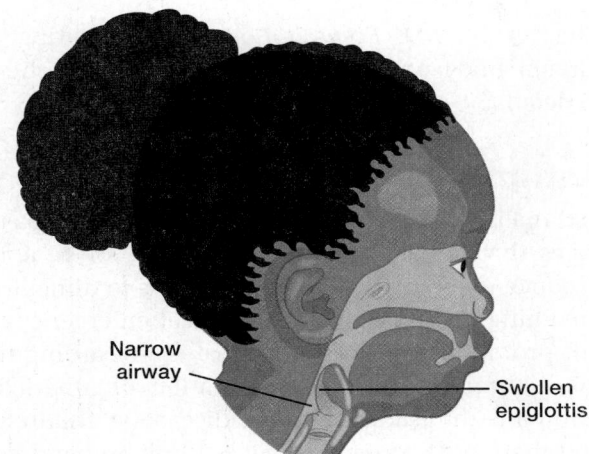

Narrow airway

Swollen epiglottis

**FIGURE 35-23** Epiglottitis is an infection that can cause airway obstruction in pediatric patients.

© Jones & Bartlett Learning.

## Special Populations

Pediatric patients who have a tracheostomy tube to assist in breathing are at risk of tracheostomy dysfunction. This is usually caused by an airway obstruction that results from an accumulation of thick mucus at the opening of the tracheostomy tube. These patients require urgent care and transport.

anaphylaxis if hives, hypotension, nausea, or vomiting accompany a sudden onset of dyspnea.

Obstruction by a foreign object may involve the upper or the lower airway, and may be partial or

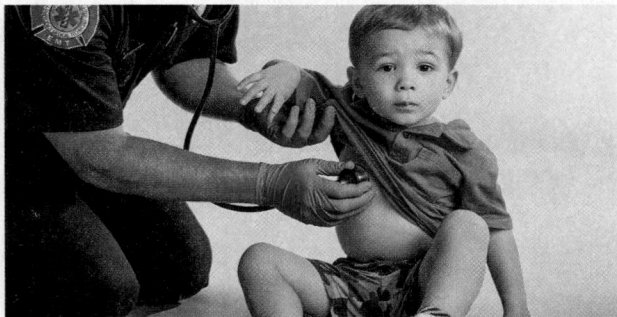

**FIGURE 35-24** The best way to auscultate breath sounds in pediatric patients is to listen on both sides of the chest at the level of the armpit.

© Jones & Bartlett Learning.

complete. Signs and symptoms that are frequently associated with a partial upper airway obstruction include a hoarse voice, decreased or absent breath sounds, and stridor. Stridor is usually caused by swelling of the area surrounding the vocal cords or upper airway obstruction. Infants or children with a complete airway obstruction will have absent breath sounds and become rapidly cyanotic.

Signs and symptoms of a lower airway obstruction include wheezing. The best way to auscultate breath sounds in a pediatric patient is to listen on both sides of the chest at the level of the armpit (**FIGURE 35-24**).

Immediately begin treatment of the child with an airway obstruction. If the patient is conscious and coughing forcefully and you know for sure that there is a foreign body in the airway—that is, if someone witnessed the object go into the child's mouth—encourage the child to cough to clear the airway. If the material in the airway does not completely block the flow of air, the child may be able to breathe adequately on his or her own without any intervention. In such cases, do not intervene except to provide supplemental oxygen (**FIGURE 35-25**). Allow the patient to remain in whatever position is most comfortable and monitor his or her condition during transport.

If you see signs of a severe airway obstruction, however, you must attempt to clear the airway immediately. The signs include the following:

- Ineffective cough (no sound)
- Inability to speak or cry
- Increasing respiratory difficulty, with stridor
- Cyanosis
- Loss of consciousness

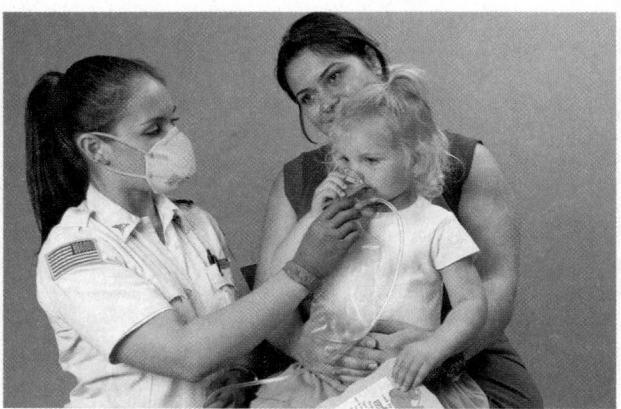

**FIGURE 35-25** If a pediatric patient has a partial airway obstruction, do not intervene except to give supplemental oxygen. Allow the child to remain in whatever position is most comfortable during transport.

© Jones & Bartlett Learning. Photographed by Glen E. Ellman.

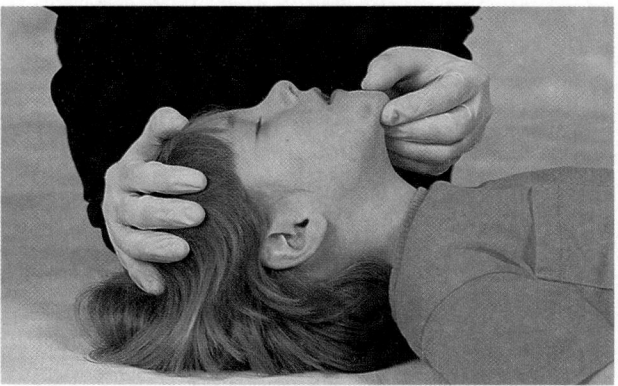

**FIGURE 35-26** Open the airway and look inside the mouth of an unconscious pediatric patient with a possible airway obstruction.

© Jones & Bartlett Learning. Courtesy of MIEMSS.

If an infant is conscious with a complete airway obstruction, perform up to five back blows followed by five chest thrusts. First, position the infant face down on your forearm. Support the infant's jaw and head with your hand. Next, use the heel of your other hand to slap the back forcefully five times (between the shoulder blades). If the airway does not clear, flip the infant onto his or her back, using your hand to support the head. Perform up to five chest thrusts in the same manner you would provide chest compressions for CPR. Repeat the process until the obstruction clears or until the infant becomes unconscious.

If a child (older than 1 year) is conscious with a complete airway obstruction, perform abdominal thrusts (Heimlich maneuver). Continue until the obstruction clears or until the child becomes unconscious.

If there is reason to believe that an unconscious child has a foreign body obstruction, open the airway using the head tilt–chin lift maneuver and look inside the mouth to see whether the obstructing object is visible (**FIGURE 35-26**). If the object is visible, try to remove it using a finger sweep motion. Never use finger sweeps if you cannot see the object because you may push it farther into the airway.

Chest compressions are recommended to relieve a severe airway obstruction in an unconscious pediatric patient. Chest compressions increase the pressure in the chest, creating an artificial cough that may force a foreign body from the airway.

Chapter 14, *BLS Resuscitation*, covers clearing a foreign body obstruction in an infant and child in detail.

## Asthma

Asthma is a condition in which the smaller air passages (bronchioles) become inflamed, swell, and produce excessive mucus, which leads to difficulty breathing. Asthma is a true medical emergency if not promptly identified and treated. According to the Asthma and Allergy Foundation of America, asthma is the leading chronic disease in children, and there are currently about 6.2 million children younger than 18 years with asthma. Common causes (triggers) for an asthma episode include upper respiratory infection, exercise, exposure to cold air or smoke, and emotional stress. Asthma is rare in children younger than 1 year.

Children with asthma will wheeze as they attempt to exhale through partially obstructed lower air passages; you may be able to hear loud wheezing without a stethoscope. In other cases, the airways are completely blocked and no air movement is heard. In severe cases, cyanosis and/or respiratory arrest may quickly develop. Asthma patients in respiratory distress will typically assume a position of comfort, such as the tripod position, to allow for maximum respiratory effort.

If possible, allow the child to assume a position of comfort in the parent's or caregiver's lap. Avoid overexciting the child because this may worsen the condition. Administer supplemental oxygen via a route that is tolerated by the child. Allow the parent or caregiver to assist the team by gathering any medications, calming the patient, or holding blow-by oxygen or a nonrebreathing mask.

A bronchodilator such as albuterol alone or with ipratropium via a metered-dose inhaler (MDI) with a spacer-mask device or by nebulizer may be administered based on local agency protocols. Often the parents or caregivers have attempted multiple dosages of albuterol. In this case, administer an additional dose while ALS providers are dispatched to meet you en route for additional medication administration and advanced care.

If you must assist ventilations in a child who is having an asthma attack, use slow, gentle breaths. Remember, the problem in asthma is getting the air out of the lungs, not into them. Resist the temptation to squeeze the reservoir bag hard and fast.

A prolonged asthma attack that is unrelieved may progress into a condition known as status asthmaticus. The child is likely to be frightened, frantically trying to breathe, and using all the accessory muscles. Status asthmaticus is a true emergency. Administer oxygen, ventilate if needed, and provide rapid transport to the ED.

The effort to breathe during an asthma attack is very tiring, and the patient may be exhausted by the time you arrive. An exhausted pediatric patient may have stopped feeling anxious or even struggling to breathe. It may look as if this patient is recovering; however, he or she is at a critical stage and is likely to stop breathing. Aggressive airway management, oxygen administration, and prompt transport are essential in this situation. Consider calling for ALS backup, if available rapidly. Follow local protocol.

## Pneumonia

According to the World Health Organization, pneumonia is the leading cause of death for children worldwide annually. Pneumonia kills an estimated 1.4 million children younger than 5 years. Pneumonia is a general term that refers to an infection of the lungs. Pneumonia is often a secondary infection; it occurs during or after treatment for a preexisting infection such as a cold. It can also be caused by direct lung injuries, such as from an accidental ingestion of a chemical or a submersion incident. Children with diseases causing immunodeficiency

are at increased risk for pneumonia. You will notice that the incidence of this type of virus is greatest during the fall and winter months, affecting a large swathe of the pediatric population.

Often pediatric patients will present with unusually rapid breathing or will breathe with grunting or wheezing sounds. Additional signs and symptoms include nasal flaring, tachypnea, and hypothermia or fever. The patient may also exhibit unilateral diminished breath sounds or crackles over the infected lung segments. Assess the work of breathing by observing for signs of accessory muscle usage. Pneumonia is particularly serious in infants because they have an increased oxygen demand and less respiratory reserve than older children or adults. For a pediatric patient with suspected pneumonia, your primary treatment will be supportive. Monitor the patient's airway and breathing status and administer supplemental oxygen if required. If the child is wheezing, administer a bronchodilator if permitted in your EMS system. A diagnosis of pneumonia must be confirmed in the hospital setting with a chest radiograph, followed by the administration of antibiotics as the primary treatment.

## Croup

Croup (laryngotracheobronchitis) is an infection of the airway below the level of the vocal cords, usually caused by a virus. This disease is typically seen in children between ages 6 months and 3 years. It is easily passed between children. The disease starts with a cold, cough, and a low-grade fever that develops over 2 days. The hallmark signs of croup are stridor and a seal-bark cough, which is a signal of significant narrowing of the air passage of the trachea that may progress to significant obstruction. Peak seasonal outbreaks of this disease occur in the late fall and during the winter. Croup often responds well to the administration of humidified oxygen. Bronchodilators are not indicated for croup and can make the child worse.

## Epiglottitis

Epiglottitis (supraglottitis) is an infection of the soft tissue in the area above the vocal cords. Bacterial infection is the most common cause. Epiglottitis occurs in patients of all ages. Since the development of a vaccine against one organism that causes epiglottitis, the incidence of this disease has dramatically decreased. In preschool- and school-aged children especially, the epiglottis can swell to two to three times its normal size. This puts the airway at risk of complete obstruction. The condition usually develops in otherwise healthy children, and symptoms are relatively sudden in onset. Children with this infection look very sick, report a very sore throat, and have a high fever. They will often be found in the tripod position and drooling.

## Bronchiolitis

Bronchiolitis is a specific viral illness of newborns and toddlers, often caused by respiratory syncytial virus (RSV) that leads to inflammation of the bronchioles. RSV is highly contagious. It is spread through droplets when the pediatric patient coughs or sneezes. RSV is more common in premature infants and results in copious secretions that may require suctioning of the nose. The virus can also survive on surfaces, including hands and clothing. The infection tends to spread rapidly in schools and day care centers.

Bronchiolitis occurs during the first 2 years of life and is more common in boys. These infections are most widespread in the winter and early spring. Bronchioles become inflamed, swell, and fill with mucus. The airways of infants and young children can easily become blocked.

When assessing a pediatric patient, look for signs of dehydration—infants with RSV often refuse liquids. If the RSV has progressed to bronchiolitis, shortness of breath and fever may be present.

Approach the pediatric patient with a calm demeanor and allow for a position of comfort. Treat airway and breathing problems as appropriate. Humidified oxygen is helpful if available. Consider calling for ALS backup and transport to the appropriate hospital.

## Pertussis

Pertussis (whooping cough) is a communicable disease caused by a bacterium that is spread through respiratory droplets. As the result of vaccination, this potentially deadly disease is less common in the United States. The typical signs and symptoms are similar to a common cold: coughing, sneezing, and a runny nose. As the disease progresses, the coughing becomes more severe and is characterized by the distinctive whoop sound heard during inspiration. Infants infected with pertussis may develop pneumonia or respiratory failure. To treat pediatric patients, keep the airway patent (open) and transport. Because pertussis is contagious, follow standard precautions, including wearing a mask and eye protection.

## YOU are the Provider

The child's father carries the child to the ambulance, where you appropriately secure her to the stretcher. You reassess her condition prior to transport and note that it has changed. On appearance, you note that her retractions have markedly weakened, she has a blank stare, and she is listless. Your partner quickly secures the child's mother in the front seat of the ambulance and begins rapid transport.

| Recording Time: 10 Minutes | |
| --- | --- |
| Level of consciousness | Decreased activity; blank stare; listless |
| Respirations | 18 breaths/min; weak retractions |
| Pulse | 90 beats/min; weak and regular |
| Skin | Perioral cyanosis; cool and dry; capillary refill time, 3 seconds |
| Blood pressure | 76/56 mm Hg |
| Spo$_2$ | 85% (on oxygen) |

**7.** How has this child's condition changed? What should you do next?

**8.** How could an ALS intercept benefit this child?

## Airway Adjuncts

In children with inadequate ventilation, use an airway adjunct to maintain an open airway. Airway adjuncts are devices that help to maintain the airway or assist in providing artificial ventilation, including oropharyngeal and nasopharyngeal airways, and bag-mask devices. Placing the adjuncts correctly starts with choosing the appropriate-size equipment (**TABLE 35-10**).

## Oropharyngeal Airway

An oropharyngeal (oral) airway is designed to keep the tongue from blocking the airway, and it makes suctioning the airway, if necessary, easier. An oropharyngeal airway should be used for pediatric patients who are unconscious and in respiratory failure. This adjunct should not be used in either conscious pediatric patients or those who have a gag reflex. Pediatric patients with a gag reflex do not tolerate an oropharyngeal airway. In addition, this adjunct should not be used in children who may have ingested a caustic or petroleum-based product because it may induce vomiting.

**SKILL DRILL 35-2** shows the steps for inserting an oropharyngeal airway in a child:

1. Determine the appropriate-size airway by placing the airway next to the face with the flange at the level of the central incisors and the bite block segment parallel to the hard palate. The tip of the airway should reach the angle of the jaw (**Step 1**). Or, use length-based resuscitation tape to determine the appropriate-size airway.
2. Position the pediatric patient's airway. If the emergency is medical, use the head tilt–chin lift maneuver. Avoid hyperextension; you may place a towel under the child's shoulders. If the patient has a traumatic injury, use the jaw-thrust maneuver and provide manual in-line stabilization (**Step 2**).
3. Open the mouth by applying pressure on the chin with your thumb.
4. Insert the airway by depressing the tongue with a tongue blade applied to the base of the tongue and inserting the airway directly over the tongue blade (**Step 3**). If a tongue blade is unavailable, point the airway tip toward the

---

| **TABLE 35-10** Pediatric Equipment: Getting the Size Right |
| --- |

One method to identify the appropriate-size equipment for a pediatric patient is to use **length-based resuscitation tape** (Broselow tape). This color-coded tool can estimate weight as well as height in pediatric patients weighing up to 75 lb (34 kg) (**FIGURE 35-27**). The proper sequence for using the tape is as follows:

1. Place the pediatric patient supine on a flat surface.
2. Lay the tape next to the pediatric patient with the multicolored side facing up.
3. Place the red end of the tape at the top of the pediatric patient's head (red to head).
4. Place one hand with its side down at the top of the pediatric patient's head, covering the red box at the end of the tape.
5. Starting from the pediatric patient's head, run the side of your free hand down the tape.
6. Stretch the tape out the full length of the child, stopping at the heel. If the child is longer than the tape, stop here and use the appropriate adult equipment.
7. Place your free hand, side down, at the bottom of the child's heel.
8. Note the color or letter block and weight range on the edge of the tape where your hand is. Say the color or letter out loud.
9. Select the appropriate-size equipment by matching the color or letter on the tape to the color or letter on the equipment.

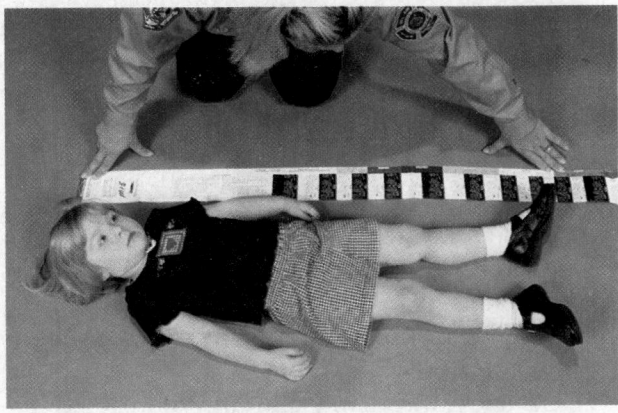

**FIGURE 35-27** Length-based resuscitation tape is the best way to estimate the correct size for airway adjuncts in children.

## Skill Drill 35-2 Inserting an Oropharyngeal Airway in a Pediatric Patient

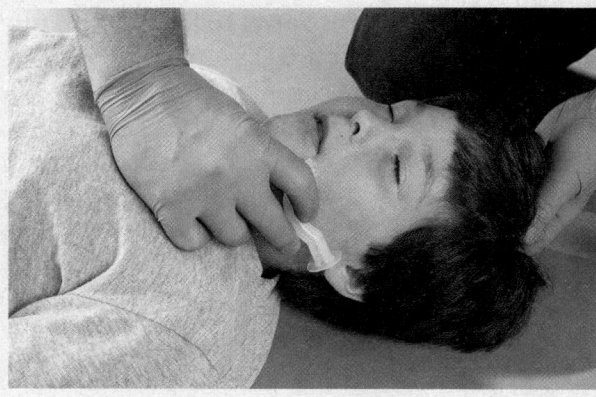

### Step 1

Determine the appropriate-size airway. Confirm the correct size visually, by placing it next to the pediatric patient's face.

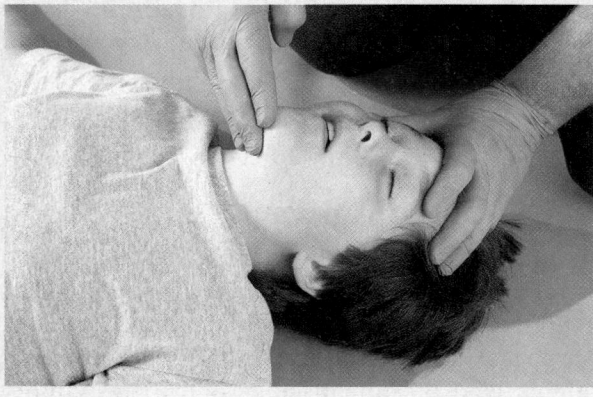

### Step 2

Position the pediatric patient's airway using the appropriate method.

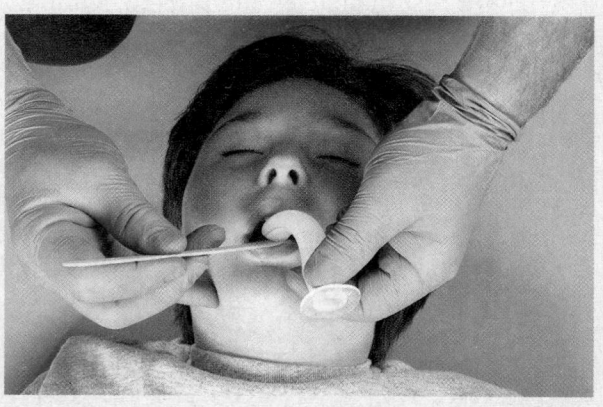

© Jones & Bartlett Learning.

### Step 3

Open the mouth. Insert the airway until the flange rests against the lips. Reassess the airway.

roof of the mouth to depress the tongue. Gently rotate the airway into position as it passes through the mouth toward the curve of the tongue. Insert the airway until the flange rests against the lips.

5. Reassess the airway after insertion. Take care to avoid injuring the hard palate as you insert the airway. Rough insertion can cause bleeding, which can aggravate airway problems and may even cause vomiting. Note also that

if the pediatric patient's airway is too small, the tongue may be pushed back into the pharynx, obstructing the airway. If the airway is too large, it may obstruct the larynx.

## Nasopharyngeal Airway

A nasopharyngeal (nasal) airway is usually well tolerated and is not as likely as the oropharyngeal airway to cause vomiting. Unlike the oropharyngeal

## Skill Drill 35-3 Inserting a Nasopharyngeal Airway in a Pediatric Patient

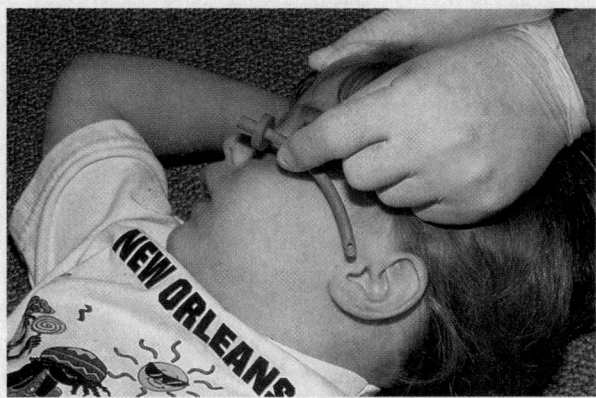

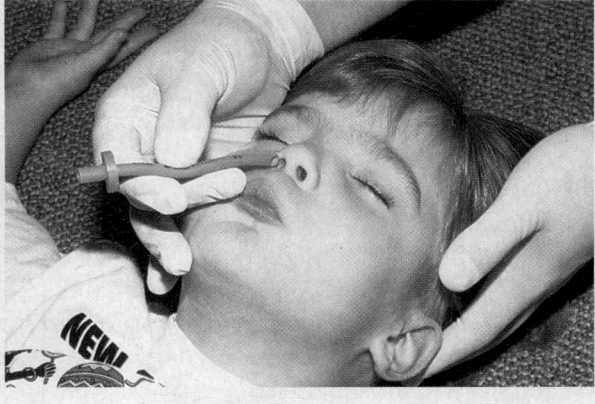

### Step 1

Determine the correct airway size by comparing its diameter to the opening of the nostril (nare). Place the airway next to the pediatric patient's face to confirm correct length. Position the airway.

### Step 2

Lubricate the airway. Insert the tip into the right naris with the bevel pointing toward the septum.

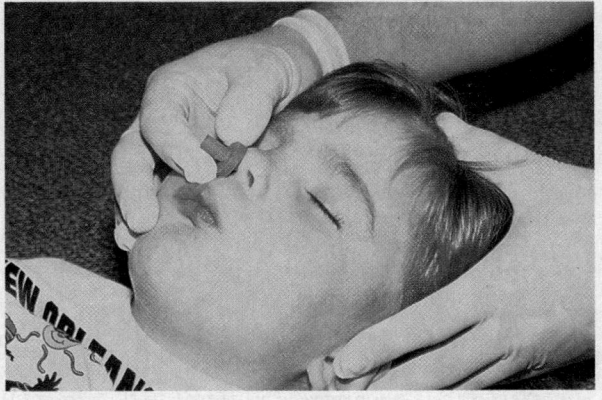

### Step 3

Carefully move the tip forward until the flange rests against the outside of the nostril. Reassess the airway.

airway, the nasopharyngeal airway is used for children who are responsive. In pediatric patients, the nasopharyngeal airway is typically used in association with possible respiratory failure. It is rarely used in infants younger than 1 year.

A nasopharyngeal airway should not be used in pediatric patients with nasal obstruction or head trauma (possible basilar skull fracture) or in children with moderate to severe head trauma because this adjunct could increase intracranial pressure.

Follow the steps in **SKILL DRILL 35-3** to insert a nasopharyngeal airway in a pediatric patient:

1.  Determine the appropriate-size airway. The external diameter of the airway should not be larger than the diameter of the nares, and

there should be no blanching of the nares after insertion.

2. Place the airway next to the child's face to make sure the length is correct. The airway should extend from the tip of the nose to the tragus of the ear. The tragus is the small cartilaginous projection in front of the opening of the ear.

3. Position the patient's airway, using the techniques described earlier for the oropharyngeal airway (**Step 1**).

4. Lubricate the airway with a water-soluble lubricant.

5. Insert the tip into the right naris (nostril opening) with the bevel pointing toward the septum, or central divider in the nose (**Step 2**). The right naris is commonly larger than the left naris in most patients.

6. Carefully move the tip forward, following the roof of the mouth, until the flange rests against the outside of the nostril (**Step 3**). If you are inserting the airway on the left side, insert the tip into the left naris upside down, with the bevel pointing toward the septum. Move the airway forward slowly approximately 1 inch (2.5 cm) until you feel a slight resistance, and then rotate the airway 180°.

7. Reassess the airway after insertion.

As with the oropharyngeal airway, there can be problems with the nasopharyngeal airway. An airway with a small diameter may easily become obstructed by mucus, blood, vomitus, or the soft tissues of the pharynx. If the airway is too long, it may stimulate the vagus nerve and slow the heart rate or enter the esophagus, causing gastric distention. Inserting the airway in responsive patients may cause a spasm of the larynx and result in vomiting. Nasopharyngeal airways should not be used when pediatric patients have facial trauma because the device may tear soft tissues and cause bleeding into the airway.

## Oxygen Delivery Devices

When treating infants and children who require more than the usual 21% oxygen found in room air, you have several options:

- Blow-by technique at 6 L/min provides more than 21% oxygen concentration.
- Nasal cannula at 1 to 6 L/min provides 24% to 44% oxygen concentration.

- Nonrebreathing mask at 10 to 15 L/min provides up to 95% oxygen concentration (unassisted ventilations).
- Bag-mask device (with oxygen reservoir) at 15 L/min provides nearly 100% oxygen concentration (assisted ventilations).

Pediatric patients need enough air to be delivered for adequate gas exchange in the lungs. Therefore, use of a nonrebreathing mask, a nasal cannula, or a simple face mask is indicated only for pediatric patients who have adequate respirations and/or tidal volumes. The tidal volume is the amount of air that is delivered to the lungs and airways in one inhalation. Children with respirations of less than 12 breaths/min or more than 60 breaths/min, an altered level of consciousness, and/or an inadequate tidal volume should receive assisted ventilation with a bag-mask device.

Blow-by oxygen is not as effective as a face mask or nasal cannula for delivering oxygen. In the blow-by technique, an oxygen tube is held near the infant or child's nose and mouth. It is often used after childbirth to deliver a small amount of oxygen to the neonate. On rare occasions when other adjuncts cannot be used or the child will not tolerate any other adjunct, this technique may be necessary. The blow-by technique does not provide a high concentration of oxygen but is better than no oxygen. Take the following steps to administer blow-by oxygen:

1. Place oxygen tubing through a small hole in the bottom of an 8-oz (237-mL) cup (**FIGURE 35-28**). A cup is a familiar object that is less likely to frighten young children than is an oxygen mask.

2. Connect the tubing to an oxygen source set at 6 L/min.

3. Hold the cup approximately 1 to 2 inches (2 to 5 cm) away from the child's nose and mouth.

## Nasal Cannula

Some pediatric patients prefer the nasal cannula, whereas others find it uncomfortable. Take the following steps to apply a nasal cannula:

1. Choose the appropriate-size pediatric nasal cannula. The prongs should not fill the nares entirely (**FIGURE 35-29**). If the nares blanch, select a smaller cannula.

2. Connect the tubing to an oxygen source set at 1 to 6 L/min.

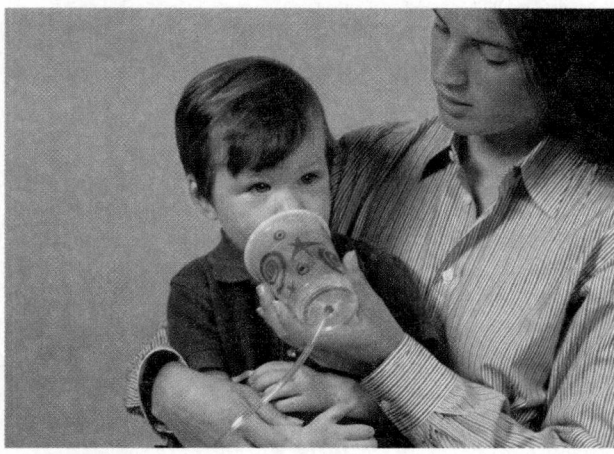

**FIGURE 35-28** The blow-by technique may be less frightening to a child than an oxygen mask. Make a small hole in an 8-oz (237-mL) cup, or use a funnel inserted into the end of the oxygen tubing. Connect tubing to an oxygen source, and hold the cup approximately 1 to 2 inches (2 to 5 cm) from the child's face.

© Jones & Bartlett Learning.

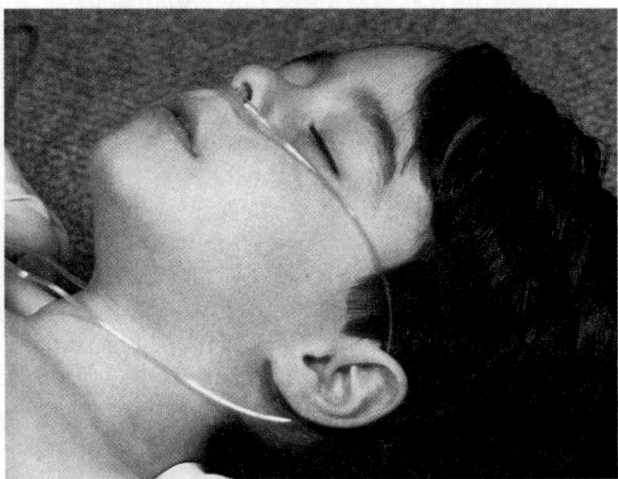

**FIGURE 35-29** The prongs of a pediatric nasal cannula should not fill the nares entirely.

© Jones & Bartlett Learning.

## Nonrebreathing Mask

A nonrebreathing mask delivers up to 95% oxygen to the pediatric patient and allows the pediatric patient to exhale all carbon dioxide without rebreathing it (**FIGURE 35-30**). To apply a nonrebreathing mask:

1. Select the appropriate-size pediatric nonrebreathing mask. The mask should extend from the bridge of the nose to the cleft of the chin.

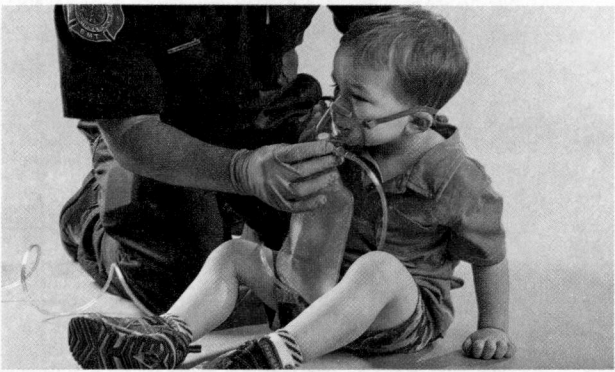

**FIGURE 35-30** A pediatric nonrebreathing mask delivers up to 95% oxygen and allows the patient to exhale carbon dioxide without rebreathing it.

© Jones & Bartlett Learning.

2. Connect the tubing to an oxygen source set at 10 to 15 L/min.
3. Adjust oxygen flow as needed to match the pediatric patient's respiratory rate and depth. The reservoir bag should neither deflate completely nor fill to bulging during the respiratory cycle.

## Bag-Mask Device

Assisting ventilations with a bag-mask device is indicated for pediatric patients who have respirations that are either too slow or too fast to provide an adequate volume of inhaled oxygen, who are unresponsive, or who do not respond in a purposeful way to painful stimuli.

Assist ventilation of an infant or child using a bag-mask device in the following way:

1. Ensure that you have the appropriate-size equipment. The proper-size mask will extend from the bridge of the nose to the cleft of the chin, avoiding compression of the eyes (**FIGURE 35-31**). The mask is transparent, so you can watch for cyanosis and vomiting. In addition, mask volume should be small to decrease dead space and avoid rebreathing; however, the bag should contain at least 450 mL of air. Use an infant bag, not a neonatal bag, for infants younger than 1 year; use a pediatric bag for children older than 1 year. Older children and adolescents may need an adult bag. Make sure that there is no pop-off

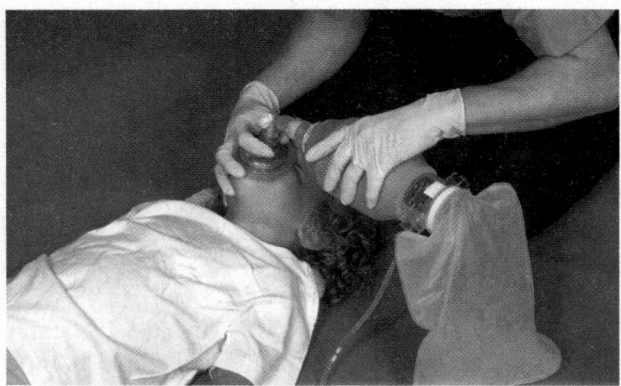

**FIGURE 35-31** Proper mask size for bag-mask ventilation is critical. The mask should extend from the bridge of the nose to the cleft of the chin, avoiding compression of the eyes.

© Jones & Bartlett Learning. Courtesy of MIEMSS.

valve on the bag; if the bag has a pop-off valve, make sure that you can hold it shut as necessary to achieve chest rise. Proper mask size for bag-mask ventilation is critical.

2. Maintain a good seal with the mask on the face.

3. Ventilate at the appropriate rate and volume using a slow, gentle squeeze, not a sharp, quick one. Stop squeezing and begin to release the bag as soon as the chest wall begins to rise, indicating that the lungs are filled to capacity. To keep from ventilating too rapidly, use the phrase "Squeeze, release, release." Say "Squeeze" as you squeeze the bag; when you see the chest start to rise, release pressure on the bag and slowly say "Release, release."

## Words of Wisdom

Remember that one-person bag-mask device ventilation is difficult; the International Liaison Committee on Resuscitation (ILCOR) guidelines do not recommend this method. Errors in technique—such as providing too much volume with each breath, squeezing the bag too forcefully, or ventilating at a rate that is too fast—can result in gastric distention or overinflation of the lung, resulting in a pneumothorax. An inadequate mask seal or improper head position can lead to hypoventilation or hypoxia.

## Special Populations

One of the problems associated with abdominal injuries in children is the presence of air in the stomach. Pediatric patients, especially those who have had a traumatic injury, tend to swallow air. Air in the stomach can cause distention and increase the risk of vomiting. Air can also accumulate in the stomach with artificial ventilation, pushing on the diaphragm and making it harder to ventilate adequately.

## One-Person Bag-Mask Ventilation on a Pediatric Patient

Perform one-person bag-mask ventilation according to these steps (**SKILL DRILL 35-4**):

1. Open the airway, and insert the appropriate airway adjunct (**Step 1**).

2. Hold the mask on the pediatric patient's face with a one-handed head tilt–chin lift maneuver (EC clamp technique). Form a *C* with the thumb and index finger along the mask while the other three fingers form an *E* along the mandible. With infants and toddlers, support the jaw with only your third fingertip. Be careful not to compress the area under the chin because you may push the tongue into the back of the mouth and block the airway. Keep fingers on the mandible.

3. Make sure the mask forms an airtight seal on the face. Maintain the seal while checking that the airway is open (**Step 2**).

4. Squeeze the bag using the correct ventilation rate of 1 breath every 2 to 3 seconds, or 20 to 30 breaths/min.

5. Each ventilation (squeeze of the bag) should last 1 second. Allow adequate time for exhalation (**Step 3**).

6. Assess the effectiveness of ventilation by watching for adequate bilateral rise and fall of the chest (**Step 4**).

## Two-Person Bag-Mask Ventilation on a Pediatric Patient

This procedure is similar to one-person ventilation except that it requires two EMTs—one to hold the mask to the pediatric patient's face and maintain

## Skill Drill 35-4 One-Person Bag-Mask Ventilation on a Pediatric Patient

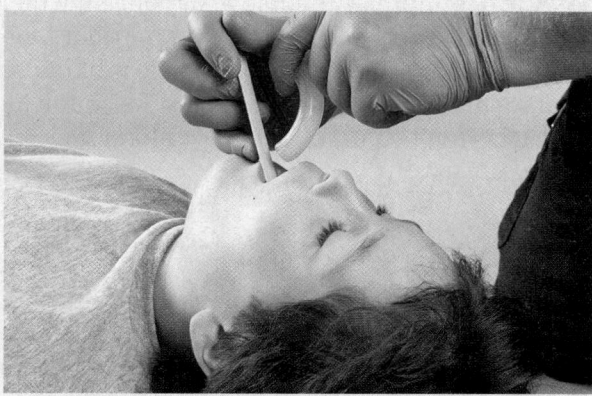

### Step 1

Open the airway and insert the appropriate airway adjunct.

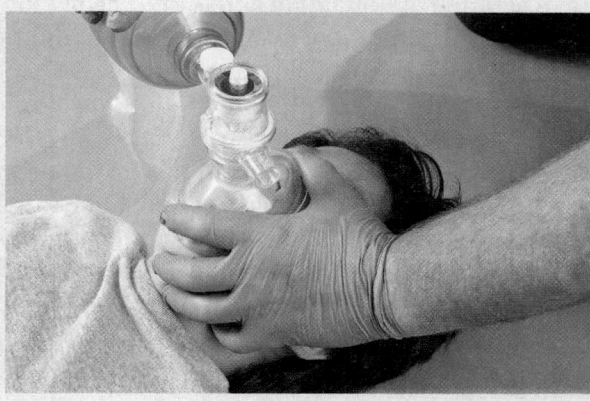

### Step 2

Hold the mask on the pediatric patient's face with a one-handed head tilt–chin lift maneuver (EC clamp method). Ensure a good mask–face seal while maintaining the airway.

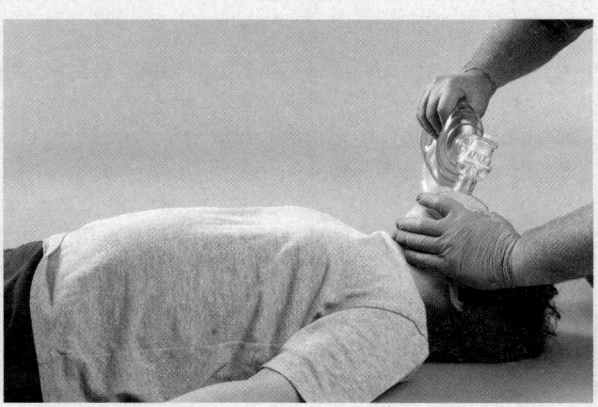

### Step 3

Squeeze the bag using the correct ventilation rate of 1 breath every 2 to 3 seconds, or 20 to 30 breaths/min. Allow adequate time for exhalation.

© Jones & Bartlett Learning.

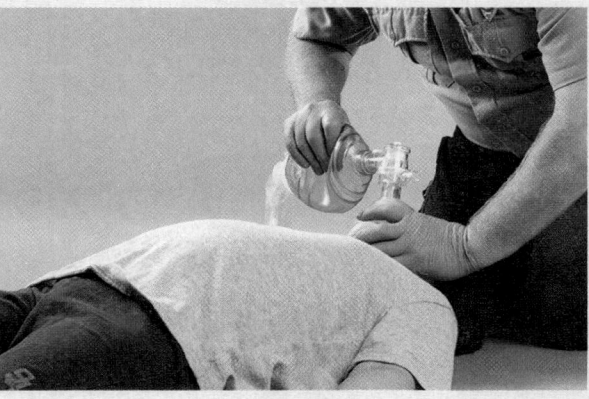

### Step 4

Assess the effectiveness of ventilation by watching bilateral rise and fall of the chest.

the pediatric patient's head position, the other to ventilate the pediatric patient. This technique is usually more effective in maintaining a tight seal, as it provides an open airway due to proper body position.

## Cardiopulmonary Arrest

As previously discussed, cardiac arrest in infants and children is most often associated with respiratory failure and respiratory arrest. Compared with adults, children are affected differently when it comes to decreasing oxygen concentrations. An adult becomes hypoxic and the heart develops a dysrhythmia that leads to sudden cardiac death. This is often in the form of ventricular fibrillation and is the reason that an AED is the treatment of choice. Children, on the other hand, become hypoxic and their hearts slow down, becoming more and more bradycardic. The heart will beat more slowly and more weakly until no pulse is felt. Any child who is breathing very poorly with a slowing heart rate must be ventilated with high concentrations of oxygen early to try to oxygenate the heart before cardiac arrest occurs. Chapter 14, *BLS Resuscitation*, covers providing CPR to pediatric patients in detail.

The pit-crew team approach to resuscitation is equally important in pediatric cardiac arrest. This approach is described in Chapter 14, *BLS Resuscitation*, and Chapter 17, *Cardiovascular Emergencies*. The focus should not be on scoop and run, but rather on effective CPR, early use of an AED, and then transport in an orderly manner to the closest ED or to meet the ALS intercept.

## Circulation Emergencies and Management

The pediatric cardiovascular system is not all that different from that of an adult. Although pediatric patients have a larger proportional amount of circulating blood volume than adults, they are more dependent on the actual cardiac output of the heart (amount of blood being pumped out of the heart in 1 minute). A pediatric patient may be in a state of shock while displaying a normal blood pressure. Infants and children have less blood circulating in their bodies than adults do, so the loss of even a small volume of fluid or blood may lead to shock.

## Shock

Shock is a condition that develops when the circulatory system is unable to deliver sufficient blood to the organs of the body. Chapter 13, *Shock*, covers this condition in greater detail. This results in organ failure and eventually cardiopulmonary arrest. The early stage of shock, while the body can still compensate for blood loss, is called compensated shock. The late stage, when blood pressure is falling, is called decompensated shock.

In pediatric patients, the most common causes include the following:

- Traumatic injury with blood loss (especially abdominal)
- Dehydration from diarrhea and vomiting
- Severe infection
- Neurologic injury, such as severe head trauma

## YOU are the Provider

The closest ALS ambulance is 8 miles across town in heavy traffic and your estimated transport time is about 5 minutes, so you make the decision to continue transport. Your partner notifies the hospital and informs them of your impending arrival. Following additional treatment, you reassess the child's condition.

| Recording Time: 18 Minutes | |
| --- | --- |
| **Level of consciousness** | Eyes are open; still appears listless |
| **Respirations** | 20 breaths/min and shallow (baseline); assisted ventilations |
| **Pulse** | 110 beats/min; stronger |
| **Skin** | Cyanosis is resolving; capillary refill time 2 seconds |
| **Blood pressure** | 84/54 mm Hg |
| **SpO₂** | 96% (on oxygen) |

**9.** Are you providing adequate ventilations? How can you tell?

**10.** Why is it especially important to avoid hyperventilating infants and children?

- A severe allergic reaction to an allergen (anaphylaxis), such as an insect bite or food allergy
- Diseases of the heart
- A collapsed lung (tension pneumothorax)
- Blood or fluid around the heart (cardiac tamponade or pericarditis)

Children respond differently than adults to fluid loss. They may respond by increasing their heart rate, increasing respirations, and showing signs of pale skin (pallor) or blue skin (cyanosis).

Signs of shock in infants and children are as follows:

- Tachycardia
- Poor capillary refill time (>2 seconds)
- Mental status changes

Begin treating shock by assessing the patient for the XABCs, intervening immediately as required; do not wait until you have performed the complete assessment to take action. If there is an obvious life-threatening external hemorrhage, the order becomes XCAB, because bleeding control is the most critical step. If cardiac arrest is suspected, the order also becomes XCAB because chest compressions are essential. Pediatric patients in shock often have increased respirations but do not demonstrate a fall in blood pressure until shock is severe.

When you assess circulation, pay particular attention to the following:

- **Pulse.** Assess both the rate and the quality of the pulse. A weak, thready pulse is a sign that there is a problem. The appropriate rate depends on age; generally, except in the case of a newborn, anything over 160 beats/min suggests shock.
- **Skin signs.** Assess the temperature and moisture of the hands and feet. How does this compare with the temperature of the skin on the trunk of the body? Is the skin dry and warm, or cold and clammy?
- **Capillary refill time.** Squeeze a finger or toe for several seconds until the skin blanches, and then release it. Does the fingertip return to its normal color within 2 seconds, or is it delayed?
- **Color.** Assess the patient's skin color. Is it pink, pale, ashen, or blue? This sign is less valuable in children with dark skin pigmentation. Reliance on other signs is necessary.

- **Changes.** Changes in pulse rate, color, skin signs, and capillary refill time are all important clues suggesting shock.

Blood pressure is the most difficult vital sign to measure in pediatric patients. The cuff must be the proper size: two-thirds the length of the upper arm. The value for normal blood pressure is also age-specific. Remember that blood pressure may be normal with compensated shock. Low blood pressure is a sign of decompensated shock, requiring care from an ALS team and rapid transport.

Part of your assessment should also include talking with the parents or caregivers to determine when the signs and symptoms first appeared and whether any of the following has occurred:

- Decrease in urine output (with infants, are there fewer than 6 to 10 wet diapers per day?)
- Absence of tears, even when the child is crying
- A sunken or depressed fontanelle (infant patient)
- Changes in level of consciousness and behavior

Limit your management to these simple interventions. Do not waste time performing field procedures. Ensure that the airway is open, prepare for artificial ventilation, control bleeding, and give supplemental oxygen by mask or blow-by method as tolerated. Continue to monitor the airway and breathing. Place the child in a position of comfort. Keep the child warm with blankets and by turning up the heat in the patient compartment. Provide rapid transport to the nearest appropriate facility and continue monitoring vital signs en route. Call for ALS backup as needed. Allow a parent or caregiver to accompany the child whenever possible.

## Anaphylaxis

Anaphylaxis, also called anaphylactic shock, is a life-threatening allergic reaction that involves a generalized, multisystem response to an antigen (foreign substance). Anaphylaxis is characterized by airway swelling and the dilation of blood vessels. Common causes include insect bites or stings, medications, and food.

A pediatric patient in anaphylactic shock will have hypoperfusion as well as additional signs such as stridor and/or wheezing, with increased work of breathing. The pediatric patient will also have an altered appearance with restlessness, agitation, and sometimes a sense of impending doom. Hives, an intensely itchy skin rash, are usually present.

Maintain the airway and administer oxygen via a route that is tolerated. Increased agitation and crying, combined with an increased work of breathing, may lead to increased bronchoconstriction. Based on local protocol, assist the parent or caregiver with administering a prescribed epinephrine auto-injector, if available. The administration of epinephrine is the highest priority in infants and children with signs and symptoms of anaphylaxis. Administration of epinephrine is discussed in Chapter 20, *Endocrine and Hematologic Emergencies*. The pediatric epinephrine auto-injector (EpiPen Jr) is supplied in a dose of 0.15 mg and is given intramuscularly in the lateral thigh. Provide rapid transport to the hospital.

## Bleeding Disorders

Hemophilia is a congenital condition in which the patient lacks one or more of the normal clotting factors of blood. There are several forms of hemophilia, most of which are hereditary and some of which are severe. Hemophilia is predominantly found in the male population. Sometimes bleeding may occur spontaneously. Because the blood of a child with hemophilia does not clot properly, all injuries, no matter how minor, are potentially serious. Transport a pediatric patient with hemophilia immediately, and do not delay tourniquet application for life-threatening hemorrhage.

## Neurologic Emergencies and Management

There are several causes of altered mental status in children. Some of the most common causes are hypoglycemia, hypoxia, seizure, and drug or alcohol ingestion. The parent or caregiver is an important resource for you when you are gathering information regarding the baseline neurologic status of the pediatric patient. A pediatric patient with altered mental status may appear sleepy, lethargic, combative, or even unresponsive to tactile stimulus. Be diligent about assessing and managing the airway because children may be susceptible to airway obstructions from their large tongues.

## Altered Mental Status

An altered mental status is an abnormal neurologic state in which the pediatric patient is less alert and interactive than is age appropriate. Sometimes, the concern of the parent or caregiver is vague, stating that the child is "not acting right." Therefore, it is key that you understand normal developmental or age-related changes in behavior and listen carefully to the parent's or caregiver's opinion about a child's baseline behavior. For instance, a 4-month-old infant should be active, have the ability to track a toy or light with his or her eyes, smile, and make eye contact. As discussed at the beginning of this chapter, if the child is not behaving in a developmentally appropriate manner, then this could indicate an altered mental status.

The mnemonic AEIOU-TIPS reflects the major causes of altered mental status (**TABLE 35-11**).

The signs and symptoms of altered mental status vary widely, from simple confusion to coma. Management of altered mental status focuses on the ABCs and transport. If the child's level of consciousness is low, then the patient may not be able to protect his or her airway. Ensure a patent airway and adequate breathing through a nonrebreathing mask or a bag-mask device. Pediatric patients with an altered level of consciousness may have inadequate breathing despite spontaneous respiratory effort, based on an inadequate respiratory rate or inadequate tidal volume. Transport to the hospital.

## Seizures

A seizure is the result of disorganized electrical activity in the brain, causes of which are listed in

| **TABLE 35-11** Mnemonic to Assess Causes of Altered Mental Status |
| --- |
| **A** Alcohol |
| **E** Epilepsy, endocrine, electrolytes |
| **I** Insulin |
| **O** Opiates and other drugs |
| **U** Uremia (kidney failure) |
| **T** Trauma, temperature |
| **I** Infection |
| **P** Poisoning, psychogenic causes |
| **S** Shock, stroke, seizure, syncope, space-occupying lesion, subarachnoid hemorrhage |

© Jones & Bartlett Learning.

TABLE 35-12. It can be frightening to witness a seizure in a child. Therefore, it is important to reassure the family and to approach assessment and management in a calm, step-by-step manner.

Seizures in children may manifest in a wide variety of ways, depending on the age of the child. Seizures in infants can be subtle, consisting only of an abnormal gaze, sucking motions, or "bicycling" motions. In older children, seizures are more obvious and typically consist of repetitive muscle contractions and unresponsiveness. Once a seizure has stopped, the patient's muscles relax, becoming almost flaccid (floppy), and the breathing becomes labored (fast and deep). This is the postictal state. The longer and more intense a seizure is, the longer it will take for the imbalance to correct itself. Likewise, longer and more severe seizures will result in longer postictal unresponsiveness and confusion. Once the child regains a normal level of consciousness, the postictal state is over.

Seizures that continue every few minutes without regaining consciousness or last longer than 30 minutes are referred to as status epilepticus. Recurring or prolonged seizures should be considered potentially life-threatening situations in which children need emergency medical care. If the child does not regain consciousness or continues to seize, protect the the child from harming himself or herself and call for ALS backup. These children need advanced airway management and medication to stop the seizure.

Securing and protecting the airway are your priorities. Position the head to open the airway.

Consider inserting a nasopharyngeal airway. Clear the mouth with suction. Consider placing the child in the recovery position if the child is actively vomiting and suction is inadequate to control the airway (**FIGURE 35-32**). Provide 100% oxygen by nonrebreathing mask or blow-by method. If there are no signs of improvement, begin bag-mask ventilation with appropriate-size equipment with supplemental oxygen. Some parents or caregivers will have given the child a rectal dose of diazepam (Diastat) to stop the seizure prior to your arrival. Monitor breathing and level of consciousness carefully in these patients. Transport the child to the appropriate facility.

Pediatric seizures caused by fever (febrile seizures) are discussed later in the chapter.

## Meningitis

**Meningitis** is an inflammation of the tissues called the meninges, which cover the spinal cord and brain. It is caused by an infection by bacteria, viruses, fungi, or parasites. If left untreated, meningitis can lead to permanent brain damage or death. You must be able to recognize a pediatric patient who may have meningitis.

Meningitis can occur in both children and adults, but some pediatric patients are at greater risk than others, as follows:

- Males
- Newborn infants
- Children with compromised immune systems (such as HIV/AIDS or cancer)

| TABLE 35-12 Common Causes of Seizures |
| --- |
| • Child abuse (with head trauma) |
| • Electrolyte imbalance |
| • Fever |
| • Hypoglycemia (low blood glucose level) |
| • Infection |
| • Ingestion |
| • Lack of oxygen |
| • Medications |
| • Poisoning |
| • Seizure disorder |
| • Recreational drug use |
| • Head trauma |
| • No cause can be found |

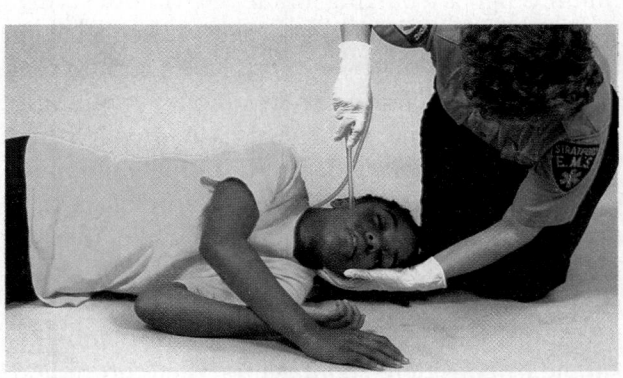

**FIGURE 35-32** Position the head to open the airway, and clear the airway with suction. If suction is inadequate or the patient is vomiting, consider placing the patient in the recovery position.

- Children who have any history of brain, spinal cord, or back surgery
- Children who have had head trauma
- Children with shunts, pins, or other foreign bodies within their brain or spinal cord

At especially high risk are children with a ventriculoperitoneal (VP) shunt. VP shunts drain excess fluids from around the brain into the abdomen. These patients are children with special needs who have tubing that can usually be seen and felt just under the scalp.

The signs and symptoms of meningitis vary, depending on the age of the patient. Fever and altered level of consciousness are common symptoms of meningitis in patients of all ages. Changes in the level of consciousness can range from a mild or severe headache to confusion, lethargy, and/or an inability to understand commands or interact appropriately. The child may also experience a seizure, which may be the first sign of meningitis. Infants younger than 2 to 3 months can have apnea, cyanosis, fever, a distinct high-pitched cry, or hypothermia.

In describing children with meningitis, physicians often use "meningeal irritation" or "meningeal signs" to describe pain that accompanies movement. Bending the neck forward or back increases the tension within the spinal canal and stretches the meninges, causing a great deal of pain. This results in the characteristic stiff neck of children with meningitis, who will often refuse to move their neck, lift their legs, or curl into a *C* position, even if coached to do so. One sign of meningitis in an infant is increasing irritability, especially when being handled. Another sign is a bulging fontanelle without crying.

One form of meningitis deserves special attention. *Neisseria meningitidis* is a bacterium that causes a rapid onset of meningitis symptoms, often leading to shock and death. Children infected with *N meningitidis* typically have small, pinpoint, cherry-red spots or a larger purple or black rash (**FIGURE 35-33**). This rash may be on part of the face or body. These children are at serious risk of sepsis, shock, and death.

All pediatric patients with possible meningitis should be considered contagious. Therefore, follow standard precautions whenever you suspect meningitis and follow up with the hospital to learn the patient's final diagnosis. If you have been exposed to saliva and respiratory secretions from a child infected with *N meningitidis*, you should receive

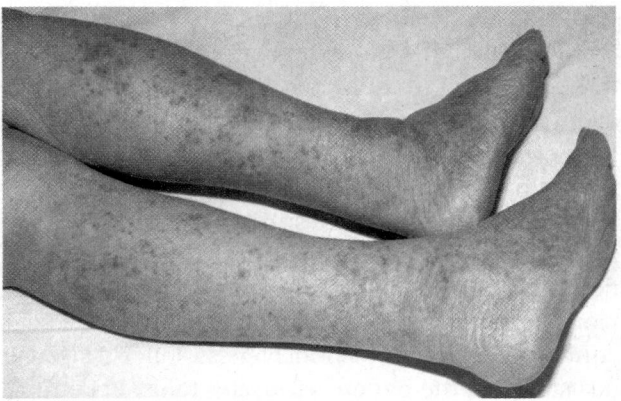

**FIGURE 35-33** Children infected with *Neisseria meningitidis* typically have small, pinpoint, cherry-red spots or a larger purple or black rash.

© Mediscan/Alamy Stock Photo.

antibiotics to protect yourself and others from the bacteria. This is particularly true if you managed the patient's airway. If you were not in close contact with the child or his or her respiratory secretions, you do not need treatment.

Provide these patients with supplemental oxygen and assist with ventilations if needed. Reassess the child's vital signs frequently as you transport the patient to the highest level of service available.

## Gastrointestinal Emergencies and Management

As with any injury or complaint in the abdominal region, the signs and symptoms of a gastrointestinal emergency in a pediatric patient may be vague in nature. The abdominal wall muscles are not as developed, which leaves this region more susceptible to injury. Pediatric patients may not be able to pinpoint the exact site where the pain or discomfort originates, but will have complaints of diffuse tenderness. Never take a complaint of abdominal pain and discomfort lightly because a large amount of bleeding may occur within the abdominal cavity without any outward signs of shock. Remember that liver and splenic injuries are common among this age group and may result in life-threatening emergencies. The patient needs to be monitored for signs and symptoms of shock, which include an altered mental status; pale, cool skin; tachypnea; tachycardia; and bradycardia (late sign).

Complaints of gastrointestinal origin are common in the pediatric population. A common source of gastrointestinal upset is the ingestion of certain foods or unknown substances, such as milk or ice cream (lactose intolerance). In most cases, you will be faced with a pediatric patient who is experiencing abdominal discomfort with nausea, vomiting, and/or diarrhea. This can become a concern because both vomiting and diarrhea can cause dehydration in children.

Appendicitis is also common in pediatric patients and, if untreated, can lead to peritonitis (inflammation of the peritoneum, which lines the abdominal cavity) or shock. Appendicitis will typically present with a fever and pain on palpation of the right lower abdominal quadrant. Rebound tenderness is a common sign associated with appendicitis. Remember that constipation also can be a cause of abdominal pain in children. If you suspect appendicitis, promptly transport the child to the hospital for further evaluation.

Because children are sensitive to fluid loss, obtain a thorough history from the parent or primary caregiver. Specifically, ask questions such as the following:

- How many wet diapers has your child had today?
- Is your child tolerating liquids and is he or she able to keep them down?
- How many times has your child had diarrhea and for how long?
- Are tears present when your child cries?

These questions can help to determine how dehydrated the patient may be. If the child is dehydrated, transport to the hospital for further care.

## Poisoning Emergencies and Management

Poisoning is common among children, and the most common sources of poisoning in children are listed in **TABLE 35-13**. It can occur by ingesting, inhaling, injecting, or absorbing a toxic substance.

The signs and symptoms of poisoning vary widely, depending on the substance and the age and weight of the pediatric patient. The child may appear normal at first, even in serious cases, or he or she may be confused, sleepy, or unconscious. With some substances, one pill may be enough to cause death in a small child.

Infants may be poisoned as a result of being fed a harmful substance by a sibling, parent, or caregiver, or as a result of child abuse. Infants can be exposed to drugs and poisons left on floors and carpeting. They can also be exposed in a setting in which harmful drugs are being smoked. Toddlers are curious and often ingest poisons when they find them in the home or garage (**FIGURE 35-34**). For example, some people store petroleum products in

| **TABLE 35-13** Common Sources of Poisoning in Children |
| --- |
| • Alcohol |
| • Aspirin and acetaminophen |
| • Cosmetics |
| • Household cleaning products (such as bleach and furniture polish) |
| • Houseplants |
| • Iron (prenatal vitamins) |
| • Prescription medications |
| • Illicit (street) drugs (such as crack, cocaine, or PCP) |
| • Vitamins |

© Jones & Bartlett Learning.

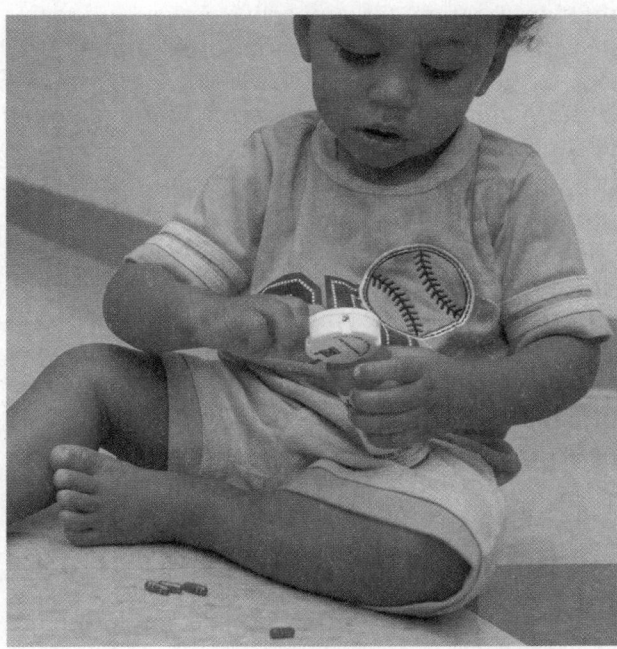

**FIGURE 35-34** A curious child will try to taste or swallow almost any substance. A common victim of accidental ingestion of dangerous compounds is the unwatched toddler.

© Jones & Bartlett Learning.

soda bottles. Toddlers may believe the substance to be soda. Adolescents are more likely to have ingested alcohol and street drugs while partying or during a suicide attempt.

After you have completed your primary assessment, ask the parent or caregiver the following questions:

- What is the substance or substances involved?
- Approximately how much of the substance was ingested or involved in the exposure (eg, number of pills, amount of liquid)?
- What time did the incident occur?
- Are there any changes in behavior or level of consciousness?
- Was there any choking or coughing after the exposure? (These can be signs of airway involvement.)

Contact the national Poison Control hotline for assistance in identifying poisons at 1-800-222-1222. This free service is available 24 hours per day, 7 days per week.

To treat a pediatric patient exposed to a poisonous substance, first perform an external decontamination. Remove tablets or fragments from the patient's mouth, and wash or brush poison from the skin. Treatment is supportive: Assess and maintain the child's ABCs and monitor breathing. Provide oxygen and perform ventilations if necessary. If the patient demonstrates signs and symptoms of shock, position the child supine, keep the child warm, and transport promptly to the nearest appropriate hospital.

In some cases, you will give activated charcoal to pediatric patients who have ingested poison, if approved by medical control or local protocol. Activated charcoal is not indicated for children who have ingested an acid, an alkali, or a petroleum product; who have a decreased level of consciousness and cannot protect their airway; or who are unable to swallow. If local protocol permits, you will likely carry plastic bottles of premixed suspension, each containing up to 50 g of activated charcoal. Some common trade names for the suspension form are InstaChar, Actidose, and LiquiChar. The usual dose for a child is 1 g of activated charcoal per kilogram of body weight. The usual pediatric dose is 12.5 to 25 g. Chapter 22, *Toxicology*, discusses the administration of activated charcoal in detail.

> **Words of Wisdom**
>
> When you respond to a poisoning, remember to remain calm and control the scene. Poisonings can be emotional for the parents or caregivers involved because of the potential for self-blame.

## Dehydration Emergencies and Management

Dehydration occurs when fluid losses are greater than fluid intake. The most common cause of dehydration in pediatric patients is vomiting and diarrhea. If left untreated, dehydration can lead to shock and eventually death. Infants and children are at greater risk than adults for dehydration because their fluid reserves are smaller than those in adults. Life-threatening dehydration can overcome an infant in a matter of hours.

Dehydration can be mild, moderate, or severe. The severity of the dehydration can be gauged by looking at several clues (**TABLE 35-14**). For example, an infant with mild dehydration may have dry lips and gums, decreased saliva, and fewer wet diapers throughout the day. As the dehydration grows more severe, the lips and gums may become very dry, the eyes may look sunken, and the infant may be sleepy and/or irritable, refusing bottles. The skin may be loose and have no elasticity; this is called poor skin turgor (**FIGURE 35-35**). Also, infants may have sunken fontanelles.

Young children can compensate for fluid losses by decreasing blood flow to the extremities and directing blood flow to vital organs such as the brain and heart. Children who are moderately to severely dehydrated may have mottled, cool, clammy skin and delayed capillary response time. Respirations will usually be increased. Be aware that blood pressure may remain within a normal range while the pediatric patient is in shock, because the compensatory mechanisms are still in place.

Emergency medical care should include assessing the ABCs and obtaining baseline vital signs. However, if the dehydration is severe, ALS backup may be necessary so that intravenous (IV) access can be obtained and rehydration can begin. All pediatric patients with signs and symptoms of moderate to severe dehydration should be transported to the ED for further evaluation and treatment.

**TABLE 35-14** Vital Signs and Symptoms of Dehydration

|  | Mild Dehydration | Moderate Dehydration | Severe Dehydration |
|---|---|---|---|
| **Pulse** | Normal | Increased | Increased; >160 beats/min is sign of impending shock in pediatric patients, except newborns |
| **Level of activity** | Normal or slowed | Slowed | Variable, weak to unresponsive |
| **Urine output** | Decreased | Decreased | No output |
| **Skin** | Normal | Cool, mottled; poor turgor | Cool, clammy; poor turgor; delayed capillary refill time |
| **Mouth** | Decreased saliva | Dry mucous membranes | Dry mucous membranes |
| **Eyes** | Normal | No tears | Sunken eyes |
| **Anterior fontanelle** | Normal to sunken | Sunken | Very sunken |
| **Level of consciousness** | Normal | Altered | Altered; lethargic |
| **Blood pressure** | Normal | Normal | Normal to low |

© Jones & Bartlett Learning.

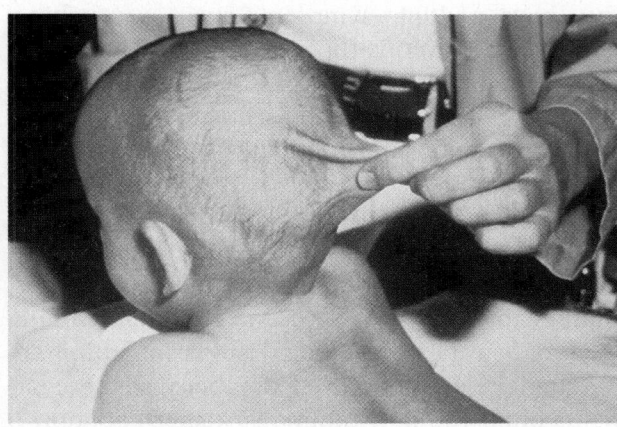

**FIGURE 35-35** An infant with dehydration may exhibit "tenting" or poor skin turgor.

Courtesy of Ronald Dieckmann, MD.

# Fever Emergencies and Management

Fever is a common reason why parents or caregivers call 9-1-1. Simply defined, a fever is an increase in body temperature, usually in response to an infection. Body temperatures of 100.4°F (38°C) or higher are considered abnormal. A fever may have many causes and is rarely life threatening. However, do not underestimate the potential seriousness of a fever that occurs in conjunction with a rash, which is a sign of serious illness, such as meningitis. Common causes of a fever in pediatric patients include the following:

- Infection, such as pneumonia, meningitis, or urinary tract infection
- Status epilepticus
- Cancer
- Drug ingestion (aspirin)
- Arthritis and systemic lupus erythematosus (rash across nose)
- High environmental temperature

Fever is the result of an internal body mechanism in which heat generation is increased and heat loss is decreased. Note that there are other conditions in which the core body temperature also increases. Hyperthermia differs from fever in that it is an increase in body temperature caused by an inability of the body to cool itself. Hyperthermia is typically seen in warm environments, such as a closed vehicle on a hot day.

An accurate body temperature is a valuable vital sign for pediatric patients. A rectal temperature is the most accurate for infants to toddlers. Older children will be able to follow directions if placing a thermometer under the tongue or under the arm.

A fever can have several causes, such as a viral or a bacterial infection. Depending on the source of infection, the pediatric patient may have additional signs, including respiratory distress, shock, stiff neck, rash, skin that is hot to the touch, flushed cheeks, seizures, and bulging fontanelles in an infant. Assess the patient for other signs and symptoms such as nausea, vomiting, diarrhea, decreased feedings, and headache. A fever that is accompanied by a stiff neck, sensitivity to light, and a rash may be an indication that the patient has either bacterial or viral meningitis.

A child with a fever may require only minimal interventions in the field. Provide rapid transport and manage the patient's ABCs. Follow standard precautions if you suspect that the patient may have a communicable disease such as meningitis.

### Febrile Seizures

Febrile seizures are common in children between the ages of 6 months and 6 years. Most pediatric seizures are the result of fever alone, which is why they are called febrile seizures.

These seizures typically occur on the first day of a febrile illness, are characterized by **generalized (tonic-clonic) seizure** activity, and last less than 15 minutes with a short postictal phase or none at all. They may be a sign of a more serious problem, such as meningitis. Obtain a history from the parent or caregiver because these children may have had a febrile seizure in the past.

If you are called to care for a child who has had a febrile seizure, you often will find that the pediatric patient is awake, alert, and fully interactive when you arrive. Keep in mind that a persistent fever can lead to another seizure. Carefully assess the ABCs, begin cooling measures with tepid (not cold) water, and provide prompt transport. All pediatric patients with febrile seizures need to be seen in the hospital setting.

### Drowning Emergencies and Management

In drowning emergencies, you must always ensure your own safety when rescuing the patient from the water. Do not become a victim yourself!

According to the Centers for Disease Control and Prevention (CDC), drowning is the second most common cause of unintentional death among children aged 1 to 4 years in the United States. At this age, children often fall into swimming pools and lakes, but many drown in bathtubs and even puddles or buckets of water. Older adolescents drown when swimming or boating; alcohol is frequently a factor.

The principal condition that results from drowning is lack of oxygen. Drowning is discussed in Chapter 33, *Environmental Emergencies*. Even a few minutes (or less) without oxygen affects the heart, lungs, and brain, causing life-threatening problems such as cardiac arrest, respiratory failure, and coma. Submersion in icy water can lead to hypothermia. Although it is possible for victims of submersion hypothermia to survive long periods in cardiac arrest, most people in this situation die. Diving into the water, of course, increases the risk of neck and spinal cord injuries.

Signs and symptoms of a drowning patient will vary based on the type and length of submersion. A pediatric patient involved in a drowning emergency may have multiple symptoms such as coughing; choking; airway obstruction; difficulty breathing; altered mental status; seizure activity; unresponsiveness; fast, slow, or no pulse noted; pale, cyanotic skin; and vomiting or abdominal distention from ingestion of fluids.

Request ALS support for these calls whenever feasible. Once the child has been successfully removed from the water, assess and manage the ABCs. Administer oxygen at 100% via a nonrebreathing mask or bag-mask device if assisted ventilations are required. Be prepared to suction because these patients often vomit. If trauma is suspected, apply a

### Words of Wisdom

Swimming pool and water hazards are major contributors to pediatric injury and death. Pool safety begins with educating children and parents or caregivers on the risks of playing around a pool. All swimming pools should be surrounded by a fence that is at least 6 feet (2 m) high, with slats no more than 3 inches (8 cm) apart. Additional precautions include pool covers and alarm systems. Children should also take water safety and swim lessons to help ensure their safety around pools and other bodies of water.

cervical collar and place the pediatric patient on a backboard. Pad all open spaces under the pediatric patient before securing the patient onto the backboard. If the pediatric patient is unresponsive and in cardiopulmonary arrest, perform CPR.

## Pediatric Trauma Emergencies and Management

According to the CDC, unintentional injuries are the number one killer of children in the United States. As an EMT, you will frequently treat injured children; therefore, you must have a thorough understanding of how trauma affects them. The quality of care in the first few minutes after a child has been injured can have an enormous effect on that child's chances for complete recovery.

The muscles and bones of children continue to grow well into adolescence. For this reason, coupled with their risk-taking approach to activities, adolescents are susceptible to fractures of the extremities. The younger the child, the more flexible the bone structures are to trauma. If a pediatric patient is unable to place weight on an extremity or favors an extremity, suspect injury until proven otherwise. Sprains are less common in this age group because the ligaments are more developed than the growth plates of the bones.

A fracture of the femur is rare in children, but when it does occur, it can be a source of major blood loss. Older children and adolescents are susceptible to long bone fractures (femur and humerus) because they tend to take more risks during physical activities. The goal for care and treatment in this circumstance is to immobilize the injured extremity and to provide transport to an appropriate facility.

### Physical Differences

As discussed, children are smaller than adults; therefore, when they are hurt in the same type of crash

as an adult, the location of their injuries may differ from those in an adult. For example, the bumper of a motor vehicle will strike an adult pedestrian in the lower leg, whereas that same bumper will strike a child in the pelvis. In a crash involving sudden deceleration, an adult might injure a ligament in the knee; in that same crash, a child might injure the bones in the leg.

Children's bones and soft tissues are less well developed than those of adults; therefore, the force of an injury affects these structures somewhat differently than it does in an adult. Because a child's head is proportionately larger than that of an adult, it exerts greater stress on the neck structures during a deceleration injury. Because of these anatomic differences, always carefully assess children for head and neck injuries.

### Psychological Differences

Children are also less mature psychologically than adults; therefore, they are often injured because of their undeveloped judgment and their lack of experience. For example, children are more likely than adults to cross the street without looking for oncoming traffic. As a result, children are more likely than adults to be struck by motor vehicles. Children and adolescents are also more likely to sustain injuries from diving into shallow water because they forget to check the depth of the water before they dive. In such situations, always assume that the child has serious head and neck injuries.

### Injury Patterns

Although you are not responsible for diagnosing injuries in children, your ability to recognize and report serious injuries will provide critical information to hospital staff. For this reason, it is important for you to understand the special physical and psychological characteristics of children and what makes them more likely to sustain certain kinds of injuries.

### Vehicle Collisions

Children playing or riding a bicycle can dart out in front of motor vehicles without looking. In such a situation, the driver may have very little time to slow down or stop. The area of greatest injury varies, depending on the size of the child and the height of the bumper at the time of impact. When vehicles slow down at the moment of impact, the bumper dips slightly, causing the point of impact with the child to be lowered. The exact area that is struck depends on the child's height and the final position of the bumper at the time of impact. Children who are injured in these situations often sustain high-energy injuries to the head, spine, abdomen, pelvis, or legs. In addition to differences in size and anatomy, children will often turn toward an oncoming vehicle when they see it approaching and, therefore, sustain different injuries than an adult who turns away.

## Sports Activities

Children, especially those who are older or adolescents, are often injured in organized sports activities. Head and neck injuries can occur after high-speed collisions in contact sports such as football, wrestling, ice hockey, field hockey, soccer, or lacrosse. Remember to immobilize the cervical spine when caring for children with sports-related injuries when indicated. Familiarize yourself with local protocols related to helmet removal. Guidelines are presented in Chapter 29, *Head and Spine Injuries.*

## Injuries to Specific Body Systems
### Head Injuries

Head injuries are common in children. This is because the size of a child's head, in relation to the body, is larger than that of an adult. An infant also has a softer, thinner skull, which may result in injury to the underlying brain tissues. The scalp and facial vessels can bleed easily and may cause significant blood loss if the bleeding is not controlled. The signs and symptoms of head injury in a child are similar to those in an adult, but there are some important differences. Nausea and vomiting are common signs and symptoms of head injury in children; however, it is easy to mistake these for an abdominal injury or illness. You should suspect a serious head injury in any child who experiences nausea and vomiting after a traumatic event. Pediatric patients are managed in the same manner as adults. Chapter 29, *Head and Spine Injuries,* discusses head injuries in detail.

### Immobilization

Spinal immobilization is recommended for all children who have possible head or spinal injuries after a traumatic event. Follow these steps (**SKILL DRILL 35-5**):

1. Maintain the child's head in a neutral position by placing a towel under the shoulders and torso (**Step 1**).
2. Place an appropriate-size cervical collar on the pediatric patient (**Step 2**).
3. Carefully log roll the child onto the short backboard or pediatric immobilization device (**Step 3**).
4. Secure the pediatric patient's torso to the short backboard or pediatric immobilization device first (**Step 4**).
5. Secure the child's head to the short backboard or pediatric immobilization device (**Step 5**).
6. Complete immobilization by ensuring that the child is strapped in properly (**Step 6**).

Immobilization can be difficult to perform because of the child's body proportions. Young children require padding under the torso to maintain a neutral position. Beginning at ages 8 to 10 years, children no longer require padding underneath the torso to create a neutral position. Instead, they can simply lie supine on the backboard. However, another complication may occur if a child is immobilized on an adult-size backboard. A child's body is narrower than an adult's; therefore, padding will be required along the sides of the adult-size backboard so that the child can be effectively secured.

Many infants and children will be in a car seat when you approach them. The patient must be removed to a short backboard or pediatric immobilization device prior to transport. Follow these steps to immobilize a patient in a car seat (**SKILL DRILL 35-6**):

1. Carefully stabilize the patient's head in a neutral position (**Step 1**).
2. Lay the seat down into a reclined position on a hard surface. Position a short backboard or pediatric immobilization device between the patient and the surface on which the patient is resting (**Step 2**).
3. Carefully slide the patient into position on the short backboard or pediatric immobilization device (**Step 3**).

## Skill Drill 35-5 Immobilizing a Pediatric Patient

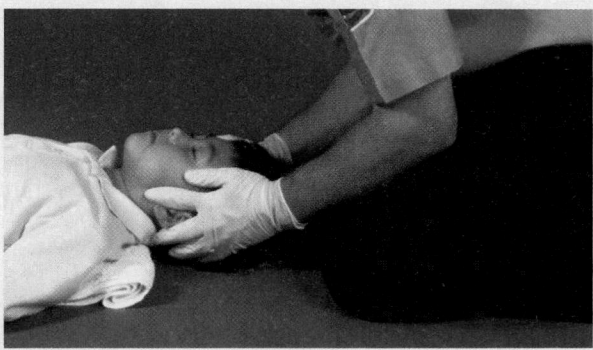

### Step 1

Use a towel under the back, from the shoulders to the hips, to maintain the head in a neutral position.

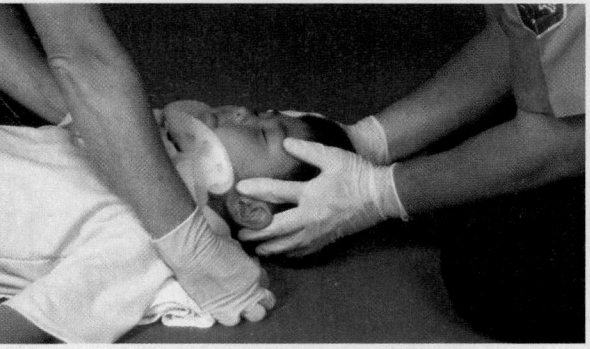

### Step 2

Apply an appropriate-size cervical collar.

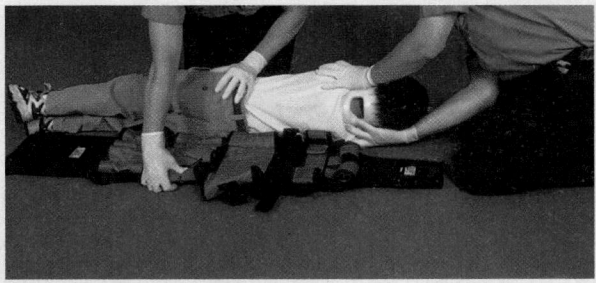

### Step 3

Log roll the child onto the short backboard or pediatric immobilization device.

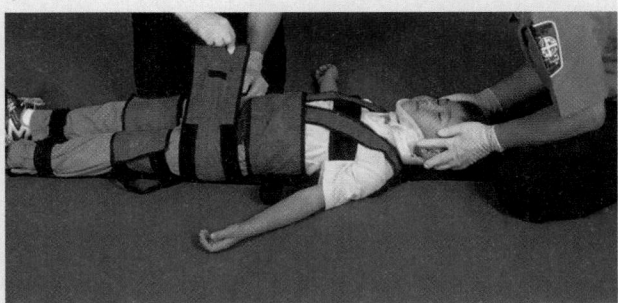

### Step 4

Secure the torso first.

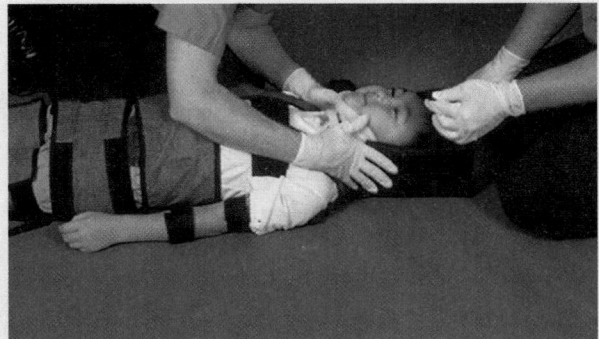

### Step 5

Secure the head.

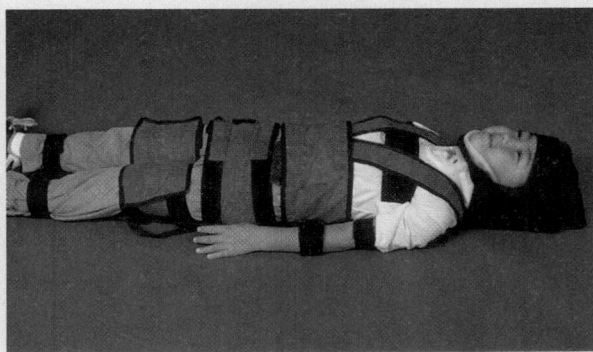

### Step 6

Ensure that the child is strapped in properly.

## Skill Drill 35-6 Immobilizing a Patient in a Car Seat

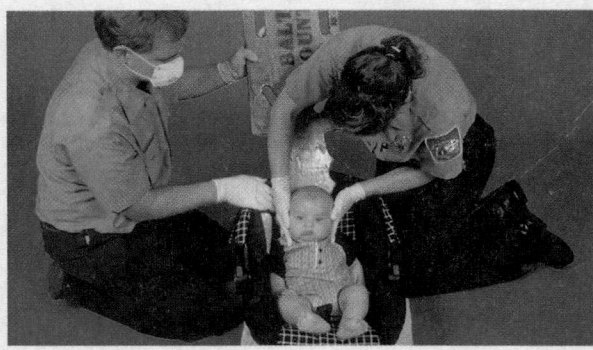

### Step 1

Stabilize the head in neutral position.

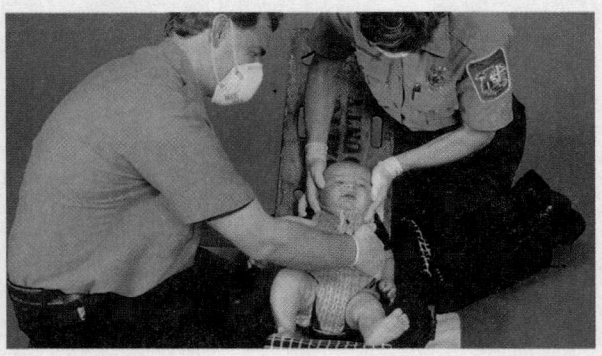

### Step 2

Place a short backboard or pediatric immobilization device between the patient and the surface he or she is resting on.

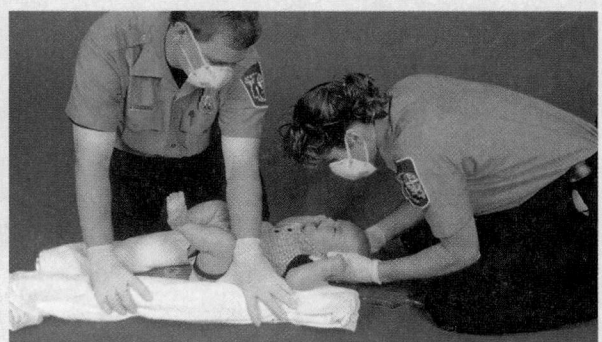

### Step 3

Slide the patient onto the short backboard or pediatric immobilization device.

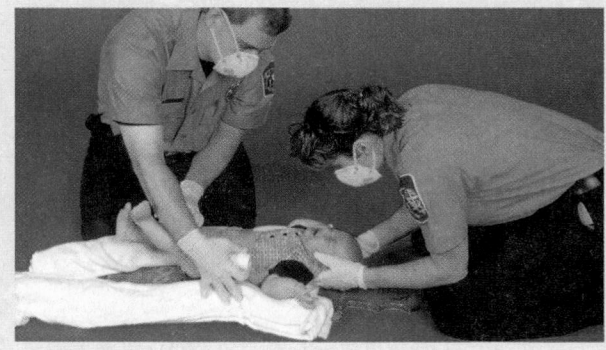

### Step 4

Place a towel under the back, from the shoulders to the hips, to ensure neutral head position.

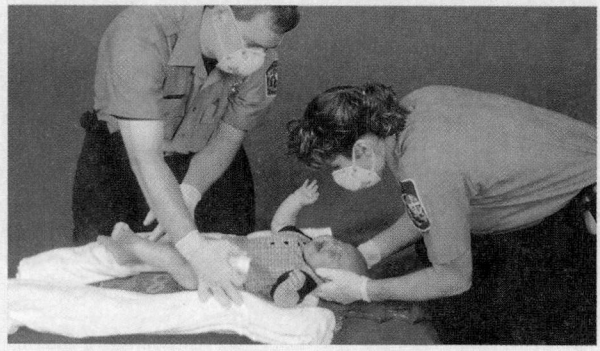

### Step 5

Secure the torso first; pad any voids.

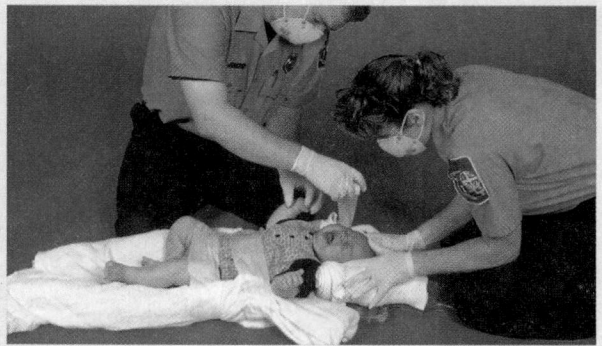

### Step 6

Secure the head to the short backboard or pediatric immobilization device.

4. Make sure the patient's head is in a neutral position by placing a towel under the back, from the shoulders to the hips (**Step 4**).
5. Secure the torso first and place padding to fill any voids (**Step 5**).
6. Secure the patient's head to the short backboard or pediatric immobilization device (**Step 6**).

## Chest Injuries

Chest injuries in children are usually the result of blunt trauma rather than penetrating objects. Remember that children have soft, flexible ribs that can be significantly compressed without breaking. This chest wall flexibility can produce a flail chest. Keep this in mind as you assess a child who has sustained high-energy blunt trauma to the chest. Although there may be no external sign of injury, such as broken ribs, contusions, or bleeding, there may be significant injuries within the chest (**FIGURE 35-36**). Pediatric patients are managed in the same manner as adults. Chapter 30, *Chest Injuries*, discusses the treatment of chest injuries in detail.

## Abdominal Injuries

Abdominal injuries are common in children. Remember, though, that children can compensate

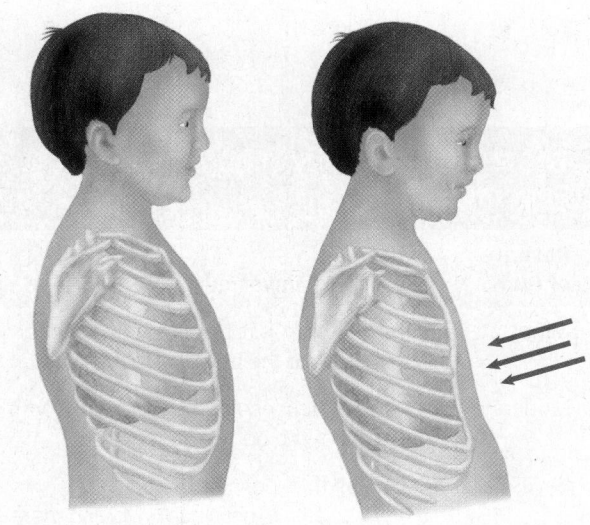

**FIGURE 35-36** A child's ribs are softer and more flexible than an adult's. As a result, they may compress the lungs and heart if there is blunt trauma, causing serious injury with no obvious external damage.

© Jones & Bartlett Learning.

for significant blood loss better than adults without signs or symptoms of shock developing (**FIGURE 35-37**). They can also have a serious injury without early external evidence of a problem. All children with abdominal injuries should be monitored for signs and symptoms of shock, including a weak, rapid pulse; cold, clammy skin; decreased capillary refill time (an early sign); confusion; and decreased systolic blood pressure (a late sign). Even in the absence of signs and symptoms of shock, or with only very few signs and symptoms, you should remain cautious about the possibility of internal injuries.

Pediatric patients are managed in the same manner as adults. Chapter 31, *Abdominal and Genitourinary Injuries*, discusses abdominal injuries in detail. If the patient shows signs and symptoms of shock, prevent hypothermia by keeping the patient warm with blankets. If the patient has bradycardia, ventilate. Monitor the patient's condition during transport.

## Burns

Burns to children are generally considered more serious than burns to adults. This is because infants and children have more surface area relative to total body mass, which means greater fluid and heat loss. In addition, children do not tolerate burns as well as adults do. Children are also more likely to go into shock, develop hypothermia, and experience airway problems because of the unique differences of their ages and anatomy.

Children can be burned in a variety of ways. The most common involve exposure to hot substances such as scalding water in a bathtub, hot items on a stove, or exposure to caustic substances such as cleaning solvents or paint thinners (**FIGURE 35-38**). According to the CDC, older children are more likely to be burned by flames from fire. You should suspect possible internal injuries from chemical ingestion when you see a child who has burns, particularly around the face and mouth.

One common problem following burn injuries in children is infection. Burned skin cannot resist infection as effectively as normal skin can. For this reason, sterile techniques should be used in handling the skin of children with burn wounds, if possible.

**TABLE 35-15** provides some general guidelines to follow in assessing a pediatric patient who has

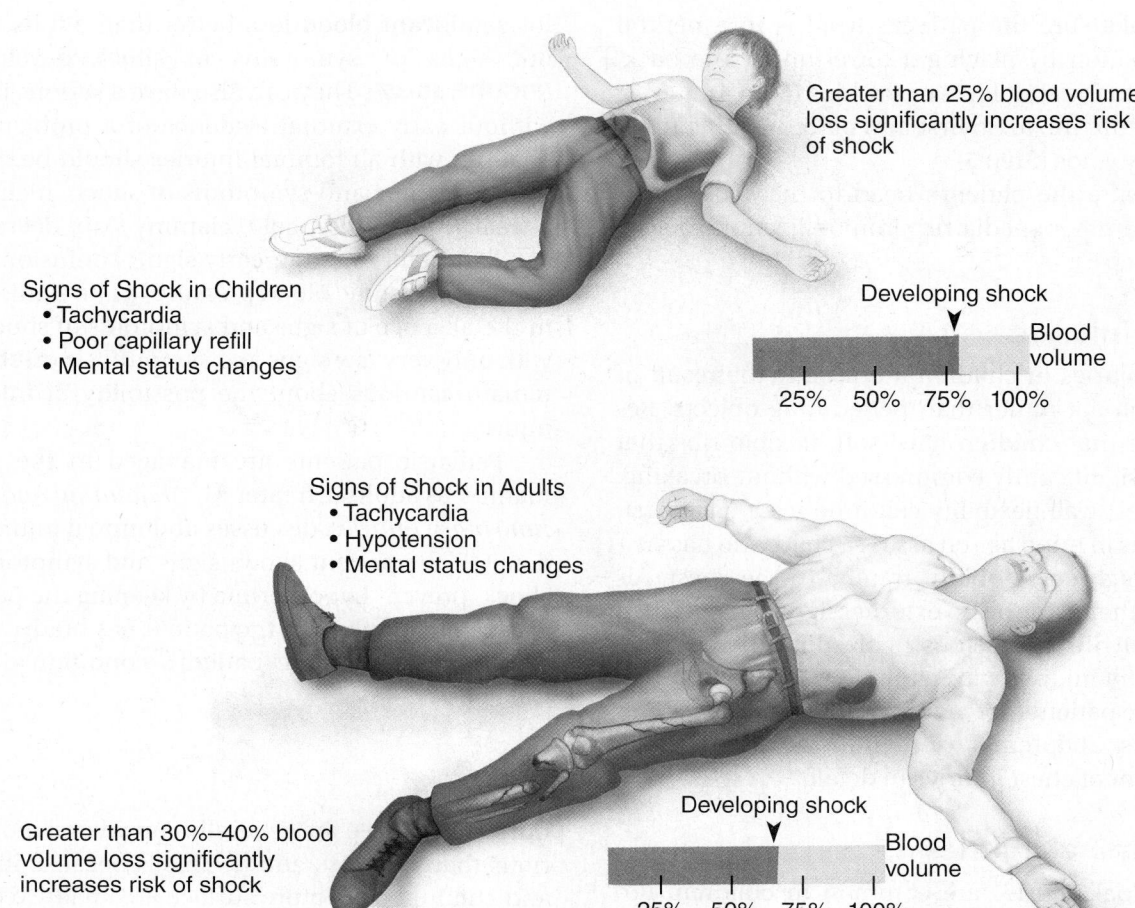

Greater than 25% blood volume loss significantly increases risk of shock

**Signs of Shock in Children**
- Tachycardia
- Poor capillary refill
- Mental status changes

Developing shock

Blood volume

25%  50%  75%  100%

**Signs of Shock in Adults**
- Tachycardia
- Hypotension
- Mental status changes

Greater than 30%–40% blood volume loss significantly increases risk of shock

Developing shock

Blood volume

25%  50%  75%  100%

**FIGURE 35-37** All children with abdominal injuries should be monitored closely for signs of shock. Although children may compensate for significant blood loss better than adults, shock develops in children after proportionally smaller blood losses.

© Jones & Bartlett Learning.

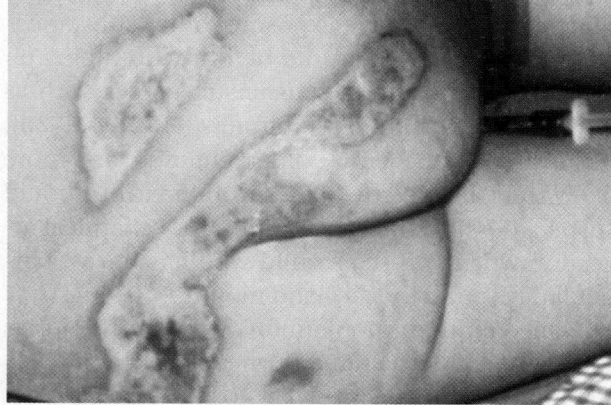

**FIGURE 35-38** Some burns in children involve exposure to hot surfaces. This child's buttocks were placed against a hot heating grate.

© Charles Stewart MD, EMDM, MPH.

| **TABLE 35-15** Severity of Burns in Pediatric Patients | |
|---|---|
| **Severity of Burn** | **Body Area Involved** |
| Minor | Partial-thickness burns involving less than 10% of the body surface area |
| Moderate | Partial-thickness burns involving 10% to 20% of the body surface area |
| Severe | Any full-thickness burn<br>Any partial-thickness burn involving more than 20% of the body surface area<br>Any burn involving the hands, feet, face, airway, or genitalia |

© Jones & Bartlett Learning.

been burned. These guidelines may help you to determine which pediatric patients should be treated primarily at specialized burn centers. Also consider the possibility of child abuse in any burn situation. Make sure you report any information about your suspicions to the appropriate authorities.

Pediatric patients are managed in the same manner as adults. Chapter 27, *Soft-Tissue Injuries*, discusses burn care in detail. If the patient shows signs and symptoms of shock, prevent hypothermia by keeping the child warm with blankets. If the patient has bradycardia, ventilate. Monitor the child's condition during transport.

## Injuries of the Extremities

Children have immature bones with active growth centers. Growth of long bones occurs from the ends at specialized growth plates. These growth plates are potential weak spots in the bone and are often injured as a result of trauma. In general, children's bones bend more easily than adults' bones. As a result, greenstick (incomplete) fractures can occur.

Extremity injuries in pediatric patients are generally managed in the same manner as those in adults. Painful, deformed limbs with evidence of broken bones should be splinted. Specialized splinting equipment, such as a traction splint for fractures of the femur, should be used only if it fits the pediatric patient. Do not attempt to use adult immobilization devices on a pediatric patient unless the child is large enough to properly fit in the device.

## Pain Management

The first step in pain management is recognizing that the patient is in pain. Since some pediatric patients will be nonverbal or have a limited vocabulary, remember to look for visual clues and use the Wong-Baker FACES scale (see Figure 35-20).

When dealing with pain management issues in children, you are limited to the following interventions: positioning, ice packs, and extremity elevation. These interventions will decrease the pain and swelling to the site of an injury. However, additional interventions (medications) from an ALS provider may be available. Another important tool is simple kindness and providing emotional support to the patient and the parent or caregiver. This act alone can decrease pediatric patient anxiety and allow for

a more soothing environment for all involved. Pediatric patients can sense fear and frustration from adults, so it is important to maintain a calm, professional, and trusting relationship with your patient and the family during the course of treatment.

## Disaster Management

The JumpSTART triage system was developed for pediatric patients because the original START triage system did not account for the developmental and physiologic differences in children (**FIGURE 35-39**). This system is intended for pediatric patients

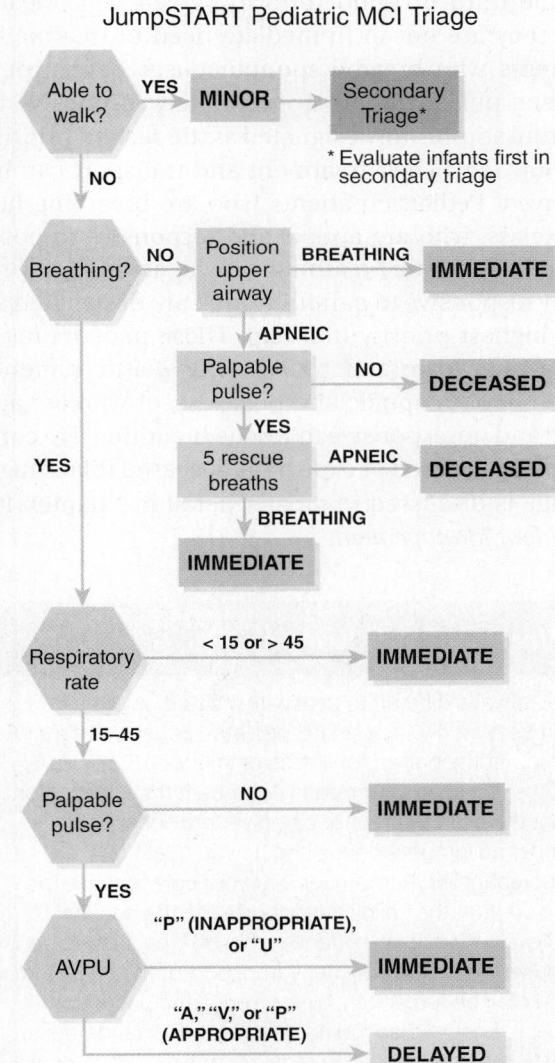

JumpSTART Pediatric MCI Triage

**FIGURE 35-39** The JumpSTART triage system.

© Lou Romig, MD, 2002.

younger than 8 years or who appear to weigh less than 100 pounds (45 kg). Because infants and children may not be able to walk or follow commands (including children with special needs) during a disaster event, they must be considered for immediate delivery to the treatment area.

There are four triage categories in the Jump-START system, designated by colors corresponding to different levels of urgency for treatment. Decision points include ability to walk (except in infants); presence of spontaneous breathing; respiratory rate of less than 15 or greater than 45 breaths/min; palpable peripheral pulse; and appropriate response to painful stimuli on the AVPU scale.

Children who are able to walk are designated as the third or minor priority (green tag), meaning they are not in immediate need of treatment. Patients who breathe spontaneously, have a peripheral pulse, and are appropriately responsive to painful stimuli are designated as the second priority (yellow tag). Their treatment and transport can be delayed. Pediatric patients who are breathing but pulseless, who are apneic and responsive to positioning or rescue breathing, or who are inappropriately responsive to painful stimuli are designated as the highest priority (red tag). These patients need immediate care and transport. Pediatric patients who are both apneic and pulseless, or who are apneic and unresponsive to rescue breathing, are considered deceased or expectant deceased (black tag). Triage is discussed in greater detail in Chapter 40, *Incident Management*.

### Words of Wisdom

It is always difficult to deal with a situation of child abuse. When you assess a pediatric patient, you may find that the pattern of illness or injury, or the severity of the illness or injury, does not match the information that the child's parent or caregiver provides to you. Under no circumstances should you question the discrepancies. Remember that your sole focus is to ensure that the child is transported to the hospital for an evaluation. If you offend or "tip off" the suspected abuser, he or she may deny transport of the child and you may be forced to leave the pediatric patient on scene. Ensure that you are familiar with mandated state laws and reporting requirements per your local protocols. Privately inform the hospital staff of your findings.

## Child Abuse and Neglect

The term child abuse means any improper or excessive action that injures or otherwise harms a child or infant; it includes physical abuse, sexual abuse, neglect, and emotional abuse. The intentional injury of a child, whether physical or emotional, unfortunately is not rare in our society. According to the report *Child Maltreatment 2017* from the US Department of Health and Human Services, more than 500,000 children are victims of child abuse annually. Many of these children sustain life-threatening injuries, and some die. If suspected child abuse is not reported, the child is likely to be abused again and again, which can lead to permanent injury or death. Therefore, you must be aware of the signs of child abuse and neglect, and it is your responsibility to report suspected abuse to law enforcement or child protection agencies.

### Signs of Abuse

As an EMT, you will be called to homes because of a reported injury to a child. Child abuse occurs in every socioeconomic status, so be aware of the patient's surroundings and document your findings objectively. EMTs are commonly called to testify in abuse cases, so it is essential to record all findings, including any statements made by parents or caregivers or others on the scene. If you suspect that physical or sexual abuse is involved, ask yourself the following questions:

- Is the injury typical for the developmental level of the child?
- Is the method of injury reported by the parent or caregiver consistent with the child's injury?
- Is the parent or caregiver behaving appropriately (concerned about the child's well-being)?
- Is there evidence of drinking or drug use at the scene?
- Was there a delay in seeking care for the child?
- Is there a good relationship between the child and the parent or caregiver?
- Does the child have multiple injuries at different stages of healing?
- Does the child have any unusual marks or bruises that may have been caused by cigarettes, heating grates, or branding injuries?
- Does the child have several types of injuries, such as burns, fractures, and bruises?

- Does the child have any burns on the hands or feet that involve a glove distribution (marks that encircle a hand or foot in a pattern that looks like a glove)?
- Is there an unexplained decreased level of consciousness?
- Is the child clean and an appropriate weight for his or her age?
- Is there any rectal or vaginal bleeding?
- What does the home look like? Clean or dirty? Is it warm or cold? Is there adequate food?

Your assessment in the field will allow a better assessment by the medical staff later. An easy way to remember these points for the pediatric population is the mnemonic CHILD ABUSE, shown in **TABLE 35-16**.

As you assess the pediatric patient, look for and pay particular attention to the following signs (**FIGURE 35-40**).

### Words of Wisdom

In children, bumps and bruises are a common occurrence. You should be concerned when bruises are found in uncommon locations or in patterns. Elbow and knee bruising, or injuries that follow the patterns of falls or rough play, match the nature of a playing child, but bruises to the back, buttocks, or backs of the arms and legs are much less common. Also be mindful of bruises in various stages of healing, which can also be an indicator of abuse. If the bruises have a unique pattern, as if a child was struck with an object once or repeatedly, this may be a sign of abuse.

**TABLE 35-16** Mnemonic for Assessing Possible Child Abuse

| | |
|---|---|
| **C** | Consistency of the injury with the child's developmental age |
| **H** | History inconsistent with injury |
| **I** | Inappropriate parental concerns |
| **L** | Lack of supervision |
| **D** | Delay in seeking care |
| **A** | Affect |
| **B** | Bruises of varying ages |
| **U** | Unusual injury patterns |
| **S** | Suspicious circumstances |
| **E** | Environmental clues |

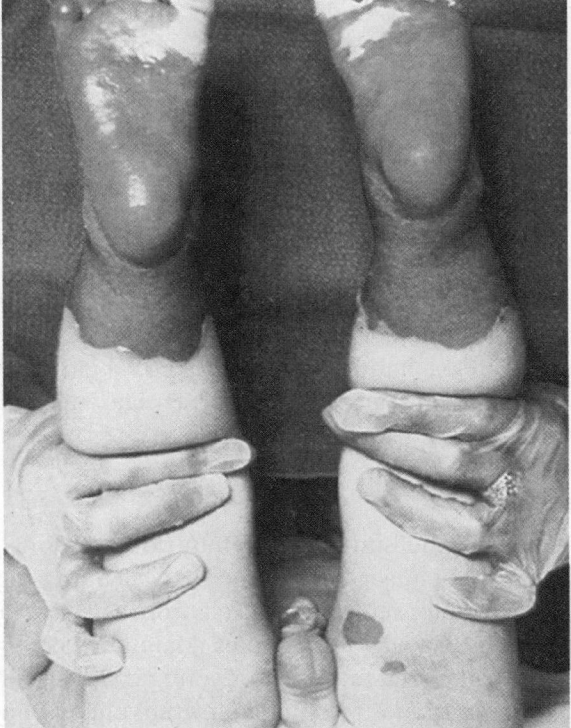

**A**

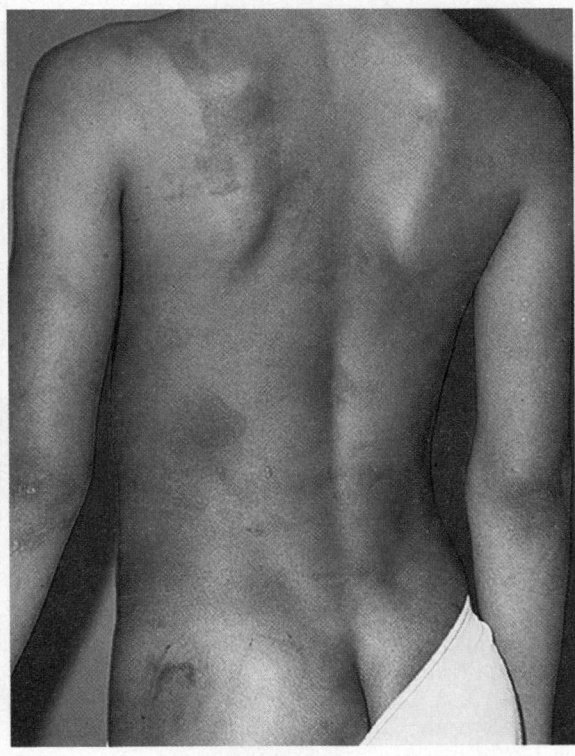

**B**

**FIGURE 35-40** Signs of child abuse. **A.** A scald. **B.** Multiple injuries at different stages of healing.

A, B: Courtesy of Ronald Dieckmann, MD.

## Bruises

Observe the color and location of any bruises. New bruises are pink or red. Over time, bruises turn blue, then green, then yellow-brown and faded. Note the location. Bruises to the back, buttocks, ears, or face are suspicious and are usually inflicted by a person.

## Burns

Burns to the penis, testicles, vagina, or buttocks are usually inflicted by someone else, as are burns that encircle a hand or foot to look like a glove. You should suspect abuse if the child has cigarette burns or grid pattern burns.

## Fractures

Fractures of the humerus or femur do not normally occur without major trauma, such as a fall from a high place or a motor vehicle crash. Falls from a bed are not usually associated with fractures. Maintain some index of suspicion if an infant or young child sustains a femur fracture or a complete fracture of any bone. As discussed, children are more likely to experience greenstick (incomplete) fractures, as opposed to complete fractures, due to their soft and pliable bones. A complete fracture in a pediatric patient indicates that the child was exposed to significant traumatic force.

## Shaken Baby Syndrome

Infants may sustain life-threatening head trauma by being shaken or struck on the head, a condition called shaken baby syndrome. With this condition, there is bleeding within the head and damage to the cervical spine as a result of intentional,

### Words of Wisdom

It is normal to have concerns about the care of children, but do not let your personal judgments cloud the true nature of a situation. You may feel upset by challenging socioeconomic factors that impact where a child lives, the condition of the home environment, and the child's sources of food. However, the parents or caregivers may have the best of intentions and may be doing everything possible for the child. In these situations, let the hospital staff or a supervisor know that the child and his or her family may need some assistance or community support. When in doubt, report the situation to the appropriate abuse and neglect authorities and the receiving facility.

forceful shaking. The infant will often be found unconscious, often without evidence of external trauma. The call for help may be for an infant who has stopped breathing or is unresponsive. The infant may appear to be in cardiopulmonary arrest, but what has likely occurred is that the shaking tore blood vessels in the brain, resulting in bleeding around the brain. The pressure from the blood results in an increased intracranial pressure, leading to coma and/or death.

## Neglect

Neglect is refusal or failure on the part of the parent or caregiver to provide life necessities, such as food, water, clothing, shelter, personal hygiene, medicine, comfort, and personal safety.

Children who are neglected are often dirty or too thin or appear developmentally delayed because of a lack of stimulation. You may observe such children when you are making calls for unrelated problems. Report all cases of suspected neglect.

## Symptoms and Other Indicators of Abuse

An abused child may appear withdrawn, fearful, or hostile. Be particularly concerned if the child refuses to discuss how an injury occurred. Occasionally, the parent or caregiver will reveal a history of several "accidents." Be alert for conflicting stories or a marked lack of concern from the parents or caregiver. Remember, the abuser may be a parent, caregiver, relative, or friend of the family. Sometimes the abuser is an acquaintance of a single parent.

EMTs in all states must report all cases of suspected abuse, even if the ED fails to do so. Most states have special forms for reporting. Supervisors are generally forbidden to interfere with the reporting of suspected abuse, even if they disagree with the assessment. You do not have to prove that there has been abuse. Law enforcement and child protection agencies are mandated to investigate all reported cases. Take all necessary precautions to protect yourself, your team, and the pediatric patient involved in this situation.

## Sexual Abuse

Children of any age or gender can be victims of sexual abuse. Maintain an index of suspicion regardless of the patient's social or economic situation.

This type of sexual abuse is often the result of long-standing abuse by relatives.

Your assessment of a child who has been sexually abused should be limited to determining the type of dressing any injuries require. Sometimes, a sexually abused child has also been beaten. Therefore, treat any bruises or fractures as well. Do not examine the genitalia of a young child unless there is evidence of bleeding or there is an injury that must be treated.

In addition, if you suspect that a child is a victim of sexual abuse, encourage the child not to wash, urinate, or defecate before a physician completes a physical examination. Although this step can be difficult for the victim, it is important to preserve evidence. If possible, ensure that an EMT or police officer of the same gender remains with the child, unless locating one will delay transport.

You must maintain professional composure the entire time you are assessing and caring for a sexually abused child. Assume a concerned, caring approach, and shield the child from onlookers and curious bystanders. Obtain as much information as possible from the child and any witnesses. The child may be hysterical or unwilling to say anything at all, especially if the abuser is a relative or family friend. You are in the best position to obtain the most accurate firsthand information about the incident. Therefore, record any information carefully and completely on the patient care report. Transport all children who are victims of sexual assault. Sexual abuse of a child is a crime. Cooperate fully with law enforcement officials in their investigations.

# Sudden Unexpected Infant Death and Sudden Infant Death Syndrome

The sudden unexpected infant death (SUID) refers to a sudden unexpected death where the cause is not known until an investigation is conducted. Causes of death may include suffocation, infection, poisoning, cardiac problems, and trauma. One of the causes of SUID is sudden infant death syndrome (SIDS), which results in death that cannot be explained by another cause. According to the CDC, about 3,500 infants die of SIDS annually. To reduce the risk of SIDS, the American Academy of Pediatrics recommends that an infant (younger than 1 year)

be placed on his or her back on a firm mattress to sleep, in a crib that is free of bumpers, blankets, and toys. The CDC recommends having the baby sleep in the same room, but not in the same bed, chair, or sofa, as an adult. Breastfeeding and use of a pacifier are also associated with a lower risk of SIDS.

Although it is impossible to predict SIDS, the following are several known risk factors:

- Mother younger than 20 years
- Mother smoked during pregnancy or after birth
- Mother used alcohol or illicit drugs during pregnancy or after birth
- Low birth weight

Deaths as the result of SIDS can occur at any time of the day; however, these children are often discovered in the morning when the parents or caregivers go in to check on the infant. If you are the first provider at the scene of suspected SIDS, you will face three tasks: assessment of the scene, assessment and management of the patient, and communication and support of the family.

## Patient Assessment and Management

SIDS is a diagnosis of exclusion. All other potential causes must first be ruled out, a process that can be time-consuming for physicians. An infant who has been a victim of SIDS will be pale or blue, not breathing, and unresponsive. Other causes for SUID include the following:

- Overwhelming infection
- Child abuse
- Airway obstruction from a foreign object or as a result of infection
- Meningitis
- Accidental or intentional poisoning
- Hypoglycemia (low blood glucose level)
- Congenital metabolic defects

Regardless of the cause, assessment and management of the infant remain the same. Remember that what you find in assessing the infant and the scene may provide important diagnostic information.

Begin with an assessment of the XABCs, and provide interventions as necessary. Depending on how much time has passed since the child was discovered, he or she may show signs of postmortem changes. These include stiffening of the body, called rigor mortis, and dependent lividity, which is the pooling of blood in the lower parts of the body or those that are in contact with the floor or bed.

If the child shows such signs, call medical control. In some EMS systems, a victim of SUID may be declared dead on the scene. Deciding whether to start CPR on a child who shows clear signs of rigor mortis or dependent lividity can be very difficult. Family members may consider anything less as withholding critical care. In this situation, the best course of action may be to initiate CPR and transport the patient and the family to the nearest ED, where the family can receive more extensive support (follow local protocols). If there is no evidence of postmortem changes, begin CPR immediately.

As you assess the infant, pay special attention to any marks or bruises on the child before performing any procedures, including CPR. Also note any intervention such as CPR that was done by the parents or caregivers before you arrived.

## Scene Assessment

Carefully inspect the environment, following local protocols, noting the condition of the scene where the parents or caregivers found the infant. Your assessment of the scene should concentrate on the following:

- Signs of illness, including medications, humidifiers, or thermometers
- The general condition of the house
- Signs of poor hygiene
- Family interaction. Do not allow yourself to be judgmental about family interactions at this time. Note and report any behavior that is clearly not within the acceptable range, such as physical and verbal abuse.
- The site where the infant was discovered. Note all items in the infant's crib or bed, including pillows, stuffed animals, toys, and small objects.

## Communication and Support of the Family After the Death of a Child

The death of a child, whether sudden death of an infant or otherwise, is a devastating event for a family; it also tends to evoke strong emotional responses among health care providers, including EMS personnel. Part of your job at this point is to allow the family to express their grief in ways that may differ from your own cultural, religious, and personal practices. Provide emotional support in whatever ways you can.

In addition to any medical treatment the child may require, you must be prepared to offer the family a high level of empathy and understanding as they begin the grieving process. First, the family may want you to initiate resuscitation efforts, which may or may not conflict with your EMS protocols. If the child is clearly deceased and, under protocol, can be declared dead in the field, but family members are so distraught that they insist that resuscitation efforts be made, initiate CPR and consult with medical control or transport the child, unless there is rigor or the safety of the crew is jeopardized.

The extent of your interaction with the family will depend, to some degree, on the number of providers available at the scene. Always introduce yourself to the child's parents or caregivers and ask about the child's date of birth and medical history. If and when the decision is made to start or stop resuscitation efforts, inform the family immediately. Find a place for family members to watch resuscitation without being in the way. Do not, in any case, speculate on the cause of the child's death. The family will want to see the child and should be asked whether they want to hold the child and say good-bye. Parents and caregivers may be experiencing strong feelings of denial.

The following interventions are helpful in caring for the family at this time:

- Learn and use the child's name rather than the impersonal "your child."
- Speak to family members at eye level, and maintain good eye contact with them.
- Use the word "dead" or "died" when informing the family of the child's death; euphemisms such as "passed away" or "gone" are ineffective.
- Acknowledge the family's feelings ("I know this is devastating for you"), but never say "I know how you feel," even if you have experienced a similar event; the statement will anger many people.
- Offer to call other family members or clergy if the family wishes.
- Keep any instructions short, simple, and basic. Emotional distress may limit their ability to process information.
- Ask each adult family member individually whether he or she wants to hold the child.

- Wrap the dead child in a blanket, as you would if he or she were alive, and stay with family members while they hold the child. Ask them not to remove tubes or other equipment that was used in an attempted resuscitation.

**TABLE 35-17** lists additional guidelines for helping the family of a deceased child.

### TABLE 35-17 How You Can Help the Family of a Deceased Child

**When Arriving on Site**
- Introduce yourself quickly.
- Obtain a brief history.
- When possible, one EMT should stay with the family.
- Ask the child's name and refer to the child by that name.

**If Resuscitation Is Attempted**
- Give brief, frequent updates and explanations.
- Allow family members to stay within viewing distance if they wish.
- Allow family members to accompany the child to the hospital when possible.

**If No Resuscitation Is Performed**
- Sit down with the family.
- Inform the family immediately.
- Explain why no resuscitation will be attempted.
- Offer to arrange for religious support, including baptism or last rites.

**Beginning the Grieving Process**
- Learn and use the child's name.
- Allow the family to express emotions; be nonjudgmental.
- Give brief explanations and answers.
- Explain to the family that the cause of death is still unknown.
- Allow time for questions.

**DO**
- Tell the family how sorry you are.
- Tell the family whom they can call if they have questions later.
- Give written instructions and referrals.

**DO NOT**
- Say, "I know how you feel."
- Say, "You have other children" or "You can have other children."
- Attempt to answer the question "Why did this happen?"
- Try to tell the family that they will feel better in time.

Remember that each individual and each culture expresses grief in a different way, some more visibly than others. Some will require intervention; others will not. Most parents or caregivers feel directly or indirectly responsible for the death of a child and may express this immediately; this does not mean that they are responsible. Although you should keep the possibility of abuse or neglect in mind, your role is not that of investigator. Any further inquiry is the responsibility of law enforcement.

Often, family members will ask specific questions about the event: Why did this happen? How did this happen? Let them know their concerns will be addressed but answers are not immediately available (**TABLE 35-18**). Remember to always use the child's name when speaking to family members. If possible, allow the family to spend time with the child and to ride in the ambulance to the hospital.

Some EMS systems arrange for home visits after the death of a child so that EMS providers and family members can come to some sort of closure together. This also gives the family an opportunity to ask any remaining questions about the event. However, you need special training for such visits.

### TABLE 35-18 Common Questions Following the Death of a Child

**Q:** Was there pain?
**A:** This often can be answered by a simple "No." If you are uncertain, you may give an indirect answer, such as "We really don't know what patients feel in these circumstances."

**Q:** What did the child die of?
**A:** Do not answer this question; you would probably be guessing.

**Q:** Why did this happen?
**A:** Do not answer this question either, as the answer depends on one's own individual philosophy or religion. "I wish I had an answer for you" is usually the most appropriate response.

**Q:** What happens now?
**A:** This question usually concerns the next few minutes or the next hour. If you know, give the family a general idea of what will happen. For example, if there is no history of illness, you can say, "A medical examination will be done, and then [child's name] will be taken to the mortuary."

Coping with the death of a child can be very stressful. You may find yourself with unexpected feelings of pain and loss. It is helpful to take some time before going back on the job to work through your feelings and to talk about the event with your EMS colleagues. Be alert for signs of posttraumatic stress in yourself and others, including nightmares, restlessness, difficulty sleeping, and changes in appetite. Consider the need for professional help if these signs or symptoms continue. Arrange for a proper debriefing after your involvement with the case comes to a close. This can be a session with a trained counselor or a group discussion with your colleagues or the entire health care team. As discussed in Chapter 2, *Workforce Safety and Wellness,* all EMS programs should have critical incident stress management protocols and debriefing teams available for traumatic incidents.

Although you may consider the death of a child to be a failure, your skill at coping with this kind of emotional event can be a great comfort to the family, helping them to accept their loss and begin the long process of grieving.

### Words of Wisdom

Most parents or caregivers of children who die suddenly will experience extremely strong emotional responses for a long time after the death. Counseling and support services begin with your care, including immediate referral to longer-term services. You can usually make this referral through social services personnel in a hospital you work with; familiarize yourself with available resources. Many communities also have support groups for grieving families. Make sure the parents or caregivers are aware of available services, offer to put them in touch while you are there, and leave the contact information in written form for their later reference even if you have helped them make the contact.

## Apparent Life-Threatening Event

Infants who have cyanosis and apnea, and are unresponsive when found by their families, sometimes resume breathing and color with stimulation. These children have had what is called an **apparent life-threatening event (ALTE)**, called near-miss SIDS in the past. In addition to cyanosis and apnea, a classic ALTE is characterized by a distinct change in muscle tone (limpness) and choking or gagging. Given the limited understanding of ALTEs and the inability to identify subtle causes in the field, parents and caregivers should be encouraged to have their infant promptly transported to an appropriate facility for a full evaluation. After the ALTE, you may find a child who appears healthy and shows no signs of illness or distress. Nevertheless, you must complete a careful assessment and provide rapid transport to the ED.

Pay strict attention to management of the airway. Assess the infant's history and, if possible, the environment. Be aware the ALTE might be the result of abuse. Allow parents or caregivers to ride in the ambulance, if appropriate. If asked, explain that you cannot say what caused the event and that the physicians will have to determine the cause at the hospital.

## Brief Resolved Unexplained Event

Occasionally, EMS systems receive a call for a possible pediatric cardiac arrest, but providers arrive on the scene to find an apparently healthy, normal infant. This circumstance is referred to as a brief resolved unexplained event (BRUE) and may occur in an infant less than 1 year of age. Signs and symptoms reported by parents or caregivers in BRUE include brief changes in color such as pale skin or cyanosis; choking; absent, slow, or irregular breathing; abnormal muscle tone (limp or stiff); and decreased level of consciousness. On assessment, the EMT will be unable to find any abnormality. Despite the appearance of an apparently normal infant, transport is required so the baby can have a full evaluation to rule out any possible life-threatening condition. If at the hospital there is no explanation for the signs and symptoms reported by the caregiver, the infant's diagnosis will be BRUE.

# YOU are the Provider SUMMARY

### 1. How does a child's airway and respiratory system differ from that of an adult?

Proportionately, infants and children have a larger, rounder occiput (back of the head). Because the tracheal cartilages are soft and easily compressed, hyperextension or flexion of the neck can cause collapse of the upper airway, which is the reason that an infant or young child's head should be maintained in a neutral (sniffing) position, especially when trying to ventilate the patient. The child's tongue is proportionately larger than an adult's tongue and larger relative to the small mandible, which makes it easier to block the airway. In addition, the pediatric airway is narrower with a proportionately larger and floppier epiglottis when compared to an adult. Because of their relatively smaller lungs, infants and children need to breathe faster to adequately exchange oxygen and carbon dioxide. Children have both a higher metabolic rate and a higher demand for oxygen due in part to the actual size of the lung tissues and the volume of air that can be exchanged in addition to the increased metabolic demands. Finally, breathing in children also requires use of both the diaphragm and intercostal muscles. Infants and young children depend much more on the diaphragm for breathing because the intercostal muscles are underdeveloped. Therefore, children quickly become fatigued when their breathing is labored, which may lead to respiratory failure. Additionally, anything that affects the diaphragm's efforts, such as abdominal distension, further compromises a child's respiratory efforts.

### 2. What are some airway and breathing problems that are unique to pediatric patients?

Foreign body airway obstruction is common in children; it often occurs when children put a small toy or other object in their mouths. Many respiratory illnesses are unique to the pediatric population, including bacterial tracheitis, croup (laryngotracheobronchitis), epiglottitis, asthma, bronchiolitis, and pertussis (whooping cough). Because of the anatomy of the child's airway (ie, larger, more anterior epiglottis and tongue and smaller mandible), the swelling due to the respiratory illnesses can quickly cause significant airway compromise. Infants and young children also have immature immune systems and may or may not have an adequate history of immunizations, making them more susceptible to infectious disease.

### 3. Why did you not immediately perform a hands-on assessment of this child?

If an infant or child is clearly experiencing a life-threatening condition, such as unconsciousness or major trauma, then an immediate hands-on assessment is indicated. However, since this child is conscious, you can use the pediatric assessment triangle (PAT) to quickly form a general impression of the child without touching her. Based on the findings of the PAT, you should be able to determine whether the child is in stable condition, in which case you can continue with your assessment, or in unstable condition, in which case you should begin immediate treatment and prepare for transport. Also consider that rushing to assess a child who is fearful may cause her to cry or struggle, further increasing her respiratory effort and potentially making her symptoms worse.

### 4. On the basis of your initial observations, is this child experiencing respiratory distress or respiratory failure?

Although the child appears fearful of your presence—a normal reaction for a young child—she is alert, exhibiting age-appropriate behavior, and maintaining eye contact with you. Her skin is pink and appears to be dry; however, she is experiencing increased work of breathing, as noted by an increased respiratory rate, obvious breathing difficulty, nasal flaring, and prominent retractions. This clinical presentation is consistent with respiratory distress.

### 5. What is the most likely cause of this child's respiratory distress?

On the basis of the child's clinical presentation and the progression of her symptoms, you should suspect that she has croup. This general impression is further reinforced by the presence of a high-pitched barking, seal-like cough, a low-grade fever, and preceding cold symptoms. Her breath sounds are clear to auscultation bilaterally; this makes a lower airway problem highly unlikely. In addition, it is autumn; croup most commonly occurs during the autumn and early winter.

### 6. Should you separate this child from her parents to provide further treatment? Why or why not?

The decision to separate a sick or injured child from his or her parents is based on the child's condition and the parents' reaction to the situation. Although this child is experiencing respiratory distress, she is clinically stable and is clinging to her mother, who is showing no evidence of emotional distress. For these reasons, do not separate the child from her mother. If you do, you will likely find that the child will become more anxious. Anxiety can easily worsen the child's condition by making her breathe harder and making her heart beat faster. It may also make the child less cooperative with further assessment or treatment.

## YOU are the Provider SUMMARY *continued*

**7. How has this child's condition changed? What should you do next?**

Compared with earlier assessments, the child's condition has obviously deteriorated; she is now in respiratory failure. When infants and children decompensate, they often do so with alarming speed. In this case, the child decompensated in the time it took to move her from the residence to the back of your ambulance! Clinical signs of this child's deterioration include a decreased level of activity; she was previously conscious and maintaining eye contact. She is breathing more slowly and her retractions have markedly weakened; this indicates chest wall muscle fatigue from prolonged increased work of breathing. She is developing cyanosis around her mouth (perioral cyanosis), indicating a decreased level of oxygen in her blood. This sign is further verified by the marked decrease in her oxygen saturation level. Perhaps the most ominous sign is the marked decrease in her heart rate. When the body is no longer able to compensate, the heart rate begins to fall; this is a sign of impending cardiopulmonary arrest.

You must act immediately to prevent this child from developing respiratory or cardiac arrest. Begin assisting her ventilations with a bag-mask device and high-flow oxygen and transport immediately. If possible, coordinate an intercept with an ALS unit en route to the hospital. If her condition continues to deteriorate, she may require advanced airway management or medication therapy.

**8. How could an ALS intercept benefit this child?**

You are caring for a child who, at a minimum, requires assisted ventilation. In some cases, children with respiratory failure require more than oxygen and assisted ventilations. Certain medications that ALS can administer (eg. nebulized epinephrine) may also be required to prevent the child's condition from deteriorating to cardiopulmonary arrest. If her condition continues to deteriorate, she may require CPR. ALS providers can perform advanced airway management, administer cardiac medications, and monitor the patient's cardiac rhythm. Because these interventions would clearly benefit the child—especially if she experiences cardiac

arrest—consider an ALS intercept if it will lead to faster access to advanced care, but do not delay transport if ALS cannot be intercepted in a timely fashion.

**9. Are you providing adequate ventilations? How can you tell?**

The child's level of consciousness (still listless) and slow, shallow respirations are clear indicators for the continued use of assisted ventilation. However, she is showing signs of improvement, indicating that your ventilations are adequate.

The child's heart rate has increased from 90 beats/min to 110 beats/min; as with any patient, an improvement in the heart rate is a sign of adequate artificial ventilation. The child's oxygen saturation has also improved significantly (from 85% to 96%); this indicates that you are adequately oxygenating her blood. The cyanosis around her mouth is resolving; this is also an indicator of adequate ventilation.

Although you have noted clinical improvement with assisted ventilation, this does not mean that you can stop. The child is still breathing at a slow rate, and the depth of her breathing is shallow. Also, she is not resisting your treatment, thus indicating that her level of consciousness is still depressed, and she is still fatigued. Continue to assist her ventilations.

**10. Why is it especially important to avoid hyperventilating infants and children?**

In the unprotected airway (ie, in the patient who is not intubated), hyperventilation forces excess air into the stomach, which causes gastric distention. Gastric distention increases the risk of aspiration if vomiting occurs. In infants and small children, an additional risk exists of air filling the stomach, pushing the diaphragm upward into the thoracic cavity and therefore limiting expansion of the chest cavity and lungs during inspiration, which may reduce the effectiveness of your ventilations. In infants and small children, there is the additional risk of pushing the diaphragm into the thoracic cavity, which may reduce the effectiveness of your ventilations. It takes much less air in the stomach of an infant or child to inhibit adequate positive pressure ventilations than it does in an adult.

### EMS Patient Care Report (PCR)

| Date: 1-15-20 | Incident No.: 013210 | Nature of Call: Respiratory distress | | Location: 545 W. San Antonio St. | |
|---|---|---|---|---|---|
| Dispatched: 2323 | En Route: 2324 | At Scene: 2330 | Transport: 2340 | At Hospital: 2353 | In Service: 0029 |

#### Patient Information

**Age:** 4
**Sex:** F
**Weight (in kg [lb]):** 16 kg (35 lb)

**Allergies:** No known drug allergies
**Medications:** None
**Past Medical History:** Recent cold
**Chief Complaint:** Respiratory distress

## YOU **are the Provider SUMMARY** *continued*

### Vital Signs

| Time: 2335 | BP: 86/56 | Pulse: 124 | Respirations: 34 | Spo$_2$: 95% |
|---|---|---|---|---|
| Time: 2340 | BP: 76/56 | Pulse: 90 | Respirations: 18 | Spo$_2$: 85% |
| Time: 2348 | BP: 84/54 | Pulse: 110 | Respirations: 20 | Spo$_2$: 96% |

### EMS Treatment (circle all that apply)

| Oxygen @ _12_ L/min via:<br><br>NC (NRM) (Bag mask) | (Assisted Ventilation) | Airway Adjunct | CPR |
|---|---|---|---|
| **Defibrillation** | **Bleeding Control** | **Bandaging** | **Splinting** | **Other** |

### Narrative

EMS dispatched to a residence for a 4-year-old child with respiratory distress.

Chief Complaint: Respiratory distress

History: Patient's mother states that she has had a cold for the past 2 days and slowly developed a low-grade fever and high-pitched cough, which she described as a "barking seal." Mother denies that her child has any significant past medical history; she has been giving her ibuprofen as needed for her low-grade fever.

Assessment: Arrived on scene and found the patient sitting on the couch next to her mother. She was conscious, maintained eye contact, and began clinging to her mother. Her airway was patent; however, her breathing was obviously labored. Visual assessment revealed that her skin was pink and appeared dry. She had prominent supraclavicular retractions and nasal flaring during inhalation.

Treatment (Rx): Administered blow-by oxygen via pediatric nonrebreathing mask and performed further assessment. Auscultation of breath sounds revealed that they were clear and equal bilaterally, but prominent intercostal retractions were noted on exposure of the chest. Capillary refill time, 1 second. Continued blow-by oxygen as patient's father carried her to the ambulance. Shortly after securing the child to the stretcher, reassessment revealed that her level of consciousness had markedly decreased. Her respiratory rate also decreased, her retractions were weak, and her oxygen saturation level markedly decreased.

Transport: Began assisting the child's ventilations with a bag-mask and high-flow oxygen and began rapid transport. Attempted to coordinate ALS intercept; however, the closest ALS unit was too far away and would have resulted in unnecessary delay in transport. Notified receiving facility of the patient's condition and of our estimated arrival time and continued assisting ventilations. Reassessment revealed that the child was still listless and was not resistant to treatment; however, her heart rate, skin color, and oxygen saturation improved. Continued ventilatory assistance and delivered child to the emergency department. Verbal report was given to staff physician Roberts. Cleared the hospital and returned to service at 0029.

**End of report**

# Prep Kit

## Ready for Review

- Children are not only smaller than adults and more vulnerable, but are also anatomically, physiologically, and psychologically different from adults in important ways.
- Infancy is the first year of life. If possible, allow the parent or caregiver to hold the infant during the assessment.

- The toddler (age 1 to 3 years) may experience separation or stranger anxiety but may be able to be distracted by a special object (blanket) or toy.
- Preschool-age children (age 3 to 6 years) can understand directions and can identify painful areas when questioned. Tell these children what you are going to do before you do it

to prevent the development of frightening fantasies.

- School-age children (age 6 to 12 years of age) are familiar with the physical examination process. Talk with them about their interests to distract them during a procedure.
- Adolescents (age 12 to 18 years) are physically similar to adults, but are still children on an emotional level. Respect the adolescent's modesty at all times.
- General rules for dealing with pediatric patients of all ages include appearing confident, being calm, remaining honest, and keeping parents or caregivers together with the pediatric patient as much as possible.
- The growing body of the pediatric patient creates some special considerations.
- The tongue is large relative to other structures, so it poses a higher risk of airway obstruction than in an adult.
- An infant breathes faster than an older child.
- Breathing requires the use of chest muscles and the diaphragm.
- The airway in a child has a smaller diameter than the airway in an adult and is therefore more easily obstructed.
- A rapid heartbeat and blood vessel constriction help pediatric patients to compensate for decreased perfusion.
- Children's internal organs are not as insulated by fat and may be injured more severely, and children have less circulating blood. Therefore, children exhibit the signs of shock more slowly, but they go into shock more quickly, with less blood loss.
- Children's bones are more flexible and bend more with injury, and the ends of the long bones, where growth occurs, are weaker and may be injured more easily.
- Because a young child might not be able to speak, your assessment of his or her condition must be based largely on what you can see and hear. Families may be able to provide vital information about an incident or illness.
- Use the pediatric assessment triangle (PAT) to obtain a general impression of the infant or child.
- You will need to carry special sizes of airway equipment for pediatric patients.
- Use length-based resuscitation tape to determine the appropriate-size equipment for children.

- The three keys to successful use of the bag-mask device in a child are: (1) have the appropriate equipment in the right size; (2) maintain a good face-to-mask seal; and (3) ventilate at the appropriate rate and volume.
- Signs of shock in children are tachycardia, poor capillary refill time (>2 seconds), and mental status changes. You must be alert for signs of shock in pediatric patients because they can decompensate rapidly.
- Begin treating shock by assessing the XABCs. In pediatric patients with obvious life-threatening external hemorrhage, always address this first.
- Febrile seizures may be a sign of a more serious problem such as meningitis.
- The most common cause of dehydration in children is vomiting and diarrhea. Life-threatening diarrhea can develop in an infant in a matter of hours.
- Fever is a common reason why parents or caregivers call 9-1-1. Body temperatures of 100.4°F (38°C) or higher are considered abnormal.
- Trauma is the number-one killer of children in the United States.
- A victim of sudden infant death syndrome (SIDS) will be pale or blue, not breathing, and unresponsive. He or she may show signs of postmortem changes, including rigor mortis and dependent lividity; if so, call medical control to report the situation.
- Carefully inspect the environment where a SIDS victim was found, looking for signs of illness, abusive family interactions, and objects in the child's crib.
- Provide emotional support for the family in whatever way you can, but do not make judgmental statements.
- The death of a child is devastating for family members and for health care providers. In dealing with family members, acknowledge their feelings, keep any instructions short and simple, use the child's name, and maintain eye contact.
- Be prepared to respond to philosophical as well as medical questions. Indicate concern and understanding; do not be specific about the cause of death.
- Be alert for signs of posttraumatic stress in yourself and others after dealing with the death of a child. It can help to talk about the event and your feelings with your EMS colleagues.

# Vital Vocabulary

**adolescents** Children between ages 12 and 18 years.

**apparent life-threatening event (ALTE)** An event that causes unresponsiveness, cyanosis, and apnea in an infant, who then resumes breathing with stimulation.

**blanch** To turn white.

**bradypnea** Slow respiratory rate; ominous sign in a child that indicates impending respiratory arrest.

**bronchiolitis** Inflammation of the bronchioles that usually occurs in children younger than 2 years and is often caused by the respiratory syncytial virus.

**central pulses** Pulses that are closest to the core (central) part of the body where the vital organs are located; include the carotid, femoral, and apical pulses.

**child abuse** A general term applying to all forms of abuse and neglect of children.

**croup** A viral inflammatory disease of the upper respiratory system that may cause a partial airway obstruction and is characterized by a barking cough; usually seen in children.

**epiglottitis** A bacterial infection in which the epiglottis becomes inflamed and enlarged and may cause an upper airway obstruction.

**fontanelles** Areas where the neonate's or infant's skull has not fused together; usually disappear at approximately 18 months of age.

**generalized (tonic-clonic) seizure** A seizure that features rhythmic back-and-forth motion of an extremity and body stiffness.

**grunting** An "uh" sound heard during exhalation; reflects the child's attempt to keep the alveoli open; a sign of increased work of breathing.

**infancy** The first year of life.

**length-based resuscitation tape** A tape used to estimate an infant's or child's weight on the basis of body length; appropriate drug doses and equipment sizes are listed on the tape.

**meningitis** An inflammation of the meningeal coverings of the brain and spinal cord; it is usually caused by a virus or a bacterium.

**nares** The external openings of the nostrils. A single nostril opening is called a naris.

**neglect** Refusal or failure on the part of the parent or caregiver to provide life necessities.

*Neisseria meningitides* A form of bacterial meningitis characterized by rapid onset of symptoms, often leading to shock and death.

**pediatric assessment triangle (PAT)** A structured assessment tool used to rapidly form a general impression of the infant or child without touching him or her; consists of assessing appearance, work of breathing, and circulation to the skin.

**pediatrics** A specialized medical practice devoted to the care of the young.

**pertussis (whooping cough)** An airborne bacterial infection that affects mostly children younger than 6 years, in which the patient is feverish and exhibits a "whoop" sound on inspiration after a coughing attack; highly contagious through droplet infection.

**preschool-age** Children between ages 3 and 6 years.

**school-age** Children between ages 6 and 12 years.

**shaken baby syndrome** A syndrome seen in abused infants and children; the patient has been subjected to violent, whiplash-type shaking injuries inflicted by the abusing individual that may cause coma, seizures, and increased intracranial pressure due to tearing of the cerebral veins with consequent bleeding into the brain.

**sniffing position** An upright position in which the patient's head and chin are thrust slightly forward to keep the airway open.

**sudden infant death syndrome (SIDS)** Death of an infant or young child that remains unexplained after a complete autopsy.

**tachypnea** Rapid respirations.

**toddler** A child age 1 to 3 years.

**tracheitis** Inflammation of the trachea.

**tripod position** An upright position in which the patient leans forward onto outstretched arms with the head and chin thrust slightly forward.

**work of breathing** An indicator of oxygenation and ventilation; reflects the child's attempt to compensate for hypoxia.

# References

1. About SUID and SIDS. Centers for Disease Control and Prevention website. https://www.cdc.gov/sids/about/index.htm. Reviewed December 31, 2018. Accessed April 17, 2020.

2. Accident statistics. Stanford Children's Health website. https://www.stanfordchildrens.org/en/topic/default?id=accident-statistics-90-P02853. Accessed April 16, 2020.

3. Acute spinal cord injury in children. Children's Hospital of Philadelphia website. https://www.chop.edu/conditions-diseases/acute-spinal-cord-injury-children. Accessed April 16, 2020.

4. American Academy of Pediatrics Task Force on Sudden Infant Death Syndrome. SIDS and other sleep-related infant deaths: updated 2016 recommendations for a safe infant sleeping environment. *Pediatrics* 2016;138(5):e20162938. https://doi.org/10.1542/peds.2016-2938.

5. Asthma facts and figures. Asthma and Allergy Foundation of America website. https://www.aafa.org/asthma-facts/. Updated June 2019. Accessed April 16, 2020.

6. Burn prevention. Centers for Disease Control and Prevention website. http://www.cdc.gov/safechild/burns/. Reviewed February 6, 2019. Accessed April 16, 2020.

7. Carll KE, Park AE, Tortolani RJ. Epidemiology of catastrophic spine injuries in high school, college, and professional sports. *Semin Spine Surg* 2010;22(4):168–172.

8. Chameides L, Samson RA, Schexnayder SM, et al. *Pediatric Advanced Life Support Provider Manual*. Dallas, TX: American Heart Association; 2015.

9. Facts on pediatric spinal cord injury. American Spinal Injury Association website. https://asia-spinalinjury.org/committees/pediatric/pediatric-committee-news-and-resources/pediatric-spinal-cord-injury-facts/. Accessed April 17, 2020.

10. Highlights of the 2019 American Heart Association guideline update for CPR and ECC. American Heart Association website. https://eccguidelines.heart.org/circulation/cpr-ecc-guidelines/. Published 2019. Accessed April 16, 2020.

11. Holmberg M, Wiberg S, Ross C, et al. Trends in survival after pediatric in-hospital cardiac arrest in the United States. *Circulation* 2019;140:1398–1408.

12. Jayaram N, McNally B, Tang F, Chan PS. Survival after out-of-hospital cardiac arrest in children. *J Am Heart Assoc* 2015;4(10):e002122. https://doi.org/10.1161/JAHA.115.002122.

13. National Association of State EMS Officials. *National EMS Scope of Practice Model 2019*. Washington, DC: National Highway Traffic Safety Administration; February 2019. Report No. DOT HS 812-666. https://www.ems.gov/pdf/National_EMS_Scope_of_Practice_Model_2019.pdf. Accessed July 6, 2020.

14. *National Emergency Medical Services Education Standards*. US Department of Transportation. National Highway Traffic Safety Administration. DOT HS 811 077A. January 2009. www.ems.gov/pdf/811077a.pdf. Accessed April 16, 2020.

15. *National Emergency Medical Services Education Standards*. Emergency Medical Technician Instructional Guidelines. US Department of Transportation. National Highway Traffic Safety Administration. DOT HS 811 077C. January 2009. www.ems.gov/pdf/811077c.pdf. Accessed April 16, 2020.

16. Pneumonia is the leading cause of death in children. World Health Organization website. https://www.who.int/maternal_child_adolescent/news_events/news/2011/pneumonia/en/. Accessed April 16, 2020.

17. Ralston M. Pediatric basic life support for health care providers. UpToDate website. https://www.uptodate.com/contents/pediatric-basic-life-support-for-health-care-providers. Updated April 13, 2020. Accessed April 16, 2020.

18. Sudden unexpected infant death and sudden infant death syndrome: data and statistics. Centers for Disease Control and Prevention website. https://www.cdc.gov/sids/data.htm. Reviewed September 13, 2019. Accessed April 16, 2020.

19. Tieder JS, Bonkowsky, JL, Etzel RA, et al.; Subcommittee on Apparent Life-Threatening Events. Brief resolved unexplained events (formerly apparent life-threatening events) and evaluation of lower-risk infants. *Pediatrics* 2016;137(5):e20160590. https://doi.org/10.1542/peds.2016-0590.

20. US Department of Health and Human Services, Administration for Children and Families, Administration of Children, Youth and Families, Children's Bureau. *Child Maltreatment 2017*. Washington DC: Department of Health and Human Services; 2019.

21. US Department of Transportation, National Highway Traffic Safety Administration. *Working Group Best-Practice Recommendations for the Safe Transportation of Children in Emergency Ground Ambulances*. DOT HS 811 677. September 2012. https://webcache.googleusercontent.com/search?q=cache:3nAnpjU77v8J:https://www.nhtsa.gov/staticfiles/nti/pdf/811677.pdf+&cd=1&hl=en&ct=clnk&gl=us&client=safari. Accessed April 16, 2020.

22. Web-based Injury Statistics Query and Reporting System (WISQARS). Centers for Disease Control and Prevention website. http://www.cdc.gov/injury/wisqars. Reviewed March 30, 2020. Accessed April 16, 2020.

23. Welcome to the Wong-Baker FACES Foundation: the official home of the Wong-Baker FACES pain rating scale. Wong Baker FACES website. http://www.wongbakerfaces.org. Accessed April 16, 2020.

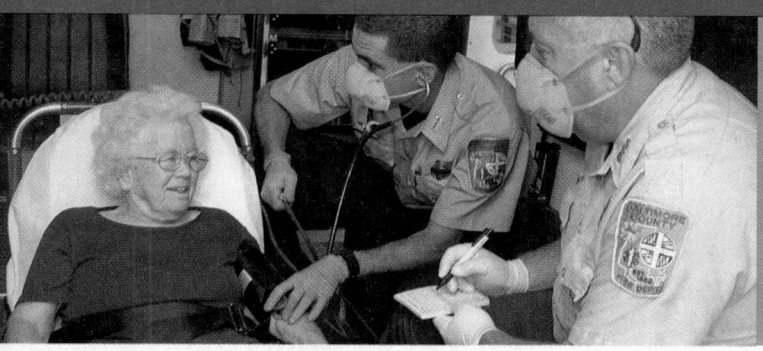

# Chapter 36

# Geriatric Emergencies

## NATIONAL EMS EDUCATION STANDARD COMPETENCIES

### Special Patient Populations

Applies a fundamental knowledge of growth, development, and aging and assessment findings to provide basic emergency care and transportation for a patient with special needs.

### Geriatrics

- Impact of age-related changes on assessment and care (pp 1368–1373)
- Changes associated with aging, psychosocial aspects of aging, and age-related assessment and treatment modifications for the major or common geriatric diseases and/or emergencies
  - Cardiovascular diseases (pp 1354–1357, 1368–1373)
  - Respiratory diseases (pp 1353–1354, 1368–1373)
  - Neurologic diseases (pp 1357–1360, 1368–1373)
  - Endocrine diseases (pp 1363, 1368–1373)
  - Alzheimer disease (pp 1358–1359, 1368–1373)
  - Dementia (pp 1358–1359, 1368–1373)

### Patients With Special Challenges

- Recognizing and reporting abuse and neglect (pp 1381–1383 and Chapter 35, *Pediatric Emergencies*)
- Health care implications of
  - Abuse (pp 1381–1383 and Chapter 35, *Pediatric Emergencies*)
  - Neglect (pp 1381–1383 and Chapter 35, *Pediatric Emergencies*)
  - Homelessness (Chapter 37, *Patients With Special Challenges*)
  - Poverty (Chapter 37, *Patients With Special Challenges*)

- Bariatrics (Chapter 37, *Patients With Special Challenges*)
- Technology dependent (Chapter 37, *Patients With Special Challenges*)
- Hospice/terminally ill (Chapter 37, *Patients With Special Challenges*)
- Tracheostomy care/dysfunction (Chapter 37, *Patients With Special Challenges*)
- Homecare (Chapter 37, *Patients With Special Challenges*)
- Sensory deficit/loss (Chapter 37, *Patients With Special Challenges*)
- Developmental disability (Chapter 37, *Patients With Special Challenges*)

### Trauma

Applies fundamental knowledge to provide basic emergency care and transportation based on assessment findings for an acutely injured patient.

### Special Considerations in Trauma

- Recognition and management of trauma in the:
  - Pregnant patient (Chapter 34, *Obstetrics and Neonatal Care*)
  - Pediatric patient (Chapter 35, *Pediatric Emergencies*)
  - Geriatric patient (pp 1375–1378)
- Pathophysiology, assessment, and management of trauma in the:
  - Pregnant patient (Chapter 34, *Obstetrics and Neonatal Care*)
  - Pediatric patient (Chapter 35, *Pediatric Emergencies*)
  - Geriatric patient (pp 1375–1378)
  - Cognitively impaired patient (Chapter 37, *Patients With Special Challenges*)

1. Define the term *geriatrics*. (p 1350)
2. Recognize some of the special aspects of the lives of older people. (p 1350)
3. Know generational considerations when communicating with a geriatric patient. (pp 1350–1351)
4. Describe the common complaints and the leading causes of death in older people. (p 1352)
5. Discuss the physiologic changes associated with the aging process and the age-related assessment and treatment modifications that result. (pp 1352–1365)
6. Define polypharmacy and the toxicity issues that can result. (pp 1365–1367)
7. Discuss the effect of aging on behavioral emergencies. (pp 1367–1368)
8. Explain the GEMS diamond and its role in the assessment and care of the geriatric patient. (p 1368)
9. Explain special considerations when performing the patient assessment process on a geriatric patient with a medical condition. (pp 1368–1373)
10. Discuss the effects of aging on environmental emergencies. (p 1375)
11. Explain special considerations when performing the patient assessment process on a geriatric patient with a traumatic injury. (pp 1375–1378)
12. Explain special considerations when responding to calls at nursing and skilled care facilities. (pp 1379–1380)
13. Define an advance directive and considerations with older patients. (pp 1380–1381)
14. Discuss the prevalence of elder abuse and neglect; include why the extent of elder abuse is not well known. (pp 1381–1383)
15. Recognize acts of commission or omission by a caregiver that result in harm, potential harm, or threat of harm to a geriatric patient. (p 1381)
16. Explain the assessment and care of a geriatric patient who has potentially been abused or neglected. (pp 1382–1383)

# Introduction

**Geriatrics** is the assessment and treatment of disease in someone who is 65 years or older. In this chapter, 65 years is used as the threshold age to be consistent with the definition used by other medical groups and governmental agencies. How fast one ages, though, is a function of genetics, lifestyle, and, perhaps, attitude.

Geriatric patients present a unique challenge for health care providers because the classic presentations of injuries and illness are often altered by chronic conditions, multiple medications, and the physiology of aging. To provide effective treatment for this growing population, you must understand the issues related to aging and modify some of your assessment and treatment approaches accordingly.

Being a patient advocate for an older patient involves much more than management of medical and traumatic emergencies. As the older population increases, communities, companies, and hospitals are encouraging awareness of geriatric issues through the media and creating programs that promote prevention of injuries. EMTs who respond to the homes of geriatric patients are in an ideal position to provide key information to others in health care and social services systems. Interventions for geriatric patients may include reviewing the home environment to ensure that safe and tolerable living conditions exist, providing information on how to prevent falls, and making referrals to appropriate social service agencies when a patient needs assistance. Often, simple preventive measures can help older people avoid further injury, costly medical treatment, and death. You are in a position to not only recognize and manage a serious emergency, but also to help prevent problems before they occur.

# Generational Considerations

It is important to understand and appreciate how the life of an older person might differ from yours. You will see older people who have recently lost a spouse and are struggling to fill the spouse's role,

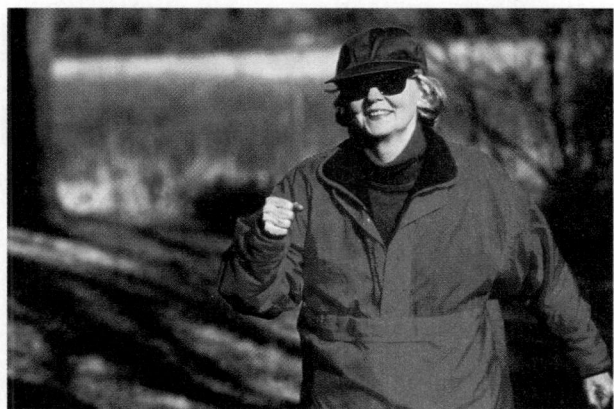

**FIGURE 36-1** Physical activity can help older people reduce their risk of illness and injury.

Courtesy of the National Cancer Institute.

such as by managing the finances or doing the housework. Many older people also live on a fixed income, which can be very challenging. Some older people may not take all of their medications in an effort to save money. Many fear losing their independence and not being able to live in their own home.

Sometimes, it takes time and patience to interact with an older person. Always treat the patient with respect. Make every attempt to avoid ageism, which is a stereotyping of older people that can lead to poor patient assessment and care. Common stereotypes include assuming that the patient has dementia, is hard of hearing, has a sedentary lifestyle, or is immobile. Older people can stay fit and be active, even though they are not able to perform at the same level as they did in their youth (**FIGURE 36-1**).

## Communication and Older Adults

Effective verbal communication skills are essential to the successful assessment and treatment of older patients. Communication with older people can be challenging. The aging process brings with it changes in vision, hearing, taste, smell, touch, and pain sensation. Also, there are changes in communication abilities that accompany aging, such as dementia and other diseases. These challenges are consequences of aging for some older adults and should be expected, but not assumed.

### Words of Wisdom

Older patients who learned English as a second language may revert back to their native language when stressed or in a crisis situation. Do not assume that the patient cannot understand you just because he or she is speaking another language.

## Communication Techniques

When caring for older individuals, use their name to communicate with them. If you do not know their name, use "sir" or "ma'am." Asking the patient how he or she prefers to be addressed can build trust. Never use familiar or casual terms such as "honey" or "dear" when addressing your patient unless he or she has invited you to do so.

When you interview an older patient, the following techniques should be used:

- **Identify yourself.**
- **Be aware of how you present yourself.** Avoid showing frustration and impatience through body language, such as crossed arms.
- **Look directly at the patient at eye level and ensure good lighting.**
- **Speak slowly and distinctly.** Do not raise your voice. Try to talk in a lower tone; some older people can hear certain pitches better than others.

- **Have one person talk to the patient and ask only one question at a time.** Do not answer questions for patients out of frustration or impatience.
- **Do not assume that all older patients are hard of hearing.** Ask the patient if he or she can hear you, and verify by asking him or her to confirm understanding of what you just said. Be aware of the presence of hearing aids.
- **Give the patient time to respond unless the condition appears urgent.**
- **Listen to the answer the patient gives you.**
- **Explain what you are going to do before you do it.** Use simple terms to explain the use of medical equipment and procedures; avoid using medical jargon or slang.
- **Do not talk about the patient in front of him or her as though the patient was not there.** This gives the patient the feeling that he or she does not have a say in decisions about his or her care.

Keep in mind the patient may be very nervous about going to the hospital. This may be due to fears of dying, loss of independence, or being placed in a care center. By using effective communication skills, you can earn the patient's trust and help him or her feel more at ease.

### Words of Wisdom

Remember, as with patients of any age, older patients may have more difficulty communicating clearly when they are stressed by an emergency or personal crisis.

## Common Complaints and the Leading Causes of Death in Older People

The changing physiology of geriatric patients can predispose this population to a host of problems not seen in youth (**TABLE 36-1**). A simple rib fracture in a 30- or 40-year-old patient can be inconsequential in the long term. The same injury in a geriatric patient who is age 80 or 90 years can result in pneumonia and even death. A hip fracture from a low-mechanism fall is common in older people and may have dire consequences. Hip fractures are more likely to occur when bones are weakened by osteoporosis. Sedentary behavior while healing can predispose the patient to pneumonia and

### TABLE 36-1 Common Conditions and the Leading Causes of Death in Geriatric Patients

**Common Conditions**

- Hypertension
- Arthritis
- Heart disease
- Cancer
- Diabetes mellitus
- Asthma
- Chronic bronchitis or emphysema
- Stroke

**Leading Causes of Death**

- Heart disease
- Cancer
- Injury
- Chronic lower respiratory disease
- Stroke
- Alzheimer disease
- Diabetes mellitus
- Injury
- Influenza and pneumonia

Heron M. Division of Vital Statistics. Deaths: leading causes for 2017. *Natl Vital Stat Rep.* 2019 June 24;68. https://www.cdc.gov/nchs/data/nvsr/nvsr68/nvsr68_06-508.pdf. Accessed May 8, 2020.

blood clots that may interfere with healing and can cause death. Many older patients who experience hip fractures do not return to their preinjury levels of activity. Many older patients are well aware of this and may be frightened. All of these factors make assessment and treatment decisions more complex and patient complaints potentially more serious.

## Changes in the Body

The process of aging is gradual and starts much earlier than most people realize. Human growth and development peaks in the late 20s and early 30s, at which point the aging process begins. A 35-year-old is aging just as fast as an 85-year-old, but the older person exhibits the cumulative results of a longer process. Of course, the aging process can vary dramatically from one person to another. You have probably seen 60-year-olds who look frail and 80-year-olds who can and do run marathons.

The aging process is inevitably accompanied by changes in physiologic function, such as a decline in the function of the liver and kidneys. All tissues in the body undergo aging, albeit not at the same rate. The decrease in the functional capacity of various organ systems is normal, and it can affect the way a patient responds to illness.

As a health care professional, you need to be knowledgeable about decreased function in organ systems in older people because this knowledge will enable you to correctly respond to a patient's illness. At the other end of the spectrum, there is a widespread—and unfortunate—tendency to attribute genuine disease symptoms to "just getting old", and to neglect their treatment.

## Changes in the Respiratory System

### Anatomy and Physiology

Age-related changes in the respiratory system can predispose an older adult to respiratory illness. Even a minor lung infection can become a life-threatening event. One of the conditions contributing to breathing problems is the weakening of the airway musculature that can cause decreased breathing capacity. This decreased muscle mass means that older patients have less help from muscles in the chest wall when they have trouble breathing. As one gets older, the alveoli in lung tissue can become enlarged and the elasticity decreases, making it harder to expel used air (air trapping). This change in lung tissue quality is comparable to a balloon that has been expanded and then deflated; the balloon loses some of its ability to contract to its original state. The lack of elasticity results in a decreased ability to bring in oxygen and push out carbon dioxide. The body's chemoreceptors, which monitor the changes in oxygen and carbon dioxide levels in the blood, become less sensitive with age. This can make the body respond more slowly to hypoxia, a dangerous condition in which the body tissues and cells do not have enough oxygen.

In addition, loss of mechanisms that protect the upper airway include decreased cough and gag reflexes. There is also a decrease in the cilia that line the bronchial tree; this lessens an older person's ability to cough and clear secretions, therefore increasing the chance of infection.

### Pathophysiology

#### Pneumonia

Because of the changes in lung physiology and decreased immune response, chronic lower respiratory disease, influenza, and pneumonia remain in the top 10 causes of geriatric deaths. In fact, one of the most common causes of death in older patients is infection with pneumococcus bacteria.

**Pneumonia** is an inflammation of the lung from bacterial, viral, or fungal causes. Pneumonia is the leading cause of death from infection in Americans older than 65 years. It especially affects people who are chronically and terminally ill. The process of aging causes some degree of immune suppression and increases the risk of contracting infections such as pneumonia. Increased mucus production, pulmonary secretions, and the inflammatory effects of infection all interfere with the ability of the alveoli to oxygenate the blood. Your management of pneumonia remains the same; however, it is important to maintain a high index of suspicion for any geriatric patient with signs and symptoms of possible pneumonia. Management of pneumonia is described in Chapter 16, *Respiratory Emergencies*. Remember to wear appropriate eye and respiratory protection including an N95 mask when you are assessing a patient with a potentially infectious respiratory disease. If you suspect an infectious lung disease process or communicable disease, you can also place a surgical mask on the patient.

---

### Street Smarts

Placing a mask on a patient with a respiratory infection such as pneumonia, tuberculosis, or COVID-19 helps stop the transmission of the pathogen, but it can also increase the patient's difficulty breathing and produce anxiety. Consider placing the mask over the nonrebreathing mask.

---

### Pulmonary Embolism

Another condition that can cause respiratory distress in older people is a **pulmonary embolism**. Pulmonary embolism is a condition that causes a sudden blockage of an artery in the lung by a venous clot. Clots develop in the veins of the legs or pelvis and then break off and embolize (move) through the heart to a pulmonary artery or one of its branches, where they lodge. A patient with a pulmonary embolism will present with shortness of breath and sometimes chest pain; thus, the pulmonary embolism can be confused with a cardiac, lung, or musculoskeletal condition. The top risk factors for a pulmonary embolism include recent hospitalization for medical illness or surgery (especially in a lower extremity) leading to sedentary behavior. Other factors include trauma, cancer, history of blood clots or heart failure, presence of a pacemaker or central venous catheter, paralyzed extremities, obesity, use of birth control pills, smoking, infection with COVID-19, and recent long-distance travel.

The presentation can be subtle or dramatic depending on how large the clot is and how much lung tissue is damaged. Patients present with tachycardia; sudden onset of dyspnea (shortness of breath, which differentiates this from an infection such as pneumonia); shoulder, back, or chest pain; cough; syncope; anxiety, which may be communicated as a sense of impending doom; apprehension; and possibly a low-grade fever or hemoptysis (the coughing up of blood). Also look for leg pain, redness, and swelling in just one ankle and foot for the source of the clot. The patient may present with profound fatigue and may go into cardiac arrest in a worst-case scenario.

Treatment should focus on airway, ventilatory, and circulatory support. Hemoptysis is usually not severe, but any blood that has been coughed up should be cleared from the airway. Because a considerable amount of lung tissue may not be able to off-load oxygen to the blood, supplemental oxygen is mandatory in a patient with a pulmonary embolism. Place the patient in a comfortable position and apply high-flow oxygen via a nonrebreathing mask. Ventilatory support may be necessary because a large pulmonary embolus may cause significant impairment of the patient's ability to breathe and could result in cardiac arrest. In this situation, ventilate with a bag-mask device, using an oropharyngeal or nasopharyngeal airway. When a patient is in respiratory and/or cardiac arrest, treat according to current emergency cardiovascular care guidelines and local protocol.

# Changes in the Cardiovascular System

## Anatomy and Physiology

Various changes occur in the cardiovascular system as a person ages, with the net effect of a decrease in the efficiency of the system. Specifically, the heart hypertrophies (enlarges) with age, usually in response to the chronically increased afterload imposed by stiffening blood vessels. However, bigger is not better for the heart. Over time, cardiac output declines, mostly as a result of a decreasing stroke volume, but the heart rate also has less ability to quickly respond to changes in preload.

Arteriosclerosis—a disease that causes the arteries to thicken, harden, and calcify—contributes to systolic hypertension in many older Americans, which places an extra burden on the heart. This phenomenon may be a consequence of disease states such as diabetes, atherosclerosis, and renal compromise, and it is associated with an increased risk of cardiovascular disease, dementia, and death. Compliance of the vascular walls depends on the production of collagen and elastin, proteins that are the primary components of muscle and connective tissue. An increase in pressure (normal hypertension seen with aging) leads to overproduction of abnormal collagen and decreased quantities of elastin, contributing to vascular stiffening. The result is a widening pulse pressure, decreased coronary artery perfusion, and changes in cardiac ejection efficiency.

Some changes in cardiovascular performance are probably not a direct consequence of aging, but rather reflect the deconditioning effect of a sedentary lifestyle. Whether because of other disabilities (such as arthritis) or for behavioral reasons, many people tend to limit physical activity and exercise as they grow older. The phrase "use it or lose it" applies just as much to the cardiac muscle as to the biceps muscle.

## Pathophysiology

Cardiac output is a measure of the workload of the heart. A younger person's body normally compensates for an increased demand on the cardiovascular system by increasing the heart rate, increasing the contraction of the heart, and constricting the blood vessels to nonvital organs. However, with aging, a person's ability to speed up contractions, increase contraction strength, and constrict or narrow blood vessels (vasoconstriction) is decreased because of stiffer vessels. As stroke volume is reduced, cardiac output decreases. The heart may lose its ability to increase cardiac output to meet the needs of the body. Older patients may also be taking beta blockers for hypertension that prevents them from having the ability to increase their heart rate.

Geriatric patients are at risk for **atherosclerosis**, an accumulation of fat and cholesterol in the arteries (**FIGURE 36-2**). Major complications of atherosclerosis include myocardial infarction (heart attack) and stroke. Atherosclerotic disease originates in the teen years and affects more than 60% of people older than 65 years. The presence of atherosclerosis makes stroke, heart disease, hypertension, and bowel infarction more likely.

Older people are also at an increased risk for formation of an **aneurysm**, an abnormal, blood-filled dilation of the wall of a blood vessel. Severe blood loss can occur when an aneurysm ruptures.

With aging, the blood vessels themselves become stiff, which results in a higher systolic blood pressure. As a result, the left ventricle, which pushes blood out into the body, becomes thicker and eventually loses elasticity, resulting in decreased filling of the left ventricle, which in turn causes decreased cardiac output.

Other anatomic changes include stiffening and degeneration of the heart valves, which may impede normal blood flow in and out of the heart. Aging also alters the heart's electrical conduction system. The sinoatrial node is the normal pacemaker of the heart, but by age 75 years, the number of the cells in the sinoatrial node will decrease by 90%. This event, combined with fibrosis and fatty deposits attaching to the electrical pathway, makes it likely that the patient will have some kind of heart rhythm

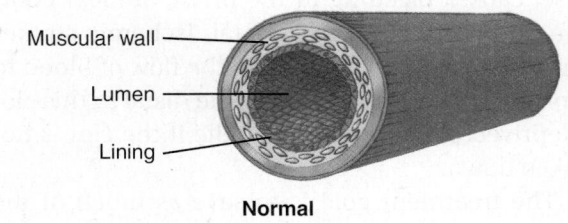

Muscular wall —
Lumen —
Lining —

**Normal**

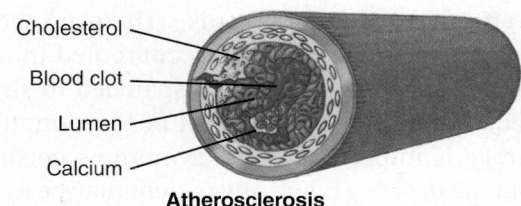

Cholesterol —
Blood clot —
Lumen —
Calcium —

**Atherosclerosis**

**FIGURE 36-2** Atherosclerosis is characterized by the buildup of fat and cholesterol on arterial walls.

© Jones & Bartlett Learning.

disturbance, or dysrhythmia. This can cause a heart rate that is too fast, too slow, or too erratic to provide effective blood flow to the body.

Another condition that affects older people is orthostatic hypotension (postural hypotension), which is a decrease in blood pressure caused by a change in position. When a person moves from a sitting to a standing position, gravity pulls blood down, away from the brain. This causes heart rate and contractility to increase. In younger people, the body's ability to compensate keeps them from passing out. Because older people become less sensitive to rapid changes in blood pressure, you may see a drop in the systolic blood pressure of 20 mm Hg when an older patient moves from a sitting position to a standing position. The body, therefore, is less able to adapt to rapid postural changes.

Another vessel-related problem is called venous stasis. Stasis means motionless state and, in this context, refers to loss of proper function of the veins in the legs that would normally carry blood back to the heart. This condition creates problems such as blood clots in the superficial veins (superficial phlebitis) and blood clots in the deep veins, known as **deep venous thrombosis**. Deep venous thrombosis is a serious concern because it can lead to pulmonary embolism.

People with venous stasis usually exhibit edema, or swelling, of the legs and ankles. Patients will report a feeling of fullness, aching, or tiredness in their legs, especially when standing. This condition eventually causes a red-brown discoloration on the skin and, in some cases, skin ulcers.

## Myocardial Infarction (Heart Attack)

Chest pain is a common complaint of older people and can often mean heart-related issues such as myocardial infarction. It is important to remember that the classic symptoms of a heart attack are often not present in geriatric patients. As many as one-third of older patients have "silent" heart attacks in which the usual chest pain is not present. This is particularly common in women and people with diabetes. Do not assume that your patient is not having a myocardial infarction because he or she is not reporting the classic, pressure-type, substernal chest pain. Any of the following symptoms may be a manifestation of acute cardiac disease in the older patient and should be evaluated by advanced life support (ALS) personnel for an underlying cardiac disorder: dyspnea; epigastric and abdominal pain; loss of bladder and bowel control; nausea and vomiting; weakness, dizziness, lightheadedness, and syncope; fatigue; and confusion.

Other signs and symptoms in older people that can indicate a cardiovascular problem include issues with circulation; diaphoresis (profound sweating); pale, cyanotic (blue), or mottled skin; abnormal or decreased breath sounds; and increased peripheral edema (swelling).

It is essential to obtain baseline vital signs because this information will provide you with a primary picture of the severity of your patient's condition, and you can use these findings to measure against in your ongoing assessment of the patient. Pulse rates can be too slow, too fast, weak, or irregular. A blood pressure reading can show hypertension or hypotension, either of which is significant in the presence of cardiac chest pain. The respiratory rate may be higher as the body attempts to take in and use more oxygen to aid an ailing heart.

At the EMT level, treatment of an older patient's cardiac problem mostly consists of airway, ventilatory, and circulatory support. Most EMS system protocols allow EMTs to administer aspirin or assist patients with the administration of medications, such as nitroglycerin, with a physician's order. Continue to evaluate your patient treatment through reassessment.

## Heart Failure

The signs and symptoms of heart failure will differ depending on the extent to which the right and/or left side of the heart is not functioning correctly.

Right-side heart failure occurs when the fluid in the blood backs up into the body. You will see jugular vein distention (visual bulging of the jugular veins in the neck), ascites (fluid in the abdomen), and peripheral edema in the body tissues. An enlarged liver may also be present from blood backing up through the portal vein. This may be determined by palpation. Right-side heart failure is often caused by left-side heart failure, so it is common to see signs of both when assessing the patient who has left-side heart failure.

With left-side heart failure, fluid backs up into the lungs. The excess fluid in the lungs causes pulmonary edema, and the patient will have severe shortness of breath and hypoxia with crackles in the lungs.

Paroxysmal nocturnal dyspnea is a condition that is characterized by sudden respiratory distress that awakens the person at night when the patient is in a reclining position. The respiratory distress is caused by fluid accumulation in the lungs. Patients report coughing, feeling suffocated, and cold sweats, and you will notice tachycardia. The term for not being able to breathe while lying down is orthopnea. One indication that your patient may be experiencing heart failure is that he or she sleeps sitting up.

Treatment should consist of airway, ventilatory, and circulatory support.

## Stroke

Stroke (cerebrovascular accident) is a leading cause of death in older people, and the likelihood of experiencing a stroke becomes greater as a person gets older. Causes of strokes can be preventable or nonpreventable. Preventable risk factors include smoking, hypertension, diabetes, atrial fibrillation, obesity, and a sedentary lifestyle. Uncontrollable factors include age, race, and sex.

Signs and symptoms of stroke include acute altered level of consciousness; numbness, weakness, or paralysis on one side of the body; slurred speech; difficulty speaking or understanding speech (aphasia); visual disturbances; headache and dizziness; incontinence; and, in the worst cases, seizure. See Chapter 18, *Neurologic Emergencies*, for more information on stroke assessment.

Hemorrhagic strokes, in which a broken blood vessel causes bleeding in the brain, are less common and more likely to be fatal. Ischemic strokes occur when a blood clot blocks the flow of blood to a portion of the brain. Brain tissue distal to this clot is deprived of oxygen and will die if the clot is not broken down.

The treatment goal is to save as much of the surrounding brain tissue as possible. Many communities now have stroke centers that specialize in fast, effective treatment of stroke. There are even a few ambulances equipped with computed tomography (CT) scanners that are dispatched to stroke patients. Determining the onset of the symptoms of stroke is important. If the symptoms occurred within the past few hours, the patient may be a candidate for stroke center therapy and has a higher chance for recovery. In some centers with very advanced capabilities, efforts to restore perfusion to brain tissue by removing the clot can be helpful in limiting long-term disability as long as 24 hours after initial onset of symptoms. Remember that a transient ischemic attack can have the same signs and symptoms as a stroke. Always manage the patient as if he or she is experiencing a stroke unless medical control directs otherwise.

## Changes in the Nervous System

### Anatomy and Physiology

Aging produces changes in the nervous system that are reflected in the neurologic examination. Changes in thinking speed, memory, and posture stability are the most common normal findings in older people. Studies have documented age-associated declines in mental function, especially slower central processing of sensory stimuli and language, and longer retrieval times for short- and long-term memory.

The brain decreases in weight (10% to 20%) and volume as a person ages. This increases the amount of space in the cranium, thus increasing the chance for brain injuries. In addition, there is a 5% to 50% loss of neurons in older people. Neurons are responsible for transmission of impulses, so the motor and sensory neural networks slow down with age. This affects the control of the rate and depth of breathing, heart rate, blood pressure, hunger, thirst, and body temperature. However, the functional significance of these changes is not clear. The human brain has an enormous reserve capacity, and having a smaller, lighter brain does not necessarily interfere with the mental capabilities of all older people, as evidenced by older people who remain active and productive.

The senses can deteriorate with age, which can be detrimental to the patient's overall health. Visual changes may begin as early as age 40 years, such that as many as 50% of patients older than 65 years have vision problems. Causes of visual impairment in older people may include diabetic retinopathy and age-related macular degeneration.

### Vision

Visual acuity, depth perception, and the ability of the eyes to accommodate to light are factors that change with age. The pupils require more time to adjust, which can make driving and even walking more hazardous (**FIGURE 36-3**). Cataracts, clouding of the lenses or their surrounding membranes, interfere with vision and make it difficult to distinguish colors and see clearly, increasing the likelihood of falls, accidents, and mistakes in taking medications. Decreased tear production leads to drier eyes. An inability to differentiate colors and decreased night vision develop in older people, affecting their ability to drive.

## YOU are the Provider

You arrive at the scene and are met at the door by the patient's daughter. She advises you that her mother has emphysema and that her respiratory distress has worsened during the past few days. You find the patient sitting in a chair in her living room; she has a blanket wrapped around her and is in mild respiratory distress. You introduce yourself to the patient and perform a primary assessment.

| Recording Time: 0 Minutes | |
| --- | --- |
| **Appearance** | Obvious respiratory distress; chills |
| **Level of consciousness** | Conscious but confused |
| **Airway** | Open; clear of secretions and foreign bodies |
| **Breathing** | Increased rate; labored |
| **Circulation** | Radial pulse irregular and weak; skin pink, warm, and dry; no obvious bleeding |

The patient is using home oxygen at 2 L/min via nasal cannula. She lives alone, but her daughter visits daily. The patient's home appears to be well kept, and you can see numerous medication containers on a nearby table.

**3.** What is the GEMS diamond? How can it facilitate your overall care of an older patient?

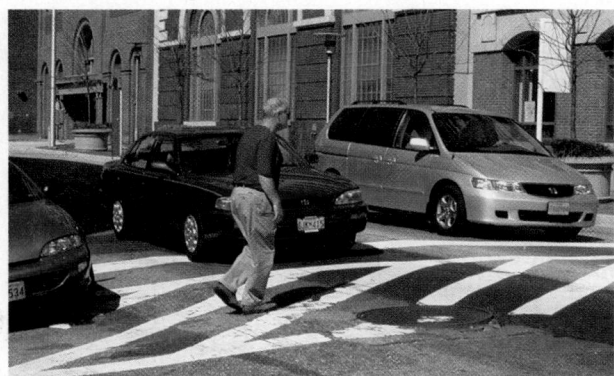

**FIGURE 36-3** Changes in vision, hearing, posture, and motor ability predispose older people to a greater risk of being struck by a vehicle or being involved in a motor vehicle crash.

© Jones & Bartlett Learning. Courtesy of MIEMSS.

Many other disease processes affect the vision of older adults. These can include glaucoma, macular degeneration, and retinal detachment. Increased intraocular pressure is a risk factor for glaucoma, which can cause damage to the optic nerve. It sometimes causes headache with nausea and vomiting and visual disturbances. Macular degeneration is a deterioration of the macula, which is in the central portion of the retina; this condition generally affects adults older than 50 years. It causes a vision loss in the central part of the visual field. Retinal detachment is a medical emergency requiring prompt surgical treatment to preserve vision. In retinal detachment, the retina is pulled away from the choroid, a thin layer of blood vessels that supply nutrients and oxygen to the retina. This condition leaves the retinal cells deprived of oxygen; therefore, there is a potential for permanent vision loss. The patient may report floaters, debris in the visual field, sudden flashes of light or shadow, or visual blurring.

## Hearing

Hearing is the sensory change that affects most older people. Typical hearing problems cause changes in the inner ear and make high-frequency sounds difficult to detect. Changes in the ear can also cause problems with balance and make falls more likely. Presbycusis is age-related hearing loss. Over time, the wear and tear on the ears from noise damages the inner ear. Heredity and long-term exposure to loud noises are the main factors that contribute to hearing loss. When assessing your patient, check for the use of hearing aids. If the patient wears hearing aids, ensure that the aids are properly in place and turned on. If the patient's condition warrants, allow the patient to put in his or her hearing aids, or at least consider bringing them to the hospital so the patient can communicate with the health care staff.

### Street Smarts

Some older patients with hearing loss may direct you to their "good ear" when you speak to them. Be patient and work to facilitate communication. If the patient has difficulty hearing, consider writing your questions.

## Taste

Even the sense of taste can be diminished for an older person because of a decrease in the number of taste buds. The negative result might be lessened interest in eating, which can lead to weight loss, malnutrition, and complaints of fatigue.

## Touch

An older person may have a decreased sense of touch and pain perception from the loss of the end nerve fibers. This loss, in conjunction with the slowing of the peripheral nervous system, can create situations in which an older person may be injured and not feel it. Specifically, there is a decreased sensation of hot and cold. An older person may be slow to react when touching something hot. This delayed response to pain could result in a more severe burn. This is an especially acute problem in people with diabetes, who also lose sensation because of diabetic neuropathy or nerve damage.

## Pathophysiology
### Dementia

You may come across an older patient who is exhibiting delusions, hallucinations, or aggressive behavior. This patient may have dementia. Dementia is the gradual onset of progressive disorientation, shortened attention span, and loss of cognitive function. It is a chronic, generally irreversible condition that causes a progressive loss of cognitive abilities, psychomotor skills, and social skills. Dementia develops slowly over a period of years rather than a few days. Dementia is the result of many neurologic diseases. Alzheimer disease, Parkinson disease, cerebrovascular accidents, and genetic factors may cause dementia.

To help you determine the patient's normal mental status, question family members or friends if present at the scene. You should also evaluate the history, risk factors, and current medications. Never assume confusion is a normal state for the patient unless the family provides evidence to believe so. In addition, never assume confusion is just a normal part of growing old.

Other aspects of dementia can complicate your ability to assess and treat the patient. Sometimes patients are not only confused, but angry as well. They may be poor historians and have impaired judgment. Patients may be unable to vocalize areas of pain and current symptoms, or they may be unable to follow commands. Patients may exhibit disorganized thoughts: inattention, memory loss, disorientation, hallucinations, delusions, and a reduced level of consciousness.

Patients with dementia may express anxiety over movement from their current residence. They may not understand why they need to go to the hospital and often express anxiety and fear of treatment. Their level of tolerance to changes in their routine may be very low. You have to exercise tolerance and patience with patients who have altered mental status or are experiencing dementia.

## Special Populations

Alzheimer disease is a common cause of dementia. Although its cause is unknown, the disease results in loss of brain tissue. Symptoms include memory loss, lack of spontaneity, subtle personality changes, disorientation, impaired thinking, restlessness, agitation, wandering, impaired judgment, and inappropriate social behavior. In late stages of the disease, the patient shows indifference to food, an inability to communicate, incontinence, and seizures. Patients with Alzheimer disease may live at home with a spouse or child who is also the caregiver or they may live in a specialized nursing facility. As with all patients, you must treat patients with Alzheimer disease with patience and respect.

## Delirium

Delirium is a sudden change in mental status, consciousness, or cognitive processes, and is marked by the inability to focus, think logically, and maintain attention.

Acute anxiety may be present in addition to the other symptoms. Usually, memory remains intact. Delirium is commonly marked by acute or recent onset and is a red flag for some type of new health problem. This condition is generally the result of a reversible physical ailment, such as a tumor, fever, or medication change. However, delirium can also have metabolic causes. Anytime a patient has an acute onset of delirious behavior, consider the evaluation of pathophysiology through history, possible risk factors, and current medications.

Other important things to look for in the history are intoxication or withdrawal from alcohol; withdrawal from sedatives; medical conditions such as a urinary tract infection (UTI) (caused by bacteria), bowel obstruction, dehydration, fever, cardiovascular disease, and hyperglycemia or hypoglycemia; psychiatric disorders such as depression; malnutrition or vitamin deficiencies; and environmental emergencies.

Assess the patient for the following specific conditions that can be managed at the prehospital level:

- Hypoxia
- Hypovolemia
- Hypoglycemia
- Hypothermia

Any of these four conditions, if unrecognized or untreated, can be fatal. With these conditions, delirium has a rapid onset and is usually curable if identified early. The onset may be described in terms of minutes, hours, or days. Critical basic life support and ALS interventions may include supplemental oxygen, treatment of shock, administration of glucose, and rewarming measures.

During the physical examination, you may see changes in circulation, breath sounds, motor function, and pupillary response. Hypotension can be an indication of hypovolemia. Dilated pupils may suggest brain damage from hypoxia; earlier hypoxia can lead to pupil constriction. Wheezing, crackles, and rhonchi are the result of disease processes that impair breathing and oxygenation.

Treatment will depend on the results of your assessment but should include airway, ventilatory, and circulatory support appropriate to the patient's condition if tolerated by the patient. ALS personnel will attempt venous access to introduce fluids that will help correct hypovolemia.

## Syncope

You should always assume that syncope, or fainting, in an older patient is caused by a life-threatening problem. Syncope is caused by an interruption of blood flow to the brain. Syncope has many causes: some are serious and others are not. Regardless, an older person who has a period of unconsciousness should be examined by a physician to determine the cause of the syncope. **TABLE 36-2** shows some of the causes of syncope in geriatric patients.

## Neuropathy

Your patient could be experiencing a neuropathy, a disorder of the nerves of the peripheral nervous system in which function and structure of the peripheral motor, sensory, and autonomic neurons are impaired. Symptoms depend on whether the nerves affected are motor, sensory, or autonomic as well as where the nerves are located.

- **Motor nerves:** muscle weakness, cramps, spasms, loss of balance, and loss of coordination
- **Sensory nerves:** tingling, numbness, itching, and pain; burning, freezing, or extreme sensitivity to touch
- **Autonomic nerves:** affect involuntary functions that could include changes in blood pressure and heart rate, sensation of hunger, and the fight-or-flight reflex.

# Changes in the Gastrointestinal System
## Anatomy and Physiology

Changes in the mouth include a reduction in the volume of saliva, with a resulting dryness of the mouth. Dental loss is not a normal result of the aging process, but rather the result of disease of the teeth and gums; nevertheless, dental loss is widespread in the geriatric population and can contribute to nutritional and digestive problems. Both of these oral changes increase the risk of choking.

Like oral secretions, gastric secretions are reduced as a person ages—although enough acid is still present to produce ulcers under certain conditions. Changes in gastric motility also occur, which may lead to slower gastric emptying—a factor of some importance when assessing the risk of aspiration.

Small and large bowel function changes little because of aging, although the incidence of certain diseases involving the bowel (such as diverticulosis) increases as a person grows older. In addition, nutrients from food are not as readily absorbed.

Blood flow to the liver declines. There are changes in hepatic enzyme systems, with some systems declining in activity and others increasing. Notably, the ability of the liver to detoxify and remove drugs from the bloodstream declines as a person ages.

## Pathophysiology

Gastrointestinal issues in older people are attributable to changes related to age or to the diseases that come with advanced age. Age-related changes in the gastrointestinal system include poor muscle

| **TABLE 36-2** Possible Causes of Syncope in Geriatric Patients | |
|---|---|
| **Cause** | **Description** |
| Dysrhythmias and heart attack | The heart is beating too fast or too slowly, the cardiac output drops, and blood flow to the brain is interrupted. A heart attack can also cause syncope. |
| Vascular and volume changes | Medication interactions can cause venous pooling and vasodilation, the widening of a blood vessel that results in a drop in blood pressure and inadequate blood flow to the brain. Another cause of syncope can be a drop in blood volume because of hidden bleeding (such as an aneurysm). |
| Neurologic cause | Syncope can be a sign of transient ischemic attack or stroke. |

tone of the smooth muscle sphincter between the esophagus and stomach that can cause regurgitation and lead to heartburn and acid reflux. Other changes include a decrease in hydrochloric acid in the stomach and alterations in absorption of nutrients and slowing peristalsis (motion that moves feces through the colon), which can cause constipation. The rectal sphincter may also become weak, resulting in fecal incontinence, or lack of bowel control.

Changes in the liver predispose older people to many problems. The liver, which is responsible for removing toxins and breaking down drugs in the body, shrinks with age. Blood flow to the liver declines, and there is decreased metabolism. This has a direct effect on how medications may affect the patient.

Serious gastrointestinal issues that affect older people are gastrointestinal bleeding caused by disease processes, inflammation, infection, and obstruction of the upper and lower intestinal tract. Gastrointestinal bleeding can include hematemesis (the vomiting of blood) or coffee ground–like vomitus. Bleeding that travels through the lower digestive tract usually manifests as melena (black, tarry stools), whereas red blood usually means a local source of bleeding, such as hemorrhoids. A patient with gastrointestinal bleeding may experience weakness, dizziness, or syncope. Bleeding into the gastrointestinal system can be life threatening because of the potential for blood loss and shock.

Specific gastrointestinal problems that are more common in older patients include diverticulitis, bleeding in the upper and lower gastrointestinal system, peptic ulcer disease, gallbladder disease, and bowel obstruction. Diverticulosis is a condition in which the walls of the gut weaken and small pouches protrude from the colon along those weakened segments. When inflammation usually associated with infection develops in one of these pouches, the condition is called diverticulitis. A geriatric patient with diverticulitis generally presents with left lower quadrant pain and fever. Fever suggests a condition that requires immediate attention.

Upper gastrointestinal bleeding occurs in the esophagus, stomach, or duodenum. These bleeding episodes are sometimes seen in people who are long-term users of nonsteroidal anti-inflammatory drugs (NSAIDs), such as celecoxib (Celebrex), ibuprofen, and naproxen, or people who are long-term alcohol users. Irritation of the lining of the stomach or ulcers can cause forceful vomiting that tears the esophagus. Hepatitis and cancer can also contribute to bleeding problems.

Lower gastrointestinal bleeding occurs in the colon or rectum. Lower gastrointestinal bleeding can be serious, especially in cases where the patient presents with tachycardia and hypotension.

Peptic ulcer disease is more common in older adults, especially people who use NSAIDs. The patient will report a gnawing, burning pain in the upper abdomen that improves after eating but returns later. Complications of peptic ulcer disease include bleeding, anemia, and bowel perforation, which are medical emergencies.

Gallbladder disease is more common in older adults, and they have a higher risk of complications from gallstones. The risk of death from surgery to remove the gallbladder increases with age. Patients with inflammation of the gallbladder, or cholecystitis, will have fever and right upper quadrant pain that may radiate to the shoulder. Patients may also have jaundice, which is a yellow appearance of the eyes and skin. This condition is dangerous because the infection can spread to the blood, causing sepsis and shock.

Bowel obstructions occur frequently in the geriatric population. The ability of the gastrointestinal tract to move feces through the system slows with aging, and patients can experience problems having bowel movements. When patients strain to have a bowel movement, they can stimulate the vagus nerve, which can cause a vasovagal response; this is a condition in which the heart rate drops dramatically and the patient becomes dizzy or passes out. The patient will usually be in stable condition on your arrival but requires transport to rule out other conditions.

In general, patients with gastrointestinal issues are agitated and are unable to find a comfortable position. When assessing patients with gastrointestinal problems, ask about NSAID and alcohol use. Presentation can include pale or yellow, thin skin; frail musculoskeletal system; peripheral, sacral, and periorbital edema; hypertension; fever; tachycardia; and dyspnea.

Orthostatic vital signs can help determine if a patient is hypovolemic. Blood pressure and pulse rates are taken with the patient lying down, and again after standing for 2 minutes. Note any drop in blood pressure and increase in heart rate that occur as the patient moves to an upright position if these values do not normalize after 2 minutes. Do not attempt to assess orthostatic vitals on a patient with obvious signs of shock, hypotension, altered level of consciousness, or possible spinal injury.

Treatment consists of airway, ventilatory, and circulatory support.

## The Acute Abdomen— Nongastrointestinal Complaints

Because of an aging nervous system, abdominal complaints in geriatric patients may be more difficult to assess. Several life-threatening problems are common in older patients. In the prehospital setting, the most serious threat from abdominal complaints is blood loss, which can lead to shock and death. Abdominal aortic aneurysm (AAA) is one of the most rapidly fatal conditions. An AAA tends to develop in people who have a history of hypertension and atherosclerosis. The walls of the aorta weaken, and blood begins to leak into the layers of the vessel, causing the aorta to bulge like a bubble on a tire. If enough blood loss occurs into the vessel wall itself, shock occurs. If the vessel wall bursts, it rapidly leads to fatal blood loss. When the problem is found early, there is a chance to repair the vessel before rupture, and fatal blood loss is less likely to occur.

A patient with an AAA most commonly reports abdominal pain radiating through to the back. If the AAA becomes large enough, it can be felt as a pulsating mass just above and slightly to the left of the navel during your physical examination, though this is rare. If you see or palpate a pulsating mass, do not continue manipulation or allow other providers to palpate the mass. Occasionally, the AAA causes a decrease in blood flow to one of the legs, and the patient reports some discomfort in the affected extremity. Assessment may also reveal diminished or absent pulses in the extremity. Compensated shock (early shock) and decompensated shock (late shock) as a result of blood loss are common occurrences. Because of a decrease in blood volume and decreased blood flow to the brain, the patient may experience syncope. You should treat the patient for shock, including high-flow oxygen and thermal regulation, and ensure prompt transport to the hospital.

# Changes in the Renal System
## Anatomy and Physiology

The genitourinary system includes the reproductive organs and the urinary system. The largest component of the urinary system is the kidneys, or renal organs. Age-related changes in the genitourinary system specific to the kidney include a reduction in renal function, a reduction in renal blood flow, and tubule degeneration. For the genitourinary system in general, there is decreased bladder capacity, decline in sphincter muscle control, decline in voiding senses, increase in nocturnal voiding, and, in men, benign prostatic hypertrophy (enlarged prostate).

Age brings changes in the kidneys as well. The kidneys are responsible for maintaining the body's fluid and electrolyte balance and have important roles in maintaining the body's long-term acid–base balance and eliminating drugs from the body. In a young adult, the kidneys weigh 8 to 9 oz (250 to 270 g); in a healthy 70-year-old, they weigh 6 to 7 oz (180 to 200 g). This decline in weight results from a loss of functioning nephron units, or tubule degeneration, translating into a smaller effective filtering surface. At the same time, renal blood flow decreases by as much as 50% as a person ages.

## Pathophysiology

Although the kidneys of an older person may be capable of dealing with day-to-day demands, they may not be able to meet unusual challenges, such as those imposed by illness. For that reason, acute illness in older patients is often accompanied by derangements in fluid and electrolyte balance. Aging kidneys, for example, respond sluggishly to sodium deficiency. An older patient may experience substantial sodium loss before the kidneys halt urinary sodium excretion, a problem that is exacerbated by the markedly decreased thirst mechanism in older people. The net result may be a rapid development of severe dehydration.

Bowel and bladder continence require anatomically correct gastrointestinal and genitourinary tracts, functioning and intact sphincters, and properly working cognitive and physical functions. Urinary incontinence (involuntary loss of urine) can have significant social and emotional effects, but relatively few people admit to the problem and even fewer seek treatment. Incontinence is not a normal part of aging and can lead to skin irritation, skin breakdown, and UTIs. As people age, the capacity of the bladder decreases. Therefore, an older person may find it difficult to postpone voiding or may have involuntary bladder contractions. An increase in nocturnal voiding is common. Two major types of incontinence are distinguished: stress and urge. Stress incontinence occurs during activities such as coughing, laughing, sneezing, lifting, and exercise. Urge incontinence occurs when you have a sudden urge to urinate. In urge incontinence, the urinary bladder contracts when it shouldn't, causing some urine to leak through the sphincter muscles holding the bladder closed. Treatment of incontinence consists of medications, physical therapy, and possibly surgery.

The opposite of incontinence is urinary retention or difficulty urinating. Patients may have difficulty voiding or absence of voiding as a result of many medical causes. In men, enlargement of the prostate can place pressure on the urethra, making voiding difficult. Bladder infections and UTIs can also cause inflammation. In severe cases of urinary retention, patients may experience renal failure.

## Changes in the Endocrine System

### Anatomy and Physiology

The endocrine system functions as the control center of the body. It uses hormones to control physiologic processes. A significant change that occurs in an older person is decreased metabolism of thyroxine. This is a thyroid hormone that affects the body's metabolism, temperature, growth, and heart rate. A reduction in thyroid hormones can cause a condition called hypothyroidism. Most of the signs and symptoms people experience are attributed to the process of aging and include slower heart rate, fatigue, drier skin and hair, cold intolerance, and weight gain.

Other endocrine system changes include an increase in the secretion of antidiuretic hormone, causing fluid imbalance; hyperglycemia; and an increase in the levels of norepinephrine, possibly having a harmful effect on the cardiovascular system.

### Pathophysiology

Hyperosmolar hyperglycemic nonketotic syndrome (HHNS) is a diabetic complication in older people, and occurs more often in people with type 2 diabetes than in those with type 1 diabetes. Unlike diabetic ketoacidosis (DKA), the resulting high blood glucose level does not cause ketosis; instead, it leads to osmotic diuresis and a shift of fluid to the intravascular space that results in dehydration. The signs and symptoms of HHNS and DKA often overlap. Associated signs and symptoms include hyperglycemia, polydipsia (thirst), polyuria (urination), and polyphagia (hunger), as well as dizziness, confusion, altered mental status, and possibly seizures.

On assessment, you may see changes in circulation such as warm, flushed skin; poor skin turgor; pale, dry oral mucosa; and a furrowed tongue. The patient may present with signs and symptoms of hypotension and shock, including tachycardia. The blood glucose level will vary in DKA, whereas in HHNS, the value is typically 600 mg/dL or higher. Another assessment difference is that patients with DKA will present with Kussmaul respirations (deep and labored), and patients with HHNS will not.

Assessment of the patient should include obtaining blood pressure, distal pulses, auscultation of breath sounds, temperature, and assessment of blood glucose level if permitted by local protocol.

Treatment should include airway, ventilatory, and circulatory support.

## Changes in the Immune System

Infections are commonly seen in older people because they generally have an increased risk of infection and are less able to fight infections once they occur. With age, systemic and cellular immune responses become less effective at fighting infection. Fevers are unable to develop in many older patients, but these patients may in fact be hypothermic as a manifestation of severe systemic infection. Anorexia, fatigue, weight loss, falls, or changes in mental status may be the primary symptoms of infection in these patients. Pneumonia and UTI are common in patients who are bedridden. When infection occurs, signs and symptoms may be decreased or minimized by the patient because of the loss of sensation, lack of awareness, or fear of being hospitalized.

# Changes in the Musculoskeletal System
## Anatomy and Physiology

Aging brings a widespread decrease in bone mass in men and women, but especially among post-menopausal women. Bones become more brittle and tend to break more easily. The disks between the vertebrae of the spine begin to narrow, and a decrease in height of between 2 and 3 inches (5 and 8 cm) may occur through the lifespan, along with changes in posture. Joints lose their flexibility and motion may be further affected by arthritic changes. In fact, more than one-half of all older people have some form of arthritis. A decrease in the amount of muscle mass often results in less strength.

## Pathophysiology

Changes in physical abilities can affect older adults' confidence in their mobility. The muscle system atrophies and weakens with age. Muscle fibers become smaller and fewer, motor neurons decline in number, and strength declines. The ligaments and cartilage of the joints lose their elasticity. Cartilage also goes through degenerative changes with aging, contributing to arthritis.

The stooped posture of older people comes from atrophy of the supporting structures of the body. Two of every three older patients will show some degree of kyphosis (a forward curling of the spine, also called humpback or hunchback). A loss of height in older adults generally results from compression in the spinal column, first in the disks and then from the process of osteoporosis in the vertebral bodies.

Osteoporosis, a condition that affects both men and women, is characterized by a decrease in bone mass leading to reduction in bone strength and greater susceptibility to fracture. The extent of bone loss that a person undergoes is influenced by numerous factors, including genetics, smoking, level of activity, diet, alcohol consumption, hormonal factors, and body weight. The most rapid loss of bone occurs in women during the years following menopause, and many postmenopausal women use hormone replacement therapy to reduce bone loss. Calcium and vitamin D supplementation is another treatment of the condition, and many other medications, such as diphosphonates, are available to improve bone strength. Older people should remain active and engage in a low-impact exercise program to maintain bone and muscle strength.

## YOU are the Provider

Further assessment of the patient reveals that she has a fever and has not been eating lately. She has a weak cough, which is producing thick, green sputum. Auscultation of her breath sounds reveals coarse rhonchi in all fields. Your partner takes her vital signs as you ask additional questions regarding her past medical history.

| Recording Time: 5 Minutes | |
| --- | --- |
| **Respirations** | 22 breaths/min; labored |
| **Pulse** | 68 beats/min; weak and irregular |
| **Skin** | Hot to the touch; pink and dry |
| **Blood pressure** | 158/88 mm Hg |
| **Oxygen saturation (Spo₂)** | 92% on 2 L/min oxygen via nasal cannula |

The patient's daughter advises you that in addition to emphysema, her mother has hypertension, atrial fibrillation, rheumatoid arthritis, and Alzheimer disease. You inquire about her confusion, and her daughter tells you that it has worsened in the past couple of days. She hands you a list of medications and states that she personally gives her mother her medications every day.

**4.** Based on the patient's current condition, how appropriate is the current oxygen therapy?

**5.** What should concern you about patients who take numerous medications?

**6.** What other assessments, if any, should be performed for this patient?

Osteoarthritis is a progressive disease of the joints that destroys cartilage, promotes the formation of bone spurs in joints, and leads to joint stiffness. This type of arthritis is thought to result from "wear and tear" and, in some cases, from repetitive trauma to the joints. It affects 35% to 45% of the population older than 65 years. Typically, osteoarthritis affects several joints of the body, most commonly those in the hands, knees, hips, and spine. Patients report pain and stiffness that gets worse with exertion. The end result is often substantial disability and disfigurement. Patients are typically treated first with anti-inflammatory medications and physical therapy to improve the range of motion. Joint replacement surgery is often effective for arthritis of the hip, knee, ankle, and shoulder when nonsurgical treatment fails.

## Changes in Skin

The proteins that make the skin pliable decline with age. The layer of fat under the skin also becomes thinner because of the redistribution of fluids and proteins. As the elasticity of the skin declines, bruising becomes more common because the skin can tear more easily. Exocrine (sweat) glands do not respond as readily to heat because of atrophy and because of changes to the tissues in the dermal layer of the skin.

Another problem that affects the skin is pressure ulcers, sometimes referred to as bedsores or decubitus ulcers. Pressure ulcers form when a patient is lying or sitting in the same position for a long time. The pressure from the weight of the body cuts off the blood flow to the area of skin. With no blood flow to the skin, a sore develops. These sores can develop in as little as 45 minutes. To help prevent these ulcers, take special care to pad under any bony prominences and in the voids under a patient. Placing a geriatric patient on a backboard can cause significant injury to the patient's skin.

You may see these ulcers in the following various stages of development:

- **Stage I:** Nonblanching redness with damage under the skin
- **Stage II:** Blister or ulcer that can affect the dermis and epidermis
- **Stage III:** Invasion of the fat layer through to the fascia
- **Stage IV:** Invasion to muscle or bone

Decubitus ulcers can be painful and cause complications such as bleeding, sepsis, and bone infection, called osteomyelitis.

## Toxicology

Several pathophysiologic changes cause older people to be susceptible to toxicity. These changes include decreased kidney function, altered gastrointestinal absorption, and decreased vascular flow in the liver that alters metabolism and excretion. The kidneys undergo many changes with age. The rate of filtration decreases an average of 50% between the ages of 50 and 90 years. Decreased liver function makes it harder for the liver to detoxify the blood and eliminate substances such as medications and alcohol. These metabolic issues can also make it difficult for physicians to find the appropriate dosage for new medications.

The use of medications by older people accounts for one-fourth of the prescribed medications and one-third of the over-the-counter (OTC) medications sold in the United States. Typical OTC medicines used by older people include aspirin, antacids, cough syrups, and decongestants (**FIGURE 36-4**). Many people believe OTC medications cannot be dangerous, but these medications can have negative effects when mixed with each other and/or with alcohol, and prescription medications.

The use of herbal supplements is common. Much like with OTC medications, many people believe that herbal supplements are safe and commonly will not mention taking them when asked about medications. The EMT should specifically ask about any supplements a patient takes, either alone or in addition to prescribed and OTC medications. Many supplements are safe, but some can pose a risk to patients. For example, St. John's wort can create serious symptoms when mixed with antidepressants, and ginkgo biloba should not be taken with blood thinners such as warfarin due to a potential increased risk of bleeding.

Polypharmacy refers to the use of multiple prescription medications by one patient. For example, a single patient may have more than one physician—for example, a primary physician for everyday care, a cardiologist for the heart, and an endocrinologist for the care of diabetes. All of them may prescribe medication. This problem can be less of an issue if the patient receives all of his or her

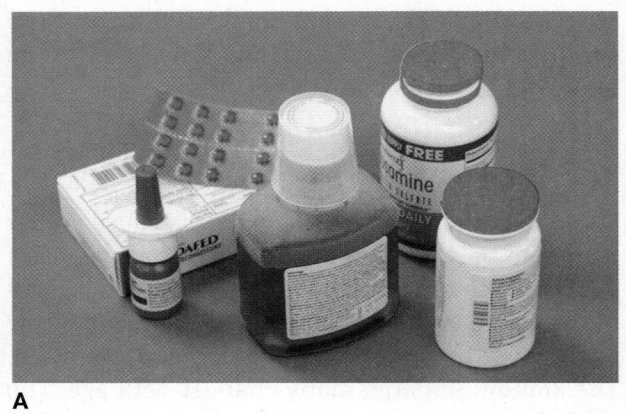

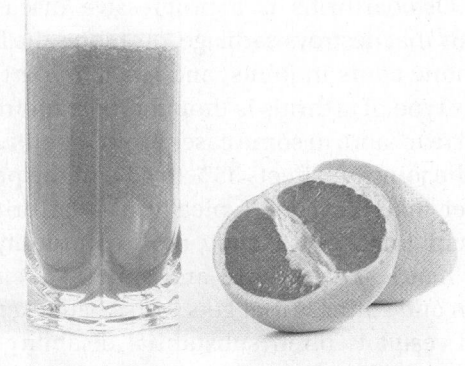

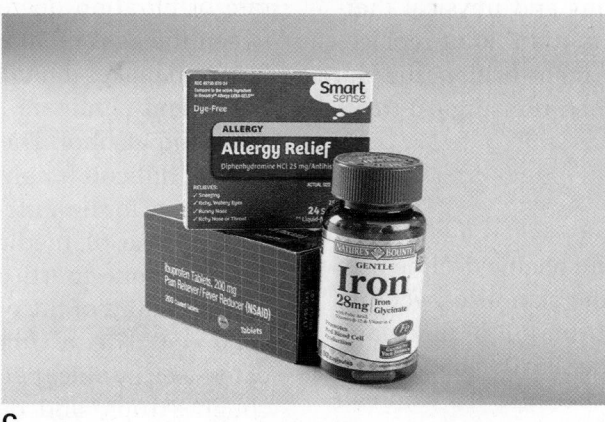

**FIGURE 36-4 A.** Over-the-counter medications such as aspirin, antacids, cough syrups, and decongestants can interact negatively with some prescription medications. **B.** Grapefruit juice cannot be taken with several medications because it can significantly increase the levels of those medications in the blood. **C.** Over-the-counter medicines such as diphenhydramine (Benadryl), nonsteroidal anti-inflammatory drugs, iron preparations, and mineral oil (used for constipation) were once thought to be harmless, but are now known to be potentially harmful in older adults.

care within an integrated health system that maintains an electronic medical record that includes information from multiple physicians and health care providers, but this is not always the case. In addition, many drugstore chains have a computerized database that can recognize multiple prescriptions, but this setup is helpful only if the patient deals exclusively with that one drugstore chain. Some states have developed health information exchanges to facilitate exchange of information between providers and pharmacies and decrease risk to the patients.

Negative effects of polypharmacy can include overdosing and negative medication interactions. Adverse reactions occur when medications taken together change the absorption, distribution, or excretion of medications in the body or the effects of the medications on the body.

Another complication associated with polypharmacy is the fact that a patient may have multiple prescriptions of different amounts that need to be taken at different times of the day. Patients can easily forget what they have taken and overdose or forget to take them at all and underdose. Both scenarios can lead to serious problems.

Medication noncompliance in older patients is also an issue and may occur because of financial challenges; inability to open containers; or impaired cognitive, vision, and hearing ability. If you suspect medication noncompliance, you should check prescription dates and the number of pills available.

The geriatric population is more likely to have cases of polypharmacy because older people are affected most by the process of aging. Physiologic factors known to be true about the hepatic and renal functions of excretion and metabolism of medications can change in the face of multiple prescriptions being consumed at once. Always be mindful of this issue when obtaining the patient's medication history.

# Behavioral Emergencies

For most older people, the later years are ones of fulfillment and satisfaction with a lifetime of accomplishments. For some older adults, however, later life is characterized by physical pain, emotional distress, doubts about the significance of life's accomplishments, financial concerns, loss of loved ones, dissatisfaction with living conditions, and seemingly unbearable disability. When these factors lead to hopelessness about the possibility for positive change in their lives, depression and, unfortunately, even suicide are possible outcomes. You are often the first health care professional to have contact with older adults who are depressed and, for some older patients, the only health care contact.

## Depression

Depression is not part of normal aging, but rather a medical disease. This common, often debilitating psychiatric disorder affects millions of older Americans. Older adults residing in skilled nursing facilities are even more likely to be depressed. Depression is diagnosed three times more commonly in women than in men. In contrast with the normal emotional experiences of sadness, grief, loss, and temporary bad moods, depression is extreme and persistent and can interfere significantly with an older adult's ability to function.

The good news is that depression is treatable with medication and therapy. The bad news is that if depression goes unrecognized or untreated, it is associated with a higher suicide rate in the geriatric population than in any other age group. Depression in older patients can mimic the effects of many other medical problems (such as dementia). Risk factors for depression in older people include a history of depression, chronic disease, and loss (function, independence, or significant others).

It is impossible to predict which older adults will have depression, but studies indicate that substance abuse, isolation, prescription medication use, and chronic medical conditions all contribute to the onset of significant depression. Treatment of severe depression in older adults usually consists of behavioral counseling, medication, or a combination of both. For many older adults, simply reestablishing relationships with the community or with family is enough to lessen the severity of the illness.

## Suicide

Depression may be difficult to recognize in older people because many do not want to complain about feeling sad, worthless, or unwanted. Disturbingly, most suicides involving older people occur in people in whom depression has recently been diagnosed. In addition, most suicide victims have seen their primary care physician within the month before the event.

Older men have the highest suicide rate of any age group in the United States. Caucasian men older than 65 years are eight times more likely to kill themselves than women of the same age. The suicide rate among older Caucasian men is almost twice the rate of all other male groups. At highest risk are white men age 85 years and older, who use firearms as their suicide method of choice. Older people who attempt suicide choose much more lethal means than younger victims and generally have diminished recuperative capacity to survive an attempt. Unlike younger people, geriatric patients typically do not make suicidal gestures or attempt to get help. Instead, the rate of completed suicide is disproportionately high in the geriatric population. Many geriatric patients see no other way out when they have a terminal illness or debilitating cardiac or neurologic condition (such as severe heart disease or stroke).

Suicide can happen in any family, regardless of socioeconomic class, culture, race, or religious affiliation. Some common predisposing events and conditions include death of a loved one, physical illness, depression and hopelessness, alcohol abuse, alcohol dependence, and loss of meaningful life roles. Keep in mind that only a small percentage of older people pursue medical treatment for behavioral issues. Not only do many older adults fail to seek care, but they also frequently deny the problem when asked about it. When assessing the patient who is displaying signs of depression, it is appropriate to ask if he or she is considering suicide. If the answer is "yes," the next question should be "Do you have a plan?" Include this information in your documentation and in your report as you transfer care at the hospital. It is vital that all members of the health care team be aware of these issues and take appropriate steps to ensure their own safety, as well as patient safety.

> ### Street Smarts
>
> A geriatric patient who has taken too much of a medication may have simply made an error, but it is possible that the patient was attempting suicide. Consider the possibility of depression and suicidal thoughts when conducting your assessment.

## The GEMS Diamond

When you are called on to care for older patients, it is important to remember certain key concepts. The GEMS diamond (**TABLE 36-3**) was created to help you remember differences in older patients compared with the rest of the population. The GEMS diamond is not intended to be a format for your approach to geriatric patients, nor is it intended to replace the XABCs of care. Instead, it is an acronym for the issues to be considered when assessing every older patient.

The "G" of the GEMS diamond stands for "geriatric patients." When responding to an emergency involving an older patient, you should consider that older patients are different from younger patients and may present as such. Be familiar with the normal changes of aging and treat older patients with compassion and respect.

The "E" of the GEMS diamond stands for an environmental assessment. Assessment of the environment can help give clues to the patient's condition and the cause of the emergency. Is the home too hot or too cold? Is it well kept? Is it secure from intruders? Are there hazardous conditions, such as trip hazards or loose (or absent) railings? Preventive care is also very important for a geriatric patient, who may not carefully study the environment or may not realize where risks exist.

The "M" of the GEMS diamond stands for medical assessment. As stated, older patients tend to have a variety of medical problems and may be taking numerous prescriptions, and OTC and herbal medications. Obtaining a thorough medical history is very important in older patients.

The "S" stands for social assessment. Older people may have a smaller social network because of the death of a spouse, family members, and friends. Older people may also need assistance with activities of daily living (ADLs), such as dressing and eating. There are numerous social agencies that are readily available to help geriatric patients. Consider obtaining information pamphlets about some of the agencies for older people in your area. If you have these brochures with you and encounter a person in need, you can provide this valuable information. Social agencies that deal with the older population will be more than happy to share a listing of the services they provide.

The GEMS diamond provides an organized way to remember the important issues for older patients. Using this concept will help you make appropriate referrals, and, as a result, you will help older patients maintain their quality of life.

## Special Considerations in Assessing a Geriatric Medical Patient

Assessing an older person can be challenging because of communication issues, hearing and vision deficits, alteration in consciousness, complicated medical histories, and the effects of medications. Previous injury or illnesses that are not associated with the current problem may also alter the assessment findings. These may include medications that mask changes in vital signs that you might expect, such as tachycardia in shock. A previous stroke may have changed a patient's baseline level of consciousness and neurologic status.

> ### Words of Wisdom
>
> Medical and trauma conditions are often superimposed on each other. A simple fall may have been preceded by weakness and dizziness, suggesting a serious medical condition. What looks like an obvious trauma call could easily have been caused by a serious medical emergency.

## TABLE 36-3 The GEMS Diamond

### G Geriatric Patients

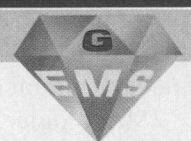

- Present atypically
- Deserve respect
- Experience changes with age

### E Environmental Assessment

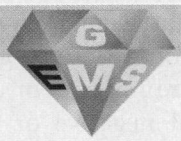

- What is the physical condition of the living space? Is the interior or exterior of the home in need of repair? Is the home secure?
- Are hazardous conditions present (eg, poor wiring, uneven floors, unventilated gas heaters, broken window glass, clutter that prevents adequate egress)?
- Are smoke detectors present and functional?
- Is the home too hot or too cold?
- Is there a fecal or urine odor in the home?
- Are pets well cared for?
- Is food present in the home? Is it adequate and unspoiled?
- Are liquor bottles present (lying empty)?
- Is bedding soiled or dirty?
- If the patient has a disability, are appropriate assistive devices (such as a wheelchair or walker) present and in adequate condition?
- Does the patient have access to a telephone?
- Are medications prescribed, expired, unmarked, or from multiple physicians?
- If the patient is living with others, is he or she confined to one part of the home?
- If the patient is residing in a nursing facility, does the care appear to be adequate to meet the patient's needs?

### M Medical Assessment

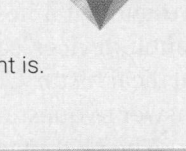

- Older patients tend to have a variety of medical problems, making assessment more complex. Keep this in mind in all cases—that is, both trauma and medical. A trauma patient may have an underlying medical condition related to the traumatic event.
- Obtaining a medical history is very important in older patients—no matter what the primary complaint is.
- Primary assessment
- Reassessment

### S Social Assessment

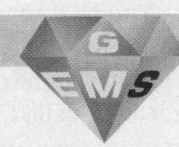

- Assess the activities of daily living (ADLs):
  - Eating
  - Dressing
  - Bathing
  - Toileting
- Are these activities being provided for the patient? If so, by whom?
- Are there delays in obtaining food, medication, or hygiene? The patient may report this, or the environment may be suggestive of this.
- Does the patient have regular visits from family members, live with family members, or live with a spouse?
- If in an institutional setting, is the patient able to feed himself or herself? If not, is food still sitting on the food tray? Has the patient been lying in his or her own urine or feces for prolonged periods of time?
- Does the patient have a social network? Does the patient have ways to interact socially with others on a daily basis?

National Association of Emergency Medical Technicians NAEMT. *Geriatric Education for Emergency Medical Services, Second Edition.* Burlington, MA: Jones & Bartlett Learning, 2014.

## Scene Size-up

Every emergency call begins with a thorough scene size-up. Is the scene safe? How many patients do you have? What is the nature of illness (NOI)? Have you taken proper standard precautions?

Geriatric patients are commonly found in their own homes, retirement homes, or skilled nursing facilities, but calls for assistance can come from any location. Many older people live alone. Access to them may be hampered if their condition prevents them from getting to the door to let you in. Police or fire department assistance may be required.

Many older people try to maintain their independence as long as they can. They may or may not have someone who checks on their welfare. You will find some people living in conditions that are not safe or appropriate. You need to take note of negative or unsafe environmental conditions. Is the home well maintained and sanitary? Are the utilities working? Look for clues that might explain the patient's medical history or current problem: Is it too hot or too cold? A geriatric patient can have hypothermia or heatstroke in temperatures that are not considered extreme. Is there food available? Is the refrigerator stocked? Is there evidence of abuse or alcohol or illegal drug use? Are there medications on the nightstand in the bedroom?

In a nursing home or residential care facility, you will need to locate the patient's room and find a staff member who can explain why you were called. In any case in which the patient's mental status is altered, you need to find someone who can tell you the patient's history and whether the patient's behavior or level of consciousness is normal or altered. The presence of a hospital bed, oxygen tanks, or therapeutic devices can give you a clue to the patient's medical history. The environment may give you the answer to questions when the patient cannot.

The NOI may be difficult to determine in older people who may have an altered mental status or dementia. Often it is someone other than the patient who called, so you must ask the family member, caregiver, or bystander why he or she called. Multiple and chronic disease processes may also complicate the determination of the NOI. Complaints from an older person may be vague, such as weakness, dizziness, or fatigue. These could be indicators of a more serious problem and require more assessment. You may need to specifically ask why the person called to determine acute versus chronic complaints. Chest pain, shortness of breath, and an altered level of consciousness should always be considered serious. You also may find that the patient's complaint is a symptom of something more serious. For example, sudden changes in the ability to talk could indicate a stroke, or the need to sleep on five pillows could suggest early congestive heart failure.

## Primary Assessment

Once you have confirmed that the scene is safe, perform the primary assessment to address life threats such as problems with airway, breathing, and circulation. Determine the priority of your patient based on his or her condition. The priority of your patient may limit on-scene time and/or treatment. Maintain a high index of suspicion for serious injuries even with mechanisms of injury that might seem minor in younger patients.

The general impression is an important aspect of all patient assessment. As you approach the patient, you should be able to tell if the patient is generally in a stable or unstable condition. You will use this information to help you with your further assessment. Use the AVPU scale to determine the patient's level of consciousness.

Remember that anatomic changes that occur as a person ages predispose geriatric patients to airway problems. Aging and disease can compromise a patient's ability to protect his or her airway with loss of a gag reflex and normal swallowing mechanisms. Changes in level of consciousness, dementia, and post-stroke weakness or paralysis can cause airway obstruction or aspiration. Ensure that the patient's airway is open and is not obstructed by dentures, vomitus, fluids, or blood. Suction may be necessary.

Anatomic changes with aging also affect a person's ability to breathe effectively. Increased chest wall stiffness, brittle bones, weakening of the airway musculature, and decreased muscle mass contribute to breathing problems. Loss of mechanisms that protect the upper airway, such as cough and gag reflexes, cause a decreased ability to clear secretions. A decrease in the number of cilia that line the bronchioles results in the inability of the patient to remove material from the lungs, which can cause infection. In some patients, the alveoli are damaged, and a lack of elasticity results in a decreased ability to exchange oxygen and carbon dioxide. Superimposed on the physiologic changes are the chronic respiratory diseases common in older people that affect the ability of the patient to breathe effectively. Airway and breathing issues should be treated rapidly and monitored constantly.

Poor perfusion is a serious issue in an older adult. People who normally live with compromised circulation have little in the way of reserves during a circulatory crisis. Physiologic changes may negatively affect circulation. Less responsive nerve stimulation may lower the rate and strength of the heart's contractions, so lower heart rates and weaker and irregular pulses are common in older patients. Vascular changes and circulatory compromise might make it difficult to feel a radial pulse on an older patient. If choosing an alternative pulse point such as the carotid, press gently. Another option is to listen to the apical pulse right over the heart. The pulse may be irregular because of common heart rhythm problems. It is important to determine if cardiac abnormalities in an older patient indicate an acute emergency or a chronic condition. Acute emergencies should be managed rapidly.

### Words of Wisdom

Dentures should be left in place unless they obstruct the airway or interfere with ventilation when bag-mask ventilation is needed.

Patient assessment is more complicated in an older adult, and multiple problems can exist. Any complaints that compromise airway, breathing, or circulation should result in transportation of the patient as a priority patient. Priority patients include patients who have a poor general impression, airway or breathing problems, acute altered level of consciousness, shock, any severe pain, or uncontrolled bleeding. Your most important task is to determine conditions that are life threatening, treat them to the best of your ability, and provide transport. Older people do not have the reserves that younger people do, and they can easily decompensate. Even a general complaint of weakness and dizziness can be an indication of something more serious such as a heart problem or pneumonia. Consider early on if ALS treatment and immediate transport is appropriate and available. If possible, try to take the patient to a facility where the patient has been treated before and has an established relationship.

### Words of Wisdom

Because of fear related to hospitalization, many older people will delay calling 9-1-1 until their problem is life threatening. Be prepared for a worst-case scenario.

## History Taking

Begin by inquiring about the chief complaint or history of the present illness. Find and account for all medications. If a patient lives alone, look for a list of medications on the refrigerator or a notice by the front door. The Vial of Life Project is one program that recommends creating a medication history for caregivers or EMS personnel. There may also be similar local programs in your area.

Communication may be more complicated with an older adult, but it is critical that you obtain a thorough patient history. It is best to obtain what information you can directly from the patient, but family or caregivers may need to assist.

The determination should be made early on as to whether an altered level of consciousness is acute or chronic. Remember that chronic mental status impairment is not a normal process of aging but is caused by a pathologic or disease process. You should never accept confusion as normal. It is important for you to determine your patient's baseline mental status; question family members, if available.

Multiple disease processes and multiple and/or vague complaints can make assessment complicated, and older people may not show severe symptoms even if they are very ill. Ask questions to assess the nature of the problem, and determine whether it may or may not be life threatening. Obtain a full set of vital signs, and ask what is normal for that patient. You may be able to determine the exact nature of the problem and will need to use your general impression to guide you.

Getting an accurate SAMPLE history can also be complicated. The chances are good that the chief complaint is related to a chronic medical problem and the patient may have experienced it before. Symptoms should be determined to be acute or chronic. Also note the signs you observe and your general impression. Allergies to food and medications are important. Is the patient taking any new medications? Make sure you have a list of the patient's medications or take the medications with you to the hospital if possible. Patient medications can reveal much information about a patient's history. The hospital will also need to determine if the patient has been taking the medications as instructed. If time and opportunity allow, check the patient's pill sorter. Has the patient taken every dose this week? Has the patient taken the medications that are scheduled for tomorrow or the next day?

The last meal is particularly important in a patient with diabetes. A history of last oral intake can indicate that the patient may be dehydrated. Last, what is the event that prompted the call? Again, it is advantageous to provide transport to a facility that "knows" the patient's medical history if the patient's condition and other factors allow.

## Street Smarts

Some geriatric patients may appear angry and will be curt in their responses. Remember, as they are approaching the end of their life, their hearing and eyesight may be failing and they may be frustrated by having lost much of their independence. Be patient and do not take it personally if a geriatric patient seems upset or seems to be yelling at you.

## Secondary Assessment

The secondary assessment may be performed on scene, en route to the emergency department (ED), or in some cases, not at all. The priority of the patient will determine this for you.

Perform a physical examination when appropriate. You may find that your older patient is not comfortable with being exposed. Protect his or her modesty. Older people are often cold, and you may have to remove several layers of clothing. Consider the need to keep your patient warm during the exam.

Vital signs may be different in older adults because of the physiologic changes that come with aging, chronic disease, and the effects of medications. The heart rate should be in the normal adult range but may be compromised by medications such as beta blockers. These medications keep the heart rate low and prevent the tachycardia that might be typically seen in dehydration or shock. Weak and irregular pulses are common in older patients. The pulse may be irregular secondary to atrial fibrillation. Circulatory compromise may make it difficult to feel a radial pulse on an older patient, and other pulse points may need to be considered.

Blood pressure tends to be higher in older people. A geriatric patient who has a blood pressure in a normal adult range could be hypotensive. Hypertension could signal impending stroke. Try to confirm if the patient has missed taking any medications for hypertension.

Capillary refill is not a good assessment tool in older adults because of skin changes and reduced circulation to the skin.

The respiratory rate should be in the same range as in a younger adult, but remember that chest rise will be compromised by increased chest wall stiffness. Be sure to auscultate breath sounds to listen for crackles associated with pulmonary edema, rhonchi associated with pneumonia, and wheezes associated with asthma.

Careful interpretation of pulse oximetry data is necessary in older adults because the pulse oximetry device requires adequate perfusion to get an accurate reading. Older adults may have poor circulation, vasoconstriction, hypotension, hypothermia, lack of red blood cells, or carbon monoxide poisoning that could result in an inaccurate reading.

## Reassessment

Reassess the geriatric patient based on his or her condition and chief complaint. Repeat the primary assessment. Reassess the vital signs and the patient's complaint. Recheck interventions. Identify and treat changes in the patient's condition.

An older patient with a complaint of shortness of breath will want to sit up or assume the tripod position. Accommodate positioning requests when possible. The position in which you found the patient may be maintaining a patent airway. Forcing a patient who is short of breath into a supine position may result in respiratory distress or failure. Allow the patient to maintain a position of comfort unless contraindicated. Assist ventilation as needed.

Other interventions include administration of glucose in a patient with diabetes who has altered mental status and a manageable airway. In specific cases, you may also assist with nitroglycerin, aspirin, or inhalers. Pharmacologic interventions require medical direction and are based on local protocol (see Chapter 12, *Principles of Pharmacology*).

Administration of oxygen may be a useful therapy for many geriatric problems, including vague complaints of weakness or dizziness if the $Spo_2$ level indicates hypoxia. When administering oxygen, be mindful of monitoring the level of consciousness in a patient with chronic obstructive pulmonary disease and the risks of providing a prolonged high concentration of oxygen. Be prepared to ventilate if breathing becomes inadequate.

## Words of Wisdom

In general, allow the patient to maintain a position of comfort unless contraindicated. If spinal motion restriction is necessary, remember to pad the void spaces or use a vacuum mattress, which is softer on bony prominences. You may have to weigh the risk of supine motion restriction versus respiratory distress or failure. Be sure to document the reasons for your decision.

Last, and critically important in older adults, is providing emotional support. An older person is often fearful of what may be happening and that he or she may never return home from the hospital. Listen to your patient, respond to your patient, and provide reassurance. This is an important component of patient advocacy.

Communicate your findings and the interventions you used to ED personnel. Remember to document all history, medication, assessment, and intervention information.

A summary of the special considerations to keep in mind when assessing a geriatric patient can be found in **TABLE 36-4**.

### TABLE 36-4 Geriatric Patient Assessment Guidelines

- When entering the home, take note of issues that would make it environmentally unsafe.
- Introduce yourself, show respect, and use patience to gain an older patient's confidence.
- Assessment of an older patient can be complicated by multiple medical or traumatic conditions, alterations in level of consciousness, and hearing and vision impairments.
- Airway, breathing, circulation, and vital signs are changed by the normal process of aging.
- Many older patients use multiple medications. Be aware of the possibility of overdose, underdose, and drug interactions.
- An older person's body does not have the flexibility or reserves of a younger person's body when facing illness or injury.
- Older people are more easily affected by poor nutrition.
- Older people cannot thermoregulate easily and tend to be cold.
- The memory and cognition of an older person may be impaired.
- The skin of an older adult may be fragile and can tear easily. Consider patient transfer options that are safe and appropriate.

© Jones & Bartlett Learning.

## YOU are the Provider

You advise the patient that she should be transported to the hospital for evaluation; however, she is reluctant to go. Her daughter reassures her that everything will be okay and that she will meet her at the hospital. After several minutes of deliberation, the patient consents to transport. Your partner increases the oxygen flow rate to 15 L/min by nonrebreathing mask as you reassess the patient's vital signs.

| Recording Time: 15 Minutes | |
|---|---|
| **Level of consciousness** | Conscious but confused |
| **Respirations** | 22 breaths/min; labored |
| **Pulse** | 84 beats/min; weak and irregular |
| **Skin** | Hot to the touch; pink and dry |
| **Blood pressure** | 152/90 mm Hg |
| **Spo$_2$** | 94% on 15 L/min via nonrebreathing mask |

The patient's blood glucose level is assessed and is noted to read 145 mg/dL. You place her onto the stretcher, place her in a position of comfort, load her into the ambulance, and begin transport to the hospital. Her daughter tells you that she will follow you to the hospital in her own vehicle.

7. What concerns would an older patient have about being transported to the hospital?

8. On the basis of the patient's past medical history and signs and symptoms, what do you suspect as the cause of her problem?

# Trauma and Geriatric Patients

In general, the risk of serious injury or death is more common in older patients who experience trauma than in younger patients. Slower homeostatic compensatory mechanisms, limited physiologic reserves, normal effects of aging on the body, and existing medical issues create risk and complicate the assessment of geriatric patients. Physical findings in an older adult may be more subtle and therefore easier to miss. The mechanisms that cause serious injury in older people are often less than what would result in similar injury in younger people. There is also the consideration that recuperation from trauma is longer and often less successful in older people. For that reason, many injuries in older people are undertriaged and undertreated.

Older pedestrians are more likely to have life-threatening complications after being struck by a vehicle because of changes in the body, such as more fragile bones. Although older pedestrians commonly sustain injury to the legs and arms, other injuries can be caused by a secondary crash onto the street, often involving the head. Any of these mechanisms can cause fractures, traumatic brain injury, spinal injury, and paralysis.

Older people are more likely to experience burns because of altered mental status, inattention, and a compromised neurologic status. Their risk of mortality from burns is increased when preexisting medical conditions are present, the immune system is weakened, and fluid replacement is complicated by renal compromise.

There is higher mortality from penetrating trauma in older adults, especially in the case of gunshot wounds. Penetrating trauma can easily cause serious internal bleeding. An older patient's limited physiologic reserves and more subtle presentation can complicate treatment.

Finally, falls are the leading cause of fatal and nonfatal injuries in older adults. Nearly one-half of fatal falls in geriatric patients are associated with traumatic brain injury. This highlights the importance of the environmental assessment and assisting your patient in recognizing trip hazards. Unfortunately, physical abuse is another common cause of trauma in older adults. Elder abuse is discussed later in the chapter.

# Anatomic Changes and Fractures

Changes in pulmonary, cardiovascular, neurologic, and musculoskeletal systems make older patients more susceptible to trauma. The brain shrinks, leading to higher risk of cerebral bleeding following head trauma. Skeletal changes cause curvature of the upper spine that often requires additional padding during spinal immobilization. Loss of strength, sensory impairment, and medical illness all increase the risk of falls.

A geriatric patient's overall physical condition may lessen the ability of the patient's body to compensate for the effects of even simple injuries. For example, the aging body has a heart that no longer can beat faster when it needs to compensate for blood loss, vessels that cannot constrict due to atherosclerosis, and lungs that do not exchange oxygen as well. Additional changes in the circulatory system leave the geriatric patient's body unable to maintain normal vital signs during hemorrhage. Also, a geriatric patient's blood pressure drops sooner than in a younger adult patient during a traumatic emergency.

## Words of Wisdom

The inability of the blood to clot normally can become a big issue in trauma and will be seen in patients who take warfarin (Coumadin), apixaban (Eliquis) or other blood-thinning medications.

As a result of bone loss from osteoporosis, older patients are prone to fractures, especially of the hip. Hip fractures are much more common among women. People with osteoporosis may fracture a hip as a result of a fall from a standing position. Contributing factors to osteoporosis and the risk of fracture include vitamin D and calcium deficiencies, metabolic bone diseases, and tumors. Injuries to the hip can also be recurring. A previous fracture increases the likelihood of a future injury.

Older people with osteoporosis are also at risk for pelvic fractures (**FIGURE 36-5**). A pelvic fracture may also be caused by a low-energy mechanism or a standing fall. The person may sustain this injury when getting out of the bathtub or descending stairs. These injuries do not usually damage the

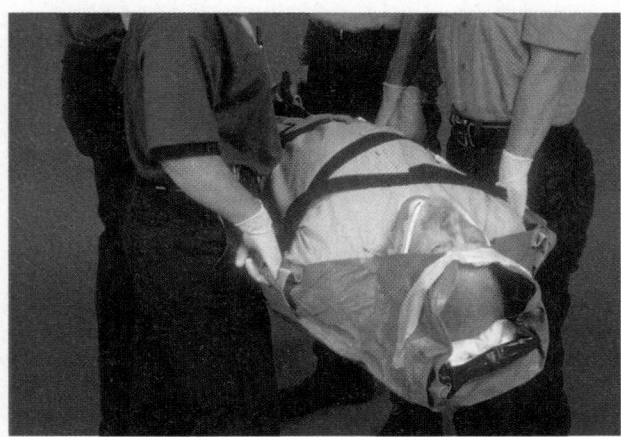

**FIGURE 36-5** Vacuum mattresses that conform to body contours can be a good choice for immobilizing geriatric patients with possible pelvic fractures.

© Jones & Bartlett Learning. Courtesy of MIEMSS.

structural integrity of the pelvic ring but may fracture an individual bone.

Recovering from these kinds of injuries can be complicated for an older person, especially one with a compromised immune system or diabetes. The fact that the person may be bedridden for a considerable amount of time may inhibit his or her ability to continue to live independently.

With age, the spine stiffens as a result of shrinkage of disk spaces, and vertebrae become brittle. Compression fractures of the spine are more likely to occur. As with a head injury, you must be suspicious of the possibility of other fractures and complicating issues.

Because brain tissue shrinks with age, older patients are more likely to sustain certain types of traumatic brain injuries, such as subdural hematomas. This is where tiny veins between the surface of the brain and its outer covering (the dura) stretch and tear, allowing blood to collect. In older people, the veins are often already stretched because of brain atrophy (shrinkage) and are more easily injured.

Acute subdural hematomas are among the deadliest of all head injuries. Blood fills the skull rapidly, compressing brain tissue, which often results in brain injury. This type of bleeding can go unnoticed initially because the blood has a void to fill before it can produce pressure in the skull; only then will the familiar signs of brain injury appear. Also, serious head injuries are often missed in older patients because the mechanism may seem relatively minor or health care providers consider the altered mental status as "part of getting old." These chronic subdural hematomas may go unnoticed for many days to weeks.

Other factors that predispose an older patient to a serious head injury include long-term abuse of alcohol, recurrent falls or repeated head injury, and/or anticoagulant medication (blood thinners, including aspirin).

## Environmental Injury

Internal temperature regulation slows with age because of a slowed endocrine system. Heat gain or loss in response to environmental changes is delayed by slowed circulation and decreased sweat production in the skin. In addition, thermoregulation can be adversely affected by chronic disease, medication use, and alcohol use, all of which are more common in older people.

Approximately one-half of all deaths from hypothermia occur in older people, and most indoor hypothermia deaths involve geriatric patients. The death rates from hyperthermia more than double in older people compared with younger people; people older than 85 years are at highest risk. Arizona has an abnormally high rate of heat-related deaths due to its long, hot summers and large geriatric population. Older people should also be checked on during very hot and very cold spikes in temperature to ensure they are sheltered from the extremes in temperature.

## Special Considerations in Assessing Geriatric Trauma Patients

Trauma is never isolated to a single issue when you are assessing and caring for a geriatric patient. An isolated hip fracture in a healthy 25-year-old adult is rarely associated with overall decline. However, the same injury in an 85-year-old patient can produce a wide-ranging, systemic effect that results in deterioration, shock, and life-threatening hypoxia.

### Scene Size-up

As with all scenes, ensure your own safety first. Take standard precautions. Consider the number of patients, especially in the case of a motor vehicle crash. Determine if you need additional or specialized resources.

Gather information on the mechanism of injury (MOI). As with any call, look for clues that indicate your patient's traumatic incident may have been preceded by a medical incident such as syncope, a cardiac problem, or an issue related to diabetes. Bystander information may help determine if a loss of consciousness occurred before the incident. You should use the same thought processes when you have a patient who has fallen. Was the fall mechanical, or was an episode of weakness or dizziness a factor?

The MOI is also important in establishing whether an injury is considered critical, and it affects treatment and transport considerations.

## Primary Assessment

During the primary assessment you will address life threats. Determine whether this is a priority patient and to which facility the patient will be transported. Because patients older than 55 years have an increased risk of major injury and death, it may make good sense to transport older trauma patients to a trauma center. Once you have determined that the patient has a potentially life-threatening condition, limit any on-scene treatment to that which is absolutely necessary for patient stabilization. Follow your local protocols.

The general impression is an important aspect of all patient assessments. As you approach the patient, note if he or she is generally in stable or unstable condition. Determining neurologic status may be difficult if you do not know the patient's baseline. Try to get information from someone familiar with the patient, if possible. Use the AVPU mnemonic and the Glasgow Coma Scale to determine mental status. An important consideration with any patient is the inability to remember the event.

If the patient is talking to you, the airway is patent. Patients who have noisy respirations may have airway compromise. Suction any blood or foreign material. Dentures can cause an airway obstruction, so assess for the presence of dentures but do not remove them unless they are creating an airway patency problem. It is more difficult to ventilate a patient who has no teeth.

In an unresponsive patient, open the airway with a modified jaw-thrust maneuver. Use an oropharyngeal or nasopharyngeal airway as appropriate, and ventilate with a bag-mask device if the patient's respiratory effort is inadequate or absent. Any curvature of the patient's spine will require padding to keep the patient supine and the airway open.

Breathing problems caused by trauma can be made worse by preexisting respiratory disease and the compromised respiratory effort that comes with aging. Remember that minor chest trauma can cause lung injury. Perform a thorough respiratory assessment and physical assessment of the chest, and treat accordingly. Use pulse oximetry to monitor oxygenation.

Manage any external bleeding immediately. Be suspicious of signs and symptoms of internal bleeding. Drinking alcohol and taking anticoagulant medications can make internal bleeding worse, or make external bleeding more difficult to control. Remember that physiologic changes due to aging can worsen the effects of trauma, and older people do not heal as easily as do younger adults. Older patients can more easily go into shock. Also, remember that patients who were hypertensive prior to injury may have a normal blood pressure when they are actually in shock.

### Words of Wisdom

#### Geriatric Patients With Head Trauma

Older people are more predisposed to head injuries, such as subdural hematomas. The mechanism may be minor; thus the severity of these injuries is often underestimated. Consider that the signs and symptoms of brain injury can sometimes mimic the signs and symptoms of a stroke. Be sure to ask about these risk factors during your assessment of a patient with a potential brain injury:

- Long-term abuse of alcohol
- Recurrent falls
- Repeated head injury
- Use of anticoagulant medication (blood thinners, including aspirin)

## History Taking

Considerations in your assessment of the patient's condition and stability must include past medical conditions, even if they are not currently acute or symptomatic. For example, you respond to a call for a patient with a history of unstable angina who has sustained a simple isolated fracture of the ankle. You must consider this patient to have the potential for an unstable condition and provide prompt transport before the stress of the simple trauma worsens the angina and an unstable overall scenario develops. In these patients, the remainder of the assessment can be performed en route to the ED.

Be sure to get a history of risk factors when you assess a geriatric patient with a potential brain injury. If a patient shows signs and symptoms of increased intracranial pressure, ask about recent head trauma.

## Secondary Assessment

The physical examination should be performed on a geriatric trauma patient in the same manner as for any adult but with consideration of the higher likelihood of damage from trauma. Remember that any head injury can be life threatening in an older adult. When examining the chest, consider that breathing may be impaired. Check lung sounds and look for any evidence of a pacemaker or previous cardiac surgery. Even though it may appear that the patient has only experienced trauma, keep in mind that this does not mean he or she may not also be having medical problems (**FIGURE 36-6**). When assessing the abdomen, remember that older patients have a flaccid abdominal wall and may not present with pain and rigidity in the abdomen when trauma has

been sustained. Decreased muscle size in the abdomen may mask abdominal trauma. Look for bruising and other evidence of trauma. Injury to the liver or spleen may present with diffuse abdominal pain, or pain may refer to the left shoulder.

Assess the pulse, blood pressure, and skin signs. Capillary refill is unreliable in older people because of compromised circulation. Remember that some older people take beta blockers, which inhibit their heart from becoming tachycardic, as you would expect in shock. Even a heart rate in normal ranges may be high for someone taking beta blockers. Try to determine if the patient's blood pressure is normal for him or her. Remember that a blood pressure that may be normal for an older adult could indicate shock in a younger patient.

## Reassessment

Repeating the primary assessment, level of consciousness, vital signs, and interventions should be performed and documented as with any patient, but remember that a geriatric patient has a higher likelihood of decompensating after trauma.

## Safety Tips

Falls in the geriatric population, even those with apparently minor mechanisms, can cause life-threatening or debilitating problems. Assess the patient's environment for potential hazards, and recommend changes.

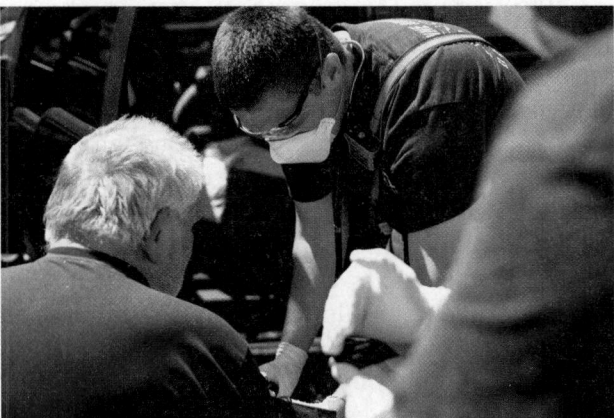

**FIGURE 36-6** Remember that when you treat a geriatric trauma patient, you must assess the injuries and carefully look for the cause of the incident. Always consider medical causes that may have led to syncope.

© ALEX EDELMAN/Contributor/AFP/Getty Images.

Broken bones are common and should be splinted in a manner appropriate to the injury. Because of the amount of flexion that occurs in the spinal column, hips, and knees of older patients, effective application of conventional splints and backboards to immobilize them may be difficult or impossible unless a large amount of padding is used. What is considered a normal anatomic position for children and adults is often abnormal for some geriatric trauma patients. Trying to force a patient into a normal anatomic position can cause harm. Some devices, such as traction splints, simply do not work on patients with flexed hips and knees and should not routinely be used to treat hip fractures. Splinting devices, such as vacuum mattresses that conform to body contours, may be a good choice for immobilization when indicated.

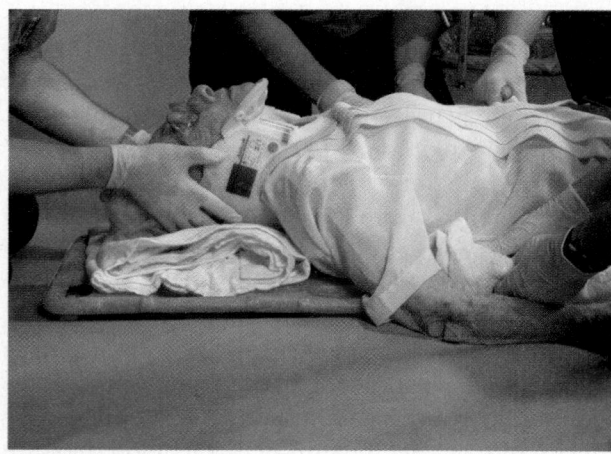
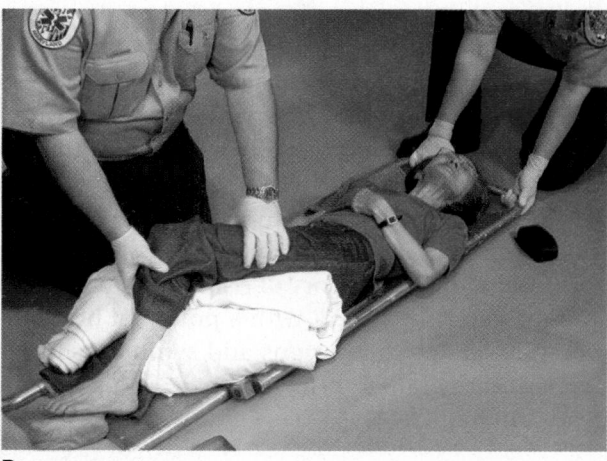

**A**    **B**

**FIGURE 36-7** Placing padding in the void space between the patient's body and the backboard is an important component of achieving spinal motion restriction in a geriatric patient. **A.** Pad the void space below the kyphotic spine. The pillows and blankets should be as wide as the backboard to allow for effective immobilization and support. **B.** Place blankets and pillows under an injured extremity to provide support to a fracture site.

**A, B:** © Jones & Bartlett Learning. Courtesy of MIEMSS.

In hip and pelvic fractures, avoid log rolling the patient because you risk causing the patient increased pain. When immobilization is indicated, patients with kyphosis will often need padding (**FIGURE 36-7**). In general, padding should be provided for comfort and to help decrease the likelihood of decubitus ulcer formation. Consider also that patients with chronic cardiac or respiratory disorders, particularly congestive heart failure, may have immense difficulty lying supine; thus, do not force them into an uncomfortable position or some other manner of achieving effective spinal motion restriction. An alternative solution may be to consider a spinal immobilization device such as a Kendrick Extraction Device, which is intended for a patient in a seated position.

Remember that older people do not have the mechanisms that help keep them warm. Provide blankets and heat to prevent hypothermia.

Communication with older people can be challenging in any situation, but it can become even more complicated when the patient is in pain or is experiencing fear from trauma. Older people also tend to fear that trauma may end their mobility and independence. Remember to provide psychological support, as well as medical treatment. Document assessment, treatment, and reassessment, including any changes in the patient's status.

## Assessment of Falls

As mentioned, falls are a leading cause of injury in geriatric patients. Falls can be caused by a medical condition such as fainting, a cardiac rhythm disturbance, or a medication interaction. Safety and environmental factors such as poor lighting, loose floor coverings, and lack of handrails are often responsible for falls. Physiologic factors include vision and balance issues, decreased visual acuity, and decreased strength.

Whenever you assess a geriatric patient who has fallen, it is critically important to find out why the fall occurred. Was it simply a mechanical fall, or was it preceded by a medical event (pathologic)? Was the patient dizzy before the fall? Does the patient remember the fall? Did a fainting episode cause the fall and injury, or did the patient trip on something and lose his or her balance? Cardiac, neurologic, and metabolic issues can create weakness, dizziness, or syncope, resulting in a fall. Traumatic and medical factors are much more interconnected in older people. Sometimes, a recent history of starting or stopping blood pressure medication is enough to cause a patient to become dizzy and fall.

Consider that the fall may have been caused by a life-threatening medical condition, and look carefully for clues from the patient, bystanders, and the environment. In motor vehicle crashes, be alert to the possibility that a medical emergency may have caused the incident, especially in single-vehicle crashes with no apparent cause.

## Response to Nursing and Skilled Care Facilities

For many of the geriatric patients with whom you interact, the call will occur at a nursing home or other skilled care facility. Relatively healthy and active seniors often live in age-restricted active adult communities. A less expensive option is age-restricted apartments that provide seniors with the physical and emotional security that comes with living with other seniors. A similar type of facility, but one that also provides communal meals, social events, and other types of support, is an independent living facility. Assisted-living residential facilities support residents with ADLs and provide 24-hour assistance. Residents get assistance with daily medication administration, and some facilities address specialized patient issues such as Alzheimer disease and dementia.

Nursing homes, also called skilled nursing facilities or long-term care facilities, are facilities that serve patients who need 24-hour care and are sometimes a step down from an acute care hospital. Patients require assistance with daily living and need therapeutic or rehabilitation services.

Calls to these types of facilities can sometimes be challenging. Patients often have an altered level of consciousness and may not be able to give you an NOI or MOI. The staff is usually spread thin and may not be familiar with what needs to be done to assist you when transport is necessary. The most important piece of information you need to establish immediately is, "What is wrong with the patient that is new or different today that made you call 9-1-1?" As soon as possible, establish the baseline status of the patient by talking to the staff who directly care for the patient on a daily basis.

With potentially limited information, you need to do an assessment to determine if the patient's problem is life threatening and/or requires ALS-level care. Optimally, the facility will provide you with a transfer record that provides critical information on the patient's history, medications, allergies, and current complaint. This information is critical because the ED staff need to know how to best treat the patient. Ideally, and when appropriate, transport the patient to the acute care facility where the patient has been treated before and where his or her records will be readily available.

Infection control needs to be a high priority when you visit these facilities. You not only need to protect yourself, but good handwashing and standard precautions can inhibit the spread of infectious pathogens to older people who already have compromised immune systems. You should also be cognizant of potential airborne pathogens. Something as simple as a cold or flu virus could result in a life-threatening pneumonia for a compromised older adult. An infection in an older patient can lead to life-threatening sepsis. Be sure to mask yourself if you have an upper respiratory infection, and mask the patient if he or she has one. Some risks to these patients and EMTs are described next.

**Methicillin-resistant** *Staphylococcus aureus* **(MRSA)** infections are common among people who live in close quarters such as nursing homes. The organism can be found in decubitus ulcers (bedsores), on feeding tubes, and on indwelling urinary catheters. The symptoms of MRSA depend on the type of infection. It can cause mild infections on the skin or invade the bloodstream, lungs, or the urinary tract. MRSA is primarily spread by broken skin-to-skin contact but is also acquired by touching objects that have the bacteria on them. To protect yourself and reduce the spread of MRSA infections, you should wash your hands before and after every patient contact, properly dispose of or disinfect all medical equipment, and take appropriate standard precautions with every patient.

Similarly, many infections in hospitals are caused by **vancomycin-resistant enterococci (VRE)**. Enterococci are bacteria that are normally present in the human intestines and the female reproductive tract. Under the right circumstances, these bacteria can cause infection. Some of the enterococci have become resistant to vancomycin, the antibiotic commonly used to treat these infections.

The **respiratory syncytial virus (RSV)** causes an infection of the upper and lower respiratory tracts. Although more typically seen in children, the virus can also cause serious illness in older people, especially those with lung disease or weakened immune systems. The symptoms are similar to the common cold but can be more severe and last longer. The virus is highly contagious and is found in discharges from the nose and throat of an infected person. RSV is also transmitted by direct contact with droplets from coughs or sneezes and by touching a contaminated surface.

MRSA and RSV infections can be life threatening, especially in an immunocompromised patient. Look for isolation signs or ask about contagious disease when you approach a patient. Be sure to wear appropriate personal protective equipment and decontaminate your ambulance and diagnostic equipment after contact with nursing home residents whether a history of infectious disease is known or not. Be sure to document the infection control issue; advise the receiving facility; and, depending on local protocol, report an infectious disease to your company or the local health department.

*Clostridium difficile* (sometimes referred to as *C diff*) is a bacterium responsible for the most common cause of hospital-acquired infectious diarrhea and regularly causes sporadic cases of diarrhea in nursing homes. It is a bacterium that normally grows in the intestines. Antibiotic use may account for the rapid increase in toxic strains that ultimately cause illness. Health care workers may carry this bacterium following contact with contaminated feces. It can also be found on environmental surfaces such as furniture, floors, toilets, sinks, and bedding. The symptoms from the resultant colitis can range from minor diarrhea to a life-threatening inflammation of the colon. Typical alcohol-based hand sanitizers do not inactivate or kill *C difficile*. Contact precautions with gowns and gloves and handwashing with soap and water after each patient contact are essential to prevent transmission.

SARS-CoV-2 is a strain of coronavirus that causes the disease COVID-19, a respiratory illness that may affect older, more vulnerable people, especially those with preexisting medical conditions such as diabetes. The virus spreads from person to person through airborne droplets created by speaking, coughing, and sneezing. When you are in contact with a patient you suspect may have COVID-19, personal protective equipment includes N95 masks, gloves, and eyewear.

## Dying Patients

As older patients are living longer, more terminally ill patients are choosing to die at home rather than in a hospital. Many have family support and/or hospice support. Often the patient comes to terms with his or her impending death before the family does. Dying patients receive what is called palliative, or comfort, care. Palliative care recognizes that death

is a normal part of the life cycle. Palliative care does not hasten or prolong death, but focuses on relieving pain and providing emotional support and comfort for the patient and his or her loved ones.

You may be called on to interact with a dying patient. One thing to remember is that this interaction will have a long-term effect on the family. Be understanding, sensitive, and compassionate, even though the situation may be uncomfortable for you as well. Determine if the family wishes the patient to go to the hospital or stay in the home.

## Advance Directives

Many people currently make use of an **advance directive**. Also called living wills, advance directives are specific legal papers that direct relatives and caregivers about what kind of medical treatment may be given to patients who cannot speak for themselves. Dealing with advance directives has become more common for EMS providers because more people are electing to use hospice services and spend their final days at home.

Advance directives may also take the form of a do-not-resuscitate (DNR) order. A DNR order gives you permission not to attempt resuscitation for a patient in cardiac arrest. However, for a DNR order to be valid, the form must be signed by the patient or legal surrogate and by one or more physicians or other licensed health care providers. In the presence of a DNR order, if the patient is still alive, you are obligated to provide supportive measures that may include oxygen delivery, pain relief, and comfort. DNR does not mean do not treat. Basic airway, breathing, and circulatory support should be provided; however, cardiopulmonary resuscitation may not. Remember a DNR was completed by the patient in a time when the patient was healthy, in consultation with his or her physician, and should be honored.

Another type of order is the Physician Orders for Life Sustaining Treatment, or POLST, which gives medical orders in addition to the advance directives. The orders may be specific to a person who has a life-threatening condition or is in frail health.

A health care power of attorney is an advance directive that is exercised by a person who has been authorized by the patient to make medical decisions for him or her. Be sure to follow your service's protocol when faced with any advance directive.

Although advance directives may be in place, family members or caregivers who are faced with the final moments of life or worsening of the patient's condition often become alarmed and call

9-1-1. If a DNR is in place, it is important to have a conversation with the family, recognizing the patient's wishes when in better health.

Another common situation is the transportation of patients from nursing facilities. Specific guidelines vary from state to state; however, you should consider the following general guidelines:

- Patients have the right to refuse treatment, including resuscitative efforts, provided that they are able to communicate their wishes.
- A DNR order is valid in a health care facility only if it is in the form of a written order by a physician.
- You should periodically review state and local protocols and legislation regarding advance directives.
- When you are in doubt or when there are no written orders, you should try to resuscitate the patient.

Every service should also provide training on the actions providers should take when presented with advance directives. You should also review the DNR orders of patients when you are provided with them, even if the patient is not dying. This review can give you insight into the form used by certain health care providers. When in doubt, your best course of action is to provide appropriate medical care until you can determine if a DNR is present and valid.

## Elder Abuse and Neglect

Trauma in older people can also be caused by abuse. Reports and complaints of abuse, neglect, and other related problems among the nation's older population are on the rise. Elder abuse is defined as any action on the part of an older person's family member, caregiver, or other associated person that takes advantage of the older person's person (for example, physical abuse), property, or emotional state. Abuse can result from acts of commission (words or actions that cause harm), such as verbal, physical, or sexual assault. Abuse can also result from acts of omission (failure to act), such as denying an older person adequate nutrition or medical care.

The exact extent of elder abuse is often not known for several reasons, including the following:

- Elder abuse is a problem that has been largely hidden from society.
- The definitions of abuse and neglect among the geriatric population vary.
- Victims of elder abuse are often hesitant to report the problem to law enforcement agencies or human and social welfare personnel.

The abused person may feel traumatized by the situation or be afraid that the abuser will punish him or her for reporting the abuse. The abused person may be frail and have multiple chronic medical

---

## YOU are the Provider

During transport, the patient remains conscious, although confused. You reassess her vital signs and then call your radio report to the hospital. During your radio report, the nurse asks you if the patient is normally confused. You inform her that the patient has Alzheimer disease and that this is her baseline mental status.

| Recording Time: 30 Minutes | |
|---|---|
| **Level of consciousness** | Conscious, but confused |
| **Respirations** | 22 breaths/min; labored |
| **Pulse** | 70 beats/min; weak and irregular |
| **Skin** | Hot to the touch; pink and dry |
| **Blood pressure** | 148/88 mm Hg |
| **Spo$_2$** | 95% on 15 L/min via nonrebreathing mask |

During the remainder of the transport, you reassure the patient that the hospital staff will take good care of her. Although confused, she looks at you and smiles. You deliver her to the hospital, transfer patient care to the emergency department staff, and return to service.

**9.** How does dementia differ from delirium? Is dementia a normal part of the aging process?

**10.** What strategies should you use when communicating with older patients?

conditions or dementia. The person may sleep-walk, have an impaired sleep cycle, and periodically shout at others. The person may also be incontinent and may depend on others for ADLs.

Elder abuse occurs most often in women older than 75 years. The physical and emotional signs of abuse, such as rape, spousal physical abuse, and nutritional deprivation, are often overlooked or not accurately identified. Older women are particularly not likely to report incidents of sexual assault to law enforcement agencies. Patients with sensory deficits, dementia, and other forms of altered mental status, such as drug-induced depression, may not be able to report abuse.

Abusers of older people are sometimes products of child abuse, and the abuse that is inflicted on the older person may be retaliatory. Most of these abusers are not trained in the particular care that older people require and have little relief time from the constant care demands of their own family, children, and spouse. Their lives are significantly complicated by the constant, demanding needs of the older person they have to care for.

The abuser may also have marked fatigue, be unemployed with financial difficulties, or abuse one or more substances. With a careful eye, you can recognize the clues to these stressful situations and help guide the family toward programs in their community that are geared to helping the whole family. Programs such as adult day care, Meals on Wheels, and many local individualized programs help to decrease the stress put on the family and lower the chances of abuse.

Abuse is not restricted to the home. Environments such as nursing and convalescent homes and continuing care centers are also sites where older people sustain physical, psychological, financial, or pharmacologic harm. Care providers in these environments can consider older people to be management problems or categorize them as obstinate and undesirable patients. Consult local authorities, but in general you should assume that you have the same obligation to report suspected elder abuse as you do suspected child abuse. Notify receiving hospital personnel of your concerns, report to the proper authorities based on local protocols, and factually document your findings. If you are in doubt, err on the side of caution and make a report. Note that it is not your responsibility to prove that the abuse occurred, only to report your findings according to protocols.

## Assessment of Elder Abuse

Abuse comes in many forms and may include physical assault. Be aware of the environment and conditions a patient lives in, and take note of soft-tissue injuries that cannot be explained by the person's lifestyle and physical condition.

While assessing the patient, try to obtain an explanation of what happened. You should suspect abuse when answers to questions about what caused the injury are concealed or avoided or inconsistent with medical findings.

You must also suspect abuse when you are given unbelievable answers. Be suspicious if you think "Does this make sense?" or "Do I really believe this story?" while reviewing the patient's history. As an EMT, you may be the first health care provider to observe the signs of possible abuse. Information that may be important in assessing possible abuse includes the following:

- Caregiver apathy about the patient's condition
- Overly defensive reaction by the caregiver to your questions
- Caregiver does not allow the patient to answer questions
- Repeated visits to the ED or clinic
- A history of being accident-prone
- Unexplainable soft-tissue injuries
- Unbelievable, vague, or inconsistent explanations of injuries
- Psychosomatic complaints
- Chronic pain without medical explanation
- Self-destructive behavior
- Eating and sleep disorders
- Depression or a lack of energy
- A history of substance and/or sexual abuse

You should remember that many patients who are being abused are so afraid of retribution that they make false statements. A geriatric patient who is being abused by family members may lie about the origin of abuse for fear of being thrown out of the home. In other cases of elder abuse, sensory deprivation or dementia may hinder adequate explanation.

Repeated abuse can lead to a high risk of death. As an EMT, you can help to reduce additional maltreatment of the patient by identifying the abuse (**TABLE 36-5**). This important measure may allow for referral to services of human, social, and public safety agencies and your state ombudsman.

| **TABLE 36-5** Categories of Elder Abuse | |
| --- | --- |
| Physical | • Assault<br>• Neglect or abandonment<br>• Dietary (malnutrition)<br>• Poor maintenance of home<br>• Poor personal hygiene<br>• Sexual assault |
| Psychological | • Benign neglect<br>• Verbal<br>• Treating the person as an infant<br>• Deprivation of sensory stimulation |
| Financial | • Theft of valuables<br>• Embezzlement |

© Jones & Bartlett Learning.

## Signs of Physical Abuse

Signs of abuse can be obvious or subtle. Injuries may be the result of acute or chronic abuse or neglect. Inflicted bruises are usually found on the buttocks and lower back, genitals and inner thighs, cheeks or earlobes, neck, upper lip, and inside the mouth. Pressure bruises caused by the human hand may be identified by oval grab marks, pinch marks, or handprints. Human bites are typically inflicted on the upper extremities and can cause lacerations and infection. You should inspect the patient's ears for indications of twisting, pulling, or pinching and evidence of frequent blows to the outer ears. You should also investigate multiple bruises in various states of healing by asking the patient and reviewing the patient's ADLs.

Burns are a common form of abuse. If you see burns, especially cigarette burns or physical marks that indicate that certain parts of the patient's body have been scalded systematically, you must suspect abuse. Typical abuse from burns is caused by contact with cigarettes, matches, heated metal, forced immersion in hot liquids, chemicals, and electrical power sources.

It may be difficult to see a failure to thrive in an older patient who has been abused. You should observe the patient's weight and try to determine whether the patient appears undernourished or has been unable to gain weight in the current environment. Does the patient have a ravenous appetite? Has medication been withheld? Is money

being withheld, so the patient cannot buy food or medicine? You should also check for signs of neglect, such as evidence of a lack of hygiene, poor dental hygiene, poor temperature regulation, or lack of reasonable amenities in the home (**FIGURE 36-8**).

You must regard injuries to the genitals or rectum with no reported trauma as evidence of sexual abuse in any patient. Geriatric patients with altered mental status may not be able to report sexual abuse. In addition, many women do not report cases of sexual abuse because of shame and the pressure to remain silent and forget.

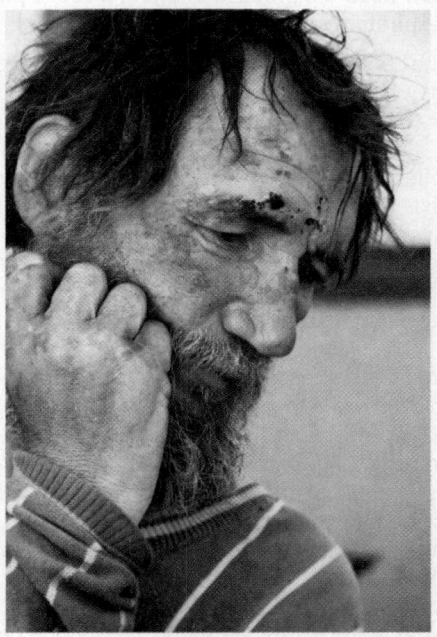

**FIGURE 36-8** Signs of neglect include evidence of a lack of hygiene, poor dental hygiene, poor temperature regulation, or lack of reasonable amenities in the home.
© wrangler/Shutterstock.

**1. As an EMT, why is it important for you to understand the anatomic and physiologic changes that occur with aging?**

Understanding the normal anatomic and physiologic changes that occur with aging is important when you are assessing and treating an older patient who is experiencing an illness or injury. You do not want to mistake these changes for signs of illness and provide treatment when it is not indicated, nor do you want to attribute them to "just getting old" and fail to provide treatment when it is indicated. Additionally, older adults may have chronic illnesses that can change their anatomic makeup (eg, osteoporosis) or physiologic functions (eg, diabetes, chronic lung diseases). They may also be taking medications that affect their vital signs and other body functions, and it is important to recognize how that may affect your assessment, and what effect an illness or injury may have on the patient. For example, some medications taken for hypertension, a common finding in older adults, may not only keep the blood pressure at a more normal level, but also keep the patient's heart rate low, so that it cannot increase as it would in younger people to compensate for dehydration, blood loss, or other stressors to the patient's body.

**2. How does the process of aging affect a person's respiratory system?**

The decreased muscle mass in older patients means they have less help from the muscles in the chest wall during respiratory distress.

Airway mechanisms, such as the cough and gag reflexes, decrease with age, resulting in a decreased ability of older adults to clear secretions from the airway. These upper and lower airway changes decrease the patient's ability to cough, which increases the risk of a respiratory infection as well as increases the risk of aspiration.

The elasticity and number of the alveoli in older patients decreases, making it harder for the patient to exhale and in some cases causing trapping of air in the lungs. This also decreases the surface area for gas exchange between alveoli and red blood cells. As a result, pulmonary respiration—the exchange of oxygen and carbon dioxide in the lungs—decreases. In some patients, fluid may collect in the alveoli (pulmonary edema).

**3. What is the GEMS diamond? How can it facilitate your overall care of an older patient?**

The GEMS diamond serves as a useful mnemonic for the issues to consider when assessing every older patient. The four components of the GEMS diamond are: G, geriatric patients; E, environmental assessment; M, medical assessment; and S, social assessment. It provides an organized way for you to remember the important considerations when assessing older patients.

**4. Based on the patient's current condition, how appropriate is the current oxygen therapy?**

The amount of oxygen being delivered to the patient should be increased. The patient reports dyspnea and has abnormal lung sounds. Despite being placed on 2 L/min of oxygen, the $SpO_2$ level is only 92% and respirations are labored. Current guidelines for oxygen therapy state the $SpO_2$ level should be maintained at or above 94%, so the oxygen being administered should be increased to achieve that level.

**5. What should concern you about patients who take numerous medications?**

The risks of inadvertent overdosing or negative medication interactions increase when patients take numerous medications. Furthermore, the physiologic changes that occur with aging make an older patient susceptible to drug toxicity—even if the patient takes all of his or her medications as prescribed. Medications tend to stay in the body for longer periods.

When numerous medications are combined, it is impossible to predict how they may interact with each other. Some medication interactions can produce acute, life-threatening emergencies. When caring for a patient who takes numerous medications, consider the possibility of an interaction as the underlying cause of, or a contributor to, his or her problem.

**6. What other assessments, if any, should be performed for this patient?**

The patient history revealed she has not been eating lately. The daughter stated her mother's level of consciousness has been altered more than usual over the past couple of days. Based on the patient's fever, multiple medications, decreased appetite, and altered level of consciousness, you should assess her blood glucose level if consistent with your local protocol.

**7. What concerns would an older patient have about being transported to the hospital?**

Fear is the most common reason why older patients are resistant to EMS transport. They often fear that when they are loaded into an ambulance and leave

## YOU are the Provider SUMMARY *continued*

the safety of their own home, they will eventually be moved to a nursing home or, even worse, never leave the hospital. Patients with Alzheimer disease or other forms of dementia may also become more confused or agitated when taken out of their familiar surroundings. As an EMT, you are always obligated to treat the patient to the best of your abilities, but you must acknowledge and respect the older patient's need for independence and the emotional attachment that he or she may have to the home.

**8. On the basis of the patient's past medical history and signs and symptoms, what do you suspect as the cause of her problem?**

On the basis of the patient's past medical history, which includes emphysema, and her current presentation—fever, chills, worsened shortness of breath, and coarse rhonchi—you should suspect pneumonia.

The presence of a preexisting lower respiratory disease (eg, chronic obstructive pulmonary disease), coupled with age-related deterioration of the respiratory and immune systems, makes older patients especially susceptible to pneumonia.

**9. How does dementia differ from delirium? Is dementia a normal part of the aging process?**

Dementia is a slow onset of progressive disorientation, as well as a progressive loss of cognitive function, psychomotor skills, and social skills. It is a chronic, generally irreversible condition that develops slowly—typically over a period of years—and is the result of a progressive deterioration in cerebral function. There are many causes of dementia, such as Alzheimer disease. In contrast, delirium is an *acute* change in mental status or cognitive function. It is marked by the inability to focus, think logically, and maintain attention, and signals the onset of a

new health problem. Unlike dementia, many causes of delirium are reversible. In older patients, delirium is commonly the result of a UTI, hypoglycemia or hyperglycemia, dehydration, bowel obstruction, fever, and vitamin deficiencies. Other causes include acute alcohol intoxication, drug overdose, withdrawal from drugs or alcohol, hypoxia, and hypovolemia, among others.

Any change in a patient's level of consciousness or mentation, regardless of his or her age, is abnormal. Confusion, abnormal behavior, and other changes in cognitive function do not come automatically with age; they should be regarded as an indicator of an underlying illness or injury.

**10. What strategies should you use when communicating with older patients?**

Speak respectfully when you introduce yourself, and identify yourself as a medical professional. This helps establish a rapport with the patient. Asking the patient how he or she prefers to be addressed is a trust-building technique.

Look directly at the patient and speak slowly and distinctly. Do not assume that the patient is hearing-impaired simply because of his or her age.

When you ask the patient a question, allow adequate time to respond, unless the condition is urgent or critical. When the patient responds, listen carefully.

Explain what you are going to do before you do it. Use simple terms to explain the use of medical equipment and procedures and avoid medical jargon and slang.

Do not talk about the patient in front of him or her as though he or she was not there. This can potentially give the patient the feeling that he or she does not have a say in care or treatment decisions.

### EMS Patient Care Report (PCR)

| Date: 11-28-20 | Incident No.: 013309 | Nature of Call: Shortness of breath | | Location: 200 Hawkins Drive | |
|---|---|---|---|---|---|
| Dispatched: 0625 | En Route: 0626 | At Scene: 0630 | Transport: 0652 | At Hospital: 0705 | In Service: 0716 |

#### Patient Information

| | |
|---|---|
| **Age:** 82 <br> **Sex:** F <br> **Weight (in kg [lb]):** 48 kg (105 lb) | **Allergies:** Erythromycin <br> **Medications:** Plavix, Digoxin, Aricept, Verapamil, Celebrex, Albuterol, Flovent <br> **Past Medical History:** Emphysema, atrial fibrillation, Alzheimer disease, rheumatoid arthritis, hypertension <br> **Chief Complaint:** Difficulty breathing |

**YOU**   are the Provider **SUMMARY** *continued*

| Vital Signs | | | | |
|---|---|---|---|---|
| **Time:** 0635 | **BP:** 158/88 | **Pulse:** 68 | **Respirations:** 22 | **Spo$_2$:** 92% |
| **Time:** 0645 | **BP:** 152/90 | **Pulse:** 84 | **Respirations:** 22 | **Spo$_2$:** 94% |
| **Time:** 0700 | **BP:** 148/88 | **Pulse:** 70 | **Respirations:** 22 | **Spo$_2$:** 95% |

| EMS Treatment (circle all that apply) | | | | |
|---|---|---|---|---|
| **Oxygen @ _15_ L/min via:**<br><br>NC (NRM) Bag mask | | **Assisted Ventilation** | **Airway Adjunct** | **CPR** |
| **Defibrillation** | **Bleeding Control** | **Bandaging** | **Splinting** | **Other:** Position of comfort; emotional support |

**Narrative**

Dispatched to a residence for a woman with respiratory distress.

Chief complaint: Difficulty breathing

History: Her daughter, who was present at the scene, advised that the patient has a history of emphysema and that her usual shortness of breath has worsened during the past few days. The patient was currently receiving home oxygen at 2 L/min via nasal cannula. The daughter further stated that the patient has been running a fever, 101°F (38°C), and has had a cough, which is producing thick, green sputum. Other past medical history significant for A-Fib, Alzheimer disease, hypertension, and rheumatoid arthritis. Inquired about patient's current mental status (confused) and was advised by the daughter that her mother has been more confused than normal over the past couple of days.

Assessment: Arrived on scene and found the patient, an 82-year-old woman, sitting in a chair in her living room. She was conscious but confused. Her airway was patent, and her breathing was labored. The patient had a blanket wrapped around her and was shivering. Further assessment revealed bilateral basilar rhonchi on auscultation of breath sounds.

Treatment (Rx): Obtained vital signs, and increased oxygen flow rate to 15 L/min by nonrebreathing mask. Advised patient that transport to the hospital for evaluation was necessary; however, she stated that she did not want to go. The patient's daughter reassured her and advised that she would follow the ambulance to the hospital. After reassurance by the daughter and EMS, the patient consented to transport.

Transport: Placed patient onto stretcher in a position of comfort, loaded her into the ambulance, and began transport. En route, patient's condition remained unchanged; she remained confused and short of breath, and her vital signs remained stable. Continued to provide emotional support and reassurance to the patient; she was able to answer some questions but had difficulty with others. Delivered patient to emergency department staff, gave verbal report to staff nurse Jacobs, and transferred patient care. Returned to service at 0716.

**End of report**

# Prep Kit

## Ready for Review

- With changes in the respiratory system, such as a decreased ability to cough, geriatric patients are more likely to present with pneumonia or upper airway infections.
- Changes in the cardiovascular system can lead to atherosclerosis, aneurysm, stiffening heart valves, orthostatic hypotension, venous stasis, deep venous thrombosis, heart attack, heart failure, and stroke.
- Many patients do not present with the classic symptom of chest pain when experiencing a heart attack. Atypical presentations are seen mostly in women, older patients, and patients with diabetes.
- Dementia and delirium are both abnormal processes and must be carefully evaluated in geriatric patients.
- As the body ages, the bones become more fragile. This leads to a higher risk of fracture in geriatric patients.
- Polypharmacy and changes in medications can cause serious problems for geriatric patients.
- Depression is treatable with medication and therapy but is a risk factor for suicide if it remains untreated in geriatric patients.
- Although assessment of geriatric patients involves the same basic approach as that for any other patient, you must take a more wary approach.

- Assessing an older person can be challenging because of communication issues, hearing and vision deficits, alteration in consciousness, complicated medical history, and the effects of multiple medications.
- To obtain an accurate history for a geriatric patient, patience and good communication skills are essential. A slow, deliberate approach to the patient history, with one EMT asking questions, is generally the best strategy.
- The risk of serious injury or death is more common in geriatric patients who experience a traumatic injury.
- When you treat a geriatric trauma patient, assess the injuries and carefully look for the cause of the injury. A medical condition such as fainting could be the actual cause of a fall. The injuries from the fall and the medical condition will need to be addressed.
- When responding to nursing and skilled care facilities, you should determine the patient's chief complaint on that day and what initial problem caused the patient to be admitted to the facility.
- Be aware of signs of abuse and neglect. Carefully document these signs, and report suspected elder abuse or neglect according to your local protocols.

## Vital Vocabulary

**abdominal aortic aneurysm (AAA)** A rapidly fatal condition in which the walls of the aorta in the abdomen weaken and blood leaks into the layers of the vessel, causing it to bulge.

**advance directive** Written documentation that specifies medical treatment for a competent

patient should the patient become unable to make decisions; also called a living will or health care directive.

**aneurysm** A swelling or enlargement of the wall of a blood vessel that results from weakening of the vessel wall.

**arteriosclerosis** A disease that causes the arteries to thicken, harden, and calcify.

**ascites** An abnormal accumulation of excess fluid in the peritoneal cavity.

**atherosclerosis** A disorder in which cholesterol and calcium build up inside the walls of the blood vessels, forming plaque, which eventually leads to a partial or complete blockage of blood flow.

**cataracts** Clouding of the lens of the eye or its surrounding transparent membranes.

**decubitus ulcers** Sores caused by the pressure of skin against a surface for long periods; can range from a discoloration of the skin to a deep wound that may invade into bone or organs; also known as bedsores.

**deep venous thrombosis** The formation of a blood clot within the larger veins of an extremity, typically following a period of prolonged immobilization.

**delirium** A temporary change in mental status characterized by disorganized thoughts, inattention, memory loss, disorientation, striking changes in personality and affect, hallucinations, delusions, or a decreased level of consciousness.

**dementia** The slow onset of progressive disorientation, shortened attention span, and loss of cognitive function; this condition is generally chronic and irreversible.

**dyspnea** Shortness of breath or difficulty breathing.

**elder abuse** Any action on the part of an older person's family member, caregiver, or other associated person that takes advantage of the older person's person, property, or emotional state.

**geriatrics** The assessment and treatment of disease in someone who is age 65 years or older.

**hemoptysis** The coughing up of blood.

**jugular vein distention** A visual bulging of the jugular veins in the neck that can be caused by fluid overload, pressure in the chest, cardiac tamponade, or tension pneumothorax.

**kyphosis** A forward curling of the back caused by an abnormal increase in the curvature of the spine.

**melena** Black, foul-smelling, tarry stool containing digested blood.

**methicillin-resistant *Staphylococcus aureus* (MRSA)** A bacterium that causes infections in different parts of the body and is often resistant to commonly used antibiotics; can be found on the skin and in surgical wounds, the bloodstream, lungs, and urinary tract.

**neuropathy** A group of conditions in which the nerves leaving the spinal cord are damaged, resulting in distortion of signals to or from the brain.

**osteoporosis** A generalized bone disease, commonly associated with postmenopausal women, in which there is a reduction in the amount of bone mass leading to fractures after minimal trauma in either sex.

**peptic ulcer disease** An abrasion of the stomach or small intestine.

**pneumonia** An infectious disease of the lung that damages lung tissue.

**polypharmacy** The use of multiple medications on a regular basis.

**presbycusis** An age-related condition of the ear that produces progressive bilateral hearing loss that is most noted at higher frequencies.

**pulmonary embolism** A blood clot that breaks off of a large vein that travels to the blood vessels of the lung, causing obstruction of blood flow.

**respiratory syncytial virus (RSV)** A virus that causes an infection of the lungs and breathing passages; can lead to other serious illnesses that affect the lungs or heart, such as bronchiolitis and pneumonia; it is highly contagious and spread through droplets.

**syncope**  A fainting spell or transient loss of consciousness.

**urinary tract infection (UTI)**  An infection, usually of the lower urinary tract (urethra and bladder),

that occurs when normal flora bacteria enter the urethra and grow.

**vancomycin-resistant enterococci (VRE)**  A bacterium that is normally present in the human intestines and the female reproductive tract, but which can cause infection and which is resistant to the antibiotic vancomycin.

## References

1. American Academy of Orthopaedic Surgeons (AAOS). *Nancy Caroline's Emergency Care in the Streets*. 8th ed. Burlington, MA: Jones & Bartlett Learning; 2018.

2. American Geriatrics Society, Snyder DR. *Geriatric Education for Emergency Medical Services*. 2nd ed. Burlington, MA: Jones & Bartlett Learning; 2016.

3. American Heart Association, American Stroke Association. *FACTS: Preventable. Treatable. Beatable.: Stroke in the U.S.* Washington, DC: American Heart Association; 2013. http://www.heart.org/idc/groups/heart-public/@wcm /@adv/documents/downloadable/ucm_305054.pdf. Accessed July 11, 2020.

4. Arizona Department of Health Services. *Trends in Morbidity and Mortality From Exposure to Excessive Natural Heat in Arizona, 2012 report*. Phoenix, AZ: Arizona Department of Health Services; 2014. https://pub.azdhs.gov/health -stats/report/heat/excessive-heat-2012.pdf. Accessed July 11, 2020.

5. Atherosclerosis. National Heart, Lung, and Blood Institute website. http://www.nhlbi.nih.gov/health/health-topics /topics/atherosclerosis. Updated November 13–14, 2018. Accessed July 11, 2020.

6. Berko J, Ingram DD, Saha S, Parker JD. *Deaths Attributed to Heat, Cold, and Other Weather Events in the United States, 2006–2010*. National Health Statistics Reports No, 76. Hyattsville, MD: National Center for Health Statistics; 2014. www.cdc.gov/nchs/data/nhsr/nhsr076.pdf. Accessed July 11, 2020.

7. Federal Interagency Forum on Aging-Related Statistics. *Older Americans 2012: Key Indicators of Well-Being*. Washington, DC: U.S. Government Printing Office; 2012. https://agingstats.gov/docs/PastReports/2012/OA2012 .pdf. Accessed July 11, 2020.

8. Fick DM, Cooper JW, Wade WE, Waller JL, Maclean JR, Beers MH. Updating the Beers criteria for potentially inappropriate medication use in older adults: results of a US consensus panel of experts. *Arch Intern Med* 2003;163(22):2716–2724.

9. Goldhaber SZ, Morrison RB. Pulmonary embolism and deep vein thrombosis. *Circulation*. 2002;106:1436–1438. http://circ.ahajournals.org/content/106/12/1436.full. Accessed July 11, 2020.

10. Grapefruit juice and some drugs don't mix. U.S. Food and Drug Administration website. http://www.fda.gov /ForConsumers/ConsumerUpdates/ucm292276.htm. Updated July 25, 2015. Accessed July 11, 2020.

11. Heron M. Deaths: leading causes for 2017. *Natl Vital Stat Rep*. 2019 June 24;68(6). https://www.cdc.gov/nchs /data/nvsr/nvsr68/nvsr68_06-508.pdf. Accessed July 11, 2020.

12. Huang J. Delirium. Merck Manual website. https://www .merckmanuals.com/home/brain,-spinal-cord,-and-nerve -disorders/delirium-and-dementia/delirium. Accessed July 11, 2020.

13. Important facts about falls. Centers for Disease Control and Prevention website. www.cdc.gov/homeand recreationalsafety/falls/adultfalls.html. Updated January 20, 2016. Accessed July 11, 2020.

14. *National Emergency Medical Services Education Standards*. US Department of Transportation. National Highway Traffic Safety Administration. DOT HS 811 077A. January 2009. www.ems.gov/pdf/811077a.pdf. Accessed July 11, 2020.

15. *National Emergency Medical Services Education Standards. Emergency Medical Technician Instructional Guidelines*. US Department of Transportation. National Highway Traffic Safety Administration. DOT HS 811 077C. January 2009. www.ems.gov/pdf/811077c.pdf. Accessed July 11, 2020.

16. National model EMS clinical guidelines. National Association of State EMS Officials website. https://www .nasemso.org/Projects/ModelEMSClinicalGuidelines /index.asp. Accessed July 11, 2020.

17. National Vital Statistics System, National Center for Health Statistics, CDC. *10 Leading Causes of Death by Age Group, United States—2012*. Centers for Disease

Control and Prevention National Center for Injury Prevention and Control. https://www.cdc.gov/injury/wisqars/pdf/leading_causes_of_death_by_age_group_2012- a.pdf. Accessed July 11, 2020.

18. Ortman JM, Velkoff VA, Hogan H. *Aging Nation: The Older Population in the United States.* Current Population Reports, P25-1140. Washington, DC: U.S. Census Bureau; 2014. www.census.gov/prod/2014pubs/p25-1140.pdf. Accessed July 11, 2020.

19. Small intestinal ischemia and infarction. Medline Plus website. http://www.nlm.nih.gov/medlineplus/ency/article/001151.htm. Updated July 2, 2020. Accessed July 11, 2020.

20. Yin S. Elderly white men afflicted by high suicide rates. Population Reference Bureau website. https://www.prb.org/elderlywhitemenafflictedbyhighsuiciderates/. Published August 2006. Accessed July 11, 2020.

21. Young J, Inouye SK. Delirium in older people. *BMJ.* 2007;334(7598):842–846.

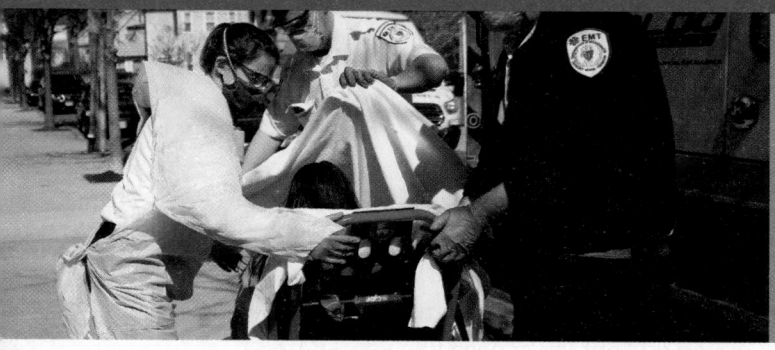

# Chapter 37

# Patients With Special Challenges

## NATIONAL EMS EDUCATION STANDARD COMPETENCIES

### Special Patient Populations

Applies fundamental knowledge of growth, development, and aging and assessment findings to provide basic emergency care and transportation for a patient with special needs.

### Patients With Special Challenges

Recognizing and reporting abuse and neglect (Chapter 35, *Pediatric Emergencies*, and Chapter 36, *Geriatric Emergencies*)
Health care implications of
- Abuse (Chapter 35, *Pediatric Emergencies*, and Chapter 36, *Geriatric Emergencies*)
- Neglect (Chapter 35, *Pediatric Emergencies*, and Chapter 36, *Geriatric Emergencies*)
- Homelessness (pp 1412–1413)
- Poverty (pp 1412–1413)
- Bariatrics (p 1402)
- Technology dependent (pp 1403–1410)
- Hospice/terminally ill (pp 1411–1412)
- Tracheostomy care/dysfunction (pp 1403–1405)
- Home care (p 1411)
- Sensory deficit/loss (pp 1396–1400)
- Developmental disability (pp 1393–1396)

### Trauma

Applies fundamental knowledge to provide basic emergency care and transportation based on assessment findings for an acutely injured patient.

### Special Considerations in Trauma

Recognition and management of trauma in
- Pregnant patient (Chapter 34, *Obstetrics and Neonatal Care*)
- Pediatric patient (Chapter 35, *Pediatric Emergencies*)
- Geriatric patient (Chapter 36, *Geriatric Emergencies*)

Pathophysiology, assessment, and management of trauma in the
- Pregnant patient (Chapter 34, *Obstetrics and Neonatal Care*)
- Pediatric patient (Chapter 35, Pediatric Emergencies)
- Geriatric patient (Chapter 36, *Geriatric Emergencies*)
- Cognitively impaired patient (pp 1393–1396)

## KNOWLEDGE OBJECTIVES

1. Give examples of patients with special challenges EMTs may encounter during a medical emergency. (p 1392)
2. Explain the special patient care considerations required when providing emergency medical care to patients with intellectual disabilities, including patients with autism spectrum disorder (ASD), Down syndrome, or prior brain injuries. (pp 1393–1396)

3. Describe the different types of visual impairments and the special patient care considerations required when providing emergency medical care for visually impaired patients, depending on the level of their disability. (pp 1396–1397)

4. Describe the various types of hearing impairments and the special patient care considerations required when providing emergency medical care for hard-of-hearing patients, including tips for effective communication. (pp 1397–1398)

5. Describe the various types of hearing aids worn by patients; include strategies to troubleshoot a hearing aid that is not working. (pp 1398–1400)

6. Explain the special patient care considerations required when providing emergency medical care to patients who have cerebral palsy, spina bifida, or paralysis. (pp 1400–1402)

7. Define obesity. (p 1402)

8. Explain the special patient care considerations required when providing emergency medical care to bariatric patients; include the best way to move bariatric patients. (pp 1402–1403)

9. Explain the special patient care considerations required when providing emergency medical care to patients who rely on a form of medical technological assistance, including the following: (pp 1403–1410)
   - Tracheostomy tube
   - Home oxygen
   - Mechanical ventilator
   - Apnea monitor
   - Internal cardiac pacemaker
   - Left ventricular assist device (LVAD)
   - External defibrillator vest
   - Central venous catheter
   - Gastrostomy tube
   - Ventricular peritoneal shunt
   - Vagus nerve stimulator
   - Colostomy bag, ileostomy bag, or urostomy bag

10. Describe home care, the types of patients it serves, and the services it encompasses. (p 1411)

11. Contrast hospice and palliative care with curative care. (pp 1411–1412)

12. Explain the responsibilities of EMTs when responding to calls for terminally ill patients who have do not resuscitate (DNR) orders. (p 1411)

13. Discuss the issues of poverty and homelessness in the United States, their negative effects on a person's health, and the role of EMTs as patient advocates. (pp 1412–1413)

## SKILLS OBJECTIVES

1. Demonstrate different strategies to communicate effectively with a patient who has a hearing impairment. (pp 1397–1398)

# Introduction

The approach to health care in the United States continues to focus on increasing value by improving quality and decreasing relative cost. One commonly employed method of achieving cost reduction is decreasing the length of hospitalization. At the same time, medicine and medical technology continue to improve. As a result, the number of children and adults with chronic diseases and injuries who live at home or in environments outside of a hospital setting continues to grow. You should be familiar with the special challenges of patients with chronic diseases and conditions.

Some examples of patients with special challenges include:

- Children who were born prematurely and who have associated respiratory problems

- Infants or small children with congenital heart disease
- Patients with neurologic disease (occasionally caused by hypoxemia at the time of birth, as with cerebral palsy)
- Patients with congenital or acquired diseases resulting in altered body function that requires medical assistance for breathing, eating, urination, or bowel function
- Patients with sensory deficits such as hearing or visual impairments
- Geriatric patients with chronic diseases requiring visitation from a home health care service

You may be called to treat children and adults who live at home and depend on mechanical ventilators, intravenous pumps, or other devices to maintain their lives. You should assess and care for patients with special challenges the same way you care for your other patients. Your priority is the assessment and treatment of the XABCs. Do not be distracted by the noise and mechanics of the medical equipment; focus on the patient the medical equipment may be assisting. If the emergency is the result of medical equipment failure, use the equipment on the ambulance. Some families will have a "go bag," which is a collection of spare equipment and supplies for such situations.

## Developmental Disability

The term developmental disability refers to a group of conditions that may impair development in the areas of physical ability, learning, language development, or behavioral coping skills. Intellectual disability is a subset of developmental disability, where patients have significant limitations in both intellectual functioning and skills needed for daily living. The diagnosis of intellectual disability is made before age 18 years. Intellectual disability spans a spectrum from mild to profound. The level of care and support these patients may need varies greatly.

Intellectual and developmental disabilities may be caused by genetic factors, congenital infections, complications at birth, malnutrition, or environmental factors. Prenatal exposure to drugs or alcohol use may also cause intellectual disability. Other causes that may occur after birth include traumatic brain injury and poisoning (such as from lead or other toxins).

Because patients with intellectual disabilities may have difficulty adjusting to change or a break in routine, an emergency call that generates a roomful of strangers can be overwhelming. A patient may become more difficult to interact with as his or her anxiety level increases. Make every effort to respect the patient's wishes and concerns. Take as much time as necessary to calmly and clearly explain the treatment the patient is about to receive.

Ask family members or caregivers what methods the patient uses to communicate. Some patients may communicate verbally, whereas others may use pictures or be completely noncommunicative. These individuals may be able to describe how the patient communicates feelings of pain or discomfort and provide you with additional information regarding the patient's medical history.

Patients with intellectual disabilities are susceptible to the same disease processes as other patients, including diabetes, heart attack, and respiratory difficulties. Assess and treat the patient according to the chief complaint. During transport, keep the patient as calm as possible.

## Autism Spectrum Disorder

Autism spectrum disorder (ASD) is an intellectual disability characterized by deficits in social communication and interactions along with restricted, repetitive patterns of behavior, interests, and activities. The causes of ASD are not completely understood and likely multifactorial. The overall prevalence of autism in the United States is approximately 1 in 40 individuals. ASD is three to four times more common in males than it is in females and in those who have an older sibling with the condition.

Patients with autism often have abnormal sensory responses. They may not feel cold, heat, or pain as others do. They may respond to pain by laughing, humming, singing, or removing clothing. Likewise, applying bandages or tape can cause anxiety or aggression. When possible, examine the patient beginning at the feet and moving upward, while explaining each step of your exam. Even when these patients cannot speak, they often understand speech.

Patients with autism may have increased sensitivity to noise or physical stimulation. Keep the transport environment calm and minimize stimulation to help with these issues. Limit the use of emergency lights and siren when practical and safe. Allowing a patient to wear sound-dampening devices may also help. The use of distraction techniques while applying a blood pressure cuff or listening with a stethoscope may be necessary. Patients may have a short phrase, item, or particular routine they use that provides comfort. Allowing their routine to be carried out when practical may avoid triggering outbursts or escalating behavior. If departmental policy permits, allow a family member or trusted caregiver to ride in the transport compartment with the patient to facilitate

care. Demonstration of examination techniques on a trusted individual may help comfort the patient. Use short, direct, and simple phrases when communicating, and allow extra time for the patient to process the communication if possible.

### Words of Wisdom

According to the CDC, vaccines do not cause ASD.

## Down Syndrome

Down syndrome is characterized by a genetic chromosomal defect resulting in mild to severe intellectual impairment (**FIGURE 37-1**). The normal human somatic cell contains 23 pairs of chromosomes. In most cases, Down syndrome, also known as trisomy 21, occurs when the two 21st chromosomes fail to separate, so that the ovum or sperm contains 24 chromosomes. When fertilization occurs, a triplication (trisomy) of chromosome 21 occurs. The extra chromosome disrupts the normal course of development.

Increased maternal age and a family history of Down syndrome are known risk factors for this condition. Various physical abnormalities are associated with Down syndrome—a round head with a flat occiput; an enlarged, protruding tongue; slanted, wide-set eyes; folded skin on either side of the nose, covering the inner corners of the eye; short, wide hands; a small face and features; congenital heart

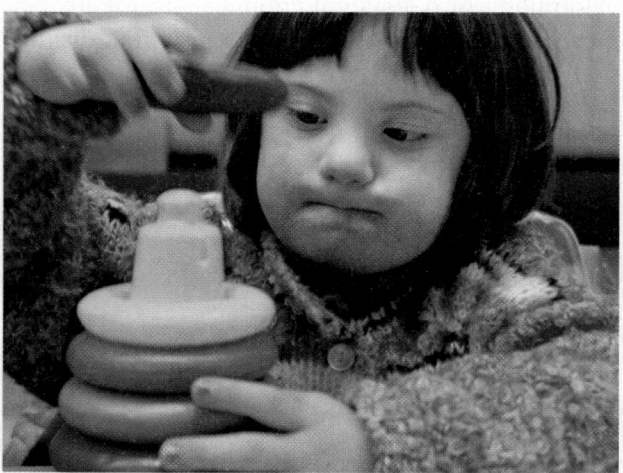

**FIGURE 37-1** A child with Down syndrome.
© PhotoCreate/ShutterStock.

defects; thyroid problems; and hearing and vision problems. People with Down syndrome usually do not have all of these signs, but a diagnosis can be made at birth because several of the signs can be seen. Depending on their level of intellectual disability, people with Down syndrome may lead independent lives. They may be employed, vote, and get involved in their communities.

Patients with Down syndrome are at increased risk for medical complications, including leukemia and conditions that affect the cardiovascular, sensory, endocrine, musculoskeletal, dental, and gastrointestinal systems as well as neurologic development. As many as 40% of these patients have heart conditions and hearing and vision problems.

Because people with Down syndrome often have large tongues and small oral and nasal cavities, airway management may be difficult. These patients may also have misaligned teeth and other dental problems. The enlarged tongue and dental problems can lead to speech abnormalities as well. In an emergency situation, if airway management is necessary, bag-mask ventilation can be challenging. In the case of airway obstruction, a jaw-thrust maneuver may be all that is needed to clear the airway. In an unconscious patient, either the jaw-thrust maneuver or a nasopharyngeal airway may be necessary.

Some people with Down syndrome have epilepsy. Most of the seizures are generalized. Patient management is the same as with other patients with seizures. Chapter 18, *Neurologic Emergencies*, discusses the emergency management of seizures in detail.

According to the National Down Syndrome Society, the atlantoaxial joint—where the first two cervical vertebrae meet—is unstable in approximately 15% of people with Down syndrome. This is termed atlantoaxial instability. Most patients with atlantoaxial instability do not show symptoms; however, they are at increased risk of complications when they experience trauma. Keep this in mind when you receive a call for a musculoskeletal problem or possible neurologic problem in a patient with Down syndrome. If the atlantoaxial joint becomes dislocated, as may occur with trauma, the patient may experience difficulty walking, neck pain or decreased neck mobility, and sensory deficits. Such a dislocation can even cause spinal cord injury. Atlantoaxial instability is diagnosed with a radiograph of the cervical vertebrae.

## Patient Interaction

It is normal to feel uncomfortable when initiating contact with a patient with an intellectual disability, especially if you have not encountered such situations frequently. The best plan of action is to treat the patient as you would any other patient.

Approach the patient in a calm, friendly manner, watching for signs of increased anxiety or fear. Remember, you are a stranger and are approaching with a group of people. The patient may not understand your uniform or realize that you and your team are there to help. It may be helpful to have your team members wait until you can establish a rapport with the patient. You can then introduce the team members and explain what they are going to do as you slowly bring them forward.

You might interact with a patient with an intellectual disability as follows: "Hello, Mr. Pemberton. My name is Jerry Booker." Shake Mr. Pemberton's hand if he will allow it. "We're here to help you. Your sister called us. She says you're not feeling well today, and we're here to help you feel better. My partner, Tina, is going to take your blood pressure. Do you remember having that done before?" Allow Mr. Pemberton to see and touch the blood pressure cuff as your partner moves forward. Move slowly but deliberately. Explain beforehand what you are going to do, just as with any other patient. Watch carefully for signs of fear or reluctance from the patient. Make sure you are at eye level with the patient. If the patient is sitting, kneel or sit down. This is important in communicating with all patients; however, it is even more important in making the patient with special challenges comfortable.

Do your best to soothe the patient's anxiety and discomfort as you work through your assessment and provide treatment. By initially establishing trust and communication, you will have a much better chance for a successful outcome.

## Brain Injury

A patient with a prior brain injury may be difficult to assess and treat. Chapter 29, *Head and Spine Injuries*, discusses traumatic brain injuries in detail. Patients with brain injuries may face a complex array of challenges related to the injury. In such cases, gathering a complete medical history from the patient, family, and friends will be helpful. Your interaction with patients with brain injuries should be tailored to their specific abilities. Take the time to speak with the patient and family to establish what is considered normal for the patient; for example, determine whether the patient has cognitive, sensory, communication, motor, behavioral, or psychological deficits.

When you care for a patient with a prior brain injury, talk in a calm, soothing tone, and watch the patient closely for signs of anxiety or aggression. In some cases, the patient may need to be specially positioned or restrained to ensure your safety and the safety of the patient. Do not expect the patient to walk to the ambulance or stretcher. As always, treat the patient with respect, use his or her name, explain procedures, and reassure the patient throughout the process.

## Sensory Disabilities
### Visual Impairment

Visual impairments may result from many different causes—a congenital defect; disease; injury; or degeneration of the eyeball, optic nerve, or nerve pathway (eg, with aging). The degree of visual impairment may range from partial to total. Some patients have a loss of peripheral or central vision; others can distinguish light from dark or identify general shapes.

Visual impairments may be difficult to recognize. During your scene size-up, look for signs that indicate the patient is visually impaired, such as the presence of eyeglasses, a cane, or a service animal (**FIGURE 37-2**). Immediately introduce yourself when you enter the room. Have your team members introduce themselves so that the patient can identify their voices and locations. In addition, retrieve any visual aids and give them to your patient to make the interaction more comfortable.

A visually impaired patient may feel vulnerable, especially during the chaos of a crash scene. The patient may have learned to use other senses such as hearing, touch, and smell to compensate for the loss of sight, and the sounds and smells of the scene may be disorienting. Remember to tell the patient what is happening, identify noises, and describe the situation and surroundings, especially if you must move the patient.

The patient may use a cane or walker to ambulate safely. Even if the patient will be carried on a gurney, remember to take the patient's cane or walker. Unless the patient is in critical condition, a service animal should remain with the patient in the patient compartment of the ambulance and will provide reassurance for the patient and prevent delays in transport; however, in some cases you may need to make arrangements for the care or

## YOU are the Provider

You arrive at the scene and find the patient lying supine in a hospital-style bed in the living room. He immediately looks at you when you approach him but does not talk to you. The patient's mother tells you that he began running a fever earlier in the day. She further advises you that the patient's home health nurse was present earlier and contacted his physician, who requested that EMS transport him to the hospital. While your partner gathers additional information, you perform a primary assessment.

| Recording Time: 0 Minutes | |
| --- | --- |
| Appearance | Eyes open |
| Level of consciousness | Conscious and alert; this is his baseline mental status |
| Airway | Tracheostomy tube in place; upper airway clear of secretions and foreign bodies |
| Breathing | 14 breaths/min via mechanical ventilator |
| Circulation | Increased pulse rate (strong and regular); skin is pink, hot, and moist; no gross bleeding |

**3.** What are some conditions that would cause a patient to become dependent on a mechanical ventilator?

**4.** How does a tracheostomy tube affect a patient's ability to communicate? How can you determine whether your patient is alert?

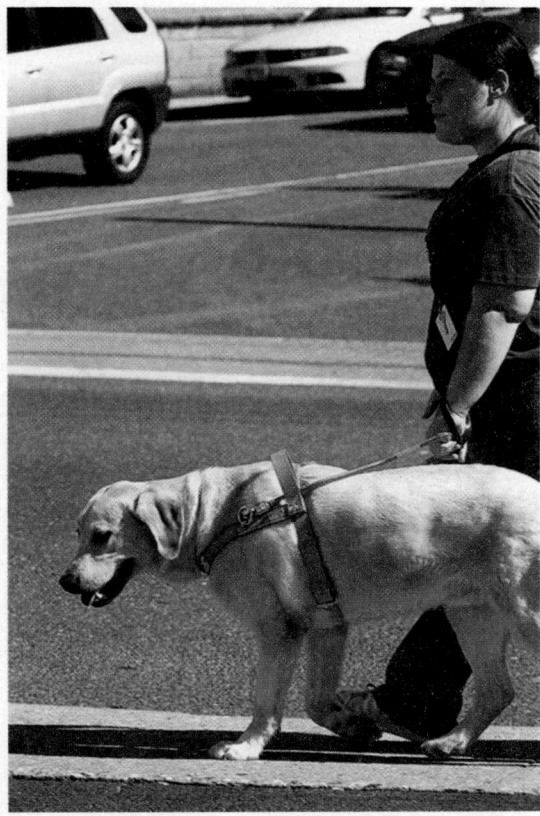

**FIGURE 37-2** Service dogs can often be identified by their harnesses or other special devices such as a vest.

Courtesy of the Guide Dog Foundation for the Blind. Photographed by Christopher Appoldt.

accompaniment of the animal. A friend of the patient or an animal control officer can be helpful in this situation. You should avoid separating the patient and the animal whenever possible, however.

An ambulatory patient may be led by a light touch on the arm or elbow. Alternatively, you may allow the patient to rest his or her hand on your shoulder, as this may enhance the patient's sense of balance and security while moving. Ask patients which method they prefer to use. Patients should be gently guided but never pulled or pushed. Obstacles

## Words of Wisdom

Service animals are not classified as pets and should, by law, be permitted to accompany the patient unless the animal is injured or out of control. Review the Service Animals section in the Americans With Disabilities Act for further information.

need to be communicated in advance. Statements such as "You're approaching the stairs. We're going to take five steps down," will allow the patient to anticipate and navigate the obstacles safely.

## Hearing Impairment

Hearing impairment can range from a slight hearing loss to total deafness. Chapter 4, *Communications and Documentation*, discusses hearing loss in further detail. Patients who are hard of hearing may have difficulty with pitch, volume, and speaking distinctly. Some patients learn to speak even though they have never heard sounds. Other patients may have heard speech and learned to speak, but have since sustained partial or total hearing loss, leading them to speak too loudly. Many older people will have some degree of hearing loss.

The two most common forms of hearing loss are sensorineural deafness and conductive hearing loss. **Sensorineural deafness**, or nerve damage, results from a lesion or damage to the inner ear. **Conductive hearing loss** is caused by a faulty transmission of sound waves, which can occur when a person has an accumulation of wax inside the ear canal or a perforated eardrum.

## Words of Wisdom

As with all interventions for barriers to communication, you should document the use of an interpreter. Also remember that conclusions based on the information from interpreters may not be valid. Ask the interpreter to report exactly what the patient signs and not to add any commentary, however well intentioned.

During your scene size-up, look for clues that a person could be hard of hearing, including the presence of hearing aids, poor pronunciation of words, or failure to respond to your presence or questions. Patients may not have their hearing aids in place. Assist the patient with finding and inserting any hearing aids as appropriate, or ask family members to help you. It may be helpful to communicate by writing until the hearing aids are located. Most patients who are hard of hearing can also read lips to some extent. Therefore, face the patient while you communicate so that he or she can see your mouth; do not exaggerate your lip movements or look away.

Position yourself approximately 18 inches (46 cm) in front of the patient. Because patients who are hard of hearing typically have more difficulty hearing higher frequency sounds, never shout; instead, try lowering the pitch of your voice.

Ask the patient, "How would you like to communicate with me?" Some patients may prefer written communication or the use of gestures or pictures. American Sign Language may be the patient's preferred method of communication (**FIGURE 37-3**). An interpreter, family member, or friend may be a valuable teammate. If needed, ask the interpreter to accompany the patient to the hospital, because this may decrease the stress of communication on the patient, EMS crew, and the hospital staff. If an interpreter is not readily available, call the receiving facility to request one as soon as you are aware of the need.

Here are some helpful hints for working with patients with hearing impairments:

- Speak slowly and distinctly into the less impaired ear, or position yourself on that side.
- Change speakers. Given that 80% of hearing loss is related to an inability to hear high-pitched sounds, it may be helpful to have a team member with a low-pitched voice communicate with the patient.
- Provide paper and a pencil so that you can write your questions and the patient can write responses.
- Have only one EMT ask interview questions, to avoid confusing the patient.
- Try the "reverse stethoscope" technique: Put the earpieces of your stethoscope in the patient's ears and speak softly into the diaphragm of the stethoscope to amplify your voice.

## Hearing Aids

A hearing aid is essentially a device that makes sound louder. Hearing aids cannot restore hearing to normal, but they do improve hearing and listening ability. Hearing aids can be either external or internal, depending on the type of hearing damage. Several types of hearing aids are available (**FIGURE 37-4**):

- **Behind-the-ear.** The working parts are contained in a plastic case that rests behind the ear.
- **Conventional body.** This older style is generally used by people with profound hearing loss.

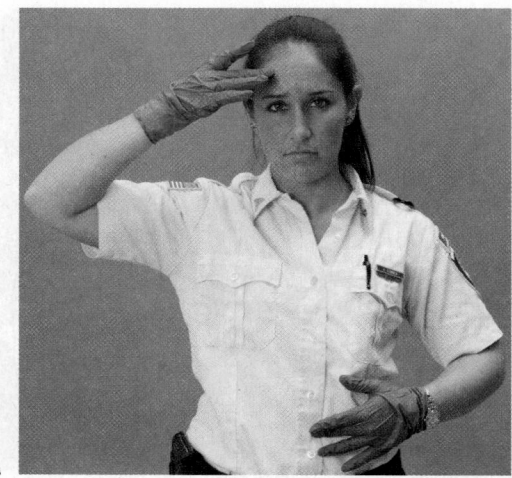

A

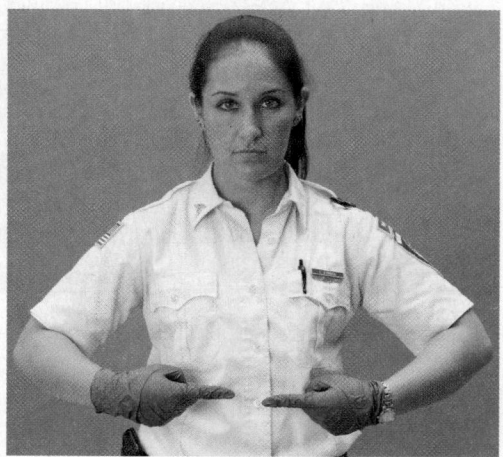

B

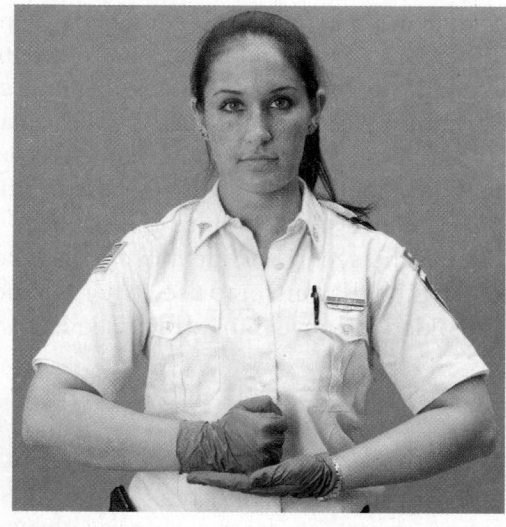

C

**FIGURE 37-3** Consider learning common terms in American Sign Language related to illness and injury. **A.** Sick. **B.** Hurt. **C.** Help.

A, B, C: © Jones & Bartlett Learning. Photographed by Glen E. Ellman.

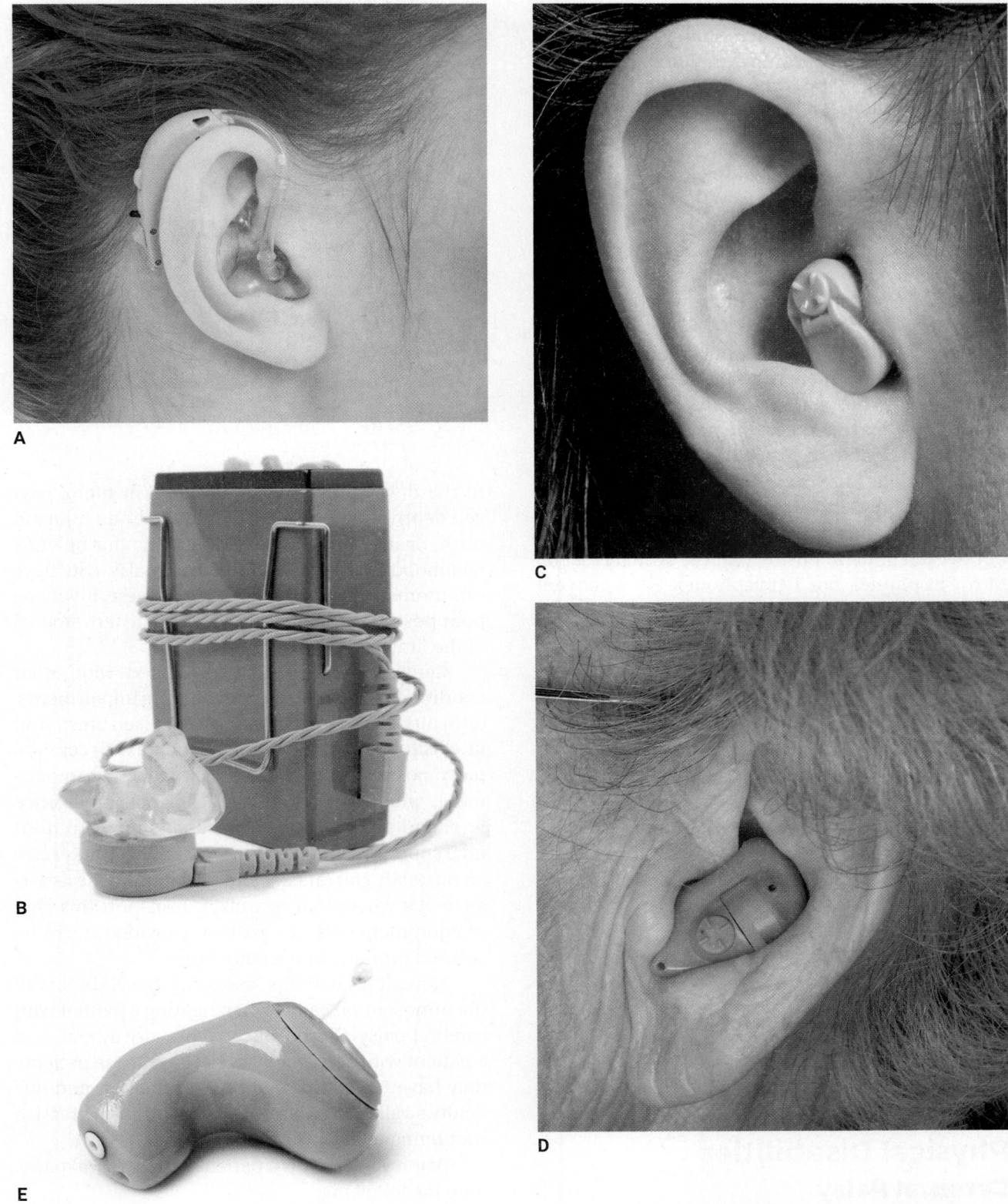

**FIGURE 37-4** Different types of hearing aids. **A.** Behind-the-ear. **B.** Conventional body. **C.** In-the-canal. **D.** In-the-ear. **E.** Completely in-the-canal.

- **In-the-canal and completely in-the-canal.** These hearing aids are contained in a tiny case that fits partly or completely into the ear canal.
- **In-the-ear.** All parts are contained in a shell that fits in the outer part of the ear.

Implantable hearing aids are also an option for patients with less profound hearing loss.

To insert a hearing aid, follow the natural shape of the ear. The device needs to fit snugly without forcing. If you hear a whistling sound, the hearing aid may not be in far enough to create a seal or the volume may be too loud. Try repositioning the hearing aid, or remove it and turn down the volume. If you cannot insert the hearing aid after two tries, put it in its box, take it with you, and document the transport and transfer of hearing aids to hospital personnel. Never try to clean hearing aids, and do not get them wet.

If you are able to insert the hearing aid but it is not working, try troubleshooting the problem. First, make sure the hearing aid is turned on. Try a fresh battery, and check the tubing to make sure it is not twisted or bent. Ensure that the switch is set on M (microphone), not T (telephone). For a conventional body-type aid, try a spare cord; the old one may be broken or shorted. Finally, make sure the ear mold is not clogged with wax.

### Words of Wisdom

Many patients with borderline hearing impairments may not be aware of the extent of their problem. The distracting and noisy EMS environment may worsen the situation. If a patient frequently asks you to repeat things, suspect a hearing impairment.

### Words of Wisdom

Some patients who are hard of hearing are sensitive to loud noises close to their ears. Remember to use a normal tone of voice when speaking to these patients.

## Physical Disabilities
### Cerebral Palsy

**Cerebral palsy** is a term for a group of disorders characterized by poorly controlled body movement (**FIGURE 37-5**). This disorder is a result of damage

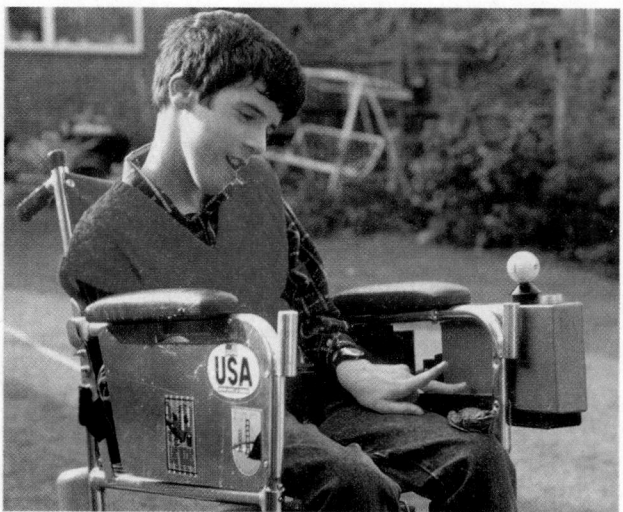

**FIGURE 37-5** A person with cerebral palsy.
© Sally and Richard Greenhill/Alamy Stock Photo.

to the developing fetal brain while in utero, oxygen deprivation at birth, a traumatic brain injury at birth, or infection such as meningitis during early childhood. Patients with cerebral palsy can have symptoms that range from mild to severe, involving poor posture and uncontrolled, spastic movements of the limbs.

Cerebral palsy is also associated with other conditions such as visual and hearing impairments, difficulty communicating, epilepsy (seizures), and intellectual disabilities. Many patients with cerebral palsy possess some degree of intellectual impairment, whereas others have a normal intelligence level and are able to live independently with minimal support. Patients with cerebral palsy may have an unsteady gait (ataxia) and may require the assistance of a wheelchair or walker. Transport this type of equipment with the patient, provided it can be secured properly in the ambulance.

As with all patients, assessing the XABCs is of the utmost importance when treating a patient with cerebral palsy. Closely observe the airway status of a patient with cerebral palsy because these patients may have increased secretion production and difficulty swallowing (dysphagia), requiring aggressive suctioning to clear the airway.

When you care for a patient with cerebral palsy, note the following:

- Do not assume that patients with cerebral palsy have an intellectual disability. Although 75% of patients have some intellectual disability, many people with cerebral palsy have a normal IQ or only slight intellectual impairment.

- Limbs are often underdeveloped and are prone to injury (eg, a fall from a wheelchair).
- Patients who have the ability to walk may have an unsteady gait and be prone to falls.
- If the patient has a specially made pillow or chair (as many pediatric patients do), the patient may prefer to use it during transport. Remember to pad the patient to ensure his or her comfort, and never force a patient's extremities into any position.
- Whenever possible, transport walkers or wheelchairs with the patient.
- Approximately 25% of patients with cerebral palsy have a seizure disorder. Be prepared to address a seizure if one occurs, and keep a suctioning unit available. Consider requesting additional advanced life support (ALS).

## Spina Bifida

Spina bifida is a birth defect caused by the incomplete closure of the spinal column during embryonic or fetal development, resulting in an exposed portion of the spinal cord (**FIGURE 37-6**). The opening can be closed surgically, but the child is often left with spinal and neurologic damage. Adequate maternal intake of vitamin B9 (folic acid) reduces the

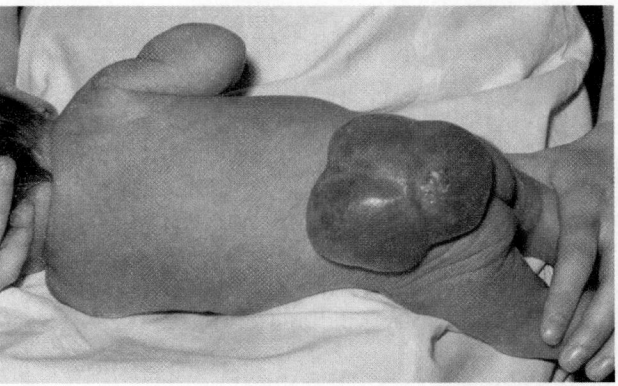

**FIGURE 37-6** Spina bifida is one of the most common disabling birth defects in the United States.
© Biophoto Associates/Science Source.

risk of spina bifida. Most defects occur before the woman knows she is pregnant, so since 1992, the US government has mandated that foods such as breads, cereals, and grains be fortified with vitamin B9. This effort has decreased the incidence of spina bifida, but, unfortunately, it is still one of the most common disabling birth defects in the United States. Some patients with spina bifida also have hydrocephalus, which requires the placement of a shunt to drain excessive amounts of cerebrospinal fluid from the brain.

Be aware that some patients with spina bifida have partial or full paralysis of the lower extremities,

## YOU are the Provider

The patient's axillary temperature reads 101.2°F (38.4°C). The patient has a gastrostomy tube and his mother tells you that she administered an appropriate dose of acetaminophen through the tube about an hour ago. Your partner assesses the patient's vital signs while you perform a physical examination, which reveals no obvious abnormalities. You note that the patient has a colostomy bag and an indwelling urinary catheter.

| Recording Time: 5 Minutes | |
|---|---|
| **Respirations** | 14 breaths/min; provided by mechanical ventilator |
| **Pulse** | 110 beats/min; strong and regular |
| **Skin** | Pink, hot, and moist |
| **Blood pressure** | 118/62 mm Hg |
| **Oxygen saturation (SpO$_2$)** | 99% (on oxygen) |

**5.** What are some potential complications that may result from your patient's condition? What can you do to prevent them or minimize the risks?

**6.** What do you suspect is the patient's underlying problem? What specific treatment should you provide to him?

loss of bowel and bladder control, and an extreme allergy to latex products. Latex-free products should be kept on the ambulance to avoid a severe anaphylactic reaction in patients with spina bifida.

Patients with spina bifida will benefit from the same considerations that you offer when you treat a patient with paralysis or a patient who has difficulty moving. Ask patients how to best move them before you transport them. It is highly likely that a patient in your community will have spina bifida.

## Paralysis

Paralysis is the inability to voluntarily move one or more body parts. It may be caused by stroke, trauma, or birth defects. Paralysis does not always involve a loss of sensation. Some patients will have normal sensation or even hyperesthesia (increased sensitivity), which may cause the patient to experience touch as pain in the affected area. Paralysis of one side of the face may cause communication challenges.

The diaphragm of some paralyzed patients may not function correctly, requiring the use of a ventilator. Patients may also rely on specialized equipment such as urinary catheters, tracheostomy tubes, colostomy bags, or feeding tubes, which are discussed later in this chapter. Some patients may have difficulty swallowing, creating the need for suctioning. Each type of spinal cord paralysis requires its own equipment and may have its own complications.

Patients who have partial or total loss of sensation in a limb cannot tell you when you are injuring them. Always use a gentle touch and take great care when lifting or moving a paralyzed patient. Ask patients how best to move them before you transport them.

## Bariatric Patients

Obesity is a complex condition in which a person has an excessive amount of body fat. It is the result of an imbalance between calories consumed and calories used. The solution to the obesity problem may sound simple—reestablish the caloric balance—but, unfortunately, the causes of obesity are not fully understood. Many cases of obesity may be attributed to a low metabolic rate or genetic predisposition.

According to the Mayo Clinic, the term *obese* is used when someone is 30% or more over his or her ideal body weight. This is a good general guideline, except in cases where body weight does not correlate to excess fat, such as in very muscular people. In severe obesity (also called extreme or morbid obesity), the person is two or three times over the ideal weight. The person's quality of life is often negatively affected, and the extra weight can cause a variety of problems, such as mobility difficulties, diabetes, hypertension, heart disease, and stroke.

### Interaction With Patients With Obesity

People with obesity are often ridiculed publicly and sometimes become targets of discrimination. Patients with obesity may be embarrassed by their condition or fearful of scorn as a result of past experiences. Some of those negative interactions may have occurred with an insensitive health care professional. As with any patient, work hard to put these patients at ease. Establish the patient's chief complaint and then communicate your plan to help. Many patients with severe obesity have a complex and extensive medical history, so mastering the art of conducting a patient interview will serve you well in your patient interactions.

If transport is necessary, plan early for extra help and do not be afraid to call for additional providers and/or specialized equipment if necessary. In particular, send a member of your team to find the easiest and safest exit to use. Remember, everyone's safety is at stake! You do not want to risk dropping the patient or injuring a team member by trying to lift too much weight. Moves, no matter how simple they may seem, become far more complex when handling a patient with obesity.

### Interaction With Patients With Morbid Obesity

Morbid obesity affects approximately nine million adult Americans. These patients may overcome mobility difficulties by pulling, rocking, or rolling into a position. The constant strain on their body's structures may leave them with chronic joint injuries or osteoarthritis. When you move a patient with morbid obesity, follow these tips:

- Treat the patient with dignity and respect.
- Be aware if you have a bias toward people with obesity. Recognizing this bias can help ensure you deliver the same care, including transport

to the hospital, for these patients as you would for others.

- Ask the patient how best to move him or her before attempting to do so.
- Avoid lifting the patient by only one limb, which would risk injury to overtaxed joints.
- Coordinate and communicate all moves to all team members prior to starting to lift.
- If the move becomes uncontrolled at any point, stop, reposition, and resume.
- Look for pinch or pressure points from equipment because this could cause significant soft-tissue injuries or deep vein thrombosis.
- Large patients will often have difficulty breathing in a supine position. When safe and appropriate to do so, elevate the head of the stretcher when transporting patients with obesity.
- There are many types of specialized equipment for patients with obesity, and some areas have specially equipped bariatric ambulances for such patients. Become familiar with the resources available in your area.
- Plan egress routes to accommodate large patients, equipment, and the lifting team members. Remember: Do no harm!
- Notify the receiving facility early to allow special arrangements to be made prior to your arrival to accommodate the patient's needs.

## Patients With Medical Technology Assistance
### Tracheostomy Tubes

A tracheostomy is a surgical procedure that creates a stoma, or opening, through a patient's anterior neck, providing a pathway directly into the trachea where a tracheostomy tube may be placed to allow for a patent airway (**FIGURE 37-7**).

Tracheostomy tubes are generally placed in patients who have anatomic abnormalities or who require long-term mechanical ventilation, require frequent tracheal suctioning, or have recurrent pulmonary infections due to the inability to adequately control oral and airway secretions. The tracheostomy may be permanent, or temporary depending on the condition that required its placement. Because these tubes are foreign to the respiratory tract, the body reacts by building up secretions in or around the tube. The tubes are prone to obstruction by mucus plugs or foreign bodies. Routine care that is provided by caregivers includes keeping the inner cannula of the tracheostomy tube clean and dry and suctioning any secretions.

Some patients who have a tracheostomy tube in place may be dependent on an automatic ventilator to provide ventilation. Almost all patients with a tracheostomy tube in place can still be ventilated

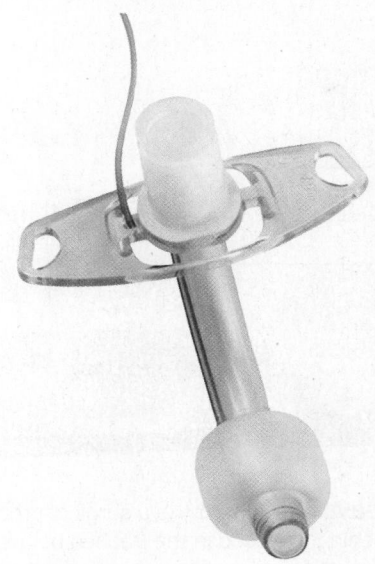

**FIGURE 37-7** Some patients require a tracheostomy tube to breathe.

Portex® Blue Line® Ultra Tracheostomy courtesy of Smiths Medical.

manually with a bag-mask device, either attached to the tracheostomy tube itself or over the mouth and nose with a standard mask.

The standard tracheostomy tube has three main components (**FIGURE 37-8**). There is an outer cannula with a flange that helps support and stabilize the device as it passes through the neck. The outer cannula may have a cuff that seals the trachea off from the upper airway. This cuff is inflated through a pilot balloon and valve on the outside of the device. Within the outer cannula is a slightly smaller inner cannula through which the patient is ventilated. The inner cannula has a 15-mm adapter that allows for a bag-mask device or ventilator circuit to be attached. Most, but not all, inner cannulas are capable of being removed for cleaning or in case a plug has developed. The final component of a tracheostomy tube setup is a rigid obturator. This blunt-tipped (rounded) device is curved and long enough to reach to the distal end of the outer cannula. It is used when reinserting the flexible inner cannula. It may also be used to occlude the tracheostomy tube when ventilations are being provided by mask over the nose and mouth during an emergency. Some patients use a valve attached to the end of the tracheostomy to help them speak. This valve needs to be removed to suction or ventilate the tracheostomy.

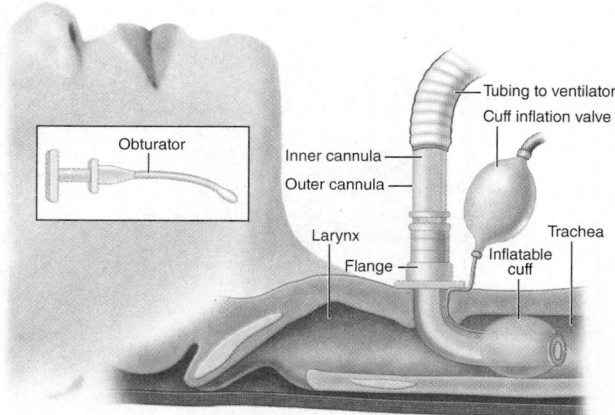

**FIGURE 37-8** A tracheostomy is a surgical procedure in which an opening is placed in the trachea below the cricoid ring. A tracheostomy tube can be inserted into the opening to maintain it. The tube can also be attached to a ventilator or bag-mask device to assist with ventilations.

© Jones & Bartlett Learning.

An obstruction of the tracheostomy tube is an emergency that requires you to intervene immediately. This type of emergency can be stressful to deal with, so it is imperative to remember the XABCs and airway management. A useful mnemonic in these situations is DOPE (**TABLE 37-1**). The DOPE mnemonic can help you remember the possible causes of an airway obstruction and correct the problem. Failure to clear an obstructed tracheostomy tube could lead to cardiopulmonary arrest.

There may be bleeding or air leaking around the tube. This is more likely to happen with new tracheostomies. The tube can become loose or dislodged. Occasionally, the opening around the tube may become infected. Your care of a patient with a tracheostomy tube includes maintaining an open airway, maintaining the patient in a position of comfort, administering supplemental oxygen as needed, and providing transport to the hospital.

Some patients with tracheostomy tubes and special health care needs may have muscle contractions that will not allow you to place them in the typical semi-Fowler position; in these cases, suction the patient in a position of comfort. If trauma is involved, protect the cervical spine.

If suctioning of the tracheostomy tube is necessary, first attempt to use the patient's suction device. It is probably already sized correctly and

**TABLE 37-1** DOPE Mnemonic

- **D** Displaced, dislodged, or damaged tube
- **O** Obstructed tube (secretions, blood, mucus, vomitus)
- **P** Pneumothorax
- **E** Equipment failure (kinked tubing, ventilator malfunction, empty oxygen supply)

© Jones & Bartlett Learning.

readily available. If the size of the suction catheter is unknown, estimate the size by doubling the inner diameter of the tracheostomy tube. To determine the length of the suction device, ask a family member or measure the length of a spare tracheostomy tube. If the length of the patient's tracheostomy tube cannot be determined, insert the suction device no more than 1 to 2 inches (3 to 6 cm) deep. The suction unit should be set to 100 mm Hg. You may need to instill 2 to 3 mL of saline before suctioning thick tracheal secretions. Do not suction for more than 10 seconds, and do not force the suction catheter into the cannula. Oxygenate before and after the procedure. Call for ALS backup.

### Words of Wisdom

If a tracheostomy tube becomes plugged, encourage the caregiver to remove the tube and reinsert a new one. Caregivers should be trained to do this and should have a spare tracheostomy tube in a "go bag" with the patient. A completely obstructed tracheostomy tube results in hypoxia and leads to cardiac arrest if not opened quickly.

## Home Oxygen

Patients with certain chronic lung diseases (such as chronic obstructive pulmonary disease) may require long-term home oxygen use. Two types of oxygen delivery systems are used for these patients. The first option is the use of oxygen from compressed gas cylinders, similar to what is available on an ambulance, only smaller and more convenient for home use. The second option is to use a machine that concentrates oxygen from the ambient air and then compresses it for delivery to the patient.

Compressed oxygen cylinders do not require electricity or complex machinery. If the power is out, the oxygen from a compressed cylinder will still flow, as long as the supply in that cylinder remains adequate. Additionally, the liter flow per minute of oxygen cylinders is limited only by the regulator attached to the cylinder and the amount of gas left in the cylinder. The drawbacks of using compressed gas cylinders mainly center around portability and limited supply. Oxygen cylinders can be heavy, bulky, and difficult to transport. Although small cylinders are available that can be carried more easily,

the amount of oxygen available in these small cylinders may be suitable for a short duration only. Additionally, regardless of the size of the oxygen cylinder, it will run out of oxygen eventually. Thus, patients using compressed gas cylinders must have multiple cylinders in the home and must coordinate with an oxygen supplier for regular delivery and pickup of these cylinders. Although oxygen is not flammable, it will cause items that are already on fire to burn at much higher temperatures and with much greater intensity.

A home oxygen concentrator takes ambient air and scrubs the nitrogen from the atmospheric air, leaving behind almost 100% oxygen (**FIGURE 37-9A**). After the oxygen has been concentrated, it is compressed so that it can be delivered to the patient via an oxygen delivery device, such as a nasal cannula or face mask. The compression that home oxygen concentrators are able to achieve varies by machine but is generally limited to 10 L/min. The main benefit of the oxygen concentrator machine is that it can provide an unlimited supply of oxygen as long as it is functioning properly and has a reliable source of electrical power. There are also smaller, more portable oxygen concentrators that can provide patients with increased mobility and freedom of travel, although these units are usually able to provide only 1 to 3 L/min of flow in most cases (**FIGURE 37-9B**). In the event of a power failure, the patient must have a backup compressed gas cylinder to use until power is restored.

When caring for patients who are on home oxygen, you should ask them why they are on home oxygen, how long they have been on home oxygen, what their baseline home oxygen requirement is (ie, how many liters per minute, how many hours a day), and whether their home oxygen requirement has changed recently. It is also important to establish these patients' baseline oxygen saturation levels. Many patients with chronic lung disease will have baseline oxygen saturations that are lower than normal. Regardless of their baseline oxygen saturation level, any patient who is in respiratory distress should be placed on supplemental oxygen at a level appropriate for his or her level of distress and work of breathing.

## Mechanical Ventilators

Patients who are on a mechanical ventilator at home cannot breathe without assistance (**FIGURE 37-10**).

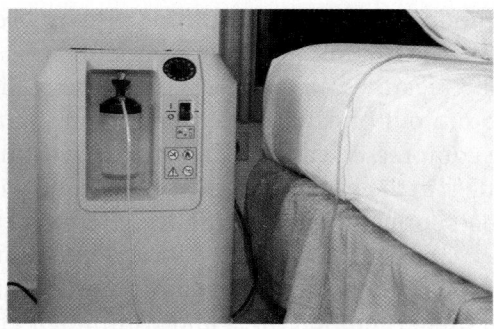

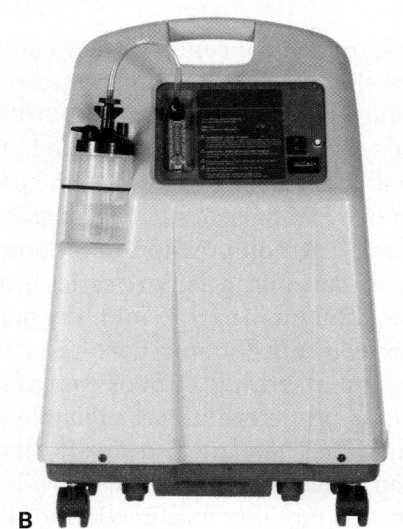

**FIGURE 37-9 A.** Home oxygen concentrator. **B.** Portable oxygen concentrator.

**A:** © abalcazar/iStock/Getty Images Plus/Getty Images; **B:** © HKPNC/E+/Getty Images.

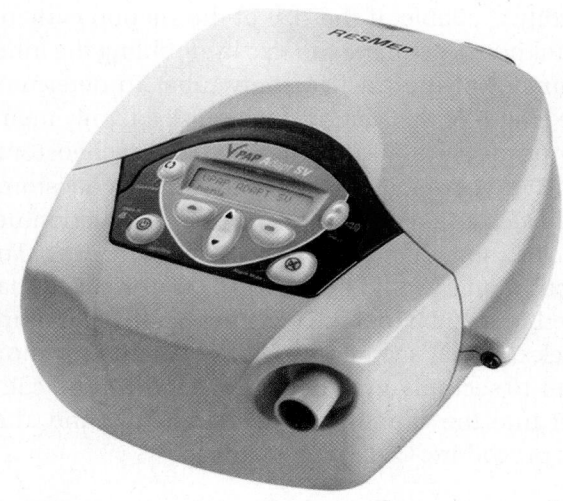

**FIGURE 37-10** A home ventilator.

© ResMed 2010. Used with permission.

Patients requiring a mechanical ventilator may not have an underlying respiratory drive because of a congenital defect or a chronic lung disease process. Other patients may have a traumatic brain injury, muscular dystrophy, or another disease process that weakens their ability to breathe and requires a permanent tracheostomy and mechanical ventilator.

Remember that patients with tracheostomies typically do not breathe through the mouth and nose; therefore, a face mask or nasal cannula cannot

## YOU are the Provider

You consult with medical control and receive instructions on how to proceed. The mechanical ventilator is too large to fit in your ambulance, so you prepare the bag-mask device, detach the ventilator circuit from the tracheostomy tube, and begin manual ventilations at 12 breaths/min. You request ALS support, which is severely delayed due to traffic. You carefully move the patient to your stretcher, secure him properly, and load him into the ambulance. Following medical control's direction, you continue to manually ventilate the patient, reassess his vital signs, and begin transport to the hospital.

| Recording Time: 15 Minutes | |
| --- | --- |
| **Level of consciousness** | Conscious and alert |
| **Respirations** | 12 breaths/min; provided by bag-mask device |
| **Pulse** | 118 beats/min; strong and regular |
| **Skin** | Pink, hot, and dry |
| **Blood pressure** | 120/60 mm Hg |
| **Spo$_2$** | 98% (on oxygen) |

**7.** What is the benefit of allowing the patient's mother to accompany her son to the hospital?

be used to treat them. If the ventilator malfunctions and the patient can breathe on his or her own, remove the patient from the ventilator and apply a tracheostomy collar. This oxygen-delivery device is specifically designed to cover the tracheostomy stoma and features a strap that goes around the neck. Tracheostomy collars are usually available in intensive care units, where many patients have tracheostomies, and may not be available in a pre-hospital setting. If you do not have a tracheostomy collar, you can improvise by placing a face mask over the stoma (**FIGURE 37-11**). Even though the mask is shaped to fit the face, you can usually achieve an adequate fit over the patient's neck by adjusting the strap. If the patient's own ventilations are absent or inadequate, ventilate the patient using a bag-mask device.

Patients on home mechanical ventilators require assisted ventilation throughout transport. Remember that the patient's caregivers will know how the mechanical ventilator works and can help you attach the bag and valve from a bag-mask device to the tracheostomy tube in preparation for transport.

### Words of Wisdom

Several states have adopted laws that require a backup generator or other devices to prevent the loss of electric supply to the homes of families or institutions that have patients using mechanical ventilators.

## Apnea Monitors

While caring for an infant with special challenges, you may come across an apnea monitor (**FIGURE 37-12**). The apnea monitor is typically used when there is a family history of sudden infant death syndrome or when an infant is born prematurely, has severe gastroesophageal reflux that causes choking episodes, or has experienced an apparent life-threatening event. Chapter 35, *Pediatric Emergencies*, discusses sudden infant death syndrome and apparent life-threatening events in detail. Because the central nervous system is not mature in pediatric patients with special challenges, an apnea monitor is used for 2 weeks to 2 months after birth of these high-risk infants to monitor the respiratory system. A typical episode of apnea may last for approximately 15 to 20 seconds, during periods of sleep. The apnea monitor is designed to sound an alarm if the infant experiences bradycardia or an episode of apnea occurs.

The apnea monitor is attached with electrodes or a belt wrapped around the infant's chest or stomach. A pulse oximeter may also be used. The apnea monitor will provide a pulse oximetry reading that will help you assess the patient's respiratory status.

The parents or caregivers of pediatric patients with special challenges will be a useful resource when obtaining the patient's medical history and a history of the events leading to the call for assistance. Parents and caregivers become knowledgeable regarding the use of apnea monitors and may be able to provide you and your partner with a computerized printout to share with ALS providers or

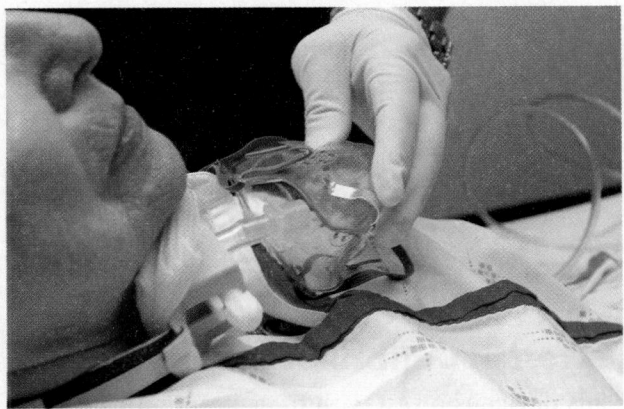

**FIGURE 37-11** If you do not have a tracheostomy collar, use a face mask instead.

© Jones & Bartlett Learning.

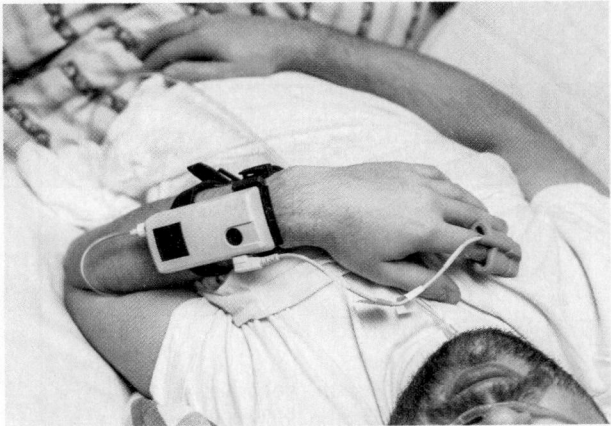

**FIGURE 37-12** An apnea monitor.

© Koldunova/iStock/Getty Images Plus/Getty Images.

ED personnel. If possible, bring the apnea monitor to the receiving hospital with the infant so that it may be evaluated and any stored information may be retrieved for further analysis.

## Internal Cardiac Pacemakers

An internal cardiac pacemaker is a device implanted under the patient's skin to regulate the heart rate. These devices are typically placed on the nondominant side of the patient's chest so that normal activities are not hindered. In small or extremely thin patients, the device may be implanted in the abdomen. Some pacemakers include an automated implanted cardioverter defibrillator, which monitors the patient's heart rhythm and is able to slow accelerated heart rates.

Never place defibrillator patches directly over the implanted device. It can be helpful for the hospital staff if you gather information about the cardiac pacemaker while you obtain the patient's history during the patient assessment process (**TABLE 37-2**). Sometimes a patient will have a pacemaker identification card in his or her wallet that contains information specific to the device.

## Ventricular Assist Devices

A ventricular assist device (VAD) is a special piece of medical equipment that takes over the function of one or both heart ventricles. These types of devices are typically used as a bridge to heart transplantation while a donor heart is being located or as a permanent solution for patients who do not qualify for a transplant. A left ventricular assist device (LVAD) is the most common VAD and all VADs

are more common in adults. There is one VAD that has been appropriate for use in patients aged 5 to 16 years. It may be difficult to palpate a pulse in patients who use a VAD. In such cases, assess perfusion by noting level of consciousness, skin color, temperature, moisture, and blood pressure.

If you encounter a patient with a VAD, you will primarily provide support measures and basic care. The parents or caregivers should be knowledgeable about the device, so use them as a resource during transport. The patient should have a "go bag" that must always be transported with him or her. Risk factors associated with the implantation of a VAD include excessive bleeding following the surgery, infection, blood clots leading to strokes, and acute heart failure. Be prepared to provide CPR. Keep in mind that the VAD may be functioning in the absence of a palpable pulse so you will have to use other assessment techniques to determine adequate perfusion. Assess the patient's level of consciousness, skin color, and capillary refill. If you encounter a patient with this device, call the number of the patient's support team, contact medical control, or follow your local protocols. If the device's alarm is sounding, check all connections and be sure the batteries are fully charged. Notify ALS personnel as soon as possible so that other supportive measures may be initiated.

---

**TABLE 37-2** Questions for Patients With Pacemakers

- What type of heart disorder do you have?
- How long has this device been implanted?
- What is your normal baseline rhythm and heart rate?
- Is your heart completely dependent on the pacemaker device?
- At what heart rate will the defibrillator fire?
- How many times has the defibrillator delivered a shock?

© Jones & Bartlett Learning.

---

### Words of Wisdom

Special equipment such as a VAD often includes a toll-free number to call for information specific to patient care. Patients and family members typically carry identification cards with necessary phone numbers and may be able to share this information with you. Make every reasonable effort to bring these patients to the hospital where the VAD was implanted to facilitate management of any problems with the device. This will obviously be a function of distance and patient condition. Seek online medical direction early, as these are among the most complicated patients you will care for.

## External Defibrillator Vest

This device is a vest with built-in monitoring electrodes and defibrillation pads, which is worn by the patient under his or her clothing. The vest is attached to a monitor that provides alerts and voice prompts when it recognizes a dangerous rhythm and before it delivers a shock. The device uses high-energy shocks similar to an AED, so avoid contact with the patient if the device warns that it is about to deliver a shock.

If the patient is in cardiac arrest, the vest should remain in place while you perform CPR unless it interferes with compressions. Any patient who is wearing a device that has already delivered a shock should be transported to an appropriate hospital for further evaluation. See Chapter 17, *Cardiovascular Emergencies,* for further information.

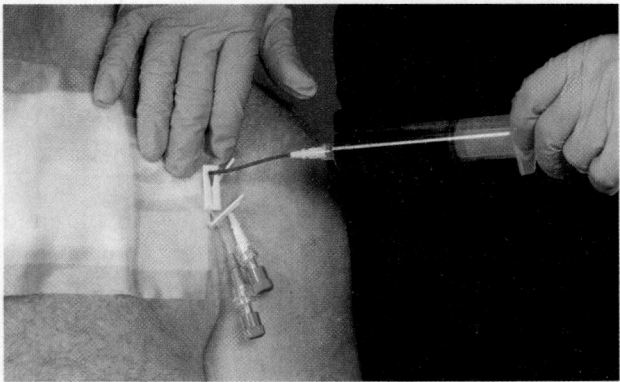

**FIGURE 37-13** Patients who require frequent intravenous medications may have a central line in place.

© Jones & Bartlett Learning. Courtesy of MIEMSS.

> ### Words of Wisdom
>
> If the patient is unresponsive and you are unsure whether the external defibrillator vest has already delivered a shock, look for blue gel on the patient's upper back. The electrodes on the vest release the gel immediately before the shock is delivered.

## Central Venous Catheter

A central venous catheter, or central line, is a catheter that has its tip placed in the vena cava to provide venous access. It is used for many types of home care patients, including those receiving chemotherapy, long-term antibiotic therapy, pain management, total parenteral nutrition, and hemodialysis (**FIGURE 37-13**). Central venous catheters are often located in the chest, upper arm, or subclavicular area.

Problems associated with central venous catheters include broken lines, infections around the lines, clotted lines, and bleeding around the line or from the tubing attached to the line. If bleeding occurs, apply direct pressure to the tubing and provide prompt transport to the hospital.

## Gastrostomy Tubes

Gastrostomy tubes, sometimes referred to as gastric tubes or G-tubes, are placed into the stomach of patients who cannot adequately ingest fluids, food, or medication by mouth (**FIGURE 37-14**). These tubes may be inserted through the nose or mouth into the stomach (using a nasogastric or orogastric tube) or inserted surgically directly into the stomach through the abdominal wall. Gastric tubes may

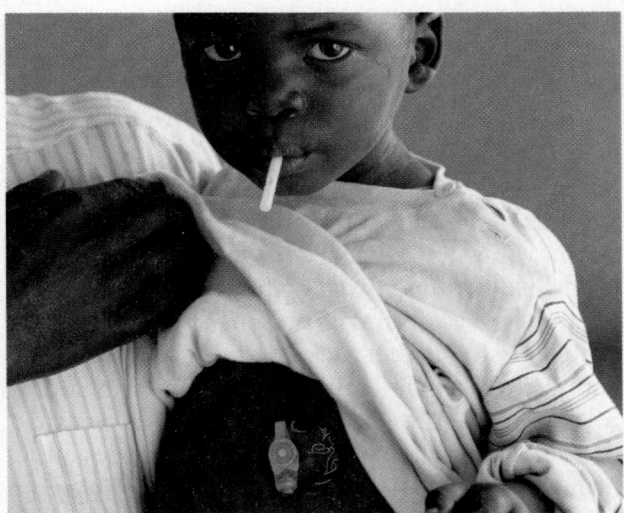

**FIGURE 37-14** Gastric tubes may be placed through the skin into the stomach for children or adults who cannot be fed by mouth.

© DELOCHE/age fotostock.

become dislodged during the patient's normal daily activities. If such a situation arises, immediately stop the flow of any fluids being infused through the tube, and assess the patient for signs or symptoms of bleeding into the stomach, such as vague abdominal discomfort, nausea, and vomiting (especially emesis with a "coffee-ground" appearance [older blood] or with bright red blood).

Patients who have a gastric tube in place may still be at increased risk of aspiration. Always have suction readily available to clear any materials from the patient's mouth. Stop the flow of any fluids if signs of aspiration are present. Patients with gastric tubes who have difficulty breathing should be transported while sitting or lying on the right side with the head elevated 30° to prevent the contents of the stomach from passing into the lungs. Give supplemental oxygen if the patient has any difficulty breathing.

Patients with diabetes who receive insulin and gastric tube feedings may become hypoglycemic quickly if the gastric tube feedings are discontinued for any reason. Be alert for an altered mental status or a change in the baseline behavior of your patient. Unless the tube is dysfunctional, dislodged, or partially dislodged, continue the tube feeding and transport the pump with you.

## Shunts

Some patients with chronic neurologic conditions may have shunts in place. For example, a patient with hydrocephalus will have a shunt. Shunts are tubes that drain excess cerebrospinal fluid from the ventricles of the brain to keep pressure from building up in the brain.

During your assessment of a patient with a shunt, you will likely feel a device beneath the skin on the side of the head, behind the ear. The device is a fluid reservoir, and its presence should alert you to the possibility that the patient has an underlying shunt. There are different types of shunts, including a ventriculoperitoneal (VP) shunt and a ventriculoatrial (VA) shunt. A VP shunt drains excess fluid from the ventricles of the brain into the peritoneum of the abdomen. A VA shunt drains excess fluid from the ventricles of the brain into the right atrium of the heart. A shunt may become blocked or an infection may result in the surrounding tissue. Infections as a result of shunt placement may occur within the first 2 months after shunt insertion. A blocked shunt may present as a medical emergency. If the shunt is unable to drain properly, intracranial pressure may increase, affecting the patient's mental status, and respiratory arrest may occur.

The signs that a patient is in distress include a high-pitched cry or bulging fontanelles (in infants), headache, projectile vomiting, altered mental status, irritability, fever, nausea, difficulty with coordination (walking), blurred vision, seizures, redness along the shunt track, bradycardia, and heart dysrhythmias. Emergency medical care includes airway management and artificial ventilation during transport.

## Vagus Nerve Stimulators

According to the Epilepsy Foundation, epilepsy is diagnosed in approximately 150,000 patients each year in the United States. Vagus nerve stimulation is a form of treatment used for seizures that are not controlled with antiepileptic medications or if the patient is not a good candidate for brain surgery. Vagus nerve stimulators stimulate the vagus nerve at predetermined intervals to prevent seizure activity. Some devices deliver an extra burst if an impending seizure is detected by a fast increase in the patient's heart rate. These devices are used in conjunction with medication to reduce the frequency of seizures. They are not meant to replace medications and are not currently used in children younger than 4 years. Further studies are being done regarding their effectiveness for seizure disorders. The device, which is approximately the size of a silver dollar, is surgically implanted under the patient's skin. The stimulator can last for up to 6 years or until the battery runs out. If you encounter a patient with this device, contact medical control or follow your local protocols.

## Colostomies, Ileostomies, and Urostomies

A colostomy or ileostomy is a surgical procedure that creates an opening from the small or large intestine to the surface of the body that allows for elimination of waste products. The special opening is referred to as a stoma. Feces are expelled and collected into a clear external bag or pouch, which is emptied or changed frequently.

If you encounter a patient with a colostomy or ileostomy bag, assess for signs and symptoms of dehydration if the patient reports diarrhea or vomiting. The area around the stoma is prone to infection, so patients and caregivers must be diligent with daily hygiene. Signs of infection include redness, warm skin around the stoma, and tenderness with palpation over the colostomy or ileostomy site.

A urostomy is a surgically created connection between the urinary system to the surface of the skin that allows urine to drain through a stoma in the abdominal wall instead of through the urethra. For example, a patient who has had his or her bladder removed due to cancer requires a urostomy.

Contact medical control or follow your local protocols for the care of a patient with a colostomy, ileostomy, or urostomy bag.

# Patient Assessment Guidelines

Interaction with the parents or caregivers of a child or adult with special challenges will be an important part of the patient assessment process. The parents, caregivers, or home health care staff members have become experts on the illness or disability and are trained to use and troubleshoot problems with medical equipment on a daily basis. Assess the patient's baseline vital signs, note any allergies (eg, to medications or latex), medications, and other pertinent medical history. You must first determine the patient's normal baseline status before an assessment of the current condition can be made. It is often helpful to ask, "What is different today?"

## Home Care

Home care occurs within a patient's home environment. Patients requiring home services represent a spectrum of special health care populations, including infants and older adults, patients with chronic illnesses, and patients with developmental disabilities. These services are commonly needed among patients older than 65 years.

Services offered by home care agencies include, but are not limited to, meal delivery, house cleaning, laundry, yard maintenance, physical therapy, and personal care, including bathing and wound care. Often, EMS is called to a residence when a home care provider has found the patient injured or has recognized a change in the patient's health status. Home care personnel are an important resource for you when you are obtaining the patient's baseline health status and the history of the present illness or condition. Home care personnel are usually familiar with the patient's surroundings and can obtain any health care documentation or medications that need to be transported with the patient to the hospital.

## Hospice Care and Terminally Ill Patients

Unfortunately, not all illnesses can be cured. As health care providers, you and your team may be called on to assist a patient who has a terminal illness. The patient may be receiving hospice care at a hospice facility or at home.

Patients receiving hospice care are terminally ill, commonly with diseases such as cancer, heart and lung failure, end-stage Alzheimer disease, or AIDS. The patient's physician will have determined that the illness is terminal and in most cases has completed a do not resuscitate (DNR) order or given medical orders for the scope of treatment, outlining the care agreed upon by the patient and/or the family. Hospice care provides comfort care, or palliative care (eg, treatment for pain, nausea, difficulty breathing), during a person's last days. Comfort care improves the patient's quality of life before death and allows the patient to be with family and friends. If you are called to a facility that provides hospice care or a home with a patient receiving hospice care, you will need to follow your local protocols, the patient's wishes, or legal documents such as a DNR order. All necessary documentation must be brought to the hospital if the patient is to be transported to the hospital and must be noted in the patient care report.

If you are called to the home of a terminally ill patient, the care you give will have a lasting effect on the family. This is a time when respect, empathy, and sensitivity are most needed. Some homes with patients receiving hospice care may be chaotic. Family members may be having a difficult time coping with the situation, and they may be angry and hostile. Treat everyone with compassion and understanding. Members of your team may be able to separate family members to speak with them privately to defuse intense emotions and restore order.

Some terminally ill patients who are at home may be receiving outpatient care from a hospice or a home health nurse. You may be called to the home because of a delay in the arrival of the regular care provider or for transport so that a physician can address an immediate need, such as increasing pain. Because terminally ill patients may use a complex variety of pain medications, transdermal patches, or self-administered pain management devices, you may need to consult medical control for guidance.

Even if a DNR order is in place, family members may not understand what to do, and they may not be ready to face the death of a loved one. In such cases, obtain a thorough history and compassionately discuss the patient's wishes. Ask to review the DNR order, and contact medical control.

Ascertain the family's wishes about having the patient remain in the home or having the patient transported to the hospital. If a family member asks to accompany the patient, he or she should be allowed to do so. If the family wishes the patient to remain at home, this request should be honored, provided it is in accordance with your local or state protocol.

Local protocols for handling the death of a patient vary, so be familiar with your local or state regulations. The protocols identify whether the coroner needs to be called to report the death and, if so, who is responsible for contacting the coroner. Also determine whether a pronouncement of death is required and, if so, who is responsible for the determination.

## Poverty and Homelessness

According to a US Bureau of the Census report, in 2018, 11.8% of the overall US population lived in poverty. Children younger than 18 years have the highest rate of poverty, at 16.2%. People who live in poverty are often unable to provide for all of their own basic needs such as housing, food, child care, health insurance, and medication. An impoverished person or family may have housing but may go without food or medication in order to pay for that housing. Disease prevention strategies such as dental care, good nutrition, and exercise are likely lacking, which increases the probability of disease.

Homelessness occurs when people are unable to acquire and/or maintain affordable housing.

According to the National Alliance to End Homelessness, approximately 550,000 people experience homelessness on any given night in the United States. Individual persons make up two-thirds of the homeless population in the United States, with families making up the remaining one-third. Chronically homeless individuals (people who are homeless for an extended time or who are repeatedly homeless) make up approximately 18% of the homeless population. Veterans and individuals younger than 25 years each account for 7% of the homeless population. Racial minorities are proportionally overrepresented among the homeless population in comparison to their numbers in the general population. Another subgroup at high risk for homelessness is LGBTQ youth, who are at 120% higher risk to report homelessness or housing insecurity compared to age- and sex-matched heterosexual populations. The homeless population also includes people with mental illness, people with prior brain trauma, victims of domestic violence, people with addiction disorders, and impoverished families. Homeless individuals are significantly more likely to use EMS and the ED than are individuals who have secure housing.

You are an advocate for all patients. Your job is to provide emergency medical care and transport patients to the appropriate facility. Remember that under the Emergency Medical Treatment and Active Labor Act, all hospital emergency departments *must* provide a medical assessment and required treatment, regardless of the patient's ability to pay. You can also be an

## YOU are the Provider

You call in your radio report to the ED. During your reassessment, you note that the patient is moving his head around and appears to be fighting your attempts to assist ventilations. You also note an acute change in his vital signs. His mother, who is riding in the back of the ambulance with you, asks you if you know what to do.

| Recording Time: 25 Minutes | |
| --- | --- |
| Level of consciousness | Conscious; moving his head around; mother advises that he is agitated |
| Respirations | 12 breaths/min; provided by bag-mask device |
| Pulse | 130 beats/min; strong and regular |
| Skin | Pink, hot, and moist |
| Blood pressure | 134/74 mm Hg |
| SpO$_2$ | 87% (on oxygen) |

**8.** What has most likely happened to your patient? What should you do next?

## Street Smarts

Some homeless patients may be uncomfortable with certain portions of the physical examination because of shame or embarrassment over their appearance or poor hygiene. It is important to communicate therapeutically with these individuals and use language and terms that normalize their condition. Reassuring these patients that you will care for them regardless of how they appear, by using phrases such as "This is a safe place, and I will take care of you no matter how you are dressed," will help facilitate care. Some homeless patients may have an odor because of an inability to access hygiene supplies or facilities. Some will have poor dentition and may mumble or not speak because of embarrassment about how their teeth look. It is important to consider these factors while caring for them. Allow these patients to guide what level of care and examination they are comfortable with when appropriate. Most importantly, reassure them that they are in a safe place and have no need to be apologetic or embarrassed about their condition or appearance.

advocate by becoming familiar with the social services resources within your community so you can refer patients to these lifelines. Depending on the community in which you work, there may be alternatives to the ED for transport consideration. Some hospitals have set up partnerships with homeless shelters to provide routine medical care and treatment for non–life-threatening conditions at the shelter in order to avoid tying up ED resources. Your knowledge of these community resources is crucial to facilitating efficient flow of the EMS network, as EMS is often the first to encounter homeless individuals on their way to the ED.

The evolution of mobile integrated health care and community paramedicine will benefit many patient populations, including patients with special challenges. As EMS systems around the United States continue to implement these new positions, patients with low-acuity (nonemergency) conditions may be able to be assessed and treated on scene without transport. In addition, EMS roles may expand to include providing telephone advice to 9-1-1 callers, preventive care, chronic disease management, and postdischarge follow-up.

## YOU are the Provider SUMMARY

**1. How will your assessment and treatment of this patient differ from that of a patient who is not dependent on a ventilator?**

The principles of patient assessment and treatment are the same, regardless of the patient's special health care needs and any medical equipment that he or she requires to function or live. As with any patient you encounter, your goal is to maintain the XABCs and safely transport the patient to an appropriate medical facility.

**2. What role do the parents or caregivers of patients with special health care needs have in the prehospital setting?**

When you care for a patient with special health care needs, it is imperative to listen to the people who take care of the patient. The parents or caregivers provide for the medical needs of the patient every day; therefore, they are aware of the patient's medical and/or

surgical history, his or her baseline mental status, and the names and doses of any medications the patient may be taking.

Parents or caregivers of this patient population are also trained and experienced in the use of any special equipment the patient requires. In many cases, the parent or caregiver will have performed certain interventions prior to calling 9-1-1. It is important to determine what interventions were performed, why they were performed, and what effect they had on the patient's condition.

**3. What are some conditions that would cause a patient to become dependent on a mechanical ventilator?**

When a person has any acute or chronic condition that impairs his or her respiratory muscles or injures the respiratory centers in the brain, he or she will require the use of a mechanical ventilator.

Your patient has quadriplegia secondary to a spinal injury. If the spinal cord is injured above the level of the fourth cervical vertebra (C4), paralysis of the respiratory muscles will also occur. Without a mechanical ventilator, your patient is unable to breathe at all.

Other conditions that often require mechanical ventilation include traumatic brain injury, muscular dystrophy, cystic fibrosis, and spina bifida. Regardless of why a patient requires mechanical ventilation, the most important thing for you to remember is that without it, he or she is unable to breathe!

**4. How does a tracheostomy tube affect a patient's ability to communicate? How can you determine if your patient is alert?**

Most patients with tracheostomy tubes are unable to speak. This is especially true if the patient requires mechanical ventilation, because he or she will be unable to breathe if the ventilator is detached from the tracheostomy tube. Patients with a tracheostomy tube who are not dependent on ventilators may be able to speak—although not as clearly—if they occlude the opening of the tube or use a special valve that fits over the end of the tracheostomy.

If patients cannot speak, they may communicate in other ways, such as by nodding the head or blinking the eyes. The parent or caregiver should be able to tell you whether the patient is communicating as he or she typically does and whether he or she is responding to questions appropriately. If the patient responds to questions appropriately, it can be said that he or she is alert.

**5. What are some potential complications that may result from your patient's condition? What can you do to prevent them or minimize the risks?**

Patients with quadriplegia who are dependent on a ventilator are typically confined to a bed for prolonged periods. Prolonged immobilization can cause potentially serious complications, including pressure sores and pulmonary embolism.

Patients who are paralyzed are particularly susceptible to urinary tract infections and pneumonia. Urinary tract infections are typically related to indwelling urinary catheters (Foley catheters). Pneumonia often occurs because of decreased or absent cough reflexes and prolonged immobilization, which increases the risk of pulmonary secretions settling in the lungs and becoming infected.

In patients with indwelling urinary catheters, always maintain the catheter collection bag below the level of the bladder; this position will prevent urine from flowing back into the bladder and therefore minimizes the risk of infection.

Thick mucus plugs can develop in the tubes of patients with tracheostomy tubes, such as your patient, which can impair oxygenation and ventilation. Ask the parent or caregiver when the tube was last suctioned and observe for signs that indicate it may need to be suctioned (eg, restlessness, signs of hypoxemia). Many mechanical ventilators will sound an alarm if there is any obstruction in the ventilator circuit, such as a mucus plug in the tracheostomy tube.

After you have transferred the patient to the ambulance stretcher, ensure that there are no wrinkles or lumps in the sheet or blanket under the patient. This simple step can help prevent pressure sores.

**6. What do you suspect is the patient's underlying problem? What specific treatment should you provide to him?**

The presence of fever suggests infection. In this patient the infection could have several causes. Furthermore, it may be the result of more than one underlying problem.

Fever is often the only presenting sign of pneumonia in paralyzed patients. This is especially true in patients with quadriplegia because their respiratory muscles are also paralyzed; therefore, outward signs of respiratory distress, such as retractions, are not present. Another possibility is a urinary tract infection.

Infection requires antibiotic therapy, which can be administered only in a hospital setting. Treatment of a patient with a possible infection is mainly supportive: monitor the patient's XABCs, observe standard precautions (eg, gloves, mask if necessary), and transport the patient to the hospital.

**7. What is the benefit of allowing the patient's mother to accompany her son to the hospital?**

The patient's mother should be allowed to accompany her son in the ambulance if she prefers. She can continue to be a source of information en route to the hospital, and could alert you to any changes in the patient's status, which may be obvious only to her.

The patient's mother can also bring supplies that the patient needs that you may or may not carry on your ambulance.

You must also consider the emotional needs of the patient. Unnecessarily separating a patient with special health care needs from his or her primary caregiver can be a source of emotional distress for the patient and the caregiver.

## YOU are the Provider SUMMARY *continued*

If the mother prefers to follow the ambulance in her own vehicle, assure her that you will take good care of her son.

**8. What has most likely happened to your patient? What should you do next?**

Your patient's clinical condition has changed. He appears to be fighting the ventilator, which is a sign of agitation. Furthermore, his heart rate has increased and his oxygen saturation level has decreased. You should suspect that he is not receiving adequate ventilation.

Tracheostomy tube obstruction is an emergency that requires immediate intervention; suction the tube and reassess the patient for signs of adequate oxygenation and ventilation.

The DOPE mnemonic can be used to troubleshoot acute deterioration in a patient with a tracheostomy tube. It is critical for you to recognize which problems you can correct and which problems require ALS. For example, if the tracheostomy tube has become dislodged, it must be replaced by a trained caregiver, paramedic, or physician; EMTs typically are not trained or permitted to perform this procedure. If the patient has a pneumothorax, the patient may require a needle chest decompression, which EMTs are not trained to perform, although nothing in the history suggests that this is the case.

---

### EMS Patient Care Report (PCR)

| Date: 1-20-20 | Incident No.: 013410 | Nature of Call: Fever | | Location: 575 Ranger Drive |
|---|---|---|---|---|

| Dispatched: 1435 | En Route: 1435 | At Scene: 1440 | Transport: 1501 | At Hospital: 1526 | In Service: 1540 |
|---|---|---|---|---|---|

#### Patient Information

| | |
|---|---|
| **Age:** 19<br>**Sex:** M<br>**Weight (in kg [lb]):** 52 kg (115 lb) | **Allergies:** Aspirin<br>**Medications:** Acetaminophen (as needed)<br>**Past Medical History:** Quadriplegia from spinal cord injury 2 years ago; ventilator-dependent<br>**Chief Complaint:** Fever |

#### Vital Signs

| Time: 1445 | BP: 118/62 | Pulse: 110 | Respirations: 14 | Spo$_2$: 99% |
|---|---|---|---|---|
| Time: 1500 | BP: 120/60 | Pulse: 118 | Respirations: 12 | Spo$_2$: 98% |
| Time: 1510 | BP: 134/74 | Pulse: 130 | Respirations: 12 | Spo$_2$: 87% |
| Time: 1520 | BP: 124/64 | Pulse: 116 | Respirations: 12 | Spo$_2$: 96% |

#### EMS Treatment (circle all that apply)

| Oxygen @ _15_ L/min via:<br>NC   NRM   (Bag mask) | (Assisted Ventilation) | Airway Adjunct | CPR |
|---|---|---|---|
| **Defibrillation** | **Bleeding Control**     **Bandaging** | **Splinting** | **Other:** (Emotional support, tracheostomy tube suctioning) |

## YOU are the Provider SUMMARY *continued*

| Narrative |
| --- |

Medic 53 dispatched to a residence for a 19-year-old man with a fever.

Chief Complaint: Fever

History: The patient has quadriplegia and is ventilator-dependent secondary to a spinal injury he experienced 2 years ago. According to the patient's mother, he began running a fever earlier in the day, and the last reading was 101.2°F (38.4°C). She administered 500 mg of acetaminophen via his gastrostomy tube about an hour before EMS arrival. The patient's physician, who was contacted by the home health agency that assists the patient's mother in his care, requested transport via ambulance to the ED.

Assessment: On arrival, found the patient lying supine in a hospital-style bed in the living room of his home. On presentation, the patient's eyes were open and he acknowledged EMS presence by nodding his head. According to his mother, who is his primary caregiver, his current mental status is consistent with his baseline. The patient has a tracheostomy tube and is receiving mechanical ventilation at 14 breaths/min. Secondary assessment revealed no gross abnormalities. Breath sounds were auscultated and found to be clear and equal bilaterally. Patient also has an indwelling urinary catheter and a colostomy bag. Assessment of these devices revealed no bleeding, redness around the area of the devices, or any other abnormalities.

Treatment (Rx): Not applicable

Transport: After consulting with medical control, moved the patient to the ambulance stretcher using a soft stretcher, disconnected him from the mechanical ventilator circuit, and resumed ventilations with a bag-mask at 12 breaths/min. Moved patient to ambulance, continued bag-mask ventilations, and reassessed his vital signs. Patient's mother accompanied her son in the back of the ambulance. Began transport to the hospital and continued to monitor the patient en route. Shortly after calling radio report to receiving facility, noted that patient became acutely agitated; his heart rate markedly increased and his oxygen saturation decreased. Suspected obstruction of the tracheostomy tube; provided suctioning one time and reassessed patient. He was now calm and his heart rate and oxygen saturation stabilized. Remainder of transport was uneventful. Delivered patient to ED and gave verbal report to Dr. Lee. Medic 53 cleared the hospital and returned to service at 1523.

**End of report**

# Prep Kit

## Ready for Review

- Medicine and medical technology continue to improve, and the number of children and adults with chronic diseases or injuries who are living at home or in environments outside of the hospital setting continues to grow.
- You may find children and adults who are living at home dependent on mechanical ventilators, intravenous pumps, or other medical devices to maintain their lives.
- Assess and care for patients with special challenges in the same manner as all other patients.
- Intellectual disability is caused by insufficient development of the brain, resulting in the inability to learn and socially adapt at a normal developmental rate.
- People with Down syndrome often have large tongues and small oral and nasal cavities, so intubation of these patients may be difficult.
- Visual impairments may be difficult to recognize. During your scene size-up, look for signs that indicate the patient is visually impaired, such as the presence of eyeglasses, a cane, or a service animal. Immediately introduce yourself when you enter the room, and have your team members introduce themselves so that the patient can identify their locations and voices.

- Hearing impairment may range from a slight hearing loss to total deafness. Clues that a person could be hard of hearing include the presence of hearing aids, poor pronunciation of words, or failure to respond to your presence or questions.
- Cerebral palsy is associated with other conditions such as visual and hearing impairments, difficulty communicating, epilepsy, and intellectual disability. Patients may also have an unsteady gait (ataxia) and may require the assistance of a wheelchair or walker.
- Patients with spina bifida will have either partial or full paralysis of the lower extremities, and loss of bowel and bladder control; they are often extremely allergic to latex products.
- Patients with obesity may be embarrassed by their condition or fearful of scorn as a result of past experiences. If transport is necessary, plan early for extra help and do not be afraid to call for more providers or special equipment if necessary. In particular, send a member of your team to find the easiest and safest exit.
- Patients who depend on home automatic ventilators or those who have chronic pulmonary medical conditions may breathe through a tracheostomy tube.
- When caring for patients who are on home oxygen, you must be able to assess their oxygen needs with consideration of their baseline status.
- Patients who are on a mechanical ventilator at home cannot breathe without assistance. If the ventilator malfunctions, remove the patient from the mechanical ventilator and begin ventilations with a bag-mask device.
- An apnea monitor is typically used when there is a family history of sudden infant death syndrome or when an infant is born prematurely, has severe gastroesophageal reflux that causes episodes of choking, or has experienced an apparent life-threatening event. The apnea monitor is designed to sound an alarm if the infant experiences bradycardia or if apnea occurs.
- An internal cardiac pacemaker is a device implanted under the patient's skin to regulate the heart rate.
- A ventricular assist device (VAD) is a special piece of medical equipment that takes over the function of one or both heart ventricles. These types of devices are used as a bridge to transplantation while a donor heart is being located or as a permanent solution for patients who do not qualify for a transplant.
- Gastrostomy tubes are placed into the stomach for feeding in patients who cannot ingest fluids, food, or medication by mouth. These tubes may be inserted through the nose or mouth or placed through the abdominal wall surgically.
- External defibrillation vests are worn under a patient's clothing. They monitor the patient's cardiac rhythm and provide an audible warning before administering a shock to correct the dysrhythmia.
- Shunts are tubes that extend from the ventricles in the brain to the abdomen to drain excess cerebrospinal fluid that may accumulate near the brain.
- A colostomy or ileostomy is a surgical procedure that creates an opening from the small or large intestine to the surface of the body to allow for elimination of waste products. Feces are expelled and collected into a clear external bag or pouch, which is emptied or changed frequently. Similarly, a urostomy drains urine.
- You and your team may be called on to assist a patient who is terminally ill. Terminally ill patients may be in a hospice facility or at home.
- Under the Emergency Medical Treatment and Active Labor Act, all health care facilities *must* provide a medical assessment and required treatment, regardless of the patient's ability to pay.

## Vital Vocabulary

**autism spectrum disorder (ASD)** A group of complex disorders of brain development, characterized by difficulties in social interaction, repetitive behaviors, and verbal and nonverbal communication.

**cerebral palsy** A group of disorders characterized by poorly controlled body movement.

**colostomy** A surgical procedure to create an opening (stoma) between the colon and the surface of the body.

**conductive hearing loss** Hearing loss caused by a faulty transmission of sound waves.

**developmental disability** Insufficient development of the brain, resulting in some level of dysfunction or impairment.

**Down syndrome** A genetic chromosomal defect that can occur during fetal development and that results in intellectual impairment as well as certain physical characteristics, such as a round head with a flat occiput and slanted, wide-set eyes.

**ileostomy** A surgical procedure to create an opening (stoma) between the small intestine and the surface of the body.

**intellectual disability** A subset of developmental disability characterized by significant limitations in both intellectual functioning and skills needed for daily living.

**obesity** A complex condition in which a person has an excessive amount of body fat.

**sensorineural deafness** A permanent lack of hearing caused by a lesion or damage of the inner ear.

**shunts** Tubes that drain excess cerebrospinal fluid from the brain to another part of the body outside of the brain, such as the abdomen; lowers pressure in the brain.

**spina bifida** A development defect in which a portion of the spinal cord or meninges may protrude outside of the vertebrae and possibly even outside of the body, usually at the lower third of the spine in the lumbar area.

**stoma** An opening through the skin and into an organ or other structure.

**tracheostomy** A surgical procedure to create an opening (stoma) into the trachea; a stoma in the neck connects the trachea directly to the skin.

**tracheostomy tube** A plastic tube placed within the tracheostomy site (stoma).

**urostomy** A surgical procedure to create an opening (stoma) that connects the urinary system to the surface of the skin and allows urine to drain through the abdominal wall.

## References

1. American Psychiatric Association. Autism spectrum disorder. In *Diagnostic and Statistical Manual of Mental Disorders*. 5th ed. Arlington, VA: American Psychiatric Association; 2013:50.

2. Autism Speaks. What is autism? https://www.autism-speaks.org/what-autism. Accessed February 20, 2020.

3. Baggett TP, Singer DE, Pao SR, O'Connell JJ, Bharel M, Rigotti NA. Food insufficiency and health services utilization in a national sample of homeless adults. *J Gen Intern Med*. 2011;26(6):627-634.

4. Bai D, Yip BHK, Windham GC, et al. Association of genetic and environmental factors with autism in a five-country cohort. *JAMA Psychiatry*. July 17, 2019. doi:10.1001/jamapsychiatry.2019.1411. [Epub ahead of print].

5. Baxter AJ, Brugha TS, Erskine HE, Scheurer RW, Vos T, Scott JG. The epidemiology and global burden of autism spectrum disorders. *Psychol Med*. 2015;45(3):601-613.

6. Bharel M, Lin WC, Zhang J, O'Connell E, Taube R, Clark RE. Health care utilization patterns of homeless individuals in Boston: preparing for Medicaid expansion under the Affordable Care Act. *Am J Public Health*. 2013;103(Suppl 2):S311-S317.

7. Bishaw A, Fontenot K. *Poverty: 2012 and 2013: American Community Survey Briefs*. Washington, DC: US Census Bureau; 2014.

8. Dachew BA, Mamun A, Maravilla JC, Alati R. Pre-eclampsia and the risk of autism-spectrum disorder in offspring: meta-analysis. *Br J Psychiatry*. 2018;212(3):142-147.

9. Dashow J. New report on youth homeless affirms the LGBTQ youth disproportionately experience homelessness. Human Rights Campaign website. https://www.hrc.org/blog/new-report-on-youth-homeless-affirms-that-lgbtq-youth-disproportionately-ex. Published November 15, 2017. Accessed February 20, 2020.

10. Deer B. How the case against the MMR vaccine was fixed. *BMJ*. 2011;342:c5347. doi:10.1136/bmj.c5347.

11. Deer B. More secrets of the MMR scare. Who saw the "histological findings"? *BMJ*. 2011;343:d7892. doi:10.1136/bmj.d7892.

12. Deer B. Pathology reports solve "new bowel disease" riddle. *BMJ*. 2011;343:d6823. doi:10.1136/bmj.d6823.

13. Deer B. Secrets of the MMR scare. How the vaccine crisis was meant to make money. *BMJ*. 2011;342:c5258. doi:10.1136/bmj.c5258.

14. Deer B. Secrets of the MMR scare. *The Lancet*'s two days to bury bad news. *BMJ*. 2011;342:c7001. doi:10.1136/bmj.c7001.

15. DeStefano F, Bodenstab HM, Offit PA. Principal controversies in vaccine safety in the United States. *Clin Infect Dis*. 2019;69(4):726-731.

16. Gadad BS, Li W, Yazdani U, et al. Administration of thimerosal-containing vaccines to infant rhesus macaques does not result in autism-like behavior or neuropathology. *Proc Natl Acad Sci USA*. 2015;112(40):12498-12503.

17. Goin-Kochel RP, Mire SS, Dempsey AG, et al. Parental report of vaccine receipt in children with autism spectrum disorder: do rates differ by pattern of ASD onset? *Vaccine*. 2016;34(11):1335-1542.

18. Hisle-Gorman E, Susi A, Stokes T, Gorman G, Erdie-Lalena C, Nylund CM. Prenatal, perinatal, and neonatal risk factors of autism spectrum disorder. *Pediatr Res*. 2018;84(2):190–198.

19. Hviid A, Hansen JV, Frisch M, Melbye M. Measles, mumps, rubella vaccination and autism: a nationwide cohort study. *Ann Intern Med*. 2019;170(8):513-520.

20. Institute of Medicine. *Immunization Safety Review: Vaccines and Autism*. Washington, DC: National Academies Press; 2004.

21. Jain A, Marshall J, Buikema A, Bancroft T, Kelly P, Newschaffer CJ. Autism occurrence by MMR vaccine status among US children with older siblings with and without autism. *JAMA*. 2015;313(15):1534-1540.

22. Kogan MD, Vladutiu CJ, Schieve LA, et al. The prevalence of parent-reported autism spectrum disorder among US children. *Pediatrics*. 2018;142(6):pii:e20174161. doi:10.1542/peds.2017-4161.

23. Kong A, Frigge ML, Masson G, et al. Rate of de novo mutations and the importance of father's age to disease risk. *Nature*. 2012;488(7412):471-475.

24. Krakowiak P, Walker CK, Bremer, et al. Maternal metabolic conditions and risk for autism and other neurodevelopmental disorders. *Pediatrics*. 2012;129(5):e1121-e1128.

25. Kushel MB, Perry S, Bangsberg D, Clark R, Moss AR. Emergency department use among the homeless and marginally housed: results from a community-based study. *Am J Public Health*. 2002;92(5):778-784.

26. Kushel MB, Vittinghoff E, Haas JS. Factors associated with the health care utilization of homeless persons. *JAMA*. 2001;285(2):200-206.

27. Loomes R, Hull L, Mandy WPL. What is the male-to-female ratio in autism spectrum disorder? A systematic review and meta-analysis. *J Am Acad Child Adolesc Psychiatry*. 2017;56(6):466-474.

28. Lopez-Rangel E, Lewis ME. Loud and clear evidence for gene silencing by epigenetic mechanisms in autism spectrum and related neurodevelopmental disorders. *Clin Genet*. 2006;69(1):21-22.

29. Mayo Clinic Staff. Diseases and conditions: obesity: symptoms. Mayo Clinic website. http://www.mayoclinic.org/diseases-conditions/obesity/basics/symptoms/con-20014834. Updated June 10, 2015. Accessed February 20, 2020.

30. Morris GL, Gloss D, Buchhalter J, Mack KG, Nickels K, Harden C. Evidence-based guideline update: vagus nerve stimulation for the treatment of epilepsy; report of the Guideline Development Subcommittee of the American Academy of Neurology. *Neurology*. 2013;81(16):1453-1459.

31. Mrozek-Budzyn D, Kieltyka A, Majewska R. Lack of association between measles-mumps-rubella vaccination and autism in children: a case-control study. *Pediatr Infect Dis J*. 2010;29(5):397-400.

32. Muhle R, Trentacoste SV, Papin I. The genetics of autism. *Pediatrics*. 2004;113(5):e472-e486.

33. National Association of State EMS Officials. *National EMS Scope of Practice Model 2019*. DOT HS 812-666. Washington, DC: National Highway Traffic Safety Administration. https://www.ems.gov/pdf/National_EMS_Scope_of_Practice_Model_2019.pdf. Accessed February 20, 2020.

34. National Center on Birth Defects and Developmental Disabilities, Centers for Disease Control and Prevention. Autism spectrum disorder (ASD): data & statistics. Centers for Disease Control and Prevention website. http://www.cdc.gov/ncbddd/autism/data.html. Reviewed September 3, 2019. Accessed February 20, 2020.

35. National Down Syndrome Society. Atlantoaxial instability and Down syndrome. https://www.ndss.org/resources/atlantoaxial-instability-syndrome/. Accessed February 20, 2020.

36. Ozonoff S, Young GS, Carter A, et al. Recurrence risk for autism spectrum disorders: a Baby Siblings Research Consortium study. *Pediatrics*. 2011;128(3):e488-e495. doi:10.1542/peds.2010-2825.

37. Raven MC, Tieu L, Lee CT, Ponath C, Guzman D, Kushel M. Emergency department use in a cohort of older homeless adults: results from the HOPE HOME study. *Acad Emerg Med*. 2017;24(1):63-74.

38. Salhi BA, White MH, Pitts SR, Wright DW. Homelessness and emergency medicine: a review of the literature. *Acad Emerg Med*. 2018;25(5):577-593.

39. Samaco RC, Nagarajan RP, Braunschweig D, LaSalle JM. Multiple pathways regulate MeCP2 expression in normal brain development and exhibit defects in autism-spectrum disorders. *Hum Mol Genet*. 2004;13(6):629-639.

40. Schaefer GB, Mendelson NJ; Professional Practice and Guidelines Committee. Clinical genetics evaluation in identifying the etiology of autism spectrum disorders: 2013 guideline revisions. *Genet Med*. 2013;15(5):399-407.

41. Semega J, Kollar M, Creamer J, Mohanty A. Income and poverty in the United States: 2018. US Census Bureau website. https://www.census.gov/library /publications/2019/demo/p60-266.html. Published September 10, 2019. Accessed February 20, 2020.

42. Sgouros S. Spina bifida hydrocephalus and shunts. *Medscape* website. http://emedicine.medscape.com /article/937979-overview. Updated October 12, 2015. Accessed February 20, 2020.

43. Shafer PO. About epilepsy: the basics. Epilepsy Foundation website. http://www.epilepsy.com/learn/about -epilepsy-basics. Updated April 1, 2019. Accessed February 20, 2020.

44. Shafer PO, Dean PM. Vagus nerve stimulation (VNS). Epilepsy Foundation website. https://www.epilepsy .com/learn/treating-seizures-and-epilepsy/devices /vagus-nerve-stimulation-vns. Reviewed March 12, 2018. Accessed February 20, 2020.

45. Stewart AM, Kanak MM, Gerald AM, et al. Pediatric emergency department visits for homelessness after shelter eligibility policy change. *Pediatrics.* 2018;142(5):pii:e20181224. doi:10.1542/peds.2018-1224.

46. Stratton K, Gable A, McCormick MC. *Immunization Safety Review: Thimerosal-Containing Vaccines and Neurodevelopmental Disorders.* Washington, DC: National Academy Press; 2001.

47. Tsai J, Doran KM, Rosenheck RA. When health insurance is not a factor: national comparison of homeless and nonhomeless US veterans who use Veterans Affairs Emergency Departments. *Am J Public Health.* 2013;103(Suppl 2):S225-S231.

48. Uno Y, Uchiyama T, Kurosawa M, Aleksic B, Ozaki N. Early exposure to the combined measles-mumps-rubella vaccine and thimerosal-containing vaccines and risk of autism spectrum disorder. *Vaccine.* 2015;33(21):2511-2516.

49. Uno Y, Uchiyama T, Kurosawa M, Aleksic B, Ozaki N. The combined measles, mumps, and rubella vaccines and the total number of vaccines are not associated with development of autism spectrum disorder: the first case-control study in Asia. *Vaccine.* 2012;30(28):4292-4298.

50. Xiang AH, Wang X, Martinez MP, et al. Association of maternal diabetes with autism in offspring. *JAMA.* 2015;313(14):1425-1434.

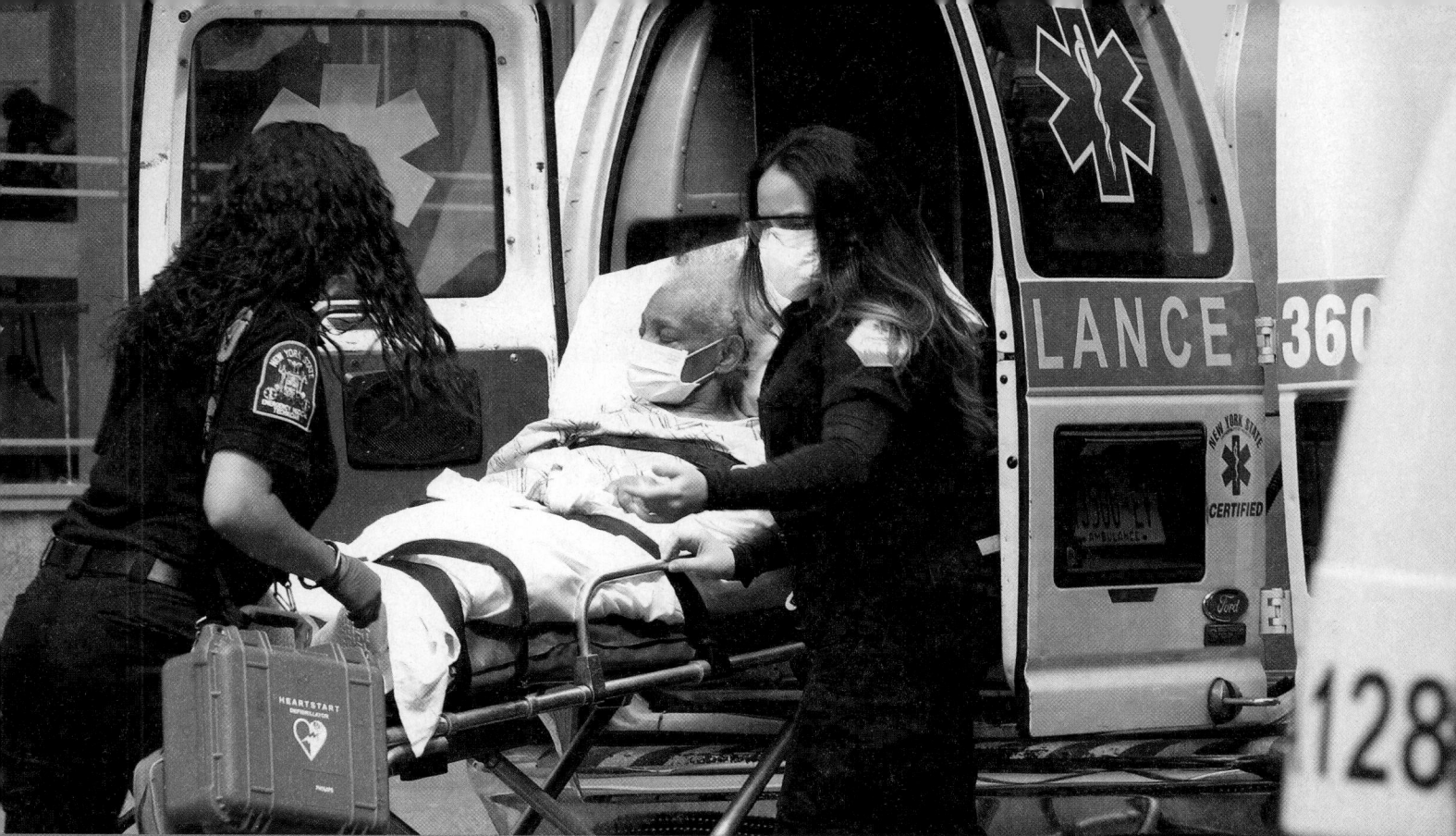

# SECTION

# 9

# EMS Operations

**38** Transport Operations

**39** Vehicle Extrication and Special Rescue

**40** Incident Management

**41** Terrorism Response and Disaster Management

# Chapter 38

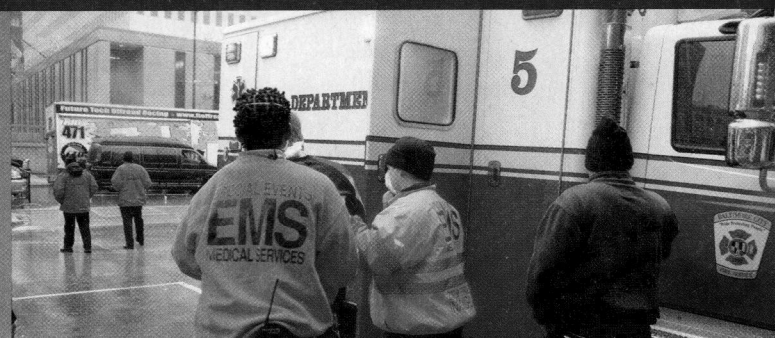

# Transport Operations

## NATIONAL EMS EDUCATION STANDARD COMPETENCIES

### EMS Operations

Knowledge of operational roles and responsibilities to ensure patient, public, and personnel safety.

### Principles of Safely Operating a Ground Ambulance

- Risks and responsibilities of emergency response (pp 1437–1453)
- Risks and responsibilities of transport (pp 1440–1453)

### Air Medical

- Safe air medical operations (pp 1453–1458)
- Criteria for utilizing air medical response (pp 1453–1454)

### Medicine

Applies fundamental knowledge to provide basic emergency care and transportation based on assessment findings for an acutely ill patient.

### Infectious Diseases

Awareness of
- How to decontaminate equipment after treating a patient (pp 1442–1443)
- How to decontaminate the ambulance and equipment after treating a patient (pp 1442–1443)

## KNOWLEDGE OBJECTIVES

1. List the nine phases of an ambulance call; include examples of key tasks EMTs perform during each phase. (pp 1426–1443)
2. Name the medical equipment carried on an ambulance; include examples of supplies that are included in each main category of the ambulance equipment checklist. (p 1428)
3. Name the safety and operations equipment carried on an ambulance; include examples of how each item might be used by EMTs in an emergency. (pp 1433–1434)
4. Discuss the importance of performing regular vehicle inspections; include the specific parts of an ambulance that should be inspected daily. (p 1435)
5. List the minimum dispatch information required by EMS to respond to an emergency call. (p 1436)
6. Describe some high-risk situations and hazards during both pretransport and transport that may affect the safety of the ambulance and its passengers. (pp 1436–1441, 1443–1453)
7. Discuss the specific considerations required to ensure scene safety; include personal safety, patient safety, and traffic control. (pp 1437–1440)
8. Describe the key elements that must be included in the written patient care report upon patient delivery to the hospital. (p 1441)
9. Summarize the tasks EMTs must complete in the postrun phase. (pp 1442–1443)
10. Define the terms cleaning, disinfection, high-level disinfection, and sterilization. (p 1442)
11. Discuss the guidelines for safely and defensively driving an ambulance. (pp 1443–1445)

12. Identify key steps EMTs should take to improve safety while en route to the scene, the hospital, and the station. (pp 1443–1453)

13. List the three factors that dictate the use of lights and siren to the scene and to the hospital; include the risk-versus-benefit factors regarding their use. (pp 1450–1451)

14. Describe the specific, limited privileges that are provided to emergency vehicle operators by most state laws and regulations. (p 1450)

15. Explain the additional risks and special considerations posed by the use of police escorts, and the hazards and special considerations posed by crossing intersections. (pp 1451–1452)

16. Describe the capabilities, protocols, and methods for accessing air ambulances. (pp 1453–1457)

17. Describe key scene safety considerations when preparing for helicopter emergency medical services, such as a helicopter medevac, including establishing a landing zone, securing loose objects, reducing onsite hazards, and approaching the aircraft. (pp 1455–1458)

## SKILLS OBJECTIVES

1. Demonstrate how to perform a daily inspection of an ambulance. (pp 1435–1436)

2. Demonstrate how to present a verbal report that would be given to receiving personnel at the hospital upon patient transfer. (p 1441)

3. Demonstrate how to write a written report that includes all pertinent patient information following patient transfer to the hospital. (p 1441)

4. Demonstrate how to clean and disinfect the ambulance and equipment during the postrun phase. (pp 1442–1443)

# Introduction

During the late 1700s, Napoleon Bonaparte commissioned the development of horse-drawn carts and a corps of soldiers trained to remove injured personnel from the battlefield and initiate treatment, establishing what was one of the more advanced professional emergency medical patient care systems in the world. Horse-drawn ambulances were also being used in major cities throughout the United States (**FIGURE 38-1**). American hospitals initiated their own professional ambulance services during the late 1860s. Ambulance attendants traveled with limited medical supplies, including brandy, a few tourniquets, several assorted bandages and sponges, basic splinting material, and blankets.

Many of today's ambulances are equipped with state-of-the-art technology, including defibrillators and monitors that can transmit information directly to the emergency department (ED), video-assisted equipment for use with airway management or telemedicine, blood and oxygen testing equipment, mechanical ventilators, automated CPR machines, global positioning systems (GPS), and computer-aided dispatch consoles. Even when following all safety guidelines, the emphasis on decreasing response times places the EMT in great danger while responding to calls. Although technology can greatly aid in directing the route and providing important information from the scene, it is also distracting and, therefore, potentially places the crew at higher risk for crashes. The driver who

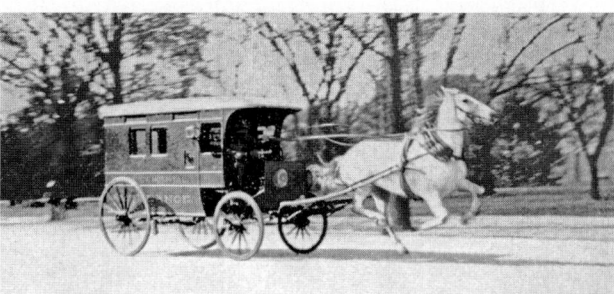

**FIGURE 38-1** Horse-drawn ambulances were used in major cities throughout the United States during the 1800s.

© National Library of Medicine.

## Safety Tips

The dangers of texting and driving are well known. However, we often downplay the cognitive workload placed on emergency responders who are operating a vehicle. We ask responders to safely operate the vehicle in an emergency situation, but we place multiple distractors within arm's reach that could draw their focus away from their primary role. From reading call notes from a computer-aided dispatch to requesting information regarding scene safety over the radio, these necessary distractions can all prove dangerous, if not fatal.

is operating the ambulance should focus solely on the road and maintaining safe driving habits, especially during lights and siren responses. In addition to assisting the driver, the EMT in the passenger's seat should be the person responsible for operating the mobile data terminal (MDT) or GPS device and communicating via radio or cell phone while en route to the scene. Anything that takes the driver's attention away from the road for even a second greatly increases the risk of a crash.

This chapter discusses ambulance design and how to equip and maintain an ambulance. It focuses on the techniques and judgment that you will need to drive an ambulance or other emergency vehicle. Topics covered include parking considerations, emergency vehicle control and operation, the effects of weather on driving, and common hazards that are encountered while driving an ambulance. Finally, the chapter describes how to work safely with air ambulances.

## Emergency Vehicle Design

An **ambulance** is a vehicle that is used for treating and transporting patients who need emergency medical care. The first use of motor-powered ambulances occurred in the late 1800s. For many decades after that, a hearse was the vehicle typically used as an ambulance. While a hearse had enough room for someone to lie down, it left little room for supplies or medical attendants.

Currently, ambulance designs are based on *NFPA 1917, Standard for Automotive Ambulances*, and, in large part, on suggestions from the ambulance industry and from EMS personnel (**FIGURE 38-2**). One of the most significant developments in ambulance design has been the emphasis on creating the safest

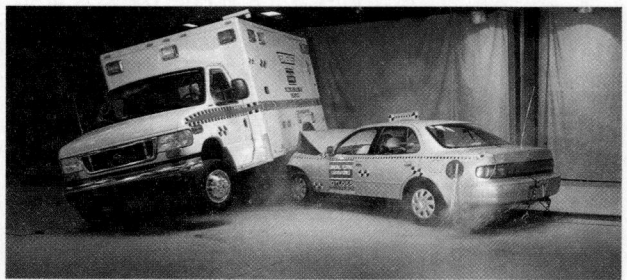

**FIGURE 38-2** Ambulances are crash tested by manufacturers while being designed.

Courtesy of AEV. Used with permission.

environment possible in the driver's compartment and the patient compartment. Another development is the use of **first-responder vehicles** (**FIGURE 38-3**), which respond initially to the scene with personnel and equipment to treat the sick and injured.

The modern ambulance is a vehicle for emergency medical care that has the following features:

- A driver's compartment
- A patient compartment that can accommodate two EMTs and at least one patient in a supine position (Additional patients may be seated on a bench seat or swivel seat with appropriate safety restraints.)
- Equipment and supplies to provide emergency medical care at the scene and during transport, to safeguard personnel and patients from hazardous conditions, and to carry out light extrication procedures
- Two-way radio communication so ambulance personnel can speak with the dispatcher, the hospital, public safety authorities, and online medical control
- Design and construction that ensure maximum safety, efficiency, and comfort

## YOU are the Provider

You are completing your morning vehicle checkoff. This is your first shift at your new station following successful completion of your new hire orientation, which included your mandatory emergency vehicle operator course. At 0800 hours, you are dispatched to 1800 Main Road for an "assault." It is a cold, rainy morning, and there is heavy traffic in front of your station. You pull the ambulance out of the bay. Your partner informs you that the scene of the call is only a few miles away from your station.

**1.** What attributes should an emergency vehicle operator possess?

**2.** What factors should you consider before responding to the scene?

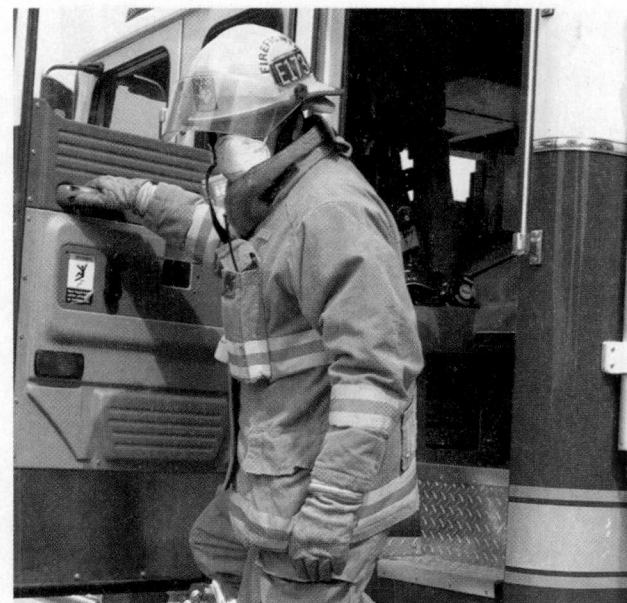

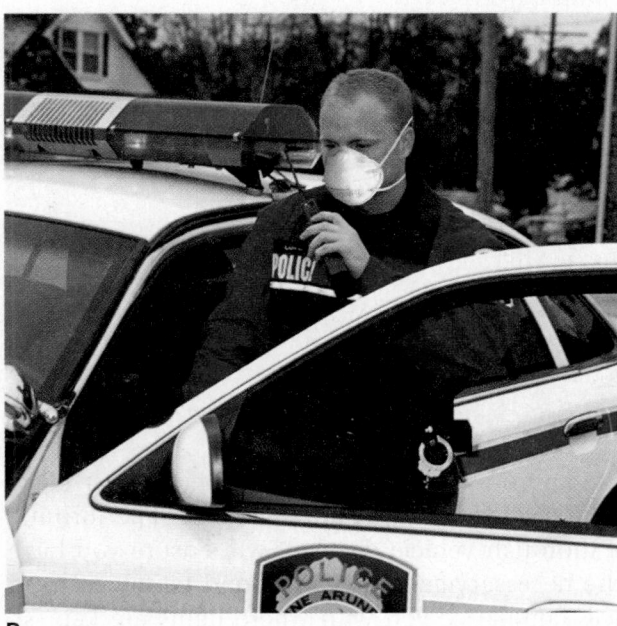

**FIGURE 38-3** First responders, such as firefighters (**A**) and law enforcement personnel (**B**), are often the first to arrive at a scene.

A, B: © Jones & Bartlett Learning. Courtesy of MIEMSS.

Each state establishes its own standards for licensing or certifying ambulance operators. Many agencies now use the federal specifications (NFPA 1917) that cover the three types of basic ambulance designs (**FIGURE 38-4** and **TABLE 38-1**).

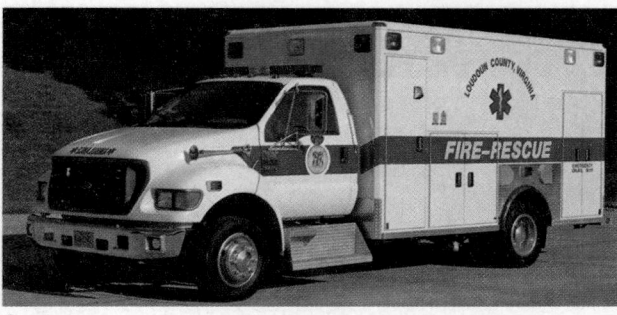

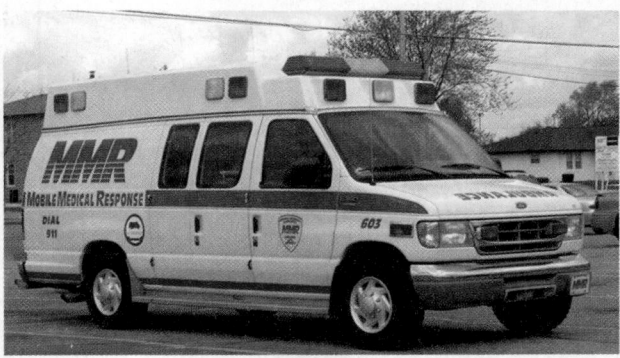

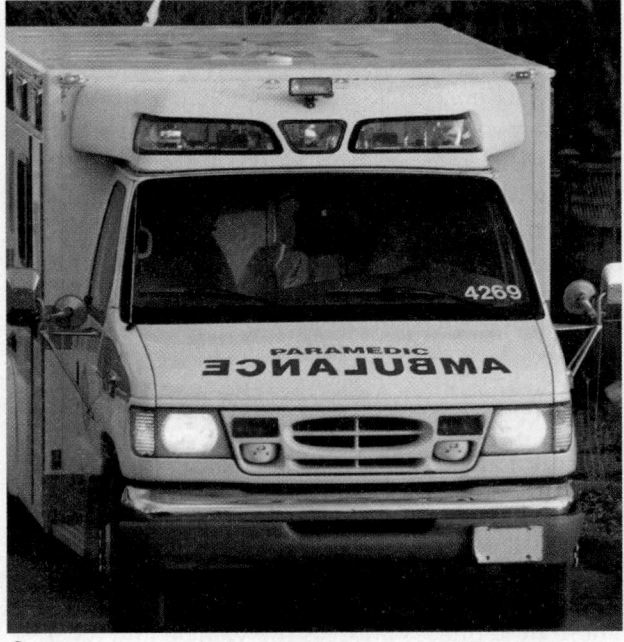

**FIGURE 38-4 A.** The conventional, truck cab-chassis has a modular ambulance body that can be transferred to a newer chassis (type I). **B.** The standard van ambulance has a forward-control integral cab body (type II). **C.** The specialty van ambulance has a cab that is mounted on a cut-away van chassis (type III).

A: © Jones & Bartlett Learning; B: Courtesy of Captain David Jackson, Saginaw Township Fire Department; C: © Kevin Norris/ShutterStock.

| TABLE 38-1 Basic Ambulance Designs | |
|---|---|
| Type I | Conventional, truck cab-chassis with a modular ambulance body that can be transferred to a newer chassis as needed |
| Type II | Standard van, forward-control integral cab-body ambulance |
| Type III | Specialty van cab with a modular ambulance body that is mounted on a cut-away van chassis |

© Jones & Bartlett Learning.

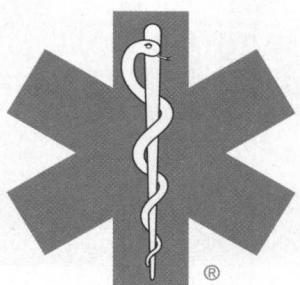

**FIGURE 38-5** The Star of Life.

Courtesy of National Highway Traffic Safety Administration.

The six-pointed **Star of Life** emblem (**FIGURE 38-5**) identifies vehicles as ambulances. It is often affixed to the sides, rear, and roof of the ambulance. Local or state regulatory authorities determine what emblems may be displayed on the side of a prehospital care ambulance. **FIGURE 38-6** illustrates some of the required features of a licensed or certified ambulance.

## Phases of an Ambulance Call

An ambulance call has nine phases: preparation, dispatch, en route, arrival at scene, transfer of patient to ambulance, en route to receiving facility (transport), at receiving facility (delivery), en route to station, and postrun, as shown in **TABLE 38-2**. These nine phases address the vehicle and its crew and their roles when responding to a medical emergency. The details of patient care are not included in these nine phases.

### The Preparation Phase

During the preparation phase, you will check to make sure all of your equipment is functional and

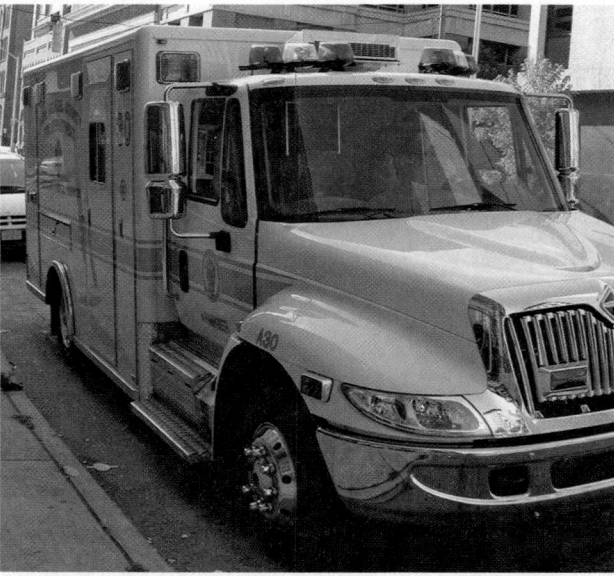

**FIGURE 38-6** Warning lights and public address systems are necessary on licensed or certified ambulances.

© Jones & Bartlett Learning. Courtesy of MIEMSS.

| TABLE 38-2 Phases of an Ambulance Call |
|---|
| 1. Preparation for the call |
| 2. Dispatch |
| 3. En route |
| 4. Arrival at scene |
| 5. Transfer of the patient to the ambulance |
| 6. En route to the receiving facility (transport) |
| 7. At the receiving facility (delivery) |
| 8. En route to the station |
| 9. Postrun |

© Jones & Bartlett Learning.

the appropriate supplies are in their proper place on the vehicle. Getting into the habit of performing a thorough vehicle checkoff will ensure you have the necessary supplies to respond to any call and will familiarize you with where items are kept so that you may quickly provide appropriate care without having to search for equipment. New equipment should be placed on an ambulance only after proper instruction is given on its use and care, and, additionally, after approval by the medical director.

Equipment and supplies should be durable and, to the extent possible, standardized. This makes it easy to quickly exchange equipment with other ambulances or restock after responding to a call.

Store equipment and supplies in the ambulance according to how urgently and how often they

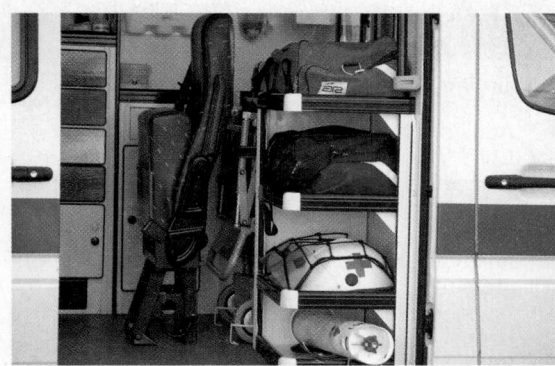

**FIGURE 38-7** Store equipment and supplies in the ambulance according to how urgently and how often they are used.

© Silvia Massacote/Shutterstock.

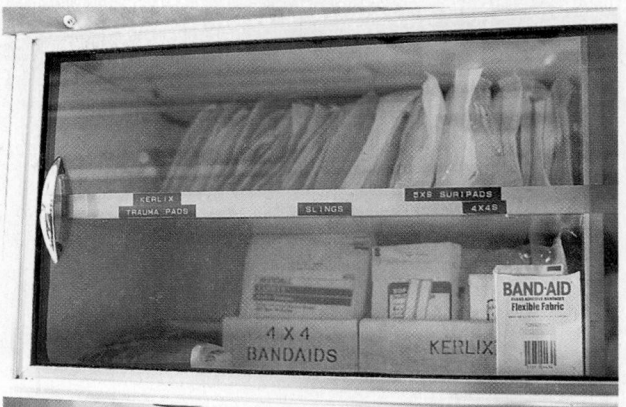

**FIGURE 38-8** Containers should be placed in cabinets and drawers with transparent fronts for quick identification.

© Jones & Bartlett Learning. Courtesy of MIEMSS.

are used (**FIGURE 38-7**). Consider grouping equipment required for critical interventions in a similar location so that you do not have to waste valuable time retrieving these items from multiple locations. For example, package equipment for airway management, artificial ventilation, and oxygen delivery together and within easy reach of the head of the primary stretcher. Place items for cardiac care, control of external bleeding, and monitoring blood pressure at the side of the stretcher. Make sure batteries are fresh and equipment is functioning properly. The most common cause of automated external defibrillator (AED) malfunction is a dead battery.

Storage cabinets and kits should open easily. They should also close securely so they do not fly open while the ambulance is in motion. The fronts of cabinets and drawers should be transparent so you can quickly identify the contents inside; if they are not, be sure to label each container (**FIGURE 38-8**). During this phase, all hard equipment and gear bags should be securely fastened in an appropriate mounting bracket or secured with webbing or straps. Loose items in the back of an ambulance can become lethal projectiles in the event of a collision.

## Medical Equipment

As an EMT, you have access to a large variety of medical equipment and supplies, far more than can be described here. Certain items on the ambulance must be available at all times, as dictated by state and jurisdictional requirements.

### Basic Supplies

**TABLE 38-3** lists the common supplies carried on ambulances. These include basic items such as personal protective equipment (PPE) and sharps containers, airway and ventilation equipment, basic wound care and bleeding control supplies, splinting supplies, childbirth supplies, an AED, patient transfer equipment, medications, communication equipment, and other regionally appropriate supplies.

### Airway and Ventilation Equipment

As listed in Table 38-3, the following airway management equipment should be carried on ambulances:

- Oropharyngeal airways for adults, children, and infants
- Nasopharyngeal airways for adults and children
- CPAP equipment
- Equipment for advanced airway procedures if your service is authorized by state regulation and the medical director to perform these procedures

It is important that two portable artificial ventilation devices that operate independently of an oxygen supply be carried on the ambulance: one for use in the ambulance and one for use outside the ambulance or as a spare. These devices include disposable pocket masks and bag-mask devices. In addition, bag-mask devices capable of oxygen enrichment and, when attached to an oxygen supply

## TABLE 38-3 Ambulance Equipment Checklist

### Basic Supplies

- Pillows and pillowcases
- Sterile sheets
- Blankets
- Towels
- Disposable emesis bags or basins
- Boxes of disposable tissue
- Bedpan (optional)
- Urinals (one each for men and women; optional)
- Blood pressure cuffs (pediatric, adult, large adult)
- Blood glucose monitor
- Stethoscope
- Disposable drinking cups
- Unbreakable container of water
- Wet wipes
- Chemical cold/hot packs
- Sterile irrigation fluid
- Restraining devices
- Plastic bags for waste or severed parts
- Hypoallergenic nitrile, vinyl, or other disposable hypoal-lergenic gloves (various sizes)
- Sharps container
- Set of hearing protectors

### Airway and Ventilation Equipment

- Infection control kits (goggles, masks, waterproof gowns)
- Oropharyngeal airways and nasopharyngeal airways of various sizes
- Continuous positive airway pressure (CPAP) equipment
- Advanced airway supplies, if local protocol permits (laryngeal mask airway, Combitube, King airways), with secondary placement confirmation devices
- Bag-mask devices (adult, child, and infant)
- Mounted suction unit and portable suction unit
- Assorted oxygen delivery devices (adult and pediatric)
- Oxygen supply units (both portable and installed)
- Pulse oximeter

### Basic Wound Care Supplies

- Trauma shears
- Sterile sheets
- Sterile burn sheets
- Adhesive tape in several widths
- Self-adhering, soft roller bandages, 4 in. × 5 yd (10 cm × 5 m)
- Self-adhering, soft roller bandages, 2 in. × 5 yd (5 cm × 5 m)
- Sterile dressings, gauze, 4 × 4 in. (10 × 10 cm)
- Sterile dressings, abdominal or laparotomy pads, usu-ally 6 × 9 in. (15 × 23 cm) or 8 × 10 in. (20 × 25 cm)
- Sterile universal trauma dressings, usually 10 × 36 in. (25 × 91 cm), folded into 9 × 10 in. (23 × 25 cm) packages
- Sterile, occlusive, nonadherent dressings (aluminum foil sterilized in original package)
- Occlusive dressings or chest seals
- Assortment of adhesive bandages
- Wound packing
- Tourniquets

### Splinting Supplies

- Adult-size traction splint
- Child-size traction splint
- A variety of arm and leg splints, such as vacuum, cardboard, plastic, foam-covered wire-ladder or aluminum alloy, or padded board (the number and type of splints should be determined by state regulations and your medical director)
- A variety of triangular bandages and roller bandages
- Short backboard/short immobilization device
- Long backboard
- Cervical collars in an adjustable size or a variety of sizes
- Head immobilization devices

### Childbirth Supplies

Emergency obstetric kit, including:
- Surgical scissors
- Hemostats or special cord clamps
- Umbilical tape or sterilized cord
- Small rubber bulb syringe
- Towels
- Gauze sponges
- Sterile gloves
- Sanitary napkins
- Plastic bag
- Baby blanket
- Baby stocking cap

### Automated External Defibrillator

Semiautomated defibrillation equipment

### Patient Transfer Equipment

- Wheeled ambulance stretcher
- Wheeled stair chair
- Other devices also carried on ambulances include:
  - Scoop stretcher
  - Binder Lift
  - Portable/folding stretcher
  - Flexible stretcher
  - Transfer tarp or slide board
  - Basket stretcher

### Medications and Other Supplies

- Activated charcoal (in some areas)
- Drinkable water and cups
- Oral glucose
- Oxygen
- Supplies for irrigating the skin and eyes
- Aspirin and epinephrine (in some areas)
- DuoDote or other regional equipment, depending on the area and local protocol
  - Inhaled beta agonist/bronchodilator/anticho-linergic (in some areas)
  - Naloxone (Narcan) (in some areas)
- Portable radio or cell phone

with the oxygen reservoir in place, able to supply almost 100% oxygen should also be carried on the ambulance. Masks for these devices come in a variety of sizes, from neonatal to adult, and are necessary materials to carry on the ambulance. Oxygen-powered devices are also available to provide ventilation to a patient but may quickly deplete available oxygen sources. You should follow local guidelines to identify the specific ventilation equipment carried on the ambulance.

The *National EMS Scope of Practice Model 2019* includes EMT administration of beta agonists and anticholinergic agents for patients who are wheezing. This administration requires use of a nebulizer mask. The use of CPAP is also included and can be administered using a variety of devices.

The ambulance should carry portable and mounted suctioning units (**FIGURE 38-9**). These units must be powerful enough to generate a vacuum of 300 mm Hg when the tube is clamped. The suctioning force must be adjustable for use on infants and children. The units should include large-bore suction tubing with semirigid tips available. The installed unit should include a suction yoke, a durable collection canister, suction catheters, sterile water for rinsing the suction tips, and suction tubing. As mentioned earlier, this equipment should be easily accessible when you are sitting at the head of the stretcher. The tubing must reach the patient's airway, regardless of the patient's position. All components of the suctioning unit must be

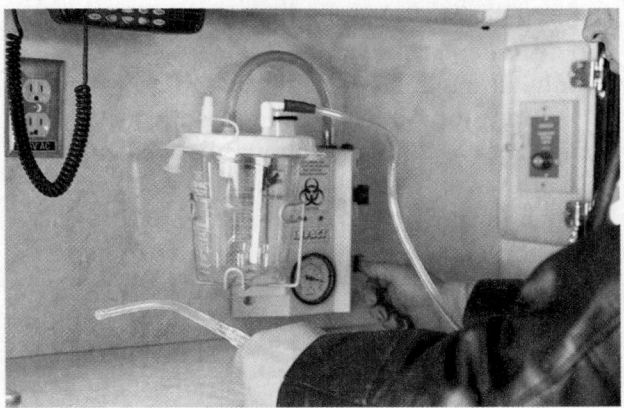

**A**

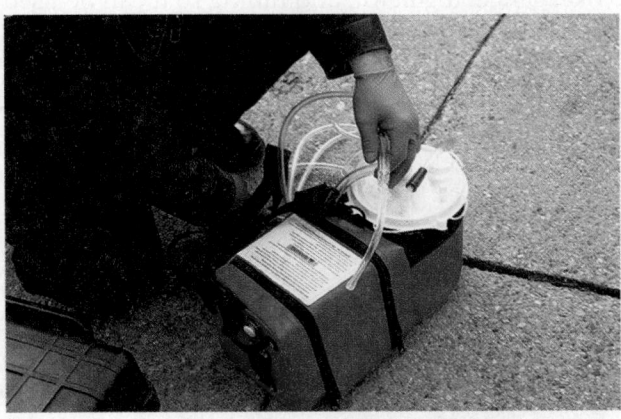

**B**

**FIGURE 38-9** The ambulance should carry both a mounted suctioning unit (**A**) and a portable unit (**B**).

**A, B:** © Jones & Bartlett Learning.

## YOU are the Provider

Law enforcement officials have arrived on scene and it is safe for you to enter. On arrival, you are led to the back porch of a house where a 42-year-old woman is lying at the base of a set of three steps, holding her left knee. She tells you that her neighbor struck her in the left leg with a baseball bat following a verbal disagreement. You see obvious swelling and deformity to the patient's left knee.

| Recording Time: 0 Minutes | |
|---|---|
| **Appearance** | Appears healthy; holding left leg; grimacing in pain |
| **Level of consciousness** | Alert and oriented |
| **Airway** | Open; clear of secretions or foreign bodies |
| **Breathing** | Normal rate; adequate depth |
| **Circulation** | Increased pulse rate, but strong and regular; skin pink, warm, and dry |

**3.** Based on the mechanism of injury (MOI) and patient presentation, what equipment do you anticipate needing?

disposable or made of material that is easy to clean and **decontaminate**.

The ambulance should carry at least two oxygen supply units: one portable and one installed on board. The portable unit should be located near a door or in the jump kit, for easy use outside the ambulance. It should have a minimum capacity of 425 L of oxygen and be equipped with a yoke, pressure gauge, flowmeter, oxygen supply tubing, nonrebreathing mask, and nasal cannula. This unit must be able to deliver oxygen at a variable rate between 1 and 15 L/min. At least one extra portable 500-L cylinder should be kept on the ambulance. Many services equip the backup cylinder with its own yoke, gauge, regulator, and tubing so it can be used for a second patient.

The mounted oxygen unit should have a capacity of 3,000 L of oxygen (**FIGURE 38-10**). It should

also be equipped with visible flowmeters that are capable of delivering 1 to 15 L/min that are accessible when you are at the head of the stretcher. Oxygen masks, with and without nonrebreathing bags, should be transparent, disposable, and in sizes for adults, children, and infants.

Ambulance services that often transport patients on runs lasting longer than 1 hour should consider using a disposable, single-use humidifier for the mounted oxygen system. On runs of less than 1 hour, humidification is not usually necessary. Humidification equipment is disposable and should be used only on a single patient to prevent the spread of infection. Humidification is less desirable in the context of a pandemic as it may increase droplet burden in the passenger compartment of the ambulance when it is in use.

> ## Words of Wisdom
>
> Regardless of their location, portable oxygen tanks must always be secured by fixed clasps or housings to prevent accidental damage and to prevent the cylinder from becoming a projectile.

### CPR Equipment

A **CPR board** provides a firm surface under the patient's torso so you can give effective chest compressions (**FIGURE 38-11A**). It also assists in establishing an appropriate degree of head tilt (**FIGURE 38-11B**). Only a few ambulances across the country carry this item. Use a tightly rolled sheet or towel to raise the patient's shoulders 3 to 4 inches (8 to 10 cm); this will also keep the patient's head in a position of maximum backward tilt and keep the shoulders and chest in a straight position. *Caution:* Do not use this roll to hyperextend the neck if you suspect a spinal injury.

Mechanical devices that operate on compressed gas or battery power and deliver chest compressions and ventilations are also available. These devices may be helpful to provide chest compressions during transport in selected circumstances.

### Basic Wound Care Supplies

Basic supplies for dressing open wounds should be carried on the ambulance. These include a pair of trauma shears; sterile sheets; sterile burn sheets; adhesive tape in several widths; self-adhering, soft

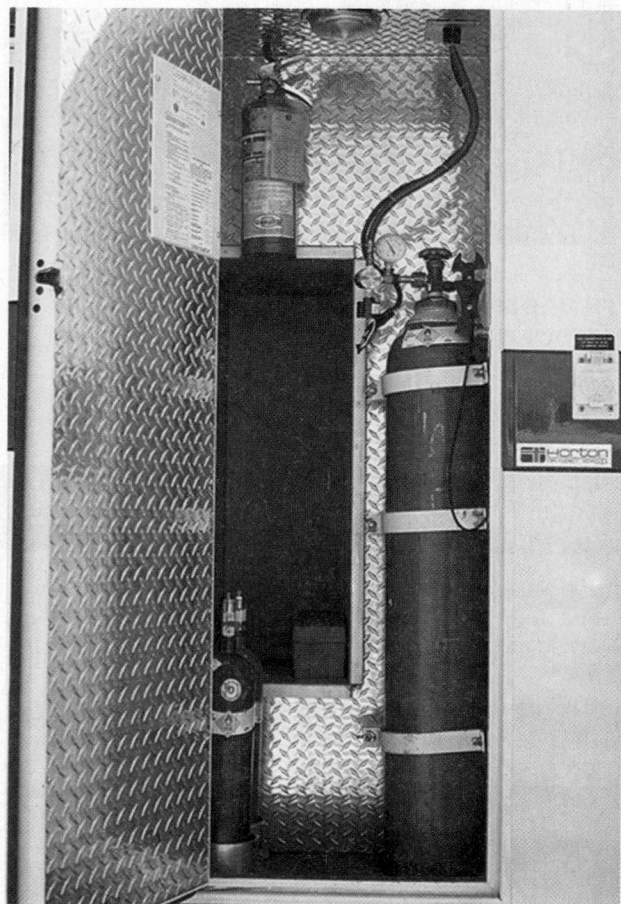

**FIGURE 38-10** An oxygen unit with a capacity of 3,000 L of oxygen should be mounted on the ambulance.

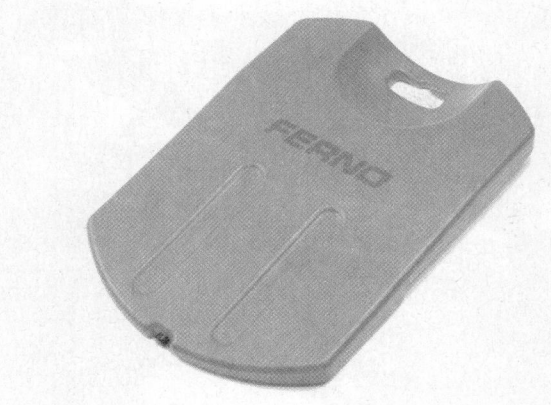

**A**

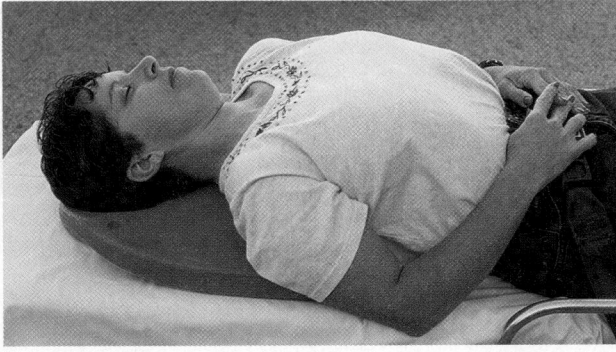

**B**

**FIGURE 38-11 A.** A CPR board may be carried on the ambulance. **B.** A patient on a CPR board has the appropriate degree of head tilt for effective artificial ventilation.

**A:** © Courtesy of Ferno Washington, Inc.; **B:** © Jones & Bartlett Learning. Courtesy of MIEMSS.

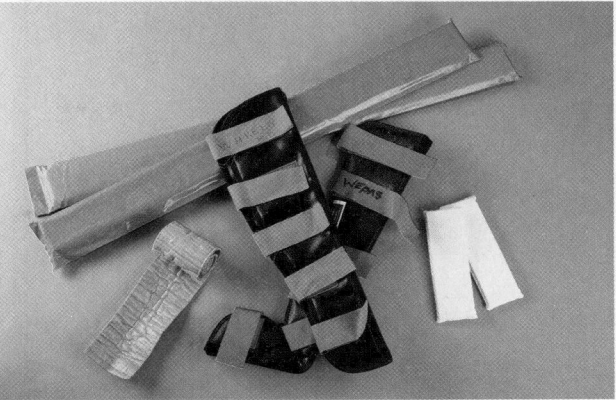

**FIGURE 38-12** Supplies for splinting fractures and dislocations should be carried on the ambulance.

© Jones & Bartlett Learning.

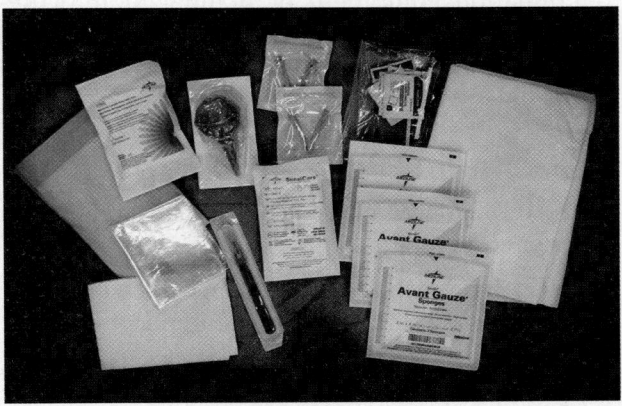

**FIGURE 38-13** A sterile emergency obstetric kit must be carried on the ambulance.

© Mark C. Ide.

roller bandages; sterile dressings; gauze; abdominal or laparotomy pads; sterile universal trauma dressings; sterile, occlusive, nonadherent dressings (aluminum foil sterilized in original package); an assortment of adhesive bandages; and tourniquets.

## Splinting Supplies

Examples of supplies for splinting fractures and dislocations that may be carried on ambulances are shown in **FIGURE 38-12**. These include an adult-size and a child-size traction splint; a variety of arm and leg splints, such as inflatable, vacuum, cardboard, plastic, foam wire-ladder, or padded board; a variety of triangular bandages and roller bandages; a short backboard; a long backboard; head immobilization devices; and cervical collars in an adjustable size or a variety of sizes.

## Childbirth Supplies

You must carry at least one sterile emergency obstetric kit (**FIGURE 38-13**) that includes the supplies listed in Table 38-3, including a pair of surgical scissors, hemostats or special cord clamps, umbilical tape or sterilized cord, a small rubber bulb syringe, towels, gauze sponges, pairs of sterile gloves, plastic wrap, sanitary napkins, a plastic bag, a baby stocking cap, and a baby blanket.

## Automated External Defibrillator

Modern-day EMS was ushered in by the first-ever prehospital use of the defibrillator by a St. Vincent's Hospital ambulance in New York City under the direction of Dr. William Grace in the early 1970s. Now a prehospital standard of care, semiautomated

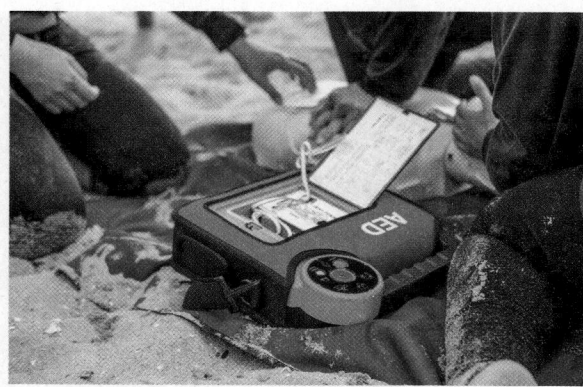

**FIGURE 38-14** Every ambulance should carry an automated external defibrillator.

© ihooyahphoto/Stock/Getty Images Plus/Getty Images.

defibrillation equipment or manual monitor/defibrillators that have AED capability, as permitted by regulation and the local medical director, should always be carried on the ambulance (**FIGURE 38-14**).

### Patient Transfer Equipment

Each ambulance should carry the following patient transfer equipment:

- A primary wheeled ambulance stretcher
- A wheeled stair chair for use in narrow spaces
- A long backboard
- A short backboard or short immobilization device

You should be able to tilt the head of the stretcher upward to at least a 60° angle, placing the patient in a semi-sitting position. Stretchers must be provided with fasteners to secure them firmly to the floor or side of the ambulance during transport. Locking mechanisms should be capable of holding the stretcher in place in case the vehicle rolls over. Make certain that the wheeled stretcher is properly locked into position, because injuries can occur to the patient and you if the stretcher becomes loose while the ambulance is in motion (**FIGURE 38-15**). Make sure there are at least three restraining devices for the patient, with deceleration or stopping straps over the shoulders, to prevent the patient from continuing to move forward in case the ambulance suddenly slows or stops. Regardless of the equipment used, it is important to use proper lifting techniques to avoid injuries. Chapter 8, *Lifting and Moving,* discusses proper lifting and moving of patients.

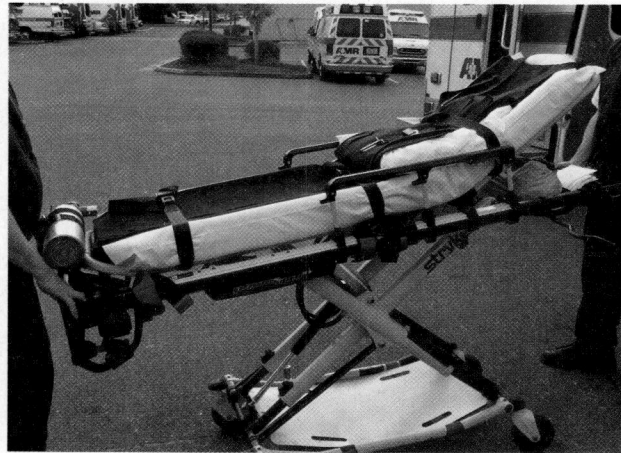

**FIGURE 38-15** The wheeled ambulance stretcher should be locked into place at an appropriate height.

Courtesy of Angulo, Raul A.

### Street Smarts

In some cases, it may seem inconvenient or time consuming to apply shoulder straps when securing the patient to the ambulance stretcher. While you are securing the patient, explain how important it is for his or her safety. Using all straps to secure the patient is an essential habit, much like applying your own seat belt when riding in the cab.

Other patient transfer devices that can be used include the following:

- A scoop stretcher
- A vacuum mattress
- A portable/folding stretcher
- A flexible stretcher
- A basket stretcher
- A Binder Lift

### Medications

It is important that the ambulance carry valid and appropriate medications. Keep the telephone number and radio frequency of online medical control or the local poison control center with you on the ambulance. The back of your clipboard is a good place to keep this information.

### The Jump Kit

The ambulance must be equipped with a portable, durable, and waterproof jump kit that you can carry

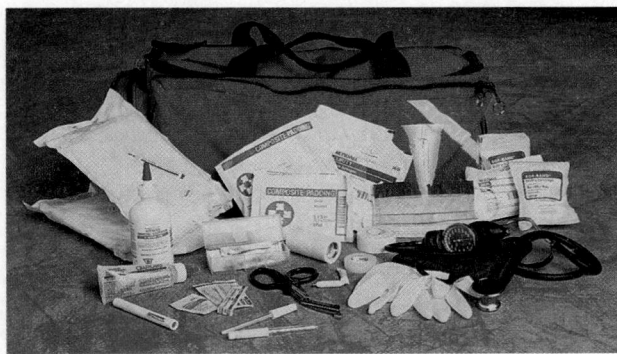

**FIGURE 38-16** A portable jump kit should contain practically anything you will need during the first 5 minutes with the patient.

© Jones & Bartlett Learning. Courtesy of MIEMSS.

to the patient (**FIGURE 38-16**). Think of the **jump kit** as the *5-minute kit,* containing anything you might need in the first 5 minutes with the patient except for the semiautomated external defibrillator, possibly the oxygen cylinder, and portable suctioning unit. The jump kit must be easy to open and secure.

**TABLE 38-4** lists the items that are typically contained in a jump kit.

## Safety and Operations Equipment

In addition to medical equipment, a properly stocked ambulance carries several kinds of equipment for responder safety, rescue operations, and locating emergency scenes. To do the job effectively, your team will need the following equipment:

- PPE
- Equipment for work areas
- Preplanning/navigation guides
- Extrication equipment

### *Personal Safety Equipment*

Along with your ANSI Class 2 reflective vest, you should always carry PPE that allows you to work safely in a limited variety of hazardous or contaminated situations. These situations include the edges of a structural fire or explosion, vehicle extrication, and in crowds. The equipment should protect you from exposure to blood and other potentially infectious body fluids. You will not be equipped to face all hazardous materials (hazmat) and other exposure situations that you may encounter; this is the job of specifically trained hazmat technicians and

| **TABLE 38-4** Items Carried in a Jump Kit |
| --- |
| • Nitrile, vinyl, or other disposable gloves |
| • Face shield or mask with goggles |
| • Triangular bandages |
| • Tourniquet |
| • Trauma shears |
| • Adhesive tape in various widths |
| • Universal trauma dressings |
| • Self-adhering soft roller bandages, 4 in. × 5 yd (10 cm × 5 m) and 2 in. × 5 yd (5 cm × 5 m) |
| • Oropharyngeal airways in adult, child, and infant sizes* |
| • Bag masks for adults, children, and infants* |
| • Blood pressure cuff |
| • Stethoscope |
| • Penlight |
| • Sterile gauze dressings, 4 × 4 in. (10 × 10 cm) |
| • Sterile dressings (abdominal pads), 6 × 9 in. (15 × 23 cm) or 8 × 10 in. (20 × 25 cm) |
| • Adhesive strips |
| • Oral glucose |
| • Naloxone |
| • Other medications allowed by local protocols |
| • Oxygen saturation monitor* |

*These might be carried in a separate airway kit, along with the portable oxygen cylinder.

© Jones & Bartlett Learning.

response teams. Your equipment might include the following:

- Face shields
- N95 masks
- Gowns, shoe covers, caps
- Turnout gear
- Helmets with face shields or safety goggles
- Safety shoes or boots
- Tactical vest

### *Equipment for Work Areas*

A weatherproof compartment that you can reach from outside the patient compartment should hold equipment for safeguarding patients and EMTs, controlling traffic and bystanders, and illuminating work areas (**FIGURE 38-17**). The following items are recommended:

- Warning devices that flash intermittently or have reflectors (Road flares can pose an additional hazard, such as ignition of flammable liquids or gases.)

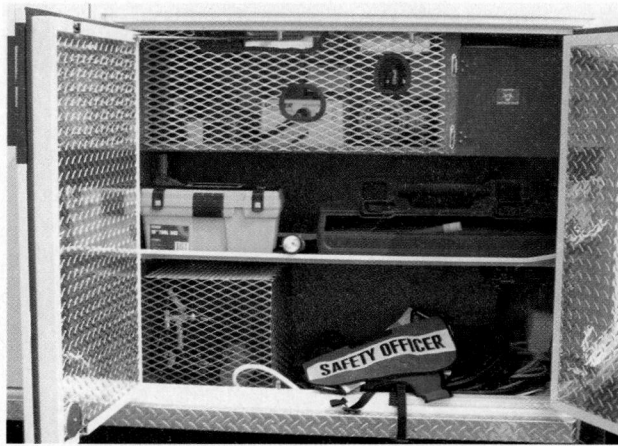

**FIGURE 38-17** The ambulance should have a weatherproof compartment that can be reached from outside the patient compartment. It should hold equipment for safeguarding patients and EMTs, controlling traffic, and illuminating work areas.

© Jones & Bartlett Learning. Courtesy of MIEMSS.

- Two high-intensity halogen, 20,000-candle power flashlights of the recharging battery-powered, standup type
- Fire extinguisher, type ABC, dry chemical, 5-lb (2.3 kg) minimum
- Hard hats or helmets with face shields or safety goggles
- Portable floodlights

### Preplanning and Navigation Equipment

GPS devices and MDTs are standard equipment in modern ambulances. The addresses of area hospitals and nursing homes should be stored for easy access. Enter the location of the hospital into the GPS device before initiating transport to the hospital and review the route that you plan to take. You should never turn your attention away from driving to use a device of any type. Your partner should assist with providing updates from the MDT or GPS devices when responding to a call, especially when using lights and siren. Make sure you also have detailed street and area maps in the driver's compartment of the ambulance. Maps can serve as a backup if there are any technical issues with the GPS device or data transmission.

Familiarize yourself with the roads and traffic patterns in your town or city so you can plan alternate routes to frequent destinations. Pay particular attention to alternate routes that may provide you

| **TABLE 38-5** Extrication Equipment |
|---|
| - 12-in. (30.5-cm) wrench, adjustable, open-end |
| - 12-in. (30.5-cm) screwdriver, standard square bar |
| - 8-in. (20-cm) screwdriver, Phillips head #2 |
| - Hacksaw with 12-in. (30.5-cm) carbide wire blades |
| - Vise-grip pliers, 10 in. (25 cm) |
| - 5-lb. (2.3-kg) hammer with 15-in. (38-cm) handle |
| - Fire axe, butt, 24-in. (61-cm) handle |
| - Wrecking bar with 24-in. (61-cm) handle. This may be a combination tool with a hammer and axe. |
| - 51-in. (130-cm) crowbar, pinch point |
| - Bolt cutter with 1- to 1.25-in. (25- to 32-mm) jaw opening |
| - Folding shovel, pointed blade |
| - Tin snips, double action, 8 in. (15-cm) minimum |
| - Gauntlets (reinforced leather covering past midforearm), one pair per crew member |
| - Rescue blanket |
| - Ropes, 5,400-lb. (2,449-kg) tensile strength in 50-ft. (15-m) lengths in protective bags |
| - Mastic knife (able to cut seat belt webbing) |
| - Spring-loaded center punch |
| - Roll of duct tape (for window application prior to center punch use) |
| - Pruning saw |
| - Heavy-duty 2 × 4–in. (5 × 10–cm) and 4 × 4–in. (10 × 10–cm) shoring (cribbing) blocks, various lengths |

© Jones & Bartlett Learning.

with ways around frequently raised bridges, congested traffic, and blocked railroad crossings. Often, switching to an alternate route will save more time than driving faster. You should be familiar with special facilities and locations within your regional operating area, such as other medical facilities, airports, arenas and stadiums, detention facilities, and chemical or research facilities that might pose unusual problems (staging areas may be predefined for emergency operations).

### Extrication Equipment

A weatherproof compartment outside the patient compartment should contain equipment that is needed for simple, light extrication, even if an extrication and rescue unit is readily available. **TABLE 38-5** lists the items that may be included in the compartment.

If rescue and extrication services are not readily available, additional equipment may be needed.

## Personnel

Every ambulance must be staffed with at least one EMT in the patient compartment whenever a patient is being transported. Certain situations may require more assistance, such as performing CPR. Some EMS systems may allow non-EMT drivers to operate the ambulance when warranted by patient condition with two EMTs in the patient compartment. In these instances, the driver is usually a firefighter or law enforcement official who is properly trained to operate the vehicle in emergency situations.

## Daily Inspections

Being fully prepared means you and your team must inspect both the ambulance and equipment daily to ensure all items are in proper working order. Because your vehicle may be required to operate during bad weather or during emergency situations, you must ensure it is in proper working condition at all times. There is no margin for error when it comes to vehicle performance in an emergency. Inspections can help to minimize the risk that your ambulance experiences a preventable mechanical failure. The ambulance inspection should include the following:

- Fuel level
- Oil level
- Transmission fluid level
- Engine cooling system and fluid levels
- Batteries
- Brake fluid
- Engine belts
- Wheels and tires, including the spare, if there is one. Check inflation pressure and look for signs of unusual or uneven wear.
- All interior and exterior lights
- Windshield wipers and fluid
- Horn
- Siren
- Air conditioners and heaters
- Ventilating system
- Doors. Make sure they open, close, latch, and lock properly.
- Communication systems, vehicle and portable
- All windows and mirrors. Check for cleanliness and position.

Check all medical equipment and supplies daily, including all the oxygen supplies; the jump

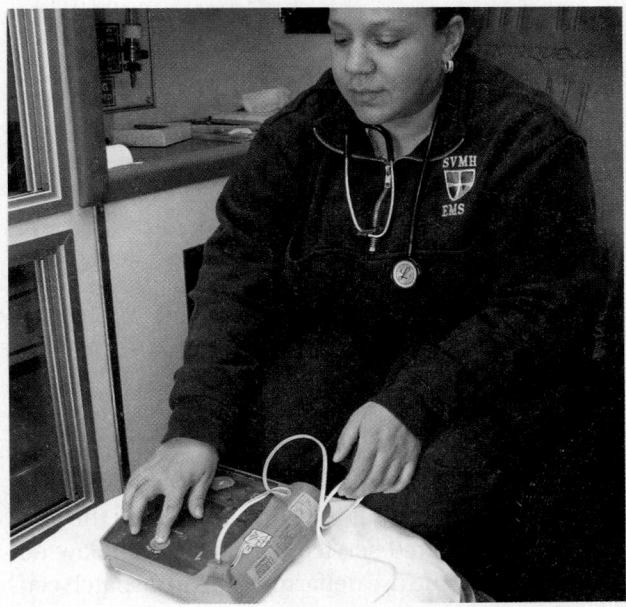

**FIGURE 38-18** Always check the defibrillator at the beginning of each day.
© Jones & Bartlett Learning. Courtesy of MIEMSS.

kit; splints, dressings and bandages; backboards and other immobilization equipment; and the emergency obstetrics kit. Is the equipment functioning properly? Are the supplies clean? Are there enough of them? All battery-operated equipment, including the defibrillator, should be operated and checked each day (**FIGURE 38-18**). Rotate the batteries according to an established schedule and ensure that any charging cables are connected.

## Safety Precautions

A final part of the preparation phase is reviewing safety precautions. These precautions, which include standard traffic safety rules and regulations, should be followed on every call. Check safety devices, such as seat belts (in the cab and patient compartment), to ensure they are in proper working order. All equipment in the cab and in the patient compartment needs to be secured appropriately. Regardless of their location, portable oxygen tanks must always be secured by fixed clasps or housings. Never attempt to secure a tank to the stretcher or bench, unless you are using a commercially manufactured device specifically designed for this purpose. All equipment, including oxygen tanks, may become projectiles if the ambulance is involved in a motor vehicle crash.

## The Dispatch Phase

Dispatch must be easy to access and in service 24 hours a day (**FIGURE 38-19**). It may be operated by the local EMS or by a shared service that also covers law enforcement and the fire department. The dispatch center might serve only one jurisdiction, such as a single city or town, or it might be an area or regional center serving several communities or an entire county. In either case, it should be staffed by trained personnel who are familiar with the agencies they are dispatching and the geography of the service area. For every emergency request, the dispatcher should gather and record the following minimum information:

- The nature of the call
- The name, current location, and call-back telephone number of the caller

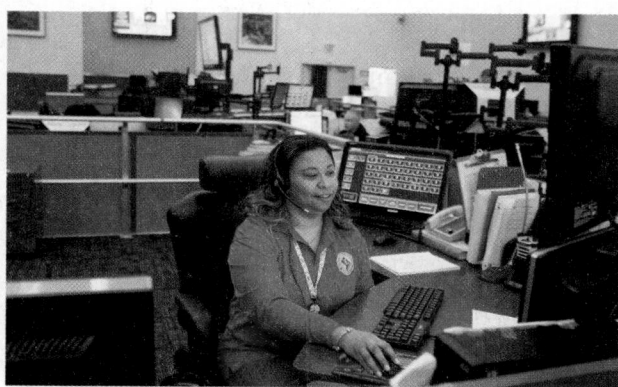

**FIGURE 38-19** The dispatcher is the key communications link throughout all phases of the ambulance run.
© Marvin Joseph/The Washington Post/Getty Images.

- The location of the patient or patients
- The number of patients and some idea of the severity of their conditions
- Any other special problems or pertinent information about hazards or weather conditions

Many areas implement emergency medical dispatching, which provides the caller with prearrival instructions for patient care before the ambulance arrives. The emergency medical dispatcher follows a set of guidelines to determine the type of information given and then guides the caller through basic care such as bleeding control or initiating CPR.

## YOU are the Provider

After assessing the patient, you determine that she is hemodynamically stable. She did not have a loss of consciousness. She has deformity to her left knee with severe pain and tenderness on palpation. She has a history of hypertension and is allergic to penicillin. There was no fall associated with the event, and she was struck only once on the knee. There is no need for spinal motion restriction.

**Recording Time: 5 Minutes**

| | |
|---|---|
| **Respirations** | 20 breaths/min; adequate depth |
| **Pulse** | 98 beats/min; strong and regular |
| **Skin** | Pink, warm, and dry |
| **Blood pressure** | 138/86 mm Hg |
| **Oxygen saturation (Spo$_2$)** | 99% (on room air) |

4. What assessment and treatment should be performed on scene and what should be delayed until you are in the ambulance and en route to the hospital?

5. How would you determine whether to use lights and siren during transport of this patient?

## En Route to the Scene

In many ways, the en route or response phase of the call is the most dangerous for responders. Crashes between motor vehicles and emergency vehicles cause many serious injuries among EMS personnel. As you and your partner prepare to respond to the scene, make sure you fasten your seat belts and shoulder harnesses before you move the ambulance. Quickly review the most appropriate route that you intend to travel while responding to the call. You should also consider what alternate routes are available if your ambulance should encounter a raised bridge or traffic congestion. You should inform dispatch that your unit is responding and confirm the nature and location of the call. This is also an excellent time to ask for any other available information about the location. For example, you might learn that the patient is on the third floor or that the best door to use is around the side of the house.

In the event that you are responding to a violent crime or your dispatcher has detected the possibility that the scene is not safe for you to enter, you may be requested to stage your ambulance away from the scene while law enforcement officers respond to secure the scene. If you are requested to stage your ambulance, make sure it is a safe distance away from the scene. Bystanders or family members who see your ambulance stopped and not proceeding immediately to the scene may become agitated or violent because they want you

to respond and render immediate care, even if the scene is not safe. Consider staging out of sight of the scene, even a few streets away. If there is only one road into or out of the neighborhood to which you are responding, do not stage on that road. If the person who originally assaulted a patient is fleeing the scene, you do not want to provide this person with the opportunity to delay or harm emergency responders. Follow local protocols and be aware of how your agency responds to possible unsafe scenes.

While en route to the call, the team should prepare to assess and care for the patient. Review dispatch information about the nature of the call and the location of the patient. Assign specific initial duties and scene management tasks to each team member and determine what type of equipment you will take with you when you first arrive on scene. Depending on the location of the patient, you may choose to take your primary stretcher or another patient transfer device with you immediately if access to the patient is limited. Make sure you follow your local operating procedures regarding the minimum equipment required for every call.

If the location of the patient changes or there are obstacles along your primary response route that could cause a significant delay, the person who is not operating the ambulance should be responsible for using the GPS or a map book to help determine an alternate route. Arriving at the scene safely and safely transporting the patient are two of the most challenging aspects of being an EMT. Refer to the *Defensive Ambulance Driving Techniques* section in this chapter for techniques on safely driving and operating an ambulance.

## Arrival at the Scene

On arrival at the incident, you will perform a scene size-up. This scene size-up begins from inside the ambulance. You begin by evaluating the safety and stability of the scene. Do you see any hazards, or is the scene safe? Is this a medical call with only one patient, who is sitting in clear view on the front porch? Is this a traffic accident with people entrapped in a vehicle? Is there a fight erupting on scene? As you gather more information, provide a brief report to your dispatch center with an update of the incident to which you have responded. This update will help to ensure that the appropriate

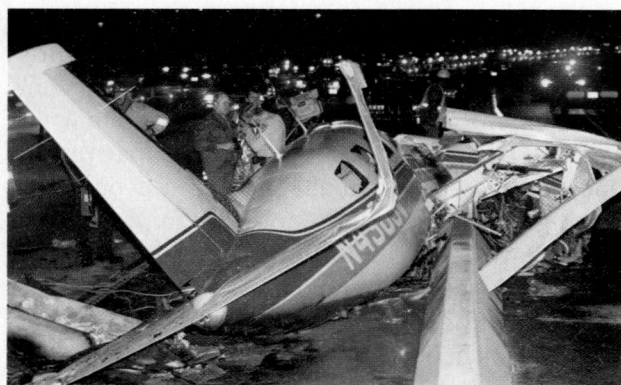

**FIGURE 38-20** If you are the first to arrive on the scene of a mass-casualty incident, you should report to dispatch and ask for additional units, such as heavy rescue or hazmat units as needed.

© Mark Terrill/AP Photos.

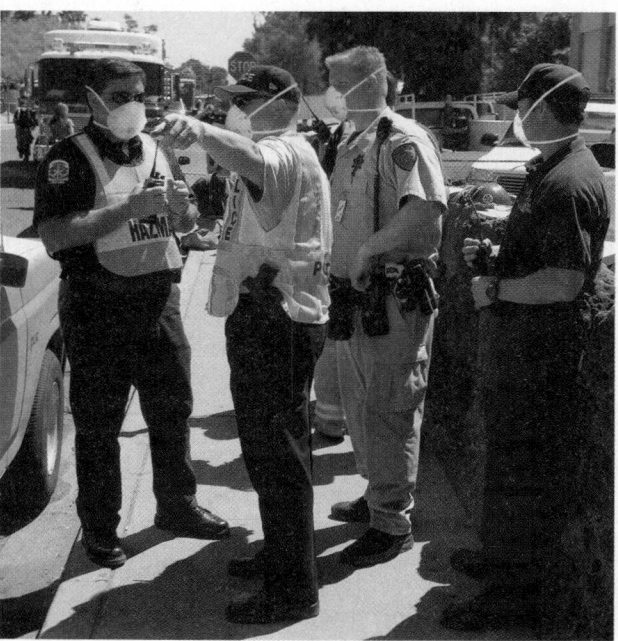

**FIGURE 38-21** At a mass-casualty incident, follow instructions from the incident commander assigning your roles, which may include assisting with triage, treating patients, or loading patients for transport to the hospital.

© John Sartin/ShutterStock.

resources are responding to the incident or possibly cancel additional resources that are not needed.

Report any unexpected situations, such as the need for specialized units, a heavy rescue unit, or a hazmat team (**FIGURE 38-20**). Do not enter the scene if there are any hazards to you. If there are hazards at the scene, the patient should be moved somewhere safe before you begin care. The patient may have to be moved by others if you are not appropriately equipped.

Immediately size up the scene by using the following guidelines:

- Look for safety hazards to yourself, your partner, bystanders, and your patient or patients.
- Evaluate the need for additional units or other assistance.
- Determine the MOI in trauma patients or the nature of the illness on medical calls.
- Evaluate the need to immobilize the spine.
- Follow standard precautions. The type of care that you expect to give will dictate the PPE you should wear.

If you are the first EMT at the scene of a mass-casualty incident, quickly estimate the number of patients, and communicate with your dispatch center or the incident commander if this person has arrived simultaneously (**FIGURE 38-21**). An accurate estimation of the number of patients will help to mobilize the appropriate number of resources to the scene. Remember that your initial estimation will be revised throughout the evolution of the incident. Mass-casualty incidents involve complex organization of personnel under the incident command system (see Chapter 40, *Incident Management*). In this system, individual EMTs may be assigned roles, such as beginning the triage process, assisting in treating patients, and loading patients for transport to a hospital.

## Safe Parking

In assessing the situation, you must decide where to park the ambulance. When parking, always use your parking brake. Pick a position that will allow for safe operations on scene, efficient traffic control, and a clear path for departing the scene. Always remember to leave yourself an exit. Whether initiating transport or retreating from a violent scene, you should park your vehicle with a clear departure path. It is best to park uphill and/or upwind of the scene if smoke or hazardous materials are present. Always leave your warning lights or devices engaged, and use extra caution if you must park on the back side of a hill or curve.

When operating on a roadway, if other responders, such as firefighters or law enforcement

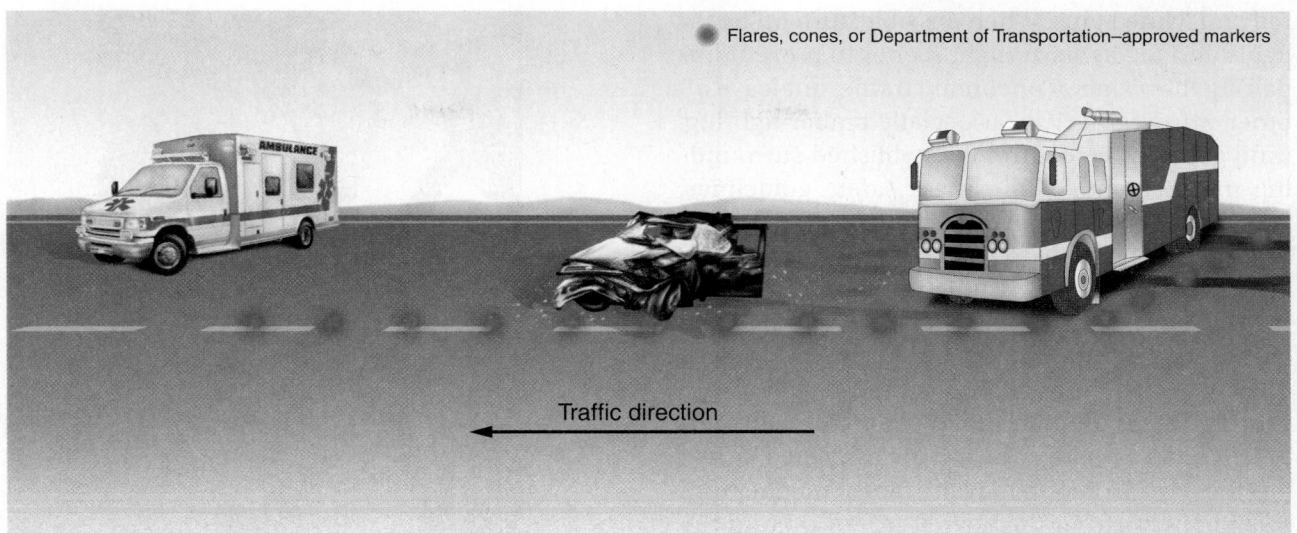

Flares, cones, or Department of Transportation–approved markers

Traffic direction

**FIGURE 38-22** If other responders, such as firefighters or law enforcement officers, are on scene first, park the ambulance about 100 feet (30 m) past the scene on the same side of the road so as to allow an unobstructed departure path.

© Jones & Bartlett Learning.

officers, are on scene first, they should position their vehicles before the scene. The first emergency vehicle should create a barrier between the scene and traffic traveling in the same direction as the lane of traffic you are occupying. If arriving after other emergency vehicles, the ambulance should be positioned about 100 ft (30 m) beyond the scene, thereby preventing your vehicle from being blocked in when transporting a patient. If the street has not been completely closed and there is a driveway or parking lot adjacent to the scene, consider parking the ambulance there.

If you are the first vehicle to arrive on scene, you should park about 100 ft (30 m) before the scene on the same side of the road in the fend-off position (**FIGURE 38-22**). In the fend-off position, the ambulance is parked at a diagonal angle with the front wheels turned away from the scene. This position helps to block the scene and create a safety barrier within which you can operate. If a vehicle strikes the rear of an ambulance parked in the fend-off position, it is more likely to be deflected outward than directly into the area of the crash, where emergency personnel are working. Distracted drivers or poor weather conditions may create dangerous scenarios in which a vehicle may inadvertently drive into the scene at full speed. Assume someone may collide with your vehicle and strike personnel on the

scene. Having a large emergency vehicle as a safety barrier may provide you with a cushion of space that could save your life.

Stay away from any fires, explosive hazards, downed wires, and structures that might collapse. Be sure to set the parking brake. If your vehicle is blocking part of the roadway, leave on the emergency warning lights. Some motorists tend to drive toward emergency vehicles with flashing red or

## Safety Tips

When operating at an incident on any roadway, use caution when exiting the ambulance, wear protective equipment, and maintain a high level of situational awareness. Even with all of the emergency vehicles parked appropriately on a scene, distracted drivers may still drive straight into an emergency vehicle. Try to operate primarily within safe areas that use signage and large vehicles as barriers from the flow of traffic. Minimize your time on the scene. Whenever you are on a roadway, it is important to wear reflective safety vests or turnout gear. If you are retrieving equipment from the side compartment of your ambulance, you may be virtually invisible if you do not have a reflective vest on. Even attentive drivers may have difficulty seeing areas around the emergency vehicles that have all warning lights on.

red and white lights. When possible, turn off headlights and fog lights at night scenes to prevent impairing the vision of oncoming traffic, but leave on other warning devices, especially amber lighting, until good traffic control is established surrounding the incident. Within these safety guidelines, you should try to park your ambulance as close to the scene as possible to facilitate emergency medical care. If necessary, you can temporarily block traffic to unload equipment and to load patients quickly and safely. If you must do this, try to do it quickly so traffic is not blocked any longer than necessary. Depending on the incident, lock the ambulance doors and ensure the designated driver has the keys. Doing so may prevent someone from stealing items from the ambulance or theft of the vehicle itself.

## Traffic Control

After you ensure your safety, your next responsibility at a crash scene is to care for the patients. Only after all the patients have been treated and the emergency situation is under control should you be concerned with restoring the flow of traffic. If the police have a delayed response to the scene, you might then need to take action to control the scene and limit access by other vehicles. It is important to ensure a safe environment for your crew and your patients.

The purposes of traffic control are to ensure an orderly traffic flow and to prevent a secondary crash. Under ordinary circumstances, traffic control is difficult. A crash or disaster scene presents serious additional problems. Passing motorists often slow down and stare, paying little attention to the roadway in front of them. Some curiosity seekers may park down the road and return on foot, creating additional hazards. As soon as possible, place appropriate warning devices, such as reflectors, on both sides of the crash.

Remember, the main objectives in directing traffic are to warn other drivers, to prevent secondary crashes, and to keep vehicles moving in an orderly manner so care of injured people is not interrupted.

## The Transfer Phase

During the transfer phase, you must package the patient for transport, safely securing him or her to the wheeled ambulance stretcher. Then move to the

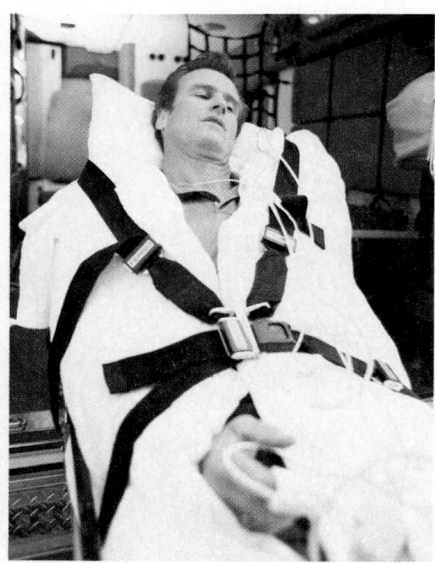

**FIGURE 38-23** Secure the patient appropriately for protection during transport.
© Jim Craigmyle/Corbis/Getty Images.

ambulance, and properly lift the patient into the patient compartment.

No matter how careful the ambulance driver may be, riding to the hospital while lying down on a stretcher can be uncomfortable and even dangerous. Be sure to secure the patient with all manufacturer-approved straps (**FIGURE 38-23**). Use deceleration or stopping straps over the shoulders to prevent the patient from continuing to move forward in case the ambulance suddenly slows or stops. This is especially important if the patient is supine.

## The Transport Phase

Inform dispatch when you are ready to leave with the patient. Report the number of patients you have, the name of the receiving hospital, and, in some jurisdictions, the beginning mileage of the ambulance. Even though you have already assessed and treated the patient, you should continue to monitor the patient's condition en route. These ongoing assessments may reveal changes in the patient's vital signs and overall condition. Recheck the patient's vital signs en route. The frequency of checking vital signs depends on the patient's acuity, but checking them every 15 minutes for a stable patient and every 5 minutes for an unstable patient is a practice that many services use. In addition, it is important that you continually reassess the patient's clinical situation, address new problems, and note the patient's responses to earlier treatment.

During the transport phase, contact the receiving hospital. Inform online medical control about the patient or patients and the nature of the problem or problems. Depending on the number of EMTs and how much care the patient needs, you may be able to begin documenting your patient care report (PCR) while en route.

Most important, do not abandon the patient emotionally. Do not become so involved in paperwork and ongoing assessments that you ignore the patient. The prehospital phase may be the only time that the patient will have one provider dedicated solely to his or her care. Remember that you may be caring for the patient immediately after a tragic event or during life-threatening illness. Do not ignore how important compassion and caring can be during this phase. You are there to help the patient, so use this time to reassure him or her. Sometimes small talk and conversation are appropriate, while other times just a quiet presence may be appreciated. Some patients, such as very young or older people, may benefit from added attention during transport. Be aware of your patient's level of need.

The use of lights and siren when transporting a patient to the hospital has been debated in recent years and has evolved as a result. Anecdotally, people believed in the past that transporting with lights and siren saved a significant amount of time and offered patients the best chance of survival. Rarely, however, is such a ride lifesaving or even close. Research suggests that there is no significant improvement in patient outcomes, and this practice may be a detriment to the patient because the quality of clinical care provided may be worse when transported with lights and siren and the overall environment for the patient is clearly less safe. Mode of transport is often not at the discretion of the crew operating the ambulance. Many jurisdictions and medical directors specifically define which situations warrant use of emergency lights and sirens for transport. Ignoring those directives could result in penalties or liability for any injuries caused.

Use common sense and defensive driving techniques at all times. In almost every case, you will provide lifesaving care right where you find the patient. You may perform less critical measures, such as bandaging and splinting, en route to the hospital.

## The Delivery Phase

Inform dispatch as soon as you arrive at the hospital and, depending on your jurisdiction, identify your ending mileage as well. Then follow these steps to transfer the patient to the receiving hospital:

1. Report your arrival to the triage nurse or other arrival personnel.
2. Physically transfer the patient from the stretcher to the bed directed for your patient.
3. Present a complete verbal report at the bedside to the nurse or physician who is taking over the patient's care. Include all pertinent information regarding your assessment and treatment. Answer any questions from the receiving staff.
4. Complete a detailed written report, obtain the required signatures, and leave a copy with an appropriate staff member. Electronic reports are commonly used. Your service should have a method for printing or sending electronic reports as well as obtaining electronic signatures.

The PCR should include a summary of the history of the patient's current illness or injury with pertinent positives and negatives, MOI, and findings on your arrival. In addition, list vital signs, relevant past medical or surgical history, and information regarding medication and allergies. Also, be sure to document any treatment and the patient's response to treatment during the prehospital setting.

While at the hospital, you may be able to restock any items that were used during the call, such as oxygen masks or dressings and bandages (**FIGURE 38-24**). Remember that your priority is transfer of the patient and patient information to the hospital staff; restocking the ambulance comes second.

### Street Smarts

As a prehospital emergency provider, your verbal report and written documentation provide a vital portion of the patient's story. You hold the key to unlocking details of everything that occurred prior to the patient arriving at the hospital. You are the only one who can help provide details from the prehospital environment that can have a significant effect on the patient's course of care at the hospital. Never forget the importance of your role in the continuum of care.

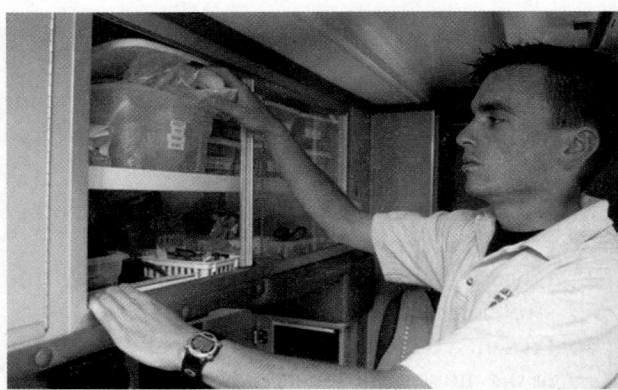

**FIGURE 38-24** After transferring the patient and relating patient information to the hospital staff, you should restock any items that were used during the run.

© Jones & Bartlett Learning. Courtesy of MIEMSS.

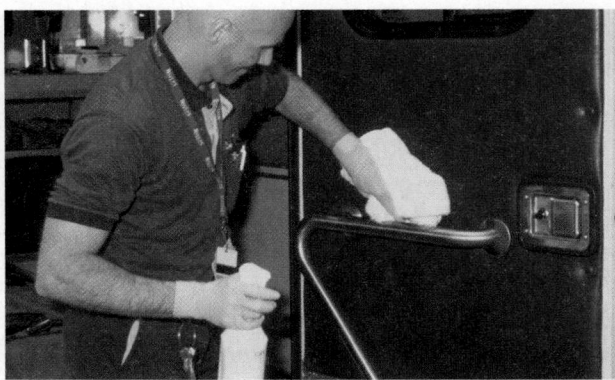

**FIGURE 38-25** Clean and disinfect the ambulance and equipment at the station if you did not do so at the hospital.

© Jones & Bartlett Learning. Courtesy of MIEMSS.

## En Route to the Station

Once you leave the hospital, inform dispatch whether you are in service and your intended destination. Depending on the call you just completed, your ambulance may not be prepared for another call until you return to your station. As soon as you are back at the station, you should do the following:

- Clean and disinfect the ambulance and any equipment that was used, if you did not do so before leaving the hospital (**FIGURE 38-25**).
- Restock any supplies you did not get at the hospital.

## The Postrun Phase

During the postrun phase, complete and file any additional reports and again inform dispatch of the unit status, location, and availability. This is also the appropriate time to debrief following the call. You should discuss the initial situation encountered on scene, strengths identified by the team's performance during the call, and opportunities for improvement regarding clinical knowledge, assessment, and skill proficiency. This debriefing process ideally should occur following every call in a professional, nonjudgmental manner while respecting each team member's input.

Each crew member is responsible for maintaining the ambulance so it is available at a moment's notice. This means you should perform routine inspections and refuel the vehicle. Use a written checklist to document needed repairs or replacement of equipment and supplies.

You should know the meanings of the terms *cleaning, disinfection, high-level disinfection,* and *sterilization,* as follows:

- **Cleaning.** The process of removing dirt, dust, blood, or other visible contaminants from a surface or equipment
- **Disinfection.** The killing of pathogenic agents by directly applying a chemical made for that purpose to a surface or equipment
- **High-level disinfection.** The killing of pathogenic agents by using potent means of disinfection and use of thorough application processes
- **Sterilization.** A process, such as the use of heat, which removes all microbial contamination

A basic rule is to do the following after every call:

1. Immediately strip used linens from the stretcher after use, and place them in a plastic bag or in the designated receptacle in the ED.
2. Discard in an appropriate receptacle all disposable equipment used for care of the patient that meets your state's definition of medical waste. Most items will be considered general trash. Discard disposable equipment that is bloody or contaminated by body fluids in an OSHA-approved biohazard container. Discard noncontaminated disposable equipment used for care of the patient following OSHA and local guidelines.
3. Wash contaminated areas with soap and water. For disinfection to be effective, cleaning must be done first.

4. Disinfect all nondisposable equipment used in the care of the patient. For example, properly clean and disinfect stethoscopes, nondisposable blood pressure cuffs, pulse oximetry probes, and other reusable equipment.

5. Clean the stretcher with an EPA-registered germicidal/virucidal solution or bleach and water at 1:100 dilution. Follow manufacturer recommendations on minimum contact time, as most will require the surface to remain visibly wet with a solution for a specified amount of time.

6. Clean up any spillage or other contamination that occurred in the ambulance, with the same germicidal/virucidal or bleach/water solution.

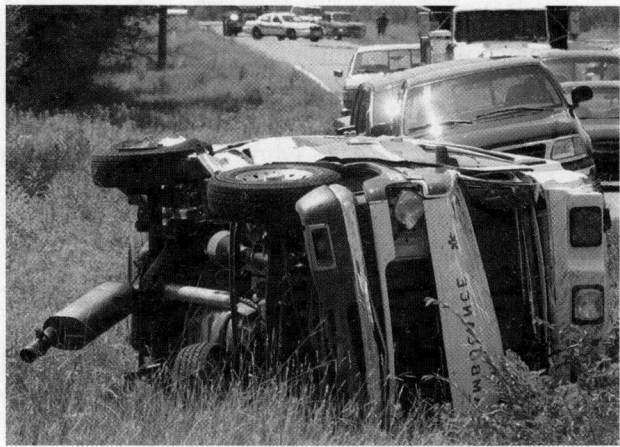

**FIGURE 38-26** Each year, ambulance crashes are the cause of thousands of injuries to pedestrians, motorists, ambulance passengers, and EMS personnel.

© Gary Lloyd, *The Decatur Daily*/AP Photos.

# Defensive Ambulance Driving Techniques

According to the National Highway Traffic Safety Administration, there has been an annual average of 29 fatal accidents involving an ambulance for the past 20 years. The average number of injuries resulting from those accidents is more than 1,500 per year. These statistics show the effect of these crashes on pedestrians, motorists, ambulance passengers, and EMS personnel (**FIGURE 38-26**). Learning how to properly operate your vehicle is just as important as learning how to care for patients when you arrive on the scene. An ambulance that is involved in a crash delays patient care, at a minimum, and may take the lives of the EMTs, patients in the ambulance, other motorists, or pedestrians. The following section is provided to introduce you to safe driving techniques; however, you cannot become a proficient and safe ambulance driver without specialized training and practice. You are strongly encouraged to participate in a certified defensive driving program, such as those offered through your EMS organization, before attempting to operate an emergency vehicle.

## Driver Characteristics

Not everyone who drives a motor vehicle is qualified to drive an emergency vehicle. In some states, you must successfully complete an approved emergency vehicle operations course before you are allowed to drive the ambulance on emergency calls. In any state, due diligence and caution are important characteristics, as are a positive attitude about your ability and tolerance of other drivers.

A crash may occur as a result of physical impairment of the driver. Do not drive if you are taking medications that may cause drowsiness or slow your reaction time. These include cold remedies, and analgesic and anxiolytic drugs. And, of course, you should never drive or provide medical care after drinking alcohol. Although most employers have guidelines that require an employee to stop drinking at least 10 to 12 hours prior to the start of his or her shift, many factors affect the rate of alcohol metabolism, so it is possible to stop drinking for this period of time and still be impaired.

Working long shifts or multiple consecutive shifts also puts drivers at risk for significant fatigue that may cause delayed reaction time and/or falling asleep behind the wheel. Although many services have regulations against working beyond a specific number of hours, all services do not take into consideration EMTs who may work for more than one service. It is your responsibility to notify your employer if you have previously worked a shift and feel unable to safely operate an emergency vehicle.

### Words of Wisdom

Driving an ambulance does not automatically give you the authority to ignore basic traffic laws or operate the vehicle without due regard for the safety of others. The good judgment needed to drive an ambulance requires practice—even for the best drivers.

Another requirement is emotional fitness. Emotions should not be taken lightly. A driver's personality often changes once he or she gets behind a steering wheel. You must remain calm and keep a clear train of thought. Whether through blatant disregard or a panicked response to an emergency vehicle behind their vehicle, other drivers on the road may have wildly different reactions when they encounter your ambulance. It is up to you to operate the vehicle in a safe fashion and never make any judgments or maneuvers based on an emotional response. Emotional maturity and stability are closely related to the ability to operate under stress.

Having the proper attitude is very important for the driver of an ambulance. Never get behind the wheel of an emergency vehicle thinking you can drive in any manner that pleases you simply because lights and siren are on. The ambulance is

### Words of Wisdom

Ambulance crashes that kill EMTs, patients, or occupants of other vehicles are common (annual average of 29 fatal accidents for the past 20 years). Many of them could have been prevented by the driver of the ambulance. Thoroughly attending to your own driving skills, driving according to established standards, and addressing any obvious lack of skills in your partner's driving all are crucial to your safety on the job.

likely much larger than your personal vehicle, and it will handle much differently, even under the best driving conditions. You must operate the vehicle with due regard for the safety of others and preservation of property. A greater responsibility is placed on the driver of an ambulance, and generally a lower burden of proof is needed to find that an EMT has caused a crash. As a rule, whenever lights and siren are used on an emergency call and there is a crash, the actions of the emergency vehicle operator fall under the most scrutiny.

## Safe Driving Practices

The first rule of safe driving in an emergency vehicle is that speed does not save lives; good care does. The second rule is that the driver and all passengers must wear seat belts and shoulder restraints at all times. These are the most important safety equipment items on every ambulance. You should wear restraints en route to the scene and whenever you are not performing direct patient care. Manufacturers are developing new ways to secure crew members in the patient compartment, enabling direct patient care while restrained in a harness. Patients should also be properly restrained. Studies show that fewer than one-half of all EMTs wear seat belts while the vehicle is in emergency mode, and few wear lap belts in the rear compartment while patient care is being rendered. If you must remove your seat belt to care for the patient, fasten the belt again as soon as possible. Also, unrestrained or improperly restrained patients and medical equipment (especially defibrillators and portable oxygen tanks) may become airborne during a crash and place you and your patient at an additional risk. All equipment and cabinets must be secured, as well as the patient and any passengers accompanying the patient.

Learn how your vehicle accelerates, corners, sways, and stops. Understand exactly how each particular vehicle will respond to steering, braking, and accelerating under various conditions.

Getting a feel for the proper brake pressure comes with experience and practice. Each vehicle has a different braking action. For example, the brakes on types I and III vehicles have a heavier feel than the brakes on a type II vehicle. The braking system on a diesel-powered unit will be different from the braking system on an identically equipped gasoline-powered unit. Certain heavy vehicles use air brakes, which have yet another feel. Get to know each vehicle you drive. It is important to understand the braking characteristics under various conditions.

When driving an ambulance during an emergency response on a multilane highway, you should usually stay in the extreme left-hand (fast) lane. This allows other motorists to move over to the right when they see or hear the ambulance approach.

**TABLE 38-6** lists further guidelines to follow when en route to a call.

## Siren Risk-Benefit Analysis

Whether responding to a call or transporting a patient from the scene to the hospital, the decision to activate the emergency lights and siren will depend on several factors, such as local protocols, patient condition, and the anticipated clinical outcome of the patient. In the past, other factors that encouraged the use of lights and siren included attempts to meet national standards regarding response times and public perception that all emergency vehicles should use lights and siren. Most systems incorporate recommendations for response modes based on the information received from dispatch. A patient who has fallen and needs assistance getting back into bed would merit a nonemergent response, and a patient who has collapsed in a mall and is receiving CPR from bystanders would merit a lights and siren response. Regardless of your jurisdictional requirements, as the driver of the ambulance, you need to evaluate the risk versus benefit of your response mode. Numerous studies have been conducted to determine whether the use of emergency lights and siren saves time getting to the patient or getting the patient from the scene to the hospital. The findings of these studies show that the time that you do save is minimal. Of the time-sensitive patients, including those suffering from trauma, heart attack, or stroke, who are generally transported with lights and siren, there is ongoing debate as to whether the time saved from using lights and siren during transport actually contributes to a decrease in overall morbidity and mortality. Many other factors that are out of the EMT's control also affect patient outcomes. We have to remember that our role is but one link in the chain of survival. Our goal should always be to

## YOU are the Provider

The hospital you are transporting to is 12 miles away. The patient's vital signs are normal and she states her pain is a 5 on a scale of 1 to 10. After traveling approximately 5 miles, you realize the ambulance is slowing down. Your partner tells you he has just heard on the radio that there is a motor vehicle crash a couple of miles ahead, and traffic is at a standstill. He says he can turn on the lights and siren and try to get through.

| Recording Time: 12 Minutes | |
| --- | --- |
| Level of consciousness | Alert and oriented |
| Respirations | 18 breaths/min; adequate depth |
| Pulse | 98 beats/min; strong and regular |
| Skin | Pink, warm, and dry |
| Blood pressure | 136/88 mm Hg |
| Spo₂ | 100% (on room air) |

**6.** What should you consider when deciding whether it is appropriate to turn on the lights and siren to maneuver through traffic?

**7.** If you are in an unfamiliar area and do not know an alternate route, what are your options?

**TABLE 38-6** Guidelines for Safe Ambulance Driving

1. Select the shortest and least congested route to the scene at the time of the dispatch.
2. Avoid routes with heavy traffic congestion; know alternate routes to each hospital during rush hours.
3. Avoid one-way streets; they may become clogged. Do not go against the flow of traffic on a one-way street, unless absolutely necessary.
4. Watch carefully for bystanders as you approach the scene. Curious bystanders may be focused on the scene and not aware of approaching vehicles.
5. Park the ambulance in a safe place once you arrive at the scene. If you park facing into traffic, turn off your headlights so they do not blind oncoming motorists unless they are needed to illuminate the scene. If the vehicle is blocking part of the road, keep your warning lights on to alert oncoming motorists.
6. Drive within the speed limit while transporting patients, except in the rare extreme emergency.
7. Go with the flow of the traffic.
8. Always drive defensively.
9. Always maintain a safe following distance. Use the 4-second rule: stay at least 4 seconds behind another vehicle in the same lane.
10. Maintain an open space or cushion in the lane next to you as an escape route in case the vehicle in front of you stops suddenly.
11. Use your siren if you turn on the emergency lights.
12. Always assume other drivers will not hear the siren or see your emergency lights.
13. Always exercise due regard for person and property.

© Jones & Bartlett Learning.

do no harm and to safely deliver the patient to the appropriate facility.

As an EMT, you should also consider the patient's condition before activating emergency lights and siren. Emergency lighting and siren noise may increase the patient's anxiety level. If you are transporting a patient having a heart attack who is already anxious, the use of lights and siren could lead to more anxiety and an increase in heart rate, blood pressure, and oxygen demand. In such cases, it may be better to transport your patient without lights and siren activated to minimize external stimuli and to prevent worsening your patient's condition.

## Driver Anticipation

Never assume other drivers see you or will respond predictably when they encounter an emergency vehicle. People's responses can vary widely when they see an emergency vehicle approaching. Learn to expect the unexpected. Motorists may indeed pull over to the right and stop or drive as close to the curb as possible, but you cannot take this behavior for granted. Operate the ambulance in a manner that allows you adequate time and space to safely maneuver around vehicles that may have suddenly stopped or pulled over in the wrong direction. Aggressive ambulance driving is never appropriate. You may not allow enough time for motorists to respond to your vehicle, or they may become nervous and not react in a rational manner. You can also look at the direction of the other vehicle's front tires to get an early indication of which way the vehicle will turn.

The acoustic glass and increased insulation in many modern vehicles provide a quieter environment for motorists but decrease their ability to hear noises from outside of the vehicle, such as emergency sirens or instructions called out over the ambulance's public address (PA) system. The PA system may worsen the situation because motorists may hesitate or make unexpected moves while attempting to hear or follow instructions. Moreover, when the driver of the ambulance is shouting to motorists and pedestrians over the PA system, he or she is now distracted from the business of driving and forced to handle the microphone when both hands should be on the steering wheel. You should avoid using the ambulance's PA system during emergency driving.

Most important, you must always drive defensively. Never rely on what another motorist will do unless you get a clear visual signal. Even then, you must be prepared to take defensive action in the case of a misunderstanding, panic, or careless driving on the part of the other driver.

## The Cushion of Safety

To safely operate an emergency vehicle, you must maintain a safe distance between your vehicle and any vehicles around you, referred to as a cushion of safety. The primary considerations in ensuring this cushion are keeping a safe distance between your vehicle and the one in front of you, checking for tailgaters behind the ambulance, and remaining aware of vehicles potentially hiding in the mirrors' blind spots.

To ensure you have enough reaction time and stopping distance from the vehicle in front of you, follow at a safe distance, which can be defined as driving about 4 or 5 seconds behind a vehicle traveling at an average speed. This distance allows the motorist enough time to move over to the right. If the motorist does not move, you will need to allow for enough time to avoid the vehicle.

While operating in emergency mode, tailgaters may follow your vehicle dangerously close in congested areas simply to use your ambulance to get through traffic. Doing so poses a threat to the crew and patient. If the ambulance has to slow down or stop suddenly to avoid a crash, the tailgating vehicle could collide with the rear of the ambulance, possibly causing you to lose control and strike other vehicles or pedestrians. Always scan the mirrors for vehicles following too closely. Instruct your partner to stay alert for such vehicles while he or she is in the rear compartment rendering care and to inform you about any tailgaters.

If you are being tailgated, never speed up to create more distance. The tailgater may, in turn, increase his or her speed to continue to follow you through traffic. Your increased speed will be counterproductive as it will increase the distance needed to avoid a crash, thereby decreasing your cushion of safety and reaction time. Slamming on your brakes to scare the other driver usually does not work either and may also cause a crash. The best method for distancing yourself from the vehicle is to slow down. Generally, tailgaters are impatient and will speed up to pass you. You can also have your dispatcher contact the local police to let them know that someone is driving recklessly behind you.

Never, under any circumstance, get out of the ambulance to confront a driver. This will only delay your response or transport of the patient and can lead to a dangerous situation. It is also unprofessional for you to become involved in a verbal argument with any member of the public and may lead to disciplinary actions or termination, depending on your service's conduct regulations.

Finally, to avoid blind spots, adjust your vehicle's side mirrors to help see vehicles or pedestrians on either side of the ambulance. Even with well-positioned mirrors, however, there are three blind spots around the ambulance that you cannot see with side or rearview mirrors:

- The rearview mirror creates a blind spot, obstructing the view ahead and preventing the driver from seeing objects such as a pedestrian or vehicle. Many new ambulance drivers will not be used to the larger mirrors on ambulances, which create a special hazard of which the driver should be aware. If your ambulance has a GPS, MDT, or dash camera mounted near the dashboard, this may also contribute to a blind spot. To eliminate this blind spot, you should lean forward in your seat, so the equipment does not obstruct the view, especially when making turns at intersections.
- The rear of the vehicle cannot be seen fully through the mirror and is therefore a blind spot. Because of the configuration of today's ambulances and the relative height of the vehicle, the rearview mirror generally gives the driver only a view of the patient compartment. It is not intended to be used for alerting the driver of a vehicle behind the ambulance. Because of this blind spot, many crashes occur when the ambulance driver is backing up. It is highly recommended, and required in many jurisdictions, that a spotter be used to help when backing up the vehicle. Rear-facing cameras are also helpful and much more common; however, these cameras may still have a limited view and be unable to provide an adequate view of the corners of the back of the ambulance. For this reason, rear-facing cameras do not replace the use of a spotter if one is available.
- The side of the vehicle often cannot be seen through the side view mirrors at a certain angle. Even when mirrors are adjusted properly, there will be spots around the sides of the vehicle that you cannot see. Entire vehicles may not be seen in the mirror, even though they are right next to the ambulance. To eliminate this problem, many EMS systems have smaller convex spot mirrors in addition to the

side mirrors to help you see this blind spot. However, if these mirrors are not available, you need to lean forward or backward in the seat to help eliminate the blind spot. This is an especially important technique to use when shifting lanes or making turns. When making a turn from an appropriate lane or across multiple lanes, be aware that other motorists, bicyclists, or pedestrians may have traveled alongside the ambulance as you are beginning your turn.

Scan your mirrors frequently for any new hazards and maintain your cushion of safety. Keep in mind that the mirrors can provide a misleading view and may block people or vehicles. Properly adjust the mirrors before operating the vehicle, and adjust your position in the driver's seat to avoid blind spots. Always use a spotter whom you can see from the driver's side mirror and agreed-on hand signals when backing up the ambulance.

## The Problem of Excessive Speed

Even in extreme life-and-death emergencies, excessive speed is not indicated. In most cases, if you properly assess and render appropriate treatments at the scene, speeding during transport is unnecessary, undesirable, and unsafe. No matter what the situation, you should never travel at a speed that is unsafe for the given road conditions. In almost every situation, slower means safer.

Excessive speeds do not increase a patient's chance of survival. More often, using excessive speed while driving to and from the scene has resulted in crashes in which the EMT, the patient, and occupants of other vehicles have been killed. It also makes it very difficult for the EMT attending to the patient to be able to provide any level of care because of the rough ride typically created by the excessive speed and maneuvering. Excessive speed also cuts down on the driver's reaction time and increases the time and distance needed to stop the ambulance. Operating at or beyond the speed limit can be viewed as operating the vehicle recklessly and without due regard. Although many state laws allow emergency vehicles to travel beyond the posted speed limits in emergencies, they offer little or no protection against prosecution should the driver become involved in a motor vehicle crash. The legal ramifications of driving

an emergency vehicle will be covered later in this section.

## Recognition of Siren Syndrome

The siren may have a physiologic and a psychological effect on EMS providers as well as on other drivers. Driving emergently in an ambulance with the lights and siren activated, at least in the early phases of your career, will likely cause you to experience a rush of adrenaline. Your respiratory rate and heart rate will increase, and your palms may become sweaty. This physiologic response is natural, but it may limit your focus and also interfere with your ability to judge distance or the potential actions of others. Understanding your body's response to driving with lights and siren can help you to mitigate the associated risks. Take a deep breath and proceed with caution, remembering the guidelines for safe ambulance operation.

The siren may also increase the anxiety of other drivers or other drivers' tendencies to drive faster in the presence of sirens. Although a siren signifies a request for drivers to yield the right-of-way, drivers do not always do so. One of the biggest mistakes you can make as an EMT is to assume motorists will hear the siren and take proper action.

## Vehicle Size and Distance Judgment

Vehicle length and width are critical factors when maneuvering, driving, and parking an emergency vehicle. They are especially important with types I and III vehicles, which are wider than they look from behind the steering wheel. To brake and pass effectively, you must know the width and length of your vehicle. Preventable accidents often occur when the driver is backing up the vehicle. Use someone outside the ambulance as a spotter when you are backing up to avoid any incidents. Vehicle size and weight greatly influence acceleration, braking, and stopping distances. Good peripheral vision and depth perception will help you judge distances, but they are no substitute for intensive training, experience, and frequent evaluation of the vehicle.

## Road Positioning and Cornering

Road position means the position of the vehicle on the roadway relative to the inside or outside edge of the paved surface. To corner efficiently, you must

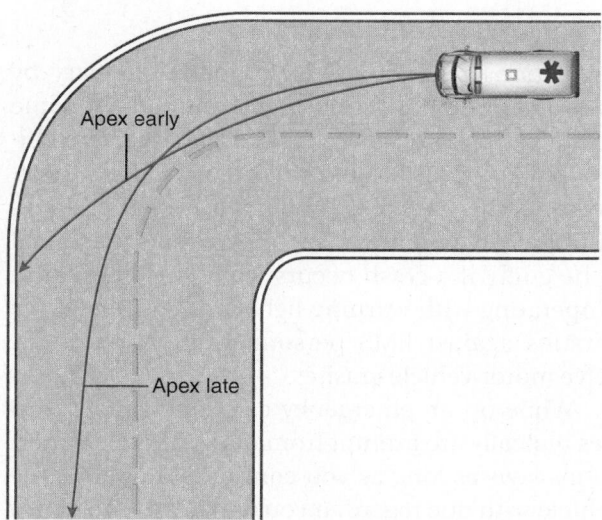

**FIGURE 38-27** To keep the ambulance in the proper lane on a curve, you must know the vehicle's current position and projected path and take the corner at the correct speed.

© Jones & Bartlett Learning.

know the vehicle's current position and its projected path. The aim is to take the corner at the speed that will put you in the proper road position as you exit the curve (**FIGURE 38-27**). When driving an ambulance, focus on safely maneuvering through a corner as opposed to taking the fastest route. The safest path is to enter high in the lane (to the outside) and exit low (to the inside). This allows room for error if you enter the turn too fast.

## Weather and Road Conditions

Certain conditions can limit your ability to control the vehicle and can contribute to a crash. Ambulances do not handle the same as small motor vehicles. Ambulances are heavier than most vehicles and will have a longer braking time and stopping distance. In addition, the weight of the ambulance is unevenly distributed, which makes it more susceptible to rolling over. These factors, in addition to bad environmental conditions, greatly increase the chance that a crash may occur. Therefore, you should remain alert to changing weather, road, and driving conditions (**FIGURE 38-28**). Whether traveling to or from an emergency, you must modify your speed according to road conditions. Take warnings of ice or hazardous conditions seriously, and be prepared to take an alternate route, if necessary. If you run into unexpected traffic congestion or deteriorating travel conditions, notify the dispatcher

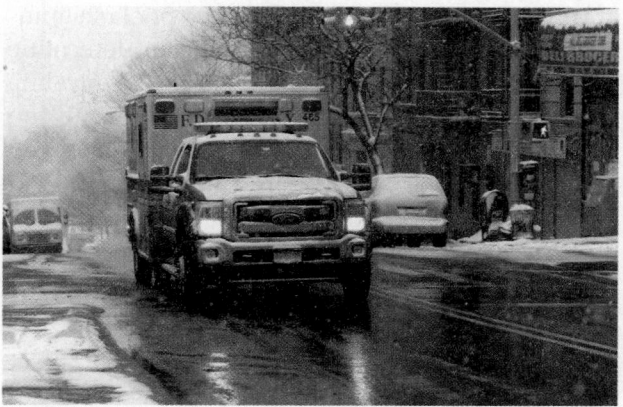

**FIGURE 38-28** Modify your speed according to changing weather, road, and driving conditions.

© eddtoro/Shutterstock.

so other emergency vehicles can select alternate routes. In the event of a major disaster or severe weather events, all public safety and emergency services should be coordinated.

Even the most careful drivers will occasionally run into unexpected situations that may require special driving skills. However, if you drive at a speed that is appropriate for the weather and road conditions and maintain an adequate cushion of safety, you will minimize the occurrence of crashing during these situations. You should decrease your speed in bad weather conditions such as fog, rain, snow, or ice. The following are examples of conditions that require the emergency vehicle operator to decrease speed, increase following distance, and be alert.

### Hydroplaning

On a wet road surface, tires are designed to move the water out of the way and stay in direct contact with the road. However, at speeds in excess of 30 mph, tires may be lifted off the road as water accumulates underneath; the vehicle may then feel as if it is floating. This problem is known as **hydroplaning**. At higher speeds on wet roadways, the front wheels may be riding on a sheet of water, robbing the driver of directional control of the vehicle. If hydroplaning occurs, you should gradually slow down without jamming on the brakes.

### Water on the Roadway

Wet brakes will not slow the vehicle as efficiently as dry brakes, and the vehicle may pull to one side or the other. If you encounter a large pool of standing water, you will likely be unable to determine how deep the water is. You should avoid traveling through standing water if at all possible. If you must drive through standing water, slow down and turn on the windshield wipers. After driving out of the water, lightly tap the brakes several times until they are dry. If the vehicle is equipped with anti-lock brakes, apply a steady, light pressure to dry the brakes. Driving through moving water should be avoided at all times.

### Decreased Visibility

In areas where there is fog, smog, snow, or heavy rain, slow down to a safe operating speed. Be cautious with activating your emergency lights, as they may be disorienting to you or other motorists. At night, use only low headlight beams for maximum visibility without reflection. You should always use headlights during the day to increase your visibility to other drivers. Also, watch carefully for stopped or slow-moving vehicles.

### Ice and Slippery Surfaces

A light mist on an oily, dusty road can be just as slippery as a patch of ice. Good all-weather tires and an appropriate speed will significantly reduce traction problems. If you are in an area that often has snowy or icy conditions, consider using studded snow tires or tire chains, if they are permitted by law. You should be especially careful on bridges and overpasses when temperatures are close to freezing. These road surfaces will freeze much faster than surrounding road surfaces because they lack the warming effect of the ground underneath.

Although preventing skids and sliding is ideal, you are likely to skid or slide occasionally, especially if you live in climates with ice and snow. Your training should include the technique for correcting slides during turns. If you are likely to drive on ice and snow, practice control maneuvers until they become automatic—at low speeds in an area where there is no danger of crashes. Remember that four-wheel-drive and front-wheel-drive vehicles behave differently than rear-wheel-drive vehicles when sliding. It is also important to remember that although four-wheel-drive vehicles have better traction for acceleration in slippery conditions, they do not stop any faster than two-wheel-drive vehicles.

## Laws and Regulations

Regulations regarding vehicle operations vary by state and by city, but some regulations are the same regardless of location. Drivers of emergency vehicles have certain limited privileges in every state. However, these privileges do not lessen their liability in a crash. In many cases, the driver is presumed to be guilty if a crash occurs while the ambulance is operating with warning lights and a siren. Many lawsuits against EMS personnel and services involve motor vehicle crashes.

While on an emergency call, emergency vehicles typically are exempt from normal vehicle operations laws as long as you continue to operate the vehicle with due regard. If you are on an emergency call and you are using your warning lights and siren, you may be allowed to do the following:

- Park or stand in an otherwise illegal location
- Proceed through a red traffic light or stop sign, but never without stopping first
- Drive above the posted speed limit
- Drive against the flow of traffic on a one-way street or make a turn that is normally illegal
- Travel left of center to make an otherwise illegal pass

Remember that these exemptions vary by state and local jurisdiction. Therefore, you should check your local statutes or regulations in your area.

An emergency vehicle is *never* allowed to pass a school bus that has stopped to load or unload children and is displaying its flashing red lights or extended stop arm. If you approach a school bus that has its lights flashing, you should stop before reaching the bus and turn off your siren. Next, you should wait for the bus driver to make sure the children are safe, close the bus door, and turn off the flashing lights. Only then may you carefully proceed past the stopped school bus.

### Use of Warning Lights and Siren

Three basic principles govern the use of warning lights and siren on an ambulance:

1. The unit, to the best of your knowledge, must be responding to a true emergency call as defined by local protocol.
2. Audible and visual warning devices must be used simultaneously.
3. The unit must be operated with due regard for the safety of all others, on and off the roadway.

EMS systems should evaluate their overall response plan with a goal of minimizing the use of lights and siren. As discussed earlier, there is a significant risk to EMTs, their partners, patients, and the general public when an ambulance is operating with lights and siren. This decision is complicated and multifaceted. Each scenario should be evaluated independently to gauge whether the use of lights and siren is necessary. Some EMS systems already incorporate algorithms into their dispatching practices with guidelines or protocols for response mode based on information obtained in the 9-1-1 call. Most systems allow the crew to upgrade or downgrade their response based on their assessment of the current situation, including dispatch information, weather, traffic, and distance to be traveled. When transporting a patient, a general guideline is that lights and siren should be used only when the highest-trained provider caring for the patient believes there to be a true benefit to the patient based on possible time saved by a shorter transport time and the patient's clinical condition. Be sure to understand your own agency's protocols with regard to use of lights and siren for transport of patients to the hospital.

As mentioned previously, thanks to advances in automotive design, including soundproofing, motorists who drive at the speed limit with the windows up and the radio on may not hear the siren until the ambulance is very close. If the radio is loud, they may not hear the siren at all. Effective siren distances are much shorter than you might think. Keep in mind that as you increase the speed of your ambulance, you decrease the amount of time and space that people in vehicles in front of you have to hear your siren and react appropriately. Some ambulances are equipped with a specialized siren (eg, the Rumbler) that emits low-frequency siren sound waves that produce a vibration and may penetrate vehicles better than traditional sirens, allowing motorists to feel the siren.

If you do have to turn on the siren, tell the patient before you do so to prevent unnecessary anxiety. Be especially mindful not to increase the speed of the ambulance just because the siren is in use. Always travel at a speed that allows you to stop safely; this will enable you to be prepared for drivers who do not yield the right of way. Never assume that warning lights and siren will allow you to drive through a congested area without stopping or slowing down.

Slow down to ensure all drivers are stopping as you approach an intersection and proceed with caution. Remember, the siren is a request that other drivers give you the right of way—it does not magically clear traffic. If you encounter a red traffic light or stop sign, come to a complete stop before proceeding through the intersection. In these high-risk situations, use all tools at your disposal to ensure nearby traffic is aware of your presence and that the danger is decreased to the greatest degree possible.

### Right-of-Way Privileges

State motor vehicle statutes or codes often grant an emergency vehicle such as an ambulance the right to disregard the rules of the road when responding to an emergency. However, the operator of an emergency vehicle must still continue to operate in a safe fashion so as not to endanger people or property under any circumstances.

Consider this case: An ambulance is approaching an intersection that is controlled by a four-way stop sign. The ambulance, with lights and siren turned on, proceeds through the intersection without slowing or stopping and crashes into a vehicle coming from its right. Did the operator of the ambulance act appropriately by going through the intersection in this manner?

Right-of-way privileges for ambulances vary by state. Some states allow you to proceed through a red light or stop sign after you stop and make sure it is safe to go on. Other states allow you to proceed through a controlled intersection with due regard, using flashing lights and siren. This means you may proceed only if you consider the safety of all people who are using the highway. If you fail to use due regard, your service may be sued. If you are found to be at fault, you may personally have to pay punitive damages or face civil and criminal sanctions.

Get to know your local right-of-way privileges. Exercise them only when it is absolutely necessary for the patient's well-being. The use of lights and audible warning devices is a matter of state and local practice and protocol.

### Use of Escorts

Using a police escort is an extremely dangerous practice. When other motorists hear a siren and see a police vehicle passing, they might assume the police vehicle is the only emergency vehicle and not see the ambulance. The only time an escort is justified is when you are in an unfamiliar area and truly need a guide more than an escort. In such cases, vehicles using warning lights or siren should use different tones to alert other motorists and be prepared to stop if needed. If you are being guided, follow at a safe distance. Assume nearby traffic will not be aware of your presence.

### Intersection Hazards

Intersection crashes are the most common and usually the most serious type of crash in which ambulances are involved. Always be alert and careful when approaching an intersection. Change the siren tone before you reach the intersection. If you are on an urgent call and cannot wait for traffic lights to change, you should still come to a brief stop at the light; look around for other motorists and pedestrians before proceeding into the intersection. Scan the intersection and your mirrors for hazards and clear each lane before you proceed. Direct your full attention to the road while proceeding through the intersection; this is not the time to talk on the radio or consult the automatic vehicle location system map.

Motorists who time the traffic lights present a serious hazard. You may arrive at an intersection while the light is green. At the same time, a motorist who is timing the lights on the cross street arrives at the intersection. The motorist has a red light but knows it is about to turn green and is expecting to go through. This creates the possibility for a serious crash to occur.

Another common intersection hazard occurs when multiple emergency vehicles are responding through the same intersection. Having convoys of emergency vehicles is not uncommon because multiple resources respond from a similar location. This is a dangerous practice. A motorist who has yielded the right of way to the first vehicle may proceed into the intersection without expecting a second vehicle. You should exercise extreme caution in these situations. To signal motorists that a second unit is approaching, use a siren tone that is different from that of the first vehicle.

You must also be aware that additional emergency vehicles responding to the same call or to a different emergency call may be coming through the same intersection from a different direction. Serious accidents could occur when two emergency vehicles enter the same intersection unless both of the drivers are operating with due regard, allowing them the time to recognize the other vehicle and safely proceed through the intersection.

### Highways

When you are responding to an emergency call and you must travel on the highway, you should turn off your emergency lights and siren until you have reached the far left lane. Turning off your emergency devices minimizes the possibility that other drivers will get confused and not know what to do or where to go.

When driving on a highway with your emergency devices activated, you should always travel in the far left-hand lane, also known as the "passing lane." This allows the ambulance to safely pass vehicles, while still leaving a safety corridor on the left side of the ambulance in case of emergency or unexpected obstacles.

When you exit the highway, you should follow the same procedures as when you entered the highway: turn off all emergency devices, move onto the off-ramp, and then turn on the emergency lights and siren if necessary.

### Unpaved Roadways

When you are required to drive the ambulance on an unpaved roadway, special care must be taken. Unpaved roadways often have uneven surfaces, as well as large potholes. While responding on this type of roadway, operate the vehicle at a lower speed and maintain a firm grip on the steering wheel to maintain complete control of the ambulance at all times. During the transport phase, these practices will help to provide a smoother ride for the EMT and patient on the stretcher.

### School Zones

When you respond through a school zone with your emergency lights turned on, it is important to remember that the lights and siren tend to attract children to the roadway and create a potential hazard. In many states, it is unlawful for an emergency vehicle to exceed the speed limit in school zones, regardless of the condition of the patient.

## Distractions

As technology progresses, so will the distractions you will face while operating the ambulance.

Although MDTs and GPS devices are necessary to assist EMTs in determining the location of the call, these devices, along with using the vehicle's mounted mobile radio, listening to the stereo, talking on your cell phone, and eating or drinking, create additional driving hazards. While the ambulance is in motion, you should focus solely on driving and anticipate roadway hazards. Your partner should operate the MDT, GPS device, and portable radios or turn on the siren. Minimizing distractions allows for a safer response and minimizes the potential for mishaps.

### Driving Alone

Although driving alone is not a standard practice or even allowable in certain systems, there may be an occasion when you need to respond to a scene by yourself in the ambulance and meet your partner at the scene. When presented with this situation, you have additional duties and responsibilities, such as figuring out the safest route to the call, operating the radios and emergency warning devices, and mentally preparing for the call. Situations such as these demand your complete attention and focus.

### Fatigue

Fatigue has many causes, such as stress, working the night shift, and lack of quality sleep in accordance with your body's circadian rhythms. Operating an emergency vehicle while feeling the effects of fatigue creates a dangerous risk to yourself and others. You must be able to recognize when you are fatigued. Do not be ashamed to admit it to yourself, your partner, or your supervisor. If you feel fatigued, you should be placed out of service for the remainder of the shift or until the fatigue has passed and you feel capable of safely operating the vehicle.

## Air Medical Operations

**Air ambulances** are used to evacuate medical and trauma patients. They are capable of landing at or near the scene to provide rapid transport of patients to an appropriate hospital, including trauma centers, stroke centers, or cardiac centers. There are two basic types of air medical units: fixed-wing and rotary-wing, otherwise known as helicopters (**FIGURE 38-29**). Fixed-wing aircraft generally are used for interhospital patient transfers over

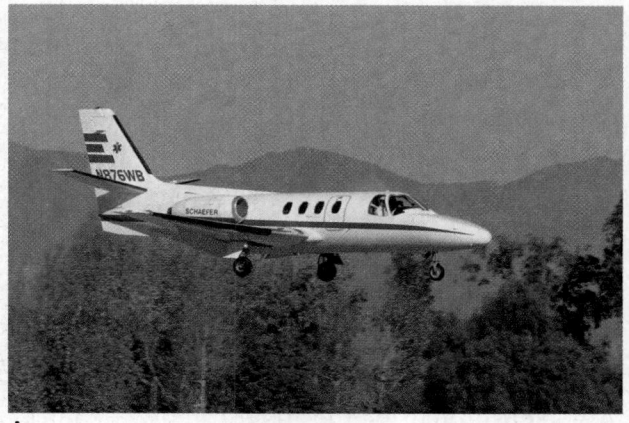

A

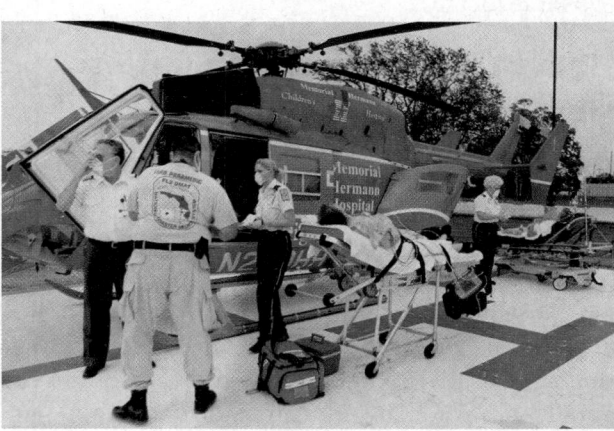

B

**FIGURE 38-29 A.** Fixed-wing aircraft are generally used to transfer patients from one hospital to another over distances greater than 200 to 250 miles. **B.** A rotary-wing aircraft, or helicopter, is used to help provide emergency medical care to patients who need to be transported quickly over shorter distances.

distances greater than 200 to 250 miles. For shorter distances, rotary-wing aircraft are more efficient.

Specifically trained medical flight crews accompany all air ambulance flights. Your role in fixed-wing aircraft transfers probably will be limited to providing ground transport for the patient and medical flight crew between the hospital and the airport.

Rotary-wing aircraft have become an important tool in providing emergency medical care. In most cases, they are capable of bringing a higher level of care or specialized supplies, such as blood products, to the patient. Trauma patient survival is directly related to the time that elapses between injury and definitive treatment. Most helicopters that are used for emergency medical operations fly well in excess of 100 mph in a straight line, without road or traffic hazards, straight to a hospital helipad. The crew may include flight paramedics, flight nurses, specialty providers such as respiratory therapists, perfusionists, or physicians.

Familiarize yourself with the capabilities, protocols, and methods for accessing helicopters in your area. Helicopter services provide training in ground operations and safety for EMS systems, fire services, and first responders. The following discussion is an introduction to safe operations and is not intended to be substituted for the more extensive courses available locally.

## Helicopter Medical Evacuation Operations

A medical evacuation is commonly known as a **medevac** and is generally performed exclusively by helicopters. Most rural and suburban EMS jurisdictions and many urban systems have the capability to perform helicopter medevacs or have a mutual aid agreement with another agency such as police or hospital-based medevac service to provide such service. Familiarize yourself with the medevac capabilities, protocols, and procedures of your particular EMS system because they vary by agency. The following are some general guidelines that you should be familiar with when considering whether to initiate a medevac operation.

### Calling for a Medevac

Every agency has specific criteria for the type of patient who may receive medical evacuation and how and when to call for a medevac. These basic guidelines will help you understand the process better.

- **Why call for a medevac?**
  - The transport time to the hospital by ground ambulance is too long considering the patient's condition. This benefit in transport time could be greater in mountainous areas or other difficult terrain.
  - The patient requires urgent initiation of specialized treatment that is not locally available. Road, traffic, or environmental conditions limit or completely prohibit the use of a ground ambulance.
  - The patient requires advanced care that you are unable to provide, such as inserting

advanced airways or placing a chest tube. There are multiple patients who will overwhelm local prehospital resources or the resources at the hospital reachable by ground transport. The helicopter may respond directly to the scene or it may be called to the hospital to transfer a patient to a facility with the capacity to provide definitive care for the patient's condition.

- **Who receives a medevac?**
  - Medical evacuations should be used for patients with time-dependent injuries or illnesses. Patients suspected of having a stroke, heart attack, or serious traumatic injuries may benefit from evacuation via helicopter.
  - Serious conditions that may require the use of helicopter medevacs may be found in remote areas and involve scuba diving accidents, near drownings, or skiing and wilderness accidents.
  - Other patients who may require medical evacuation are high-risk obstetric patients, candidates for limb replantation (for amputations), and patients requiring air transport to a burn center, a hyperbaric chamber center, or a venomous bite center. Because specific criteria vary by service, familiarize yourself with the criteria in your system used to call for this lifesaving service.

- **Whom do you call?**
  - Generally, your dispatcher must be notified first.
  - In some regions, after the medevac has been initiated, the ground EMS crew may be able to access the flight crew on a specifically designated radio frequency for one-on-one communications. If available, it is important to keep this frequency clear of chatter and lengthy communications. You may be asked to give a brief report including the patient's weight, clinical condition, and an update on the patient's condition. In this case, you should gather your thoughts and speak clearly and concisely, avoiding information that is not pertinent. Another important topic of communication between the ground and flight EMS crews will be where to land the helicopter. This will be covered in the next section.

## Establishing a Landing Zone

A benefit of helicopter medevac is that helicopters do not need an airport to land. An important part of conducting a medevac is choosing the best location to establish a landing zone. Establishing a landing zone is the responsibility of either the ground EMS crew or a local fire department. It involves more than simply looking for a clear space. You must be prepared to take action to ensure the flight crew is able to land and take off safely. Similar to an airplane, a helicopter's approach and departure involve the aircraft descending or climbing at a consistent rate at a slight angle. Keeping in mind that the helicopter is unlikely to fly straight down or straight up, you should consider the following when selecting and establishing a landing zone:

- Ensure the area is a hard or grassy level surface that measures 100 × 100 ft (30 × 30 m) (recommended) and no less than 60 × 60 ft (18 × 18 m) (**FIGURE 38-30**). If the site is not level, notify the flight crew of the steepness and direction of the slope. The slope should not exceed 5 to 7 degrees.

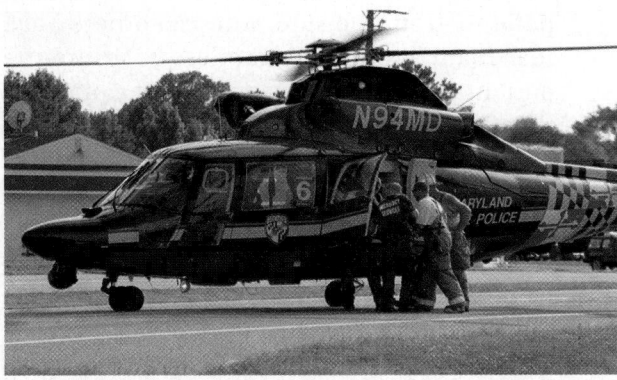

**FIGURE 38-30** A landing area for an EMS helicopter should be a level surface measuring 100 ft × 100 ft (30 m × 30 m).

© Mark C. Ide.

- Ensure the area is clear of any loose debris that could become airborne and strike the helicopter, the patient, bystanders, or the EMS crew. This includes branches, trash bins, flares, sheets, caution tape, and medical equipment.
- Examine the immediate area for any overhead or tall hazards such as power lines, telephone cables, antennas, and tall or leaning trees. If you see any of these hazards, immediately inform the flight crew because an alternative landing site may be required. It is imperative to communicate what you can see from the ground. At altitude, the flight crew may not be able to see hazards that you can see easily from the ground, especially at night. The flight crew may request that the hazard be marked or illuminated by weighted cones or that an emergency vehicle with its lights turned on be positioned next to or under the potential hazard.
- To mark the landing site, use weighted cones or position emergency vehicles at the corners of the landing zone with the headlights facing inward to form an "X." This procedure may be valuable during night landings as well. It is common for fire suppression personnel to help mark the landing site because they are often called to the scene to stand by. Never use caution tape or people to mark the site. Flares should not be used because they can become airborne, and they have the potential to start a fire or cause an explosion.
- Move all nonessential people and vehicles to a safe distance outside of the landing zone.
- Both the approach and departure will be performed into the wind. If the wind is strong, communicate the direction of the wind to the flight crew. They may request that you create some form of wind directional device to aid their approach.

## Landing Zone Safety and Patient Transfer

Helicopter safety is a combination of using good sense and maintaining a constant awareness of the need for personal safety. You should stay away from the helicopter and go only where the pilot or flight crew member directs you. The most important rule is to keep a safe distance from the aircraft whenever it is on the ground and hot, which means when the helicopter blades are spinning. The engines will usually stay on and the rotor blades remain spinning because the flight crew does not generally expect to remain on the ground for a long time. This means all EMTs should stay outside the landing zone perimeter unless directed to come to the aircraft by the pilot or a member of the flight crew. Usually, the flight crew will come to the EMTs; they will carry their own equipment and do not require any assistance inside the landing zone. If you are asked to enter the landing zone, stay away from the rear of the aircraft, where the tail rotor is located; the tips of its blades move so rapidly that they are essentially invisible. Remove any loose items from yourself or the stretcher, including baseball hats, sheets, or loose medical supplies. Always approach a helicopter from the front, even if it is not running, and you should approach only after the pilot or a flight crew member signals it is clear to do so. If you imagine the front of the helicopter as the number 12 on a clock, then you should enter only the area between the 10 o'clock and 2 o'clock positions. If you must move from one side of the helicopter to another, go around the front. Never duck under the body, the tail boom, or the rear section of the helicopter. The pilot cannot see you in these areas.

Another area of concern is the height of the main rotor blade. On many aircraft, it is flexible and may dip as low as 4 ft (1.2 m) off the ground (**FIGURE 38-31**). When you approach the aircraft, walk in a crouched position. Wind gusts can alter the blade height without warning, so protect yourself and your equipment as you carry it under the blades.

When accompanying a flight crew member, you must follow directions exactly. Never open any aircraft door or move equipment unless instructed by a crew member. When told to approach the aircraft, use extreme caution and pay constant attention to hazards.

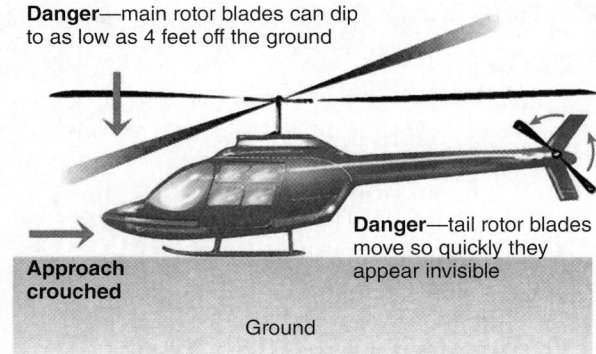

**FIGURE 38-31** The main rotor blade of the helicopter is flexible and may dip as low as 4 feet (1.2 m) off the ground depending on the type of helicopter.

© Jones & Bartlett Learning.

Keep the following guidelines in mind when operating at a landing zone:

- Familiarize yourself with helicopter hand signals used within your jurisdiction (**FIGURE 38-32**).
- Do not approach the helicopter unless instructed and accompanied by flight crew.
- Ensure all patient care equipment is properly secured to the stretcher and that the patient is fastened as well. This includes oxygen tanks, cervical collars, and head stabilizers. Any loose articles or belongings such as hats, coats, or bags that belong to the patient or crew should not be brought into the landing zone and will likely need to be transported to the hospital by ground.
- Be aware that some helicopters may load patients from the side, whereas others have rear-loading doors. Regardless of where the patient is being loaded, always approach the aircraft from the front unless otherwise instructed by the flight crew. It is very important that the pilot be able to see anyone who comes near the aircraft. Always take the same path when exiting and moving away from the helicopter, and move the patient headfirst.
- Smoking, open flames, and flares are prohibited within 50 ft (15 m) of the aircraft at all times.
- Wear eye protection during approach and takeoff.

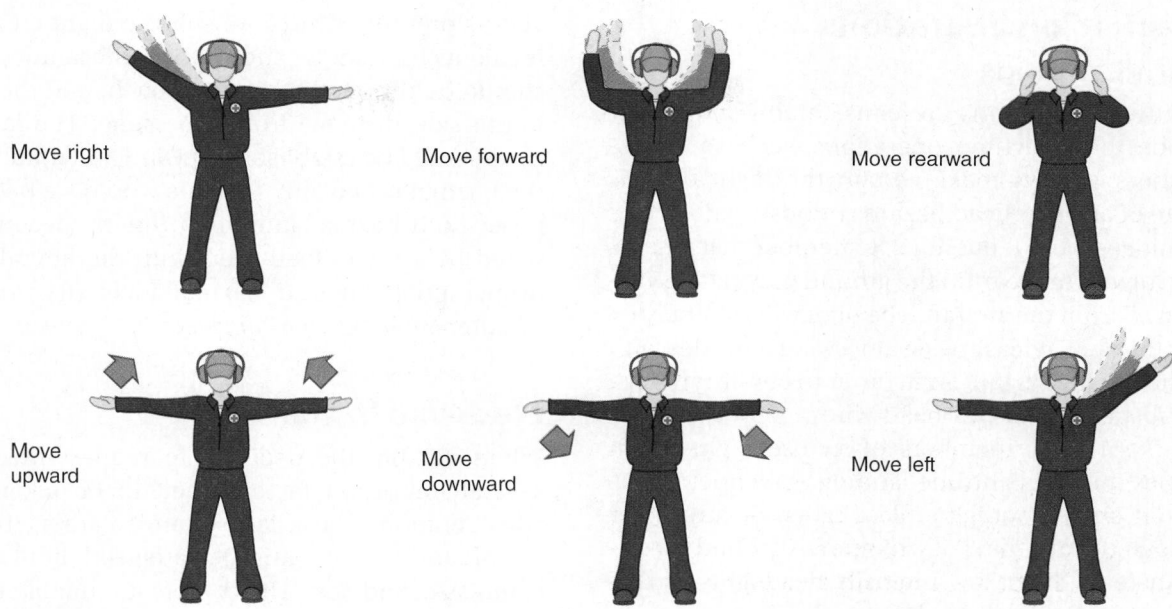

Move right

Move forward

Move rearward

Move upward

Move downward

Move left

**FIGURE 38-32** Some examples of helicopter hand signals. Be familiar with those used within your jurisdiction.

© Jones & Bartlett Learning.

## Communication Issues

When interacting with other agencies, there is always the possibility of communication issues. Medevacs are no exception. Although the typical EMS system has a specific and well-defined jurisdiction, medevacs respond to service requests throughout a large, multijurisdictional area. Because of this large area with numerous jurisdictions, the medevac interacts with many services on a multitude of different radio frequencies.

To prevent miscommunication, when the request is made for a medevac response, the request should include a ground contact radio channel (typically a preestablished mutual aid channel), as well as a call sign of the unit with which the medevac should make contact.

## YOU are the Provider

After turning around and determining a new route, your partner advises you there is now a 25-minute transport time. Your partner also warns that you are approaching a stopped school bus with its stop sign out, and children are exiting the bus.

| Recording Time: 22 Minutes | |
| --- | --- |
| **Level of consciousness** | Alert and oriented |
| **Respirations** | 20 breaths/min; adequate depth |
| **Pulse** | 94 beats/min; strong and regular |
| **Skin** | Pink, warm, and dry |
| **Blood pressure** | 142/90 mm Hg |
| **Spo$_2$** | 97% (on room air) |

**8.** When traveling in the emergency mode, how do you respond to a stopped school bus?

**9.** Where do most serious ambulance crashes occur, and what should you do to help avoid a crash?

# Special Considerations

## Night Landings

Nighttime operations are considerably more hazardous than daytime operations because of the darkness. Always make certain the flight crew is aware of any overhead hazards or obstructions and illuminate these if possible. Remember that what is easy for you to see from the ground may not be visible at all from the aircraft. The pilot will generally fly over the area at least twice at varying altitudes with the helicopter's lights on in order to confirm potential obstacles and overhead wires. Medevac pilots and flight crew members often use night-vision goggles during nighttime landing zone operations. Do not shine spotlights, flashlights, or any other lights in the air; they may temporarily blind the pilot. Instead, direct low-intensity headlights or lanterns toward the ground at the landing site from opposite corners to form an "X" at the center of the landing zone.

## Landing on Uneven Ground

If the helicopter must land on a grade (uneven surface), extra caution is advised. The slope should not exceed 5 to 7 degrees. The main rotor blade will be closer to the ground on the uphill side. In this situation, approach the aircraft only from the downhill side or as directed by the flight crew (**FIGURE 38-33**). Do not move the patient to the helicopter until the crew has signaled that they are ready to receive you.

## Medevacs at Hazmat Incidents

Notify the flight crew immediately of the presence of hazmat at the scene. The aircraft generates tremendous wind and may easily spread any hazmat

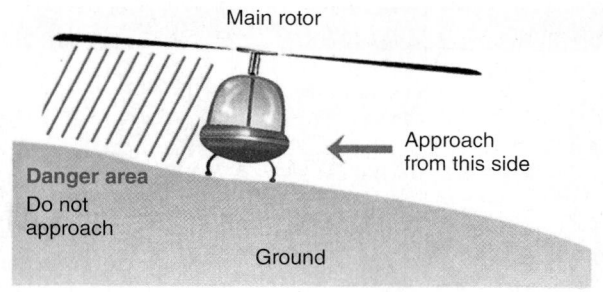

**FIGURE 38-33** Approach a helicopter on a grade only from the downhill side.

© Jones & Bartlett Learning.

vapors present. Always consult the flight crew and incident commander about where the landing zone should be set up, the best approach, and the minimum safe distance from the scene. The landing zone should be established upwind and uphill from the hazmat scene. Any patients who have been exposed to a hazmat must be properly decontaminated before you load them into the aircraft. For proper procedures at hazmat incidents, refer to Chapter 40, *Incident Management.*

# Medevac Issues

When making the decision to request medevac, several important factors need to be taken into consideration. These factors are weather, the environment/terrain, altitude, airspeed limitations, cabin size, and cost. Helicopters are unable to operate in severe weather conditions such as thunderstorms, blizzards, and heavy rain. The environment may pose a risk as well. In mountainous or desert terrain, there may be too many hazards in the immediate vicinity to safely land the helicopter in the desired location.

As elevation increases, the air thins, which makes it more difficult for pilots and patients to breathe. Because of this danger, helicopters have a maximum limit on flight elevations. Most helicopter services are limited to flying at 10,000 feet above sea level. This could create a problem if your patient is located at 13,500 feet above sea level. Remember that medevac helicopters are not jets, so it takes time for them to arrive on the scene, because of limitations in airspeed. Typically, medevac helicopters fly between 130 and 150 mph.

Because of the helicopter cabin's confined space, helicopters are limited in the number of patients who can be safely transported and by the size of the patient whom they can safely transport. Although a helicopter may be able to safely lift off with a 500-lb (227-kg) patient, because of his or her size and girth, it may be impossible to safely fit and secure the patient into the cabin area.

Typical medevac flights are extremely expensive compared to local ambulance transports. However, they can provide a truly lifesaving service if utilized correctly. The decision to request a medevac should not be based on the perceived ability of the patient to pay the bill, but rather on the medical necessity.

# YOU are the Provider SUMMARY

**1. What attributes should an emergency vehicle operator possess?**

The EMT who is serving as an emergency vehicle operator should possess good situational awareness, be able to make reasonable decisions, and maintain a calm demeanor in stressful situations. Operating an emergency vehicle requires the driver's undivided attention and constant awareness of possible dangers. From deteriorating weather conditions to inattentive drivers on the roadway, many threats may be encountered while responding to an emergency. The driver will have to account for all of these factors while ensuring safe operation of the vehicle. Emergency vehicle operator courses are often required before personnel are cleared to operate an emergency vehicle. These courses are beneficial in teaching best practices specific to ambulance operation, including maintaining a safe distance from other vehicles, passing through an intersection, and driving with lights and siren activated. You must always operate the vehicle in a safe fashion. Remember, you will be unable to help anyone if you do not reach the scene or the hospital safely.

**2. What factors should you consider before responding to the scene?**

Before you begin your response, you need to consider several factors to ensure a safe, quick response. First, you must identify the location of the scene and the route you intend to take. Notify your dispatch center that you are responding. Given that the nature of the call involves the potential for violence (assault), you should ask your dispatch center if the scene has been secured by law enforcement officers and is safe for you to enter. With the scene being close to your station, you want to take the time to make sure the scene is safe. You do not want to rush into the scene only to realize you are in imminent danger. Stage your ambulance in a safe location that is close to the scene, but far enough away from any danger, until law enforcement has secured the scene.

You must also consider the weather conditions and traffic when deciding how you will respond to the scene. When there are poor weather conditions or heavy traffic, you will need to be extra vigilant and cautious when responding. It may be most appropriate to respond without lights and siren due to the weather conditions and the need to wait for law enforcement to secure the scene. It may be appropriate to respond cautiously with lights and siren if the scene has already been secured by law enforcement and there is heavy traffic through which you will need to travel. You must make a reasonable decision after looking at the specific circumstances and factors involved in the call. Remember that safety should always remain at the forefront.

**3. Based on the MOI and patient presentation, what equipment do you anticipate needing?**

For this patient, you would need the jump kit, which should contain anything you might need within the first 5 minutes after making contact with any patient, including splinting and bandaging supplies. If she were unstable, splinting and bandaging would be delayed until you are en route and all other necessary assessments and treatments are completed.

**4. What assessment and treatment should be performed on scene and what should be delayed until you are in the ambulance and en route to the hospital?**

This patient is stable, with only an isolated injury to the left lower extremity. There was no loss of consciousness, and vital signs are within normal limits. Because this is not a priority load-and-go patient, you should complete your secondary assessment on scene and take the time to splint her leg.

Once you are en route to the hospital, repeat the primary assessment, including taking vital signs, and reassess the effectiveness of any interventions. Now would also be the time to manage any minor secondary injuries. Remember that stable patients should be reassessed every 15 minutes, and critical or unstable patients should be reassessed every 5 minutes.

**5. How would you determine whether to use lights and siren during transport of this patient?**

The transport mode (ie, lights and siren [emergency mode] versus no lights and siren [nonemergency mode]) is determined by the patient's current condition and his or her anticipated clinical outcome. In this case, the patient is stable; she is alert and oriented, her vital signs are stable, and she has no life-threatening conditions (ie, airway problems, uncontrolled bleeding). Therefore, the use of lights and siren during transport is not indicated.

**6. What should you consider when deciding whether it is appropriate to turn on the lights and siren to maneuver through traffic?**

Regulations regarding vehicle operations vary by state and by city, but some regulations are the same regardless of location. Emergency vehicle operators have certain limited privileges in every state. However, these privileges do not reduce your liability in the event of a crash.

## YOU are the Provider SUMMARY *continued*

Three basic principles govern the use of warning lights and siren on an ambulance:

1. The unit must be, to the best of your knowledge, on a true emergency call.
2. The use of lights and sirens must be authorized by your agency and medical director for the category and condition of the patient you are transporting.
3. Audible and visual warning devices must be used simultaneously.

The unit must be operated with due regard for the safety of all others, on and off the roadway.

In this situation, the patient's condition clearly does not warrant the use of lights and siren. If you choose to use an emergency transport, you will put yourself, your partner, your patient, and other motorists at risk. You could also face possible litigation. You have time to take an alternate route and avoid creating more hazards as other drivers try to move out of the way.

**7.** **If you are in an unfamiliar area and do not know an alternate route, what are your options?**

The best option would be to use a GPS device to navigate through an unfamiliar area. Another option is to call the dispatcher via radio and ask for street-by-street directions. As a last resort, you can wait for the traffic to clear.

**8.** **When traveling in the emergency mode, how do you respond to a stopped school bus?**

Although state motor vehicle statutes or codes often grant an emergency vehicle certain privileges when responding to an emergency, special privileges are not given to emergency vehicles when driving through a school zone or approaching a stopped school bus that is loading or unloading children. In these situations, the emergency vehicle operator is required to obey the law like any other motorist.

An emergency vehicle operator is never allowed to pass a school bus that has stopped to load or unload children and is displaying its red warning lights and extended stop arm. If you approach a school bus that is loading or unloading children, you should stop before you reach the bus and turn off your siren. Wait for the bus driver to make sure the children are safe, the bus door has been closed, and its red warning lights are turned off. Only then may you cautiously proceed past the stopped school bus.

**9.** **Where do most serious ambulance crashes occur, and what should you do to help avoid a crash?**

Intersection crashes are the most common and usually the most serious type of crash involving ambulances. Therefore, the emergency vehicle operator must be especially careful and alert when approaching an intersection. If you are operating the vehicle in emergency mode and cannot wait for traffic lights to change, you should still come to a complete stop, look around for other motorists and pedestrians, and then cautiously proceed. The same applies if you approach an intersection with stop signs.

### EMS Patient Care Report (PCR)

| **Date:** 11-16-2019 | **Incident No.:** 19-49843 | **Nature of Call:** Assault | | **Location:** 1800 Main Road | |
|---|---|---|---|---|---|
| **Dispatched:** 0800 | **En Route:** 0801 | **At Scene:** 0809 | **Transport:** 0820 | **At Hospital:** 0856 | **In Service:** 0911 |

#### Patient Information

| **Age:** 42<br>**Sex:** F<br>**Weight (in kg [lb]):** 66 kg (145 lb) | **Allergies:** Penicillin<br>**Medications:** Hydrochlorothiazide<br>**Past Medical History:** Hypertension<br>**Chief Complaint:** Left knee pain |
|---|---|

#### Vital Signs

| **Time:** 0814 | **BP:** 138/86 | **Pulse:** 98 | **Respirations:** 20 | **Spo$_2$:** 99% RA |
|---|---|---|---|---|
| **Time:** 0821 | **BP:** 136/88 | **Pulse:** 98 | **Respirations:** 18 | **Spo$_2$:** 100% RA |
| **Time:** 0831 | **BP:** 142/90 | **Pulse:** 94 | **Respirations:** 20 | **Spo$_2$:** 97% RA |
| **Time:** 0841 | **BP:** 140/88 | **Pulse:** 100 | **Respirations:** 20 | **Spo$_2$:** 98% RA |
| **Time:** 0851 | **BP:** 136/86 | **Pulse:** 94 | **Respirations:** 18 | **Spo$_2$:** 98% RA |

## YOU are the Provider SUMMARY *continued*

| EMS Treatment (circle all that apply) | | | | |
|---|---|---|---|---|
| Oxygen @ __ L/min via:<br><br>NC   NRM   Bag mask | | Assisted Ventilation | Airway Adjunct | CPR |
| Defibrillation | Bleeding Control | Bandaging | (Splinting) | **Other:** Emotional support |

| Narrative |
|---|

Dispatched to a residence for an "assault."

Chief Complaint: Left knee pain

History: Arrived on scene to find a 42-year-old female with isolated knee injury and no other complaints voiced. Patient states she was struck in the left knee with a baseball bat. Patient reports left knee pain. Pt. denies falling.

Assessment: The patient is alert and oriented and denies any loss of consciousness. Swelling and deformity to the left knee noted on exam. Vital signs are within normal limits, and other secondary assessment was normal. Patient has good pulse, movement, and sensation in left lower leg. Breath sounds are clear and equal bilaterally, and pupils are equal and reactive to light.

Treatment (Rx): Splinted left leg, immobilizing the leg above and below the knee, and reassessed pulse, motor, and sensory functions.

Transport: Patient was lifted onto the stretcher and loaded into the ambulance. En route monitored vital signs and level of consciousness. Prior to reaching the destination, medic unit was forced to detour due to a motor vehicle crash, and transport time was extended by 25 minutes. Closely monitored the patient's condition for the duration of the transport and provided emotional support as needed. Her condition remained unchanged. Arrived at the hospital, gave verbal report to the staff nurse Smith, and transferred patient care.

**End of report**

# Prep Kit

## Ready for Review

- Today's ambulances are designed according to strict government regulations based on national standards.
- The six-pointed Star of Life emblem identifies vehicles that meet federal specifications as licensed or certified ambulances.
- An ambulance call has nine phases:
  - Preparation for the call
  - Dispatch
  - En route
  - Arrival at scene
  - Transfer of the patient to the ambulance
  - En route to the receiving facility (transport)
  - At the receiving facility (delivery)
  - En route to the station
  - Postrun
- Certain items, such as sterile gloves, must be available on the ambulance at all times, as dictated by state and jurisdictional requirements.
- Every ambulance must be staffed with at least one EMT in the patient compartment whenever a patient is being transported. However, two EMTs are strongly recommended. Some services may operate with a non-EMT driver and a single EMT in the patient compartment.
- Check all medical equipment and supplies daily, including all the oxygen supplies, the jump kit, splints, dressings and bandages, backboards and other immobilization equipment, and the emergency obstetric kit.
- During the postrun phase, you should complete and file any additional written reports and inform dispatch of your status, location, and availability. Perform a routine inspection to ensure the ambulance is ready to respond to the next call.

- Learning how to properly operate your vehicle is just as important as learning how to care for patients when you arrive on the scene.
  - The first rule of safe driving in an emergency vehicle is that speed does not save lives; good care does.
  - The second rule is that the operator and all passengers must wear seat belts and shoulder restraints at all times.

- Air ambulances are used to evacuate medical and trauma patients.
  - There are two basic types of air medical units: fixed-wing and rotary-wing, otherwise known as helicopters.
  - A medical evacuation is commonly known as a medevac and is generally performed exclusively by helicopters.

## Vital Vocabulary

**air ambulances** Fixed-wing and rotary-wing (known as helicopters) aircraft that have been modified for medical care; used to evacuate and transport patients with life-threatening injuries to treatment facilities.

**ambulance** A specialized vehicle for treating and transporting sick and injured patients.

**blind spots** Areas of the road that are blocked from your view by your vehicle or mirrors.

**cleaning** The process of removing dirt, dust, blood, or other visible contaminants from a surface.

**CPR board** A device that provides a firm surface under the patient's torso.

**cushion of safety** A safe distance between your vehicle and any vehicles around you.

**decontaminate** To remove or neutralize radiation, chemical, or other hazardous material from clothing, equipment, vehicles, and personnel.

**disinfection** The killing of pathogenic agents by direct application of chemicals.

**first-responder vehicles** Specialized vehicles used to transport EMS equipment and personnel to the scenes of medical emergencies.

**high-level disinfection** The killing of pathogenic agents by using potent means of disinfection.

**hydroplaning** Occurs when the tires of a vehicle are lifted off the road surface as a result of water piling up underneath them, making the vehicle feel as though it is floating.

**jump kit** A portable kit containing items that are used in the initial care of the patient.

**medevac** Medical evacuation of a patient by helicopter.

**spotter** A person who assists a driver in backing up an ambulance to help adjust for blind spots at the back of the vehicle.

**Star of Life** The six-pointed star emblem that identifies vehicles that meet federal specifications as licensed or certified ambulances.

**sterilization** A process, such as heating, that removes microbial contamination.

## References

1. Kupas DF. *Lights and Siren Use by Emergency Medical Services (EMS): Above All Do No Harm*. US Department of Transportation, National Highway Traffic Safety Administration, Office of Emergency Medical Services. www.ems.gov/pdf/Lights_and_Sirens_Use_by_EMS_May_2017.pdf. Published May 2017. Accessed February 21, 2020.

2. Murray B, Kue R. The use of emergency lights and sirens by ambulances and their effect on patient outcomes and public safety: a comprehensive review of the literature. *Prehosp Disaster Med*. 2017;32(2):209-216.

3. National Association of State EMS Officials. *National EMS Scope of Practice Model 2019*. DOT HS 812-666. https://www.ems.gov/pdf/National_EMS_Scope_of_Practice_Model_2019.pdf. Accessed February 15, 2020.

4. National Fire Protection Association. *NFPA 1917: Standard for Automotive Ambulances*. Quincy, MA: NFPA; 2019.

5. National Highway Traffic Safety Administration. Fatality Analysis Reporting System (FARS). https://www.nhtsa.gov/research-data/fatality-analysis-reporting-system-fars. Accessed February 21, 2020.

6. National Highway Traffic Safety Administration. *The National Highway Traffic Safety Administration and Ground Ambulance Crashes*. Washington, DC: National Highway Traffic Safety Administration; 2014.

7. Poole K, Couper K, Smyth MA, Yeung J, Perkins GD. Mechanical CPR: Who? When? How? *Crit Care*. 2018;22(1):140.

8. US Fire Administration. *Traffic Incident Management Systems*. FA 330. https://www.usfa.fema.gov/downloads/pdf/publications/fa_330.pdf. Published March 2012. Accessed February 21, 2020.

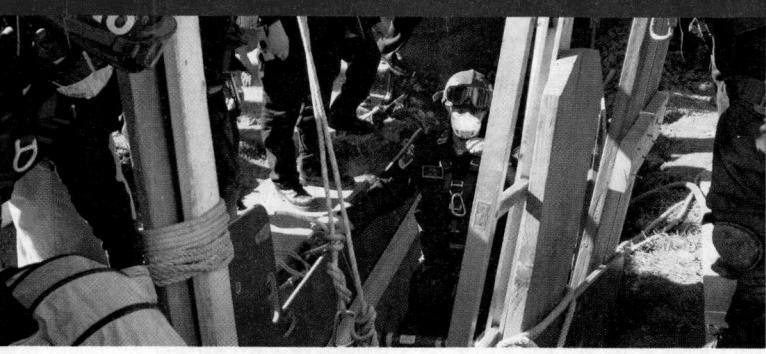

# Chapter 39

# Vehicle Extrication and Special Rescue

## NATIONAL EMS EDUCATION STANDARD COMPETENCIES

### EMS Operations

Knowledge of operational roles and responsibilities to ensure patient, public, and personnel safety.

### Vehicle Extrication

- Safe vehicle extrication (pp 1464–1475)
- Use of simple hand tools (p 1472)

## KNOWLEDGE OBJECTIVES

1. Explain the responsibilities of an EMT in patient rescue and vehicle extrication. (p 1464)
2. Discuss how to ensure safety at the scene of a rescue incident, including scene size-up and the selection of the proper personal protective equipment and additional necessary gear. (pp 1464–1469)
3. Describe examples of vehicle safety components that may be hazardous to both EMTs and patients following a collision and how to mitigate their dangers. (pp 1464–1465)
4. Define the terms extrication and entrapment. (p 1465)
5. Describe the 10 phases of vehicle extrication and the role of the EMT during each one. (pp 1466–1475)
6. Discuss the various factors related to ensuring situational safety at the site of a vehicle extrication, including controlling traffic flow, performing a 360° assessment, stabilizing the vehicle, dealing with unique hazards, and

evaluating the need for additional resources. (pp 1466–1470)

7. Describe the special precautions the EMT should follow to protect the patient during a vehicle extrication. (pp 1470–1472)
8. Explain the different factors that must be considered before attempting to gain access to the patient during an incident that requires extrication. (pp 1470–1472)
9. Explain the difference between simple access and complex access in vehicle extrication. (p 1472)
10. Discuss patient care considerations related to assisting with rapid extrication, providing emergency care to a trapped patient, and removing and transferring a patient. (pp 1473–1475)
11. Describe examples of situations that would require special technical rescue teams and the EMT's role in these situations. (pp 1475–1479)

## SKILLS OBJECTIVES

There are no skills objectives for this chapter.

## Introduction

As an EMT, you will usually not be responsible for rescue, though you may assist with extrication. Rescue involves many different processes and environments, including vehicle, water, and wilderness rescue. These incidents require training beyond the level of the EMT. You must understand the basic concepts of extrication in order to function effectively as part of a team during a rescue incident. In some cases, you may be the first emergency unit to arrive at the scene, and your initial actions may determine how efficiently the rescue is completed.

The chapter begins with a discussion of safety at the scene of a rescue incident, followed by the 10 phases of extrication. This includes how to gain access to patients and how to keep yourself, your partner, patients, and bystanders safe in the process. In most cases, once you have reached the patient, extrication will occur around you and the patient. Communication between you and the personnel performing the extrication is vital.

## Safety

You must always be prepared, mentally and physically, for any incident that requires rescue or extrication. Your priority as an EMT is to provide patient care. However, your personal safety and the safety of your team are paramount and must be addressed before patient care is initiated. Safety begins with the proper mindset and the proper protective equipment.

The equipment that you use and the gear that you wear will depend on the hazards you expect to encounter, as well as what you observe during your scene size-up (**FIGURE 39-1**). Such protective gear

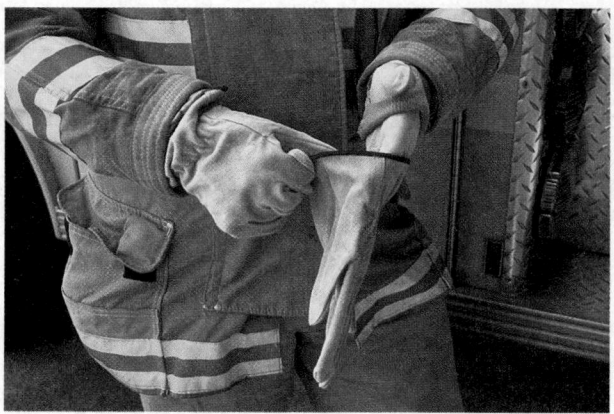

**FIGURE 39-1** Proper protective equipment varies depending on the anticipated hazards.
© Jones & Bartlett Learning. Courtesy of MIEMSS.

may include turnout gear, a helmet, hearing protection, and a fire extinguisher. However, the importance of wearing blood- and fluid-impermeable gloves at all times during patient contact cannot be overemphasized. If you will be involved with extrication, wear a pair of leather gloves over your disposable gloves to protect you from injury when handling ropes, tools, broken glass, hot or cold objects, or sharp metal.

## Vehicle Safety Systems

A variety of safety systems are used in modern vehicles. Although many of these devices are useful when the vehicle is in motion, they can become hazards after the vehicle has been involved in a crash.

Shock-absorbing bumpers provide vehicle protection from low-speed impact. Following a frontal or rear-end crash, the shock absorbers within these bumpers may be compressed or loaded. Avoid standing directly in front of such bumpers, and always approach vehicles from the side, because the shock absorbers can release and injure your knees and legs.

Manufacturers are now mandated to incorporate supplemental restraint systems, or airbags, into all vehicles. These airbags fill with a nonharmful gas on impact and quickly deflate after the crash. Although they were present in some older vehicles, federal legislation mandated in 1998 that newly manufactured cars and light trucks be equipped with front airbags. Since that time, additional airbags have been added as standard or optional equipment on passenger vehicles. In addition to the standard front airbags located in the steering wheel and upper dashboard, it is important to remember that there may be airbags located at multiple points inside of the passenger compartment. Side airbags may be located in the door or the roof rail with the intention of protecting occupants in the event of a side-impact collision with another vehicle or a tree. The lower portion of the dashboard may have airbags designed to lessen the extent of injury to the patient's lower extremities and pelvis. Some vehicles even have airbags located in the seat belts or the front middle area to lessen seat belt injuries or injuries occurring when two front occupants strike one another.

Airbags should normally deploy and deflate before your arrival on the scene. However, airbags that have not deployed may spontaneously inflate while you or other rescue personnel are in the vehicle, causing injury. Use caution when working in damaged vehicles in which airbags have not inflated. Generally, you should maintain at least a 5-inch (13-cm) clearance around side-impact airbags, a 10-inch (25-cm) clearance around driver-side airbags, and a 20-inch (51-cm) clearance around passenger-side airbags.

> ### Words of Wisdom
>
> A vehicle crash scene can present many hazards to emergency responders and patients, including fuel spills that pose fire and explosion risks, downed power lines that pose electric hazards, broken glass and torn metal, and exposure to potentially infectious body fluids. Your safety at every type of emergency scene begins with, and depends on, your scene size-up. What you see at the scene helps you determine which personal protective equipment to use and whether to call for additional resources or specialized assistance.

You may notice a haze similar to smoke inside vehicles in which airbags have deployed. This haze is caused by the cornstarch or talcum powder that manufacturers used to place on the airbags to prevent minor skin irritations by reducing the friction between the occupant's skin and the airbag. Appropriate protective gear, including eye protection, will reduce the risk of eye or lung irritation from this substance.

> ### Street Smarts
>
> After an airbag deploys, the powder from the airbag may trigger medical conditions such as asthma. Patients may also be anxious, mistaking the powder from the bag for smoke and thinking their vehicle is on fire. Be thorough in your assessment, and reassure patients.

## Fundamentals of Extrication

As an EMT, your primary concern during all phases of a rescue is safety, and your primary roles are to provide emergency medical care and prevent further injury to the patient. You will provide care to the patient as extrication goes on around you unless this proves to be too dangerous for you or the patient. **Extrication** is the removal from entrapment or from a dangerous situation or position (also called disentanglement).

**Entrapment** is a condition in which a person is caught within a closed area with no way out or has a limb or other body part trapped. In the context of this chapter, extrication means removal of a patient from a wrecked vehicle. However, the same principles and concepts apply to other situations, such as a collapsed building.

> ### Words of Wisdom
>
> Extended entrapment of a limb or other body part can lead to crush syndrome in a patient. Crush syndrome requires specific and specialized care. This is discussed in greater detail in Chapter 27, *Soft-Tissue Injuries*.

Each emergency responder has a distinct role at a vehicle extrication scene. EMS providers assess patients, provide immediate medical care,

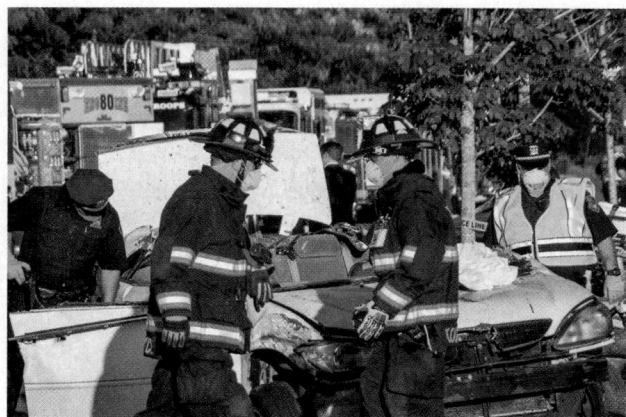

**FIGURE 39-2** EMS providers, the rescue team, law enforcement officers, and firefighters have distinct responsibilities at a rescue scene and must cooperate to manage the incident.

© Brian Logan Photography/Shutterstock.

| **TABLE 39-1** Ten Phases of Extrication |
| --- |
| **1.** Preparation |
| **2.** En route to the scene |
| **3.** Arrival and scene size-up |
| **4.** Hazard control |
| **5.** Support operations |
| **6.** Gaining access |
| **7.** Emergency care |
| **8.** Removal of the patient |
| **9.** Transfer of the patient |
| **10.** Termination |

© Jones & Bartlett Learning.

triage and package patients, provide additional assessment and care as needed once patients are removed, and provide transport to the emergency department.

The rescue team secures and stabilizes the vehicle, provides safe entrance and **access** to the patients (the ability to reach the patients), safely extricates patients, and provides adequate room so that patients can be removed properly.

Law enforcement officers control traffic, maintain order at the scene, establish and maintain a perimeter so that bystanders are kept at a safe distance, and ultimately investigate the crash or crime scene. Firefighters extinguish fire, prevent additional ignition, ensure that the scene is safe, and remove spilled fuel (**FIGURE 39-2**).

Roles and responsibilities often vary based on jurisdiction and the available agencies. For example, the fire department may take primary responsibility for traffic control in certain situations. An incident commander (discussed later in the chapter) should take command of the scene and coordinate the response, ensuring the agencies work seamlessly together. Good communication among team members and clear leadership are essential to safe, efficient provision of proper emergency care.

There are 10 phases of the extrication process (**TABLE 39-1**). Many are similar to the phases of an ambulance call (discussed in Chapter 38, *Transport Operations*). Each will be discussed, with emphasis on the phases in which you will participate.

## Safety Tips

Just as in patient care, the first priority in rescue is *personal safety*. The scene of an extrication is dynamic, meaning it constantly changes. Be alert to new dangers, and plan an escape route.

## Preparation

Preparing for an incident requiring extrication involves preincident training with rescue personnel for the various types of rescue situations to which you might respond. Tabletop discussions and mock scenarios conducted during training evolutions offer valuable insight and practice so that all personnel understand the operational capabilities and tactics that may be used during a real rescue. Just as they must check the equipment carried on the ambulance, rescue personnel must also check their extrication tools and response vehicles to ensure proper operation on a daily basis. If you notice that any of the extrication equipment on your ambulance is damaged or nonfunctional, find an appropriate replacement or request one from your service. Such preparations reduce the possibility of equipment failure at an emergency scene.

## En Route to the Scene

Procedures and safety precautions similar to those discussed in the phases of an ambulance call are used when responding to a rescue incident. Review dispatch information about the nature of the call and the location of the patient. If initial dispatch information includes keys that specialized resources may be necessary, ensure with your dispatcher that those resources have been assigned to the incident. Assign specific initial duties and scene management tasks to each team member and determine what type of equipment you will take with you when you first arrive on scene.

## Words of Wisdom

Your dispatcher may be busy fielding multiple calls and assigning resources to separate events. If you identify the need for additional resources early in your response, ensure that those resources are en route. This is a team sport, and your vigilance can help identify information that may have slipped through the cracks. Early recognition and mobilization of resources can make a huge difference for the patient.

## Arrival and Scene Size-up

If you are the first unit to arrive on the scene, position the ambulance to block traffic and create a safety barrier within which you can safely begin to assess the scene. Use only essential warning lights, because too many lights tend to distract or confuse motorists. Many emergency responders have been injured on scenes when they were struck by passing vehicles. In some areas, policies indicate that emergency lighting for stationary vehicles can be reduced or turned off after the scene is secured, leaving only the first vehicle parked before the incident with emergency lighting activated; this practice may reduce the risk of a secondary crash.

If you are not the first to arrive, choose a location that will allow safe access to the scene while leaving a way to drive your ambulance out. This area is typically located at the very front of the accident scene in the same lane of traffic as the accident. Do not park in an area where you will be blocked in. If law enforcement or fire units have blocked the roadway, position your unit so that the back of the ambulance is pointing toward the scene to facilitate patient transport. Avoid parking alongside the incident on an active roadway; doing so could increase the risk of your vehicle or responders being struck.

Sometimes the scene at a crash is complicated by the presence of **hazardous materials**. A

hazardous material is any substance that is toxic, poisonous, radioactive, flammable, or explosive and can cause injury or death with exposure. If there is a hazardous material present at the scene, always park uphill and upwind from the hazard.

Before exiting your vehicle at an emergency scene, put on proper protective gear. At a minimum, this should include a high-visibility reflective safety vest. Be alert for any vehicles that might cause injury to you. Do not assume that motorists will always see you or heed the warning lights. Even during daylight hours, drivers may be distracted by the warning lights or trying to catch a glimpse of the scene. Inattentive drivers pose a serious threat to you, your partner, the patients, and all emergency responders working the scene.

Before proceeding, make sure that the scene is properly marked and protected. Request assistance from law enforcement and/or fire personnel (**FIGURE 39-3**), who should close the road or divert traffic safely around the scene with cones, flares, or barricade tape. Remember, your job is to provide patient care. You may be forced to direct traffic until other units arrive, but ultimately, traffic control is usually handled by other public safety units.

## Words of Wisdom

When responding to incidents at night, use your headlights and spotlights to illuminate the scene. Wear a high-visibility reflective safety vest so that you will be seen by fellow emergency responders and motorists.

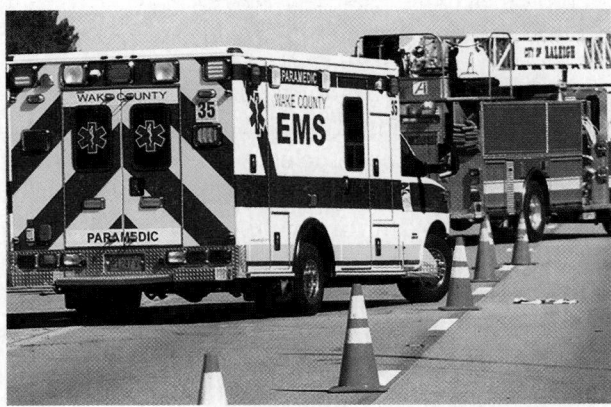

**FIGURE 39-3** The scene of a crash should be marked properly, and traffic should be diverted so that responders have enough room to work.

**Size-up** is the ongoing process of information gathering and scene evaluation to determine appropriate strategies and tactics to manage an emergency, while paying attention to hazards such as downed power lines, leaking fluids, fire, and broken glass. One of the important responsibilities of scene size-up is to determine what, if any, additional resources will be needed. If you are first on the scene, you may need to initiate a rescue response or call for additional EMS units, law enforcement, utility departments, or specialized crews such as hazardous materials (hazmat) personnel.

A 360° walk around the scene will allow you to evaluate the hazards and potential injuries and determine the number of patients. If there is a large group of patients, implement local mass-casualty incident protocols as necessary. During your walk, look for the following:

- The mechanism of injury
- Downed power lines
- Leaking fuels or fluids
- Smoke or fire
- Broken glass
- Trapped or ejected patients
- The number of patients and vehicles involved

## Words of Wisdom

Practice situational awareness. Situational awareness is the ability to understand and react to the threats around you. Remember that scenes are dynamic; you always should be alert for changing situations. Consider weather and environmental conditions, and be aware of traffic, patients, and bystanders.

On the scene of a motor vehicle crash, it is important to note the physical damage to the structure of the vehicle or vehicles. A bent steering wheel is a mechanism of injury for significant face and/or thoracic trauma. Imprints in the dashboard, which are usually the result of the knees striking it, indicate the potential for serious lower extremity injuries such as hip dislocations and fractures. Always lift deployed airbags to see if there is deformity to the steering wheel or dashboard, which indicates that the patient struck the structure after the airbag deflated. Determine if the patient was restrained or not. An unrestrained patient may have contact injuries as well as secondary injuries. If the unrestrained patient is thrown forward, he or she may strike the windshield with the head, resulting in a spiderweb pattern of shattered glass and possible head, face, or neck injuries. Include any findings in your documentation and maintain a high index of suspicion, even if the patient does not present with significant obvious injuries. For a detailed discussion of the kinematics of trauma, see Chapter 25, *Trauma Overview*.

Use the information you have gathered to evaluate the need for additional resources such as the following:

- Extrication equipment
- Fire department
- Law enforcement
- Hazmat unit
- Utility company
- Advanced life support unit or units
- Air transport

Look for spilled fuel and other flammable substances. Motor vehicles carry a variety of fuels and lubricants that pose a fire hazard. Sometimes postcrash fires are started when sparks created during the crash ignite spilled fuel. A short in a vehicle's electric system or a damaged battery may also cause a postcrash fire. These fires may trap the occupants of the vehicle and require fire suppression. Rescue operations may also create sparks that could ignite spilled fuel. It is important to recognize these hazards as soon as possible during your scene size-up.

Environmental conditions can lead to unique hazards at a crash scene. Crashes that occur in rain, sleet, or snow, for example, present an added hazard for rescue personnel and patients. Crashes that occur on hills are harder to handle than those that occur on level ground. Uneven terrain increases the potential for the vehicle to roll over, requiring stabilization of the vehicle prior to gaining access. Remember that the conditions responsible for the crash may also cause other motorists to lose control of their vehicles and injure you.

Some crash scenes may present threats of violence if the vehicle's occupants are intoxicated, have an altered mental status, or are upset with other motorists. If they suddenly regain consciousness or are significantly confused, patients may perceive a threat during rescue operations. This may pose a threat to you or to others on the scene. Be alert for weapons that are carried in civilian vehicles.

You will need to coordinate your efforts with the rescue teams and with law enforcement officials. If you respect their jobs, they will respect yours. You should communicate with members of the rescue team throughout the extrication process. Report to the incident commander as soon as you arrive at the scene. Under the incident command system (described in Chapter 40, *Incident Management*), rescue operations are integrated as a separate group. You become a member of this group and will enter the vehicle and provide care for the patient or patients when approved by the incident commander.

## Hazard Control

A variety of hazards may be present at the extrication scene. Downed power lines are a common example. Never attempt to move downed power lines. If power lines are touching or located in proximity to a vehicle involved in the crash, patients should be instructed to remain in the vehicle until power is shut off by a utility company representative.

If you are not the first on scene, in most incidents, there will be an area designated as the **safe zone**. You and the ambulance should remain in that area, outside of the danger zone (**FIGURE 39-4**). A **danger zone (hot zone)** is an area where people can be exposed to sharp metal edges, broken glass, toxic substances, radiation, or explosion of hazardous materials.

Bystanders and family members can also create hazards. If they are allowed to get too close, they are at risk of injury and may also interfere with the overall management of the incident. For these reasons, the danger zone is off-limits to bystanders (**FIGURE 39-5**). You should help to set up and enforce this zone. If you arrive before the rescue team, coordinate crowd control with law enforcement officials.

The vehicle itself can be a hazard. A vehicle that came to rest on its side or roof is unstable and can

---

## YOU are the Provider

As you approach the wreckage of the aircraft, you see a badly damaged aluminum body with a twisted tubular frame protruding through sections of the body. There is a single small door at the front of the aircraft with additional aluminum bars over the top of the passenger compartment. The door is bent and cannot be opened manually. A rescue team member is able to cut through the bars with bolt cutters and use a hydraulic cutter to allow better access to the patient. Your partner is able to reach through the bars and manually stabilize the patient's head. You access the patient through the opposite side and perform a primary assessment. The woman is approximately 55 years old and is unresponsive but breathing. Her legs and chest are pinned by twisted aluminum bars, and she has large lacerations to her left temple and right arm. The bones at the elbow are exposed.

| Recording Time: | 0 Minutes |
|---|---|
| **Appearance** | Unresponsive with snoring respirations |
| **Level of consciousness** | Unresponsive |
| **Airway** | Open with a modified jaw thrust; clear of secretions or foreign bodies |
| **Breathing** | Decreased rate; shallow depth |
| **Circulation** | Radial pulses weak and rapid; skin cool, clammy, and pale; laceration to the forehead from the temple through the left orbit with minimal bleeding; laceration to right arm with the bones of the elbow exposed and bleeding controlled |

Because of the mechanism of injury, the patient's clinical condition, and the possibility of a prolonged extrication, you request air transport to respond to the scene and to transport the patient to a trauma center located 35 miles away. You apply high-flow oxygen via nonrebreathing mask, cover the laceration on her forehead, apply a cervical collar, and attempt to shield the patient from debris during the extrication process.

**3.** How should you initially attempt to gain access to a crash victim?

**4.** What treatment should you provide to a patient who is entrapped in wreckage?

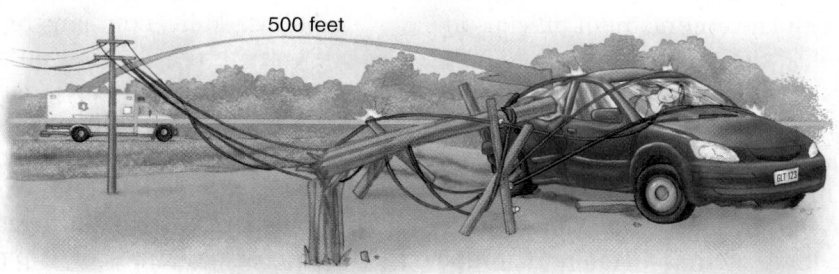

**FIGURE 39-4** Remain outside the danger zone (hot zone).

© Jones & Bartlett Learning.

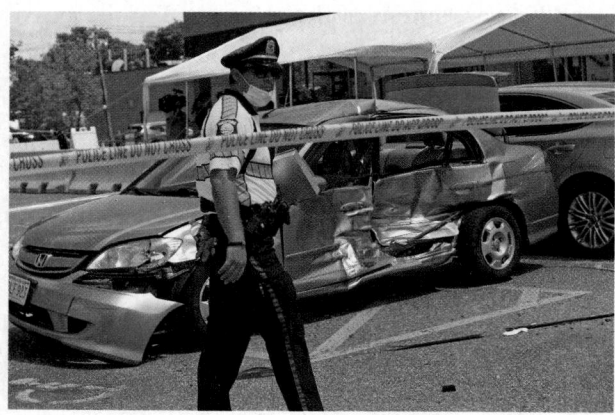

**FIGURE 39-5** Establish a danger zone to prevent bystanders from entering the incident area.

© Boston Globe/Contributor/Getty Images.

be dangerous to you. Rescue personnel can stabilize the vehicle with a variety of jacks or cribbing (wooden blocks). Prior to attempting to gain access to the vehicle, the vehicle gear should be set in park with the parking brake set and the ignition turned off. Both battery cables should be disconnected, negative side first, to minimize the possibility of sparks or fire.

### Safety Tips

Always assume that oncoming traffic cannot see you and take appropriate steps to keep yourself safe. Rubberneckers are gawking at the crash, not looking at you!

## Alternative Fuel Vehicles

Currently, with advances in automotive technology, some vehicles on the road use alternative fuel. Vehicles may be powered by electricity or electricity/

gasoline hybrids, or fuels such as propane, natural gas, methanol, or hydrogen. One feature is common throughout all alternative vehicles—the need for rescue personnel to disconnect the battery to prevent further fire or explosion. In many of the currently available alternate fuel vehicles, the batteries are not located in the engine compartment, but in other areas, such as the trunk or under the seats. Furthermore, there may be more than one battery or capacitor present used to store energy. Be aware that tanks used to store alternative fuel may also be located in different places than in traditional gas-powered vehicles. You must remain vigilant when presented with alternative fuel vehicles and be aware of their inherent dangers. For example, hybrid batteries have a higher voltage than traditional automotive batteries, and it may take up to 10 minutes for a high-voltage system to deenergize after the main battery is turned off. Avoid contact with high-voltage cables (typically orange) and components throughout the rescue. Damaged high-voltage batteries may also give off toxic fumes. Do not approach the vehicle if you detect an unusual odor, and retreat if you experience burning in your eyes or throat until the scene is safe. If not previously notified, call dispatch to request additional assistance from the fire department and/or hazmat team.

## Support Operations

Support operations include lighting the scene, establishing tool and equipment staging areas, and marking helicopter landing zones. Fire and rescue personnel will work together on these functions.

## Gaining Access

A critical phase of extrication is gaining access to the patient. Remember, do not attempt to gain access to the patient or enter the vehicle until you are sure that the vehicle is stable and that any hazards have been identified and properly controlled or eliminated. When an incident commander is present, you will be authorized to enter the scene or the vehicle only when these conditions have been met.

The safest, most efficient way to reach the patient or patients depends on the situation. It is up to you and the team to identify the best way to gain access. Darkness, uneven terrain, tall grass, shrubbery, and wreckage may make patients hard to find (**FIGURE 39-6**). Multiple vehicles with multiple patients may be involved. If this is the situation, you should locate and rapidly triage each patient to determine who needs urgent care before you proceed with any treatment and patient packaging. Triage is discussed in Chapter 40, *Incident Management.*

### Words of Wisdom

Remember that scene size-up is a dynamic and ongoing process, because the situation often changes. As a result, you may need to change your plans for gaining access and providing treatment.

To determine the exact location and position of the patient, consider the following questions:

- Is the patient in a vehicle or in some other structure?
- Is the vehicle or structure severely damaged?
- What hazards exist that pose a risk to the patient and responders?

- In what position is the vehicle? On what type of surface? Is the vehicle stable or is it likely to roll over?

You must also consider the severity of the patient's injuries and change your course of action as you learn more about the patient's condition. What if you have to quickly remove a patient from a vehicle because the environment is threatening or you need to perform CPR? Chest compressions and airway management may be ineffective if the patient is upside down or pinned to the seat by the dashboard. Depending on the patient's condition and scene safety, you and your team may have to use the rapid extrication technique (discussed in Chapter 8, *Lifting and Moving Patients*) to move a patient who is not entrapped from a sitting position inside a vehicle to a supine position on a long backboard. A team of experienced EMTs should be able to perform rapid extrication of an untrapped patient in 1 minute or less.

During the access and extrication phases, make sure that the patient remains safe. For example, cover the patient with a heavy, fire-resistant blanket or place a backboard between the windshield and the patient to protect the patient from breaking glass, flying particles, tools, or other hazards. In addition, maintain good communication with the patient. Reassure the patient that everything possible is being done to remove him or her from the situation. Always describe what you are going to do before you do it and as you are doing it, even if you think the patient is unresponsive (**FIGURE 39-7**).

In many cases, you or your partner may need to provide cervical spine stabilization or other care

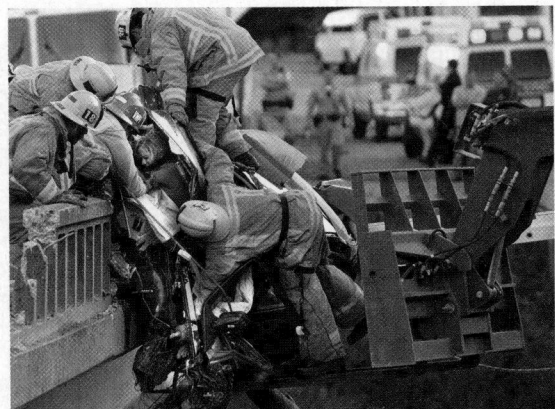

**FIGURE 39-6** The exact way to gain access depends on many factors, including the terrain, the way in which the vehicle is situated, and the weather.

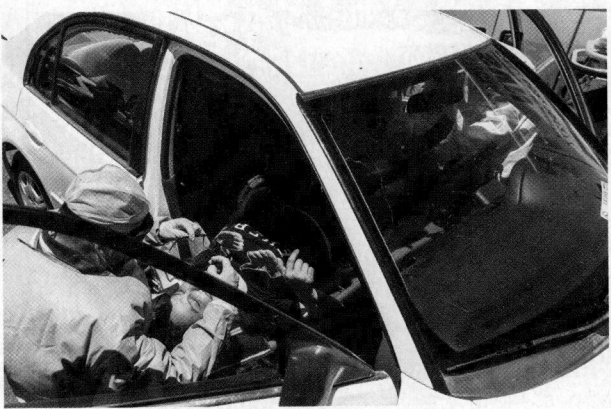

**FIGURE 39-7** Always explain to the patient why you are there and what you are doing.

during extrication. The rescue team should try to keep heat, noise, and force to a minimum and use only what is necessary to extricate the patient safely.

## Simple Access

The first step is simple access, trying to get to the patient as quickly and simply as possible without using any tools or force. Motor vehicles are built for easy entry and exit; however, it may be necessary to use forcible entry methods. The rescue team is responsible for providing the entrance you need to gain access to the patient. In situations where the rescue team has not yet arrived and delayed access to the patient could be life threatening, simple hand tools, such as hammers, center punches (to break side or rear windows), pry bars, and hacksaws, are usually stored on the ambulance for you to use. Whenever possible, you should first try to unlock the doors (or ask the patient to unlock them) or roll down the windows. Try to open every door using the door handles to gain access before breaking any windows or using other methods of forced entry (**FIGURE 39-8**).

### Street Smarts

Always try before you pry. Just like when resuscitating a patient, start with the basics. Try to open the door before resigning to the idea that it must be removed using large hydraulic devices.

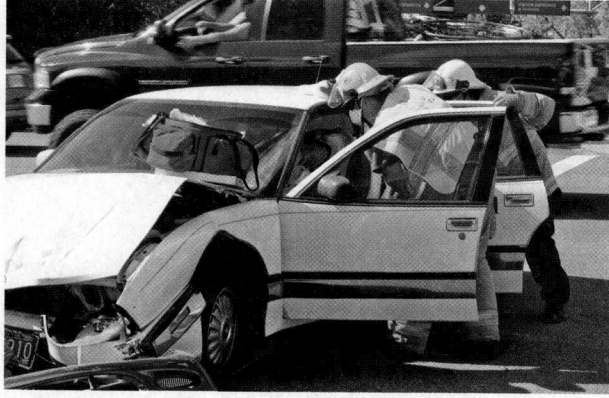

**FIGURE 39-8** Get to the patient as quickly and simply as possible by opening the door without using tools or breaking any glass.
© TFoxFoto/Shutterstock.

## Complex Access

Complex access requires the use of special tools, such as pneumatic and/or hydraulic devices, and special training that includes breaking the windshield or removing the roof (**FIGURE 39-9**). These advanced skills are typically performed by a specialized team rather than EMS providers and are listed in **TABLE 39-2**.

## Emergency Care

Providing medical care to a patient who is trapped in a vehicle is essentially the same as for any other patient. Unless there is an immediate threat of fire, explosion, or other danger, once entrance and access to the patient have been provided and the

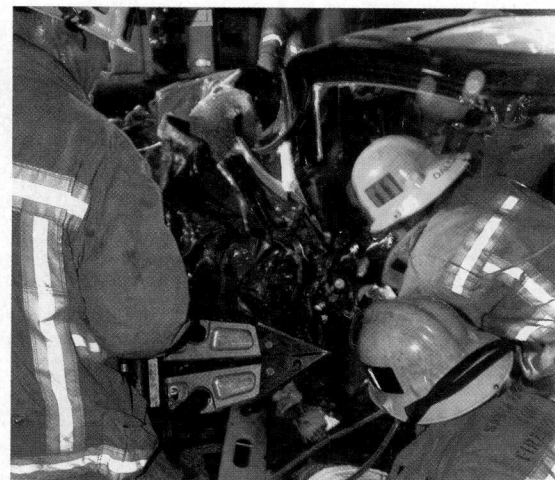

**FIGURE 39-9** Complex access often requires the use of pneumatic and/or hydraulic devices.
© Keith D. Cullom.

| **TABLE 39-2** Vehicle Extrication Techniques (Complex Access) |
|---|
| • Brake and gas pedal displacement |
| • Dashboard roll-up |
| • Door removal |
| • Roof opening and removal |
| • Seat displacement |
| • Steering column displacement |
| • Steering wheel cutting |

© Jones & Bartlett Learning.

scene is safe, you should perform a primary assessment and provide care before further extrication begins, as follows:

1. Address any exsanguinating hemorrhage with direct pressure or a tourniquet if appropriate.
2. Provide manual stabilization to protect the cervical spine, as needed.
3. Open the airway.
4. Provide high-flow oxygen, if indicated.
5. Assist or provide for adequate ventilation.
6. Control any significant external bleeding.
7. Treat all critical injuries.

If the patient has obvious, life-threatening external hemorrhage, address it first (even before airway and breathing) and control it quickly.

## Removal of the Patient

In the case of a vehicle extrication, work with rescue personnel to determine the best route to remove the patient from the vehicle. This should be a collaborative effort with consideration given to the specific details of the entrapment, the patient's condition, and the expertise of the crews on scene. Whereas one crash may require removal of the patient through the driver's door, a similar crash may require complete removal of the vehicle's roof. Removal of a patient from a motor vehicle is a multistep process that is intensive in the number of

rescue personnel involved, the equipment used, and the effort required to prevent further injury or harm.

As a part of your assessment, participate in the preparation for patient removal. Determine how urgently the patient must be extricated, where you should be positioned to best protect the patient during extrication, and, once the patient has been freed, how you will best move the patient from within the vehicle onto the backboard and onto the stretcher. Carefully examine the exposed area of the limb or other part of the patient that is trapped to determine the extent of injury and whether there is a possibility of hidden bleeding. If you have concerns about significant hemorrhage from a peripheral vascular injury, work swiftly to control the hemorrhage. Consider placing a tourniquet on the entrapped limb or limbs. Tourniquet use is independently associated with a sixfold decrease in overall mortality of patients with peripheral vascular injury. If possible, evaluate sensation in the trapped area so that you will know whether increased pain indicates that an object is pressing on or has impaled the patient during extrication.

During this time, the rescue team assesses exactly how the patient is trapped and determines the safest, easiest way to extricate him or her. Your input is essential so that the rescue team plans an extrication that protects the patient from further harm.

## YOU are the Provider

As your partner continues to manually stabilize the patient's head, she begins to respond to voice and moans loudly. As the rescue team prepares to remove enough wreckage to allow her to be pulled free, you quickly assess the patient's vital signs.

| Recording Time: 7 Minutes | |
|---|---|
| Respirations | 15 breaths/min; shallow |
| Pulse | 138 beats/min; weak at the radial artery |
| Skin | Cool, clammy, and pale |
| Blood pressure | 98/40 mm Hg |
| Oxygen saturation (Spo₂) | 93% (on oxygen) |

A rescue team member informs you that the medical helicopter will arrive in approximately 4 minutes. A landing zone has been established about 500 yards (457 m) away.

5. Is it appropriate to obtain the vital signs of a patient who is entrapped? Why or why not?
6. What should you do as the patient is being extricated from the wreckage?

Reevaluate whether the patient needs to be immediately removed by using manual stabilization and the rapid extrication technique, or whether a spinal motion restriction device (such as a vest-style extrication device or short backboard) can be applied before he or she is moved further. In most cases, it is impractical and difficult to properly apply extremity splints within the vehicle. Extremity injuries can generally be rapidly supported and stabilized while the patient is being removed by securing an injured arm to the body and, if a leg is injured, securing one leg to the other. This will be adequate until the patient is placed on the stretcher or until time permits a more detailed assessment and splinting of each injury.

Once the extrication plan has been devised and everyone understands what will be done, determine how best to protect the patient. Often, you or your partner will be placed in the vehicle alongside the patient to monitor his or her condition as the vehicle is being forcibly cut, bent, or disassembled. Be sure to wear proper protective clothing. You should have a helmet on with an impact-resistant visor down to protect your face.

Remember, your safety and that of the patient are paramount during this process. Extrication is often extremely noisy, and appropriate hearing protection should be worn by you and the patient. Be sure that you can communicate effectively with the patient and the rescue team so that you can instantly let the rescue personnel know if they need to stop.

## Transfer of the Patient

Once the patient has been freed, rapidly assess any other patients who were previously inaccessible, and then perform a complete primary assessment. Provide critical interventions, if required. Make sure the patient's spine is manually stabilized and apply a cervical collar if this was not previously done (**FIGURE 39-10**).

To avoid injuring yourself, your team members, or the patient, ensure that each EMT is positioned so that he or she can lift and carry properly at all times. Move the patient in a series of smooth, slow, controlled steps, with designated stops to allow for repositioning and adjustments. Make sure that sufficient team members are available for the move. One EMT should be in charge; this EMT will

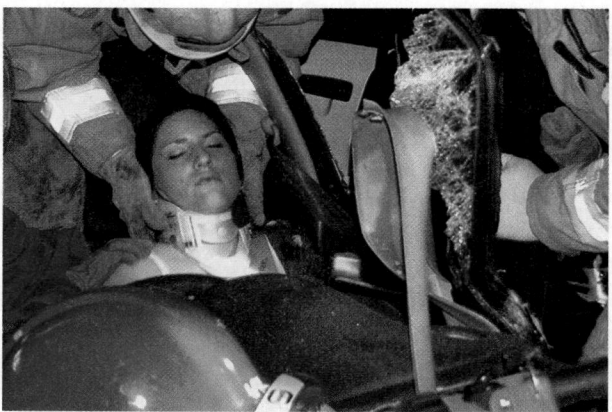

**FIGURE 39-10** Once the patient has been accessed, rapidly assess the patient and make sure that the spine is manually stabilized. Apply a cervical collar if this was not previously done.
© Keith D. Cullom.

plan and verbalize the exact steps that you will follow to move the patient from a sitting position in the vehicle to lying supine on the backboard or stretcher. Choose a path that requires the least manipulation of the patient and equipment. Once you are sure that everyone understands the steps and is ready, you can safely transfer the patient. Move only on the team leader's command and move the patient as a unit. While transferring the patient, continue to protect the patient from any hazards.

### Street Smarts

There are often several different ways a patient can be extricated from a vehicle or other entrapment. The team leader must determine the appropriate method. Team members should listen to determine their individual roles; offer closed-loop communication, acknowledging they understand their roles; and bring to the team leader's attention any circumstance that could injure the team or further injure the patient.

Once the patient has been placed on the stretcher, continue with any additional assessment and treatment that was deferred. If it is extremely cold or hot, raining, or snowing, load the stretcher and patient into the climate-controlled ambulance before continuing assessment and treatment. If the patient's condition requires immediate transport, provide only the additional care that is necessary to package the patient. Perform the remaining steps en route to the hospital.

## Termination

Termination involves returning the emergency units to service. For rescue units, this process may be time-consuming. All equipment used on the scene, including hydraulic, electric, and hand tools, must be cleaned, repacked, and checked before reloading them on the vehicle.

You will also be required to check the ambulance thoroughly, replacing used supplies and decontaminating the unit as required by bloodborne pathogen standards.

Finally, rescue units and medical units will be required to complete all necessary reports.

## Specialized Rescue Situations

On most calls, you can drive the ambulance to or within a short distance of the patient's location. However, in some situations, the patient can be reached only by teams trained in special technical rescues. Specialized skills of these teams include the following:

- Cave rescue
- Confined space rescue
- Cross-field and trail rescue (park rangers)
- Dive rescue
- Missing person search and rescue
- Mine rescue
- Mountain-, rock-, and ice-climbing rescue
- Ski slope and cross-country or trail snow rescue (ski patrol)
- Structural collapse rescue
- Special weapons and tactics (SWAT) team
- Technical rope rescue (low- and high-angle rescue)
- Trench rescue
- Water and small craft rescue
- White water rescue

## Technical Rescue Situations

A technical rescue situation requires specialized skills and equipment to safely enter and move around. These situations may contain hidden dangers, and it is unsafe to include personnel who do not have the necessary training and experience. A technical rescue group is made up of people from one or more departments in a region who are trained and on call for certain types of technical rescues. Many members of a technical rescue group are also trained as emergency medical responders (EMRs) or EMTs so that they can provide the necessary immediate care when they safely reach the patient. Even when the technical rescue group includes a paramedic or physician, generally only essential care is provided until the group members can bring the patient to the nearest safe and stable setting, known as the staging area.

If a technical rescue group is necessary but is not present when you arrive, immediately check with the incident commander to make sure that the group has been summoned and is en route to your location. The incident commander is the individual who has overall command of the scene in the field (**FIGURE 39-11**). Although every team member's input at the scene is important, one person must be clearly in charge. A lack of identifiable leadership at the scene hinders the rescue effort and patient care. The incident commander's assessment of the patient and the scene will dictate how medical care, packaging, and transport will proceed. Usually, the

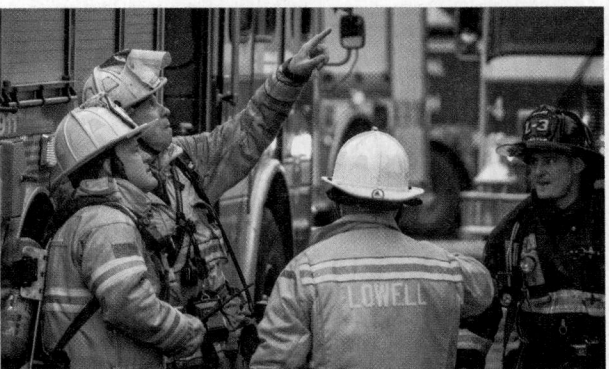

**FIGURE 39-11** The incident commander is the individual who has overall command of the scene. On February 24, 2019, command strategy is discussed at a large fire in an apartment building.

© Ted Pendergast/Shutterstock.

senior medical official is responsible for this role. If no incident commander is present, follow local guidelines. (Chapter 40, *Incident Management*, discusses this in more detail.)

When you arrive at a scene where a technical rescue is in progress, you will usually be met by a member of the technical rescue group and directed or led to the staging area. If the staging area is some distance from the road, you may need to leave the ambulance on the road. The use of the ambulance stretcher is impractical in these situations; instead take a backboard and/or basket stretcher (or similar rescue stretcher) to carry the patient back to the ambulance. Be sure that you take all of the jump kits and other equipment you may need to treat and stabilize the patient at the staging area.

When you arrive at the rescue site, identify the designated staging area and set up your equipment there. As soon as the technical rescue group brings the patient to the staging area, perform a primary assessment and, after providing the treatment indicated, package the patient without delay. Although you are responsible for the patient's care, it usually requires a cooperative effort by the technical rescue group and the EMTs to carry the patient to the waiting ambulance. Consider using air transport if the patient will need to be carried or transported an extensive distance.

## Safety Tips

Do not endanger yourself, your partner, or the patient by attempting a technical rescue if you do not have the appropriate training. Await the arrival of appropriately trained resources to implement the rescue. You are not helping the patient by getting yourself into danger (and potentially needing to be rescued yourself).

## Search and Rescue

When someone is missing outdoors and a search effort is initiated, an ambulance is usually summoned to the incident **command post** (location of the incident commander) or staging area. Each search team will be organized to include a member who is trained at the EMR or EMT level and who carries the essential equipment to provide essential, immediate care. Your role, and that of the other EMTs who arrive with the ambulance, is to stand by at the command post until the missing person or people have been found.

As soon as you arrive at the scene and have been briefed on the situation, you should isolate and prepare the equipment you will need to carry to the patient's location; this will save time once the patient has been found or if a member of the search team is

## YOU are the Provider

The side of the ultralight has been cut away using hydraulic tools, and the patient's seat has been cut to allow access. The patient's legs are freed by moving the back of the seat. You remove the patient from the wreckage using the rapid extrication technique and perform a rapid secondary assessment as your partner reassesses her vital signs.

| Recording Time: 18 Minutes | |
| --- | --- |
| Level of consciousness | Responsive to voice |
| Respirations | 14 breaths/min |
| Pulse | 148 beats/min; weak radial pulses |
| Skin | Cool, clammy, and pale |
| Blood pressure | 80/58 mm Hg |
| Spo$_2$ | 94% (on oxygen) |

You note a large, open wound just distal to her right knee with obvious deformity of the tibia. There is no active bleeding. After securing the patient to the long spine board, you cover her with a blanket.

**7.** How does the rapid extrication technique differ from other methods of patient removal? When is it indicated?

injured. The carry-in equipment, including a backboard or other devices you will need to immobilize the patient, should be left in the back of the ambulance until it is needed, so that it is protected from the weather. In addition, if the ambulance should need to be relocated, the equipment will not need to be reloaded and will not be left behind. You will usually be given a portable radio that is tuned to the search frequency so that you can monitor the progress of the search and communicate with those in charge of the search operation.

Sometimes, you may be asked to stay with relatives of the missing individual who are at the scene. Find out from relatives whether the missing person has any medical history that may need to be addressed and pass this information on to those who are in charge of the search. Unless you have been instructed otherwise, only the incident commander should communicate any news or progress of the search to the family. For this reason, be sure that your radio is set at a discreet volume.

Once the missing person has been found, you will be guided by search personnel to that location or to a prearranged meeting point where the patient will be carried, which allows you to begin treatment more quickly. Consider relocating the ambulance or, if one is available, using a four-wheel drive, all-terrain vehicle (ATV), or snowmobile to decrease the time and effort needed to reach and carry out the patient. In some cases, helicopter rescue may be the best method of removing the patient to a safe location. Be sure that equipment is evenly distributed among personnel and that the pace is such that all can stay together easily. Remember that although EMS will assume the responsibility for patient care once they are at the patient's side, a cooperative effort between the EMS and search teams is necessary to safely carry the patient to the staging area and waiting ambulance.

## Trench Rescue

Because of the physical forces involved, many cave-ins and trench collapses have poor outcomes for victims. Collapses usually involve large areas of falling dirt that weigh approximately 100 pounds per cubic foot (1,602 kg per cubic meter). Victims with thousands of pounds of dirt resting on their chests cannot fully expand their lungs and will become hypoxic.

The risk of a secondary collapse during the rescue operation is a concern for rescue personnel and EMTs. Safety measures can reduce the potential for injury from this and other hazards. When arriving on the scene of a cave-in or trench collapse, response vehicles should park at least 500 feet (150 m) from the scene. Because vibration is a primary cause of secondary collapse, all vehicles, including on-scene construction equipment, should be turned off. In addition, all road traffic should be diverted from the 500-foot (150-m) safety area. Other hazards include exposed or downed electric wires and broken gas or water lines. In addition, construction equipment at the collapse may be unstable and could fall into the cave-in or trench site.

Identify any witnesses to the incident. They may provide valuable information on the number of victims and their location within the collapsed area. Assist all uninjured people and nonessential personnel away from the area. At no time should medical or rescue personnel enter a trench deeper than 4 feet (1 m) without proper shoring (temporary supports to prevent collapse) in place.

During the extrication of any survivors from a cave-in or trench collapse site, trained medical personnel will provide most medical care. Be prepared to receive patients once they have been extricated from the site.

## Tactical Emergency Medical Support

A steady increase in violence throughout the country has resulted in EMTs taking precautions to ensure personal safety. Normally, when the potential for violence exists—as in shootings, stabbings, and attempted suicides—responding units should wait until the scene is secured by law enforcement officers. However, some incidents pose an increased risk to emergency responders. Hostage incidents, barricaded subjects, and snipers require the use of specialized law enforcement tactical units or the special weapons and tactics (SWAT) team.

Because of the high potential for injuries at these volatile incidents, many communities have incorporated specially trained EMTs, paramedics, nurses, and even physicians into their SWAT units. These EMS providers provide a special level of care to the sick and injured, and their training goes well beyond the practices seen in standard emergency medical care. Thus, the techniques used may seem inappropriate or inadequate. For example, spinal motion restriction is not used within an unsecured area where gunfire is a risk. The time and manpower necessary to completely secure a victim to a backboard may expose EMS providers and SWAT officers to injury or death from gunfire (**FIGURE 39-12**). Such altered standards of care are similar to those used by military EMS providers on the battlefield and are *not* used in the standard situations you will encounter as an EMT.

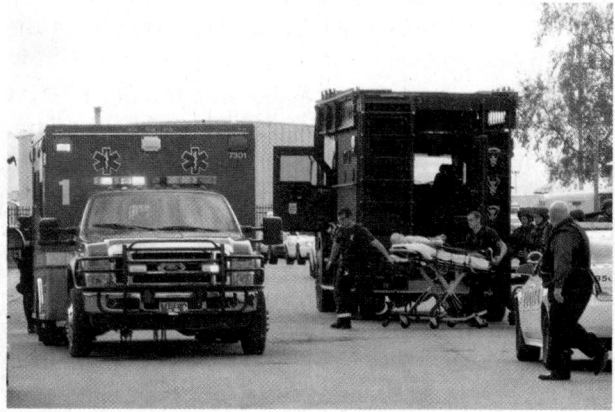

**FIGURE 39-12** Tactical EMS providers move a downed officer; only the most basic medical care is provided in an unsecured area.

© Rachel D'Oro/AP Photo.

When called to the scene of a law enforcement tactical situation, determine the location of the command post and report to the incident commander for instructions. Lights and siren should be turned off when nearing the scene, and outside radio speakers should not be used. The command post is usually located in an area that cannot be seen by the suspect and is out of range of possible gunfire. Remain in this area and do not roam beyond this site. Nearby areas may be visible to the suspect, and you could be injured.

Several planning measures will reduce the potential for chaos should a mass-casualty incident occur at the scene. First, have the incident commander identify the specific location of the incident, including the street address and the side of the street on which the house or building is located. The incident commander should determine a safe location (staging area) where you can meet SWAT team members or tactical EMS providers should an injury occur. The incident commander should also determine a safe route to this point. Tactical EMS providers or officers will remove the patient to this area for continued treatment and transport to a medical facility.

To save valuable time in critical situations, designate primary and secondary helicopter landing zones if your region uses aeromedical evacuation. The closest hospital, burn center, and trauma center should be identified. The route of travel to

## YOU are the Provider

A rescue team member drives the ambulance to the landing zone as your partner applies a rigid splint to the patient's right leg and covers the open wounds with a bulky dressing. You continue to attempt to obtain a brief medical history while you reassess her vital signs.

| Recording Time: 40 Minutes | |
| --- | --- |
| Level of consciousness | Responsive to voice |
| Respirations | 16 breaths/min; adequate |
| Pulse | 128 beats/min; weak radial pulse |
| Skin | Cool, clammy, and pale |
| Blood pressure | 84/60 mm Hg |
| Spo$_2$ | 96% (on oxygen) |

The medical helicopter is waiting, and you give a verbal report to the flight paramedic. You assist in the loading of the patient onto the helicopter. You then return to the scene to retrieve any equipment you may have left and to assist with removal of the pilot's body from the wreckage.

**8.** What are your considerations when calling for air transport?

## Words of Wisdom

The topic of active shooter and mass-casualty incidents has received a great deal of attention in recent years. In response, some EMS providers are being trained to enter the area directly around the hazard (the warm zone) with appropriate law enforcement cover. Their role is to identify patients, provide targeted lifesaving interventions, and perform extraction. Because it is impractical for EMS providers to carry large bags or heavy equipment, they generally provide only essential, specific care, including applying a tourniquet for hemorrhage control or maintaining an open airway with basic airway adjuncts and maneuvers.

Such policies should only be implemented in collaboration with local law enforcement and must include appropriate training. Training related to shooting incidents is an excellent resource for you; take advantage of these opportunities. However, traditional continuing education that focuses on high-quality CPR and other skills that have the greatest potential to save lives on a regular basis should receive the highest emphasis.

## Words of Wisdom

### F-A-I-L-U-R-E

The reasons for rescue failure can be summarized by the mnemonic FAILURE:

- **F** Failure to understand the environment or underestimating it
- **A** Additional medical problems not considered
- **I** Inadequate rescue skills
- **L** Lack of teamwork or experience
- **U** Underestimating the logistics of the incident
- **R** Rescue versus recovery mode not considered
- **E** Equipment not mastered

these facilities should also be noted. Many of these measures are incorporated into the operational plan used by tactical EMS providers. If tactical EMS providers are used in your jurisdiction, coordinate with them on your arrival at the command post.

## Structure Fires

In most areas, an ambulance is dispatched with the fire department to any **structure fire**, whether or not injuries are reported. A fire in a house or other building is considered a structure fire. When responding to a major fire scene, determine whether any special route will be necessary to reach the scene. Once you arrive at the scene, ask the incident commander where the ambulance should be staged. It is essential that the ambulance be staged in a visible location but parked far enough from the active scene to be safe from the fire itself or a collapsing building. You must also ensure that the ambulance will not block other arriving units or be blocked in by other equipment or hose lines. The fire officer who is the incident commander will help to determine this location.

After parking your ambulance, your next step is to determine whether there are any injured patients at the scene or whether you have been called to stand by. When you check in with the incident commander, you should be able to obtain this information. It is common for multiple ambulances to be dispatched to a structure fire. This practice allows for transport of any patients who are immediately found to require medical attention, as well as a resource to stand by during the firefighting operations. An ambulance should be available to assist with any rehabilitation efforts for firefighters. For further discussion of scene management, such as rehabilitation considerations for providers, see Chapter 40, *Incident Management*.

As with other specialized rescue situations, search and rescue in a burning building requires special training and equipment. Search and rescue operations are performed by teams of firefighters wearing full turnout gear and **self-contained breathing apparatus (SCBA)** and carrying tools and fully charged hose lines. These teams will bring patients out of the burning building to the area where the ambulance is staged. Therefore, unless otherwise ordered, you should always stay with the ambulance. Do not leave the scene even after the fire is out because you may need to treat a firefighter who has been injured during salvage and overhaul. The ambulance should leave the scene only if transporting a patient or if the incident commander has released it.

Sometimes the scene at a fire is complicated by the presence of hazardous materials. In addition to posing a threat to you and others at the immediate scene, hazardous materials may pose a threat to a larger population. Whenever there is a possibility that a hazardous material is involved, you will have to follow several additional special procedures. Chapter 40, *Incident Management*, covers the specifics of hazardous material procedures.

## YOU are the Provider SUMMARY

**1. What information is obtained from a 360° assessment of an aircraft crash?**

The 360° assessment of an aircraft crash focuses on hazards unique to this type of incident. Common safety hazards include leaking fuels or other fluids, smoke or fire, broken glass, twisted metal, and aircraft instability. Safety issues must be addressed by the appropriate personnel before anyone attempts to gain access to the patient or patients.

Other information obtained during the 360° assessment of a plane crash includes the mechanism of injury, the position of the patient or patients in the aircraft, and whether patients are entrapped or have been ejected.

**2. How would your approach change if leaking fuel were present?**

A scene with leaking fuel cannot be made 100% safe unless the plane's fuel tank can be emptied. Safely emptying a fuel tank may not be possible before the patient's condition deteriorates. Therefore, it is imperative that you understand the capabilities of the fire department and rescue team and that all efforts be efficiently coordinated. The approach to extricating the patient and the speed with which this is accomplished may change based on the hazards present and the capabilities of the resources. Your safety and the safety of fellow responders comes first. Understand the risks of attempting such a rescue and plan an exit route in the event the scene becomes more unstable. Fuel spills must also be handled appropriately by qualified personnel. Rescue attempts may ignite the fuel. If the fuel spills onto the patient, he or she will have to be decontaminated prior to transport. Avoid walking through fuel spills, which will contaminate your own boots and then the ambulance.

**3. How should you initially attempt to gain access to a crash victim?**

Do not attempt to gain access to the patient until you are sure that the wreckage is stable and that any hazards have been identified and properly controlled or eliminated. The incident commander will inform you when it is safe to gain access to the patient.

Whenever possible, you should use simple access techniques to get to the patient. Try to unlock and open all of the doors, starting with the least damaged door. Using simple techniques can often save you valuable time, as extrication with hydraulic tools can take several minutes or longer. If the patient's condition requires immediate care and you cannot access the passenger compartment, attempt to provide basic care through windows or openings as the extrication is performed. Be on constant alert for dangers to yourself, your partner, and the patient.

If you must break a window to gain access, try to break one that is farthest away from the patient. However, if the patient's condition warrants immediate entry (ie, airway compromise, severe bleeding), do not hesitate to break the closest window. If you cannot gain access to the patient by opening a door or breaking a window, pneumatic and/or hydraulic rescue tools will be necessary to gain access to the patient and allow extrication of the patient from the vehicle.

**4. What treatment should you provide to a patient who is entrapped in wreckage?**

Treatment should occur only if there is no immediate threat of fire, explosion, or other danger. Once entry and access to the patient have been provided, perform a primary assessment and begin immediate emergency care before the process of extrication begins. Focus on identifying and correcting immediate life threats. A lengthy, detailed assessment is inappropriate because this delays the process of patient extrication. Pass on any information that you obtain about the type or degree of entrapment to the extrication team.

In the case of this patient, you can access only her head and upper extremities. Her legs and torso are pinned by the wreckage. Your partner is manually stabilizing the patient's head and maintaining an open airway with a modified jaw thrust. The airway is clear, and she is breathing, although the rate is a little slow and shallow. There is not enough room to ventilate the patient with a bag-mask device, but you can apply a nonrebreathing mask to facilitate oxygenation until you have full access to her airway. You have already determined that her pulse is weak and rapid, and her skin is cool, clammy, and pale. You note lacerations to her forehead and right arm.

On the basis of your findings, you should apply high-flow oxygen, control the bleeding from her forehead and arm, and control any other bleeding to the areas of her body that you can access. It would be appropriate to apply a cervical collar—after assessing the back of the neck for any deformities—to help maintain cervical spine alignment and stability. Cover as much of the patient as you can with a blanket to preserve body heat and to protect the patient from broken glass or metal fragments during the extrication process.

The patient is showing signs of shock; therefore, after correcting problems with airway, breathing, and circulation, she must be extricated so that you can complete your assessment and provide additional treatment including spinal motion restriction.

**5. Is it appropriate to obtain the vital signs of a patient who is entrapped? Why or why not?**

It is not always appropriate or practical to obtain a complete set of vital signs while a patient is

## YOU are the Provider SUMMARY *continued*

entrapped. Your primary focus should be to provide immediate lifesaving care and then have the patient extricated as quickly and safely as possible. While providing lifesaving care or if extrication is delayed, it is reasonable to obtain pertinent vital signs to help you determine the patient's status and overall acuity. For example, you may be able to palpate a radial pulse or note whether the patient is breathing slowly or rapidly as well as the quality of the respirations and presence of any respiratory distress. Noting a weak, rapid pulse in this scenario may help strengthen your suspicions of hemorrhagic shock. This check will not constitute a complete set of vital signs; however, it may help to identify acute changes in the patient's condition throughout extrication.

Do not delay extrication to assess the patient's vital signs. The longer the patient remains trapped in the vehicle, the longer the delay to definitive care.

### 6. What should you do as the patient is being extricated from the wreckage?

During the coordinated extrication process, your input is essential. Communication with the patient and fellow rescuers is extremely important. If you notice that the patient has life-threatening hemorrhage after her legs are freed from underneath the wreckage, you should communicate the need for immediate treatment before allowing further efforts at removing the patient. If the patient suddenly screams in pain, instruct the rescue team to stop extrication if possible while you determine where the patient is hurting; it may be necessary for the rescue team to take a different extrication approach.

Once a plan has been devised and all team members understand what will be done, you have a role in protecting the patient. Be sure you are all wearing the appropriate protective clothing (ie, a bunker coat, heavy-duty gloves [over your exam gloves], a rescue helmet with goggles and mask or full face shield, and hearing protection). You may also be able to shield the patient with a fire safety blanket. When possible, position yourself alongside the patient to monitor his or her condition as the wreckage is being cut, bent, or disassembled. In the case of this patient, you and your partner are positioned on opposite sides of the aircraft. Your partner should continue to provide manual stabilization of the cervical spine if it can be managed safely while you continue assessment and treatment of life-threatening injuries.

### 7. How does the rapid extrication technique differ from other methods of patient removal? When is it indicated?

The main difference between the rapid extrication technique and other methods of patient removal (ie, short backboard, vest-style extrication device) is that it is fast and requires minimal preparation of the patient in the vehicle before he or she is removed. For example, it takes between 6 and 8 minutes—and in some cases, even longer—to properly apply a spinal immobilization device. This is clearly too long when your patient is critically injured and needs immediate treatment and transport. The rapid extrication technique can be performed in 1 minute or less, but should be done carefully with as little spinal motion as possible while moving the patient onto a backboard for transfer to the ambulance stretcher.

### 8. What are your considerations when calling for air transport?

Air transport is an excellent consideration when a patient is in critical condition. Patients with time-sensitive conditions or who require a higher level of care, such as advanced airway management or blood product administration in trauma, may benefit from the expertise and available resources that can be provided by a critical care flight team. Medical helicopters can quickly access remote locations and provide rapid transport to definitive care. You must locate an area that is large enough and obstacle-free to allow for a landing zone. If the rescue site is not accessible as a landing zone, identify the nearest safe location and transport the patient by ambulance to the alternative location. To save valuable time in critical situations, designate primary and secondary helicopter landing zones.

### EMS Patient Care Report (PCR)

| Date: 11-30-20 | Incident No.: 013210 | Nature of Call: Aircraft crash | | Location: 24 Palm Blvd. | |
|---|---|---|---|---|---|
| Dispatched: 1400 | En Route: 1401 | At Scene: 1408 | Transport: 1448 | At Landing Zone: 1450 | In Service: 1530 |

### Patient Information

**Age:** Approximately 55
**Sex:** F
**Weight (in kg [lb]):** 68 kg (150 lb)

**Allergies:** Unknown
**Medications:** Unknown
**Past Medical History:** Unknown
**Chief Complaint:** Altered mental status and multiple traumatic injuries

# YOU are the Provider SUMMARY *continued*

### Vital Signs

| | | | | |
|---|---|---|---|---|
| **Time:** 1415 | **BP:** 98/40 | **Pulse:** 138 | **Respirations:** 15 | **Spo$_2$:** 93% |
| **Time:** 1420 | **BP:** 94/50 | **Pulse:** 142 | **Respirations:** 15 | **Spo$_2$:** 93% |
| **Time:** 1426 | **BP:** 80/58 | **Pulse:** 148 | **Respirations:** 14 | **Spo$_2$:** 94% |
| **Time:** 1438 | **BP:** 82/60 | **Pulse:** 136 | **Respirations:** 14 | **Spo$_2$:** 94% |
| **Time:** 1448 | **BP:** 84/60 | **Pulse:** 128 | **Respirations:** 16 | **Spo$_2$:** 96% |

### EMS Treatment (circle all that apply)

| Oxygen @ _15_ L/min via:  NC (NRM) Bag mask | | Assisted Ventilation | Airway Adjunct | CPR |
|---|---|---|---|---|
| **Defibrillation** | **Bleeding Control** | (**Bandaging**) | **Splinting:** (Right lower extremity) | **Other:** (Spinal motion restriction; maintain warmth) |

### Narrative

EMS was dispatched to beach access at 24 Palm Blvd for an ultralight aircraft crash involving two passengers.

Chief Complaint: Altered mental status and multiple traumatic injuries

History: Medical history unknown. Passenger in an ultralite airplane that crashed.

Assessment: On arrival, fire rescue on scene advised that the scene was safe. The aircraft was stabilized, and fire personnel were preparing equipment for extrication. A 360° assessment of the victims showed that the pilot had massive trauma to the head and chest that was incompatible with life. An unresponsive female passenger, approximately 55 years, occupied the second seat. There were no windows in the aircraft, only the windshield in front of the pilot. The patient's head and upper extremities were accessible through bars along the portion of the plane next to the patient, but her lower extremities were not visible under the wreckage. Laceration to the forehead from the temple through the left orbit with minimal bleeding; laceration to right arm with the bones of the elbow exposed.

Treatment (Rx): Cervical spine immobilization was established, and the patient's airway opened using the jaw thrust. Respirations were shallow, radial pulses were present but weak, and her skin was pale, cool, and diaphoretic. Unable to use a bag mask device to ventilate the patient because of space restrictions, so she was placed on a nonrebreathing mask at 15 L/min. Patient had a large laceration superior to her left orbit and laceration to her right arm; both were bandaged, and the patient was covered with a blanket to preserve heat and provide protection. Side bars were removed, and a side flap was created by rescue team to allow access to the patient. Patient responding to voice at this time. Seat was disassembled, and the patient was extricated onto a backboard. The patient's clothing was removed, and she was covered with blankets.

Transport: Patient fully immobilized and moved to ambulance on a backboard for transport to the helicopter landing zone. Reassessed vital signs and splinted fracture of right lower extremity in the ambulance with long board splints. Transferred to air transport team, and gave verbal report to flight paramedic. Medic 8 returned to service at 1530.

**End of report**

# Prep Kit

## Ready for Review

- You must always be prepared, mentally and physically, for any incident that requires rescue or extrication.
- As an EMT, your first priority in a rescue incident is personal safety.
- EMS personnel are responsible for the assessment, care, triage, packaging, and transport of patients.
- The rescue team secures and stabilizes the vehicle, provides safe access to patients, and safely extricates patients.
- Law enforcement officers control traffic, maintain order at the scene, establish and maintain a perimeter, and ultimately investigate the crash or crime scene.
- Firefighters extinguish fire, prevent additional ignition, ensure scene safety, and remove spilled fuel. Variations in responsibilities are possible, depending on jurisdictional protocols.
- Vehicle safety systems, such as shock-absorbing bumpers and airbags, protect your patients but also have the potential to injure you.
- Simple access is easily achieved without the use of tools or force. Complex access requires heavy-duty tools and special training.
- The 10 phases of extrication are:
  - Preparation
  - En route to the scene
  - Arrival and scene size-up
  - Hazard control
  - Support operations
  - Gaining access
  - Emergency care
  - Removal of the patient
  - Transfer of the patient
  - Termination
- In some situations, the patient can only be reached by teams trained in special technical rescues. Situations requiring specialized teams include:
  - Cave rescue
  - Confined space rescue
  - Cross-field and trail rescue (park rangers)
  - Dive rescue
  - Missing person search and rescue
  - Mine rescue
  - Mountain-, rock-, and ice-climbing rescue
  - Ski slope and cross-country or trail snow rescue (ski patrol)
  - Structural collapse rescue
  - Special weapons and tactics (SWAT) team
  - Technical rope rescue (low- and high-angle rescue)
  - Trench rescue
  - Water and small craft rescue
  - White water rescue

## Vital Vocabulary

**access** Gaining entry to an enclosed area and reaching a patient.

**command post** The location of the incident commander at the scene of an emergency and where command, coordination, control, and communication are centralized.

**complex access** Entry that requires special tools and training and includes the use of force.

**danger zone (hot zone)** An area where people can be exposed to hazards such as electric wires, sharp metal edges, broken glass, toxic substances, radiation, or fire.

**entrapment** To be caught (trapped) within a vehicle, room, or container with no way out or to have a limb or other body part trapped.

**extrication** Removal of a patient from entrapment or a dangerous situation or position, such as removal from a wrecked vehicle, industrial incident, or collapsed building.

**hazardous materials** Any substances that are toxic, poisonous, radioactive, flammable, or explosive and cause injury or death with exposure.

**incident commander** The individual who has overall command of the incident in the field.

**safe zone** An area of protection providing safety from the danger zone (hot zone).

**self-contained breathing apparatus (SCBA)** Respirator with independent air supply used by firefighters to enter toxic and otherwise dangerous atmospheres.

**simple access** Access that is easily achieved without the use of tools or force.

**size-up** The ongoing process of information gathering and scene evaluation to determine appropriate strategies and tactics to manage an emergency.

**special weapons and tactics (SWAT) team** A specialized law enforcement tactical unit.

**structure fire** A fire in a house, apartment building, office, school, plant, warehouse, or other building.

**tactical situation** A hostage, robbery, or other situation in which armed conflict is threatened or shots have been fired and the threat of violence remains.

**technical rescue group** A team of emergency responders from one or more departments in a region who are trained and on call for certain types of technical rescue.

**technical rescue situation** A rescue that requires special technical skills and equipment in one of many specialized rescue areas, such as technical rope rescue, cave rescue, and dive rescue.

## References

1. Long RT Jr, Blum AF, Bress TJ, Cotts BRT. *Best Practices for Emergency Response to Incidents Involving Electric Vehicles Battery Hazards: A Report on Full-Scale Testing Results.* Bowie, MD: Fire Protection Research Foundation; 2013.

2. National Highway Traffic Safety Administration. Air bag deployment. http://www.safercar.gov/Vehicle+Shoppers /Air+Bags/Air+Bag+Deployment. Accessed March 2, 2020.

3. National Highway Traffic Safety Administration. *National Emergency Medical Services Education Standards.* DOT HS 811 077A. www.ems.gov/pdf/811077a.pdf. Published January 2009. Accessed March 2, 2020.

4. National Highway Traffic Safety Administration. *National Emergency Medical Services Education Standards. Emergency Medical Technician Instructional Guidelines.* DOT HS 811 077C. www.ems.gov/pdf/811077c.pdf. Published January 2009. Accessed March 2, 2020.

5. Teixeira PGR, Brown CVR, Emigh B, et al. Civilian prehospital tourniquet use is associated with improved survival in patients with peripheral vascular injury. *J Am Coll Surg.* 226(5);2018:769–776.

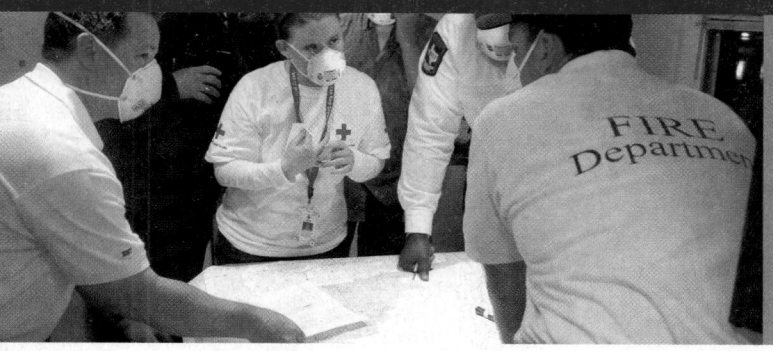

# Chapter 40

# Incident Management

## NATIONAL EMS EDUCATION STANDARD COMPETENCIES

### EMS Operations

Knowledge of operational roles and responsibilities to ensure patient, public, and personnel safety.

### Incident Management

- Establish and work within the incident management system. (pp 1486–1495)

### Multiple-Casualty Incidents*

- Triage principles (pp 1497–1499)
- Resource management (pp 1486–1487, 1491–1495)

- Triage (pp 1497–1502)
  - Performing (pp 1497–1502)
  - Retriage (p 1498)
  - Destination decisions (pp 1501–1502)
  - Posttraumatic and cumulative stress (pp 1495, 1502)

### Hazardous Materials Awareness

- Risks and responsibilities of operating in a cold zone at a hazardous material or other special incident. (pp 1514–1515)

## KNOWLEDGE OBJECTIVES

1. Describe the purpose of the National Incident Management System (NIMS) and its major components. (pp 1486–1487)
2. Describe the purpose of the incident command system (ICS) and its organizational structure. (pp 1487–1491)
3. Explain the role of EMS response within the ICS. (pp 1491–1493)
4. Describe how the ICS assists EMS in ensuring both personal safety and the safety of bystanders, health care professionals, and patients during an emergency. (pp 1492–1493)
5. Describe the role of the EMT in establishing command under the ICS. (p 1493)
6. Describe the purpose of the medical branch of the ICS and its organizational structure. (pp 1493–1495)
7. Describe the specific conditions that would define a situation as a mass-casualty incident (MCI); include examples. (pp 1496–1497)

8. Describe what occurs during primary and secondary triage, how the four triage categories are assigned to patients on the scene, and how destination decisions regarding triaged patients are made. (pp 1497–1499)
9. Explain how to perform the START and JumpSTART triage methods. (pp 1499–1501)
10. Contrast a disaster with a mass-casualty incident. (p 1502)
11. Describe the role of EMTs during a disaster operation. (p 1502)
12. Recognize the entry-level training or experience requirements identified by the HAZWOPER regulation for EMTs to respond to a hazmat incident. (p 1503)
13. Define hazardous material; include the classification system used by the National Fire Protection Association (NFPA). (pp 1503, 1516)

---

*This text uses the term mass-casualty incident.

14. Discuss the specific reference materials that EMTs use to recognize a hazmat incident. (pp 1510–1513)

15. Explain the role of EMTs during a hazmat incident both before and after the hazmat team arrives; include the precautions required to ensure the safety of civilians and responders. (pp 1514–1515)

16. Describe how the three control zones are established at a hazmat incident, the characteristics of each zone, and the responders who work within each one. (pp 1514–1515)

17. Describe the four levels of personal protective equipment (PPE) required at a hazmat incident to protect responders from injury by or contamination from a particular substance. (pp 1516–1517)

18. Explain patient care at a hazmat incident; include the special requirements that are necessary for those patients who require immediate treatment and transport prior to full decontamination. (pp 1517–1519)

## SKILLS OBJECTIVES

1. Demonstrate how to perform triage based on a fictional scenario that involves a mass-casualty incident. (pp 1497–1501)

2. Using a reference, correctly identify Department of Transportation (DOT) labels, placards, and markings that are used to designate hazardous materials. (pp 1508–1509)

3. Demonstrate the ability to use a variety of reference materials to identify a hazardous material. (pp 1510–1514)

# Introduction

Some of the most challenging situations you will encounter are disasters and mass-casualty incidents. In this text, a disaster refers to any situation that overwhelms your resources. A single incident with two critical patients can constitute a disaster if there is only one EMS unit available to respond. A mass-casualty incident (MCI) refers to any call that involves three or more patients, any situation that places such a great demand on available equipment or personnel that the system would require a mutual aid response (an agreement between neighboring EMS systems to respond when local resources are insufficient to handle the response), or any incident that has the potential to create one of the previously mentioned situations. Bus or train crashes and earthquakes are obvious examples of MCIs. These incidents can be overwhelming because you will encounter a large number of patients and not enough resources.

When you respond to an event with a large number of patients, you must use a systematic approach to manage the incident efficiently. By learning to use the principles of the incident command system (ICS), you will be able to do the greatest good for the greatest number of people. As an EMT, you will typically be assigned to work within the EMS/medical branch under an ICS, but you may be asked to function in other areas, which will be discussed later in this chapter. The National Incident Management System (NIMS) was developed to promote more efficient coordination between emergency responders at the regional, state, and national levels. To reduce on-scene problems and to increase your efficiency, you need a solid understanding of the basics of the NIMS. Training courses may also be accessed through the Federal Emergency Management System (FEMA) website.

# National Incident Management System

The Department of Homeland Security implemented the National Incident Management System (NIMS) in 2004. Most incidents are handled at the local level, but major incidents require the involvement of multiple jurisdictions, agencies, and emergency response disciplines. The NIMS provides a comprehensive framework to enable federal, state, and local governments, as well as private-sector and nongovernmental organizations, to work together effectively. The NIMS is used to prepare for, prevent, respond to, mitigate, and recover from domestic incidents, regardless of cause, size, or complexity, including acts of catastrophic terrorism and hazardous materials (hazmat) incidents.

Two important underlying principles of the NIMS are flexibility and standardization. The organizational structure must be flexible enough to be rapidly adapted for use in any situation. The NIMS provides standardization in terminology, resource classification, personnel training, certification, and more. This standardization allows for unity of effort, which is a third guiding principle of NIMS. Unity of effort allows various agencies to achieve common objectives by supporting each other while maintaining individual authorities. In other words, multiple agencies can work together toward the same goal, while maintaining their autonomy. The unity of effort is possible due, in part, to the NIMS concept of interoperability, which refers to the ability of agencies of different types or from different jurisdictions to communicate with each other. Interoperability can be accomplished by maintaining a shared frequency or by having radio systems programmed to other agencies' frequencies.

The ICS is one component of the NIMS. The three major NIMS components are as follows:

1. **Communications and information management.** Effective communications, information management, and information sharing are critical aspects of domestic incident management. The NIMS communications and information management systems enable the essential functions needed to assess available information, provide interoperability, and ensure appropriate communication of decisions.
2. **Resource management.** The NIMS sets up mechanisms to describe, inventory, track, and dispatch resources before, during, and after an incident. The NIMS also defines standard procedures to recover equipment used during the incident.
3. **Command and coordination.** The NIMS standardizes incident management for all hazards and across all levels of government. It provides comprehensive frameworks and recommended organizational structures. The NIMS standard incident command structures are based on three key constructs: ICS, multiagency coordination systems, and public information systems.

## Incident Command System

It is important for you to be familiar with the terminology and concepts of the incident command system (ICS). (Some agencies refer to the incident command system as the incident management system.) The purpose of the ICS is to ensure responder and public safety, achieve incident management goals, and ensure the efficient use of resources.

As you know, communication is the building block of good patient care. Common terminology and the use of clear text communications (plain English as opposed to 10-codes) help responders from multiple agencies work efficiently together.

Using the ICS gives you a modular organizational structure that can be applied to all hazards. The ICS can be activated for incidents ranging from a single vehicle crash with one patient to a natural gas pipeline explosion involving multiple communities and numerous injuries. The goal of the ICS is to make the best use of your resources to manage the environment around the incident and to treat patients during an emergency. The ICS is designed to avoid duplication of effort and freelancing, in which individual units or different organizations make independent and often inefficient decisions about the next appropriate action. Follow your local standard operating procedures for establishing the ICS.

One of the organizing principles of the ICS is to limit the span of control of any one individual. This principle refers to keeping the supervisor/worker ratio at one supervisor for five subordinates. A supervisor who has more than five people reporting to him or her is exceeding an effective span of control and needs to divide tasks and delegate the supervision of some tasks to another person. The NIMS does acknowledge that this is a guideline. Incident personnel may evaluate the actual incident and use their best judgment to determine the appropriate span of control.

The organizational levels may include sections, branches, divisions, and groups **FIGURE 40-1**:

- **Sections** are responsible for a major functional area such as finance/administration, logistics, planning, or operations.
- **Branches** are managed by the branch director and may be functional or geographic in nature. These tend to be established when span of control is a problem—for example, at larger incidents, where more oversight may be needed. Branches are in charge of activity directly related to the section (ie, fire, law enforcement, EMS, operations, etc.).
- **Divisions and groups** serve to align resources and/or crews under one supervisor. Divisions usually refer to crews working in the same geographic area. Groups usually refer to crews working in the same functional area, but possibly in different locations. To better visualize how divisions and groups work, think about an incident involving a mid-air collision between two commercial aircraft. With two scenes separated by almost a mile, Division A, composed of a fire suppression group, a rescue group, and an EMS group, may be assigned to work the site where the first aircraft came down.

Generally, the larger the incident, the more divisions there will be. A small incident may require

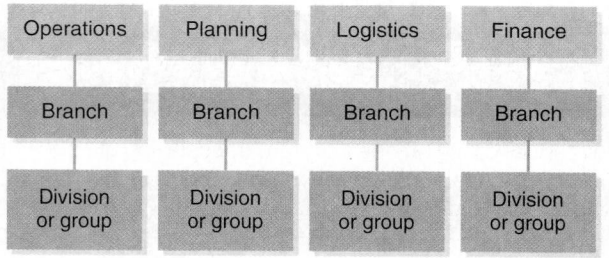

**FIGURE 40-1** The ICS organizational structure may include sections, branches, divisions, and groups.

only an incident commander and support from fire, EMS, and law enforcement. An incident on a much larger scale, such as the Boston Marathon bombing in 2013, will require massive efforts and many agencies working together.

In some regions, emergency operations centers may exist. The centers are usually operated by the city, state, or federal government. These centers will usually be activated only in a catastrophic event that may go on for days, or a pandemic that may be problematic for weeks or months. Such events can involve hundreds of patients and tax the entire system. Most emergency operating centers were activated during the COVID-19 pandemic to coordinate resources between government resources and prehospital care, healthcare, and public health.

The responders who will participate in an MCI or a disaster should use the ICS. When an incident occurs, find out from your service who is in charge, how it is activated, and what your expected role will be.

## ICS Roles and Responsibilities

There are many roles defined in the ICS. The general staff includes command, finance/administration, logistics, operations, and planning. It is important for you to understand the specific duties of each and how they work to coordinate the response. Command staff include the public information officer (PIO), safety officer, and liaison officer.

### Command

The incident commander (IC) is the person in charge of the overall incident. The IC will assess the incident, establish the strategic objectives and priorities, and develop a plan to manage the incident (**FIGURE 40-2**). The number of command duties the IC takes on often varies by the size of the incident. Small incidents often mean the IC will assume responsibility for all command duties. In an incident of medium size or complexity, the IC may delegate some functions but retain others. For example, at a motor vehicle crash site with multiple patients, the IC may designate a safety officer or assign a PIO but maintain responsibility for the other command functions. In a complex situation, the IC may appoint team members to all command roles.

Large MCIs, such as a hazmat incident, require a multiagency or multijurisdictional response and need to use a unified command system. In this case, plans are drawn up in advance by all agencies that

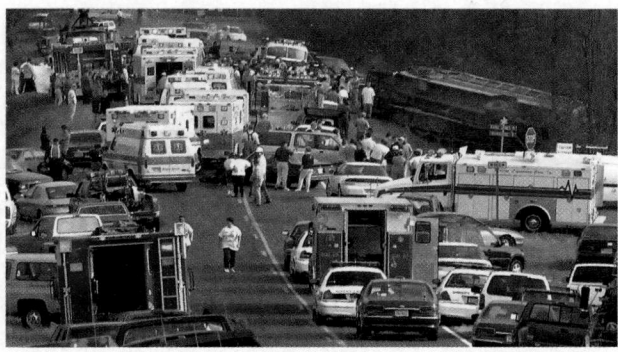

**FIGURE 40-2** The person in command at a mass-casualty incident oversees the incident and develops a plan for the response.

© David Crigger/Bristol Herald Courier/AP Images.

assume a shared responsibility for decision making. The response plan should designate the lead and support agencies in several types of MCIs. (For example, the hazmat team will take the lead in a chemical leak, whereas the medical team will take the lead in a multivehicle crash.) Agencies that share a border should train often with each other to ensure that a unified command system will function well and that communication among the responders is well established before a real incident occurs.

A single command system is one in which one person is in charge, even if multiple agencies respond. It is generally used with incidents in which one agency has the most responsibility for incident management. Ideally, it is used for short-duration, limited incidents that require the services of a single agency.

Your IC should be on or near the scene, where he or she can easily communicate with all emergency responders. It is important that you know who the IC is, how to communicate with the IC, and where the command post is located. If the incident is very large, you will report to a supervisor working under the IC. This will help to maintain a manageable span of control. To make the IC easily identifiable, some type of garment is worn, such as a brightly colored vest labeled with the word COMMAND. The command post may be set up at a vehicle, and it may be identified by a placard or unique color strobe (green is commonly used to identify a command post). Make sure your supervisor or the IC knows of any plans or operations before they are initiated.

Communication is particularly important if a transfer of command takes place. Because an incident can rapidly change in size and complexity, an IC may turn over command to someone with more experience in a critical area. This change, or transfer of command, must take place in an orderly manner and, if possible, face-to-face. In extreme situations, it could be done by phone, radio, or email, although these methods are not recommended. It is imperative that the transfer of command be communicated to those involved in the incident, especially the command staff and general staff. Your agency should have standard operating procedures that govern the transfer of command. Make certain to follow the standard operating procedures. When an incident draws to a close, there should be a termination of command. Your agency should implement demobilization procedures as the situation deescalates or comes to an end.

## Finance/Administration

The finance/administration section chief is responsible for documenting all expenditures at an incident for reimbursement. Finance personnel are not usually needed at smaller incidents, but at larger incidents it is necessary to keep track of personnel hours and expenditures for materials and supplies. Ultimately, that information is reported at meetings of the general staff. Responding agencies and organizations may be eligible for reimbursement after the incident, and an efficient finance/administration section chief will help your agency to succeed in the reimbursement process. Finance personnel should be trained in the process of assessing expenditures long before an actual incident.

The various functions within the finance/administration section include (1) the time unit, (2) the procurement unit, (3) the compensation and claims unit, and (4) the cost unit. The time unit is responsible for ensuring the daily recording of personnel time and equipment use. The procurement unit deals with all matters concerning vendor contracts. The compensation and claims unit has two major purposes: dealing with claims as a result of the incident, and injury compensation. Finally, the cost unit is responsible for collecting, analyzing, and reporting the costs related to an incident.

## Logistics

The logistics section is responsible for communications equipment, facilities, food and water, fuel, lighting, and medical equipment and supplies for patients and emergency responders. Local standard operating procedures will list the medical equipment needed for the incident, depending on the type of incident. Logistics personnel are trained to find food, shelter, fuel, and health care for you and the other responders at the scene of an MCI. In a large incident, it is often necessary for many people to handle logistics, but only the section chief will report to the IC.

## Operations

At a large or complex incident, the IC should appoint an operations section chief, who is responsible for managing the tactical operations usually handled by the IC on routine EMS calls. This frees the IC to coordinate with other agencies and the media, engage in strategic planning, and ensure that logistics are functioning effectively. The operations section chief will supervise the people working at the scene of the incident, who will be assigned to branches, divisions, and groups. Operations personnel often have experience in management within EMS.

## Planning

The planning section solves problems as they arise during the incident. Planners obtain data about the problem, analyze the previous incident plan, and predict what or who is needed to make the new plan work. They need to work closely with the operations, finance/administration, and, especially, logistics sections. Planners can and should call on technical experts to help with the planning process. They should document their decisions and what they learned from the incident and set out a course for demobilizing the response when necessary.

Another function of the planning section is the development of an incident action plan, which is the central tool for planning during a response to a disaster emergency. The incident action plan is prepared by the planning section chief with input from the appropriate sections and units of the incident command team. The purpose of an incident action plan is to provide clear, concise information about incident activities, including objectives, tactics, and assignments. It should be written at the outset of the response and revised continually throughout the response. In an initial response for an incident that is readily controlled, a written plan may not be necessary. Larger, more complex incidents will require an incident action plan to coordinate activities. The level of detail required in an incident action plan will vary according to the size and complexity of the response.

## Command Staff

Three important positions that help the general staff (described previously) and the IC are the safety officer, the PIO, and the liaison officer. The safety officer monitors the scene for conditions or operations that may present a hazard to responders and patients. The safety officer may need to work with environmental health and hazmat specialists. The importance of the safety officer cannot be underestimated—he or she has the authority to stop an emergency operation whenever a rescuer is in danger. A safety officer should remove hazards to EMS personnel and patients before the hazards cause injury.

The public information officer (PIO) provides the public and media with clear and understandable information. A wise PIO positions his or her headquarters well away from the incident command post and, most important, away from the incident, to minimize distractions. Also, the PIO must keep the media safe and from becoming part of the incident. The designated PIO may cooperate with PIOs from other agencies in a joint information center (JIC). In some circumstances, the PIO/JIC may be responsible for distributing a message designed to help a situation, prevent panic, and provide evacuation directions.

The liaison officer relays information and concerns among command, the general staff, and other agencies. If an agency is not represented in the command structure, questions and input should be given through the liaison officer.

## Communications and Information Management

Communications has historically been the weak point at most major incidents. To minimize the effects of communications problems, it is recommended that communications be integrated. This means that all agencies involved should be able to communicate quickly and effortlessly via radios. Communications allow for accountability throughout the incident, as well as instant communication between recipients. As always, and more so during a large incident, you must maintain professionalism on all radio communications, and remember to communicate clearly and concisely using plain language (not 10-codes or language specific to just your system).

## Mobilization and Deployment

When an incident has been declared and the need for additional resources has been identified, a request is made for additional resources. Once a request is made, these resources are mobilized and deployed to the scene. It is important to wait until the request is made before you depart for the scene, to minimize the potential for freelancing.

## Check-in at the Incident

On arrival at an incident, first check in with the IC at the base, staging area, or other location designated by the IC. If the incident is large in size or complexity, you will be assigned to a supervisor working under the IC. Check-in also allows for personnel tracking throughout the incident, and ensures that costs, wages, and reimbursement can be calculated accurately. Should a building collapse or secondary incident occur, it is vital for the IC to have an accurate report of what resources and personnel were on scene prior to that secondary event.

## Initial Incident Briefing

After the check-in process is complete, report to your supervisor for an initial briefing that will allow you to obtain information regarding the incident, as well as your specific job functions and responsibilities.

## Incident Record Keeping

Record keeping is important for financial reasons and for documentation purposes. If a large piece of equipment becomes inoperable, it may be possible for the agency to be reimbursed for replacement costs. Record keeping also allows for tracking of time spent on the incident for reimbursement purposes.

## Accountability

Because of the large number of responders at a large incident, accountability is important. Accountability means keeping your supervisor advised of your location, actions, and completed tasks. It also includes advising your supervisor of the tasks that you have been unable to complete and what tools you need to complete them.

## Incident Demobilization

Once the incident has been stabilized and all of the hazards mitigated, the IC will determine which resources are needed or not needed and when to begin demobilization. This process allows for a prompt return of resources to their parent organizations to be placed back in service.

### Words of Wisdom

Preplanning is crucial to the success of an MCI response, as is participating in mock or practice MCI drills. Once a disaster plan is in place, it should be run as a simulation event. Multiple agencies should be invited to participate, including police, fire, EMS, helicopter services, and hospitals. After the drill, a debriefing allows responders to review the plan's effectiveness and make any necessary changes.

## EMS Response Within the ICS
### Preparedness

Preparedness involves the decisions made and basic planning done before an incident occurs. Every state is at risk for natural disasters, such as hurricanes, tornadoes, earthquakes, and wildfires. Therefore, preparedness in a given area involves anticipating the most likely natural disasters for that specific area, among other disasters.

Your EMS agency should have written disaster plans that you are regularly trained to carry out. A copy of the disaster plan should be kept in each EMS vehicle. EMS facilities should have disaster supplies for at least a 72-hour period of self-sufficiency. Your EMS service should have mutual aid agreements with surrounding organizations; these will facilitate requests for help in an emergency. All groups with mutual aid agreements should practice using the plans frequently. Organizations should share a list of resources with each other so they will know early on what they can access. Also, your local EMS organizations should develop an assistance program for the families of EMS responders. If EMS responders have concerns about their families during a disaster, their effectiveness on the job could be diminished.

## Scene Size-up

Remember that scene size-up starts with dispatch. If dispatch information indicates a possible unsafe scene, stay away from the scene or get only close enough to make an assessment without putting yourself in harm's way. When you arrive first on the scene of an incident, you will make an initial assessment and some preliminary decisions. The size-up will be driven by three basic questions that you must ask yourself:

- *What do I have?*
- *What resources do I need?*
- *What do I need to do?*

These questions have a symbiotic relationship. The answer from one helps to answer the others, and each answer represents a piece to the puzzle. Work as a team when you answer these questions because overlooking just one safety issue early on can start a chain reaction of problems.

## What Do I Have?

Start with scene safety. First, assess the scene for hazards. Warn all other responders about hazardous materials, fuel spills, electrical hazards, or other safety concerns as soon as possible. Confirm the incident location.

Establish whether the incident is open or closed. An **open incident** is one that is not yet contained; there may be patients who are yet to be located and the situation may be ongoing, producing even more patients. A **closed incident** is one that is contained and in which all casualties are accounted for. However, as with any situation, a closed incident may quickly become an open incident as situations change.

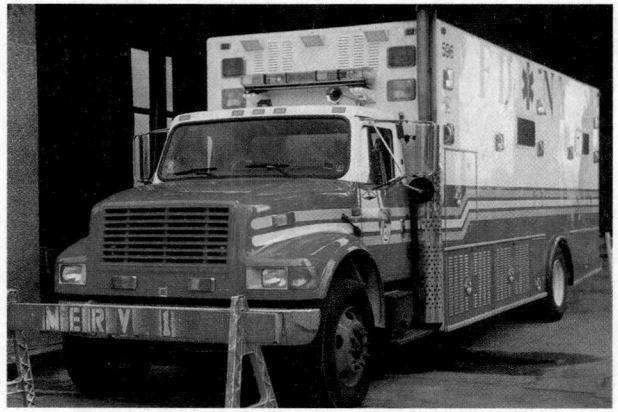

**FIGURE 40-3** This mobile emergency room is staffed by EMTs, paramedics, and physicians who are able to provide advanced life support to multiple patients simultaneously on the scene of a mass-casualty incident.

© Jones & Bartlett Learning. Courtesy of MIEMSS.

Estimate the number of casualties. Immediately provide a brief incident report to dispatch. An example of such a report would be: "EMT unit number one arriving on scene, multiple vehicles involved, full road blockage, no apparent hazards at this time, EMT unit number one is assuming command."

## What Do I Need?

Decide what resources are needed. You may need more EMS responders, ambulances, or other forms of transportation. If extrication is required, a rescue unit and fire department response may be needed. If there are hazardous materials, request a hazmat team immediately (discussed later in the chapter). Many large EMS systems deploy specialized MCI units or mobile emergency room vehicles that have the capacity to treat dozens of patients at the scene (**FIGURE 40-3**).

## YOU are the Provider

On reaching the scene, you see utter chaos. Your unit is the first to arrive, and the large crowd makes it virtually impossible to determine the number of patients or the extent of injuries. The dispatcher advises that law enforcement, fire department, and additional EMS units are en route.

**3.** How should you and your partner proceed?

**4.** Once command has been established, what are your duties?

## What Do I Need to Do?

Keep the following priorities in mind:

- Safety
- Incident stabilization
- Preservation of property and the environment

You need to consider these priorities in the order they are given. Safety is paramount. Safety includes your life, your partner's life, and other responders' lives. Then, consider the safety of the patients and any bystanders. This will be difficult for anyone dedicated to saving lives, but it is important to put yourself and your partner first—you have the skills, and bystanders usually do not; the situation can worsen if you become a victim yourself. Often, if a responder is injured, other responders will focus on "their own," removing critical resources from the incident.

Initially, you may have to work to isolate or stabilize the incident before providing care to injured people—this is another difficult concept for all emergency workers. Remember, you cannot help the injured if the scene is unstable. An unstable scene can lead to an injured EMT or additional bystanders becoming injured, thereby making your job much more difficult.

## Establishing Command

Once you have performed a good scene size-up and answered the three basic questions, command should be established by the most senior official, notification to other responders should go out, and necessary resources should be requested. Recall that a command system ensures that resources are effectively and efficiently coordinated. Command must be established early, preferably by the first-arriving, most experienced public safety official from the most relevant service. These officials may include police, fire, or EMS personnel.

## Communications

As discussed earlier, communication is often the key problem at an MCI or a disaster. The infrastructure may be damaged, or communications capabilities may be overwhelmed. If possible, use face-to-face communications to limit radio traffic. Some organizations responding to a disaster might not know how to use a radio. As mentioned previously, if you communicate via radio, do not use 10-codes or language specific to your EMS system. Doing so could be confusing for ancillary services and other personnel who are responding. Most communications problems should be worked out before a disaster happens by designating channels strictly for command during a disaster. Whatever form of communications equipment is used, it must be reliable, durable, and field-tested. Be sure there are backups in place if the primary communications system does not work. Some regions have mobile self-contained communications centers, whereas others use local radio groups such as ham radio operators to assist with communications. Most important, your plan should include a "plan B" in case of communications failure.

## The Medical Branch of Incident Command

What has traditionally been referred to as medical incident command is more commonly known as the medical (or EMS) branch of the ICS (**FIGURE 40-4**). At incidents that have a significant medical factor, the IC will designate someone as the chief of the medical branch under the operations section. This person will supervise the primary roles of the medical branch—triage, treatment, and transport of injured people. The medical branch director helps to ensure that EMS units responding to the scene are working within the ICS, each medical division or group receives a clear assignment before beginning work at the scene, and personnel remain with their vehicle in the staging area until they are assigned their duties.

### Triage Supervisor

The triage supervisor is ultimately in charge of counting and prioritizing patients. During large incidents, a number of triage personnel may be needed. The primary duty of the triage division or group is to ensure that every patient receives initial assessment of his or her condition. One of the most difficult parts of working as triage personnel is that you must not begin treatment until all patients are triaged, or you will compromise your triage efforts.

### Treatment Supervisor

The treatment supervisor will locate and set up the treatment area with a tier for each priority of patient.

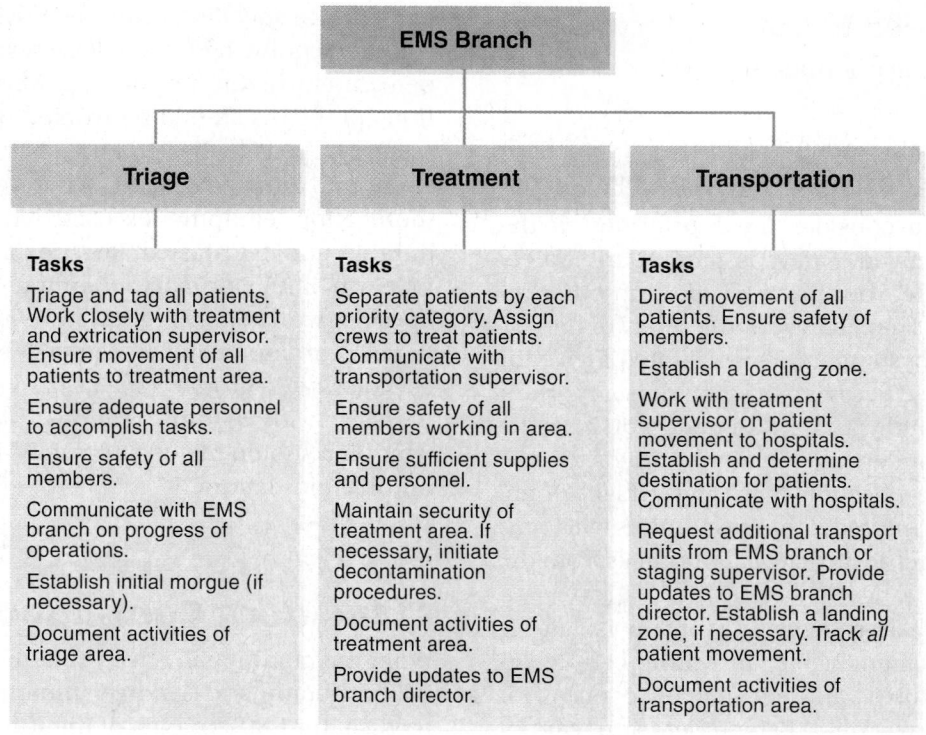

**EMS Branch**

**Triage**

**Tasks**

Triage and tag all patients. Work closely with treatment and extrication supervisor. Ensure movement of all patients to treatment area.

Ensure adequate personnel to accomplish tasks.

Ensure safety of all members.

Communicate with EMS branch on progress of operations.

Establish initial morgue (if necessary).

Document activities of triage area.

**Treatment**

**Tasks**

Separate patients by each priority category. Assign crews to treat patients. Communicate with transportation supervisor.

Ensure safety of all members working in area.

Ensure sufficient supplies and personnel.

Maintain security of treatment area. If necessary, initiate decontamination procedures.

Document activities of treatment area.

Provide updates to EMS branch director.

**Transportation**

**Tasks**

Direct movement of all patients. Ensure safety of members.

Establish a loading zone.

Work with treatment supervisor on patient movement to hospitals. Establish and determine destination for patients. Communicate with hospitals.

Request additional transport units from EMS branch or staging supervisor. Provide updates to EMS branch director. Establish a landing zone, if necessary. Track *all* patient movement.

Document activities of transportation area.

**FIGURE 40-4** Components of the medical branch within the incident command system.

© Jones & Bartlett Learning.

The treatment supervisor ensures that secondary triage of patients is completed and that adequate patient care is provided as resources allow. The treatment supervisor also assists with moving patients to the transportation area. As the treatment supervisor supervises the responders, he or she must communicate with the medical branch director to request sufficient quantities of supplies, including bandages, burn supplies, airway and respiratory supplies, and patient packaging equipment.

## Transportation Supervisor

The transportation supervisor coordinates the transportation and distribution of patients to appropriate receiving hospitals and helps to ensure that hospitals do not become overwhelmed by a patient surge. The transportation supervisor coordinates with the IC to ensure that enough personnel and ambulances are in the staging area or have been requested. Some regions may plan for a designated hospital to coordinate with area hospitals on destination decisions. An MCI typically disrupts the everyday functioning of the region's trauma system, so good coordination

is needed. The transportation supervisor documents and tracks the number of transport vehicles, patients transported, and the facility destination of each vehicle and patient.

## Staging Supervisor

A staging supervisor is assigned when an MCI or disaster requires a multivehicle or multiagency response. Emergency vehicles receive direction from the staging supervisor to enter an MCI scene and should drive only in the directed area. The staging area should be established away from the scene so that the parked vehicles are not in the way. If a staging area is located too close to a chaotic scene, patients or fellow responders may see the number of ambulances waiting and bring patients directly to the staging area as opposed to the triage area. The staging supervisor locates an area to stage equipment and responders, tracks unit arrivals, and releases vehicles and supplies when ordered by command. This position plans for efficient access to and exit from the scene and prevents traffic congestion among responding vehicles.

## Physicians on Scene

In an MCI or disaster, some areas have plans in place for physicians to respond to the scene. Sometimes this includes the EMS medical director or another physician who regularly works, trains, and interacts with your agency. Sometimes, even without a plan, the enormity of the situation may require physicians on scene. EMS physicians, especially, will have the training to make difficult triage decisions. They also provide secondary triage decisions in the treatment area, deciding which priority patients are to be transported first. Physicians can provide on-scene medical direction for EMTs, and they can provide care as appropriate. Like other fire and EMS providers, there is the possibility that physicians who are nearby may self-dispatch to respond to the scene to help. If you encounter a physician, you should ensure that he or she is assigned to the incident. This precaution will verify the physician's credentials and will ensure this new resource is factored into the ICS. As mentioned previously, the IC must be able to account for all people on scene should a secondary event occur.

## Rehabilitation Supervisor

In disasters or MCIs that will last for extended periods, a rehabilitation section for the responders should be established. The **rehabilitation supervisor** establishes an area that provides protection for responders from the elements and the situation. The **rehabilitation area** should be located away from exhaust fumes and crowds (especially members of the media) and out of view of the scene itself. Rehabilitation is where a responder's needs for rest, fluids, food, and protection from the elements are met. The rehabilitation supervisor must also monitor responders for signs of stress. These signs may include fatigue, altered thinking patterns, and complete collapse. Remember that all EMS personnel must be aware of signs of stress. Your service might consider having a defusing or debriefing team in this area. Responders should be encouraged to take advantage of these services but should never be forced to participate.

## Extrication and Special Rescue

Some MCIs or disasters require search and rescue or extrication of patients (**FIGURE 40-5**). A unit leader may need to be appointed, such as an **extrication**

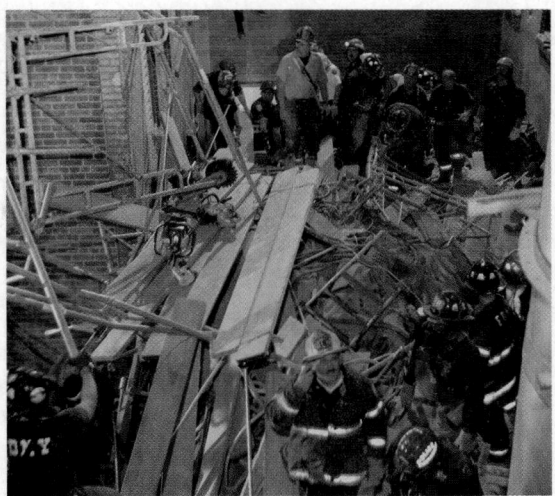

**FIGURE 40-5** Some disasters will involve search and rescue or extrication. New York City firemen, police, and rescue crews work to clear rubble and extract workers trapped after the brick facade of a 20-story building collapsed on Wednesday, October 24, 2001. Four were killed and six more were missing.

© Edward Keating/POOL/AP Photos.

supervisor or **rescue supervisor**. These officers determine the type of equipment and resources needed for the situation. In some incidents, victims may need to be extricated or rescued by specifically trained personnel before they can be triaged and treated. Extrication and rescue can be dangerous, so team member safety is of utmost importance.

## Morgue Supervisor

In some MCIs or disasters, there will be many dead patients. The **morgue supervisor** will work with area medical examiners, coroners, disaster mortuary assistance teams, and law enforcement agencies to coordinate removal of the bodies and even, possibly, body parts. The morgue supervisor should attempt to leave the dead victims in the location found, if possible, until a removal and storage plan can be determined. The location of victims may help in the identification of the dead victims in mass-fatality situations, or there may be crime scene considerations. If it is determined that a morgue area is needed, the morgue supervisor should ensure that the morgue is out of view of the living patients and other responders because the psychological impact could worsen the situation. In addition, the morgue should be secured from the public to prevent theft of any personal effects of the dead victims.

# Mass-Casualty Incidents

As discussed earlier, an MCI is an emergency situation that involves three or more patients, places great demand on the EMS system, and/or has the potential to produce multiple casualties (**FIGURE 40-6**). However, other causes of MCIs are far more common than disasters and are usually much smaller in scope. **FIGURE 40-7** is a diagrammed example of a residential building fire confined to one apartment that may only produce one patient but that has the potential to generate dozens of patients from among the responders and residents. Loss of power

to a hospital or nursing home with ventilator-dependent and nonambulatory victims is considered an MCI, although no one is injured. By using the ICS and the NIMS and understanding the various roles and responsibilities of each position, the responders and/or IC can manage the incident in a smooth, organized manner.

All systems have different protocols for when to declare an MCI and initiate the ICS; however, as an EMT, ask yourself the following questions when considering whether the call is an MCI:

- *How many seriously injured or ill patients can I care for effectively and transport in the ambulance? One? Two?*
- *What happens when I have three patients to manage?*
- *How long will it take for additional help to arrive?*
- *What happens if the number of patients exceeds the number of available ambulances?*

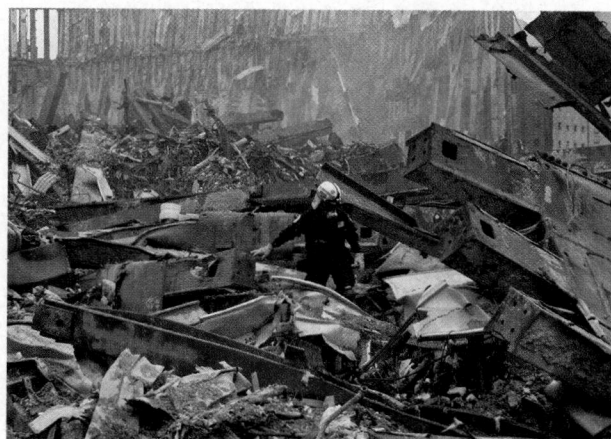

**FIGURE 40-6** Mass-casualty incidents can be large, such as the attack on September 11, 2001, or they can be much smaller in scope.

Courtesy of Michael Rieger/FEMA.

## Words of Wisdom

The terminology used to describe an incident with multiple patients varies in different communities. Many communities use *mass-casualty situation* to describe an emergency that involves more than one patient, but they will use the term *mass-casualty incident* to describe larger-scale events, such as those with more than 20 patients. In this text, the term *mass-casualty incident* is used to describe any call that involves three or more patients.

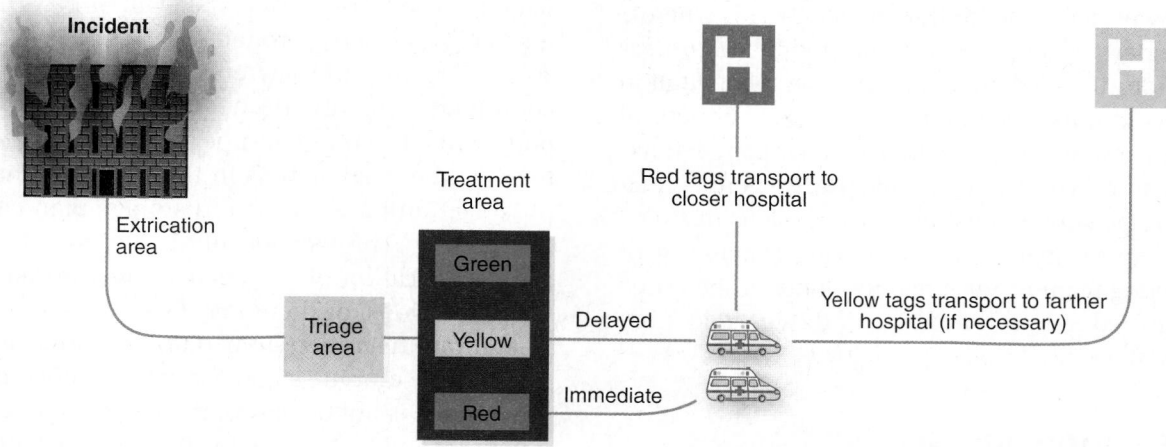

**FIGURE 40-7** Diagram of a mass-casualty incident. The incident command system established at the scene of a building fire may look similar to this diagram.

© Jones & Bartlett Learning.

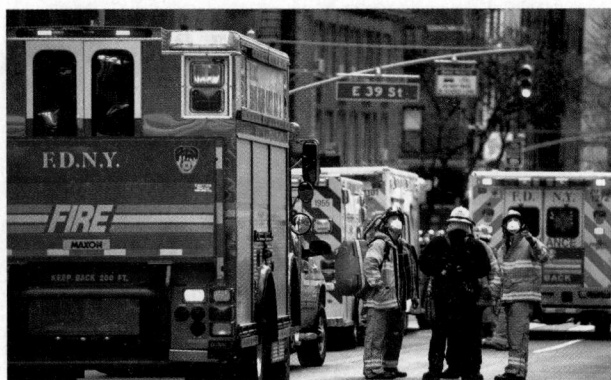

**FIGURE 40-8** Mass-casualty incidents require additional ambulances and EMS providers from the immediate region.

© NurPhoto/Getty Images.

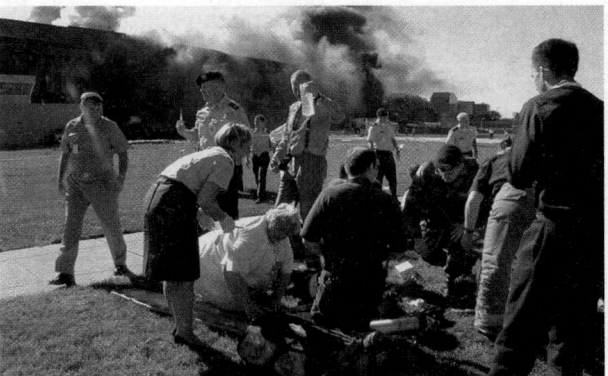

**FIGURE 40-9** Triage is the process of sorting and prioritizing patients based on severity of conditions. Medical personnel and volunteers work the first medical triage area set up outside the Pentagon after a hijacked commercial airliner crashed into the southwest corner of the building on September 11, 2001.

Courtesy of Journalist 1st Class Mark D. Faram/US Navy.

Obviously, you and your team cannot treat and transport all injured patients at the same time. At an MCI, you will often experience an increased demand for equipment and personnel. For example, you may realize that you are the only ambulance crew currently at the scene and there is a wait of 15 or more minutes before the next ambulance arrives. Never leave the scene with patients if there are still other patients present who are sick or wounded. This would leave patients at the scene without medical care and can be considered abandonment. If there are multiple patients and not enough resources to handle them without abandoning victims, you should declare an MCI (at least for the present time), request additional resources, and initiate the ICS and triage procedures (discussed next) (**FIGURE 40-8**). Although this may cause some delay in initiating treatment to all patients, it will not adversely affect the patient care. Always follow your local protocol. Many large EMS systems deploy specialized MCI units or mobile emergency room vehicles that have the capacity to treat dozens of patients on the scene.

## Triage

**Triage** simply means to sort your patients based on the severity of their injuries (**FIGURE 40-9**). The goal of doing the greatest good for the greatest number means the triage assessment is brief, and you will group the patients into basic categories based on their acuity. **Primary triage** is the initial triage done in the field, allowing you to quickly and accurately

categorize the patient's condition and transport needs, whereas **secondary triage** is done as patients are brought to the treatment area. During primary triage, patients are briefly assessed and then identified in some way, such as by attaching a triage tag or colored triage tape. The main information needed on the tag is a unique number and a triage category. Rapid and accurate triage will help bring order to the chaos of the MCI scene and allow the most critical patients to be transported first. After the primary triage, the triage supervisor should communicate the following information to the medical branch director:

- Total number of patients
- Number of patients in each of the triage categories
- Recommendations for extrication and movement of patients to the treatment area
- Resources needed to complete triage and begin movement of patients

### Words of Wisdom

For multiple victims of a lightning strike, you should use the reverse triage method. With traditional triage, an apneic and pulseless patient would typically be triaged as "black" or "expectant." In the case of a lightning strike, however, treat cardiac or respiratory arrest victims first. Lightning strike injuries are covered in detail in Chapter 33, *Environmental Emergencies*.

When the initial triage has been completed, secondary triage, or retriage, can occur, allowing you to reassess all remaining patients and, if necessary, to upgrade their triage category. In smaller MCI events, this step may not be necessary if enough resources have arrived on the scene.

## Triage Categories

There are four common triage categories. You can remember them using the mnemonic IDME, which stands for Immediate (red), Delayed (yellow), Minor or Minimal (green; hold), and Expectant (black; likely to die or dead) (**TABLE 40-1**). This is the order of priority for treatment and transport of the patients at an MCI.

Immediate (red-tag) patients are your first priority. They need immediate care and transport. They usually have problems with the ABCs, head trauma, or signs and symptoms of shock.

Delayed (yellow-tag) patients are the second priority and need treatment and transport, but it can be delayed. Patients usually have multiple injuries to bones or joints, including back injuries with or without spinal cord injury.

Minimal (green-tag) patients are the third priority. Patients may require no field treatment or only minimal treatment. In some parts of the world, this is the hold category. These patients are the "walking wounded" at the scene. If they have any apparent injuries, they are usually soft-tissue injuries such as contusions, abrasions, and lacerations.

The last priority is the expectant (black tag) patients who are dead or whose injuries are so severe that they have, at best, a minimal chance of survival. This category may include patients who are in cardiac arrest or who have an open head injury, for example. If you have limited resources, this category may also include patients in respiratory arrest. Patients in this category receive treatment and transport only after patients in the other three categories have received care.

An interesting development is the possible addition of a new, fifth triage category—the orange-tag category. This category represents an intermediate category between the critical (red tag) and noncritical, nonambulatory (yellow tag) categories of patients. During a true MCI, there may be ambulatory patients who require prompt evaluation and treatment for symptoms that are the result of medical comorbidities and not the acute traumatic injuries associated with the initial event. Consider patients who are having nontraumatic chest pain or shortness of breath following the event. In the

| **TABLE 40-1**  Triage Priorities | |
|---|---|
| **Triage Category** | **Typical Injuries** |
| **Red tag:** first priority (immediate)<br>Patients who need immediate care and transport<br>Treat these patients first, and transport as soon as possible | • Airway and breathing compromise<br>• Uncontrolled or severe bleeding<br>• Severe medical problems<br>• Signs of shock (hypoperfusion)<br>• Severe burns<br>• Open chest or abdominal injuries |
| **Yellow tag:** second priority (delayed)<br>Patients whose treatment and transport can be temporarily delayed | • Burns without airway compromise<br>• Major or multiple bone or joint injuries<br>• Back injuries with or without spinal cord damage |
| **Green tag:** third priority, minimal (walking wounded)<br>Patients who require minimal or no treatment and transport can be delayed until last | • Minor fractures<br>• Minor soft-tissue injuries |
| **Black tag:** fourth priority (expectant)<br>Patients who are already dead or have little chance for survival<br>Treat salvageable patients before treating these patients | • Obvious death<br>• Obviously nonsurvivable injury, such as major open brain trauma<br>• Respiratory arrest (if limited resources)<br>• Cardiac arrest |

past, these patients may have been undertriaged as stable, requiring little or no treatment, simply because they were ambulatory. A patient placed in this intermediate category could be more appropriately prioritized for treatment and transport if his or her condition required a specific destination that was not a trauma center (ie, cardiac catheterization center or hyperbaric chamber). The New York City Simple Triage and Rapid Treatment (FDNY-START) system now incorporates the orange tag category, and there may be ongoing developments as other systems adopt similar classifications.

## Triage Tags

Whatever triage system is used, it is vital that a patient has a tag or some type of label. Tagging patients early assists in tracking them and keeping an accurate record of their condition. Triage tags should be waterproof and easily read (**FIGURE 40-10**). The patient tags or tape should be color-coded and should clearly show the category of the patients. The use of symbols and colors to indicate the triage categories is important in case some responders are color-blind.

The tags will become part of the patient's medical record. Most have a tear-off receipt with a number correlating with the number on the tag. When torn off by the transportation officer, it will assist him or her in tracking the patient. If the patient is unconscious and cannot be identified at the scene, the tag will be an identifier for tracking purposes. Some areas use digital photography to assist in identifying patients later. The photograph is catalogued with the patient's tag number, and the patient's location is tracked with this information. When family members are brought to crisis centers to help locate loved ones, the pictures may be of assistance. This technique has been used effectively in Europe and Israel with Polaroid or digital photos. Another way of tracking and accounting for patients is to issue only 20 to 25 cards or tags at a time with a scorecard to mark how patients are triaged and their priority. When the responder returns for more tags, the scorecard will provide a patient count to help command and the staff to develop a plan to respond and ensure that appropriate resources are either available or summoned. Whatever labeling system is used, it is imperative for the transportation officer to be able to identify which patient was transported by which unit and to which destination, and the priority of the patient's condition.

## START Triage

START triage is one of the easiest methods of triage. START stands for Simple Triage And Rapid Treatment. The staff members at Hoag Memorial Hospital, Newport Beach, CA, developed this method of triage. It is easily mastered with practice and will give you the ability to rapidly categorize patients at an MCI. START triage uses a limited assessment of the patient's ability to walk, respiratory status, hemodynamic status (pulse), and neurologic status.

The first step of the START triage system is performed on arrival at the scene by calling out to patients at the disaster site, "If you can hear my voice and are able to walk..." and then directing patients to an easily identifiable landmark. You should pick a landmark that is away from your ambulance. Bringing a large number of patients toward you and your ambulance will hinder your ability to properly triage all of the patients. You can send the ambulatory patients toward a landmark, such as a lamp pole or the corner of a street. This will help to manage the chaos of an MCI. The injured people in this group are the walking wounded and are considered minimal (green) priority, or third-priority, patients.

The second step in the START process is directed toward nonwalking patients. Move to the first nonambulatory patient and assess the respiratory status. If the patient is not breathing, open the airway by using a simple manual maneuver. A patient who still does not begin to breathe is triaged as

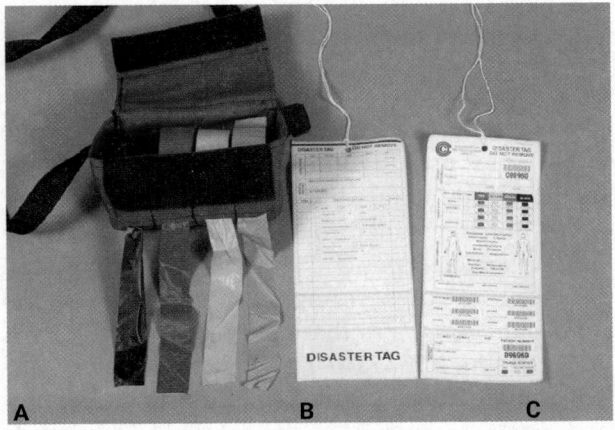

**FIGURE 40-10** Triage tags (from left to right). **A.** Waterproof triage tape. **B.** Triage tag: back. **C.** Triage tag: front.

expectant (black). If the patient begins to breathe, tag him or her as immediate (red), place in the recovery position, and move on to the next patient (**FIGURE 40-11**).

If the patient is breathing, make a quick estimation of the respiratory rate. A patient who is breathing faster than 30 breaths/min or slower than 10 breaths/min is triaged as an immediate priority (red). If the patient is breathing from 10 to 29 breaths/min, move to the next step of the assessment.

The next step is to assess the hemodynamic status of the patient by checking for bilateral radial pulses. An absent radial pulse implies the patient is likely hypotensive; tag him or her as an immediate priority. If the radial pulse is present, go to the next assessment.

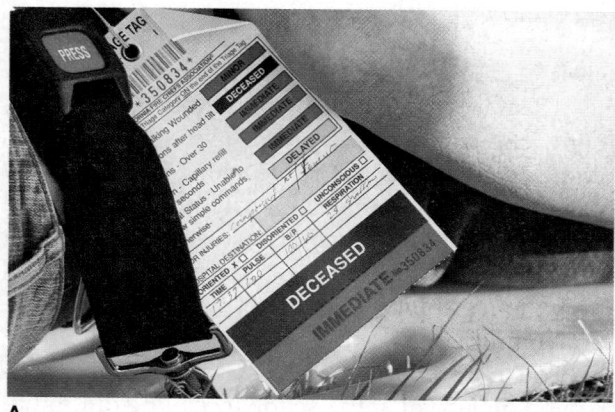

**A**

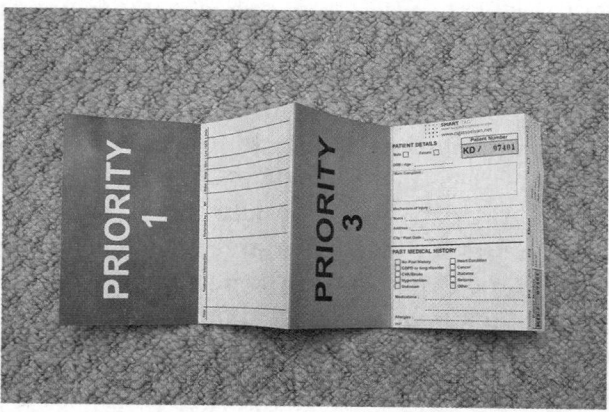

**B**

**FIGURE 40-11 A.** A START triage tag is ripped to the level of severity. **B.** A SMART triage tag folds to the level of severity.

A: Nancy G Fire Photography, Nancy Greifenhagen/Alamy Stock Photo; **B:** Courtesy of Richard Pilbery.

The final assessment in START triage is to assess the patient's neurologic status, which simply means to assess the patient's ability to follow simple commands, such as "Show me three fingers." This assessment establishes that the patient can understand and follow commands. A patient who is unconscious or cannot follow simple commands is an immediate priority patient. A patient who complies with a simple command should be triaged in the delayed category (yellow).

### Words of Wisdom

Another triage method is the Sort, Assess, Lifesaving interventions, and Treatment and/or Transport (SALT) triage system. This triage system begins with a global sorting of patients. This step identifies the patients who are able to understand verbal instructions and are therefore likely to have good systemic perfusion. Patients who can walk are asked to move to a designated area and are assigned last priority. This is an attempt to decrease the number of patients leaving the scene and overwhelming local hospital resources before EMS can begin to move highest priority patients. Once those patients have been identified and moved, each remaining patient is assessed individually. The SALT method differs from others in its lifesaving intervention steps, which include bleeding control, opening the airway, and two rescue breaths for children. It also includes needle decompression for tension pneumothorax and auto-injector antidotes for ALS providers. These interventions may be all that is needed to upgrade the patient's condition on the SALT triage scale. The final step is treatment and/or transport.

## JumpSTART Triage for Pediatric Patients

Lou Romig, MD, recognized that the START triage system does not take into account the physiologic and developmental differences of pediatric patients. She developed the JumpSTART triage system for pediatric patients. JumpSTART is intended for use in children younger than 8 years or who appear to weigh less than 100 pounds (45 kg). As in START, the JumpSTART system begins by identifying the walking wounded. Infants or children not developed enough to walk or follow commands (including children with special needs) should be taken as soon as possible to the treatment area for immediate secondary triage. This action assists in getting children who cannot take care of their own basic needs to a health care provider. There are several differences within the respiratory status assessment compared with that in START. First, if you find that a pediatric patient is not breathing, immediately check the pulse. If there is no pulse, label the patient as expectant (black). If the patient is not breathing but has a pulse, open the airway with a manual maneuver. If the patient does not begin to breathe, give five rescue breaths and check respirations again. A child who does not begin to breathe should be labeled expectant. The primary reason for this difference is that the most common cause of cardiac arrest in children is respiratory arrest.

The next step of the JumpSTART process is to assess the approximate rate of respirations. A child who is breathing fewer than 15 breaths/min or more than 45 breaths/min is tagged as an immediate priority (red), and you move on to the next patient. If the respirations are within the range of 15 to 45 breaths/min, the patient is assessed further.

The next assessment in JumpSTART triage is also the hemodynamic status of the patient. Just like in START, you are simply checking for a distal pulse. This does not need to be the brachial pulse; assess the pulse that you feel the most competent and comfortable checking. If there is an absence of a distal pulse, label the child as an immediate priority and move to the next patient. If the child has a distal pulse, move on to the next assessment.

The final assessment is for neurologic status. Because of the developmental differences in children, their responses will vary. For JumpSTART, a modified AVPU score is used. A child who is unresponsive or responds to pain by posturing or with incomprehensible sounds or is unable to localize pain is tagged as an immediate priority. A child who responds to pain by localizing it or withdrawing from it or is alert is considered a delayed-priority patient (yellow).

## Triage Special Considerations

There are a few special situations in triage. Patients who are hysterical and disruptive to rescue efforts may need to be handled as an immediate priority and transported off the site, even if they are not seriously injured. Panic breeds panic, and this type of behavior could have a negative effect on other patients and on the responders.

A responder who becomes sick or injured during the rescue effort should be handled as an immediate priority and be transported off the site as soon as possible to avoid negative effect on the morale of remaining responders.

Hazmat and weapons of mass destruction incidents force the hazmat team to identify patients as contaminated or decontaminated before the regular triage process. Contamination by chemicals or biologic weapons in a treatment area, hospital, or trauma center could obstruct all systems and organizations coping with the MCI or disaster. Bear in mind that some incidents may require multiple triage areas or teams because the victims are located far apart.

## Destination Decisions

All patients triaged as immediate (red) or delayed (yellow) should preferably be transported by ground ambulance or air ambulance, if available, to the most appropriate facility (trauma, burn, or pediatric center). In extremely large situations, a bus may transport the walking wounded. If a bus is used for minimal-priority patients, it is strongly suggested that they be transported to a hospital or clinic distant from the MCI or disaster site to avoid overwhelming the local area hospital resources. Refer to the Centers for Disease Control and Prevention 2011 decision scheme for field triage of injured patients. This scheme is presented in Chapter 25, *Trauma Overview*. If a bus is used, plan for at least one EMT or paramedic to ride on board and to have an ambulance follow the bus. If a minimal-priority patient's condition worsens, the patient could be moved to the ambulance and transported to a closer facility. The EMT or paramedic can stay with the minimal-priority patients until their arrival at the designated hospital. Any worsening of a patient's condition must be relayed to the receiving hospital as soon as possible in whatever manner the incident dictates.

Immediate-priority patients should be transported two at a time until all are transported from the site. Then patients in the delayed category can be transported two or three at a time until all are at a hospital. Finally, the walking wounded are transported. Expectant patients who are still alive would receive treatment and transport at this time. Dead victims are handled or transported according to the standing operating procedure for the area.

It is important to remember that during an MCI, local hospitals may have their resources overwhelmed. Early notification to receiving facilities will allow for hospitals to increase staffing and move patients within their facility as required. Typically, EMS agencies will know a hospital's surge capacity, which will tell the agency how many patients of each category the hospital is able to safely handle and care for.

## Disaster Management

A **disaster** is a widespread event that disrupts functions and resources of a community and threatens lives and property. Many disasters do not necessarily result in personal injuries—for example, droughts causing widespread crop damage. However, many disasters such as floods, fires, and hurricanes will result in widespread injuries. Unlike an MCI, which generally lasts no longer than a few hours, emergency responders will generally be on the scene of a disaster for days to weeks and sometimes months (as in the events following Hurricane Katrina in 2005). Although you can declare an MCI as an EMT, only an elected official can declare a disaster.

Your role in a disaster is to respond when requested and to report to the IC for assigned tasks. In a disaster with an overwhelming number of casualties, area hospitals may decide that they cannot treat all patients at their facility. In this case, they may mobilize medical and nursing teams with equipment and set up a **casualty collection area** at a facility near the disaster scene, such as a warehouse. Once at the casualty collection area, the teams can perform triage, provide medical care, and transport patients to the hospital on a priority basis.

If a casualty collection area is established, it will be coordinated through the ICS in the same way as all other branches and areas of the operation. This is usually done only in a major disaster such as an earthquake when transportation to a hospital facility is impossible or involves prolonged delays. It may take several hours to establish a casualty collection area.

### Street Smarts

MCIs and disasters take a physical and emotional toll on emergency responders. Make certain that you are medically evaluated if you have been injured, come in contact with any hazardous substance, or inhale any dust, fumes, or smoke. Often the health effects of such exposures do not manifest for years and are difficult to link back to a specific event. In addition, you should be aware of the signs of stress in yourself and in your coworkers. Consider taking advantage of critical incident stress debriefing (CISD)/critical incident stress management (CISM) opportunities after an incident if you feel they may be valuable. Chapter 2, *Workforce Safety and Wellness*, covers stress and CISD/CISM in detail.

### Words of Wisdom

Urban Search and Rescue teams (USARs) and Disaster Medical Assistance Teams (DMATs) may be mobilized in the event of a natural disaster or MCI. USARs typically provide rescue and initial medical stabilization to patients entrapped in confined spaces, such as from a structural collapse. DMATs provide medical care during an incident; they include providers such as physicians, paramedics, nurses, and EMTs who work at the federal level. DMATs are typically activated for periods of 2 weeks, and they arrive with sufficient supplies and equipment to provide care for 3 days.

### YOU are the Provider

Using the ambulance's public address system, you ask for anyone who can walk to come to the front gate, where a bus will be positioned to transport them. Next, you approach a supine middle-aged woman who is unresponsive with slow respirations. She has weak radial pulses. The next patient you encounter is a teenage boy who is apneic with a weak carotid pulse and no radial pulses. You note exposed brain matter. The third patient is an older woman with a severe laceration through the neck and chest; the neck injury has caused near-decapitation. She is apneic and pulseless.

**5.** What are your considerations in determining whether you should stop and provide treatment for the first patient?

**6.** What triage categories should you assign to the second and third patients?

# Introduction to Hazardous Materials

Your training has taught you that rapid response to the scene of a crash can save lives. However, when you arrive at the scene of a possible hazmat incident, you must first step back and assess the situation. It can be very difficult to stop yourself from immediately engaging in patient care, particularly if you can see a patient. However, rushing into an unsafe scene can have catastrophic results. If you are overcome by a hazardous substance, not only will patients suffer because you will be unable to assist them, but you will also place a strain on the system because you will require emergency care.

## Words of Wisdom

Methamphetamine (meth) is an illegal substance that has gained in popularity due to its increased accessibility, highly addictive properties, and relatively low cost. Meth is manufactured in illegal labs with highly volatile chemicals in a process known as cooking. The toxic fumes from meth labs not only create respiratory hazards, but may also ignite, causing fires or explosions. Exposure to the toxic fumes may cause irritation to the nose and throat, headaches, confusion, altered mental status, dizziness, nausea and/or vomiting, and respiratory problems.

You may find meth labs anywhere in the country, including homes, garages, abandoned trailers, or the trunk of a vehicle. People who cook meth are often exposed to the toxins or have burn injuries because the risk of explosion is high. Therefore, your potential for contact with a meth lab is high.

When responding to a general medical call, you may not realize that you are responding to a hazardous area. A house with all windows covered, glass cookware with a powdery residue, or a strong smell of an unusual odor such as ammonia, cat urine, or nail polish remover is a sign of a potential meth lab. If you have any suspicions that you may be in the presence of a meth lab, leave the area immediately and notify law enforcement to secure the scene and arrange for decontamination and cleanup.

Because of the unique aspects of responding to and working at a **hazardous materials (hazmat) incident**, the Occupational Safety and Health Administration (OSHA) has published a set of guidelines known as the Hazardous Waste Operations and Emergency Response (HAZWOPER). All providers, including EMTs, must meet specific additional training requirements before becoming involved in hazmat incidents. As an EMT, you need training at the First Responder Awareness Level. This text does not include the skills and information necessary to meet those requirements. You need to check with your agency for information about specific awareness-level training.

On the basis of the HAZWOPER regulation, first responders at the awareness level should have sufficient training or experience to demonstrate competency in the following areas:

- An understanding of what hazardous substances are and the risks associated with them
- An understanding of the potential outcomes of an incident
- The ability to recognize the presence of hazardous substances
- The ability to identify the hazardous substances, if possible
- An understanding of the role of the first responder awareness individual in the emergency response plan
- The ability to determine the need for additional resources and to notify the communication center

# Recognizing a Hazardous Material

A **hazardous material** is any material that poses an unreasonable risk of damage or injury to people, property, or the environment if it is not properly controlled during handling, storage, manufacture, processing, packaging, use and disposal, and transportation. Recognizing a hazmat incident, determining the identity of the material or materials, and understanding the hazards involved often require some detective work. You must train yourself to take the time to look at the whole scene so that you can identify the critical visual indicators and fit them into what you know about the problem.

Hazardous materials may be involved in any of the following situations (**FIGURE 40-12**):

- A truck or train crash in which a substance is leaking from a tank truck or railroad tank car

- A leak, fire, or other emergency at an industrial plant, refinery, or other complex where chemicals or explosives are produced, used, or stored
- A leak or rupture of an underground natural gas pipe
- Deterioration of underground fuel tanks and seepage of oil or gasoline into the surrounding ground

- Buildup of methane or other by-products of waste decomposition in sewers or sewage-processing plants
- A motor vehicle crash in which a gas tank has ruptured

Initially, it is important to approach the scene from a safe location and direction. The traditional rules of staying uphill and upwind are a good place to start. In addition, it may be wise to use binoculars and view the scene from a safe distance. Be sure to question anyone involved in the incident—a wealth of information may be available to you if you simply ask the right person. Take enough time to assess the scene and interpret other clues such as dead animals near the point of release, discolored pavement, dead grass, visible vapors or puddles, or labels that may help identify the presence of a hazardous material. Once you have a basic idea of what happened or determine that danger may be present, you can begin to formulate a plan for addressing the incident.

## Occupancy and Location

A wide variety of chemicals are stored in warehouses, hospitals, laboratories, industrial complexes, residential garages, bowling alleys, home improvement centers, garden supply stores, restaurants, and scores of other facilities or businesses in your response area. So many different chemicals exist in so many different locations that you could encounter almost anything during any type of emergency situation. The location and type of building are two good indicators of the possible presence of a hazardous material. For example, a biomedical laboratory is more likely than a preschool to have chemicals that could be hazardous on site. However, it is important to remember that many common buildings may have materials, like large amounts of cleaning supplies, that could be hazardous in the right scenario.

## Senses

Another way to detect the presence of hazardous materials is to use your senses, although this technique must be used carefully to avoid exposure. The senses you can safely use are sight and sound. As a general rule, the farther you are from the incident, the safer you will be. When it comes to hazmat

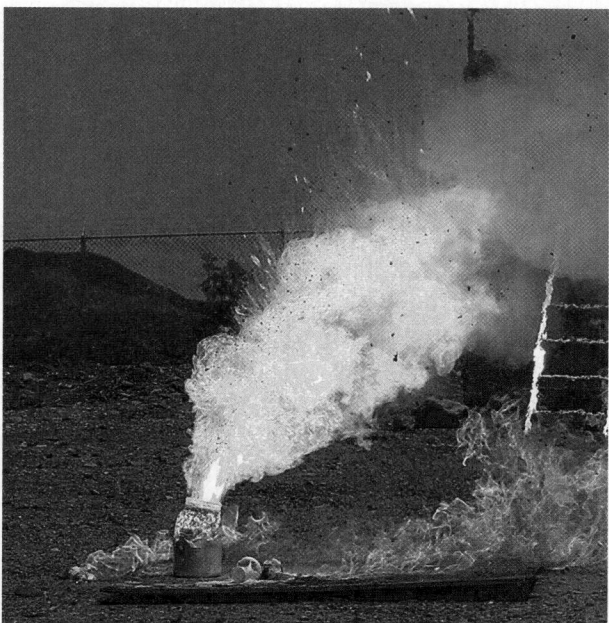

**A**

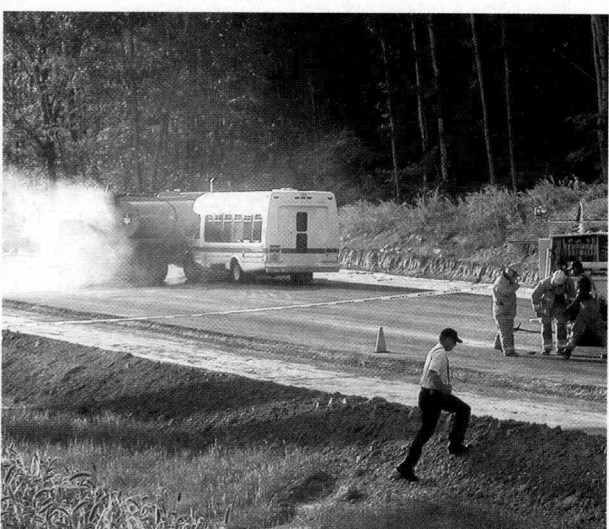

**B**

**FIGURE 40-12** Two examples of hazardous materials incidents. **A.** Burning container of flammable liquid. **B.** Crashed tanker truck.

**A:** Courtesy of Rob L. Jackson/US Marines; **B:** Courtesy of George Roarty/Virginia Department of Emergency Management.

incidents, "leading with your nose" is not a good tactic—but using binoculars from a distance is.

Clues that are seen or heard from a distance may enable you to take precautionary steps. Vapor clouds at the scene, for example, are a signal to move yourself and others away to a place of safety; the sound of an alarm from a toxic gas sensor in a chemical storage room or laboratory may also serve as a warning to retreat. Some highly vaporous and odorous chemicals—chlorine and ammonia, for example—may be detected by smell a long way from the actual point of release.

## Containers

In basic terms, a **container** is any vessel or receptacle that holds a material. Often the container's type, size, and material of construction provide important clues about the nature of the substance inside. Nevertheless, do not rely solely on the type of container when making a determination about hazardous materials.

Red phosphorus from a drug laboratory, for example, might be found in an unmarked plastic container. In this case, there may not be legitimate markings to alert you to the possible contents. Gasoline or waste solvents may be stored in 55-gallon (208-L) steel drums. Sulfuric acid, at 97% concentration, could be found in a polyethylene drum that might be colored black, red, white, or blue. In most cases, there is no correlation between the color of the drum and the possible contents. The same sulfuric acid might also be found in a 1-gallon (3.8-L) amber glass container. Steel or polyethylene drums, bags, high-pressure gas cylinders, railroad tank cars, plastic buckets, aboveground and underground storage tanks, cargo tanks, and pipelines all are examples of how hazardous materials are packaged, stored, and transported (**FIGURE 40-13**).

Some recognizable chemical containers, such as 55-gallon (208-L) drums and compressed gas cylinders, can be found in almost every type of manufacturing facility. Materials stored in a cardboard drum are usually in solid form. Stainless steel containers hold particularly dangerous chemicals, and cold liquids are kept in containers designed to maintain the appropriate temperature (**FIGURE 40-14**).

One way to distinguish containers is to divide them into two categories based on their capacity: bulk and nonbulk storage containers.

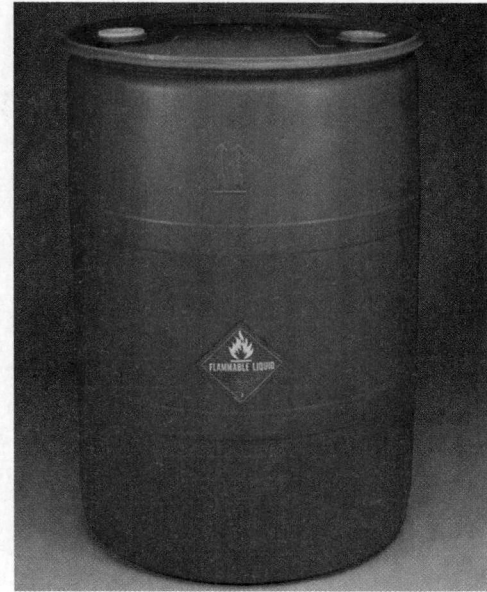

**FIGURE 40-13** Drums may be constructed of many different types of materials, including cardboard, polyethylene, and stainless steel. The drum shown here is made of polyethylene.

Courtesy of EMD Chemicals, Inc.

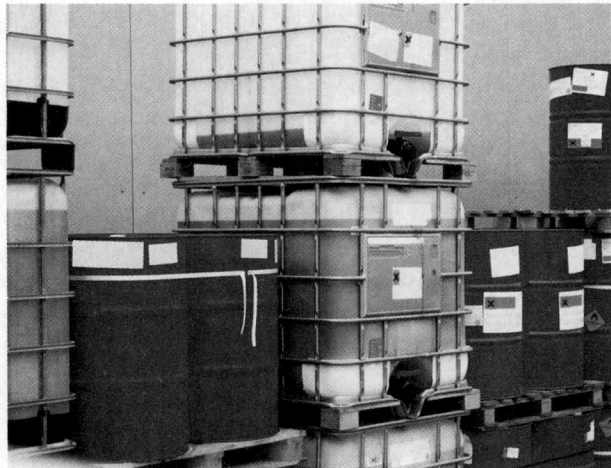

**FIGURE 40-14** A series of chemical storage containers.

© Ulrich Mueller/Shutterstock.

## Safety Tips

When you consider locations for possible hazardous materials incidents, do not limit your thinking. You may be surprised at how many different kinds of containers you may find in your area.

## Container Volume

**Bulk storage containers** include fixed tanks, highway cargo tanks, rail tank cars, totes, and intermodal tanks. In general, bulk storage containers are found in buildings that rely on and need to store large quantities of a particular chemical. Most manufacturing facilities have at least one type of bulk storage container. Often these bulk storage containers are surrounded by a secondary containment system to help control an accidental release. **Secondary containment** is an engineered method to control spilled or released product if the main containment vessel fails. A 5,000-gallon (18,927-L) vertical storage tank, for example, may be surrounded by a series of short walls that form a catch basin around the tank.

Large-volume horizontal tanks are also common. When stored above ground, these tanks are referred to as aboveground storage tanks; if they are placed underground, they are known as underground storage tanks. These tanks can hold a few hundred gallons to several million gallons of product and are usually made of aluminum, steel, or plastic.

Another commonly encountered bulk storage vessel is the tote, also referred to as an intermediate bulk container. Totes are found in a variety of shapes and sizes, with the most common sizes being 275 and 330 gallons (1,041 and 1,249 L). These portable plastic tanks are surrounded by a stainless steel web that adds both structural stability and protection to the container. They can contain any type of chemical, including flammable liquids, corrosives, food-grade liquids, or oxidizers (**FIGURE 40-15**).

Shipping and storing totes can be hazardous. These containers often are stacked atop one another and moved with a forklift, and a mishap with the loading or moving process can damage the tote. Because totes have no secondary containment system, any leak has the potential to create a large puddle. In addition, the steel webbing around the tote may make it difficult to access and patch leaks.

**Intermodal tanks** are both shipping and storage vessels. They hold between 4,000 and 6,000 gallons (15,142 and 22,712 L) of product and can be pressurized or nonpressurized. Intermodal tanks can also be used to ship and store gaseous substances that have been chilled until they liquefy, such as

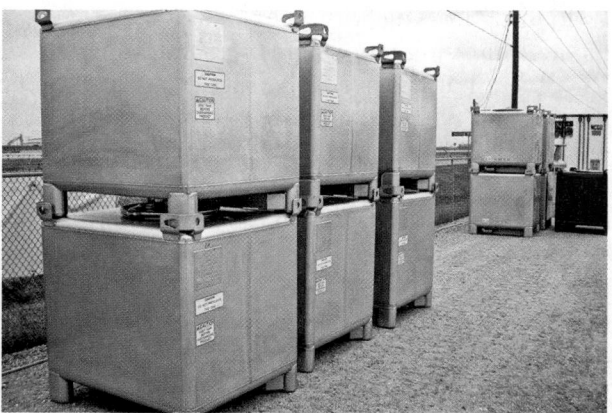

**FIGURE 40-15** A tote is a commonly encountered bulk storage vessel.
Courtesy of Tank Service, Inc.

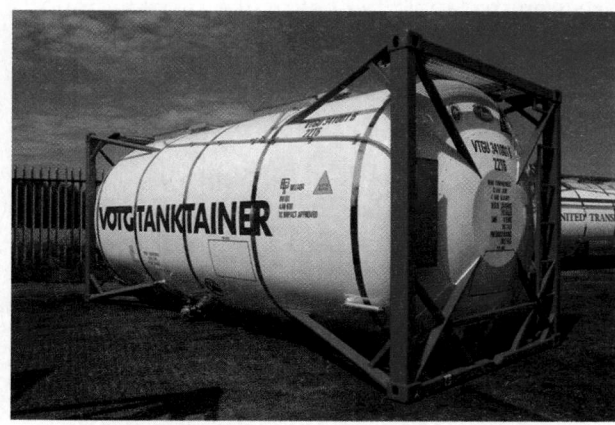

**FIGURE 40-16** An intermodal tank.
Courtesy of UBH International Ltd.

liquid nitrogen. In most cases, an intermodal tank is shipped to a facility, where it is stored and used and then returned to the shipper for refilling. Intermodal tanks can be shipped by all methods of transportation—air, sea, and land (**FIGURE 40-16**).

## Nonbulk Storage Vessels

Essentially, **nonbulk storage vessels** are all types of containers other than bulk containers. Nonbulk storage vessels can hold a few ounces to 119 gallons (450 L) of product and include vessels such as drums, bags, compressed gas cylinders, cryogenic containers, and more. Nonbulk storage vessels hold commonly used commercial and industrial chemicals such as solvents, industrial cleaners, and compounds. This section describes the most commonly encountered types of nonbulk storage vessels.

### Drums

Drums are easily recognizable, barrellike containers. They are used to store a wide variety of substances, including food-grade materials, corrosive substances, flammable liquids, and grease. Drums may be constructed of low-carbon steel, polyethylene, cardboard, stainless steel, nickel, or other materials. Generally, the nature of the chemical determines the construction of the storage drum. Steel utility drums, for example, hold flammable liquids, cleaning fluids, oil, and other noncorrosive chemicals. Polyethylene drums are used for corrosives such as acids, bases, oxidizers, and other materials that cannot be stored in steel containers. Cardboard drums hold solid materials such as soap flakes, sodium hydroxide pellets, and food-grade materials. Stainless steel or other heavy-duty drums generally hold materials too aggressive (ie, too reactive) for either plain steel or polyethylene.

### Bags

Bags are commonly used to store solids and powders such as cement powder, sand, pesticides, soda ash, and slaked lime. Storage bags may be constructed of plastic, paper, or plastic-lined paper. Bags come in different sizes and weights, depending on their contents.

Pesticide bags must be labeled with specific information (**FIGURE 40-17**). You can learn a great deal from the label, including the following details:

- Name of the product
- Active ingredients
- Hazard statement
- The total amount of product in the container
- The manufacturer's name and address
- The Environmental Protection Agency (EPA) registration number, which provides proof that the product was registered with the EPA
- The EPA establishment number, which shows where the product was manufactured
- Signal words to indicate the relative toxicity of the material:
  - Danger—Poison: Highly toxic by all routes of entry

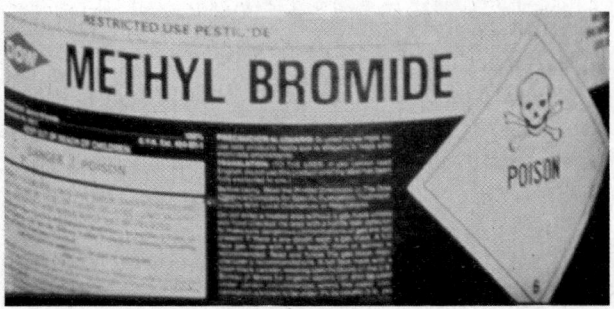

**FIGURE 40-17** A pesticide bag must be labeled with the appropriate information.
Courtesy of the USDA.

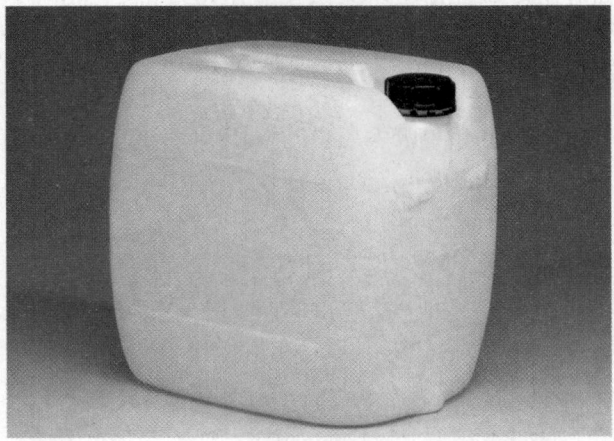

**FIGURE 40-18** A carboy is used to transport and store corrosive chemicals.
Courtesy of EMD Chemicals, Inc.

  - Danger: Severe eye damage or skin irritation
  - Warning: Moderately toxic
  - Caution: Minor toxicity and minor eye damage or skin irritation
- Practical first-aid treatment description
- Directions for use
- Agricultural use requirements
- Precautionary statements such as mixing directions or potential environmental hazards
- Storage and disposal information
- Classification statement on who may use the product

In addition, every pesticide label must carry the statement, "Keep out of reach of children."

### Carboys

Some corrosives and other types of chemicals are transported and stored in carboys (**FIGURE 40-18**).

A carboy is a glass, plastic, or steel container that holds 1 to 15 gallons (4 to 57 L) of product. Glass carboys are often placed in a protective wood, foam, fiberglass, or steel box to help prevent breakage. For example, nitric acid, sulfuric acid, and other strong acids are often transported and stored in thick glass carboys protected by a wooden or polystyrene (Styrofoam) crate to shield the glass container from damage during normal shipping.

### Cylinders

Several types of **cylinders** are used to hold liquids and gases. Uninsulated compressed gas cylinders are used to store substances such as nitrogen, argon, helium, and oxygen. They come in a range of sizes. As an EMT, you are already familiar with the shape of a cylinder; it holds the oxygen for your patients.

## The Department of Transportation Marking System

The presence of labels, placards, and other markings on buildings, packages, boxes, and containers can often enable you to identify a released chemical. When used correctly, marking systems indicate the presence of a hazardous material from a safe distance and provide clues about the substance.

The US Department of Transportation (DOT) marking system is an identification system characterized by labels, placards, and markings (**FIGURE 40-19**). This marking system is used in the United States when materials are being transported from one location to another. The same marking system is also used in Canada by Transport Canada.

**Placards** are diamond-shaped indicators (at least 9.8 inches [250 mm] per side) that are placed on all four sides of highway transport vehicles,

Table of placards and initial response guide to use on scene. Use this table only if materials cannot be specifically identified by using the shipping document, numbered placard, or orange panel number.

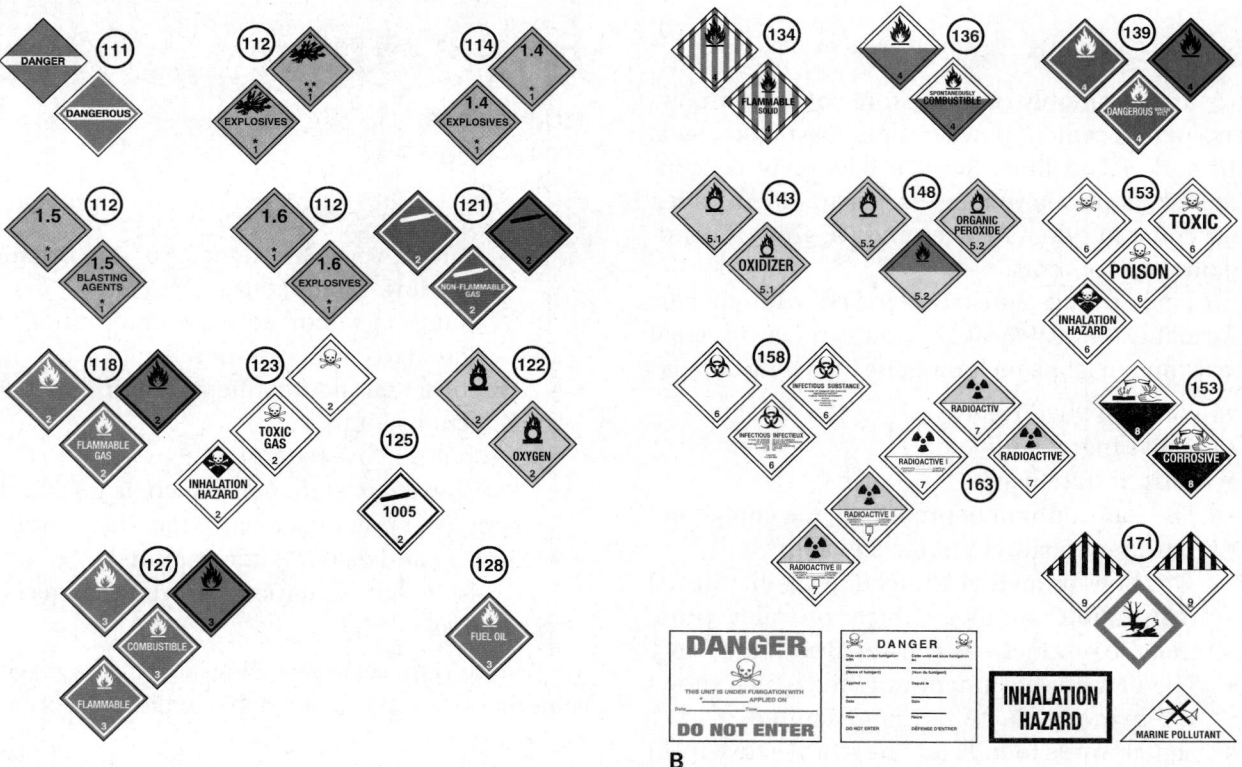

**FIGURE 40-19** The Department of Transportation uses labels, placards, and markings (such as these found in the *Emergency Response Guidebook*) to give a general idea of the hazard inside a particular container or cargo tank.

Courtesy of the US Department of Transportation.

railroad tank cars, and other forms of transportation carrying hazardous materials (**FIGURE 40-20**). Labels are smaller versions (3.9 inches [100 mm] per side) of placards; they are placed on the four sides of individual boxes and smaller packages being transported.

Placards, labels, and markings are intended to give a general idea of the hazard inside each container or cargo tank. A placard identifies the broad hazard class (flammable, poison, corrosive) to which the material inside belongs. A label on a box inside a delivery truck, for example, relates only to the potential hazard inside that particular package (**FIGURE 40-21**).

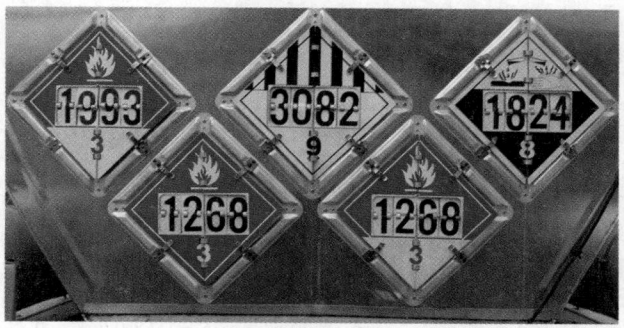

**FIGURE 40-20** A placard is a large diamond-shaped indicator that is placed on all sides of transport vehicles that carry hazardous materials.

© Mark Winfrey/Shutterstock.

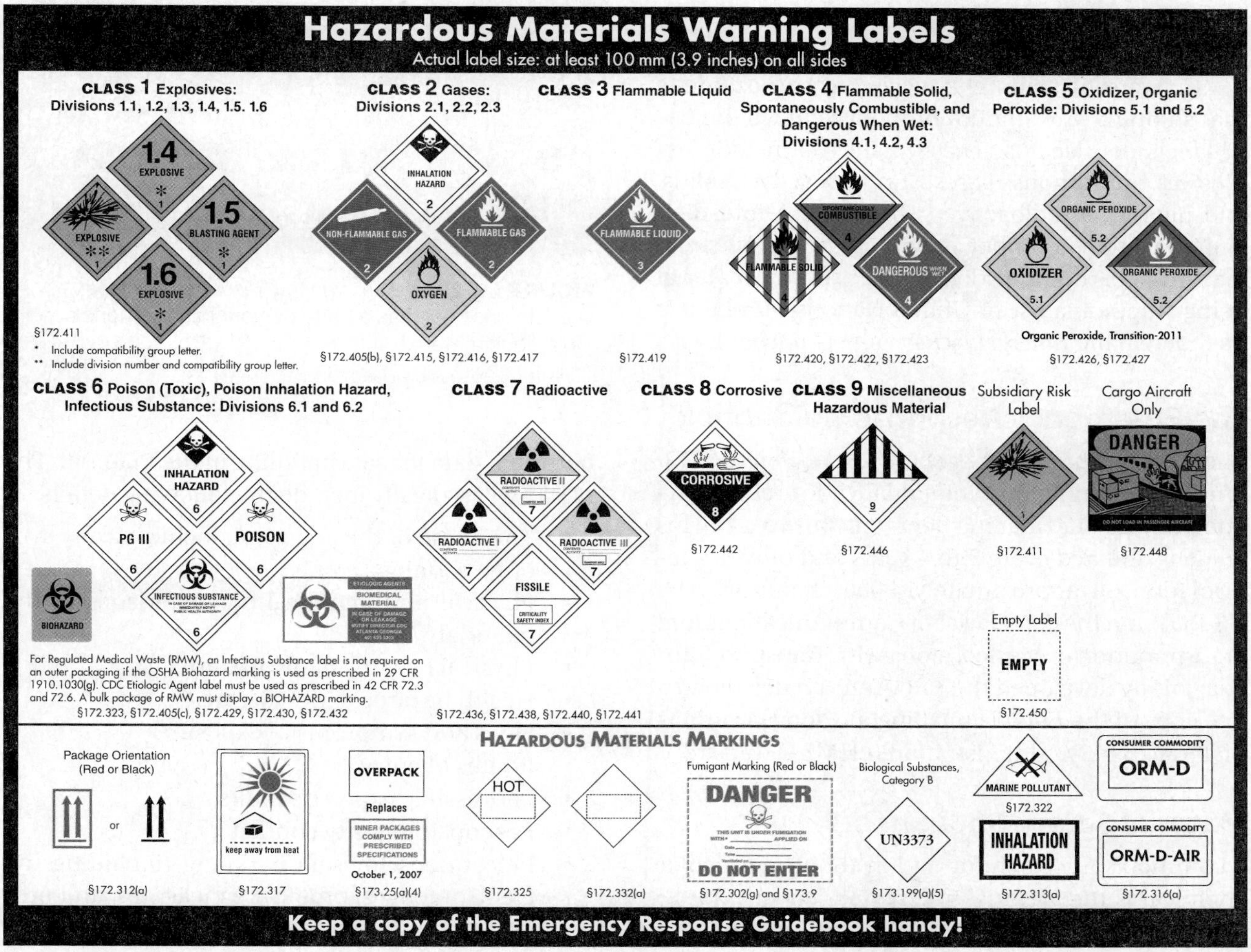

**FIGURE 40-21** A label is a smaller version of the placard and is placed on boxes or smaller packages that contain hazardous materials.

Courtesy of the US Department of Transportation.

## Other Considerations

The DOT system does not require that all chemical shipments be marked with placards or labels. In most cases, the package or cargo tank must contain a certain amount of hazardous material before a placard is required. For example, the "1,000-pound rule" applies to blasting agents (a substance that contains a fuel and oxidizer that is intended for blasting, but is not classified as an explosive), flammable and nonflammable gases, flammable/combustible liquids, flammable solids, air-reactive solids, oxidizers and organic peroxides, poison solids, corrosives, and miscellaneous (class 9) materials. Placards are required for these materials only when the shipment weighs more than 1,000 pounds (454 kg). Commercial package delivery services often carry small amounts of hazardous materials that fall below that weight limit. The vehicle exterior will not display placards to warn you of the danger.

Conversely, some chemicals are so hazardous that shipping any amount of them requires the use of labels or placards. These materials include explosives, poisonous gases, water-reactive solids, and high-level radioactive substances. A four-digit United Nations number may be required on some placards. This number identifies the specific material being shipped; a list of United Nations numbers is included in the *Emergency Response Guidebook*.

## The Emergency Response Guidebook

The DOT's *Emergency Response Guidebook (ERG)* offers a certain amount of guidance for responders operating at a hazmat incident (**FIGURE 40-22**). This guide is updated every 3 to 4 years and provides information on approximately 4,000 chemicals. The US DOT and the Secretariat of Communications and Transportation of Mexico, along with Transport Canada, jointly developed the *ERG*. You can download a free copy of the *ERG* via the Pipeline and Hazardous Materials Safety Administration (PHMSA) website.

## Material Safety Data Sheets

A common source of information about a particular chemical is the material safety data sheet (MSDS) (or safety data sheet [SDS]) specific to that substance (**FIGURE 40-23**). Essentially, the MSDS provides basic information about the chemical makeup of a substance, the potential hazards it presents, appropriate first aid in the event of an exposure, and other

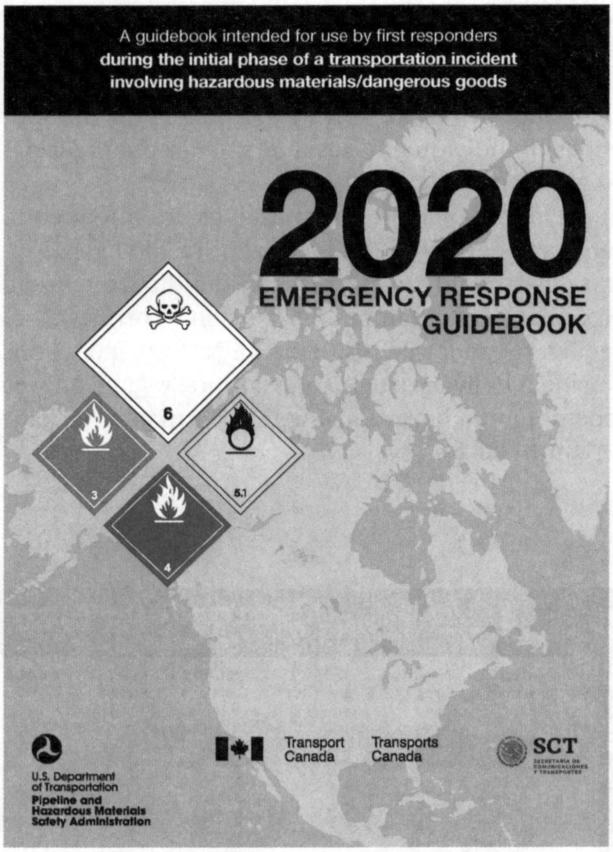

**FIGURE 40-22** The *Emergency Response Guidebook* is a reference used as a base for your initial actions at a hazardous materials incident.
Courtesy of the US Department of Transportation.

pertinent data for safe handling of the material. The MSDS will typically include the following details:

- The name of the chemical, including any synonyms for it
- Physical and chemical characteristics of the material
- Physical hazards of the material
- Health hazards of the material
- Signs and symptoms of exposure
- Routes of entry
- Permissible exposure limits
- Responsible-party contact
- Precautions for safe handling (including hygiene practices, protective measures, and procedures for cleaning up spills or leaks)
- Applicable control measures, including personal protective equipment
- Emergency and first-aid procedures
- Appropriate waste disposal

**MATERIAL SAFETY DATA SHEET**
**ANHYDROUS AMMONIA**

TI

**DISTRIBUTORS:**

**TANNER INDUSTRIES, INC.**

**DIVISIONS:**

| | |
|---|---|
| NATIONAL AMMONIA | NORTHEASTERN AMMONIA |
| HAMLER INDUSTRIES | BOWER AMMONIA & CHEMICAL |

735 Davisville Road, Third Floor, Southampton, PA 18966; 215-322-1238
**CORPORATE EMERGENCY TELEPHONE NUMBER: 800-643-6226 CHEMTREC: 800-424-9300**

**DESCRIPTION**

**CHEMICAL NAME**: Ammonia, Anhydrous — **CAS REGISTRY NO**: 7664-41-7
**SYNONYMS**: Ammonia — **CHEMICAL FAMILY**: Inorganic Nitrogen Compound
**FORMULA**: $NH_3$ — **MOL. WT**: 17.03 ($NH_3$) — **COMPOSITION**: 99+% Ammonia

**STATEMENT OF HEALTH HAZARD**

**HAZARD DESCRIPTION**:
Ammonia is an irritant and corrosive to the skin, eyes, respiratory tract and mucous membranes. Exposure to liquid or rapidly expanding gases may cause severe chemical burns and frostbite to the eyes, lungs and skin. Skin and respiratory related diseases could be aggravated by exposure.

Not recognized by OSHA as a carcinogen.
Not listed in the National Toxicology Program.
Not listed as a carcinogen by the International Agency for Research on Cancer.

**EXPOSURE LIMITS FOR AMMONIA**: Vapor

| | | | |
|---|---|---|---|
| OSHA | 50 ppm, | 35 mg / m$^3$ PEL | 8 hour TWA |
| NIOSH | 35 ppm, | 27 mg / m$^3$ STEL 15 minutes | |
| | 25 ppm, | 18 mg / m$^3$ REL | 10 hour TWA |
| | 300 ppm, | IDLH | |
| ACGIH | 25 ppm, | 18 mg / m$^3$ TLV | 8 hour TWA |
| | 35 ppm, | 27 mg / m$^3$ STEL 15 minutes | |

**TOXICITY**: LD 50 (Oral / Rat) 350 mg / kg

**PHYSICAL DATA**

**BOILING POINT**: -28°F at 1 Atm.
**PH**: N/A
**SPECIFIC GRAVITY OF GAS (air = 1):** 0.596 at 32°F
**SPECIFIC GRAVITY OF LIQUID (water = 1):** 0.682 at 28°F (Compared to water at 39°F).
**PERCENT VOLATILE**: 100% at 212°F
**APPEARANCE AND ODOR**: Colorless liquid or gas with pungent odor.
**CRITICAL TEMPERATURE:** 271.4°F
**GAS SPECIFIC VOLUME:** 20.78 Ft$^3$/Lb at 32°F and 1 Atm.
**VAPOR DENSITY:** 0.0481 Lb/Ft$^3$ at 32°F
**LIQUID DENSITY:** 38.00 Lb/Ft$^3$ at 70°F
**APPROXIMATE FREEZING POINT**: -108°F
**WEIGHT (per gallon):** 5.15 pounds at 60°F
**VAPOR PRESSURE**: 114 psig at 70°F
**SOLUBILITY IN WATER (per 100 pounds of water)**: 86.9 pounds at 32°F, 51 pounds at 68°F
**SURFACE TENSION**: 23.4 Dynes / cm at 52°F
**CRITICAL PRESSURE:** 111.5 atm

Revision: September 2005 Page 1 of 4 Prepared By: JRP

**FIGURE 40-23** An example of a material safety data sheet for anhydrous ammonia.

Courtesy of Tanner Industries, Inc., Southampton, PA.

All facilities that use or store chemicals are required by law to have an MSDS on file for each chemical used or stored in the facility. Many sites, especially those that stock many different chemicals, may keep this information archived on a computer database. Although the MSDS is not a definitive response tool, it is a key piece of the puzzle. The MSDS can also be obtained from the transporting vehicle.

## Shipping Papers

Shipping papers are required whenever hazardous materials are transported from one place to another. They include the names and addresses of the shipper and the receiver, identify the material being shipped, and specify the quantity and weight of each part of the shipment. Shipping papers for road and highway transportation are called **bills of lading** or **freight bills** and are located in the cab of the vehicle (**FIGURE 40-24**). Drivers transporting chemicals are required by law to have a set of shipping papers on their person or within easy reach inside the cab at all times.

## CHEMTREC

Located in Falls Church, VA, the **Chemical Transportation Emergency Center (CHEMTREC)**, now operated by the American Chemistry Council, is an agency that provides invaluable technical information for first responders of all disciplines who

**STRAIGHT BILL OF LADING**
ORIGINAL - NOT NEGOTIABLE

BOL/Reference No.
RSI82715

CARRIER: NORFOLK SOUTHERN

Date: 12/23/2008

Shipper: RSI LOGISTICS, INC (OKEMOS, MI US)

The property described below, in apparent good order, except as noted (contents and condition of packages unknown), marked, consigned, and destined as indicated below, which said carrier (the word carrier being understood throughout this contract as meaning any person or corporation in possession of the property under the contract) agrees to carry to its usual place of delivery at said destination, if on its route, otherwise to deliver to another carrier on the route to said destination. It is mutually agreed, as to each carrier of all or any said property, that every service to be performed hereunder shall be subject to all the terms and conditions of the Uniform Domestic Straight Bill of Lading set forth (1) in Offcial, Southern, Western and Illionis Freight Classification in effect on the date hereof, if this is a rail or a rail-water shipment, or (2) in the applicable motor carrier classification or tariff if this is a motor carrier shipment
Shipper herby certifies that he is familiar with all the terms and conditions or the said bill of lading, including those on the back thereof, set forth in the classification or tariff which governs the transportation of this shipment, and the said terms and conditions are hereby agreed to by the shipper and accepted for himself and his assigns.

| | |
|---|---|
| Consignee Information: CONSIGNEE DEER PARK, TX<br>Address:<br>City: DEER PARK, TX US | |
| Route: NS-ESTL-BNSF | |
| Origin Switch Route: | |
| Destination Switch Route: HUSTN-PTRA | Rail Car No: GATX290861 |

*For assistance in any transportation emergency involving chemicals, phone CHEMTREC, day or night, oll Free 1-800-424-9300*

| DESCRIPTION | | *THGIEW |
|---|---|---|
| ONE<br>TANK<br>CAR | Contains:<br>Methyl Esters<br>STCC#2899415<br>BIODIESEL-15, Biodiesel<br><br>Sales Order Contract No: RSI82715<br>Sales Order Contract No: AAT122308-4<br>Purchase Order Contract No: AAT122308-4 | (Sub. To Correction)<br>204400 Lbs. |

SEAL NUMBERS: Gross

Tare

Net

Weighed By: ____________________

If charges are to be prepaid, write or stamp here, "To be Prepaid"
**Prepaid**

Subject to Section 7 of the conditions of applicable bill of lading, if this shipment is to be delivered to the consignee witho ut recourse on the consignor, the consignor shall sign the following statement:: *The carrier shall not make delivery of this shipment without payment of freight and all other lawful charges.*

Not In Effect

* This is to certify that the above named materials are properly classified, described, packaged, marked, and labeled, and are in proper condition for transportation, according to the applicable regulations of the Department of Transportation.

**FIGURE 40-24** A bill of lading or freight bill.

Courtesy of RSI Logistics.

are called on to respond to chemical incidents. The toll-free number for CHEMTREC is 1-800-262-8200. CHEMTREC can provide you with technical chemical information via telephone, fax, or other electronic media. It also offers a phone conferencing service to connect you with thousands of shippers, subject matter experts, and chemical manufacturers.

When you call CHEMTREC, be sure to have the following basic information ready:

- The name of the chemical(s) involved in the incident (if known)
- Name of the caller and callback telephone number
- Location of the incident or problem

## YOU are the Provider

While you are triaging the patients, several other ambulances and other pieces of fire department equipment arrive on the scene, as well as a battalion chief who assumes command. You update him on your findings and the status of your EMS personnel and ambulances. There are 37 walking wounded (green) patients who will need to be loaded onto a bus for transport. Of the three remaining patients, two have been tagged expectant (black) and one is immediate (red).

**7.** What changes, if any, should you make in your initial triage assignments with the arrival of additional responders?

**8.** What should you consider in deciding whether to set up a treatment area at this incident?

- Shipper or manufacturer of the chemical (if known)
- Container type
- Railcar or vehicle markings or numbers
- The shipping carrier's name
- Recipient of material
- Local conditions and exact description of the situation

When you are speaking with CHEMTREC personnel, spell out all chemical names; if using a third party, such as a dispatcher, it is vital that you confirm all spellings to avoid misunderstandings. One number or letter out of place could throw off all subsequent research. When in doubt, be sure to obtain clarification.

## Identification

Unfortunately, even with all of these resources, identifying materials can still be difficult. Little consistency is used on labels and placards, and sometimes dishonest transporters will not label containers or vessels appropriately. The laws and regulations that cover labeling of packages and transport vehicles can also be misleading. As discussed previously, in most cases, the package or tank must contain a certain amount of a hazardous material before a placard is required. For example, because of the small quantities of hazardous materials that are involved, a truck carrying 99 pounds (45 kg) of hazmat No. 1 and 99 pounds (45 kg) of both hazmat No. 2 and hazmat No. 3 may not be required by law to display any labels or placards. The truck may show only a "Please drive carefully" placard, implying that it does not carry hazardous materials. Therefore, a crash involving this truck is a serious situation, but you would not necessarily know this if you relied on labels and placards. Always maintain a high index of suspicion when approaching the scene of a truck or train tanker crash.

Some substances are not hazardous; however, when mixed with another substance, they may become highly toxic. There may not be regulations against carrying such substances together on one truck or railroad car (or adjacent tank cars). The driver of a commercial truck and the conductor of a train, however, must carry shipping papers that identify what is being transported in their care. These shipping papers may be your first clue that there is a possible hazmat problem, although,

depending on the nature of the incident, the papers may not be available to you.

In the event of a leak or spill, a hazmat incident is often indicated by the presence of the following:

- A visible cloud or strange-looking smoke resulting from the escaping substance
- A leak or spill from a tank, container, truck, or railroad car with or without hazmat placards or labels
- An unusual, strong, noxious (harmful), harsh odor in the area

To indicate the presence of normally odorless toxic gases or fluids during a leak or spill, manufacturers may add a substance that produces a strong noxious odor. However, a large number of hazardous gases and fluids are essentially odorless (or do not have a distinctive unpleasant smell) even when a substantial leak or spill has occurred. In some incidents, many people are exposed and may be injured or killed before the presence of a hazmat incident is identified. If you approach a scene where more than one person has collapsed or is unconscious or in respiratory distress, you should assume that there has been a hazmat leak or spill and that it is unsafe to enter the area.

It is important for you to understand the potential danger of hazardous materials and know how to operate safely at a hazmat incident. If you do not follow the proper safety measures, you and many others could end up needlessly injured or dead. The safety of you and your team, the other responders, and the public must be your most important concern.

There will be times when the ambulance is the first to arrive at the scene. If, as you approach, any signs suggest that a hazmat incident has occurred, stop at a safe distance and park upwind or uphill

---

### Words of Wisdom

Safety considerations at hazmat scenes differ considerably from those involved in emergency response in general. A hazmat scene requires you to have an even higher degree of alertness than usual to avoid entering a dangerous environment and to help others avoid it. There is also a need to prevent the spread of contamination to yourself and your ambulance. Understanding these two concepts is a good start toward safe operations in the presence of hazardous materials.

from the incident. After rapidly sizing up the scene, call for a hazmat team. If you are already too close by the time you first recognize the danger, immediately leave the area. Once you have reached a safe place, try to rapidly assess the situation and provide as much information as possible when calling for the hazmat team, including your specific location, the size and shape of the containers of the hazardous material, and what you have observed and have been told has occurred. Do not reenter the scene, and do not leave the area until you have been cleared by the hazmat team, or you may contribute to the situation by spreading hazardous materials. Finally, do not allow civilians to enter the scene, if possible. No one should enter the area without the proper protective equipment, respiratory protection, or training.

Above all, avoid any contact with the material!

## Hazmat Scene Operations

Once you have recognized the incident as one involving hazardous materials and have called for the hazmat team, focus your efforts on activities that will ensure the safety and survival of the greatest number of people. Use the ambulance's public address system to alert people who are near the scene and direct them to move to a location where they will be sufficiently far from danger. With the aid of others on your team, try to set up a perimeter to stop traffic and people from entering the area.

### Establishing Control Zones

Setting control zones and limiting access to the incident site helps reduce the number of civilians and responders who may be exposed to the released substance. Control zones are established at a hazmat incident based on the chemical and physical properties of the released material, the environmental factors at the time of the release, and the general layout of the scene. Of course, isolating a city block in the busy downtown area of a large city presents far different challenges than isolating the area around a rolled-over cargo tank on an interstate highway. Each situation is different, requiring flexibility and thoughtfulness. Securing access to the incident helps ensure that no one will accidentally enter a contaminated area.

If the incident takes place inside a structure, the best place to control access is at the normal points of ingress and egress (entry and exit)—doors. Once the doors are secured so that no unauthorized

personnel can enter, appropriately trained emergency response crews can begin to isolate other areas as appropriate.

The same concept applies to outdoor incidents. The goal is to secure logical access points around the hazard. Begin by controlling intersections, on and off ramps, service roads, and other access routes to the scene. Law enforcement officers should assist by diverting traffic at a safe distance outside the hazard area. They should block off streets, close intersections, and redirect traffic as needed.

During a long-term incident, highway department or public works department employees may be called on to set up traffic barriers. Whatever methods or devices are used to restrict access, they should not limit or prevent a rapid withdrawal of responders from the area.

It is not uncommon to set large control zones at the onset of an incident, only to discover that the zones may have been established too liberally. At the same time, control zones should not be defined too narrowly (**FIGURE 40-25**). As the IC gets more information about the specifics of the chemical or material involved, the control zones may be expanded or reduced. Ideally, the control zones will be established in the right place the first time. Wind shifts are a common reason why control zones are modified during the incident. If there is a prevailing wind pattern and you are in the area, that should be factored into any decision making when it comes to control zones.

Typically, control zones at hazmat incidents are labeled as *hot, warm,* or *cold*. You may also discover that other terms are used, such as *exclusionary zone* (hot zone), *contamination reduction zone* (warm zone), and *outer perimeter* (cold zone). In any case, make sure you understand the terminology used in your jurisdiction. Be aware that

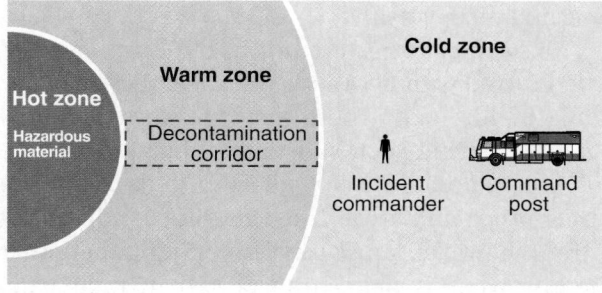

**FIGURE 40-25** Control zones spread outward from the center of a hazardous materials incident.

© Jones & Bartlett Learning.

different jurisdictions may use terminology and setup procedures unlike the ones used in your agency. As long as you understand the concepts behind the actions and remember that safety is the main focus, the act of setting up and naming zones can remain flexible.

The **hot zone** is the area immediately surrounding the release, which is also the most contaminated area. Its boundaries should be set large enough that adverse effects from the released substance will not affect people outside of the hot zone. An incident involving a gaseous substance or a vapor, for example, may require a larger hot zone than one involving a solid or nonvolatile liquid leak. In some cases, atmospheric monitoring, plume modeling, or reference sources such as the *Emergency Response Guidebook* may prove useful in helping to establish the perimeters of a hot zone. Specifically trained responders, in accordance with their level of training, should be tasked with using these tools. Keep in mind that the physical characteristics of the released substance will significantly affect the size and layout of the hot zone. In addition, all specifically trained responders entering the hot zone should avoid contact with the product to the greatest extent possible. Adhering to this important policy makes the job of decontamination easier and reduces the risk of cross-contamination.

Personnel accountability is important, so access into the hot zone must be limited to only the responders necessary to control the incident. All personnel and equipment must be decontaminated when they leave the hot zone. This practice ensures that contamination is not inadvertently spread to clean areas of the scene.

The **warm zone** is where personnel and equipment transition into and out of the hot zone. It contains control points for access to the hot zone as well as the decontamination area. Only the minimum number of personnel and the equipment necessary to perform decontamination or support those operating in the hot zone should be permitted in the warm zone.

A patient's skin and clothing may contain hazardous material, so the **decontamination area** is set up in the warm zone. The decontamination area is the designated area where contaminants are removed before an individual can go to another area. **Decontamination** is the process of removing or neutralizing and properly disposing of hazardous materials from equipment, patients, and rescue personnel.

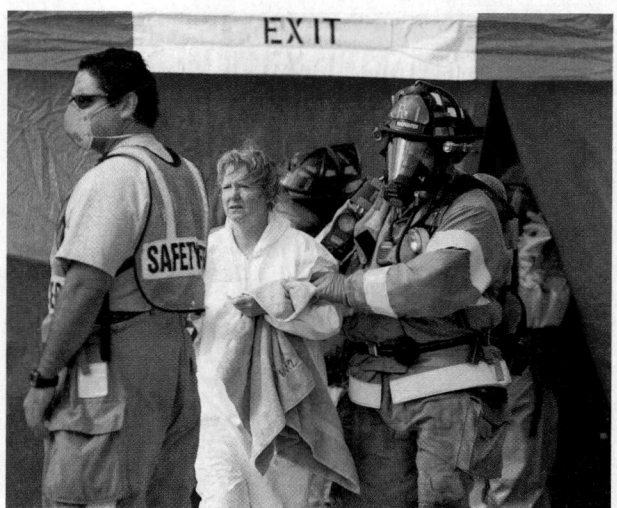

**FIGURE 40-26** Patients should be decontaminated before they are taken to treatment areas.

© ZUMA Press Inc/Alamy Stock Photo.

The decontamination area must include special containers for contaminated clothing and special bags to isolate each patient's personal effects safely until they can be decontaminated (**FIGURE 40-26**). The area will also contain several special facilities to thoroughly wash and rinse patients and backboards. The water that is used must be captured and delivered into special sealable containers.

Anyone who leaves the hot zone must pass through the decontamination area. Firefighters' and hazmat team members' outer protective gear is rinsed and washed in the decontamination area before it is removed (**FIGURE 40-27**). To prevent needless contact and transmission of splash or residues, different personnel are used in the decontamination and treatment areas. Do not move into the decontamination area unless you are properly trained and equipped. Wait for the patients to be brought to you.

Beyond the warm zone is the **cold zone**. The cold zone is a safe area where personnel do not need to wear any special protective clothing for safe operation. Personnel staging, the command post, EMS providers, and the area for medical monitoring, support, and/or treatment after decontamination are all located in the cold zone.

## Role of the EMT

As an EMT, your job is to report to a designated area outside of the hot and warm zones and provide triage, treatment, transport, or rehabilitation when hazmat team members bring patients to you.

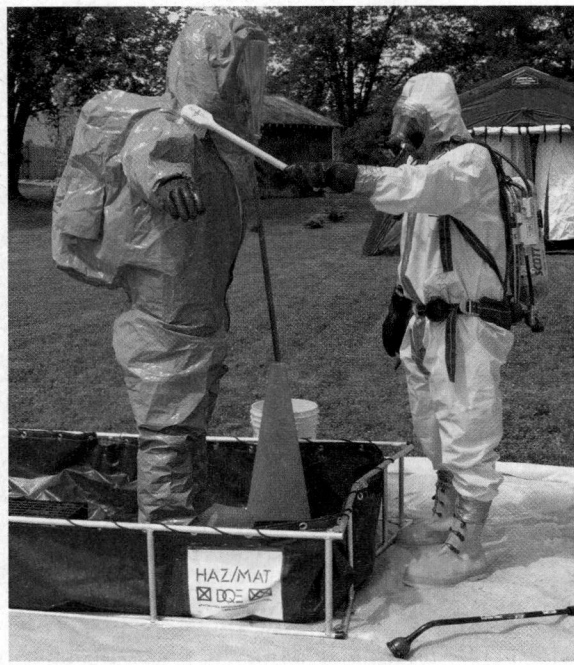

**FIGURE 40-27** The decontamination zone is where firefighters' and hazmat team members' outer protective gear is rinsed and washed before removal.

Courtesy of Airman 1st Class Scherrie Gates/US Air Force.

## Classification of Hazardous Materials

The National Fire Protection Association (NFPA) 704 hazardous materials classification standard is a system for the identification of hazardous materials according to health hazard or toxicity levels, fire hazard, chemical reactive hazard, and special hazards (such as radiation and acids) for fixed facilities that store hazardous materials. Toxicity protection levels are also classified according to the level of personal protection required. For your safety, you must know the type and degree of health, fire, and reactive hazard protection you need to operate safely near these substances before you enter the scene.

### Toxicity Level

Toxicity levels are measures of the health risk that a substance poses to someone who comes in contact with it. There are five toxicity levels: 0, 1, 2, 3, and 4. The higher the number, the greater the toxicity, as follows:

- **Level 0** includes materials that would cause little, if any, health hazard if you came in contact with them.

- **Level 1** includes materials that would cause irritation on contact but only mild residual injury, even without treatment.
- **Level 2** includes materials that could cause temporary damage or residual injury unless prompt medical treatment is provided. Both levels 1 and 2 are considered slightly hazardous but require use of self-contained breathing apparatus (SCBA) if you are going to come in contact with them.
- **Level 3** includes materials that are extremely hazardous to health. Contact with these materials requires full protective gear so that none of your skin surface is exposed.
- **Level 4** includes materials that are so hazardous that minimal contact will cause death. For level 4 substances, you need specialized gear that is designed for protection against that particular hazard.

Note that all health hazard levels, with the exception of 0, require respiratory and chemical protective gear that is not standard on most ambulances and specialized training. **TABLE 40-2** further describes the four hazard classes.

## Personal Protective Equipment Level

Personal protective equipment (PPE) levels indicate the amount and type of protective gear that you need to prevent injury from a particular substance. The four recognized protection levels, A, B, C, and D, are as follows (**FIGURE 40-28**):

- **Level A**, the most hazardous, requires fully encapsulated, chemical-resistant protective clothing that provides full body protection, as well as SCBA and special, sealed equipment.
- **Level B** requires nonencapsulated protective clothing or clothing that is designed to protect against a particular hazard (**FIGURE 40-29**).
- **Level C**, like Level B, requires the use of nonpermeable clothing and eye protection. In addition, face masks that filter all inhaled outside air must be used.
- **Level D** requires a work uniform, such as coveralls, that affords minimal protection.
- All levels of protection require the use of gloves. Two pairs of rubber gloves are needed for protection in case one pair must be removed because of heavy contamination.

**TABLE 40-2** Toxicity Levels of Hazardous Materials

| Level | Health Hazard | Protection Needed |
|---|---|---|
| 0 | Little or no hazard | None |
| 1 | Slightly hazardous | SCBA (level C suit) only |
| 2 | Slightly hazardous | SCBA (level C suit) only |
| 3 | Extremely hazardous | Full protection, with no exposed skin (level A or B suit) |
| 4 | Minimal exposure causes death | Special hazmat gear (level A suit) |

© Jones & Bartlett Learning.

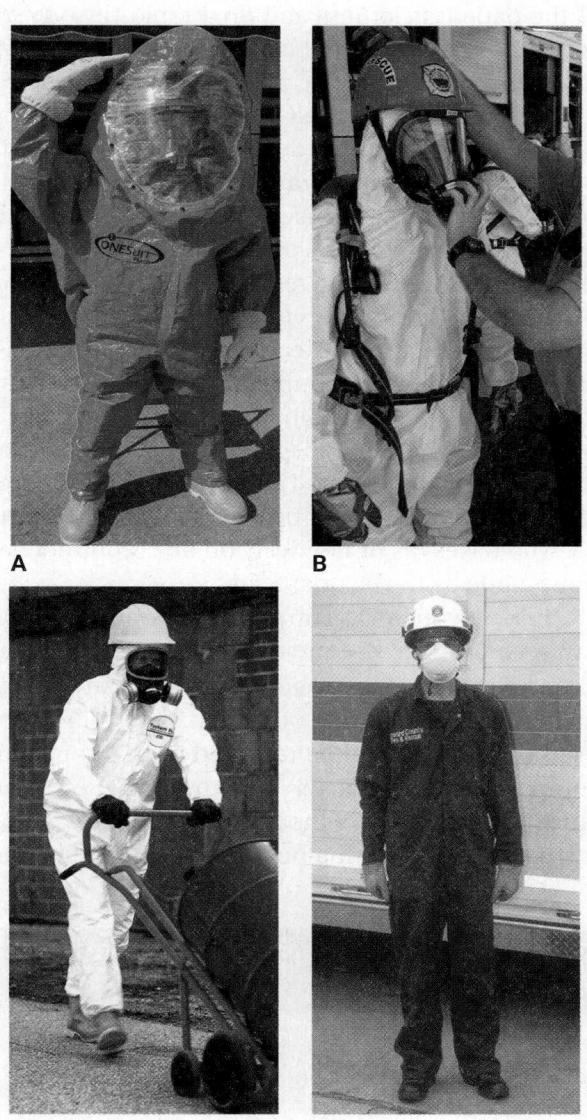

**A** **B**

**C** **D**

**FIGURE 40-28** Four levels of protection. **A.** Level A protection. **B.** Level B protection. **C.** Level C protection. **D.** Level D protection.

A, B: © Jones & Bartlett Learning. Photographed by Glen E. Ellman. C: Courtesy of The DuPont Company. D: © Jones & Bartlett Learning. Courtesy of MIEMSS.

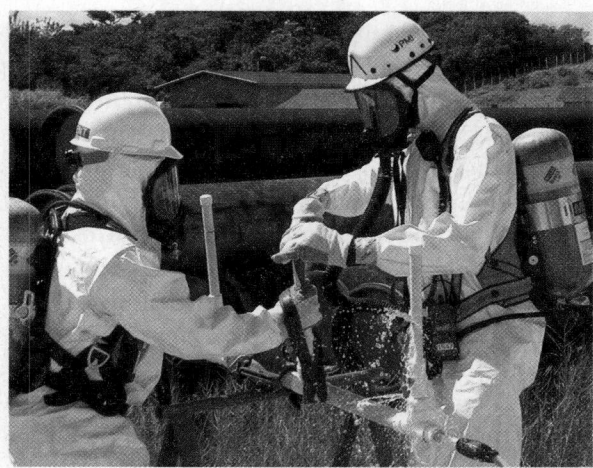

**FIGURE 40-29** Workers in Level B protection.

© Jones & Bartlett Learning. Courtesy of MIEMSS.

Usually, this clothing is made of material that will only allow limited amounts of moisture and vapor pass through (nonpermeable). Level B also requires eye protection and breathing devices that contain their own air supply, such as SCBA.

## Caring for Patients at a Hazmat Incident

Generally, hazmat team members who are trained in prehospital emergency care will initiate emergency care for patients who have been exposed to a hazardous material. However, because of the dangers, time constraints, and bulky protective gear that team members wear, it is practical only to provide the simplest assessment and essential care in the hazard zone and the decontamination area. In addition, to avoid entrapment and spread of contaminants, no bandages or splints are applied—except pressure dressings that are needed to control bleeding—until the clean (decontaminated) patient has been moved to the treatment area. Therefore, when you are providing care in the treatment area, assess and treat the patient in the same way as you would a patient who has not been previously assessed or treated.

Your care of patients at a hazmat incident must address the following two issues:

- Any trauma that has resulted from other related mechanisms, such as vehicle crash, fire, or explosion
- Injury and harm that have resulted from exposure to the hazardous substance

Most serious injuries and deaths from hazardous materials result from airway and breathing problems. Therefore, be sure to maintain the airway, and, if the patient appears to be in distress, give oxygen at 12 to 15 L/min with a nonrebreathing mask. Monitor the patient's breathing at all times. If you see signs that indicate respiratory distress is increasing, you may need to provide assisted ventilation with a bag-mask device and high-flow oxygen.

Treat the patient's injuries in the same way that you would treat any injury. There are few specific antidotes or treatments for exposure to most hazardous materials. Different people may respond differently to contact with the same hazardous material. Therefore, your treatment for the patient's exposure to the toxic substance should focus mainly on supportive care and initiating prompt transport to the hospital.

If antidotes or other special treatments need to be initiated in the field, they will be ordered by medical control and relayed to the officer in charge of EMS operations at the scene. If special treatment includes medications, intravenous fluids, or other advanced care, paramedics or other advanced personnel will be sent to work with you at the treatment area.

## Special Care

In some cases, before the decontamination area has been completely set up, the hazmat team will find one or two patients who need immediate treatment and transport without delay if they are to survive. Even if the decontamination area is set up and functioning, some patients may have such respiratory distress or otherwise urgent critical condition that the time necessary for full decontamination may prove fatal. If additional delay for proper decontamination seems life threatening in nontoxic exposure situations, it may be necessary to simply cut away all of the patient's clothing and do a rapid rinse to remove the majority of the contaminating matter before transport.

If you must treat and transport a patient who has not been properly decontaminated, you will need to increase the amount of protective clothing you wear, including the use of SCBA. At the least, this should include two pairs of gloves, goggles or a face shield, a protective coat, respiratory protection, and a disposable fluid-impervious apron or similar outfit. Many hazmat teams carry lightweight, easy-to-use, disposable, fluid-impervious protective suits for such a purpose. Remember, however, that transporting a contaminated patient merely increases the scope of the event. The decision to transport even one patient with critical injuries rests with the IC, who bases his or her decision on recommendations made by the hazmat team.

Prior to your arrival on scene, there are steps you can take to make decontaminating the ambulance easier. First, tape the cabinet doors shut. Any equipment kits, monitors, and other items that will not be used en route should be removed from the patient compartment and placed in the front of the ambulance or in outside compartments. Before loading the patient, turn on the power vent ceiling fan and

## YOU are the Provider

As the patients are being retriaged and treated, the IC contacts the local trauma center to advise staff of the situation and to determine how many of the walking wounded they can handle in addition to the one critically injured patient. Hospital staff advises him that they can handle 10 of the patients. You reassess a boy whom you originally triaged as expectant. He is now apneic and pulseless. Your partner begins CPR as you contact medical control. Based on the patient's injuries, medical control determines that resuscitation is not indicated.

**9.** What factors should be considered when determining the appropriate transport destination?

**10.** Why did medical control advise termination of resuscitation?

patient compartment air-conditioning unit fan. Unless the weather is too severe, the windows in the driver's area and sliding side windows in the patient compartment should also be partially opened to prevent creating a "closed box" inside the ambulance and to ensure that it is properly ventilated for the safety of the patient, you, and your team members.

When you leave the scene, inform the hospital that you are transporting a critically injured patient who has not been fully decontaminated at the scene. This will allow the hospital to prepare to receive the patient. Many emergency departments have decontamination facilities and trained personnel for such an event. You may be diverted to a facility with these capabilities if the receiving hospital is not so equipped. On arrival, one EMT enters the emergency department and, after giving hospital staff the report and advising them again of the incomplete decontamination, obtains directions before the patient is unloaded and brought inside. If there are enough ambulances at a hazmat scene, one may be isolated and used only to transport such patients. Remember, the ambulance needs to be decontaminated before transporting another patient.

## YOU are the Provider SUMMARY

**1. How will you decide whether to declare this an MCI?**

In this case, you are responding to an incident potentially involving many patients, and the severity of their injuries is unknown. One ambulance and two EMTs can effectively treat and transport only two stable patients *or* one critical patient at a time. In addition, there will likely be a crowd at the scene, which may hinder responder access and pose a possible danger to them, so law enforcement should be dispatched to control bystanders.

An MCI involves three or more patients, places great demand on the equipment or personnel of the EMS system, or has the potential to produce multiple casualties. On the basis of the information provided by dispatch, you should request additional EMS units. It is arguably better to call for help earlier, rather than wait until you arrive at the scene and find yourself overwhelmed by patients—some of whom may be critically injured. This holds true for all types of resources. The longer it takes to call for help, the longer it will take for help to arrive. Some centralized dispatch systems automatically send multiple EMS units and fire or law enforcement units depending on the information received from callers. In other cases, however, dispatch is dependent on input from the first responding agency. Other dispatched units can be cancelled if you determine they are not needed after you arrive on scene.

**2. How will the ICS facilitate operations at this scene?**

You have requested the assistance of other EMS units because you have determined that there are more patients than you can effectively care for. When the other units arrive, the ICS will facilitate the processes of triage, treatment, and transport; it will also help control the duplication of efforts and freelancing, in which individual units or different organizations make independent and often inefficient decisions that could compromise the effectiveness of the entire operation.

**3. How should you and your partner proceed?**

Once you have conducted a good scene size-up and answered the three basic questions—*What do I have? What resources do I need? What do I need to do?*—command should be established by the highest-ranking public safety provider present, notification to other responders should go out, and necessary resources should be requested. In this instance, you and your partner will need to establish command until more senior personnel arrive. If not already done, one of your first actions as you establish command of the scene should be to immediately request additional resources. Keep in mind that this number may change throughout the evolution of the incident, but you should not delay requesting additional resources just to make sure you have an idea of the perfect number of resources needed.

**4. Once command has been established, what are your duties?**

Once an IC and safety officer have been identified, you and your partner should begin the process of locating the patients and triaging them.

Because you and your partner are the only EMTs at the scene, you will initially need to function as the triage and treatment officer, and the primary and secondary triage will likely occur in the same area. If you have triaged all patients and additional help has still not arrived, begin treating the most critically injured patients first. As additional EMTs and ambulances arrive, they should be assigned accordingly—again, with priority given to the most critically injured patients. Depending on which units have arrived and what has been accomplished already, you will typically pass command to another person and continue performing triage or begin treating patients. In some systems that have a well-developed ICS or MCI plan, these roles will automatically evolve as personnel arrive.

**5. What are your considerations in determining whether you should stop and provide treatment for the first patient?**

Major treatment is not allowed during the triage process; however, because this patient is breathing—although slowly—and has a pulse, it is acceptable to stop and roll her to the recovery position. This may facilitate her breathing and possibly improve her condition. Due to her altered mental status, respiratory status, and weak pulses, she should be categorized as immediate (red). You should return to treat her as soon as you have completed triage or assign her to one of the first units responding to the scene.

**6. What triage categories should you assign to the second and third patients?**

Both patients should be categorized as expectant (black tag). The boy is unresponsive; is not breathing; has a slow, weak carotid pulse; and has no radial pulses. He also has exposed brain matter indicating injury that is highly likely to be incompatible with life. If adequate help was available at the scene, this patient would be categorized as immediate. The near-decapitation injury in the older woman is also likely to be incompatible with life. Compared with others encountered during your triage, these two patients have the least likely chance of survival. If you and your partner were to focus on treating these two patients, the condition of the patient you categorized as red could deteriorate further, potentially resulting in her death also.

**7. What changes, if any, should you make in your initial triage assignments with the arrival of additional responders?**

One patient was initially triaged as immediate (red tag); her triage category should stay the same.

When you and your partner were the only EMTs at the scene, you had to decide which patients were the most critical, yet the most likely to survive with immediate treatment and prompt transport. The nonbreathing teenage boy and the older woman with near-decapitation were initially triaged as expectant (black tag) because they were the least likely to survive and your available resources were limited. However, now that you have a sufficient number of EMTs and ambulances at the scene, you may reconsider their triage categories. Patients triaged as red and yellow should still receive the most immediate treatment and transport.

If you leave the teenager in the expectant category, he will die. However, if you provide immediate treatment and prompt transport, there is a chance that he will survive. Because he is apneic, begin ventilations and if he loses his pulse, begin CPR and contact medical control; treatment and transport may still be indicated. Because the third patient has already been pulseless for a while and had an injury incompatible with life, beginning treatment would be futile, so she should remain triaged as black.

**8. What should you consider in deciding whether to set up a treatment area at this incident?**

Initially, there were only two EMTs at the scene and three critically injured patients. It would be more practical and time-saving to triage and treat the patients in the same area. Taking the time to set up a treatment area would delay patient care and would require more personnel. Once more EMS resources arrive at the scene, there may be a need for a designated treatment area if transport will be delayed for any of the patients or if any of the patients initially triaged as green begin to show symptoms or need treatment for minor injuries.

**9. What factors should be considered when determining the appropriate transport destination?**

As soon as you declare an MCI, area hospitals should be notified as early as possible, informing them of the situation and determining their surge capacity; this information will tell the incident commander how many patients in each category are able to receive safe and effective care. It will also allow the hospitals to increase their staffing and, if needed, move patients within the facility.

The basic principles of transport that apply to any other patient also apply to MCIs; the most critically injured (red-tagged) patients should be transported to a designated trauma center, whereas yellow-tagged patients can be transported to hospitals that are located farther away. In cases where the closest trauma center is located a great distance away, air medical transport should be considered. Incident command or a designated transport officer should coordinate the transport, particularly when many patients are being transported, to prevent one receiving site from being overwhelmed. The receiving hospital for each patient should be notified.

**10.** **Why did medical control advise termination of resuscitation?**

He is a poor candidate because he is apneic and pulseless with exposed brain matter. A patient who is critically injured will require more resources than are available and will pull valuable resources from others who may benefit from less time-consuming care. Multiple other patients may be saved in the amount of time required to treat this one individual. Even though it would be ideal to save everyone, the purpose of triage is to do the most good for the greatest number.

However, once all other patients are treated, or if there is enough manpower, even those patients who are considered poor candidates may receive treatment. This patient's age is a consideration for attempting resuscitation. Although an older person is more likely to have a more extensive medical history, a younger person may respond well to minimal treatment. If you are unsure whether to resuscitate, it is acceptable to initiate treatment and contact medical control for further direction, which in this case was to terminate the resuscitation.

**Patient No. 1**

Triage Tag
No. 239351

| | |
|---|---|
| Move the Walking Wounded | **MINIMAL** |
| NO respirations after head tilt | **EXPECTANT** |
| | **IMMEDIATE** |
| ☐ Respirations–under 10 | |
| ☐ Perfusion–capillary refill over 2 seconds /radial pulse absent | **IMMEDIATE** |
| ☐ Mental status–unresponsive | **IMMEDIATE** |
| Otherwise | **DELAYED** |

MAJOR INJURIES: None
HOSPITAL DESTINATION : Trauma Center
ORIENTED × ☑4  DISORIENTED ☐  UNCONSCIOUS ☒

| TIME | PULSE | B/P | RESPIRATION |
|------|-------|-----|-------------|
| 1425 | 132 | N/A | 6 |
| N/A | N/A | N/A | N/A |

PERSONAL INFORMATION:
NAME : Unknown
MALE ☐  FEMALE ☒    AGE: N/A  WEIGHT : N/A
MEDICAL COMPLAINTS/HISTORY
Unknown medical history

**EXPECTANT**    No  239351

**IMMEDIATE**    No  239351

## YOU are the Provider SUMMARY *continued*

### Patient No. 2
Triage Tag
No. 239352

Move the Walking Wounded.                          **MINIMAL**

No respirations after head tilt                    **EXPECTANT**

☐ Respirations—under 10                            **IMMEDIATE**

☐ Perfusion—capillary refill over                  **IMMEDIATE**
  2 seconds /radial pulse absent

☐ Mental status—unresponsive                       **IMMEDIATE**

Otherwise                                          **DELAYED**

MAJOR INJURIES: Open skull fx with exposed brain matter
HOSPITAL DESTINATION : No transport
ORIENTED × ☐   DISORIENTED ☐   UNCONSCIOUS ☒

| TIME | PULSE | B/P | RESPIRATION |
|------|-------|-----|-------------|
| 1427 | 174 | N/A | 0 |
| N/A | N/A | N/A | N/A |

PERSONAL INFORMATION:
NAME : Not available
MALE ☒   FEMALE ☐   AGE: N/A   WEIGHT : N/A
MEDICAL COMPLAINTS/HISTORY
Apneic, absent radials/weak carotid pulse, exposed brain matter, unknown medical hx

**EXPECTANT**   No   239352

### Patient No. 3
Triage Tag
No. 239353

Move the Walking Wounded                           **MINIMAL**

NO respirations after head tilt                    **EXPECTANT**

☐ Respirations—under 10                            **IMMEDIATE**

☐ Perfusion—capillary refill over                  **IMMEDIATE**
  2 seconds /radial pulse absent

☐ Mental status—unresponsive                       **IMMEDIATE**

Otherwise                                          **DELAYED**

MAJOR INJURIES: Chest and head
HOSPITAL DESTINATION : No transport
ORIENTED × ☐   DISORIENTED ☐   UNCONSCIOUS ☒

| TIME | PULSE | B/P | RESPIRATION |
|------|-------|-----|-------------|
| 1428 | N/A | N/A | N/A |
| N/A | N/A | N/A | N/A |

PERSONAL INFORMATION:
NAME : Not available
MALE ☐   FEMALE ☒   AGE: N/A   WEIGHT : N/A
MEDICAL COMPLAINTS/HISTORY
Unconscious, apneic, pulseless, unknown medical history

**EXPECTANT**   No   239353

# Prep Kit

## Ready for Review

- The NIMS provides a comprehensive framework to enable federal, state, and local governments, as well as private-sector and nongovernmental organizations, to work together effectively. The NIMS is used to prepare for, prevent, respond to, mitigate, and recover from domestic incidents, regardless of cause, size, or complexity, including acts of catastrophic terrorism and hazardous materials (hazmat) incidents.
- The three major NIMS components are command and coordination, communication and information management, and resource management.
- The purpose of the ICS is to ensure responder and public safety, achieve incident management goals, and ensure the efficient use of resources.
- Preparedness involves the decisions made and basic planning done before an incident occurs.
- Your agency should have written disaster plans that you are regularly trained to carry out.
- At incidents that have a significant medical factor, the IC will designate someone as the

chief of the medical (or EMS) branch under the operations section. This person will supervise the primary roles of the medical group: triage, treatment, and transport of the injured.

- An MCI refers to any call that involves three or more patients, any situation that places such a great demand on available equipment or personnel that the system would require a mutual aid response, or any incident that has a potential to create one of the previously mentioned situations.
- The goal of triage is to do the greatest good for the greatest number of people. This means that the triage assessment is brief and the patient condition categories are basic.
- There are four basic triage categories that can be recalled using the mnemonic IDME:

- Immediate (red)
- Delayed (yellow)
- Minimal (green; hold)
- Expectant (black; likely to die or dead)
- A disaster is a widespread event that disrupts functions and resources of a community and threatens lives and property.
- Many disasters, such as a drought, may not involve personal injuries.
- When you arrive at the scene of a hazmat incident, you must first step back and assess the situation. This can be very stressful, particularly if you see a patient.
- CHEMTREC is a valuable resource for determining what the hazardous material is and what you should do.

## Vital Vocabulary

**bills of lading** The shipping papers used for transport of chemicals over roads and highways; also referred to as freight bills.

**bulk storage containers** Any container other than nonbulk storage containers, such as fixed tanks, highway cargo tanks, rail tank cars, totes, and intermodal tanks. These are typically found in manufacturing facilities and are often surrounded by a secondary containment system to help control an accidental release.

**carboys** Glass, plastic, or steel containers, ranging in volume from 5 to 15 gallons (19 to 57 L).

**casualty collection area** An area set up by physicians, nurses, and other hospital staff near a major disaster scene where patients can receive further triage and medical care.

**Chemical Transportation Emergency Center (CHEMTREC)** An agency that assists emergency responders in identifying and handling hazardous materials transport incidents.

**closed incident** An incident that is contained; all casualties are accounted for.

**cold zone** A safe area at a hazardous materials incident for the agencies involved in the operations. The incident commander, the command post, EMS providers, and other support functions necessary to control the incident should be

located in this zone. Also referred to as the clean zone or the support zone.

**command** In incident command, the position that oversees the incident, establishes the objectives and priorities, and develops a response plan.

**command post** The designated field command center where the incident commander and support staff are located.

**container** Any vessel or receptacle that holds material, including storage vessels, pipelines, and packaging.

**control zones** Areas at a hazardous materials incident that are designated as hot, warm, or cold, based on safety issues and the degree of hazard found there.

**cylinders** Portable, compressed gas containers used to hold liquids and gases such as nitrogen, argon, helium, and oxygen. They have a range of sizes and internal pressures.

**decontamination** The process of removing or neutralizing and properly disposing of hazardous materials from equipment, patients, and responders.

**decontamination area** The designated area in a hazardous materials incident where all patients and responders must be decontaminated before going to another area.

**demobilization** The process of directing responders to return to their facilities when work at a disaster or mass-casualty incident has finished, at least for those particular responders.

**disaster** A widespread event that disrupts community resources and functions, in turn threatening public safety, citizens' lives, and property.

**drums** Barrel-like containers used to store a wide variety of substances, including food-grade materials, corrosives, flammable liquids, and grease. May be constructed of low-carbon steel, polyethylene, cardboard, stainless steel, nickel, or other materials.

**Emergency Response Guidebook (ERG)** A preliminary action guide for first responders operating at a hazardous materials incident in coordination with the US Department of Transportation's labels and placards marking system. Jointly developed by the DOT, the Secretariat of Communications and Transportation of Mexico, and Transport Canada.

**extrication supervisor** In incident command, the person appointed to determine the type of equipment and resources needed for a situation involving extrication or special rescue; also called the rescue officer.

**finance/administration** In incident command, the position in an incident responsible for accounting of all expenditures.

**freelancing** When individual units or different organizations make independent and often inefficient decisions about the next appropriate action.

**freight bills** The shipping papers used for transport of chemicals along roads and highways; also referred to as bills of lading.

**hazardous material** Any substance that is toxic, poisonous, radioactive, flammable, or explosive and causes injury or death with exposure.

**hazardous materials (hazmat) incident** An incident in which a hazardous material is no longer properly contained and isolated.

**hot zone** The area immediately surrounding a hazardous materials spill or incident site that endangers life and health. All responders working in this zone must wear appropriate protective clothing and equipment. Entry requires approval by the incident commander or other designated officer.

**incident action plan** An oral or written plan stating general objectives reflecting the overall strategy for managing an incident.

**incident commander (IC)** The overall leader of the incident command system to whom commanders or leaders of incident command system divisions report.

**incident command system (ICS)** A system implemented to manage disasters and mass-casualty incidents in which section chiefs, including finance/administration, logistics, operations, and planning, report to the incident commander.

**intermodal tanks** Shipping and storage vessels that can be either pressurized or nonpressurized.

**joint information center (JIC)** An area designated by the incident commander, or a designee, in which public information officers from multiple agencies distribute information about the incident.

**JumpSTART triage** A sorting system for pediatric patients younger than 8 years or weighing less than 100 pounds (45 kg). There is a minor adaptation for infants because they cannot ambulate on their own.

**liaison officer** In incident command, the person who relays information, concerns, and requests among responding agencies.

**logistics** In incident command, the position that helps procure and stockpile equipment and supplies during an incident.

**mass-casualty incident (MCI)** An emergency situation involving three or more patients or that can place great demand on the equipment or personnel of the EMS system or has the potential to produce multiple casualties.

**material safety data sheet (MSDS)** A form, provided by manufacturers and compounders (blenders) of chemicals, containing information about chemical composition, physical and chemical properties, health and safety hazards, emergency response, and waste disposal of a specific material; also known as safety data sheet (SDS).

**morgue supervisor** In incident command, the person who works with area medical examiners, coroners, and law enforcement agencies to coordinate the disposition of dead victims.

**mutual aid response** An agreement between neighboring EMS systems to respond to mass-casualty incidents or disasters in each other's region when local resources are insufficient to handle the response.

**National Incident Management System (NIMS)** A Department of Homeland Security system designed to enable federal, state, and local governments and private-sector and nongovernmental organizations to effectively and efficiently prepare for, prevent, respond to, and recover from domestic incidents, regardless of cause, size, or complexity, including acts of catastrophic terrorism.

**nonbulk storage vessels** Any container other than bulk storage containers, such as drums, bags, compressed gas cylinders, and cryogenic containers. These hold commonly used commercial and industrial chemicals such as solvents, industrial cleaners, and compounds.

**open incident** An incident that is not yet contained; there may be patients to be located and the situation may be ongoing, producing more patients.

**operations** In incident command, the position that carries out the orders of the commander to help resolve the incident.

**personal protective equipment (PPE) levels** Indicates the amount and type of protective equipment that an individual needs to avoid injury during contact with a hazardous material.

**placards** Signage required to be placed on all four sides of highway transport vehicles, railroad tank cars, and other forms of hazardous materials transportation; the sign identifies the hazardous contents of the vehicle, using a standardization system with diamond-shaped indicators.

**planning** In incident command, the position that ultimately produces a plan to resolve any incident.

**primary triage** A type of patient sorting used to rapidly categorize patients; the focus is on speed in locating all patients and determining an initial priority as their conditions warrant.

**public information officer (PIO)** In incident command, the person who keeps the public informed and relates any information to the media.

**rehabilitation area** The area that provides protection and treatment to firefighters and other responders working at an emergency. Here, workers are medically monitored and receive any needed care as they enter and leave the scene.

**rehabilitation supervisor** In incident command, the person who establishes an area that provides protection for responders from the elements and the situation.

**rescue supervisor** In incident command, the person appointed to determine the type of equipment and resources needed for a situation involving extrication or special rescue; also called the extrication officer.

**safety officer** In incident command, the person who monitors the scene for conditions or operations that may present a hazard to responders and patients; he or she may stop an operation when responder safety is an issue.

**secondary containment** An engineered method to control spilled or released product if the main containment vessel fails.

**secondary triage** A type of patient sorting used in the treatment area that involves retriage of patients.

**single command system** A command system in which one person is in charge; generally used with small incidents that involve only one responding agency or one jurisdiction.

**span of control** In incident command, the subordinate positions under the commander's direction to which the workload is distributed; the ideal supervisor/worker ratio is one supervisor for five subordinates.

**staging supervisor** In incident command, the person who locates an area to stage equipment and personnel and tracks unit arrival and deployment from the staging area.

**START triage** A patient sorting process that stands for Simple Triage And Rapid Treatment and uses a limited assessment of the patient's ability to walk, respiratory status, hemodynamic status, and neurologic status.

**termination of command** The end of the incident command structure when an incident draws to a close.

**toxicity levels** Indicates the risk that a hazardous material poses to the health of an individual who comes into contact with it.

**transportation area** The area in a mass-casualty incident where ambulances and crews are organized to transport patients from the treatment area to receiving hospitals.

**transportation supervisor** In incident command, the person in charge of the transportation sector in a mass-casualty incident who assigns patients from the treatment area to waiting ambulances in the transportation area.

**treatment area** The location in a mass-casualty incident where patients are brought after being triaged and assigned a priority, where they are reassessed, treated, and monitored until transport to the hospital.

**treatment supervisor** In incident command, the person, usually a physician, who is in charge of and directs EMS providers at the treatment area in a mass-casualty incident.

**triage** The process of sorting patients based on the severity of injury and medical need to establish treatment and transportation priorities.

**triage supervisor** In incident command, the person in charge of the incident command triage sector who directs the sorting of patients into triage categories in a mass-casualty incident.

**unified command system** A command system used in larger incidents in which there is a multiagency response or multiple jurisdictions are involved.

**warm zone** The area located between the hot zone and the cold zone at a hazardous materials incident. The decontamination corridor is located in this zone.

# References

1. Arshad FH, Williams A, Asaeda G, et al. A modified simple triage and rapid treatment algorithm from the New York City (USA) Fire Department. *Prehosp Disaster Med.* 2015;30(2):199-204.

2. Department of Homeland Security. *National Incident Management System, 3rd ed.* Washington, DC: US Department of Homeland Security; 2017. https://www.fema.gov/media-library-data/1508151197225-ced8c60378c3936adb92c1a3ee6f6564/FINAL_NIMS_2017.pdf. Accessed March 3, 2020.

3. National EMS Management Association. *Operational Templates and Guidance for EMS Mass Incident Deployment.* Emmitsburg, MD: US Fire Administration; 2012. https://www.usfa.fema.gov/downloads/pdf/publications/templates_guidance_ems_mass_incident_deployment.pdf. Accessed March 3, 2020.

4. National Highway Traffic Safety Administration. *National Emergency Medical Services Education Standards.* DOT HS 811 077A. www.ems.gov/pdf/811077a.pdf. Published January 2009. Accessed March 3, 2020.

5. National Highway Traffic Safety Administration. *National Emergency Medical Services Education Standards. Emergency Medical Technician Instructional Guidelines.* DOT HS 811 077C. www.ems.gov/pdf/811077c.pdf. Published January 2009. www.ems.gov/pdf/811077c.pdf. Accessed March 3, 2020.

6. SALT mass casualty triage: concept endorsed by the American College of Emergency Physicians, American College of Surgeons Committee on Trauma, American Trauma Society, National Association of EMS Physicians, National Disaster Life Support Education Consortium, and State and Territorial Injury Prevention Directors Association. *Disaster Med Public Health Prep.* 2008;2(4):245-246.

7. Chemical Hazards Emergency Medical Management. START adult triage algorithm. US Department of Health and Human Services. https://chemm.nlm.nih.gov/startadult.htm. Updated June 26, 2019. Accessed March 3, 2020.

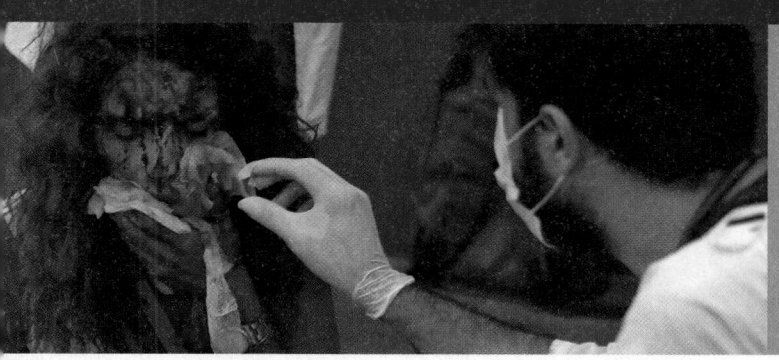

# Chapter 41

# Terrorism Response and Disaster Management

## NATIONAL EMS EDUCATION STANDARD COMPETENCIES

### EMS Operations

Knowledge of operational roles and responsibilities to ensure patient, public, and personnel safety.

### Mass-Casualty Incidents Due to Terrorism and Disaster

- Risks and responsibilities of operating on the scene of a natural or man-made disaster. (pp 1528–1553)

## KNOWLEDGE OBJECTIVES

1. Define international terrorism and domestic terrorism; include examples of incidents that have been caused by each one. (p 1528)

2. Name four different types of goals that commonly motivate terrorist groups to carry out terrorist attacks. (p 1529)

3. Define weapon of mass destruction (WMD) and weapon of mass casualty (WMC); include examples of weapons considered WMDs. (p 1531)

4. Explain how the Department of Homeland Security (DHS) National Terrorism Advisory System (NTAS) relates to the actions and precautions EMTs must take while performing their daily activities. (pp 1532–1533)

5. Name the key observations EMTs must make on every call to determine the potential of a terrorist attack. (pp 1532–1533)

6. Explain the critical response actions related to establishing and reassessing scene safety, personnel protection, notification procedures,

and establishing command that EMTs must perform at a suspected terrorist event. (pp 1532–1535)

7. Discuss the history of chemical agents, their four main classifications, routes of exposure, and the effects on patient care. (pp 1535–1542)

8. List three categories of biologic agents, their routes of exposure, effects on the patient, and patient care. (pp 1542–1548)

9. Explain the role of EMS in relation to syndromic surveillance and points of distribution (PODs) during a biologic event. (pp 1548–1549)

10. Discuss the history of nuclear/radiologic devices, sources of radiologic materials and dispersal devices, medical management of patients, and protective measures EMTs must take during a nuclear/radiologic incident. (pp 1549–1552)

11. Describe the mechanisms of injury caused by incendiary and explosive devices; include the types and severity of wounds. (pp 1552–1553)

# Introduction

With the increasing number of terrorist attacks every year, you must be mentally and physically prepared for the possibility of a terrorist event. Both international groups and domestic terrorists have attacked, with an alarming trend toward targeting civilian populations. From coordinated attacks with firearms and homemade explosives to large-scale events targeting hundreds or thousands, it is no longer a question of *if* another attack will occur, but when and where it will occur.

The use of weapons of mass destruction (WMDs), or weapons of mass casualty (WMCs), further complicates the management of the terrorist incident and places you in greater danger. Although it is difficult to plan and anticipate a response to many terrorist events, there are several key principles that apply to every response. This chapter discusses the types of terrorist events, personnel safety, and patient management and gives you tools to prepare to respond to these events. You will learn the signs, symptoms, and treatment of patients who have been exposed to nuclear, chemical, or biologic agents or an explosive attack. At the end of this chapter, you will be able to answer the following key questions:

- What are my initial actions?
- Whom should I notify, and what should I tell them?
- What type of additional resources do I require?
- How should I proceed to address the needs of the victims?
- How do I ensure the safety of myself, my partner, and the victims?
- What is the clinical presentation of a victim exposed to a WMD?
- How do I assess and treat patients who have been affected by WMD?
- How should I avoid becoming contaminated or cross-contaminated with a WMD agent?

For the EMT working in today's society, these new challenges all translate to the need to maintain a high degree of situational awareness, prepare yourself mentally and physically to respond to these types of events, and support educating immediate responders to assist in saving lives.

# What Is Terrorism?

Terrorist forces have been at work since early civilization. Used to instill fear in the hearts of others, terrorist attacks have targeted small groups and large societies alike. Currently, terrorists pose a threat to nations and cultures everywhere. International and domestic terrorism has brought a new fear into the lives of many American citizens.

The US Department of Justice defines both **international terrorism** and **domestic terrorism** with these points:

- Involves violent acts or acts dangerous to human life that violate federal or state law
- Appears to be intended (i) to intimidate or coerce a civilian population; (ii) to influence the policy of a government by intimidation or coercion; or (iii) to affect the conduct of a government by mass destruction, assassination, or kidnapping

One difference between the two is location. International terrorism occurs primarily outside the territorial jurisdiction of the United States, and domestic terrorism occurs primarily within the territorial jurisdiction of the United States.

Modern-day terrorism is common in the Middle East, where terrorist groups frequently attack civilian populations. In Central and South America, political terrorist groups target oil resources as a means to instill fear.

In the United States, domestic terrorists have carried out multiple attacks. The destruction of the Alfred P. Murrah Federal Building in Oklahoma City in 1995 and the Boston Marathon bombing in 2013 are examples (**FIGURE 41-1**). Terrorist organizations are often categorized based on their beliefs and goals. Only a small percentage of groups turn toward terrorism as a means to achieve their goals, such as the following:

1. **Religious extremist groups/doomsday cults.** These include groups such as Aleph (formerly Aum Shinrikyo), which carried out chemical attacks in Tokyo in 1994 and 1995. Some of these groups may participate in apocalyptic violence.
2. **Extremist political groups.** They may include violent separatist groups and those who seek political, religious, economic, and social freedom.
3. **Cyber terrorists.** They attack a population's technological infrastructure to draw attention to their cause.
4. **Single-issue groups.** These include antiabortion groups, animal rights groups, anarchists, racists, and even ecoterrorists who threaten or use violence to protect the environment (**FIGURE 41-2**).

## Active Shooter Events

An alarming new trend in domestic terrorism involves the concept of the lone wolf terrorist attack. This method has quickly become a frequent threat in the United States and has resulted in some of the most devastating attacks on US soil in recent years.

In *Report: Lone Wolf Terrorism*, the National Security Critical Issue Task Force defines lone wolf terrorism as "the deliberate creation and exploitation of fear through violence or threat of violence committed by a single actor who pursues political change linked to a formulated ideology, whether his own or that of a larger organization, and who does not receive orders, direction, or material support from outside sources."

The motives of the lone wolf terrorist are not always clear. These attacks may target schools, music festivals, or even shopping centers and have been difficult to predict. Examples of lone wolf terrorist attacks include the 2015 Emanuel Church shooting in Charleston, South Carolina, the Pulse nightclub shooting of 2016 in Orlando, Florida (**FIGURE 41-3**), and the 2017 Las Vegas, Nevada, shooting at the Route 91 Harvest music festival. The combined

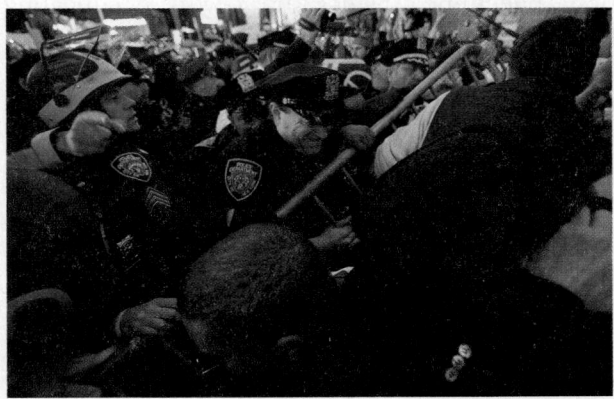

**FIGURE 41-2** Demonstrators being held back by police in Times Square in 2011.

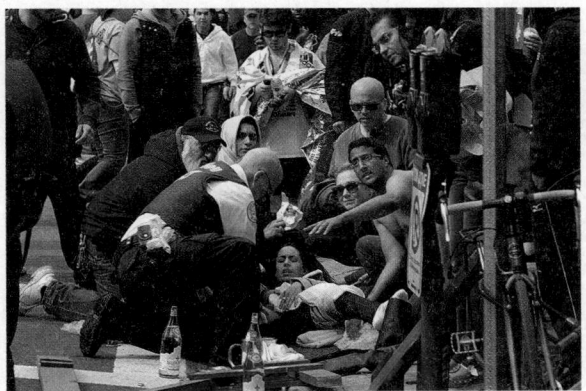

**FIGURE 41-1** The bombing at the Boston Marathon in 2013 was an example of domestic terrorism.

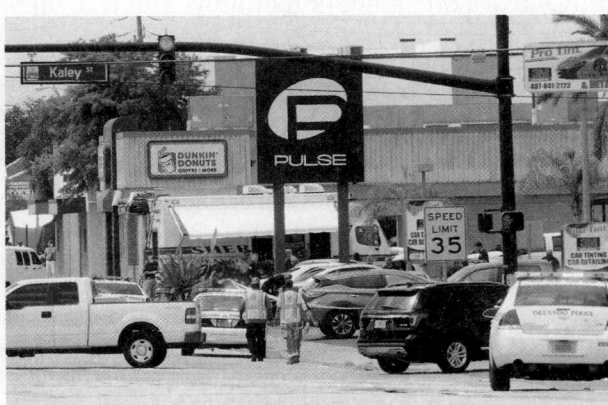

**FIGURE 41-3** The Pulse nightclub shooting in Orlando in 2016 was an example of a lone wolf terrorist attack.

death toll from just those three events is over 110 people, with the total number of injured people close to 1,000.

Many lone wolf terrorist attacks involve firearms and not explosives; thus this type of event can be further classified as an **active shooter event**. The alarming increase in the frequency of these attacks has prompted discussion of gun laws, mental health, and education of the public and first responders on how to treat casualties of active shooter events. In 2013, a committee of the American College of Surgeons that included law enforcement, EMS, fire, military and federal agencies produced recommendations for best practices aimed at improving survival during active shooter and intentional mass-casualty events. The committee's recommendations are known as the Hartford Consensus. The Hartford Consensus consists of four reports that have helped to shape national policy and provides a framework for educating both the public and first responders.

The Hartford Consensus recommends that a response plan designed for active shooter response should include the acronym THREAT: Threat suppression, Hemorrhage control, Rapid Extrication to safety, Assessment by medical providers, and Transport to definitive care. This plan encourages a continuum of care that begins with immediate responders: those who are present at the time and place of the attack. The continuum of care progresses with professional responders arriving at the scene and trauma professionals at the hospital.

The Hartford Consensus highlights the importance of early hemorrhage control. Although education and training can help immediate responders truly make a difference and improve survival, there may not always be uninjured people available to help the injured. The Hartford Consensus recommends reevaluating the practice of staging away from the scene and having patients brought to the ambulance. Traditionally, it may take a significant amount of time for professional responders to reach injured patients after the threat has been neutralized and the scene has been declared safe for all responders to enter. To provide care sooner, many EMS organizations have revised the roles and responsibilities of personnel responding to an active shooter event. EMS crews may be equipped with ballistic vests and helmets so that they can potentially be paired with law enforcement to assist with treatment and evacuation of injured people from an active scene. A key component to safely incorporating EMS crews with law enforcement teams who are moving forward into an active shooter scene is interagency training. This remains a controversial topic because it forces EMS systems to question how much risk to providers is acceptable to save the lives of others.

## Safety Tips

An ideal scenario would involve complete threat elimination before any additional responders would enter the scene. Following a shooting at a large high school, the process of law enforcement searching the facility room by room and ensuring there are no threats to additional responders could take hours. This delay may be fatal for many of the injured. There has not been a universally accepted solution to this debate, so make sure you discuss this topic with your agency and follow your local protocols and policies.

## YOU are the Provider

You and your partner are on standby at a local holiday parade. Due to many parades in the area, you are the only medical resource assigned to this parade. As the parade is nearing the midway point, your unit is requested to respond to an injured law enforcement officer who was found with multiple stab wounds in an alley along the parade route. As you near the officer's location, you suddenly see dozens of people frantically running away from the parade route. Your partner stops the ambulance immediately. An event worker rushes up to your unit and says event staff had reports of a trash can that was smoking heavily about two blocks up. As he was walking to investigate the report, a man stepped out of the crowd and began to shoot a large rifle into the crowd. He said there were lots of people lying on the ground bleeding, and he believes the suspected shooter was shot and killed by police.

**1.** On the basis of the information you have received, how should you approach this incident?

**2.** What indicators suggest that an incident is the result of terrorism?

The recommendations from the Hartford Consensus also paved the way for the Stop the Bleed campaign. Launched in 2015 by the Department of Defense, this nationwide campaign promotes offering education on hemorrhage control to the public to help improve the willingness and effectiveness of immediate responders who are able to help save lives at the point of injury. As of September 2019, over one million people around the world have been trained to save a life through the Stop the Bleed campaign.

Some terrorist attacks require the coordination of multiple terrorists or "actors" working together. Nineteen hijackers worked together to commit the worst act of terrorism in US history on September 11, 2001 (**FIGURE 41-4**). At least four terrorists worked together to commit the London Subway bombings on July 7, 2005. However, in a few instances a single terrorist has been responsible for causing devastating results. A single person who acted alone carried out each of the Atlanta abortion clinic attacks in 1996 and the 1996 Summer Olympics attack.

# Weapons of Mass Destruction

A **weapon of mass destruction (WMD)**, or **weapon of mass casualty (WMC)**, is any agent designed to bring about mass death, casualties, and/or massive damage to property and infrastructure (bridges, tunnels, airports, and seaports). To help remember the different kinds of weapons of mass destruction, use the mnemonic **B-NICE**: **b**iologic, **n**uclear, **i**ncendiary, **c**hemical, and **e**xplosive weapons; or CBRNE for **c**hemical, **b**iologic, **r**adiologic, **n**uclear, and **ex**plosive weapons.

To date, the preferred WMD for terrorists has been explosive devices. Terrorist groups have favored tactics that use truck bombs or car or pedestrian suicide bombers. Many previous attempts by terrorists to use either chemical or biologic weapons to their full capacity have been unsuccessful. Nonetheless, as an EMT, you must ensure that you understand the destructive potential of these weapons.

The motives and tactics of the new-age terrorist groups have begun to change. As with the doomsday cults, many terrorist groups participate in indiscriminate killing. This doctrine of total carnage would make the use of WMDs highly desirable. WMDs are relatively easy to obtain or create and are specifically geared toward killing a lot of people. Had the proper techniques been used during the 1995 Aum Shinrikyo attack on the Tokyo subway, there might have been tens of thousands of casualties. Since the fall of the Soviet Union, the technology and expertise to produce WMDs may be available to terrorist groups with sufficient funding. Moreover, the technical recipes for making B-NICE weapons can be readily found on the Internet; in fact, they have even been published on terrorist group websites.

> ## Words of Wisdom
>
> Chemical warfare may consist of agents in the form of a liquid, powder, or vapor.

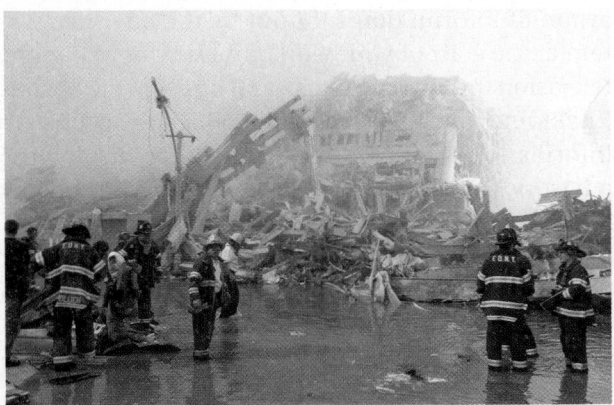

**FIGURE 41-4** The September 11, 2001, attack on the World Trade Center in New York City accounted for most of the deaths caused by terrorists in 2001.

© Ron Agam/Stringer/Getty Images News/Getty Images.

## Chemical Terrorism/Warfare

Chemical agents are manufactured substances that can have devastating effects on living organisms. They can be produced in liquid, powder, or vapor form depending on the desired route of exposure and dissemination technique. Developed during World War I (WWI), these agents have been implicated in thousands of deaths since being introduced on the battlefield, and they have been used to terrorize civilian populations. These agents consist of the following types:

- Vesicants (blister agents)
- Respiratory agents (choking agents)
- Nerve agents
- Metabolic agents (cyanides)

## Biologic Terrorism/Warfare

Biologic agents are organisms that cause disease. They are generally found in nature; however, for terrorist use, they are cultivated, synthesized, and mutated in a laboratory. The **weaponization** of biologic agents is performed to artificially maximize the target population's exposure to the germ, thereby exposing the greatest number of people and achieving the desired result.

The primary types of biologic agents that you may come in contact with during a biologic event include the following:

- Viruses
- Bacteria
- Toxins

## Nuclear/Radiologic Terrorism

There have been only two publicly known uses of a nuclear device, both occurring during wartime. During World War II (WWII), Hiroshima and Nagasaki were devastated when they were targeted with nuclear bombs. The awesome destructive power demonstrated by the attack ended WWII and has served as a deterrent to nuclear war.

There are nations that hold close ties with terrorist groups (known as **state-sponsored terrorism**) and have obtained some degree of nuclear capability.

It is also possible for a terrorist to secure radioactive materials or waste to perpetrate an act of terror. These materials are far easier for a terrorist to acquire than are nuclear weapons and require less expertise to use. The difficulties in developing a nuclear weapon are well documented. Radioactive materials, however, such as those in radiologic dispersal devices (RDDs), also known as "dirty bombs," can cause widespread panic and civil disturbances. These devices are covered later in this chapter.

## EMT Response to Terrorism

When you respond to a terrorist event, the basic foundations of patient care remain the same; however, the treatment can and will vary. Terrorist events can produce a single casualty, hundreds of casualties, or even thousands of casualties. In all cases, you must remember situational awareness is key. You must do everything in your power to be as safe as possible while caring for the sick and injured. Your response in one situation may not be appropriate for another situation. In large-scale terrorist events, it is important to use triage and base patient care on available resources.

## Recognizing a Terrorist Event (Indicators)

The planning of most acts of terror is **covert**, which means that the public safety community generally has no prior knowledge of the time, location, or nature of the attack. This element of surprise makes responding to an event more complex. You must constantly be aware of your surroundings and understand the possible risks for terrorism associated with certain locations, at certain times. Therefore, it is important that you know the current threat level issued by the federal government through the Department of Homeland Security (DHS).

In April 2011, the color-coded Homeland Security Advisory System was replaced by the National Terrorism Advisory System (NTAS). Alerts from the NTAS contain a summary of the threat and the actions that first responders, government agencies, and the public can take to maintain safety. On the basis of threat information, make sure you take the appropriate actions and precautions while you continue to perform your daily duties and respond to calls.

The DHS has not issued specific recommendations for EMS personnel to follow in response to specific threats. Follow your local protocols, policies, and procedures.

It is your responsibility to make sure you are aware of information sent out by the advisory system at the start of your workday. Daily newspapers, television news programs, and multiple websites (including the DHS website) all give up-to-date information. Many EMS organizations display the advisory system on boards where it can be seen by staff when they arrive for a shift.

Understanding and being aware of the current threat is only the beginning of responding safely to calls. To determine the potential for a terrorist attack, make the following observations on every call:

- **Type of location.** Is the location a monument, infrastructure, government building, or a specific type of location, such as a temple? Is there a large gathering? Is there a special event taking place?

- **Type of call.** Is there a report of an explosion or suspicious device nearby? Are there reports of people fleeing the scene?
- **Number of patients.** Are there multiple victims with similar signs and symptoms? This is probably the single most important clue that a terrorist attack or an incident involving a WMD has occurred.
- **Victims' statements.** This is probably the second-best indication of a terrorist or WMD event. Are the victims fleeing the scene giving statements such as "Everyone is passing out," "There was a loud explosion," or "There are a lot of people shaking on the ground"? If so, something is occurring that you do not want to rush into, even if it is questionable as to whether it is a terrorist event.
- **Preincident indicators.** Has there been a recent increase in violent political activism? Are you aware of any credible threats made against the location, gathering, or occasion?

## Response Actions

Once you suspect that a terrorist event has occurred or a WMD has been used, there are certain actions you must take to ensure you will be safe and properly prepared to help the community.

## Scene Safety

Remember to stage your vehicle a safe distance (usually 1 to 2 blocks) from the incident, and wait for law enforcement personnel to advise you that the scene has been made secure. If you think that it may not be safe, do not enter. When dealing with a WMD scene, assume you will not be able to enter the scene where the event has occurred—nor do you want to. The best location for staging is upwind and uphill from the incident. Wait for assistance from those who are trained in assessing and managing WMD scenes (**FIGURE 41-5**). Expect that a perimeter will be created, usually by law enforcement personnel, to isolate the scene, prevent further contamination of evidence, and protect rescuers and the public from further danger. In addition, remember the following rules:

- Failure to park your vehicle at a safe location can place you and your partner in danger (**FIGURE 41-6**). Always have an escape plan

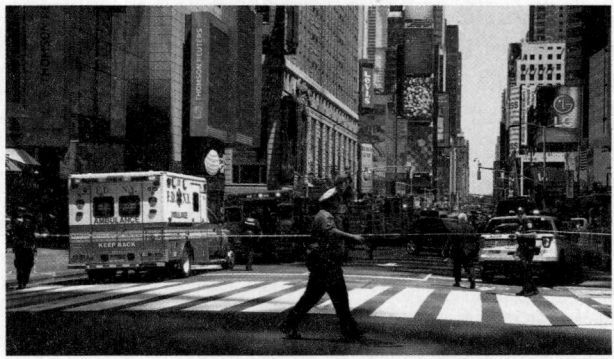

**FIGURE 41-5** Improper staging of a mass-casualty scene can lead to injury or even death of EMS personnel. Wait for trained personnel to assist in assessing and managing such scenes. This scene shows an incident in 2017 in New York City. A person drove a vehicle into multiple pedestrians on a busy sidewalk.

© Volkan Furuncu/Anadolu Agency/Getty Images.

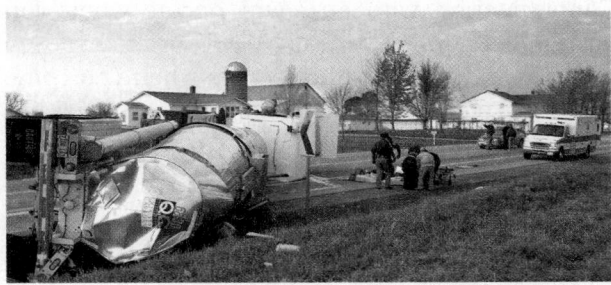

**FIGURE 41-6** Park your vehicle at a safe location.

© Dennis MacDonald/Alamy Stock Photo.

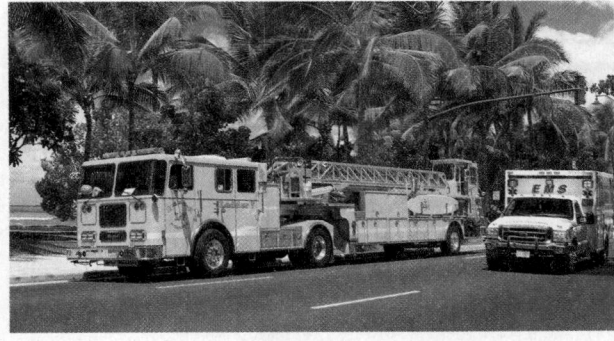

**FIGURE 41-7** Make sure your vehicle is not blocked in by other emergency vehicles.

© pbpgalleries/Alamy Stock Photo.

determined beforehand, in case the scene becomes unsafe.
- If your vehicle is blocked in by other emergency vehicles or damaged by a secondary device (or event), you will be unable to provide transportation for victims (**FIGURE 41-7**) or escape yourself.

Terrorists have been known to plant additional explosives that are set to explode after the initial bomb. This type of **secondary device** is intended primarily to injure responders and to secure media coverage because the media generally arrive on scene just after the initial response. Secondary devices may include various types of electronic equipment such as cell phones or pagers that are designed to detonate the secondary device on activation.

## Responder Safety (Personnel Protection)

The best form of protection from a WMD agent is preventing yourself from coming in contact with the agent. The greatest threats facing you in a WMD attack are contamination and **cross-contamination**. Contamination with an agent occurs when you have direct contact with the WMD or are exposed to it. Cross-contamination occurs when you come in contact with a contaminated person who has not yet been decontaminated.

## Notification Procedures

When you suspect a terrorist or WMD event has taken place, notify the dispatcher. Vital information needs to be communicated effectively if you are to receive the appropriate assistance. (See Chapter 4, *Communications and Documentation*, for information on effective communication.) Inform dispatch of the nature of the event, any additional resources that may be required, the estimated number of patients, and the upwind route of approach or optimal route of approach.

It is extremely important to establish a staging area, where additional arriving units will converge. Be mindful of access and exit routes when you direct units to respond to a location. It is unwise to have units respond to the front entrance of a hotel or apartment building that has sustained an explosion. (See Chapter 38, *Transport Operations*, for more on vehicle positioning.) Last, trained responders in the proper protective equipment are the only people equipped to handle the WMD incident. These specialized units, traditionally hazardous materials (hazmat) teams, must be requested as early as possible because of the time required to assemble and dispatch the team and their equipment. Many jurisdictions share hazmat teams, so the team may have to travel a long distance to reach the location of the event. It is always better to be safe than sorry; call the team early, and the outcome of the call may be more favorable.

Keep in mind that there may be more than one type of device or agent present.

### Words of Wisdom

#### Weapons of Mass Destruction

On September 11, 2001, communications were severely affected by the collapse of the World Trade Center. The primary communications repeater was located on top of one of the towers. In addition, excess radio traffic made transmitting and receiving messages extremely difficult. Not only were radio communications affected, but most cell phones and most radio and television stations were disabled. The lesson learned from this event is to have multiple backups to your ability to communicate with your dispatcher. In the event of a terrorist or WMD event, refrain from using the radio unless you have something important to transmit. If you do transmit, gather your thoughts and speak in as calm a tone as possible, avoiding unnecessary chatter. Remember, while you are transmitting, others may be unable to call for help.

## YOU are the Provider

Several law enforcement officers run past your ambulance toward the scene of the shooting. You are told that the suspect is down, and they need immediate assistance at the scene of the shooting. Two blocks away, additional officers are evacuating the area around the trash can that was smoking heavily.

**3.** What should you consider when determining if the scene is safe for you and other EMS personnel to enter?

**4.** What immediate actions should you perform prior to proceeding into the scene?

## Establishing Command

The first provider on the scene must begin to sort out the chaos and define his or her responsibilities under the incident command system (ICS). As the first person on scene, you may need to establish command until additional personnel arrive. Depending on the circumstances and stage of the operation, you and other EMTs may function as medical branch directors, triage supervisors, treatment supervisors, transportation supervisors, logistic officers, or command and general staff. If the initial ICS is already in place, then immediately find the medical staging officer to receive your assignment. Chapter 40, *Incident Management*, discusses in detail how to work within the ICS and the National Incident Management System.

## Reassessing Scene Safety

Do not rely on others to secure your safety. It is your responsibility to constantly assess and reassess the scene for safety. This is an important component of situational awareness. It is easy to overlook a suspicious package while you are treating casualties. Stay alert. Something as subtle as a change in the wind direction during a gas attack or an increase in the number of contaminated patients can place you in danger. Never become so involved with the tasks you are performing that you do not look around and make sure the scene remains safe. Remember that as a responder, you may represent a prime target for those meaning to cause harm and incite chaos.

### Words of Wisdom

Although it may be difficult for you because of ethical or moral reasons to treat a suspected criminal or suspected terrorist, it is important that this patient receive the same care as any other patient. You are not the judge or jury. It is up to the legal system to prove in a court of law that someone is guilty.

# Chemical Agents

Chemical agents are liquids or gases that are dispersed to kill or injure. Modern-day chemicals were first developed during WWI and WWII. During the Cold War, many of these agents were perfected and stockpiled. Whereas the United States has long renounced the use of chemical weapons, many nations still develop and stockpile them. These agents are deadly and pose a threat if they are acquired by terrorists.

Chemical weapons have several classifications. The properties or characteristics of an agent can be described as liquid, gas, or solid material. **Persistency** and **volatility** describe how long the agent will stay on a surface before it evaporates. Persistent, or nonvolatile agents can remain on a surface for long periods, usually longer than 24 hours. Nonpersistent, or volatile agents evaporate relatively fast when left on a surface in the optimal temperature range. An agent that is described as highly persistent (such as VX, a nerve agent) can remain in the environment for weeks to months, whereas an agent that is highly volatile (such as sarin, also a nerve agent) will turn from liquid to gas (evaporate) within minutes to seconds.

**Route of exposure** is how the agent most effectively enters the body. Chemical agents can have either a vapor or contact hazard. Agents with a **vapor hazard** enter the body through the respiratory tract in the form of vapors. Agents with a **contact hazard** (or skin hazard) give off very little vapor or no vapors and enter the body through the skin.

## Vesicants (Blister Agents)

The primary route of exposure of blister agents, or **vesicants**, is the skin (contact); however, if vesicants are left on the skin or clothing long enough, they produce vapors that can enter the respiratory tract. Vesicants cause burn-like blisters to form on the victim's skin and in the respiratory tract. The vesicant agents consist of sulfur mustard (H), lewisite (L), and phosgene oxime (CX) (the symbols H, L, and CX are military designations for these chemicals). The vesicants usually cause the most damage to damp or moist areas of the body, such as the armpits, groin, and respiratory tract. Signs of vesicant exposure on the skin include the following:

- Skin irritation, burning, and reddening
- Immediate, intense skin pain (with L and CX)
- Formation of large blisters
- Gray discoloration of skin (a sign of permanent damage seen with L and CX)
- Swollen and closed or irritated eyes
- Permanent eye injury (including blindness)

If vapors were inhaled, the patient may experience the following signs and symptoms:

- Hoarseness and stridor
- Severe cough
- Hemoptysis (coughing up blood)
- Severe dyspnea

Sulfur mustard (H), commonly known as mustard gas, is a brownish, yellowish oily substance that is generally considered very persistent. When released, mustard gas has the distinct smell of garlic or mustard and is quickly absorbed into the skin and/or mucous membranes. As the agent is absorbed into the skin, it begins an irreversible process of damage to the cells. Absorption through the skin or mucous membranes usually occurs within seconds, and damage to the underlying cells takes place within 1 to 2 minutes.

Mustard gas is considered a mutagen, which means that it mutates, damages, and changes the structures of cells. Eventually, cellular death will occur. On the surface, the patient will generally not show any signs or symptoms until 4 to 6 hours after exposure (depending on concentration and amount of exposure) (**FIGURE 41-8**).

The patient will experience a progressive reddening of the affected area, which will gradually develop into large blisters. These blisters are very similar in shape and appearance to those associated with thermal second-degree burns. The fluid within the blisters does not contain any of the agent; however, the skin covering the area is considered contaminated until trained personnel have decontaminated the patient.

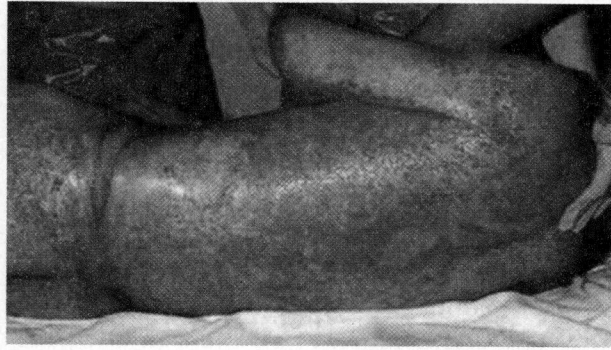

**FIGURE 41-8** Skin damage resulting from exposure to sulfur mustard (H).

Courtesy of Dr. Saeed Keshavarz/RCCI, Research Center of Chemical Injuries/IRAN.

Mustard gas also attacks vulnerable cells within the bone marrow and depletes the body's ability to reproduce white blood cells. Like other burns, the primary complication associated with vesicant blisters is secondary infection. If the patient survives the initial direct injury from the agent, the depletion of the white blood cells leaves the patient with a decreased resistance to infections. Although sulfur mustard is regarded as persistent, the vapors it releases when dispersed can be inhaled. This creates upper and lower airway compromise. The result is damage and swelling of the airways. The airway compromise makes the patient's condition far more serious.

Lewisite (L) and phosgene oxime (CX) produce blister wounds very similar to those caused by mustard gas. They are highly volatile and have a rapid onset of symptoms, compared with the delayed onset seen with mustard gas. These agents produce immediate intense pain and discomfort when contact is made. The patient's skin may have a gray discoloration at the contaminated site. Although tissue damage also occurs with exposure to these agents, they do not cause the secondary cellular injury that is associated with mustard gas.

## Vesicant Agent Treatment

There are no antidotes for mustard gas or CX exposure. British anti-lewisite is the antidote for agent L; however, it is not carried by civilian EMS. Ensure the patient has been decontaminated before you initiate any treatment. If any agent has been inhaled, the patient may require prompt airway support as soon as decontamination is completed. Initiate transport as soon as possible. Generally, burn centers are best equipped to handle the wounds and subsequent infections produced by vesicants. Follow your local protocols when determining the transport destination.

## Pulmonary Agents (Choking Agents)

The pulmonary agents are gases that cause immediate harm to people exposed to them and include chlorine (Cl) and phosgene. These agents produce respiratory-related symptoms such as dyspnea and tachypnea. The primary route of exposure for these agents is through the respiratory tract, which makes them an inhalation or vapor hazard. Once inside the lungs, they damage the lung tissue and fluid leaks into the lungs. Pulmonary edema develops in the patient, resulting in difficulty breathing because of severely impaired gas exchange.

Chlorine (Cl) was the first chemical agent ever used in warfare. It has a distinct odor of bleach and creates a green haze when released as a gas. Initially, it produces upper airway irritation and a choking sensation. The patient may later experience the following signs and symptoms:

- Shortness of breath
- Tightness in chest
- Hoarseness and stridor as the result of upper airway constriction
- Gasping and coughing

With serious exposures, patients may experience pulmonary edema, complete airway constriction, and death. The fumes from a mixture of household bleach and ammonia create an acid gas that produces similar effects. According to the American Association of Poison Control Centers' 2017 data report, human exposure involving household cleaning substances was the second most frequently reported exposure.

Do not confuse phosgene with phosgene oxime, a blistering agent, or vesicant. Not only has phosgene been produced for chemical warfare, but it is also a product of combustion that might be produced as a result of a fire involving other chemicals, such as at a textile factory or house, or from metalwork or burning Freon (a liquid chemical used in refrigeration). Therefore, you may encounter a victim of exposure to this gas during a normal call or at a fire scene. Phosgene is a very potent agent that has a delayed onset of symptoms, usually hours. Unlike Cl, when phosgene enters the body, it generally does not produce severe irritation that would possibly cause the victim to leave the area or hold his or her breath. In fact, the odor produced by the chemical is similar to that of freshly mowed grass or hay. The result is that much more of the gas may enter the body unnoticed. Initially, a mild exposure may include the following signs and symptoms:

- Nausea
- Tightness in chest
- Severe cough
- Dyspnea on exertion

The victim of a severe exposure may present with dyspnea at rest and excessive pulmonary edema. The pulmonary edema may be so severe that the patient continually coughs up white or pink-tinged fluid. A severe exposure produces such large amounts of fluid in the lungs that the patient may become hypovolemic and subsequently hypotensive.

## Pulmonary Agent Treatment

The best initial treatment of any patient who has been exposed to a pulmonary agent is to remove the patient from the contaminated atmosphere. This should be done by trained personnel in the proper personal protective equipment (PPE). Aggressively manage the ABCs, paying attention to oxygenation, ventilation, and suctioning, if required. Do not allow the patient to be active because this will worsen the condition. There are no antidotes to counteract the pulmonary agents. The primary goals for basic life support prehospital emergency care are to perform the ABCs, allow the patient to rest in a position of comfort with his or her head elevated, and initiate rapid transport. If the patient's condition does not improve with basic airway support, consider requesting an advanced life support (ALS) intercept. Continuous positive airway pressure may benefit some of these patients, but others will require more advanced airway management.

## Nerve Agents

The nerve agents are among the deadliest chemicals developed. They are classified as WMDs. Nerve agents are not readily available to the general public and are extremely toxic and rapidly fatal with any route of exposure. Designed to kill a large number of people by using small quantities, nerve agents can cause cardiac arrest within seconds to minutes of exposure. Nerve agents, discovered while in search of a superior pesticide, are a class of chemical called organophosphates, which are found in household bug sprays, agricultural pesticides, and some industrial chemicals at much lower strengths than in the weaponized form. Organophosphates block an essential enzyme in the nervous system, causing the body's organs to become overstimulated and burn out.

G agents came from the early nerve agents, the G-series, which were developed by German scientists (hence the G) in the period after WWI and during WWII. There are three G-series agents, which are all designed with the same basic chemical structure with slight variations to produce different properties. The two variations of these agents are lethality and volatility. The following G agents are listed from high volatility to low volatility:

- **Sarin (GB)**. Highly volatile colorless and odorless liquid. Turns from liquid to gas within seconds to minutes at room temperature. The lethal concentration of sarin in air is approximately 28 to 35 mg/m$^3$ per minute for a 2-minute exposure time by a healthy adult breathing normally. Sarin is primarily a vapor hazard, with the respiratory tract as the main route of entry. This agent is especially dangerous in enclosed environments such as office buildings, shopping malls, and subway cars. When this agent comes into contact with the skin, it is quickly absorbed and evaporates. When sarin is on clothing, it has the effect of **off-gassing**, which means that the vapors are continuously released over time (similar to perfume). This renders the victim and the victim's clothing contaminated.
- **Soman (GD)**. Twice as persistent as sarin and five times as lethal. It has a fruity odor as a result of the type of alcohol used in the agent and generally has no color. This agent is a contact and inhalation hazard that can enter the body through skin absorption and through the respiratory tract. A unique additive in GD causes it to bind to the cells that it attacks faster than any other agent. This irreversible binding is called **aging**, which makes it more difficult to treat patients who have been exposed.
- **Tabun (GA)**. Approximately one-half as lethal as sarin and 36 times more persistent. Under the proper conditions it will remain present for several days. It has a fruity smell and an appearance similar to sarin. The components

used to manufacture GA are easy to acquire, and the agent is easy to manufacture, which makes it unique. GA is a contact and inhalation hazard that can enter the body through skin absorption and through the respiratory tract.

- **V agent (VX)**. Clear, oily agent that has no odor and looks like baby oil. V agent was developed by the British after WWII and has chemical properties similar to the G-series agents. The difference is that VX is more than 100 times more lethal than sarin and is extremely persistent (**FIGURE 41-9**). In fact, VX is so persistent that given the proper conditions, it will remain relatively unchanged for weeks to months. These properties make VX primarily a contact hazard because it lets off very little vapor. It is easily absorbed into the skin, and the oily residue that remains on the skin's surface is extremely difficult to decontaminate.

Nerve agents all produce similar symptoms but have varying routes of entry. Nerve agents differ slightly in lethal concentration or dose and also differ in their volatility. Some agents are designed to quickly become a gas (nonpersistent or highly volatile), whereas others remain a liquid for a period of time (persistent or nonvolatile). These agents have been used successfully in warfare and, until recently, were the only type of chemical agent that had been used successfully in a terrorist act. Once the agent has entered the body through skin contact or through the respiratory system, the patient will begin to exhibit a pattern of predictable symptoms. Like all chemical agents, the severity of the patient's symptoms will depend on the route of exposure of the agent and the amount of exposure.

The symptoms are described in **TABLE 41-1** using the military mnemonic SLUDGEM and the medical mnemonic DUMBELS. The medical mnemonic is

## YOU are the Provider

As you approach the scene of the shooting, a law enforcement officer informs you that the source of the smoke from the trash can was a smoke grenade used to create a diversion. That area has been secured by law enforcement and there are no additional patients at that location.

**5.** Given the situation, what are some unique concerns about this incident?

**6.** What types of injuries should you expect to encounter?

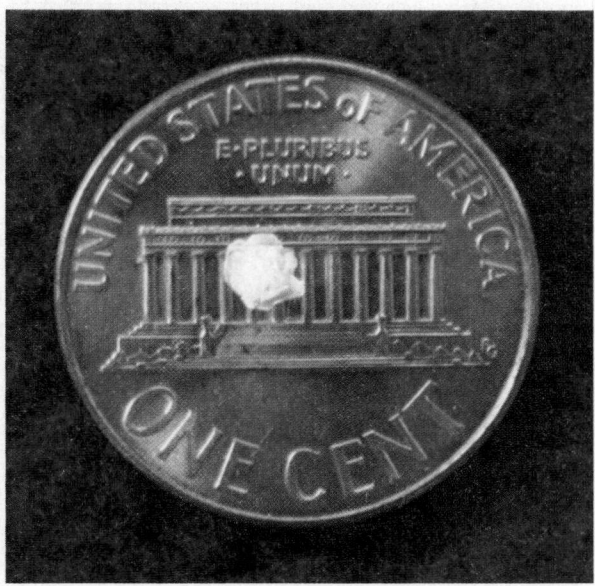

**FIGURE 41-9** VX is the most toxic chemical ever created. The dot on the penny demonstrates the amount needed to achieve the lethal dose.

© Jones & Bartlett Learning. Photographed by Kimberly Potvin.

| Military Mnemonic: SLUDGEM | Medical Mnemonic: DUMBELS (all age groups) |
|---|---|
| **TABLE 41-1** Symptoms of Exposure to Nerve Agents | |
| **S**alivation, **S**weating, **S**eizures | **D**iarrhea |
| **L**acrimation (excessive tearing) (also rhinorrhea) | **U**rination |
| **U**rination | **M**iosis (pinpoint pupils), **M**uscle weakness |
| **D**efecation, **D**rooling, **D**iarrhea | **B**radycardia, **B**ronchospasm, **B**ronchorrhea |
| **G**astric upset and cramps | **E**mesis (vomiting) |
| **E**mesis (vomiting) | **L**acrimation (excessive tearing) (also rhinorrhea) |
| **M**uscle twitching/**M**iosis (pinpoint pupils) | **S**eizures, **S**alivation, **S**weating |

© Jones & Bartlett Learning.

more useful to you because it lists the more dangerous symptoms associated with exposure to nerve agents.

There are only a handful of medical conditions that are associated with the bilateral pinpoint constricted pupils (**miosis**) seen with nerve agent exposure. Conditions such as a cerebrovascular accident, direct light to both eyes, and a drug overdose all can cause bilaterally constricted pupils. Therefore, assess the patient for all of the SLUDGEM/DUMBELS signs and symptoms to determine whether the patient has been exposed to a nerve agent.

Miosis is the most common symptom of nerve agent exposure and can persist for days to weeks. This symptom, along with the others listed in Table 41-1, will help you recognize exposure to a nerve agent early. Miosis will be seen quickly in a vapor exposure but may occur later after an isolated skin exposure. In some cases, the patient may have been exposed to both.

The seizures that are associated with nerve agent exposure are unlike those found in patients with a history of seizure. The seizure will continue until the patient dies or until treatment is given with a nerve agent antidote kit (DuoDote Auto-Injector or Antidote Treatment Nerve Agent Auto-Injector [ATNAA]).

## Nerve Agent Treatment

Fatalities from severe exposure to a nerve agent occur as a result of respiratory complications, which lead to respiratory arrest. Once the patient has been decontaminated, be prepared to treat aggressively, if the patient is to be saved. You can greatly increase the patient's chances of survival simply by providing airway and ventilatory support. As with all emergencies, securing the ABCs is the best and most important treatment that you can provide. Often in patients exposed to these agents, seizures will begin and will not stop. These patients will require administration of nerve agent antidote kits in addition to support of the ABCs.

Medical treatment for nerve agent exposure may include the DuoDote Auto-Injector. The DuoDote Auto-Injector contains 2.1 mg of atropine and 600 mg of pralidoxime chloride (2-PAM) and is delivered as a single dose through one needle. Atropine is used to block the nerve agent. However, because the nerve agent may remain in the body for long periods, 2-PAM is used to eliminate the agent from the body. Many of the symptoms described in the DUMBELS mnemonic can begin to be reversed with the use of atropine; however, many doses may be necessary to see total cessation of the symptoms. The military form of this combination injector is the Antidote Treatment Nerve Agent Auto-Injector (ATNAA).

In some regions, EMTs may carry DuoDote kits on the unit and will be called on to administer the antidotes to themselves or their patients. If your service carries a nerve agent antidote, refer to your local protocols for dosage and usage information. These medications are delivered using the same technique as the EpiPen auto-injector; however, multiple doses may need to be administered. Activated antidote kits need to be properly disposed of in a sharps container.

TABLE 41-2 provides a quick reference and comparison of the nerve agents.

## Words of Wisdom

On March 20, 1995, members of Aum Shinrikyo, a Japanese cult, released sarin (GB) in the Tokyo subway. The first arriving medical responders were met with chaos as thousands of people fled the subway system (**FIGURE 41-10**). Many were contaminated and showed signs and symptoms of nerve agent exposure. In the end, more than 5,000 people sought medical care for exposure to sarin, and 12 people died. None of the EMS personnel wore protective clothing, so most became cross-contaminated. Remember, you can avoid becoming exposed. Do not become a victim.

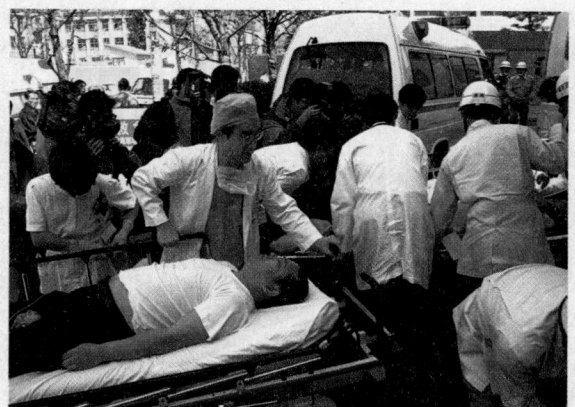

**FIGURE 41-10** Medical professionals responding to an attack in 1995, where cult members released sarin in the Tokyo subway.

© Chiaki Tsukumo/AP/Shutterstock.

## Metabolic Agents (Cyanides)

Hydrogen cyanide (AC) and cyanogen chloride (CK) are both agents that affect the body's ability to use oxygen. Cyanide is a colorless gas that has an odor similar to that of bitter almonds. The effects of the cyanides begin on the cellular level and are very rapidly seen at the organ and system levels. Unlike nerve agents, however, these deadly gases are commonly found in many industrial settings. Cyanides are produced every year in massive quantities throughout the United States for industrial uses such as gold and silver mining, photography, and plastics processing. The combustion of household goods such as insulation, carpeting, upholstery, plastic, and synthetic rubber can release a significant amount of cyanide. In fact, cyanide is naturally found in the pits of many fruits in very low quantities.

There is very little difference in the symptoms found between AC and CK. In low doses, these chemicals are associated with dizziness, lightheadedness, headache, and vomiting. Higher doses will produce symptoms that include the following:

- Shortness of breath and gasping respirations
- Respiratory distress or arrest
- Tachypnea
- Flushed skin (may be difficult to detect in dark-skinned people)
- Tachycardia
- Altered mental status
- Seizures

**TABLE 41-2** The Nerve Agents

| Name | Military Designation | Odor | Special Features | Onset of Symptoms | Volatility | Route of Exposure |
|------|---------------------|------|-----------------|-------------------|-----------|-------------------|
| Tabun | GA | Fruity | Easy to manufacture | Immediate | Low | Skin contact and vapor hazard |
| Sarin | GB | None (if pure) or strong | Will off-gas while on victim's clothing | Immediate | High | Primarily respiratory vapor hazard; skin exposure is extremely lethal |
| Soman | GD | Fruity | Ages rapidly; difficult to treat | Immediate | Moderate | Skin contact; minimal vapor hazard |
| V agent | VX | None | Most lethal chemical agent; difficult to decontaminate | Immediate | Very low | Skin contact; no vapor hazard (unless aerosolized) |

© Jones & Bartlett Learning.

- Coma
- Apnea
- Cardiac arrest

The symptoms associated with the inhalation of a large amount of cyanide will all appear within several minutes. Death is likely unless the patient is treated promptly.

## Words of Wisdom

Patients who are exposed to cyanide and who have shortness of breath will have a normal pulse oximetry reading. This is because cyanide impairs the body's ability to offload the oxygen molecules at a cellular level. Cyanide will create true hypoxia at a cellular level despite the presence of oxygen circulating through the bloodstream.

## Cyanide Agent Treatment

Cyanide binds with the body's cells, preventing oxygen from being used. Several medications act as antidotes, but most services do not carry them. After trained personnel wearing the proper PPE have removed the patient from the source of exposure, even if there is no liquid contamination, all of the patient's clothes must be removed to prevent off-gassing in the ambulance. Trained and protected personnel must decontaminate any patients who may have been exposed to liquid contamination before you can initiate treatment. Then you can support the patient's ABCs. Mild effects of cyanide exposure will generally resolve by simply removing the victim from the source of contamination and administering supplemental oxygen. Severe exposure, however, will require aggressive oxygenation and perhaps ventilation with supplemental oxygen. Always use a bag-mask device or oxygen-powered ventilator device to ventilate a victim of a metabolic agent. The agent can easily be passed on from the patient to you through mouth-to-mouth or mouth-to-mask ventilations. Initiate transport immediately if administration of an antidote by ALS is not available.

## Words of Wisdom

Always make sure your patients have been thoroughly decontaminated by trained personnel before you come in contact with them. Chemical agents are primarily a vapor hazard, and all of the patient's clothing must be removed prior to treatment to prevent off-gassing to you. Protect yourself as you manage the airway of a patient exposed to a vapor hazard. Many of the vapors may linger in the patient's airway, and cross-contamination may occur.

**TABLE 41-3** Chemical Agents

| Name | Military Designations | Odor | Lethality | Onset of Symptoms | Volatility | Primary Route of Exposure |
|---|---|---|---|---|---|---|
| Nerve agents | Tabun (GA) Sarin (GB) Soman (GD) VX | Fruity or none | Highly lethal chemical agents; kill within minutes; effects are reversible with antidotes | Immediate | Moderate (GA, GD) Very high (GB) Low (VX) | GA—both GB—vapor hazard GD—both VX—contact hazard |
| Vesicants | Mustard (H) Lewisite (L) Phosgene oxime (CX) | Garlic (H) Geranium (L) | Cause large blisters to form; inhalation severely damages upper airway; severe, intense pain and gray skin discoloration (L and CX) | Delayed (H) Immediate (L, CX) | Very low (H, L) Moderate (CX) | Primarily contact, with some vapor hazard |
| Pulmonary agents | Chlorine (Cl) Phosgene (CG) | Bleach Cut grass (CG) | Cause irritation choking (Cl); severe pulmonary edema (CG) | Immediate (Cl) Delayed (CG) | Very high | Vapor hazard |
| Cyanide agents | Hydrogen cyanide (AC) Cyanogen chloride (CK) | Almonds (AC) Irritating (CK) | Highly lethal chemical gases; kill within minutes; effects are reversible with antidotes | Immediate | Very high | Vapor hazard |

© Jones & Bartlett Learning.

**TABLE 41-3** summarizes the chemical agents. The odors of the particular chemicals are provided for informational purposes only. The sense of smell is a poor tool to use to determine whether there is a chemical agent present. Many people are unable to smell the agents, and the odor could be derived from another source. This information is useful to you if you receive reports from victims who claimed to smell bleach or garlic, for example. Never enter a potentially hazardous area and "sniff the air" to determine whether a chemical agent is present.

## Biologic Agents

Biologic agents pose many difficult issues when used as WMDs. Biologic agents can be almost completely undetectable. Also, most of the diseases caused by these agents will be similar to the other minor illnesses commonly seen by EMS providers.

Biologic agents are grouped as viruses, bacteria, and neurotoxins and may be spread in various ways. **Dissemination** is the means by which a terrorist spreads the agent—for example, poisoning the water supply or aerosolizing the agent into the air or ventilation system of a building. A **disease vector** is an animal that spreads disease, once infected, to another animal. For example, bubonic plague can be spread by infected rats; smallpox by infected humans; and West Nile virus by infected mosquitoes. How easily the disease spreads from one human to another human is called *communicability*. Some diseases, such as those caused by the human immunodeficiency virus (HIV), are difficult to spread by routine contact. Therefore, communicability is considered low. In other instances when communicability is high, such as with smallpox, the person is considered contagious. Typically, routine standard precautions are enough to prevent contamination from contagious biologic organisms.

Incubation is the time between the person becoming exposed to the agent and the appearance of the first symptoms. The incubation period is especially important for you to understand. Although your patient may not exhibit signs or symptoms, he or she may be contagious.

Be aware of when you should suspect the use of biologic agents. If the agent is in the form of a powder, as was the case in the October 2001 terrorist attacks involving letters laced with anthrax powder appearing in the US mail, the incident must be handled by hazmat specialists. Patients who come into direct contact with the agent need to be decontaminated before you make any contact with them or initiate treatment.

## Viruses

Viruses are germs that require a living host to multiply and survive. A virus is a simple organism and cannot thrive outside of a host (living body). Once in the body, the virus invades healthy cells and replicates itself to spread through the host. As the virus spreads, so does the disease that it carries. Viruses spread from host to host by direct methods, such as through respiratory droplets, or through vectors. A *vector* is any agent that acts as a carrier or transporter.

Viral agents that may be used during a biologic terrorist release pose an extraordinary problem for health care providers, especially those in EMS. Although some viral agents do have vaccines, there is often no treatment for a viral infection other than antiviral medications for some agents. Because of this characteristic, the following viruses have the potential to be used as terrorism agents.

### Smallpox

Smallpox is a highly contagious disease. Use all forms of standard precautions to prevent cross-contamination. Simply by wearing examination gloves, a HEPA-filtered respirator, and eye protection, you will greatly reduce your risk of contamination. The last natural case of smallpox in the world was seen in 1977. Before the rash and blisters show, the illness will start with a high fever and body aches and headaches. The patient's temperature is usually in the range of 101°F to 104°F (38.3°C to 40°C).

An easy, quick way to differentiate the smallpox rash from other skin disorders is to observe the size, shape, and location of the lesions. In smallpox, all the lesions are identical in their development. In other skin disorders, the lesions will be in various stages of healing and development. Smallpox blisters begin on the face and extremities and eventually move toward the chest and abdomen. The disease is in its most contagious phase when the blisters begin to form (**FIGURE 41-11**). Unprotected contact with these blisters will promote transmission of the disease (**TABLE 41-4**). There is a vaccine to prevent smallpox; however, it has been linked to medical complications and, in rare cases, death. Should an outbreak occur, the US government has enough vaccine to vaccinate every person in the United States.

### Viral Hemorrhagic Fevers

Viral hemorrhagic fevers consist of a group of diseases caused by viruses that include the Ebola, Rift

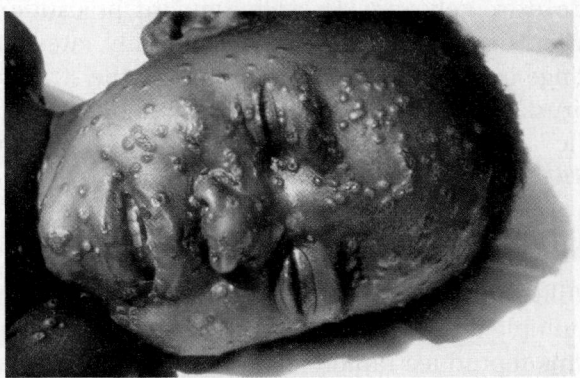

**FIGURE 41-11** In smallpox, all the lesions are identical in their development. In other skin disorders, the lesions will be in various stages of healing and development.
Courtesy of CDC.

| TABLE 41-4 Characteristics of Smallpox | |
|---|---|
| **Dissemination** | Aerosolized for warfare or terrorist uses |
| **Communicability** | High from infected patients or contaminated items (such as blankets); person-to-person transmission possible |
| **Route of entry** | Inhalation of coughed droplets or direct skin contact with blisters |
| **Signs and symptoms** | Severe fever, malaise, body aches, headaches, small blisters on the skin, bleeding of the skin and mucous membranes; incubation period 10 to 12 days; duration of the illness, approximately 4 weeks |
| **Medical management** | Standard precautions; no specific treatment; provide supportive care (ABCs) |

© Jones & Bartlett Learning.

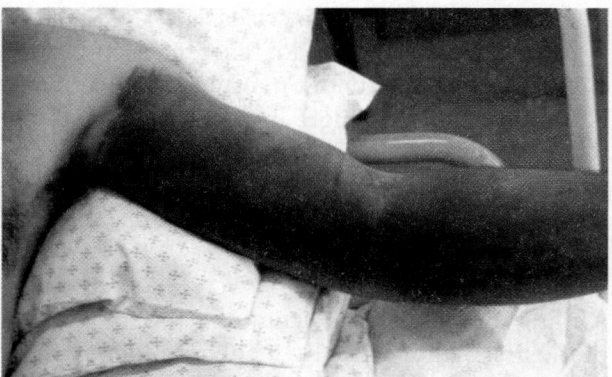

**FIGURE 41-12** Viral hemorrhagic fevers cause the blood vessels and tissues to seep blood. The end result is ecchymosis, bloody sputum, and blood in the patient's stool. Notice the severe discoloration in the arm of this patient with Crimean Congo hemorrhagic fever, indicating internal bleeding.

Courtesy of Professor Robert Swanepoel/National Institute for Communicable Disease, South Africa.

| TABLE 41-5 Characteristics of Viral Hemorrhagic Fevers | |
|---|---|
| **Dissemination** | Direct contact with infected body fluids; can be aerosolized for use in an attack |
| **Communicability** | Moderate from person to person or contaminated items |
| **Route of entry** | Direct contact with infected body fluids |
| **Signs and symptoms** | Sudden onset of fever, weakness, muscle pain, headache, and sore throat; all followed by vomiting and, as the virus runs its course, internal and external bleeding |
| **Medical management** | Standard precautions; no specific treatment; provide supportive care (ABCs) and treat for shock and hypotension, if present |

© Jones & Bartlett Learning.

Valley, Marburg, and yellow fever viruses, among others. This group of viruses causes the blood in the body to seep out from the tissues and blood vessels (**FIGURE 41-12**). Initially, the patient will have flulike symptoms, progressing to more serious symptoms such as internal and external hemorrhaging. Outbreaks are not uncommon in Africa and South America; however, outbreaks in the United States are extremely rare. Use all standard precautions when treating these illnesses. Mortality rates can range from 5% to 90%, depending on the strain of virus, the victim's age and health condition, and the availability of a modern health care system (**TABLE 41-5**).

## Bacteria

Unlike viruses, bacteria do not require a host to multiply and live. These single-celled microorganisms reproduce rapidly and are much more complex and larger than viruses. They can grow up to 100 times larger than the largest virus. Bacteria contain all the cellular structures of a normal cell and are completely self-sufficient. Most bacterial infections can be treated with antibiotics.

Most bacterial infections will generally begin with flulike symptoms, which can make it quite difficult for health care providers to identify whether the cause is a biologic attack or a natural infection.

## Inhalation and Cutaneous Anthrax (*Bacillus anthracis*)

**Anthrax** is caused by deadly bacteria that lie dormant in a spore (protective shell). When exposed to the optimal temperature and moisture, the germ will be released from the spore. The routes of entry for anthrax bacteria are inhalation, cutaneous, and gastrointestinal (from consuming food that contains spores) (**FIGURE 41-13**). The inhalational form, or pulmonary anthrax, is the deadliest and often presents as a severe cold. Pulmonary anthrax is associated with a 90% death rate if untreated. Antibiotics can be used to treat anthrax successfully. There is also a vaccine to prevent anthrax infections (**TABLE 41-6**).

## Plague (Bubonic/Pneumonic)

The 14th-century plague that ravaged Asia, the Middle East, and finally Europe (the Black Death) killed an estimated 33 to 42 million people (50% of the European population at the time). In the early 19th century, almost 20 million people in India and China died due to plague. The plague's natural vectors are infected rodents and fleas. When a person is

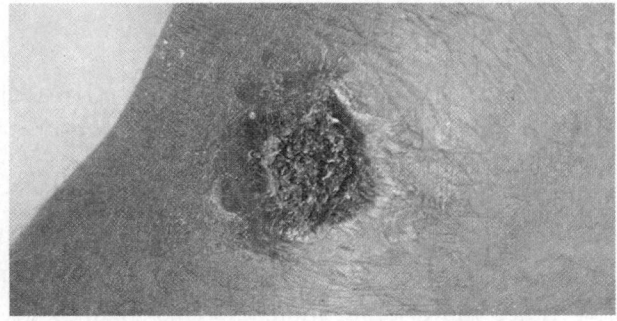

**FIGURE 41-13** Cutaneous anthrax.

Courtesy of James H. Steele/CDC.

| TABLE 41-6 Characteristics of Anthrax | |
|---|---|
| **Dissemination** | Aerosol |
| **Communicability** | Only in the cutaneous form (rare) |
| **Route of entry** | Inhalation of spore, skin contact with spore, or direct contact with skin wound (cutaneous) |
| **Signs and symptoms** | Flulike symptoms, fever, respiratory distress with tachycardia, shock, pulmonary edema, and respiratory failure after 3 to 5 days of flulike symptoms |
| **Medical management** | Inhalation: Standard precautions, oxygen, ventilatory support if patient has pulmonary edema or respiratory failure, and transport<br>Cutaneous: Standard precautions, apply dry sterile dressing to prevent accidental contact with wound and fluids |

© Jones & Bartlett Learning.

bitten by an infected flea or comes in contact with an infected rodent (or the waste of the rodent), the person can contract bubonic plague.

**Bubonic plague** infects the **lymphatic system** (a passive circulatory system in the body that bathes the tissues in lymph and works with the immune system). When this occurs, the patient's **lymph nodes** (area of the lymphatic system where infection-fighting cells are housed) become infected and grow. The glands of the nodes will grow large (up to the size of a tennis ball) and round, forming **buboes** (**FIGURE 41-14**). If left untreated, the infection may spread through the body, leading to sepsis and possibly death. This form of plague is not contagious and is not likely to be seen in a bioterrorist incident.

**Pneumonic plague** is a lung infection, also known as plague pneumonia, that results from inhalation of plague bacteria. This form of the disease is contagious and has a much higher death rate than the bubonic form (**TABLE 41-7**).

## Neurotoxins

**Neurotoxins** are the most deadly substances known to humans. The strongest neurotoxin is 15,000 times

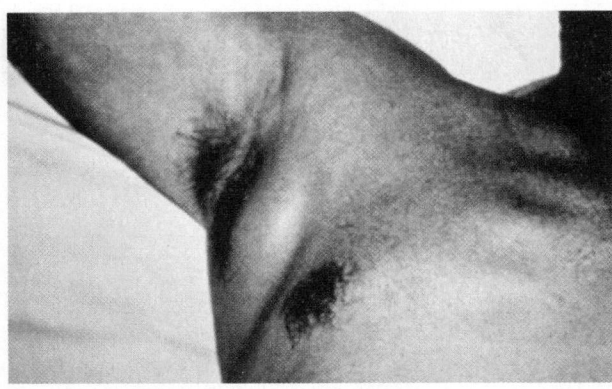

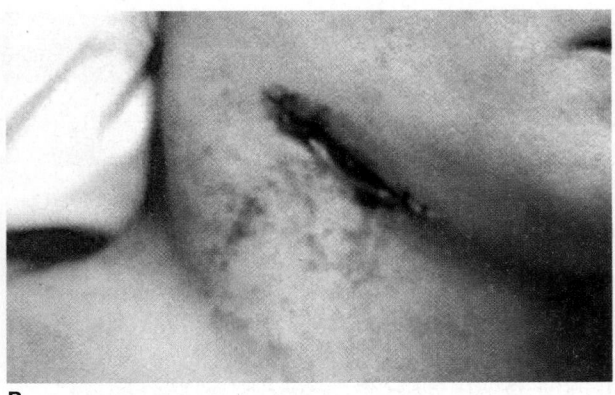

**FIGURE 41-14 A.** Plague bubo at lymph node under arm. **B.** Plague bubo at lymph node on neck.

**A, B:** Courtesy of CDC.

| TABLE 41-7 Characteristics of Plague | |
| --- | --- |
| **Dissemination** | Aerosol |
| **Communicability** | Bubonic: Low, only from contact with fluid in buboes<br>Pneumonic: High, from person to person |
| **Route of entry** | Ingestion, inhalation, or cutaneous |
| **Signs and symptoms** | Fever, headache, muscle pain and tenderness, pneumonia, shortness of breath, extreme lymph node pain and enlargement (bubonic) |
| **Medical management** | Standard precautions, provide supportive care (ABCs), oxygen if indicated, and transport |

© Jones & Bartlett Learning.

| TABLE 41-8 Characteristics of Botulinum Toxin | |
| --- | --- |
| **Dissemination** | Aerosol or food supply sabotage or injection |
| **Communicability** | None |
| **Route of entry** | Ingestion, inhalation |
| **Signs and symptoms** | Dry mouth, intestinal obstruction, urinary retention, constipation, nausea and vomiting, abnormal pupil dilation, blurred vision, double vision, drooping eyelids, difficulty swallowing, difficulty speaking, and respiratory failure as the result of paralysis |
| **Medical management** | Provide supportive care (ABCs), oxygen, and transport; provide ventilatory support in case of paralysis of the respiratory muscles; vaccine available |

© Jones & Bartlett Learning.

more lethal than VX and 100,000 times more lethal than sarin. These toxins are produced from plants, marine animals, molds, and bacteria. The route of entry for these toxins is through ingestion, inhalation from aerosols, or injection. Unlike viruses and bacteria, neurotoxins are not contagious and have a faster onset of symptoms. Although these biologic toxins have immense destructive potential, they have not been used successfully as a WMD.

## Botulinum Toxin

The most potent neurotoxin is botulinum, which is produced by bacteria. When introduced into the body, this neurotoxin affects the nervous system's ability to function. Voluntary muscle control diminishes as the toxin spreads. Eventually the toxin causes muscle paralysis that begins at the head and face and spreads downward throughout the body.

The patient's accessory muscles and diaphragm will become paralyzed, and the patient will go into respiratory arrest (**TABLE 41-8**).

## Ricin

Although not as deadly as botulinum, ricin is still five times more lethal than VX. This toxin is derived from mash that is left from the castor bean (**FIGURE 41-15**). When introduced into the body, ricin causes pulmonary edema and respiratory and circulatory failure leading to death (**TABLE 41-9**).

The clinical picture depends on the route of exposure. The toxin is quite stable and extremely toxic

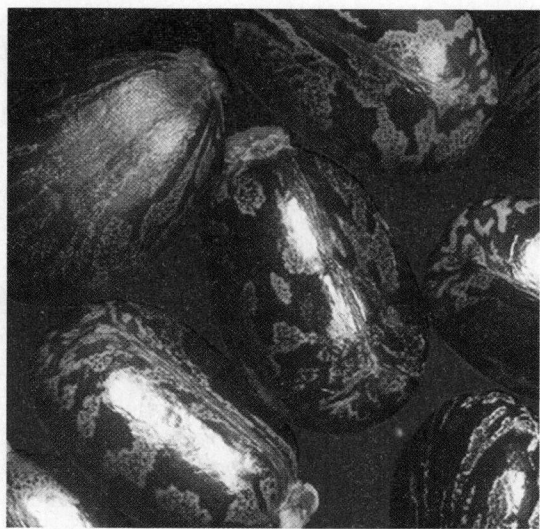

**FIGURE 41-15** These seemingly harmless castor beans contain the key ingredient for ricin, one of the most potent toxins known to humans.

Courtesy of Brian Prechtel/USDA.

by many routes of exposure, including inhalation. It is likely that 0.5 to 3 mg of ricin can kill an adult, and the ingestion of one seed can most likely kill a child.

Although all parts of the castor bean are poisonous, it is the seeds that are the most toxic. Castor bean ingestion causes a rapid onset of nausea, vomiting, abdominal cramps, and severe diarrhea, followed by vascular collapse. Death usually occurs on the third day in the absence of appropriate medical intervention.

Ricin is least toxic by the oral route. This is probably a result of poor absorption in the gastrointestinal tract, some digestion in the gut, and, possibly, some expulsion of the agent as caused by the rapid onset of vomiting. Ingestion causes local hemorrhage and necrosis of the liver, spleen, kidneys, and gastrointestinal tract. Signs and symptoms appear 4 to 8 hours after exposure.

| TABLE 41-9 Characteristics of Ricin | |
| --- | --- |
| **Dissemination** | Released into indoor or outdoor air (aerosol) Food and water contamination |
| **Communicability** | None |
| **Route of exposure** | Inhalation, ingestion, injection |
| **Signs and symptoms** | Inhaled: Cough, difficulty breathing, tightness in chest, nausea, muscle aches, pulmonary edema, and hypoxia Ingested: Nausea and vomiting, internal bleeding, and death Injected: No signs except swelling at the injection site and death |
| **Medical management** | Provide supportive care (ABCs); no treatment or vaccine available |

© Jones & Bartlett Learning.

Signs and symptoms of ricin ingestion are as follows:

- Fever
- Chills
- Headache
- Muscle aches
- Nausea
- Vomiting
- Diarrhea
- Severe abdominal cramping
- Dehydration
- Gastrointestinal bleeding
- Necrosis of the liver, spleen, kidneys, and gastrointestinal tract

## YOU are the Provider

On arriving at the scene, you establish medical command. You see eight people lying in the street, including the suspect and two police officers. There are a few bystanders who are attempting to help the injured. You see several people applying makeshift tourniquets to bleeding extremities and one person performing CPR on a teenage girl. After triaging the patients, you have three patients who are in the expectant category (black tags), three patients in the immediate category (red tags), and two patients in the delayed category (yellow tags).

**7.** On the basis of the number of patients and their apparent conditions, how many ambulances and EMTs should be present at the scene?

Inhaling ricin will cause nonspecific weakness, cough, fever, hypothermia, and hypotension. Symptoms occur about 4 to 8 hours after inhalation, depending on the inhaled dose. The onset of profuse sweating some hours later signifies the termination of the symptoms.

Signs and symptoms of ricin inhalation are as follows:

- Fever
- Chills
- Nausea
- Local irritation of eyes, nose, and throat
- Profuse sweating
- Headache
- Muscle aches
- Nonproductive cough
- Chest pain
- Dyspnea
- Pulmonary edema
- Severe lung inflammation
- Cyanosis
- Seizures
- Respiratory failure

Treat with both respiratory support and cardiovascular support as needed. ALS support along with rapid transport to the ED for early intubation and ventilation, combined with treatment of pulmonary edema, are appropriate. ALS support can also initiate the intravenous fluids and electrolyte replacement that are essential to treat the dehydration caused by profound vomiting and diarrhea.

**TABLE 41-10** summarizes the biologic agents.

## Words of Wisdom

In a mass-casualty incident, it is important to frequently communicate with your patient. Remember, your patient is probably scared and does not know what is going on. Explain to your patient any delays that are occurring, as well as the actions you are taking, so you may alleviate the patient's fears.

## Other EMT Roles During a Biologic Event

### Syndromic Surveillance

Syndromic surveillance is the monitoring, usually by local or state health departments, of patients presenting to emergency departments and alternative care facilities, the recording of EMS call

| **TABLE 41-10** Biologic Agents | | | | |
|---|---|---|---|---|
| **Disease** | **Person-Person Transmission** | **Incubation Period** | **Duration of Illness** | **Lethality (approximate case fatality rates)** |
| **Inhalation anthrax** | No | 1 to 6 d | 3 to 5 d (usually fatal if untreated) | High |
| **Pneumonic plague** | High | 2 to 3 d | 1 to 6 d (usually fatal) | High unless treated within 12 to 24 h |
| **Smallpox** | High | 7 to 17 d (average, 12 d) | 4 wk | High to moderate |
| **Viral hemorrhagic fevers** | Moderate | 4 to 21 d | Death within 7 to 16 d | High to moderate, depending on type of fever |
| **Botulinum poisoning** | No | 1 to 5 d | Death within 24 to 72 h; lasts months if patient does not die | High without respiratory support |
| **Ricin poisoning** | No | 18 to 24 h | Death within 10 to 12 d for ingestion | High |

volume, and the use of over-the-counter medications. Patients with signs and symptoms that resemble influenza are particularly important. Local and state health departments monitor for an unusual influx of patients with these symptoms in hopes of discovering an outbreak early. The role of EMS in syndromic surveillance is valuable in the overall tracking of a biologic terrorist event or infectious disease outbreak. Quality assurance and dispatch operations need to be aware of an unusual number of calls from patients with unexplainable symptom clusters coming from a particular region or community.

### Points of Distribution (Strategic National Stockpile)

**Points of distribution (PODs)** are existing facilities that are used as mass distribution sites for antibiotics, antidotes, vaccinations, and other medications and supplies during an emergency.

These medications may be released in deliveries called "push packs" by the Centers for Disease Control and Prevention (CDC) Strategic National Stockpile (**FIGURE 41-16**). These push packs have a delivery time of 12 hours anywhere in the country and contain antibiotics, chemical antidotes, antitoxins, life-support medications, intravenous administration supplies, airway maintenance supplies, and medical/surgical items. In some

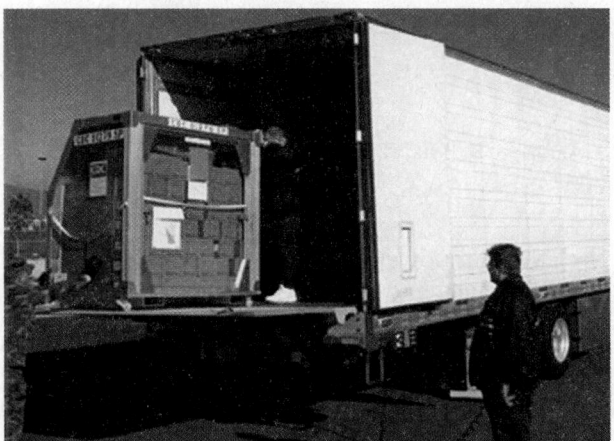

**FIGURE 41-16** The Centers for Disease Control and Prevention Strategic National Stockpile can deliver one of many push packs to any location in the country within 12 hours of an emergency.

Courtesy of the Strategic National Stockpile/CDC.

regions, local and state municipalities have started to stockpile their own supplies to reduce the time delay.

EMTs, AEMTs, and paramedics may be called on to assist in the delivery of the medications to the public (depending on local emergency management planning). Your role may include triage, treatment of seriously ill patients, and patient transport to the hospital. Most plans for PODs include at least one ambulance on standby to transport seriously ill patients.

## Radiologic/Nuclear Devices
### What Is Radiation?

**Ionizing radiation** is energy that is emitted in the form of rays, or particles. This energy can be found in **radioactive material**, such as rocks and metals. Radioactive material is any material that emits radiation. This material is unstable, and it attempts to stabilize itself by changing its structure in a natural process called **decay**. As the substance decays, it emits radiation until it stabilizes. The process of radioactive decay can take from as little as seconds to billions of years; meanwhile, the substance remains radioactive.

The energy that is emitted from a strong radiologic source is released in one or more of several forms, which are termed **alpha radiation**, **beta radiation**, **gamma (x-ray) radiation**, or **neutron radiation**. Alpha radiation is the least harmful penetrating type of radiation and cannot penetrate through most objects. In fact, a sheet of paper or the body's skin can easily stop it. Beta radiation is slightly more penetrating than alpha radiation and requires a layer of clothing to stop it. Gamma rays travel faster and have more energy than alpha and beta rays. These rays easily penetrate through the human body and require lead or several inches of concrete to prevent penetration. Neutron particles are among the most powerful forms of radiation. Neutrons easily penetrate through lead and require several feet of concrete to stop them (**FIGURE 41-17**).

### Sources of Radiologic Material

There are thousands of radioactive materials found on the earth. These materials are generally used for purposes that benefit humankind, such as

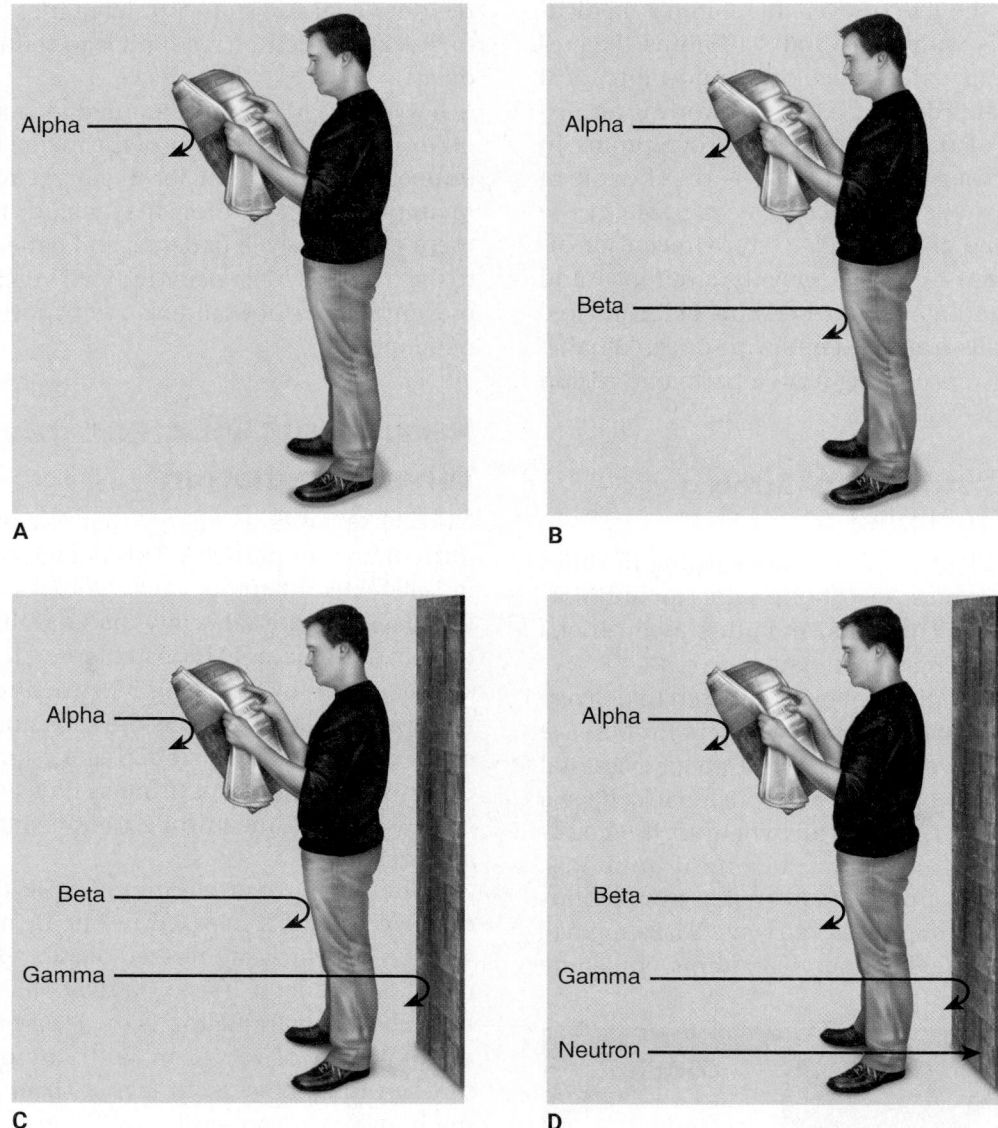

**FIGURE 41-17** The penetrating potential of radiation. **A.** Alpha. **B.** Beta. **C.** Gamma. **D.** Neutron.

A-D: © Jones & Bartlett Learning.

medicine, killing germs in food (irradiating), and construction. Once radiologic material has been used for its purpose, the material remaining is called radiologic waste. Radiologic waste remains radioactive but is no longer useful for its original purpose. These materials can be found at the following locations:

- Hospitals and other health care facilities with radiology departments
- Colleges and universities

- Nuclear power plants
- Chemical and industrial sites

Not all radioactive material is tightly guarded, and the waste is often not guarded at all. This makes radioactive material and substances appealing to terrorists.

## Radiologic Dispersal Devices

A radiologic dispersal device (RDD) is any container that is designed to disperse radioactive material. This would generally require the use of a bomb—hence the nickname dirty bomb. A dirty bomb has the potential to cause injury not only as a result of the radioactive material, but also from the explosive material used to deliver it. Just the thought of an RDD creates fear in a population, and so the ultimate goal of some terrorists—fear—is accomplished. However, the actual destructive capability of a dirty bomb is limited to the explosives that are attached to it. Therefore, if the explosive is sufficient to kill 10 people without radioactive material, it will also kill 10 people with the radioactive material added. There may be long-term injuries and illness associated with the use of an RDD, yet not much more than the bomb by itself would create. In short, the dirty bomb is an ineffective WMD.

## Nuclear Energy

Nuclear energy is artificially made by altering (splitting) radioactive atoms. The result is an immense amount of energy that usually takes the form of heat. Nuclear material is used in medicine, weapons, naval vessels, and power plants. Nuclear material gives off all forms of radiation, including neutrons (the deadliest type). Like radioactive material, when nuclear material is no longer useful it becomes waste that remains radioactive.

## Nuclear Weapons

The destructive energy of a nuclear explosion is unlike any other weapon in the world. That is why nuclear weapons are kept in only secure facilities throughout the world. There are nations that have ties to terrorists and that have actively attempted to build nuclear weapons. However, these nations do not have the capability to deliver a nuclear weapon, such as a missile or bomb.

There is also the deterrent of complete mutual annihilation. Therefore, the likelihood of a nuclear attack is extremely remote.

Unfortunately, since the collapse of the Soviet Union, the whereabouts of many small nuclear devices have become unknown. These small suitcase-sized nuclear weapons are called Special Atomic Demolition Munitions (SADM). The SADM, or "suitcase nuke," was designed to destroy individual

| **TABLE 41-11** Common Signs of Acute Radiation Toxicity | |
|---|---|
| **Low exposure** | Nausea, vomiting, diarrhea, dizziness, headache |
| **Moderate exposure** | First-degree burns, hair loss, compromised immune system (death of white blood cells), and cancer |
| **Severe exposure** | Second- and third-degree burns, cancer, and death |

© Jones & Bartlett Learning.

targets, such as important buildings, bridges, tunnels, and large ships. Some of these are believed to be missing. Information or updates on the whereabouts of these devices has not been made public.

## Symptomatology

Patients exposed to a known or suspected source of excessive radiation are considered victims of acute radiation toxicity. The effects of radiation exposure will vary depending on the amount of radiation received and the route of entry. Radiation can be introduced into the body by all routes of entry as well as through the body (irradiation). Patients can inhale radioactive dust from nuclear fallout or from a dirty bomb or have radioactive liquid absorbed into their body through their skin. Once inside the body, the radiation source will irradiate the person from within rather than from an external source (such as radiography equipment). Some common signs of acute radiation sickness are listed in **TABLE 41-11**. Additional injuries will occur with a nuclear blast, such as thermal and blast trauma, trauma from flying objects, and eye injuries.

## Medical Management

Being exposed to a radiation source does not make a patient contaminated or radioactive. However, when patients have a radioactive source on their bodies (such as debris from a dirty bomb), they are contaminated and must be initially cared for by a hazmat responder. Once the patient is decontaminated and there is no threat to you, you may begin treating the ABCs and treat the patient for any burns or trauma. As always, wear appropriate PPE. Any body fluids obtained from the patient should be secured in plastic bags. Place all body fluids in containers and properly dispose of them with other potentially radioactive waste.

## Protective Measure

There are no suits or protective gear designed to completely shield you from radiation. The people who work in high-risk areas wear specific protection such as lead-lined suits; however, this equipment is not available to EMTs. The best ways to protect yourself from the effects of radiation are to use time and distance and shield yourself using buildings and walls for protection. Do not enter a hazmat area unless you are trained as a hazmat responder and have proper training in the use of self-contained breathing apparatus.

- **Time.** Radiation has a cumulative effect on the body. The less time that you are exposed to the source, the less the effects will be. If you realize the patient is near a radiation source, leave the area immediately.
- **Distance.** Radiation is limited as to how far it can travel. Depending on the type of radiation, moving only a few feet is often enough to remove you from immediate danger. Alpha radiation cannot travel more than a few inches but gamma rays can travel hundreds or thousands of meters. Take this into account when responding to a nuclear or radiologic incident and make certain that responders are stationed far enough away from the incident.
- **Shielding.** Remember, the path of all radiation can be stopped by a specific object. It will be

impossible for you to recognize the type of radiation being emitted or even from which direction it is coming. Therefore, always assume you are dealing with the strongest form of radiation and use concrete shielding (such as buildings or walls) between yourself and the incident. The importance of shielding cannot be overemphasized.

## Incendiary and Explosive Devices

Incendiary and explosive devices come in various shapes and sizes. Incendiary devices are weapons used to start fires. Terrorists use flamethrowers, chemicals, Molotov cocktails, or other explosive devices for this purpose. Although you are not required to recognize all of the possible types of explosive devices, including improvised explosive devices, it is important for you to be able to identify an object you believe is a potential device, notify the proper authorities, and safely evacuate the area. Always remember that there is the possibility of a secondary device when you are responding to the scene of an incendiary or explosive device call.

## Mechanisms of Injury

The type and severity of wounds sustained from incendiary and explosive devices primarily depend on the patient's distance from the epicenter of the explosion. Patients close to the epicenter of the explosion are likely to sustain injury from all wound-causing agents of the munitions. Patients who are farther away from the epicenter are likely to experience a combination of blast injuries from the explosion and

**YOU** are the Provider

The patients have been triaged and appropriately treated. After the transportation officer notifies the receiving facilities about the patients' injuries, the final patient is transported. She is an unresponsive adult who is breathing and has no radial pulse. You glance at an adjacent patient with a large gunshot wound to the head and confirm that he is not breathing even after a head tilt. After decontaminating yourselves and the ambulance, you and your crew discuss the incident, including terrorism in general.

**8.** What type of terrorist group was most likely responsible for this incident?

**9.** What level of knowledge of terrorism and weapons of mass destruction should you possess?

penetrating trauma injuries from primary and secondary projectiles created by the explosion.

Blast injuries occur in a number of ways.

- **Primary blast injury.** Due solely to the direct effects of the pressure wave on the body. The injury from the primary blast is seen almost exclusively in the hollow organs of the body—the lungs, intestines, and ears. An injury to the lungs causes the greatest morbidity and mortality.
- **Secondary blast injury.** Penetrating or nonpenetrating injury that results from being struck by flying debris, such as ordnance projectiles or secondary missiles, that has been set in motion by the explosion. Objects are propelled by the force of the blast and strike the victim, causing injury.
- **Tertiary blast injury.** Results from whole-body displacement and subsequent traumatic impact with environmental objects (eg, trees, buildings, and vehicles). Other indirect effects include crush injury from the collapse of structures (buildings, bunkers, or tunnels).
- **Quaternary blast injury.** Any other injury caused by a blast occurs in this way. This includes toxic inhalation of combustion gases, burns, a medical emergency (such as a myocardial infarction) sustained while fleeing the scene of an explosion, and even a mental health disorder that develops immediately after or days to weeks after detonation of an explosive device.

## The Physics of an Explosion

When a substance is detonated, a solid or liquid is chemically converted into large volumes of gas under high pressure with resultant explosive energy release. Propellants, like gunpowder, are explosives designed to release energy relatively slowly compared with high-energy explosives, which are designed to detonate very quickly. This generates a pressure pulse in the shape of a spherical blast wave that expands in all directions from the point of explosion. Flying debris and high winds commonly cause conventional blunt and penetrating trauma.

## Tissues at Risk

Hollow organs such as the middle ear, lungs, and gastrointestinal tract are most susceptible to pressure changes. The junction between tissues of different densities and exposed tissues such as the head and neck are prone to injury as well. The ear is the organ system most sensitive to blast injuries. The patient may report ringing or pain in the ears or some loss of hearing, and blood may be visible in the ear canal. Permanent hearing loss is possible.

Primary **pulmonary blast injuries** occur as contusions and hemorrhages. When the explosion occurs in an open space, the patient's side that is toward the explosion is usually injured, but the injury can be bilateral when the patient is in a confined space. The patient may report tightness or pain in the chest and may cough up blood and have tachypnea or other signs of respiratory distress. Subcutaneous emphysema (air trapped under the skin) over the chest may be palpated, indicating the presence of a pneumothorax. Pneumothorax is common and may require emergency decompression if there are signs of severe respiratory distress or hemodynamic compromise.

Solid organs are relatively protected from shockwave injury but may be injured by secondary missiles or a hurled body. Hollow organs, however, may be injured by mechanisms similar to those that injure lung tissue. Petechiae, or pinpoint hemorrhages that show up on the skin, to large hematomas are the most visible sign.

According to the CDC, blast lung is the most common cause of death from blast injury. Neurologic injuries and head trauma are also common causes of fatality from blast injury. Subarachnoid (beneath the arachnoid layer covering the brain) and subdural (beneath the outermost covering of the brain) hematomas are often seen. Permanent or transient neurologic deficits may occur secondary to concussion, intracerebral bleeding, or air embolism. Instant but transient unconsciousness, with or without retrograde amnesia, may be initiated not only by head trauma, but also by cardiovascular problems. Bradycardia and hypotension are common after an intense pressure wave from an explosion.

Extremity injuries, including traumatic amputations, are common, and patients may die of massive hemorrhage without the rapid application of a tourniquet.

## YOU are the Provider SUMMARY

**1. On the basis of the information you have received, how should you approach this incident?**

This incident calls for your highest level of alertness and vigilance. Your life and the lives of others depend on your ability to quickly and accurately sort through the information. You must process the information, determine what is pertinent, and create a plan of action. Given that frantic bystanders often provide some of the early reports in these types of incidents, it is reasonable to consider that some of the information may be confusing or inaccurate. Do not become distracted. Focus on reports that provide any information about immediate threats to your safety and the location of injured personnel.

From the information you have received, there has been a possible mass-casualty event involving multiple scenes within close proximity to your current location. You are not able to determine if there is a hazmat component to this call, but that thought should be in your mind, given the reports of smoke coming from a trash can followed by a shooting. While we often consider staging away from a dangerous scene, you have been thrust into the middle of this incident. You should make sure you are in a safe location. With possible multiple events and/or attackers in your proximity, retreating could be as dangerous as advancing toward the injured. Do your best to get your bearings and stay calm. Ensure that adequate resources are dispatched, including those with the capacity to asses and manage potential safety threats.

**2. What indicators suggest that an incident is the result of terrorism?**

Information from dispatch such as the location and type of incident, the number of patients, and victims' statements may be the first indicators that an incident is the result of terrorism. For example, is the incident location a government building, a festival, or a specific structure? Are there multiple patients with similar injuries or symptoms, such as difficulty breathing? Are victims fleeing the scene and making statements such as "There was a loud explosion?" There may be incidents involving terrorism that are on a small scale and some that are on a much larger scale. Some terrorist attacks may be designed in a strategic way to create maximum chaos or try to lure more people to a certain area to maximize the number of injured. If there are separate reports of multiple unusual events near each another, you must consider the possibility of terrorism. For example, if

you are responding to reports of an unconscious person and separate 9-1-1 calls come in about an explosion at a church across the street from the initial dispatch location, you must consider the possibility of terrorism.

**3. What should you consider when determining if the scene is safe for you and other EMS personnel to enter?**

Due to the unique circumstances of this incident, you will have to weigh the risks and benefits of continuing to stage versus continuing into the scene. You should evaluate what the current threat level is at your precise location. Can you hear active gunfire? Are you near the location of a recent explosion or active fire? Is there any threat of hazardous materials where you are or where you are planning to go? Are there any reports from law enforcement or bystanders that a threat is headed in your direction? Remember that there may be secondary devices that specifically target both responders rushing to help the injured and anyone who is fleeing the initial scene. A good resource in this incident would be the closest law enforcement official. This person should be able to provide current information about known or suspected threats to your safety and report whether the scene is secured for you to begin treating the injured.

**4. What immediate actions should you perform prior to proceeding into the scene?**

As discussed with regard to recommendations from the Hartford Consensus, EMS systems must reevaluate the practice of staging away from the scene and waiting for patients to be brought to the ambulance. You have already been thrust into the middle of this incident. While requesting additional resources, communicate your location to dispatch. Ask if they have any information about the scene. If your agency supplies any ballistic vests or helmets for EMTs, you should put this equipment on immediately. Find the closest law enforcement officer. This person may be able to provide some protection from threats as you maintain your current position or advance toward injured personnel when it is determined to be appropriate for you to do so. If you are going to move toward the injured, do not worry about bringing every piece of medical equipment. Your initial role will likely be triage and basic treatment to control life-threatening hemorrhage. Carry your triage tape or tags and basic trauma equipment. Do not weigh yourself down with unnecessary items. You want to be able to move quickly if another threat emerges.

**5. Given the situation, what are some unique concerns about this incident?**

In the past, terrorists have been known to plant additional explosives (secondary devices) that were set to detonate after the initial device. Secondary devices are primarily intended to injure emergency responders or bystanders who have gathered in attempts to help or flee the scene. These devices may not be in the same location as the primary device. The secondary device could be a package or briefcase that has been planted across the street or it could be an electronic device, such as a cell phone, that is designed to detonate on activation.

Although the scene may be secured initially, you must realize that the scene can easily become unsafe. Do not rely on others to keep you safe; it is *your* responsibility to constantly reassess the scene for indicators of danger. A subtle change in wind direction during an incident involving radiation or an increase in the number of patients who are contaminated can place you in danger.

**6. What types of injuries should you expect to encounter?**

Given this scenario, you would expect to find that the majority of injuries involve penetrating trauma. The initial report of a police officer who was stabbed will present differently than someone who was shot with a high-velocity rifle, but both patients are at risk for catastrophic injuries and life-threatening hemorrhage. The severity of the injuries can depend on the type of gun that was used, the number of times the person was shot, and the anatomic location of the injuries. Penetrating trauma to the extremities may produce significant hemorrhage that may require the use of a tourniquet. Penetrating trauma to the head, neck, and chest is often rapidly fatal if not immediately treated with appropriate airway management, ventilatory support, and hemorrhage control.

**7. On the basis of the number of patients and their apparent conditions, how many ambulances and EMTs should be present at the scene?**

Your general impression of the scene has revealed that there are eight total patients, with five of them

considered salvageable. Assume all five patients have critical injuries until they have been triaged and treatment has begun. One ambulance and two EMTs can effectively care for only one critically injured patient at a time. You will likely need at least 5 ambulances and 10 EMTs to transport the five critical patients.

However, remember that some patients who were initially triaged in the expectant category may ultimately be upgraded to the immediate category as more resources arrive on scene. Therefore, there should be a total of eight ambulances and 16 EMTs at the scene—two EMTs and one ambulance per patient. It is better to have enough resources to treat every patient than to have a patient who requires treatment and no available resources.

This scenario demonstrates how the resources required to manage an incident due to terrorism could easily overwhelm the available sources for a single EMS system.

**8. What type of terrorist group was most likely responsible for this incident?**

In this incident, a single actor created a diversion to push the crowd in his direction before he began shooting into the crowd. This behavior suggests a lone wolf terrorist. The motive may not always be clear in these types of attacks. There may be a personal grievance or motive that relates to a larger group, but lone wolf terrorists, by definition, do not receive any assistance from outside sources in planning or implementing their attack.

**9. What level of knowledge of terrorism and weapons of mass destruction should you possess?**

You are not expected to be an expert in terrorism and weapons of mass destruction (WMDs). However, you are expected to be aware of the various types of threats—just like any other citizen—and recognize certain indicators of terrorism when responding to an incident. As an EMT, you should possess a basic working knowledge of the different types of WMDs that terrorists could use, signs and symptoms and treatment of victims of WMDs, measures to take to ensure personal safety and safety of the patient, and knowledge of the ICS.

## YOU are the Provider SUMMARY continued

### Patient No. 1
Triage Tag
No. 240351

Move the Walking Wounded

NO Respirations after head tilt

[X] Respirations—over 30

[ ] Perfusion—capillary refill over 2 seconds

[ ] Mental status—unable to follow simple commands

Otherwise

MINIMAL
EXPECTANT
IMMEDIATE
IMMEDIATE
IMMEDIATE
DELAYED

MAJOR INJURIES: Open chest and abdominal injuries
HOSPITAL DESTINATION: Harbor Bay Trauma Center
ORIENTED × [ ]   DISORIENTED [X]   UNCONSCIOUS [ ]

| TIME | PULSE | B/P | RESPIRATION |
|------|-------|------|-------------|
| 1025 | 118 | 80/60 | 26 (labored) |
| 1030 | 110 | 94/64 | 24 (labored) |

PERSONAL INFORMATION:
NAME: Lisa Malone
MALE [ ]   FEMALE [X]   AGE: 41   WEIGHT: 57 kg (126 lb)
MEDICAL COMPLAINTS/HISTORY
Penetrating injuries to chest and abdomen; shard of glass impaled in chest; abdominal evisceration; history of high blood pressure

EXPECTANT   No   240351

IMMEDIATE   No   240351

### Patient No. 2
Triage Tag
No. 240352

Move the Walking Wounded

NO respirations after head tilt

[ ] Respirations—over 30

[X] Perfusion—capillary refill over 2 seconds

[ ] Mental status—unable to follow simple commands

Otherwise

MINIMAL
EXPECTANT
IMMEDIATE
IMMEDIATE
IMMEDIATE
DELAYED

MAJOR INJURIES: Possible pneumothorax, deformed left femur
HOSPITAL DESTINATION: Harbor Bay Trauma Center
ORIENTED × [4]   DISORIENTED [ ]   UNCONSCIOUS [ ]

| TIME | PULSE | B/P | RESPIRATION |
|------|-------|------|-------------|
| 1026 | 112 | 100/58 | 28 (labored) |
| 1031 | 118 | 98/60 | 28 (labored) |

PERSONAL INFORMATION:
NAME: Stanley Green
MALE [X]   FEMALE [ ]   AGE: 34   WEIGHT: 75 kg (165 lb)
MEDICAL COMPLAINTS/HISTORY
Difficulty breathing; multiple abrasions and lacerations; left femur deformity; no medical history

EXPECTANT   No   240352

IMMEDIATE   No   240352

# Prep Kit

## Ready for Review

- As a result of the increase in terrorist activity, it is possible that you, as an EMT, could witness a terrorist event. You must be mentally and physically prepared for the possibility of a terrorist event.
- Types of groups that tend to use terrorism include religious extremist groups/doomsday cults, extremist political groups, cyber terrorists, and single-issue groups.
- Lone wolf terrorist attacks, particularly active shooter events, are a growing threat in the United States. EMS systems should incorporate the Hartford Consensus recommendations and the Stop the Bleed campaign to guide care at these scenes.
- A weapon of mass destruction (WMD) is any agent designed to bring about mass death, casualties, and/or massive damage to property and infrastructure (bridges, tunnels, airports, and seaports). These can be biologic, nuclear, incendiary, chemical, and explosive weapons (B-NICE).
- Indicators that may give you clues as to whether the emergency is the result of a terrorist attack include the type of location, type of call, number of patients, victims' statements, and preincident indicators.
- If you suspect that a terrorist or an event involving a WMD has occurred, ensure that the scene is safe. If you have any doubt that it may not be safe, do not enter. Wait for assistance.
- Terrorists may set secondary devices that are designed to explode after the initial bomb, thus injuring responders and increasing media coverage. Constantly assess and reassess the scene for safety.
- Chemical agents are manufactured liquid, gas, or solid substances that can have devastating effects on living organisms.
- Persistency and volatility describe how long the agent will stay on the surface before it evaporates, and the route of exposure is how the agent most effectively enters the body.
- Biologic agents include viruses such as smallpox and those that cause viral hemorrhagic fevers; bacteria such as those that cause anthrax and plague; and neurotoxins such as botulinum toxin and ricin.
- Nuclear or radiologic weapons produced from radioactive waste material can create a massive amount of destruction.
- Ionizing radiation is energy that can enter the human body and cause damage.
- Explosive and incendiary devices come in various shapes and sizes. It is important to be able to identify an object you believe is a potential device and notify the proper authorities, while safely evacuating the area.

## Vital Vocabulary

**active shooter event** An act of terror in which firearms are used in an ongoing assault of multiple people.

**aging** The process by which the temporary bond between an organophosphate and acetylcholinesterase undergoes hydrolysis, resulting in a permanent covalent bond.

**alpha radiation** A type of energy that is emitted from a strong radiologic source; it is the least harmful penetrating type of radiation and cannot travel more than a few inches or penetrate most objects.

**anthrax** A disease caused by a deadly bacterium (*Bacillus anthracis*) that lies dormant in a spore (protective shell); the germ is released from the spore when exposed to the optimal temperature and moisture. The routes of entry are inhalation, cutaneous, and gastrointestinal (from consuming food that contains spores).

**Antidote Treatment Nerve Agent Auto-Injector (ATNAA)** A nerve agent antidote kit containing atropine and pralidoxime chloride; delivered as a single dose through one needle.

**bacteria** Microorganisms that reproduce by binary fission. These single-cell creatures reproduce rapidly. Some can form spores (encysted variants) when environmental conditions are harsh.

**beta radiation** A type of energy that is emitted from a strong radiologic source; it is slightly more penetrating than alpha radiation and requires a layer of clothing to stop it.

**B-NICE** A memory device to recall the types of weapons of mass destruction: biologic, nuclear, incendiary, chemical, and explosive.

**botulinum** Produced by bacteria, this is the most potent neurotoxin known. When introduced into the body, this neurotoxin affects the nervous system's ability to function and causes botulism.

**buboes** Enlarged lymph nodes (up to the size of a tennis ball) that are characteristic in people infected with the bubonic plague.

**bubonic plague** Bacterial infection that affects the lymphatic system. It is transmitted by infected rodents and fleas and characterized by acute malaise, fever, and the formation of tender, enlarged, inflamed lymph nodes that appear as lesions, called buboes. Also called the Black Death.

**chlorine (Cl)** The first chemical agent ever used in warfare. It has a distinct odor of bleach and creates a green haze when released as a gas. Initially it produces upper airway irritation and a choking sensation.

**contact hazard** The term used to describe the danger posed by a chemical whose primary route of entry into the body is through the skin; posed by a hazardous agent that gives off very little or no vapors; also called a skin hazard.

**contagious** An infectious disease that spreads from one human to another; communicable.

**covert** An act in which the public safety community generally has no prior knowledge of the time, location, or nature of the attack.

**cross-contamination** Occurs when a person is contaminated by an agent as a result of coming in contact with another contaminated person.

**cyanide** An agent that affects the body's ability to use oxygen. It is a colorless gas that has an odor similar to almonds. The effects begin on the cellular level and are very rapidly seen at the organ and system levels.

**decay** A natural process in which a material that is unstable attempts to stabilize itself by changing its structure.

**dirty bomb** Name given to an explosive radiologic dispersal device.

**disease vector** An animal that, once infected, spreads a disease to another animal.

**dissemination** The means by which a terrorist will spread an agent; for example, by poisoning the water supply or aerosolizing the agent into the air or ventilation system of a building.

**domestic terrorism** Terrorism that is carried out by people in their own country.

**DuoDote Auto-Injector** A nerve agent antidote kit containing atropine and pralidoxime chloride; delivered as a single dose through one needle.

**G agents** Early nerve agents that were developed by German scientists in the period after World War I and into World War II. There are three such agents: sarin, soman, and tabun.

**gamma (x-ray) radiation** A type of energy that is emitted from a strong radiologic source that travels faster and has more energy than alpha and beta rays. These rays easily penetrate through the human body and require lead or several inches of concrete to prevent penetration.

**incubation** The period of time between a person being exposed to an agent and the time when symptoms appear.

**international terrorism** Terrorism that is carried out by people in a country other than their own; also known as cross-border terrorism.

**ionizing radiation** Energy that is emitted in the form of rays, or particles.

**lewisite (L)** A blistering agent that has a rapid onset of symptoms and produces immediate, intense pain and discomfort on contact.

**lone wolf terrorist attack** An act of terror carried out by a single person to further an ideological goal.

**lymphatic system** A passive circulatory system in the body that transports a plasmalike liquid called lymph, a thin fluid that bathes the tissues of the body.

**lymph nodes** The area of the lymphatic system where infection-fighting cells are housed.

**miosis** Excessively constricted pupil; often bilateral after exposure to nerve agents.

**mutagen** A substance that mutates, damages, and changes the structures of DNA in the body's cells.

**nerve agents** A class of chemical called organophosphates; they function by blocking an essential enzyme in the nervous system, which causes the body's organs to become overstimulated and burn out.

**neurotoxins** Biologic agents that are the deadliest substances known to humans; they include botulinum toxin and ricin.

**neutron radiation** The type of energy that is emitted from a strong radiologic source, involving particles that are among the most powerful forms of radiation; the particles easily penetrate through lead and require several feet of concrete to stop them.

**off-gassing** The release of an agent after exposure—for example, from a person's clothes that have been exposed to the agent.

**pandemic** An outbreak that occurs on a global scale.

**persistency** How long a chemical agent will stay on a surface before it evaporates.

**phosgene** A pulmonary agent that is a product of combustion, resulting from a fire at a textile factory or house, or from metalwork or burning Freon. It is a very potent agent that has a delayed onset of symptoms, usually hours.

**phosgene oxime (CX)** A blistering agent that has a rapid onset of symptoms and produces immediate, intense pain and discomfort on contact.

**pneumonic plague** A lung infection, also known as plague pneumonia, that is the result of inhalation of plague-causing bacteria.

**points of distribution (PODs)** Existing facilities used as mass distribution sites for antibiotics, antidotes, vaccinations, and other medications and supplies during an emergency.

**primary blast injury** Injuries caused by an explosive pressure wave to the hollow organs of the body.

**pulmonary blast injuries** Pulmonary trauma resulting from short-range exposure to the detonation of high-energy explosives.

**quaternary blast injury** A blast injury that falls into one of the following categories: burns, crush injuries, toxic inhalation, medical emergencies, or mental health disorders.

**radioactive material** Any material that emits radiation.

**radiologic dispersal device (RDD)** Any container that is designed to disperse radioactive material.

**ricin** A neurotoxin derived from mash that is left from the castor bean; causes pulmonary edema and respiratory and circulatory failure leading to death.

**route of exposure** The manner by which a toxic substance enters the body.

**sarin (GB)** A nerve agent that is one of the G agents; a highly volatile colorless and odorless liquid that turns from liquid to gas within seconds to minutes at room temperature.

**secondary blast injury** A penetrating or nonpenetrating injury caused by ordnance projectiles or secondary missiles.

**secondary device** A secondary explosive used by terrorists, set to explode after the initial bomb.

**smallpox** A highly contagious viral disease; it is most contagious when blisters begin to form.

**soman (GD)** A nerve agent that is one of the G agents; twice as persistent as sarin and five times as lethal; it has a fruity odor as a result of the type of alcohol used in the agent, and is a contact and an inhalation hazard that can enter the body through skin absorption and through the respiratory tract.

**Special Atomic Demolition Munitions (SADM)** Small suitcase-sized nuclear weapons that were designed to destroy individual targets, such as important buildings, bridges, tunnels, and large ships.

**state-sponsored terrorism** Terrorism that is funded and/or supported by nations that hold close ties with terrorist groups.

**sulfur mustard (H)** A vesicant; it is a brown-yellow oily substance that is generally considered very persistent; has the distinct smell of garlic or mustard and, when released, is quickly absorbed into the skin and/or mucous membranes and begins an irreversible process of damaging the cells. Also called mustard gas.

**syndromic surveillance** The monitoring, usually by local or state health departments, of patients presenting to emergency departments and alternative care facilities, the recording of EMS call volume, and the use of over-the-counter medications.

**tabun (GA)** A nerve agent that is one of the G agents; 36 times more persistent than sarin and approximately one-half as lethal; has a fruity smell and is unique because the components used to manufacture the agent are easy to acquire and the agent is easy to manufacture.

**tertiary blast injury** An injury from whole-body displacement and subsequent traumatic impact with environmental objects.

**V agent (VX)** One of the G agents; it is a clear, oily agent that has no odor and looks like baby oil; more than 100 times more lethal than sarin and extremely persistent.

**vapor hazard** The term used to describe danger posed by an agent that enters the body through the respiratory tract.

**vesicants** Blister agents; the primary route of entry for such agents is through the skin.

**viral hemorrhagic fevers** A group of diseases caused by viruses that include the Ebola, Rift Valley, and yellow fevers, among others. This group of viruses causes the blood in the body to seep out from the tissues and blood vessels.

**viruses** Germs that require a living host to multiply and survive.

**volatility** How long a chemical agent will stay on a surface before it evaporates.

**weaponization** The creation of a weapon from a biologic agent that is generally found in nature and that causes disease; the agent is cultivated, synthesized, and/or mutated to maximize the target population's exposure to the germ.

**weapon of mass casualty (WMC)** Any agent designed to bring about mass death, casualties, and/or massive damage to property and infrastructure (bridges, tunnels, airports, and seaports); also known as a weapon of mass destruction (WMD).

**weapon of mass destruction (WMD)** Any agent designed to bring about mass death, casualties, and/or massive damage to property and infrastructure (bridges, tunnels, airports, and seaports); also known as a weapon of mass casualty (WMC).

## References

1. Alfaro-Gonzalez L, Barthelmes RJ, Bartol C, et al.; Security Studies Program. *Report: Lone Wolf Terrorism.* Georgetown Security Studies Review website. georgetownsecuritystudiesreview.org/wp-content/uploads/2015/08/NCITF-Final-Paper.pdf. Published June 27, 2015. Accessed April 18, 2020.

2. American College of Surgeons. Out of great tragedy, a life-saving response begins around the world. Stop the Bleed website. www.stopthebleed.org/our-story. Accessed April 18, 2020.

3. Gummin DD, Mowry JB, Spyker DA, Brooks DE, Osterthaler KM, Banner W. 2017 annual report of the American Association of Poison Control Centers' National Poison Data System (NPDS): 35th annual report. *Clin Toxicol (Phila)* 2018;56(12):1213–1415.

4. Joint Committee to Create a National Policy to Enhance Survivability From Intentional Mass-Casualty Shooting Events. Active shooter and intentional mass-casualty events: the Hartford Consensus II. *The Bulletin* website. bulletin.facs.org/2013/09/hartford-consensus-ii/. Published September 1, 2013. Accessed April 18, 2020.

5. Joint Committee to Create a National Policy to Enhance Survivability From Mass-Casualty Shooting Events. Improving survival from active shooter events: the Hartford Consensus. *Bull Am Coll Surg* 2013;98(6):14–16.

# Glossary

**abandonment:** Unilateral termination of care by the EMT without the patient's consent and without making provisions for transferring care to another medical professional with the skills and training necessary to meet the needs of the patient.

**abdomen:** The body cavity that contains many of the major organs of digestion and excretion. It is located below the diaphragm and above the pelvis.

**abdominal aortic aneurysm (AAA):** A rapidly fatal condition in which the walls of the aorta in the abdomen weaken and blood leaks into the layers of the vessel, causing it to bulge.

**abdominal thrust maneuver:** The preferred method to dislodge a severe airway obstruction in adults and children; also called the Heimlich maneuver.

**abduction:** Motion of a limb away from the midline.

**abrasion:** Loss of or damage to the superficial layer of skin as a result of a body part rubbing or scraping across a rough or hard surface.

**abruptio placentae:** Premature separation of the placenta from the wall of the uterus.

**absorption:** The process by which medications travel through body tissues until they reach the bloodstream.

**access:** Gaining entry to an enclosed area and reaching a patient.

**accessory muscles:** The secondary muscles of respiration. They include the neck muscles (sternocleidomastoids), the chest pectoralis major muscles, and the abdominal muscles.

**acetabulum:** The depression on the lateral pelvis where its three component bones join, in which the femoral head fits snugly.

**acidosis:** The buildup of excess acid in the blood or body tissues that can result from a primary illness.

**acromioclavicular (AC) joint:** A simple joint where the bony projections of the scapula and the clavicle meet at the top of the shoulder.

**action:** The therapeutic effect of a medication on the body.

**active compression-decompression CPR:** A technique that involves compressing the chest and then actively pulling it back up to its neutral position or beyond (decompression); may increase the amount of blood that returns to the heart and, thus, the amount of blood ejected from the heart during the compression phase.

**active shooter event:** An act of terror in which firearms are used in an ongoing assault of multiple people.

**activities of daily living:** The basic activities a person usually accomplishes during a normal day, such as eating, dressing, and bathing.

**acute abdomen:** A condition of sudden onset of pain within the abdomen, usually indicating peritonitis; immediate medical or surgical treatment is necessary.

**acute coronary syndrome (ACS):** A group of symptoms caused by myocardial ischemia; includes angina and myocardial infarction.

**acute myocardial infarction (AMI):** A heart attack; death of heart muscle following obstruction of blood flow to it. "Acute" in this context means "new" or "happening right now."

**acute stress reactions:** Reactions to stress that occur during a traumatic situation.

**addiction:** A state of overwhelming obsession or physical need to continue the use of a substance.

**adduction:** Motion of a limb toward the midline.

**adenosine triphosphate (ATP):** The nucleotide involved in energy metabolism; used to store energy.

**adolescent:** A young person age 12 to 18 years.

**adrenal glands:** Endocrine glands located on top of the kidneys that release adrenaline when stimulated by the sympathetic nervous system.

**adrenergic:** Pertaining to nerves that release the neurotransmitter norepinephrine, or noradrenaline (eg, adrenergic nerves, adrenergic response); also pertains to the receptors acted on by norepinephrine.

**advanced EMT (AEMT):** An individual who has training in specific aspects of advanced life support, such as intravenous therapy, and the administration of certain emergency medications.

**advance directive:** Written documentation that specifies medical treatment for a competent patient should the patient become unable to make decisions; also called a living will or health care directive.

**advanced life support (ALS):** Advanced life-saving procedures, some of which are now being provided by the EMT.

**adventitious breath sounds:** Abnormal breath sounds such as wheezing, stridor, rhonchi, and crackles.

**adverse effects:** Any unwanted clinical results of a medication.

**aerobic metabolism:** Metabolism that can proceed only in the presence of oxygen.

**aerosol-generating procedure:** Any airway manipulation that induces the production of aerosols that may present a risk for airborne transmission of pathogens, such as CPR.

**afterload:** The force or resistance against which the heart pumps.

**aging:** The process by which the temporary bond between an organophosphate and acetylcholinesterase undergoes hydrolysis, resulting in a permanent covalent bond.

**agonal gasps:** Abnormal breathing pattern characterized by slow, gasping breaths, sometimes seen in patients in cardiac arrest.

**agonist:** A medication that causes stimulation of receptors.

**air ambulances:** Fixed-wing and rotary-wing (known as helicopters) aircraft that have been modified for medical care; used to evacuate and transport patients with life-threatening injuries to treatment facilities.

**airborne transmission:** The spread of an organism via droplets or dust.

**air embolism:** The presence of air in the veins, which can lead to cardiac arrest if it enters the heart.

**airway:** The upper airway tract or the passage above the larynx, which includes the nose, mouth, and throat.

**algor mortis:** Cooling of the body after death until it matches the ambient temperature.

**alkalosis:** The buildup of excess base (lack of acids) in the body fluids.

**allergen:** A substance that causes an allergic reaction.

**allergic reaction:** The body's exaggerated immune response to an internal or surface agent.

**alpha-adrenergic receptors:** Portions of the nervous system that, when stimulated, can cause constriction of blood vessels.

**alpha radiation:** A type of energy that is emitted from a strong radiologic source; it is the least harmful penetrating type of radiation and cannot travel more than a few inches or penetrate most objects.

**altered mental status:** A change in the way a person thinks and behaves that may signal disease in the central nervous system or elsewhere in the body.

**alveolar minute volume:** The volume of air moved through the lungs in 1 minute minus the dead space; calculated by multiplying tidal volume (minus dead space) and respiratory rate.

**alveolar ventilation:** The volume of air that reaches the alveoli. It is determined by subtracting the amount of dead space air from the tidal volume.

**alveoli:** The air sacs of the lungs in which the exchange of oxygen and carbon dioxide takes place.

**ambient temperature:** The temperature of the surrounding environment.

**ambulance:** A specialized vehicle for treating and transporting sick and injured patients.

**American Standard Safety System:** A safety system for large oxygen cylinders, designed to prevent the accidental attachment of a regulator to a cylinder containing the wrong type of gas.

**Americans With Disabilities Act (ADA):** Comprehensive legislation that is designed to protect people with disabilities against discrimination.

**amniotic sac:** The fluid-filled, baglike membrane in which the fetus develops.

**amputation:** An injury in which part of the body is completely severed.

**anaerobic metabolism:** Metabolism that takes place in the absence of oxygen; the main by-product is lactic acid.

**anaphylactic shock:** Severe shock caused by an allergic reaction.

**anaphylaxis:** An extreme, life-threatening, systemic allergic reaction that may include shock and respiratory failure.

**anatomic position:** The position of reference in which the patient stands facing forward, arms at the side, with the palms of the hands forward.

**anatomy:** The study of the physical structure of the body and its components.

**anemic:** Describes a condition in which the patient has too few red blood cells, resulting in a decreased ability to transport oxygen throughout the body via the bloodstream.

**aneurysm:** A swelling or enlargement of the wall of a blood vessel that results from weakening of the vessel wall.

**angina pectoris:** Transient (short-lived) chest discomfort caused by partial or temporary blockage of blood flow to the heart muscle; also called angina.

**angioedema:** Localized areas of swelling beneath the skin, often around the eyes and lips, but can also involve other body areas as well.

**anisocoria:** Naturally occurring uneven pupil size.

**antagonist:** A medication that binds to a receptor and blocks other medications.

**anterior:** The front surface of the body; the side facing you in the standard anatomic position.

**anterograde (posttraumatic) amnesia:** Inability to remember events after an injury.

**anthrax:** A disease caused by a deadly bacterium (*Bacillus anthracis*) that lies dormant in a spore (protective shell); the germ is released from the spore when exposed to the optimal temperature and moisture. The routes of entry are inhalation, cutaneous, and gastrointestinal (from consuming food that contains spores).

**antibiotic:** A medication used to treat infections caused by a bacterium.

**anticoagulant:** A medication that impairs the ability of blood to clot.

**antidote:** A substance that is used to neutralize or counteract a poison.

**Antidote Treatment Nerve Agent Auto-Injector (ATNAA):** A nerve agent antidote kit containing atropine and pralidoxime chloride; delivered as a single dose through one needle.

**antifungal:** A medication used to treat infections caused by a fungus.

**antiplatelet:** A medication that prevents blood platelets from clumping or sticking together.

**antipyretics:** Medications that treat or reduce a fever.

**antivenin:** A serum that counteracts the effect of venom from an animal or insect.

**aorta:** The main artery leaving the left side of the heart and carrying freshly oxygenated blood to the body.

**aortic aneurysm:** A weakness in the wall of the aorta that makes it susceptible to rupture.

**aortic valve:** The one-way valve that lies between the left ventricle and the aorta and keeps blood from flowing back into the left ventricle after the left ventricle ejects its blood into the aorta; one of four heart valves.

**apex (plural apices):** The pointed extremity of a conical structure.

**Apgar score:** A scoring system for assessing the status of a newborn that assigns a number value to each of five areas.

**aphasia:** The inability to understand and/or produce speech.

**apnea:** Absence of spontaneous breathing.

**apneic oxygenation:** A technique in which oxygen administered via a high-flow nasal cannula is left in place during an intubation attempt, allowing for continuous oxygen delivery into the airways during all phases of the procedure.

**apparent life-threatening event (ALTE):** An event that causes unresponsiveness, cyanosis, and apnea in an infant, who then resumes breathing with stimulation.

**appendicitis:** Inflammation or infection of the appendix.

**appendicular skeleton:** The portion of the skeletal system that comprises the arms, legs, pelvis, and shoulder girdle.

**appendix:** A small, tubular structure that is attached to the lower border of the cecum in the lower right quadrant of the abdomen.

**applied ethics:** The manner in which principles of ethics are incorporated into professional conduct.

**arterial air embolism:** Air bubbles in the arterial blood vessels.

**arterioles:** The smallest branches of arteries leading to the vast network of capillaries.

**arteriosclerosis:** A disease that causes the arteries to thicken, harden, and calcify.

**artery:** A blood vessel, consisting of three layers of tissue and smooth muscle, that carries blood away from the heart.

**articular cartilage:** A pearly white layer of specialized cartilage covering the articular surfaces (contact surfaces on the ends) of bones in synovial joints.

**artifact:** A tracing on an electrocardiogram that is the result of interference, such as patient movement, rather than the heart's electrical activity.

**ascites:** An abnormal accumulation of excess fluid in the peritoneal cavity.

**aspiration:** In the context of the airway, the introduction of vomitus or other foreign material into the lungs.

**aspirin (acetylsalicylic acid or ASA):** A medication that is an antipyretic (reduces fever), analgesic (reduces pain), anti-inflammatory (reduces inflammation), and a potent inhibitor of platelet aggregation (clumping).

**assault:** Unlawfully placing a patient in fear of bodily harm.

**asthma:** An acute spasm of the smaller air passages, called bronchioles, associated with excessive mucus production and with swelling of the mucous lining of the respiratory passages.

**asystole:** The complete absence of all heart electrical activity.

**ataxic respirations:** Irregular, ineffective respirations that may or may not have an identifiable pattern.

**atelectasis:** Collapse of the alveolar air spaces of the lungs.

**atherosclerosis:** A disorder in which cholesterol and calcium build up inside the walls of the blood vessels, forming plaque, which eventually leads to a partial or complete blockage of blood flow.

**atrium:** One of the two upper chambers of the heart.

**aura:** A sensation experienced before a seizure; serves as a warning sign that a seizure is about to occur.

**auscultate:** To listen to sounds within an organ with a stethoscope.

**autism spectrum disorder (ASD):** A group of complex disorders of brain development, characterized by difficulties in social interaction, repetitive behaviors, and verbal and nonverbal communication.

**automated external defibrillator (AED):** A device that detects treatable life-threatening cardiac dysrhythmias (ventricular fibrillation and ventricular tachycardia) and delivers the appropriate electrical shock to the patient.

**automaticity:** The ability of cardiac muscle cells to contract without stimulation from the nervous system.

**automatic transport ventilator (ATV):** A ventilation device attached to a control box that allows the variables of ventilation to be set. It frees the EMT to perform other tasks while the patient is being ventilated.

**autonomic nervous system:** The part of the nervous system that controls the involuntary activities of the body such as the heart rate, blood pressure, and digestion of food.

**AVPU scale:** A method of assessing the level of consciousness by determining whether the patient is awake and alert, responsive to verbal stimuli or pain, or unresponsive; used principally early in the assessment process.

**avulsion:** An injury in which soft tissue is torn completely loose or is hanging as a flap.

**axial loading injuries:** Injuries in which load is applied along the vertical or longitudinal axis of the spine, which results in load being transmitted along the entire length of the vertebral column; for example, falling from a height and landing on the feet in an upright position.

**axial skeleton:** The part of the skeleton comprising the skull, vertebral column, and rib cage.

**axons:** Extensions of a neuron that carry impulses away from the nerve cell body to the dendrites (receivers) of another neuron.

**backboard:** A long, flat board made of rigid, rectangular material that is used to provide support to a patient who is suspected of having a hip, pelvic, spinal, or lower extremity injury; also called a spine board, trauma board, and longboard.

**bacteria:** Microorganisms that reproduce by binary fission. These single-cell creatures reproduce rapidly. Some can form spores (encysted variants) when environmental conditions are harsh.

**bacterial vaginosis:** An overgrowth of bacteria in the vagina; characterized by itching, burning, or pain, and possibly a "fishy"-smelling discharge.

**bag-mask device:** A device with a one-way valve and a face mask attached to a ventilation bag; when attached to a reservoir and connected to oxygen, it delivers more than 90% supplemental oxygen.

**ball-and-socket joint:** A joint that allows internal and external rotation, as well as bending.

**bariatrics:** A branch of medicine concerned with the management (prevention or control) of obesity and allied diseases.

**barotrauma:** Injury caused by pressure to enclosed body surfaces, for example, from too much pressure in the lungs.

**barrier device:** A protective item, such as a pocket mask with a valve, that limits exposure to a patient's body fluids.

**base station:** Any radio hardware containing a transmitter and receiver that is located in a fixed place.

**basic life support (BLS):** Noninvasive emergency life-saving care that is used to treat medical conditions, including airway obstruction, respiratory arrest, and cardiac arrest.

**basilar skull fractures:** Fractures that usually occur following diffuse impact to the head (eg, falls, motor vehicle crashes); generally result from extension of a linear fracture to the base of the skull and can be difficult to diagnose with a radiograph.

**basket stretcher:** A rigid stretcher commonly used in technical and water rescues that surrounds and supports the patient yet allows water to drain through holes in the bottom; also called a Stokes litter.

**battery:** Unlawfully touching a patient or providing emergency care without consent.

**Battle sign:** Bruising behind an ear over the mastoid process that may indicate a skull fracture.

**behavior:** How a person functions or acts in response to his or her environment.

**behavioral crisis:** The point at which a person's reactions to events interfere with activities of daily living; this becomes a psychiatric emergency when it causes a major life interruption, such as attempted suicide.

**behavioral health emergency:** An emergency in which abnormal behavior threatens a person's own health and safety or the health and safety of another person—for example, when a person becomes suicidal or homicidal, or has a psychotic episode.

**bends:** A common name for decompression sickness.

**beta-adrenergic receptors:** Portions of the nervous system that, when stimulated, can cause an increase in the force of contraction of the heart, an increased heart rate, and bronchial dilation.

**beta radiation:** A type of energy that is emitted from a strong radiologic source; it is slightly more penetrating than alpha radiation and requires a layer of clothing to stop it.

**biceps:** The large muscle that covers the front of the humerus.

**bilateral:** A body part or condition that appears on both sides of the midline.

**bile ducts:** The ducts that convey bile between the liver and the intestine.

**bills of lading:** The shipping papers used for transport of chemicals over roads and highways; also referred to as freight bills.

**bioethics:** The study of ethics related to issues that arise in health care.

**birth canal:** The vagina and cervix.

**blanch:** To turn white.

**blind spots:** Areas of the road that are blocked from your view by your vehicle or mirrors.

**bloodborne pathogens:** Pathogenic microorganisms that are present in human blood and can cause disease in humans. These pathogens include, but are not limited to, hepatitis B virus and human immunodeficiency virus (HIV).

**blood pressure (BP):** The pressure that the blood exerts against the walls of the arteries as it passes through them.

**bloody show:** A small amount of blood in the vagina that appears at the beginning of labor and may include a plug of pink-tinged mucus that is discharged when the cervix begins to dilate.

**blowout fracture:** A fracture of the orbit or of the bones that support the floor of the orbit.

**blunt trauma:** An impact on the body by objects that cause injury without penetrating soft tissues or internal organs and cavities.

**B-NICE:** A memory device to recall the types of weapons of mass destruction: biologic, nuclear, incendiary, chemical, and explosive.

**body mechanics:** The relationship between the body's anatomic structures and the physical forces associated with lifting, moving, and carrying; the ways in which the body moves to achieve a specific action.

**botulinum:** Produced by bacteria, this is the most potent neurotoxin known. When introduced into the body, this neurotoxin affects the nervous system's ability to function and causes botulism.

**brachial artery:** The major vessel in the upper extremities that supplies blood to the arm.

**bradycardia:** A slow heart rate, less than 60 beats/min.

**bradypnea:** Slow respiratory rate; an ominous sign in a child that indicates impending respiratory arrest.

**brain:** The controlling organ of the body and center of consciousness; functions include perception, control of reactions to the environment, emotional responses, and judgment.

**brainstem:** The area of the brain between the spinal cord and cerebrum, surrounded by the cerebellum; controls functions that are necessary for life, such as respiration.

**breach of confidentiality:** Disclosure of information without proper authorization.

**breath-holding syncope:** Loss of consciousness caused by a decreased breathing stimulus.

**breath sounds:** An indication of air movement in the lungs, usually assessed with a stethoscope.

**breech presentation:** A delivery in which the buttocks come out first.

**bronchial breath sounds:** Normal breath sounds made by air moving through the bronchi.

**bronchioles:** Subdivision of the smaller bronchi in the lungs; made of smooth muscle and dilate or constrict in response to various stimuli.

**bronchiolitis:** Inflammation of the bronchioles that usually occurs in children younger than 2 years and is often caused by the respiratory syncytial virus.

**bronchitis:** An acute or chronic inflammation of the lung that may damage lung tissue; usually associated with cough and production of sputum and, depending on its cause, sometimes fever.

**buboes:** Enlarged lymph nodes (up to the size of a tennis ball) that are characteristic in people infected with the bubonic plague.

**bubonic plague:** Bacterial infection that affects the lymphatic system. It is transmitted by infected rodents and fleas and characterized by acute malaise, fever, and the formation of tender, enlarged, inflamed lymph nodes that appear as lesions, called buboes. Also called the Black Death.

**bulk storage containers:** Any container other than nonbulk storage containers, such as fixed tanks, highway cargo tanks, rail tank cars, totes, and intermodal tanks. These are typically found in manufacturing facilities and are often surrounded by a secondary containment system to help control an accidental release.

**burnout:** A combination of exhaustion, cynicism, and reduced performance resulting from long-term job stresses in health care and other high-stress professions.

**burns:** Injuries in which soft-tissue damage occurs as a result of thermal heat, frictional heat, toxic chemicals, electricity, or nuclear radiation.

**calcaneus:** The heel bone.

**capillaries:** The small blood vessels that connect arterioles and venules; various substances pass through capillary walls, into and out of the interstitial fluid, and then on to the cells.

**capillary refill:** A test that evaluates distal circulatory system function by squeezing (blanching) blood from an area such as a nail bed and watching the speed of its return after releasing the pressure.

**capillary vessels:** The tiny blood vessels between the arterioles and venules that permit transfer of oxygen, carbon dioxide, nutrients, and waste between body tissues and the blood.

**capnography:** A noninvasive method to quickly and efficiently provide information on a patient's ventilatory status, circulation, and metabolism; effectively measures the concentration of carbon dioxide in expired air over time.

**capnometry:** The use of a capnometer, a device that measures the amount of expired carbon dioxide.

**carbon dioxide:** A component of air that typically makes up 0.03% of air at sea level; also a waste product exhaled during expiration by the respiratory system.

**carbon dioxide retention:** A condition characterized by a chronically high blood level of carbon dioxide in which the respiratory center no longer responds to high blood levels of carbon dioxide.

**carbon monoxide:** An odorless, colorless, tasteless, and highly poisonous gas that results from incomplete oxidation of carbon in combustion.

**carboys:** Glass, plastic, or steel containers, ranging in volume from 5 to 15 gallons (19 to 57 L).

**cardiac arrest:** When the heart fails to generate effective and detectable blood flow; pulses are not palpable in cardiac arrest, even if muscular and electrical activity continues in the heart.

**cardiac muscle:** The heart muscle.

**cardiac output (CO):** A measure of the volume of blood circulated by the heart in 1 minute, calculated by multiplying the stroke volume by the heart rate.

**cardiac tamponade (pericardial tamponade):** Compression of the heart as the result of buildup of blood or other fluid in the pericardial sac, leading to decreased cardiac output.

**cardiogenic shock:** A state in which not enough oxygen is delivered to the tissues of the body, caused by low output of blood from the heart. It can be a severe complication of a large acute myocardial infarction, as well as other conditions.

**cardiopulmonary resuscitation (CPR):** The combination of chest compressions and rescue breathing used to establish adequate ventilation and circulation in a patient who is not breathing and has no pulse.

**carina:** Point at which the trachea bifurcates (divides) into the left and right main stem bronchi.

**carotid artery:** The major artery that supplies blood to the head and brain.

**carpals:** Small bones that comprise the wrist.

**cartilage:** The smooth connective tissue that forms the support structure of the skeletal system and provides cushioning between bones; also forms the nasal septum and portions of the outer ear.

**casualty collection area:** An area set up by physicians, nurses, and other hospital staff near a major disaster scene where patients can receive further triage and medical care.

**cataracts:** Clouding of the lens of the eye or its surrounding transparent membranes.

**cavitation:** A phenomenon in which speed causes a bullet to generate pressure waves, which cause damage distant from the bullet's path.

**cecum:** The first part of the large intestine, into which the ileum opens.

**cellular metabolism:** A set of chemical reactions that supplies cells with energy. Includes both anaerobic and aerobic metabolism.

**cellular telephone:** A low-power portable radio that communicates through an interconnected series of repeater stations called cells.

**Centers for Disease Control and Prevention (CDC):** The primary federal agency that conducts and supports public health activities in the United States. The CDC is part of the US Department of Health and Human Services.

**central nervous system (CNS):** The brain and spinal cord.

**central neurogenic hyperventilation:** An abnormal breathing pattern associated with increased intracranial pressure that is characterized by deep, rapid breathing; this pattern is similar to Kussmaul respirations, but without an acetone breath odor.

**central pulses:** Pulses that are closest to the core (central) part of the body where the vital organs are located; include the carotid, femoral, and apical pulses.

**cerebellum:** One of the three major subdivisions of the brain, sometimes called the little brain; coordinates the various activities of the brain, particularly fine body movements.

**cerebral edema:** Swelling of the brain.

**cerebral palsy:** A group of disorders characterized by poorly controlled body movement.

**cerebrospinal fluid (CSF):** Fluid produced in the ventricles of the brain that flows in the subarachnoid space and bathes the meninges.

**cerebrovascular accident (CVA):** An interruption of blood flow to the brain that results in the loss of brain function; also called a stroke.

**cerebrum:** The largest part of the three subdivisions of the brain, sometimes called the gray matter; made up of several lobes that control movement, hearing, balance, speech, visual perception, emotions, and personality.

**certification:** A process in which a person, an institution, or a program is evaluated and recognized as meeting certain predetermined standards to provide safe and ethical care.

**cervical spine:** The portion of the vertebral column consisting of the first seven vertebrae that lie in the neck.

**cervix:** The lower third, or neck, of the uterus.

**channel:** An assigned frequency or frequencies that are used to carry voice and/or data communications.

**Chemical Transportation Emergency Center (CHEMTREC):** An agency that assists emergency responders in identifying and handling hazardous materials transport incidents.

**chemoreceptors:** Monitor the levels of oxygen, carbon dioxide, and pH of the cerebrospinal fluid and then provide feedback to the respiratory centers to modify the rate and depth of breathing based on the body's needs at any given time.

**chest compression fraction:** The total percentage of time during a resuscitation attempt in which active chest compressions are being performed.

**Cheyne-Stokes respirations:** A cyclical pattern of abnormal breathing that increases and then decreases in rate and depth, followed by a period of apnea.

**chief complaint:** The reason a patient called for help; also, the patient's response to questions such as "What's wrong?" or "What happened?"

**chief concern:** The condition requiring the most urgent intervention as determined by the provider's assessment of the patient; it is not always the same as the chief complaint.

**child abuse:** A general term applying to all forms of abuse and neglect of children.

**chlamydia:** A sexually transmitted disease caused by the bacterium *Chlamydia trachomatis*.

**chlorine (Cl):** The first chemical agent ever used in warfare. It has a distinct odor of bleach and creates a green haze when released as a gas. Initially it produces upper airway irritation and a choking sensation.

**cholecystitis:** Inflammation of the gallbladder.

**chordae tendineae:** Thin bands of fibrous tissue that attach to the valves in the heart and prevent them from inverting.

**chronic bronchitis:** Irritation of the major lung passageways from long-term exposure to infectious disease or irritants such as smoke.

**chronic obstructive pulmonary disease (COPD):** A lung disease characterized by chronic obstruction of lung airflow that interferes with normal breathing and is not fully reversible.

**chyme:** The substance that leaves the stomach. It is a combination of all of the eaten foods with added stomach acids.

**circulatory system:** The complex arrangement of connected tubes, including the arteries, arterioles, capillaries, venules, and veins, that moves blood, oxygen, nutrients, carbon dioxide, and cellular waste throughout the body.

**clavicle:** The collarbone; it is lateral to the sternum and anterior to the scapula.

**cleaning:** The process of removing dirt, dust, blood, or other visible contaminants from a surface.

**closed abdominal injury:** An injury in which there is soft-tissue damage inside the body but the skin remains intact.

**closed chest injury:** An injury to the chest in which the skin is not broken, usually caused by blunt trauma.

**closed-ended questions:** Questions that can be answered in short or single-word responses.

**closed fracture:** Any break in a bone in which the overlying skin is not broken.

**closed head injury:** Injury in which the brain has been injured but the skin has not been broken and there is no obvious bleeding.

**closed incident:** An incident that is contained; all casualties are accounted for.

**closed injuries:** Injuries in which damage occurs beneath the skin or mucous membrane but the surface of the skin remains intact.

**coagulation:** The formation of clots to plug openings in injured blood vessels and stop blood flow.

**coccyx:** The last three or four vertebrae of the spine; the tail bone.

**cold zone:** A safe area at a hazardous materials incident for the agencies involved in the operations. The incident commander, the command post, EMS providers, and other support functions necessary to control the incident should be located in this zone. Also referred to as the clean zone or the support zone.

**colostomy:** A surgical procedure to create an opening (stoma) between the colon and the surface of the body.

**coma:** A state of profound unconsciousness from which the patient cannot be roused.

**combining vowel:** The vowel used to combine two word roots or a word root and suffix.

**command:** In incident command, the position that oversees the incident, establishes the objectives and priorities, and develops a response plan.

**command post:** The designated field command center where the incident commander and support staff are located.

**commotio cordis:** A blunt chest injury caused by a sudden, direct blow to the chest that occurs only during the critical portion of a person's heartbeat.

**communicable disease:** A disease that can be spread from one person or species to another.

**communication:** The transmission of information to another person—verbally or through body language.

**community paramedicine:** A health care model in which experienced paramedics receive advanced training to equip them to provide additional services in the prehospital environment, such as health evaluations, monitoring of chronic illnesses or conditions, and patient advocacy.

**compartment syndrome:** Swelling in a confined space that produces dangerous pressure; may cut off blood flow or damage sensitive tissue.

**compassion fatigue:** A stress disorder characterized by gradual lessening of compassion over time.

**compensated shock:** The early stage of shock, in which the body can still compensate for blood loss.

**compensatory damages:** Damages awarded in a civil lawsuit that are intended to restore the plaintiff to the same condition that he or she was in prior to the incident.

**competent:** Able to make rational decisions about personal well-being.

**complex access:** Entry that requires special tools and training and includes the use of force.

**compliance:** The ability of the alveoli to expand when air is drawn in during inhalation.

**concealment:** The use of objects to limit a person's ability to see you.

**concussion:** A temporary loss or alteration of part or all of the brain's abilities to function without actual physical damage to the brain.

**conduction:** The loss of heat by direct contact (eg, when a body part comes into contact with a colder object).

**conductive hearing loss:** Hearing loss caused by a faulty transmission of sound waves.

**congestive heart failure (CHF):** A disorder in which the heart loses part of its ability to effectively pump blood, usually as a result of damage to the heart muscle and usually resulting in a backup of fluid into the lungs.

**conjunctiva:** The delicate membrane that lines the eyelids and covers the exposed surface of the eye.

**conjunctivitis:** Inflammation of the conjunctiva.

**consent:** Permission to render care.

**contact burn:** A burn caused by direct contact with a hot object.

**contact hazard:** The danger posed by a chemical whose primary route of entry into the body is through the skin; posed by a hazardous agent that gives off very little or no vapors; also called a skin hazard.

**contagious:** An infectious disease that spreads from one human to another; communicable.

**container:** Any vessel or receptacle that holds material, including storage vessels, pipelines, and packaging.

**contamination:** The presence of infectious organisms on or in objects such as dressings, water, food, needles, wounds, or a patient's body.

**continuous positive airway pressure (CPAP):** A method of ventilation used primarily in the treatment of critically ill patients with respiratory distress; can prevent the need for endotracheal intubation.

**continuous quality improvement (CQI):** A system of internal and external reviews and audits of all aspects of an EMS system aimed at improving outcomes.

**continuum of care:** The concept of consistent patient care across the entire health care team from first patient contact to patient discharge; working together with a unified goal results in improved individual and team performance, better patient and provider safety, and improved patient outcome.

**contraindications:** Conditions that make a particular medication or treatment inappropriate because it would not help, or may actually harm, a patient.

**contributory negligence:** A legal defense that may be raised when the defendant thinks that the conduct of the plaintiff somehow contributed to any injuries or damages that were sustained by the plaintiff.

**control zones:** Areas at a hazardous materials incident that are designated as hot, warm, or cold, based on safety issues and the degree of hazard found there.

**contusion:** A bruise from an injury that causes bleeding beneath the skin without breaking the skin; also see *ecchymosis*.

**convection:** The loss of body heat caused by air movement (eg, a breeze blowing across the body).

**conventional reasoning:** A type of reasoning in which a child looks for approval from peers and society.

**core temperature:** The temperature of the central part of the body (eg, the heart, lungs, and vital organs).

**cornea:** The transparent tissue layer in front of the pupil and iris of the eye.

**coronal (frontal) plane:** An imaginary plane where the body is divided into front and back parts.

**coronary arteries:** The blood vessels that carry blood and nutrients to the heart muscle.

**coup-contrecoup brain injury:** A brain injury that occurs when force is applied to the head and energy transmission through brain tissue causes injury on the opposite side of original impact.

**cover:** The tactical use of an impenetrable barrier for protection.

**covert:** An act in which the public safety community generally has no prior knowledge of the time, location, or nature of the attack.

**COVID-19:** A respiratory disease caused by the virus SARS-CoV-2. The virus is a coronavirus, similar to the one that causes the common cold.

**coxae:** The hip bones (singular: coxa).

**CPR board:** A device that provides a firm surface under the patient's torso.

**crackles:** Crackling, rattling breath sounds that signal fluid in the air spaces of the lungs.

**cranium:** The part of the skull that encloses the brain and is composed of eight bones.

**credentialing:** An established process to determine the qualifications necessary to be allowed to practice a particular profession, or to function as an organization.

**crepitus:** A grating or grinding sensation or sound caused by fractured bone ends or joints rubbing together.

**crew resource management (CRM):** A set of procedures for use in environments where human error can have disastrous consequences. It empowers people within a team to communicate effectively with one another with a goal of improving team situational awareness, patient and crew safety, and overall communication.

**cricoid cartilage:** A firm ridge of cartilage that forms the lower part of the larynx.

**cricothyroid membrane:** A thin sheet of fascia that connects the thyroid and cricoid cartilages that make up the larynx.

**critical incident stress management (CISM):** A process that confronts the responses to critical incidents and defuses them, directing the emergency services personnel toward physical and emotional equilibrium.

**cross-contamination:** Occurs when a person is contaminated by an agent as a result of coming in contact with another contaminated person.

**croup:** A viral inflammatory disease of the upper respiratory system that may cause a partial airway obstruction and is characterized by a barking cough; usually seen in children.

**crowning:** The appearance of the fetus's head at the vaginal opening during labor.

**crushing injury:** An injury that occurs when a great amount of force is applied to the body.

**crush syndrome:** Significant metabolic derangement that develops when crushed extremities or body parts remain trapped for prolonged periods. This can lead to renal failure and death.

**cultural imposition:** When one person imposes his or her beliefs, values, and practices on another because he or she believe his or her ideals are superior.

**cumulative stress reactions:** Prolonged or excessive stress.

**cushion of safety:** A safe distance between your vehicle and any vehicles around you.

**cyanide:** An agent that affects the body's ability to use oxygen. It is a colorless gas that has an odor similar to almonds. The effects begin on the cellular level and are very rapidly seen at the organ and system levels.

**cyanosis:** A blue skin discoloration that is caused by a reduced level of oxygen in the blood. Although paleness, or a decrease in blood flow, can be difficult to detect in dark-skinned people, it may be observed by examining mucous membranes inside the inner lower eyelid and capillary refill. On general observation, the patient may appear ashen or gray.

**cylinders:** Portable, compressed gas containers used to hold liquids and gases such as nitrogen, argon, helium, and oxygen. They have a range of sizes and internal pressures.

**cystitis:** Inflammation of the bladder.

**danger zone (hot zone):** An area where people can be exposed to hazards such as electric wires, sharp metal edges, broken glass, toxic substances, radiation, or fire.

**DCAP-BTLS:** A mnemonic for assessment in which each area of the body is evaluated for Deformities, Contusions, Abrasions, Punctures/penetrations, Burns, Tenderness, Lacerations, and Swelling.

**dead space:** Any portion of the airway that does contain air and cannot participate in gas exchange, such as the trachea and bronchi.

**decay:** A natural process in which a material that is unstable attempts to stabilize itself by changing its structure.

**deceleration:** The slowing of an object.

**decision-making capacity:** Ability to understand and process information and make a choice regarding appropriate medical care.

**decompensated shock:** The late stage of shock when blood pressure is falling.

**decompression sickness:** A painful condition seen in divers who ascend too quickly, in which gas, especially nitrogen, forms bubbles in blood vessels and other tissues; see *bends*.

**decontaminate:** To remove or neutralize radiation, chemical, or other hazardous material from clothing, equipment, vehicles, and personnel.

**decontamination:** The process of removing or neutralizing and properly disposing of hazardous materials from equipment, patients, and responders.

**decontamination area:** The designated area in a hazardous materials incident where all patients and responders must be decontaminated before going to another area.

**decubitus ulcers:** Sores caused by the pressure of skin against a surface for long periods; can range from a discoloration of the skin to a deep wound that may invade into bone or organs; also known as bedsores.

**dedicated line:** A special telephone line that is used for specific point-to-point communications; also known as a *hotline*.

**deep:** Farther inside the body and away from the skin.

**deep venous thrombosis:** The formation of a blood clot within the larger veins of an extremity, typically following a period of prolonged immobilization.

**defamation:** The communication of false information about a person that is damaging to that person's reputation or standing in the community.

**defibrillate:** To shock a fibrillating (chaotically shaking) heart with specialized electric current in an attempt to restore a normal, rhythmic beat.

**dehydration:** Loss of water from the tissues of the body.

**delayed stress reactions:** Reactions to stress that occur after a stressful situation.

**delirium:** A temporary change in mental status characterized by disorganized thoughts, inattention, memory loss, disorientation, striking changes in personality and affect, hallucinations, delusions, or a decreased level of consciousness.

**delirium tremens (DTs):** A severe withdrawal syndrome seen in individuals with alcoholism who are deprived of ethyl alcohol; characterized by restlessness, fever, sweating, disorientation, agitation, and seizures; can be fatal if untreated.

**dementia:** The slow onset of progressive disorientation, shortened attention span, and loss of cognitive function; this condition is generally chronic and irreversible.

**demobilization:** The process of directing responders to return to their facilities when work at a disaster or mass-casualty incident has finished, at least for those particular responders.

**denitrogenation:** The process of replacing nitrogen in the lungs with oxygen to maintain a normal oxygen saturation level during advanced airway management.

**dependent edema:** Swelling in the part of the body closest to the ground, caused by collection of fluid in the tissues; a possible sign of congestive heart failure.

**dependent lividity:** Blood settling to the lowest point of the body, causing discoloration of the skin; a definitive sign of death.

**depositions:** Oral questions asked of parties and witnesses under oath.

**depression:** A persistent mood of sadness, despair, and discouragement; may be a symptom of many different mental and physical disorders, or may be a disorder on its own.

**dermis:** The inner layer of the skin, containing hair follicles, sweat glands, nerve endings, and blood vessels.

**designated officer:** The individual in the department who is charged with the responsibility of managing exposures and infection control issues.

**developmental disability:** Insufficient development of the brain, resulting in some level of dysfunction or impairment.

**diabetes mellitus:** A metabolic disorder in which the ability to metabolize carbohydrates (sugars) is impaired, usually because of a lack of insulin.

**diabetic ketoacidosis (DKA):** A form of hyperglycemia in uncontrolled diabetes in which certain acids accumulate when insulin is not available.

**diamond carry:** A carrying technique in which one provider is located at the head end of the stretcher or backboard, one at the foot end, and one at each side of the patient; each of the two providers at the sides uses one hand to support the stretcher or backboard so that all are able to face forward as they walk.

**diaphoretic:** Characterized by light or profuse sweating.

**diaphragm:** A muscular dome that forms the undersurface of the thorax, separating the chest from the abdominal cavity. Contraction of this (and the chest wall muscles) brings air into the lungs. Relaxation allows air to be expelled from the lungs.

**diastole:** The relaxation, or period of relaxation, of the heart, especially of the ventricles.

**diastolic pressure:** The pressure that remains in the arteries during the relaxing phase of the heart's cycle (diastole) when the left ventricle is at rest.

**diffusion:** Movement of a gas from an area of higher concentration to an area of lower concentration.

**digestion:** The processing of food that nourishes the individual cells of the body.

**dilation:** Widening of a tubular structure such as a coronary artery.

**diphtheria:** An infectious disease in which a pseudo-membrane forms, lining the pharynx; this lining can severely obstruct the passage of air into the larynx.

**direct contact:** Exposure or transmission of a communicable disease from one person to another by physical contact.

**direct ground lift:** A lifting technique that is used for patients who are found lying supine on the ground with no suspected spinal injury.

**direct laryngoscopy:** Visualization of the airway with a laryngoscope.

**dirty bomb:** Name given to an explosive radiologic dispersal device.

**disaster:** A widespread event that disrupts community resources and functions, in turn threatening public safety, citizens' lives, and property.

**discovery:** The phase of a civil lawsuit where the plaintiff and defense obtain information from each other that will enable the attorneys to have a better understanding of the case and which will assist in negotiating a possible settlement or in preparing for trial. Discovery includes depositions, interrogatories, and demands for production of records.

**disease vector:** An animal that, once infected, spreads a disease to another animal.

**disinfection:** The killing of pathogenic agents by direct application of chemicals.

**dislocation:** Disruption of a joint in which ligaments are damaged and the bone ends are no longer in contact.

**displaced fracture:** A fracture in which bone fragments are separated from one another, producing deformity in the limb.

**dissecting aneurysm:** A condition in which the inner layers of an artery, such as the aorta, become separated, allowing blood (at high pressures) to flow between the layers.

**dissemination:** The means by which a terrorist will spread an agent; for example, by poisoning the water supply or aerosolizing the agent into the air or ventilation system of a building.

**distal:** Farther from the trunk or nearer to the free end of the extremity.

**distracting injury:** Any injury that prevents the patient from noticing other injuries he or she may have, even severe injuries; for example, a painful femur or tibia fracture that prevents the patient from noticing back pain associated with a spinal fracture.

**distress:** A negative response to a stressor.

**distributive shock:** A condition that occurs when there is widespread dilation of the small arterioles, small venules, or both.

**diverticulitis:** Inflammation in small pockets at weak areas in the muscle walls of the intestines.

**diving reflex:** The slowing of the heart rate caused by submersion in cold water.

**documentation:** The recorded portion of the EMT's patient interaction, either written or electronic. This becomes part of the patient's permanent medical record.

**domestic terrorism:** Terrorism that is carried out by people in their own country.

**do not resuscitate (DNR) order:** Written documentation by a physician giving permission to medical personnel not to attempt resuscitation in the event of cardiac arrest.

**dorsal:** The posterior surface of the body, including the back of the hand.

**dorsalis pedis artery:** The artery on the anterior surface of the foot between the first and second metatarsals.

**dose:** The amount of medication given on the basis of the patient's size and age.

**Down syndrome:** A genetic chromosomal defect that can occur during fetal development and that results in intellectual impairment as well as certain physical characteristics, such as a round head with a flat occiput and slanted, wide-set eyes.

**drag:** Resistance that slows a projectile, such as air.

**drowning:** The process of experiencing respiratory impairment from submersion or immersion in liquid.

**drums:** Barrel-like containers used to store a wide variety of substances, including food-grade materials, corrosives, flammable liquids, and grease. May be constructed of low-carbon steel, polyethylene, cardboard, stainless steel, nickel, or other materials.

**DuoDote Auto-Injector:** A nerve agent antidote kit containing atropine and pralidoxime chloride; delivered as a single dose through one needle.

**duplex:** The ability to transmit and receive simultaneously.

**durable power of attorney for health care:** A type of advance directive executed by a competent adult that appoints another individual to make medical treatment decisions on his or her behalf, in the event that the person making the appointment loses decision-making capacity.

**duration:** The amount of time that clinical effects of a medication last.

**duty to act:** A medicolegal term relating to certain personnel who either by statute or by function have a responsibility to provide care.

**dysarthria:** Slurred speech.

**dysbarism injuries:** Any signs and symptoms caused by the difference between the surrounding atmospheric pressure and the total gas pressure in various tissues, fluids, and cavities of the body.

**dyspnea:** Shortness of breath or difficulty breathing.

**dysrhythmia:** An irregular or abnormal heart rhythm.

**early adult:** A young adult age 19 to 40 years.

**ecchymosis:** A buildup of blood beneath the skin that produces a characteristic blue or black discoloration as the result of an injury.

**eclampsia:** A pregnancy complication that is characterized by new-onset hypertension (systolic blood pressure >140 mm Hg or diastolic blood pressure >90 mm Hg) with seizure activity and preceding systemic effects, such as blurred vision, headache, or protein in the urine. It is differentiated from preeclampsia by the presence of seizure activity.

**ectopic pregnancy:** A pregnancy that develops outside the uterus, typically in a fallopian tube.

**edema:** The presence of abnormally large amounts of fluid between cells in body tissues, causing swelling of the affected area.

**elder abuse:** Any action on the part of an older person's family member, caregiver, or other associated person that takes advantage of the older person's person, property, or emotional state.

**elimination:** The process of removing a medication or chemical from within the body.

**emancipated minor:** A person who is under the legal age in a given state but, because of other circumstances, is legally considered an adult.

**embolus:** A blood clot or other substance in the circulatory system that travels to a blood vessel where it causes a blockage of blood flow.

**embryo:** The early stage of development after the fertilization of the egg (first 10 weeks).

**emergency:** A serious situation, such as injury or illness that threatens the life or welfare of a person or group of people and requires immediate intervention.

**emergency doctrine:** The principle of law that permits a health care provider to treat a patient in an emergency situation when the patient is incapable of granting consent because of an altered level of consciousness, disability, the effects of drugs or alcohol, or the patient's age.

**emergency medical care:** Immediate care or treatment.

**emergency medical dispatch (EMD):** A system that assists dispatchers in selecting appropriate units to respond to a particular call for assistance and provides callers with vital instructions until the arrival of EMS crews.

**emergency medical responder (EMR):** A trained professional, such as police officer, firefighter, lifeguard, or other rescuer, who may arrive first at the scene of an emergency to provide initial medical assistance.

**emergency medical services (EMS):** A multidisciplinary system that represents the combined efforts of several professionals and agencies to provide prehospital emergency care to the sick and injured.

**emergency medical technician (EMT):** An individual who has training in basic life support, including automated external defibrillation, use of a definitive airway adjunct, and assisting patients with certain medications.

**emergency move:** A move in which the patient is dragged or pulled from a dangerous scene before assessment and care are provided.

*Emergency Response Guidebook* **(ERG):** A preliminary action guide for first responders operating at a hazardous materials incident in coordination with the US Department of Transportation's labels and placards marking system. Jointly developed by the US Department of Transportation, the Secretariat of Communications and Transportation of Mexico, and Transport Canada.

**emesis:** Vomiting.

**emotional intelligence:** The ability to understand and manage one's own emotions and properly respond to the emotions of others.

**emphysema:** A disease of the lungs in which there is extreme dilation and eventual destruction of the pulmonary alveoli with poor exchange of oxygen and carbon dioxide; it is one form of chronic obstructive pulmonary disease.

**EMT-administered medication:** Administration of a medication by the EMT directly to the patient.

**endocrine glands:** Glands that secrete or release chemicals that are used inside the body.

**endocrine system:** The complex message and control system that integrates many body functions, including the release of hormones.

**endometrium:** The lining of the inside of the uterus.

**endotracheal (ET) intubation:** Insertion of an endotracheal tube directly through the larynx between the vocal cords and into the trachea to maintain and protect an airway.

**end-tidal $CO_2$:** The amount of carbon dioxide present at the end of an exhaled breath.

**enteral medications:** Medications that enter the body through the digestive system.

**entrapment:** To be caught (trapped) within a vehicle, room, or container with no way out or to have a limb or other body part trapped.

**envenomation:** The act of injecting venom.

**enzymes:** Substances designed to speed up the rate of specific biochemical reactions.

**epidemic:** Occurs when new cases of a disease in a human population substantially exceed the number expected based on recent experience.

**epidermis:** The outer layer of skin, which is made up of cells that are sealed together to form a watertight protective covering for the body.

**epidural hematoma:** An accumulation of blood between the skull and the dura mater.

**epiglottis:** A thin, leaf-shaped valve that allows air to pass into the trachea but prevents food and liquid from entering.

**epiglottitis:** A bacterial infection in which the epiglottis becomes inflamed and enlarged and may cause an upper airway obstruction.

**epilepsy:** A disorder in which abnormal electrical discharges occur in the brain, causing seizures and possible loss of consciousness; a medication that increases heart rate and blood pressure but also eases breathing problems by decreasing muscle tone of the bronchiole tree.

**epinephrine:** A medication that increases heart rate and blood pressure but also eases breathing problems by decreasing muscle tone of the bronchiole tree; a substance produced by the body (commonly called adrenaline), and a drug produced by pharmaceutical companies that increases pulse rate and blood pressure; the drug of choice for an anaphylactic reaction.

**epistaxis:** A nosebleed.

**esophageal intubation:** Improper placement of an advanced airway device into the esophagus rather than into the trachea.

**esophagus:** A collapsible tube that extends from the pharynx to the stomach; muscle contractions propel food and liquids through it to the stomach.

**ethics:** The philosophy of right and wrong, of moral duties, and of ideal professional behavior.

**ethnocentrism:** When a person considers his or her own cultural values as more important when interacting with people of a different culture.

**eustachian tube:** A tube that connects the middle ear to the oropharynx.

**eustress:** A beneficial response to a stressor.

**evaporation:** The conversion of water or another fluid from a liquid to a gas.

**evidence-based medicine (EBM):** An approach to medicine where decisions are based on well-conducted research, classifying recommendations based on the strength of the scientific evidence; also called science-based medicine.

**evisceration:** The displacement of organs outside of the body.

**excited delirium:** A serious behavioral condition in which a person exhibits agitated behavior combined with disorientation, hallucinations, or delusions; also called agitated delirium or exhaustive mania.

**exhalation:** The passive part of the breathing process in which the diaphragm and the intercostal muscles relax, forcing air out of the lungs.

**expiratory reserve volume:** The amount of air that can be exhaled following a normal exhalation; average volume is about 1,200 mL in the average adult male.

**exposure:** A situation in which a person has had contact with blood, body fluids, tissues, or airborne particles in a manner that suggests disease transmission may occur.

**expressed consent:** A type of consent in which a patient gives verbal or nonverbal authorization for provision of care or transport.

**extension:** The straightening of a joint.

**external auditory canal:** The ear canal; leads to the tympanic membrane.

**external respiration:** The exchange of gases between the lungs and the blood cells in the pulmonary capillaries; also called pulmonary respiration.

**extremity lift:** A lifting technique that is used for patients who are supine or in a sitting position with no suspected extremity or spinal injuries.

**extrication:** Removal of a patient from entrapment or a dangerous situation or position, such as removal from a wrecked vehicle, industrial incident, or collapsed building.

**extrication supervisor:** In incident command, the person appointed to determine the type of equipment and resources needed for a situation involving extrication or special rescue; also called the rescue officer.

**eyes-forward position:** A head position in which the patient's eyes are looking straight ahead and the head and torso are in line.

**fallopian tubes:** The tubes that connect each ovary with the uterus and are the primary location for fertilization of the ovum.

**false imprisonment:** The confinement of a person without legal authority or the person's consent.

**false motion:** Movement that occurs in a bone at a point where there is no joint, indicating a fracture; also called free movement.

**fascia:** The fiberlike connective tissue that covers arteries, veins, tendons, and ligaments.

**febrile seizures:** Seizures that result from sudden high fevers; most often seen in children.

**Federal Communications Commission (FCC):** The federal agency that has jurisdiction over interstate and international telephone and telegraph services and satellite communications, all of which may involve EMS activity.

**femoral artery:** The major artery of the thigh, a continuation of the external iliac artery. It supplies blood to the lower abdominal wall, external genitalia, and legs. It can be palpated in the groin area.

**femoral head:** The proximal end of the femur, articulating with the acetabulum to form the hip joint.

**femur:** The thighbone; the longest and one of the strongest bones in the body.

**fetal alcohol syndrome:** A condition caused by the consumption of alcohol by a pregnant woman; characterized by growth and physical problems, mental retardation, and a variety of congenital abnormalities in her child.

**fetus:** The developing, unborn infant inside the uterus, from 10 weeks after fertilization until birth.

**fibula:** The smaller of the two bones that form the lower leg, located on the lateral side.

**field impression:** The conclusion about the cause of the patient's condition after considering the situation, history, and examination findings.

**finance/administration:** In incident command, the position in an incident responsible for accounting of all expenditures.

**first-responder vehicles:** Specialized vehicles used to transport EMS equipment and personnel to the scenes of medical emergencies.

**flail chest:** A condition in which two or more adjacent ribs are fractured in two or more places or in association with a fracture of the sternum so that a segment of the chest wall is effectively detached from the rest of the thoracic cage.

**flame burn:** A burn caused by an open flame.

**flank:** The region below the rib cage and above the hip.

**flash burn:** A burn caused by exposure to very intense heat, such as in an explosion.

**flexible stretcher:** A stretcher that is a rigid carrying device when secured around a patient but can be folded or rolled when not in use.

**flexion:** The bending of a joint.

**flutter valve:** A one-way valve that allows air to leave the chest cavity but not return; formed by taping three sides of an occlusive dressing to the chest wall, leaving the fourth side open as a valve; may also be part of a commercial vented occlusive dressing.

**focal seizure:** A seizure affecting a limited portion of the brain.

**focused assessment:** A type of physical assessment typically performed on patients who have sustained nonsignificant mechanisms of injury or on responsive medical patients. This type of examination is based on the chief complaint and focuses on one body system or part.

**fontanelles:** Areas where the neonate's or infant's skull has not fused together; usually disappear at approximately 18 months of age.

**foodborne transmission:** The contamination of food or water with an organism that can cause disease.

**foramen magnum:** A large opening at the base of the skull through which the brain connects to the spinal cord.

**forcible restraint:** The act of physically preventing an individual from initiating any physical action.

**four-person log roll:** The recommended procedure for moving a patient with a suspected spinal injury from the ground to a long backboard or other spinal precaution device.

**Fowler position:** An inclined position in which the head of the bed is raised.

**fracture:** A break in the continuity of a bone.

**freelancing:** When individual units or different organizations make independent and often inefficient decisions about the next appropriate action.

**freight bills:** The shipping papers used for transport of chemicals along roads and highways; also referred to as bills of lading.

**frontal bones:** The bones of the cranium that form the forehead.

**frostbite:** Damage to tissues as the result of exposure to cold; frozen or partially frozen body parts are frostbitten.

**full-thickness (third-degree) burns:** Burns that affect all skin layers and may affect the subcutaneous layers, muscle, bone, and internal organs, leaving the area dry, leathery, and white, dark brown, or charred.

**functional disorder:** A disorder in which there is no known physiologic reason for the abnormal functioning of an organ or organ system.

**fundus:** The dome-shaped top of the uterus.

**G agents:** Early nerve agents that were developed by German scientists in the period after World War I and into World War II. There are three such agents: sarin, soman, and tabun.

**gag reflex:** A normal reflex mechanism that causes retching; activated by touching the soft palate or the back of the throat.

**gallbladder:** A sac on the undersurface of the liver that collects bile from the liver and discharges it into the duodenum through the common bile duct.

**gamma (x-ray) radiation:** A type of energy that is emitted from a strong radiologic source that travels faster and has more energy than alpha and beta rays. These rays easily penetrate through the human body and require lead or several inches of concrete to prevent penetration.

**gastric distention:** A condition in which air fills the stomach, often as a result of high volume and pressure during artificial ventilation.

**gastroesophageal reflux disease (GERD):** A condition in which the sphincter between the esophagus and the stomach opens, allowing stomach acid to move up into the esophagus, usually resulting in a burning sensation within the chest; also called acid reflux.

**gel:** A semiliquid substance that is administered orally in capsule form or through plastic tubes.

**general adaptation syndrome:** The body's response to stress that begins with an alarm response, followed by a stage of reaction and resistance, and then recovery or, if the stress is prolonged, exhaustion.

**general impression:** The overall initial impression that determines the priority for patient care; based on the patient's surroundings, the mechanism of injury, signs and symptoms, and the chief complaint.

**generalized (tonic-clonic) seizure:** A seizure characterized by severe twitching of all of the body's muscles that may last several minutes or more; formerly known as a grand mal seizure.

**generic name:** The original chemical name of a medication (in contrast to one of its proprietary or trade names); the name is not capitalized.

**genital system:** The reproductive system in men and women.

**geriatrics:** The assessment and treatment of disease in someone who is age 65 years or older.

**germinal layer:** The deepest layer of the epidermis, where new skin cells are formed.

**gestational diabetes:** Diabetes that develops during pregnancy in women who did not have diabetes before pregnancy.

**gestational hypertension:** A blood pressure greater than or equal to 140 mm Hg systolic or 90 mm Hg diastolic in a pregnant female in whom hypertension has not previously been diagnosed.

**Glasgow Coma Scale (GCS) score:** An evaluation tool used to determine level of consciousness, which evaluates and assigns point values (scores) for eye opening, verbal response, and motor response, which are then totaled; effective in helping predict patient outcomes.

**glenoid fossa:** The part of the scapula that joins with the humeral head to form the glenohumeral joint.

**globe:** The eyeball.

**glottis:** The space in between the vocal cords that is the narrowest portion of the adult's airway; also called the glottic opening.

**glucose:** One of the basic sugars; it is the primary fuel, in conjunction with oxygen, for cellular metabolism.

**Golden Hour:** The time from injury to definitive care, during which treatment of shock and traumatic injuries should occur because survival potential is best; also called the Golden Period.

**gonorrhea:** A sexually transmitted disease caused by *Neisseria gonorrhoeae*.

**good air exchange:** A term used to distinguish the degree of distress in a patient with a mild airway obstruction. With good air exchange, the patient is still conscious and able to cough forcefully, although wheezing may be heard.

**Good Samaritan laws:** Statutory provisions enacted by many states to protect citizens from liability for errors and omissions in giving good-faith emergency medical care, unless there is wanton, gross, or willful negligence.

**governmental immunity:** Legal doctrine that can protect an EMS provider from being sued or that may limit the amount of the monetary judgment that the plaintiff may recover; generally applies only to EMS systems that are operated by municipalities or other governmental entities.

**greater trochanter:** A bony prominence on the proximal lateral side of the thigh, just below the hip joint.

**gross negligence:** Conduct that constitutes a willful or reckless disregard for a duty or standard of care.

**group:** In the context of EMS, a collection of individual health care providers working independently to help the patient.

**grunting:** An "uh" sound heard during exhalation; reflects the child's attempt to keep the alveoli open; a sign of increased work of breathing.

**guarding:** Involuntary muscle contractions (spasm) of the abdominal wall to minimize the pain of abdominal movement; a sign of peritonitis.

**gum elastic bougie:** A flexible device that is inserted between the glottis under direct laryngoscopy; the endotracheal tube is threaded over the device, facilitating its entry into the trachea.

**hair follicles:** The small organs that produce hair.

**hallucinogen:** An agent that produces false perceptions in any one of the five senses.

**handover:** The transfer of pertinent patient information and the responsibility for the patient's care; often involves the physical movement of the patient and associated equipment; also known as handoff.

**hay fever:** An allergic response, usually to outdoor airborne allergens such as pollen or sometimes indoor allergens such as dust mites or pet dander; also called allergic rhinitis.

**hazardous material:** Any substance that is toxic, poisonous, radioactive, flammable, or explosive and causes injury or death with exposure.

**hazardous materials (hazmat) incident:** An incident in which a hazardous material is no longer properly contained and isolated.

**head tilt–chin lift maneuver:** A combination of two movements to open the airway by tilting the forehead back and lifting the chin; not used for trauma patients.

**health care directive:** A written document that specifies medical treatment for a competent patient, should he or she become unable to make decisions. Also known as an advance directive or a living will.

**health care proxy:** A type of advance directive executed by a competent adult that appoints another individual to make medical treatment decisions on his or her behalf in the event that the person making the appointment loses decision-making capacity. Also known as a durable power of attorney for health care.

**health information exchange (HIE):** A system that allows EMS providers to access relevant health data (eg, past medical problems, medications, allergies, end-of-life decisions), avoid unnecessary duplication of effort in data entry, and view patient outcomes related to hospital care.

**Health Insurance Portability and Accountability Act (HIPAA):** Federal legislation passed in 1996. Its main effect in EMS is in limiting availability of patients' health care information and penalizing violations of patient privacy.

**heart:** A hollow muscular organ that pumps blood throughout the body.

**heart rate (HR):** The number of heartbeats during a specific time (usually 1 minute).

**heat cramps:** Painful muscle spasms usually associated with vigorous activity in a hot environment.

**heat exhaustion:** A heat emergency in which a significant amount of fluid and electrolyte loss occurs because of heavy sweating; also called heat prostration or heat collapse.

**heatstroke:** A life-threatening condition of severe hyperthermia caused by exposure to excessive natural or artificial heat, marked by warm, dry skin; severely altered mental status; and often irreversible coma.

**hematemesis:** Vomiting blood.

**hematology:** The study and prevention of blood-related disorders.

**hematoma:** A mass of blood that has collected within damaged tissue beneath the skin or in a body cavity.

**hematuria:** Blood in the urine.

**hemiparesis:** Weakness on one side of the body.

**hemoglobin:** An oxygen-carrying protein found in red blood cells.

**hemophilia:** A hereditary condition in which the patient lacks one or more of the blood's normal clotting factors.

**hemopneumothorax:** The accumulation of blood and air in the pleural space of the chest.

**hemoptysis:** The coughing up of blood.

**hemorrhage:** Bleeding.

**hemorrhagic stroke:** A type of stroke that occurs as a result of bleeding inside the brain.

**hemostatic dressing:** A dressing impregnated with a chemical compound that slows or stops bleeding by assisting with clot formation.

**hemothorax:** A collection of blood in the pleural cavity.

**hepatitis:** Inflammation of the liver, usually caused by a viral infection, that causes fever, loss of appetite, jaundice, fatigue, and altered liver function.

**hernia:** The protrusion of an organ or tissue through an abnormal body opening.

**herpes simplex:** A common virus that is asymptomatic in 80% of people carrying it, but characterized by small blisters on the lips or genitals in symptomatic infections.

**high-level disinfection:** The killing of pathogenic agents by using potent means of disinfection.

**hinge joints:** Joints that can bend and straighten but cannot rotate; they restrict motion to one plane.

**histamines:** Chemical substances released by the immune system in allergic reactions that are responsible for many of the symptoms of anaphylaxis, such as vasodilation.

**history taking:** A step within the patient assessment process that provides details about the patient's chief complaint and an account of the patient's signs and symptoms.

**hollow organs:** Structures through which materials pass, such as the stomach, small intestines, large intestines, ureters, and urinary bladder.

**homeostasis:** A balance of all systems of the body.

**hormones:** Substances formed in specialized organs or glands and carried to another organ or group of cells in the same organism; they regulate many body functions, including metabolism, growth, and body temperature.

**host:** The organism or individual that is attacked by the infecting agent.

**hot zone:** The area immediately surrounding a hazardous materials spill or incident site that endangers life and health. All responders working in this zone must wear appropriate protective clothing and equipment. Entry requires approval by the incident commander or other designated officer.

**human immunodeficiency virus (HIV):** Acquired immunodeficiency syndrome (AIDS) is caused by HIV, which damages the cells in the body's immune system so that the body is unable to fight infection or certain cancers.

**humerus:** The supporting bone of the upper arm.

**hydroplaning:** Occurs when the tires of a vehicle are lifted off the road surface as a result of water piling up underneath them, making the vehicle seem as if it is floating.

**hydrostatic pressure:** The pressure of water against the walls of its container.

**Hymenoptera:** A family of insects that includes bees, wasps, ants, and yellow jackets.

**hypercapnia:** An abnormally high level of carbon dioxide in the bloodstream; also called hypercarbia.

**hypercarbia:** Increased carbon dioxide level in the bloodstream.

**hyperglycemia:** An abnormally high blood glucose level.

**hyperosmolar hyperglycemic nonketotic syndrome (HHNS):** A life-threatening condition resulting from high blood glucose that typically occurs in older adults and which causes altered mental status, dehydration, and organ damage.

**hypertension:** Blood pressure that is higher than the normal range.

**hypertensive emergency:** An emergency situation created by excessively high blood pressure, which can lead to serious complications such as stroke or aneurysm.

**hyperthermia:** A condition in which the body core temperature rises to 101°F (38.3°C) or higher.

**hyperventilation:** Rapid or deep breathing that lowers the blood carbon dioxide level below normal; may lead to increased intrathoracic pressure, decreased venous return, and hypotension when associated with bag-mask device use.

**hyperventilation syndrome:** This syndrome occurs in the absence of physical problems. The respirations of a person who is experiencing hyperventilation syndrome may be as high as 40 shallow breaths/min or as low as only 20 very deep breaths/min. This syndrome is often associated with panic attacks.

**hypnotic:** A sleep-inducing effect or agent.

**hypoglycemia:** An abnormally low blood glucose level.

**hypoperfusion:** A condition in which the circulatory system fails to provide sufficient circulation to maintain normal cellular function; also called shock.

**hypotension:** Blood pressure that is lower than the normal range.

**hypothermia:** A condition in which the internal body temperature falls below 95°F (35°C).

**hypovolemic shock:** A condition in which low blood volume, due to massive internal or external bleeding or extensive loss of body water, results in inadequate perfusion.

**hypoxia:** Deficient oxygen concentration in the tissues.

**hypoxic drive:** A condition in which chronically low levels of oxygen in the blood stimulate the respiratory drive; seen in patients with chronic lung diseases.

**ileostomy:** A surgical procedure to create an opening (stoma) between the small intestine and the surface of the body.

**ileus:** Paralysis of the bowel, arising from any one of several causes; stops contractions that move material through the intestine.

**ilium:** One of three bones that fuse to form the pelvic ring.

**immune:** The body's ability to protect itself from acquiring a disease.

**immune response:** The body's response to a substance perceived by the body as foreign.

**immune system:** The body system that includes all of the structures and processes designed to mount a defense against foreign substances and disease-causing agents.

**immunology:** The study of the body's immune system.

**impaled objects:** Objects that penetrate the skin but remain in place.

**impedance threshold device (ITD):** A valve device placed between the endotracheal tube and a bag-mask device that limits the amount of air entering the lungs during the recoil phase between chest compressions.

**implied consent:** Type of consent in which a patient who is unable to give consent is given treatment under the legal assumption that he or she would want treatment.

**incident action plan:** An oral or written plan stating general objectives reflecting the overall strategy for managing an incident.

**incident commander (IC):** The individual who has overall command of the incident in the field.

**incident command system (ICS):** A system implemented to manage disasters and mass-casualty incidents in which section chiefs, including finance/administration, logistics, operations, and planning, report to the incident commander.

**incision:** A sharp, smooth cut in the skin.

**incontinence:** Loss of bowel and/or bladder control; may be the result of a generalized seizure.

**incubation:** The period of time between a person being exposed to an agent and the time when symptoms appear.

**index of suspicion:** Awareness that unseen life-threatening injuries may exist when determining the mechanism of injury.

**indications:** The therapeutic uses for a specific medication.

**indirect contact:** Exposure or transmission of disease from one person to another by contact with a contaminated object.

**induced abortion:** The elective termination of a pregnancy prior to the time of viability.

**infancy:** The first year of life.

**infant:** A young child age 1 month to 1 year.

**infarction:** Death of a body tissue, usually caused by interruption of its blood supply.

**infection:** The abnormal invasion of a host or host tissues by organisms such as bacteria, viruses, or parasites, with or without signs or symptoms of disease.

**infection control:** Procedures to reduce transmission of infection among patients and health care personnel.

**infectious disease:** A medical condition caused by the growth and spread of small, harmful organisms within the body.

**inferior:** Below a body part or nearer to the feet.

**inferior vena cava:** One of the two largest veins in the body; carries blood from the lower extremities and the pelvis and the abdominal organs to the heart.

**influenza:** A virus that has crossed the animal/human barrier and infected humans and that kills thousands of people every year.

**influenza type A:** Virus that has crossed the animal/human barrier and has infected humans, recently reaching a pandemic level with the H1N1 strain.

**informed consent:** Permission for treatment given by a competent patient after the potential risks, benefits, and alternatives to treatment have been explained.

**ingestion:** Swallowing; taking a substance by mouth.

**inhalation:** The active, muscular part of breathing that draws air into the airway and lungs; a medication delivery route.

**in loco parentis:** Refers to the legal responsibility of a person or organization to take on some of the functions and responsibilities of a parent.

**inspiratory reserve volume:** The amount of air that can be inhaled after a normal inhalation; the amount of air that can be inhaled in addition to the normal tidal volume.

**insulin:** A hormone produced by the islets of Langerhans (endocrine gland located throughout the pancreas) that enables glucose in the blood to enter cells; used in synthetic form to treat and control diabetes mellitus.

**intellectual disability:** A subset of developmental disability characterized by significant limitations in both intellectual functioning and skills needed for daily living.

**intermodal tanks:** Shipping and storage vessels that can be either pressurized or nonpressurized.

**internal respiration:** The exchange of gases between the blood cells and the tissues.

**international terrorism:** Terrorism that is carried out by people in a country other than their own; also known as cross-border terrorism.

**interoperable communications system:** A communication system that uses voice-over-Internet Protocol (VoIP) technology to allow multiple agencies to communicate and transmit data.

**interrogatories:** Written questions that the defense and plaintiff send to one another.

**interstitial space:** The space in between the cells.

**intervertebral disks:** Tough, elastic structures between adjoining vertebrae that act as shock absorbers.

**intracellular space:** The space within a cell or cells.

**intracerebral hematoma:** Bleeding within the brain tissue (parenchyma) itself; also referred to as an intraparenchymal hematoma.

**intracranial pressure (ICP):** The pressure within the cranial vault.

**intramuscular (IM) injection:** An injection into a muscle; a medication delivery route.

**intranasal (IN):** A delivery route in which a medication is pushed through a specialized atomizer device called a mucosal atomizer device (MAD) into the naris.

**intraosseous (IO) injection:** An injection into the bone; a medication delivery route.

**intrapulmonary shunting:** Bypassing of oxygen-poor blood past nonfunctional alveoli to the left side of the heart.

**intravenous (IV) injection:** An injection directly into a vein; a medication delivery route.

**intravenous (IV) therapy:** The delivery of medication directly into a vein.

**involuntary activities:** Actions of the body that are not under a person's conscious control.

**involuntary muscle:** The muscle over which a person has no conscious control. It is found in many automatic regulating systems of the body.

**ionizing radiation:** Energy that is emitted in the form of rays, or particles.

**iris:** The muscle and surrounding tissue behind the cornea that dilate and constrict the pupil, regulating the amount of light that enters the eye; pigment in this tissue gives the eye its color.

**irreversible shock:** A condition defined by the inability to successfully achieve resuscitation regardless of the methods employed.

**ischemia:** A lack of oxygen that deprives tissues of necessary nutrients, resulting from partial or complete blockage of blood flow; potentially reversible because permanent injury has not yet occurred.

**ischemic stroke:** A type of stroke that occurs when blood flow to a particular part of the brain is cut off by a blockage (eg, a blood clot) inside a blood vessel.

**ischium:** One of three bones that fuse to form the pelvic ring.

**jaundice:** Yellow skin or sclera that is caused by liver disease or dysfunction.

**jaw-thrust maneuver:** Technique to open the airway by placing the fingers behind the angle of the jaw and bringing the jaw forward; used for patients who may have a cervical spine injury.

**joint:** The place where two bones come into contact.

**joint capsule:** The fibrous sac that encloses a joint.

**joint information center (JIC):** An area designated by the incident commander, or a designee, in which public information officers from multiple agencies distribute information about the incident.

**jugular vein distention:** A visual bulging of the jugular veins in the neck that can be caused by fluid overload, pressure in the chest, cardiac tamponade, or tension pneumothorax.

**jump kit:** A portable kit containing items that are used in the initial care of the patient.

**JumpSTART triage:** A sorting system for pediatric patients younger than 8 years or weighing less than 100 pounds (45 kg). There is a minor adaptation for infants because they cannot ambulate on their own.

**junctional tourniquet:** A device that provides proximal compression of severe bleeding near the axial or inguinal junction with the torso.

**kidnapping:** The seizing, confining, abducting, or carrying away of a person by force, including transporting a competent adult for medical treatment without his or her consent.

**kidneys:** Two retroperitoneal organs that excrete the end products of metabolism as urine and regulate the body's salt and water content.

**kidney stones:** Solid crystalline masses formed in the kidney, resulting from an excess of insoluble salts or uric acid crystallizing in the urine; may become trapped anywhere along the urinary tract.

**kinetic energy:** The energy of a moving object.

**Kussmaul respirations:** Deep, rapid breathing; usually the result of an accumulation of certain acids when insulin is not available in the body.

**kyphosis:** A forward curling of the back caused by an abnormal increase in the curvature of the spine.

**labia majora:** Outer fleshy "lips" covered with pubic hair that protect the vagina.

**labia minora:** Inner fleshy "lips" devoid of pubic hair that protect the vagina.

**labored breathing:** The use of muscles of the chest, back, and abdomen to assist in expanding the chest; occurs when air movement is impaired.

**laceration:** A deep, jagged cut in the skin.

**lacrimal glands:** The glands that produce fluids to keep the eye moist; also called tear glands.

**lactic acid:** A metabolic by-product of the breakdown of glucose that accumulates when metabolism proceeds in the absence of oxygen (anaerobic metabolism).

**large intestine:** The portion of the digestive tube that encircles the abdomen around the small bowel, consisting of the cecum, the colon, and the rectum. It helps regulate water balance and eliminate solid waste.

**larynx:** A complex structure formed by many independent cartilaginous structures that all work together; where the upper airway ends and the lower airway begins; also called the voice box.

**lateral:** Parts of the body that lie farther from the midline; also called outer structures.

**length-based resuscitation tape:** A tape used to estimate an infant's or child's weight on the basis of body length; appropriate drug doses and equipment sizes are listed on the tape.

**lens:** The transparent part of the eye through which images are focused on the retina.

**lesser trochanter:** The projection on the medial/superior portion of the femur.

**leukotrienes:** Chemical substances that contribute to anaphylaxis; released by the immune system in allergic reactions.

**lewisite (L):** A blistering agent that has a rapid onset of symptoms and produces immediate, intense pain and discomfort on contact.

**liaison officer:** In incident command, the person who relays information, concerns, and requests among responding agencies.

**libel:** False and damaging information about a person that is communicated in writing.

**licensure:** The process whereby a competent authority, usually the state, allows people to perform a regulated act.

**life expectancy:** The average number of years a person can be expected to live.

**ligaments:** Bands of fibrous tissue that connect bones to bones. Ligaments support and strengthen a joint.

**lightening:** The movement of the fetus down into the pelvis late in pregnancy.

**limb presentation:** A delivery in which the presenting part is a single arm or leg.

**linear skull fractures:** Fractures that commonly occur in the temporoparietal region of the skull and that are not associated with deformities to the skull; account for 80% of skull fractures; also referred to as nondisplaced skull fractures.

**liver:** A large, solid organ that lies in the right upper quadrant immediately below the diaphragm; it produces bile, stores glucose for immediate use by the body, and produces many substances that help regulate immune responses.

**load-distributing band (LDB):** A circumferential chest compression device composed of a constricting band and backboard that is either electrically or pneumatically driven to compress the heart by putting inward pressure on the thorax.

**logistics:** In incident command, the position that helps procure and stockpile equipment and supplies during an incident.

**lone wolf terrorist attack:** An act of terror carried out by a single person to further an ideological goal.

**lumbar spine:** The lower part of the back, formed by the lowest five nonfused vertebrae; also called the dorsal spine.

**lumen:** The inside diameter of an artery or other hollow structure.

**lymph:** A thin, straw-colored fluid that carries oxygen, nutrients, and hormones to the cells and carries waste products of metabolism away from the cells and back into the capillaries so that they may be excreted.

**lymph nodes:** Tiny, oval-shaped structures located in various places along the lymph vessels that filter lymph.

**lymphatic system:** A passive circulatory system in the body that transports a plasmalike liquid called lymph, a thin fluid that bathes the tissues of the body.

**malleolus:** A rounded bony prominence on either side of the ankle; also called the ankle bone.

**mandible:** The bone of the lower jaw.

**manubrium:** The upper quarter of the sternum.

**mass-casualty incident (MCI):** An emergency situation involving three or more patients or that can place great demand on the equipment or personnel of the EMS system or has the potential to produce multiple casualties.

**mastoid process:** The prominent bony mass at the base of the skull about 1 inch (2.5 cm) posterior to the external opening of the ear.

**material safety data sheet (MSDS):** A form, provided by manufacturers and compounders (blenders) of chemicals, containing information about chemical composition, physical and chemical properties, health and safety hazards, emergency response, and waste disposal of a specific material; also known as a safety data sheet (SDS).

**maxillae:** The upper jawbones that assist in the formation of the orbit, the nasal cavity, and the palate and hold the upper teeth.

**mean arterial pressure (MAP):** The average pressure in the circulatory system during one cardiac cycle.

**mechanical piston device:** A device that depresses the sternum via a compressed gas-powered or electric-powered plunger mounted on a backboard.

**mechanism of injury (MOI):** The forces, or energy transmission, applied to the body that cause injury.

**meconium:** Fetal stool. When appearing as a dark green material in the amniotic fluid, it can indicate distress or disease in the newborn; it can be aspirated into the fetus's lungs during delivery.

**MED channels:** VHF and UHF channels that the Federal Communications Commission has designated exclusively for EMS use.

**medevac:** Medical evacuation of a patient by helicopter.

**medial:** Parts of the body that lie closer to the midline; also called inner structures.

**mediastinum:** Space within the chest that contains the heart, major blood vessels, vagus nerve, trachea, major bronchi, and esophagus; located between the two lungs.

**medical control:** Physician instructions given directly by radio or cell phone (online/direct) or indirectly by protocol/guidelines (offline/indirect), as authorized by the medical director of the service program.

**medical director:** The physician who authorizes or delegates to the EMT the authority to provide medical care in the field.

**medical emergencies:** Emergencies that are not caused by an outside force; illnesses or conditions.

**medication:** A substance that is used to treat or prevent disease or relieve pain.

**medication error:** Inappropriate use of a medication that could lead to patient harm.

**medicolegal:** A term relating to medical jurisprudence (law) or forensic medicine.

**medulla oblongata:** Nerve tissue that is continuous inferiorly with the spinal cord; serves as a conduction pathway for ascending and descending nerve tracts; coordinates heart rate, blood vessel diameter, breathing, swallowing, vomiting, coughing, and sneezing.

**melena:** Black, foul-smelling, tarry stool containing digested blood.

**menarche:** The first menstrual cycle or onset of the first menstrual bleeding in females.

**meninges:** Three distinct layers of tissue that surround and protect the brain and the spinal cord within the skull and the spinal canal.

**meningitis:** An inflammation of the meningeal coverings of the brain and spinal cord; it is usually caused by a virus or a bacterium.

**meningococcal meningitis:** An inflammation of the meningeal coverings of the brain and spinal cord; can be highly contagious.

**menopause:** The cessation of menstruation, typically in the fourth or fifth decade of life.

**mental model:** The picture an individual has in his or her head of "what's going on" in a given situation.

**metabolism:** The biochemical processes that result in production of energy from nutrients within the cells; also called cellular respiration.

**metacarpals:** Bones of the hand, situated between the carpals and phalanges.

**metatarsals:** Bones of the foot, situated between the tarsals and phalanges.

**metered-dose inhaler (MDI):** A miniature spray canister used to direct medications through the mouth and into the lungs.

**methicillin-resistant** *Staphylococcus aureus* **(MRSA):** A bacterium that can cause infections in different parts of the body and is often resistant to commonly used antibiotics; it is transmitted by different routes, including the respiratory route, and can be found on the skin, in surgical wounds, and in the bloodstream, lungs, and urinary tract.

**midbrain:** The part of the brain that is responsible for helping to regulate the level of consciousness.

**middle adult:** An adult age 41 to 60 years.

**midsagittal (midline) plane:** An imaginary vertical line drawn from the middle of the forehead through the nose and the umbilicus (navel) to the floor, dividing the body into equal left and right halves.

**mild airway obstruction:** Occurs when a foreign body partially obstructs the patient's airway. The patient is able to move adequate amounts of air, but also experiences some degree of respiratory distress.

**minute volume:** The volume of air that moves in and out of the lungs per minute; calculated by multiplying the tidal volume and respiratory rate; also called minute ventilation.

**miosis:** Excessively constricted pupil; often bilateral after exposure to nerve agents.

**miscarriage:** The spontaneous passage of the fetus and placenta before 20 weeks; also called spontaneous abortion.

**mission-critical communications:** Any communications where disruption will result in the failure of the mission at hand.

**mobile data terminal (MDT):** A small computer terminal inside the ambulance that directly receives data from the dispatch center.

**mobile integrated health care (MIH):** A method of delivering health care that involves providing health care within the community rather than at a physician's office or hospital.

**morality:** A code of conduct that can be defined by society, religion, or a person, affecting character, conduct, and conscience.

**morgue supervisor:** In incident command, the person who works with area medical examiners, coroners, and law enforcement agencies to coordinate the disposition of dead victims.

**Moro reflex:** An infant reflex in which, when an infant is caught off guard, the infant opens his or her arms wide, spreads the fingers, and seems to grab at things.

**motor nerves:** Nerves that carry information from the central nervous system to the muscles of the body.

**mucosal atomizer device (MAD):** A device that is used to change a liquid medication into a spray and push it into a nostril.

**mucous membranes:** The linings of body cavities and passages that communicate directly or indirectly with the environment outside the body.

**mucus:** The watery secretion of the mucous membranes that lubricates the body openings.

**multigravida:** A woman who has had previous pregnancies.

**multiplex:** The ability to transmit audio and data signals through the use of more than one communications channel.

**multisystem trauma:** Trauma that affects more than one body system.

**musculoskeletal system:** The bones and voluntary muscles of the body.

**mutagen:** A substance that mutates, damages, and changes the structures of DNA in the body's cells.

**mutual aid response:** An agreement between neighboring EMS systems to respond to mass-casualty incidents or disasters in each other's region when local resources are insufficient to handle the response.

**myocardial contractility:** The ability of the heart muscle to contract.

**myocardial contusion:** Bruising of the heart muscle.

**myocardium:** The heart muscle.

**narcotic:** A drug that produces sleep or altered mental consciousness.

**nares:** The external openings of the nostrils. A single nostril opening is called a naris.

**nasal cannula:** An oxygen-delivery device in which oxygen flows through two small, tubelike prongs that fit into the patient's nostrils; delivers 24% to 44% supplemental oxygen, depending on the flow rate.

**nasal flaring:** Widening of the nostrils, indicating that there is an airway obstruction.

**nasopharyngeal (nasal) airway:** Airway adjunct inserted into the nostril of an unresponsive patient or a patient with an altered level of consciousness who is unable to maintain airway patency independently.

**nasopharynx:** The part of the pharynx that lies above the level of the roof of the mouth, or palate.

**National EMS Scope of Practice Model:** A document created by the National Highway Traffic Safety Administration (NHTSA) that outlines the skills performed by various EMS providers.

**National Incident Management System (NIMS):** A Department of Homeland Security system designed to enable federal, state, and local governments and private-sector and nongovernmental organizations to effectively and efficiently prepare for, prevent, respond to, and recover from domestic incidents, regardless of cause, size, or complexity, including acts of catastrophic terrorism.

**nature of illness (NOI):** The general type of illness a patient is experiencing.

**neglect:** Refusal or failure on the part of the parent or caregiver to provide life necessities.

**negligence:** Failure to provide the same care that a person with similar training would provide.

**negligence per se:** A theory that may be used when the conduct of the person being sued is alleged to have occurred in clear violation of a statute.

*Neisseria meningitides:* A form of bacterial meningitis characterized by rapid onset of symptoms, often leading to shock and death.

**neonate:** A newborn age birth to 1 month.

**nephrons:** The basic filtering units in the kidneys.

**nerve agents:** A class of chemicals called organophosphates; they function by blocking an essential enzyme in the nervous system, which causes the body's organs to become overstimulated and burn out.

**nervous system:** The system that controls virtually all activities of the body, both voluntary and involuntary.

**neurogenic shock:** Circulatory failure caused by paralysis of the nerves that control the size of the blood vessels, leading to widespread dilation; seen in patients with spinal cord injuries.

**neurons:** The functional units of the nervous system; also called nerve cells.

**neuropathy:** A group of conditions in which the nerves leaving the spinal cord are damaged, resulting in distortion of signals to or from the brain.

**neurotoxins:** Biologic agents that are the deadliest substances known to humans; they include botulinum toxin and ricin.

**neutron radiation:** The type of energy that is emitted from a strong radiologic source, involving particles that are among the most powerful forms of radiation; the particles easily penetrate through lead and require several feet of concrete to stop them.

**nitroglycerin:** A medication that increases cardiac perfusion by causing blood vessels to dilate; EMTs may be allowed to assist the patient to self-administer this medication.

**noise:** Anything that dampens or obscures the true meaning of a message.

**nonbulk storage vessels:** Any container other than bulk storage containers, such as drums, bags, compressed gas cylinders, and cryogenic containers. These hold commonly used commercial and industrial chemicals such as solvents, industrial cleaners, and compounds.

**nondisplaced fracture:** A simple crack in the bone that has not caused the bone to move from its normal anatomic position; also called a hairline fracture.

**nonrebreathing mask:** A combination mask and reservoir bag system that is the preferred way to give oxygen in the prehospital setting; delivers up to 90% inspired oxygen and prevents inhaling the exhaled gases (carbon dioxide).

**norepinephrine:** A neurotransmitter and drug sometimes used in the treatment of shock; produces vasoconstriction through its alpha-stimulator properties.

**nuchal cord:** An umbilical cord that is wrapped around the fetus's neck.

**obesity:** A complex condition in which a person has an excessive amount of body fat.

**obstructive shock:** Shock that occurs when there is a block to blood flow in the heart or great vessels, causing an insufficient blood supply to the body's tissues.

**occipital bone:** The most posterior bone of the cranium.

**occlusion:** A blockage, usually of a tubular structure such as a blood vessel.

**occlusive dressing:** An airtight dressing that protects a wound from air and bacteria; a commercial vented version allows air to passively escape from the chest, while an unvented dressing may be made of petroleum jelly–based (Vaseline) gauze, aluminum foil, or plastic.

**Occupational Safety and Health Administration (OSHA):** The federal regulatory compliance agency that develops, publishes, and enforces guidelines concerning safety in the workplace.

**off-gassing:** The release of an agent after exposure—for example, from a person's clothes that have been exposed to the agent.

**older adult:** An adult age 61 years or older.

**oncotic pressure:** The pressure of water to move, typically into the capillary, as the result of the presence of plasma proteins.

**onset of action:** The amount of time from the administration of a medication to the onset of clinical effects.

**open abdominal injury:** An injury in which there is a break in the surface of the skin or mucous membrane, exposing deeper tissue to potential contamination.

**open-book pelvic fracture:** A life-threatening fracture of the pelvis caused by a force that displaces one or both sides of the pelvis laterally and posteriorly.

**open chest injury:** An injury to the chest in which the chest wall itself is penetrated by a fractured rib or, more frequently, by an external object such as a bullet or knife.

**open-ended questions:** Questions for which the patient must provide detail to give an answer.

**open fracture:** Any break in a bone in which the overlying skin has been broken.

**open head injury:** Injury to the head often caused by a penetrating object in which there may be bleeding and exposed brain tissue.

**open incident:** An incident that is not yet contained; there may be patients to be located and the situation may be ongoing, producing more patients.

**open injuries:** Injuries in which there is a break in the surface of the skin or the mucous membrane, exposing deeper tissue to potential contamination.

**open pneumothorax:** An open or penetrating chest wall wound through which air passes during inspiration and expiration, creating a sucking sound; also referred to as a sucking chest wound.

**operations:** In incident command, the position that carries out the orders of the commander to help resolve the incident.

**opiate:** A subset of the opioid family, referring to natural, nonsynthetic opioids.

**opioid:** A synthetically produced narcotic medication, drug, or agent similar to the opiate morphine, but not derived from opium; used to relieve pain.

**OPQRST:** A mnemonic used in evaluating a patient's pain: Onset, Provocation/palliation, Quality, Region/radiation, Severity, and Timing.

**optic nerve:** A cranial nerve that transmits visual information to the brain.

**oral:** By mouth; a medication delivery route.

**oral glucose:** A simple sugar that is readily absorbed by the bloodstream; it is carried on the EMS unit.

**orbit:** The eye socket, made up of the maxilla and zygoma.

**organic brain syndrome:** Temporary or permanent dysfunction of the brain, caused by a disturbance in the physical or physiologic functioning of brain tissue.

**orientation:** The mental status of a patient as measured by memory of person (name), place (current location), time (current year, month, and approximate date), and event (what happened).

**oropharyngeal (oral) airway:** Airway adjunct inserted into the mouth of an unresponsive patient to keep the tongue from blocking the upper airway and to facilitate suctioning the airway, if necessary.

**oropharynx:** A tubular structure that extends vertically from the back of the mouth to the esophagus and trachea.

**orthopnea:** Severe dyspnea experienced when lying down and relieved by sitting up.

**osteoporosis:** A generalized bone disease, commonly associated with postmenopausal women, but that can occur in either sex, in which there is a reduction in the amount of bone mass, leading to fractures after minimal trauma.

**ovaries:** The primary female reproductive organs that produce an ovum, or egg, that, if fertilized, will develop into a fetus.

**overdose:** An excessive quantity of a drug that, when taken or administered, can have toxic or lethal consequences.

**over-the-counter (OTC) medications:** Medications that may be purchased directly by a patient without a prescription.

**ovulation:** The process in which an ovum is released from a follicle.

**oxygen:** A gas that all cells need for metabolism; the heart and brain, especially, cannot function without oxygen.

**oxygenation:** The process of delivering oxygen to the blood by diffusion from the alveoli following inhalation into the lungs.

**oxygen toxicity:** A condition of excessive oxygen consumption resulting in cellular and tissue damage.

**paging:** The use of a radio signal and a voice or digital message that is transmitted to pagers ("beepers") or desktop monitor radios.

**palmar:** The forward-facing part of the hand in the anatomic position.

**palmar grasp reflex:** An infant reflex that occurs when something is placed in the infant's palm; the infant grasps the object.

**palpate:** To examine by touch.

**pancreas:** A flat, solid organ that lies below the liver and the stomach; it is a major source of digestive enzymes and produces the hormone insulin.

**pancreatitis:** Inflammation of the pancreas.

**pandemic:** An outbreak that occurs on a global scale.

**paradoxical motion:** The motion of the portion of the chest wall that is detached in a flail chest; the motion—in during inhalation, out during exhalation—is exactly the opposite of normal chest wall motion during breathing.

**paramedic:** An individual who has extensive training in advanced life support, including endotracheal intubation, emergency pharmacology, cardiac monitoring, and other advanced assessment and treatment skills.

**parasympathetic nervous system:** The part of the autonomic nervous system that controls vegetative functions such as digestion of food and relaxation.

**parenteral medications:** Medications that enter the body by a route other than the digestive tract, skin, or mucous membranes.

**parietal bones:** The bones that lie between the temporal and occipital regions of the cranium.

**parietal pleura:** Thin membrane that lines the chest cavity.

**paroxysmal nocturnal dyspnea:** Severe shortness of breath, especially at night after several hours of reclining; the person is forced to sit up to breathe.

**partial pressure:** The term used to describe the amount of gas in air or dissolved in fluid, such as blood.

**partial-thickness (second-degree) burns:** Burns that affect the epidermis and some portion of the dermis but not the subcutaneous tissue, characterized by blisters and skin that is white to red, moist, and mottled.

**passive ventilation:** The act of air moving into and out of the lungs during chest compressions.

**patella:** The knee cap; a specialized bone that lies within the tendon of the quadriceps muscle.

**patent:** Open, clear of obstruction.

**pathogen:** A microorganism that is capable of causing disease in a susceptible host.

**pathophysiology:** The study of how normal physiologic processes are affected by disease.

**patient-assisted medication:** When the EMT assists the patient with the administration of his or her own medication.

**patient autonomy:** The right of a patient to make informed choices regarding his or her health care.

**patient care report (PCR):** The legal document used to record all patient care activities. This report has direct patient care functions but also administrative and quality control functions. PCRs are also known as *prehospital care reports*.

**peak:** The point or period when the maximum clinical effect of a drug is achieved.

**pectoral girdle:** The supporting structure for the arms, which attaches the arms to the axial skeleton. It comprises the clavicles and scapulae; also called the shoulder girdle.

**pediatric assessment triangle (PAT):** A structured assessment tool used to rapidly form a general impression of the infant or child without touching him or her; consists of assessing appearance, work of breathing, and circulation to the skin.

**pediatrics:** A specialized medical practice devoted to the care of the young.

**peer-assisted medication:** When the EMT administers medication to himself or herself or to a partner.

**pelvic binder:** A device to splint the bony pelvis to reduce hemorrhage from bone ends, venous disruption, and pain.

**pelvic girdle:** The supporting structure for the legs, which serves to connect the legs to the axial skeleton.

**pelvic inflammatory disease (PID):** An infection of the fallopian tubes and the surrounding tissues of the pelvis.

**penetrating trauma:** Injury caused by objects, such as knives and bullets, that pierce the surface of the body and damage internal tissues and organs.

**penetrating wound:** An injury resulting from a sharp, piercing object.

**peptic ulcer disease:** An abrasion of the stomach or small intestine.

**perfusion:** The flow of blood through body tissues and vessels.

**pericardial effusion:** A collection of fluid between the pericardial sac and the myocardium.

**pericardium:** The fibrous sac that surrounds the heart.

**perineum:** The area of the skin between the vagina and the anus.

**peripheral nervous system (PNS):** The part of the nervous system that consists of 31 pairs of spinal nerves and 12 pairs of cranial nerves; these may be sensory nerves, motor nerves, or connecting nerves.

**peristalsis:** The wavelike contraction of smooth muscle by which the ureters or other tubular organs propel their contents.

**peritoneal cavity:** The abdominal cavity.

**peritoneum:** The membrane lining the abdominal cavity (parietal peritoneum) and covering the abdominal organs (visceral peritoneum).

**peritonitis:** Inflammation of the peritoneum.

**per os (PO):** Through the mouth; a medication delivery route; same as oral.

**per rectum (PR):** Through the rectum; a medication delivery route.

**persistency:** How long a chemical agent will stay on a surface before it evaporates.

**personal protective equipment (PPE):** Protective equipment that blocks exposure to a pathogen or a hazardous material.

**personal protective equipment (PPE) levels:** Indicates the amount and type of protective equipment that an individual needs to avoid injury during contact with a hazardous material.

**pertinent negatives:** Negative findings that warrant no care or intervention.

**pertussis (whooping cough):** An airborne bacterial infection that affects mostly children younger than 6 years. Patients will be feverish and exhibit a "whoop" sound on inspiration after a coughing attack; highly contagious through droplet infection.

**phalanges:** The bones of the fingers and toes.

**pharmacodynamics:** The process by which a medication works in the body.

**pharmacokinetics:** The processes that the body performs on a medication, including how it is absorbed, distributed, possibly changed, and eliminated.

**pharmacology:** The study of the properties and effects of medications.

**phosgene:** A pulmonary agent that is a product of combustion, resulting from a fire at a textile factory or house, or from metalwork or burning Freon. It is a very potent agent that has a delayed onset of symptoms, usually hours.

**phosgene oxime (CX):** A blistering agent that has a rapid onset of symptoms and produces immediate, intense pain and discomfort on contact.

**phrenic nerves:** The two nerves that innervate the diaphragm; necessary for adequate breathing to occur.

**physiology:** The study of the normal functions of living organisms and their parts.

**pin-indexing system:** A system established for portable cylinders to ensure that a regulator is not connected to a cylinder containing the wrong type of gas.

**pinna:** The external, visible part of the ear.

**placards:** Signage required to be placed on all four sides of highway transport vehicles, railroad tank cars, and other forms of hazardous materials transportation; the sign identifies the hazardous contents of the vehicle, using a standardization system with diamond-shaped indicators.

**placenta:** The tissue attached to the uterine wall that nourishes the fetus through the umbilical cord.

**placenta previa:** A condition in which the placenta develops over and covers the cervix.

**planning:** In incident command, the position that ultimately produces a plan to resolve any incident.

**plantar:** The bottom surface of the foot.

**plasma:** A sticky, yellow fluid that carries the blood cells and nutrients and transports cellular waste material to the organs of excretion.

**platelets:** Tiny, disc-shaped elements that are much smaller than the cells; they are essential in the initial formation of a blood clot, the mechanism that stops bleeding.

**pleura:** The serous membranes covering the lungs and lining the thorax, completely enclosing a potential space known as the pleural space.

**pleural effusion:** A collection of fluid between the lung and chest wall that may compress the lung.

**pleural space:** The potential space between the parietal pleura and the visceral pleura; described as "potential" because under normal conditions, the space does not exist.

**pleuritic chest pain:** Sharp, stabbing pain in the chest that is worsened by a deep breath or other chest wall movement; often caused by inflammation or irritation of the pleura.

**pneumonia:** An infectious disease of the lung that damages lung tissue.

**pneumonic plague:** A lung infection, also known as plague pneumonia, that is the result of inhalation of plague-causing bacteria.

**pneumothorax:** An accumulation of air or gas in the pleural cavity.

**points of distribution (PODs):** Existing facilities used as mass distribution sites for antibiotics, antidotes, vaccinations, and other medications and supplies during an emergency.

**point tenderness:** Tenderness that is sharply localized at the site of the injury, found by gently palpating along the bone with the tip of one finger.

**poison:** A substance whose chemical action could damage structures or impair function when introduced into the body.

**polydipsia:** Excessive thirst that persists for long periods despite reasonable fluid intake; often the result of excessive urination.

**polyphagia:** Excessive eating; in diabetes, the inability to use glucose properly can cause a sense of hunger.

**polypharmacy:** The use of multiple medications on a regular basis.

**polyuria:** The passage of an unusually large volume of urine in a given period; in diabetes, this can result from the wasting of glucose in the urine.

**pons:** An organ that lies below the midbrain and above the medulla and contains numerous important nerve fibers, including those for sleep, respiration, and the medullary respiratory center.

**poor air exchange:** A term used to describe the degree of distress in a patient with a mild airway obstruction. With poor air exchange, the patient often has a weak, ineffective cough, increased difficulty breathing, or possible cyanosis and may produce a high-pitched noise during inhalation (stridor).

**portable stretcher:** A stretcher with a strong, rectangular, tubular metal frame and rigid fabric stretched across it.

**positional asphyxia:** Restriction of chest wall movements and/or airway obstruction; can rapidly lead to sudden death.

**position of function:** A hand position in which the wrist is slightly dorsiflexed and all finger joints are moderately flexed.

**postconventional reasoning:** A type of reasoning in which a child bases decisions on his or her conscience.

**posterior:** The back surface of the body; the side away from you in the standard anatomic position.

**posterior tibial artery:** The artery just behind the medial malleolus; supplies blood to the foot.

**postictal state:** The period following a seizure that lasts 5 to 30 minutes; characterized by labored respirations and some degree of altered mental status.

**posttraumatic stress disorder (PTSD):** A delayed stress reaction to a prior incident. Often the result of one or more unresolved issues concerning the incident, and may relate to an incident that involved physical harm or the threat of physical harm.

**potential energy:** The product of mass, gravity, and height, which is converted into kinetic energy and results in injury, such as from a fall.

**power grip:** A technique in which the stretcher or backboard is gripped by inserting each hand under the handle with the palm facing up and the thumb extended, fully supporting the underside of the handle on the curved palm with the fingers and thumb.

**power lift:** A lifting technique in which the EMT's back is held upright, with legs bent, and the patient is lifted when the EMT straightens the legs to raise the upper body and arms.

**preconventional reasoning:** A type of reasoning in which a child acts almost purely to avoid punishment or to get what he or she wants.

**preeclampsia:** A pregnancy complication that is characterized by new-onset hypertension (systolic blood pressure >140 mm Hg or diastolic blood pressure >90 mm Hg) along with systemic effects, such as blurred vision, headache, or protein in the urine. Differentiated from eclampsia by the lack of seizure activity.

**prefix:** Part of a term that appears before a word root, changing the meaning of the term.

**preload:** The precontraction pressure in the heart as the volume of blood builds up.

**preoxygenation:** The process of providing oxygen, often in combination with ventilation, prior to intubation in order to raise the oxygen levels of body tissues; a critical step in advanced airway management. This extends the time during which an advanced airway can be placed in an patient with apnea, because the more oxygen that is available in the alveoli, the longer the patient can maintain adequate gas exchange in the lungs during the procedure.

**presbycusis:** An age-related condition of the ear that produces progressive bilateral hearing loss that is most noted at higher frequencies.

**preschool-age:** Children between ages 3 and 6 years.

**preschooler:** A child age 3 to 6 years.

**prescription medications:** Medications that are distributed to patients only by pharmacists according to a physician's order.

**presentation:** The position in which an infant is born; defined by the part of the body that appears first.

**primary assessment:** A step within the patient assessment process that identifies and initiates treatment of immediate and potential life threats.

**primary blast injury:** Injuries caused by an explosive pressure wave to the hollow organs of the body.

**primary (direct) injury:** An injury to the brain and its associated structures that is a direct result of impact to the head.

**primary prevention:** Efforts to prevent an injury or illness from ever occurring.

**primary service area:** The designated area in which the EMS agency is responsible for the provision of prehospital emergency care and transportation to the hospital.

**primary triage:** A type of patient sorting used to rapidly categorize patients; the focus is on speed in locating all patients and determining an initial priority as warranted by their conditions.

**primigravida:** A woman who is experiencing her first pregnancy.

**projectile:** Any object propelled by force, such as a bullet by a weapon.

**prolapse of the umbilical cord:** A situation in which the umbilical cord comes out of the vagina before the fetus.

**prone:** Lying face down.

**prostate gland:** A small gland that surrounds the male urethra where it emerges from the urinary bladder; it secretes a fluid that is part of the ejaculatory fluid.

**protected health information (PHI):** Any information about health status, provision of health care, or payment for health care that can be linked to an individual. This is interpreted rather broadly and includes any part of a patient's medical record or payment history.

**proximal:** Closer to the trunk.

**proximate causation:** When a person who has a duty abuses it, and causes harm to another individual, the EMT, the agency, and/or the medical director may be sued for negligence.

**psychiatric disorder:** An illness with psychological or behavioral symptoms and/or impairment in functioning caused by a social, psychological, genetic, physical, chemical, or biologic disturbance.

**psychogenic shock:** Shock caused by a sudden, temporary reduction in blood supply to the brain that causes fainting (syncope).

**psychosis:** A mental disorder characterized by the loss of contact with reality.

**pubic symphysis:** A hard, bony, and cartilaginous prominence found at the midline in the lowermost portion of the abdomen where the two halves of the pelvic ring are joined by cartilage at a joint with minimal motion.

**pubis:** One of three bones that fuse to form the pelvic ring.

**public health:** The branch of medicine that is focused on examining the health needs of entire populations with the goal of preventing health problems.

**public information officer (PIO):** In incident command, the person who keeps the public informed and relates any information to the media.

**public safety access point:** A call center, staffed by trained personnel who are responsible for managing requests for police, fire, and ambulance services.

**pulmonary artery:** The major artery leading from the right ventricle of the heart to the lungs; carries oxygen-poor blood.

**pulmonary blast injuries:** Pulmonary trauma resulting from short-range exposure to the detonation of high-energy explosives.

**pulmonary circulation:** The flow of blood from the right ventricle through the pulmonary arteries and all of their branches and capillaries in the lungs and back to the left atrium through the venules and pulmonary veins; also called the lesser circulation.

**pulmonary contusion:** Injury or bruising of lung tissue that results in hemorrhage.

**pulmonary edema:** A buildup of fluid in the lungs, often as a result of congestive heart failure.

**pulmonary embolism:** A blood clot that breaks off from a large vein and travels to the blood vessels of the lung, causing obstruction of blood flow.

**pulmonary veins:** The four veins that return oxygenated blood from the lungs to the left atrium of the heart.

**pulse:** The wave of pressure created as the heart contracts and forces blood out the left ventricle and into the major arteries.

**pulse oximetry:** An assessment tool that measures oxygen saturation of hemoglobin in the capillary beds.

**pulse pressure:** The difference between the systolic and diastolic pressures.

**punitive damages:** Damages that are sometimes awarded in a civil lawsuit when the conduct of the defendant was intentional or constituted a reckless disregard for the safety of the public.

**pupil:** The circular opening in the middle of the iris that admits light to the back of the eye.

**putrefaction:** Decomposition of body tissues; a definitive sign of death.

**quadrants:** The sections of the abdominal cavity, in which two imaginary lines intersect at the umbilicus, dividing the abdomen into four equal areas.

**quality control:** Oversight by the medical director to ensure the appropriate medical care standards are met by EMTs on each call.

**quaternary blast injury:** A blast injury that falls into one of the following categories: burns, crush injuries, toxic inhalation, medical emergencies, or mental health disorders.

**rabid:** Infected with rabies.

**raccoon eyes:** Bruising under the eyes that may indicate a skull fracture.

**radial artery:** The major artery in the forearm; it is palpable at the wrist on the thumb side.

**radiation:** The transfer of heat to colder objects in the environment by radiant energy; for example, heat gain from a fire.

**radioactive material:** Any material that emits radiation.

**radiologic dispersal device (RDD):** Any container that is designed to disperse radioactive material.

**radius:** The bone on the thumb side of the forearm.

**rape:** Sexual intercourse forcibly inflicted on another person, against that person's will.

**rapid extrication technique:** A technique to move a patient from a sitting position inside a vehicle to supine on a backboard in less than 1 minute when conditions do not allow for standard immobilization.

**rapport:** A trusting relationship that you build with your patient.

**reassessment:** A step within the patient assessment process performed at regular intervals during the assessment process to identify and treat changes in a patient's condition. A patient in unstable condition should be reassessed every 5 minutes, whereas a patient in stable condition should be reassessed every 15 minutes.

**recovery position:** A side-lying position used to maintain a clear airway in unresponsive patients who are breathing adequately and do not have suspected injuries to the spine, hips, or pelvis.

**rectum:** The lowermost end of the colon.

**red blood cells:** Cells that carry oxygen to the body's tissues; also called erythrocytes.

**reduce:** To return a dislocated joint or fractured bone to its normal position; to set.

**referred pain:** Pain felt in an area of the body other than the area where the cause of pain is located.

**rehabilitation area:** The area that provides protection and treatment to firefighters and other responders working at an emergency. Here, workers are medically monitored and receive any needed care as they enter and leave the scene.

**rehabilitation supervisor:** In incident command, the person who establishes an area that provides protection for responders from the elements and the situation.

**renal pelvis:** A cone-shaped area that collects urine from the kidneys and funnels it through the ureter into the bladder.

**repeater:** A special base station radio that receives messages and signals on one frequency and then automatically retransmits them on a second frequency.

**rescue supervisor:** In incident command, the person appointed to determine the type of equipment and resources needed for a situation involving extrication or special rescue; also called the extrication officer.

**residual volume:** The air that remains in the lungs after maximal expiration.

**resilience:** The capacity of an individual to cope with and recover from distress.

**res ipsa loquitur:** When the EMT or an EMS system is held liable even when the plaintiff is unable to clearly demonstrate how an injury occurred.

**respiration:** The process of exchanging oxygen and carbon dioxide.

**respiratory compromise:** The inability of the body to move gas effectively.

**respiratory syncytial virus (RSV):** A virus that causes an infection of the lungs and breathing passages; can lead to other serious illnesses that affect the lungs or heart, such as bronchiolitis and pneumonia. RSV is highly contagious and spread through droplets.

**respiratory system:** All the structures of the body that contribute to the process of breathing, consisting of the upper and lower airways and their component parts.

**responsiveness:** The way in which a patient responds to external stimuli, including verbal stimuli (sound), tactile stimuli (touch), and painful stimuli.

**reticular activating system (RAS):** Located in the upper brainstem; responsible for maintenance of consciousness, specifically one's level of arousal.

**retina:** The light-sensitive area of the eye where images are projected; a layer of cells at the back of the eye that changes the light image into electric impulses, which are carried by the optic nerve to the brain.

**retinal detachment:** Separation of the retina from its attachments at the back of the eye.

**retractions:** Movements in which the skin pulls in around the ribs during inspiration.

**retrograde amnesia:** The inability to remember events leading up to a head injury.

**retroperitoneal:** Behind the abdominal cavity.

**retroperitoneal space:** The space between the abdominal cavity and the posterior abdominal wall, containing the kidneys, certain large vessels, and parts of the gastrointestinal tract.

**retroperitoneum:** The potential space located posterior to the peritoneal cavity of the abdomen.

**return of spontaneous circulation (ROSC):** The return of a pulse and effective blood flow to the body in a patient who previously was in cardiac arrest.

**reverse triage:** A triage process used in treating multiple victims of a lightning strike, in which efforts are focused on those who are in respiratory and cardiac arrest. Reverse triage is different from conventional triage, where such patients would be classified as deceased.

**Revised Trauma Score (RTS):** A scoring system used for patients with head trauma.

**rhonchi:** Coarse, low-pitched breath sounds heard in patients with chronic mucus in the upper airways.

**ricin:** A neurotoxin derived from mash that is left from the castor bean; causes pulmonary edema and respiratory and circulatory failure leading to death.

**rigor mortis:** Stiffening of the body muscles; a definitive sign of death.

**rooting reflex:** An infant reflex that occurs when something touches an infant's cheek, and the infant instinctively turns his or her head toward the touch.

**route of exposure:** The manner by which a toxic substance enters the body.

**rule of nines:** A system that assigns percentages to sections of the body, allowing calculation of the amount of skin surface involved in the burn area.

**sacroiliac joint:** The connection point between the pelvis and the vertebral column.

**sacrum:** One of three bones (sacrum and two pelvic bones) that make up the pelvic ring; consists of five fused sacral vertebrae.

**safety officer:** In incident command, the person who monitors the scene for conditions or operations that may present a hazard to responders and patients; he or she may stop an operation when responder safety is an issue.

**safe zone:** An area of protection providing safety from the danger zone (hot zone).

**sagittal (lateral) plane:** An imaginary line where the body is divided into left and right parts.

**salivary glands:** The glands that produce saliva to keep the mouth and pharynx moist.

**SAMPLE history:** A brief history of a patient's condition to determine signs and symptoms, allergies, medications, pertinent past history, last oral intake, and events leading to the injury or illness.

**sarin (GB):** A nerve agent that is one of the G agents; a highly volatile colorless and odorless liquid that turns from liquid to gas within seconds to minutes at room temperature.

**scald burn:** A burn caused by hot liquids.

**scalp:** The thick skin covering the cranium, which usually bears hair.

**scanner:** A radio receiver that searches or scans across several frequencies until the message is completed; the process is then repeated.

**scapula:** The shoulder blade.

**scene size-up:** A step within the patient assessment process that involves a quick assessment of the scene and the surroundings to provide information about scene safety and the mechanism of injury or nature of illness before you enter and begin patient care.

**schizophrenia:** A complex, difficult-to-identify mental disorder whose onset typically occurs during early adulthood. Symptoms typically become more prominent over time and include delusions, hallucinations, a lack of interest in pleasure, and erratic speech.

**school age:** A person who is 6 to 12 years of age.

**sciatic nerve:** The major nerve to the lower extremities; controls much of muscle function in the leg and sensation in most of the leg and foot.

**sclera:** The tough, fibrous, white portion of the eye that protects the more delicate inner structures.

**scoop stretcher:** A stretcher that is designed to be split into two or four sections that can be fitted around a patient who is lying on the ground or other relatively flat surface; also called an orthopaedic stretcher.

**scope of practice:** Most commonly defined by state law; outlines the care that the EMT is able to provide for the patient.

**scuba gear:** A system that delivers air to the mouth and lungs at various atmospheric pressures, increasing with the depth of the dive; self-contained underwater breathing apparatus.

**sebaceous glands:** Glands that produce an oily substance called sebum, which discharges along the shafts of the hairs.

**secondary assessment:** A step within the patient assessment process in which a systematic physical examination of the patient is performed. The examination may be a systematic exam or an assessment that focuses on a certain area or region of the body, often determined through the chief complaint.

**secondary blast injury:** A penetrating or nonpenetrating injury caused by ordnance projectiles or secondary missiles.

**secondary containment:** An engineered method to control a spilled or released product if the main containment vessel fails.

**secondary device:** A secondary explosive used by terrorists, set to explode after the initial bomb.

**secondary (indirect) injury:** The aftereffects of the primary injury; includes abnormal processes such as cerebral edema, increased intracranial pressure, cerebral ischemia and hypoxia, and infection; onset is often delayed following the primary brain injury.

**secondary prevention:** Efforts to limit the effects of an injury or illness that you cannot completely prevent.

**secondary triage:** A type of patient sorting used in the treatment area that involves retriage of patients.

**sedative:** A substance that decreases activity and excitement.

**seizure:** A neurologic episode caused by a surge of electrical activity in the brain; can be a convulsion characterized by generalized, uncoordinated muscular activity, and can be associated with loss of consciousness.

**self-contained breathing apparatus (SCBA):** Respirator with independent air supply used by firefighters to enter toxic and otherwise dangerous atmospheres.

**semen:** Fluid ejaculated from the penis and containing sperm.

**seminal vesicles:** Storage sacs for sperm and seminal fluid, which empty into the urethra at the prostate.

**sensitization:** Developing a sensitivity to a substance that initially caused no allergic reaction.

**sensorineural deafness:** A permanent lack of hearing caused by a lesion or damage of the inner ear.

**sensory nerves:** The nerves that carry sensations such as touch, taste, smell, heat, cold, and pain from the body to the central nervous system.

**septic shock:** Shock caused by severe infection, usually a bacterial infection.

**severe airway obstruction:** Occurs when a foreign body completely obstructs the patient's airway. The patient cannot breathe, talk, or cough.

**sexual assault:** An attack against a person that is sexual in nature, the most common of which is rape.

**shaken baby syndrome:** A syndrome seen in abused infants and children; the patient has been subjected to violent, whiplash-type shaking injuries inflicted by the abusing individual that may cause coma, seizures, and increased intracranial pressure due to tearing of the cerebral veins with consequent bleeding into the brain.

**shallow respirations:** Respirations characterized by little movement of the chest wall (reduced tidal volume) or poor chest excursion.

**shock:** A condition in which the circulatory system fails to provide sufficient circulation to maintain normal cellular functions; also called hypoperfusion.

**shunts:** Tubes that drain excess cerebrospinal fluid from the brain to another part of the body outside of the brain, such as the abdomen; lowers pressure in the brain.

**sickle cell disease:** A hereditary disease that causes normal, round red blood cells to become oblong, or sickle shaped.

**sign:** Objective finding that can be seen, heard, felt, smelled, or measured.

**simple access:** Access that is easily achieved without the use of tools or force.

**simple pneumothorax:** Any pneumothorax that is free from significant physiologic changes and does not cause drastic changes in the vital signs of the patient.

**simplex:** Single-frequency radio; transmissions can occur in either direction but not simultaneously; when one party transmits, the other can only receive, and the party that is transmitting is unable to receive.

**single command system:** A command system in which one person is in charge; generally used with small incidents that involve only one responding agency or one jurisdiction.

**situational awareness:** Knowledge and understanding of one's surroundings and the ability to recognize potential risks to the safety of the patient or EMS team.

**size-up:** The ongoing process of information gathering and scene evaluation to determine appropriate strategies and tactics to manage an emergency.

**skeletal muscle:** Muscle that is attached to bones and usually crosses at least one joint; striated, or voluntary, muscle.

**skeletal system:** The framework of the body, composed of bones and other connective tissues, that supports and protects internal organs and other body tissues.

**slander:** False and damaging information about a person that is communicated by spoken word.

**sling:** A bandage or material that helps to support the weight of an injured upper extremity.

**small intestine:** The portion of the digestive tube between the stomach and the cecum, consisting of the duodenum, jejunum, and ileum.

**smallpox:** A highly contagious viral disease; it is most contagious when blisters begin to form.

**small-volume nebulizer:** A respiratory device that holds liquid medicine that is turned into a fine mist. The patient inhales the medication into the airways and lungs as a treatment for conditions such as asthma.

**smooth muscle:** Involuntary muscle; it constitutes the bulk of the gastrointestinal tract and is present in nearly every organ to regulate automatic activity.

**sniffing position:** An upright position in which the patient's head and chin are thrust slightly forward to keep the airway open.

**solid organs:** Solid masses of tissue where much of the chemical work of the body takes place (eg, the liver, spleen, pancreas, and kidneys).

**solution:** A liquid mixture that cannot be separated by filtering or allowing the mixture to stand.

**soman (GD):** A nerve agent that is one of the G agents; twice as persistent as sarin and five times as lethal; it has a fruity odor as a result of the type of alcohol used in the agent, and is a contact and an inhalation hazard that can enter the body through skin absorption and through the respiratory tract.

**somatic nervous system:** The part of the nervous system that regulates activities over which there is voluntary control.

**span of control:** In incident command, the subordinate positions under the commander's direction to which the workload is distributed; the ideal supervisor/worker ratio is one supervisor for five subordinates.

**Special Atomic Demolition Munitions (SADM):** Small suitcase-sized nuclear weapons that were designed to destroy individual targets, such as important buildings, bridges, tunnels, and large ships.

**special weapons and tactics (SWAT) team:** A specialized law enforcement tactical unit.

**sphincters:** Muscles that encircle and, by contracting, constrict a duct, tube, or opening. Examples are found within the rectum, bladder, and blood vessels.

**sphygmomanometer:** A device used to measure blood pressure.

**spina bifida:** A development defect in which a portion of the spinal cord or meninges may protrude outside of the vertebrae and possibly even outside of the body, usually at the lower third of the spine in the lumbar area.

**spinal cord:** An extension of the brain, composed of virtually all the nerves carrying messages between the brain and the rest of the body. It lies inside of and is protected by the spinal canal.

**splint:** A flexible or rigid device used to protect and maintain the position of an injured extremity.

**spontaneous abortion:** The loss of a pregnancy prior to 20 weeks of gestation without any preceding surgical or medical intervention. Often called a miscarriage.

**spontaneous pneumothorax:** A pneumothorax that occurs when a weak area on the lung ruptures in the absence of major injury, allowing air to leak into the pleural space.

**spontaneous respirations:** Breathing that occurs without assistance.

**spotter:** A person who assists a driver in backing up an ambulance to help adjust for blind spots at the back of the vehicle.

**sprain:** A joint injury involving damage to supporting ligaments, and sometimes partial or temporary dislocation of bone ends.

**staging supervisor:** In incident command, the person who locates an area to stage equipment and personnel and tracks unit arrival and deployment from the staging area.

**stair chair:** A lightweight folding device that is used to carry a conscious, seated patient up or down stairs.

**standard of care:** Written, accepted levels of emergency care expected by reason of training and profession; written by legal or professional organizations so that patients are not exposed to unreasonable risk or harm.

**standard precautions:** Protective measures that have traditionally been developed by the Centers for Disease Control and Prevention (CDC) for use in dealing with objects, blood, body fluids, and other potential exposure risks of communicable disease.

**standing orders:** Written documents, signed by the EMS system's medical director, that outline specific directions, permissions, and sometimes prohibitions regarding patient care; also called protocols.

**Star of Life:** The six-pointed star emblem that identifies vehicles that meet federal specifications as licensed or certified ambulances.

**START triage:** A patient sorting process that stands for Simple Triage And Rapid Treatment and uses a limited assessment of the patient's ability to walk, respiratory status, hemodynamic status, and neurologic status.

**state-sponsored terrorism:** Terrorism that is funded and/or supported by nations that hold close ties with terrorist groups.

**status epilepticus:** A condition in which seizures recur every few minutes or last longer than 30 minutes.

**statute of limitations:** The time within which a legal case must be commenced.

**steam burn:** A burn caused by exposure to hot steam.

**sterilization:** A process, such as heating, that removes microbial contamination.

**sternocleidomastoid muscles:** The muscles on either side of the neck that allow movement of the head.

**sternum:** The breast bone.

**stimulant:** An agent that produces an excited state.

**stoma:** An opening through the skin and into an organ or other structure.

**strain:** Stretching or tearing of a muscle; also called a muscle pull.

**strangulation:** Complete obstruction of blood circulation in a given organ as a result of compression or entrapment; an emergency situation causing death of tissue.

**stratum corneum:** The outermost or dead layer of the skin.

**stridor:** A harsh, high-pitched respiratory sound, generally heard during inspiration, that is caused by partial blockage or narrowing of the upper airway; may be audible without a stethoscope.

**stroke:** An interruption of blood flow to the brain that results in the loss of brain function; also called a cerebrovascular accident (CVA).

**stroke volume (SV):** The volume of blood pumped forward with each ventricular contraction.

**structure fire:** A fire in a house, apartment building, office, school, plant, warehouse, or other building.

**subarachnoid hemorrhage:** Bleeding into the subarachnoid space, where the cerebrospinal fluid circulates.

**subcutaneous emphysema:** A characteristic crackling sensation felt on palpation of the skin, caused by the presence of air in soft tissues.

**subcutaneous injection:** Injection into the fatty tissue between the skin and muscle; a medication delivery route.

**subcutaneous tissue:** Tissue, largely fat, that lies directly under the dermis and serves as an insulator of the body.

**subdural hematoma:** An accumulation of blood beneath the dura mater but outside the brain.

**sublingual (SL):** Under the tongue; a medication delivery route.

**substance abuse:** The misuse of any substance to produce a desired effect.

**sucking chest wound:** An open or penetrating chest wall wound through which air passes during inspiration and expiration, creating a sucking sound. See also *open pneumothorax*.

**sucking reflex:** An infant reflex in which the infant starts sucking when his or her lips are stroked.

**suction catheter:** A hollow, cylindrical device used to remove fluid from the patient's airway.

**sudden infant death syndrome (SIDS):** Death of an infant or young child that remains unexplained after a complete autopsy.

**suffix:** The part of a term that comes after the word root, at the end of the term.

**sulfur mustard (H):** A vesicant; it is a brown-yellow oily substance that is generally considered very persistent; has the distinct smell of garlic or mustard and, when released, is quickly absorbed into the skin and/or mucous membranes and begins an irreversible process of damaging the cells. Also called mustard gas.

**superficial:** Closer to or on the skin.

**superficial (first-degree) burns:** Burns that affect only the epidermis, characterized by skin that is red but not blistered or actually burned through.

**superior:** Above a body part or nearer to the head.

**superior vena cava:** One of the two largest veins in the body; carries blood from the upper extremities, head, neck, and chest into the heart.

**supine:** Lying face up.

**supine hypotensive syndrome:** Low blood pressure resulting from compression of the inferior vena cava by the weight of the pregnant uterus when the woman is supine.

**surfactant:** A liquid protein substance that coats the alveoli in the lungs, decreases alveolar surface tension, and keeps the alveoli expanded; a low level in a premature infant contributes to respiratory distress syndrome.

**suspension:** A mixture of ground particles that are distributed evenly throughout a liquid but do not dissolve.

**swathe:** A bandage that passes around the chest to secure an injured arm to the chest.

**sweat glands:** The glands that secrete sweat, located in the dermal layer of the skin.

**sympathetic nervous system:** The part of the autonomic nervous system that controls active functions such as responding to fear (also known as the fight-or-flight system).

**symphyses:** Joints that have grown together to form a very stable connection.

**symptom:** Subjective findings that the patient feels but that can be identified only by the patient.

**symptomatic hyperglycemia:** A state of unconsciousness resulting from several problems, including ketoacidosis, dehydration because of excessive urination, and hyperglycemia.

**symptomatic hypoglycemia:** Severe hypoglycemia resulting in changes in mental status.

**syncope:** A fainting spell or transient loss of consciousness.

**syndromic surveillance:** The monitoring, usually by local or state health departments, of patients presenting to emergency departments and alternative care facilities, the recording of EMS call volume, and the use of over-the-counter medications.

**synovial fluid:** The small amount of liquid within a joint used as lubrication.

**synovial membrane:** The lining of a joint that secretes synovial fluid into the joint space.

**systemic circulation:** The portion of the circulatory system outside of the heart and lungs.

**systemic vascular resistance (SVR):** The resistance that blood must overcome to be able to move within the blood vessels; related to the amount of dilation or constriction in the blood vessel.

**systole:** The contraction, or period of contraction, of the heart, especially that of the ventricles.

**systolic pressure:** The increased pressure in an artery with each contraction of the ventricles (systole).

**tabun (GA):** A nerve agent that is one of the G agents; 36 times more persistent than sarin and approximately one-half as lethal; has a fruity smell and is unique because the components used to manufacture the agent are easy to acquire and the agent is easy to manufacture.

**tachycardia:** A rapid heart rate, more than 100 beats/min.

**tachypnea:** Rapid respirations.

**tactical situation:** A hostage, robbery, or other situation in which armed conflict is threatened or shots have been fired and the threat of violence remains.

**tarsals:** The group of bones situated between the lower leg bones (ie, tibia and fibula) and the metatarsal bones of the foot.

**team:** In the context of EMS, a group of health care providers who are assigned specific roles and are working interdependently in a coordinated manner under a designated leader.

**team leader:** The team member who provides role assignments, coordination, oversight, centralized decision making, and support for the team to accomplish their goals and achieve desired results.

**technical rescue group:** A team of emergency responders from one or more departments in a region who are trained and on call for certain types of technical rescue.

**technical rescue situation:** A rescue that requires special technical skills and equipment in one of many specialized rescue areas, such as technical rope rescue, cave rescue, and dive rescue.

**telemetry:** A process in which electronic signals are converted into coded, audible signals; these signals can then be transmitted by radio or telephone to a receiver with a decoder at the hospital.

**temporal bones:** The lateral bones on each side of the cranium; the temples.

**temporomandibular joint:** The joint formed where the mandible and cranium meet, just in front of the ear.

**tendons:** The fibrous connective tissue that attaches muscle to bone.

**tension pneumothorax:** An accumulation of air or gas in the pleural cavity that progressively increases pressure in the chest and that interferes with cardiac function, with potentially fatal results.

**termination of command:** The end of the incident command structure when an incident draws to a close.

**tertiary blast injury:** An injury from whole-body displacement and subsequent traumatic impact with environmental objects.

**testicle:** A male genital gland that contains specialized cells that produce hormones and sperm.

**therapeutic communication:** Verbal and nonverbal communication techniques that encourage patients to express their feelings and to achieve a positive relationship.

**therapeutic effect:** The desired or intended effect a medication is expected to have on the body.

**thermal burn:** A burn caused by heat.

**thoracic cage:** The chest or rib cage.

**thoracic spine:** The 12 vertebrae that lie between the cervical vertebrae and the lumbar vertebrae. One pair of ribs is attached to each of these vertebrae.

**thorax:** The chest cavity that contains the heart, lungs, esophagus, and great vessels.

**thromboembolism:** A blood clot that has formed within a blood vessel and is floating within the bloodstream.

**thrombophilia:** A tendency toward the development of blood clots as a result of an abnormality of the system of coagulation.

**thrombosis:** A blood clot, either in the arterial or venous system. When the clot occurs in a cerebral artery, it may result in the interruption of cerebral blood flow and subsequent stroke.

**thyroid cartilage:** A firm prominence of cartilage that forms the upper part of the larynx; the Adam's apple.

**tibia:** The shinbone; the larger of the two bones of the lower leg.

**tidal volume:** The amount of air (in milliliters) that is moved into or out of the lungs during one breath.

**toddler:** A child age 1 to 3 years.

**tolerance:** The need for increasing amounts of a drug to obtain the same effect.

**tonsil tips:** Large, semirigid suction tips recommended for suctioning the pharynx.

**topical medications:** Lotions, creams, and ointments that are applied to the surface of the skin and affect only that area; a medication delivery route.

**topographic anatomy:** The superficial landmarks of the body that serve as guides to the structures that lie beneath them.

**torts:** Wrongful acts that give rise to a civil lawsuit.

**tourniquet:** The bleeding control method used when a wound continues to bleed despite the use of direct pressure; useful if a patient is bleeding severely from a partial or complete amputation.

**toxicity levels:** Indicates the risk that a hazardous material poses to the health of an individual who comes into contact with it.

**toxicology:** The study of toxic or poisonous substances.

**toxin:** A poison or harmful substance.

**trachea:** The windpipe; the main trunk for air passing to and from the lungs.

**tracheitis:** Inflammation of the trachea.

**tracheostomy:** A surgical procedure to create an opening (stoma) into the trachea; a stoma in the neck connects the trachea directly to the skin.

**tracheostomy tube:** A plastic tube placed within the tracheostomy site (stoma).

**traction:** Longitudinal force applied to a structure.

**trade name:** The brand name that a manufacturer gives a medication; the name is capitalized.

**tragus:** The small, rounded, fleshy bulge that lies immediately anterior to the ear canal.

**trajectory:** The path a projectile takes once it is propelled.

**transcutaneous (transdermal):** Through the skin; a medication delivery route.

**transient ischemic attack (TIA):** A disorder of the brain in which brain cells temporarily stop functioning because of insufficient oxygen, causing strokelike symptoms that resolve completely within 24 hours of onset.

**transmission:** The way in which an infectious disease is spread: contact, airborne, by vehicles, or by vectors.

**transportation area:** The area in a mass-casualty incident where ambulances and crews are organized to transport patients from the treatment area to receiving hospitals.

**transportation supervisor:** In incident command, the person in charge of the transportation sector in a mass-casualty incident who assigns patients from the treatment area to waiting ambulances in the transportation area.

**transverse (axial) plane:** An imaginary line where the body is divided into top and bottom parts.

**trauma emergencies:** Emergencies that are the result of physical forces applied to the body; injuries.

**trauma score:** A score calculated from 1 to 16, with 16 being the best possible score. It relates to the likelihood of patient survival, with the exception of a severe head injury. It takes into account the Glasgow Coma Scale (GCS) score, respiratory rate, respiratory expansion, systolic blood pressure, and capillary refill.

**traumatic asphyxia:** A pattern of injuries seen after a severe force is applied to the chest, forcing blood from the great vessels back into the head and neck.

**traumatic brain injury (TBI):** A traumatic insult to the brain capable of producing physical, intellectual, emotional, social, and vocational changes.

**treatment area:** The location in a mass-casualty incident where patients are brought after being triaged and assigned a priority, where they are reassessed, treated, and monitored until transport to the hospital.

**treatment supervisor:** In incident command, the person, usually a physician, who is in charge of and directs EMS providers at the treatment area in a mass-casualty incident.

**triage:** The process of establishing treatment and transportation priorities according to severity of injury and medical need.

**triage supervisor:** In incident command, the person in charge of the incident command triage sector who directs the sorting of patients into triage categories in a mass-casualty incident.

**triceps:** The muscle in the back of the upper arm.

**tripod position:** An upright position in which the patient leans forward onto two arms stretched forward and thrusts the head and chin forward.

**trunking:** Telecommunication systems that allow a computer to maximize utilization of a group of frequencies.

**trust versus mistrust:** The stage of development from birth to approximately 18 months of age, during which infants gain trust in their parents or caregivers if their world is planned, organized, and routine.

**tuberculosis (TB):** A chronic bacterial disease, caused by *Mycobacterium tuberculosis*, that usually affects the lungs but can also affect other organs such as the brain and kidneys; it is spread by cough and can lie dormant in a person's lungs for decades and then reactivate.

**tunica media:** The middle and thickest layer of tissue of a blood vessel wall, composed of elastic tissue and smooth muscle cells that allow the vessel to expand or contract in response to changes in blood pressure and tissue demand.

**turbinates:** Layers of bone within the nasal cavity.

**turgor:** The ability of the skin to resist deformation; tested by gently pinching skin on the forehead or back of the hand.

**two- to three-word dyspnea:** A severe breathing problem in which a patient can speak only two to three words at a time without pausing to take a breath.

**tympanic membrane:** The eardrum; a thin, semi-transparent membrane in the middle ear that transmits sound vibrations to the internal ear by means of auditory ossicles.

**type 1 diabetes:** An autoimmune disorder in which the individual's immune system produces antibodies to the pancreatic beta cells, and therefore the pancreas cannot produce insulin; onset in early childhood is common.

**type 2 diabetes:** A condition in which insulin resistance develops in response to increased blood glucose levels; can be managed by exercise and diet modification, but is often managed by medications.

**UHF (ultra-high frequency):** Radio frequencies between 300 and 3,000 MHz.

**ulna:** The inner bone of the forearm, on the side opposite the thumb.

**umbilical cord:** The structure that connects the pregnant woman to the fetus via the placenta; contains two arteries and one vein.

**umbilicus:** The navel; also called the belly button.

**unified command system:** A command system used in larger incidents in which there is a multiagency response or multiple jurisdictions are involved.

**unintended effects:** Actions that are undesirable but pose little risk to the patient.

**untoward effects:** Actions that can be harmful to the patient.

**uremia:** Severe kidney failure resulting in the buildup of waste products within the blood. Eventually brain functions will be impaired.

**ureter:** A small, hollow tube that carries urine from the kidneys to the bladder.

**urethra:** The canal that conveys urine from the bladder to outside the body.

**urinary bladder:** A sac behind the pubic symphysis made of smooth muscle that collects and stores urine.

**urinary system:** The organs that control the discharge of certain waste materials filtered from the blood and excreted as urine.

**urinary tract infection (UTI):** An infection, usually of the lower urinary tract (urethra and bladder), that occurs when normal flora bacteria enter the urethra and grow.

**urostomy:** A surgical procedure to create an opening (stoma) that connects the urinary system to the surface of the skin and allows urine to drain through the abdominal wall.

**urticaria:** Small areas of generalized itching and/or burning that appear as multiple raised areas on the skin; hives.

**uterus:** The muscular organ where the fetus grows; also called the womb; responsible for contractions during labor.

**V agent (VX):** One of the G agents; it is a clear, oily agent that has no odor and looks like baby oil; more than 100 times more lethal than sarin and extremely persistent.

**vagina:** The outermost cavity of a woman's reproductive tract; the lower part of the birth canal.

**vancomycin-resistant enterococci (VRE):** Bacteria that are normally present in the human intestines and the female reproductive tract, but which can cause infection and which are resistant to the antibiotic vancomycin.

**vapor hazard:** The term used to describe danger posed by an agent that enters the body through the respiratory tract.

**vasoconstriction:** Narrowing of a blood vessel.

**vasoocclusive crisis:** Ischemia and pain caused by sickle-shaped red blood cells that obstruct blood flow to a portion of the body.

**vector-borne transmission:** The use of an animal to spread an organism from one person or place to another.

**veins:** The blood vessels that carry blood from the tissues to the heart.

**vented chest seal:** An occlusive dressing designed to allow air to escape through the dressing but not be drawn back in.

**ventilation:** The exchange of air between the lungs and the environment; occurs spontaneously by the patient or with assistance from another person, such as an EMT.

**ventral:** The anterior surface of the body.

**ventricle:** One of the two lower chambers of the heart.

**ventricular fibrillation:** Disorganized, ineffective quivering of the ventricles, resulting in no blood flow and a state of cardiac arrest.

**ventricular tachycardia:** A rapid heart rhythm in which the electrical impulse begins in the ventricle (instead of the atria), which may result in inadequate blood flow and eventually deteriorate into cardiac arrest.

**venules:** Very small, thin-walled blood vessels.

**vernix caseosa:** A white, cheesy substance that covers the body of the fetus.

**vertebrae:** The bones of the vertebral column.

**vertebral column:** The structure formed by the 33 vertebrae, separated by intervertebral disks. It houses and protects the spinal cord; also called the spinal column.

**vertex presentation:** A delivery in which the head of the newborn comes out first.

**vesicants:** Blister agents; the primary route of entry for such agents is through the skin.

**vesicular breath sounds:** Normal breath sounds made by air moving in and out of the alveoli.

**VHF (very high frequency):** Radio frequencies between 30 and 300 MHz; the VHF spectrum is further divided into high and low bands.

**video laryngoscopy:** Visualization of the vocal cords, and thereby placement of the endotracheal tube, that is facilitated by use of a video camera and monitor.

**viral hemorrhagic fevers:** A group of diseases caused by viruses that include the Ebola, Rift Valley, and yellow fever viruses, among others. This group of viruses causes the blood in the body to seep out from the tissues and blood vessels.

**virulence:** The strength or ability of a pathogen to produce disease.

**viruses:** Germs that require a living host to multiply and survive.

**visceral pleura:** Thin membrane that covers the lungs.

**vital capacity:** The amount of air that can be forcibly expelled from the lungs after breathing in as deeply as possible.

**vital signs:** The key signs that are used to evaluate the patient's overall condition, including respirations, pulse, blood pressure, level of consciousness, and skin characteristics.

**vocal cords:** Thin white bands of tough muscular tissue that are lateral borders of the glottis and serve as the primary center for speech production.

**volatility:** How long a chemical agent will stay on a surface before it evaporates.

**voluntary activities:** Actions that we consciously perform, in which sensory input or conscious thought determines a specific muscular activity.

**voluntary muscle:** Muscle that is under direct voluntary control of the brain and can be contracted or relaxed at will; skeletal, or striated, muscle.

**V̇/Q̇ ratio:** A measurement that examines how much gas is being moved effectively and how much blood is flowing around the alveoli where gas exchange (perfusion) occurs.

**warm zone:** The area located between the hot zone and the cold zone at a hazardous materials incident. The decontamination corridor is located in this zone.

**weaponization:** The creation of a weapon from a biologic agent that is generally found in nature and that causes disease; the agent is cultivated, synthesized, and/or mutated to maximize the target population's exposure to the germ.

**weapon of mass casualty (WMC):** Any agent designed to bring about mass death, casualties, and/or massive damage to property and infrastructure (bridges, tunnels, airports, and seaports); also known as a weapon of mass destruction (WMD).

**weapon of mass destruction (WMD):** Any agent designed to bring about mass death, casualties, and/or massive damage to property and infrastructure (bridges, tunnels, airports, and seaports); also known as a weapon of mass casualty (WMC).

**wellness:** The active pursuit of a state of good health.

**wheal:** A raised, swollen, well-defined area on the skin resulting from an insect bite or allergic reaction.

**wheeled ambulance stretcher:** A specially designed stretcher that can be rolled along the ground. A collapsible undercarriage allows it to be loaded into the ambulance; also called an ambulance stretcher.

**wheezing:** A high-pitched, whistling breath sound that is most prominent on expiration, and which suggests an obstruction or narrowing of the lower airways; occurs in asthma and bronchiolitis.

**white blood cells:** Blood cells that have a role in the body's immune defense mechanisms against infection; also called leukocytes.

**word root:** The main part of a term that contains the primary meaning.

**work:** The measure of force over distance.

**work of breathing:** An indicator of oxygenation and ventilation; reflects the child's attempt to compensate for hypoxia.

**xiphoid process:** The narrow, cartilaginous lower tip of the sternum.

**zone of injury:** The area of potentially damaged soft tissue, adjacent nerves, and blood vessels surrounding an injury to a bone or a joint.

**zygomas:** The quadrangular bones of the cheek, articulating with the frontal bone, the maxillae, the zygomatic processes of the temporal bone, and the great wings of the sphenoid bone.

# Index

## A

AAA. See abdominal aortic aneurysm
abandonment, 101–102, 113
abbreviations, medical terminology,
    174–175
ABCs assessment. See under specific
    emergencies
abdomen, 226–228
    anatomy, 756f, 756–758
    emergencies, 760t
    focused assessment, 379, 379f
    hollow organs in, 1119–1121, 1120f
    injuries. See abdominal injuries
    pain, sudden onset of. See acute
        abdomen
    physical examination, 769, 769f, 1305
    postdelivery massage, 1264, 1265f
    quadrants, 1119, 1119f
    solid organs, 1119–1121, 1120f
abdominal aortic aneurysm (AAA)
    definition of, 1387
    in elderly, 1362
abdominal injuries. See also specific
    abdominal injuries
    assessment, 920–922, 1135–1137
        chief complaint investigation, 1126
        history taking, 1126–1127
        mechanism of injury/nature of
            illness, 1125
        primary, 1135–1136
        reassessment, 1129
        scene size-up, 1135
        secondary, 1127–1128
        of vital signs, 1128
    closed/blunt, 1121–1122, 1121f
    emergency medical care,
        1121–1122, 1130f
    interventions, 1129
    open/penetrating, 1122–1123, 1122f,
        1129–1131, 1130f
    pathophysiology, 1121
    pediatric, 1333, 1334f
    safety, on-scene, 1135
    from seat belts and airbags,
        1121–1122, 1122f
    transport decisions, 1126–1127
    wounds, emergency medical care,
        977–978, 978f
abdominal-thrust maneuver (Heimlich
    maneuver)
    definition of, 600

technique, 588, 588f, 600
abduction, definition of, 172, 187, 1171
abortion, spontaneous. See miscarriage,
    spontaneous abortion
abrasion, 967, 967f, 1002
abruptio placenta, 1249, 1249f, 1251
absorption, 498
    definition of, 35
    of toxins, 827–828, 828f
abuse
    of children. See child abuse
    of elderly. See elder abuse
    sexual. See sexual abuse
acceptance, in grieving process, 68
access
    definition of, 1466, 1483
    for extrication, 1470–1472, 1471f
        complex, 1472, 1483
        simple, 1472, 1472f
accessory muscles, 356, 410
Accidental Death and Disability: The
    Neglected Disease of Modern
    Society, 8
acetaminophen poisoning, 843
acidosis, 646, 671
    definition of, 434, 789, 801
    hyperventilation and, 646
    metabolic. See metabolic acidosis
acquired immunodeficiency syndrome
    (AIDS), 614–615
acromioclavicular (AC) joint,
    1170, 1196
acromioclavicular joint separation, 1170
ACS (acute coronary syndrome),
    685–688, 720
action, definition of, 496
active compression-decompression
    CPR, 573–575, 600
active shooter, 1479
active shooter event, 1530, 1557
activities of daily living (ADLs),
    855, 878, 1368
acute abdomen
    causes of, 758–759
    definition of, 758, 775
    gynecologic problems and, 766
    physical examination, 768, 769f
    signs/symptoms, 769
acute chest syndrome, 794
acute coronary syndrome (ACS),
    685–688, 720
acute kidney injury (AKI), 765

acute myocardial infarction (AMI)
    consequences, 687
    definition of, 685, 720
    pain of, 686–687
    physical findings, 687
    signs/symptoms, 686–688
    silent, 687
acute psychosis, 862–863
acute stress reactions, 70
Adam's apple, 1007
addiction, 834, 851
adduction, definition of, 172, 187, 1172
ADLs (activities of daily living),
    855, 878, 1368
adolescents
    assessment, 1289–1290, 1289f
    with behavioral disorders, 869
    definition of, 261, 271, 1289, 1347
    interviews with, 262
    physical changes, 261, 261f
    psychosocial changes, 262, 262f
    sexually transmitted diseases
        and, 885
    vital signs, 261
adrenaline. See epinephrine
adults
    early
        definition of, 263, 271
        physical changes, 263, 263f
        psychosocial changes, 263
        vital signs, 263
    late. See also elderly
        psychosocial changes, 268f
    middle
        definition of, 263, 271
        physical changes, 263–264, 263f
        psychosocial changes, 264
    older
        cardiovascular system, 264
        definition of, 271
        digestive systems, 266
        endocrine system of, 266
        nervous systems, 266–267, 267f
        psychosocial changes, 267–268
        renal systems, 266
        respiratory system, 265–266
        sensory changes, 267
Advair (fluticasone), 658t
advance directives, 93, 113,
    1380–1381, 1387
advanced life support (ALS), definition
    of, 4, 27, 558, 600

adventitious breath sounds, 650, 651*t*, 671

adverse effects, 497

AEIOU-TIPS mnemonic, 736

aerobic metabolism
  definition of, 488
  internal respiration and, 428

afterload
  definition of, 536, 552

age/aging
  communication and, 119
  of nerve agents, 1537–1540, 1557
  related changes
    cardiovascular system, 264–265, 1354–1357, 1355*f*
    endocrine system, 1363
    gastrointestinal system, 1360–1362
    immune system, 1363
    moving elderly patients and, 307
    musculoskeletal system, 1364–1365
    nervous system, 1357–1360
    renal system, 1362–1363
    respiratory system, 1353–1354

agitated delirium, 864

agonal gasps, 433, 488

agonist, 496

AHA (American Heart Association), basic life support standards, 99, 100*f*

AICD (automatic implantable cardiac defibrillator), 704, 704*f*

AIDS (acquired immunodeficiency syndrome), 614–615

air ambulances, definition of, 1453, 1453*f*, 1462

airbags, 1465
  abdominal injuries from, 1121–1122, 1122*f*
  vehicular collisions and, 907

airborne diseases. *See also specific airborne diseases*
  transmission, definition of, 39, 82

air embolism
  in ascent injuries, 1222
  causes, 1032
  definition of, 1037, 1222, 1239
  pathophysiology, 979, 980*f*

air medical operations
  air ambulances, 1453–1454, 1453*f*, 1462
  communication with other agencies, 1457, 1457*f*
  hand signals, 1456, 1457*f*
  landings
    at night, 1458
    on uneven ground, 1458, 1458*f*
  landing zones
    establishing, 1455–1456
    patient transfer in, 1456–1457
    safety considerations, 1456–1457, 1457*f*
  medical evacuations, 1454–1455

air splints, 1167

airway
  anatomy
    in adults, 265–266
    in children, 1290–1292, 1291*f*
  artificial. *See* airway adjuncts
  assessment, 431–439, 432*t*, 433*f*, 434*f*
  assessment, patient position for, 1297–1298, 1297*f*
  assisting with ALS procedures, 477–482
  breathing and. *See* breathing
  definition of, 488
  emergency medical care
    head injuries, 1062
    spinal injuries, 1064
  evaluation/assessment, 354–355
    in ABCDEs assessment. *See under specific emergencies*
    of infants, 255–256
    in infants/children, 582–583
    of restrained patient, 865–866
  infections
    management of, 662
  inhalation injury, 987–988
  lower, 629*f*
    anatomy of, 420–423, 422*f*
    infection of, 632*t*
    inhalation injuries, 992
    obstruction of, 634
  management, 418, 449–451
    artificial ventilation. *See* artificial ventilation
    in brain-injured patient, 1062
    with continuous positive airway pressure or CPAP, 469–474
    dentures and, 477
    with gastric distention, 467
    recovery position for, 449
    stomas and, 474
    suctioning. *See* suctioning
    supplemental oxygen for. *See* oxygen, supplemental
    supraglottic devices for, 480*f*
    tracheostomy tubes and, 474, 474*f*
  management equipment, in ambulances, 1427–1430, 1428*t*, 1429*f*
  obstruction. *See* airway obstruction
  opening, 439–442
    in adults, 566–569, 566*f*
    head tilt–chin lift maneuver for, 440, 566, 566*f*
    jaw-thrust maneuver for, 441–442
    in unresponsive patient, 439
  problems, 354
  suctioning
    equipment for, 443, 444*f*
    techniques for, 444–446
  upper, 628, 629*f*
    anatomy of, 418–420, 419*f*
    infection of, 632*t*
    obstruction of, 634

airway adjuncts, 446–449, 446*f*
  nasal. *See* nasopharyngeal (nasal) airway
  oropharyngeal, 446–448, 446*f*
  for pediatric emergencies, 1313–1316, 1313*t*

airway obstruction
  causes, 645*f*
  from facial fractures, 1030–1031
  from foreign body. *See* foreign bodies, airway obstruction
  in infants/children, 1308–1310
  management, 662
  mild, 587
  in responsive patients, 587
  in unresponsive patients, 355, 439, 440*f*, 587–588, 589–590

AKI (acute kidney injury), 765

albuterol
  indications/contraindications, 658*t*
  pediatric dose, 1311

alcohol
  consumption, history taking, 370–371, 370*f*
  intoxication, history taking and, 374
  poisoning from, 834–836, 843
  workplace abuse, 77

alcoholism, 834–836

algorithms
  automated external defibrillation, 715*f*
  life-threatening opioid overdose, 837*f*
  neonatal resuscitation, 1267*f*

algor mortis, 96, 113

alkalosis, 646, 671
  causes of, 646

allergens, 804
  categories of, 806–808
  definition of, 642, 671, 819

allergic reactions, 804
  *vs.* anaphylaxis, 804
  definition of, 819
  epinephrine administration for, 813–816
  to medication, 806, 806*f*
  severe, categories of, 538
  signs/symptoms, 810*t*
  source, 808

alpha radiation, 1549, 1557

altered mental status, 353, 410, 735, 752, 857, 878. *See also* mental status, alteration

alternative fuel vehicles, 1470

Alupent (metaproterenol), 658*t*

alveolar minute volume, 425*t*, 488

alveolar ventilation, 488

alveoli (air sacs), during respiration, 629, 629*f*

Alzheimer disease, 860, 1359

ambient temperature, 1202, 1239

ambulance calls, phases, 1426*t*
  arrival at scene, 1437–1440, 1438*f*
  delivery, 1441, 1442*f*
  dispatch, 1436, 1436*f*

en route to scene, 1437
en route to station, 1442, 1442*f*
postrun, 1442–1443
preparation. *See* ambulances,
    preparation
safe parking, 1438–1440, 1439*f*
traffic control, 1440
transfer, 1440, 1440*f*
ambulance drivers
    characteristics, 1443–1444
    fatigue, 1453
ambulances
    air. *See* air ambulances
    cleaning, 1442, 1462
    crashes, 1447
    daily inspections, 1435
    defensive driving techniques,
        1443–1453, 1446*t*
    definition of, 1424, 1462
    designs, 1424, 1424*f*, 1426*t*
    disinfection, 1442, 1462
    driving
        backing up, 1448
        road positioning and cornering,
            1448–1449, 1449*f*
        size and distance judgment, 1448
    extrication equipment, 1434, 1434*t*
    features, 1424
    jump kit, 1432–1433, 1433*f*, 1433*t*,
        1462
    licensing specifications, 1425, 1425*f*
    loading wheeled stretcher onto,
        290–291, 290*f*
    personnel, 1435
    police escorts, 1451–1452
    preparation
        medical equipment, 1427–1433,
            1428*t*, 1429–1433*f*, 1433*t*
        storage of equipment/supplies,
            1427, 1427*f*
        preplanning/navigation equipment,
            1434
    right-of-way privileges, 1451
    safety/operations equipment,
        1433–1434
    safety precautions, 1435
    work areas, equipment for,
        1433–1434, 1434*f*
American Heart Association (AHA),
    basic life support standards,
    99, 100*f*
American National Standards Institute
    (ANSI), 61
American Sign Language, 1398, 1398*f*
American Standard Safety System,
    453, 488
Americans With Disabilities Act of 1990,
    7, 27
AMI. *See* acute myocardial infarction
amniotic fluid, 1245
amniotic sac, 1245
    definition of, 1245, 1278
    unruptured, 1263
amphetamines, 839–840

amputations, 1158, 1196
    bleeding control, 1191
    definition of, 968, 1002, 1191
anaerobic metabolism
    definition of, 488
    internal respiration and, 428
anaphylactic reactions,
    643–644, 663
anaphylactic shock
    causes, 544*t*
    definition of, 538, 552
    pediatric, 1321–1322
    signs/symptoms, 539*t*, 544*t*
    treatment, 544*t*, 546
anaphylaxis, 538, 643, 671, 804
    *vs.* allergic reaction, 804
    definition of, 552, 804, 819
    epinephrine administration for,
        813–816
    in infants/children, 1321–1322
    sequence of events in, 805*f*
    signs/symptoms, 632*t*, 810*t*
anatomic position, 173–174
anatomy of organ systems. *See under*
    *specific organ systems*
anemia, 796
anemic, 1246, 1278
aneurysm, 729, 752
aneurysms
    definition of, 553, 1387
    dissecting, 691, 721
    elderly and, 1355
    hemorrhagic stroke and, 729–730
    syncope and, 539
anger
    of critically ill/injured patient, 68
    in grieving process, 68–69
    of patient, during history taking,
        372–373
angina pectoris
    definition of, 685–686, 720
    pain, 685–686
angioedema, 805, 819
angioplasty, 703
angular collision, motorcycle, 912
angulation, 1189
animal bites, 980–981, 980*f*
anisocoria, 395, 1009, 1037
ankle
    bones, 1150, 1150*f*
    injuries, 1189, 1190*f*
ANS. *See* autonomic nervous system
ANSI. *See* American National Standards
    Institute
antagonist, 496
anterior portion, definition of,
    172, 187
anterograde (posttraumatic) amnesia,
    1051, 1088
anthrax, 1545, 1545*f*, 1545*t*, 1548*t*, 1557
antibiotic, 496
antibody, 805*f*
anticholinergics, 824*t*
antidote, 824, 851

Antidote Treatment Nerve Agent Auto-
    Injector (ATNAA), 1539, 1557
antifungal, 496
antigen, 805*f*
antipyretics, 498
antivenin, 1228, 1239
ant stings, 1229
anus, 882, 882*f*
anxiety
    of critically ill/injured patient, 65
    disorders, 856
    history taking and, 372–373
anxious-avoidant attachment, 257
aorta, 935, 959
    definition of, 677, 720
aortic aneurysm, 691, 720, 760*t*
aortic valve, 679, 720
apex portion, 172, 187
Apgar score, 1264, 1269–1270, 1269*t*,
    1278
aphasia, 730
apnea, 434, 488
apnea monitors, 1407–1408
apneic oxygenation, 477, 488
apparent life-threatening event (ALTE),
    1342, 1347
appearance, in pediatric assessment
    triangle, 1294, 1294*f*, 1295*t*
appendicitis, 760*t*, 761–762,
    775, 1325
appendicular skeleton, 195
appendix, 229, 761
applied ethics, definition of, 106, 113
aqueous humor, 1009
arachnoid, of meninges, 1042
arm, anatomy, 1148
arm drag, 294*f*
arm-to-arm drag, 294*f*
arterial air embolism, 918, 930
arteries, 211–213
    in extremities, 1147*f*
    function, 679
    *vs.* veins, 1245
arterioles, 679, 935
arteriosclerosis, 1354, 1388
articular cartilage, 1150, 1196
articulations. *See* joints
artifact, ECG, 700, 720
artificial eyes, 1026–1027
artificial ventilation
    gastric distention and, 569
    methods, order of preference, 461
    normal *vs.* positive pressure
        ventilation, 461–462, 462*t*
    of pediatric patients, 463
    precautions, 461
    stoma ventilation, 569*f*
ascites, 1356, 1388
ASD (autism spectrum disorder),
    1394, 1418
aspiration, 385, 420, 488, 665
aspirin, 511
    poisoning, 843
assault, definition of, 102, 113

assessment. *See under specific emergencies*
in EMT training, 6
flowchart, 343, 350, 366, 377, 404
focused. *See* focused assessment
history taking. *See* history taking
importance of, 341
in medical emergencies, 605–606
overview, 342–343
primary survey. *See* primary survey
reassessment. *See* reassessment
respiratory system emergencies, 648
scene size-up. *See* size-up
secondary assessment. *See* secondary assessment
assisted ventilation. *See* artificial ventilation
asthma
definition of, 671
in elderly, 1372
management, 663–664
medications, 658*t*
pathophysiology, 642–643, 642*f*
pediatric, 1310–1311
signs/symptoms, 632*t*
triggers, 652
asystole, 688, 720
ataxic respirations, 434, 488
atelectasis, definition of, 633, 671
atherosclerosis, 264, 271
definition of, 720, 728, 753, 1388
in elderly, 1355, 1355*f*
ischemic stroke and, 728–729, 728*f*
pathophysiology, 684–685, 684*f*
atherosclerotic disease, 264
ATNAA (Antidote Treatment Nerve Agent Auto-Injector), 1539, 1557
atrial fibrillation, 1356
atrioventricular node (AV node), 678
atrium, 677, 720
atropine, 1540
attachment
anxious-avoidant, 257
secure, 257
aura, definition of, 732, 753
auscultation, 378, 410
autism spectrum disorder (ASD), 1394, 1418
automated external defibrillator (AED)
aftercare, 714
algorithm, 715*f*
in ambulances, 1428*t*, 1431–1432, 1432*f*
for cardiac arrest, 705–710, 715*f*
with cardiopulmonary resuscitation, 707–708
for children, 562
definition of, 10, 27
description, 705–710, 705*f*
early, rationale for, 707, 707*f*
inspection checklist, 709*f*
maintenance, 708–710, 709*f*
medical direction, 710

with pacemaker, 562
performance, 711–716
preparation, 710–711
safety precautions, 711
transdermal medication patches and, 562
wet patients and, 562
automatic implantable cardiac defibrillator (AICD), 704, 704*f*
automaticity, 678, 720
automatic transport ventilator (ATV), 468–469, 488
autonomic nervous system (ANS)
definition of, 553, 679, 720
functions, 533, 679, 936, 1044
regulation of heart function, 679
in shock, 533
AV node (atrioventricular node), 678
AVPU scale, definition, 410
AVPU test for responsiveness
definition, 648
description, 352, 353*f*
primary assessment and, 607–608
avulsions
definition of, 1002
facial, 1016*f*
pathophysiology, 967, 968*f*
axial loading injuries, 1053, 1088
axial skeleton, 193–195

### B

back
focused assessment, 401
physical examination, 1305
backboards, 1062
definition of, 318
description, 276, 276*f*, 311, 311*f*
KED vest-type immobilization device for, 311*f*
log rolling onto, 282, 282*f*
placement for extrication, 1473–1474
short-boards, 311
bacteria, as biologic warfare agents, 1544–1545, 1545*f*, 1545*t*, 1558
bacterial infections, 615
bacterial vaginosis, 885, 897
bag-mask device
advantages, 463–467, 463*f*
components, 463–464
definition of, 463, 488
pediatric, 463, 1317–1318, 1318*f*
for infants, 256
one-person technique, 1318
two-person technique, 1318–1319
technique
two-person, 464, 466*f*
using EC clamp, 464
for ventilating patient with plugged tracheostomy tube, 1404
bag-mask ventilation, for newborn, 1266
bags, for hazardous materials, 1507
balloon angioplasty, 703
bandages/bandaging, 998
barbiturates, 837

bargaining, in grieving process, 68
bariatric patients, 1402–1403
bariatrics, 307, 318, 1402–1403
bariatric stretchers, 309*f*
barotrauma, 256, 271
barrier devices
definition of, 488
for infectious disease risk reduction, 45–46, 46*f*
types, 462, 462*f*
base stations
definition of, 146, 160
licensing, 150
basic life support (BLS)
airway assessment. *See* airway, assessment
automated external defibrillation. *See* automated external defibrillation
basic principles of, 561
breathing assessment. *See* breathing, assessment
cardiopulmonary resuscitation. *See* cardiopulmonary resuscitation
chain of survival, 559, 559*f*
definition of, 557, 600
elements, 557–559, 558*f*, 559*f*
external chest compressions, 563, 563*f*, 565*f*
for infants/children, 577–583, 578*t*
circulation assessment, 582–583, 582*f*
responsiveness determination, 578–579, 579*f*
introduction of, 556–557
needs assessment, 560–561, 561*f*
positioning patient for, 562–563
principles, 561
pulse, checking for, 563–565, 563*f*
stopping, 586–587
when not to start, 584–586, 585*f*
basilar skull fractures, 1027, 1047, 1048*f*, 1088
basket stretcher, 311–312, 312*f*, 318
bath salts, 840–841
battery
definition of, 102, 113
example of, 102
Battle sign, 1047, 1047*f*, 1088
beclomethasone (Beclovent), 658*t*
beestings, 1229
behavior
definition of, 855, 878
emergencies. *See* psychiatric/behavioral emergencies; *specific emergencies*
normal, 855
problems, in elderly, 855
behavioral crisis, 855, 879
behavioral health emergencies, 855, 879
belly breathing (diaphragmatic breathing), 256, 421
bends, 1222, 1239
benzodiazepines, 837
beta radiation, 1549, 1558

bilateral
  breath sounds, 480
  definition of, 488
  structure, definition of, 172, 187
bills of lading, 1511, 1512f, 1523
bioethics, definition, 106, 113
biologic terrorism/warfare
  agents, 1532, 1548t
    bacteria, 1544–1545, 1545f,
      1545t, 1558
    neurotoxins, 1545–1548, 1546f,
      1546t, 1548t, 1559
    viruses, 1543–1544, 1543f,
      1544t, 1560
birth canal, 1244, 1278
bites, 1228–1234
  emergency medical care, 980–981
  insect
    allergens from, 806
    allergic reactions to, 807
    as poisoning by injection, 829
  snake, 1230–1223, 1230–1231f
  spider, 1228–1229, 1228f
  tick, 1234, 1234f
black eye, 1024f
black widow spider bites,
  1228–1229, 1228f
bladder, urinary. See urinary bladder
blanch, 1300, 1316
blanket drag, 294f
blast injuries
  categories of, 915–918
  definition of, 915
  eye, 1026
  mechanism of injury, 969
  mechanisms of, 915–917, 915f
  tissues at risk, 917–918, 1553
  types, 1553
blast lung, 1553
bleeding. See also hemorrhage
  assessment
    chief complaint investigation,
      942–943
    history taking, 942–943
    primary, 942
    reassessment, 944
    scene size-up, 941–942
    secondary, 943–944
    of vital signs, 943
    XABCs, 942
  in brain, 731
  from capillary vessels, 939, 939f
  control
    in facial injuries, 1015, 1015f
    in neck injuries, 1032–1033
    in pelvic injuries, 1178–1179
  from ears, 951–954, 954f
  emergency medical care,
    944–956
  external
    assessment of, 360–361
    control of, 360–361
  gastrointestinal, 1361
  internal
    emergency care for, 955–956

mechanisms of injury/nature of
  illness, 940
  signs/symptoms of, 940–941
interventions, 944
from mouth, 951–954
from nose, 951–954
pediatric disorders, 1322
safety precautions, 938
significance of, 938
subdural, 731, 731f
transport decisions, 942
vaginal, 1248–1250
blind spots, 1447, 1462
blister agents, 1535–1536
blood
  deoxygenated arterial, 424
  function of, 217–218
  in perfusion triangle, 532, 533f
bloodborne pathogens, 39, 82
blood cells. See also specific types of
    blood cells
  age-related effects, 265
blood clotting, 537, 685
blood composition, 214–215
blood disorders emergencies. See
    hematologic emergencies
blood flow, regulation, 533
blood glucose
  determination methods,
    402–404, 403f
  levels, normal range, 780
  monitor (glucometer), 788
  regulation, in elderly, 1363
  self-monitoring, 782f
blood pressure
  in acute myocardial infarction, 687
  of adolescents, 261
  of adults, 263
  of children, infants, 254
  control, 533
  decrease, 388
  definition of, 410
  diastolic, 388, 411
  elevated, 388
  measurement, 378, 389
    by auscultation, 390
    by palpation, 392
    units of, 682
  normal, 391
  in pediatric emergencies, 1306
  in shock, 540
  systolic, 388, 413
    age and, 1306
blood supply, of musculoskeletal
    system, 1146
blood vessels. See also specific types of
    blood vessels
  in perfusion triangle, 532, 533f
  walls of, 684, 684f
bloody show, 1244, 1278
blow-by oxygen technique,
  1311, 1316, 1317f
blow-out fracture, 1025, 1037
BLS. See basic life support
blunt myocardial injury, 1109

blunt trauma
  to chest, 1092
  definition of, 904, 930
  eye, 1024–1025, 1025f
  from falls, 912–913, 913f
  as mechanism of injury, 346
  neck, 1031–1032, 1032f
  in vehicular collisions, 904–911,
    905–906f
B-NICE, 1531, 1558
body armor, for injury prevention, 65
body drags, 282f
  emergency moves, 294–295, 294f, 318
  one-rescuer, 294f, 295f
  two-rescuer, 282
body heat loss, from cold exposure, 1202
body language
  in dealing with patient, 125
  as nonverbal communication,
    120–121, 121f
body mechanics, 277–280
  definition, 318
body temperature
  assessment, 1202
  core, 1203, 1204t, 1240
  of infants, 254
body weight, of infants, 254
bonding, definition of, 257
bones, 191–192
  exposed, as fracture sign, 1155, 1155f
  of leg, 1150, 1150f
  long, architecture of, 1149f
boots, for injury prevention,
    63–64, 64f
botulinum, 1546, 1546t, 1548t, 1558
Bourdon-gauge flowmeter, 454
bowel obstructions, in elderly, 1361
brachial plexus, 1043f
brachial pulse, palpation, 357–358, 358f,
    1299, 1299f
bradycardia
  definition of, 410, 688, 721
  pulse rate, 387
bradypnea, 1299
  definition of, 1347
  in pediatric emergencies, 1299
  in respiratory failure, 357t
brain, 220–222
  anatomy, 724–725, 725f, 1041, 1041f
  bleeding in, 731
  cerebrospinal fluid, 221
  circulation in the head, 221–222
  damage, from hypoglycemia, 786
  depressed function, 395
  of elderly, 266–267, 267f
  injuries
    patient interaction and, 1395–1396
    traumatic. See traumatic brain
      injury
  left hemisphere problems, 730
  physiology, 724–725, 725f
  protective coverings, 1042, 1042f
  right hemisphere problems, 730–731
brain attack. See stroke
brain death, 95

brainstem, anatomy, 725, 725f, 1041–1042
breach of confidentiality, 91, 113
breach of duty, 101
    in determining negligence, 101
breath-holding syncope, 1226, 1239
breathing, 1297
    adequate
        recognition of, 432
        signs of, 631
    assessment, 355–357
        in ABCDEs assessment. See under specific emergencies
        in infants/children, 583, 583f
        of quality of breathing, 384–385
        of respiratory rate, 384, 384f, 385t
        of respiratory rhythm, 384
    depth of, 385
    diaphragmatic or belly, 256
    emergency medical care
        head injuries, 1062
        spinal injuries, 1064
    inadequate or hypoventilation
        recognition of, 432–434
        signs/symptoms of, 631t
    labored, 432, 433f
    normal, 356
    physiology of, 423–428, 425–428f, 425t
breath sounds
    assessment, 385–387, 386f
    definition of, 411
    normal, 386
    in pediatrics, 1309, 1309f
    in respiratory system emergencies, 650–651, 650f
    wheezing, 387
breech presentation, 1270, 1271f, 1278
brief resolved unexplained event (BRUE), 1342
bronchial breath sounds, 650, 671
bronchioles, 422, 488
bronchiolitis, 636, 671, 1312, 1347
    signs/symptoms, 632t
bronchitis, 639, 671
    dyspnea and, 632t
    medications for, 658t
    signs/symptoms, 632t
brown recluse spider bites, 1229, 1229f
bruising
    in child abuse, 1338
    as fracture signs, 1154–1155, 1155f
buboes, 1545, 1546f, 1558
bubonic plague, 1545, 1546f, 1546t, 1558
building collapse, as hazard in fires, 58
bulk storage container, 1506, 1523
bullets, penetrating trauma from, 914, 915f
burn depth, 984–985
burn injuries
    airway assessment, 986
    assessment, vital signs, 989
    breathing assessment, 986
burnout, definition of, 72, 82
burns
    assessment, 986–989
        chief complaint investigation, 986

communication/documentation of, 989
        general impressions, 986
        history taking, 987–988
        primary, 986–987
        reassessment, 989
        scene size-up, 986
        secondary, 988–989
    in child abuse, 1338
    circumferential, compartment syndrome and, 982
    classification
        by depth, 984–985, 984f
        by severity, 983–986, 983t
    complications, 982
    deaths from, 982
    definition of, 964, 1002
    extent, 985–986, 985f
    to eye, 1021–1023, 1021–1023f
    in infants/children, 986
    interventions, 989
    pathophysiology, 982
    pediatric, 1333–1335, 1334f, 1334t
    safety, on-scene, 986
    thermal, emergency medical care, 991–992
    transport decisions, 987
burn severity, 983–986, 983t
bystanders, 100
    duty to act and, 100
    managing, at vehicle crash scene, 1469
    presence during patient interview, 123

**C**

CAAHEP (Commission on Accreditation of Allied Health Education Programs), 19
calcaneus, 1150, 1196
cannabis compounds, 841
capillaries, 213, 679
capillary hydrostatic pressure, 533
capillary refill time
    definition of, 411
    estimating, 1296, 1300f
    evaluation, 360
capnography, 402, 411, 437, 489
capnometer, 437f
capnometry, 411, 437, 489
car-versus-bicycle collisions, 911, 911f
carbon dioxide ($CO_2$)
    definition of, 402, 411
    as hazard in fires, 58
    during inspiration, 629
    during respiration, 629, 630f
    retention
        definition of, 633, 671–672
        hypoxic drive and, 633
carbon monoxide (CO), 647, 672
    as hazard in fires, 58
    intoxication, 992
    poisonings, 826, 831
carboys, 1507–1508, 1507f, 1523

cardiac arrest
    automated external defibrillation for, 705–710, 705f, 709f
    definition of, 687, 721
    emergency medical care, 710–716, 715f
    in pregnancy, 593–594
    sudden death and, 687–688
    during transport, 714–715
cardiac asthma, 640, 641t
cardiac compromise, physical findings, 687
cardiac cycle, 682
cardiac medications, overdose, 843. See also specific cardiac medications
cardiac monitoring, 700–702
cardiac muscle, 1146
cardiac output, 535, 1095
    definition of, 535, 721
    formula, 682
cardiac surgery, for cardiovascular emergencies, 703–704, 703f
cardiac tamponade, 536, 553
    pathophysiology, 1105–1106
cardiac tamponade (pericardial tamponade)
    definition of, 1115
    pathophysiology, 536, 1107f
    signs/symptoms, 1105–1106
    treatment, 546
cardiogenic shock
    causes, 535f, 544t
    definition of, 534, 553, 688, 721
    signs/symptoms, 544t, 688
    treatment, 543–545, 544t, 688
cardiopulmonary arrest, pediatric, 1319–1320
cardiopulmonary resuscitation (CPR)
    with automated external defibrillation, 707–708
    cardiac arrest in pregnancy, 593–594
    in chain of survival, 559, 559f
    for children, 577–583, 578t, 579
    components of, 559–560
    definition of, 557, 600
    education and training, 595
    equipment, in ambulance, 1430, 1431f
    external chest compressions, 563, 563f, 565f
    grief support, 594–595
    indications, 358
    for infants, 577–583, 578t
    interrupting, 583–584
    one-rescuer, adult, 569–571
    opioid overdose, 593–594
    special circumstances, 593–594
    steps, 557–558
    switching positions during, 571–573
    timing, 558, 558f
    two-rescuer, adult, 571–573
cardiovascular emergencies
    assessment, 692–696
        chief complaint investigation, 693
        communication/documentation of, 696
        general impressions, 692

history taking, 693–695
mechanism of injury/nature of
    illness, 692
primary, 692–693
reassessment, 696
scene size-up, 692
secondary, 695–696
vital signs, 696
atherosclerosis, 684–685, 684*f*
cardiac arrest. *See* cardiac arrest
cardiac surgery for, 703–704, 703*f*
cardiogenic shock, 688
hypertensive, 690–692
interventions, 696
pacemakers for, 703–704, 703*f*
pathophysiology, 684–688, 684*f*
pulmonary edema, 690
safety, on-scene, 692
sudden death, 687–688
transport decisions, 693, 696
cardiovascular system
age-related changes,
    1354–1357, 1355*f*
anatomy, 677–684, 678*f*, 680–681*f*
breathing physiology and, 423–428,
    425–428*f*, 425*t*
of elderly, 264–265
emergencies. *See* cardiovascular
    emergencies
focused assessment, 387–393
of infants, 255
medical emergencies, 605, 605*t*
perfusion triangle, 532, 533*f*
physiology, 677–684, 678*f*, 680–681*f*
carina, 420, 422*f*, 489
carotid arteries, 1007
carotid pulse
in child, 357
palpation of, 357–358, 358*f*
carpopedal spasm, 646
carrying of patients
diamond carry, 284, 284*f*, 318
directions/commands, 291–293
guidelines, 283*t*
one-handed technique, 284, 286
by one rescuer, 296*f*
on stairs, 289
using scoop stretcher, 305–306
car seat, immobilization of child in,
    1331–1332
cartilage, definition of, 1150
castor beans, ricin poisoning
    from, 846*f*, 1546–1548,
    1547*f*, 1548*t*
casualty collection area, 1502, 1523
cataracts, 1357, 1388
cathinones, synthetic, 840–841
cavitation, 914, 915*f*, 930, 1122
CBRNE mnemonic, 1531
cells, 191
cellular telephone, 148, 160
cellular transport mechanisms,
    diffusion. *See* diffusion
Centers for Disease Control and
    Prevention (CDC), 37, 82

central cyanosis, 1269
central nervous system (CNS), 220–223.
    *See also specific central nervous
    system structures*
anatomy, 1041–1042, 1041*f*
definition of, 1040
protection, 1042
central neurogenic hyperventilation,
    1049, 1089
central pulses, 1299, 1347
central venous catheters, 1409, 1409*f*
cerebellum
anatomy, 724–725, 725*f*
functions, 1041
cerebral cortex, 1050
cerebral edema, 1049, 1089
cerebral embolism, 729
cerebral palsy, 1400–1401, 1400*f*, 1418
cerebrospinal fluid (CSF), 1042
cerebrovascular accident (CVA), 727,
    753. *See also* stroke
cerebrum
anatomy, 725, 725*f*, 1041–1042, 1041*f*
function, 1041–1042
certification, 3, 27, 100
cervical collars, 1061–1063, 1065–1067
cervical spine
focused assessment, 398
stabilization, 1064–1066
cervix, 882*f*, 883, 897, 1244, 1278
chain of survival, 559, 559*f*, 707, 707*f*
channel, radio, definition of, 146, 160
charcoal, activated, 833, 843
CHART method, 138–139
cheek injuries, 1031
chemical burns
emergency medical care,
    993–994, 993*f*
eye, 1021, 1021*f*
chemical mediators, 805*f*
chemicals, as allergens, 806
chemical terrorism/warfare, 1531
agents, 1531
    biological, 1542–1549, 1543–1544*f*,
        1544*t*
    contact hazard, 1535
    metabolic or cyanides, 1540–1542,
        1542*t*
    nerve agents, 1537–1540,
        1539*t*, 1541*t*
    persistency, 1535
    respiratory or choking, 1536–1537
    route of exposure, 1535
    vapor hazard, 1535
    vesicants, 1535–1536
    volatility, 1535, 1560
description, 1531
Chemical Transportation Emergency
    Center (CHEMTREC), 1511, 1523
chemoreceptors
definition of, 429, 489
functions
    in respiration, 429
CHEMTREC (Chemical Transportation
    Emergency Center), 1511, 1523

chest
focused assessment, 398–399
injuries. *See* chest injuries
physical examination, 1305
chest compressions
external, 563, 563*f*, 565*f*
    hand position, 563–565, 565*f*
    technique, 563–565, 565*f*
fraction, 584, 600
for infants, 578
for newborn, 1266
chest injuries. *See also specific chest
    injuries*
assessment, 921, 1097–1102
    chief complaint investigation, 1099
    communication/documentation,
        1102
    general impressions, 1098
    history taking, 1099–1100
    mechanism of injury/nature of
        illness, 1097
    primary, 1098–1099
    reassessment, 1101–1102
    scene size-up, 1097–1098
    secondary, 1100–1101
    vital signs, 1100
    XABCs, 1098
closed, 1095, 1095*f*
emergency medical care, 1103
in infants/children, 1333, 1333*f*
interventions, 1101
open, 1095, 1096*f*
pathophysiology, 1095–1096, 1095*f*
safety, on-scene, 1097–1098
signs/symptoms, 1096–1097
transport decisions, 1099
chest pain
in angina pectoris, 685–686
in elderly, 1370
pleuritic, 644, 673
chest thrusts, 588–589, 589*f*
Cheyne-Stokes respirations, 434, 434*f*,
    489, 1049
CHF. *See* congestive heart failure
chief complaint, 139, 160
definition of, 346, 411
investigation, 367–368, 367*f*, 368*f*
chief concern, 139, 160
child abuse
burn injuries, 986
definition of, 1347
sexual, 1338–1339
signs/symptoms, 1336–1338,
    1337*f*, 1337*t*
thermal burns and, 991
CHILD ABUSE mnemonic, 1337, 1337*t*
childbirth
abnormal/complicated, 1270–1274,
    1271*f*
multiple births, 1272
normal, 1256–1265
    delivering the newborn,
        1258–1264
    delivery field preparation,
        1256–1258, 1259*f*

childbirth *(Continued)*
  preparation for delivery,
    1256–1258, 1259*f*
  stages of labor, 1255–1256
  placenta, delivery of, 1264
  postdelivery care, 1264–1265
  supplies, in ambulances, 1428*t*,
    1431, 1431*f*
children
  abdominal injuries, 766
  abdominal pain, 766
  adolescent. *See* adolescents
  airway opening
    head tilt–chin maneuver, 582
    jaw-thrust maneuver, 582–583
  anatomy, 1291*t*
    airway, 421, 421*f*
    musculoskeletal system, 1292–1293
    nervous system, 1292
    respiratory system, 1290–1292,
      1291*f*, 1291*t*
  assessment, 1293–1307
    primary, 1294–1303
    scene size-up, 1293
  automated external defibrillation, 562
  basic life support, 577–583, 578*t*
  with behavioral disorders, 869
  blood loss, from skull region, 1061
  cardiopulmonary resuscitation,
    577–583, 578*t*, 579
  communication with, 128–129, 129*f*
  consent in critical situations,
    88–89, 89*f*
  with diabetes, 786
  foreign body obstructions,
    590–593, 591*f*
  gastrointestinal system, anatomy
    of, 1292
  immunizations, recommended, 52
  infants. *See* infants
  integumentary system, anatomy
    of, 1293
  oropharyngeal airway insertion, 447
  poisonings, 822
  preschool-age
    assessment, 1287–1288, 1287*f*
    definition of, 1287, 1347
  school-age
    assessment of, 1288–1289, 1288*f*
    definition of, 260, 271, 1288, 1347
    physical changes, 260, 261*f*
    psychosocial changes, 260–261
    vital signs, 260
  shock, 540
  with type 1 diabetes, 782
chlamydia, 885, 897
chlorine (Cl), in chemical terrorism/
  warfare, 1537, 1542*t*, 1558
choking, universal sign for, 587, 587*f*
choking agents, in chemical terrorism/
  warfare, 1536–1537
cholecystitis
  definition of, 759, 775
  localization of pain, 760*t*
  referred pain from, 760, 760*f*

signs/symptoms, 761
cholinergics, 824*t*
chronic bronchitis, 639, 672
chronic diseases, 1392
chronic kidney disease, 765
chronic obstructive pulmonary disease
  (COPD), 639, 672
  assessment, 652
  *vs.* congestive heart failure,
    639–641, 641*t*
  definition of, 672
  management, 663
    medications for, 658*t*
    oxygen therapy for, 639
  pathophysiology, 639–641, 640*f*
  signs/symptoms, 640*f*, 652
  types, 639
Cincinnati Prehospital Stroke Scale,
  741, 742*t*
circulation
  assessment, 357–361, 358–360*f*
    in ABCDEs assessment. *See under
      specific emergencies*
    capillary refill, 360, 360*f*
    in infants/children, 582–583, 582*f*
    in pediatric assessment triangle,
      1294*f*, 1295*f*, 1296, 1299
    pulse. *See* pulse
    of restrained patient, 865–866, 866*f*
    skin assessment and, 358–360, 360*f*
  devices and techniques to assist,
    573–577, 575*f*
  emergency medical care, head
    injuries, 1062–1063
  fetal, 1245
  pediatric emergencies
    anaphylactic shock, 1321–1322
    bleeding disorders, 1322
    shock, 1320–1322
circulatory compromise, 431
circulatory system
  anatomy, 207–215
    arteries, 211–213
    blood composition, 214–215
    capillaries, 213
    heart, 208–210
    spleen, 215
    veins, 213–214
  physiology, 215–220
    blood, function of, 217–218
    inadequate circulation, 216–217
    nervous system control, CNS and,
      218–220
    normal circulation, 215–216
  signs, of anaphylactic shock, 539*t*
circumflex coronary arteries, 680*f*
CISM (critical incident stress
  management), 71, 71*f*, 82
civil lawsuit, 100
clarification, 123*t*
clavicle (collarbone)
  injuries, 1170, 1170*f*
clavicle fractures, 1109
cleaning
  of ambulance, 1442, 1462

disinfectant solution for, 50
  practices, for infection control
    plan, 47*t*
  products, poisonings from, 844
clitoris, 882
clonic phase, 732
closed-ended questions
  definition of, 122, 160
  in patient interview, 122, 123*t*
closed incident, 1492, 1523
closed injuries
  abdominal, 1121–1122, 1122*f*
    definition of, 1143
    signs/symptoms, 1122*f*
  assessment, 970–976
  chest, 1095, 1095*f*, 1115
  definition of, 964, 1003
  emergency medical care of, 976
  fractures, 1153, 1196
  head, definition of, 1089
  scene size-up, 970–971
*Clostridium botulinum*, 844*t*
*Clostridium difficile*, 1380
clothing
  removal, in pediatric
    emergencies, 1300
  socks, 64
  of toxin-exposed patient, 826
clothing drag, 294*f*
CO. *See* carbon monoxide
$CO_2$. *See* carbon dioxide
CoAEMSP (Committee on Accreditation
  of Education Programs for the
  Emergency Medical Services
  Profession), 19
coagulation, 939, 959
cocaine, 840
cold injuries
  assessment, 1206–1209
    ABCs, 1206
    chief complaint investigation, 1207
    communication/documentation,
      1209
    history taking, 1207–1208
    mechanism of injury/nature of
      illness, 1207
    primary, 1207
    reassessment, 1208–1209
    scene size-up, 1206–1207
    secondary, 1209
    of vital signs, 1208
  emergency medical care,
    1209–1210, 1209*f*
  hypothermia, 1203–1205, 1204*f*, 1204*t*
  interventions, 1209–1210
  local, 1205–1206, 1205*f*
  prevention, 1209–1210
  transport decisions, 1208
  underlying factors, 1205
cold weather clothing, for injury
  prevention, 62
cold zone, 1514*f*, 1515, 1523
Colles fracture, 1175
colon, 757
colors, medical terminology, 169

colostomy, 1410, 1418
coma, 725, 753
combat veteran, 871–873
combining form, medical terminology, 176–178t
combining vowels, medical terminology, 166–167, 187
command, establishing, at terrorism event, 1535
command, in incident command system, 1488–1489, 1523
command post, 1476, 1483, 1488, 1523
Commission on Accreditation of Allied Health Education Programs (CAAHEP), 19
Committee on Accreditation of Education Programs for the Emergency Medical Services Profession (CoAEMSP), 19
common cold, characteristics, 632t
commotion cordis, 1109, 1115
communicable disease, 613, 626
    definition of, 38, 82
    vs. infectious disease, 38
    risk reduction and prevention, 41–50
communication
    age and, 119
    of assessment findings. See under specific emergency situations
    with children, 128–129, 129f
    culture and, 119
    definition of, 118, 161
    with elderly, 127–128, 127f
    en route, 152t
    factors/strategies for, 119t
    with family
        in pediatric emergencies, 1284
        in sudden infant death syndrome, 1340–1342, 1341t
    with hearing-impaired patients, 129–130, 129f
    importance of, 118
    during labor/delivery, 1258
    at mass-casualty incident, 1493
    with medical control and hospitals, 153–156, 153f
    noise and, 121
    with non–English-speaking patients, 131
    nonverbal
        body language, 120–121, 121f
        eye contact, 120–121
        facial expressions, 120–121
        physical factors and, 121–122, 122t
    with older patients, 1351–1352
    with other agencies, during air medical operations, 1457, 1457f
    with other health care professionals, 132, 133f
    with patient, in pediatric emergencies, 1284
    patient care handover, 132–133
    personal experience and, 120
    radio. See radio communications
    respect and, 120

Shannon–Weaver model of, 119f
    with special needs patients, 119
    telephones, cell/satellite, 148–149
    therapeutic, 119, 162
    verbal, 118, 122–126
    with visually impaired patients, 130–131
    written, 118, 133–146
        documenting refusal of care, 143, 144f, 146t
        special reporting situations, 146
communication systems
    base station radios, 146–147
    cellular/satellite telephones, 148–149
    digital equipment, 148
    equipment, 149–150
    mobile and portable radios, 147, 147f
    mobile data terminals, 149, 149f
    repeater-based, 147–148, 148f
    technology for, 12–13
communication techniques, 123t
community paramedicine, 15, 27, 321
compartment syndrome, 966, 982, 1003, 1191–1192, 1196
compensated (nonprogressive) shock, 540, 540t, 553
compensatory damages, 108, 113
competent, definition of, 93, 113
complex access, 1472, 1483
complex carbohydrates, as energy source, 34
compliance, 468, 489
compliance monitoring, for infection control plan, 48t
compressed gas cylinders. See gas cylinders
concussion
    definition of, 1089
    signs/symptoms, 1051
    spinal cord, 1051, 1089
conduction, 1202, 1239
    system, 678
conductive hearing loss, 1397, 1418
confidentiality, disclosure of information, 91
confrontation
    definition of, 123t
    example of, 123t
congestive heart failure (CHF)
    vs. chronic obstructive pulmonary disease, 639–641, 641t
    definition of, 688, 721
    left-side, 690
    right-side, 690
    signs/symptoms, 632t, 640, 688–690
    treatment, 689t
conjunctiva, 359, 411, 1009, 1037
conjunctivitis, 1017, 1037
connecting nerves, 1043, 1043f
consent
    in behavioral emergencies, 873–874
    definition of, 86, 113
    expressed, 87, 114
    implied, 88, 114
    informed, 87, 114

involuntary, 88
    minors and, 88–89, 89f
    for organ donation, 97, 97f
    refusal of, 90–91
contact burn, 991, 1003
contact hazard, 1535, 1558
contact lenses, 1026–1027
contagious, 1543, 1558
containers, for hazardous materials, 1505–1508, 1505f, 1506f, 1507f
contamination
    definition of, 38, 82, 1003
    in soft-tissue injuries, 966
    standard precautions, 41, 42t
continuous positive airway pressure (CPAP), 662, 672
    application, 470–473
    complications, 473–474
    for congestive heart failure, 662, 689t
    contraindications, 470
    definition of, 489
    indications, 461, 470
continuous quality improvement (CQI)
    definition of, 16, 27
    methods for, 16
continuum of care, 321
contractility, 684
contraindications, definition of, 496, 497
contributory negligence, 108
    decision-making capacity, definition, 113
controlled motorcycle crash, 912
controlled substances. See specific controlled substances
control zones, 1514–1515, 1514f, 1523
contusion, 965, 965f, 1003
    cerebral, 1051
    definition of, 940, 959
    pulmonary, 1108
    spinal cord, 1051
convection, 1202, 1240
conventional reasoning, 260, 271
COPD. See chronic obstructive pulmonary disease (COPD)
coral snake bites, 1230f, 1232–1233
core temperature, 1203
    definition of, 1240
    falling, 1203
cornea, 1008f, 1009, 1037
coronal plane, definition of, 190
coronary arteries, 679, 721
coronary artery disease, 685
coronary sinus, 680f
coroner (medical examiner), 96, 96f
corticosteroids, 656
coughing techniques, to avoid contamination, 39–40, 40f
coup-contrecoup brain injury, 905, 906f, 930
coup-contrecoup injury, 1049, 1089
cover, definition of, 82, 1532, 1558
COVID-19, 620, 637, 672
    characteristics, 632t
    signs/symptoms, 632t

CPAP. *See* continuous positive airway pressure
CPR. *See* cardiopulmonary resuscitation
CPR board, 1430, 1431*f*, 1462
CQI. *See* continuous quality improvement
crackles (rales), 387, 411, 650, 651*t*, 672
credentialing, 27
credentialing, definition, 4
crepitus, 399, 411, 1115, 1155, 1196
crew resource management (CRM), 325
cricoid cartilage, 1007–1008
critical incident stress, 70
critical incident stress management (CISM), 71, 71*f*, 82, 1342
critically ill/injured patients
anger/hostility of, 68
anxiety of, 65
working with, 66
cromolyn (Intal), 658*t*
cross-contamination, 1534, 1558
croup
characteristics, 632*t*, 634–635
in children, 1311
definition of, 672, 1347
signs/symptoms, 632*t*
crowning, 1256, 1278
crushing injury, 966, 1003
crush syndrome, 966, 1003
crying patients, history taking and, 374
CSF. *See* cerebrospinal fluid
cultural considerations, during pregnancy, 1252–1253
cultural diversity, in workplace, 75–76
cultural imposition, 120, 161
culture, communication and, 119
cumulative stress reactions, 70, 82
Cushing triad, 1063
cushion of safety, 1446–1448, 1462
custody, involuntary consent and, 88
CVA (cerebrovascular accident), 727, 753
CX (phosgene oxime), 1536
cyanides
in chemical terrorism/warfare, 1540–1542, 1541*t*, 1558
poisonings, 831
cyanosis
in anaphylactic shock, 538
causes, 359, 359*f*
in chest injuries, 1097
definition of, 411, 553
skin color and, 608*f*
cylinders
gas, 451–452, 453*f*
for hazardous materials, 1508, 1523
cystic fibrosis (CF), 666–667
cystitis, 764, 775
localization of pain, 760*t*

**D**

danger zone (hot zone), 1469, 1483, 1514*f*, 1515
date rape drugs, 838

DCAP-BTLS mnemonic
definition of, 361, 411
in trauma assessment, 1013
dead space, 206, 425, 425*t*, 489
death/dying, 67–69
of child, 1339–1342
critically ill or injured patient, working with, 66
definitive signs of, 95–96, 96*f*
grieving process, 68
hypothermia and, 95
medical examiner cases, 96–97, 96*f*
medical identification insignia and, 97, 97*f*
organ donation, consent for, 97, 97*f*
physical signs of, 95–97
presumptive signs of, 95, 95*t*
working with family members, 66
debriefing sessions, for critical incident stress management, 71
decay, of radiological material, 1549, 1558
deceased patient, immediate actions for, 95
deceleration, 930
decision-making capacity, definition, 86
decompensated shock, 540, 540*t*, 553
decompression sickness, 1222–1223, 1240
decontaminated, 1462
decontamination
area, 1515, 1516*f*, 1523
definition of, 1523
of equipment for moving of patients, 312
in hazmat incidents, 1515, 1516*f*
decubitus ulcers, 1365, 1388
dedicated line (hotline), 147, 161
deep portion, definition of, 171, 187
deep vein thrombosis, 795–796
deep venous thrombosis, 1355, 1388
defamation, 102–103, 113
defendant, 107
defibrillation, 688, 710, 721
deformity, as fracture signs, 1154, 1154*f*
dehydration, 539, 553
definition of, 539
in elderly, 1359, 1372
pediatric, 1325–1327, 1327*f*, 1327*t*
delayed stress reactions, 70, 82
delirium, 736, 753
agitated, 864
causes, 1359–1360
definition of, 1359, 1388
signs/symptoms, 1359–1360
delirium tremens (DTs), 835, 851
delivery
abnormal/complicated, 1270–1274
preparation for, 1259*f*
dementia, 860, 1358–1359, 1388
demobilization, 1488, 1524
denial, in grieving process, 67
denitrogenation, 467, 489
dental appliances
causing airway obstruction, 477

dentures, airway maintenance and, 477
dental injuries
emergency medical care, 1031
with facial fractures, 1031, 1031*f*
traumatic, 1010–1011
dentures, airway maintenance and, 477
Department of Transportation (DOT)
*Emergency Response Guidebook*, 55, 57*f*
marking system for hazardous materials, 1508–1509, 1508*f*
National Standard Curriculum, 8
dependent edema, 721
dependent lividity, 95, 96*f*, 113, 584, 585*f*, 600
depressed skull fracture, 1047, 1048*f*
depression, 874
definition of, 855, 879
in elderly, 855, 1367
in grieving process, 68
history taking, 374
dermis
anatomy, 963–964, 963*f*
definition of, 963, 1003
designated officer, 41, 82
developmental disabilities
autism spectrum disorder, 1394, 1418
characteristics, 1393–1394
definition of, 1393, 1418
Down syndrome, 1394–1395, 1394*f*, 1418
patient interactions, 1395–1396
diabetes mellitus
blood glucose self-monitoring, 782*f*
in children, 786
definition of, 801
insulin and, 780–781
pathophysiology, 782–784
type 1, 782–784
type 2, 784
undiagnosed, 783
diabetic ketoacidosis (DKA), 783, 801
dialysis, renal, 771–772
diamond carry, 284, 284*f*, 318
diaphoretic, 360, 411
diaphragm
during inspiration, 628
in spinal cord injury, 1092, 1092*f*
diaphragmatic breathing (belly breathing), 256
diarrhea, in elderly, 1380
diastole, 680
diastolic pressure, 388, 411
dieffenbachia, 846, 846*f*
diet, healthy, 33, 34*f*
diffusion, 427, 489
digestive system
anatomy, 226–229
abdomen, 226–228
appendix, 229
esophagus, 228
large intestine, 229
liver, 228–229

mouth, 228
oropharynx, 228
pancreas, 228
rectum, 229
small intestine, 229
stomach, 228
in elderly, 266
physiology, 229–230
digital equipment, for communication
systems, 148–149
dilation, 679, 721
diphtheria
characteristics, 632*t*
definition of, 672
signs/symptoms, 632*t*
direct carry method, 302–304
direct contact, 39, 40*f*, 82
direct ground lift, 300–302, 318
directional terms, medical terminology,
170–173, 171*f*, 171*t*
anterior, 172
apex, 172
deep, 171
distal, 171
inferior, 170–171
lateral, 171
medial, 171
palmar, 172
plantar, 172
posterior, 172
proximal, 171
superficial, 171
superior, 170–171
direct laryngoscopy, 478, 489
direct pressure
for external bleeding, 939, 945*f*
for external hemorrhage, 945
dirty bomb, 1532, 1558
disability
developmental, 1393
long-term, from musculoskeletal
injuries, 1170
Disaster Medical Assistance Teams
(DMATs), 1502
disasters
casualty collection area, 1502
children in, 1335–1336, 1335*f*
definition of, 1486, 1502, 1524
management, 1502
disease prevention, wellness and,
36–38
disease vector, 1542, 1558
disinfection
of ambulance, 1442, 1462
high-level, 1442, 1462
infection control practices, 47*t*
dislocations
definition of, 1155, 1197
elbow, 1173, 1174*f*
knee, 1187–1188, 1187*f*
patellar, 1188–1189, 1189*f*
shoulder, 1171–1172, 1174*f*
signs/symptoms, 1155–1156, 1156*f*
dispatch phase of EMS, 151
displaced fracture, 1153, 1197

dissecting aneurysm, 691, 721
dissemination, 1542, 1558
distal portion, 171, 187
distal radius fractures, 1175, 1176*f*
distracting injury, 354*t*, 411
distributive shock, 537–539, 553
diverticulitis, 759, 760*t*, 764, 775
diving emergencies
assessment, 1220–1222, 1223–1225
ABCs, 1224
communication/documentation
of, 1224
history taking, 1224
primary, 1223–1224
reassessment, 1224–1225
scene size-up, 1223
secondary, 1224
of vital signs, 1224
at bottom, 1222
chief complaint investigation, 1224
descent problems, 1220–1222
emergency medical care,
1225–1226
interventions, 1224
prevention, 1226
safety, on-scene, 1223
transport decisions, 1226
upon ascent, 1222
water rescue, 1219
diving reflex, 1220, 1240
dizziness, in elderly, 1371
DKA (diabetic ketoacidosis), 783
DNR orders, 93, 97, 114, 1380, 1411
documentation
of assessment findings. *See under
specific emergency situations*
definition of, 118, 161
during labor/delivery, 1255
of pain, 368
of refusal of care, 143, 144*f*, 146*t*
domestic terrorism, 1558
DOPE mnemonic, 1404, 1404*t*
dorsal portion, 172, 187
dose/doses, 496
DOT. *See* Department of Transportation
Down syndrome, 1394–1395,
1394*f*, 1418
drag (air resistance), 915, 930
draw sheet method, 304–305
dressings
bandaging and, 998
occlusive, 977, 1003
sterile, 980, 998
driving, of emergency vehicles
cushion of safety for, 1446–1448, 1462
driver anticipation, 1446
intersection hazards, 1452
laws/regulations, 1450–1452
safety guidelines, 1444–1453, 1446*t*
in school zones, 1452
siren risk/benefit analysis,
1445–1446
speed, 1448
weather/road conditions and,
1449–1450

drowning
assessment, 1223–1225
ABCs, 1224
chief complaint investigation, 1224
communication/documentation
of, 1225
history taking, 1224
primary, 1223–1224
reassessment, 1224–1225
scene size-up, 1223
secondary, 1224
of vital signs, 1224
definition of, 1218, 1240
events in, 1218–1220
interventions, 1224
*vs.* near drowning, 1218
pediatric, 1328–1329
prevention, 1226
recovery techniques, 1220
transport decisions, 1224
water rescue, 1219, 1219*f*
drug abuse, 77
drugs/medications
absorption. *See* absorption
administration, 495
as allergens, 806
allergic reaction to, 806, 806*f*
in ambulances, 1428*t*, 1432
cardiac. *See specific cardiac
medications*
definition of, 495
interactions in elderly, 1365–1367
names of, 497–498
noncompliance, in elderly, 1366
overdose, 843
polypharmacy, 1365, 1388
prescription, 497
rape, 890
respiratory inhalation, 658*t*
drug use, history taking, 370–371
drums, for hazardous materials,
1507, 1507*f*
dry lungs, *vs.* wet lungs, 640, 641*t*
DTs (delirium tremens), 835
DUMBELS mnemonic, 1539*t*, 1540
duodenal ulcer, 760*t*
duodenum, 757
DuoDote kit, 843, 1540, 1558
duplex, 149, 161
durable power of attorney for health
care, 93, 114
dura mater, 1042
duty to act, 100, 114
dysarthria, 730, 753
dysbarism injuries, 1226, 1240
dysphagia, 1033, 1400
dyspnea, 1354, 1388
causes, 633–634, 1097
definition of, 489, 628, 672
paroxysmal nocturnal, 632
signs/symptoms, 426
dysrhythmia
definition of, 721
in elderly, 1360*t*
sudden death and, 687–688

# E

ear
  anatomy, 1007, 1007*f*
  Battle sign, 1047, 1047*f*
  bleeding from, 951–954, 954*f*
  injuries, 1028–1030, 1029*f*
  physical examination, 1305
  protection, for injury prevention, 64
early adults. *See* adults, early
Ebola, 620
ecchymosis
  definition of, 959, 1003, 1197
  as fracture sign, 1154
  internal bleeding and, 940
  pathophysiology, 965
eclampsia, 1248, 1278
ectopic pregnancy
  assessment, 1249
  definition of, 1278
  pathophysiology, 884
  signs/symptoms, 885–886
edema
  definition of, 535, 553
  dependent, 690, 721
  pulmonary. *See* pulmonary edema
ejection, in motorcycle collision, 912
elbow
  dislocation, 1174, 1174*f*
  injuries, 1174, 1174*f*
  sprain, 1174
elder abuse
  categories, 1381–1383, 1383*t*
  definition of, 1388
  signs/symptoms, assessment and
    management of, 1381–1383
  thermal burns and, 991
elderly
  abuse/neglect. *See* elder abuse
  age-related changes
    endocrine system, 1363
    gastrointestinal system, 1360–1362
    immune system, 1363
    musculoskeletal system, 1364–1365
  airway opening, 566–567
  alcohol use, subdural hematoma
    and, 1050
  anatomy, physiology and
    pathophysiology, 1353–1367
  behavioral problems, 855, 860
  cardiovascular system, 264–265
    anatomy, physiology and
      pathophysiology, 1354–1357
  communication with, 127–128, 127*f*,
    1351–1352
  death, leading causes of, 1352, 1352*t*
  emergencies, patient assessment of,
    1368–1373
  emergency medical care, 1374–1378
  endocrine system, 266
  falls, 913
  GEMS diamond, 1368, 1369*t*
  hip fracture, 1179
  history taking and, 373, 739–741
  internal hemorrhages, 942

joint pain, 1152
moving, considerations for, 307
nervous system, anatomy, physiology
  and pathophysiology, 1357–1360
renal failure, 1363
renal system, anatomy, physiology
  and pathophysiology, 1362–1363
respiratory system, anatomy,
  physiology and pathophysiology,
  1353–1354
response to nursing and skilled care
  facilities, 1379–1380
in shock, treatment of, 548
stereotypes, 1351
terminology, 1350
trauma, 1375–1378
  assessment of, 1375–1378
  causes of, 1375
urinary tract infections, 1359
working with, 1350
electrical burns, 994–996, 995*f*
electrical hazards, at scene, 57–58
electrocardiogram (ECG)
  electrodes, 699–700, 699*f*
  transmission over UHF
    frequencies, 149
electrolytes, 1211. *See also specific*
  *electrolytes*
emancipated minors, 88, 114
embolus, 645, 672, 728, 729*f*, 753
embryo
  definition of, 1244, 1278
  implantation, 1244
emergency, definition of, 98, 99*f. See*
  *also specific emergencies*
emergency medical care. *See under*
  *specific emergencies*
  in absence of DNR orders, 95
  in behavioral emergencies, 873–874
  of burn injuries, 989–997
  of closed injuries, 976
  cold injuries, 1209–1210
  consent for, 88
  considerations for, 86
  definition of, 86, 114
  for drowning and diving emergencies,
    1225–1226
  for elderly, 1374–1378
  endocrine system emergencies, 791
  external hemorrhaging, 944–954, 945*f*
  for extrication, 1472–1473
  gastrointestinal emergencies,
    770–771
  head injuries, 1061–1063
  heat-related emergencies,
    1215–1217, 1216*f*
  hematologic emergencies, 797
  for lightning injuries, 1227
  neurologic emergencies, 745–749, 746*t*
  for respiratory system emergencies,
    656–662
  scope of practice, 98
  for shock, 543–548
  thoracic/chest injuries, 1103
  toxicologic emergencies, 833

emergency medical dispatch
  definition of, 13, 27
  purpose of, 13
emergency medical dispatcher (EMD),
    paging of EMS personnel, 152
emergency medical responder (EMR)
  definition of, 4, 27
  training, 10–11, 11*f*
    National EMS Scope of Practice
      Model guidelines, 9*t*
emergency medical service (EMS)
  as career, 6
  components of, 12–21
    communications systems, 12–13
    evaluation, 16
    human resources, 13–14
    information systems, 15–16
    legislation/regulation, 14
    medical direction, 14
    prevention, 19–20
    public access, 12–13
    public education, 19–20
    research, 20–21
    system finance, 18
  definition of, 3, 27
  history of, 7–9
  in incident command system. *See*
    incident command system (ICS),
    EMS branch
  notification, 153
  personnel, 4
  research, 20–21
  response, dispatch, 151
Emergency Medical Services
    Development Act of 1973, 8
emergency medical technician (EMT)
  certification, 3, 27
  definition of, 4, 27
  dependent groups, 323
  effective performance, team, 323–326
  generally, 320
  group *vs.* team, 322–323
  independent groups, 323
  interdependent groups, 323
  National EMS Scope of Practice Model
    guidelines, 9*t*
  professional attributes, 22, 22*t*
  roles/responsibilities, 21–22, 21*t*
    in biologic terrorism/warfare event,
      1548–1549
  teams, types of, 321–322
  training, 6, 11
  training for, 4
emergency moves, 294–295, 294*f*, 318
emergency responders, safety, at
    terrorism events, 1534
emergency responders stress, signs
    of, 1502
*Emergency Response Guidebook*
    (US DOT), 55, 57*f*, 1510, 1510*f*
emergency vehicles
  ambulances. *See* ambulances
  first-responder, 1424, 1462
emesis, 775, 835, 851
emotional crisis, 854

emotional intelligence, 126, 161
empathy
    definition of, 123*t*
    example of, 123*t*
emphysema
    definition of, 672
    lung destruction in, 639
    signs/symptoms, 632*t*
employer, infection control
        responsibilities, 46–47, 48*t*
EMR. *See* emergency medical responder
EMS Agenda for the Future, 9
EMT. *See* emergency medical technician
EMT-assisted medication, 506
endocrine emergencies
    airway assessment, 787
    assessment, 786–791
        chief complaint investigation, 787
        communication/documentation
            of, 790
        history taking, 787
        primary, 786–787
        reassessment, 788–791
        scene size-up, 786
        secondary, 787–788, 788*f*
    breathing assessment, 787
    communication, 797
    documentation, 790
    emergency medical care, 791
    interventions, 788
    safety, on-scene, 786
    transport decisions, 787
endocrine glands, definition of, 778, 801
endocrine system, 230–232, 778, 801
    age-related changes, 1363
    anatomy, 778–780, 779*f*
    in elderly, 266
    emergencies. *See* endocrine
        emergencies
    medical emergencies, 605, 605*t*
    pathophysiology, 780–786
        diabetes. *See* diabetes mellitus
        symptomatic hypoglycemia,
            785–786
    physiology, 778–780
endocrine system emergencies
    assessment, vital signs, 788
    general impressions, 786–787
endometrium, 1244, 1278
end-organ perfusion, 1300
endotracheal (ET) intubation, 477, 489
end-stage renal disease (ESRD), 771
end-tidal carbon dioxide (ETCO$_2$), 437, 489
    in airway management, 437
energy
    kinetic, 902
    nuclear, 1551
    potential, 902
    sources
        complex carbohydrates, 34
        glucose, 34
    trauma and, 901–904, 901*f*
enroute communications, 152*t*
enteral medications, 498
entrance wound, 915

electrical burns, 995, 995*f*
entrapment, 1465, 1483
envenomations, 806, 819, 1228–1234
environmental conditions
    ambient temperature, 1202, 1239
    assessment, in GEMS diamond,
        1368, 1369*t*
    exposure and, 1201–1202
environmental emergencies
    bites and envenomations,
        1228–1234
    definition of, 1200
    exposure
        to cold temperatures, 1202–1203
        factors affecting, 1201–1202
    heat exposure. *See* heat exposure
    from heat exposure, 1210–1213
    heat-related, emergency medical care,
        1215–1217, 1216*f*
    from high altitude, 1226–1227
    lightning injuries, 1227
    marine animal injuries, 1235,
        1235*f*, 1235*t*
    radiation exposure, 1211
    risk factors, 1201
    water-related, 1218–1222
        diving emergencies. *See* diving
            emergencies
        drowning. *See* drowning
        patient assessment, 1223–1225
        water rescue, 1219, 1219*f*
environmental exposure, factors
        affecting, 1201–1202
environmental/industrial exposures,
        647–648, 665
epidemic, 613–614, 625
epidermis, 963, 963*f*, 1003
epidural bleeding, 731, 731*f*
epidural hematoma, 1049–1050,
        1050*f*, 1089
epiglottis
    adult *vs.* child, 421, 421*f*
    in children, 1311–1312
    definition of, 1347
    function, 420
epiglottitis
    characteristics, 632*t*, 635
    in children, 662*f*
    definition of, 672
    signs/symptoms, 632*t*
epilepsy, 753
epinephrine (adrenaline), 513
    administration, 813–816
    for anaphylactic shock, 547*f*
    contraindications, 813*t*
    definition of, 812, 819
    dosage/administration, 812–816
    effects, 533–534
    indications, 813*t*
    side effects, 813*t*
EpiPen administration, 812–816
epiphyseal (growth) plate
    definition of, 1292
    fracture, 1153
    injuries, in children, 1175

epistaxis (nosebleeds)
    controlling, 951–954
    definition of, 959
    emergency medical care, 1028
    nasal fractures and, 1027
equipment, for moving patients, 288*f*,
        309–312, 309*f*, 310*f*, 312*f*
errors
    prevention, 16
    reporting of, 142–143, 142*f*
esophageal intubation, 481, 489
esophageal varices, 762
esophagitis, 762
esophagus, 228
    anatomy, 1093
    functions, 756–757
ESRD (end-stage renal disease), 771
ethical responsibilities, for health care
        providers, 106–107
ethics
    applied, 106, 113
    definition of, 106, 114
    guidelines for decision making,
        106, 107*t*
ethnocentrism, 120, 161
eustachian tube, 1028, 1037
eustress, definition of, 32, 82
evaluation, of emergency medical
        services, functions of, 16
evaporation, 1202, 1240
evidence-based medicine (EBM),
        20, 27
evisceration
    abdominal, emergency medical care,
        1130, 1131*f*
    definition of, 1003, 1143
        abdominal, 1123, 1131*f*
    pathophysiology, 977, 978*f*
excited delirium, 864, 879, 996, 1003
exercise, for wellness, 35, 35*f*
exhalation, 425, 489
external respiration
        (pulmonary), 489
exit wound, 915
    electrical burns, 995, 995*f*
expiration, 425, 629
explanation
    definition of, 123*t*
    example of, 123*t*
explosions
    blast injuries, 1553
    tissues at risk, 1553
exposure
    of children, 1300
    definition of, 38, 82
    determination of, 47*t*
expressed consent, 87, 114
exsanguinations, 1032
extension, definition of, 172, 187
external auditory canal, 1028,
        1029*f*, 1037
external chest compressions
    hand position, 563–565, 565*f*
    technique, 563–565, 565*f*
external defibrillator vest, 1408–1409

external genitalia
female, injuries to, 1134–1135
male, injuries to, 1134
external respiration (pulmonary),
427–428, 427*f*
extremities
focused assessment, 400–401, 400*f*
injuries
pediatric, 1335
that impair circulation, 1162
lower, anatomy of, 1148–1151
physical examination, 1305
upper, anatomy, 1148, 1149*f*
extremity lift, 302, 318
extrication
definition of, 1465, 1483
at mass-casualty incident,
1495, 1495*f*
phases, 1466*t*
arrival and scene size-up,
1467–1469, 1467*f*
emergency care, 1472–1473
en route to scene, 1466–1467
gaining access, 1470–1472, 1471*f*
hazard control, 1469–1470, 1470*f*
preparation, 1466
removal of patient, 1473–1474
support operations, 1470
termination, 1475
transfer of patient, 1474–1475, 1474*f*
extrication supervisor, 1495, 1524
eye
age-related changes, 267
anatomy, 1008–1009, 1008*f*
artificial, 1026–1027
chemical agents in, 827, 828*f*
chemical burns, emergency medical
care, 993–994, 993*f*, 994*f*
contact, as nonverbal
communication, 120–121
contact lenses, 1026–1027
injuries, 1016–1027, 1017*f*
blast injuries, 1026
blunt trauma, 1024–1025, 1025*f*
burns, 1021–1023, 1021–1023*f*
following head trauma,
1025–1026, 1025*f*
foreign objects, 1016–1021
impaled foreign object,
1016–1021
initial examination, 1016*f*
lacerations, 1023–1024, 1024*f*
irrigation, 1017, 1021, 1022*f*
orbit of, 1008
postexposure management, 53–54
protection
for injury prevention, 64
for risk reduction and prevention,
45, 45*f*
raccoon, 1047, 1047*f*, 1089
eyelid, removal of foreign object
from, 1018
eyes-forward position, 1064, 1089

**F**

face
anatomy, 1006–1009, 1007*f*
bleeding, causing airway obstruction,
477, 477*f*
expressions
as nonverbal communication,
120–121
smiling, 121
facial injuries. *See also specific facial
injuries*
assessment, 1011–1015
ABCs, 1014
chief complaint investigation,
1012–1013
communication/documentation
of, 1015
general impressions, 1011
history taking, 1012–1013
primary, 1011–1012
scene size-up, 1011
secondary, 1013–1014
of vital signs, 1013
emergency medical care, 1015–1033,
1015*f*
fractures, 1030–1031, 1031*f*
emergency medical care, 1030–
1031, 1030*f*
maxillary, 1011
nasal, 1027–1028
interventions, 1014
safety, on-scene, 1011
soft-tissue, 1010, 1010*f*
transport decisions, 1012
facilitation, 123*t*
fainting. *See* syncope
fallopian tubes
anatomy, 882*f*, 883, 1244
definition of, 897
falls, accidental
abdominal injuries from, 1121
blunt trauma from, 912–913, 913*f*
in elderly, 1378–1379
during pregnancy, 1251
false imprisonment, 102, 114
false motion, 1155, 1197
as fracture sign, 1155
family
balancing with work and health, 38
members of patient who has died,
working with, 69
presence during patient
interview, 123
fascia, 967, 1003
definition of, 1147, 1197
compartment syndrome and,
1191–1192
FCC (Federal Communications
Commission), 150, 161
febrile seizures
in children, 1323
definition of, 732, 753

Federal Communications Commission
(FCC), 150, 161
The Federal Food, Drug, and Cosmetic
Act of 1938, 497
female reproductive system
acute abdomen, causes of, 766
anatomy, 757, 882–883, 882*f*, 1131,
1133*f*, 1243–1245, 1244*f*
external genitalia, 882*f*
genitalia injuries, 1134–1135, 1138
pathophysiology, 884–886
physiology, normal, 882–883
femoral shaft fractures, 1181–1186
fertilization, 1244–1245*f*
fetal alcohol syndrome, 1251, 1278
fetal death, 1273–1274
fetal distress, 1251
fetus, 1244, 1278
fever
in elderly, 1363
pediatric, 1327–1328
fibula, 1150, 1150*f*, 1197
injuries, 1189, 1189*f*
field impression, 342, 411
finance and administration, in incident
command system, 1488, 1524
finger injuries, 1176, 1176*f*
fire, hazards in, 58–59, 58*f*
fire ant stings, 807, 807*f*
firefighter's carry, 296*f*
firefighter's drag, 296*f*
firefighting gloves, for injury prevention,
63, 63*f*
first-responder vehicles, 1424, 1462
flail chest, 1107–1108, 1107*f*, 1115
flame burn, 991, 1003
flank, of human body, 1128, 1143
flash burn, 991, 1003
flexible stretchers, 310–311, 311*f*, 318
flexion
definition of, 172, 187
injuries, of spine, 1052
Flovent Diskus (fluticasone), 658*t*
flowchart, patient assessment, 343, 350,
366, 377, 404
fluticasone (Flovent Diskus), 658*t*
flutter valve, 1103, 1115
focal seizures, definition of,
732, 753
focused assessment
abdomen, 399, 399*f*
back, 401
cardiovascular system, 387–393
cervical spine, 398
chest, 398–399
in chief complaint investigation, 385*t*
definition of, 411
extremities, 400–401, 401*f*
head, 398, 398*f*
neck, 398, 398*f*
neurologic system, 394
neurovascular status, 396–398
respiratory system, 383–384

fontanelles
  anatomy, 256*f*
  assessment, 1293
  definition of, 271, 1347
  functions, 256
food, as allergen, 806
foodborne transmission, 40, 82
food poisoning, 843–845
foot
  bones, 1150, 1150*f*
  injuries, 1190–1191, 1191*f*
force
  causing musculoskeletal
      injuries, 1151
  in determining mechanism of
      injury, 346
forcible restraint
  definition of, 89, 114
  local laws and, 89–90, 89*f*
forearm fractures, 1175–1176, 1176*f*
foreign bodies
  airway obstruction
    in infants/children, 590–593, 591*f*
    recognizing, 587, 587*f*, 645, 645*f*
  in eye, 1016–1021
  impaled
    in abdomen, 1128
    emergency medical care, 978
    in eye, 1020
  obstruction
    recognition, 475, 475*f*
  removal
    from airway, 588–590, 588*f*, 591*f*
    in airway obstruction, 588–590,
        588*f*, 591*f*
    in responsive infants, 590–591, 591*f*
    in unresponsive infants, 593
  in vagina, 889
foreign body aspiration, 665
foreign body aspiration and obstruction
      in infants/children, 1308–1310,
      1309*f*
four-person log roll, 1067
Fowler position, 173–174, 173*f*, 187
  definition of, 173
fractures
  blood loss from, 1178
  in child, through growth plate, 1175
  in child abuse, 1338
  clavicle, 1109
  closed, 1153, 1196
  definition of, 1152, 1197
  in elderly, 1374
  facial. *See* facial injuries, fractures
  greenstick, 1335
  humerus, 1172–1173, 1172*t*
  injuries associated with, 1152–1155
  open, 1153, 1197
  osteoporosis and, 1180
  pathologic, 1153
  rib, 1107
  signs/symptoms, 1154*f*, 1155
  skull, 1046–1048, 1048*f*

basilar, 1047, 1048*f*
  depressed, 1047, 1048*f*
  linear, 1047, 1047*f*
  open, 1047–1048, 1048*f*
  sternal, 1108–1109
  types, 1153, 1153*f*
freelancing, 1487, 1524
free movement, as fracture sign, 1155
freight bills, for hazardous materials,
      1511, 1512*f*, 1524
French catheter, 443, 444*f*
frequency, definition of, 147
friends, presence during patient
      interview, 123
front cradle carry, 296*f*
frostbite, 360, 411
  definition of, 1206, 1240
  emergency medical care, 1210
  signs/symptoms, 1206, 1206*f*
frostnip, 1205–1206
full-thickness (third-degree) burns,
      984–985, 984*f*, 1003
functional disorders, 857, 879
fundus, 1244*f*, 1278
fungal infections, 615

## G

G agents, 1537, 1558
gag reflex, 446, 446*f*, 489
gallstones, 761
gamma (x-ray) radiation, 1549, 1558
gangrene, 1206
gas cylinders
  flowmeters, 454, 454*f*
  pressure regulators, 454
  safety considerations, 453
gases. *See specific gases*
gas transfer, in lungs, 628
gastric distention
  airway management and, 467
  artificial ventilation and, 569
  definition of, 601
gastroenteritis, 763–764
gastroesophageal reflux disease (GERD),
      762, 775
gastrointestinal bleeding, 1361
gastrointestinal emergencies
  assessment, 766–770
    communication/documentation
        of, 768
    general impressions, 768
    history taking, 768
    mechanism of injury/nature of
        illness, 767
    primary, 767–768
    reassessment, 770
    scene size-up, 766–767
    secondary, 768–770, 769*f*
    of vital signs, 770
  safety, on-scene, 766–767
  transport decisions, 768
gastrointestinal hemorrhage, 762

gastrointestinal system
  age-related changes, 1360–1362
  anatomy, 756–757, 756*f*
  bleeding. *See* gastrointestinal
      hemorrhage
  in children, 1292
  emergencies. *See* gastrointestinal
      emergencies
  medical emergencies, 605, 605*t*
  pathophysiology, 758–766
  pediatric emergencies,
      1324–1325
gastrostomy tubes (gastric tubes;
      G-tubes), 1409–1410, 1409*f*
GA (tabun), 1538, 1541*t*
GB (sarin), 1538, 1541*t*
GCS. *See* Glasgow Coma Scale
GD (soman), 1538, 1541*t*
gel, definition of, 503
GEMS diamond, 1368, 1369*t*
general adaptation syndrome, 69, 82
general impressions. *See also under
      specific emergencies*
  definition of, 351, 411
  formation, 351, 351*f*
generalized anxiety disorder, 856
generalized seizures, definition of,
      732, 753
generalized (tonic-clonic) seizure,
      1328, 1347
generic name, definition of, 497
genital system, 233–234
  female, 234. *See also* female
      reproductive system
  male, 233–234. *See also* male
      reproductive system
genitourinary injuries. *See also specific
      genitourinary injuries*
  anatomy, 1133–1135
  assessment, 1135–1137
    chief complaint investigation, 1136
    history taking, 1136
    primary, 1135–1136
    reassessment, 1137
    scene size-up, 1135
    secondary, 1136–1137
    of vital signs, 1137
  emergency medical care, 1137–1138
  interventions, 1137
  rape, 1138–1139
  safety, on-scene, 1135
  sexual assault, 1138-1139
  transport decisions, 1136
GERD (gastroesophageal reflux disease),
      762, 775
geriatric emergencies
  assessment, 1368–1373
    chief complaint investigation, 1371
    general impressions, 1370
    history taking, 1371–1372
    primary, 1370–1371
    reassessment, 1372–1373
    scene size-up, 1369–1370

geriatric emergencies *(Continued)*
  secondary, 1372
  of vital signs, 1372
  XABCs, 1368
geriatric patients. *See* elderly
geriatrics, 1388
geriatric trauma, 1375–1378
  assessment
    falls assessment, 1378–1379
    history taking, 1376–1377
    primary, 1376
    reassessment, 1377–1378
    scene size-up, 1375–1376
    secondary, 1377
gestation, 1245
gestational diabetes, 780, 1247, 1278
gestational hypertension, 1247, 1279
glands. *See specific glands*
Glasgow Coma Scale (GCS), 395*t*, 1058
  definition, 930–931
  modified, 1059
  in neurologic emergencies, 745*t*
  in pediatric emergencies, 1300, 1301*t*
  scoring, 395*t*, 745*t*, 924, 926*t*
  trauma score and, 924, 926*t*
glaucoma, 1358
glenoid fossa, 1171, 1197
globe, 1009, 1037
glottic opening, 420
glottis, 420, 489
gloves
  for cleaning/disinfecting, 43–45, 43*f*
  double, 43
  firefighting, 63, 63*f*
  latex, 43
  removal technique, 43–44
  vinyl, 43
glucagon, 779
  for hypoglycemia, 784
glucometer (blood glucose monitor),
    404, 788
glucose
  blood levels. *See* blood glucose
  definition of, 779, 801
  as energy source, 34
  function, 779–780
  oral administration, 746, 791, 791*f*
Golden Period (Golden Hour), 364, 364*f*,
    411, 543, 1158
gonorrhea, 885, 897
good air exchange, 475, 489
Good Samaritan laws, 103–104, 114
governmental immunity, definition,
    108, 114
grand mal seizures. *See* tonic-clonic
    seizures
greenstick fractures, 1153, 1153*f*, 1335
grieving process, 68
gross negligence, 103, 114
group, definition of, 322
grunting, 1295, 1347
guarding
  abdominal, 399
  definition of, 411, 775, 1143
  disorders associated with, 769

as fracture sign, 1154
signs/symptoms, 1126
gum elastic bougie, 478, 489
gunshot wounds, penetrating trauma
    from, 915, 915*f*
gynecologic emergencies, 605*t*. *See also*
    *specific gynecologic emergencies*
  assessment, 886–889
    ABCs, 889
    chief complaint investigation, 887
    communication/documentation
      of, 889
    general impressions, 886
    history taking, 887
    mechanism of injury/nature of
      illness, 886
    physical examinations, 887
    primary, 886–887
    reassessment, 889
    scene size-up, 886
    secondary, 887–889
    of vital signs, 888
  emergency medical care, 889
  interventions, 889
  transport decisions, 888

**H**

hallucinogens
  definition of, 841–842, 851
  overdose, 841–842
hand
  anatomy, 1148, 1149*f*
  injuries, 1176–1177, 1176*f*
  position, for external chest
    compressions, 563–565, 565*f*
hand signals, for air medical operations,
    1456, 1457*f*
handwashing, proper technique for,
    41, 43
HAPE (high-altitude pulmonary
    edema), 1226–1227
hay fever, 663, 672
hazard control, at extrication scene,
    1469–1470, 1470*f*
hazardous materials
  containers, 1505–1508, 1505*f*,
    1506*f*, 1507*f*
  definition of, 1467, 1484, 1503
  Department of Transportation marking
    system, 1508–1509, 1508*f*
  detection by senses, 1504–1505
  identification, 1513–1514
  occupancy/location, 1504
  references
    CHEMTREC, 1511, 1523
    *Emergency Response Guidebook,*
      1510, 1510*f*
    safety data sheets, 1510–1511, 1511*f*
    shipping papers/bills of lading,
      1511, 1511*f*, 1523
  safety placards, 56*f*
  situations with. *See* hazardous
    materials incidents

hazardous materials incidents (hazmat
    incidents)
  definition of, 1503, 1524
  examples, 1503–1504, 1504*f*
  scene operations, 1514–1515
    establishing control zones,
      1514–1515, 1515*f*
    patient care, 1517–1519
    personal protective equipment
      levels, 1516–1517, 1517*f*
hazards, on-scene evaluation of, 54–61,
    54*f*, 344–345, 345*f*
hazmat incidents. *See* hazardous
    materials incidents
HAZWOPER regulations, 1503
head. *See also specific structures of*
  anatomy, 1006–1009, 1007*f*
  focused assessment, 398, 398*f*
  injuries. *See* head injuries
  physical examination, 1305
  trauma, eye injuries from,
    1025–1026, 1025*f*
headache
  emergency medical care, 747
  types of, 747
head injuries. *See also* traumatic brain
    injury (TBI)
  assessment, 920, 1053–1061
    chief complaint investigation, 1056
    communication/documentation
      of, 1061
    history taking, 1056–1057
    primary, 1054–1056
    reassessment, 1060–1061
    scene size-up, 1053–1054
    secondary, 1057–1060
    of vital signs, 1060
    XABCs, 1054
  definition of, 1045
  emergency medical care,
    1061–1063
  helmet removal, 1079–1084, 1080*f*
  interventions, 1060
  safety, on-scene, 1053–1054
  transport
    decision making for, 1056
    of sitting patients, 1075–1077
    of supine patients, 1067–1075
  traumatic
    eye injuries from, 1025–1026, 1025*f*
    pediatric, immobilization
      techniques for, 1330–1333
head-on collision, motorcycle, 912
head tilt–chin lift maneuver
  definition of, 489, 601
  technique
    for adult, 440, 566, 566*f*
    for child, 582
head trauma, definition of, 1045
health, balancing with work and
    family, 38
health care directive, 93, 114
health care professionals. *See specific
    health care professionals*
health care proxy, 93, 114

Health Insurance Portability and
    Accountability Act (HIPAA), 18,
    27, 91–92, 125
hearing, age-related changes, 267, 1358
hearing aids, 1398–1400, 1399f
hearing-impaired patients, 1397–1400,
    1399f
    communication with, 129–130, 129f
    dealing with, 129–130
    hearing aids for, 1398–1400, 1399f
hearing impairments
    age-related, 1358
    history taking and, 375
heart, 208–210
    blood flow, 680f
    circulation, 679–684, 681f
    definition of, 677
    electrical conduction system, 678, 678f
    in perfusion triangle, 532, 533f
    structures of, 677f
    valves of, 677f
heart failure in elderly, 1370
heat cramps
    definition of, 1211, 1240
    emergency medical care, 1215, 1215f
    pathophysiology, 1211
heat exhaustion
    definition of, 1211, 1240
    emergency medical care, 1215–1217
    pathophysiology, 1211–1212
    signs/symptoms, 1211–1212
heat exposure illnesses
    assessment, 1213–1215, 1214t
        chief complaint investigation, 1214
        communication/documentation
            of, 1215
        history taking, 1214
        primary, 1213–1214, 1214t
        reassessment, 1214–1215
        scene size-up, 1213
        secondary, 1214
        of vital signs, 1214
    interventions, 1215
    pathophysiology, 1211–1212
    safety, on-scene, 1213
    transport decisions, 1214
    types of. See specific heat-related
        illnesses
heat index, 1212f
heatstroke
    definition of, 1212, 1240
    emergency medical care,
        1217, 1217f
    pathophysiology, 1212–1213
    signs/symptoms, 1212–1213
Heimlich maneuver (abdominal-thrust
    maneuver), 588f, 600
Helicobacter pylori, 760
helmets
    for injury prevention, 63, 63f
    motorcycle collisions and, 911
    removal, 1079–1084, 1080f
        alternate method, 1083–1084, 1083f
        car-versus-bicycle collision and,
            911, 911f
    in head and spinal injuries,
        1079–1084, 1083f
    preferred method, 1081–1083
helminthic infections, 615
hematemesis, 761, 775, 835, 851, 941,
    959, 1361, 1388
hematologic disorder, 793
hematologic emergencies. See also
    specific hematologic emergencies
    assessment, 796–797
        chief complaint investigation, 796
        communication/documentation
            of, 797
        general impressions, 796
        history taking, 796–797
        mechanism of injury/nature of
            illness, 796
        primary, 796
        reassessment, 797
        scene size-up, 796
        secondary, 797
        of vital signs, 797
    emergency medical care, 797
    as medical emergencies, 605, 605t
    pathophysiology, 793–796, 794f
    safety, on-scene, 796
    transport decisions, 797
hematology, 793, 801
    anatomy, 793, 794f
    blood-forming organs, 793, 794f
    definition of, 783
    physiology, 793, 794f
hematomas
    definition of, 959, 1003
    in elderly, 1050
    epidural, 1049–1050, 1050f
    facial, 1010, 1010f
    internal bleeding and, 941
    pathophysiology, 965, 965f
    subdural, 1050, 1050f, 1089
hematopoietic system
    emergencies. See hematologic
        emergencies
hematuria, 941, 959
    definition of, 1143, 1179, 1197
    pelvic fractures and, 1178–1179
    urinary tract infections and, 765
hemiparesis
    definition of, 753
    postictal state and, 735
hemoglobin, 427
hemophilia, 794–795, 801, 939, 959
    pediatric, 1322
hemopneumothorax, 1106f, 1115
hemoptysis, 941, 959, 1097
hemorrhage
    definition of, 938, 959
    external
        emergency medical care for,
            944–954, 945f
        types of, 938–940, 939f
    gastrointestinal, 762
    internal, 940–941
    in elderly, 942
    postpartum, 1264
subarachnoid, 1050–1051, 1089
hemorrhagic shock, 539
hemorrhagic stroke
    causes, 729–730
    definition of, 753
hemorrhoids, 764
hemostatic dressing, 946, 959
hemothorax, 431, 489
    definition of, 1105, 1115
    pathophysiology, 1105
hepatitis
    characteristics, 617t
    definition of, 39, 82, 615
    signs/symptoms, 615–618, 616f
    transmission, 39, 617t
hepatitis A immunization, 51
hepatitis B vaccine program, 47t
herbicides, absorption of, 827
hernia, 765, 775
heroin, 836
herpes simplex, 614, 625
high-altitude pulmonary edema
    (HAPE), 1226–1227
high-level disinfection, 1442, 1462
high-visibility public safety vest, 61
highways, driving emergency vehicles
    on, 1452
Highway Safety Act of 1966, 8
HIPAA (Health Insurance Portability
    and Accountability Act), 18, 27,
    91–92, 125
hip dislocation, 1179–1180, 1180f
histamine, definition of, 804, 819
history taking, 366–376. See also
    assessment for specific
    emergencies
    anger and, 373–374
    with confusing behavior and
        history, 374
    with crying patients, 374
    definition of, 366, 411
    with depressed patients, 374
    history of present illness. See chief
        complaint investigation
    hostility and, 373–374
    identifying pertinent negatives, 369
    language barrier in, 375
    multiple symptoms and, 372–373
    OPQRST, 368–369
    OPQRST-I. See OPQRST-I
    for patients with limited cognitive
        abilities, 374–375
    SAMPLE history. See SAMPLE history
    on sensitive topics, 370–372, 371f
    silent patients and, 372
    for visually impaired patients, 376
HIV. See human immunodeficiency
    virus
H1N1 virus (swine flu), 614
hollow organs, 1120f, 1123–1124, 1143
homelessness, 1412–1413
homeostasis, 1200, 1240
    definition of, 553
    in shock, 531
home remedies, 695

honeybee stings, 807, 812*f*
hormones, definition of, 778, 801
hornet stings, 807
hospice care, 1411–1412
hospital, EMS provider communication
    with, 153–156, 153*f*
host, 51, 82
hostility
    in grieving process, 68
    of patient, history taking and, 373–374
hot zone (danger zone), 1469, 1514*f*,
    1515, 1524
household cleaning products,
    poisonings from, 844
human bite wounds, 980–981, 981*f*
human body
    cells, 191
    cellular metabolism, alteration of, 240
    circulatory system. *See* circulatory
        system
    digestive system. *See* digestive system
    endocrine system, 230–232
    genital system, 233–234
        female, 234
        male, 233–234
    integumentary system. *See*
        integumentary system
    life support chain, 235
    lymphatic system, 230
    musculoskeletal system. *See*
        musculoskeletal system
    nervous system. *See* nervous system
    pathophysiology, 236–238
    planes of body, 190–191, 190*f*
    respiratory system. *See* respiratory
        system
    shock, 238–240
    skeletal system. *See* skeletal system
    topographic anatomy, 190–191
    urinary system, 232–233
human immunodeficiency virus (HIV)
    definition of, 39, 82
    immune response, 51
    signs/symptoms, 614–615
    transmission of, 39
humerus
    distal, fracture of, 1172–1173
    fracture, 1172–1173, 1172*t*
hydration, proper, 34–35
hydrocarbons, 839
hydrogen cyanide inhalation injury, 992
hydroplaning, 1449, 1462
hymenoptera, 1229–1230, 1240
hypercarbia, 430, 489
hyperextension of spine, 1052
hyperglycemia
    characteristics, 781*t*
    definition of, 733, 753, 780, 801
    interventions, 788
    signs/symptoms, 780–781, 781*t*
hyperosmolar hyperglycemic
        nonketotic syndrome (HHNS),
        785, 801, 1363
hyperosmolar hyperglycemic syndrome
        (HHS), 1363

hypersensitivity to drugs, 511
hypertension
    definition of, 392, 411
    in elderly, 1372
    during pregnancy, 1247–1248
hypertensive emergency
    aortic/dissecting aneurysm, 691
    definition of, 690, 721
hyperthermia, 1211, 1214, 1240
hyperventilation, 568, 601, 646–647,
    664–665, 672
hyperventilation syndrome (panic
    attack), 646, 672
hyphema, 1024, 1025*f*
hypnotic, 834, 851
hypoglycemia, 507
    altered mental state and, 736, 736*f*
    altered mental status, 857
    characteristics, 781*t*
    definition of, 733, 753, 801
    emergency medical care, 792–793
    interventions, 788
    pathophysiology (symptomatic),
        785–786
    signs/symptoms, 780–781, 781*t*
hypoperfusion, 936, 959
hypotension, 392, 411, 1061
hypothermia, 360, 411
    death and, 95
    definition of, 553, 1203, 1240
    emergency medical care, 1209*f*, 1210
    mild, 1203
    neurogenic shock and, 538
    prevention, 1209–1210
    severe, 1204
    signs/symptoms, 1203–1205, 1204*t*
    submersion and, 1220
hypothermia thermometer, 1203
hypovolemic shock, 539
    causes, 539, 544*t*
    circulatory compromise and, 431
    definition of, 553, 959
    development, 941
    in open injuries, 977
    signs/symptoms, 544*t*
    treatment, 544*t*, 547–548
hypoxemia, 435
hypoxia
    death from, 426
    definition of, 489, 633, 672
    in elderly, 1375
    mental status alteration and, 857
    signs of, 128
hypoxic drive
    carbon dioxide retention and, 633
    definition of, 489, 633, 672
    physiology, 426

**I**

IC. *See* incident commander
ICP. *See* intracranial pressure
ICS. *See* incident command system
i-gel airway device, 480*f*
ileostomy, 1410, 1418

ileus, 758, 775
illness prevention, 77
IM injections. *See* intramuscular
    injections
immediate care or treatment. *See*
    emergency medical care
immersion foot, 1205–1206
immobilization
    of cervical spine, 1064
    of children, 1083, 1083*f*
    of infant in car seat, 1084
    for pediatric head injuries, 1330–1333
        in car seat, 1331–1332
    in sitting position, 1075–1077
immobilization devices, 1064–1067
    cervical collars, 1065–1067, 1067*f*
    KED vest-type, for backboards, 311*f*
    long backboards, 1079*f*
immune. *See* immunity
immune response, 804, 819
immune system, 804
    age-related changes, 1363
    definition of, 804, 819
    emergencies. *See* immunologic
        emergencies
    infants, 257
    pathophysiology, 804–806, 805*f*
    physiology, 804, 805*f*
immunity
    definition of, 51, 82
    Good Samaritan laws and, 103–104
    to infectious disease, 51–53, 52*t*
immunizations, 51–53
immunologic emergencies
    assessment, 808–812
        chief complaint investigation, 809
        communication/documentation
            of, 812
        emergency medical care, 812–816
        history taking, 809–810
        interventions, 812
        as medical emergencies, 605, 605*t*
        primary, 808–809
        reassessment, 811–812
        safety, on-scene, 808
        scene size-up, 808
        secondary, 810–811
        transport decisions, 811–812
        of vital signs, 811
immunology, 804, 819
impaled objects, 968, 1003
impedance threshold device (ITD), 575,
    576*f*, 601
implied consent
    definition of, 88, 114
    emergency doctrine of, 88
    for treating children in critical
        situations, 88
inadequate breathing, 207
incarcerated hernia, 765
incendiary/explosive devices, in
    terrorism, 1552–1553
incident action plan, 1490, 1524
incident commander (IC)
    definition of, 1484, 1488, 1524

roles/responsibilities, 1475–1476, 1475*f*, 1488–1489
incident command system (ICS)
   command, 1488–1489, 1524
   command staff, 1490
   communications and information management, 1487, 1490–1491
   definition of, 411, 1487, 1524
   EMS branch
      communications, 1493
      establishing command, 1493
      organization of, 1493*f*
      preparedness of, 1491–1492
      response within, 1491–1493, 1492*f*
   equipment, 1491–1492
   finance and administration, 1489, 1524
   logistics, 1489–1490, 1524
   medical branch. *See* medical incident command
   mobilization/deployment, 1491
   with multiple patients, 348, 348*f*
   operations, 1490
   organizational divisions, 1487, 1488*f*
   planning, 1490
   roles/responsibilities, 1487–1490, 1489*f*
incident management, 1486–1518
incision, 967, 1003
incomplete fracture, 1153
incontinence
   definition of, 734, 753
   generalized seizures and, 734
incubation period, 1543, 1558
index of suspicion, 607, 625, 901, 931
indications, definition of, 496, 497
indirect contact, 39, 83
induced abortion, 1250, 1279
industrial/environmental exposures, 647–648, 665
infancy, definition of, 1285, 1347
infants
   airway, 421, 421*f*
   assessment, 1285–1286
   bag-mask ventilation, 256
   basic life support, 577–583, 578*t*
   blood loss, from skull region, 1061
   burn injuries, 986*t*
   cardiovascular system, 255
   chest compressions, 578
   definition of, 254, 255*f*, 271
   falling accidents, 255
   falls/injuries in, 255
   foreign body airway obstruction, 590–593, 591*f*
   growth/development, 1285–1286, 1286*f*
   immobilization in car seat, 1084
   immune system, 257
   immunizations, recommended, 51
   neonates
      definition of, 271, 354
      pulmonary system, 255–256
   nervous system, 256–257
   physical changes, vital signs, 254
   psychosocial changes, 257–258, 257*t*
   pulmonary system, 255–256
   weight, 254
infarction, 685, 721
infection
   definition
      definition of, 38, 83
      risk reduction, 41
infection control
   definition of, 48, 83
   employer responsibilities for, 46–47, 48*t*
   establishing routine for, 48–49
   plan, components of, 47–48*t*
infectious disease, 613, 625
   AIDS, 614–615
   causes of, 615
   *vs.* communicable diseases, 38
   COVID-19, 620
   definition of, 38, 83
   Ebola, 620
   epidemic and pandemic considerations, 613–614
   general assessment principles, 613
   immunity to, 51–53, 52*t*
   management principles, general, 613
   MERS-CoV, 620
   postexposure management, 53–54
   risk reduction and prevention, 41–50
      employer responsibilities, 46–47, 48*t*
      establishing infection control routine, 48–49
      eye protection, 45, 45*f*
      gloves, 43–44, 43*f*
      gowns, 45
      handwashing, proper technique for, 41, 43
      masks, respirators, and barrier devices, 45–46, 45*f*
      sharps disposal, proper, 46, 46*f*
      standard precautions, 41, 42*t*
   routes of transmission, 38–40, 39*f*
   travel medicine and, 620–621
inferior, definition of, 679, 721
inferior portion, definition of, 170–171, 187
inferior vena cava, 677, 677*f*
influenza, 614, 625
   definition of, 614
   type A
      characteristics, 632*t*
      definition of, 637, 672
informed consent, 87, 114
ingestion, 804, 822, 852
   of toxins, 822, 825*f*
inhalation, 499, 806
   definition of, 424, 489
   physiology, 424–425
inhalation injury, 992
inhalation medications, 515–518
injury patterns, in vehicle collisions, pediatric, 1329–1330
injury prevention, 77
   body armor, 65
   ear protection for, 64
   eye protection for, 64
   protective clothing for, 61–65, 62*f*, 64*f*
   skin protection for, 64

*in loco parentis*, definition, 89, 114
insecticides, absorption of, 827
insect stings
   allergens from, 806–808
   allergic reactions to, 807
   removal of stinger, 812, 812*f*
inspiration, 424, 629
institutional standards, standards of care and, 99–100
insulin
   definition of, 779, 801
   diabetes mellitus and, 780–781
   pumps, for diabetes, 782
   role of, 779–780
Intal (cromolyn), 658*t*
integumentary system
   anatomy, 224–225
      in children, 1294
   physiology, 225–226
intellectual disability, 1393, 1418
intended effect, 497
intermodal tanks, 1506, 1524
internal cardiac pacemakers, 1408
internal respiration, 428, 428*f*, 489
International Liaison Committee on Resuscitation (ILCOR), 21
international terrorism, 1528. *See also* terrorism
interoperable communications system, 149, 161
interpretation
   definition of, 123*t*
   example of, 123*t*
interrogatories, definition, 108, 114
interventions in OPQRST. *See under* *specific emergencies*
intervertebral disks, 1045, 1089
interviews, patient
   with adolescents, 262
   communication techniques, 123
   with elderly, 127–128, 127*f*
   presence of family, friends or bystanders during, 123
   questions for, 122
   techniques to avoid, 124*t*
   therapeutic rapport for, 125–126, 125*f*
intestine, 757
intoxicated patients, history taking and, 374
intracerebral hematoma, 1050, 1050*f*, 1089
intracranial pressure (ICP)
   definition of, 1049, 1089
   increase, with hemorrhagic stroke, 727
   increased, in infant, 257
   in traumatic brain injury, 1049–1051
intramuscular (IM) injection, 499
intramuscular medications, 513–515
intranasal (IN), 500
intranasal medications, 515
intraosseous (IO) injection, 499
intrapulmonary shunting, 431, 490
intravenous access, pediatric, 1326
intravenous (IV) injection, 499

intravenous (IV) therapy, 28
involuntary activities, 1043, 1089
involuntary consent, 88
ionizing radiation, 1549, 1558
ipratropium (Atrovent), 658*t*
iris, 1009, 1009*f*, 1037
irreversible shock, 540, 540*t*
irrigation, of eye, 1017, 1021, 1022*f*
ischemia, 577, 601, 684, 721, 728, 753
ischemic stroke
    definition of, 728, 753
    pathophysiology, 728–729, 728*f*
islets of Langerhans
    definition of, 779
    function, 779
isolette, 312, 312*f*
ITD (impedance threshold device), 575,
    576*f*, 601
IV administration. *See* intravenous
    administration
IV fluid therapy. *See* intravenous fluid
    therapy
IV solutions. *See* intravenous solutions

## J

jaundice, 359, 411, 616, 616*f*
jaw-thrust maneuver
    definition of, 490, 601
    purpose, 441–442
    technique, 566, 567*f*, 1055, 1064*f*
        for adult, 441–442
        for child, 582–583
jellyfish stings, 1235, 1235*f*
JIC (joint information center),
    1490, 1524
joint information center (JIC),
    1490, 1524
joints, 192–193
    anatomy, 1150, 1150*f*
    definition of, 1150, 1197
    functions, 1150*f*
jugular vein distention, 1356, 1388
jugular vein distention (JVD), 1098
jump kit, 1432–1433, 1433*f*, 1433*t*, 1462
JumpSTART triage system, 1335, 1335*f*,
    1500–1501, 1524
junctional tourniquet, 951, 959
JVD (jugular vein distention), 1098

## K

KED vest-type immobilization device,
    for backboards, 311*f*
ketamine (Special K), 838
kidnapping, 114
kidney/kidneys
    anatomy, 1124
    definition of, 764
    infection, localization of pain, 760*t*
    injuries, 1124, 1137
kidney stones
    characteristics, 764–765
    definition of, 775
    localization of pain, 760*t*

kinetic energy, 902, 931
King LT airway device, 480*f*
knee
    dislocation, 1187–1188
    ligament injuries, 1187
Kübler-Ross, Elisabeth, 68
Kussmaul respirations, 434, 783,
    787, 801
kyphosis, 1364, 1388

## L

labels, for hazardous materials,
    1508–1509, 1508*f*
labia majora, 882, 882*f*, 897
labia minora, 882, 882*f*, 897
labor, stages, 1255–1256
labored breathing, 356, 411, 432, 433*f*,
    490
lacerations
    definition of, 1003
    ear, 1028, 1030*f*
    emergency medical care, 1023, 1024*f*
    eye, 1023–1024, 1024*f*
    facial, 1023
    fractures and, 1161
    pathophysiology, 967, 967*f*
    scalp, 1046, 1046*f*
lacrimal glands, 1009, 1009*f*, 1037
lactic acid, 1146
landing zones, for air medical
        operations, patient transfer,
        1456–1457
    establishing, 1455
    safety considerations, 1456–1457,
        1457*f*
landline phone, 149
language
    barriers, in history taking, 375
    tone, pace and volume of, 120
    understandable, in dealing with
        patient, 125
large intestine, 229
laryngectomy, 474
laryngopharynx (hypopharynx), 419,
    419*f*
laryngospasm, 446
larynx
    anatomy, 420, 1008, 1008*f*
    definition of, 490
    fracture, 1033
    injuries, 1033
lateral portion, definition of, 171, 187
law enforcement personnel, scene
    safety and, 61
laws/regulations
    for driving emergency vehicles,
        1450–1452
    standards of care imposed by, 98–99
LDB (load-distributing band), 576–577,
    577*f*, 601
12-lead ECG electrodes, 699, 699*f*
left ventricular assist devices, 575,
    704, 1408
leg, anatomy, 1150, 1150*f*

legal authority, limited in behavioral
        emergencies, 874
legislation, EMS, 14. *See also specific
    legislation*
length-based resuscitation tape,
    1313*t*, 1347
lens, 1008*f*, 1009, 1037
leukocytes, 793. *See also* white blood
    cells
leukotrienes, 804, 819
level A protection, 1516, 1517*f*
level B protection, 1516, 1517*f*
level C protection, 1516, 1517*f*
level D protection, 1516–1517, 1517*f*
level of consciousness
    AVPU test for, 352, 353*f*
    categories of, 352–353
    in pediatric emergencies, 1300
lewisite (L), 1536, 1541*t*, 1558
liaison officer, 1490, 1524
libel, definition of, 102, 115
licensing standards, for radio
        equipment, 151
licensure
    definition of, 4, 28, 100
    requirements, 6–7
life expectancy, 264, 271
life support chain, 235
lifting of patients
    directions/commands, 291–293
    equipment, 284
    from ground, 300–302
    guidelines, 283*t*
    of obese patients, 307
    by one rescuer, 294*f*, 296*f*
    personal considerations, 313
    positioning, 312–313
    restraints, 313
    technique, 274–275, 275*f*
        for power lift, 278, 318
        proper hold for, 317
    vacuum mattresses, 311
ligaments, definition of, 1150, 1197
light burns, to eye, 1023
lightening, of fetus, 1256, 1279
lightning, as scene hazard, 58
lightning injuries, 1227
limb lead placement, 699, 699*f*
limb presentation, 1271, 1271*f*, 1279
linear skull fracture, 1047, 1048*f*, 1089
linens, contaminated, removal of, 50, 51*f*
liquid oxygen, 452
lithium, 833
liver, 228–229
    physiology, 757
living will. *See* advance directives
L (lewisite), 1536, 1541*t*, 1558
load-distributing band (LDB), 576–577,
    577*f*, 601
locked joint, as fracture sign, 1155
logistics, in incident command system,
    1489–1490, 1524
log rolling, for moving patients
    technique, 282, 282*f*, 1074
lone wolf terrorist attack, 1529, 1558

Los Angeles Prehospital Stroke Scale, 741, 743*t*
lower airway, 200–201
lower extremities, 196–197
LSD (lysergic acid diethylamide), 841
lumen, 684, 721
lungs
    assessment, in respiratory system emergencies, 650–651
    compliance, 468
    wet *vs.* dry, 640, 641*t*
lung sounds, adventitious, 650, 651*t*
Lyme disease, 1234, 1234*f*
lymphatic system, 230
    bubonic plague and, 1545
    definition of, 1558
lymph nodes
    bubonic plague and, 1545
    definition of, 1559
lysergic acid diethylamide (LSD), 841

## M

macular degeneration, 1357–1358
male reproductive system
    anatomy, 757, 1132, 1132*f*
    external genitalia, injuries to, 1134
    genitalia injuries, emergency medical care, 1137–1138
Mallory-Weiss tear, 763
mandatory reporting, 104
mandibular fractures, 1011
manual left displacement of the uterus, 594*f*
marijuana, 841
marine animal injuries, 1235, 1235*f*, 1235*t*
masks
    for infectious disease risk reduction, 45–46, 45*f*
    nonbreathing. *See* nonbreathing masks
mass-casualty incidents (MCIs)
    accountability, 1491
    definition of, 1486, 1496, 1524
    demobilization, 1491
    diagram, 1496, 1496*f*
    disasters, 1502
    initial briefing, 1491
    mutual aid response, 1486, 1525
    record keeping, 1491
    reporting, 146
    scene, check-in, 1491
    transport decisions, 1501–1502
mast cells, 805*f*
mastoid process, 1007, 1038
material safety data sheet (MSDS), 828, 852
maternal age, Down syndrome and, 1394
maxillary fractures, 1011
MCIs. *See* mass-casualty incidents
MDI. *See* metered-dose inhaler
mean arterial pressure (MAP), 394, 412
mechanical piston device, 575–576, 576*f*, 601

mechanical ventilator, 1405–1407, 1406*f*
mechanics of breathing, 201–202
mechanism of injury (MOI). *See also under specific emergencies*
    in blunt *vs.* penetrating trauma, 345–346
    definition of, 346, 411, 901, 931
    determination, 345–347
    from incendiary/explosive devices, 1552–1553
    in internal bleeding, 938
    profiles, 904
    significant, 904
meconium, 1254, 1268, 1279
    staining, 1268
MED channels, 149, 161
medevac, 1454–1455, 1462
    at hazard incidents, 1458
medial portion, definition of, 171, 187
mediastinum, 422, 490, 1093
    definition of, 490
    structures in, 422, 1104
medical assessment, in GEMS diamond, 1368, 1369*t*
medical control
    calling, 155–156
    definition of, 14, 28
    EMS provider communication with, 153–156, 153*f*
    off-line or indirect, 14
    online or direct, 14
    role of, 154–155
medical director, 14, 28
medical emergencies, 901, 931
    assessment, 605–606
        history taking, 608–609, 609*f*
        mechanism of injury/nature of illness, 606
        primary, 607–608, 608*f*
        reassessment, 611
        scene size-up, 606–607
        secondary, 609–610
        of vital signs, 610
    definition of, 605, 625
    infectious diseases, 613–614
        general assessment principles, 613
        management principles, general, 613
    interventions, 605
    transport, 611–613, 612*f*
        decision making, 608
        destination selection and, 613
        time on scene and, 611
        types, 611–612, 612*f*
    types of, 605, 605*t*
medical equipment, in ambulances, 1427–1433, 1427*t*, 1429–1433*f*, 1433*t*
medical evacuation operations, 1454–1455, 1458*f*
medical examiner (coroner), 96, 96*f*
medical identification insignia, 97, 97*f*
medical identification tags, 366
medical incident command, 1493, 1494*f*

extrication supervisor, 1495, 1524
morgue supervisor, 1495, 1525
physicians on scene, 1495
rehabilitation supervisor, 1495, 1525
rescue supervisor, 1495, 1525
staging supervisor, 1494
transportation supervisor, 1494, 1526
treatment supervisor, 1493–1494, 1526
triage, 1497–1502, 1498*t*, 1499*f*
triage supervisor, 1493, 1526
medical necessity, 140–141
Medical Practices Act, 100
medical technology assistance, patients with
    apnea monitors, 1407–1408
    assessment, 1411
    central venous catheters, 1409, 1409*f*
    colostomy, 1410, 1418
    external defibrillator vest, 1408–1409
    gastrostomy tubes, 1409–1410, 1409*f*
    home care, 1411
    ileostomy, 1410, 1418
    internal cardiac pacemakers, 1408, 1408*t*
    left ventricular assist devices, 575, 704, 1408
    mechanical ventilator, 1405–1407, 1406*f*
    shunts, 1410, 1418
    tracheostomy tubes, 1403–1410, 1403*f*
    urostomy, 1410
    vagus nerve stimulators, 1410
medical terminology
    abbreviations, 174–175, 180–185*t*
    anatomy of, 165–168
    in calling medical control, 156
    colors, 169
    combining form, 176–178*t*
    combining vowels, 166–167
    components, 165–168
    directional terms, 170–172, 171*f*, 171*t*
        anterior, 172
        apex, 172
        deep, 171
        distal, 171
        inferior, 170–171
        lateral, 171
        medial, 171
        palmar, 172
        plantar, 172
        posterior, 172
        proximal, 171
        superficial, 171
        superior, 170–171
    Fowler, 173–174
    introduction, 165
    master tables, 176–185*t*
    movement and positional terms, 172*f*
    movement terms, 172
    pharmacology, related to abbreviations, 180–185*t*
    plural endings, 168
    position of the patient, 173–174, 173*f*
        Fowler, 173–174, 173*f*
        prone, 173, 173*f*

medical terminology (*Continued*)
  recovery position, 173*f*
  supine, 173, 173*f*
  prefixes, 165–166, 179*t*
    medication administration, 179*t*
    numerical, 168–169*t*
    position, direction, and location, 169, 170*t*
  suffixes, 166, 180*t*
  symbols, 175, 175*t*
  word roots, 165, 166*t*, 176–178*t*
medication error, 522
medications. *See also* drugs/
      medications; *specific medications*
  inhalation, 515–518
  intramuscular, 513–515
  intranasal, 515
  oral, 507–511
  patient, 518–522
  sublingual, 511–513
medicolegal, definition of, 88, 115
medicolegal considerations, in
      behavioral emergencies, 873–874
melena, 761, 775, 1361
  definition of, 960, 1143, 1388
  internal bleeding and, 941
menarche, 883, 1244, 1279
meninges
  anatomy, 1042, 1042*f*
  definition of, 1089
meningitis
  in children, 1323–1324, 1324*f*
  definition of, 625, 1347
  diagnosis, 618
meningococcal meningitis, 618, 625
menopause, 1244, 1279
  definition of, 883
  signs/symptoms, 264
menstrual cycle, 1244
menstruation, 883
mental disorder, definition of, 856
mental health problems
  causes of, 854
  emergencies. *See* psychiatric/
      behavioral emergencies
  involuntary consent for mentally ill
      patients, 88
  magnitude of, 856
  misconceptions about mental
      illness, 854
  pathophysiology, 856–857
mental model, 131, 161
mental status
  in acute myocardial infarction, 687
  alteration
    as behavioral emergency, 857
    causes, 724, 736–737
    in elderly, 1375
    in hypoglycemia, 736, 736*f*
    as neurologic emergency, 735–737, 736*f*
    pediatric, 1322
MERS-CoV, 620
mescaline, 841*t*
metabolic acidosis, causes, 434

metabolic agents, in chemical
      terrorism/warfare, 1540–1542, 1541*t*
metabolism, 402, 412, 427, 490
metaproterenol (Alupent), 658*t*
metered-dose inhaler (MDI), 502
  administration, 787–788
  contraindications, 657
  definition of, 672
  medications for, 656, 657, 658*t*
  spacer, 659, 659*f*
methamphetamine, 839–840
methicillin-resistant *Staphylococcus aureus* (MRSA)
  definition of, 625–626, 1388
  in elderly, 1379
  transmission, 619–620
middle adults. *See* adults, middle
migraine headaches, 747
mild airway obstruction, 475, 490
military time, 136*t*
ministroke. *See* transient ischemic
      attack
minute volume, 90, 425*t*, 1095
miosis, 1539, 1559
miscarriages (spontaneous abortions), 885, 1279
  definition of, 1250
  signs/symptoms, 1250
mission-critical communications, 131, 161
mitral valve, 677*f*
mobile data terminals, 149, 149*f*, 161
mobile integrated health care (MIH), 15, 28, 321
mobile radio, 147, 147*f*
monitoring devices, for vital signs. *See*
      vital signs; *specific monitoring devices*
morality, 106, 115
morbid obesity, 1402
morgue supervisor, 1495, 1525
Moro reflex (startle reflex), 256, 271
morphine, 836, 836*t*
motorcycle collisions, 911–912
motor function assessment, 401
motor nerves, 224, 1043
motor vehicle accidents
  airbags and, 907
  with bicycles, 911, 911*f*
  collisions, pediatric injury patterns, 1329
  crash scenes, 1465
  death from, 906
  extrication of passengers. *See*
      extrication
  frontal collision injuries, 907–909, 909*f*
  frontal impact, types of, 906*f*, 907–909
  lateral, 910
  motorcycle, 911–912
  with pedestrians, 911
  during pregnancy, 1251
  rear-end, 909, 910*f*

rollover crashes, 910–911, 910*f*
  rotational, 911
  scene of, 59–60
  seat belts and, 907
  "star" on windshield, 1053*f*
motor vehicles
  alternative fuel-type, 1470
  safety systems, 1470
mouth, 228
  bleeding from, 951–954
  physical examination, 1305
mouth-to-mask ventilation
  advantages, 462–463
  barrier device, 462, 462*f*
  technique, 462–463
moving of patients
  across bed, 304
  body drags, 280–282, 282*f*
    emergency moves, 294–295, 294*f*, 318
    one-rescuer, 294*f*, 295*f*
  by carrying. *See* carrying of patients
  elderly, considerations for, 307
  emergency moves, 294–295, 294*f*, 318
  equipment for, 288*f*, 309–312, 309*f*, 310*f*, 311*f*
  by log rolling, 282, 282*f*
  nonurgent, 300–307
    direct carry method, 302–304
    direct ground lift, 300–301, 318
    draw sheet method, 304–305
    extremity lift, 302, 318
    for transfer, 302–304
  obesity and, 307
  personal considerations, 313
  planning, 293
  positioning, 312–313
  reaching/pulling, safety principles for, 280–282, 281–282*f*, 281*f*
  restraints, 313
  safety considerations, 280–291
  urgent, methods of, 295–300, 296*t*
  vacuum mattresses, 311, 311*f*
  weight distribution and, 280
MRSA. *See* methicillin-resistant
      Staphylococcus aureus
mucosal atomizer device (MAD), 500
mucous membranes, 964, 1003
multigravida, 1255, 1279
multiple births, 1272
multiple-casualty incident. *See* mass-
      casualty incidents
multiplex communications, 149, 161
multisystem trauma, 918–920, 931
muscles, types, 1146, 1147*f*. *See also*
      *specific types of muscles*
muscles of breathing, 202–203
muscular dystrophy, 1406
musculoskeletal injuries
  assessment, 1159–1162
    chief complaint investigation, 1161
    communication/documentation of, 1162
    history taking, 1161

mechanism of injury/nature of illness, 1151–1152
  primary, 1159–1160
  reassessment, 1162–1163
  scene size-up, 1159
  secondary, 1161–1162
  of vital signs, 1162
  XABCs, 1159
complications, 1158
emergency medical care, 1163–1169
interventions, 1162
mechanism of injury, 1151–1152
pathophysiology, 1151–1158, 1152–1357f
severity, grading of, 1158, 1158t
specific. *See specific musculoskeletal injuries*
transport
  considerations for, 1162
  decision making, 1159
musculoskeletal system
  age-related changes, 1364–1365
  anatomy, 197–198, 1146–1147, 1147f
    skeletal muscle, 198
  blood supply, 1146
  in children, 1293–1294
  injuries. *See* musculoskeletal injuries
  physical examination, in burn injuries, 988–989
  physiology, 198
mustard (sulfur mustard), 1536, 1541t
mutagens, 1536, 1559
mutual aid response, 1486, 1491, 1525
*Mycobacterium tuberculosis*, 618
myocardial contractility, 536, 553
myocardial contusion, 1099t, 1109, 1115
myocardial infarction
  signs/symptoms, in elderly, 1355–1356
myocardial ischemia, 685
myocardium, 679, 721

## N

narcotics, 836
  definition of, 836, 852
  poisonings, 836
nares, 1296, 1347
nasal cannulas, 458, 458f, 490
  pediatric, 1316–1317, 1317f
nasal flaring, 356, 412
nasopharyngeal (nasal) airway
  contraindications, 449
  definition of, 490
  indications, 449
  insertion, 449
  for pediatric emergencies, 1314–1316
  types, 449, 449f
nasopharynx, 418–420, 419, 419f, 490
National EMS Education Standards, 3
National EMS Information System (NEMSIS), 133
National EMS Scope of Practice Model, 3, 9t, 28
  definition of, 3, 28

guidelines, 9t
purpose of, 3
National Fire Protection Association (NFPA), 1516
National Highway Traffic Safety Administration (NHTSA)
  EMS Agenda for the Future, 9
  EMS Education Standards, 5
National Incident Management System (NIMS)
  components, 1486–1487
    communications and information management, 1487
    incident command system. *See* incident command system
  definition of, 1486, 1525
  principles, 1487
National Registry of EMTs (NREMT), 3
nature of illness (NOI), 345–347, 346, 412, 606, 626. *See also under specific illnesses/disorders*
near-miss SIDS. *See* brief resolved unexplained event (BRUE)
nebulizers, small-volume, 656, 657, 673
neck
  anatomy, 1007–1008, 1008f
  focused assessment, 398, 398f
  injuries. *See* neck injuries
  physical examination, 1305
neck injuries
  assessment, 920–921, 1011–1015
    ABCs, 1014
    chief complaint investigation, 1012–1013
    communication/documentation of, 1015
    general impressions, 1011
    history taking, 1012–1013
    primary, 1011–1012
    scene size-up, 1011
    secondary, 1013–1014
    of vital signs, 1013
  emergency medical care, 1015, 1015f, 1031–1032, 1032f
  interventions, 1014
  open wounds, emergency medical care, 978, 980f
  safety, on-scene, 1011
  soft-tissue, 1010, 1010f
  transport decisions, 1012
neglect
  of children, 1338, 1347
  of elderly, 1381–1383
negligence
  categories, 101
  contributory, 108
  definition of, 115
negligence per se, 101, 115
*Neisseria gonorrhoeae*, 885
*Neisseria meningitidis*, 1324, 1324f, 1347
neonatal resuscitation
  algorithm, 1267f
  performing, 1265–1269
    chest compressions, 1266

    positive-pressure ventilation, 1266
    steps, 1266t
  rapid assessment, 1265–1269
neonates
  definition of, 271, 354
  pulmonary system, 255–256
nephrons, 266, 271
nerve agents, 1537, 1559
nervous system
  age-related changes, 1357–1360
  anatomy, 724–725, 726f
    in children, 1293
  anatomy and physiology
    central nervous system, 220–223
  brain, 220–222
    cerebrospinal fluid, 221
    circulation in the head, 221–222
  central, anatomy of, 1041–1042, 1041f, 1042f
  of elderly, 266–267, 267f
  emergencies. *See* neurologic emergencies
  emergency medical care
    headache, 747
  focused assessment, 394
  of infants, 256–257
  injuries, from explosions, 1553
  motor nerves, 224
  pathophysiology, 725–731
    stroke, 727–728, 728f
  peripheral, anatomy of, 1042–1043, 1043f
  physiology, 724–725, 725f, 1040–1043
  sensory nerves, 223–224
  spinal cord, 222–223
nervous system control, CNS and, 218–220
neurogenic shock
  causes, 544t
  definition of, 553
  signs/symptoms, 544t
  treatment, 544t, 546
neurologic emergencies
  altered mental state, 735–737, 736f
  assessment, 737–745
    communication/documentation, 746
    focused, 394
    history taking, 739–741, 740f
    mechanism of injury/nature of illness, 737
    primary, 738–739, 738f
    reassessment, 744–745
    scene size-up, 737–738
    secondary, 741
  communication, 746
  documentation, 745, 746
  emergency medical care, 745–749, 746t
  interventions, 745
  as medical emergencies, 605, 605t
  pediatric, 1322–1324, 1323f, 1324f
  safety, on-scene, 737–738
  transport decisions, 737

neuromuscular growth, toddlers/
  preschoolers, 259
neuropathy
  definition of, 1388
  in elderly, 1360
neurotoxins, as biological warfare
    agents, 1545–1548, 1546f, 1546t,
    1547f, 1548t, 1559
neurovascular compromise, 1169
neurovascular status assessment,
    396–398, 1162
neutron radiation, 1549, 1559
newborn
  assessment, 1265–1269
  crying, 1269
  delivering, 1258–1264
    of body, 1263–1264
    of head, 1263
  premature, 1273, 1273f
  skin color, 1269
Newton's first law, 903
Newton's second law, 903
Newton's third law, 903
NFPA (National Fire Protection
    Association), 1516
NIMS. See National Incident
    Management System
9-1-1 calls, 151, 151f
9-1-1 system, enhanced, 12
nitroglycerin, 511
  dosage/administration, 697–699
  elderly and, 1372
  forms of, 697–699
Nitrostat. See nitroglycerin
NOI (nature of illness), 345–347. See also
    under specific emergencies
noise
  communication and, 121
  definition of, 121, 161
nonbulk storage vessels,
    1506–1508, 1507f
nondisplaced fracture, 1153, 1197
nonhemorrhagic shock, 539
nonprogressive (compensated) shock,
    540, 540t, 553
nonrebreathing masks
  definition of, 490
  pediatric, 1317, 1317f
  usage, 458, 458f
norepinephrine, effects, 533–534
nose
  anatomy, 1027–1028, 1028f
  bleeding from, 951–954
  fractures, 1027–1028
  injuries, 1027–1028, 1028f
  physical examination, 1305
nosebleeds (epistaxis), 951–954, 959
notification
  of hospital, 153, 153f
  procedures, for terrorism events, 1534
NREMT (National Registry of EMTs), 3
nuchal cord, 1263, 1279
nuclear terrorism/warfare
  exposure
    medical management, 1551–1552

protective measures, 1552
symptomatology, 1551, 1551t
weapons/devices, 1551
nutrition, for wellness, 33–35, 34f

**O**

obesity, 1402–1403, 1418
objective information, 134
oblique fracture, 1153, 1153f
obstetric kit, emergency, 1257
obstructive shock, 536–537
  causes, 544t
  definition of, 553
  signs/symptoms, 544t
  treatment, 544t, 546
occiput, 1290
occlusion
  of coronary artery, 684
  definition of, 721
occlusive dressings, 977, 1003,
    1103–1104, 1115
Occupational Safety and Health
    Administration (OSHA)
  definition of, 41, 83
  infection control guidelines, 47
off-gassing, 1538, 1559
older patients. See elderly
olecranon process fracture, 1170
onset of problem, in OPQRST, 368
open-book pelvic fracture, 951, 960
open-ended questions
  definition of, 122, 161
  in patient interview, 122, 123t
open fractures, 1153, 1155, 1155f, 1197
open incident, 1492, 1525
open injuries
  abdominal
    definition of, 1143
    emergency medical care,
        1129–1131, 1130f
    signs/symptoms, 1122–1123, 1122f
  assessment, 970–976
    scene size-up, 970–971
  chest, 1095, 1096f, 1115
  definition of, 964, 1003
  emergency medical care, 976–981, 980f
  head, 1047–1048, 1089
  types of, 967–969, 967–969f
open pneumothorax, 1103, 1103f, 1115
open skull fractures, 1047–1048, 1048f
operations, in incident command
    system, 1490, 1525
opiate
  definition of, 836, 852
  poisonings, 836–837
opioid
  definition of, 836, 852
  poisonings, 836–837
opioid overdose
  algorithm, life-threatening, 837f
  CPR and, 593
OPQRST, 768, 1161
  definition of, 368–369, 412
  for pain assessment, 695, 695t

optic nerve, 1009, 1037
oral glucose, 510, 746
oral medications, 507–511
organ donation, consent for, 97, 97f
organic brain syndrome, 857, 879
organophosphates, 842–843
orientation, 352, 412
oropharyngeal (oral) airway
  definition of, 446, 490
  insertion
    in adult, 447–448
    in children, 447
    with 90 degree rotation, 447–448
  for pediatric emergencies,
      1313–1314
  for unresponsive patients, 446, 446f
oropharynx, 228, 419–420, 419f, 490
orthopnea, 632t, 672
OSHA (Occupational Safety and Health
    Administration), 41, 83
osteoporosis
  definition of, 1388
  in elderly, 1364
  fracture risk, 1180
OTC (over-the-counter)
    medications, 497
ovaries
  anatomy, 882–883, 882f, 1243–1244
  definition of, 897
overdose
  cardiac medications, 843
  definition of, 822, 852
over-the-counter (OTC) medications
  definition of, 497
  overdosage, 835
over-the-counter (OTC)
    medications, 497
ovulation, 883, 897, 1244
oxygen
  deficiency, as hazard in fires, 58, 58f
  during inspiration, 424, 629
  during respiration, 629, 630f
  supplemental, 451–457
    equipment for, 451–454, 451f,
        452t, 453f
    hazards, 457
    nasal cannula, 458
  supply units, in ambulance,
      1427–1430, 1430f
oxygenation, 639, 672
  definition of, 423, 490
  physiology, 427
  respiration and, 531
oxygen cylinders
  flowmeters, 454, 454f
  hazards, 457
  pin-indexing system, 453–454, 453f
  placing into service, 455–457
  pressure regulators, 454
  safety precautions/considerations,
      453, 456
  sizes, 451, 452t
oxygen-delivery devices, 457–460
  nasal cannulas, 458, 458f
  nonrebreathing mask, 458, 458f

oxygen humidifiers, 460, 460*f*
partial rebreathing mask, 459
for pediatric emergencies,
1316–1319, 1317*f*
tracheostomy mask, 459–460, 460*f*
Venturi mask, 459, 459*f*
oxygen humidifiers, 460, 460*f*
oxygen saturation (Spo₂), 435
oxygen therapy. *See* oxygen,
supplemental
oxygen toxicity, 457, 490

**P**

pacemakers
automated external defibrillation
and, 562
for cardiovascular emergencies,
703–704, 703*f*
packaging, 11
in EMT training, 11
pack strap, for lifting/carrying, 296*f*
paging, 152, 161
pain
of acute myocardial infarction,
686–687
in angina, 685
assessment, in pediatric emergencies,
1300, 1301*f*
as fracture sign, 1155
localization
in appendicitis, 760*t*
in diverticulitis, 760*t*
in duodenal ulcer, 760*t*
management, pediatric, 1334
quality, in OPQRST, 368
radiation, 368
referred, 760, 760*f*, 760*t*, 775
responsiveness to, 353*f*
palliating factors, in OPQRST, 368
palmar grasp, 256
palmar grasp reflex, 271
palmar portion, definition of, 188
palmar surface, definition of, 172
palpate, 357, 412
pancreas, 228
physiology, 779–780
pancreatitis, 760*t*, 761, 775
pandemic, 613–614, 626, 637, 672
panic attack (hyperventilation
syndrome), 646
panic disorder, 856
paradoxical motion, 399, 412, 1108, 1115
paralysis
definition of, 1402
paramedic
definition of, 4, 28
training, 9*t*, 11
parasitic infections, 615
parasympathetic nervous system, 679,
721, 1044
parenteral medications, 498
parietal pleura, 421, 490
Parkinson disease, 1359
paroxysmal nocturnal dyspnea, 632*t*, 672

partial pressure, 424
partial pressure of oxygen (Pao₂), 424
partial rebreathing mask, 459
partial-thickness (second-degree)
burns, 984, 984*f*, 1003
passive ventilation, 467, 490
PAT. *See* pediatric assessment
triangle (PAT)
patella, dislocation, 1188–1189, 1189*f*
patent, airway, 425, 426*f*, 490
pathogen, definition of, 38, 83
pathologic fracture, 1153*f*
pathophysiology. *See under specific
emergency disorders*
patient
anxious, history taking and, 372–373
assessment of. *See* assessment
autonomy, 86, 115
carrying. *See* carrying of patients
determining number at scene,
348–349, 348*f*
geriatric. *See* elderly
high-priority, 363–365
interviews with. *See* interviews,
patient
moving. *See* moving of patients
nutrition/hydration, exposure and,
1201
over talkative, dealing with, 372
physical condition, exposure and,
1201
silent, dealing with, 372
transfer of. *See* transfer of patients
unresponsive, removal from vehicle
by one rescuer, 295*f*
violent
potential, assessment of, 868–869
risk factors for, 868–869
wet, automated external defibrillation
and, 562
patient assessment. *See* assessment
patient assessment flowchart, 343, 350,
366, 377, 404
patient-assisted medication, 506
patient care handover, 132–133
patient care report (PCR)
administration information gathered
from, 134
CHART method, 138–139
confidentiality of, 139
data collection, 134
definition of, 133, 134, 161
electronic, 138*f*
example of, 135*f*
functions, 134
legal issues, 134
narrative section, 137
patient information in, 134
purpose of, 134–137
quoting patient in, 137*t*
refusal form, 90
requirements for, 135, 137*t*
significant negative findings in, 137
SOAP method, 139–140
types of, 137–138

patient medications, 518–522
patient name, using when dealing with
patient, 125
patient position
for basic life support, 562–563
for delivery, 1258, 1259*f*
for pediatric airway assessment,
1297–1298, 1297*f*
recovery position, in seizure
disorders, 1323*f*
standing, 278
patient rights, to refuse treatment, 90
patients age, exposure and, 1201
PAT (pediatric assessment triangle),
1294–1297, 1347
pause
definition of, 123*t*
example of, 123*t*
PCP (phencyclidine), 841
PCR. *See* patient care report
pectoral girdle, anatomy, 1148, 1149*f*
pedestrians, collisions with vehicles, 911
pediatric assessment triangle (PAT),
1294–1297, 1347
pediatric emergencies
abdominal injuries, 1119
assessment
chief complaint investigation, 1303
hands-on XABCs, 1297–1302
history taking, 1303–1304
reassessment, 1306–1307
scene size-up, 1293
secondary, 1304–1306
child abuse, 1336–1338, 1337*f*, 1337*t*
circulatory, 1320–1322
shock, 1320–1322
communication, with patient/
family, 1284
death of child, 1339–1342, 1341*t*
dehydration, 1325–1327, 1327*f*, 1327*t*
disaster management,
1335–1336, 1335*f*
drowning, 1328–1329
fever, 1327–1328
gastrointestinal, 1324–1325
neurologic, 1322–1324, 1323*f*, 1324*f*
poisonings, 1325–1327, 1327*f*
respiratory, 1308–1320
airway adjuncts, 1313–1316, 1313*t*
anaphylaxis, 1321–1322
asthma, 1310–1311
bronchiolitis, 1312
cardiopulmonary arrest, 1319–1320
croup, 1311
epiglottis, 1311–1312
foreign body aspiration and
obstruction, 1308–1310, 1309*f*
oxygen delivery devices for,
1316–1319, 1317*f*
pertussis, 1312
pneumonia, 1311
signs/symptoms of, 1308
sudden infant death syndrome,
1339–1342, 1341*t*
transport decisions, 1302–1303

pediatric emergencies *(Continued)*
  trauma, 1329–1335
    abdominal injuries, 1333, 1334*f*
    burns, 1333–1335, 1334*f*, 1334*t*
    chest injuries, 1333, 1333*f*
    extremity injuries, 1335
    head injuries, immobilization of,
      1330–1333
    injury patterns, 1329–1330
    pain management, 1335
    physical differences, 1329
    psychological differences, 1329
pediatric emergencies respiratory
  SAMPLE components for, 1304*t*
  signs/symptoms of, 1304*t*
pediatrics, 1284, 1347
PEEP (positive end-expiratory
    pressure), 473
peer-assisted medication, 506
pelvic binder, 951, 960, 1168–1169,
    1169*f*, 1197
pelvic compression device, 951
pelvic fractures
  care of, 1178–1179, 1179*f*
  open, 1178
  types, 1178–1179
  with urinary bladder injuries, 1134
pelvic girdle anatomy, 1149
pelvic inflammation, localization of
    pain, 760*t*
pelvic inflammatory disease (PID)
  assessment and management, 889–890
  cause, 884–885
  definition of, 897
pelvic region, assessment of, 1179*f*
pelvis, 196
  focused assessment, 399–400, 400*f*
  fractures, 1178–1179
penetrating trauma
  definition of, 904, 931
  low-energy, 913, 914*f*
  as mechanism of injury, 346
  medium-velocity and high-velocity, 915
  neck injuries from, 1032, 1033*f*
  wounds
    definition of, 1003
penetrating wound, 968, 1003
peptic ulcer disease, 760, 1361, 1388
  in elderly, 1361
perfusion, 650
  components, 683
  definition of, 354, 412, 531, 553, 683,
    721, 937, 960
  physiology, 531–534, 937, 937*f*
perfusion triangle, 532, 533*f*
pericardial effusion, 536, 553
pericardial sac. *See* pericardium
pericardial tamponade. *See* cardiac
    tamponade
pericardium (pericardial sac)
  definition of, 1115
  function, 1105
perineum
  anatomy, 882, 882*f*, 1244
  definition of, 897, 1279

peripheral nerve injury, 1042–1043
peripheral nervous system (PNS)
  anatomy, 1042–1043, 1043*f*
  definition of, 1042
peristalsis, 757
peritoneal cavity, 1120, 1143
peritoneum, 758, 775, 1120, 1143
peritonitis, 758, 775, 1126
per os (PO), 498
per rectum (PR), 498
persistency, 1535, 1559
personal experience, communication
    and, 120
personal protection, at scene, 54–61
personal protective equipment (PPE)
  boots, for injury prevention, 63–64, 64*f*
  definition of, 38, 83, 412
  face shields, 45
  glasses, 45, 45*f*
  gloves. *See* gloves
  gowns, 45
  helmets, for injury prevention, 63, 63*f*
  in infection control plan, 47–48*t*
  levels for hazmat incidents,
    1516–1517, 1517*f*
  masks, 45–46, 45*f*
  as safety precaution, 347
personal safety equipment in
    ambulances, 1433
pertinent negatives, 369, 412
pertussis (whooping cough)
  characteristics, 632*t*, 636–637
  definition of, 672–673, 1347
  signs/symptoms, 619, 632*t*, 1312
pesticides
  absorption of, 827
  bags for, 1507
pharmacodynamics, 495
pharmacokinetics, 496
pharmacology, principles of, 495–527
Phencyclidine (PCP), 841
phobias, 856
phosgene, in chemical terrorism/
    warfare, 1536, 1541*t*, 1559
phosgene oxime (CX), 1536, 1541*t*, 1559
phrenic nerve, 423, 490
physical abuse
  elderly, 1381–1382
  history taking, 371, 371*f*
physical disabilities
  cerebral palsy, 1400–1401, 1400*f*, 1418
  muscular dystrophy, 1406
  paralysis, 1402
  spina bifida, 1401–1402, 1401*f*, 1418
physical examinations. *See* assessment,
    *under specific emergencies*
physical factors, in nonverbal
    communication, 121–122, 122*t*
physician orders for life-sustaining
    treatment (POLST), 93
physicians
  at mass-casualty incident scene, 1495
  medical control and, 14
pia mater, 1042
PID. *See* pelvic inflammatory disease

pin-indexing system, 453–454, 453*f*, 490
pinna, 1007, 1007*f*, 1037
PIO (public information officer),
    1490, 1525
pit vipers, 1231–1232, 1231*f*
placards, for hazardous materials,
    1508, 1508*f*
placenta
  definition of, 1245, 1279
  delivery of, 1264
placenta previa, 1249, 1249*f*, 1279
plaintiff, 101
planes of body, 190–191, 190*f*
planning, in incident command system,
    1490, 1525
plantar portion, definition of, 188
plantar surface, definition of, 172
plants
  as allergens, 806
  poisonous, 846–847, 846*t*, 847*f*
plasma
  components, 680
  definition of, 793
platelets (thrombocytes)
  definition of, 793
  functions, 680
platinum 10 minutes, 919, 922
play, importance for toddlers/
    preschoolers, 259
pleural effusion, 644–645, 645*f*,
    664, 673
pleural space, 1105
pleuritic chest pain, 644, 673
plural endings, medical
    terminology, 168
pneumonia, 1353, 1388
  characteristics, 632*t*, 636
  definition of, 673
  in elderly, 1353, 1372
  management, 665
  pathophysiology, 639
  pediatric, 1311
  signs/symptoms, 632*t*
pneumonic plague, 1545, 1546*t*, 1548*t*,
    1559
pneumothorax
  causes, 431
  definition of, 490, 673
  management, 664
  open, 1103, 1103*f*, 1115
  pathophysiology, 644, 644*f*
  signs/symptoms, 632*t*
  simple, 1104, 1115
  spontaneous, 644, 1104, 1115
  tension. *See* tension pneumothorax
PODs (points of distribution),
    1549, 1559
points of distribution (PODs),
    1549, 1559
point tenderness, 1154, 1197
poison, definition of, 822, 852
poison centers, 826
poisonings
  by absorption, 827–828, 828*f*
  food, 843–845

by ingestion, 825f, 828–829
by inhalation, 826–827
by injection, 829–830
pediatric, 1325–1327, 1327f
from plant ingestions, 846–847,
    846t, 847f
signs/symptoms, 830
treatment, 833
police escorts, for ambulances,
    1451–1452
polydipsia, 783, 801
polyphagia, 783, 802
polypharmacy, 1365, 1388
polyuria, definition of, 783, 802
poor air exchange, 475, 490
portable radio, 147, 147f
portable stretchers, 310, 310f, 318
Portuguese man-of-war stings,
    1235, 1235f
positional asphyxia, 864, 879
position of function, 1197
positive end-expiratory pressure
    (PEEP), 473
positive pressure ventilation
    neonatal, 1267f
    vs. normal ventilation, 461–462, 462t
postconventional reasoning, 260, 271
posterior, definition, 679, 721
posterior portion, definition of, 172, 188
postexposure management
    general considerations for, 53–54
    for infection control plan, 47t
postictal state
    definition of, 731, 753
    hemiparesis and, 735
    safety during, 735
postpartum complications, 1274
postterm pregnancy, 1273
posttraumatic (anterograde)
        amnesia, 1051
posttraumatic stress disorder (PTSD),
    871, 879
    critical incident stress management,
        71, 71f
    definition of, 71, 83
postural hypotension, 1355
potential energy, 902, 931
poverty, 1412
power grip, 280, 280f, 318
power lift, 278, 318
power lines, downed at scene, 57
PPE. See personal protective equipment
preconventional reasoning, 260, 271
preeclampsia
    definition of, 1248, 1279
    signs/symptoms, 1248
    transport precautions, 1248
    treatment, 1248
prefixes, medical terminology, 165–166,
        179t, 188
    definition of, 165–166
    medication administration, 179t
    numerical, 168–169t
    position, direction, and location,
        169, 170t

pregnancy
    assessment, 1252
        chief complaint investigation, 1254
        primary, 1253–1254
        reassessment, 1255
        secondary, 1254–1255
    cardiac arrest in, 593–594
    cultural considerations, 1252–1253
    ectopic, 884, 1249, 1279
    emergencies
        mechanism of injury/nature of
            illness, 1253
    fetal death, 1273–1274
    general impressions, 1253
    history taking, 1254
    hypertension during, 1247–1248
    interventions during, 1255
    normal maternal changes, 1246–1247
    pathophysiology, 1247–1252
    postpartum complications, 1274
    postterm, 1273
    trauma during, 1251–1252
    vital signs during, 1255
pregnancy emergencies
    assessment
        scene size-up, 1253–1254
        transport decisions, 1254
    preload, 536, 553, 684
    premature birth, 1273, 1273f
    premature rupture of the
            membranes, 1256
    preoxygenation, 477, 490–491
    presbycusis, 1358, 1388
    preschool-age children
        assessment of, 1287–1288, 1287f
        definition of, 258, 271, 1287, 1347
        examination of, 258–259
        physical changes, 258–259, 259f
        psychosocial changes, 260
        vital signs, 259
    prescription medications, 497. See also
            drugs/medications; specific
            medications
        definition of, 497
    pressure regulators, for gas
            cylinders, 454
    pressure ulcers, 1365
    presumptive negligence, 98
    prevention
        primary, 19, 28
        secondary, 20, 28
    primary assessment, 350–365
        of airway, 354–355
        bleeding control and assessment,
            360–361
        of breathing, 355–357
        of circulation, 357–361, 358–360f
        definition, 412
        definition of, 350
        in determining patient care and
                transport priorities,
            363–365, 364f
        general impression, 351, 351f
        level of consciousness assessment,
            352–353

life threats, identifying and treating,
        361–363
    of orientation, 352, 412
    questions for, 352
    of responsive patients, 354–355
    of unresponsive patients, 355
    vital signs evaluation, 350, 351f
primary blast injuries, 915, 1553, 1559
primary brain injury, 1048, 1089
primary prevention, 19, 28
primary service area, 14, 28
primary survey. See under specific
        assessments of specific emergency
        situations; specific emergencies
primary triage, 1497, 1525
primigravida, 1255, 1279
professional standards, standards of
        care and, 99–100, 100f
projectile, 913, 931
prolapsed umbilical cord, 1271f,
        1272f, 1279
prone
    definition of, 188
    position, 173, 173f
protected health information, 92, 115
protective clothing, for injury
        prevention, 61–65, 62f, 63f
protocols, for forcible restraint, 89–90
protozoan infections, 615
provoking factors, in OPQRST, 368
proximal femur fractures, 1180–1181
proximal portion, definition of, 171, 188
proximate causation, 101, 115
pruritus, in anaphylaxis, 805f
psilocybin mushrooms, 841t
psychiatric/behavioral emergencies. See
        also specific emergencies
    assessment, 857–862
        communication/documentation
            of, 861
        history taking, 859–860
        mechanism of injury/nature of
            illness, 857
        physical examinations, 860–861
        primary, 858–859
        reassessment, 861–862
        scene size-up, 857
        secondary, 860–861
        of vital signs, 860–861
    interventions, 859
    as medical emergencies, 605, 605t
    medicolegal aspects, 862, 873–874
    safety considerations, 858t
    transport decisions, 861
psychiatric disorder, 856, 879
psychogenic shock
    causes, 544t
    definition of, 539, 553
    signs/symptoms, 544t
    treatment, 544t, 546–547
psychosis, 862–863, 879
PTSD (posttraumatic stress disorder),
        871, 879
public access, to emergency medical
        services, 11

public education, 19–20
public health, 19, 28
public information officer (PIO), 1490, 1525
public safety access point, 12, 28
pulling, when moving patients, 280–282, 281f
pulmonary blast injuries, 918, 931, 1553, 1559
pulmonary contusion, 1108, 1115
pulmonary edema, 535f, 690
  definition of, 673
  high-altitude, 1226–1227
  management, 662–663
  pathophysiology, 638–639, 638f
  respiration and, 431
pulmonary embolism
  definition of, 673, 1388
  in elderly, 1353–1354
  management, 664
  pathophysiology, 645–646, 646f
  risk factors, 1353–1354
  signs/symptoms, 632t, 645–646, 1353–1354
pulmonic valve, 677f
pulsation, 682
pulse oximetry
  in airway management, 435–436
  of children, 1307f
  definition of, 412, 491
  description of, 401, 401f, 435–436, 435f
  in geriatric emergencies, 1376
  performing, 435–436
  purpose, 401
pulse pressure, 553
  definition of, 533, 553
pulse rate
  of adolescents, 261
  of adults, 263
  of children, 1292t
   infants, 254
  normal ranges, 388t
pulses
  in acute myocardial infarction, 687
  central, 1299, 1347
  checking for, 563–565, 565f
  definition of, 357, 412
  distal, 400f
  palpation, 357
  quality of, 388
  rhythm, 388
punitive damages, 108, 115
pupils
  assessment
   with eye injuries, 1016, 1016f
   in head injuries, 1060
   methods of, 394–396, 395f
  definition of, 1037
  physical examination, 1305
putrefaction, 96, 115, 584

**Q**

quadrants
  abdominal, 1119, 1119f

definition of, 172
quality assurance. *See* continuous quality improvement
quality control
  definition of, 16, 28
  medical director and, 16
quaternary blast injuries, 917, 1553, 1559

**R**

rabid animals, 981, 1003
raccoon eyes, 1047, 1047f, 1089
radial head fracture, 1174
radial pulse palpation, 357, 358f
radiation, 1202, 1240
radiation, body heat loss from, 1202
radiation burns, 996–997
radiation of pain, 368
radioactive material
  definition of, 1549, 1559
  sources, 1549–1550
radio communications, 150–151
  notification, 150
  systems
   base station radios, 146–147
   mobile and portable radios, 147, 147f
radio frequencies, allocation of, 150
radiologic dispersal device (RDD), 1550–1551, 1559
radiologic terrorism/warfare
  devices, 1550–1551
  exposure
   medical management, 1551–1552
   protective measures, 1552
   symptomatology, 1551, 1551t
  previous incidents, 1532
radius, anatomy, 1148, 1149f
rales (crackles), 650, 651t, 672
range of motion, definition of, 188
rape, 890–892, 897, 1138–1139
rapid extrication technique, 295–300
  definition of, 318
  performing, 295–300
  situations for, 296t
rapport
  definition of, 125, 161
  therapeutic, Golden Rules for, 125–126
RBCs (red blood cells), 680
RDD (radiologic dispersal device), 1550–1551, 1559
reaching, when moving patients, 280–282, 281f
reassessment. *See also under specific emergency situations*
  definition of, 405, 412
rebound tenderness
  in appendicitis, 761
  assessment, 399, 1126
reciprocity, 14
records/recordkeeping
  for infection control plan, 48t
  legal considerations, 92

for mass-casualty incident, 1491
recovery position, 173f
  for child, 579, 579f
  definition of, 491, 601
  purpose, 451, 567–568, 567f
  in seizure disorders, 1322–1323
recovery techniques, for drowning, 1220
rectum, 229
red blood cells (RBCs)
  functions, 680
  production, 793, 794f
red phosphorus, containers for, 1505
reducible hernia, 765
Reel splint, 1182, 1182f
referred pain
  in abdominal conditions, 760, 760f, 760t
  definition of, 775
reflection, 123t
refusal form, 143, 144f, 146t
refusal of care, documenting, 143, 144f, 146t
regulation, of EMS system, 14
rehabilitation area, 1495, 1525
rehabilitation supervisor, 1495, 1525
relaxation, for wellness, 35
renal dialysis, 771–772
renal failure
  in elderly, 1363
renal system
  age-related changes, 1362–1363
  of elderly, 266
  emergencies, 764–765
  of toddlers/preschoolers, 259
repeaters, 147–148, 148f, 161
reports/reporting
  of errors, 142–143, 142f
  of evidence at scene of crime, 105
  honesty in, 107
  legal considerations, 92
  mandatory requirements, 104–105
  obligation for, 104
  patient, standard format for, 154
  special situations, 146
  submission of, 146
rescue situations
  extrication. *See* extrication
  specialized
   search and rescue, 1476–1477
   structure fires, 1479
   tactical, 1477–1478, 1478f
   technical rescue situations, 1475–1476
   trench rescue, 1477
rescue supervisor, 1495, 1525
research, emergency medical service, 21
residual volume, 425t, 491
resilience
  definition of, 32, 83
*res ipsa loquitur*, 101, 115
respiration, 203–205
  in acute myocardial infarction, 687
  assessment, 434–439
  body heat loss from, 1202, 1240
  definition of, 423, 491, 673

external, 489
external or pulmonary, 427, 427f
factors affecting, 430–431
    external, 430
    internal, 430–431
oxygenation and, 531
pathophysiology, 428–431
physiology, 427–428, 427f, 629–631, 630f
*vs.* ventilation, 633
respiration rate, normal range, 432t
respirators, for infectious disease risk reduction, 45–46, 46f
respiratory agents, in chemical terrorism/ warfare, 1536–1537, 1541t
respiratory arrest, 1308
respiratory distress, 1308
definition of, 357
in elderly, 1372
pediatric, 1308
signs/symptoms, 433–434, 1308
respiratory effort easing, supine position for, 809
respiratory emergencies
    airway obstruction, 645, 645f
    anaphylactic reactions, 643–644
    assessment, 648
        ABCs, 648–650
        chronic conditions, 652
        general impressions, 648
        history taking, 651–653
        mechanism of injury/nature of illness, 648
        primary, 648–651, 650f
        questioning patient, 652–653
        reassessment, 655–656
        SAMPLE history, 652
        scene size-up, 648
        secondary, 653–655
        of vital signs, 653–655
    asthma. *See* asthma
    COPD. *See* chronic obstructive pulmonary disease (COPD)
    cystic fibrosis, 666–667
    emergency medical care, 656–662
    environmental/industrial exposure, 647–648
    interventions, 655
    pleural effusion, 644–645, 645f, 673
    pulmonary edema, 638–639, 638f
    safety, on-scene, 648
    spontaneous pneumothorax, 644, 644f
respiratory failure, 1308
definition of, 357
pediatric, 1308
respiratory (mechanical ventilator), 1405–1407, 1406f
respiratory rate, 432t
of adolescents, 261
of adults, 263
in children, 1291t, 1292t
determination, 384, 384f
of infants, 254
of toddlers/preschoolers, 259

respiratory syncytial virus (RSV)
    characteristics, 632t, 635–636
    definition of, 673, 1388–1389
    in elderly, 1379
    pediatric bronchiolitis, 1312
    signs/symptoms, 632t
respiratory system
    age-related changes, 1353–1354
    airway adjuncts, for pediatric emergencies, 1312, 1313t
    anatomy, 418–423, 419–423f, 628–629, 630f
        in children, 1290–1292, 1291f, 1292t
        lower airway, 200–201
        mechanics of breathing, 201–202
        muscles of breathing, 202–203
        upper airway, 198–200
    disorders. *See also specific respiratory system disorders*
        signs/symptoms of, 632t
    of elderly, 265–266
    emergencies. *See* respiratory emergencies
    focused assessment, 383–384
    medical emergencies, 605, 605t
    pathophysiology, 631–633
    pediatric emergencies, 1308–1320
        anaphylaxis, 1321
        asthma, 1310–1311
        bronchiolitis, 1312
        cardiopulmonary arrest, 1319–1320
        croup, 1311
        epiglottis, 1311–1312
        foreign body aspiration and obstruction, 1308–1310, 1309f
        oxygen delivery devices for, 1316–1319, 1317f
        pertussis, 1312
        pneumonia, 1311
        signs/symptoms of, 1308
    physical examination, in burn injuries, 988
    physiology, 203–207, 629–631, 630f
        inadequate breathing, 207
        normal breathing, characteristics of, 207
        respiration, 203–205
        ventilation, 205–207
    physiology of breathing and, 423–428, 425–428f, 425t
    signs, of anaphylactic shock, 539t
responsiveness
    definition of, 352, 412
    determination, in infants/children, 578–579, 579f
restraints, patient
    in behavioral emergencies, 864–867, 866f
    for moving/lifting patients, 313
resuscitation equipment, for pediatric emergencies, 1313f
retina, 1008f, 1009, 1038
retinal detachment, 1009, 1038
retractions, 356, 412, 433, 491

retrograde amnesia, 1051, 1089
retroperitoneal space, 1178, 1197
retroperitoneal structures, 758
retroperitoneum, 1121, 1143
return of spontaneous circulation (ROSC), 559, 601, 713, 721
reverse triage, 1240
revised Trauma Score, (RTS), 924, 926t, 931
rhonchi, 387, 412, 651, 651t, 673
rib fractures, 1107
RICES mnemonic, 976, 1191
ricin, 1546–1548, 1547f, 1547t, 1548t, 1559
right-of-way privileges, for ambulances, 1451
rigor mortis, 96, 115, 584, 601
roads
    conditions, driving of emergency vehicles and, 1449–1450
    unpaved, driving emergency vehicles on, 1452
Rocky Mountain spotted fever, 1234
rooting reflex, 256, 271
ROSC (return of spontaneous circulation), 559, 601
rotation-flexion injuries, 1052
route of exposure, 1535, 1559
RSV. *See* respiratory syncytial virus
RTS (Revised Trauma Score), 924, 926t
rule of nines, 985, 985f, 1003
rule of palms, 985
rupture of the membranes, 1256

# S

SADM (Special Atomic Demolition Munitions), 1551, 1559
safety
    at behavioral emergencies, 858t
    with compressed gas cylinders, 453
    on-scene. *See under specific emergency situations*
    systems, for motor vehicles, 1470
    when pulling and reaching to move patients, 280–282, 281f
safety data sheet (SDS), 1510–1511, 1511f
safety officer, 1490, 1525
safety/operations equipment, in ambulances, 1433–1434
safety placards, for hazardous materials, 56f
safe zone, 1469, 1484
Sager splint, 1182, 1185
salmeterol (Serevent), 658t
*Salmonella* food poisoning, 844
SALT triage system, 1500
SAMPLE history
    definition of, 412
    information in, 369
    obtaining, 369
    as part of history taking. *See* history taking
SA node (sinoatrial node), 678
sarin (GB), 1538, 1541t, 1559

SARS-CoV-2. *See* COVID-19
SARS (severe acute respiratory
  syndrome), 614, 620
SBAT format, 133
scald burn, 991, 1003
scalp
  lacerations
    description of, 1046, 1046*f*
    emergency medical care, 1062
scanner, radio receiver, 148, 161
scapula
  injuries, 1170, 1170*f*
SCBA (self-contained breathing
  apparatus), 1479, 1484
scene
  assessment, in sudden infant death
    syndrome, 1340
  of crime, evidence, reporting on, 105
  en route to, safety precautions, 54
  environmental considerations, 345
  hazards, 55–60, 58*f*
    electrical, 57–58
    fire, 58–59, 58*f*
  of mass-casualty incident, check-in
    at, 1491
  personal protection at, 54–61, 54*f*
  safety, 54–61, 55*f*
  size-up of. *See* size-up
  terrain considerations, 344
  traffic at, 344
  of vehicle crashes, 59–60
scene size-up, definition, 343, 412
schizophrenia, 863, 879
school-age children. *See* children,
  school-age
school zones, driving emergency
  vehicles in, 1452
sciatic nerve, 1179, 1197
SC injections. *See* subcutaneous
  injections
sclera, 359, 412, 1008*f*, 1009, 1038
scoop stretcher, 305–306, 306*f*, 318, 1071
scope of practice, 3, 10*f*, 98, 115
scorpion stings, 1233–1234, 1233*f*
scuba gear, 1220, 1240
SDS (safety data sheet), 1510–1511, 1511*f*
seat belts, 54, 54*f*
  abdominal injuries from,
    1121–1122, 1122*f*
  in vehicular collisions, 907
secondary assessment. *See also under
  specific assessments of specific
  emergency situations; specific
  emergencies*
  components, 377–404
  definition of, 377, 412
  focused assessment, 379–401. *See also*
    focused assessment
  Glasgow Coma Scale, 395*t*
  vital signs, monitoring devices for. *See
    specific monitoring devices*
secondary blast injuries, 916–917,
  1553, 1559
secondary brain injury, 1048, 1089
secondary containment, 1506, 1525

secondary device, 1534, 1559
secondary prevention, 20, 28
secondary triage, 1497, 1525
secure attachment, 257
sedative, 834, 852
sedative-hypnotics, 837–838
seizures, 732–733
  causes, 724
  definition of, 732, 753
  emergency medical care, 748–749
  febrile, 1328
  pediatric, 1322–1323, 1323*t*
  recognizing, importance of, 734–735
  tonic-clonic, 1328, 1347
  types of, 732–733, 733*t*
selective serotonin reuptake inhibitors
  (SSRIs), 844*t*
self-contained breathing apparatus
  (SCBA), 1479, 1484
sensitization, 538, 553
sensorineural deafness, 1397, 1418
sensory disabilities, 1396–1400, 1397*f*
sensory function
  age-related changes, 267, 1357–1358
  assessment, 401
sensory nerves, 223–224, 1043
separation anxiety
  in infants, 258, 1285
  in toddlers/preschoolers, 258
sepsis, 394
September 11, 2001, terrorism event,
  1531*f*, 1534
septic shock
  causes, 544*t*
  definition of, 537, 553
  signs/symptoms, 544*t*
  treatment, 544*t*, 546
Serevent (salmeterol), 658*t*
service dogs, for visually impaired
  patients, 1397*f*
severe acute respiratory syndrome
  (SARS), 614, 620
severe airway obstruction, 475, 491
severity, in OPQRST, 369
sexual abuse, of children, 1338–1339
sexual assault, 890–892, 893*t*
  drugs used, 890
sexual development, adolescent, 261
sexual harassment, avoiding, 76–77
sexual history, 371–372
sexually transmitted diseases
  (STDs), 885
shaken baby syndrome, 1338, 1347
shallow respiration, 356, 412
Shannon–Weaver communication
  model, 119*f*
sharps, proper disposal of, 46, 46*f*
shipping papers, for hazardous
  materials, 1511, 1511*f*
shivering, 1202–1203, 1204*t*
shock, 238–240
  assessment, 540–542
    ABCs, 541
    chief complaint investigation, 541
    general impressions, 541

history taking, 542
    primary, 541–542
    reassessment, 542
    SAMPLE history, 542
    scene size-up, 540–541
    secondary, 542
    of vital signs, 542
  from blood loss, pediatric, 1333, 1334*f*
  causes, 534, 534*f*
  definition of, 531, 553, 936, 960
  emergency medical care, 543–548
  fluid administration, 539
  hypovolemic, signs/symptoms of, 941
  interventions, 542
  neurogenic, 1061
  pathophysiology, 531–534, 532*f*, 533*f*
  pediatric, 1320–1322
  progression, 540, 540*t*
    compensated, 540, 540*t*
    decompensated, 540
    irreversible, 540, 540*t*
  safety, on-scene, 540
  signs/symptoms, 539*t*, 938
  supportive measures, 544*t*
  transport decisions, 542
  types of, 534–539
shortening, as fracture signs, 1154
shortness of breath, in elderly, 1372
shoulder joint, dislocation,
  1171–1172, 1171*f*
shunts, 771–772, 1410, 1418
sickle cell disease, 793–794, 794*f*, 802
side effects. *See under specific drugs/
  medications*
SIDS (sudden infant death syndrome),
  1339–1342, 1341*t*, 1347
sight impairment. *See* visually impaired
  patients
significant negative findings, 137
sign language, for communicating with
  hearing-impaired patients, 130,
  130*f*, 1398*f*
signs. *See also under specific disorders*
  definition of, 342, 412
  *vs.* symptoms, 342
signs of death, 95–97
silver fork deformity, 1175, 1176*f*
simple access, 1472, 1472*f*, 1484
simplex system, 149, 161
single command system, 1489, 1525
Singulair (montelukast), 658*t*
sinoatrial node (SA node), 678
sinus headaches, 726
situational awareness, 325, 343, 412, 1468
six Ps of musculoskeletal
  assessment, 1162
size, of extrication scene, 1467–1469
size-up
  definition of, 1468, 1484
  of emergency scene, 343–349
    considering additional or
      specialized resources, 349
    definition of, 345, 412
    in EMT training, 6
    ensuring scene safety, 344–345, 345*f*

mechanism of injury/nature of illness determination, 345–347
nature of illness determination, 345–347
number of patients, determination of, 348–349, 348*f*
questions, for mass-casualty incident, 1492–1493
safety assessment, 344–345
standard precautions for, 347–348, 347*f*
of extrication scene, 1467*f*
skeletal muscle, 198
definition of, 1146, 1147*f*
skeletal system, 191–197
anatomy, 191–197, 1044–1045, 1044*f*
appendicular skeleton, 195
axial skeleton, 193–195
bones, 191–192
joints, 192–193
lower extremities, 196–197
pelvis, 196
physiology, 197
skeleton, anatomy, 1148–1151, 1149–1151*f*
skilled care facilities, response to nursing and, 1379–1380
skin. *See also* integumentary system
anatomy, 963–964, 963*f*
assessment, 358–360, 360*f*
color, 359, 359*f*, 608, 608*f*
condition, in heat exposure illnesses, 1214*t*
functions, 358–359, 962–964, 1153
moisture, 360
protection, for injury prevention, 64
signs, of anaphylactic shock, 539*t*
temperature, 359–360
turgor, 1214, 1240
skin turgor, 1214
skull
anatomy, 1044–1045, 1044*f*, 1148
fractures, 1046–1047, 1048*f*
basilar, 1047, 1048*f*
depressed, 1047, 1048*f*
linear, 1047, 1048*f*
open, 1047–1048, 1048*f*
slander, 102, 115
sleep, wellness and, 35–36
slings
application, 1170*f*, 1171, 1172*f*
definition of, 1170, 1197
SLUDGEM mnemonic, 842, 1538, 1539
small intestine, 229
smallpox, 1543–1544, 1543*f*, 1544*t*, 1548*t*, 1559
small-volume nebulizers
administration of, 656, 659
definition of, 656, 673
smell, sense of, 1358
smiling, importance of, 121
smoke, as fire hazard, 58–59, 58*f*
smoking cessation, wellness and, 37
smooth muscle, 1146, 1147*f*
snake bites, 1230–1231*f*, 1230–1233

coral, 1230*f*, 1232–1233
pit vipers, 1231–1233, 1231*f*
types, 1230*f*
sneezing techniques, to avoid contamination, 39–40, 40*f*
sniffing position, 356, 412, 1294, 1347
newborns, 1266
SOAP method, 139–140
social assessment, in GEMS diamond, 1368, 1369*t*
socks, 64
soft-tissue injuries
assessment, 970–976
communication/documentation of, 976
general impressions, 971
history taking, 973–974
primary, 971–973
reassessment, 974–976
SAMPLE history, 973
scene size-up, 970–971
secondary, 974
transport decisions, 971
of vital signs, 974
XABCs, 974–975
from blunt trauma, 965
burns. *See* burns
closed, 964
definition of, 964
emergency medical care of, 976
death from, 964
emergency medical care, 976–981
of face and neck, 1010, 1010*f*, 1015–1016, 1015–1016*f*
interventions, 974
open wounds, 970
definition of, 970
emergency medical care of, 976–981, 980*f*
pathophysiology, 964–970
prevention, 962
safety, on-scene, 970–971
solid organs. *See also specific solid organs*
abdominal, 1119–1121, 1120*f*
definition of, 1143
solution, 501
soman (GD), 1538, 1541*t*, 1559
somatic (voluntary) nervous system, 1044
sovereign immunity, 103
spacer, 659
span of control, 1487, 1525
Special Atomic Demolition Munitions (SADM), 1551, 1559
special K (ketamine), 838
special populations
children. *See* children
geriatric. *See* elderly
infants. *See* infants
special situations, calling medical control and hospitals, 156
special weapons and tactics (SWAT) teams, 1477, 1484
sperm, 1244

sphincters, 533, 553
sphygmomanometer, 389, 389*f*
spice, synthetic marijuana, 841
spider bites, 1228–1229, 1228*f*, 1229*f*
spina bifida, 1272, 1279, 1401–1402, 1401*f*, 1418
spinal column anatomy, 1045, 1045*f*
vertebrae, 1045, 1045*f*
spinal cord, 222–223
functions, 725, 726*f*
injuries. *See* spinal cord injuries
spinal cord injuries, 1045, 1052
assessment, 1053–1061
ABCs, 1054
chief complaint investigation, 1060
communication/documentation of, 1061
history taking, 1056–1057
primary, 1054–1056
reassessment, 1060–1061
scene size-up, 1053–1054
secondary, 1057–1060
of vital signs, 1060
concussion, 1051, 1089
contusion, 1051–1052
emergency medical care, 1064–1067
with face and neck injuries, 1032
helmet removal, 1079–1081, 1083*f*
interventions, 1060
safety, on-scene, 1053–1054
signs/symptoms, 1052
in submersion incidents, 1218–1220
transport decisions, 1056
spinal motion restriction, 1054, 1064
spine injuries. *See* spinal cord injuries
spiral fracture, 1154
spleen, 215
splints/splinting
definition of, 1164, 1197
distal circulation and, 1168
formable, 1167–1168
general principles, 1164–1165
of hand and wrist, 1176–1177
improper, hazards of, 1169
in-line traction, 1181
pelvic binder, 1168, 1169*f*, 1197
with pillow, 1189, 1191*f*
purpose
to control bleeding, 946, 948*f*, 976
rigid, 1165–1166
supplies, in ambulances, 1428*t*, 1431, 1431*f*
traction, 1181–1186, 1197
spontaneous abortion, 1250
spontaneous pneumothorax, 644, 664, 1104
spontaneous respiration, 355, 413
spotter, 1447, 1462
sprains
definition of, 1156–1157, 1197
elbow, 1174
management, 1191
signs/symptoms, 1157

sputum types, 651*t*
SSRIs (selective serotonin reuptake
    inhibitors), 844*t*
staging supervisor, 1494, 1525
stair chair
    definition of, 287, 287*f*, 318
    description, 287
    technique for using, 287–288
standard of care
    definition of, 98, 115
    establishment of, 98, 98*f*
        imposed by law, 98–99
        imposed by local custom, 98
        imposed by professional and
            institutional standards, 99–100
        imposed by state, 100
    minimum, 99
standard precautions
    definition of, 41, 83, 347, 413
    types of protection in, 42*t*, 347–348,
        347*f*
standing orders, 98, 156, 161
Star of Life, 1426, 1426*f*, 1462
startle reflex (Moro reflex), 256, 271
START triage, 1499–1500, 1525
state government, standard of care
    for, 100
state-sponsored terrorism, 1532, 1559
status asthmaticus, 663
status epilepticus, 733, 753
statute of limitations, 108, 115
STD (sexually transmitted disease), 885
steam burn, 991, 1003
sterile dressings, 980, 998, 1015
sterilization, 1442, 1462
sternal fracture, 1108–1109
sternocleidomastoid muscles, 1008, 1038
stimulants, definition of, 839, 852
stings
    hymenoptera, 1229–1230, 1240
    scorpion, 1233–1234, 1233*f*
stomach, 228, 757
stomas, 1410
    airway management and, 474
    artificial ventilation, 569, 569*f*
    catheters for, 443, 444*f*
    definition of, 491, 1418
strains, 1157, 1191, 1197
strangulation, 766, 775
stress
    causes of, 69–75
    critical incident, 70
    management, 69–70, 72*t*
    peer support, 38
    physiologic responses to, 69
    posttraumatic stress disorder,
        71–72, 83
    reactions
        acute, 70, 82
        cumulative, 70, 82
        delayed, 70, 82
    suicide and, 72–73
    warning signs, 72*t*
stretchers
    bariatric, 309, 309*f*

basket, 311–312, 312*f*, 318
    flexible, 311, 311*f*, 318
    guidelines for carrying patients, 283*t*
    moving patient onto, draw sheet
        method for, 304–305
    portable/folding, 310, 310*f*, 318
    wheeled. *See* wheeled ambulance
        stretchers
stridor, 475, 491, 587, 601, 805
    definition of, 413, 651, 673, 805, 819
    diseases associated with, 651, 651*t*
    sound of, 355, 651
stroke (cerebrovascular accident)
    assessment, 741–742*t*, 741–744, 742*t*
    conditions mimicking, 731
    death from, 724
    definition of, 753
    emergency medical care, 747–748
    ischemic, 728*f*, 728–729
    signs/symptoms, 731
stroke volume (SV), 682
structure fire, 1479, 1484
structure fires, 1479
study tips, 5*t*
subarachnoid hemorrhage,
    1050–1051, 1089
subcutaneous emphysema, 398, 413,
    1032, 1038
subcutaneous injection, 499
subdural bleeding, 731, 731*f*
subdural hematomas, 1050,
    1050*f*, 1089
sublingual medications, 511–513
sublingual (SL), 499
submersion
    hypothermia and, 1220
    with suspected spinal injury,
        1218–1220
substance abuse, 822, 852
    terminology, 822
    workplace, 77
sucking chest wound, 1103, 1103*f*, 1115
sucking reflex, 256, 271
suction catheter, 443, 491
suctioning
    equipment, 443, 444*f*
    techniques, 444–446
suctioning units, in ambulances,
    1429, 1429*f*
sudden death, 687–688
sudden infant death syndrome (SIDS),
    1339–1342, 1341*t*, 1347
suffixes, medical terminology, 166,
    180*t*, 188
    definition of, 166
suicide, 869–871, 1367–1368
    stress and, 72–73
sulfuric acid, containers for, 1505
sulfur mustard (H), 1536, 1541*t*,
    1559–1560
summary, definition/example of, 123*t*
sunlight exposure, excessive, 1215
superficial (first-degree) burns, 984,
    984*f*, 1003
superficial portion, 172, 188

superior, definition, 679, 721
superior portion, 170–171, 188
superior vena cava, 679
supine, definition of, 173, 188
supine hypotensive syndrome,
    1134, 1248
supine position, 173, 173*f*, 188
supplies, medical. *See also specific
    medical supplies*
    in ambulances, 1427, 1428*t*
surfactant, 427, 491
suspension, 501
SV (stroke volume), 682, 721
swathe, 1170, 1170*f*, 1197
SWAT teams (special weapons and
    tactics teams), 1477
swelling, as fracture signs, 1154
swine flu (H1N1 virus), 614
symbols, medical terminology,
    162–175, 175*t*
sympathetic nervous system,
    679, 721, 1044
sympathomimetics, 824*t*, 839–840
symptomatic hyperglycemia, 784, 802
    definition of, 784
symptomatic hypoglycemia, 785, 802
symptoms. *See also under specific
    disorders*
    definition of, 342, 413
    multiple, history taking and, 372–373
    *vs.* signs, 342
syncope, 686, 721
    definition of, 735, 753
syncope (fainting episode)
    breath-holding, 1226
    causes, in elderly, 1376
    definition of, 539, 553, 1389
syndromic surveillance, 1548–1549,
    1560
synthetic cathinones, 840–841
syphilis, 890
systemic reaction, 811
systole, 680
systolic pressure, definition of, 388, 413


**T**

tabun (GA), 1538, 1541*t*, 1560
tachycardia
    definition of, 387, 413, 688, 721
    in pediatric emergencies, 1300
tachypnea, 1097, 1115
    in chest injuries, 1097
    definition of, 1347
    increased work of breathing and, 1296
    in respiratory failure, 357*t*
tactical medicine, 1478, 1478*f*
tactical situation, 1477–1478,
    1478*f*, 1484
tactile stimulation, 1266
Taser injuries, 996
TBI. *See* traumatic brain injury
TCAs. *See* tricyclic antidepressants
team, health care and
    assisting with ALS skills, 328–329

BLS and ALS providers, 328
conflicts, troubleshooting, 331
critical thinking and clinical decision
    making, 329–330
defined, 322
dependent groups, 323
effective performance, team, 323–326
    collaboration and
        communication, 325
    crew resource management,
        325–326
    diverse and competent skill sets,
        323–324
    roles and responsibilities, 323
    shared goal, 323
    supportive and coordinated
        leadership, 325
    team membership, 325
generally, 320
independent groups, 323
interdependent groups, 323
transfer of patient care, 326–327
types of, 321–322
team leader, 325
technical rescue group, 1475–1476,
    1475f, 1484
technical rescue situation,
    1475–1476, 1484
teenage pregnancy, 1253
teenagers. *See* adolescents
teeth
    avulsed, 1011
    fractured, 1011
teething, 257
telemetry, 148, 161–162
telephones, cellular/satellite, 148–149
temperature, high ambient, as hazard in
    fires, 58
temporomandibular joint (TMJ),
    1007, 1038
tenderness, as fracture sign, 1154
tension headache, 726
tension pneumothorax, 431, 491
    definition of, 536, 1115
    pathophysiology, 1104–1105
    signs/symptoms, 632t, 1104–1105
    treatment, 546
    tenting, 1327f
term gestation, 1250, 1279
terminal illness, 1411
termination of command, 1489, 1526
terrorism
    biologic warfare. *See* biologic
        terrorism/warfare
    chemical warfare. *See* chemical
        terrorism/warfare
    definition of, 1528
    events
        establishing command, 1535
        indicators of, 1532–1533
        notification procedures, 1534
        responder safety, 1534
        scene safety, 1533–1534, 1535
    incendiary/explosive devices,
        1552–1553

nuclear/radiologic warfare, 1549–1552
tertiary blast injuries, 917, 1553, 1560
tetanus, 980
therapeutic communication, 119, 162
therapeutic effect, 496
therapeutic rapport, for patient
    interview, 125–126, 125f
thermal burns
    definition of, 991–992, 1003
    to eye, 1021–1023, 1023f
third-degree (full-thickness) burns, 984,
    984f, 1003
thoracic cavity
    anatomy, 420–423, 422f, 1093, 1094f
    physiology, 1092–1093, 1094f
throat injuries, assessment of, 920–921
thrombocytes (platelets), 793
thromboembolism, 685, 721
thrombophilia, 795, 802
thrombosis, 728, 753, 802
thyroid cartilage, 420
TIA (transient ischemic attack), 730,
    746, 753
tibia, 1150, 1197
    injuries, 1189, 1189f
tick bites, 1234, 1234f
TICLS mnemonic, 1295, 1295t
tidal volume, 385, 413, 425, 491, 1316
time/timing
    for cardiopulmonary resuscitation,
        558, 558f
    in OPQRST, 369
toddlers
    assessment, 1286–1287
    definition of, 258, 271, 1286, 1347
    examination of, 258–259
    growth/development, 1286–1287, 1286f
    physical changes, 258–259, 259f
    psychosocial changes, 260
    vital signs, 259
tolerance, 834, 852
tongue, in children, 1290, 1291f
tonic-clonic seizures, 732, 1328
tonic phase, 732
tonsil-tip catheter, 443, 444f, 491
tonsil tips, 443
topical medications, 502
topographic anatomy, 190–191
topographic anatomy, definition of, 190,
    251
tort, 101, 115
    definition of, 101
touch/touching
    sensory age-related changes, 1358
    using in patient interview, 123, 124f
tourniquet
    application method, 949–954, 949f
    definition of, 949, 960, 1159, 1197
toxicologic emergencies
    airway assessment, 833
    assessment, 830–833
        communication/documentation
            of, 833
        history taking, 831–832
        primary, 831

reassessment, 832–833
SAMPLE history, 831–832
scene size-up, 830, 831f
secondary, 832
secondary assessment, 832
of vital signs, 832
breathing assessment, 831
circulation assessment, 831
definition of, 822
emergency medical care, 833
general impressions, 831
interventions, 833
medical, 605, 605t
pathophysiology, routes of
    absorption, 824–830, 825f, 828f
patient assessment, scene size-up,
    830, 831f
safety, on-scene, 830, 831f
with specific poisons,
    organophosphates
    alcohol, 834–836
    cannabis compounds, 841
    hallucinogens, 841–842
    hypnotics, 837–838
    marijuana, 841
    narcotics, 836–837
    opiates, 836–837
    opioids, 836–837
    sedatives, 837–838
transport decisions, 831
toxicology, 822, 852
elderly, 1365–1367
toxin-induced hepatitis, 617t
toxins
    absorption of, 827–828, 828f
    definition of, 807, 819, 822, 852
    inhalation of, 826–827
    marine animal, 1235t
toys, using when communicating with
    children, 128
trachea, 420, 1093
tracheitis, 1308, 1347
tracheostomy
    collar, 1407, 1407f
    definition of, 459, 491
    dysfunction, 665
    mask, 459–460, 460f
    tubes
        airway management and, 474, 474f
        definition of, 474, 1418
traction, 1181–1186
    applying, 1183–1184
    definition of, 1197
traction splint, 1181–1186
trade name, definition of, 497
tragus, 1007, 1038, 1316
training
    focus of, 6
    infection control, 47t
    levels of, 9–11, 9t
        EMR. *See* emergency medical
            responder, training
        EMT. *See* emergency medical
            technician, training
        paramedic. *See* paramedic, training

training *(Continued)*
  public basic life support and
    immediate aid, 10
  National Standard Curriculum, 8
  requirements for, 6
trajectory, 914, 931
transcutaneous (transdermal)
    medications, 499
  patches, automated external
    defibrillation and, 562
transfer of patients
  to ambulance, 1440, 1440*f*
  equipment, in ambulances, 1428*t*, 1432
  during extrication, 1474–1475, 1474*f*
  in landing zone for air medical
    operations, 1456–1457
  moves, 302–304
  transfer moves, 302–304
transient ischemic attack (TIA), 730,
    746, 753, 1357
transmission
  definition of, 38, 83
  routes, for infectious diseases,
    38–40, 39*f*
transport
  cardiac arrest during, 714–715
  decisions. *See under specific*
    *emergencies*
  in mass-casualty incident triage,
    1501–1502
  moving patients for. *See* moving of
    patients
  musculoskeletal injuries, 1162
  of obese patients, 1402
  refusal of, 90
  of sitting patients, with head injuries,
    1075–1077
  of supine patients, with head injuries,
    1067–1075
  types of, 924–928, 925*f*
transportation area, 1494, 1526
transportation supervisor, 1494, 1526
transport layer, of cold weather
    clothing, 62
transverse (axial) plane, definition
    of, 191
transverse fracture, 1154
trauma centers, levels of, 923*t*
trauma emergencies
  blast injuries, 915–918, 915*f*
  blunt. *See* blunt trauma
  definition of, 605, 626
  destination selection, 922–924, 923*t*
  elderly and. *See* geriatric trauma
  energy and, 901–904, 905*f*
  to face. *See* facial injuries
  level II patients, care for, 923, 923*t*
  level I patients, care for, 922, 923*t*
  mechanism of injury, 901, 931
  multisystem, 918–920, 931
  to neck. *See* neck injuries
  on-scene time, 922
  patient assessment, 920–922
  pediatric. *See* pediatric emergencies,
    trauma

penetrating, 904, 913–915, 915*f*, 931
  during pregnancy, 1251–1252
  prehospital care, 919–920
  transport decisions, 919, 922
trauma score, 924, 931
traumatic asphyxia, 1109, 1115
traumatic brain injury (TBI)
  death from, 1048
  definition of, 1048, 1089
  intracranial pressure, 1049–1051
  patient assessment, 1053–1061
travel medicine, 620–621
treatment, refusal rights, 90
treatment area, 1493, 1526
treatment supervisor, 1493–1494, 1526
trench rescue, 1477
triage, 1493
  categories, 1498–1499, 1498*t*
  definition of, 349, 413, 1497
  destination decisions, 1501–1502
  JumpSTART, 1500–1501, 1524
  primary, 1497, 1525
  SALT, 1500
  secondary, 1497, 1525
  special considerations, 1501
  START triage, 1499–1500, 1525–1526
  supervisor, 1493, 1526
  tag system, 1499, 1499*f*
tricuspid valve, 677*f*
tricyclic antidepressants, 842
Tridil. *See* nitroglycerin
trimesters, 1246
tripod position, 356, 356*f*, 413, 1296, 1347
trisomy 21. *See* Down syndrome
trunking, 149, 162
trust and mistrust stage of
    development, 271
tuberculin skin testing/fit testing, for
    infection control plan, 47*t*
tuberculosis
  characteristics, 618–619, 637–638, 732*t*
  definition of, 626, 673
  signs/symptoms, 632*t*
  transmission, 618–619
turbinates
  anatomy, 1027, 1028*f*
  definition of, 1038
turgor, 1214
turnout gear (bunker gear), for injury
    prevention, 62, 62*f*
twin births, 1272
two- to three-word dyspnea,
    356, 413
tympanic membrane, 917, 931, 1028,
    1029*f*, 1038
type 1 diabetes, 782–784, 802
type 2 diabetes, 784, 802

## U

UHF (ultra-high frequency), 147, 162
ulcers, 760–761
ulna
  anatomy, 1148, 1149*f*
  olecranon process fracture, 1174

umbilical cord
  anatomy, 1245
  around newborn's neck, 1263
  clamping, 1263
  definition of, 1245, 1279
  prolapsed, 1271, 1272*f*, 1279
umbilical vein catheters (UVCs), 1245
unified command system, 1488, 1526
unilateral structure, definition of, 172
unintended effects, 497
untoward effects, 497
upper airway, 198–200
Urban Search and Rescue teams
    (USARs), 1502
uremia, 764, 776
ureters, 757
urethra, anatomy, 757, 882*f*
urinary bladder
  anatomy, 758
  definition of, 758
  injuries, 1134, 1137
urinary incontinence, in elderly, 1362
urinary retention, 764
  in elderly, 1363
urinary system, 232–233
  anatomy, 757–758, 758*f*
urinary tract emergencies
  assessment, 766–770
    general impressions, 768
    mechanism of injury/nature of
      illness, 767
    primary, 767–768
    scene size-up, 766–767
  as medical emergencies, 605, 605*t*
  safety, on-scene, 766–767
  transport decisions, 768
urinary tract infections (UTIs), 764, 776,
    1359, 1389
urine, 758
urologic system. *See* urinary system
urostomy, 1410, 1418
urticaria, 805
  characteristics, 805, 805*f*
  definition of, 819
uterine rupture, 1250
uterus
  anatomy, 882*f*, 883, 1244
  definition of, 897
  manual left displacement, 594*f*
UTIs (urinary tract infections),
    764, 776
UVC (umbilical vein catheter), 1245

## V

vacuum mattresses, 311, 311*f*, 1070
vacuum splints, 1167–1168
V agent (VX), 1538, 1541*t*, 1560
vagina
  anatomy, 882*f*, 883, 1244
  bleeding from
    causes of, 885–886
    in pregnancy, 885–886
  definition of, 897
vagus nerve stimulators, 1410

vancomycin-resistant enterococci (VRE), 1379, 1389
vapor hazard, 1535, 1560
vasoconstriction, 360, 413, 939, 1354
vasodilation, 1360*t*
vasodilatory shock, 431
vasoocclusive crisis, 794, 802
vector-borne transmission, 40, 83
vehicle assessment, 901–902
vehicles. *See* motor vehicles
veins, 213–214, 935, 960
  *vs.* arteries, 1245
  functions, 679
vented chest seal, 1098, 1115
ventilation, 205–207
  alveolar, 488
  definition of, 423, 491, 568, 601, 633, 673
  equipment, in ambulances, 1428*t*, 1429, 1431*f*
  factors affecting, 429–430
  mechanisms, 424–426, 425*f*
  mouth-to-mouth, 462–463
  normal, *vs.* positive pressure ventilation, 461–462, 462*t*
  physiology, 1092
  regulation, 426
  *vs.* respiration, 633
ventilation/perfusion ratio and mismatch (V/Q), 429
ventilation rates, for apneic patients, 462
Ventolin. *See* albuterol
ventral portion, 172, 188
ventricle, 677, 721
ventricular fibrillation (VF), 688, 721
ventricular tachycardia (VT), 688, 721
Venturi mask, 459, 459*f*
venule, 679
venules, 935, 960
verbal report, 133
vernix caseosa, 1264, 1279
vertebrae, anatomy, 1045, 1045*f*
vertebral body, 1045
vertex presentation, 1270, 1279
vesicants, 1535–1536, 1541*t*, 1560
vesicular breath sounds, 650, 673
veteran, 871–873
VF (ventricular fibrillation), 688, 721
VHF (very high frequency), 147, 162
Vial of Life, 1371
video laryngoscopy, 478
violence, safety precautions for, 60
viral hemorrhagic fevers (VHF), 1543–1544, 1544*f*, 1544*t*, 1548*t*, 1560
viral infections, 615
virulence, 616, 626

viruses, in chemical terrorism/warfare, 1543–1544, 1543*f*, 1544*f*, 1544*t*, 1560
visceral pleura, 421, 491
vision, age-related changes, 1357–1358
visually impaired patients
  communication with, 130–131
  history taking and, 376
  interaction with, 1396–1397, 1397*f*
vital capacity, 425*t*, 491
vital signs
  of adolescents, 261
  of adults, 263
  assessment, 350, 351*f*
    in emergencies. *See under specific emergencies*
    monitoring devices for. *See specific monitoring devices*
  definition of, 350, 413
  documenting, 142
  of school-age children, 260
  of toddlers/preschoolers, 258–259
vitreous humor, 1009
vocal cords, 420, 491
volatility, 1535, 1560
Volmax. *See* albuterol
volume, of hazardous material containers, 1506, 1506*f*
voluntary activities, 1043, 1044, 1089
/ ratio (ventilation/perfusion ratio and mismatch), 429
VT (ventricular tachycardia), 688, 721
VX (V agent), 1538, 1541*t*, 1560

**W**

walking assist, one-person, 296*f*
warm zone, 1514*f*, 1525
wasp stings, 807, 807*f*, 1229
water rescue, 1219, 1219*f*
WBCs. *See* white blood cells
weakness, in elderly, 1371
weaponization, 1532, 1560
weapon of mass casualty (WMC), 1531, 1560
weapon of mass destruction (WMD), 1531, 1560
weather conditions, driving of emergency vehicles and, 1449–1450
wellness
  balancing work, family and health, 38
  disease prevention and, 36–38
  exercise, 35, 35*f*
  nutrition, 33–35, 34*f*
  relaxation for, 35
  sleep, 35–36
wet lungs, *vs.* dry lungs, 641*t*

wet patients, automated external defibrillation and, 562
wheals, 807, 808*f*
wheeled ambulance stretchers (wheeled stretchers)
  definition of, 318
  description, 275–276, 275–286, 275*f*
  pneumatic and electronic powered, 309, 310*f*
  rolling, 275, 275*f*
wheezing, 475, 491, 805
  in allergic reactions, 805
  in asthma, 642
  definition of, 413, 673, 805
  respiratory diseases associated with, 651*t*
white blood cells (leukocytes; WBCs)
  definition of, 793
  functions, 680
whooping cough. *See* pertussis
WMC (weapon of mass casualty), 1531, 1560
WMD (weapon of mass destruction), 1531, 1560
Wong-Baker FACES scale, in pediatric emergencies, 1300, 1301*f*
word roots, medical terminology, 165, 166*t*, 176–178*t*, 188
work
  balancing with family and health, 38
  definition of, 902, 931
work of breathing, 1294
  definition of, 1347
  in pediatric assessment triangle, 1294*f*, 1295
workplace issues, 75–77
wound care supplies, in ambulances, 1428*t*, 1430–1431
wound healing, pathophysiology of, 964–965
wrist
  anatomy, 1148, 1149*f*
  injuries, 1176–1177

**X**

XABCs mnemonic, 942, 1339
x-ray (gamma) radiation, 1549, 1558

**Y**

yellowjacket stings, 1229

**Z**

zone of injury, 1151, 1197